CLINICAL PHARMACY

—— AND ——

THERAPEUTICS

T0175828

CLINICAL PHARMACY AND THERAPEUTICS

SIXTH EDITION

EDITED BY

CATE WHITTLESEA, BSc, MSc, PhD, MRPharmS
Professor of Pharmacy Practice and Associate Director of Clinical Education
UCL School of Pharmacy
University College London
London, UK

and

KAREN HODSON, BSc(Pharm), MSc, PhD, FRPharmS, FFRPS
Director MSc in Clinical Pharmacy and Pharmacist Independent Prescribing Programmes
School of Pharmacy and Pharmaceutical Sciences, Cardiff University
Cardiff, UK

For additional online content visit StudentConsult.com

ELSEVIER

ELSEVIER

© 2019, Elsevier Limited. All rights reserved.

First edition 1994
Second edition 1999
Third edition 2003
Fourth edition 2007
Fifth edition 2012
Sixth edition 2019

No part of this publication may be reproduced or transmitted in any form or by any means, electronic or mechanical, including photocopying, recording, or any information storage and retrieval system, without permission in writing from the publisher. Details on how to seek permission, further information about the Publisher's permissions policies and our arrangements with organizations such as the Copyright Clearance Center and the Copyright Licensing Agency, can be found at our website: www.elsevier.com/permissions.

This book and the individual contributions contained in it are protected under copyright by the Publisher (other than as may be noted herein).

Notices

Practitioners and researchers must always rely on their own experience and knowledge in evaluating and using any information, methods, compounds or experiments described herein. Because of rapid advances in the medical sciences, in particular, independent verification of diagnoses and drug dosages should be made. To the fullest extent of the law, no responsibility is assumed by Elsevier, authors, editors or contributors for any injury and/or damage to persons or property as a matter of products liability, negligence or otherwise, or from any use or operation of any methods, products, instructions, or ideas contained in the material herein.

ISBN: 978-0-7020-7012-9
International Edition   ISBN 978-0-7020-7011-2

Senior Content Strategist: Pauline Graham
Content Development Specialist: Carole McMurray
Project Manager: Beula Christopher
Design: Paula Catalano
Illustration Manager: Amy Faith Heyden
Illustrator: MPS LLC
Marketing Manager: Deborah Watkins

Printed in India
Last digit is the print number: 9   8   7   6   5   4

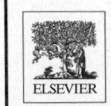

Working together
to grow libraries in
developing countries

www.elsevier.com • www.bookaid.org

Preface

In both primary and secondary health care, the use of medicines is the most common intervention. However, the use of medicines is not without risk. Selecting and prescribing drugs is increasingly complex and demanding, and it is undertaken as part of a multi-disciplinary process that involves pharmacists, some of whom are now prescribers in their own right, along with doctors, nurses and other members of the healthcare team. All must strive to promote safe, appropriate and cost-effective prescribing that respects patient choice and promotes adherence. This book was written to help the reader understand and address many of these issues. It is unashamedly written from a pharmacy perspective, although we do hope those from other disciplines will also find it of use.

We have made considerable effort to update each chapter and ensure the content is relevant to current practice. Selected website addresses have been included to assist those who want to obtain further information, and many references are now available electronically. However, knowledge in therapeutics progresses rapidly, changes to dose regimens and licensed indications are frequent, safety issues emerge with established drugs and new medicines appear at regular intervals. Yesterday another landmark study may have been published that added to, or perhaps altered, the evidence base for a specific treatment. Together with the ongoing publication of national and international guidelines and frameworks, the face of therapeutics is ever changing. It is therefore inevitable that some sections of this book will date more quickly than others.

In practice, many licensed drugs are used 'off label' or 'near label' when prescribed for a certain indication or used in a specific patient group, such as children. To omit reference to these agents in the relevant chapter would leave an apparent gap in therapeutic management. As a consequence, we have encouraged our authors to present details of all key drugs used, along with details of the prescribed regimens, even if not licensed for that specific indication. There is, however, a downside to this approach. The reader must always use this text critically and with caution. If this is done, the book will serve as a valuable learning resource and help the reader understand some of the principles of therapeutics. We hope that, in some small way, this will also assist in achieving positive patient outcomes.

Cate Whittlesea
Karen Hodson

Acknowledgements

The first edition of this book was published in 1994 by Roger Walker and Clive Edwards. We very much hope that this edition lives up to the high standards of both past editors. We acknowledge the enormous contribution Roger Walker made to all previous editions and very much hope he will look in pride at this, our first edition, without him at the helm. Like Roger, undergraduate and postgraduate students have sustained our enthusiasm and commitment while continuing to be the inspiration and the *raison d'etre* for this book. To all those who have provided feedback in the past, thank you. For those who would like to comment on this edition, we welcome your feedback; please contact us at c.whittlesea@ucl.ac.uk or hodsonkl@cardiff.ac.uk.

We remain indebted to all authors who, through their hard work, patience and tolerance, have contributed to the sixth edition of this book. We are particularly grateful to those who have again contributed to another edition of this textbook and who strive, along with us, to produce an ever-better book. To our first-time authors, we are very grateful for your contribution, that you accepted our cryptic editorial comments in good faith and still managed to submit on time. We hope that you will continue to work with us on future editions.

A textbook of this size cannot, of course, be produced without the invaluable help, support and occasional comments of numerous colleagues, particularly from the Department of Pharmacy, Durham University, UCL School of Pharmacy and the Associate Course Directors of the MSc in Clinical Pharmacy within the School of Pharmacy and Pharmaceutical Sciences, Cardiff University. It would be invidious to name individuals who have helped us, in part for fear of offending anyone we might miss. We do, however, continue to make one exception to this rule. The administrative support from Dean Routledge has been invaluable.

Finally, and on a personal note, we would like thank our close families for their support and tolerance with our indulgence in editing this text. At times it may have appeared that everything in our lives took second place to 'the book'. We are eternally grateful for their understanding, particularly when we got our priorities in life wrong. Without the unfailing support of Rob and Phil, Maddy and Logan, this book would never have materialised.

Cate Whittlesea
Karen Hodson

List of Contributors

The editors would like to acknowledge and offer grateful thanks for the input of all previous editions' contributors, without whom this new edition would not have been possible.

Tamara Ahmed Ali
Directorate Lead Pharmacist-Ophthalmology, City Hospitals Sunderland NHS Trust, Sunderland, UK
56. Glaucoma

Sotiris Antoniou
Consultant Pharmacist, Cardiovascular Medicine, Barts Health NHS Trust, St Bartholomew's Hospital, London, UK
22. Arrhythmias

Kelly Atack
Advanced Clinical Pharmacist, Medicines Management and Pharmacy, St James's University Hospital, Leeds Teaching Hospital NHS Trust, Leeds, UK
25. Asthma

Deborah Baidoo
Chief Pharmacist (Interim), West London Trust, St Bernard's Hospital, Middlesex, London, UK
27. Insomnia

David S. Baldwin
Professor of Psychiatry, Clinical and Experimental Sciences Academic Unit, Faculty of Medicine, University of Southampton, Southampton, UK
28. Anxiety disorders

Catrin Barker
Chief Pharmacist, Pharmacy Department, Alder Hey Children's NHS Foundation Trust, Liverpool, UK
10. Paediatrics

Roger Barker
Professor of Clinical Neuroscience, Honorary Consultant in Neurology, University of Cambridge and Addenbrooke's Hospital, Cambridge, UK
32. Parkinson's disease

Lee Beale
Anaesthetic Registrar ST7, University Hospital of Wales, Cardiff, UK
6. Laboratory data

Jonathan Berry
Academic Clinical Educator, School of Pharmacy, Keele University, Staffordshire, UK
14. Constipation and diarrhoea

Stephen Bleakley
Chief Pharmacist, Salisbury NHS Foundation Trust, Salisbury, UK
28. Anxiety disorders

Gonçalo Cação
UCL Institute of Neurology, London, UK
31. Epilepsy

Anthony Cadogan
Macmillan Advanced Pharmacist, Haematology and Oncology, Prince Charles Hospital (Merthyr Tydfil) and Royal Glamorgan Hospital (Llantrisant), Cwm Taf University Health Board, Wales, UK
50. Anaemia

Laura Cameron
Principal Pharmacist - Cancer Services Operational Lead, Guy's and St Thomas' NHS Foundation Trust, London, UK
52. Lymphomas

Toby Capstick
Lead Respiratory Pharmacist, Pharmacy Department, Leeds Teaching Hospitals NHS Trust, Leeds, UK
41. Tuberculosis

Neil J. B. Carbarns
Consultant Medical Microbiologist, Aneurin Bevan University Health Board, Abergavenny, Monmouthshire, UK
37. Urinary tract infections

Sheena Castelino
Principal Pharmacist, HIV and Sexual Health, Guy's and St Thomas' NHS Foundation Trust, Pharmacy Department, St Thomas' Hospital, London, UK
42. HIV infection

Ben Challocombe
Consultant Urologist, Guy's and St Thomas' NHS
Foundation Trust, London, UK
49. Prostate disease

Ian Clifton
Consultant Respiratory Physician and Honorary Senior
Lecturer, Department of Respiratory Medicine,
St James's University Hospital, Leeds Teaching Hospital
NHS Trust, Leeds, UK
25. Asthma

Paul Cockwell
Consultant Nephrologist, University Hospital
Birmingham and Professor of Nephrology, University of
Birmingham, Birmingham, UK
17. Acute kidney injury
18. Chronic kidney disease and end-stage renal disease

Katie Conway
Consultant Physician in GU/HIV Medicine, Guy's and
St Thomas' NHS Foundation Trust, Pharmacy
Department, St Thomas' Hospital, London, UK
42. HIV infection

Jonathan Cooke
Honorary Professor, Manchester Pharmacy School,
Faculty of Biology, Medicine and Health, University
of Manchester, Manchester; Visiting Professor in the
Infectious Diseases and Immunity Section, Division of
Infectious Diseases, Department of Medicine, Imperial
College London, London, UK
8. Pharmacoeconomics

Alan G. Cosslett
Lecturer, School of Pharmacy and Pharmaceutical
Sciences, Cardiff University, Cardiff, UK
7. Parenteral nutrition

Anthony R. Cox
Senior Lecturer in Clinical Pharmacy and Drug Safety,
School of Pharmacy, University of Birmingham,
Birmingham, UK
5. Adverse drug reactions

Netty (Annette) Cracknell
Specialist Oncology Pharmacist, Netty Cracknell
Consultancy; Pharmacy Manager, Springfield Hospital,
Chelmsford, UK; Executive Committee Member, British
Oncology Pharmacy Association (BOPA), UK
53. Solid tumours

Daniel Creamer
Consultant Dermatologist, Department of
Dermatology, King's College Hospital NHS Foundation
Trust, London, UK
57. Drug-induced skin disorders

Sarah Cripps
Consultant Pharmacist - Gastroenterology/Hepatology,
Oxford University Hospitals NHS Foundation Trust,
Oxford, UK
13. Inflammatory bowel disease

Emma Crosbie
NIHR Clinician Scientist, Senior Lecturer and Honorary
Consultant in Gynaecological Oncology, Division of
Molecular and Clinical Cancer Sciences, University of
Manchester, St Mary's Hospital, Manchester, UK
46. Menstrual cycle disorders
47. Menopause

Octavio Aragon Cuevas
Lead Rheumatology Pharmacist, Pharmacy Department,
Alder Hey Children's NHS Foundation Trust, Liverpool, UK
10. Paediatrics

J. Graham Davies
Professor of Clinical Pharmacy and Therapeutics, King's
College London, London, UK
1. Clinical pharmacy practice

Nemesha Desai
Consultant Dermatologist, St John's Institute of
Dermatology, Guy's and St Thomas' NHS Foundation
Trust, London, UK
58. Eczema and psoriasis

Mark D. Doherty
Consultant Ophthalmologist, Sunderland Eye Infirmary,
Sunderland, UK
56. Glaucoma

Tobias Dreischulte
Research Pharmacist, NHS Tayside, Community Health
Sciences Division, Dundee, UK
21. Chronic heart failure

Jackie Elliott
Senior Clinical Lecturer in Diabetes and Honorary
Consultant, Diabetes and Endocrine Centre, Northern
General Hospital, Sheffield, UK
45. Diabetes mellitus

Sarah Fenner
Director, West Midlands Medicines Information Service
and UK Drugs in Lactation Advisory Service, Good Hope
Hospital, Sutton Coldfield, UK
48. Drugs in pregnancy and lactation

Ray W. Fitzpatrick
Clinical Director of Pharmacy, New Cross Hospital,
Wolverhampton, UK
3. Practical pharmacokinetics

Peter Golightly
Senior Medicines Information Pharmacist, West Midlands
and Trent Regional Medicines Information Services and
UK Drugs in Lactation Advisory Service, Good Hope
Hospital NHS Trust, Sutton Coldfield, UK
48. Drugs in pregnancy and lactation

Alison Grant
Highly Specialist Pharmacist in HIV and Sexual Health,
Guy's and St Thomas' NHS Foundation Trust, St Thomas'
Hospital, London, UK
42. HIV infection

Jim Gray
Consultant Microbiologist, Department of Microbiology,
Birmingham Women's and Children's NHS Foundation
Trust, Birmingham Children's Hospital, Birmingham, UK
38. Gastro-intestinal infections
39. Infective meningitis

Dan Greer
Pharmacist Lecturer/Practitioner, Programme Manager,
Postgraduate Programme in Pharmacy Practice,
University of Leeds, Leeds, UK
12. Dyspepsia, peptic ulcer disease and
gastro-oesophageal reflux disease

Imran Hafiz
Principal Cardiovascular Pharmacist, Guy's and
St Thomas' NHS Foundation Trust; Clinical Lecturer,
King's College London, UK
20. Coronary heart disease

Keith Harding
Dean of Clinical Innovation, Professor of Wound Healing
Research, Clinical Innovation Cardiff (CIIC), College of
Biomedical and Life Sciences, Cardiff University School
of Medicine, Cardiff, UK
59. Wounds

Susanna J. Harwood
Pharmacist, Aseptic Services, University Hospital of
Wales, Cardiff, UK
7. Parenteral nutrition

Tina Hawkins
Retired Specialist Pharmacist in Rheumatology,
Leeds, UK
54. Rheumatoid arthritis and osteoarthritis
55. Gout and hyperuricaemia

Gregory J. Hobbs
Consultant in Pain Medicine, Primary Integrated
Community Solutions, Nottingham, UK
34. Pain

Samantha Holloway
Senior Lecturer/Programme Director, Centre for Medical
Education, School of Medicine, Cardiff University,
Cardiff, UK
59. Wounds

Philip Howard
NHS-Improvement AMR Project Lead, Leeds Teaching
Hospitals, Leeds, UK
40. Surgical site infection and antimicrobial prophylaxis

Gail Jones
Consultant Haematologist, Northern Centre for Cancer
Care, Freeman Hospital, Newcastle upon Tyne, UK
51. Leukaemia

Atul Kalhan
Endocrinology, Department of Diabetes and Endocrinology,
Royal Glamorgan Hospital, Ynysmaerdy, Llantrisant, UK
44. Thyroid and parathyroid disorders

Sallianne Kavanagh
Lead Pharmacist – Diabetes and Endocrinology, Sheffield
Teaching Hospital NHS Foundation Trust, Pharmacy
Department, Sheffield, UK
45. Diabetes mellitus

Patrick Kennedy
Reader in Hepatology, Blizard Institute, Barts and The
London School of Medicine and Dentristy, Queen Mary
University of London, London, UK
16. Liver disease

Roger David Knaggs
Associate Professor in Clinical Pharmacy Practice,
School of Pharmacy, University of Nottingham;
Specialist Pharmacist in Pain Management, Primary
Integrated Community Solutions, Nottingham, UK
34. Pain

Apostolos Koffas
ST4 in Gastroenterolgy and Hepatology, University
Hospital of Larisa, Larisa, Greece
16. Liver disease

Janet Krska
Professor of Clinical and Professional Practice, Medway
School of Pharmacy, Chatham, Kent, UK
5. Adverse drug reactions

Alan Lamont
Clinical Oncologist (Retired), Colchester Hospital
University Foundation Trust, Colchester, UK;
Chair, Cambridge East Research Ethics Committee,
Health Research Authority, London, UK
53. Solid tumours

Emma Lane
Senior Lecturer in Pharmacology, School of Pharmacy
and Pharmaceutical Sciences, Cardiff University, Cardiff,
UK
32. Parkinson's disease

Michelle Lannon
Post CCT Fellow, Haematology, Northern Centre for
Cancer Care, Freeman Hospital, Newcastle Upon Tyne, UK
51. Leukaemia

Catherine Loughran
Lead Pharmacist, Haematology, Pharmacy Department,
Leicester Royal Infirmary, Leicester, UK
52. Lymphomas

Katie Maddock
Director of Master of Pharmacy Learning and Teaching,
School of Pharmacy, Keele University, Keele, UK
3. Practical pharmacokinetics

Helen Marlow
Lead Pharmacist, Surrey Down CCG, Leatherhead, UK
2. Prescribing

John Marriott
School of Clinical and Experimental Medicine, College of
Medical and Dental Sciences, University of Birmingham,
Birmingham, UK
17. Acute kidney injury
18. Chronic kidney disease and end-stage renal disease

Kay Marshall
Head of the School of Health Sciences, University of
Manchester, Manchester, UK
46. Menstrual cycle disorders
47. Menopause

Emma Mason
Department of Acute Medicine, Royal Gwent Hospital,
Newport, Wales, UK
35. Nausea and vomiting

John McAnaw
Head of Pharmacy, NHS 24, South Queensferry, UK
21. Chronic heart failure

Niamh McGarry
Lead Pharmacist for Care of the Elderly/Older People
Services, Belfast Health and Social Care Trust, Belfast
City Hospital, Belfast, UK
50. Anaemia

Duncan McRobbie
Associate Chief Pharmacist – Clinical Services, Guy's
and St Thomas' NHS Foundation Trust; Clinical Reader,
Kings College London; Visiting Professor UCL School of
Pharmacy, Pharmacy Department, St. Thomas' Hospital,
London, UK
1. Clinical pharmacy practice
20. Coronary heart disease

Helen Meynell
Consultant Pharmacist/Clinical Governance Lead,
Doncaster and Bassetlaw Teaching Hospitals NHS
Foundation Trust, Doncaster, UK
26. Chronic obstructive pulmonary disease

Catherine Molyneux
Consultant Microbiologist, County Durham and
Darlington NHS Foundation Trust, Durham, UK
36. Respiratory infections

Manjusha Narayanan
Consultant Microbiologist, Department of Microbiology,
Royal Victoria Infirmary, Newcastle upon Tyne, UK
43. Fungal infections

Mike D. Page
Consultant Diabetes and Endocrinology (Retired), Royal
Glamorgan Hospital, Ynysmaerdy, Llantrisant, UK
44. Thyroid and parathyroid disorders

Caroline Parker
Consultant Pharmacist Adult Mental Health, St Charles'
Hospital for Central and North West London NHS
Foundation Trust, London, UK
30. Schizophrenia

Alan Pollard
Independent Mental Health Pharmacy Consultant,
Associate Lecturer Worcester University, Worcester, UK
29. Affective disorders

Sophie Rintoul-Hoad
Specialist Registrar in Urology, Guy's and St. Thomas'
hospital, London, UK
49. Prostate disease

Ali Robb
Consultant Microbiologist, Royal Victoria Infirmary,
Newcastle upon Tyne, UK
36. Respiratory infections

Trevor Rogers
Consultant Respiratory Physician and Director of R&D,
Chest Clinic, Doncaster Royal Infirmary, Doncaster, UK
26. Chronic obstructive pulmonary disease

Linda Ross
Highly Specialist Renal Transplant and Urology
Pharmacist, Department of Renal Transplant and
Urology, Guy's and St Thomas' NHS Foundation Trust,
Guy's Hospital, London, UK
49. Prostate disease

Philip A. Routledge
Professor Emeritus of Clinical Pharmacology, Cardiff
University; Clinical Director of the All Wales Therapeutics
and Toxicology Centre, Cardiff, UK
23. Thrombosis
35. Nausea and vomiting

Paula Russell
Principal Pharmacist (Medicines Information and NHSD
Support), Newcastle Drug and Therapeutics Centre,
Newcastle upon Tyne, UK
48. Drugs in pregnancy and lactation

Josemir W. Sander
Professor of Neurology, University College London,
London, UK
31. Epilepsy

Jonathan Sandoe
Consultant Microbiologist, St James University Hospital,
Leeds, UK
40. Surgical site infection and antimicrobial prophylaxis

Sara Sawieres
Senior Clinical Pharmacist, Liver and Private Patient
Services, King's College Hospital, London, UK
15. Adverse effects of drugs on the liver

Hamsaraj Shetty
Consultant Physician and Honorary Senior Lecturer,
University Hospital of Wales and Cardiff University,
Cardiff, UK
11. Geriatrics
23. Thrombosis

Michele Sie
Chief Pharmacist, Pharmacy Department, South West
London and St George's Mental Health NHS Trust,
Springfield University Hospital, London, UK
27. Insomnia

Ian Smith
Teaching Fellow, School of Pharmacy, Keele University,
Staffordshire, UK
14. Constipation and diarrhoea

Simon Sporton
Consultant Cardiologist, Barts and the London NHS
Trust, St Bartholomew's Hospital, London, UK
22. Arrhythmias

Stephanie Stringer
Consultant Nephrologist, Queen Elizabeth Hospital
Birmingham, Birmingham, UK
17. Acute kidney injury
18. Chronic kidney disease and end-stage renal disease

Denise Taylor
Senior Lecturer, Graduate School of Nursing, Midwifery
and Health, Victoria University of Wellington, New Zealand
33. Dementia

Ruben Thanacoody
Consultant Physician and Clinical Pharmacologist,
Newcastle upon Tyne Hospitals NHS Foundation Trust;
Honorary Clinical Senior Lecturer, Institute of Cellular
Medicine, Newcastle University, Newcastle upon Tyne, UK
4. Drug interactions

Sarah Walsh
Consultant Dermatologist, Department of Dermatology,
Kings College Hospital NHS Foundation Trust, London,
UK
57. Drug-induced skin disorders

John Warburton
Critical Care Pharmacist, Bristol Royal Infirmary,
University Hospitals Bristol NHS Foundation Trust,
Bristol, UK
6. Laboratory data

Martin P. Ward-Platt
Consultant Paediatrician and Honorary Clinical Reader in
Neonatal and Paediatric Medicine, Newcastle Neonatal
Service, Royal Victoria Infirmary, Newcastle upon Tyne,
UK
9. Neonates

David Webb
Chief Pharmacist, Guy's and St Thomas' NHS Foundation
Trust, London, UK
1. Clinical pharmacy practice

Paul Whitaker
Consultant in Respiratory Medicine, Department of
Respiratory Medicine, Leeds Teaching Hospitals NHS
Trust, Leeds, UK
41. Tuberculosis

Cate Whittlesea
Professor of Pharmacy Practice and Associate Director
of Clinical Education, UCL School of Pharmacy,
University College London, London, UK
2. Prescribing

Simon J. Wilkins
Senior Lecturer and Programme Director, Cardiff
University School of Medicine, Cardiff, UK
23. Thrombosis

Helen Williams
Consultant Pharmacist for Cardiovascular Disease, South
London; Clinical Director for Atrial Fibrillation, Health
Innovation Network; Clinical Associate for CV Disease,
Southwark CCG; Clinical Network Lead for CV Disease,
Lambeth CCG, Hosted by Southwark CCG, Medicines
Optimisation Team, Southwark CCG, London, UK
19. Hypertension
24. Dyslipidaemia

Ken Woodhouse
Professor Emeritus of Geriatric Medicine, Cardiff
University, Cardiff, UK
11. Geriatrics

Richard Woolf
Academic Clinical Lecturer and Specialist Registrar in
Dermatology, St John's Institute of Dermatology, King's
College London, Guy's Hospital, London, UK
58. Eczema and psoriasis

Laura Yates
Head of Teratology, UK Teratology Information Service,
Newcastle Drug and Therapeutics Centre, Newcastle
upon Tyne, UK
48. Drugs in pregnancy and lactation

Contents

SECTION 1

GENERAL

1 Clinical Pharmacy Practice

Duncan McRobbie, David Webb and J. Graham Davies

Key points

- Clinical pharmacy comprises a set of skills that promote the optimal use of medicines for individual patients. Optimising the use of medicines requires a patient-centred approach that is grounded in principles of safety, evidence-based and consistent practice, and an understanding of the patient's experience.
- Clinical pharmacy has enabled pharmacists to shift from a product-oriented role towards direct engagement with patients and the value they derive from, or the problems they encounter with, their medicines.
- Achieving specific and positive patient outcomes from the optimal use of medicines is a characteristic of the pharmaceutical care process. The practice of clinical pharmacy is an essential component of pharmaceutical care.
- The three main elements of the care process are assessing the patient, determining the care plan and evaluating the outcome.
- An ability to consult with patients is a key step in the delivery of pharmaceutical care and the optimal use of medicines. Consultation skills require regular review and practice, regardless of the practitioner's experience.

Clinical pharmacy encourages pharmacists and pharmacy support staff to shift their focus from product orientation to more direct engagement with patients, to maximise the benefits that individuals obtain from the medicines they take. Since the late 1980s the practice of clinical pharmacy has grown from a collection of patient-related functions to a process in which all actions are undertaken with the intention of achieving explicit outcomes for the patient. In doing so clinical pharmacy has moved forward to embrace the philosophy of pharmaceutical care (Hepler and Strand, 1990) and, more recently, the principles of medicines optimisation (Royal Pharmaceutical Society, 2013).

The aim of this chapter is to provide a practical framework within which knowledge of therapeutics and an understanding of clinical practice can best be utilised. This chapter describes a pragmatic approach to applying aspects of the pharmaceutical care process and the specific skills of clinical pharmacy to support the optimal use of medicines in a manner that does not depend on the setting of the practitioner or patient.

Development of clinical practice in pharmacy

The emergence of clinical pharmacy as a form of professional practice has been attributed to the poor medicines control systems that existed in hospitals during the early 1960s (Cousins and Luscombe, 1995). Although provoked by similar hospital-associated problems, the nature of the professional response differed between the USA and the UK.

In the USA the approach was to adopt unit dose dispensing and pursue decentralisation of pharmacy services. In the UK the unification of the prescription and the administration record meant this document needed to remain on the hospital ward and required the pharmacist to visit the ward to order medicines. Clinical pharmacy developed from the presence of pharmacists in these patient areas and their interest in promoting safer medicines use. This was initially termed 'ward pharmacy', but participation in medical ward rounds in the late 1970s signalled the transition to clinical pharmacy.

Medication safety may have been the spur, but clinical pharmacy in the 1980s grew because of its ability to promote the cost-effective use of medicines in hospitals. This role was recognised by the government, which in 1988 endorsed the implementation of clinical pharmacy services to secure value for money from medicines. Awareness that support depended to an extent on the quantification of actions and cost savings led several groups to develop ways of measuring pharmacists' clinical interventions. Coding systems were necessary to aggregate large amounts of data in a reliable manner, and many of these drew upon the eight steps (Table 1.1) of the drug use process (DUP) indicators (Hutchinson et al., 1986).

Data collected from these early studies revealed that interventions had very high physician acceptance rates, were made most commonly at the 'select regimen' and 'need for drug' stages of the DUP, and were influenced by hospital ward type (intensive care and paediatrics having the highest rates), pharmacist seniority (rates increasing with seniority) and time spent on wards (Barber et al., 1997).

Despite the level of activity that intervention monitoring revealed, coupled with evidence of cost containment and a broadly supportive healthcare system, frustrations began to

Table 1.1 Drug use process indicators

DUP stage	Action
Establish need for a drug	Ensure there is an appropriate indication for each medicine and that all medical problems are addressed therapeutically. Consider deprescribing medicines that are no longer appropriate.
Select drug	Select and recommend the most appropriate medicine based upon the ability to reach therapeutic goals, with consideration of patient variables, formulary status and cost of therapy.
Select regimen	Select the most appropriate medicines for accomplishing the desired therapeutic goals at the least cost without diminishing effectiveness or causing toxicity.
Provide drug	Facilitate the dispensing and supply process so that medicines are accurately prepared, dispensed in ready-to-administer form and delivered to the patient on a timely basis.
Administer drug	Ensure that appropriate devices and techniques are used for medicines administration.
Monitor drug therapy	Monitor medicines for effectiveness or adverse effects to determine whether to maintain, modify or discontinue.
Counsel patient	Counsel and educate the patient or caregiver about the patient's therapy to ensure proper use of medicines.
Evaluate effectiveness	Evaluate the effectiveness of the patient's medicines by reviewing all the previous steps of the DUP and taking appropriate steps to ensure that the therapeutic goals are achieved.

DUP, Drug use process.

appear. These in part stemmed from a lack of certainty about the fundamental purpose of clinical pharmacy and also from tensions between the desire for clinical specialisation and organisational goals of improving services more generally in hospitals and other care settings.

Pharmaceutical care

A need to focus on outcomes of medicines use, as opposed to the functions of clinical pharmacy, became apparent (Hepler and Strand, 1990). The launch of pharmaceutical care as the 'responsible provision of drug therapy for the purpose of achieving definite outcomes that improve a patient's quality of life' (Hepler and Strand, 1990, p. 539) was a landmark in the topography of pharmacy practice. In reality, this was a step forward rather than a revolutionary leap, as expansion of the traditional dispensing role and the acquisition of new responsibilities, in particular

Table 1.2 Definitions of clinical pharmacy, pharmaceutical care and medicines optimisation

Term	Definition
Clinical pharmacy	Clinical pharmacy comprises a set of functions that promote the safe, effective and economic use of medicines for individual patients. Clinical pharmacy process requires the application of specific knowledge of pharmacology, pharmacokinetics, pharmaceutics and therapeutics to patient care.
Pharmaceutical care	Pharmaceutical care is a cooperative, patient-centred system for achieving specific and positive patient outcomes from the responsible provision of medicines. The practice of clinical pharmacy is an essential component in the delivery of pharmaceutical care.
Medicines optimisation	Medicines optimisation aims to ensure that the right patients get the right choice of medicine at the right time. The purpose is to help patients take their medicines appropriately and, by doing so, avoid unnecessary treatment, improve safety and outcomes, and reduce wastage. Ultimately it can support patients to take greater ownership of their treatment.

the ability to be able to handle the interpersonal relationships required at the interface of the pharmacy system and the patient, had been debated for some time (Brodie, 1981).

The delivery of pharmaceutical care is dependent on the practice of clinical pharmacy, but the key feature of care is that the practitioner takes responsibility for a patient's medicines-related needs and is held accountable for that commitment. None of the definitions of pharmaceutical care is limited by reference to a specific professional group. Although pharmacists and pharmacy support staff would expect to play a central role in pharmaceutical care, it is essentially a cooperative system that embraces the contribution of other professionals and patients (Table 1.2). The philosophy of pharmaceutical care anticipated healthcare policy in which certain functions, such as the prescribing of medicines, have extended beyond their traditional professional origins to be undertaken by those trained and identified to be competent to do so.

Medication-related problems

When the outcome of medicines use is not optimal, the underlying medication-related problem (MRP) can be classified according to the criteria set out in Box 1.1 (Hepler and Strand, 1990). Some MRPs are associated with significant morbidity and mortality. Preventable medication-related hospital admissions in the UK and USA have been estimated to have a prevalence rate of 4% to 5%, indicating that gains in public health from improving prescribing, monitoring and adherence to medicines would be sizeable (Howard et al., 2003; Winterstein et al., 2002).

In prospective studies, up to 28% of accident and emergency department visits have been identified as medication related, of

---

Box 1.1   Categories of medication-related problems

- Untreated indication
- Treatment without indication
- Improper drug selection
- Too little drug
- Too much drug
- Non-adherence
- Adverse drug reaction
- Drug interaction

---

which 70% were deemed preventable (Zed, 2005). Again the most frequently cited causes were non-adherence and inappropriate prescribing and monitoring. In England adverse drug reactions (ADRs) have been identified as the cause of 6.5% of hospital admissions for patients older than 16 years. The median bed stay for patients admitted with an ADR was 8 days, representing 4% of bed capacity. The projected annual cost to the National Health Service (NHS) was £466 million, the equivalent of seven 800-bed hospitals occupied by patients admitted with an ADR. More than 70% of the ADRs were determined to have been avoidable (Pirmohamed et al., 2004).

Between 2005 and 2010 more than half a million medication incidents were reported to the National Patient Safety Agency, and 16% of these reports involved actual patient harm (Cousins et al., 2012). In 2004 the direct cost of medication errors in NHS hospitals, defined as preventable events that may cause or lead to inappropriate medicines use or harm, was estimated to lie between £200 and £400 million per year. To this should be added the costs arising from litigation (Department of Health, 2004). In care homes, one study found that more than two-thirds of residents were exposed to one or more medication errors (Barber et al., 2009), whilst in hospitals a prescribing error rate of almost 9% has been identified (Doran et al., 2010). In addition nearly a third of patients are non-adherent 10 days after starting a new medicine for a chronic condition, of whom 45% are intentionally non-adherent (Barber et al., 2004), a significant contributor to the £150 million per annum estimated avoidable medicines waste in primary care (York Health Economics Consortium and School of Pharmacy, 2010). The scale of the misadventure that these findings reveal, coupled with increasing concerns about the costs of drug therapy, creates an opportunity for a renaissance in clinical pharmacy practice, providing that it realigns strongly with the principles of medicines optimisation. Pharmacists and their teams are uniquely placed to help reduce the level of medication-related morbidity in primary care by virtue of their skills and accessibility, and by building on relationships with general practice.

Medicines optimisation

The aim of medicines optimisation is to help patients take their medicines appropriately and, by doing so, improve safety and outcomes, avoid unnecessary treatment and reduce wastage. Ultimately it supports patients in taking greater ownership of

their treatment (Royal Pharmaceutical Society, 2013). At its heart are four guiding principles:

- communicating with the patient and/or his or her carer about the patient's choice and experience of using medicines to manage his or her condition;
- supporting the most appropriate choice of clinically and cost-effective medicines (informed by the best available evidence base);
- ensuring that medicines use is as safe as possible, including safe processes and systems, effective communication between professionals and the minimising likelihood of unwanted effects and interactions;
- making medicines optimisation part of routine practice by routinely discussing with patient, carers and other health professionals how to achieve the best outcomes from medicines.

By locating clinical pharmacy skills within a pharmaceutical care philosophy, medicines optimisation seeks to be the step change that will better realise the benefits of treatment with medicines and reduce both suboptimal use and MRPs. It is a patient-centred endeavour based firmly on professionalism and partnership.

Evidence supporting the unique clinical contribution of pharmacists has been building since the launch of pharmaceutical care in the 1990s. In the USA, for example, pharmacists' participation in physician ward rounds was shown to reduce adverse drug events by 78% and 66% in general medical (Kucukarslan et al., 2003) and intensive care settings (Leape et al., 1999), respectively. A study covering 1029 US hospitals was the first to indicate that both centrally based and patient-specific clinical pharmacy services are associated with reduced mortality rates (Bond et al., 1999). The services involved were medicines information, clinical research performed by pharmacists, active pharmacist participation in resuscitation teams and pharmacists undertaking admission medication histories.

In the UK the focus also has been on prevention and management of MRPs. Recognition that many patients either fail to benefit or experience unwanted effects from their medicines has elicited two types of response from the pharmacy profession. Firstly, to put in place, and make use of, a range of postgraduate initiatives and programmes to meet the developmental needs of pharmacists working in clinical settings; secondly, the re-engineering of pharmaceutical services to introduce schemes for medicines optimisation at an organisational level. These have ranged from specific initiatives to target identified areas of medication risk, such as pharmacist involvement in anticoagulation services, to more general approaches where the intention is to ensure consistency of medicines use, particularly across care interfaces. Medicines reconciliation on hospital admission ensures that medicines prescribed to in-patients correspond to those that the patient was taking prior to admission. Guidance recommends that medicines reconciliation should be part of standard care and that pharmacists should be involved as soon as possible after the patient has been admitted (National Institute for Health and Care Excellence [NICE], 2015). The process requires the name, dosage, frequency and route of administration to be established for all medicines taken prior to admission. The information collected as part of medicines reconciliation is a prerequisite for medication review that the NICE guideline defines as a structured, critical examination of a person's medicines with the objective of reaching an agreement about treatment, optimising the impact of medicines, minimising the number of MRPs and reducing waste (NICE, 2015).

Pharmaceutical consultation

Structured postgraduate education has served to improve the knowledge of clinical pharmacists, but fully achieving the goals of pharmaceutical care has proved more challenging. Part of the difficulty has been the requirement to place the patient at the heart of the system, rather than being a relatively passive recipient of drug therapy and associated information. To deliver pharmaceutical care requires more than scientific expertise. It mandates a system that describes first the role and responsibilities of the pharmacist and provides the necessary infrastructure to support them in this role, and secondly a clear process by which the pharmacist can deliver his or her contribution to patient care.

Pharmaceutical care is predicated on a patient-centred approach to identifying, preventing or resolving medicine-related problems. Central to this aim is the need to establish a therapeutic relationship. This relationship must be a partnership in which the pharmacist works with the patient to resolve medication-related issues in line with the patient's wishes, expectations and priorities. Table 1.3 summarises the three key elements of the care process (Cipolle et al., 1998). Research in chronic diseases has shown that self-management is promoted when patients more fully participate in the goal-setting and planning aspects of their care (Sevick et al., 2007). These are important aspects to consider when pharmacists consult with patients. In community pharmacy in the UK, approaches to help patients use their medicines more effectively are the medicines use review (MUR) and the new medicines service (NMS). The MUR uses the skills of pharmacists to help patients understand how their medicines should be used, why they take them and to identify any problems patients have in relation to their medicines, providing feedback to the prescriber if necessary. Two goals of MUR are to improve the adherence of patients to prescribed medicines and to reduce medicines wastage. The NMS has been introduced to allow pharmacists to support patients with long-term conditions who have been recently started on a medicine to target medicines adherence

early. Currently the service targets four key conditions/therapies: asthma and chronic obstructive pulmonary disease, type 2 diabetes, hypertension and antiplatelet or anticoagulant therapy (Pharmaceutical Services Negotiating Committee, 2013). Clinical guidance on medicines adherence emphasises the importance of patient involvement in decisions about medicines (NICE, 2009).

Recommendations include that healthcare professionals should:

- Adapt their consultation style to the needs of individual patients.
- Consider any factors that may affect patients' involvement in the consultation.
- Establish the most effective way of communicating with each patient.
- Encourage patients to ask about their condition and treatment.
- Be aware that consultation skills can be improved to enhance patient involvement.

Medicines-taking behaviour

The need for a care process that ensures that the patient is involved at all stages has become clearer as the extent of non-adherence to medicines has been revealed. Significant proportions (between 30% and 50%) of patients with chronic conditions do not take their prescribed medicines as directed. Many factors are thought to influence a patient's decision to adhere to a prescribed regimen. These include the characteristics of the disease and the treatment used to manage it, the patient's beliefs about his or her illness and medicines, as well as the quality of the interaction between the patient and healthcare practitioners. Non-adherence can be categorised broadly into two types: intentional and unintentional. Unintentional non-adherence may be associated with physical or sensory barriers to taking medicines, for example, not being able to swallow or unable to read the labels, forgetfulness or poor comprehension. Traditionally pharmacists have played a key role in helping patients overcome these types of problems, but they have been less active in identifying and resolving intentional non-adherence.

Intentional (or deliberate) non-adherence may be because of a number of factors. Recent work in health psychology has shaped our understanding of how patients perceive health and illness, and why they often decide not to take their medicines. When people receive information about illness and its treatment, it is processed in accordance with their own belief systems. Often patients' perceptions are not in tune with the medical reality and when this occurs, taking medicines may not make sense to the individual. For example, a patient diagnosed with hypertension may view the condition as one that is caused by stress and, during periods of lower stress, may not take their prescribed medicines (Baumann and Leventhal, 1985). Consequently, a patient holding this view of hypertension may be at increased risk of experiencing an adverse outcome such as a stroke.

Research has shown that patient beliefs about the necessity of the prescribed medication and concerns about the potential long-term effects have a strong influence on medicines-taking behaviour (Horne et al., 2013). However, a patient's beliefs about the benefits and risks of medicines are rarely explored during consultation, despite evidence of an association between non-adherence

Table 1.3	Key elements of the care process
Element	Purpose
Assessment	The main goal of assessment is to establish a full medication history and highlight actual and potential medication-related problems.
Care plan	The care plan should clearly state the goals to optimise care and the responsibilities of both the pharmacist and the patient in attaining the stated goals.
Evaluation	The evaluation reviews progress against the stated patient outcomes.

and the patient's satisfaction with the consultation process adopted by practitioners (Ley, 1988). Classifying patients as intentional or unintentional non-adherers does not fully explain the reasons for such behaviour. A recently proposed psychological framework takes into account a wider range of factors. Known as the COM-B framework (Michie et al., 2011), it proposes that for people to engage in a behaviour, they must have the capability (C), opportunity (O) and motivation (M) to do so. For example, a complex treatment regimen may be beyond the planning ability of a patient (capability barrier), especially if the patient fears disclosure about a health condition that is incorrectly perceived to have a detrimental effect on his or her ability to do his or her job (opportunity barrier). Over time non-adherence may have no discernible effect on the patient's health status, so he or she makes the decision to stop treatment completely (motivation barrier). Interventions designed to support behaviour change need to address any barriers within all three key components. Jackson et al. (2014) provide more examples of the COM-B framework applied to medicines adherence.

Consultation process

There are several comprehensive accounts of the functions required to satisfy each stage of the DUP, but few go on to explore how the pharmacist can create a therapeutic relationship with his or her patient. The ability of a pharmacist to consult effectively is fundamental to pharmaceutical care, and this includes establishing a platform for achieving adherence/concordance. Nurturing a relationship with the patient is essential to understanding the patient's medication-related needs.

Descriptions of pharmaceutical consultation have been confined largely to the use of mnemonics such as WWHAM, AS METTHOD and ENCORE (Box 1.2). These approaches provide the pharmacist with a rigid structure to use when questioning patients about their symptoms, but, although useful, serve to make the symptom or disease the focus of the consultation rather than the patient. A common misconception is that healthcare professionals who possess good communication skills are also able to consult effectively with patients; this relationship will not hold if there is a failure to grasp the essential components of the consultation technique. Research into patients' perceptions of their illness and treatment has demonstrated that they are more likely to adhere to their medication regimen, and be more satisfied with the consultation, if their views about illness and treatment have been taken into account and the risks and benefits of treatment discussed (Martin et al., 2005). The mnemonic approach to consultation does not adequately address the complex interaction that may take place between a patient and a healthcare practitioner.

Undertaking a pharmaceutical consultation can be considered as a series of four interlinked phases, each with a goal and set of competencies (Table 1.4). These phases follow a problem-solving pattern, embrace relevant aspects of adherence research and attempt to involve the patient at each stage in the process. This approach forms the basis of the medication-related consultation framework, a tool shown to improve the capability of pharmacists to consult (Abdel-Tawab et al., 2011). For effective consultation the practitioner also needs to draw upon a range of communication behaviours (Box 1.3). By integrating the agendas

---

Box 1.2 Mnemonics used in the pharmacy consultation process

WWHAM
Who is it for?
What are the symptoms?
How long has it been going on?
Action taken?
Medicines taken?

AS METTHOD
Age of the patient?
Self or for someone else?
Medicines being taken?
Exactly what do you mean (by the symptom)?
Time and duration of the symptom?
Taken any action (medicine or seen a healthcare practitioner)?
History of any disease?
Other symptoms?
Doing anything to alleviate or worsen the symptom?

ENCORE
Evaluate the symptom, its onset, recurrence and duration.
No medication is always an option.
Care when dealing with specific patient groups, notably the elderly, the young, nursing mothers, pregnant women, those receiving specific medication such as methotrexate and anticoagulants, and those with a particular disease, for example, renal impairment.
Observe the patient for signs of systemic disturbance and ask about presence of fever, loss of weight and any accompanying physiological disturbance.
Refer when in doubt.
Explain any course of action recommended.

---

of both patient and pharmacist, the approach outlined earlier provides the vehicle for agreeing on the issues to be addressed and the responsibilities accepted by each party in achieving the desired outcomes.

The ability to consult with patients is a key process in the delivery of pharmaceutical care and consequently requires regular review and development, regardless of experience. To ensure these core skills are developed, individuals should use trigger questions to prompt reflection on their approach to consulting (Box 1.4).

Clinical pharmacy functions and knowledge

The following practical steps in the delivery of pharmaceutical care are based largely on the DUP. The 'select regimen' and 'drug administration' indicators have been amalgamated at step 3.

Step 1. Establishing the need for drug therapy

For independent prescribers this step includes establishing a diagnosis and then balancing the risks and benefits of treatment against the risks posed by the disease. Current practice for most pharmacists means that another professional, most frequently a

Table 1.4 Pharmaceutical consultation process

Element	Goal	Examples of associated competencies
Introduction	Building a therapeutic relationship	Invites patient to discuss medication or health-related issue
		Discusses structure and purpose of consultation
		Negotiates shared agenda
Data collection and problem identification	Identifying the patient's medication-related needs	Takes a full medication history
		Establishes patient's understanding of his or her illness
		Establishes patient's understanding of the prescribed treatment
		Identifies and prioritises patient's pharmaceutical problems
Actions and solutions	Establishing an acceptable management plan with the patient	Involves patient in designing management plan
		Tailors information to address patient's perception of illness and treatment
		Checks patient's understanding
		Refers appropriately
Closure	Negotiating safety netting strategies with the patient	Provides information to guide action when patient experiences problems with management plan
		Provides further appointment or contact point

Box 1.3 Consultation behaviours

- Apply active listening.
- Appropriately use open and closed questions.
- Respect patient.
- Avoid jargon.
- Demonstrate empathy.
- Deal sensitively with potentially embarrassing or sensitive issues.

Box 1.4 Key postconsultation questions

- Do I know more now about the patient?
- Was I curious?
- Did I really listen?
- Did I find out what really mattered to the patient?
- Did I explore the patient's beliefs and expectations?
- Did I identify the patient's main medication-related problems?
- Did I use the patient's thoughts when I started explaining?
- Did I share the treatment options with the patient?
- Did I help my patient to reach a decision?
- Did I check that my patient understood what I said?
- Did we agree?
- Was I friendly?

doctor, will have diagnosed the patient's presenting condition and any co-existing disease. The pharmacist's role, therefore, is often one of providing information to the independent prescriber on the expected benefits and risks of drug therapy by evaluating both the evidence base and individual patient factors. Pharmacists also draw on these concepts as they become more involved in prescribing and adjusting therapy for patients under their care.

The evidence for one specific mode of therapy may not be conclusive. In this circumstance the pharmacist will need to call on his or her understanding of the principles of pharmaceutical science and on clinical experience to provide the best advice possible.

Step 1.1. Relevant patient details

Without background information on the patient's health and social circumstances (Table 1.5) it is difficult to establish the existence of, or potential for, MRPs. When this information is lacking, a review solely of prescribed medicines will probably be of limited value and incurs the risk of making a flawed judgement on the appropriateness of therapy for that individual.

Current and co-existing conditions with which the patient presents can be established from various sources. In medical notes the current diagnosis (Δ) or differential diagnoses ($\Delta\Delta$) will be documented, as well as any medical history. Other opportunities to gather information come from discussion with the patient and participation in medical rounds. In primary care, primary care clinicians' computer systems carry information on the patient's diagnosis.

Once the diagnosis and past medical history (PMH) are established, it is then possible to identify the medicines that would be expected to be prescribed for each indication, based on contemporary evidence. This list of medicines may be compiled from appropriate national or international guidelines, local formularies and knowledge of current practice.

Step 1.2. Medication history

A medication history is the part of a pharmaceutical consultation that identifies and documents allergies or other serious adverse medication events, as well as information about how medicines are taken currently and have been taken in the past. It is the starting point for medicines reconciliation and medication review.

Obtaining accurate and complete medication histories has been shown to have a positive effect on patient care, and pharmacists have demonstrated that they can compile such histories with a high degree of precision and reliability as part of medicines reconciliation. The benefit to the patient is that prescribing errors of omission or transcription are identified and corrected early, reducing the risk of harm and improving care.

Discrepancies between the history recorded by the medical team and that which the pharmacist elicits fall into two categories: intentional (where the medical team has made a decision to alter the regimen) or unintentional (where a complete record was not obtained). Discrepancies should be clarified with the prescriber or referred to a more senior pharmacist. Box 1.5 lists the key components of a medication history.

Table 1.5   Relevant patient details

Factor	Implications
Age	The very young and the very old are most at risk of medication-related problems. A patient's age may indicate his or her likely ability to metabolise and excrete medicines, and has implications for step 2 of the drug use process.
Gender	This may alter the choice of the therapy for certain indications. It may also prompt consideration of the potential for pregnancy or breastfeeding.
Ethnic or religious background	Racially determined predispositions to intolerance or ineffectiveness should be considered with certain classes of medicines, for example, angiotensin-converting enzyme inhibitors in Afro-Caribbean people. Formulations may be problematic for other groups, for example, those based on blood products for Jehovah's Witnesses or porcine-derived products for Jewish patients.
Social history	This may impact on ability to manage medicines and influence pharmaceutical care needs, for example, living alone or in a care home, or availability of nursing, social or informal carers
Presenting complaint	The presenting complaint includes symptoms the patient describes and the signs identified by the doctor on examination. Pharmacists should consider whether these might be attributable to the adverse effects of prescribed or purchased medicines.
Working diagnosis	This should enable the pharmacist to identify the classes of medicines that would be anticipated on the prescription based on current evidence.
Medical history	Understanding the patient's other medical conditions and his or her history helps ensure that management of the current problem does not compromise a prior condition and guides the selection of appropriate therapy by identifying potential contraindications.
Laboratory or physical findings	The focus should be on findings that may affect therapy, such as: • renal function • liver function • full blood count • blood pressure • cardiac rhythm Results may convey a need for dosage adjustment or presence of an adverse reaction.

Step 1.3. Deprescribing

Given that many problems associated with medicines use often occur as a result of problematic polypharmacy, sometimes because of a lack of ongoing review, a new concept, namely that of deprescribing, has emerged. This has been defined by Reeve et al. (2015) as 'the process of withdrawal of an inappropriate medication, supervised by a healthcare professional with the goal

Box 1.5   Key components of a medication history

1. Introduce yourself to the patient and explain the purpose of the consultation.
2. Identify any allergies or serious adverse reactions and record these on the prescription chart, care notes or patient medication record.
3. Ascertain information about prescribed and non-prescribed treatments from:
   - the patient's recall
   - medicines in the patient's possession
   - referral letter (usually from the patient's primary care doctor)
   - copy of prescriptions issued or a repeat prescription list
   - medical notes
   - contact with the appropriate community pharmacist or primary care doctor
4. Ensure the following are recorded:
   - generic name of medicine (unless specific brand is required)
   - dose
   - frequency
   - duration of therapy
5. Ensure items such as inhalers, eye drops, topical medicines, and herbal and homeopathic remedies are included because patients often do not consider these as medicines.
6. Ascertain the patient's medication-taking behaviour.
7. Consider practical issues such as swallowing difficulties, ability to read labels and written information, container preferences, and ordering or supply problems.
8. Document the history in an appropriate format.
9. Note any discrepancies between this history and that recorded by other healthcare professionals.
10. Ascertain whether these discrepancies are intentional (from patient, nursing staff, medical staff or medical notes).
11. Communicate non-intentional discrepancies to the prescriber.
12. Document any other important medication-related information in an appropriate manner, for example, implications of chronic renal failure, dialysis and long-term steroid treatment.

of managing polypharmacy and improving outcomes' (p. 1264). This should now be seen as an important aspect of establishing the need for drug therapy to limit the adverse effects seen by the continued prescribing of inappropriate medicines.

Step 2. Selecting the medicine

The issues to be tackled at this stage include clinical and cost-effective selection of a medicine in the context of individual patient care. The list of expected treatments generated at step 1 is now scrutinised for its appropriateness for the patient. This requires three separate types of interaction to be identified: drug–patient, drug–disease and drug–drug. The interactions should be prioritised in terms of likelihood of occurrence and the potential severity of outcome should they occur.

Step 2.1. Identify drug–patient interactions

Many medicines have contraindications or cautions to their use that relate to age groups or gender. Potential drug–patient interactions should be identified that may arise with any of the medicines that could be used to treat the current and pre-existing conditions. Types of drug–patient interactions may include allergy or previous ADR, the impact of abnormal renal or hepatic function or chronic heart failure on the systemic availability of some medicines, and patients' preferences for certain treatment options, formulations or routes of administration.

Step 2.2. Identify drug–disease interactions

A drug–disease interaction may occur when a medicine has the potential to make a pre-existing condition worse. Older people are particularly vulnerable due to the co-existence of several chronic diseases and exposure to polypharmacy. Prevention of drug–disease interactions requires an understanding of the pharmacodynamic properties of medicines and an appreciation of their contraindications.

Step 2.3. Drug–drug interactions

Medicines may affect the action of other medicines in a number of ways. Those with similar mechanisms of action may show an enhanced effect if used together, whilst those with opposing actions may reduce each other's effectiveness. Metabolism of one medicine can be affected by a second that acts as an inducer or inhibitor of the cytochrome P450 enzyme system.

The practitioner should be able to identify common drug interactions and recognise those medicines with increased risk of potential interaction, such as those with narrow therapeutic indices or involving hepatic P450 metabolic pathways. It is important to assess the clinical significance of drug interactions and consider the options for effective management.

The list of potential evidence-based treatments should be reviewed for possible drug–patient, drug–disease and drug–drug interactions. The refined list can then be compared with the medicines that have been prescribed for the patient. The practitioner should explore any discrepancies to ensure the patient does not experience an MRP. This may necessitate consultation with medical staff or other healthcare professionals, or referral to a more senior pharmacist.

Step 3. Administering the medicine

Many factors influence the effect that a medicine has at its locus of action. These include the rate and extent of absorption, degree of plasma protein binding and volume of distribution, and the routes of metabolism or excretion. Factors that affect bioavailability may include the extent of absorption of the drug from the gastro-intestinal tract in relation to food and other medicines, or the amount adsorbed onto intravenous infusion bags and giving sets when used to administer medicines parenterally.

The liver has extensive capacity for drug metabolism, even when damaged. Nevertheless, the degree of hepatic impairment should be assessed from liver function tests and related to potential changes in drug metabolism. This is particularly important for medicines that require activation by the liver (prodrugs) or those whose main route of elimination is transformation into water-soluble metabolites.

Table 1.6 Pharmaceutical considerations in the administration of medicines

Dose	Is the dose appropriate, including adjustments for particular routes or formulations? Examples: differences in dose between intravenous and oral metronidazole, intramuscular and oral chlorpromazine, and digoxin tablets compared with the elixir
Route	Is the prescribed route available (is the patient nil by mouth?) and appropriate for the patient? Examples: unnecessary prescription of an intravenous medicine when the patient can swallow, or the use of a solid dosage form when the patient has dysphagia
Dosage form	Is the medicine available in a suitable form for administration via the prescribed route?
Documentation	Is documentation complete? Do nurses or carers require specific information to safely administer the medicine? Examples: appropriateness of crushing tablets for administration via nasogastric tubes, dilution requirements for medicines given parenterally, rates of administration and compatibilities in parenteral solutions (including syringe drivers)
Devices	Are devices required, such as spacers for inhalers?

Table 1.6 summarises the main pharmaceutical considerations for step 3. At this point the practitioner needs to ensure the following tasks have been completed accurately.

Step 3.1. Calculating the appropriate dose

Where doses of oral medicines require calculation, this is usually a straightforward process based on the weight of the patient. However, medicines to be administered parenterally may require more complex calculations, including knowledge of displacement values (particularly for paediatric doses) and determination of appropriate concentrations in compatible fluids and rates of infusion.

Step 3.2. Selecting an appropriate regimen

Giving medicines via the oral route is the preferred method of administration. Parenteral routes carry significantly more risks, including infection associated with vascular access. This route, however, may be necessary when no oral formulation exists or when the oral access is either impossible or inappropriate because of the patient's condition.

Although simple regimens (once- or twice-daily administration) may facilitate adherence, some medicines possess short half-lives and may need to be given more frequently. The practitioner should be familiar with the duration of action of regularly encountered medicines to ensure dosage regimens are optimally designed.

Step 4. Providing the medicine

Ensuring that a prescription is legal, legible, accurate and unambiguous contributes in large measures to the right patient receiving the right medicine at the right time. For the majority of pharmacists this involves screening prescriptions written by other professionals, but those acting as supplementary and independent prescribers need to be cognisant of guidance on prescribing, such as that contained within the British National Formulary, when generating their prescriptions.

In providing a medicine for an individual, due account must be taken of the factors that influence the continued availability and supply of the medicine within the hospital or community setting, for example, formulary and drug tariff status, primary/secondary shared care arrangements and whether the prescribed indication is within the product licence. This is particularly important with unlicensed or non-formulary medicines when information and agreement on continuation of prescribing, recommended monitoring and availability of supply are transferred from a hospital to a primary care setting.

Risks in the dispensing process are reduced by attention to products with similar names or packaging, patients with similar names, and when supplying several family members at the same time. Medicines should be labelled accurately, with clear dosage instructions and advisory labels, and presented appropriately for patients with specific needs, for example, the visually impaired, those unable to read English or those with limited dexterity.

Step 5. Monitoring therapy

Monitoring criteria for the effectiveness of treatment and its potential adverse effects can be drawn from the characteristics of the prescribed medicines used or related to specific patient needs. Close monitoring is required for medicines with narrow therapeutic indices and for the subset of drugs where therapeutic drug monitoring may be beneficial, for example, digoxin, phenytoin, theophylline and aminoglycosides. Anticoagulant therapy, including warfarin and unfractionated heparin, is associated with much preventable medication-related morbidity and always warrants close scrutiny.

Throughout this textbook, details are presented on the monitoring criteria that may be used for a wide range of medicines. Patients with renal or hepatic impairment or an unstable clinical condition need particular attention because of the likely requirement for dosage adjustment or change in therapy.

Step 6. Patient advice and education

A vast quantity of information on drug therapy is available to patients. The practitioner's contribution in this context is to provide accurate and reliable information in a manner that the patient can understand. This may require the pharmacist to convey the benefits and risks of therapy, as well as the consequences of not taking medicines.

Information about medicines is best provided at the time of, or as soon as possible after, the prescribing decision. In the hospital setting this means enabling patients to access information throughout their stay, rather than waiting until discharge. With many pharmacy departments providing medicines in patient packs, the patient can be alerted to the presence of information leaflets, encouraged to read them and ask any questions they may have. This approach enables patients to identify their own information needs and ensures that pharmacists do not create a mismatch between their own agenda and that of the patient. However, there will be a need to clearly explain the limitations of leaflets, particularly when medicines are prescribed for unlicensed indications.

Although the research on adherence indicates the primacy of information that has been tailored to the individual's needs, resources produced by national organisations, such as Diabetes UK (https://www.diabetes.org.uk) and British Heart Foundation (https://www.bhf.org.uk), may also be of help to patients and their family or carers. In addition, patients often require specific information to support their daily routine of taking medicines. All written information, including medicines reminder charts, should be dated and include contact details of the pharmacist to encourage patients to raise further queries or seek clarification.

Step 7. Evaluating effectiveness

The provision of drug therapy for the purpose of achieving definite outcomes is a fundamental objective of pharmaceutical care. These outcomes need to be identified at the outset and form the basis for evaluating the response to treatment. Practitioners delivering pharmaceutical care have a responsibility to evaluate the effectiveness of therapy by reviewing the earlier steps 1–6 and taking appropriate action to ensure the desired outcomes are achieved. Depending on the duration of direct engagement with a patient's care, this may be a responsibility the pharmacist can discharge in person, or it may necessitate transfer of care to a colleague in a different setting where outcomes can be assessed more appropriately.

Case study

The following case is provided to illustrate the application of several steps in the delivery of pharmaceutical care. It is not intended to be a yardstick against which patient care should be judged.

Case 1.1

Mr JB, a 67-year-old retired plumber, has recently moved to your area and has come to the pharmacy to collect his first prescription. He has a PMH of coronary heart disease and has recently had an elective admission where a drug-eluting coronary artery stent was inserted. He has a long history of asthma, which is well controlled with inhaled medicines.

Step 1. Establishing the need for drug therapy

What classes of medicines would you expect to be prescribed for these indications? (Answer is listed in Table 1.7.)

Table 1.7 The case of Mr JB: Potential drug interactions with the patient, the disease or other drugs

	Drug–patient interactions	Drug–disease interactions	Drug–drug interactions
Medicines that should be prescribed for coronary heart disease			
Aspirin	Previous history of dyspepsia	Aspirin should be used with caution in asthma	Combination of antiplatelet agents increases risk of bleeding
Clopidogrel	Previous history of dyspepsia		Combination of antiplatelet agents increases risk of bleeding
Statins			
β-Blockers		β-Blockers should be used with caution in asthma; if peak flows worsen, an alternative rate-controlling agent should be considered	Combination of different agents to control angina may lead to hypotension
Nitrates (glyceryl trinitrate spray)	Previous history of side effects (e.g., headache, flushing) may result in patient not using spray when required		
Medicines that may be prescribed for asthma			
β2-Agonist inhalers	Patient's ability to use inhaler devices effectively	β2-Agonists can cause tachycardia	
Corticosteroid inhaler			

Mr JB gives a complete medication history that indicates he takes his medicines as prescribed, he has no medication-related allergies, but he does suffer from dyspepsia associated with acute use of non-steroidal anti-inflammatory agents. He has a summary of his stent procedure from the hospital that indicates normal blood chemistry and liver function tests.

Step 2. Selecting the medicine

What drug–patient, drug–disease and drug–drug interactions can be anticipated? (See Table 1.7.)

Steps 3 and 4. Administering and providing the medicines

What regimen and individualised doses would you recommend for Mr JB? (Answer is listed in Table 1.8.)

This predicted regimen can be compared with the prescribed therapy and any discrepancies resolved with the prescriber. Step 4 (provision) in Mr JB's case would be relatively straightforward.

Steps 5, 6 and 7. Monitoring therapy, patient education and evaluation

What criteria would you select to monitor Mr JB's therapy, and what information would you share with the patient? What indicators would convey effective management of his condition? (Answer is listed in Table 1.9.)

Quality assurance of clinical practice

Quality assurance of clinical pharmacy has tended to focus on the review of performance indicators, such as intervention rates, or rely upon experienced pharmacists to observe and comment on the practice of others using local measures. The lack of generally agreed or national criteria raises questions about the consistency of these assessments, where they take place and the overall standard of care provided to patients. Following the Bristol Royal Infirmary Inquiry (2001) into paediatric cardiac surgery, there has been much greater emphasis on the need for regulation to maintain the competence of healthcare professionals, the importance of periodic performance appraisal coupled with continuing professional development and the introduction of revalidation.

The challenges for pharmacists are twofold: firstly, to demonstrate their capabilities in a range of clinical pharmacy functions and, secondly, to engage with continuing professional development in a meaningful way to satisfy the expectations of pharmaceutical care and maintain registration with, for example, the General Pharmaceutical Council in the UK. The pragmatic approach to practice and the clinical pharmacy process outlined throughout this chapter has been incorporated into a professional development framework, called the Foundation Pharmacy Framework (Royal Pharmaceutical Society, 2014), that can be used to develop skills, knowledge and other attributes irrespective of the setting of the pharmacist and their patients.

Table 1.8 The case of Mr JB: Possible therapeutic regimen

	Recommendation	Rationale
Medicines that should be prescribed for CHD		
Aspirin	75 mg daily orally after food	Benefit outweighs risk if used with PPI
Clopidogrel	75 mg daily orally after food	Benefit outweighs risk if used with PPI Length of course should be established in relation to previous stent
Lansoprazole	15 mg daily orally	Decreases risk of GI bleeds with combination antiplatelets Concerns about some PPIs reducing the effectiveness of clopidogrel makes selection of specific PPI important
Atorvastatin	40 mg daily orally	Higher doses are recommended if patient suffers an acute coronary event
Nitrates	2 puffs sprayed under the tongue when required for chest pain	
Bisoprolol	5 mg daily orally	Used for rate control to reduce anginal episodes; dose can be titrated against pulse and blood pressure
Ramipril	10 mg daily orally	To reduce the progression of CHD and heart failure
Medicines that may have been prescribed		
Salbutamol inhaler	2 puffs (200 micrograms) to be inhaled when required	Patient should follow asthma treatment plan if peak flow decreases
Beclometasone inhalers	2 puffs (400 micrograms) twice a day	Asthma treatment plan that may include twice a day increasing the dose of inhaled steroids if peak flow decreases

CHD, Coronary heart disease; GI, gastro-intestinal; PPI, proton pump inhibitor.

Table 1.9 The case of Mr JB: Monitoring criteria and patient advice

	Recommendation
Medicines that should be prescribed for CHD	
Aspirin	Ask patient about any symptoms of dyspepsia or worsening asthma
Clopidogrel	Ask patient about any symptoms of dyspepsia
Lansoprazole	If PPIs do not resolve symptoms, the primary care doctor should be consulted
Atorvastatin	Liver function tests 3 months after any change in dose or annually; creatine kinase only if presenting with symptoms of unexplained muscle pain; cholesterol levels 3 months after any change in dose, or annually if at target
Nitrates (GTN spray)	Frequency of use to be noted; increasing frequency that results in a resolution of chest pain should be reported to primary care doctor, and anti-anginal therapy may be increased Any use that does not result in resolution of chest pain requires urgent medical attention
Bisoprolol	Blood pressure and pulse monitored regularly, monitor peak flows on initiation
Ramipril	Renal function and blood pressure monitored within 2 weeks of any dose change or annually
Medicines that may have been prescribed for asthma	
Salbutamol inhaler	Salbutamol use should be monitored because any increase in requirements may require increase in steroid dose; monitor inhaler technique
Beclometasone inhaler	Monitor for oral candidiasis; monitor frequency of exacerbations and 'step up/step down' dose as required; monitor inhaler technique

CHD, Coronary heart disease; GTN, glyceryl trinitrate; PPI, proton pump inhibitor.

References

Abdel-Tawab, R., James, D.H., Fichtinger, A., 2011. Development and validation of the medication-related consultation framework (MRCF). Patient Educ. Couns. 83 (3), 451–457.

Barber, N., Parsons, J., Clifford, S., et al., 2004. Patients' problems with new medication for chronic conditions. Qual. Saf. Health Care 13, 172–175.

Barber, N.D., Batty, R., Ridout, D.A., 1997. Predicting the rate of physician-accepted interventions by hospital pharmacists in the United Kingdom. Am. J. Health Syst. Pharm. 54, 397–405.

Barber, N.D., Alldred, D.P., Raynor, D.K., et al., 2009. Care homes use of medicines study: prevalence, causes and potential for harm of medication errors in care homes for older people. Qual. Saf. Health Care 18, 341–346.

Baumann, L.J., Leventhal, H., 1985. I can tell when my blood pressure is up, can't I? Health Psychol. 4, 203–218.

Bond, C.A., Raehl, C.L., Franke, T., 1999. Clinical pharmacy services and hospital mortality rates. Pharmacotherapy 19, 556–564.

Bristol Royal Infirmary Inquiry, 2001. The Report of the Public Inquiry into Children's Heart Surgery at the Bristol Royal Infirmary 1984–1995. Learning from Bristol Stationery Office, London. Available at: http://webarchive.nationalarchives.gov.uk/20090811143822/; http://www.bristol-inquiry.org.uk/final_report/the_report.pdf.

Brodie, D.C., 1981. Pharmacy's societal purpose. Am. J. Hosp. Pharm. 38, 1893–1896.

Cipolle, R.J., Strand, L.M., Morley, P.C. (Eds.), 1998. Pharmaceutical Care Practice. McGraw-Hill, New York.

Cousins, D.H., Gerrett, D., Warner, B., 2012. A review of medication incidents reported to the National Reporting and Learning System in England and Wales over 6 years (2005–2010). Br. J. Clin. Pharmacol. 74, 597–604.

Cousins, D.H., Luscombe, D.K., 1995. Forces for change and the evolution of clinical pharmacy practice. Pharm. J. 255, 771–776.

Department of Health, 2004. Building a safer NHS for patients: improving medication safety. Department of Health, London. <http://www.dh.gov.uk/en/Publicationsandstatistics/Publications/PublicationsPolicyAndGuidance/DH_4071443>

Doran, T., Ashcroft, D., Heathfield, H., et al., 2010. An in depth investigation into causes of prescribing errors by foundation trainees in relation to their medical education. EQUIP study. Available at: https://www.gmc-uk.org/FINAL_Report_prevalence_and_causes_of_prescribing_errors.pdf_28935150.pdf.

Hepler, C.D., Strand, L.M., 1990. Opportunities and responsibilities in pharmaceutical care. Am. J. Hosp. Pharm. 47, 533–543.

Horne, R., Chapman, S.C.E., Parham, R., et al., 2013. Understanding patients' adherence-related beliefs about medicines prescribed for long-term conditions: a meta-analytic review of the necessity-concerns framework. PLoS One 8 (12), e80633. https://doi.org/10.1371/journal.pone.0080633.

Howard, R.L., Avery, A.J., Howard, P.D., et al., 2003. Investigation into the reasons for preventable drug related admissions to a medical admissions unit: observational study. Qual. Saf. Health Care 12, 280–285.

Hutchinson, R.A., Vogel, D.P., Witte, K.W., 1986. A model for inpatient clinical pharmacy practice and reimbursement. Drug Intell. Clin. Pharm. 20, 989–992.

Jackson, C., Eliasson, L., Barber, N., et al., 2014. Applying COM-B to medication adherence: a suggested framework for research and interventions. Eur. Health Psychol. 16 (1), 7–17.

Kucukarslan, S.N., Peters, M., Mlynarek, M., et al., 2003. Pharmacists on rounding teams reduce preventable adverse drug events in hospital general medicine units. Arch. Intern. Med. 163, 2014–2018.

Leape, L.L., Cullen, D.J., Clapp, M.D., et al., 1999. Pharmacist participation on physician rounds and adverse drug events in the intensive care unit. J. Am. Med. Assoc. 282, 267–270.

Ley, P., 1988. Communicating with Patients. Improving Communication, Satisfaction and Compliance. Croom Helm, London.

Martin, L.R., Williams, S.L., Haskard, K.B., et al., 2005. The challenge of patient adherence. Ther. Clin. Risk Manag. 1, 189–199.

Michie, S., van Stralen, M.M., West, R., 2011. The behaviour change wheel: a new method for characterising and designing behaviour change interventions. Implement. Sci. 6, 42.

National Institute for Health and Care Excellence (NICE), 2015. Medicines optimisation: the safe and effective use of medicines to enable the best possible outcomes (NG5). NICE, London. https://www.nice.org.uk/guidance/ng5.

National Institute for Health and Care Excellence (NICE), 2009. Medicines adherence: involving patients in decisions about prescribed medicines and supporting adherence. Clinical Guideline 76. NICE, London. <https://www.nice.org.uk/nicemedia/pdf/CG76NICEGuideline.pdf>

National Institute for Health and Care Excellence (NICE), 2015. Medicines optimisation: the safe and effective use of medicines to enable the best possible outcomes. NICE, London. <https://www.nice.org.uk/guidance/ng5>

Pharmaceutical Services Negotiating Committee, 2013. Service specification – new medicine service (NMS). <http://psnc.org.uk/wp-content/uploads/2013/06/NMS-service-spec-Aug-2013-changes_FINAL.pdf>

Pirmohamed, M., James, S., Meakin, S., et al., 2004. Adverse drug reactions as cause of admission to hospital: prospective analysis of 18 820 patients. Br. Med. J. 329, 15–19.

Reeve, E., Gnjidic, D., Long, J., et al., 2015. A systematic review of the emerging definition of 'deprescribing' with network analysis: implications for future research and clinical practice. Br. J. Clin. Pharmacol. 80 (6), 1254–1268.

Royal Pharmaceutical Society (RPS), 2013. Medicines optimisation: helping patients to make the most of medicines: good practice guidance for healthcare professionals in England. RPS, London. <https://www.rpharms.com/Portals/0/RPS%20document%20library/Open%20access/Policy/helping-patients-make-the-most-of-their-medicines.pdf>

Royal Pharmaceutical Society (RPS), 2014. Foundation Pharmacy Framework. RPS, London. <https://www.rpharms.com/resources/frameworks/foundation-pharmacy-framework-fpf?Search=foundation%20framework>

Sevick, M.A., Trauth, J.M., Ling, B.S., et al., 2007. Patients with complex chronic diseases: perspectives on supporting self management. J. Gen. Intern. Med. 22 (Suppl. 3), 438–444.

Winterstein, A.G., Sauer, B.C., Helper, C.D., et al., 2002. Preventable drug-related hospital admissions. Ann. Pharmacother. 36, 1238–1248.

York Health Economics Consortium and School of Pharmacy, University of London, 2010. Evaluation of the scale, causes and costs of waste medicines. YHEC/School of Pharmacy, University of London, London. <https://core.ac.uk/download/pdf/111804.pdf>

Zed, P.J., 2005. Drug-related visits to the emergency department. J. Pharm. Pract. 18, 329–335.

2 Prescribing

Helen Marlow and Cate Whittlesea

Key points

- Prescribers need to assess the potential benefits and harms of treatment to support patients to obtain the best possible outcomes from their medicines.
- Patients should receive cost-effective medication appropriate to their clinical needs, in doses that meet their requirements and for an adequate period.
- Respect for patient autonomy, obtaining consent and sharing decision making is a fundamental part of the prescribing process.
- The consultation is a fundamental part of clinical practice and requires effective interpersonal reasoning and practical skills.
- Use of a consultation framework is recommended to ensure relevant issues are covered within the consultation.
- Prescribing is influenced by a complex mix of factors including evidence, external influences and cognitive biases, and these should be recognised.

To prescribe is to authorise, by means of a written prescription, the supply of a medicine. Prescribing incorporates the processes involved in decision making undertaken by the prescriber before the act of writing a prescription. Historically prescribing has been the preserve of those professionals with medical, dental or veterinary training. As the role of other healthcare professionals, pharmacists, nurses, optometrists, physiotherapists, podiatrists and therapeutic radiographers have expanded, prescribing rights have in turn been extended to them. The premise for this development has been that it better utilises the training of these professional groups, is clinically appropriate and improves patient access to medicines.

Regardless of the professional background of the individual prescriber, the factors that motivate them to prescribe a particular medicine are a complex mix of evidence of effectiveness and harms, external influences and cognitive biases. A rational approach to prescribing uses evidence, has outcome goals and evaluates alternatives in partnership with the patient. With the advent of new professional groups of prescribers (non-medical prescribers), there is a need for a systematic approach to prescribing and an understanding of the factors that influence the decision to prescribe a medicine. These issues will be covered in the following sections. Initially the fundamentals of rational and effective prescribing will be discussed followed by a brief outline of the acquisition of prescribing rights by pharmacists and the associated legal framework. The prescribing process and factors which influence it will also be covered.

Rational and effective prescribing

Prescribing a medicine is one of the most common interventions in health care used to treat patients. Medicines have the potential to save lives and improve the quality of life, but they also have the potential to cause harm, which can sometimes be catastrophic. Therefore, prescribing of medicines needs to be rational and effective to maximise benefit and minimise harm. This is best done using a systematic process that puts the patient at the centre (Fig. 2.1).

What is meant by rational and effective prescribing?

No universally agreed-on definition of good prescribing exists. The World Health Organization (WHO) promotes the rational use of medicines, which requires that patients receive medications appropriate to their clinical needs, in doses that meet their own individual requirements, for an adequate period and at the lowest cost to them and their community (de Vries et al., 1994). However, a more widely used framework for good prescribing has been described (Barber, 1995) and identifies what the prescriber should be trying to achieve, both at the time of prescribing and in monitoring treatment thereafter. The prescriber should have the following four aims:
- maximise effective,
- minimise risks,
- minimise costs,
- respect the patient's choices.

This model links to the four key principles of biomedical ethics – beneficence, non-maleficence, justice and veracity, and respect for autonomy – and can be applied to decision making at both an individual patient level and when making decisions about medicines for a wider population, for example, in a Drug and Therapeutics Committee. One of the strengths of this model is the consideration of the patient's perspective and the recognition of the inherent tensions among the four key aims.

Another popular framework to support rational prescribing decisions is known as STEPS (Preskorn, 1994). The STEPS model includes five criteria to consider when deciding on the choice of treatment:
- safety
- tolerability
- effectiveness
- price
- simplicity

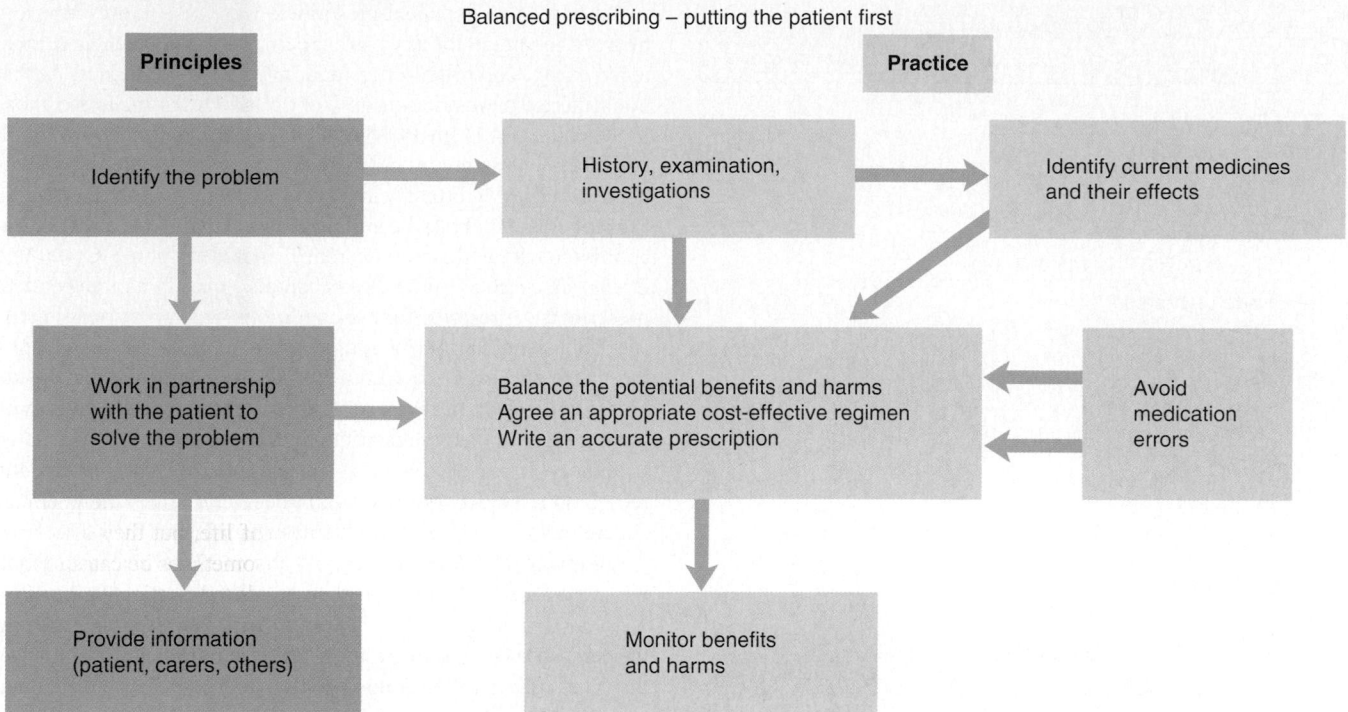

Balanced prescribing – putting the patient first

Fig. 2.1 A framework for good prescribing. (From Background Briefing. A blueprint for safer prescribing 2009 with kind permission from the British Pharmacological Society, London.)

Inappropriate or irrational prescribing

Good prescribing is sometimes defined as the lack of irrational or inappropriate prescribing. Prescribing can be described as irrational for many reasons; for example:

- poor choice of a medicine,
- inappropriate polypharmacy or co-prescribing of interacting medicine,
- prescribing for a self-limiting condition,
- prescribing without considering the risk of harm and managing the risk,
- continuing to prescribe for a longer period than necessary,
- prescribing too low a dose of a medicine,
- prescribing without taking account of the patient's wishes.

Inappropriate or irrational prescribing can result in serious morbidity and mortality, particularly when childhood infections or chronic diseases such as hypertension, diabetes, epilepsy and mental disorders are being treated. Inappropriate prescribing also represents a waste of resources and, as in the case of antimicrobials, may harm the health of the public by contributing to increased antimicrobial resistance. Finally, an over willingness to prescribe stimulates inappropriate patient demand and fails to help patients understand when they should seek out support from a healthcare professional.

Pharmacists as prescribers and the legal framework

Evolution of non-medical prescribing

In 1986 a report was published in the UK ('Cumberlege report') which recommended that community nurses should be given authority to prescribe a limited number of medicines as part

of their role in patient care (Department of Health and Social Security, 1986). Up to this point prescribing in the UK had been the sole domain of doctors, dentists and veterinarians. This was followed in 1989 by a further report (the first Crown report) which recommended that community nurses should prescribe from a limited formulary (Department of Health [DH], 1989). The legislation to permit this was passed in 1992.

At the end of the 1990s, in line with the then UK Government's desire to give patients quicker access to medicines, improve access to services and make better use of the skills of healthcare professionals, the role of prescriber was proposed for other healthcare professionals. This change in prescribing to include non-medical prescribers (e.g. pharmacists and nurses) was developed following a further review (Crown, 1999). This report suggested the introduction of supplementary prescribers, that is, non-medical healthcare professionals who could prescribe, to provide appropriate treatment within a general care plan drawn up by another professional (usually a doctor) or team (Crown, 1999). This led to pharmacists and nurses qualifying as non-medical prescribers (initially as supplementary and then independent prescribers). Subsequently optometrists, physiotherapists, podiatrists and therapeutic radiographers were also able to qualify as independent prescribers.

Supplementary prescribing

The Health and Social Care Act 2001 allowed pharmacists and other healthcare professionals to prescribe. Following this legislation, in 2003 the Department of Health outlined the implementation guide allowing pharmacists and nurses to qualify as supplementary prescribers (DH, 2003). In 2005 supplementary prescribing was extended to physiotherapists, chiropodists/

Box 2.1 Overview of the requirements for a clinical management plan for supplementary prescribing

Legal requirements

Patient details
- Name
- Patient identification, e.g. NHS number
- Patient allergies
- Difficulties patient has with medicines

Disease and treatment
- Condition
- Class or name of medicines
- Limitations on doses, strength or time of treatment
- When to seek advice from or refer back to independent prescriber
- Arrangements for notification of adverse drug reactions or incidents

Prescriber information
- Name of independent prescriber (doctor or dentist)
- Name of supplementary prescriber (pharmacist, nurse, physiotherapists, chiropodists/podiatrists, radiographers, dietitian and optometrists)
- Start date
- Review date

---

podiatrists, radiographers and optometrists (DH, 2005), with dietitians gaining prescribing rights in 2016 (National Health Service [NHS] England, 2016a). Paramedics are now awaiting legislation to become independent prescribers.

Supplementary prescribing is defined as a voluntary prescribing partnership between an independent prescriber (doctor or dentist) and a supplementary prescriber, to implement an agreed patient-specific clinical management plan with the patient's consent. Currently a supplementary prescriber can be a nurse, pharmacist, chiropodist/podiatrist physiotherapist, radiographer, optometrist or dietitian. This prescribing arrangement also requires information to be shared and recorded in a common patient file. In this form of prescribing the independent prescriber, that is, the doctor or, if appropriate, the dentist, undertakes the initial assessment of the patient, determines the diagnosis and defines the initial treatment plan. The elements of this plan which are the responsibility of the supplementary prescriber are then documented in the patient-specific clinical management plan. The legal requirements for this are detailed in Box 2.1. Supplementary prescribers can prescribe controlled drugs and also both off-label and unlicensed medicines.

Non-medical independent prescribing

Following publication of a report on the implementation of nurse and pharmacist independent prescribing within the NHS in England (DH, 2006), pharmacists were enabled to become independent prescribers as defined under the Medicines and Human Use (Prescribing) (Miscellaneous Amendments) Order of May 2006. Independent prescribing is defined as 'prescribing by a practitioner (doctor, dentist, nurse, pharmacist) who is responsible and accountable for the assessment of patients with undiagnosed or diagnosed conditions and for decisions about the clinical management required including prescribing' (DH, 2006, p. 2).

Pharmacist independent prescribers were able to prescribe any licensed medicine for any medical condition within their competence except controlled drugs and unlicensed medicines. At that point there was restriction on Controlled Drugs including those in Schedule 5 (CD Inv.POM and CD Inv. P) such as co-codamol. At the same time nurses could also become qualified as independent prescribers (formerly known as Extended Formulary Nurse Prescribers) and prescribe any licensed medicine for any medical condition within their competence, including some Controlled Drugs. Since 2008 optometrists can also qualify as independent prescribers to prescribe for eye conditions and the surrounding tissue. They cannot prescribe for parenteral administration, and they are unable to prescribe Controlled Drugs. Physiotherapists can prescribe for human movement, performance and function, with podiatrists restricted to disorders of the feet, ankle and associated structures (Human Medicines Regulation, 2013). Therapeutic radiographers can prescribe within the overarching framework of cancer treatment (Human Medicines Regulation, 2016).

Following a change in legislation in 2010, pharmacist and nurse non-medical prescribers were allowed to prescribe unlicensed medicines (DH, 2010). In 2012 changes were made to the Misuse of Drugs Regulations 2001 relating to restriction on the types of controlled drugs which could be prescribed by both pharmacist and nurse independent prescribers. This allowed them to prescribe within their area of competence any Controlled Drug listed in Schedules 2–5 except diamorphine, cocaine and dipipanone for the treatment of addiction (DH, 2012).

From the above it should be evident that in the UK suitably qualified pharmacists can prescribe as either supplementary or independent prescribers. Pharmacist prescribing has been and is being considered by a number of countries. For example, legislative changes in New Zealand allowed suitably trained specialist pharmacists to become prescribers. In Canada pharmacist prescribing has been approved by provincial governments, although the scope does vary.

Accountability

Prescribers have the authority to make prescribing decisions for which they are accountable both legally and professionally. Accountability when prescribing covers three aspects: the law, the statutory professional body and the employer.

The law of Tort, the concept of a 'civil wrong', includes clinical negligence. In such a claim the patient needs to demonstrate that the prescriber caused them injury or damage. For this allegation to be substantiated the patient needs to prove that the prescriber owed them a duty of care, that this duty of care was breached and that this caused the injury identified and also that the injury was foreseeable. The law of Tort also permits actions for breach of confidentiality and also for battery should a patient be treated without consent. Therefore, prescribers (independent and supplementary) are legally and professionally accountable for their decisions. This includes decisions not to prescribe and also ensuring that the prescription is administered as directed. The legal responsibility for prescribing always lies with the individual who signed the prescription. In addition, prescribers also have a responsibility to ensure that the instructions are clear and not open to misinterpretation.

If a prescriber is an employee, then the employer expects the prescriber to work within the terms of his or her contract, competency and within the rules and policies, standard operating procedure, guidelines and so forth laid down by the organisation. Therefore, working as a prescriber, under these conditions, ensures that the employer has vicarious liability. So should any patient be harmed through the action of the prescriber and he or she is found in a civil court to be negligent, then under these circumstances the employer is responsible for any compensation to the patient. Therefore, it is important to always work within these frameworks because working outside these requirements makes the prescriber personally liable for such compensation. To reinforce this message it has been stated that the job descriptions of non-medical prescribers should incorporate a clear statement that prescribing forms part of the duties of their post (DH, 2006).

Ethical framework

Four main ethical principles of biomedical ethics have been set out for use by healthcare staff in patient–practitioner relationships (Beauchamp and Childress, 2001): respect for autonomy, non-maleficence, beneficence, and justice and veracity. These principles need to be considered at all points in the prescribing process.

Autonomy

Autonomy recognises an individual patient's right to self-determination in making judgements and decisions for himself or herself and encompasses informed patient consent. Respect for autonomy is therefore a form of personal liberty which freely permits a patient to choose whether he or she wishes to have treatment in accordance with his or her own plans.

Confidentiality. Confidentiality is a fundamental right with respect to patient autonomy. Therefore, patients have the right to confidentiality, and consent is required to disclose information regarding their health and treatment.

Consent. Obtaining consent from a patient for treatment can be divided into three components: voluntariness, information and competency. Consent, whether this is an investigation or treatment, can only be gained if the patient understands three important aspects: nature (i.e. what), purpose (i.e. why) and consequence. It also needs to be freely obtained. Consent is invalid when it is given under pressure or coercion. Therefore, it is important that consent is obtained for each act and not assumed because this is a routine assessment or procedure and therefore can be carried out automatically. It is essential that the patient understands his or her diagnosis, potential benefit, rationale and likelihood of success of the proposed treatment, and that reasonable care has been taken to ensure that the patient is aware of any material risks involved and of any reasonable potential alternative treatments. Therefore, a prescriber needs to discuss these aspects with the patient. In particular, care should be taken to understand what aspects of treatment and the risks involved would probably be deemed of significance by this particular patient to allow the patient to make a comparison with the proposed plan (Sokol, 2015). The prognosis if no treatment is prescribed should also be discussed. Such a wide-ranging discussion may require more than one appointment and reinforces the necessity for an ongoing

patient–professional relationship focused on the needs of the patient. Since the Montgomery test case in 2015 this has now been applied in several other cases. Ethically the rulings demonstrate a shift to a more cooperative approach between patient and prescriber in the consultation (Chan et al., 2017).

Associated with this is the need to determine whether the patient has the competency to make decisions for himself or herself with respect to vulnerable groups, such as those who have learning disabilities, children and the elderly. Young people aged 16 and 17 years are normally presumed to be able to consent to their own treatment.

Gillick competence is used to determine whether children have the capacity to make healthcare decisions for themselves. Children younger than 16 years can give consent as long as they can satisfy the prescriber that they have capacity to make this decision. However, with the child's consent, it is good practice to involve the parents in the decision-making process. In addition a child younger than 16 years may have the capacity to make some decisions relating to their treatment, but not others. So it is important that an assessment of capacity is made related to each decision. There is some confusion regarding the naming of the test used to objectively assess legal capacity to consent to treatment in children younger than 16 years, with some organisations and individuals referring to Fraser guidance and others Gillick competence. Gillick competence is the principle used to assess the capacity of children younger than 16, whereas Fraser guidance refers specifically to contraception (Wheeler, 2006).

The Mental Capacity Act (2005) protects the rights of adults who are unable to make decisions for themselves. The fundamental concepts within this act are the presumption that every adult has capacity to make decisions for themselves, and that they must be given all appropriate help and support to enable them to make their own decision. To obtain valid consent, the prescriber must take practicable steps to ensure the patient understands the nature, purpose and reasonable or foreseeable consequences of the proposed investigation or treatment. Therefore, patients should be able to understand the information relevant to the decision they are making. They also need to be able to retain this information, use or assess the information as part of their decision-making process and communicate their decision. The five key principles are listed in Box 2.2. Therefore, any decision made on their behalf should be as unrestrictive as possible and must be in the patient's own interest, not biased by any other individual or organisation's benefit. Therefore, when taking consent, it is extremely important to plan and consider the information needs of the patient and to communicate this information using simple terms and basic language appropriate to the individual. This may require practical steps should the patient have problems communicating. Advice regarding patient consent is listed in Box 2.3. Although there is no statutory form to record assessment of capacity, information to record in the patient's medical record are the date, decision to be made, what information needed to be understood, practical steps taken to gain consent and confirmation that the patient did not have capacity to give consent together with the reason why this was not obtained.

Non-maleficence

At the heart of the principle of non-maleficence is the concept of not knowingly causing harm to the patient. The principle is

---

Box 2.2 Overview of the five principles of the Mental Capacity Act

- A person is assumed to have capacity unless it is established that he/she lacks capacity.
- A person should not be treated as unable to make a decision unless all practical steps to enable them to do this have been taken without success.
- A person cannot be treated as unable to make a decision because he/she makes an unwise decision.
- Acts or decisions made for or on behalf of a person who lacks capacity must be in that person's best interests.
- Before an act or decision is made, the purpose has to be reviewed to assess if it can be achieved as effectively in a way that is less restrictive of the person's rights/freedom of action.

Box 2.3 Advice on patient consent

- Take care when obtaining consent.
- Assess the patient and ensure information presented is appropriate to the patient.
- Use simple terms and basic language.
- Ensure information provided covers the nature, purpose and consequence of the investigation/treatment using the following questions (Sokol, 2015):
  - Does the patient know about the material risks of the treatment I am proposing?
    What sort of risks would a reasonable person in the patient's circumstances want to know?
    What sorts of risks would this particular patient want to know?
  - Does the patient know about reasonable alternatives to this treatment?
  - Have I taken reasonable care to ensure that the patient actually knows all this?
  - Do any of the exceptions to my duty to disclose apply here?
- Give the patient understandable information about all material risks that he or she is likely to consider significant.
- Ensure the patient has the opportunity to ask questions and consider his or her options.
- Document in the patient's notes the key elements of the discussion including advice and warnings provided.
- If higher levels of risk are involved, invite the patient to sign that they understand and accept the risks explained.
- Should your patient not have capacity to give consent, record your assessment in his or her medical record, including the reason why the patient was unable to give consent.
- Record in the patient's notes if he or she declines to undergo a procedure.

expressed in the Hippocratic Oath. This obligation not to harm is distinct from the obligation to help others. Although codes of all healthcare professionals outline obligations not to harm clients, many interventions result in some harm, however transitory. Sometimes one act can be described as having a 'double effect', that is, two possible effects: one good effect (intended) and one harmful effect (unintended). The harmful effect is allowed if proportionally it is less than the good effect. Therefore, it is important for prescribers to review both the potential positive effects of treatment (e.g. symptom control) and the negative effects (e.g.

side effects). It is also important to consider both acts of commission and omission, because a failure to prescribe can also cause harm to the patient.

Beneficence

Beneficence is the principle of doing good and refers to the obligation to act for the benefit of others that is set out in codes of professional conduct, for example, Standards for pharmacy professionals (General Pharmaceutical Council, 2017). Beneficence refers to both physical and psychological benefits of actions and also relates to acts of both commission and omission. Standards set for professionals by their regulatory bodies such as the General Pharmaceutical Council can be higher than those required by law. Therefore, in cases of negligence the standard applied is often that set by the relevant statutory body for its members.

Justice and veracity

This last principle of justice and veracity is related to the distribution of resources to ensure that such division or allocation is governed by equity and fairness. This is often linked to cost-effectiveness of treatment and potential inequalities if treatment options are not offered to a group of patients or an individual. However, as a prescriber it is important to consider the evidence base for the prescribed medicine and also to review the patient as an individual to ensure the treatment offered adheres to this principle. This principle of fairness and freedom from discrimination therefore encompasses human rights including the need for assessment of medication as part of the Equality Act (2010). Healthcare professionals have a duty under this act to make reasonable adjustments to ensure that all patients have the same opportunity for good health. Therefore, a prescriber should also assess with the patient that the medication prescribed can be accessed by them. Veracity, or 'truth telling', underpins both effective communication and patient consent.

Professional frameworks for prescribing

Each professional regulatory body has standards to which their members must adhere. Members are accountable to such bodies for their practice and can be sanctioned by these bodies if their actions do not adhere to these standards. Therefore, individuals will be held accountable by their respective statutory body for their prescribing decisions.

The professional standards for pharmacists are defined within the 'Standards for Pharmacy Professionals' (General Pharmaceutical Council, 2017). In addition the Royal Pharmaceutical Society (2017) publishes 'Medicines, Ethics and Practice', a professional guide for pharmacists which provides advice on a wide range of areas encompassing core concepts and skills in addition to underpinning knowledge, legislation and professional bodies.

Off-label and unlicensed prescribing

For a medicine to be licensed for use in a specific country the manufacturer must obtain a marketing authorisation, formerly called the 'product license'. This details the patients, conditions and purpose under which the medicine is licensed for use. Any medicine which does not have a marketing authorisation for the specific country where it is prescribed is termed 'unlicensed'. Unlicensed medicines prescribed include new medicines undergoing clinical trial and those licensed and imported from another country but not licensed in the country where they are to be used. It also includes 'specials', that is, medicines manufactured to meet a specific patient's needs, or produced when two licensed medicines are mixed together for administration to a patient.

However, if a licensed medicine is prescribed outside that specified in the marketing authorisation, then this use is described as 'off-label'. This happens in practice; for example, many medicines are not licensed for use in children but are prescribed for them. In addition some established medicines are prescribed for conditions outside their marketing authorisation (e.g. amitriptyline for neuropathic pain and azathioprine in Crohn's disease). The British National Formulary includes information on off-label use as an annotation of 'unlicensed use' to inform healthcare professionals. The details of a medicine's marketing authorisation are provided in the Summary of Product Characteristics.

The company which holds the marketing authorisation has the responsibility to compensate patients who are proven to have suffered unexpected harm caused by the medicine when prescribed and used in accordance with the marketing authorisation. Therefore, if a medicine is prescribed which is either unlicensed or off-label, then the prescriber carries professional, clinical and legal responsibility and is therefore liable for any harm caused. Best practice on the use of unlicensed and off-label medicines is described in Box 2.4. In addition all healthcare professionals have a responsibility to monitor the safety of medicines. Suspected adverse drug reactions (ADRs) should therefore be reported in accordance with the relevant reporting criteria.

Prescribing across the interface between primary and secondary care

When a patient moves between care settings, there is a risk that a 'gap' in care will take place. These 'gaps' in care are almost always as a result of poor communication and frequently involve medicines, particularly when the patient is discharged from hospital into a community setting. To date there are few evidence-based solutions to these problems. A systematic review did identify randomised controlled trials of interventions designed to improve handover between hospital and primary care when patients were discharged. However, the complexity of interventions did not allow firm conclusions about which had positive effects (Hesselink et al., 2012). The National Institute for Health Care and Excellence (2015) in their guidance on medicines optimisation recommend that complete and accurate information on medicines should be shared and acted upon in a timely manner when patients transfer between care settings. They also make recommendations on what information should be shared and who should be involved in this process. The primary care prescriber with the responsibility for the continuing management of the patient in the community may be required to prescribe medicines with which they are not familiar. The prescriber should be fully informed and competent to prescribe a particular medicine for his or her patient. Supporting information from the hospital, in the form of shared care guidelines, can help

Box 2.4 Advice for prescribing unlicensed and off-label medicines

Consider
- Before prescribing an unlicensed medicine, be satisfied that an alternative licensed medicine would not meet the patient's needs.
- Before prescribing a medicine off-label, be satisfied that such use would better serve the patient's needs than an appropriately licensed alternative.
- Before prescribing an unlicensed medicine or using a medicine off-label:
  - be satisfied that there is a sufficient evidence base and/or experience of using the medicine to show its safety and efficacy;
  - take responsibility for prescribing the medicine and for overseeing the patient's care, including monitoring and follow-up;
  - record the medicine prescribed and, where common practice is not being followed, the reason for prescribing the medicine; you may wish to record that you have discussed this with the patient.

Communicate
- You give patients, or those authorising treatment on their behalf, sufficient information about the proposed treatment, including knowing serious or common adverse drug reactions, to enable them to make an informed decision.
- Where current practice supports the use of a medicine outside the terms of its license, it may not be necessary to draw attention to the license when seeking consent. However, it is good practice to give as much information as patients or carers require or which they see as relevant.
- You explain the reasons for prescribing a medicine off-label or prescribing an unlicensed medicine where there is little evidence to support its use, or where the use of the medicine is innovative.

From Medicines and Healthcare products Regulatory Agency. 2009. Off-label use or unlicensed medicines: prescribers' responsibilities. Drug Safety Update 2:7 with kind permission from MHRA.

inform the prescriber about medicines with which he or she may not be very familiar. Overall the decision about who should take responsibility for continuing care or prescribing treatment after the initial diagnosis or assessment should be based on the patient's best interests rather than on the healthcare professional's convenience or the cost of the medicine. However, when prescribers are uncertain about their competence to prescribe, where they consider they have insufficient expertise to accept responsibility for the prescription or where the product is of a very specialised nature and/or requires complex ongoing monitoring, it is legitimate for a prescriber to refuse to prescribe and make other arrangements for continued prescribing, for example, by asking the specialist to continue to prescribe. Guidance and principles for transferring information about medicines between care settings has been published by the Royal Pharmaceutical Society in conjunction with the Royal Colleges (Royal Pharmaceutical Society, 2012).

Clinical governance

Clinical governance is defined as 'the system through which NHS organisations are accountable for continuously improving the quality of their services and safeguarding high standards of care, by creating an environment in which clinical excellence will flourish' (DH, 1998, p. 33). It is a process embraced by the NHS to ensure that the quality of health care embedded within organisations is continuously monitored and improved. Clinical governance parallels corporate governance within commercial organisations and as such provides a systematic set of mechanisms such as duties, accountabilities and rules of conduct to deliver quality health care.

Clinical governance is described as having seven pillars:
- patient, service user, carer and public involvement
- risk management
- clinical audit
- staffing and management
- education, training and continuing professional development
- research and clinical effectiveness
- use of information

Within the NHS, standards of practice have been developed and monitored to ensure risks are managed and controlled. As part of this framework, the performance of staff is also assessed and remedial action taken, if required. NHS organisations have clinical governance requirements for their staff which include requirements for non-medical prescribing.

Professional bodies have also incorporated clinical governance into their codes of practice. The four tenants of clinical governance are: to ensure clear lines of responsibility and accountability, a comprehensive strategy for continuous quality improvement, policies and procedures for assessing and managing risks, and procedures to identify and rectify poor performance in staff. Suggested indicators for good practice are detailed in Box 2.5.

Competence and competency frameworks

Competence can be described as the knowledge, skills and attributes required to undertake an activity to a specific minimum standard within a defined environment. A competency framework is a group of competencies identified as essential to effectively perform a specific task. It can be used by an individual or an organisation to assess performance in a defined area. For example, it can be used for staff selection/recruitment, training and performance review.

The National Prescribing Centre competency framework for pharmacist prescribers was published in 2006 (Granby and Picton, 2006). In 2012 a prescribing competency framework was published to encompass all prescribers (independent and supplementary) which was subsequently reviewed and updated in 2016 (Royal Pharmaceutical Society, 2016). This framework is composed of 10 competencies assigned to 2 domains, the consultation and prescribing governance. The 10 competencies are:
- assess the patient,
- consider the options,
- reach a shared decision,
- prescribe,
- provide information,
- monitor and review,
- prescribe safely,

| **Box 2.5** | Overview of clinical governance practice recommendations for prescribers |

- Ensure effective communication with patients and carers to meet the patient's needs so that the patient can make informed choices about his or her treatment.
- Prescribe within competence (scope of practice).
- Obtain patient consent for investigations and management.
- Document in the patient's medical record a comprehensive record of the consultation and the agreed treatment plan.
- Undertake full assessment of patients competently and with consent.
- Prescribe safely, legally, appropriately, clinically and cost-effectively with reference to national and local guidelines.
- Assess and manage risk of treatment and associated investigations.
- Prescribe and refer in accordance with the clinical management plan if relevant.
- Ensure the secure storage of prescriptions and follow the relevant organisational procedures if they are lost or stolen.
- Ensure wherever possible separation of prescribing and dispensing and prescribing and administration.
- Audit prescribing practice.
- Identify and report incidents and adverse drug reactions.
- Participate and record continuing professional development relating to prescribing.
- Follow organisational procedures for dealing with the pharmaceutical industry regarding gifts and hospitality.

- prescribe professionally,
- improve prescribing practice,
- prescribe as part of a team.

Each of these competencies is supported by a series of statements, all of which an individual needs to demonstrate to achieve overall competency (Table 2.1). Prescribers can review their prescribing performance using the 10 competencies and the associated 64 statements using this framework as a self-assessment tool. Unlike the previous frameworks, some aspects of applying professionalism were not included. However, seven example statements (e.g. 'adapts consultations to meet the needs of different patients/carers') were provided within a separate section to encourage prescribers to reflect on professional practice linked to prescribing (Royal Pharmaceutical Society, 2016). The framework is particularly useful when structuring ongoing continuing professional development because it also allows prescribers to identify and reflect on strengths and areas for development.

The prescribing process
Consultation

The consultation is a fundamental part of the prescribing process, and prescribers need to understand and utilise this to help them practice effectively. The medical model of disease, diagnosis and prescribing is often central to practice, but an understanding of the patient's background together with his or her medical beliefs and anxieties is equally important in helping the prescriber

Table 2.1 Overview of the competency framework for all prescribers (Royal Pharmaceutical Society, 2016)

Domain	Competency	Statements
The consultation	Assess the patient.	8 statements For example, accesses and interprets all available and relevant patient records to ensure knowledge of the patient's management to date
	Consider the options.	10 statements For example, considers all pharmacological treatment options including optimising doses, as well as stopping treatment (appropriate polypharmacy, deprescribing)
	Reach a shared decision.	6 statements For example, explores the patient/carer understanding of a consultation and aims for a satisfactory outcome for the patient/carer and prescriber
	Prescribe.	13 statements For example, prescribes a medicine only with adequate, up-to-date awareness of its actions, indications, dose, contraindications, interactions, cautions, and unwanted effects
	Provide information.	5 statements For example, ensures that the patient/carer knows what to do if there are any concerns about the management of their condition, if the condition deteriorates or if there is no improvement in a specific time frame
	Monitor and review.	4 statements For example, ensures that the effectiveness of treatment and potential unwanted effects are monitored
Prescribing governance	Prescribe safely.	6 statements For example, prescribes within own scope of practice and recognises the limits of own knowledge and skill
	Prescribe professionally.	6 statements For example, accepts personal responsibility for prescribing and understands the legal and ethical implications
	Improve prescribing practice.	3 statements For example, reflects on own and others' prescribing practice, and acts upon feedback and discussion
	Prescribe as part of a team.	4 statements For example, acts as part of a multidisciplinary team to ensure that continuity of care across care settings is developed and not compromised

Seven example behaviours identified as applying professionalism are also provided to encourage reflection of professional practice linked to prescribing, for example, undertakes the consultation in an appropriate setting taking account of confidentiality, consent, dignity and respect.

understand his or her own role and behaviours alongside those of his or her patients. Each patient's own beliefs, values, experience and expectations are important to acknowledge, explore and incorporate into all consultations. All prescribers should employ a non-judgemental approach to the consultation and listen to patients' beliefs and concerns (National Institute for Health and Care Excellence [NICE], 2012). Consideration should also be given to the consultation environment to ensure the patient's privacy is respected and also to how to maximise the patient's participation in the consultation. Some patients might like a family member or friend to be present or participate in a consultation, and this should be discussed and accommodated. A broad range of practical skills are needed in the consultation:

Interpersonal skills: the ability to communicate and make relationships with patients, considering the most effective communication method, including large print, symbols, Braille pictures, etc. and the avoidance of jargon;

summarising information, checking the patient has understood important information and giving the patient opportunities to ask questions should also be incorporated into the consultation

Reasoning skills: the ability to gather appropriate information, interpret the information and then apply it both in diagnosis and management

Practical skills: the ability to perform physical examinations and use clinical instruments

The style in which the consultation is undertaken is also important. The paternalistic prescriber–patient relationship is no longer appropriate. This has been replaced in modern health care by a more patient-centred focus that ensures patient autonomy and consent. This model is based on an equal role for both patient and prescriber and is supported by policies which promote patient empowerment and self-care/management. This uses a task-orientated approach to keep consultation times to a reasonable

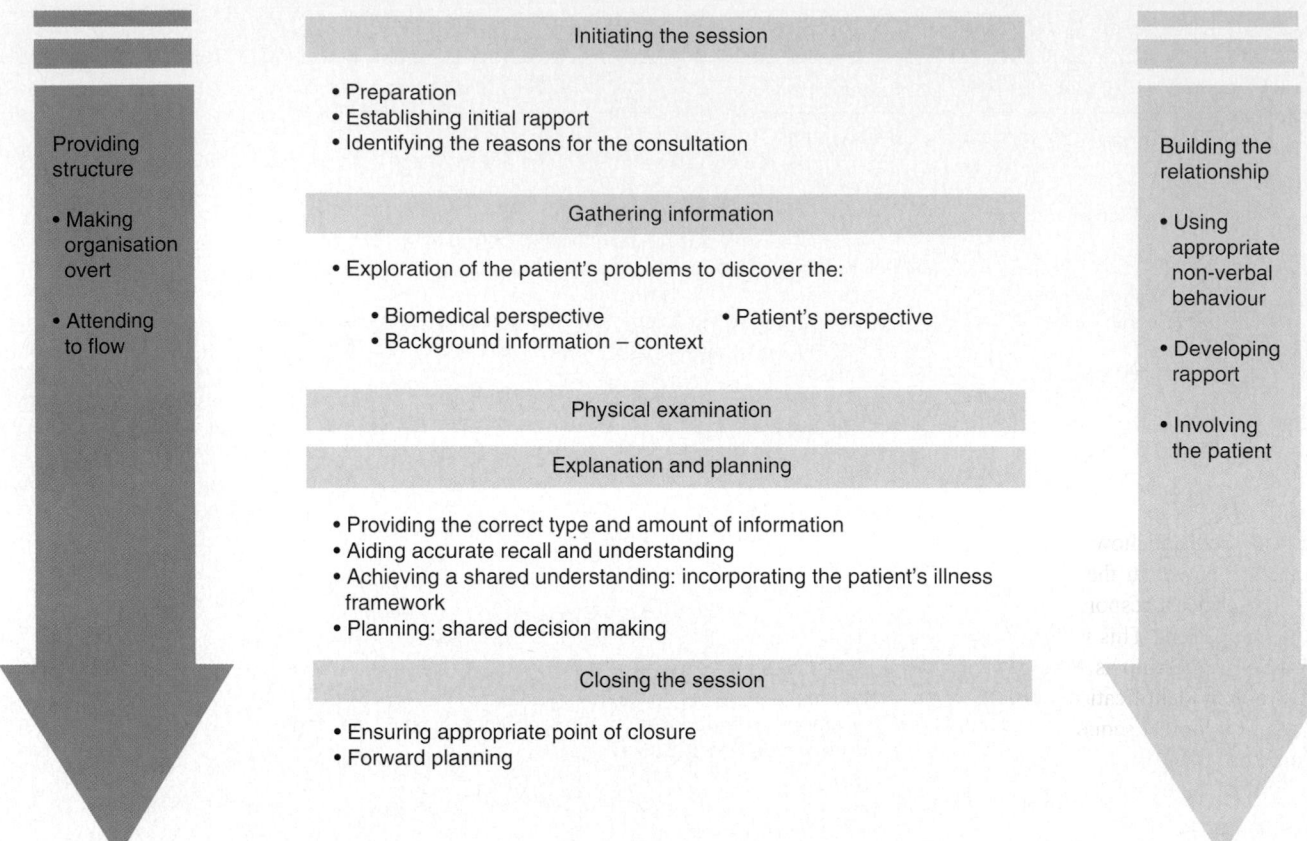

Fig. 2.2 Calgary–Cambridge consultation framework (Silverman et al., 2005). (Reproduced with kind permission from the Radcliffe Publishing Ltd., Oxford.)

duration and to set parameters to ensure a realistic expectation from the consultation.

An example of this is the Calgary Cambridge framework which can be used to structure and guide patient consultations (Silverman et al., 2005). The framework is represented in Fig. 2.2. The five key stages of the consultation are:
- initiating the session
- gathering information
- physical examination
- explanation and planning
- closing the session

In addition to these stages two key tasks are performed throughout the consultation. These are 'providing structure' and 'building the patient–prescriber relationship'. These two tasks are vital in ensuring an effective consultation. For a patient–prescriber communication to be effective, it is important that this focuses on interaction between the patient and the prescriber and is not just passive transmission of information. Feedback from the patient about the information received is essential for effective communication.

Building relationships

Non-verbal communication is important and can be used by the prescriber to gain information from the patient. Facial expressions and body posture can give clues about how the patient is feeling (e.g. anxious or tired). Proximity and eye contact are also important to determine whether the patient is actively engaged in the conversation or is distracted. Such non-verbal clues (e.g. anxiety, tiredness and pain) can then be explored verbally with the patient.

Prescribers also need to review their own non-verbal communication to ensure this reinforces the verbal message they are giving to the patient. For example, doctors who face the patient, make eye contact and maintain an open posture were regarded by their patients to be more interested and empathic (Harrigan et al., 1985). Also healthcare professionals in primary care who demonstrated non-verbal intimacy (close distance, leaning forward, appropriate body orientation and touch) had increased patient satisfaction (Larsen and Smith, 1981).

Because eye contact is an important non-verbal form of communication, obtaining information from patient records and documenting the consultation could undermine these skills. Therefore, it is important to read notes in advance of the consultation and avoid writing up the outcome while the patient is speaking. Indicating to the patient that references need to be made to their record or information documented ensures the patient is informed about the break in the consultation. This strategy should be adopted for both paper and computer-based records.

Developing rapport is also essential to building an effective patient–prescriber relationship. This can be achieved by providing an accepting response to the patient's concerns and expectations. This is achieved by acknowledging the patients' views, valuing their contribution and accepting this information in a non-judgemental way. This does not necessarily mean that the prescriber agrees with the information, but that he or she accepts that this is a legitimate view from the patient's perspective. This can be reinforced by summarising the patient's view. The prescriber should acknowledge the patient's coping efforts and self-care. Avoiding jargon and explaining complex concepts in simple terms, to enable patients to understand the diagnosis and management, is also important.

Providing structure

Providing structure is important in the patient–prescriber consultation to enable the five key stages to be effectively completed. The prescriber needs to establish the boundaries for the consultation. This includes the time available for the consultation, the topics covered and how to finish the consultation. Therefore, because the power in the consultation is with the prescriber, it is the prescriber's responsibility to guide the consultation and involve the patient. This is to ensure that a patient-centered collaborative partnership is established. This can be achieved by using problem identification, screening and agenda-setting skills. The use of a logical sequence, signposting from one part of the consultation to the next and including an initial and end summary, will provide an effective structure to the consultation.

Initiating the session

During the first stage of the consultation the prescriber needs to greet the patient and confirm his or her identity. Prescribers should also ensure that the environment for the consultation is appropriate for maintaining eye contact and ensuring confidentiality. Prescribers should also introduce themselves, their role and gain relevant consent. During this stage the prescriber must demonstrate respect for the patient and establish a patient-centered focus. Using initially open and then closed questions, the prescriber needs to identify the patient's problem and/or issues. By adopting this approach and actively listening, the prescriber is able to confirm the reason for the consultation and identify other issues. This allows the prescriber to negotiate an agenda for the next stages of the consultation through agreement with the patient, taking into account both the patient's and the prescriber's needs. This initial stage is vital for the success of the consultation because many patients have hidden agendas which if not identified at this stage can lead to these concerns not being addressed. Beckman and Frankel (1984) studied doctors' listening skills and identified that even minimal interruptions by the doctors to the initial patient's statement at the beginning of the consultation prevented the patients' concerns from being expressed. This resulted in either these issues not being identified at all, or they were raised by the patient late in the consultation.

Gathering information

The aim of this stage is to explore the problem identified from both the patient's and the prescriber's perspective to gain background information which is both accurate and complete. Britten

et al. (2000) identified that lack of patient participation in the consultation led to 14 categories of misunderstanding between the prescriber and the patient. These categories included patient information unknown to the prescriber, conflicting information from the patient and communication failure with regard to the prescriber's decision. During this stage, the illness framework, identified by exploring patients' ideas, concerns, expectations and experience of their condition and effect on their life, is combined with the information gained by the prescriber through their biomedical perspective. This encompasses signs, symptoms, investigations and underlying pathology. Assimilation of this information leads the prescriber to a differential diagnosis. By incorporating information from both viewpoints, a comprehensive history detailing the sequence of events can be obtained using questioning, listening and clarification. This ends with an initial summary where the prescriber invites the patient to comment and contribute to the information gathered.

Physical examination

At the start of the physical examination stage it is important to again obtain the patient's consent for any examination by explaining the process and rationale for the assessment. The environment (e.g. room temperature and screening for the examination) is important, and the prescriber should review this to ensure the patient's comfort. Guidance on maintaining clear sexual boundaries for pharmacy professionals has been published which includes advice on the use of chaperones (General Pharmaceutical Council, 2012).

Explanation and planning

The explanation and planning stage of the consultation incorporates three aspects: the differential diagnosis/hypothesis, the prescriber's management plan (investigations and alternative treatments), and explanation and negotiation of the plan of action with the patient.

In one UK study, doctors were found to overestimate the extent to which they completed the tasks of discussing the risk of medication, checking the ability of the patient to follow the treatment plan and obtaining the patient's input and view on the medication prescribed (Makoul et al., 1995).

To successfully accomplish this stage of the consultation, the prescriber needs to use a number of skills and also to involve the patient. Prescribers should ensure they give the correct type and amount of information. This is done by assessing the patient's prior knowledge employing both open and closed questions. By organising the information given into chunks which can be easily assimilated, the prescriber can then check that the patient understands the information given. Questioning the patient regarding additional information they require also helps to ensure the patient's involvement and to maintain rapport. The prescriber must determine the appropriate time to give explanations and also allow the patient time to consider the information provided. Signposting can also be a useful technique to employ during this stage. Once again the language used should be concise, easy to understand and avoid jargon. Using diagrams, models and written information can enhance and reinforce patient understanding.

The explanation should be organised into discreet sections with a logical sequence so that important information can be repeated and summarised.

To achieve shared understanding and shared decision making, it is important to incorporate the patient's perspective by relating the information given to the patient's illness framework. The patients also need to have the opportunity to ask questions, raise doubts and obtain clarification. This is especially important because national surveys of patients have identified that many patients, particularly those with long-term conditions, are less likely to report being involved in their own care (Care Quality Commission, 2016). Discussing with patients their beliefs, culture, abilities and lifestyle is important when discussing treatment options, for example, fasting during Ramadan or use of memory aids to support adherence. Prescribers should also explain their rational for the management plan identified and also discuss possible alternatives. By involving and negotiating with the patient in this way, a mutually acceptable treatment plan can be identified which allows patients to take responsibility for their own health.

Box 2.6 summarises the issues the prescriber should consider before prescribing a medicine.

Closing the session

The effectiveness of the end of a consultation is as important as the preceding stages. A number of steps are undertaken during the closing stage. These include agreeing to a contract with the patient as to the next steps to be taken by both patient and prescriber, for example, additional investigations and/or referral. Safety net strategies are also employed and discussed so the patient can identify unexpected outcomes or treatment failure and also understand who and how to contact the prescriber or another healthcare professional if appropriate. The end summary is an essential component of this stage and is used to briefly and accurately identify the management plan established during the previous stage in the consultation. This is followed by a final check that the patient has understood and consented to this management plan. At the end of the consultation the patient is given another opportunity to ask any final questions.

Communicating risks and benefits of treatment

Shared decision making supports patients to actively participate in their care. Before this stage of the consultation is reached, the healthcare professional has to use the best available evidence about treatment and be able to apply it to the individual patient in front of them, taking into account their needs, values and preferences. This requires the healthcare professional to discuss and provide information about the risks, benefits and consequences of treatment options, check that the patient understands the information, encourage the patient to clarify what is important to them and check that their choice is consistent with this. This ensures patient's consent to treatment is informed, and that the patient has an opportunity to participate in shared decision making about his or her treatment.

It is important to be able to communicate the risks and benefits of treatment options in relation to medicines. This should be done

---

> **Box 2.6** Issues the prescriber should reflect upon before prescribing a medicine (National Prescribing Centre, 1998)
>
> - What is the drug?
>   - Is it novel?
>   - Is it a line extension?
> - What is the drug used for?
>   - What are the licensed indications?
>   - Any restrictions on initiation?
>   - Does first line mean first choice?
> - How effective is the drug?
>   - Is there good evidence for efficacy?
>   - How does it compare with existing drugs?
> - How safe is the drug?
>   - Are there published comparative safety data?
>   - Has it been widely used in other countries?
>   - Are the details contained in the Summary of Product Characteristics understood?
>   - Are there clinically important drug interactions?
>   - Are there monitoring requirements?
>   - Can it be used long-term?
> - Who should not receive this drug?
>   - Are there patients in whom it is contraindicated?
> - Does the drug provide value for money?
>   - Is there good evidence of cost-effectiveness compared with other available interventions?
>   - What impact will this drug have on the healthcare budget?
> - What is its place in therapy?
>   - What advantages are there?
>   - Are the benefits worth the cost?
>   - Are there some patients who would particularly benefit?

---

without bias and should avoid personal anecdotal information. Most patients want to be involved in decisions about their treatment, and would like to be able to understand the risks of side effects versus the likely benefits of treatment before they commit to the inconvenience of taking regular medication. An informed patient is more likely to be concordant with treatment, reducing waste of healthcare resources including professional time and the waste of medicines which are dispensed but not taken. Healthcare professionals need to recognise that the patient's values and preferences may be different from those of the healthcare professional, and that they should avoid making assumptions about patients. This may result in the patient making a treatment decision that is different from the healthcare professional's preferred option.

Communicating risk is not simple (Paling, 2003). Many different dimensions and inherent uncertainties need to be taken into account, and patients' assessment of risk is primarily determined by emotions, beliefs and values, not facts. This is important, because patients and healthcare professionals may ascribe different values to the same level of risk. Healthcare professionals need to be able to discuss risks and benefits with patients in a context that would enable the patient to have the best chance of understanding those risks. It is also prudent to inform the patient that virtually all treatments are associated with some harm and that there is almost always a trade-off between benefit and harm. How healthcare professionals present risk and benefit can affect the patient's perception of risk.

The National Institute of Health and Care Excellence (NICE, 2012) recommends using the following principles when discussing risks and benefits with patients:

- personalise risks and benefits as far as possible;
- use absolute risk rather than relative risk (e.g. the risk of an event increases from 1 in 1000 to 2 in 1000, rather than the risk of the event doubles);
- use natural frequency (e.g. 10 in 100) rather than a percentage (10%);
- be consistent in the use of data (e.g. use the same denominator when comparing risk: 7 in 100 for one risk and 20 in 100 for another, rather than 1 in 14 and 1 in 5);
- present a risk over a defined period (months or years) if appropriate (e.g. if 100 people are treated for 1 year, 10 will experience a given side effect);
- include both positive and negative framing (e.g. treatment will be successful for 97 of 100 patients and unsuccessful for 3 of 100 patients);
- be aware that different people interpret terms such as 'rare', 'unusual' and 'common' in different ways, and use numerical data if available;
- think about using a mixture of numerical and pictorial formats (e.g. numerical rates and pictograms).

Visual patient decision aids are becoming increasingly popular as a tool that healthcare professionals can use to support discussions with patients by increasing their knowledge about expected outcomes and helping them to relate these to their personal values (National Prescribing Centre, 2008). Further information about using patient decision aids can be found at: http://ipdas.ohri.ca or http://sdm.rightcare.nhs.uk (NHS-specific information on patient decision aids and shared decision making).

Adherence

Adherence has been defined as the extent to which a patient's behaviour matches the agreed recommendation from the prescriber. When a patient is non-adherent this can be classified as intentional or unintentional non-adherence (NICE, 2009). Adherence/non-adherence is a variable behaviour, rather than a trait characteristic, and is best understood in terms of the patient's encounter with his or her specific treatment. To facilitate optimal adherence, both perceptual factors (e.g. beliefs, preferences and incentives), which are associated with intentional non-adherence, and practical factors (e.g. capacity and resources), which are associated with unintentional non-adherence, need to be addressed.

Unintentional non-adherence occurs when the patient wishes to follow the treatment plan agreed with the prescriber but is unable to do so because of circumstances beyond his or her control. Examples of this include forgetting to take the medicine at the defined time or an inability to use the device prescribed. Strategies to overcome such obstacles include medication reminder charts, use of multi-compartment medication dose systems, large print for those with poor eyesight and aids to improve medication delivery (e.g. inhaler aids, tube squeezers for ointments and creams, and eye drop administration devices). A selection of these devices is detailed in a guide to the design of dispensed medicines (National Patient Safety Agency, 2007).

Intentional non-adherence occurs when the patient decides he or she does not wish to follow the agreed treatment plan. This may occur because of the patient's beliefs, perceptions or motivation. Therefore, it is important that all of these aspects are included in the discussion between the patient and the prescriber when the treatment plan is developed. Patients need to fully appreciate their medical condition and its prognosis to understand the rationale for the treatment options discussed. The benefits of the treatment plan, the effect of not taking the treatment, as well as the side effects all need to be explicitly explored with the patient. Patient decision aids and medicine-specific patient information leaflets can be used to support this discussion. However, evidence is inconclusive as to whether written medicines information is effective in changing knowledge, attitudes and behaviours related to medicine taking (Nicolson et al., 2009). The patient's previous experience of medicines and associated side effects should be explored because this gives the prescriber vital information about perceptions and motivation. Adherence to existing prescribed medication should be explored non-judgementally. For example, asking the patient how often he or she missed taking doses at the prescribed time over the previous 7 days would enable the prescriber to assess adherence but also explore lifestyle factors or side effects which may impact on the patient. These can then be discussed and strategies developed to optimise adherence.

More than 40% of working-age adults are unable to understand or make use of everyday health information because of limited health literacy. Reduced health literacy is associated with poorer health outcomes including increased risk of morbidity, premature death, poorer understanding of how to take medicines and increased non-adherence. Prescribers need to recognise patients' health literacy needs and employ a range of communication tools and strategies to support their needs (Public Health England, 2015).

Studies have demonstrated that between 35% and 50% of medicines prescribed for chronic conditions are not taken as recommended (NICE, 2009). Therefore, it is the prescriber's responsibility to explore with patients their perceptions of medicines to determine whether there are any reasons why they may not want to or are unable to use the medicine. In addition, any barriers which might prevent the patient from using the treatment as agreed, for example, manual dexterity, eyesight and memory, should be discussed and assessed. Such a frank discussion should enable the patient and prescriber to jointly identify the optimum treatment regimen to treat the condition. In addition, information from the patient's medical records can be used to assess adherence. For example, does the frequency of requests for repeat medication equate to the anticipated duration of use?

Review of unused medicines can be undertaken, and it is also important to assess the patient's administration technique on an ongoing basis for devices (e.g. asthma inhalers) to optimise correct technique. This can be achieved, for example, by carrying out a medicines reconciliation on hospital admission when the patient's prescribed medicines are compared with what the patient was taking before admission through discussion with the patient and/or carers and review of primary care records.

Because it is likely that at some point all patients will forget to take their medicine, it is important to give all patients information on what to do should a dose be missed. For individuals who are taking medication for treatment of a chronic condition, adherence should not be assumed; therefore, assessment of adherence should form an ongoing discussion at each consultation.

Medication review

Medication review has been defined as 'a structured, critical examination of a patient's medicines with the objective of reaching an agreement with the patient about treatment, optimising the impact of medicines, minimising the number of medication-related problems and reducing waste' (NICE, 2015, p. 22).

It is important that medicines are prescribed appropriately and that patients continue to achieve benefits from their medicines. The regular review of medicines is a key part of a good prescribing process and has many potential benefits for patients, including improving the management of the patient's medical condition, optimising the use of medicines, reducing risk of ADRs and involving the patient more actively in his or her treatment and care.

Often medicines prescribed regularly on a long-term basis are for patients with multiple comorbidities. This often results in individual patients being prescribed many medicines, a term known as 'polypharmacy'. Polypharmacy is important because evidence suggests that being on multiple medicines increases a person's risk of harm and contributes to hospital admissions (NICE, 2015). Using a medication review process to reduce the number of inappropriate medicines a patient is taking (deprescribing) and optimise appropriate medication can minimise unwanted harms from medicines (including falls) and reduce costs. In UK primary care, repeat prescribing systems enable patients on long-term regular medication to obtain further supplies of their medicine without routinely having to see their primary care doctor or prescriber. Robust systems and processes are required for this repeat prescribing to ensure the safe and efficient use of medicines. Reviewing a patient's medication forms is an essential element of a robust repeat prescribing process.

Specific groups of patients are recommended for a structured medication review (NICE, 2015), including all patient groups who are taking multiple medicines (polypharmacy), patients with chronic or long-term conditions and older people. Different types of medication review are required to meet the needs of patients for different purposes. A medication review can vary from a simple review of the prescription to an in-depth structured clinical medication review. NICE (2015) recommends that a structured medication review should be carried out by a healthcare professional with a sufficient level of knowledge of processes for managing medicines and therapeutic knowledge on medicines use. The scope of this review includes the following:
- the patient's and carer's (if appropriate) views and understanding about their medicines;
- the patient's and carer's (if appropriate) concerns, questions or problems with their medicines;
- all prescribed, over-the-counter and complementary medicines that the patient is taking or using, and what these are for;
- how safe the medicines are, how well they are working, how appropriate they are and whether their use is in line with national guidance/evidence;
- whether the patient has had or has any risk factors for development of ADRs;
- what monitoring is needed.

Characteristics of the different types of medication review are described in Table 2.2.

The key elements of a structured medication review are (All Wales Medicines Strategy Group, 2014; Scottish Government, 2015):
- identify aims and objectives of drug therapy;
- identify essential drug therapy;
- assess if the patient is taking unnecessary drug therapy;
- check if the therapeutic objectives are being achieved;
- determine if the patient is at risk of ADRs or suffering an actual ADR
- consider if drug therapy is cost-effective;
- determine the patient's willingness and ability to take their drug therapy;
- agree on actions to stop, reduce dose, continue or start drug therapy;
- communicate actions with all relevant parties;
- monitor and adjust regularly.

NO TEARS (Lewis, 2004) (Table 2.3) is a simpler tool for carrying out structured medication review. There are a number of

Table 2.2 Characteristics of types of medication review

Type of review	Purpose of the review	Requires patient to be present	Access to patient's full clinical notes
Level 1 Prescription review	Technical review of patient's list of medicines, e.g. dose optimisation, anomalies, changed items, cost-effectiveness	Not essential (any resulting changes to prescribed medicines must involve the patient/carer)	Not normally (community pharmacist can use Summary Care Record)
Level 2 Treatment review	Address issues relating to the patient's medicine-taking behaviour and use of medicines, e.g. dose modification, stopping medicines	Usually (any resulting changes to prescribed medicines must involve the patient/carer)	Possibly (community pharmacist may not have access to patient's full clinical notes)
Level 3 Clinical medication review	Address issues relating to the patient's use of medicines in the context of his or her clinical condition	Yes	Yes

Medication reviews include all medicines, including prescription, complementary and over-the-counter medicines. Treatment and prescription review may relate to one therapeutic area only.
Adapted from Medicines Partnership, 2002.

Table 2.3 The NO TEARS approach to medication review

NO TEARS	Questions to think about
Need and indication	Why is the patient taking the medicine, and is the indication clearly documented in the notes? Does the patient still need the medicine? Is the dose appropriate? Has the diagnosis been confirmed or refuted? Would a non-drug treatment be better? Does the patient know what his or her medicines are for?
Open questions	Use open questions to find out what the patient understands about his or her medicines, and what problems the patient may be having with them.
Tests and monitoring	Is the illness under control? Does treatment need to be adjusted to improve control? What special monitoring requirements are there for this patient's medicines? Who is responsible for checking test results?
Evidence and guidelines	Is there new evidence or guidelines that mean I need to review the patient's medicines? Is the dose still appropriate? Do I need to do any other investigations or tests?
Adverse effects	Does the patient have any side effects? Are any of the patient's symptoms likely to be caused by side effects of medicines, including over-the-counter and complementary medicines? Are any of the patient's medicines being used to treat side effects of other medicines? Is there any new advice or warnings on side effects or interactions?
Risk reduction and prevention	If there is time, ask about alcohol use, smoking, obesity, falls risk or family history for opportunistic screening. Is treatment optimised to reduce risks?
Simplification and switches	Can the patient's medicines regimen be simplified? Are repeat medicines synchronised for prescribing at the same time? Explain any changes in medicines to the patient.

published tools and websites to support improving polypharmacy and deprescribing. These tools incorporate guidance on assessing appropriateness or need for medicines and assessing risk of medicines (e.g. anticholinergic burden score). Examples of such tools can be found at: http://www.polypharmacy.scot.nhs.uk and http://www.prescqipp.info.

Factors that influence prescribers

A prescriber is subject to various influences which may impact their decision making when deciding whether to prescribe a medicine and which medicine to prescribe. Some of these influences may result in poor decision making; therefore, it is important to have an understanding of these influences and how they may impact on prescribing decisions. A range of influences that affect the prescribing decisions made by primary care doctors have been identified (Fig. 2.3).

Patients and prescribing decisions

The prescribing and use of medicines is strongly influenced by cultural factors that affect patients and prescribers alike. Issues such as whether the patient expects a prescription or whether the prescriber thinks the patient expects a prescription both influence the decision to prescribe. Patients may want a prescription for a whole variety of reasons, some of which are more valid than others. Beyond wanting a medicine for its therapeutic effect, a prescription for a medicine may demonstrate to the patient that his or her illness is recognised, may be seen as a symbol of care, may offer legitimacy for time off work because of illness or may fit with their health beliefs. Patients who frequently consult and receive a prescription are more likely to repeat the experience and expect a prescription at the next consultation.

A number of studies have found that doctors sometimes feel under pressure from patients to prescribe, although patients may not always expect a prescription from the doctor. However, even though patients often expect to receive a medicine, they also have more complex agendas that need to be explored in the consultation. Patients may have mixed attitudes towards medicines, and reluctance to take medicines is quite common. Although a medicine may be prescribed for its pharmacological effect, there may be other associated reasons to prescribe for a patient, for example, to end the consultation, to avoid doing anything else or having to say no, to maintain contact with the patient as a response to carer anxiety or to fulfil the patient's expectation.

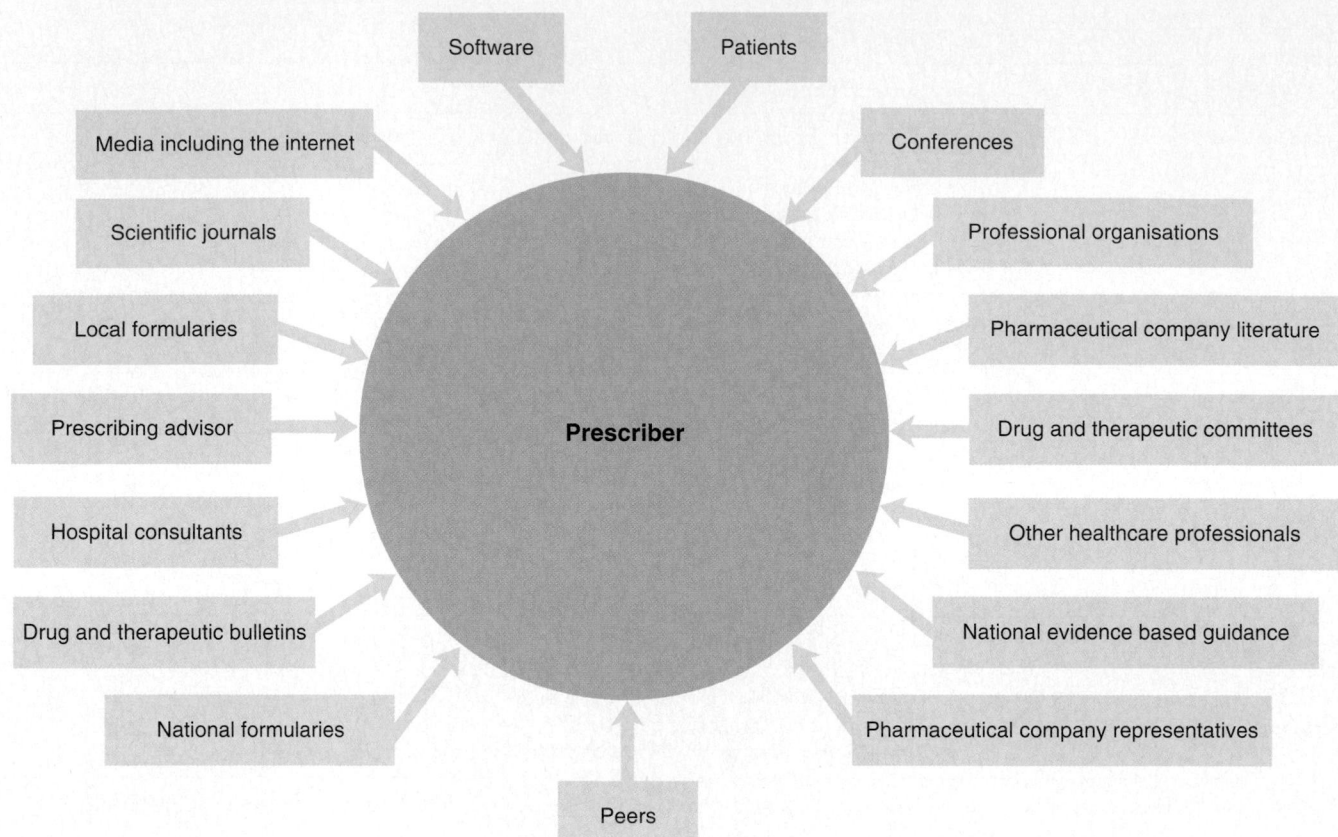

Fig. 2.3 Influences on prescribing decisions.

The informed patient

Health care is moving to a position of greater shared decision making with patients and development of the concept of patient autonomy. This is being supported through the better provision of information for patients about their prescribed medicines. The European Union directive 2001/83 (European Commission, 2001) requires that all pharmaceutical products are packaged with an approved patient information leaflet, which provides information on how to take the medicine and possible adverse effects. Patients are increasingly using the Internet and social media to learn about health and medicines. This can be challenging for healthcare professionals, particularly when the quality of information sources used may be highly variable. When media coverage does not provide balanced coverage, for example, reporting regarding the safety of measles, mumps and rubella (MMR) vaccine, this can have important consequences. In this case there was a rapid decline in MMR vaccination rates in children and a subsequent mumps outbreak (Gupta et al., 2008).

Direct advertising of medicines to patients is allowed in the USA and New Zealand, but not in Europe. Advertising medicines in this way is clearly effective in increasing sales of medicines, as evidenced by the increased spending and prescriptions for advertised drugs, compared with non-advertised drugs in these countries. This has led to concern that direct-to-consumer advertising encourages unnecessary and inappropriate use of medication. In the UK, education for patients may be provided by the manufacturer through sponsored disease awareness campaigns, but there is concern these encourage individuals to seek advice or treatment from their doctor for previously undiagnosed conditions. These campaigns may also help to raise awareness of conditions that have not been well managed in the past. However, they can also act in a way to promote prescription medicines. Such campaigns, which may be established by a drug company with or without the endorsement of a patient group, often take place at the same time as a drug's launch and may involve aggressive promotion. As a consequence there have been calls to control the influence of companies on the production of disease awareness campaigns that impact on the individual patient, who then exerts pressure on the prescriber for a specific medicine.

Healthcare policy

National policy and guidelines, for example, guidance from the NICE and Scottish Intercollegiate Guidelines Network in the UK, have a significant influence on prescribing and uptake of new medicines (NHS England, 2016b). The uptake of guidance and impact on prescribing can show considerable variation between individual clinicians and healthcare organisations. A range of complex factors have been identified that affect the impact of national guidance (Kings Fund, 2006), for example, prescriber's knowledge, attitude and behaviour, lack of staff, resources or managerial leadership, attitudes of patients, environmental factors, such as the regulatory environment, and the structure of reimbursement mechanisms.

Colleagues

Several studies have found that healthcare professionals in primary care (both doctors and nurses) rely on advice from trusted colleagues and opinion leaders as a key source of information on how to manage patients. It has been estimated that 40% of prescribing in primary care was strongly influenced by hospitals because the choice of medicine prescribed in general practice was often guided by hospital specialists through their precedent prescribing and educational advice (National Audit Office, 2007). The pharmaceutical industry recognises the value of identifying 'key opinion' leaders amongst the medical community and will try to cultivate them to influence their peers and fellow clinicians by paying them for a consultancy, lecture fees, attendance at medical conferences, supporting research and writing articles favourable to that company's products.

Pharmacists, in both primary and secondary care, themselves have an influence on prescribing through their roles as clinical pharmacists, or as part of their work advising on prescribing in primary care. Pharmacists are often regarded as trusted colleagues, and as such can have an important influence on prescribing. In whichever sector they are working, pharmacists need to be aware that their advice and decisions may be influenced by exactly the same factors that influence the prescriber.

Pharmaceutical industry

The pharmaceutical industry has a very wide and important influence on prescribing decisions affecting every level of healthcare provision, from the medicines that are initially discovered and developed through clinical trials to the promotion of medicines to the prescriber and patient groups, the prescription of medicines and the compilation of clinical guidelines. There are more than 8000 pharmaceutical company representatives in the UK who are trying to persuade prescribers to prescribe their company's product. This represents a ratio of about 1 representative for every 7.5 doctors (House of Commons Health Committee, 2005), with 1 representative for every 4 primary care doctors (National Audit Office, 2007). Whilst representatives from the pharmaceutical industry can provide useful and important new information to prescribers about medicines, the information presented is not without bias and rarely provides any objective discussion of available competitor products.

The influence of the pharmaceutical industry extends well beyond the traditional selling approach of using representatives and is increasingly sophisticated. The pharmaceutical industry spends millions on advertising, company-sponsored information in medical journals and supplements, sponsorship to attend conferences and meetings, and medical education. More than half of postgraduate education and training for doctors in the UK is sponsored by the pharmaceutical industry. The wide variety, volume and intensity of marketing activities the industry engages in is an important influence on prescribing by healthcare professionals. But when asked whether they are influenced by the pharmaceutical industry, prescribers usually deny that drug promotion affects their own prescribing practices, although they do believe that it affects other prescribers' prescribing habits. This is clearly not the case, because research has shown that even use of modest samples, gifts, and food exerts a significant influence on prescriber behaviour.

Cognitive factors

Most prescribing decisions are made using the processes our brains develop to handle large volumes of complex information quickly. This rapid decision making is aided by heuristics, strategies that provide shortcuts to quick decisions. This type of decision making largely relies on a small number of variables that we believe are important based on information collected by brief reading in summary journals (e.g. *Prescriber*, *Drug and Therapeutics Bulletin*), articles in popular doctors' and nurses' magazines mailed free of charge and talking to colleagues. However, it is important to recognise that cognitive biases affect these heuristics (or shortcuts) involved in rapid decision making, and that experts, as well as generalists, are just as fallible to cognitive biases in decision making (Makhinson, 2010). More than 50 cognitive biases and affective biases in medical decision making have been described. Some examples of cognitive biases that may affect prescribing decisions are listed in Table 2.4.

Table 2.4 Examples of types of cognitive biases which influence prescribing

Type of cognitive bias	Description
Novelty preference	The belief that the progress of science always results in improvements and that newer treatments are generally better than older treatments
Over optimism bias	Tendency of people to overestimate the outcome of actions, events, or personal attributes to a positive skew
Confirmation bias	Information that confirms one's already firmly held belief is given higher weight than refuting evidence
Mere exposure effect	More familiar ideas or objects are preferred or given greater weight in decision making
Loss aversion	To weigh the avoidance of loss more greatly than the pursuit of an equivalent gain
Illusory correlation	The tendency to perceive two events as causally related, when in fact the connection between them is coincidental or even non-existent

Strategies to influence prescribing

Healthcare organisations at local and national levels have been seeking to influence prescribing behaviour over many years, both to control expenditure on medicines and to improve quality of care. Medicines are one of the most well-researched interventions in healthcare, with a relative wealth of evidence to support their use. Despite this, there is still a wide variation in prescribing practice between clinicians and between healthcare organisations. This reflects variation in clinical practice arising from the inconsistent implementation of evidence-based medicine and the impact of the many factors that influence prescribing. Strategies to improve prescribing can be managerial and process orientated, or more supportive and educationally orientated. Strategies that use a combination of different interventions on a repeat basis are more likely to be successful at influencing prescribing.

Managerial approaches to influence prescribing

Formularies are agreed lists of medicines to which prescribers are encouraged or required to adhere. The benefits of a formulary include improving patient outcomes by optimising the use of medicines, supporting the inclusion of patient factors in decision making about medicines, improving local care pathways, reducing inappropriate variation in clinical care and ensuring more cost-effective use of resources across a health economy. In secondary care, prescribers can usually prescribe only those medicines included within the formulary, because these are the medicines stocked in the pharmacy. In primary care, a formulary is generally advisory in nature and less restrictive because community pharmacies can supply any medicine that is reimbursable on the NHS.

The NICE (2014) has published good practice recommendations on the systems and processes that should be used to develop and update local formularies. These recommendations describe best practice for how the formulary should be developed, who should be involved, how decisions should be made when including a medicine on the formulary, how the formulary should be implemented and disseminated, and how it should be updated. Some formularies are developed to cover prescribing in both primary and secondary care, which mean they can have a significant influence on prescribing patterns in the whole of a local health economy. Over recent years formularies have developed beyond just being a list of medicines and often include useful advice for prescribers; for example, they may include care pathways and guidelines for managing specific conditions or diseases.

Local and national guidelines

Guidelines for the use of a medicine, a group of medicines or the management of a clinical condition may be produced for local or national use. They can be useful tools to guide and support prescribers in choosing which medicines they should be prescribing. Ideally guidelines should make evidence-based standards of care explicit and accessible, and aid clinical decision making. The best quality guidelines are usually those produced using systematically developed evidence-based statements to assist clinicians in making decisions about appropriate health care for specific clinical circumstances. In the UK the NICE has an accreditation scheme to recognise organisations that achieve high standards in producing health or social care guidance. Examples of accredited guidelines are those produced by the NICE (http://www.nice.org.uk), some Royal Colleges and the Scottish Intercollegiate Guideline Network (http://www.sign.ac.uk). Local guidelines are often developed to provide a local context and interpretation of national guidance, and offer guidance on managing patients between primary and secondary care. However, despite the availability of good-quality accessible clinical guidelines, implementation in practice remains variable.

Clinical decision support systems are increasingly popular as a way of improving clinical practice and influencing prescribing. These often utilise interactive computer programs that help clinicians with decision-making tasks at the point of care, and also help them keep up to date and support implementation of clinical guidelines. For example, clinical knowledge summaries (https://cks.nice.org.uk) is a decision support system developed for use in primary care that includes patient information leaflets, helps with differential diagnosis, suggests investigations and referral criteria, and gives screens that can be shared between the patient and the prescriber in the surgery.

Incentives

In an effort to contain prescribing costs, some healthcare systems use direct incentives to influence clinical behaviour and, in particular, prescribing. The incentives, which are usually financial, may offer some benefits to the prescriber's patients or to the prescriber's own healthcare organisation. They can have a significant impact on prescribing practice. Typically primary care doctors are given indicative prescribing budgets and are expected to meet the prescribing needs of their patients from within this budget. Financial incentive schemes to reward good fiscal management of prescribing budgets and improve the quality of prescribing are used to encourage prescribers to change their practice or maintain good practice. Incentive schemes usually influence what is prescribed, rather than whether a prescription is written. The most effective schemes are simple to understand, have achievable targets and require information about prescribing patterns to be readily available. However, incentives schemes for prescribing need to be managed carefully in order not to create perverse incentives, such as increasing the referral of patients to another part of the healthcare system or causing an increase in overall healthcare costs.

Provision of comparative (benchmarking) information

The provision of benchmarked information on comparative prescribing patterns to clinicians is an important influence on prescribing behaviour. Using appropriate benchmarking data puts the behaviour of practices into a local and national context. Benchmarking can provide the basis for making clinicians aware of the potential for change and allows them to understand the potential outcome of any action. Various prescribing indicators have been developed both locally and nationally to measure and compare quality and cost-effectiveness of prescribing. Ideally indicators used should be evidence based, utilise available data sources and be validated.

Support and education

One of the challenges for modern healthcare organisations is to ensure consistent implementation of evidence-based interventions and the improvement of clinical practice. Simply providing prescribers with information or education about an evidence-based intervention rarely produces a change in practice. There is a need to understand the concerns that the adopting clinician may have about the change and recognise that these concerns are often legitimate. However, these may change over time, and the concerns must be addressed and overcome before successful adoption can occur. Interpersonal influence, particularly through the use of trusted colleagues or opinion leaders, is a powerful way to change practice. This is the basis for using pharmacists as prescribing advisers or 'academic detailers' to influence prescribing practice, particularly in primary care. Prescribing advisers present evidence-based tailored messages, allow the exchange of information and try to negotiate and persuade clinicians to change practice. Clinicians see pharmacists as a trusted and credible source of prescribing information who can be moderately successful in changing practice, particularly if linked with an incentive.

To change prescribing practice, pharmacists need to be aware of how to use an adoption model-based approach to convey key messages to prescribers to help them change practice. One such model is known as AIDA (Awareness, Interest, Decision, Action) (Table 2.5).

More sophisticated multifaceted educational interventions can also be effective at changing prescribing behaviour, but they need to be flexible to meet the needs of individual clinicians. This sort of combination approach includes small group learning, audit and feedback, practical support to make changes in practice and involvement and education of patients.

Table 2.5 AIDA adoption model for influencing prescribers

Awareness	Make the prescriber aware of the issues, prescribing data and evidence for the need to change.
Interest	Let the prescriber ask questions and find out more about the proposed change, what the benefits are and what the prescribers concerns are.
Decision	Help the prescriber come to a decision to make a change. They will need to apply the change to their practice, and may need further information, training and support to do this.
Action	Action refers to making a change by the prescriber. Support this with simple reminders, patient decision support, feedback data and audit.

Conclusion

While medicines have the capacity to improve health, they also have the potential to cause harm. Prescribing of medicines needs to be rational and effective in order to maximise benefit and minimise harm. Good prescribing should ensure the patient's ideas, concerns and expectations are taken into account. This can be effectively managed by adopting a consultation framework and using patient decision aids to support shared decision making with the patient as an equal partner. Prescribers need to be aware of their responsibilities and accountability, particularly when prescribing off label or unlicensed medicines. They also need to work within their organisation's clinical governance framework. The influences and biases that affect prescribing need to be recognised and minimised by utilising trusted independent sources of information to inform prescribing decisions.

References

All Wales Medicines Strategy Group, 2014. Polypharmacy: Guidance for Prescribing. All Wales Therapeutics and Toxicology Centre, Vale of Glamorgan, UK. Available at: http://www.awmsg.org/docs/awmsg/medman/Polypharmacy - Guidance for Prescribing.pdf.

Barber, N., 1995. What constitutes good prescribing? Br. Med. J. 310, 923–925.

Beauchamp, T.L., Childress, J.F., 2001. Principles of Biomedical Ethics, fifth ed. Oxford University Press, Oxford.

Beckman, H.B., Frankel, R.M., 1984. The use of videotape in internal medicine training. J. Gen. Intern. Med. 9, 517–521.

Britten, N., Stevenson, F.A., Barry, C.A., Barber, N., Bradley, C.P., 2000. Misunderstandings in prescribing decision in general practice: qualitative study. Br. Med. J. 320, 484–488.

Care Quality Commission, 2016. Better care in my hands: a review of how people are involved in their care. Available at: http://www.cqc.org.uk/content/better-care-my-hands-review-how-people-are-involved-their-care.

Chan, S.W., Tulloch, E., Cooper, E.S., 2017. Montgomery and informed consent: where are we now? Br. Med. J. 357, j2224. https://doi.org/10.1136/bmj.j2224.

Crown, J., 1999. Review of prescribing, supply and administration of medicines. Department of Health, London. Available at: http://webarchive.nationalarchives.gov.uk/20130107105354/http://www.dh.gov.uk/prod_consum_dh/groups/dh_digitalassets/@dh/@en/documents/digitalasset/dh_4077153.pdf.

de Vries, T.P., Henning, R.H., Hogerzeil, H.V., et al., 1994. Guide to good prescribing. A practical manual. World Health Organization Action Programme on Essential Drugs, Geneva. Available at: http://apps.who.int/medicinedocs/pdf/whozip23e/whozip23e.pdf.

Department of Health (DH), 1989. Review of prescribing, supply and administration of medicines (The Crown Report). Department of Health, London.

Department of Health, 1998. A first class service: quality in the New NHS Department of Health, London

Department of Health (DH), 2003. Supplementary prescribing by nurses and pharmacists with the NHS in England a guide for implementation. Department of Health, London. Available at: http://webarchive.nationalarchives.gov.uk/20130107105354/http://www.dh.gov.uk/prod_consum_dh/groups/dh_digitalassets/@dh/@en/documents/digitalasset/dh_4068431.pdf.

Department of Health (DH), 2005. Supplementary prescribing by nurses, pharmacists, chiropodists/podiatrists, physiotherapists and radiographers within the NHS in England: a guide for implementation. Department of Health, London. Available at: http://webarchive.nationalarchives.gov.uk/20130107105354/http://dh.gov.uk/prod_consum_dh/groups/dh_digitalassets/@dh/@en/documents/digitalasset/dh_4110033.pdf.

Department of Health (DH), 2006. Improving patients' access to medicines. A guide to implementing nurse and pharmacist independent prescribing within the NHS in England. Department of Health, London. Available at: http://www.dh.gov.uk/prod_consum_dh/groups/dh_digitalassets/@dh/@en/documents/digitalasset/dh_4133747.pdf.

Department of Health (DH), 2010. Changes to medicines legislation to enable mixing of medicines prior to administration in clinical practice. Department of Health, London. Available at: http://webarchive.nationalarchives.gov.uk/+/www.dh.gov.uk/en/Healthcare/Medicinespharmacyandindustry/Prescriptions/TheNon-MedicalPrescribingProgramme/DH_110765.

Department of Health (DH), 2012. Nurse and pharmacist independent prescribing changes announced Department of Health, London. Available at: https://www.gov.uk/government/news/nurse-and-pharmacist-independent-prescribing-changes-announced.

Department of Health and Social Security, 1986. Neighborhood nursing. A focus for care. Report of the Community Nursing Review. HMSO, London.

European Commission, 2001. Proposal for a directive of the European Parliament and of the Council amending directive 2001/83/EC on the community code relating to medicinal products for human use. Available at: http://www.ema.europa.eu/docs/en_GB/document_library/Regulatory_and_procedural_guideline/2009/10/WC500004481.pdf.

General Pharmaceutical Council, 2012. Guidance on maintaining clear sexual boundaries. General Pharmaceutical Council, London. Available at: https://www.pharmacyregulation.org/sites/default/files/gphc_guidance_on_sexual_boundaries_14.pdf.

General Pharmaceutical Council, 2017. Standards for Pharmacy Professionals. General Pharmaceutical Council, London. Available at: https://www.pharmacyregulation.org/sites/default/files/standards_for_pharmacy_professionals_may_2017_0.pdf.

Granby, T., Picton, C., 2006. Maintaining competency in prescribing. An outline framework to help pharmacists prescribers. Available at: https://www.webarchive.org.uk/wayback/archive/20140627112002/http://www.npc.nhs.uk/non_medical/resources/competency_framework_oct_2006.pdf.

Gupta, R., Best, J., MacMahon, E., 2008. Mumps and the UK Epidemic 2005. Br. Med. J. 330, 1132–1135.

Harrigan, J.A., Oxman, T.E., Rosenthal, R., 1985. Rapport expressed through non-verbal behavior. J. Nonverbal Behav. 9, 95–110.

Hesselink, G., Schoonhoven, L., Barach, P., et al., 2012. Improving patient handovers from hospital to primary care: a systematic review. Ann. Intern. Med. 157, 417–428.

House of Commons Health Committee, 2005. The Influence of the Pharmaceutical Iindustry HC 42-I. The Stationery Office, London.

Human Medicines Regulation, 2013. SI 2013 No. 1855 Medicines, The Human Medicines (Amendment) Regulations 2013. Available at: http://www.legislation.gov.uk/uksi/2013/1855/pdfs/uksi_20131855_en.pdf.

Human Medicines Regulation, 2016. S1 2016 No. 186, Medicines, The Human Medicines (Amendment) Regulations 2016. Available at: http://www.legislation.gov.uk/uksi/2016/186/pdfs/uksi_20160186_en.pdf.

Kings Fund, 2006. Interventions that change clinician behaviour: mapping the literature. Available at: https://www.nice.org.uk/Media/Default/About/what-we-do/Into-practice/Support-for-service-improvement-and-audit/Kings-Fund-literature-review.pdf.

Larsen, K.M., Smith, C.K., 1981. Assessment of non-verbal communication in patient-physician interview. J. Fam. Pract. 12, 481–488.

Lewis, T., 2004. Using the NO TEARS tool for medication review. Br. Med. J. 329, 434.

Makhinson, M., 2010. Biases in medication prescribing: the case of second-generation antipsychotics. J. Psychiatr. Pract. 16, 15–21.

Makoul, G., Arnston, P., Scofield, T., 1995. Health promotion in primary care physician-patient communication and decision about prescription medicines. Soc. Sci. Med. 41, 1241–1254.

Medicines and Healthcare products Regulatory Agency, 2009. Off-label use or unlicensed medicines: prescribers' responsibilities. Drug Saf. Update 2, 7.

Medicines Partnership, 2002. Room for review. A guide to medication review: the agenda for patients, practitioners and managers. Medicines Partnership, London. Available at: http://myweb.tiscali.co.uk/bedpgme/CG/Room%20for%20Review%20-%20Medication%20review.pdf.

National Audit Office, 2007. Prescribing Costs in Primary Care. The Stationery Office, London.

National Health Service (NHS) England, 2016a. Summary of the responses to the public consultation on proposals to introduce supplementary prescribing by dietitians across the United Kingdom. Available at: https://www.england.nhs.uk/wp-content/uploads/2016/02/dietitians-summary-consult-responses.pdf.

National Health Service (NHS) England, 2016b. NHS England Innovation Scorecard. Available at: https://www.england.nhs.uk/ourwork/innovation/innovation-scorecard/.

National Institute for Health and Care Excellence (NICE), 2009. Medicines adherence: involving patients in decisions about prescribed medicines and supporting adherence. Clinical Guideline 76. NICE, London. Available at: https://www.nice.org.uk/guidance/cg76.

National Institute for Health and Care Excellence (NICE), 2012. Patient experiences in adult NHS services: improving the experience of care for people using adult NHS services. Clinical Guideline 138. NICE, London. Available at: https://www.nice.org.uk/guidance/cg138.

National Institute for Health and Care Excellence (NICE), 2014. Developing and updating local formularies. Medicines Practice Guideline MPG1. NICE, London. Available at: https://www.nice.org.uk/guidance/mpg1.

National Institute for Health and Care Excellence (NICE), 2015. Medicines optimisation: the safe and effective use of medicines to enable the best possible outcomes. NICE Guideline NG5. NICE, London. Available at: https://www.nice.org.uk/guidance/ng5.

National Patient Safety Agency, 2007. Design for patient safety: a guide to the design of dispensed medicines. NPSA, London.

National Prescribing Centre, 1998. Prescribing new drugs in general practice. MeReC Bull. 9 (6), 21–22.

National Prescribing Centre, 2008. Using patient decision aids. MeReC Extra No. 36. Available at: https://www.webarchive.org.uk/wayback/archive/20140627112837/http://www.npc.nhs.uk/merec/mastery/mast4/merec_extra_no36.php.

Nicolson, D.J., Knapp, P., Raynor, D.K., et al., 2009. Written information about individual medicines for consumers. Cochrane Database Syst. Rev. 2009 (2), CD002104. https://doi.org/10.1002/14651858.CD002104.pub3.

Paling, J., 2003. Strategies to help patients understand risks. Br. Med. J. 327, 745–748.

Preskorn, S.H., 1994. Antidepressant drug selection: criteria and options. J. Clin. Psychiatry 55 (Suppl. A), 6–22, discussion 23–24, 98–100.

Public Health England, 2015. Improving health literacy to reduce health inequalities. Public Health England and UCL Institute of Health Equity. Available at: https://www.gov.uk/government/publications/local-action-on-health-inequalities-improving-health-literacy.

Royal Pharmaceutical Society, 2012. Keeping patients safe when they transfer between care providers – getting the medicines right. Good practice guidance for healthcare professions. Available at: https://www.rpharms.com/Portals/0/RPS%20document%20library/Open%20access/Publications/Keeping%20patients%20safe%20transfer%20of%20care%20report.pdf.

Royal Pharmaceutical Society, 2016. A Competency Framework for All Prescribers. Royal Pharmaceutical Society, London. Available at: https://www.rpharms.com/Portals/0/RPS%20document%20library/Open%20access/Professional%20standards/Prescribing%20competency%20framework/prescribing-competency-framework.pdf.

Royal Pharmaceutical Society, 2017. Medicines Ethics and Practice: The Professional Guide for Pharmacists, forty first ed. Royal Pharmaceutical Society, London.

Scottish Government, 2015. Model of Care Polypharmacy Working Group. Polypharmacy Guidance, second ed. Scottish Government. Available at: http://www.sehd.scot.nhs.uk/publications/DC20150415polypharmacy.pdf.

Silverman, J., Kurtz, S., Draper, J., 2005. Skills for Communicating with Patients, second ed. Radcliffe Publishing, Oxford.

Sokol, D.K., 2015. Update on the UK law on consent. Br. Med. J. 350, h1481. https://doi.org/10.1136/bmj.h1481.

Wheeler, R., 2006. Gillick or Fraser? A plea for consistency over competence in children. Br. Med. J. 332, 807.

Further reading

Appelbe, G.E., Wingfield, J., 2013. Dale and Appelbe's Pharmacy and Medicines Law, tenth ed. Pharmaceutical Press, London.

Bond, C., Blenkinsopp, A., Raynor, D.K., 2012. Prescribing and partnership with patients. Br. J. Clin. Pharmacol. 47 (4), 581–588.

Duerden, M., Millson, D., Avery, A., et al., 2011. The quality of GP prescribing. Kings Fund, London. Available at: https://www.kingsfund.org.uk/sites/files/kf/field/field_document/quality-gp-prescribing-gp-inquiry-research-paper-mar11.pdf.

General Pharmaceutical Council, 2012. Guidance on consent. General Pharmaceutical Council, London. Available at: https://www.pharmacyregulation.org/sites/default/files/guidance_on_consent_08.09.14_0.pdf.

General Pharmaceutical Council, 2017. In practice guidance on confidentiality. General Pharmaceutical Council, London. Available at: https://www.pharmacyregulation.org/sites/default/files/in_practice-_guidance_on_confidentiality_may_2017.pdf.

Horne, R., Weinman, J., Barber, N., et al., 2005. Concordance, adherence and compliance in medicine taking. Report for the National Co-ordinating Centre for NHS Service Delivery and Organisation R&D, London. Available at: http://www.netscc.ac.uk/hsdr/files/project/SDO_FR_08-1412-076_V01.pdf.

Jansen, J., Naganathan, V., Carter, S., et al., 2016. Too much medicine in older people? Deprescribing through shared decision making. Br. Med. J. 353, i2893.

NHS Litigation Authority, 2003. Clinical negligence. A very brief guide for clinicians. NHS Litigation Authority, London.

Silverman, J., Kurtz, S., Draper, J., 2013. Skills for Communicating with Patients, third ed. CRC Press, London.

Useful websites

PolyPharmacy Guidance: 7 steps' approach, http://www.polypharmacy.scot.nhs.uk

Patient trusted medical information and support, https://www.patient.info

International Patient Decision Aid Standards Collaboration, http://ipdas.ohri.ca

NHS Patient decision aids, http://sdm.rightcare.nhs.uk (Account access is required for this site)

PolyPharmacy Guidance: Tools to support improving polypharmacy, http://www.polypharmacy.scot.nhs.uk

PrescQIPP: Tools to support improving polypharmacy, https://www.prescqipp.info

3 Practical Pharmacokinetics

Ray W. Fitzpatrick and Katie Maddock

Key points

- Pharmacokinetics can be applied to a range of clinical situations with or without therapeutic drug monitoring (TDM).
- TDM can improve patient outcomes but is necessary only for drugs with a narrow therapeutic index, where there is a good concentration response relationship and where there is no easily measurable physiological parameter.
- Sampling before steady state is reached or before distribution is complete leads to erroneous results.
- The volume of distribution (V_d) can be used to determine the loading dose.
- The elimination half-life determines the time to steady state and the dosing interval.
- Kinetic constants determine the rate of absorption and elimination.
- Clearance determines the maintenance dose.
- Creatinine clearance can be reliably estimated from population values.
- Use of actual blood level data wherever possible to assist dose adjustment is advisable. However, population pharmacokinetic values can be used for digoxin, theophylline and gentamicin.
- Once-daily dosing of gentamicin is used as an alternative to multiple dosing.
- TDM is essential in the dose titration of vancomycin, lithium and phenytoin, but of little value for valproate or the newer anticonvulsants.

Clinical pharmacokinetics may be defined as the study of the time course of the absorption, distribution, metabolism and excretion of drugs and their corresponding pharmacological response. In practice, pharmacokinetics makes it possible to model what may happen to a drug after it has been administered to a patient. Clearly this science may be applied to a wide range of clinical situations, hence the term 'clinical pharmacokinetics'. However, no matter how elegant or precise the mathematical modelling, the relationship between concentration and effect must be established before pharmacokinetics will be of benefit to the patient.

General applications

Clinical pharmacokinetics can be applied in daily practice to drugs with a narrow therapeutic index, even if drug level monitoring is not required.

Time to maximal response

By knowing the half-life of a drug, the time to reach a steady state may be estimated (Fig. 3.1), and also when the maximal therapeutic response is likely to occur, irrespective of whether drug level monitoring is needed.

Need for a loading dose

The same type of information can be used to determine whether the loading dose of a drug is necessary, because drugs with longer half-lives are more likely to require loading doses for acute treatment.

Dosage alterations

Clinical pharmacokinetics can be useful in determining dosage alteration if the route of elimination is impaired through end-organ failure, for example, renal failure or drug interaction. Quantitative dosage changes can be estimated using limited pharmacokinetic information, such as the fraction that should be excreted unchanged (f_e value), which can be found in most pharmacology textbooks.

Choosing a formulation

An understanding of the pharmacokinetics of absorption may also be useful in evaluating the appropriateness of particular formulations of a drug in a patient.

Application to therapeutic drug monitoring

Clinical pharmacokinetics is usually associated with therapeutic drug monitoring (TDM) and its subsequent utilisation. When TDM is used appropriately, it has been demonstrated that patients suffer fewer side effects than those who are not monitored (Reid et al., 1990). Although TDM is a proxy outcome measure, a study with aminoglycosides (Crist et al., 1987) demonstrated shorter hospital stays for patients when TDM was used. Furthermore, a study on the use of anticonvulsants (McFadyen et al., 1990) showed better epilepsy control in those patients for whom TDM was used. A literature review of the cost-effectiveness of TDM concluded that emphasis should not be placed solely on cost-effectiveness, but how TDM can be applied in a cost-effective and clinically useful way (Touw et al., 2005). There are various levels of sophistication for the application of pharmacokinetics to TDM. Knowledge of the distribution time and an understanding of the concept of steady state can facilitate determination of appropriate sampling times.

For most drugs that undergo first-order elimination, a linear relationship exists between dose and concentration, which can be used for dose adjustment purposes. However, if the clearance of the drug changes as the concentration changes (e.g. phenytoin), then an understanding of the drug's pharmacokinetics will assist in making correct dose adjustments.

More sophisticated application of pharmacokinetics involves the use of population pharmacokinetic data to produce initial dosage guidelines, for example, nomograms for digoxin and gentamicin, and to predict drug levels. Pharmacokinetics can also assist in complex dosage individualisation using actual patient-specific drug level data.

Given the wide range of clinical situations in which pharmacokinetics can be applied, pharmacists must have a good understanding of the subject and of how to apply it to maximise their contribution to patient care.

Basic concepts

Volume of distribution

The apparent V_d may be defined as the size of a compartment which will account for the total amount of drug in the body (A)

if it were present in the same concentration as in plasma. This means that it is the apparent volume of fluid in the body which results in the measured concentration of drug in plasma (C) for a known amount of drug given, that is:

$$C = \frac{A}{V_d}$$

This relationship assumes that the drug is evenly distributed throughout the body in the same concentration as in the plasma. However, this is not the case in practice because many drugs are present in different concentrations in various parts of the body. Thus, some drugs which concentrate in muscle tissue have a very large apparent V_d, for example, digoxin. This concept is better explained in Fig. 3.2.

The apparent V_d may be used to determine the plasma concentration after an intravenous (i.v.) loading dose:

$$C = \frac{\text{loading dose}}{V_d} \quad (1)$$

Conversely, if the desired concentration is known, the loading dose may be determined:

$$\text{loading dose} = \text{desired } C \times V_d \quad (2)$$

In the previous discussion, it has been assumed that after a given dose a drug is instantaneously distributed between the various tissues and plasma. In practice this is seldom the case. For practical purposes it is reasonable to generalise by referring to plasma as one compartment and tissue as if it were another single separate compartment. However, in reality there will be many tissue subcompartments. Thus, in pharmacokinetic terms the body may be described as if it were divided into two compartments: the plasma and the tissues.

Fig. 3.3 depicts the disposition of a drug immediately after administration and relates this to the plasma concentration–time graph.

Initially, the plasma concentration falls rapidly, due to distribution and elimination (α phase). However, when an equilibrium is reached between the plasma and tissue, that is, the distribution is complete, the change in plasma concentration is only due to elimination from the plasma (β phase), and the plasma concentration falls at a slower rate. The drug is said to follow a two-compartment model. However, if distribution is completed

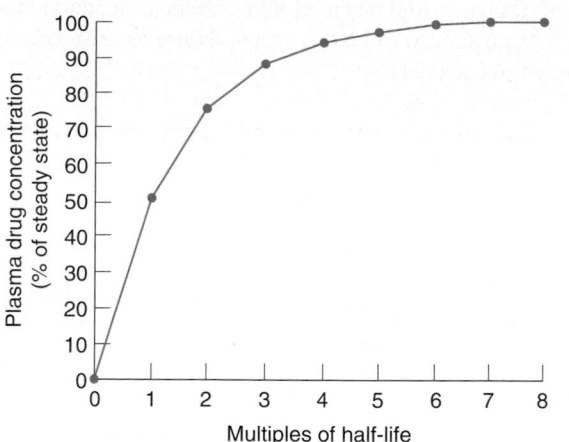

Fig. 3.1 Time to steady state.

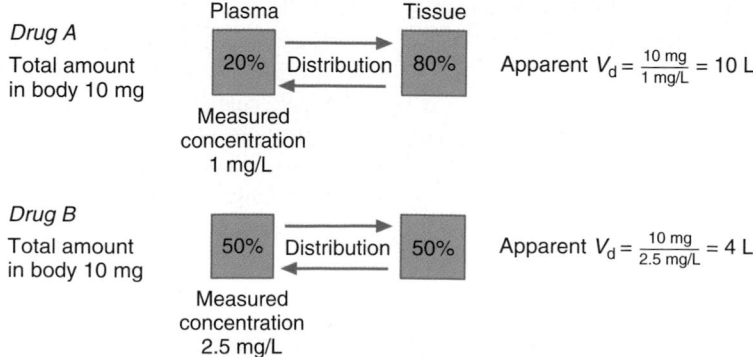

Fig. 3.2 Distribution: more of drug A is distributed in the tissue compartment, resulting in a higher apparent volume of distribution than for drug B, where more remains in the plasma.

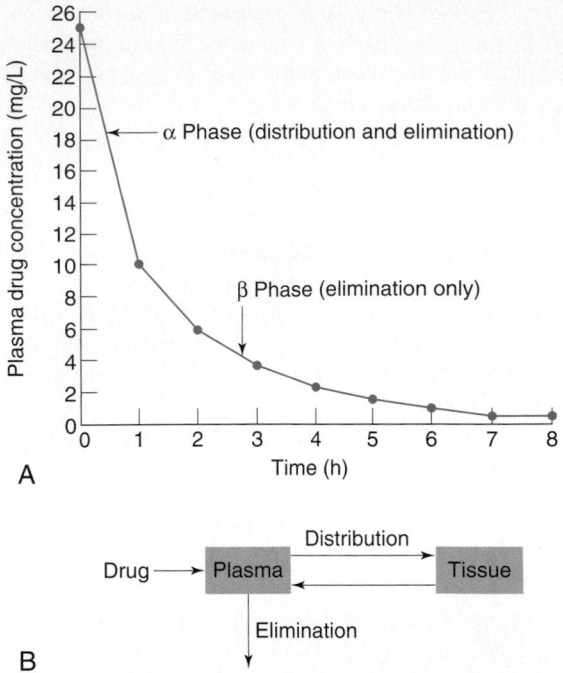

A

B

Fig. 3.3 (A) Two-compartment plasma concentration–time graph showing two phases in the plasma concentration–time profile. (B) Representation of a two-compartment model showing distribution of drug between plasma and tissue compartments.

quickly (within minutes), then the α phase is not seen, and the drug is said to follow a one-compartment model.

The practical implications of a two-compartment model are that any sampling for monitoring purposes should be carried out after distribution is complete. In addition, i.v. bolus doses are given slowly to avoid transient side effects caused by high peak concentrations.

Elimination

Drugs may be eliminated from the body by a number of routes. The primary routes are excretion of the unchanged drug in the kidneys or metabolism (usually in the liver) into a more water-soluble compound for subsequent excretion in the kidneys, or a combination of both.

The main pharmacokinetic parameter describing elimination is clearance (CL). This is defined as the volume of plasma completely emptied of drug per unit time. For example, if the concentration of a drug in a patient is 1 g/L and the clearance is 1 L/h, then the rate of elimination will be 1 g/h. Thus, a relationship exists:

$$\text{rate of elimination} = \text{CL} \times C \qquad (3)$$

Total body elimination is the sum of the metabolic rate of elimination and the renal rate of elimination. Therefore:

$$\text{total body clearance} = \text{CL (metabolic)} + \text{CL (renal)}$$

Thus, if the fraction eliminated by the renal route is known (f_e), then the effect of renal impairment on total body clearance (TBC) can be estimated.

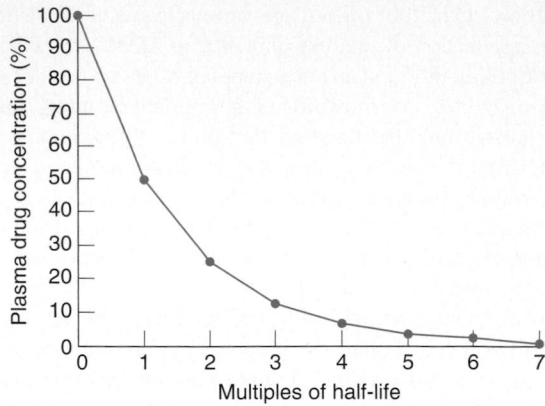

Fig. 3.4 First-order elimination.

The clearance of most drugs remains constant for each individual. However, it may alter in cases of drug interactions, changing end-organ function or auto-induction. Therefore, it is clear from Eq. (3) that as the plasma concentration changes so will the rate of elimination. However, when the rate of administration is equal to the rate of elimination, the plasma concentration is constant (C^{ss}) and the drug is said to be at a steady state; that is:

$$\text{rate in} = \text{rate out}$$

At the beginning of a dosage regimen the plasma concentration is low. Therefore, the rate of elimination from Eq. (3) is less than the rate of administration, and accumulation occurs until a steady state is reached (see Fig. 3.1):

$$\text{rate of administration} = \text{rate of elimination} = \text{CL} \times C^{ss} \qquad (4)$$

It is clear from Eq. (3) that as the plasma concentration falls (e.g. on stopping treatment or after a single dose), the rate of elimination also falls. Therefore, the plasma concentration–time graph follows a non-linear curve characteristic of this type of first-order elimination (Fig. 3.4). This is profoundly different from a constant rate of elimination irrespective of plasma concentration, which is typical of zero-order elimination.

For drugs undergoing first-order elimination, there are two other useful pharmacokinetic parameters in addition to the V_d and clearance. These are the elimination rate constant and elimination half-life.

The elimination rate constant (k_e) is the fraction of the amount of drug in the body (A) eliminated per unit time. For example, if the body contains 100 mg of a drug and 10% is eliminated per unit time, then $k_e = 0.1$. In the first unit of time, 0.1×100 mg, or 10 mg is eliminated, leaving 90 mg. In the second unit of time, 0.1×90 mg, or 9 mg is eliminated, leaving 81 mg. Elimination continues in this manner. Therefore:

$$\text{rate of elimination} = k_e \times A \qquad (5)$$

Combining Eqs. (3) and (5) gives:

$$\text{CL} \times C = k_e \times A$$

and because

$$C = \frac{A}{V_d}$$

then

$$CL \times \frac{A}{V_d} = k_e \times A$$

Therefore:

$$CL = k_e \times V_d \tag{6}$$

Elimination half-life ($t_{1/2}$) is the time it takes for the plasma concentration to decay by half. In five half-lives the plasma concentration will decline to approximately zero (see Fig. 3.4).

The equation which is described in Fig. 3.4 is:

$$C_2 = C_1 \times e^{-k_e \times t} \tag{7}$$

where C_1 and C_2 are plasma concentrations and t is time.

If half-life is substituted for time in Eq. (7), C_2 must be half of C_1. Therefore:

$$0.5 \times C_1 = C_1 \times e^{-k_e \times t_{1/2}}$$

$$0.5 = e^{-k_e \times t_{1/2}}$$

$$\ln 0.5 = -k_e \times t_{1/2}$$

$$0.693 = -k_e \times t_{1/2}$$

$$t_{1/2} = \frac{0.693}{k_e} \tag{8}$$

There are two ways of determining k_e: either by estimating the half-life and applying Eq. (8) or by substituting two plasma concentrations in Eq. (7) and applying natural logarithms:

$$\ln C_2 = \ln C_1 - (k_e \times t)$$

$$k_e \times t = \ln C_1 - \ln C_2$$

$$k_e = \frac{\ln C_1 - \ln C_2}{t}$$

In the same way as it takes approximately five half-lives for the plasma concentration to decay to zero after a single dose, it takes approximately five half-lives for a drug to accumulate to the steady state on repeated dosing or during constant infusion (see Fig. 3.1).

This graph may be described by Eq. (9):

$$C = C^{ss} \left(1 - e^{-k_e \times t}\right) \tag{9}$$

where C is the plasma concentration at time t after the start of the infusion and C^{ss} is the steady-state plasma concentration. Thus, if the appropriate pharmacokinetic parameters are known, it is possible to estimate the plasma concentration any time after a single dose or the start of a dosage regimen.

Absorption

In the preceding sections, the i.v. route has been discussed, and with this route all of the administered drug is absorbed. However, if a drug is administered by any other route it must be absorbed into the bloodstream. This process may or may not be 100% efficient.

The fraction of the administered dose which is absorbed into the bloodstream is the bioavailability (F). Therefore, when applying pharmacokinetics for oral administration, the dose or rate of administration must be multiplied by F. Bioavailability, F, is determined by calculating the area under the concentration time curve (AUC). The rationale for this is described below.

The rate of elimination of a drug after a single dose is given by Eq. (3). By definition the rate of elimination is the amount of drug eliminated per unit time:

Amount eliminated in any one unit of time:

$$dt = CL \times C \times dt$$

Total amount of drug eliminated $= \sum_0^\infty CL \times C \times dt$

As previously explained, CL is constant. Therefore:

Total amount eliminated $= CL \times \Sigma C \times dt$

from start until C is zero.

$\Sigma C \times dt$ is actually the area under the plasma concentration–time curve (Fig. 3.5).

After a single i.v. dose, the total amount eliminated is equal to the amount administered, D i.v. Therefore:

$$D \text{ i.v.} = CL \times AUC \text{ i.v.} \quad \text{or} \quad CL = D \text{ i.v.}/AUC.$$

However, for an oral dose, the amount administered is

$$F \times D \text{ p.o.}$$

Because CL is constant in the same individual:

$$CL = F \times D \text{ p.o.}/AUC \text{ p.o.} = D \text{ i.v.}/AUC \text{ i.v.}$$

Rearranging gives:

$$F = (D \text{ i.v.} \times AUC \text{ p.o.})/(D \text{ p.o.} \times AUC \text{ i.v.})$$

In this way, F can be calculated from plasma concentration–time curves.

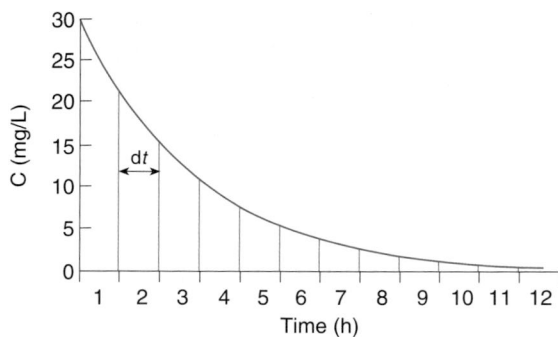

Fig. 3.5 The area under the concentration time curve is the sum of the individual areas which are $= C \times dt$.

Dosing regimens

From the preceding sections, it is possible to derive equations which can be applied in clinical practice.

From Eq. (1) we can determine the change in plasma concentration ΔC immediately after a single dose:

$$\Delta C = \frac{S \times F \times \text{dose}}{V_d} \qquad (10)$$

where F is bioavailability and S is the salt factor, which is the fraction of active drug when the dose is administered as a salt; for example, aminophylline is 80% theophylline, therefore, $S = 0.8$.

Conversely, to determine a loading dose:

$$\text{loading dose} = \frac{\text{desired change in } C \times V_d}{S \times F} \qquad (11)$$

At the steady state it is possible to determine maintenance dose or steady-state plasma concentrations from a modified Eq. (4):

$$\text{rate in} = \frac{S \times F \times \text{dose}}{T} = \text{CL} \times \text{average } C^{ss} \qquad (12)$$

where T is the dosing interval.

Peak and trough levels

For oral dosing and constant i.v. infusions, it is usually adequate to use the term 'average steady state plasma concentration' (average C^{ss}). However, for some i.v. bolus injections it is sometimes necessary to determine peak and trough levels, for example, gentamicin.

At the steady state, the change in concentration due to the administration of an i.v. dose will be equal to the change in concentration due to elimination over one dose interval:

$$\Delta C = \frac{S \times F \times \text{dose}}{V_d} = C_{max} - C_{min}$$

Within one dosing interval the maximum plasma concentration (C^{ss}_{max}) will decay to the minimum plasma concentration (C^{ss}_{min}) as in any first-order process.

Substituting C^{ss}_{max} for C_1 and C^{ss}_{min} for C_2 in Eq. (7):

$$C^{ss}_{max} = C^{ss}_{max} \times e^{-k_e \times t}$$

where t is the dosing interval.

If this is substituted into the preceding equation:

$$\frac{S \times F \times \text{dose}}{V_d} = C^{ss}_{max} - \left(C^{ss}_{max} \times e^{-k_e \times t} \right)$$

Therefore:

$$C^{ss}_{max} = \frac{S \times F \times \text{dose}}{V_d \left(1 - e^{-k_e \times t}\right)} \qquad (13)$$

$$C^{ss}_{min} = \frac{S \times F \times \text{dose}}{V_d \left(1 - e^{-k_e \times t}\right)} \times e^{-k_e \times t} \qquad (14)$$

Interpretation of drug concentration data

The availability of the technology to measure the concentration of a drug in plasma should not be the reason for monitoring. A number of criteria should be fulfilled before TDM is undertaken:
- The drug should have a narrow therapeutic index.
- There should be a good concentration–response relationship.
- There are no easily measurable physiological parameters.

In the absence of these criteria being fulfilled, the only other justification for undertaking TDM is to monitor adherence or to confirm toxicity. When interpreting TDM data, a number of factors need to be considered.

Sampling times

In the preceding sections, the time to reach the steady state has been discussed. When TDM is carried out as an aid to dose adjustment, the concentration should be at steady state. Therefore, approximately five half-lives should elapse after initiation or after changing a maintenance regimen, before sampling. The only exception to this rule is when toxicity is suspected. When the steady state has been reached, it is important to sample at the correct time. It is clear from the discussion above that this should be done when distribution is complete (see Fig. 3.3).

Dosage adjustment

Under most circumstances, provided the preceding criteria are observed, adjusting the dose of a drug is relatively simple, because a linear relationship exists between the dose and concentration if a drug follows first-order elimination (Fig. 3.6, A). This is the case for most drugs.

Capacity limited clearance

If a drug is eliminated by the liver, it is possible for the metabolic pathway to become saturated because it is an enzymatic system. Initially the elimination is first-order, but once saturation of the system occurs, elimination becomes zero-order. This results in the characteristic dose–concentration graph shown in Fig. 3.6 (B). For the majority of drugs eliminated by the liver, this effect is

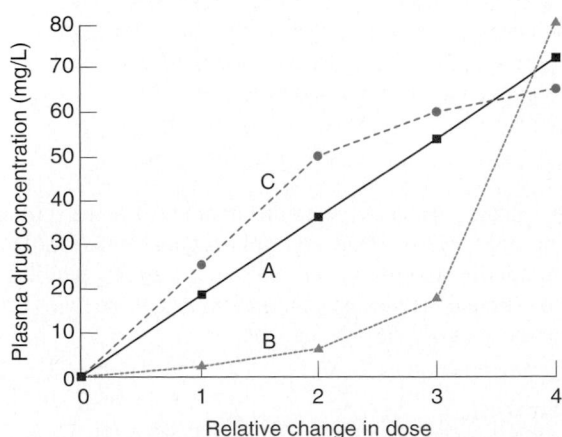

Fig. 3.6 Dose–concentration relationships: (A) first-order elimination, (B) capacity-limited clearance, and (C) increasing clearance.

not seen at normal therapeutic doses and occurs only at very high supratherapeutic levels, which is why the kinetics of some drugs in overdose is different from normal. However, one important exception is phenytoin, where saturation of the enzymatic pathway occurs at therapeutic doses. This will be dealt with later in the Phenytoin section.

Increasing clearance

The only other situation where first-order elimination is not seen is where clearance increases as the plasma concentration increases (see Fig. 3.6, C). Under normal circumstances, the plasma protein binding sites available to a drug far outnumber the capacity of the drug to fill those binding sites, and the proportion of the total concentration of drug which is protein bound is constant. However, this situation is not seen in one or two instances, for example, valproate and disopyramide. For these particular drugs, as the concentration increases the plasma protein binding sites become saturated and the ratio of unbound drug to bound drug increases. The elimination of these drugs increases disproportionately to the total concentration because elimination is dependent on the unbound concentration.

Therapeutic range

Wherever TDM is carried out, a therapeutic range is usually used as a guide to the optimum concentration. The limits of these ranges should not be taken as absolute. Some patients may respond to levels above or below these ranges, whereas others may experience toxic effects within the so-called therapeutic range. These ranges are only adjuncts to dose determination, which should always be done in light of the clinical response.

Clinical applications

Estimation of creatinine clearance

Because many drugs are renally excreted, and the most practical marker of renal function is creatinine clearance (CrCL), it is often necessary to estimate this to undertake dosage adjustment in renal impairment. The usual method is to undertake a 24-hour urine collection coupled with a plasma creatinine measurement. The laboratory then estimates the patient's CrCL. The formula used to determine CrCL is based upon the pharmacokinetic principles in Eq. (3).

The rate of elimination is calculated from the measurement of the total amount of creatinine contained in the 24-hour urine sample divided by 24, that is:

$$\frac{\text{amount of creatinine}}{24} = \text{rate of excretion (mg/h)}$$

Using this rate of excretion and substituting the measured plasma creatinine for C^{ss} in Eq. (4), the CrCL can be calculated.

However, there are practical difficulties with this method. The whole process is cumbersome and there is an inevitable delay in obtaining a result. The biggest problem is the inaccuracy of the 24-hour urine collection.

An alternative approach is to estimate the rate of production of creatinine (i.e. rate in) instead of the rate of elimination (rate out). Clearly this has advantages because it does not involve 24-hour urine collections and requires only a single measure of plasma creatinine. There are data in the literature that relate creatinine production to age, weight and sex because the primary source of creatinine is the breakdown of muscle.

Therefore, equations have been produced which are rearrangements of Eq. (4), that is:

$$\text{creatinine clearance} = \frac{\text{rate of production}}{C^{ss}}$$

Rate of production is replaced by a formula which estimates this from physiological parameters of age, weight and sex.

It has been shown that the equation produced by Cockcroft and Gault (1976) appears to be the most satisfactory. A modified version using SI units is shown as:

$$\frac{\text{creatinine clearance}}{\text{(mL/min)}} = \frac{F \times [(140 - \text{age in years}) \times \text{weight (kg)}]}{\text{plasma creatinine (mmol/L)}}$$

where $F = 1.04$ (females) or 1.23 (males).

There are limitations using only plasma creatinine to estimate renal function. The modification of diet in renal disease (MDRD) formula can be used to estimate glomerular filtration rate (eGFR). This formula uses plasma creatinine, age, sex and ethnicity (Department of Health, 2006):

$$\begin{aligned} \text{eGFR} = {}& 175 \times [\text{plasma creatinine (mmol/L)} \times 0.011312]^{-1.154} \\ & \times [\text{age in year}]^{-0.203} \times [1.212 \text{ if patient is black}] \\ & \times [0.742 \text{ if female}] \end{aligned}$$

eGFR = glomerular filtration rate (mL/min/1.73 m^2)

The MDRD should be used with care when calculating doses of drugs because most of the published dosing information is based on the Cockcroft and Gault formula. In patients with moderate-to-severe renal failure, it is best to use the Cockcroft and Gault formula to determine drug dosing.

Digoxin

Action and uses

Digoxin is the most widely used of the digitalis glycosides. Its primary actions on the heart are those of increasing the force of contraction and decreasing conduction through the atrioventricular node. Currently, its main role is in the treatment of atrial fibrillation by slowing down the ventricular response, although it is also used in the treatment of heart failure in the presence of sinus rhythm. The primary method of monitoring its clinical effect in atrial fibrillation is by measurement of heart rate, but knowledge of its pharmacokinetics can be helpful in predicting a patient's dosage requirements.

Plasma concentration–response relationship

- <0.5 microgram/L: no clinical effect
- 0.7 microgram/L: some positive inotropic and conduction blocking effects

- 0.8–2 micrograms/L: optimum therapeutic range (0.5–0.9 microgram/L in patients >65-years-old)
- 2–2.5 micrograms/L: increased risk of toxicity, although tolerated in some patients
- >2.5 micrograms/L: gastro-intestinal, cardiovascular system, and central nervous system toxicity

Distribution

Digoxin is widely distributed and extensively bound in varying degrees to tissues throughout the body. This results in a high apparent V_d. Digoxin V_d can be estimated using the equation 7.3 L/kg x (ideal body weight [BWt]), which is derived from population data. However, distribution is altered in patients with renal impairment, and a more accurate estimate in these patients is given by:

$$V_d = 3.8 \times \text{ideal BWt} + (3.1 \times \text{creatinine clearance (mL/min)})$$

A two-compartment model best describes digoxin disposition (see Fig. 3.3), with a distribution time of 6–8 hours. Clinical effects are seen earlier after i.v. doses, because the myocardium has a high blood perfusion and affinity for digoxin. Sampling for TDM must be done no sooner than 6 hours post-dose; otherwise, an erroneous result will be obtained.

Elimination

Digoxin is eliminated primarily by renal excretion of unchanged drug (60–80%), but some hepatic metabolism occurs (20–40%). The population average value for digoxin clearance is:

$$\text{digoxin clearance (mL/min)} = 0.8 \times \text{BWt} + (\text{creatinine clearance (mL/min)})$$

However, patients with severe congestive heart failure have a reduced hepatic metabolism and a slight reduction in renal excretion of digoxin:

$$\text{digoxin clearance (mL/min)} = 0.33 \times \text{BWt} + (0.9 \times \text{creatinine clearance (mL/min)})$$

Ideal body weight should be used in these equations.

Absorption

Digoxin is poorly absorbed from the gastro-intestinal tract, and dissolution time affects the overall bioavailability. The two oral formulations of digoxin have different bioavailabilities:

$$F \text{(tablets)} = 0.65$$

$$F \text{(liquid)} = 0.8$$

Practical implications

Using population averages, it is possible to predict plasma concentrations from specific dosages, particularly because the time to reach the steady state is long. Population values are only averages, and individual values may vary. In addition a number of diseases and drugs affect digoxin disposition.

As can be seen from the preceding discussion, congestive heart failure, hepatic diseases and renal diseases all decrease the elimination of digoxin. In addition, hypothyroidism increases the plasma concentration (decreased metabolism and renal excretion) and increases the sensitivity of the heart to digoxin. Hyperthyroidism has the opposite effect. Hypokalaemia, hypercalcaemia, hypomagnesaemia and hypoxia all increase the sensitivity of the heart to digoxin. Numerous drug interactions have been reported of varying clinical significance. The usual cause is either altered absorption or clearance.

Theophylline

Theophylline is an alkaloid related to caffeine. It has a variety of clinical effects including mild diuresis, central nervous system stimulation, cerebrovascular vasodilatation, increased cardiac output and bronchodilatation. It is the last which is the major therapeutic effect of theophylline. Theophylline does have some serious toxic effects. However, there is a good plasma concentration–response relationship.

Plasma concentration–response relationship

- <5 mg/L: no bronchodilatation[1]
- 5–10 mg/L: some bronchodilatation and possible anti-inflammatory action
- 10–20 mg/L: optimum bronchodilatation, minimum side effects
- 20–30 mg/L: increased incidence of nausea, vomiting[2] and cardiac arrhythmias
- >30 mg/L: cardiac arrhythmias, seizures

Distribution

Theophylline is extensively distributed throughout the body, with an average V_d based on population data of 0.48 L/kg.

Theophylline does not distribute very well into fat, and estimations should be based on ideal body weight. A two-compartment model best describes theophylline disposition, with a distribution time of approximately 40 minutes.

Elimination

Elimination is a first-order process primarily by hepatic metabolism to relatively inactive metabolites.

The population average for theophylline clearance is 0.04 L/h/kg, but this is affected by a number of diseases, drugs and pollutants. Therefore, this value should be multiplied by:

- 0.5, where there is cirrhosis, or when cimetidine, erythromycin, clarithromycin, ciprofloxacin or norfloxacin is being taken concurrently due to enzyme inhibition in the liver;
- 0.4, where there is congestive heart failure with hepatomegaly due to reduced hepatic clearance;

---

[1] Some patients exhibit a clinical effect at these levels which has been attributed to possible anti-inflammatory effects.
[2] Nausea and vomiting can occur within the therapeutic range.

- 0.8, where there is severe respiratory obstruction [forced expiratory volume in 1 second (FEV_1) < 1 L];
- 1.6, for patients who smoke (defined as >10 cigarettes/day), because smoking stimulates hepatic metabolism of theophylline.

Neonates metabolise theophylline differently, with 50% being converted to caffeine. Therefore, when it is used to treat neonatal apnoea of prematurity, a narrower therapeutic range is used (usually 5–10 mg/L) because caffeine contributes to the therapeutic response.

Product formulation

Aminophylline (the ethylenediamine salt of theophylline) is only 80% theophylline. Therefore, the salt factor (S) is 0.8. Most sustained-release (SR) preparations show good bioavailability, but not all SR preparations are the same, which is why advice in the British National Formulary (BNF) recommends patients are maintained on the same brand.

Practical implications

Intravenous bolus doses of aminophylline need to be given slowly (preferably by short infusion) to avoid side effects caused by transiently high blood levels during the distribution phase. Oral doses with SR preparations can be estimated using population average pharmacokinetic values and titrated proportionately according to blood levels and clinical response. In most circumstances SR preparations may be assumed to provide 12-hour cover. However, more marked peaks and troughs are seen with fast metabolisers (smokers and children). In these cases the SR preparation with the lowest k_a value may be used twice daily [e.g. Uniphyllin (k_a = 0.22)]. Alternatively, thrice-daily dosage is required if a standard (k_a = 0.3–0.4) SR product is used [e.g. Phyllocontin (k_a = 0.37) or Nuelin SA (k_a = 0.33)].

Gentamicin

Clinical use

The spectrum of activity of gentamicin is similar to other aminoglycosides, but its most significant activity is against *Pseudomonas aeruginosa*. It is still regarded by many as first choice for this type of infection.

Therapeutic range

Gentamicin has a narrow therapeutic index, producing dose-related side effects of nephrotoxicity and ototoxicity. The use of TDM to aid dose adjustment is essential if these toxic effects which appear to be related to peak and trough plasma levels are to be avoided. It is generally accepted that the peak level (drawn 1 hour post-dose after an i.v. bolus or intramuscular injection) should not exceed 12 mg/L and the trough level (drawn immediately pre-dose) should not exceed 2 mg/L.

The above recommendations relate to multiple daily dosing of gentamicin. Once-daily dosing has superseded multiple-dose gentamicin except for certain conditions. Therefore, when once-daily dosing is used, different monitoring and interpretation parameters apply as described at the end of this section.

Distribution

Gentamicin is relatively polar and distributes primarily into extracellular fluid. Thus, the apparent V_d is only 0.3 L/kg. Gentamicin follows a two-compartment model, with distribution being complete within 1 hour.

Elimination

Elimination is by renal excretion of the unchanged drug. Gentamicin clearance is approximately equal to CrCL.

Practical implications

Because the therapeutic range is based on peak (1 hour post-dose to allow for distribution) and trough (pre-dose) concentrations, it is necessary to be able to predict these from any given dosage regimen.

Initial dosage. Initial dosage may be based on the patient's physiological parameters. Gentamicin clearance may be determined directly from CrCL. The V_d may be determined from ideal body weight. The elimination constant k_e may then be estimated using these parameters in Eq. (6). By substituting k_e and the desired peak and trough levels into Eq. (7), the optimum dosage interval can be determined (add on 1 hour to this value to account for sampling time). Using this value (or the nearest practical value) and the desired peak or trough value substituted into Eq. (13) or (14), it is possible to determine the appropriate dose.

Changing dosage. Changing dosage is not as straightforward as for theophylline or digoxin, because increasing the dose will increase the peak and trough levels proportionately. If this is not desired, then use of pharmacokinetic equations is necessary. By substituting the measured peak and trough levels and the time between them into Eq. (7), it is possible to determine k_e (and the half-life from Eq. (8) if required). To estimate the patient's V_d from actual blood level data, it is necessary to know the C^{ss}_{max} immediately after the dose (time zero), not the 1-hour value which is measured. To obtain this, Eq. (7) may be used, this time substituting the trough level for C_2 and solving for C_1. Subtracting the trough level from this C^{ss}_{max} at time zero, the V_d may be determined from Eq. (10). Using these values for k_e and V_d, derived from actual blood level data, a new dose and dose interval can be determined as before.

Once-daily dosing. There are theoretical arguments for once-daily dosing of gentamicin because aminoglycosides display concentration-dependent bacterial killing and a high enough concentration to minimum inhibitory concentration (MIC) ratio may not be achieved with multiple dosing. Furthermore, aminoglycosides have a long post-antibiotic effect. Aminoglycosides also accumulate in the kidneys, and once-daily dosing could reduce renal tissue accumulation. A number of clinical trials have compared once-daily administration of aminoglycosides with conventional administration. A small number of these trials have shown less nephrotoxicity, no difference in ototoxicity and similar efficacy with once-daily administration.

Initial dosage for a once-daily regimen is 5–7 mg/kg/day for patients with a CrCL of >60 mL/min. This is subsequently adjusted on the basis of blood levels. However, monitoring of once-daily dosing of gentamicin is different from multiple dosing. One approach is to take a blood sample 6–14 hours after the first dose and plot the time and result on a standard concentration-time plot (the Hartford nomogram; Nicolau et al., 1995; Fig. 3.7). The position of the individual patient's point in relation to standard lines on the nomogram indicates what the most appropriate dose interval should be (either 24, 36 or 48 hours). Once-daily dosing of gentamicin has not been well studied in pregnant or breastfeeding women, patients with major burns, renal failure, endocarditis or cystic fibrosis. Therefore, although once-daily dosing has superseded multiple-dose gentamicin, it cannot be recommended in these groups and multiple daily dosing should be used.

Vancomycin

Vancomycin is an amphoteric glycopeptide antibiotic which has bactericidal activity against aerobic and anaerobic Gram-positive bacteria. Vancomycin is particularly useful in severe staphylococcal infections resistant to other antibiotics and has shown efficacy in endocarditis, osteomyelitis, septicaemia and soft tissue infections. Oral vancomycin is poorly absorbed for systemic use but is indicated for the treatment of *Clostridium difficile* colitis.

Concentration–response relationship

Although vancomycin has been in use since the late 1950s, there is conflicting evidence of the relationship between concentration and toxicity, particularly nephrotoxicity and ototoxicity. Early data suggested a link between high serum concentrations and ototoxicity, although a retrospective review of the literature has not identified a specific threshold level. Similarly nephrotoxicity has been associated with vancomycin treatment, but again the evidence is not strong enough to identify specific threshold levels. Although AUC-to-MIC ratio is the parameter which correlates best with vancomycin activity, it is impractical to use in routine clinical practice. Therefore, vancomycin trough concentrations are used as a surrogate marker. There is little justification for measuring peak concentrations. The BNF recommends trough levels are maintained in the range of 10–15 mg/L, but a slightly higher trough level range of 15–20 mg/L for endocarditis and less sensitive strains of meticillin-resistant *Staphylococcus aureus*.

Absorption and distribution

Although absorption following oral administration of vancomycin is poor, this increases where there is inflammation and

---

If result available within 24 h
- Use graph below to select dose interval. Use serum concentration and time interval between start of infusion and sample to plot intercept (see example given on graph).
- Give next dose (7 mg/kg by infusion as above) after interval indicated by graph.
  If result falls above upper limit for Q48 h, abandon once daily regimen. Measure gentamicin concentration after another 24 h and adopt multiple daily dose regimen if result <2 mg/L.
  If result falls on Q24 h sector it is not necessary to recheck gentamicin concentration within 5 days unless patient's condition suggests renal function may be compromised.

- **Graph:**   Use values of plasma concentration and time interval to find intercept
  (Example given of 6 mg/L after 10 h yields dose interval of 36 h)

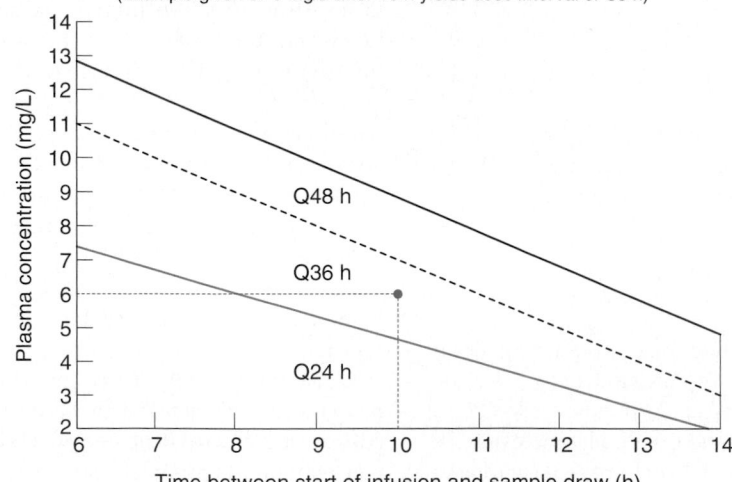

MONITORING
- Repeat U&E daily. Calculate creatinine clearance from serum creatinine to check dose interval has not changed.
- If dose interval has to be changed, check gentamicin concentration 6–4 h after start of next infusion note time of start of infusion and time of sampling and use graph to verify correct dose interval.

Fig. 3.7 Nomogram for adjustment of once-daily gentamicin dosage (Nicolau et al., 1995).

following repeated doses. Therefore, vancomycin is given by i.v. administration for systemic use and penetrates into most body spaces, but concentrations are variable and dependent on the degree of inflammation. A two-compartment pharmacokinetic model best describes vancomycin after i.v. administration (see Fig. 3.3) with a distribution phase of 30–60 minutes in patients with normal renal function. The V_d is between 0.4 and 1 L/kg.

Elimination

When given i.v. vancomycin is excreted primarily via the kidneys and follows first-order elimination kinetics with clearance (CL) = CrCL. Oral doses are excreted primarily in the faeces. Elimination half-life is approximately 6–7 hours in patients with normal function but prolonged in those with renal insufficiency.

Practical applications

Because the AUC-to-MIC ratio is not practical to use in clinical practice, trough concentrations are used as a surrogate measure to guide safe and effective dosing.

- Intravenous doses should be administered by infusion over 60 minutes to avoid infusion-related side effects due to local irritation and transient high peaks.
- Although vancomycin has a relatively short half-life, it has a long duration of action and should be administered every 12 hours to ensure appropriate trough levels are maintained and to reduce the number of i.v. administrations for the reasons outlined above.
- Trough levels should be taken at steady state (30–35 hours), which is normally just before the third or fourth dose on a 12-hour regimen.
- Because vancomycin clearance is directly related to renal function, dosage should be reduced in patients with impaired renal function and the patient carefully monitored. The Summary of Product Characteristics (SPC) contains a dosage nomogram to assist in this.

As vancomycin follows first-order elimination, adjusting the 12-hour dose will result in a proportional increase or decrease in trough levels.

Lithium

Lithium is effective in the treatment of acute mania and in the prophylaxis of manic depression. The mechanism of action is not fully understood, but it is thought that it may substitute for sodium or potassium in the central nervous system. Lithium is toxic, producing dose-dependent and dose-independent side effects. Therefore, TDM is essential in assisting in the management of the dosage.

Dose-dependent effects

The plasma concentration–response relationship derived on the basis of the 12-hour standardised lithium level (measured 12 hours after the evening dose of lithium) is as follows:

- <0.4 mmol/L: little therapeutic effect
- 0.4–1.0 mmol/L: optimum range for prophylaxis

- 0.8–1.2 mmol/L: optimum range for acute mania
- 1.2–1.5 mmol/L: causes possible renal impairment
- 1.5–3.0 mmol/L: causes renal impairment, ataxia, weakness, drowsiness, thirst, diarrhoea
- 3.0–5.0 mmol/L: causes confusion, spasticity, dehydration, convulsions, coma, death (Levels >3.5 mmol/L are regarded as a medical emergency.)

Dose-independent effects

Dose-independent effects include tremor, hypothyroidism (approximately 10% of patients on chronic therapy), nephrogenic diabetes insipidus, gastro-intestinal upset, loss in bone density, weight gain (approximately 20% of patients gain >10 kg) and lethargy.

Distribution

Lithium is unevenly distributed throughout the body, with a V_d of approximately 0.7 L/kg. Lithium follows a two-compartment model (see Fig. 3.3) with a distribution time of 8 hours (hence the 12-hour sampling criterion).

Elimination

Lithium is excreted unchanged by the kidneys. Lithium clearance is approximately 25% of CrCL because there is extensive reabsorption in the renal tubules.

In addition to changes in renal function, dehydration, diuretics (particularly thiazides), angiotensin-converting enzyme inhibitors and non-steroidal anti-inflammatory drugs (except aspirin and sulindac) all decrease lithium clearance. Conversely, aminophylline and sodium loading increase lithium clearance.

Notwithstanding the earlier factors, there is a wide interindividual variation in clearance, and the lithium half-life in the population varies between 8 and 35 hours, with an average of approximately 18 hours. Lithium clearance shows a diurnal variation, being slower at night than during the day.

Practical implications

In view of the narrow therapeutic index, lithium should not be prescribed unless facilities for monitoring plasma lithium concentrations are available. Because lithium excretion is a first-order process, changes in dosage result in a proportional change in blood levels. Blood samples should be drawn 12 hours after the evening dose, because this will allow for distribution and represent the slowest excretion rate. Population pharmacokinetic data (particularly the V_d) cannot be relied upon to make initial dosage predictions, although renal function may give an approximate guide to clearance. Blood level measurements are reported in SI units; therefore, it is useful to know the conversion factors for the various salts:

- 100 mg of lithium carbonate is equivalent to 2.7 mmol of lithium ions,
- 100 mg of lithium citrate is equivalent to 1.1 mmol of lithium ions.

Phenytoin

Phenytoin is used in the treatment of epilepsy (see Chapter 31). Use is associated with dose-independent side effects which include hirsutism, acne, coarsening of facial features, gingival hyperplasia, hypocalcaemia and folic acid deficiency. However, phenytoin has a narrow therapeutic index and has serious concentration-related side effects.

Plasma concentration–response relationship

- <5 mg/L: generally no therapeutic effect
- 5–10 mg/L: some anticonvulsant action with approximately 50% of patients obtaining a therapeutic effect with concentrations of 8–10 mg/L
- 10–20 mg/L: optimum concentration for anticonvulsant effect
- 20–30 mg/L: nystagmus, blurred vision
- >30 mg/L: ataxia, dysarthria, drowsiness, coma

Distribution

Phenytoin follows a two-compartment model with a distribution time of 30–60 minutes. The apparent V_d is 1 L/kg.

Elimination

The main route of elimination is via hepatic metabolism. However, this metabolic route can be saturated at normal therapeutic doses. This results in the characteristic non-linear dose–concentration curve shown in Fig. 3.6 (B). Therefore, instead of the usual first-order pharmacokinetic model, a Michaelis–Menten model, used to describe enzyme activity, is more appropriate.

Using the Michaelis–Menten model, the daily dosage of phenytoin can be described by:

$$\frac{S \times F \times \text{dose}}{T} = \frac{V_{max} \times C^{ss}}{K_m + C^{ss}} \quad (15)$$

where K_m is the plasma concentration at which metabolism proceeds at half the maximal rate. The population average for this is 5.7 mg/L, although this value varies greatly with age and race. V_{max} is the maximum rate of metabolism of phenytoin and is more predictable at approximately 7 mg/kg/day.

Because clearance changes with blood concentration, the half-life also changes. The usual reported value is 22 hours, but this increases as concentration increases. Therefore, it is difficult to predict when the steady state will be reached. However, as a rule of thumb, 1–2 weeks should be allowed to elapse before sampling after a dosage change.

In overdose it can be assumed that metabolism of the drug is occurring at the maximum rate of V_{max}. Therefore, the decline in plasma concentration is linear (zero-order) at approximately 7 mg/L/day.

Practical implications

Because the dose–concentration relationship is non-linear, changes in dose do not result in proportional changes in plasma concentration (see Fig. 3.6, B). Using the Michaelis–Menten model, if the plasma concentration is known at one dosage, then

V_{max} may be assumed to be the population average (7 mg/kg/day), because this is the more predictable parameter, and K_m is calculated using Eq. (15). The revised values of K_m can then be used in Eq. (15) to estimate the new dosage required to produce a desired concentration. Alternatively, a nomogram (orbit diagram) may be used to assist in dose adjustments (Bauer, 2008).

Care is needed when interpreting TDM data and making dosage adjustments when phenytoin is given concurrently with other anticonvulsants, because these affect distribution and metabolism of phenytoin. Because phenytoin is approximately 90% protein bound, in patients with a low plasma albumin and or uraemia, the free fraction increases and, therefore, an adjusted total phenytoin should be calculated or a free salivary level taken. The following equation can be applied to adjust the observed concentration in hypoalbuminaemia:

$$C_{adjusted} = \frac{C_{observed}}{0.9 \times (C_{albumin}/44) + 0.1}$$

Albumin concentration is in g/L.

In uraemic patients with severe renal failure, the unbound fraction is approximately doubled, so the target concentration needs to be half the normal concentration, or apply the adjusted concentration equation if albumin level is known.

The oral formulations of phenytoin show good bioavailability. However, tablets and capsules contain the sodium salt ($S = 0.9$), whereas the suspension and infatabs are phenytoin base ($S = 1$). Intramuscular phenytoin is slowly and unpredictably absorbed, due to crystallisation in the muscle tissue, and is therefore not recommended. Fosphenytoin, a prodrug of phenytoin, is better absorbed from the intramuscular site. Doses should be expressed as phenytoin equivalent. Fosphenytoin sodium 1.5 mg is equivalent to phenytoin sodium 1 mg.

Carbamazepine

Carbamazepine is indicated for the treatment of partial and secondary generalised tonic-clonic seizures, primary generalised tonic-clonic seizures, trigeminal neuralgia, and prophylaxis of bipolar disorder unresponsive to lithium. There are a number of dose-independent side effects, including various dermatological reactions and, more rarely, aplastic anaemia and Stevens–Johnson syndrome. However, the more common side effects are concentration related.

Plasma concentration–response relationship when used in the treatment of epilepsy

- <4 mg/L: little therapeutic benefit
- 4–12 mg/L: optimum therapeutic range for monotherapy
- >9 mg/L: possible side effects of nystagmus, diplopia, drowsiness and ataxia, particularly if patients are receiving other anticonvulsant therapy
- >12 mg/L: side effects common, even on monotherapy

Distribution

Carbamazepine is widely distributed in various organs, with the highest concentration found in liver and kidneys. Carbamazepine is 70–80% protein bound and shows a wide variation in the population average apparent V_d (0.8–1.9 L/kg). This wide variation is thought to be due to variations in absorption (because there is no parenteral form) and protein binding.

Elimination

Carbamazepine is eliminated almost exclusively by metabolism, with less than 2% being excreted unchanged in the urine. Elimination is a first-order process, but carbamazepine induces its own metabolism (auto-induction). Therefore, at the beginning of therapy, clearance is 0.01–0.03 L/h/kg, increasing to 0.05–0.1 L/h/kg on chronic therapy. Auto-induction begins in the first few days of commencing therapy and is maximal at 2–4 weeks.

Because clearance changes with time, so does half-life, with reported values as long as 35 hours after a single dose, decreasing to 5–7 hours on regular dosing.

Absorption

Absorption after oral administration is slow, with peak concentrations being reached 2–24 hours post-dose (average 6 hours). Absorption is incomplete, with bioavailability estimated at approximately 80% ($F = 0.8$). Bioavailability via rectal administration is even less, and 125 mg of suppositories is approximately equivalent to 100 mg of tablets.

Practical implications

Use of pharmacokinetic equations is limited due to the auto-induction effect. However, there are a number of important practical points:
- Blood samples should not be drawn before the steady state, which will not be achieved until 2–4 weeks after starting therapy to allow for auto-induction, or 3–4 days after subsequent dose adjustments.
- When sampling, the trough level should be measured because of the variable absorption pattern.
- Complex calculations are not helpful, but as a rule of thumb each 100 mg dose will increase the plasma concentration at steady state by approximately 1 mg/L in adults.
- A number of other drugs (including phenytoin) when given concurrently will affect carbamazepine metabolism and subsequent blood levels.

Valproate

Sodium valproate as valproic acid in the bloodstream has a broad spectrum of anticonvulsant activity, being useful in generalised absence, generalised tonic–colonic and partial seizures.

Plasma concentration–response relationship

There is no clear concentration–response relationship for valproate, although a range of 50–100 mg/L is often quoted as being optimal, with 50% of patients showing a response at levels greater than 80 mg/L. Levels greater than 100 mg/L do not confer

any additional therapeutic benefits. Although no clear relationship exists between plasma levels and toxic effects, the rare hepatotoxicity associated with valproate appears to be related to very high levels of more than 150 mg/L.

Distribution

Valproate is extensively bound to plasma protein (90–95%), and unlike other drugs it can saturate protein binding sites at concentrations greater than 50 mg/L, altering the free fraction of drug. Therefore, the apparent V_d of valproate varies from 0.1 to 0.5 L/kg.

Elimination

Elimination of valproate is almost entirely by hepatic metabolism, with less than 5% being eliminated by the kidneys.

As a result of the saturation of protein binding sites and the subsequent increase in the free fraction of the drug, clearance of the drug increases at higher concentrations. Therefore, there is a non-linear change in plasma concentration with dose, which is illustrated in Fig. 3.6 (C).

Practical implications

In view of the lack of a clear concentration–response relationship and the variable pharmacokinetics, there are limited indications for the measurement of valproate levels. In most cases dosage should be based on clinical response. Valproic acid can take several weeks to become fully active, so adjustment of doses must not be made quickly.

In a few cases where seizures are not controlled at high dosage, a plasma level may be helpful in confirming treatment failure. If monitoring is to be undertaken, levels should be drawn at steady state (2–3 days). A trough sample will be the most useful because wide fluctuations of blood levels may occur during a dose interval.

Newer epilepsy treatments

Newer epilepsy medicines include gabapentin, lamotrigine, lacosamide, vigabatrin, levetiracetam, perampanel, pregabalin, retigabine, rufinamide, tiagabine, topiramate and zonisamide. They are indicated for the treatment of a range of types of epilepsy and some with additional indications. All are used as adjunctive treatment with other anticonvulsants, and some are indicated for monotherapy.

Plasma concentration–response relationship

No clear relationship exists between plasma concentration and response for these newer anticonvulsants. The situation is further complicated because these preparations are usually used as add-on therapy with other anticonvulsants.

Practical implications

Although these newer anticonvulsants have narrow therapeutic indices and interindividual and intraindividual variation in pharmacokinetics, there is not enough evidence to support routine TDM, and dosage should be titrated to clinical response.

Ciclosporin

Ciclosporin is a neutral lipophilic cyclic undecapeptide extracted from the fungus *Tolypocladium inflatum gams*. It is a potent immunosuppressive agent, used principally to reduce graft rejection after organ and tissue transplantation. The drug has a narrow therapeutic index, with a number of toxic effects including nephrotoxicity, hepatotoxicity, gastro-intestinal intolerance, hypertrichosis and neurological problems. Efficacy in reducing graft rejection, as well as the main toxic effects of nephrotoxicity and hepatotoxicity, appear to be concentration related.

Plasma concentration–response relationship

With all drugs that are monitored, the therapeutic range is a window with limits, which are not absolute. It is even more difficult to define a therapeutic range for ciclosporin, because there are a number of influencing factors. First, the measured concentration varies depending on sampling matrix (i.e. whole blood or plasma). Second, it depends on whether the assay is specific for ciclosporin alone or non-specific to include metabolites. A target concentration varies between centres but is commonly around 100–200 ng/mL in the first 6 months after transplantation and 80–150 ng/mL from 6 months onwards. Levels below the lower limit of this window are associated with an increased incidence of graft rejection. Levels above the upper limit are associated with an increased incidence of nephrotoxicity and hepatotoxicity.

Distribution

Ciclosporin is highly lipophilic and is widely distributed throughout the body with a V_d of 4–8 L/kg. There is variable distribution of ciclosporin within blood, because the whole blood concentration is approximately twice the plasma concentration. Within plasma, ciclosporin is 98% protein bound.

Elimination

Ciclosporin is eliminated primarily by hepatic metabolism, with wide interindividual variation in clearance (0.1–2 L/h/kg). In children these values are approximately 40% higher, with a resulting increased dosage requirement on a milligram per kilogram basis. In elderly patients or patients with hepatic impairment, a lower clearance rate has been observed.

Practical implications

In addition to the wide interpatient variability in distribution and elimination pharmacokinetic parameters, absorption of standard formulations of ciclosporin is variable and incomplete (F = 0.2–0.5 in normal subjects). In transplant patients this variation in bioavailability is even greater and increases during the first few months after transplant. Furthermore, a number of drugs are known to interact with ciclosporin. All of these factors suggest that TDM will assist in optimum dose selection, but the use of population averages in dose prediction is of little benefit due to wide interpatient variation. When using TDM with ciclosporin, a number of practical points need to be considered:

* The sampling matrix should be whole blood because there is a variable distribution of ciclosporin between blood and plasma.
* Samples should represent trough levels and be drawn at the steady state, which is achieved 2–3 days after initiating or changing the dosage (average half-life is 9 hours).
* Ciclosporin concentration monitoring should be undertaken every 2–3 days in the immediate postoperative phase until the patient's clinical condition is stable. Thereafter, monitoring can be undertaken every 1–2 months.
* TDM should be performed when changing brands of ciclosporin because there are marked differences in the bioavailability of different brands.

Tacrolimus

Similar to ciclosporin, tacrolimus is a calcineurin-inhibiting immunosuppressant used to reduce graft rejection after organ and tissue transplantation. Tacrolimus has a wide range of side effects covering most of the body systems.

Plasma concentration–response relationship

A strong correlation exists between AUC and whole blood trough levels at steady state. Therefore, monitoring of whole blood trough levels provides a good estimate of systemic exposure.

Absorption

Tacrolimus has been shown to be absorbed throughout the gastro-intestinal tract. Following oral administration of a non-slow-release formulation, peak concentrations (C_{max}) of tacrolimus in blood are achieved in approximately 1–3 hours.

Distribution

Tacrolimus plasma concentration time curve after i.v. infusion follows a classic biphasic form as described in Fig. 3.3.

In the systemic circulation, tacrolimus binds strongly to erythrocytes, resulting in an approximate 20:1 distribution ratio of whole blood/plasma concentrations. Tacrolimus is extensively distributed in the body. The steady-state V_d based on plasma concentrations is approximately 1300 L (healthy subjects). Corresponding data based on whole blood averaged 47.6 L.

Elimination

Tacrolimus is widely metabolised in the liver, primarily by the cytochrome P450-3A4.

In healthy subjects, the average TBC estimated from whole blood concentrations was 2.25 L/h. In adult liver, kidney and heart transplant patients, values of 4.1, 6.7, and 3.9 L/h, respectively, have been observed. Paediatric liver transplant recipients have a TBC approximately twice that of adult liver transplant patients.

The half-life of tacrolimus is long and variable. In healthy subjects, the mean half-life in whole blood is approximately 43 hours. In adult and paediatric liver transplant patients, it averaged 11.7 and 12.4 hours, respectively, compared with 15.6 hours in adult kidney transplant recipients. Increased clearance rates contribute to the shorter half-life observed in transplant recipients.

Practical implications

The following points should be considered when using TDM for tacrolimus:
- After initial dosing and for maintenance treatment tacrolimus doses should be adjusted according to whole blood concentrations.
- Whole blood concentrations should be trough levels drawn immediately before the next dose.
- In view of the relatively short half-life in transplant recipients, steady state will be achieved in approximately 3 days.
- The majority of patients can be successfully managed if tacrolimus blood trough levels are maintained at less than 20 ng/mL. In clinical practice, whole blood trough levels have generally been in the range of 5–20 ng/mL in liver transplant recipients and 10–20 ng/mL in kidney and heart transplant patients in the early post-transplant period. Subsequently, during maintenance therapy, blood concentrations have generally been in the range of 5–15 ng/mL in liver, kidney and heart transplant recipients.
- Due to the variation in the oral formulations of tacrolimus, patients stabilised on a particular formulation of tacrolimus should be maintained on that formulation and prescription, and dispensing should be by brand name to avoid inadvertent switching.
- When strong inhibitors of CYP3A4 (such as telaprevir, boceprevir, ritonavir, ketoconazole, voriconazole, itraconazole, telithromycin or clarithromycin) or inducers of CYP3A4 (such as rifampicin and rifabutin) are prescribed with tacrolimus, tacrolimus blood levels should be monitored to adjust the tacrolimus dose appropriately.

Sirolimus

Sirolimus is a non-calcineurin-inhibiting immunosuppressant which is used for the prophylaxis of organ rejection in adult patients at low-to-moderate immunological risk receiving a renal transplant. It is recommended for use initially in combination with ciclosporin microemulsion and corticosteroids for 2–3 months and may be continued as maintenance therapy with corticosteroids only if ciclosporin microemulsion can be progressively discontinued. The most commonly reported adverse reactions to sirolimus are thrombocytopaenia, anaemia, pyrexia, hypertension, hypokalaemia, hypertriglyceridaemia, abdominal pain, lymphocoele, peripheral oedema, arthralgia, acne, diarrhoea, constipation, nausea, headache, increased blood creatinine and increased blood lactate dehydrogenase.

Concentration–response relationship

The efficacy of sirolimus decreases when the trough concentrations fall below the target ranges, and the incidence of any adverse effect increases as trough levels increase.

Following initiation of sirolimus the dose should then be individualised to obtain whole blood trough levels of 4–12 ng/mL (chromatographic assay) when used in combination with ciclosporin. Ciclosporin should be progressively discontinued over 4–8 weeks, and sirolimus dose should be adjusted to obtain whole blood trough levels of 12–20 ng/mL.

Whole blood sirolimus levels should be closely monitored in patients with hepatic impairment, when CYP3A4 inducers (rifampicin) or CYP3A4 inhibitors (ketoconazole, voriconazole, diltiazem, verapamil and erythromycin) are concurrently administered, and after their discontinuation. Levels should be closely monitored if ciclosporin dosing is markedly reduced or discontinued, because ciclosporin inhibits the metabolism of sirolimus, and consequently sirolimus levels will decrease when ciclosporin is discontinued.

Therapeutic monitoring of the medicinal product should not be the sole basis for adjusting sirolimus therapy. Careful attention should be made to clinical signs/symptoms, tissue biopsies and laboratory parameters.

Absorption and distribution

Much of the general pharmacokinetic information was obtained using the sirolimus oral solution. Following administration of the oral solution, sirolimus is rapidly absorbed, with a time to peak concentration of 1 hour in healthy subjects receiving single doses and 2 hours in patients with stable renal allografts receiving multiple doses. In healthy subjects there is a difference in bioavailability between the tablets and oral solution after a single dose, but the difference is less marked upon steady-state administration to renal transplant recipients, and therapeutic equivalence has been demonstrated.

Similar to ciclosporin, sirolimus is lipophilic and is widely distributed in lipid membranes of body tissues, as well as erythrocytes, which gives rise to a high apparent V_d of 5.6–16.4 L/kg.

Elimination

Sirolimus is primarily eliminated by hepatic metabolism and similar to ciclosporin there is wide interindividual variation in clearance (0.04–0.34 L/h/kg) due to the variability in enterocyte P-glycoprotein and CYP3A4 content. Sirolimus has a relatively long terminal half-life ranging from 44 to 87 hours, although in clinical practice effective half-life is shorter and steady state is achieved in 5–7 days.

Practical applications

As with ciclosporin the wide interpatient variability in sirolimus pharmacokinetic parameters using population averages for dose prediction is of little benefit, but TDM will assist in optimum dose selection. The following points should be considered when using TDM for sirolimus:
- The sampling matrix should be whole blood because there is a variable distribution of sirolimus between blood and plasma.
- Samples should represent trough levels and be drawn at steady state.
- When switching patients between oral solution and tablet formulations, it is recommended to give the same dose and to

Table 3.1 Summary of pharmacokinetic data

Drug	Therapeutic range	V_d (L/kg)	CL (L/h/kg)	Half-life (h)
Digoxin	0.8–2.0 micrograms/L (0.5–0.9 microgram/L in patients >65 years) 1–2.6 nmol/L (0.625–1.1 nmol/L in patients >65 years)	7.3	See text	36
Theophylline	10–20 mg/L 55–110 mmol/L	0.48	0.04	8
Gentamicin	Peak 5–12 mg/L Trough <2 mg/L	0.3	1 × CL (creatinine)	2
Vancomycin	Trough 10–15 mg/L (15–20 mg/L for endocarditis and less sensitive strains of meticillin-resistant *Staphylococcus aureus*)	0.4–1	1 × CL (creatinine)	6–7
Lithium	0.4–0.8 mmol/L	0.5–1	0.25 × CL (creatinine)	18
Phenytoin	10–20 mg/L 40–80 mmol/L	1	K_m = 5.7 mg/L V_{max} = 7 mg/kg/day	
Carbamazepine	4–12 mg/L 17–50 mmol/L	0.8–1.9	0.05–1 See text	
Valproate	<100 mg/L <693 mmol/L		See text	
Ciclosporin	Varies between centres 100–200 ng/mL (first 6 months after transplantation) 80–150 ng/mL (from 6 months onwards)	4–8	0.1–2	9
Sirolimus	Trough (whole blood) 4–12 ng/mL with ciclosporin 12–20 ng/mL without ciclosporin	5.6–16.4	0.04–0.34	44–87

Population pharmacokinetic parameters are based on averages. The degree of variability around the average is different for each drug. See text for variability. CL, Clearance; K_m, plasma concentration; V_d, volume of distribution.

verify the sirolimus trough concentration 1–2 weeks later to check that it remains within recommended target ranges. Also, when switching between different tablet strengths, verification of trough concentrations is recommended.

- The target concentration range for sirolimus is different when used alone and in combination with ciclosporin.
- Careful monitoring is particularly needed in patients with hepatic impairment and where medicines which interfere with CYP3A4 are co-prescribed.

Summary pharmacokinetic data for drugs with therapeutic plasma concentrations are listed in Table 3.1.

Case studies

Case 3.1

You are reviewing a formulary submission for a new formulation of a product, which has reportedly an improved side effect profile due to better absorption characteristics. However, there is conflicting evidence in the literature over the absorption of the new preparation. One paper, which is available to you, shows a concentration–time profile for the oral formulation after a single oral dose of 250 mg as in Table 3.2.

The paper also quotes an area under the curve after a single i.v. dose of 200 mg as 87 mg/L/h.

Questions

1. What is the area under the curve after the single oral dose of 250 mg?
2. What is the bioavailability of the new formulation?

Answers

1. Draw the concentration–time profile on a piece of paper; try to do it reasonably accurately, but it does not have to be exact. Draw down vertical lines from the curve at each 1-hour time interval to create a series of trapeziums (the first one is actually a triangle). Calculate the area of each trapezium from the formula:

   Area of trapezium = (sum of the height of each side/2) × width (1 h)

   Then add all the areas together (assume a value of 0 after 12 hours):

   AUC p.o. = 69.99 mg/L/h

2. From the equation:

$$F = \frac{D\ i.v. \times AUC\ p.o.}{D\ p.o. \times AUC\ i.v.}$$

   $F = 200 \times 69.99/250 \times 87$
   $F = 0.64$

Table 3.2 Concentration–time profile for the oral formulation after a single oral dose of 250 mg

Time after administration	1 h	2 h	3 h	4 h	5 h	6 h	7 h	8 h	9 h	10 h	11 h	12 h
Concentration (mg/L)	10	18	12.7	9	6.4	4.5	3.2	2.25	1.6	1.1	0.78	0.55

Case 3.2

An 86-year-old lady, Mrs EJ, is admitted to hospital by her primary care doctor, with increasing shortness of breath. She lives in a care home and is relatively immobile. Mrs EJ has a stable plasma creatinine of 150 mmol/L. She is 55 kg, 4' 11" (1.5 m) tall. She is known to have osteoporosis, ischaemic heart disease and recently diagnosed non-paroxysmal atrial fibrillation.

Mrs EJ's current medication is:

Calcium carbonate 1.25 g	2 tablets daily
Imdur	60 mg daily
Simvastatin	40 mg daily
Senna	7.5 mg daily
Digoxin	62.5 micrograms daily
Apixaban	5 mg twice daily

She has been taking digoxin in a dosage of 62.5 micrograms daily for the last 3 weeks.

Questions

1. Calculate the predicted digoxin level for Mrs EJ.
2. A digoxin blood level is reported to be 1.0 microgram/L. List the reasons for the difference between the measured and predicted digoxin levels.
3. The hospital doctor queries if he should increase the dose of digoxin because the blood level is on the low side. Use an evidence-based approach to reply to the clinician.

Answers

1. Her predicted glomerular filtration rate is calculated from Cockcroft and Gault equation:

$$\frac{\text{creatinine clearance}}{\text{(mL/min)}} = \frac{F \times [(140 - \text{age in years}) \times \text{weight (kg)}]}{\text{plasma creatinine (mmol/L)}}$$

$$\text{creatinine clearance (CL}_{cr}) = \frac{1.04\,(140 - 86)\,55}{150} = 20.6 \text{ mL/min}$$

On the assumption that the patient has severe congestive heart failure, the predicted digoxin level is calculated using the equation:

$$CL_{dig} = 0.33 \times IBW + 0.9 \times CL_{cr} = (0.33 \times 55) + (0.9 \times 20.6)$$
$$= 36.69 \text{ mL/min} = 2.2 \text{ L/h}$$

Ideal body weight [IBW (kg)]:

$$\text{male} = 50 + (2.3 \times \text{height in inches over 5 feet})$$

$$\text{female} = 45.5 + (2.3 \times \text{height in inches over 5 feet})$$

Eq. (4):

$$\text{rate of administration} = \text{rate of elimination} = CL \times C^{ss}$$

Rearranging Eq. (4):

$$C^{ss}_{ave} = \frac{\text{dose} \times S \times F}{CL_{dig} \times t} = \frac{62.5 \times 1 \times 0.63}{2.2 \times 24} = 0.75 \text{ micrograms/L}$$

2. The predicted level is less than the measured level, this may be because:
   - the level has been taken less than 6 hours after the oral dose,
   - non-adherence is suspected,
   - congestive heart failure has affected the renal function.
3. A subgroup analysis of the Digitalis Investigation Group suggested that participants older than 65 years who had low blood levels (0.5–0.9 microgram/L) had reductions in all-cause mortality. It has also been suggested that digoxin may be associated with an increased risk of problems in patients with atrial fibrillation (Gjesdal et al., 2008). Therefore, the dose of digoxin should not be increased.

Case 3.3

A 72-year-old man, Mr MA (80 kg, 1.70 m tall), is admitted to the medical ward with a diagnosis of infective endocarditis following an invasive dental procedure 2 weeks ago. He was commenced on i.v. vancomycin 1 g every 12 hours in accordance with the hospital protocol.

Mr MA's current laboratory results are:

Urea	9.1 mmol/L (3.2–7.5 mmol/L)
Creatinine	120 mmol/L (71–133 mmol/L)

Vancomycin levels were taken 2 and 6 hours after the first dose and reported as 28 and 25 mg/L, respectively.

Questions

1. Calculate Mr MA's elimination constant k_e.
2. Calculate the plasma concentration at C^0 immediately after the infusion.
3. Using the plasma concentration at C^0, calculate the level you would expect the patient to achieve immediately prior to his next dose.
4. Using the vancomycin dosing nomogram, calculate the recommended 12-hourly dosage for Mr MA based upon his available laboratory results.

Answers

1. Because the two plasma levels are known, the elimination constant k_e is calculated from the following equation:

$$k_e = \frac{\ln C_1 - \ln C_2}{t}$$

Using the plasma levels reported:

$$k_e = \frac{\ln 28 - \ln 25}{4}$$
$$k_e = 0.028 \text{ h}^{-1}$$

2. The plasma concentration at C^0 immediately after the first infusion is calculated as:

$$C^t = C^0 \times e^{-k_e \times t}$$
$$28 = C^0 \times e^{-0.028 \times 1}$$
$$C^0 = 28.8 \text{ mg/L}$$

3. The plasma concentration at C^0 is then used to calculate the expected level to be achieved immediately prior to his next dose:

$$C^t = C^0 \times e^{-k^e \times t}$$

$$C^t = 28.8 \times e^{-0.028 \times 12}$$

$$= 20.58 \text{ mg/L}$$

4. Mr MA's CrCL is calculated using the Cockcroft and Gault equation:

$$\text{creatinine clearance} \atop (\text{mL/min}) = \frac{F \times [(140 - \text{age in years} \times \text{weight(kg)}]}{\text{plasma creatinine (mmol/L)}}$$

$$\text{CrCL} = \frac{1.23 \times (140 - 72) \times 80}{120}$$

$$\text{CrCL} = 55.76 \text{ mL/min}$$

Convert 55.76 mL/min to mL/min/kg:

$$= \frac{55.76}{80}$$

$$= 0.7 \text{ mL/min/kg}$$

From the vancomycin dosing nomogram this equates to a dosage of 10.8 mg/kg/24 h = 864 mg/24 h = 432 mg every 12 hours. In practice the nearest practical dose would be 450 mg every 12 hours.

Case 3.4

A 34-year-old man (75 kg), Mr RP, was taken by his wife to the emergency department with symptoms of nausea, vomiting, diarrhoea and increasing confusion. He had a fall whilst out running 2 weeks before and sprained his ankle. To alleviate the pain and inflammation of his injury, Mr RP started taking his wife's ibuprofen tablets. She thought he was taking one 400 mg tablet three times a day. Mr RP was also taking lithium for bipolar disorder and his therapy was stable.

Blood samples were taken from which the following results were obtained:

Lithium	3.1 mmol/L (0.6–1 mmol/L)
Sodium	152 mmol/L (135–145 mmol/L)
Creatinine	110 mmol/L (71–133 mmol/L)

Treatment with lithium was stopped.

Questions

1. Calculate the patient's pharmacokinetic parameters: clearance (CL), V_d and elimination constant (k_e) using population data.
2. Estimate the time for the lithium level to decrease to the middle of the normal range.
3. Briefly describe the symptoms of lithium toxicity.

Answers

1. Population data suggest that the clearance of lithium can be calculated using the following equation:

$$\text{CL} = 0.25 \times \text{CrCL (L/h)}$$

The patient's CrCL is calculated using the Cockcroft and Gault equation:

$$\text{creatinine clearance} \atop (\text{mL/min}) = \frac{F \times [(140 - \text{age in years}) \times \text{weight (kg)}]}{\text{plasma creatinine (mmol/L)}}$$

$$\text{CrCL} = \frac{1.23 \times (140 - 34) \times 75}{110}$$

$$= 88.9 \text{ mL/min}$$

Convert 88.9 mL/min to L/h:

$$= \frac{88.9 \times 60}{1000} = 5.334 \text{ L/h}$$

lithium clearance $= 0.25 \times 5.334 = 1.3335 \text{ L/h}$

Population data suggest that the V_d for lithium is 0.7 L/kg. Therefore, for this patient:

$$V_d = 0.7 \times 75$$

$$V_d = 52.5 \text{ L}$$

The elimination rate constant k_e is calculated by rearranging Eq. (6):

$$\text{CL} = k_e \times V_d \text{ to give } k_e = \frac{\text{CL}}{V_d}$$

$$k_e = \frac{1.3335}{52.5}$$

$$k_e = 0.0254 \text{ h}^{-1}$$

2. The time it will take for Mr RP's lithium level to return to the middle of the normal range (0.6–1 mmol/L), that is, 0.8 mmol/L, is calculated by rearranging Eq. (7):

$$\text{time to decay} = \frac{\ln Cp^1 - \ln Cp^2}{k_e}$$

$$\text{time to decay} = \frac{\ln 3.1 - \ln 0.8}{0.0254}$$

time to decay = 53 hours = 2.2 days = approximately 2 days

3. Acute lithium toxicity tends to present with gastro-intestinal symptoms. If the toxicity is due to an increase in dose, symptoms will include neuromuscular signs, for example, ataxia and tremor. This is sometimes referred to as acute on chronic toxicity. Chronic toxicity is harder to treat due to tissue deposition and involves neurological problems.

Case 3.5

Mr BT is a 38-year-old, 63-kg man who suffers from asthma. He has been admitted to hospital and Nuelin S.A. 500 mg 12 hourly (6 am and 6 pm) has been added to his regimen. He responds well to this treatment, but unfortunately after 2 days of treatment two doses are missed (evening dose and following morning dose). The clinical team is anxious to discharge him, so it is decided to give him a loading dose of aminophylline at 10 am before restarting him on maintenance therapy.

Questions

1. Was Mr BT at steady state before the medication was omitted?
2. What is the estimated theophylline level at 10 am?
3. The levels were then checked and the theophylline level was reported as 4 mg/L. What loading dose of i.v. aminophylline would you recommend?

Answers

1. Mr BT's pharmacokinetic parameters can be calculated from population data:

$$\text{clearance} = 63\ \text{kg} \times 0.04\ \text{L/h/kg} = 2.52\ \text{L/h}$$

$$V_d = 63\ \text{kg} \times 0.45\ \text{L/kg} = 28.3\ \text{L}$$

$$k_e = \frac{CL}{V_d}$$

$$k_e = 0.089\ \text{h}^{-1}$$

Inserting this k_e value into Eq. (8) indicates that
The patient's half-life ($t_{1/2}$) = 7.8 hours.
It can therefore be assumed that Mr BT was at steady state after 48 hours of treatment (more than 5× half-life).

2. To calculate Mr BT's levels at 10 am, it is assumed that S.R. theophylline behaves like an i.v. infusion ($F = 1.0$). Although this is not strictly true, Nuelin S.A. has a good slow-release profile.
From Eq. (12):

$$\frac{S \times F \times \text{dose}}{T} = \text{average } C^{ss} \times CL$$

$$\text{average } C^{ss} = \frac{S \times F \times \text{dose}}{T \times CL}$$

$$\text{average } C^{ss} = \frac{500 \times 1}{12 \times 2.52}$$

$$\text{average } C^{ss} = 16.5\ \text{mg/L}$$

The morning dose from the previous day will have provided a steady dose of theophylline until the evening (first missed dose), the starting dose is C^{ss}. In order to calculate the theophylline concentration at 10am (C^{10am}) the dose will decay for 16 hours. Inserting this k_e value into Eq. (7) indicates that:

$$C_2 = C_1 \times e^{-k_e \times t}$$

$$C^{10\,am} = 16.5 \times e^{-k_e \times 16}$$

$$C^{10\,am} = 16.5 \times e^{-0.089 \times 16}$$

$$C^{10\,am} = 3.97\ \text{mg/L}$$

3. To calculate a loading dose, the change in theophylline concentration (C) to be achieved needs to be calculated:

$$C = \text{desired } C\ (15\ \text{mg/L}) - \text{actual}\ (4\ \text{mg/L})$$

From Eq. (1):

$$\text{loading dose} = C \times V_d$$

$$\text{loading dose} = 11 \times 28.3\ \text{L}$$

$$\text{loading dose} = 311\ \text{mg of theophylline}$$

Aminophylline is only 80% theophylline; therefore:

$$\text{loading dose} = \frac{311}{0.8}$$

Aminophylline loading dose is 390 mg to be administered by slow i.v. bolus. In practice the nearest practical loading dose of 400 mg by slow i.v. bolus would be administered.

Case 3.6

A 39-year-old woman (60 kg), Ms RM, has been taking phenytoin at a dose of 250 mg daily. At her last clinic visit topiramate was added to her regimen. Ms RM is seen in the hospital outpatient department complaining of blurred vision and exhibiting nystagmus. Her phenytoin level taken in clinic is 22 mg/L.
Ms RM's current medication is:

| Phenytoin capsules | 250 mg daily |
| Topiramate tablets | 200 mg daily in two divided doses |

Questions

1. Calculate V_{max} and K_m for this patient.
2. How long will it take for Ms RM's phenytoin level to fall within the therapeutic range if the current dose is stopped?
3. Using these parameters, calculate the new dose to achieve a level of 15 mg/L.
4. What is the most likely reason for Ms RM's phenytoin level to go out of range?

Answers

1. From population data V_{max} = 7 mg/kg/day × 60 kg = 420 mg/day. Substitute this into Eq. (15) using the measured C^{ss} of 22 mg/L and Ms RM's current dose of 250 mg/day and assuming S = 0.9, solve for K_m:

$$\frac{0.9 \times 250}{1} = \frac{420 \times 22}{K_m + 22}$$

$$K_m + 22 = \frac{420 \times 22}{0.9 \times 250}$$

$$= \frac{9240}{225}$$

$$K_m + 22 = 41$$

$$K_m = 19\ \text{mg/L}$$

2. At supra-therapeutic levels it can be assumed that metabolism is occurring at V_{max}. By dividing V_{max} (amount eliminated from the body per day) by V_d you can calculate the rate of fall of blood level. V_d from population data is 1 L/kg × 60 kg = 60 L. Therefore, the rate of fall in blood level is 420 mg/60 L/day = 7 mg/L/day. Therefore, withhold treatment for 1 day for the blood level to fall from 22 mg/L to 15 mg/L and recommence on new calculated dose.

3. Substitute these K_m and V_{max} values into Eq. (15) with a desired C^{ss} of 15 mg/L and assume S = 0.9.

$$\frac{0.9 \times \text{dose}}{1} = \frac{420 \times 15}{19 + 15}$$

$$= \frac{6300}{34}$$

$$0.9 \times \text{dose} = 185.3$$

$$\text{dose} = \frac{185.3}{0.9}$$

This gives a dose of 205.9 mg/day. This should be rounded down to 200 mg/day.

4. Interaction with topiramate which is known to increase phenytoin levels.

References

Bauer, L.A., 2008. Phenytoin in Applied Clinical Pharmacokinetics, second ed. McGraw-Hill, New York, pp. 485–548.

Cockcroft, D.W., Gault, M.H., 1976. Prediction of creatinine clearance from plasma creatinine. Nephron 16, 31–41.

Crist, K.D., Nahata, M.C., Ety, J., 1987. Positive impact of a therapeutic drug monitoring program on total aminoglycoside dose and hospitalisation. Ther. Drug Monit. 9, 306–310.

Department of Health, 2006. Estimated Glomerular Filtration Rate (eGFR). Department of Health Publications, London. Available at: http://webarc hive.nationalarchives.gov.uk/20130107105354/http://www.dh.gov.uk/en /Publicationsandstatistics/Publications/PublicationsPolicyAndGuidance/ DH_4133020.

Gjesdal, K., Feyzi, J., Olsson, S.B., 2008. Digitalis: a dangerous drug in atrial fibrillation? An analysis of the Sportif 111 and V data. Heart 94 (2), 191–196.

McFadyen, M.L., Miller, R., Juta, M., et al., 1990. The relevance of a first world therapeutic drug monitoring service to the treatment of epilepsy in third world conditions. South Afr. Med. J. 78, 587–590.

Nicolau, D.P., Freeman, C.D., Belliveau, P.P., et al., 1995. Experience with a once daily aminoglycoside program administered to 2,184 adult patients. Antimicrob. Agents Chemother. 39, 650–655.

Reid, L.D., Horn, J.R., McKenna, D.A., 1990. Therapeutic drug monitoring reduces toxic drug reactions: a meta-analysis. Ther. Drug Monit. 12, 72–78.

Touw, D.J., Neef, C., Thomson, A.H., et al., 2005. Cost-effectiveness of therapeutic drug monitoring: a systematic review. Ther. Drug Monit. 1, 7–10.

Further reading

Begg, E.J., Barclay, M.L., Duffull, S.B., 1995. A suggested approach to once daily aminoglycoside dosing. Br. J. Clin. Pharmacol. 39, 605–609.

Burton, M.E., Shaw, L.M., Schentag, J.J., 2006. Applied Pharmacokinetics and Pharmacodynamics: Principles of Therapeutic Drug Monitoring, fourth ed. Lippincott Williams & Wilkins, Baltimore.

Dhillon, S., Kostrzewski, A., 2006. Clinical Pharmacokinetics. Pharmaceutical Press, London.

Elwes, R.D.C., Binnie, C.D., 1996. Clinical pharmacokinetics of newer antiepileptic drugs. Clin. Pharmacokinet. 30, 403–415.

Jermain, D.M., Crismon, M.L., Martin, E.S., 1991. Population pharmacokinetics of lithium. Clin. Pharmacokinet. 10, 376–381.

Lemmer, B., Bruguerolle, B., 1994. Chronopharmacokinetics: are they clinically relevant? Clin. Pharmacokinet. 26, 419–427.

Luke, D.R., Halstenson, C.E., Opsahl, J.A., et al., 1990. Validity of creatinine clearance estimates in the assessment of renal function. Clin. Pharmacol. Ther. 48, 503–508.

Mahalati, K., Kahan, B.D., 2001. Clinical pharmacokinetics of sirolimus. Clin. Pharmacokinet. 40, 573–585.

Rambeck, B., Boenigk, H.E., Dunlop, A., et al., 1980. Predicting phenytoin dose: a revised nomogram. Ther. Drug Monit. 1, 325–354.

Ryback, M.J., 2006. The pharmacokinetic and pharmacodynamic properties of vancomycin. Clin. Infect. Dis. 42, S35–S39.

Tserng, K., King, K.C., Takieddine, F.N., 1981. Theophylline metabolism in premature infants. Clin. Pharmacol. Ther. 29, 594–600.

Winter, M.E., 2009. Basic Clinical Pharmacokinetics, fifth ed. Lippincott Williams & Wilkins, Baltimore.

Yukawa, E., 1996. Optimisation of antiepileptic drug therapy: the importance of plasma drug concentration monitoring. Clin. Pharmacokinet. 31, 120–130.

4

Drug Interactions

Ruben Thanacoody

Key points

- Drug interactions can cause significant patient harm and are an important cause of morbidity.
- Most clinically important drug interactions occur as a result of either decreased drug activity with diminished efficacy or increased drug activity with exaggerated or unusual effects. Drugs with a narrow therapeutic range, such as theophylline, lithium and digoxin, or a steep dose–response curve, such as anticoagulants, oral contraceptives and antiepileptics, are often implicated.
- The most important pharmacokinetic interactions involve drugs that can induce or inhibit enzymes in the hepatic cytochrome P450 system.
- Pharmacodynamic interactions are difficult to classify, but their effects can often be predicted when the pharmacology of co-administered drugs is known.
- In many cases potentially interacting drugs can be given concurrently, provided the possibility of interaction is kept in mind and any necessary changes to dose or therapy are initiated promptly. In some situations, however, concurrent use of potentially interacting drugs should be avoided altogether.
- Suspected adverse drug interactions should be reported to the appropriate regulatory authority as for other adverse drug reactions.

Drug interactions have been recognised for more than 100 years. Today, with the increasing availability of complex therapeutic agents and widespread polypharmacy, the potential for drug interactions is enormous, and they have become an increasingly important cause of adverse drug reactions (ADRs).

Despite regulatory requirements to define the safety profile of new medicines, including their potential for drug–drug interactions before marketing, the potential for adverse interactions is not always evident. This was illustrated by the worldwide withdrawal of the calcium channel blocker (CCB) mibefradil, within months of launch, following reports of serious drug interactions (Po and Zhang, 1998). Since the late 1990s, a number of medicines have either been withdrawn from the market (e.g. terfenadine, grepafloxacin and cisapride) or had their use restricted because of prolongation of the QT interval on the electrocardiogram (e.g. domperidone). Drug interactions are an important cause of QT

prolongation, which increases the risk of development of a life-threatening ventricular arrhythmia known as torsade de pointes (Roden, 2004).

The increasing availability and non-prescription use of herbal and complementary medicines has also led to greater awareness of their potential for adverse interactions. St John's wort, a herbal extract used for treatment of depression, can cause serious interactions as a result of its enzyme-inducing effects. Drug interactions with food and drink are also known to occur, exemplified by the well-known interaction between monoamine oxidase inhibitor (MAOI) antidepressants and tyramine-containing foodstuffs. Grapefruit juice is a potent inhibitor of cytochrome P450 (CYP450) 3A4 and causes clinically relevant interactions with a number of drugs, including simvastatin and atorvastatin, thereby increasing the risk of statin-induced adverse reactions such as myopathy and myositis.

Although medical literature is awash with drug interaction studies and case reports of adverse drug interactions, only a relatively small number of these are likely to cause clinically significant consequences for patients. The recognition of clinically significant interactions requires knowledge of the pharmacological mechanisms of drug interactions and a thorough understanding of high-risk drugs and vulnerable patient groups.

Definition

An interaction is said to occur when the effects of one drug are altered by the co-administration of another drug, herbal medicine, food, drink or other environmental chemical agents (Preston, 2016). The net effect of the combination may manifest as an additive or enhanced effect of one or more drugs, antagonism of the effect of one or more drugs, or any other alteration in the effect of one or more drugs.

Clinically significant interactions refer to a combination of therapeutic agents which have direct consequences on the patient's condition. Therapeutic benefit can be obtained from certain drug interactions; for example, a combination of different antihypertensive drugs may be used to improve blood pressure control, or an opioid antagonist may be used to reverse the effect of an overdose of morphine. This chapter concentrates on clinically significant interactions which have the potential for undesirable effects on patient care.

Epidemiology

Accurate estimates of the incidence of drug interactions are difficult to obtain because published studies frequently use different criteria for defining a drug interaction and for distinguishing between clinically significant and non-significant interactions.

The reported incidence of drug–drug interactions in hospital admissions ranged from 0% to 2.8% in a review which included nine studies, all of which had some design flaws (Jankel and Fitterman, 1993). In the Harvard Medical Practice Study of adverse events, 20% of events in acute hospital inpatients were drug related. Of these, 8% were considered to be due to a drug interaction, suggesting that interactions are responsible for less than 2% of adverse events in this patient group (Leape et al., 1992).

In a 1-year prospective study of patients attending an emergency department, 3.8% resulted from a drug–drug interaction, and most of these led to hospital admissions (Raschett et al., 1999). In a prospective UK study carried out on hospital inpatients ADRs were responsible for hospital admission in 6.5% of cases. Drug interactions were involved in 16.6% of adverse reactions, therefore being directly responsible for leading to hospital admission in approximately 1% of cases (Pirmohamed et al., 2004).

Few studies have attempted to quantify the incidence of drug–drug interactions in the outpatient hospital setting and in the community. In the early 1990s, a Swedish study investigated the occurrence of potential drug interactions in primary care and reported an incidence rate of 1.9% (Linnarsson, 1993). In the outpatient setting, the availability of newer drugs for a variety of chronic conditions has increased the risk of drug–drug interactions in this patient group.

Although the overall incidence of serious adverse drug interactions is low, it remains a potentially preventable cause of morbidity and mortality.

Susceptible patients

The risk of drug interactions increases with the number of drugs used. In a hospital study, the rate of ADRs in patients taking 6–10 drugs was 7%, rising to 40% in those taking 16–20 drugs, with the exponential rise being largely attributable to drug interactions (Smith et al., 1969). In a high-risk group of emergency department patients, the risk of potential adverse drug interaction was 13% in patients taking two drugs and 82% in those taking seven or more drugs (Goldberg et al., 1996).

Although polypharmacy is common and often unavoidable, it places certain patient groups at increased risk of drug interactions. Patients at particular risk include those with hepatic or renal disease, those on long-term therapy for chronic disease (e.g. HIV infection, epilepsy, diabetes), patients in intensive care, transplant recipients, patients undergoing complicated surgical procedures and those with more than one prescriber. Critically ill and elderly patients are at increased risk not only because they take more medicines but also because of impaired homeostatic mechanisms that might otherwise counteract some of the unwanted effects. Interactions may occur in some individuals, but not in others.

Box 4.1 Examples of drugs with high risk of interaction

Concentration-dependent toxicity
Digoxin
Lithium
Aminoglycosides
Cytotoxic agents
Warfarin

Steep dose–response curve
Verapamil
Sulfonylureas
Levodopa

Patient dependent on therapeutic effect
Immunosuppressives, e.g. ciclosporin and tacrolimus
Glucocorticoids
Oral contraceptives
Antiepileptics
Antiarrhythmics
Antipsychotics
Antiretrovirals

Saturable hepatic metabolism
Phenytoin
Theophylline

The effects of interactions involving drug metabolism may vary greatly in individual patients because of differences in the rates of drug metabolism and in susceptibility to microsomal enzyme induction. Certain drugs are frequently implicated in drug interactions and require careful attention (Box 4.1).

Mechanisms of drug interactions

Drug interactions are conventionally discussed according to the mechanisms involved. These mechanisms can be conveniently divided into those with a pharmacokinetic basis and those with a pharmacodynamic basis. Drug interactions often involve more than one mechanism. There are some situations where drugs interact by unique mechanisms, but the most common mechanisms are discussed in this section.

Pharmacokinetic interactions

Pharmacokinetic interactions are those that affect the processes by which drugs are absorbed, distributed, metabolised or excreted. Due to marked inter-individual variability in these processes, these interactions may be expected, but their extent cannot be easily predicted. Such interactions may result in a change in the drug concentration at the site of action with subsequent toxicity or decreased efficacy.

Absorption

Following oral administration, drugs are absorbed through the mucous membranes of the gastro-intestinal tract. A number of factors can affect the rate of absorption or the extent of absorption (i.e. the total amount of drug absorbed).

Changes in gastro-intestinal pH. The absorption of a drug across mucous membranes depends on the extent to which it exists in the non-ionised, lipid-soluble form. The ionisation state depends on the pH of its environment, the acid dissociation constant (pK_a) of the drug and formulation factors. Weakly acidic drugs, such as the salicylates, are better absorbed at low pH because the non-ionised form predominates.

An alteration in gastric pH due to antacids, histamine H_2 antagonists or proton pump inhibitors therefore has the potential to affect the absorption of other drugs. The clinical significance of antacid-induced changes in gastric pH is not certain, particularly because relatively little drug absorption occurs in the stomach. Changes in gastric pH tend to affect the rate of absorption rather than the extent of absorption, provided that the drug is acid labile. Although antacids could theoretically be expected to markedly influence the absorption of other drugs via this mechanism, in practice there are very few clinically significant examples. Antacids, histamine H_2 antagonists and proton pump inhibitors can significantly decrease the bioavailability of ketoconazole and itraconazole, which require gastric acidity for optimal absorption, but the absorption of fluconazole and voriconazole is not significantly altered by changes in gastric pH.

The alkalinising effects of antacids on the gastro-intestinal tract are transient, and the potential for interaction may be minimised by leaving an interval of 2–3 hours between the antacid and the potentially interacting drug.

Adsorption, chelation and other complexing mechanisms. Certain drugs react directly within the gastro-intestinal tract to form chelates and complexes which are not absorbed. The drugs most commonly implicated in this type of interaction include tetracyclines and the quinolone antibiotics that can complex with iron, and antacids containing calcium, magnesium and aluminium. Tetracyclines can chelate with divalent or trivalent metal cations such as calcium, aluminium, bismuth and iron to form insoluble complexes, resulting in greatly reduced plasma tetracycline concentrations.

Bisphosphonates are often co-prescribed with calcium supplements in the treatment of osteoporosis. If these are taken concomitantly, however, the bioavailability of both is significantly reduced, with the possibility of therapeutic failure.

The absorption of some drugs may be reduced if they are given with adsorbents such as charcoal or kaolin, or anionic exchange resins such as cholestyramine or colestipol. The absorption of paracetamol, digoxin, warfarin, calcitriol, thiazide diuretics, raloxifene and levothyroxine is reduced by cholestyramine.

Most chelation and adsorption interactions can be avoided if an interval of 2–3 hours is allowed between doses of the interacting drugs. For cholestyramine the advice is for the patient to take other drugs at least 1 hour before or 4–6 hours after cholestyramine to reduce possible issues with their absorption (Joint Formulary Commission, 2017).

Effects on gastro-intestinal motility. Because most drugs are largely absorbed in the upper part of the small intestine, drugs that alter the rate at which the stomach empties its contents can affect absorption. Drugs with anticholinergic effects, such as tricyclic antidepressants, phenothiazines and some antihistamines,

decrease gut motility and delay gastric emptying. The outcome of the reduced gut motility can be either an increase or a decrease in drugs given concomitantly. For example, tricyclic antidepressants can increase dicoumarol absorption, probably as a result of increasing the time available for its dissolution and absorption. Anticholinergic agents used in the management of movement disorders have been shown to reduce the bioavailability of levodopa by as much as 50%, possibly as a result of increased metabolism in the intestinal mucosa.

Opioids such as diamorphine and pethidine strongly inhibit gastric emptying and greatly reduce the absorption rate of paracetamol, without affecting the extent of absorption. Codeine, however, has no significant effect on paracetamol absorption. Metoclopramide increases gastric emptying and increases the absorption rate of paracetamol, an effect which is used to therapeutic advantage in the treatment of migraine to ensure rapid analgesic effect. Although metoclopramide also accelerates the absorption of propranolol, mefloquine, lithium and ciclosporin, this interaction is rarely clinically significant.

Induction or inhibition of drug transport proteins. The oral bioavailability of some drugs is limited by the action of drug transporter proteins, which eject drugs that have diffused across the gut lining back into the gut. At present, the most well-characterised drug transporter is P-glycoprotein. Digoxin is a substrate of P-glycoprotein, and drugs that inhibit P-glycoprotein, such as verapamil, may increase digoxin bioavailability with the potential for digoxin toxicity (DuBuske, 2005).

Malabsorption. Drugs such as neomycin may cause a malabsorption syndrome leading to reduced absorption of drugs such as digoxin. Orlistat is a specific long-acting inhibitor of gastric and pancreatic lipases, thereby preventing the hydrolysis of dietary fat to free fatty acids and triglycerides. This can theoretically lead to reduced absorption of fat-soluble drugs co-administered with orlistat. As a result, the Medicines and Healthcare products Regulatory Agency (MHRA, 2010) has advised of a possible impact on efficacy of co-administration of orlistat with levothyroxine, antiepileptic drugs such as valproate sodium and lamotrigine, and antiretroviral HIV drugs such as efavirenz and lopinavir.

Most of the interactions that occur within the gut result in reduced rather than increased absorption. It is important to recognise that the majority result in changes in absorption rate, although in some instances the total amount (i.e. extent of drug absorbed) is affected. For drugs that are given chronically on a multiple-dose regimen, the rate of absorption is usually unimportant provided the total amount of drug absorbed is not markedly altered. In contrast, delayed absorption can be clinically significant where the drug affected has a short half-life or where it is important to achieve high plasma concentrations rapidly, as may be the case with analgesics or hypnotics. Absorption interactions can often be avoided by allowing an interval of 2–3 hours between administrations of the interacting drugs.

Drug distribution

Following absorption, a drug undergoes distribution to various tissues, including to its site of action. Many drugs and their metabolites are highly bound to plasma proteins. Albumin is the main plasma protein to which acidic drugs such as warfarin are bound, whereas basic drugs such as tricyclic antidepressants, lidocaine, disopyramide and propranolol are generally bound to α_1-acid glycoprotein. During the process of distribution, drug interactions may occur, principally as a result of displacement from protein-binding sites. A drug displacement interaction is defined as a reduction in the extent of plasma protein binding of one drug caused by the presence of another drug, resulting in an increased free or unbound fraction of the displaced drug. Displacement from plasma proteins can be demonstrated in vitro for many drugs and has been thought to be an important mechanism underlying many interactions in the past. However, clinical pharmacokinetic studies suggest that, for most drugs, once displacement from plasma proteins occurs, the concentration of free drug rises temporarily, but falls rapidly back to its previous steady-state concentration due to metabolism and distribution. The time this takes will depend on the half-life of the displaced drug. The short-term rise in the free drug concentration is generally of little clinical significance but may need to be taken into account in therapeutic drug monitoring. For example, if a patient who is taking phenytoin is given a drug which displaces phenytoin from its binding sites, the total (i.e. free plus bound) plasma phenytoin concentration will fall even though the free (active) concentration remains the same.

There are few examples of clinically important interactions which are entirely due to protein-binding displacement. It has been postulated that a sustained change in steady-state free plasma concentration could arise with the parenteral administration of some drugs which are extensively bound to plasma proteins and non-restrictively cleared; that is, the efficiency of the eliminating organ is high. Lidocaine has been given as an example of a drug fitting these criteria.

Drug metabolism

Most clinically important interactions involve the effect of one drug on the metabolism of another. Metabolism refers to the process by which drugs and other compounds are biochemically modified to facilitate their degradation and subsequent removal from the body. The liver is the principal site of drug metabolism, although other organs such as the gut, kidneys, lung, skin and placenta are involved. Drug metabolism consists of phase I reactions such as oxidation, hydrolysis and reduction, and phase II reactions, which primarily involve conjugation of the drug with substances such as glucuronic acid and sulphuric acid. Phase I metabolism generally involves the CYP450 mixed function oxidase system. The liver is the major site of cytochrome 450-mediated metabolism, but the enterocytes in the small intestinal epithelium are also potentially important.

CYP450 isoenzymes. The CYP450 system comprises 57 isoenzymes, each derived from the expression of an individual gene. Because there are many different isoforms of these enzymes, a classification for nomenclature has been developed, comprising a family number, a subfamily letter, and a number for an individual enzyme within the subfamily (Wilkinson, 2005). Four main subfamilies of P450 isoenzymes are thought to be responsible for most (about 90%) of the metabolism of commonly used drugs in humans: CYP1, CYP2, CYP3 and CYP4. The most extensively studied isoenzyme is CYP2D6, also known as debrisoquine hydroxylase. Although there is overlap, each cytochrome 450 isoenzyme tends to metabolise a discrete range of substrates. Of the many isoenzymes, a few (CYP1A2, CYP2C9, CYP2C19, CYP2D6, CYP2E1 and CYP3A4) appear to be responsible for the human metabolism of most commonly used drugs.

The genes that encode specific cytochrome 450 isoenzymes can vary between individuals and, sometimes, ethnic groups. These variations (polymorphisms) may affect metabolism of substrate drugs. Interindividual variability in CYP2D6 activity is well recognised. It shows a polymodal distribution, and people may be described according to their ability to metabolise debrisoquine. Poor metabolisers tend to have reduced first-pass metabolism, increased plasma levels and exaggerated pharmacological response to this drug, resulting in postural hypotension. By contrast, ultra-rapid metabolisers may require considerably higher doses for a standard effect. About 5–10% of Caucasians and up to 2% of Asian and black people are poor metabolisers.

The CYP3A family of P450 enzymes comprises two isoenzymes, CYP3A4 and CYP3A5, so similar that they cannot be easily distinguished. CYP3A is probably the most important of all drug-metabolising enzymes because it is abundant in both the intestinal epithelium and the liver, and it has the ability to metabolise a multitude of chemically unrelated drugs from almost every drug class. It is likely that CYP3A is involved in the metabolism of more than half the therapeutic agents that undergo alteration by oxidation. In contrast with other cytochrome 450 enzymes, CYP3A shows continuous unimodal distribution, suggesting that genetic factors play a minor role in its regulation. Nevertheless, the activity of the enzyme can vary markedly among members of a given population.

The effect of a cytochrome 450 isoenzyme on a particular substrate can be altered by interaction with other drugs. Drugs may be themselves substrates for a cytochrome 450 isoenzyme and/or may inhibit or induce the isoenzyme. In most instances, oxidation of a particular drug is brought about by several CYP isoenzymes and results in the production of several metabolites. So, inhibition or induction of a single isoenzyme would have little effect on plasma levels of the drug. However, if a drug is metabolised primarily by a single cytochrome 450 isoenzyme, inhibition or induction of this enzyme would have a major effect on the plasma concentrations of the drug. For example, if erythromycin (an inhibitor of CYP3A4) is taken by a patient being given carbamazepine, which is extensively metabolised by CYP3A4, this may lead to toxicity caused by higher concentrations of carbamazepine. Table 4.1 gives examples of some drug substrates, inducers and inhibitors of the major cytochrome 450 isoenzymes.

Enzyme induction. The most powerful enzyme inducers in clinical use are the antibiotic rifampicin and antiepileptic agents such as barbiturates, phenytoin and carbamazepine. Some enzyme inducers, notably barbiturates and carbamazepine, can induce their own metabolism (auto-induction). Cigarette smoking, chronic alcohol use and the herbal preparation St John's wort can also induce drug-metabolising enzymes. Because the process of enzyme induction requires new protein synthesis, the effect usually develops over several days or weeks after starting an enzyme-inducing agent. Similarly, the effect generally persists for a similar period

Table 4.1 Examples of drug substrates, inducers and inhibitors of the major cytochrome P450 enzymes

P450 isoform	Substrate	Inducer	Inhibitor
CYP1A2	Caffeine Clozapine Imipramine Olanzapine Theophylline Tricyclic antidepressants R-warfarin	Omeprazole Lansoprazole Phenytoin Tobacco smoke	Amiodarone Cimetidine Quinolones Fluvoxamine
CYP2C9	Diazepam Diclofenac Losartan Statins Selective serotonin reuptake inhibitors S-warfarin	Barbiturates Rifampicin	Amiodarone Azole antifungals Isoniazid
CYP2C19	Cilostazol Diazepam Lansoprazole	Carbamazepine Rifampicin Omeprazole	Cimetidine Fluoxetine Tranylcypromine
CYP2D6	Amitriptyline Codeine Dihydrocodeine Flecainide Fluoxetine Haloperidol Imipramine Nortriptyline Olanzapine Ondansetron Opioids Paroxetine Propranolol Risperidone Tramadol Venlafaxine	Dexamethasone Rifampicin	Amiodarone Bupropion Celecoxib Duloxetine Fluoxetine Paroxetine Ritonavir Sertraline
CYP2E1	Enflurane Halothane	Alcohol (chronic) Isoniazid	Disulfiram
CYP3A4	Amiodarone Ciclosporin Corticosteroids Oral contraceptives Tacrolimus R-warfarin Calcium channel blockers Donepezil Benzodiazepines Cilostazol	Carbamazepine Phenytoin Barbiturates Dexamethasone Primidone Rifampicin St John's wort Bosentan Efavirenz Nevirapine	Cimetidine Clarithromycin Erythromycin Itraconazole Ketoconazole Grapefruit juice Aprepitant Diltiazem Protease inhibitors Imatinib Verapamil

following drug withdrawal. Enzyme-inducing drugs with short half-lives such as rifampicin will induce metabolism more rapidly than inducers with longer half-lives (e.g. phenytoin) because they reach steady-state concentrations more rapidly. There is evidence that the enzyme induction process is dose dependent, although some drugs may induce enzymes at any dose.

Enzyme induction usually results in a decreased pharmacological effect of the affected drug. St John's wort is now known to be a potent inducer of CYP3A (Mannel, 2004). Thus, when a patient receiving ciclosporin, tacrolimus, HIV-protease inhibitors, irinotecan or imatinib takes St John's wort, there is a risk of therapeutic failure with the affected drug. However, if the affected drug has active metabolites, this may lead to an increased pharmacological effect. The effects of enzyme induction vary considerably between patients and are dependent upon age, genetic factors, concurrent drug treatment and disease

Table 4.2 Examples of interactions due to enzyme induction

Drug affected	Inducing agent	Clinical outcome
Oral contraceptives	Rifampicin	Therapeutic failure of contraceptives
	Carbamazepine	Additional contraceptive precautions required
	Modafinil	Increased oestrogen dose required
Ciclosporin	Phenytoin Carbamazepine St John's wort	Decreased ciclosporin levels with possibility of transplant rejection
Paracetamol	Alcohol (chronic)	In overdose, hepatotoxicity may occur at lower doses
Corticosteroids	Phenytoin Rifampicin	Increased metabolism with possibility of therapeutic failure

Box 4.2 Examples of enzyme inhibitors frequently implicated in interactions

Antibacterials
Ciprofloxacin
Clarithromycin
Erythromycin
Isoniazid
Metronidazole

Antidepressants
Duloxetine
Fluoxetine
Fluvoxamine
Paroxetine
Sertraline

Antifungals
Fluconazole
Itraconazole
Ketoconazole
Miconazole
Voriconazole

Antivirals
Indinavir
Ritonavir
Saquinavir

Cardiovascular drugs
Amiodarone
Diltiazem
Quinidine
Verapamil

Gastro-intestinal drugs
Cimetidine
Esomeprazole
Omeprazole

Antirheumatic drugs
Allopurinol
Azapropazone

Other
Aprepitant
Bupropion
Disulfiram
Grapefruit juice
Imatinib
Sodium valproate

state. Some examples of interactions due to enzyme induction are shown in Table 4.2.

Enzyme inhibition. Enzyme inhibition is responsible for many clinically significant interactions. Many drugs act as inhibitors of cytochrome 450 enzymes (Box 4.2). A strong inhibitor is one that can cause ≥5-fold increase in the plasma area under the curve (AUC) value or more than 80% decrease in clearance of CYP3A substrates. A moderate inhibitor is one that can cause ≥2- but <5-fold increase in the AUC value or 50–80% decrease in clearance of sensitive CYP3A substrates when the inhibitor is given at the highest approved dose and the shortest dosing interval. A weak inhibitor is one that can cause ≥1.25- but <2-fold increase in the AUC values or 20–50% decrease in clearance of sensitive CYP3A substrates when the inhibitor is given at the highest approved dose and the shortest dosing interval.

Concurrent administration of an enzyme inhibitor leads to reduced metabolism of the drug and hence an increase in the steady-state drug concentration. Enzyme inhibition appears to be dose related. Inhibition of hepatic metabolism of the affected drug occurs when sufficient concentrations of the inhibitor are achieved in the liver, and the effects are usually maximal when the new steady-state plasma concentration is achieved. Thus, for drugs with a short half-life, the effects may be seen within a few days of administration of the inhibitor. Maximal effects may be delayed for drugs with a long half-life.

The clinical significance of this type of interaction depends on various factors, including dosage (of both drugs), alterations in pharmacokinetic properties of the affected drug, such as half-life, and patient characteristics such as disease state. Interactions of this type are again most likely to affect drugs with a narrow therapeutic range such as theophylline, ciclosporin, oral anticoagulants and phenytoin. For example, starting treatment with an enzyme inhibitor such as amiodarone in a patient who is taking warfarin could result in a marked

increase in warfarin plasma concentrations and increased bleeding risk. Some examples of interactions due to enzyme inhibition are shown in Table 4.3.

The isoenzyme CYP3A4 in particular is present in the enterocytes. Thus, after oral administration of a drug, cytochrome 450 enzymes in the intestine and the liver may reduce the portion of a dose that reaches the systemic circulation, that is, the bioavailability of the drug. Drug interactions resulting in inhibition or induction of enzymes in the intestinal epithelium can have significant consequences. For example, by selectively inhibiting CYP3A4 in the enterocyte, grapefruit juice can markedly increase the bioavailability of some oral CCBs, including felodipine (Wilkinson, 2005). Such an interaction is usually considered to be a drug

Table 4.3 Examples of interactions due to enzyme inhibition

Drug affected	Inhibiting agent	Clinical outcome
Anticoagulants (oral)	Clarithromycin Ciprofloxacin	Anticoagulant effect increased and risk of bleeding
Azathioprine	Allopurinol	Enhancement of effect with increased toxicity of azathioprine
Clopidogrel	Omeprazole	Reduced antiplatelet effect
Carbamazepine Phenytoin Sodium valproate	Cimetidine	Antiepileptic levels increased with risk of toxicity
Sildenafil	Ritonavir	Enhancement of sildenafil effect with risk of hypotension

metabolism interaction, even though the mechanism involves an alteration in drug absorption. A single glass of grapefruit juice can cause CYP3A inhibition for 24–48 hours, and regular consumption may continuously inhibit enzyme activity. Consumption of grapefruit juice is therefore not recommended in patients who are receiving drugs that are extensively metabolised by CYP3A, such as simvastatin, tacrolimus and vardenafil.

Enzyme inhibition usually results in an increased pharmacological effect of the affected drug, but in cases where the affected drug is a pro-drug which requires enzymatic metabolism to active metabolites, a reduced pharmacological effect may result. For example, clopidogrel is metabolised via CYP2C19 to an active metabolite which is responsible for its antiplatelet effect. Proton pump inhibitors such as omeprazole are inhibitors of CYP2C19 and may lead to reduced effectiveness of clopidogrel when used in combination.

Predicting interactions involving metabolism. Predicting drug interactions is not easy for many reasons. First, individual drugs within a therapeutic class may have different effects on an isoenzyme. For example, the quinolone antibiotics ciprofloxacin and norfloxacin inhibit CYP1A2 and have been reported to increase plasma theophylline levels, whereas moxifloxacin is a much weaker inhibitor and appears not to interact in this way. While atorvastatin and simvastatin are metabolised predominantly by the CYP3A4 enzyme, fluvastatin is metabolised by CYP2C9 and pravastatin is not metabolised by the CYP450 system to any significant extent.

Identification of CYP450 isoenzymes involved in drug metabolism using in vitro techniques is now an important step in the drug development process. However, findings of in vitro studies are not always replicated in vivo, and more detailed drug interaction studies may be required to allow early identification of potential interactions. Nevertheless, some interactions affect only a small proportion of individuals and may not be identified unless large numbers of volunteers or patients are studied.

Suspected drug interactions are often described initially in published case reports and are then subsequently evaluated in formal studies. For example, published case reports indicated that commonly used antibiotics such as amoxicillin may reduce the effect of oral contraceptives, although this interaction has not been demonstrated in formal studies, leading to a change in the advice provided to patients who take the oral contraceptive pill and non-enzyme-inducing antibiotics. Another factor complicating the understanding of metabolic drug interactions is the finding that there is a large overlap between the inhibitors/inducers and substrates of the drug transporter protein P-glycoprotein and those of CYP3A4. Therefore, both mechanisms may be involved in many of the drug interactions previously thought to be due to effects on CYP3A4.

Elimination interactions

Most drugs are excreted in either the bile or urine. Blood entering the kidneys is delivered to the glomeruli of the tubules where molecules small enough to pass across the pores of the glomerular membrane are filtered through into the lumen of the tubules. Larger molecules, such as plasma proteins and blood cells, are retained. The blood then flows to other parts of the kidney tubules where drugs and their metabolites are removed, secreted or reabsorbed into the tubular filtrate by active and passive transport systems. Interactions can occur when drugs interfere with kidney tubule fluid pH, active transport systems or blood flow to the kidney, thereby altering the excretion of other drugs.

Changes in urinary pH. As with drug absorption in the gut, passive reabsorption of drugs depends on the extent to which the drug exists in the non-ionised lipid-soluble form. Only the non-ionised form is lipid soluble and able to diffuse back through the tubular cell membrane. Thus, at alkaline pH, weakly acidic drugs (pK_a 3.0–7.5) largely exist as ionised lipid-insoluble molecules which are unable to diffuse into the tubule cells and will therefore be lost in the urine. The renal clearance of these drugs is increased if the urine is made more alkaline. Conversely, the clearance of weak bases (pK_a 7.5–10) is higher in acid urine. Strong acids and bases are virtually completely ionised over the physiological range of urinary pH, and their clearance is unaffected by pH changes.

This mechanism of interaction is of very minor clinical significance because most weak acids and bases are inactivated by hepatic metabolism rather than renal excretion. Furthermore, drugs that produce large changes in urine pH are rarely used clinically. Urine alkalinisation or acidification has been used as a means of increasing drug elimination in poisoning with salicylates and amphetamines, respectively.

Changes in active renal tubule excretion. Drugs that use the same active transport system in the kidney tubules can compete with one another for excretion. Such competition between drugs can be used to therapeutic advantage. For example, probenecid may be given to increase the plasma concentration of penicillins by delaying renal excretion. With the increasing understanding of drug transporter proteins in the kidneys, it is now known that probenecid inhibits the renal secretion of many other anionic drugs via organic anion transporters (Lee and Kim, 2004). Increased methotrexate toxicity, sometimes life-threatening, has been seen in some patients concurrently treated with salicylates and some other non-steroidal anti-inflammatory drugs (NSAIDs). The development of toxicity is more likely in patients treated with high-dose methotrexate and those with impaired renal function. The mechanism of this interaction may be multifactorial, but competitive inhibition of methotrexate's renal tubular secretion is likely to be involved. If patients who are taking methotrexate are given salicylates or NSAIDs concomitantly, the dose of methotrexate should be closely monitored.

Changes in renal blood flow. Blood flow through the kidney is partially controlled by the production of renal vasodilatory prostaglandins. If the synthesis of these prostaglandins is inhibited by drugs such as indometacin, the renal excretion of lithium is reduced with a subsequent rise in plasma levels. The mechanism underlying this interaction is not entirely clear, because plasma lithium levels are unaffected by other potent prostaglandin synthetase inhibitors, for example, aspirin. If an NSAID is prescribed for a patient who is taking lithium, then the plasma levels should be closely monitored.

Biliary excretion and the enterohepatic shunt. A number of drugs are excreted in the bile, either unchanged or conjugated, for example, as the glucuronide, to make them more water soluble. Some of the conjugates are metabolised to the parent compound by the gut flora and are then reabsorbed. This recycling process prolongs the stay of the drug within the body, but if the gut flora are diminished by the presence of an antibacterial, the drug is not recycled and is lost more quickly. This mechanism has been postulated as the basis of an interaction between broad-spectrum antibiotics and oral contraceptives. Antibiotics may reduce the enterohepatic circulation of ethinylestradiol conjugates, leading to reduced circulating oestrogen levels with the potential for therapeutic failure. There is considerable debate about the nature of this interaction because the evidence from pharmacokinetic studies is not convincing. Until a few years ago, due to the potential adverse consequences of pill failure, most authorities recommended a conservative approach, including the use of additional contraceptive precautions. This advice has now been changed to recommend that additional contraceptive precautions are not required for short-term use of antibiotics which do not induce liver enzymes (Joint Formulary Commission, 2017).

Drug transporter proteins. Drugs and endogenous substances are now known to cross biological membranes not just by passive diffusion but by carrier-mediated processes, often known as transporters. Significant advances in the identification of various transporters have been made and although their contribution to drug interactions is not yet clear, they are now thought to play a role in many interactions formerly attributed to cytochrome 450 enzymes (DuBuske, 2005).

P-glycoprotein is a large cell membrane protein that is responsible for the transport of many substrates, including drugs. It is a product of the *ABCB1* gene (previously known as the multidrug resistance gene, *MDR1*) and a member of the adenosine triphosphate (ATP)–binding cassette family of transport proteins (ABC transporters). P-glycoprotein is found in high levels in various tissues, including the renal proximal tubule, hepatocytes, intestinal mucosa, the pancreas and the blood–brain barrier.

Table 4.4 Examples of inhibitors and inducers of P-glycoprotein

Inhibitors	Atorvastatin
	Ciclosporin
	Clarithromycin
	Dipyridamole
	Erythromycin
	Itraconazole
	Ketoconazole
	Propafenone
	Quinidine
	Ritonavir
	Verapamil
Inducers	Rifampicin
	St John's wort

P-glycoprotein acts as an efflux pump, exporting substances into urine, bile and the intestinal lumen. Its activity in the blood–brain barrier limits drug accumulation in the central nervous system (CNS). Examples of some possible inhibitors and inducers of P-glycoprotein are listed in Table 4.4. The pumping actions of P-glycoprotein can be induced or inhibited by some drugs. For example, concomitant administration of digoxin and verapamil, a P-glycoprotein inhibitor, is associated with increased digoxin levels with the potential for digoxin toxicity. An overlap exists between CYP3A4 and P-glycoprotein inhibitors, inducers and substrates. Many drugs that are substrates for CYP3A4 are also substrates for P-glycoprotein. Therefore, both mechanisms may be involved in many of the drug interactions initially thought to be due to changes in CYP3A4. Digoxin is an example of the few drugs that are substrates for P-glycoprotein, but not CYP3A4.

Pharmacodynamic interactions

Pharmacodynamic interactions are those where the effects of one drug are changed by the presence of another drug at its site of action. Sometimes these interactions involve competition for specific receptor sites, but often they are indirect and involve interference with physiological systems. They are much more difficult to classify than interactions with a pharmacokinetic basis.

Antagonistic interactions

It is to be expected that a drug with an agonist action at a particular receptor type will interact with antagonists at that receptor. For example, the bronchodilator action of a selective β_2-adrenoreceptor agonist such as salbutamol will be antagonised by β-adrenoreceptor antagonists. There are numerous examples of interactions occurring at receptor sites, many of which are used to therapeutic advantage. Specific antagonists may be used to reverse the effect of another drug at receptor sites; examples include the opioid antagonist naloxone and the benzodiazepine antagonist flumazenil. α-Adrenergic agonists such as metaraminol may be used in the management of priapism induced by α-adrenergic antagonists such as phentolamine. There are many other examples of drug classes that

Table 4.5 Examples of additive or synergistic interactions

Interacting drugs	Pharmacological effect
Non-steroidal anti-inflammatory drugs, warfarin, clopidogrel	Increased risk of bleeding
Angiotensin-converting enzyme inhibitors and K$^+$-sparing diuretic	Increased risk of hyperkalaemia
Verapamil and β-adrenergic antagonists	Bradycardia and asystole
Neuromuscular blockers and aminoglycosides	Increased neuromuscular blockade
Alcohol and benzodiazepines	Increased sedation
Pimozide and sotalol	Increased risk of QT interval prolongation
Clozapine and co-trimoxazole	Increased risk of bone marrow suppression

have opposing pharmacological actions, such as anticoagulants and vitamin K and levodopa and dopamine antagonist antipsychotics.

Additive or synergistic interactions

If two drugs with similar pharmacological effects are given together, the effects can be additive (Table 4.5). Although not strictly drug interactions, the mechanism frequently contributes to ADRs. For example, the concurrent use of drugs with CNS-depressant effects such as antidepressants, hypnotics, antiepileptics and antihistamines may lead to excessive drowsiness, yet such combinations are frequently encountered. Combinations of drugs with arrhythmogenic potential such as antiarrhythmics, neuroleptics, tricyclic antidepressants and those producing electrolyte imbalance (e.g. diuretics) may lead to ventricular arrhythmias and should be avoided. Another example which has assumed greater importance of late is the risk of ventricular tachycardia and torsade de pointes associated with the concurrent use of more than one drug with the potential to prolong the QT interval on the electrocardiogram (Roden, 2004).

Serotonin syndrome

Serotonin syndrome (SS) is associated with an excess of serotonin that results from therapeutic drug use, overdose or inadvertent interactions between drugs. Although severe cases are uncommon, it is becoming increasingly well recognised in patients receiving combinations of serotonergic drugs (Boyer and Shannon, 2005). It can occur when two or more drugs affecting serotonin are given at the same time, or after one serotonergic drug is stopped and another started. The syndrome is characterised by symptoms including confusion, disorientation, abnormal movements, exaggerated reflexes, fever, sweating, diarrhoea and hypotension or hypertension. Diagnosis is made when three or more of these symptoms are present and no other cause can be found. Symptoms usually develop within hours of starting the second drug, but occasionally they can occur later. Drug-induced SS is generally mild and resolves when the offending drugs are stopped. Severe cases occur infrequently and fatalities have been reported.

SS is best prevented by avoiding the use of combinations of several serotonergic drugs. Special care is needed when changing from a selective serotonin reuptake inhibitor (SSRI) to an MAOI and vice versa. The SSRIs, particularly fluoxetine, have long half-lives, and SS may occur if a sufficient washout period is not allowed before switching from one to the other. When patients are being switched between these two groups of drugs, the guidance in manufacturers' Summaries of Product Characteristics should be followed. Many drugs have serotonergic activity as their secondary pharmacology, and their potential for causing the SS may not be readily recognised. For example, linezolid, an antibacterial with monoamine oxidase inhibitory activity, has been implicated in several case reports of SS.

Many recreational drugs such as amphetamines and cocaine have serotonin agonist activity, and SS may ensue following the use of other serotonergic drugs.

Drug or neurotransmitter uptake interactions

Although seldom prescribed nowadays, the MAOIs have significant potential for interactions with other drugs and foods. MAOIs reduce the breakdown of noradrenaline in the adrenergic nerve ending. Large stores of noradrenaline can then be released into the synaptic cleft in response to either a neuronal discharge or an indirectly acting amine. The action of the directly acting amines adrenaline, isoprenaline and noradrenaline appears to be only moderately increased in patients who are taking MAOIs. In contrast, the concurrent use of MAOIs and indirectly acting sympathomimetic amines such as amphetamines, tyramine, MDMA (ecstasy), phenylpropanolamine and pseudoephedrine can result in a potentially fatal hypertensive crisis. Some of these compounds are contained in proprietary cough and cold remedies. Tyramine, contained in some foods (e.g. cheese and red wine), is normally metabolised in the gut wall by monoamine oxidase to inactive metabolites. In patients who are taking MAOI, however, tyramine will be absorbed intact. If patients who are taking MAOIs also take these amines, there may be a massive release of noradrenaline from adrenergic nerve endings, causing a sympathetic overactivity syndrome, characterised by hypertension, headache, excitement, hyperpyrexia and cardiac arrhythmias. Fatal intracranial haemorrhage and cardiac arrest may result. The risk of interactions continues for several weeks after the MAOI is stopped because new monoamine oxidase enzyme must be synthesised. Patients who are taking irreversible MAOIs should not take any indirectly acting sympathomimetic amines. All patients must be strongly warned about the risks of cough and cold remedies, illicit drug use and the necessary dietary restrictions.

Drug–food interactions

It is well established that food can cause clinically important changes in drug absorption through effects on gastro-intestinal absorption or motility, hence the advice that certain drugs should not be taken with food, for example, iron tablets and antibiotics. Two other common examples already outlined include the interaction between tyramine in some foods and MAOIs, and the interaction between grapefruit juice and CCBs. With improved understanding of drug metabolism mechanisms, there is greater recognition of the effects of some foods on drug metabolism. The interaction between grapefruit juice and felodipine was discovered serendipitously when grapefruit juice was chosen to mask the taste of ethanol in a study of the effect of ethanol on felodipine. Grapefruit juice mainly inhibits intestinal CYP3A4, with only minimal effects on hepatic CYP3A4. This is demonstrated by the fact that intravenous preparations of drugs metabolised by CYP3A4 are not much affected, whereas oral preparations of the same drugs are. Some drugs that are not metabolised by CYP3A4, such as fexofenadine, show decreased levels with grapefruit juice. The probable reason for this is that grapefruit juice inhibits some drug transporter proteins and possibly affects organic anion-transporting polypeptides, although inhibition of P-glycoprotein has also been suggested. The active constituent of grapefruit juice is uncertain. Grapefruit contains naringin, which degrades during processing to naringenin, a substance known to inhibit CYP3A4. Although this led to the assumption that whole grapefruit will not interact, but that processed grapefruit juice will, some reports have implicated the whole fruit. Other possible active constituents in the whole fruit include bergamottin and dihydroxybergamottin.

Initial reports of an interaction between cranberry juice and warfarin, prompting regulatory advice that the international normalised ratio (INR) should be closely monitored in patients taking this combination, have not been confirmed by subsequent controlled studies.

Cruciferous vegetables, such as Brussels sprouts, cabbage and broccoli, contain substances that are inducers of the CYP450 isoenzyme CYP1A2. Chemicals formed by burning (e.g. barbecuing) meats additionally have these properties. These foods do not appear to cause any clinically important drug interactions in their own right, but their consumption may add another variable to drug interaction studies, thus complicating interpretation.

Drug–herb interactions

There has been a marked increase in the availability and use of herbal products in the UK, which include Chinese herbal medicines and Ayurvedic medicines. Up to 24% of hospital patients report using herbal remedies (Constable et al., 2007). Such products often contain pharmacologically active ingredients which can give rise to clinically significant interactions when used inadvertently with other conventional drugs.

Extracts of *Glycyrrhizin glabra* (liquorice) used for treating digestive disorders may cause significant interactions in patients who are taking digoxin or diuretics. It may exacerbate hypokalaemia induced by diuretic drugs and precipitate digoxin toxicity. Herbal products such as Chinese ginseng (*Panax ginseng*), Chan Su (containing bufalin) and Danshen may also contain digoxin-like compounds which can interfere with digoxin assays, leading to falsely elevated levels being detected.

A number of herbal products have antiplatelet and anticoagulant properties and may increase the risk of bleeding when used with aspirin or warfarin. Herbal extracts containing coumarin-like constituents include alfalfa (*Medicago sativa*), angelica (*Angelica archangelica*), dong quai (*Angelica polymorpha, A. dahurica, A. atropurpurea*), chamomile, horse chestnut and red clover (*Trifolium pratense*), which can potentially lead to interactions with warfarin. Herbal products with antiplatelet properties include borage (*Borago officinalis*), bromelain (*Ananas comosus*), capsicum, feverfew, garlic, ginkgo (*Ginkgo biloba*) and turmeric, amongst others.

Other examples of drug–herb interactions include enhancement of hypoglycaemic (e.g. Asian ginseng) and hypotensive (e.g. hawthorn) effects, and lowering of seizure threshold (e.g. evening primrose oil and *Shankhapushpi*). The most widely discussed drug–herb interactions are those involving St John's wort (*Hypericum* extract), an unlicensed herbal medicine used for depression which has been implicated in interactions, for example, with hormonal contraceptives including implants, ciclosporin and antiepileptic drugs. It is therefore imperative that patients are specifically asked about their use of herbal medicines because they may not volunteer this information.

Conclusion

Whilst one should acknowledge the impossibility of memorising all potential drug interactions, healthcare staff need to be alert to the possibility of drug interactions and take appropriate steps to minimise their occurrence. Drug formularies and the Summary of Product Characteristics provide useful information about interactions. Other resources that may also be of use to prescribers include drug safety updates from regulators such as the Medicines and Healthcare products Regulatory Agency (available at https://www.gov.uk/drug-safety-update), interaction alerts in prescribing software and the availability of websites which highlight interactions for specific drug classes, for example, HIV drugs (http://www.hiv-druginteractions.org).

Possible interventions to avoid or minimise the risk of a drug interaction include:

1. switching one of the potential interacting drugs;
2. allowing an interval of 2–3 hours between administration of the interacting drugs;
3. altering the dose of one of the interacting drugs, for example, reducing the dose of the drug which is likely to have an enhanced effect as a result of the interaction. In this case, the dose is generally reduced by one-third or half with subsequent monitoring for toxic effects either clinically or by therapeutic drug monitoring. Conversely, if the drug is likely to have reduced effects as a result of the interaction, the patient should be monitored similarly for therapeutic failure and the dose increased if necessary;
4. advising patients to seek guidance about their medication if they plan to stop smoking or start a herbal medicine, because they may need close monitoring during the transition.

Overall, it is important to anticipate when a potential drug interaction might have clinically significant consequences for the patient. In these situations, advice should be given on how to minimise the risk of harm, for example, by recommending an alternative treatment to avoid the combination of risk, by making a dose adjustment or by monitoring the patient closely.

Case studies

Case 4.1

Mrs C is a 72-year-old woman with a history of hypertension, atrial fibrillation and hyperlipidaemia. Her current medication comprises digoxin 62.5 micrograms daily, warfarin as per INR, simvastatin 40 mg daily and amlodipine 10 mg daily. Mrs C is suffering from a respiratory tract infection and her primary care doctor has prescribed a 7-day course of clarithromycin.

Questions

1. Are there likely to be any clinically significant drug interactions?
2. What advice do you give?

Answers

1. There is potential for interaction between simvastatin and amlodipine, between simvastatin and clarithromycin and between clarithromycin and warfarin. Some statins, particularly simvastatin and atorvastatin, are metabolised by CYP450 (CYP3A4), and co-administration of potent inhibitors of this enzyme may increase plasma levels of these statins and so increase the risk of dose-related side effects, including rhabdomyolysis. Clarithromycin is a potent CYP450 enzyme inhibitor and can also inhibit the metabolism of warfarin, leading to over-anticoagulation.
2. Current advice is that amlodipine and simvastatin may be given together provided the simvastatin dose does not exceed 20 mg daily, so it is reasonable for simvastatin to be continued at a reduced dose of 20 mg. However, clarithromycin should not be given together with simvastatin. Myopathy and rhabdomyolysis have been reported in patients who are taking the combination. Mrs C should therefore be advised not to take her simvastatin while she is taking clarithromycin and to start taking it again after she has completed the course of antibiotic. During the course of clarithromycin, the daily dose of warfarin may need to be reduced; more frequent monitoring of the INR is suggested.

Case 4.2

A 19-year-old woman, Miss P, is receiving long-term treatment with minocycline 100 mg daily for acne. She wishes to start using the combined oral contraceptive, and her doctor has prescribed a low-strength pill (containing ethinylestradiol 20 micrograms with norethisterone 1 mg). The doctor contacts the pharmacist for advice on whether the tetracycline will interfere with the efficacy of the oral contraceptive.

Question

Is there a clinically significant interaction in this situation?

Answer

Contraceptive failure has been attributed to doxycycline, lymecycline, oxytetracycline, minocycline and tetracycline in about 40 reported cases, 7 of which specified long-term antibacterial use. There is controversy about whether a drug interaction occurs, but if there is one it appears to be rare. Controlled trials have not shown any effect of tetracycline or doxycycline on contraceptive steroid levels. The postulated mechanism is suppression of intestinal bacteria resulting in a fall in enterohepatic recirculation of ethinylestradiol. Overall, there is no evidence that this is clinically important.

In the case of long-term use of tetracyclines for acne, a small number of cases of contraceptive failure have been reported. Nevertheless, the only well-designed, case–control study in dermatological practice indicated that the incidence of contraceptive failure due to this interaction could not be distinguished from the general and recognised failure rate of oral contraceptives. Current guidance advises that women who are receiving long-term antibiotic therapy that does not induce liver enzymes do not need to take additional contraceptive precautions (Joint Formulary Commission, 2017). In addition, there is some evidence that ethinylestradiol may accentuate the facial pigmentation that can be caused by minocycline.

Case 4.3

A 48-year-old man, Mr H, with a history of epilepsy is admitted to hospital with tremor, ataxia, headache, abnormal thinking and increased partial seizure activity. His prescribed medicines are phenytoin 300 mg daily, clonazepam 6 mg daily and fluoxetine 20 mg daily. It transpires that fluoxetine therapy had been initiated 2 weeks previously. Mr H's phenytoin level is found to be 35 mg/L; at the last outpatient clinic visit 4 months ago, it was 18 mg/L.

Question

What is the proposed mechanism of interaction between fluoxetine and phenytoin and how should it be managed?

Answer

Fluoxetine is believed to inhibit the metabolism of phenytoin by the CYP450 isoenzyme CYP2C9, potentially leading to increased plasma phenytoin levels. There are a number of published case reports and anecdotal observations of phenytoin toxicity occurring with the combination, but the available evidence is conflicting. A review by the US Food and Drug Administration suggested that a marked increase in plasma phenytoin levels, with accompanying toxicity, can occur within 1–42 days (mean onset time of 2 weeks) after starting fluoxetine. If fluoxetine is added to treatment with phenytoin, the patient should be closely monitored. Ideally the phenytoin plasma levels should be monitored and there may be a need to reduce the phenytoin dosage.

Case 4.4

A 79-year-old man, Mr G, presented to hospital with a 3-day history of increasing confusion and collapse. He had a history of chronic lumbosacral pain, treated with oxycodone 10 mg twice daily and amitriptyline 75 mg daily. Five days before hospital admission Mr G had been prescribed tramadol 100 mg four times daily for worsening sciatica. On admission Mr G had a Glasgow Coma Scale score of 11 and he was delirious and hallucinating. There were no focal neurological signs. Over the next 2 days he became increasingly unwell, confused and sweaty with pyrexia and muscular rigidity. Biochemical tests showed a metabolic acidosis (base deficit of 10.7) and an elevated creatine kinase level of 380 IU/L. There was no evidence of infection. At this stage a diagnosis of probable serotonin syndrome (SS) was made.

Questions

1. What is SS, and what drugs are most commonly associated with it?
2. How is SS managed?

Answers

1. SS is often described as a clinical triad of mental status changes, autonomic hyperactivity and neuromuscular abnormalities. However, not all these features are consistently present in all patients with the disorder. Symptoms arising from a serotonin excess range from diarrhoea and tremor in mild cases to delirium, neuromuscular rigidity, rhabdomyolysis and hyperthermia in life-threatening cases. Disturbance of electrolytes, transaminases and creatinine kinase may occur. Clonus is the most important finding in establishing the diagnosis of SS. The differential diagnosis includes neuroleptic malignant syndrome, sepsis, hepatic encephalopathy, heat stroke, delirium tremens and anticholinergic reactions. SS may not be recognised in some cases because of its protean manifestations. A wide range of drugs and drug combinations has been associated with SS, including MAOIs, tricyclic antidepressants, SSRIs, opioids, linezolid and serotonin receptor (5HT$_1$) agonists. Tramadol is an atypical opioid analgesic with partial μ antagonism and central reuptake inhibition of serotonin (5HT) and noradrenaline. At high doses it may also induce serotonin release. Tramadol is reported as causing SS alone (in a few case reports) and in combination with SSRIs, venlafaxine and atypical antipsychotics.
2. Management of SS involves removal of the precipitating drugs and supportive care. Many cases typically resolve within 24 hours after serotonergic drugs are stopped, but symptoms may persist in patients who are taking medicines with long half-lives or active metabolites. The 5HT$_{2A}$-antagonist cyproheptadine and atypical antipsychotic agents with 5HT$_{2A}$-antagonist activity, such as olanzapine, have been used to treat SS, although their efficacy has not been conclusively established.

Case 4.5

A 42-year-old woman, Mr M, is receiving long-term treatment with azathioprine 100 mg daily and bendroflumethiazide 2.5 mg daily. The latter was discontinued after an episode of gout, but she had three further episodes over the following year. Her doctor considers prescribing allopurinol as prophylaxis.

Question

Is this likely to cause a clinically significant interaction?

Answer

Azathioprine is metabolised in the liver to mercaptopurine and then converted to an inactive metabolite by the enzyme xanthine oxidase. Allopurinol is an inhibitor of xanthine oxidase and will lead to the accumulation of mercaptopurine, which can cause bone marrow

suppression and haematological abnormalities such as neutropenia and thrombocytopenia.

The dose of azathioprine should be reduced by at least 50%, and close haematological monitoring is required if allopurinol is used concomitantly.

Case 4.6

A 68-year-old woman, Mrs T, is receiving long-term treatment with lansoprazole for gastro-oesophageal reflux disease and warfarin for atrial fibrillation. She is admitted with haematemesis. On direct questioning, Mrs T also revealed that she takes various herbal medicines which contain chamomile, horse chestnut, garlic, feverfew, ginseng and St John's wort.

Question

What drug–herb interactions may have contributed to Mrs T's presentation to hospital?

Answer

Garlic, feverfew and ginseng all inhibit platelet aggregation by inhibiting the production or release of prostaglandins and thromboxanes. In addition, chamomile and horse chestnut contain coumarin-like constituents which can potentiate the anticoagulant effect of warfarin. St John's wort is a potent enzyme inducer and may induce the metabolism of lansoprazole via CYP2C19, thereby reducing the effectiveness of lansoprazole. Although the effects of herbs individually may be small, their combined effects may lead to serious complications.

Case 4.7

A 56-year-old man, Mr W, with ischaemic heart disease seeks advice whether he can use sildenafil for erectile dysfunction. Mr W takes aspirin, bisoprolol, isosorbide mononitrate and atorvastatin.

Question

What advice do you give?

Answer

Sildenafil is a selective inhibitor of cyclic guanosine monophosphate (cGMP)–specific phosphodiesterase-5 inhibitor which can interact with nitrates to cause increases in cGMP leading to marked hypotension. Patients using nitrates should be advised not to use sildenafil.

Case 4.8

A 68-year-old man, Mr P, with a history of atrial fibrillation is admitted with left-sided weakness and computed tomography (CT) scan of his head showed a large intracerebral haematoma. Mr P takes dabigatran etexilate for stroke thromboprophylaxis. He was recently started on verapamil for heart rate control.

Question

What is the mechanism of action for the interaction between dabigatran and verapamil? How can the effect of the interaction be minimised?

Answer

Dabigatran etexilate is an oral direct thrombin inhibitor with potent anticoagulant effects. The pro-drug dabigatran etexilate is a P-glycoprotein substrate, but the active metabolite dabigatran is not. Verapamil is a P-glycoprotein inhibitor and leads to increased intestinal absorption of dabigatran etexilate leading to increased plasma concentrations of dabigatran. In healthy volunteers, verapamil administered 1 hour before dosing with dabigatran etexilate caused increased plasma concentrations of dabigatran etexilate, but not when given 2 hours before. The combination of verapamil and dabigatran should be used with caution, but the interaction may be minimised by dosing verapamil at least 2–3 hours before dabigatran etexilate.

References

Boyer, E.W., Shannon, M., 2005. Current concepts: the serotonin syndrome. N. Engl. J. Med. 352, 1112–1120.

Constable, S., Ham, A., Pirmohamed, M., 2007. Herbal medicines and acute medical emergency admissions to hospital. Br. J. Clin. Pharmacol. 63, 247–248.

DuBuske, L.M., 2005. The role of P-glycoprotein and organic anion-transporting polypeptides in drug interactions. Drug Saf. 28, 789–801.

Goldberg, R.M., Mabee, J., Chan, L., et al., 1996. Drug–drug and drug–disease interactions in the ED: analysis of a high-risk population. Am. J. Emerg. Med. 14, 447–450.

Jankel, C.A., Fitterman, L.K., 1993. Epidemiology of drug–drug interactions as a cause of hospital admissions. Drug Saf. 9, 55–59.

Joint Formulary Committee, 2017. British National Formulary (online). BMJ Group and Pharmaceutical Press, London. Available at http://www.medicinescomplete.com.

Leape, L.L., Brennan, T.A., Laird, N., et al., 1992. The nature of adverse events in hospitalised patients: results of the Harvard Medical Practice Study II. N. Engl. J. Med. 324, 377–384.

Lee, W., Kim, R.B., 2004. Transporters and renal drug elimination. Annu. Rev. Pharmacol. Toxicol. 44, 137–166.

Linnarsson, R., 1993. Drug interactions in primary health care. A retrospective database study and its implications for the design of a computerized decision support system. Scand. J. Prim. Health Care 11, 181–186.

Mannel, M., 2004. Drug interactions with St John's Wort: mechanisms and clinical implications. Drug Saf. 27, 773–797.

Medicines and Healthcare products Regulatory Agency (MHRA), 2010. Orlistat safety update. Drug Saf. Update 3 (7), 4.

Pirmohamed, M., James, S., Meakin, S., et al., 2004. Adverse drug reactions as cause of admission to hospital: prospective analysis of 18820 patients. Br. Med. J. 329, 15–19.

Po, A.L., Zhang, W.Y., 1998. What lessons can be learnt from withdrawal of mibefradil from the market? Lancet 351, 1829–1830.

Preston, C.L., 2016. Stockley's Drug Interactions, eleventh ed. Pharmaceutical Press, London.

Raschett, R., Morgutti, M., Mennitti-Ippolito, F., et al., 1999. Suspected adverse drug events requiring emergency department visits or hospital admissions. Eur. J. Clin. Pharmacol. 54, 959–963.

Roden, D.M., 2004. Drug-induced prolongation of the QT interval. N. Engl. J. Med. 350, 1013–1022.

Smith, J.W., Seidl, L.G., Cluff, L.E., 1969. Studies on the epidemiology of adverse drug reactions v. clinical factors influencing susceptibility. Ann. Intern. Med. 65, 629.

Wilkinson, G.R., 2005. Drug therapy: drug metabolism and variability among patients in drug response. N. Engl. J. Med. 352, 2211–2221.

Further reading

Preston, C.L. (Ed.), 2016. Stockley's Drug Interactions, eleventh ed. Pharmaceutical Press, London.

5 Adverse Drug Reactions

Janet Krska and Anthony R. Cox

Key points

- An adverse drug reaction is an unintended and noxious response occurring after the use of a drug, which is suspected to be associated with the drug.
- Adverse drug reactions can be classified as type A, which are most common and related to the drug's pharmacological effect, or type B, which are rare and unpredictable, although other classes of reaction can be identified.
- Few adverse reactions are identified during pre-marketing studies; therefore, pharmacovigilance systems to detect new adverse drug reactions are essential.
- Spontaneous reporting schemes are a common method of pharmacovigilance. These depend primarily on health professionals, but patients are encouraged to report suspected adverse reactions themselves in many countries.
- Adverse drug reactions are a significant cause of morbidity and mortality, are responsible for approximately 1 in 20 hospital admissions and are a considerable financial burden on health systems.
- Predisposing factors for adverse drug reactions include age, sex, ethnicity, genetic factors, comorbidities and concomitant medication.
- Many adverse drug reactions may be preventable through rational prescribing and careful monitoring of drug therapy.
- Health professionals need to be able to identify and assess adverse drug reactions and play a major role in preventing their occurrence.
- Patients want to receive information about potential side effects of medicines; therefore, communicating the risks of using medicines is an important skill for health professionals.

Introduction

All medicines with the ability to produce a desired therapeutic effect also have the potential to cause unwanted adverse effects. Health professionals should have an awareness of the following: the burden that adverse drug reactions (ADRs) place on health services and the public, the skills to identify and reduce the risk of ADRs in the patients they care for, and the duty they have to participate in post-marketing surveillance of medicines to improve medication safety.

Risks associated with medicinal substances are documented throughout history. For example, William Withering's 1785 account of digitalis provides a meticulous description of the adverse effects of digitalis toxicity. However, the thalidomide disaster and subsequent political pressure created the modern regulatory environment for medicines. Thalidomide was first marketed by the German company Chemie Grünenthal in 1957 and distributed in the UK by Distillers Ltd., whose chief medical advisor stated, 'If all the details of this are true, then it is a most remarkable drug. In short, it is impossible to give a toxic dose' (Brynner and Stephens, 2001). Despite an absence of supporting evidence, in 1958 thalidomide was recommended for use in pregnant and nursing mothers. An Australian doctor, Jim McBride, and a German doctor, Widukind Lenz, independently associated thalidomide exposure with serious birth defects, and thalidomide was withdrawn in December 1961. Thalidomide left behind between 8000 and 12,000 deformed children and an unknown number of deaths in utero. Many still live with this legacy.

The 1970s saw another unexpected and serious adverse reaction. The cardio-selective β-adrenergic receptor blocker practolol, launched in June 1970, was initially associated with rashes, some of which were severe. A case series of psoriasis-like rashes linked to dry eyes, including irreversible scarring of the cornea, led other doctors to report eye damage, including corneal ulceration and blindness, to regulators. Cases of sclerosing peritonitis, a bowel condition associated with significant mortality, were also reported. Practolol had remained on the market for 4 years; more than 100,000 people had been treated and hundreds were seriously affected.

Some adverse effects can be more difficult to differentiate from background events occurring commonly in the population. The cyclo-oxygenase-2 selective non-steroidal anti-inflammatory drugs (NSAIDs) celecoxib (introduced in 1998) and rofecoxib (introduced in 1999) were marketed on the basis of reduced gastro-intestinal ADRs in comparison with other non-selective NSAIDs. Apparent excesses of cardiovascular events with these drugs, which were noted during clinical trials and in elderly patient groups, were ascribed to the supposed cardioprotective effects of comparator drugs. However, in September 2004 a randomised controlled trial of rofecoxib in the prevention of colorectal cancer showed the drug to be associated with a significantly increased risk of cardiovascular events (Bresalier et al., 2005). Celecoxib was also associated with a dose-related increased risk of cardiovascular events in clinical trials. Rofecoxib was voluntarily withdrawn from the market. Further research has provided evidence of thrombotic risk with non-selective NSAIDs, in particular diclofenac. This risk appears to extend to all NSAID users, irrespective of baseline cardiovascular risk.

Reports by healthcare professionals to regulatory authorities are a major source of evidence for the majority of drug withdrawals. A total of 19 drugs were withdrawn from the market in the European Union (EU) between 2002 and 2011, most frequently because of cardiovascular problems, but also due to liver problems and neurological or psychiatric disorders (McNaughton et al., 2014). Worldwide 462 medicinal products were withdrawn from the market between 1953 and 2013, with the most common reason being hepatotoxicity. Withdrawal was less frequent in Africa compared with the rest of the world.

Not all drug safety issues are related to real effects. In 1998 a widely publicised paper by Andrew Wakefield and co-authors, later retracted, which alleged a link between measles mumps and rubella (MMR) vaccine and autism led to a crisis in parental confidence in the vaccine. This had a detrimental effect on vaccination rates, resulting in frequent outbreaks of measles and mumps, despite epidemiological and virological studies showing no link between MMR vaccine and autism. The MMR vaccine controversy illustrates how media reporting of drug safety information can influence patients' views of medicines and can cause significant harm. Poor presentation of drug safety issues in the media often creates anxiety in patients about medicines that they may be using, regardless of their benefits. As an example, the complexity of the debate on the benefits and risks of statins in the literature, when viewed through the prism of media reporting, has led to public concerns about their use in the secondary prevention of cardiovascular disease.

Assessing the safety of drugs

When drugs are newly introduced to the market, their safety profile is inevitably provisional. Although efficacy and evidence of safety must be demonstrated for regulatory authorities to permit marketing, it is not possible to discover the complete safety profile of a new drug prior to its launch. Pre-marketing clinical trials involve on average 2500 patients, with perhaps a hundred patients using the drug for longer than a year. Therefore, pre-marketing trials do not have the power to detect important reactions that occur at rates of 1 in 10,000, or fewer, drug exposures. Often only pharmacologically predictable ADRs with short onset times are identified in clinical trials, nor can relatively short trials detect ADRs which occur a long time after drug exposure. For drugs subject to an accelerated assessment process under early access schemes for unmet clinical needs, there may be a further reduction in pre-marketing safety information.

Additionally, patients within trials are often relatively healthy, without the multiple disease states, multiple risk factors or complex drug histories of patients in whom the drug will be used. Furthermore the patient's perspective is also frequently excluded from safety assessment in clinical trials, with ADRs being assessed only by the clinicians who run them (Basch, 2010). Up to 60% of drugs may also experience dose reductions following marketing (Heerdink et al., 2002). For these reasons, rare and potentially serious adverse effects often remain undetected until a wider population is exposed to the drug. The vigilance of health professionals is an essential factor in discovering these new risks, together with regulatory authorities that continuously monitor reports of adverse effects throughout the lifetime of a marketed medicinal product. For so-called orphan drugs and those which are little used, careful monitoring is essential.

As a result of this monitoring, the safety profile of well-established drugs is often well-known, although new risks are occasionally identified. However, an important part of the therapeutic management of medical conditions is the minimisation of these well-known risks. This can best be achieved through rational prescribing, recording of previous ADRs and careful monitoring of drug therapy, and the involvement of patients, who need to be well-informed about the risks of drugs. Much evidence suggests that all of these could be improved.

Definitions

Having clear definitions of what constitutes an ADR is important. The World Health Organization's (WHO's) original definition of an ADR was 'a response to a drug that is noxious and unintended and occurs at doses normally used in man for the prophylaxis, diagnosis or therapy of disease, or for modification of physiological function' (WHO, 1972, p. 9). The use of the phrase 'at doses normally used in man' distinguishes the noxious effects of drugs during normal medical use from toxic effects caused by poisoning. Whether an effect is considered noxious depends on both the drug's beneficial effects and the severity of the disease for which it is being used. There is no need to prove a pharmacological mechanism for any noxious response to be termed an ADR. More recently, the EU definition of an ADR has been expanded to take into account off-label use, overdose, misuse, abuse and medication errors.

The EU definition of adverse reaction is (European Medicines Evaluation Agency [EMEA], 2014, p. 8):

A response to a medicinal product which is noxious and unintended.
[...]
Adverse reactions may arise from use of the product within or outside the terms of the marketing authorisation or from occupational exposure. Use outside the marketing authorisation includes off-label use, overdose, misuse, abuse and medication errors.

The terms *adverse drug reaction* (ADR) and *adverse drug effect* can be used interchangeably; adverse reaction applies to the patient's point of view, whereas adverse effect applies to the drug. The terms *suspected ADR* or *reportable ADR* are commonly used in the context of reporting ADRs to regulatory authorities, for example, through the UK's Yellow Card Scheme, operated by the Medicines and Healthcare products Regulatory Authority (MHRA). Although the terms *side effect* and *ADR* are often used synonymously, the term *side effect* is distinct from an ADR. A side effect is an unintended effect of a drug related to its pharmacological properties and can include unexpected benefits of treatment.

It is important also to avoid confusion with the term *adverse drug event* (ADE). An ADR is an adverse outcome in a patient that is attributed to a suspected action of a drug, whereas an ADE is an adverse outcome in a patient, which occurs after the use of a drug, but which may or may not be linked to use of the drug. It therefore follows that all ADRs are ADEs, but that not all ADEs will be ADRs. This distinction is important in the assessment of the drug safety literature, because the term *ADE* can be used when a causal link between a drug treatment and an adverse outcome has not been proven. The suspicion of a causal relationship between the drug and the adverse effect is central to the definition of an ADR.

Classification of adverse drug reactions

Classification systems for ADRs are useful for educational purposes, for those working within a regulatory environment and for clarifying thinking on the avoidance and management of ADRs.

Rawlins–Thompson classification

The Rawlins–Thompson system of classification divides ADRs into two main groups: type A and type B (Rawlins, 1981). Type A reactions are the normal, but quantitatively exaggerated, pharmacological effects of a drug. They include the primary effect of the drug, as well as any secondary effects of the drug, for example,

ADRs caused by the antimuscarinic activity of tricyclic antidepressants. Type A reactions are the most common, accounting for 80% of reactions.

Type B reactions are qualitatively abnormal effects, which appear unrelated to the drug's normal pharmacology, such as hepatoxicity from isoniazid. They are more serious in nature, more likely to cause deaths and are often not discovered until after a drug has been marketed. The Rawlins–Thompson classification has undergone further elaboration over the years (Table 5.1), to take account of ADRs that do not fit within the existing classifications (Edwards and Aronson, 2000).

The DoTS system

The DoTS classification is based on *do*se relatedness, *t*iming and patient *s*usceptibility (Aronson and Ferner, 2003). In contrast with the Rawlins–Thompson classification, which is defined only by the properties of the drug and the reaction, the DoTS classification provides a useful template to examine the various factors that both describe a reaction and influence an individual patient's susceptibility.

The DoTS system first considers the dose of the drug, because many adverse effects are clearly related to the dose of the drug used. For example, increasing the dose of a cardiac glycoside will increase the risk of digitalis toxicity. In the DoTS system reactions are divided into toxic effects (effects related to the use of drugs outside of their usual therapeutic dosage), collateral effects (effects occurring within the normal therapeutic use of the drug) and hypersusceptibility reactions (reactions occurring

Table 5.1 Extended Rawlins–Thompson classification of adverse drug reactions

Type of reaction	Features	Examples
Type A: augmented pharmacological effect	Common Predictable effect Dose dependent High morbidity Low mortality	Bradycardia associated with a β-adrenergic receptor antagonist
Type B: bizarre effects not related to pharmacological effect	Uncommon Unpredictable Not dose dependent Low morbidity High mortality	Anaphylaxis associated with a penicillin antibiotic
Type C: dose-related and time-related	Uncommon Related to the cumulative dose	Hypothalamic-pituitary-adrenal axis suppression by corticosteroids
Type D: time-related	Uncommon Usually dose-related Occurs or becomes apparent sometime after use of the drug	Carcinogenesis
Type E: withdrawal	Uncommon Occurs soon after withdrawal of the drug	Opiate withdrawal syndrome
Type F: unexpected failure of therapy	Common Dose-related Often caused by drug interactions	Failure of oral contraceptive in presence of enzyme inducer

in subtherapeutic doses in susceptible patients). Collateral effects include reactions not related to the expected pharmacological effect of the drug or off-target reactions of the expected therapeutic effect in other body systems. It is worth noting that approximately 20% of newly marketed drugs have their dosage recommendations reduced after marketing, often because of drug toxicity.

The time course of a drug's presence at the site of action can influence the likelihood of an ADR occurring. For example, rapid infusion of furosemide is associated with transient hearing loss and tinnitus, and a constant low dose of methotrexate is more toxic than equivalent intermittent bolus doses. The DoTS system categorises ADRs as either time-independent or time-dependent reactions. Time-independent reactions occur at any time within the treatment period, regardless of the length of course. Time-dependent reactions range from rapid and immediate reactions following exposure to reactions that are delayed.

The final aspect of the DoTS classification system is susceptibility, which includes factors such as genetic predisposition, age, sex, altered physiology, disease and exogenous factors such as drug interactions (Table 5.2).

Factors that affect susceptibility to adverse drug reactions

Awareness among prescribers of the factors that increase the risk of ADRs is key to reducing the burden on individual patients, and such awareness should inform all prescribing decisions. The risk that drugs pose to patients varies dependent on the population exposed and the individual characteristics of patients. Some reactions may be unseen in some populations, outside of susceptible subjects. Other reactions may follow a continuous distribution in the exposed population. Although many susceptibilities may not be known, a number of general factors that affect susceptibility to ADRs and others that affect the propensity of specific drugs to cause ADRs are well-known.

Age

Children differ from adults in their response to drugs. Neonatal differences in body composition, metabolism and other physiological parameters can increase the risk of specific adverse reactions. Higher body water content can increase the volume of distribution for water-soluble drugs, reduced albumin and total protein may result in higher concentrations of highly protein bound drugs, while an immature blood–brain barrier can increase sensitivity to drugs such as morphine. Differences in drug metabolism and elimination and end-organ responses can also increase the risk. Chloramphenicol, digoxin and ototoxic antibiotics such as streptomycin are examples of drugs that have a higher risk of toxicity in the first weeks of life.

Older children and young adults may also be more susceptible to ADRs, a classic example being the increased risk of extrapyramidal effects associated with metoclopramide. The use of aspirin was restricted in those younger than 12 years after an association with Reye's syndrome was found in epidemiological studies. Additionally, children can be exposed to more adverse effects because of the heightened probability of dosing errors and the relative lack of evidence for both safety and efficacy.

Elderly patients may be more prone to ADRs, with age-related decline in both the metabolism and elimination of drugs from the body. They also have multiple comorbidities and are therefore exposed to more prescribed drugs. Chronological age is therefore arguably a marker for altered physiological responses to drugs and for the presence of comorbidities and associated drug use rather than a risk per se. However, with an increasingly ageing population in many countries, the mitigation of preventable ADRs in older people is of great importance.

Comorbidities and concomitant medicines use

Reductions in hepatic and renal function substantially increase the risk of ADRs, because most drugs are metabolised in the liver, renally excreted or both. Factors that predict repeat admissions

Table 5.2 DoTS system of adverse drug reaction classification

Dose relatedness	Time relatedness	Susceptibility
Toxic effects: ADRs that occur at doses higher than the usual therapeutic dose	Time-independent reactions: ADRs that occur at any time during treatment	Raised susceptibility may be present in some individuals, but not others. Alternatively, susceptibility may follow a continuous distribution—increasing susceptibility with impaired renal function. Factors include genetic variation, age, sex, altered physiology, exogenous factors (interactions) and disease.
Collateral effects: ADRs that occur at standard therapeutic doses	Time-dependent reactions: *Rapid reactions* occur when a drug is administered too rapidly.	
Hypersusceptibility reactions: ADRs that occur at subtherapeutic doses in susceptible patients	*Early reactions* occur early in treatment, then abate with continuing treatment (tolerance). *Intermediate reactions* occur after some delay, but if reaction does not occur after a certain time little or no risk exists. *Late reactions,* risk of an ADR increases with continued-to-repeated exposure, including withdrawal reactions. *Delayed reactions* occur sometime after exposure, even if the drug is withdrawn before the ADR occurs.	

ADR, Adverse drug reaction.

to hospital with ADRs in older patients are comorbidities such as congestive heart failure, diabetes, and peripheral vascular, chronic pulmonary, rheumatological, hepatic, renal and malignant diseases. All are strong predictors of readmissions for ADRs, whereas advancing age alone is not. Reasons for this could be pharmacokinetic and pharmacodynamic changes associated with pulmonary, cardiovascular, renal and hepatic insufficiency, or drug interactions from prescribed multiple drug therapy (Zhang et al., 2009). Multiple medicine use, or polypharmacy, is strongly associated with increasing risk of both interactions and ADRs, and it is important to recognise that polypharmacy is not just a feature of ageing. Prescribed medicines use is increasing dramatically, with one study showing that the proportion of adults dispensed five or more drugs was almost 21% in 2010 (Guthrie et al., 2015).

Sex

Women may be more susceptible to ADRs, but they also receive more drugs than men. In addition, there are particular adverse reactions that appear to be more common in women. For example, impairment of concentration and psychiatric adverse events associated with the antimalarial mefloquine are more common in females.

Females are more susceptible to drug-induced torsade de pointes, a ventricular arrhythmia linked to ventricular fibrillation and death. Women are overrepresented in reports of torsades de pointes associated with cardiovascular drugs (such as sotalol) and erythromycin. This increased susceptibility in women is thought to be due to their longer QTc interval compared with men.

Ethnicity

Ethnicity has also been linked to susceptibility to ADRs, because of inherited traits of metabolism. It is known, for example, that the cytochrome P450 genotype, involved in drug metabolism, has varied distribution among people of differing ethnicity. For example, CYP2C9 alleles associated with poor metabolism occur more frequently in white individuals compared with black individuals. This has a potential effect on warfarin metabolism and increases the risk of toxicity.

Examples of ADRs linked to ethnicity include the increased risk of angioedema with the use of angiotensin-converting enzyme inhibitors in black patients (McDowell et al., 2006), the increased propensity of white and black patients to experience central nervous system ADRs associated with mefloquine compared with patients of Chinese or Japanese origin and differences in the pharmacokinetics of rosuvastatin in Asian patients, which may expose them to an increased risk of myopathy. However, susceptibility based on ethnicity could be associated with genetic or cultural factors, and ethnicity can be argued to be a poor marker for a patient's genotype.

Pharmacogenetics

Pharmacogenetics, the study of genetic variations that influence individuals' responses to drugs, examines polymorphisms that code for drug transporters, drug-metabolising enzymes and drug receptors. A greater understanding of the genetic basis of variations in individual responses to drug therapy is beginning to deliver

a new era of precision or stratified medicine. Although pharmacogenetics has yet to reach its full potential to reduce ADRs, there are now significant examples of severe ADRs that may be avoided with knowledge of a patient's genetic susceptibility.

As already noted, major genetic variation is found in the cytochrome CYP450 group of isoenzymes. This can result in either inadequate responses to drugs or increased risk of ADRs. Clinically relevant genetic variation has been seen in CYP2D6, CYP2C9, CYP2C19 and CYP3A5. A large effect on the metabolism of drugs can occur with CYP2C9, which accounts for 20% of total hepatic CYP450 content.

The narrow therapeutic index of warfarin, its high interindividual variability in dosing and the serious consequences of toxicity have made it a major target of pharmacogenomics research. Studies of genetic polymorphisms influencing the toxicity of warfarin have focused on CYP2C9, which metabolises warfarin, and vitamin K epoxide reductase (VKOR), the target of warfarin anticoagulant activity. Genetic variation in the *VKORC1* gene, which encodes VKOR, influences warfarin dosing by a threefold greater extent than CYP2C9 variants. In 2007 the US Food and Drug Administration (FDA) changed the labeling requirement for warfarin, advising that a lower initial dose should be considered in people with certain genetic variations. However, concerns exist that genetic variations account for only a proportion of the variability in drug response and that clinicians may obtain a false sense of reassurance from genetic testing, leading to complacency in monitoring of therapy. In addition, there appears to be little evidence of additional benefit, in terms of preventing major bleeding events, compared with careful monitoring of the INR (Laurence, 2009).

A success story for pharmacogenetics is the story of abacavir. Hypersensitivity skin reactions to this nucleoside analogue reverse transcriptase inhibitor are a particular problem in the treatment of human immunodeficiency virus (HIV) infection. Approximately 5–8% of patients who are taking abacavir develop a severe hypersensitivity reaction, including symptoms such as fever, rash, arthralgia, headache, vomiting, and other gastrointestinal and respiratory disturbances. Early reports that only a subset of patients was affected, a suspected familial predisposition, the short onset time (within 6 weeks of starting therapy) and an apparent lower incidence in African patients led to suspicion of a genetic cause. Subsequent research revealed a strong predictive association with the HLA-*B5701 allele in Caucasian and Hispanic patients. The presence of the allele can be used to stratify the predicted risk of hypersensitivity as high risk (>70%) for carriers of HLA-*B570 and low risk (<1%) for non-carriers of HLA-*B5701. Evidence from practical use of HLA-*B5701 screening has shown substantial declines in the incidence of hypersensitivity reactions, as well as a more general improved compliance with the medication (Lucas et al., 2007).

Another example involves the cutaneous ADRs, Stevens–Johnson syndrome (SJS) and toxic epidermal necrolysis (TEN), which are serious reactions associated with substantial morbidity and mortality. Forty percent of patients with TEN will die during an episode. SJS and TEN have been associated with numerous drugs, although the incidence of such reactions is rare. Antiepileptic drugs, such as carbamazepine and phenytoin, are known causes of SJS and TEN. Such reactions are more common in South East Asian populations (including those from China,

Thailand, Malaysia, Indonesia, the Philippines and Taiwan, and to a lesser extent, India and Japan). The presence of human leukocyte antigen (HLA) allele, HLA-B*1502, for which genetic testing is already available, indicates an increased risk of skin reactions for carbamazepine, phenytoin, oxcarbazepine and lamotrigine. The FDA has recommended HLA-B*1502 screening before using carbamazepine in South East Asian individuals (FDA, 2007).

Erythrocyte glucose-6-phophatase dehydrogenase deficiency

Glucose-6-phophatase dehydrogenase (G6PD) deficiency is present in more than 400 million people worldwide. It is an X-linked inherited enzyme deficiency, leading to susceptibility to haemolytic anaemia. There are many variants of the genotype, with most G6PD-deficient patients remaining asymptomatic until an oxidative stress is placed upon them. Oxidant drugs such as primaquine, sulfonamides and nitrofurantoin can act as provoking agents (Cappellini and Fiorelli, 2008).

Porphyrias

The porphyrias are a heterogeneous group of mainly autosomal dominant inherited disorders of haem biosynthesis, leading to excess porphyrin production. Patients with acute porphyrias may have life-threatening attacks precipitated by commonly prescribed drugs.

A number of drugs may induce excess porphyrin synthesis, but there is wide variation in the response, and in the dose required, between individual patients. Lists of drugs that are known to be unsafe and drugs which are thought to be safe for use in acute porphyria are available in the British National Formulary.

Table 5.3 Classification of immunological (hypersensitivity) reactions

Classification	Mechanism	Symptoms/signs and examples
Type I (immediate)	Drug/IgE complex binds to mast cells which release histamine and leukotrienes	Pruritus, urticaria, bronchoconstriction, angioedema, hypotension, shock, e.g. penicillin anaphylaxis
Type II (cytotoxic)	IgG and complement binding to (usually) red blood cell Cytotoxic T cells lyse the cell	Haemolytic anaemia and thrombocytopaenia, e.g. associated with cephalosporins, penicillins and rifampicin
Type III (immune complex)	Drug antigen and IgG or IgM form immune complex, attracting macrophages and complement activation	Cutaneous vasculitis, serum sickness, e.g. associated with chlorpromazine and sulfonamides
Type IV (delayed type)	Antigen presentation with major histocompatibility complex protein to T cells and cytokine and inflammatory mediator release	Usually occur after 7–20 days; macular rashes and organ failure, including Stevens–Johnson syndrome and toxic epidermal necrolysis, e.g. associated with neomycin, sulfonamides

Ig, Immunoglobulin.

Immunological reactions

The immune system is able to recognise drugs as foreign substances, leading to allergic reactions. Smaller drug molecules (<600 Da) can bind with proteins to trigger an immune response, or larger molecules can trigger an immune response directly. The immune response is not related to the pharmacological action of the drug and prior exposure to the drug is required. Immunological reactions are often distinct recognisable responses.

Allergic reactions range from rashes, serum sickness and angioedema to the life-threatening bronchospasm and hypotension associated with anaphylaxis. Patients with a history of atopic or allergic disorders are at higher risk. Immunological (hypersensitivity) reactions are split into four main types (Table 5.3).

Formulation issues that contribute to adverse drug reactions

Although ADRs caused by formulation problems are rare in developed countries with stringent regulation, examples have occurred and regulatory authorities remain vigilant for such problems. In 1937 the S. E. Massengill Company, in the USA, developed a liquid preparation of an early antibiotic sulfanilamide which contained 72% diethylene glycol. Over a 4-week period 353 patients received the elixir, 30% of whom died, including 34 children. Sadly, episodes of diethylene glycol poisoning have been reported in contemporary times in a number of countries including Nigeria, India, Argentina and Haiti. In 2006 cough medicines made using glycerine contaminated with diethylene glycol, sourced from China, were responsible for the suspected deaths of more than 300 people in Panama.

Osmosin was a slow-release preparation of Indometacin using a novel osmotic pump to deliver the drug through a laser-drilled hole in an impervious tablet. Osmosin was withdrawn in 1983 after 36 fatal gastro-intestinal haemorrhages were suspected to be caused by the tablet becoming lodged against the mucosa of the gastro-intestinal tract.

Adverse reactions have been associated with excipient changes. In Australia and New Zealand a decision to change the formulation of phenytoin to one in which calcium sulphate dihydrate was replaced with lactose led to previously stable patients developing severe adverse reactions, including coma. This unfortunate result was because the calcium salt had slowed phenytoin absorption, whereas the lactose in the new formulation increased absorption.

Although excipients are often referred to as inert substances, serious adverse reactions such as anaphylaxis and angioedema have been reported to these substances. Sweeteners, flavourings, colouring agents/dyes and preservatives have been all been associated with adverse reactions (Kumar, 2003). In many countries, generic prescribing is increasing, which results in patients receiving differing formulations of medicines made by different manufacturers, who may use different excipients. It is important to recognise that this can mean that patients experience a reaction to one brand of medicine and not to another, and not to dismiss such reports.

Epidemiology of adverse drug reactions

ADRs are an important public health issue. In Sweden ADRs are suggested to be responsible for 3% of deaths (Wester et al., 2008), whereas in England ADRs were shown to occur in 0.4% of all patients admitted to hospital, with mortality being higher in those experiencing an ADR than in those who did not (Davies et al., 2009). The median length of stay in patients who experience an ADR is 20 days, compared with 8 days, and costs associated with in-patient ADRs were calculated at £171 million annually for the NHS in England (Davies et al., 2009). Costs to the NHS associated with admissions due to ADRs have been estimated as £466 million annually (Pirmohamed et al., 2004).

A systematic review of European studies found the median percentage of hospital admissions due to an ADR to be 3.5% (range 0.5–12.8%), based on 22 studies, and the proportion experiencing an ADR during hospitalisation as 10.1% (range 1.7–50.9%), based on 13 studies (Bouvy et al., 2015). An observational study of more than 6000 paediatric admissions found 2.9% of admissions were associated with ADRs (Gallagher et al., 2012).

In primary care, estimates of the incidence of ADRs are more difficult to obtain, and very few well-designed studies are to be found. Prevalence rates of approximately 7% have been found in two Swedish studies using medical records and self-report (Hakkarainen et al., 2013a, 2013b), while other studies which rely on patients' reports of ADRs, either to postal questionnaires or telephone surveys, provide estimates of around 25% in the USA (Gandhi et al., 2003) and 30% in the UK (Jarernsiripornkul et al., 2002). These higher figures relate to the methodologies used and are hampered by the lack of information about non-responders. A systematic review in 2007 found an incidence of overall ADEs, including ADRs, of 14.9 per 1000 person-months in primary care settings (Thomsen et al., 2007).

Pharmacovigilance and epidemiological methods in adverse drug reaction detection

As already noted, the inherent weaknesses of pre-marketing studies mean that post-marketing surveillance of medicines is

essential to detect previously unrecognised adverse effects. This surveillance is termed *pharmacovigilance*, which is defined as 'science and activities relating to the detection, assessment, understanding and prevention of adverse effects or any other medicine-related problem' (WHO, 2002, p. 7). Pharmacovigilance supports health professionals to make rational and safe therapeutic decisions in clinical practice. Pharmacovigilance also helps to ensure that unsafe products are withdrawn from the market. However, despite the increasing importance placed on this and improvements worldwide in the systems for detecting ADRs, the time between an ADR first being reported and the date of withdrawal has not changed in 60 years, taking approximately 6 years (Onakpoya et al., 2016).

Spontaneous reporting

Pharmacovigilance uses multiple methods, but this chapter will mainly cover spontaneous reporting systems. Spontaneous reporting systems collect data about suspected ADRs in a central database. Cases are not collected in a systematic manner, but accumulate through reports submitted spontaneously by people who make a connection between a drug and a suspected drug-induced event. In the UK, the spontaneous reporting scheme is the Yellow Card Scheme. In some countries reporting is a voluntary activity; in others reporting is a legal requirement, but there is no evidence that this increases reporting rates.

Spontaneous reporting has a number of advantages. It is relatively cheap to administer, can follow a product throughout its life and can cover all products on the market, including over-the-counter and herbal products, as well as products obtained via the Internet or by illicit means. Such schemes are, however, passive surveillance systems, which rely on the ability of the reporters to recognise possible ADRs and to distinguish these from symptoms related to the underlying disease. It is important to emphasise that only a suspicion of a causal link between a drug and an adverse event is required; confirmation of the association is not required. One disadvantage of spontaneous reporting systems is their inability to quantify any particular risk associated with an individual drug. The number of reports are known, but estimates of the incidence of reactions cannot be made, because the population exposed to the drug cannot be ascertained accurately. Furthermore, only a minority of reactions are reported. Spontaneous reports are, however, an important form of evidence leading to drug withdrawals and are crucial for generating hypotheses about potential associations between a drug and an adverse event, which can then be investigated further.

Signal detection

A signal is described as a possible causal relationship between an adverse event and a drug which was previously unknown. Using statistical approaches, run automatically by computer systems, databases of spontaneous reports are scanned for 'drug-adverse event pairs' that are disproportionately present within the database as a whole. These mathematical approaches do help to develop hypotheses, but they are not conclusive evidence of an ADR in themselves. A signal could be due to causes other than the drug. Confounding factors, such as particular groups of patients being 'channelled' into receiving a drug, can influence reporting. The spontaneous reports from which signals are generated have been submitted by people with differing levels of competence, training, experience and awareness of ADRs. There is also a tendency for reporting rates to be higher with newly introduced drugs, while articles in the media, regulatory action and even legal cases can provoke reporting of particular reactions. Therefore, the strength of the signal also depends on the quality of the individual spontaneous reports. It is rare for a signal to provide strong evidence that requires immediate restriction on use of the drug or its withdrawal.

Causality assessment

Causality assessment relates to the assessment of whether a drug is responsible for a suspected ADR. This is of great importance to the regulators who license medicines and control use within a country. In the UK the regulator is the MHRA; other important regulators are the EMEA and the FDA in the USA. Such agencies exist worldwide, and most operate spontaneous reporting schemes. Many then send these reports to the WHO international monitoring centre in Uppsala, Sweden; thus, a very large database exists of spontaneous reports gathered from around the world.

A suspected ADR is rarely confirmed with a definite degree of certainty, despite the numbers of reports, the variable amounts and quality of information available in spontaneous reports, in particular the lack of any evidence derived from rechallenge with the suspected drug which is usually ethically unacceptable. Thus, causality is difficult to prove conclusively, and a high degree of suspicion is often sufficient for a regulator to take action to modify the use of the product.

One of the most common methods of causality assessment is unstructured clinical assessment, also known as global introspection. Expert review of clinical information is undertaken and a judgement is made about the likelihood of the reaction being due to drug exposure. The assessment of complex situations, often with missing information, is open to variation between different assessors, and studies have shown marked disagreements between experts. The WHO international monitoring centre uses global introspection for case assessment, assigning standardised causality categories to suspected ADRs (Table 5.4).

A number of alternative methods of assessing causality have been developed using standardised decision algorithms, in an attempt to increase objectivity and reduce assessor bias. One of the most commonly used is the Naranjo algorithm (Naranjo et al., 1981). This uses a scored questionnaire with points being added or taken away based on the response to each question, such as *'Did the adverse reaction reappear when the drug was re-administered?'* The total score is then used to place the assessed reaction on the following scale: definite, probable, possible or doubtful. Algorithms may be less open to the effects of confounding variables, such as underlying disease states or concomitant drugs, but variation in assessor judgements still occurs.

Table 5.4 World Health Organization Uppsala Monitoring Centre causality categories

Category	Description
Certain	Pharmacologically definitive, with rechallenge if necessary
Probably/likely	Reasonable temporal relationship; unlikely to be attributed to disease processes or other drugs, with reasonable dechallenge response
Possible	Reasonable temporal relationship, but could be explained by concurrent disease or drugs; no information on withdrawal
Unlikely	Temporal relationship improbable; concurrent disease or drugs provide plausible explanation
Conditional/ unclassified	An event which requires more data for assessment
Unassessable/ unclassifiable	An event that cannot be judged because of insufficient/contradictory information which cannot be supplemented or verified

Yellow Card Scheme

The UK's Yellow Card Scheme, now operated by the MHRA, was established in 1964 following the thalidomide tragedy. All healthcare professionals are encouraged to submit reports of suspected ADRs using a Yellow Card (found in the British National Formulary), online (https://yellowcard.mhra.gov.uk) or via an application for mobile phones. It is not necessary to confirm an association between the medicine and the event; a suspicion is sufficient for a report to be submitted. The MHRA requests that all serious suspected ADRS to established drugs are reported, but for newer drugs, all suspected ADRs should be reported, even minor events. Newer drugs under intensive surveillance are identified with an inverted black triangle symbol (▼) in product information, including both Summaries of Product Characteristics (SPCs) and patient information leaflets (PILs), and standard prescribing texts. Black triangle status is generally maintained for at least 2 years, but the period varies, depending on how much information is obtained about a product's continued safety.

Community pharmacists are particularly encouraged to report suspected ADRs to over-the-counter medicines and herbal products, as they are providers of these and people are most likely to inform them of any problems encountered. The Yellow Card Scheme now also includes medical devices, counterfeit products and defective medicines. Suspected ADRs to biological products are particularly desired, as the variation between brands and even between batches can be significant.

All information from Yellow Card reports is entered into a database, and the suspected reactions are categorised using the internationally accepted Medical Dictionary for Regulatory Affairs (MedDRA), which provides a hierarchical taxonomy of ADRs by system organ class. All resultant signals generated by the reports are assessed for causality. Where there is a valid signal that may be an ADR, further work is usually then required to further assess the association. This may involve requesting further details from reporters, contacting manufacturers, searching the literature for case reports and other evidence (cohort or case–control studies) or asking pharmaceutical manufacturers to carry out pharmacoepidemiological studies. The MHRA estimates that about 40% of the safety signals it investigates are generated from spontaneous reports.

When new ADRs are identified and an association confirmed, the MHRA may take action in the form of changes to the SPC and/or the PIL, restricting usage or withdrawing marketing authorisation for the medicine. Withdrawal of marketing authorisation or change in use requires that prescribers and suppliers are informed immediately, but such information is also usually publicised in the media and online; hence patients are often aware of these actions and may present with requests for information and advice.

Unfortunately all spontaneous reporting systems, including the Yellow Card Scheme, suffer from severe under-reporting. A systematic review estimated this to be between 82% and 98% (Hazell and Shakir, 2006). There are a variety of reasons for under-reporting, including lack of certainty that the medicine caused the symptom, but it is important to emphasise that such certainty is not required. There is also no requirement to provide the patient name or contact details, only those of the actual reporter, hence confidentiality, also cited as a reason for under-reporting, is not an issue. Furthermore, the MHRA has systems in place to check for duplicate reports covering the same incident; therefore, concerns about two people submitting reports about the same event in a given patient is also not a valid reason for failing to report a suspected ADR.

Direct patient reporting

It is important to recognise that a patient is frequently the first person to suspect an ADR, and given there is no requirement for causality to be confirmed in order to submit a report about a suspected ADR, patients are capable of doing so themselves. Patient reports have been accepted by the FDA for many years; since October 2005 patients have been permitted to report directly to the MHRA, and increasingly other countries are allowing direct reporting. It has been suggested that direct reporting by patients has advantages such as faster signal generation, avoiding the filtering effect of interpretation of events by health professionals and, not least, maintaining the number of reports at a time when reporting by health professionals may be reducing.

Respondents to a survey of UK patient reporters indicated that facility to report was important and most had an understanding of the purpose of reporting. Many considered it provided an opportunity to influence the content of PILs, so that other patients may be better informed. However, there remains a need to further increase awareness of direct patient reporting amongst both the public and health professionals. Despite this limited awareness of the facility, people find it relatively easy to report suspected ADRs (McLernon et al., 2009). The majority of people who reported a suspected ADR identified it through issues relating to timing, as outlined in the causality methods used by pharmacovigilance experts, or by accessing information about the medicine from the PIL (Krska et al., 2010). A comparison of the ADRs reported by patients and health professionals to the MHRA in the first 2 years of the scheme indicated that patient reports covered a wider range of drugs and ADRs than health professional reports, that patients were more likely to describe the impact of the ADR than health professionals, but that the proportion of serious reactions was similar between patients and health professionals (Avery et al., 2011). Overall, evaluations have concluded that patient reports make a useful contribution to pharmacovigilance.

Published case reports

In addition to reporting via the Yellow Card Scheme, practitioners may also report individual cases in the literature, especially when the event is previously unknown or unpredictable. As seen with thalidomide and practolol, astute and vigilant clinicians submitting case reports to the medical press has been of importance in drug safety. Case reports are less common than in the past and are now more likely to require that a causal link is established, or that a case series is gathered to form a more comprehensive article. Both this and the time taken to draft a case report for publication mean that this is a lesser used mechanism for identifying suspected ADRs. Interestingly case reports were cited as evidence in almost all 19 drug withdrawals which took place between 2002 and 2011 (McNaughton et al., 2014) and in 78% of all withdrawals between 1953 and 2013 (Onakpya et al., 2016). It may take several months for a case report about a suspected ADR to be published, during which time more patients may be exposed to the potential risk. However, published case reports can alert others to the possibility of ADRs, which may encourage them to be more observant in their own practice.

Cohort studies

Cohort studies are prospective pharmacoepidemiological studies that monitor a large group of patients who are taking a particular drug over a period of time. Ideally such studies compare the incidence of a particular adverse event in two groups of patients: those taking the drug of interest and another group, matched for all important characteristics except the use of the drug. Such studies can indicate the relative risks associated with the adverse event in people exposed to the drug being studied. A very large cohort study conducted in Denmark followed women aged 15–49 years with no history of thrombotic disease from January 2001 to December 2009 to determine the proportion who developed a deep vein thrombosis in those who used oral contraception compared with those who did not (Lidegaard et al., 2011). This study found the relative risk of developing a deep vein thrombosis associated with oral contraception was 2.9 [95% confidence interval (CI): 2.2–3.8]. Another example of cohort studies being used to investigate suspected ADRs is the risk of bleeding with selective serotonin reuptake inhibitors (SSRIs). Four cohort studies included in a meta-analysis found the odds ratio (OR) for bleeding risk was 1.68 (95% CI: 1.13–2.50), which was similar to that found in 10 case–control studies (OR 1.66; 95% CI: 1.44–1.92) (Anglin et al., 2014).

Case–control studies

Case–control studies compare the extent of drug usage in a group of patients who have experienced the adverse event with the extent of usage among a matched control group who are similar in potentially confounding factors, but have not experienced the event. By comparing the prevalence of drug taking between the groups, it may be possible to identify whether significantly more people who experienced the event also took a particular drug. Examples of associations that have been established by case–control studies are Reye's syndrome and aspirin, and the relationship between maternal diethylstilboestrol ingestion and vaginal adenocarcinoma in female offspring. Case–control studies are an effective method of confirming whether a drug causes a given reaction once a suspicion has been raised through signal generation. Being retrospective, they rely on good record-keeping about drug use and alone are not capable of detecting previously unsuspected adverse reactions. They are particularly good at investigating rare adverse events.

Roles of health professionals

Ensuring medicines are used safely is fundamental to the role of all health professionals who prescribe, supply, administer, monitor or advise on medicines. When selecting a medicine for an individual patient, whether this is to be prescribed or sold, all health professionals should take account of all relevant patient factors, which may predispose to ADRs. As outlined earlier this includes comorbidities, concomitant drugs, renal and liver function, and genetic predisposition. Importantly it is invaluable to have information about the patient's ADR history. Studies have repeatedly shown that this is poorly documented, leading to inappropriate re-use of medicines which have previously caused problems. Hence another important role of all health professionals is documentation of identified ADRs. The patient may have information about this, if documentation is insufficient; therefore, questioning the patient about his or her ability to tolerate specific medicines or extracting a full ADR history should be considered at every opportunity.

Identifying and assessing adverse drug reactions in clinical practice

As well as being of importance for pharmacovigilance, the identification of potential ADRs is an essential component of clinical practice. Although such assessments may lack the formality of expert or algorithmic assessment, they are likely to take into account similar factors, such as whether the clinical event is commonly drug-related, the temporal relationship with drug use, a dose relationship and exclusion of other possible causes. A list of such factors is set out in Box 5.1.

Many triggers could lead to the suspicion of an ADR – for example, changes in medicines, dose reduction, prescription of medicines used to treat allergic reactions or those frequently used to counteract the effects of other drugs. Simple questioning of patients could easily be incorporated into many aspects of routine care to increase the chances of detecting potential ADRs.

Box 5.1 Factors that may raise or suppress suspicions of a drug-induced event (Shakir, 2004)

The **temporal relationship** between the exposure to the drug and the subsequent event

The **clinical and pathological characteristics of the event** – events which are known to be related to drug use, rather than disease processes

The **pharmacological plausibility** – based on the observer's knowledge of pharmacology

Existing information in published drug information sources – whether the event has been noted by others

Concomitant medication – which may be considered the cause of an event

Underlying and concurrent illnesses – may alter the event or be considered the cause of the event

Dechallenge – disappearance of symptoms after dose reduction or cessation of therapy

Rechallenge – reappearance of symptoms after dose increases or recommencement of therapy

Patient characteristics and medical history – history of the patient may colour the view of the event

The potential for **drug interactions**

The process of identifying an ADR then involves making a judgement about whether a particular event, such as a symptom, condition or abnormal test result, could be related to a drug used in the patient who is experiencing the event. The prior experiences of the patient with other medicines should also be taken into consideration.

Every opportunity should be taken to question patients about their experiences, to determine whether they perceive any adverse events that could be due to medicines. While routinely asking simple questions is important, it is equally important to develop a positive attitude to patients' perceptions of suspected ADRs. There is some evidence that health professionals may dismiss patients who report that they have experienced an ADR, but recent work (Krska et al., 2010) shows that many patients identify such problems appropriately, using factors such as onset, effect of dose change, effect of dechallenge or even rechallenge, as well as the information sources freely accessible to them. To ascertain whether a symptom reported by a patient can be reasonably suspected of being an ADR requires careful questioning.

The key questions that health professionals need to ask may be summarised by the mnemonic SCOOTA. These cover:

Symptoms/severity: What exactly were the symptoms experienced and how severe are/were they?

Cause: What medicine do they suspect caused the symptoms?

Outcomes: Have the symptoms gone away, reduced or are they still causing problems?

Other causes: Could other medicines being taken, medical conditions or allergies explain the symptoms?

Timing: When did the symptoms start in relation to taking the medicine? Have they changed with changes in dose?

Actions: What actions have already been taken? Has the medicine been stopped? Has a health professional already been consulted?

As already stated, the MHRA encourages reporting of all serious suspected ADRs to established drugs and all suspected ADRs to new drugs or vaccines. This is thus an important role for all health professionals. If not reporting themselves, health professionals should consider encouraging others to report instead. For example, a community pharmacist may have insufficient information to fully complete a Yellow Card, so he or she may encourage a primary care doctor to report or a hospital pharmacist may report on behalf of a consultant clinician. Encouraging others to report also extends to providing information about reporting and educating others, including patients, to report. Community pharmacies and primary care medical practices should all have a supply of Yellow Cards for patients, but patients may require advice and support in completing these. Pharmacists in particular, because of their role in dispensing prescriptions written by others, may also be involved in educating and supporting others in preventing ADRs and in developing methods for detecting ADRs through prescription monitoring.

Preventing adverse drug reactions

The majority of ADRs are theoretically preventable; hence there is potential to dramatically reduce the costs associated with ADRs and possibly also deaths. Assessing preventability is a difficult area because it involves judgements and many different methods have been developed for making these judgements. The method developed by Hallas et al. (1990) is widely used, providing definitions of 'avoidability' which range from definite (due to a procedure inconsistent with present-day knowledge or good medical practice) to unevaluable (poor data or conflicting evidence). Recent estimates suggest that 52% of ADRs seen at admission were preventable, and 45% (95% CI: 33–58%) of ADRs in in-patients were preventable (Hakkarainen et al., 2012). However, not all ADRs are absolutely preventable, and assessments using hindsight are unlikely to replicate clinical decision making at the point of prescribing. Preventability also varies; sometimes there are clear solutions, such as avoiding prescribing a teratogenic drug to a female of child-bearing age, but others, such as a drug that increases the risk of an event occurring within a population, are less easy to prevent.

ADRs can most easily be prevented by good clinical practice and rational drug use. This means ensuring that ADRs are fully documented and this information is transferred between care settings; checking a patient's previous ADR history before prescribing, dispensing or administering drugs; minimising the use of drugs known to carry a high risk of ADRs; and tailoring drug selection to individuals based on the factors that predispose them to ADRs. Many recent initiatives have the potential to minimise the burden of ADRs. Wider use of computer systems that incorporate clinical decision support, and improved transfer and sharing of information about patients between healthcare providers, including centrally stored electronic health records, should help to ensure more accurate drug histories and avoidance of inappropriate prescribing. In addition, the increasing availability of guidance on drug selection and appropriate use, combined with increasing regular review of medicines, should also help to increase rational prescribing, which may ultimately have an effect on the incidence of ADRs.

Monitoring therapy

Monitoring the effects of drugs, either by direct measurement of plasma concentrations or by measurements of physiological markers, is another potential mechanism to reduce the risk of ADRs. For example, it has been estimated that one in four preventable drug-related hospital admissions are caused by failure to monitor renal function and electrolytes (Howard et al., 2003).

There is good evidence that monitoring can be effective. Clozapine, used for the management of treatment-resistant schizophrenia and psychosis, is associated with significant risk of agranulocytosis. Mandatory monitoring of white blood cell counts has led to more than 90% of fatal agranulocytosis cases being prevented.

Ideally guidance on monitoring should be clear and provide an evidence-based frequency of monitoring and acceptable reference values. However, robust evidence for optimal monitoring frequency is limited for many drugs, hampering specific guidance, which tends to vary between various expert bodies and drug information sources. An examination of the adequacy of manufacturers' advice on monitoring for haematological ADRs found that advice was too vague to be useful to prescribers (Ferner et al., 2005).

Even when guidance is clear, monitoring can be neglected, although practitioners may take greater care when treating the elderly and those with more comorbidities (McDowell, 2010). The need for baseline parameters to be measured before drugs are started, such as liver function tests for statins, is often ignored; thus, changes due to drug treatment become difficult to confirm. Despite a clearly defined monitoring requirement, warfarin remains one of the top 10 drugs involved in drug-induced admissions.

Explaining risks to patients

Evidence shows that patients want to receive information about side effects; however, health professionals view providing side effect information with far less importance than the patients receiving it. One of the main sources of information about ADRs is clearly the PIL, which, in the EU, must be provided every time a medicine is prescribed or supplied. Ultimately patients then have to make a decision about whether to use the medicine, and health professionals are increasingly encouraged to involve patients in this decision. Therefore, patients have both a right to, and a need for, understandable information about the potential for harm that medicines may cause, to enable them to make informed decisions. Although there may still be debate about whether the provision of information on side effects encourages reduced adherence to taking medicines or spurious reporting of adverse effects, it is clear that this information is useful to patients and its availability has increased dramatically in recent decades in most countries. Patients often use the PIL when suspected adverse events are experienced to assist in assessing the cause of the problem; therefore, as outlined earlier, side effect information should be understandable and the EU requires that information leaflets are tested with patients prior to use to ensure this is the case.

Patients increasingly also access a wider range of information sources about medicines and about ADRs themselves; indeed they are actively encouraged to do so. SPCs are easily accessed by patients, as are the Drug Analysis Prints produced by the

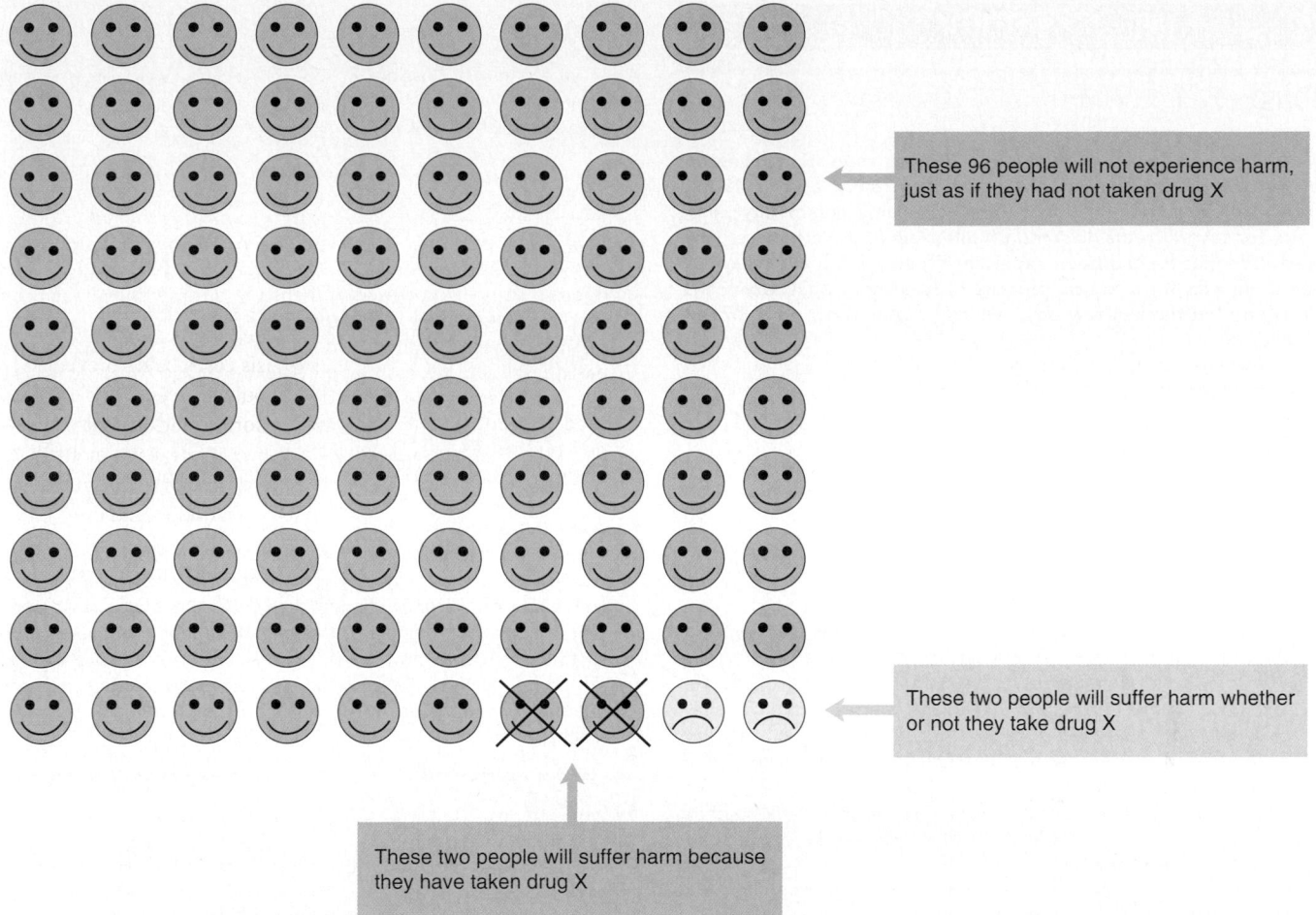

These 96 people will not experience harm, just as if they had not taken drug X

These two people will suffer harm whether or not they take drug X

These two people will suffer harm because they have taken drug X

Fig. 5.1 A Cates plot in 100 people showing how drug X doubles the risk of an unspecified harm compared with no treatment. (From Cox and Butt, 2012, with permission.)

MHRA, which summarise the data obtained from the Yellow Card reports they receive. Hence patients may question judgements about individual products they have been prescribed or sold. In this situation the health professional must be able to interpret information accessed by patients to ensure that the information they use to make decisions about whether to take a medicine is unbiased and accurate.

The EU recommends using verbal terms to describe the risk of experiencing an ADR, ranging from 'very common' (for rates of >1 in 10) to 'very rare' (for rates of <1 in 10,000). The MHRA advocates combining words with frequencies, for example, 'Common (affects >1 in 100 persons)'. Studies show that patients tend to over-estimate the risk when these are described using words only and that patients differ in their understanding of what the terms mean. Percentages, particularly those less than 1%, are also not understood by everybody. This lack of understanding of the risks of experiencing ADRs can potentially reduce willingness to use the medicine.

Another approach is the use of pictures, such as faces, graphs or charts. One example is the 'Paling palette', which is a grid of 1000 stick figures (100 × 100) to convey information on the chances of experiencing a particular outcome. A similar method is a 'Cates plot', which is a grid of 100 faces (10 × 10), coloured differently and either smiling or downcast, depending on the outcome. These types of icon grids are mainly used to convey the potential benefits and risks of a particular action, which can include the risk of getting a side effect. They are increasingly used in patient decision aids, now being produced by the National Institute for Health and Care Excellence (NICE). A generic example of a decision aid is shown in Fig. 5.1. However, there are people who do not find these easy to understand (Ancker et al., 2006).

It is important to appreciate that, when communicating information about potential ADRs, how risks are perceived will be affected by the relationship between the health professional and the patient, the patient's prior experiences and beliefs, how information is framed and the context in which it is given. Patients may also have views on the acceptability of ADRs, which should be taken into account when selecting a product for an individual. An ADR that is viewed as minor by health professionals may be considered to reduce quality of life by one patient, while another patient may be happy to accept this for the potential benefit the medicine offers. Even when drugs are withdrawn from the market for safety reasons, significant numbers of patients will feel they were willing to accept the harm-benefit of the drug. Communicating the harms and benefits of medicines is therefore an important role of health professionals.

Case studies

Case 5.1

Mr KM is a fairly active 69-year-old. He has regularly presented his repeat prescription for atenolol 50 mg daily, aspirin 75 mg daily and simvastatin 40 mg daily to the same community pharmacy for several years. Last month diltiazem SR 60 mg twice daily was added, as he had been experiencing increasing angina symptoms. He asks for a topical product to treat neck pain, which has developed in the last few days, which he puts down to a 'frozen shoulder'.

Questions

1. Could this be an ADR, and why did it develop now?
2. Is it appropriate to change to another statin?
3. What actions should the pharmacist take?

Answers

1. Neck pain, 'frozen shoulder' and such descriptions are typical of the muscular pain which is induced by statins. The onset varies from a few weeks to more than 2 years after starting treatment, the incidence is dose-related and the severity ranges from mild aches to severe pain, causing reduced mobility. Older people, who may have reduced renal function or liver function, are at greater risk of statin-induced myopathy.
   Diltiazem can inhibit the metabolism of simvastatin because of its actions on cytochrome P450 isoenzyme CYP3A4, thereby increasing the risk of myopathy.
   Statin-induced myopathy ranges from mild myopathies and myalgias, to myositis, to rare cases of potentially life-threatening rhabdomyolysis, in which muscle cell walls are disrupted and the contents leak into the systemic circulation. Muscle pain in patients who are taking statins should therefore always be taken seriously.
2. The problem is associated with all drugs in the class. Although simvastatin and atorvastatin, the most widely prescribed, are both lipophilic and metabolised by cytochrome P450 3A4 and, therefore, may be most likely to cause muscle pain, there is no reliable comparative data on different statins.
3. Creatinine kinase (CK) levels should have been measured before initiating statin therapy, but regardless of whether this was done, a CK level should be measured now, plus liver function tests. Mr KM's primary care doctor should be contacted to inform him about the suspected ADR, and the patient encouraged to report the ADR via the Yellow Card scheme. It may be appropriate to discontinue or reduce the dose of the simvastatin, depending on the result of the CK level and the severity of the symptoms. The problem may not resolve immediately on discontinuation. Because grapefruit juice can increase blood levels of simvastatin and high alcohol intake increases the risk of myopathy, the pharmacist should also warn Mr KM about avoiding these.

Case 5.2

Mr SC, a 39-year-old man who is taking varenicline for smoking cessation, reports that he has been suffering from vivid dreams and has become increasingly aggressive towards his family. Last night he had a major argument with his wife. His wife mentioned he had not been the same since he started the varenicline and he would like to know if this was a possible cause.

Questions

1. Is varenicline a possible cause of Mr SC's vivid dreams and aggression?
2. Is this a reportable ADR?

Answers

1. Varenicline has been associated with neuropsychiatric ADRs, including depression, suicidal thoughts, suicidal behaviour and aggression. Vivid dreams and other sleep disorders have also been reported. Prescribers have been warned that such reactions have been reported, although a meta-analysis and systematic review has questioned the association (Thomas et al., 2015). Assessing the cause of this reaction is difficult because smoking cessation itself is associated with exacerbations of underlying psychiatric illness and the risk of symptoms of depression. As varenicline dosing starts 1–2 weeks before stopping smoking, a key question is how long the patient has been taking the drug and if the symptoms appeared before the smoking cessation date.
2. If a health professional considers that a patient's symptoms are a possible ADR, then they should be reported to regulatory authorities (in the UK, this would be through the MHRA's Yellow Card scheme). Only a suspicion is necessary to report a reaction, not proven causality. In the case of new drugs, any reaction, no matter how trivial, should be reported. Patients can also report directly to regulatory authorities in some countries, including the UK. Neuropsychiatric reactions such as this are commonly reported by patients.

Case 5.3

Mr AG, a 65-year-old man with heart failure, is admitted to hospital with a potassium level of 7.1 mmol/L (range 3.4–5.0 mmol/L). Already stabilised on lisinopril 20 mg daily, he had recently been started on spironolactone 25 mg daily. He had a serum creatinine of 160 micromol/L (range 75–155 micromol/L).

Questions

1. What is the mechanism of any possible ADR?
2. How should future episodes of hyperkalaemia be avoided?

Answers

1. Spironolactone, an aldosterone receptor antagonist, has a beneficial effect on mortality and hospital admission in patients with heart failure. However, spironolactone can increase potassium serum levels because of its effect on aldosterone. When used in combination with angiotensin-converting enzyme inhibitors, serious hyperkalaemia can occur.
   Although clinical trials of spironolactone showed no risk, cases have been reported in the literature, and other epidemiological studies have indicated that in real-world clinical situations the incidence of hyperkalaemia is increased (MHRA, 2016).
2. Care taken should be taken when prescribing spironolactone outside of trial criteria, particularly with regard to renal function. Other susceptibilities for the development of hyperkalaemia include diabetes and the elderly due to reduced aldosterone production. Changes in other therapy should be monitored, as well as episodes of acute illness. Those with mildly increased serum potassium should have a reduced dose of spironolactone. More intensive monitoring of potassium levels at the commencement of therapy might be useful, although the hyperkalaemia can occur months after initiation.

Case 5.4

Mrs KT, a 55-year-old woman attending a warfarin outpatient clinic, has a raised INR. On questioning it is discovered that she has recently started taking glucosamine for muscle aches for the last 2 weeks.

Questions

1. What is the likelihood that glucosamine was responsible for the rise in the INR?
2. Should this reaction be reported to regulatory authorities?

Answers

1. Glucosamine is a popular supplement purchased for 'joint health'. It is commonly used by older patients. Spontaneous reports of

interactions between warfarin and glucosamine have been submitted to UK, Australian and US regulators. Additional cases have been reported in the literature (Knudsen and Sokol, 2008). While there is no known mechanism and no formal interaction studies, the published cases and spontaneous reports are sufficient evidence to suggest a potential interaction. Given the wide use of glucosamine, the interaction may be rare, although under-reporting is common.
   Assessment of this individual case requires further questioning to eliminate other confounding factors such as changes in diet or adherence issues.
2. Interactions with, or adverse reactions to, complementary and alternative remedies can be reported to spontaneous reporting schemes, such as the UK Yellow Card scheme. Collation of such reports allows regulators to gather further information on the suspected reaction and any susceptibilities that may in time provide useful information to other users.

References

Ancker, J., Senathirajah, Y., Kukafka, R., et al., 2006. Design features of graphs in health risk communication: a systematic review. J. Am. Med. Inform. Assoc. 13, 608–618.

Anglin, R., Yuan, Y., Moayyedi, P., et al., 2014. Risk of upper gastrointestinal bleeding with selective serotonin reuptake inhibitors with or without concurrent nonsteroidal anti-inflammatory use: a systematic review and meta-analysis. Am. J. Gastroenterol. 109, 811–819.

Aronson, J.K., Ferner, R.E., 2003. Joining the DoTS: new approach to classifying adverse drug reactions. Br. Med. J. 327, 1222–1225.

Avery, A.J., Anderson, C., Bond, C.M., et al., 2011. Evaluation of patient reporting of adverse drug reactions to the UK 'Yellow Card Scheme': literature review, descriptive and qualitative analyses, and questionnaire surveys. Health Technol. Assess. 15, 20.

Basch, E., 2010. The missing voice of patient in drug-safety reporting. N. Engl. J. Med. 362 (10), 865–869.

Bouvy, J.C., De Bruin, M.L., Koopmanschap, M.A., 2015. Epidemiology of adverse drug reactions in Europe: a review of recent observational studies. Drug Saf. 38 (5), 437–453.

Bresalier, R., Sandler, R., Quan, H., et al., 2005. Cardiovascular events associated with rofecoxib in a colorectal adenoma chemoprevention trial. N. Engl. J. Med. 352, 1092–1102.

Brynner, R., Stephens, T., 2001. Dark remedy: the impact of thalidomide and its revival as a vital medicine. Perseus Books, New York.

Cappellini, M.D., Fiorelli, G., 2008. Glucose-6-phosphate dehydrogenase deficiency. Lancet. 317 (9606), 64–74.

Cox, A.R., Butt, T.F., 2012. Adverse drug reactions: when the risk becomes a reality for patients. Drug Saf. 35 (11), 977–981.

Davies, E.C., Green, C.F., Taylor, S., et al., 2009. Adverse drug reactions in hospital in-patients: a prospective analysis of 3 965 patient-episodes. PLoS One. 4 (2), e4439. https://doi.org/10.1371/journal.pone.0004439.

Edwards, I.R., Aronson, J.K., 2000. Adverse drug reactions: definitions, diagnosis, and management. Lancet. 356, 1255–1259.

European Medicines Evaluation Agency (EMEA), 2014. Guideline on Good Pharmacovigilance Practices (GVP) Annex I – Definitions (Rev 4). EMA/87633/2011 Rev 4. Available at: http://www.ema.europa.eu/docs/en_GB/document_library/Scientific_guideline/2013/05/WC500143294.pdf.

Ferner, R.E., Coleman, J., Pirmohammed, M., et al., 2005. The quality of information on monitoring for haemotological adverse drug reactions. Br. J. Pharmacol. 60 (4), 448–451.

Food and Drug Administration (FDA), 2007. Information for healthcare professional: dangerous or even fatal skin reactions – Carbamazepine (marketed as Carbatrol, Equetro, Tegretol, and generics). Available at: https://www.fda.gov/drugs/drugsafety/postmarketdrugsafetyinformationforpatientsandproviders/ucm124718.htm.

Gallagher, R.M., Mason, J.R., Bird, K.A., et al., 2012. Adverse drug reactions causing admission to a paediatric hospital. PLoS One. 7 (12), e50127.

Gandhi, T.K., Weingart, S.N., Borus, J., et al., 2003. Adverse drug events in ambulatory care. N. Engl. J. Med. 348 (16), 1556–1564.

Guthrie, B., Makubate, B., Hernandez-Santiago, V., et al., 2015. The rising tide of polypharmacy and drug–drug interactions: population database analysis 1995–2010 BMC Medicine 13, 74.

Hakkarainen, K.M., Hedna, K., Petzold, M., et al., 2012. Percentage of patients with preventable adverse drug reactions and preventability of adverse drug reactions: a meta-analysis. PLoS One. 7 (3), e33236.

Hakkarainen, K.M., Hedna, K., Petzold, M., et al., 2013a. Prevalence and perceived preventability of self-reported adverse drug events: a population-based survey of 7099 adults. PLoS One. 8 (9), e73166.

Hakkarainen, K.M., Gyllensten, H., Jonsson, A.K., et al., 2013b. Prevalence, nature and potential preventability of adverse drug events: a population-based medical record study of 4970 adults. Br. J. Clin. Pharmacol. 78, 170–183.

Hallas, J., Harvald, B., Gran, L.F., et al., 1990. Drug-related hospital admissions: the role of definitions and intensity of data collection and the possibility of prevention. J. Intern. Med. 228, 83–90.

Hazell, L., Shakir, S.A., 2006. Under-reporting of adverse drug reactions: a systematic review. Drug Saf. 29, 385–396.

Heerdink, E.R., Urquhart, J., Leufkens, H.G., 2002. Changes in prescribed drug doses after market introduction. Pharmacoepidemiol Drug Saf. 11 (6), 447–453.

Howard, R., Avery, A.J., Howard, P.D., et al., 2003. Investigations into the reasons for preventable admissions to a medical admissions unit. Qual. Saf. Health Care. 12, 280–285.

Jarernsiripornkul, N., Krska, J., Capps, P.A.G., et al., 2002. Patient reporting of potential adverse drug reactions: a methodological study. Br. J. Clin. Pharmacol. 53, 318–325.

Knudsen, J.F., Sokol, G.H., 2008. Potential glucosamine-warfarin interaction resulting in increased international normalized ratio: case report and review of the literature and MedWatch database. Pharmacotherapy. 28 (4), 540–548.

Krska, J., Taylor, J., Avery, A.J., 2010. How do patients identify ADRs? A quantitative analysis in reporters to the Yellow Card Scheme. Pharmacoepidemiol. Drug Saf. 19, 652.

Kumar, A., 2003. Adverse effects of pharmaceutical excipients. Adverse Drug React. Bull. 222, 851–854.

Laurence, J., 2009. Getting personal: the promises and pitfalls of personalized medicine. Transl. Med. 154, 269–271.

Lidegaard, Ø., Nielsen, L.H., Skovlund, C.W., et al., 2011. Risk of venous thromboembolism from use of oral contraceptives containing different progestogens and oestrogen doses: danish cohort study, 2001–9. BMJ. 343, d6423.

Lucas, A., Nolan, D., Mallal, S., 2007. HLA-B*5701 screening for susceptibility to a bacavir hypersensitivity. J. Antimicrob. Chemother. 59 (4), 591–593.

McDowell, S.E., 2010. Monitoring of patients treated with antihypertensive therapy for adverse drug reactions. Adverse Drug React. Bull. 261, 1003–1006.

McDowell, S.E., Coleman, J.J., Ferner, R.E., 2006. Systematic review and meta-analysis of ethnic differences in risks of adverse reactions to drugs used in cardiovascular medicine. Br. Med. J. 332, 1177–1181.

McLernon, D., Lee, A.J., Watson, M.C., et al., 2009. Consumer reporters' views and attitudes towards the Yellow Card Scheme for Adverse Drug Reaction reports: a questionnaire study. Int. J. Pharm. Pract. 17 (Suppl. 2), B25–B26.

McNaughton, R., Huet, G., Shakir, S., 2014. An investigation into drug products withdrawn from the EU market between 2002 and 2011 for safety reasons and the evidence used to support the decision-making. Br. Med. J. Open. 4 (1) e004221.

Medicines and Healthcare products Regulatory Authority (MHRA), 2016. Spironolactone and renin-angiotensin system drugs in heart failure: risk of potentially fatal hyperkalaemia. Drug Safety Update. Available at: https://www.gov.uk/drug-safety-update/spironolactone-and-renin-angiotensin-system-drugs-in-heart-failure-risk-of-potentially-fatal-hyperkalaemia#history.

Naranjo, C.A., Busto, U., Sellers, E.M., et al., 1981. Naranjo ADR probability scale. Clin. Pharmacol. Ther. 30, 239–245.

Onakpoya, I.J., Heneghan, C.J., Aronson, J.K., 2016. Post-marketing withdrawal of 462 medicinal products because of adverse drug reactions: a systematic review of the world literature. BMC Med. 14 (1), 10.

Pirmohamed, M., James, S., Meakin, S., et al., 2004. Adverse drug reactions as cause of admission to hospital: prospective analysis of 18 820 patients. Br. Med. J. 329, 15–19.

Rawlins, M.D., 1981. Clinical pharmacology: adverse reactions to drugs. Br. Med. J. 282, 974–976.

Shakir, S.A.W., 2004. Causality and correlation in pharmacovigilance. In: Talbot, T., Waller, P. (Eds.), Stephens' Detection of New Adverse Drug Reactions, fifth ed. Wiley and Sons Ltd., Chichester, pp. 329–343.

Thomas, K.H., Martin, R.M., Knipe, D.W., et al., 2015. Risk of neuropsychiatric adverse events associated with varenicline: systematic review and meta-analysis. Br. Med. J 350, h1109 https://doi.org/10.1136/bmj.h1109.

Thomsen, L.A., Winterstein, A.G., Sondergaard, B., et al., 2007. Systematic review of the incidence and characteristics of preventable adverse drug events in ambulatory care. Ann. Pharmacother. 41, 1411–1426.

Wester, K., Jonnson, A.K., Sigset, O., et al., 2008. Incidence of fatal adverse drug reactions: a population based study. Br. J. Clin. Pharmacol 65, 573–579.

World Health Organization (WHO), 1972. International drug monitoring: the role of national centres. Technical Report Series; No 498. WHO, Geneva.

World Health Organization (WHO), 2002. The importance of pharmacovigilance: safety monitoring of medicinal products. WHO, Geneva.

Zhang, M., Homan, C.D.J., Price, S.D., et al., 2009. Co-morbidity and repeat admission to hospital for adverse drug reactions in older adults: retrospective cohort study. BMJ. 338, a2752.

Further reading

Aronson, J.K., Ferner, R.E., 2005. Clarification of terminology in drug safety. Drug Saf. 28, 851–870.

Lee, A., 2006. Adverse Drug Reactions, second ed. Pharmaceutical Press, London.

Talbot, J., Aronson, J.K., 2011. Stephens' Detection of New Adverse Drug Reactions, sixth ed. Wiley Blackwell, Chichester.

Waller, P., 2010. An Introduction to Pharmacovigilance. Wiley Blackwell, Chichester.

Useful websites

Drug Safety Update. Available at: https://www.gov.uk/drug-safety-update.

Yellow Card Reporting. Available at: https://yellowcard.mhra.gov.uk.

6 Laboratory Data

John Warburton and Lee Beale

Key points

- Haematological and biochemical tests provide useful information for the diagnosis, screening, management, prognosis and monitoring of disease and its response to treatment.

- Reference ranges are important guides which generally represent the test values from 95% of the healthy population (mean ± 2 standard deviations); however, interlaboratory difference will be observed.

- A series of values, rather than a single test value, is often required to ensure clinical relevance and eliminate erroneous values due to patient variation and analytical or sampling errors.

- A wide variety of intracellular enzymes may be released into the blood following damage to tissues such as hepatocytes and skeletal muscle. These can be measured in serum to provide useful diagnostic information. Commonly requested haematological test profiles include full blood count, differential white blood cell (WBC) count, erythrocyte sedimentation rate (ESR), serum folate and vitamin B_{12} and iron status, and clotting screen.

- Commonly requested biochemical test profiles include the so-called 'U and Es' (urea and electrolytes), liver function tests, troponins and C-reactive protein.

- Drug therapy can cause abnormal test results.

- Drugs can have an important role in preventing or treating abnormalities.

This chapter will consider the common haematological and biochemical tests that are of clinical and diagnostic importance. For convenience, each individual test will be dealt with under a separate heading, and a brief review of the physiology and pathophysiology will be given where appropriate to explain the basis of haematological and biochemical disorders.

It is usual for a reference range to be quoted for each individual test (see ranges at the start of each section). This range is based on data obtained from a sample of the general population served by the testing laboratory, which is assumed to be from healthy, disease-free individuals. The reference ranges in this chapter are intended as a guide only, and specific local reference ranges, particular to the type of assay, should be used in clinical practice. Many test values have a normal distribution, and the reference values are taken as the mean ± 2 standard deviations (SD). This includes 95% of the population. The 'normal' range must always be used with caution because it takes little account of an individual's age, sex, weight, height, muscle mass or disease state, many of which variables can influence the value obtained. Although reference ranges are valuable guides, they must not be used as sole indicators of health and disease. A series of values rather than a simple test value may be required in order to ensure clinical relevance and to eliminate erroneous values caused, for example, by spoiled specimens or interference from diagnostic or therapeutic procedures. Furthermore, a disturbance of one parameter often cannot be considered in isolation without looking at the pattern of other tests within the group.

Further specific information on the clinical and therapeutic relevance of each test may be obtained by referral to the relevant chapter in this book.

Haematology data

The haematology profile (Table 6.1) is an important part of the investigation of many patients and not just those with primary haematological disease. It is commonly termed the full blood count (FBC). The test is performed on a small quantity of anticoagulated blood; the anticoagulant used routinely is ethylenediaminetetra-acetic acid (EDTA). The FBC gives information on the different cells that together form the blood – red blood cells (RBCs), platelets and WBCs – and their differentials. All of these cells are formed from the same multipotential stem cells within the bone marrow (Fig. 6.1). Cell production is under the control of a number of growth factors, including erythropoietin and colony stimulating factor (CSF); the coagulation screen gives information with regard to haemostasis. We will consider each of these in turn. Typical measurements reported in a haematology screen, with their normal values, are shown in Table 6.1, and a list of the common descriptive terms used in haematology is presented in Table 6.2.

Red blood cells

The main role of the RBC is to deliver oxygen to the tissues and remove carbon dioxide to the lungs. The oxygen and carbon dioxide are both carried by the haemoglobin molecules attached to the red blood cell.

Red blood cell count

RBCs are produced in the bone marrow by the process of erythropoiesis under the control of erythropoietin. Erythropoietin is produced predominantly in the kidney in response to a decrease in oxygen delivery. Erythropoietin stimulates the bone marrow

Table 6.1 Normal values in haematology

Laboratory test	Reference range
FBC	
Haemoglobin	115–165 g/L
White blood cell (WBC)	$4.0–11.0 \times 10^9$/L
Platelets	$150–450 \times 10^9$/L
Red blood cell (RBC)	$3.8–4.8 \times 10^{12}$/L
Reticulocytes	$50–100 \times 10^9$/L
Packed cell volume (PCV)	0.36–0.46 L/L
Mean cell volume (MCV)	83–101 FL
Mean cell haemoglobin (MCH)	27–34 pg
Mean cell haemoglobin concentration (MCHC)	31.5–34.5 g/dL

WBC differential

Cell type	Percentage of WBC count	
Neutrophils	40–75%	$2.0–7.0 \times 10^9$/L
Lymphocytes	5–15%	$1.5–4.0 \times 10^9$/L
Monocytes	2–10%	$0.2–0.8 \times 10^9$/L
Basophils	<1%	$<0.1 \times 10^9$/L
Eosinophils	1–6%	$0.04–0.4 \times 10^9$/L
Coagulation		
PT	10–14 seconds	
APTT	35–45 seconds	
Fibrinogen	1.5–4 g/L	

APTT, activated partial thromboplastin time; FBC, full blood count; PT, prothrombin time; WBC, white blood cell.

to produce more RBCs by the conversion of immature erythroblasts to mature erythrocytes which are released into the circulation. Prior to their release the RBCs shed the nucleus and adopt a biconcave disc shape. Normally, only non-nucleated mature erythrocytes are seen in the peripheral blood:

erythroblasts
↓
normoblasts (nucleated)
↓
reticulocytes (non-nucleated)
↓
erythrocytes

The lifespan of a mature RBC is usually between 110 and 120 days, and during this time it travels 300 miles through the circulatory system. A decrease in RBC lifespan, as, for instance, in haemolysis, reduces the circulating mass of RBCs, and with it the supply of oxygen to tissues is decreased. In these circumstances, RBC production is enhanced in healthy bone marrow by an increased output of erythropoietin by the kidneys. Under normal circumstances RBCs are destroyed by lodging in the spleen due to decreasing flexibility of the cells. They are removed by the reticuloendothelial system.

A high RBC count (erythrocytosis or polycythaemia) indicates increased production by the bone marrow and may occur as a physiological response to hypoxia, as in chronic airway disease, or as a malignant condition of RBCs, such as in polycythaemia rubra vera.

Reticulocytes

Reticulocytes are the earliest non-nucleated RBCs. They owe their name to the fine, net-like appearance of their cytoplasm, which can be seen, after appropriate staining, under the microscope and contain fine threads of ribonucleic acid (RNA) in a reticular network. Reticulocytes normally represent between 1% and 2% of the total RBC count and do not feature significantly in a normal blood profile. However, increased production (reticulocytosis) can be detected in times of rapid RBC regeneration, as occurs in response to haemorrhage or haemolysis. At such times the reticulocyte count may reach 40% of the RBCs. The reticulocyte count may be useful in assessing the response of the marrow to iron, folate or vitamin B_{12} therapy. The count peaks at about 7–10 days after starting such therapy and then subsides.

Haemoglobin

The primary role of the RBC is to transport oxygen. The adult haemoglobin molecule is composed of four polypeptide chains, two alpha (α) and two beta (β). Contained within each of the four polypeptide chains is a haem molecule that consists of a ferrous iron (Fe^{2+}) and protoporphyrin. It is the iron that binds reversibly with the oxygen.

It is the haemoglobin level that is of interest and the concentration in whole blood, measured in grams/litre (g/L). Haemoglobin levels are used as a marker of anaemia, when the concentration of haemoglobin is below that expected for the person's age and sex. The haemoglobin concentration in men is normally greater than in women, reflecting in part the higher RBC count in men. Lower concentrations in women are due, at least in part, to menstrual loss. Increased haemoglobin may reflect a polycythemia (reactive or neoplastic) or be due to dehydration.

In some relatively rare genetic diseases, the haemoglobinopathies, alterations in the structure of the haemoglobin molecule can be detected by electrophoresis. Abnormal haemoglobins which can be detected in this manner include HbS (sickle haemoglobin in sickle cell disease) and HbA2 found in β-thalassaemia carriers.

Of note is that in 2013 the units of measurement of haemoglobin were standardised across Europe, with the units changing from grams/decilitre to grams/litre, a factor of 10 increase.

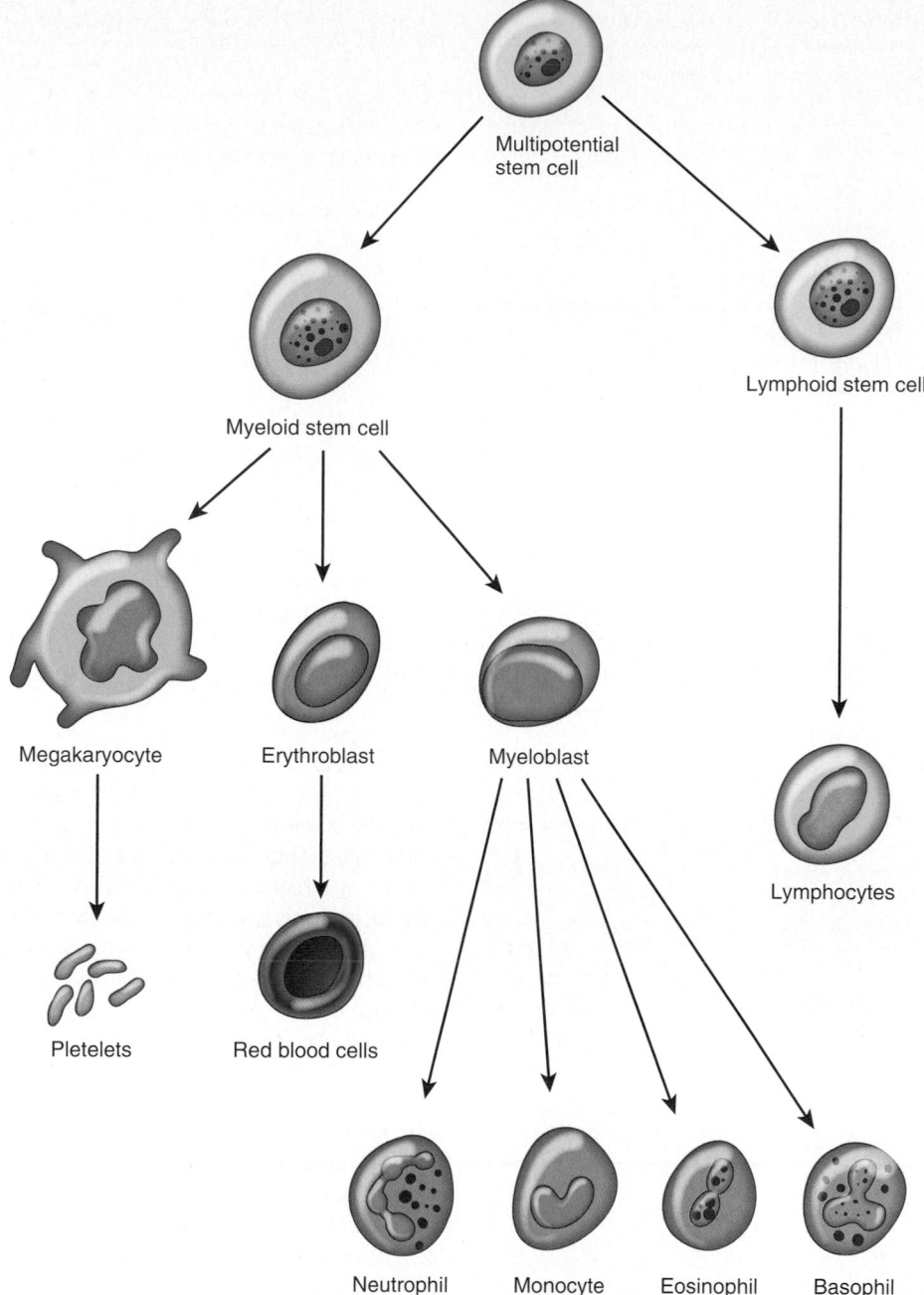

Fig. 6.1 The differentiation pathway of multipotent stem cells.

Mean cell volume

The mean cell volume (MCV) is the average volume of a single RBC and is measured in femtolitres (10^{-15} L). A RBC can be described as microcytic, normocytic or macrocytic, which are descriptive of a low, normal or high MCV, respectively. They are useful in the process of identification of various types of anaemia (Table 6.3).

Packed cell volume

The packed cell volume (PCV) or haematocrit is the ratio of the volume occupied by RBCs to the total volume of blood. It can be measured by centrifugation of a capillary tube of blood and then expressing the height of RBCs in a capillary tube to the height of the total height of the blood column. It is reported as a fraction of unity or as a percentage (e.g. 0.45 L/L or 45%). The use of modern laboratory analysers has removed the need to directly measure the PCV. PCV is now derived from the multiplication of the MCV and RBC count. The PCV often reflects the RBC count and will, therefore, be decreased in bleeding or a dilution anaemia (where excess intravenous fluid has been given) and raised in polycythaemia. It may, however, be altered irrespective of the RBC count, when the size of the RBC is abnormal, as in macrocytosis and microcytosis.

Table 6.2 Descriptive terms in commonly used in haematology

Anisocytosis	Abnormal variation in cell size (usually refers to RBCs), e.g. red cells in iron deficiency anaemia
Agranulocytosis	Lack of granulocytes (principally neutrophils)
Aplastic	Depression of synthesis of all cell types in bone marrow (as in aplastic anaemia)
Basophilia	Increased number of basophils
Hypochromic	MCHC low, red cells appear pale microscopically
Leucocytosis	Increased white cell count
Leucopenia	Reduced white cell count
Macrocytic	Large cells
Microcytic	Small cells
Neutropenia	Reduced neutrophil count
Neutrophilia	Increased neutrophil count
Normochromic	MCHC normal; red cells appear normally pigmented
Pancytopenia	Decreased number of all cell types: it is synonymous with aplastic anaemia
Poikilocytosis	Abnormal variation in cell shape, e.g. some red cells appear pear shaped in macrocytic anaemias
Thrombocytopenia	Lack of platelets

MCHC, mean cell haemoglobin concentration.

Table 6.3 Causes of anaemia according to mean cell volume

Low MCV (<83 fL)	Normal MCV (83–101 fL)	High MCV (>101 fL)
Microcytic	*Normocytic*	*Macrocytic*
Iron deficiency	*Acute blood loss*	*B_{12} deficiency*
Thalassaemic disorders	Early iron deficiency	Folate deficiency
	Chronic renal insufficiency	Alcohol abuse

MCV, mean cell volume.

Mean cell haemoglobin

The mean cell haemoglobin MCH is the average weight of haemoglobin contained in an RBC. It is measured in picograms (10^{-12} g) and is calculated from the relationship:

$$MCH = \frac{haemoglobin}{RBC\ count}$$

Box 6.1 Drugs known to cause platelet dysfunction

- Caffeine
- Colchicine
- Furosemide
- Hydroxychloroquine
- Hydralazine
- Nonsteroidal anti-inflammatory drugs
- Penicillin
- Theophylline
- Tricyclic antidepressants
- Vincristine

Cells with a reduced MCH will appear pale in comparison and are termed hypochromic, whereas those with a normal MCH are termed normochromic. The MCH is dependent on the size of the RBCs and the concentration of haemoglobin in the cells. Thus, it is usually low in iron-deficiency anaemia when there is microcytosis and there is less haemoglobin in each cell, but it may be raised in macrocytic anaemia.

Mean cell haemoglobin concentration

The mean cell haemoglobin concentration (MCHC) is a measure of the average concentration of haemoglobin per unit weight of RBCs. It is usually expressed as grams per litre but may be reported as a percentage. The MCHC will be reported as low in the same conditions that give rise to a low MCV and MCH, namely, iron-deficiency anaemia. A raised MCHC, in contrast, is associated with a range of congenital or acquired conditions. These include spherocytosis or in other congenital haemolytic anaemias, including sickle cell anaemia and haemoglobin C disease.

Platelets

Platelets (thrombocytes) are small disk-shaped cells formed in the bone marrow from megakaryocytes. Damage caused to the vascular endothelium is plugged by the aggregation of platelets to form an occlusive plug; they also act in the initiation of the coagulation process. Platelets are normally present in the circulation for 8–12 days.

A reduction in platelet number (thrombocytopenia) may reflect either a depressed synthesis in the marrow or consumption of formed platelets. A small fall in the platelet count may be seen in pregnancy and following viral infections. Severe thrombocytopenia may result in spontaneous bleeding. The short lifespan of a platelet is useful to bear in mind when evaluating a possible drug-induced thrombocytopenia because recovery should be fairly swift when the offending agent is withdrawn. An increased platelet count (thrombocytosis) occurs in malignancy, inflammatory disease and in response to blood loss.

The FBC will show the actual platelet count and gives no indication of platelet function. The function of platelets can be inhibited by many drugs (Box 6.1); the most commonly used is aspirin, which acts to inhibit the production of thromboxane A_2 for the life of the platelet.

Table 6.4 White blood cell differential

Granulocytes	Agranulocytes
Neutrophils	Lymphocytes
Eosinophils	Monocytes
Basophils	

White blood cell count

A haematology profile often reports a total WBC count and a differential count, the latter separating the composition of WBCs into the various types. WBCs (leucocytes) are of two types: the granulocytes and the agranulocytes (Table 6.4). Each of the different cells serves a particular function and will be reviewed individually in the following sections.

Neutrophils

Neutrophils or polymorphonucleocytes (PMNs) are the most abundant type of WBC. Neutrophils rapidly migrate to the sites of inflammation with the role of removing foreign material. At the site of inflammation, neutrophils engulf the foreign material through phagocytosis and the release of preformed granular enzymes to remove the pathogen. Neutrophils are formed in the bone marrow from stem cells which form myoblasts and develop through a number of stages to become a functional neutrophil. Neutrophils have a classical appearance of a multi-segmented nucleus and constitute approximately 40–75% of circulating WBCs in normal, healthy blood. They have a remarkably short lifespan with a circulating half-life of 6–8 hours and thus are produced at a high rate of up to 10×10^{10} cells per day. The neutrophil count increases in response to infection, tissue damage (e.g. infarction) and inflammation (e.g. vasculitis). Neutropenia, also described as agranulocytosis in its severest forms, is associated with malignancy and drug toxicity but may also occur in viral infections such as influenza, infectious mononucleosis and hepatitis.

The highly destructive capacity of neutrophils can lead to the damage of healthy tissues; this phenomenon is observed in inflammatory diseases such as inflammatory bowel disease and rheumatoid arthritis.

Basophils

Basophils normally constitute a small proportion of the WBC count (<1%). Their function is not well understood, but they play a role in parasitic infections and acute hypersensitivity reactions. They contain numerous vesicles within their cytoplasm that contain inflammatory mediators, including heparin and histamine. Basophilia is also observed in various malignant and premalignant disorders, including chronic myeloid leukaemia and myelofibrosis.

Eosinophils

Eosinophils normally constitute less than 6% of WBCs. Their function appears to be concerned with inactivation of mediators released from mast cells, and eosinophilia is, therefore, apparent in many allergic conditions, such as asthma, hay fever and drug sensitivity reactions, as well as some malignant diseases.

Lymphocytes

Lymphocytes are the second most abundant WBCs in the circulating blood, but the majority of them are found in the spleen and other lymphatic tissue. They are formed in the bone marrow. An increase in lymphocyte numbers occurs particularly in viral infections such as rubella, mumps, infectious hepatitis and infectious mononucleosis.

Monocytes

Monocytes circulate in the blood and have a key role during inflammation and pathogen challenge. Monocytes enter the tissues and there undergo a transformation to macrophages. Macrophages are phagocytic cells which produce numerous inflammatory cytokines and act as accessory cells to T-lymphocytes by presenting antigens to them. A monocytosis is observed in some infections, such as typhoid, subacute bacterial endocarditis, infectious mononucleosis and tuberculosis.

Coagulation

The haemostatic system is a critical defense mechanism for protecting the vascular system. Haemostasis is activated within seconds of injury to the endothelium and can be considered in two stages. Primary haemostasis is the formation of the initial 'platelet plug', and secondary haemostasis is the formation of a fibrin clot. The formation of a stable fibrin clot was classically described as a coagulation cascade, a complex biochemical cascade where inactive coagulation factors, known as zymogens (non-enzymatic precursors), are activated to enzymes. Many of the coagulation factors are referred to by Roman numerals and depicted by suffixing the letter 'a' when activated. The cascade is formed of two independent cascades, the intrinsic and extrinsic pathways that culminate in the final common pathway (Fig. 6.2).

The current model of coagulation has been updated to better represent the in vivo activity (Hoffman and Monroe, 2001). The model consists of three overlapping steps: initiation, amplification and propagation. This cellular model of normal haemostasis is shown in Fig. 6.3. The initiation phase leads to small amounts of factor IIa (thrombin) being produced by cells containing tissue factor (TF) (e.g. smooth muscle or fibroblasts). The level of thrombin production is too low to convert fibrinogen to fibrin, requiring a second phase, amplification, leading to platelet activation at the site of injury. Thrombin cleaves the factor VIII/vWF complex and activates factors V, VIII and XI, which adhere to the platelets. The third phase is propagation where the activated platelets generate large amounts of thrombin to cleave fibrinogen into fibrin and form a crosslinked clot in conjunction with factor XIIIa. To prevent inappropriate propagation of the thrombus, the process is controlled by naturally occurring

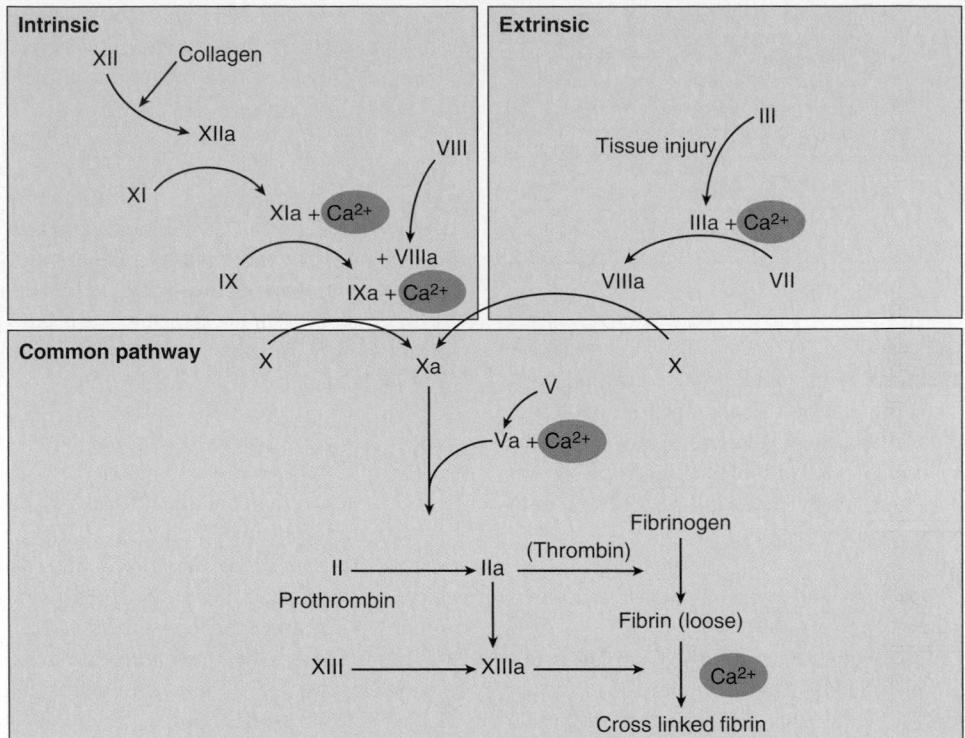

Fig. 6.2 Classical coagulation cascade. Ca, calcium.

anticoagulants and the fibrinolytic system, the final effector of which is plasmin, which cleaves fibrin into soluble degradation products.

Despite the complexity of this model, the basic coagulation tests can still be interpreted in relation to the 'intrinsic', 'extrinsic' and 'final common pathway' components of the traditional cascade.

Monitoring coagulation

The standard laboratory screening test of coagulation includes the prothrombin time (PT), activated partial thromboplastin time (APTT) and fibrinogen level and is performed on citrated platelet-poor plasma. These tests do not reflect the complexity of haemostasis in vivo or the risk of bleeding and require interpretation in relation to clinical context.

Prothrombin time

The PT tests the extrinsic and common pathways and represents the time taken to fibrin strand formation in platelet-poor plasma and is reported in seconds. The PT is measured by adding calcium and thromboplastin (tissue factor and phospholipid) to citrated plasma. The PT clotting time depends on factors I (fibrinogen), II (prothrombin), V, VII and X and is prolonged by liver disease, disseminated intravascular coagulation (DIC) and vitamin K deficiencies (factors II, VII and X are vitamin K dependent). It is most commonly employed in the monitoring of warfarin anticoagulation therapy through the International Normalised Ratio (INR).

International Normalised Ratio

The normal range for the PT varies by laboratory, reagent and equipment configuration. The INR, unlike the PT, allows for the comparison of results from different laboratories, times and locations. The INR represents the ratio of the patient's PT to a laboratory control PT obtained and the international sensitivity index (ISI) applied.

$$INR = \left[\frac{\text{patient's PT}}{\text{laboratory control PT}} \right]^{ISI}$$

The ISI is based on an international World Health Organization (WHO) reference thromboplastin reagent and represents the sensitivity of a given thromboplastin to the depression of factors II, VII and X. The more responsive a thromboplastin is to change, the lower its ISI value.

The target value varies according to the indication for the anticoagulant, but for most, including for thromboembolic prophylaxis in atrial fibrillation, it is 2.5. For some indications, including recurrent deep vein thrombosis and pulmonary embolism whilst on warfarin, the target is higher at 3.5.

The most common use of the PT and INR is to monitor oral anticoagulant therapy, but the PT is also useful in assessing liver function because of its dependence on the activity of clotting factors II, V, VII and X, which are produced in the liver.

Activated partial thromboplastin time

The activated partial thromboplastin time (APTT) tests the intrinsic and common pathways and is the time, in seconds, to fibrin formation. The APTT is measured by incubating platelet-poor

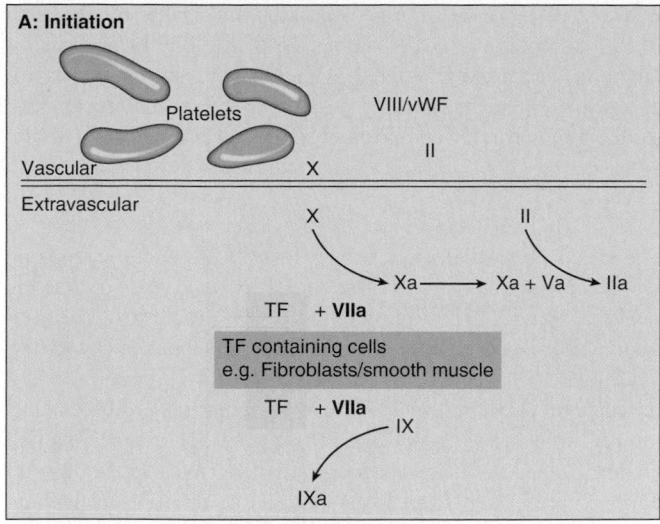

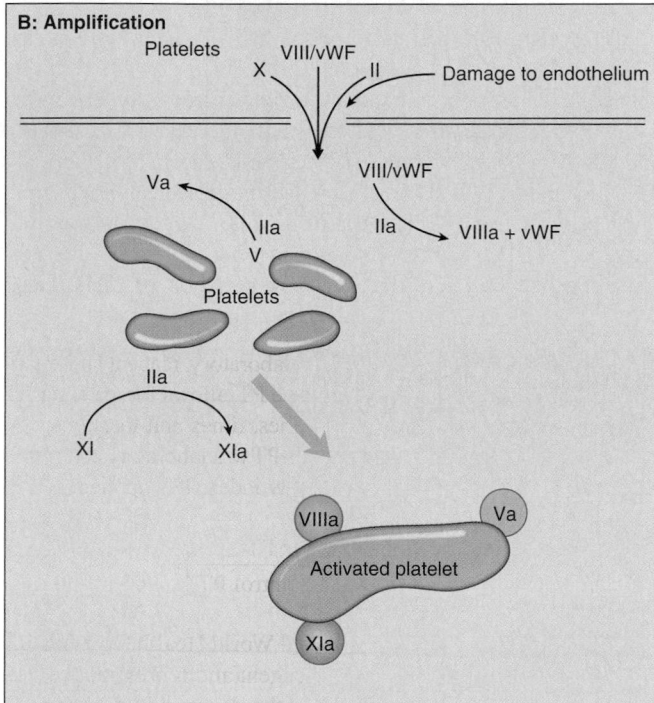

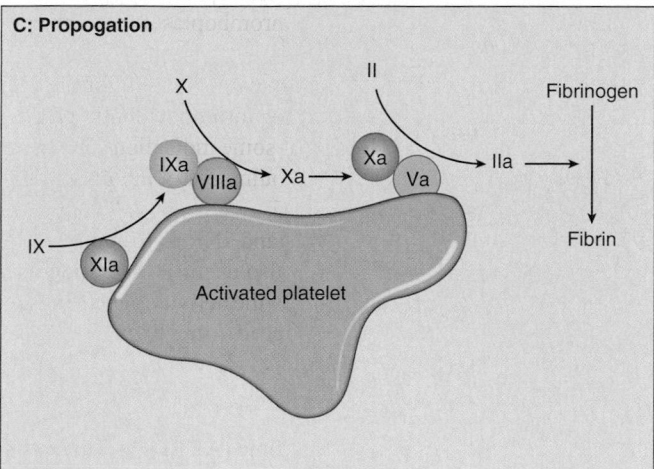

Fig. 6.3 The cell-based coagulation theory: (a) initiation, (b) amplification, (c) propagation. (Adapted from Bahuleyan, 2015.)

plasma with a phospholipid (a platelet substitute) and an activator such as kaolin. It is the lack of TF that distinguishes it from the PT. The sample is then recalcified, and the time to clot formation is the APTT. It is designed to detect deficiencies in factor VIII, IX and XI. It is the most common method for monitoring unfractionated heparin (UFH) therapy. The desirable APTT for optimal heparin therapy is between 1.5 and 2.5 times the normal control.

Low-molecular-weight heparins (LMWH) are commonly used for the prevention and treatment of venous thromboembolism, and because they provide more predictable anticoagulant activity than unfractionated heparin, it is not usually necessary to monitor them during treatment. Unlike with UFH, the APTT is considered suboptimal for monitoring LMWH. Anti-factor Xa is the gold standard and relates well with the concentration of LMWH in the blood, but it correlates less well with the effect of the drug in vivo. The APTT gives little indication of bleeding tendencies, as the presence of a lupus anticoagulant prolongs the APTT, but the patient has thrombotic tendencies. Factor XII deficiency gives rise to a long APTT but rarely a bleeding tendency.

Fibrinogen

The laboratory standard for the measurement of fibrinogen is the von Clauss assay. First, plasma is diluted to remove clotting inhibitors (e.g. heparin), and then a high concentration of thrombin is added, which allows comparison with controls to derive the fibrinogen concentration. The normal concentration in the blood (Table 6.1) varies between individuals and increases in inflammation because it is an acute-phase reactant. There is evidence to suggest that a level of over 1.0 g/L is required for sufficient clot stabilisation, and the British Committee for Standards in Haematology (BCSH) recommends the use of cryoprecipitate when fibrinogen is less than 1 g/L in severe bleeding.

Urea and electrolytes

The homeostasis of various elements, water and acid–base balance are interrelated. Standard biochemical screening includes several measurements (Table 6.5) which provide a picture of fluid and electrolyte balance and renal function. These are colloquially referred to as 'U and Es' (urea and electrolytes), and the major tests are described in the following sections.

Fluid homeostasis

In order to contextualise abnormal findings in urea and electrolyte levels, it is important to understand the movement of water in healthy individuals. Water constitutes approximately 60% of body weight in men and 55% in women (women have a greater proportion of adipose tissue, which contains little water). Approximately two-thirds of body water is found in the intracellular fluid (ICF) and one-third in the extracellular fluid (ECF), which is divided between the interstitial fluid and serum (Fig. 6.4). Total body water is regulated by the renal action of antidiuretic hormone (ADH, sometimes referred to as vasopressin), the renin–angiotensin–aldosterone system, noradrenaline and by thirst, which is stimulated by rising plasma osmolality.

Water can permeate freely from the vascular compartment to the intracellular compartment via the interstitial space. Water and solutes pass through the capillary wall and the cell wall, two semipermeable membranes, to get from one to the other. Osmotic pressure in each compartment determines the direction of movement, with water moving from low to high solute concentration. Water movement reduces as the oncotic pressure between compartments equalises; that is, they become isotonic, which ensures normal cell membrane integrity and cellular processes.

The osmolality of the ECF is largely determined by sodium and its associated anions, chloride and bicarbonate, whereas the major contributor to the osmolality of the ICF is potassium. Glucose and urea have a lesser, but nevertheless important, role in determining ECF osmolality. Protein, especially albumin, makes only a small (0.5%) contribution to the osmolality of the ECF but is a major factor in determining water distribution between the two compartments. The contribution of proteins to the osmotic pressure of serum is known as the colloid osmotic pressure or oncotic pressure.

Fluid balance

The amount of water taken in and lost by the body depends on intake, diet, activity and environmental conditions. Over time the intake of water is normally equal to that lost (Table 6.6). The minimum daily intake necessary to maintain this balance is approximately 1100 mL. Of this, 500 mL is required for normal excretion of waste products in urine, whereas the remaining volume is lost to insensible losses via the skin in sweat, via the lungs in expired air, and in faeces. The kidneys regulate water balance, with water being filtered, then reabsorbed in variable amounts depending primarily on the level of ADH.

An imbalance in the intake versus loss of water, without the intake or loss of the corresponding electrolytes, will result in changes to solute concentrations and hence osmolality. For example, a loss of water from the ECF will increase its osmolality and result in the movement of water from the ICF to the ECF. This increase in ECF osmolality will stimulate the hypothalamic thirst centres to encourage drinking while also stimulating the release of ADH, which promotes water reabsorption with subsequent concentration of the urine. The secretion of ADH is also

Table 6.5 Standard values for urea, electrolytes and associated tests

Laboratory test	Reference range
Urea and electrolytes (U & Es)	
Sodium	135–145 mmol/L
Potassium	3.4–5.0 mmol/L
Urea	3.1–7.9 mmol/L
Creatinine	75–155 mmol/L
eGFR	≥90 mL/min/1.73 m^2
Associated tests	
Magnesium	0.7–1.0 mmol/L
Osmolality	282–295 mmol/kg of water

eGFR, estimate of glomerular filtration rate.

Table 6.6 Typical daily water balance for a healthy 70-kg adult

	Input (mL)		Output (mL)
Oral fluids	1400	Urine	1500
Food	700	Lung	400
Metabolic oxidation	400	Skin	400
		Faeces	200
Total	2500		2500

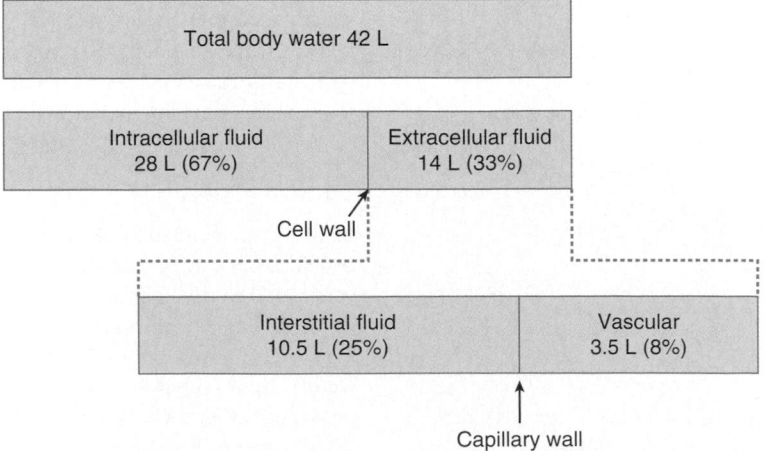

Fig. 6.4 Approximate distribution of normal fluid in a 70-kg man.

stimulated by angiotensin II, baroreceptors, volume receptors, stress (including pain), exercise and drugs, including morphine, nicotine, tolbutamide, carbamazepine and vincristine.

Water depletion

Water depletion will occur if intake is inadequate or loss excessive. Excessive loss of water through the kidney is unusual, except in diabetes insipidus or following the overuse of diuretics.

Water depletion can occur with diarrhoea and increased sweating due to fever, amongst other reasons. Such a loss is usually compensated for, in the first instance by increasing water intake if the thirst mechanism is intact or can be acted upon, but this may not occur in patients who are unconscious, have swallowing difficulties or are disabled. Severe water depletion may induce cerebral dehydration causing confusion, fits, coma and circulatory failure.

The underlying cause for the water depletion should be identified and treated. Replacement water should be given orally, where possible, or by nasogastric tube, intravenously or subcutaneously as necessary. Fluid therapy should be individualised for each patient taking in to account both the need for water and supplementation of electrolytes. These requirements will dictate which fluid is prescribed from physiologically balanced solutions like compound sodium lactate to the very rarely used hypotonic solutions.

Water excess

Water excess is usually associated with an impairment of water excretion, such as that caused by renal failure or the syndrome of inappropriate secretion of the antidiuretic hormone arginine vasopressin (SIADH). This syndrome has several causes. including pneumonia and some tumours, particularly small cell carcinoma of the lung. Excess intake is rarely a cause of water excess because the healthy adult kidney can excrete water at a rate of up to 2 mL/min. Patients affected usually present with signs consistent with cerebral overhydration, although if it is of gradual onset, over several days, they may be asymptomatic.

Sodium

Sodium distribution

The body of an average 70-kg man contains approximately 3000 mmol of sodium. Most of this sodium is freely exchangeable and is extracellular. In contrast to the normal plasma concentration (Table 6.5), the ICF concentration of sodium is only about 10 mmol/L. The ECF volume is dependent upon total body sodium because sodium is almost entirely restricted to the ECF, and water intake and loss are regulated to maintain a constant concentration of sodium in the ECF compartment.

Sodium regulation

Each day approximately 1000 mmol of sodium is secreted into the gut and 25,000 mmol filtered by the kidney. The bulk of this is recovered by reabsorption from the gut and renal tubules. Sodium balance is maintained by renal excretion. Normally, 70% of filtered sodium is actively reabsorbed in the proximal tubule, with further

reabsorption in the loop of Henle. Less than 5% of the filtered sodium load reaches the distal tubule where aldosterone can stimulate further sodium reabsorption. It should be clear, therefore, that partial failure of homeostatic control can potentially have major consequences.

Other factors, such as natriuretic peptide hormone, can affect sodium reabsorption. This hormone is secreted by the cardiac atria in response to atrial stretch following a rise in atrial pressure associated with volume expansion. It is natriuretic (increases sodium excretion in urine) and, amongst other actions, reduces aldosterone concentration.

Hyponatraemia

Inadequate oral intake of sodium is rarely the cause of sodium depletion. A fall in the serum sodium level can be the result of sodium loss, inappropriate secretion of ADH or water retention in excess of sodium, usually resulting from defects in free water excretion caused by low ECF volume. Increased water intake without corresponding sodium, also known as a dilutional hyponatraemia, may also contribute and can occur with inappropriate parenteral treatment using hypotonic solutions.

Sodium depletion commonly occurs alongside water loss, resulting in dehydration or volume depletion. The normal response of the body to the resulting hypovolaemia includes an increase in aldosterone secretion (which stimulates renal sodium reabsorption) and an increase in ADH secretion if ECF volume depletion is severe. A number of drugs have also been implicated in causing hyponatraemia (Box 6.2).

Inappropriate secretion of ADH is the mechanism underlying many drug-induced hyponatraemias. In this syndrome, the drug may augment the action of endogenous ADH (e.g. tolbutamide or lamotrigine), increase the hypothalamic production of ADH (e.g. carbamazepine) or have a direct ADH-like action on the kidney (e.g. oxytocin or, more obviously, desmopressin). Hyponatraemia can also be induced by mechanisms different from those just described. Lithium may cause renal damage and a failure to conserve sodium. Likewise, the natriuretic action of diuretics can predispose to hyponatraemia.

Clinical features. Hyponatraemia can present asymptomatically; however, vomiting, drowsiness, headache and seizures may

Box 6.2	Examples of drugs known to cause hyponatraemia

- Antidepressants – SSRIs and tricyclic derivatives
- Amphotericin
- Angiotensin-converting enzyme inhibitors
- Carbamazepine
- Cisplatin
- Cyclophosphamide
- Diuretics
- Gliclazide
- Levothyroxine
- Nonsteroidal anti-inflammatory drugs
- Proton pump inhibitors
- Tolbutamide
- Vasopressin
- Vincristine

SSRIs, selective serotonin reuptake inhibitors.

Box 6.3 Examples of drugs known to cause hypernatraemia

- Adrenocorticotrophic hormone
- Anabolic steroids
- Androgens
- Corticosteroids
- Demeclocycline
- Fosfomycin
- Lactulose
- Lithium
- Micafungin
- Oral contraceptives
- Phenytoin
- Sodium bicarbonate

be associated with rapid onset or severe hyponatraemia. These symptoms present as a result of cerebral oedema and raised intracranial pressure. Chronic hyponatraemia must be corrected slowly so as not to cause neurological damage as a result of pontine demyelination.

Hypernatraemia

Hypernatraemia, or sodium excess, can be a result of either increased intake or decreased excretion. Excessive intake is not a common cause, although hypernatraemia can be associated with excessive intravenous saline infusion or unreplaced hypotonic water excretion as a result of impaired access to free water or impaired thirst.

Sodium excess is usually attributable to impaired excretion. It may also be caused by a primary mineralocorticoid excess, for example, Cushing's syndrome or Conn's syndrome. However, it is often the result of a secondary hyperaldosteronism associated with, for example, heart failure, nephrotic syndrome, hepatic cirrhosis with ascites or renal artery stenosis. Sodium and water retention causes oedema.

Drug-induced hypernatraemia is either the result of a defect in ADH secretion (central diabetes insipidus) or poor response of the renal tubules to ADH (nephrogenic diabetes insipidus). The affected patient presents with polyuria, polydipsia or dehydration.

- Lithium causes a nephrogenic diabetes insipidus, which has been reported after only 2 weeks of therapy. The syndrome is usually reversible on discontinuation. Whilst affected, however, many patients are unresponsive to exogenous ADH.
- Demeclocycline can also cause diabetes insipidus and can be used in the management of patients with SIADH.
- Phenytoin generally has a less pronounced effect on urinary volume than lithium or demeclocycline and does not cause nephrogenic diabetes insipidus. It inhibits ADH secretion at the level of the central nervous system.

Hypernatraemia can be caused by a number of other drugs (Box 6.3) and by a variety of mechanisms; for example, hypernatraemia secondary to sodium retention is known to occur with corticosteroids, and the administration of sodium-containing drugs parenterally in high doses (e.g. benzylpenicillin) also has the potential to cause hypernatraemia.

Clinical features and management. The signs and symptoms of hypernatraemia are those associated with neuronal cell shrinkage and include irritability, lethargy, confusion and seizures. It is likely that the patient may display signs consistent with the associated dehydration, including muscle weakness and orthostatic hypotension. Hypernatraemia should be corrected slowly: not more than half of the water deficit should be corrected in the first 12 to 24 hours.

Potassium

Potassium distribution

The total amount of potassium in the body, like sodium, is 3000 mmol. About 10% of the total body potassium is bound in RBCs, bone and brain tissue and is not exchangeable. The remaining 90% of total body potassium is free and exchangeable, with the vast majority having an intracellular location, being pumped in and out by Na/K-ATPase pumps. This is controlled by mechanisms aimed at ensuring stable intracellular to extracellular ratios and hence correct muscular and neuronal excitability. Only 2% of the exchangeable total body potassium is in the ECF, the compartment from where the serum concentration is sampled and measured. Consequently, the measurement of serum potassium is not an accurate index of total body potassium, but together with the clinical status of a patient, it permits a sound, practical assessment of potassium homeostasis.

Potassium regulation

The serum potassium concentration is controlled mainly by the kidney, with the gastro-intestinal tract normally having a minor role. The potassium filtered in the kidney is almost completely reabsorbed in the proximal tubule. Potassium secretion is largely a passive process in response to the need to maintain membrane potential neutrality associated with active reabsorption of sodium in the distal convoluted tubule and collecting duct. The extent of potassium secretion is determined by a number of factors, including:

- the amount of sodium available for exchange in the distal convoluted tubule and collecting duct;
- the availability of hydrogen and potassium ions for exchange in the distal convoluted tubule or collecting duct;
- the ability of the distal convoluted tubule or collecting duct to secrete hydrogen ions;
- the concentration of aldosterone;
- tubular fluid flow rate.

As described previously, both potassium and hydrogen can neutralise the membrane potential generated by active sodium reabsorption, and consequently, there is a close relationship between potassium and hydrogen ion homeostasis. In acidosis, hydrogen ions are normally secreted in preference to potassium, and potassium moves out of cells; thus, hyperkalaemia is often associated with acidosis, except in renal tubular acidosis. In alkalosis, fewer hydrogen ions will be present, potassium moves into cells and potassium is excreted; thus, hypokalaemia is often associated with alkalosis.

The normal daily dietary intake of potassium is of the order of 60–200 mmol, which is more than adequate to replace that lost from the body. It is unusual for a deficiency in intake to account for hypokalaemia. A transcellular movement of potassium into cells, loss from the gut and excretion in the urine are the main causes of hypokalaemia.

Hypokalaemia

Transcellular movement into cells. The shift of potassium from the serum compartment of the ECF into cells accounts for the hypokalaemia reported following intravenous or, less frequently, nebulised administration of β-adrenoreceptor agonists such as salbutamol. Parenteral insulin also causes a shift of potassium into cells and is used for this purpose in the acute management of patients with hyperkalaemia. Catecholamines, for example, adrenaline and theophylline, also have this effect.

Loss from the gastro-intestinal tract. Although potassium is secreted in gastric juice, much of this, together with potassium ingested in the diet, is reabsorbed in the small intestine. Stools do contain some potassium, but in a patient with chronic diarrhoea or a fistula, considerable amounts of potassium may be lost and precipitate hypokalaemia. Likewise, the abuse of laxatives increases gastro-intestinal potassium loss and may precipitate hypokalaemia. Analogous to the situation with diarrhoea, the potassium secreted in gastric juice may be lost following persistent vomiting and can also contribute to hypokalaemia.

Loss from the kidneys. Mineralocorticoid excess, whether it be a result of primary or secondary hyperaldosteronism or Cushing's syndrome, can increase urinary potassium loss and cause hypokalaemia. Likewise, increased excretion of potassium can result from renal tubular damage. Nephrotoxic antibiotics such as gentamicin have been implicated.

Many drugs which can induce hypokalaemia do so by affecting the regulatory role of aldosterone upon potassium–sodium exchange in the distal tubule and collecting duct. Administered corticosteroids mimic aldosterone and can, therefore, increase potassium loss.

The most commonly used groups of drugs that can cause hypokalaemia are thiazide and loop diuretics. Both groups of drugs increase the amount of sodium delivered and available for reabsorption at the distal convoluted tubule and collecting ducts. Consequently, this will increase the amount of potassium excreted from the kidneys. Some of the drugs known to cause hypokalaemia are shown in Box 6.4.

Clinical features and management. The patient with moderate hypokalaemia may be asymptomatic, but the symptoms of more severe hypokalaemia include muscle weakness, hypotonia, paralytic ileus, depression and confusion. Typical changes on the electrocardiogram (ECG) are ST depression, T wave depression/inversion and prolonged P–R interval, and as a result, cardiac arrhythmias may occur. Although hypokalaemia tends to make antiarrhythmic drugs less effective, the action of digoxin, in contrast, is potentiated, leading to increased signs of toxicity. Insulin secretion in response to a rising blood glucose concentration requires potassium, and this mechanism may be impaired in hypokalaemia. Rarely there may be impaired renal concentrating ability with polyuria and polydipsia.

Box 6.4 Examples of drugs known to cause hypokalaemia

- Amphotericin
- Aspirin
- Benzylpenicillin
- Corticosteroids
- Diuretics (loop and thiazide)
- Fluconazole
- Insulin
- Laxatives
- Piperacillin/tazobactam
- Salbutamol
- Sodium bicarbonate

Hypokalaemia is managed by giving either oral potassium or suitably dilute intravenous potassium solutions, depending on its severity and the clinical state of the patient.

Hyperkalaemia

Hyperkalaemia may arise from excessive intake, decreased elimination or a shift of potassium from cells to the ECF. It is rare for excessive oral intake to be the sole cause of hyperkalaemia. The inappropriate use of parenteral infusions containing potassium is probably the most common iatrogenic cause of excessive intake. Hyperkalaemia is a common problem in patients with renal failure because of their inability to excrete a potassium load.

The combined use of potassium-sparing diuretics such as amiloride or spironolactone with an angiotensin-converting enzyme (ACE) inhibitor, which will lower aldosterone, is a recognised cause of hyperkalaemia, particularly in the elderly. Mineralocorticoid deficiency states such as Addison's disease, where there is a deficiency of aldosterone, also decrease renal potassium loss and contribute to hyperkalaemia. Those at risk of hyperkalaemia should be warned not to take dietary salt (NaCl) substitutes in the form of potassium chloride (KCl).

The majority of body potassium is intracellular. Severe tissue damage, catabolic states or impairment of the energy-dependent sodium pump, caused by hypoxia or diabetic ketoacidosis, may result in apparent hyperkalaemia as a result of potassium moving out of, and sodium moving into cells. If serum potassium rises, insulin release is stimulated, which, through increasing activity in Na/K-ATPase pumps, causes potassium to move into cells. Box 6.5 gives examples of some drugs known to cause hyperkalaemia.

Haemolysis during sampling or a delay in separating cells from serum will result in potassium escaping from blood cells into the serum causing an artefactual hyperkalaemia.

Clinical features and management. Hyperkalaemia can be asymptomatic but fatal. An elevated potassium level has many effects on the heart: notably the resting membrane potential is lowered and the action potential shortened. Characteristic changes of the ECG, reduced P wave and 'tented' T wave, precede ventricular fibrillation and cardiac arrest.

In the emergency management of a patient with hyperkalaemia (>6.5 mmol/L ± ECG changes), calcium gluconate (or chloride) at a dose of 10 mL of 10% solution is given intravenously over 5 minutes. This does not reduce the potassium concentration but

---

Box 6.5 Examples of drugs known to cause hyperkalaemia

- Angiotensin-converting enzyme inhibitors
- β-Adrenoceptor blockers
- Ciclosporin
- Diuretics (potassium sparing, e.g. amiloride and spironolactone)
- Heparins
- Nonsteroidal anti-inflammatory drugs
- Potassium supplements
- Propofol
- Suxamethonium

---

antagonises the effect of potassium on cardiac tissue particularly sodium channels. Immediately thereafter, glucose 50 g with 20 units of soluble insulin by intravenous infusion will lower serum potassium levels within 30 minutes by increasing the shift of potassium into cells. Sodium bicarbonate, in the case of acidosis, will also promote cellular uptake of potassium.

The long-term management of hyperkalaemia may involve the use of oral or rectal polystyrene cation-exchange resins which remove potassium from the body. Chronic hyperkalaemia, in renal failure, is managed by a low-potassium diet.

Urea

The catabolism of dietary and endogenous amino acids in the body produces large amounts of ammonia. Ammonia is toxic, and its concentration is kept very low by conversion in the liver to urea. Urea is eliminated in urine and represents the major route of nitrogen excretion. Urea is filtered from the blood at the renal glomerulus and undergoes significant tubular reabsorption of 40–50%. This tubular reabsorption is pronounced at low rates of urine flow but is reduced in advanced renal failure. Serum urea is a less reliable marker of glomerular filtration rate (GFR) than creatinine. Urea levels vary widely with diet, rate of protein metabolism, liver production and the GFR. A high protein intake from the diet, tissue breakdown, major haemorrhage in the gut with consequent absorption of the protein from the blood, and corticosteroid therapy may produce elevated serum urea levels (up to 10 mmol/L). Urea concentrations of more than 10 mmol/L are usually a result of renal disease or decreased renal blood flow following shock or dehydration. As with serum creatinine levels, serum urea levels do not begin to increase until the GFR has fallen by 50% or more. Elevated urea levels can influence the protein binding of some drugs, such as phenytoin, leading to a greater free fraction.

Production is decreased in situations where there is a low protein intake and in some patients with liver disease. Thus, nonrenal and renal influences should be considered when evaluating changes in serum urea concentrations.

Creatinine

Serum creatinine concentration is largely determined by its rate of production, rate of renal excretion and volume of distribution. It is frequently used to evaluate renal function.

Creatinine is produced at a fairly constant rate from creatinine and creatinine phosphate in muscle. Daily production is a function of muscle mass and declines with age from 24 mg/kg/day in a healthy 25-year-old to 9 mg/kg/day in a 95-year-old. Creatinine undergoes complete glomerular filtration with little reabsorption by the renal tubules. Its clearance is, therefore, usually a good indicator of the GFR. As a general rule, and only at the steady state, if the serum creatinine doubles this equates to a 50% reduction in the GFR and consequently renal function. The serum creatinine level can be transiently elevated following meat ingestion, but less so than urea, or strenuous exercise. Individuals with a high muscle bulk produce more creatinine and, therefore, have a higher serum creatinine level compared to an otherwise identical but less muscular individual.

The value for creatinine clearance is higher than the true GFR because of the active tubular secretion of creatinine. In a patient with a normal GFR, this is of little significance. However, in an individual in whom the GFR is low (<10 mL/min), the tubular secretion may make a significant contribution to creatinine elimination and overestimate the GFR. In this type of patient, the breakdown of creatinine in the gut can also become a significant source of elimination. Some drugs, including trimethoprim and cimetidine, inhibit creatinine secretion, possibly through competitive inhibition of active secretion, reducing creatinine clearance and elevating serum creatinine without affecting the GFR.

Measured and estimated GFR. GFR measured as the urinary or plasma clearance of an ideal filtration marker, such as inulin, is the best overall measure of kidney function, but techniques are complex and expensive. Urinary clearance of creatinine allows estimation of GFR, but blood sampling and timed urine collection have practical difficulty and are subject to error.

More commonly, laboratory-reported creatinine levels are accompanied by an estimated glomerular filtration rate. The Chronic Kidney Disease Epidemiology Collaboration (CKD-EPI) equation is the recommended calculation for adults, giving the best all-around approximation of eGFR when compared with the Modification of Diet in Renal Disease (MDRD) formula. Both are adjusted for body surface area, unlike the Cockcroft-Gault equation (Jones, 2011).

Caution should be exercised when interpreting eGFR results over 60mL/min/1.73m^2 and in people with extremes of muscle mass. A reduced muscle mass will lead to overestimation; increased muscle mass to underestimation of the GFR. In patients with a low body mass index (BMI), and the elderly, the Cockcroft–Gault estimation of creatinine clearance remains a good alternative. The Schwartz formula is a widely used, and more appropriate, alternative for calculating GFR in children (Jones, 2011).

Magnesium

Magnesium is an essential cation, found primarily in bone, muscle and soft tissue, with around 1% of the total body content in the ECF. As an important cofactor for numerous enzymes and ATP, it is critical in energy-requiring metabolic processes, protein synthesis, membrane integrity, nervous tissue conduction, neuromuscular excitability, muscle contraction, hormone secretion and in intermediary metabolism. Serum magnesium levels are usually maintained within a tight range (0.7–1.0 mmol/L). Although a serum concentration of less than this usually indicates some level of magnesium depletion, serum levels may be normal in spite of low intracellular magnesium due to magnesium depletion. Hypocalcaemia is a prominent manifestation of moderate to severe magnesium deficiency in humans.

Hypomagnesaemia

Hypomagnesaemia is frequently seen in critically ill patients. Causes include excessive gastro-intestinal losses, renal losses, surgery (particularly oesophageal), trauma, infection, malnutrition and sepsis. The drugs most likely to induce significant hypomagnesaemia are cisplatin, amphotericin B and ciclosporin, but it is also a potential complication of treatment with aminoglycosides, laxatives, pentamidine, tacrolimus and carboplatin. A hypomagnesaemic effect of furosemide and hydrochlorothiazide is questionable, and routine monitoring and treatment are not required. Use of digoxin has been associated with hypomagnesaemia, possibly by enhancing magnesium excretion, which may predispose to digoxin toxicity, for example, dysrhythmias.

Manifestations of hypomagnesaemia may include muscle tremor, cardiac arrhythmia, loss of appetite and fatigue. Where treatment is indicated, oral supplements are available, but because of their slow onset of action and gastro-intestinal intolerance, the intravenous route is often preferred and especially in critically ill patients with severe symptomatic hypomagnesaemia.

Hypermagnesaemia

Hypermagnesaemia is most commonly caused by renal insufficiency and excess iatrogenic magnesium administration. It may remain undetected for some time as around 80% remain unsymptomatic. Bradycardia, uncharacteristic ECG changes, hypotension and nausea and vomiting have been described in some cases.

Liver profile and associated tests

Routine liver function tests (LFTs), shown in Table 6.7, give information regarding the activity or concentrations of enzymes and compounds in serum, rather than quantifying specific hepatic functions. Therefore they must be interpreted in the context of the patient's characteristic and the pattern of the abnormalities. Results are useful in confirming or excluding a diagnosis of clinically suspected liver disease and monitoring its course.

Serum albumin levels and prothrombin time (PT) indicate hepatic protein synthesis; bilirubin is a marker of overall liver function. Transaminase levels indicate hepatocellular injury and death, whereas alkaline phosphatase levels estimate the amount of impedance of bile flow.

Bilirubin

At the end of their life, RBCs are broken down by the reticuloendothelial system, mainly in the spleen. The liberated haemoglobin molecules are split further into globin and haem. The

Table 6.7 Standard values in a liver profile

Laboratory test	Reference range
Liver function tests	
Albumin	34–50 g/L
Bilirubin	<19 mmol/L
ALT	<45 U/L
AST	<35 U/L
ALP	35–120 U/L
Amylase	<100 U/L
γ-GT	<70 U/L
Associated tests	
Ammonia	Male: 15–50 mmol/L Female: 10–40 mmol/L

ALT, alanine transaminase; AST, aspartate transaminase; ALP, alkaline phosphatase; γ-GT, gamma-glutamyl transpeptidase.

globin enters the general protein pool, the iron in haem is recycled, and the remaining tetrapyrrole ring of haem is degraded to bilirubin. Unconjugated bilirubin is lipophilic and is transported to the liver tightly bound to albumin. Unconjugated hyperbilirubinaemia in adults is most commonly the result of haemolysis, or Gilbert's syndrome resulting from genetic defects in UDP-glucuronyltransferase. It is actively taken up by hepatocytes, conjugated with glucuronic acid and excreted into bile. The conjugated bilirubin is water soluble and secreted rapidly into the gut, where it is broken down by bacteria into urobilinogen, a colourless compound, which is subsequently oxidised in the colon to urobilin, a brown pigment excreted in faeces. Some of the urobilinogen is absorbed, and most is subsequently re-excreted in bile (enterohepatic circulation). A small amount is absorbed into the systemic circulation and excreted in urine, where it too may be oxidised to urobilin. The presence of increased conjugated bilirubin is usually a sign of liver disease.

The liver produces 300 mg of bilirubin each day. However, because the mature liver can metabolise and excrete up to 3 g daily, serum bilirubin concentrations are not a sensitive test of liver function. As a screening test they rarely do other than confirm the presence or absence of jaundice. In chronic liver disease, however, changes in bilirubin concentrations over time do convey prognostic information.

An elevation of serum bilirubin concentration above 50 mmol/L (i.e. approximately 2.5 times the normal upper limit) will reveal itself as jaundice, seen best in the sclerae and skin. Elevated bilirubin levels can be caused by increased production of bilirubin (e.g. haemolysis, ineffective erythropoiesis), impaired transport into hepatocytes (e.g. interference with bilirubin uptake by drugs such as rifampicin or as a result of hepatitis), decreased excretion (e.g. with drugs such as rifampicin and methyltestosterone, intrahepatic obstruction caused by cirrhosis, tumours) or a combination of these factors.

The bilirubin in serum is normally unconjugated and bound to protein; it is not filtered by the glomeruli and does not normally appear in the urine. Bilirubin in the urine (bilirubinuria) is usually the result of an increase in serum concentration of conjugated bilirubin and indicates an underlying pathological disorder.

Enzymes

The enzymes measured in routine LFTs are listed in Table 6.7. Enzyme concentrations in the serum of healthy individuals are normally low. When cells are damaged, increased amounts of enzymes are detected as the intracellular contents are released into the blood.

It is important to remember that the assay of 'serum enzymes' is a measurement of catalytic activity and not actual enzyme concentration and that activity can vary depending on assay conditions. Consequently, the reference range may vary widely between laboratories.

While the measurement of enzymes may be very specific, the enzymes themselves may not be specific to a particular tissue or cell. Many enzymes arise in more than one tissue, and an increase in the serum activity of one enzyme can represent damage to any one of the tissues which contain the enzymes. In practice, this problem may be clarified because some tissues contain two or more enzymes in different proportions, which are released on damage. For example, alanine and aspartate transaminase both occur in cardiac muscle and liver cells, but their site of origin can often be differentiated because there is more alanine transaminase in the liver than in the heart. In those situations where it is not possible to look at the relative ratio of enzymes, it is sometimes possible to differentiate the same enzyme from different tissues. Such enzymes have the same catalytic activity but differ in some other measurable property and are referred to as isoenzymes.

The measured activity of an enzyme will be dependent on the time it is sampled relative to its time of release from the cell. If a sample is drawn too early after a particular insult to a tissue, there may be no detectable increase in enzyme activity. If it is drawn too late, the enzyme may have been cleared from the blood.

Transaminases

The two transaminases of diagnostic use are aspartate transaminase (AST), also known as aspartate aminotransferase, and alanine transaminase (ALT), also known as alanine aminotransferase. These enzymes catalyse the transfer of α-amino groups from aspartate and alanine to the α-keto group of ketoglutaric acid to generate oxaloacetic and pyruvic acid. They are found in many body tissues, with the highest concentration in hepatocytes and muscle cells. In the liver, ALT is localised solely in cytoplasm, whereas AST is cytosolic and mitochondrial.

Serum AST levels are increased in a variety of disorders, including liver disease, crush injuries, severe tissue hypoxia, myocardial infarction, surgery, trauma, muscle disease and pancreatitis. ALT is elevated to a similar extent in the disorders listed which involve the liver, although to a much lesser extent in the other disorders, making it more specific for liver damage. In the context of liver disease, increased transaminase activity indicates deranged integrity of hepatocyte plasma membranes and/or hepatocyte necrosis. They may be raised in all forms of viral and non-viral, acute and chronic liver disease, most markedly in acute viral, drug-induced (e.g. paracetamol poisoning), alcohol-related and ischaemic liver damage. Non-alcoholic fatty liver disease is now the most common cause of mild alteration of aminotransferase levels in the developed world.

Alkaline phosphatase

Alkaline phosphatase is an enzyme which transports metabolites across cell membranes. Alkaline phosphatases are found in the canalicular plasma membrane of hepatocytes, in bone where they reflect bone building or osteoblastic activity, and in the intestinal wall and placenta, kidneys and leucocytes. Hepatic alkaline phosphatase is also present on the surface of bile duct epithelia. Each site of origin produces a specific isoenzyme of alkaline phosphatase, which can be electrophoretically separated if concentrations are sufficiently high.

Disorders of the liver which can elevate alkaline phosphatase include intra- or extra-hepatic cholestasis, space-occupying lesions (e.g. tumour or abscess) and hepatitis. Drug-induced liver injury, for example, by ACE inhibitors or oestrogens, may present with a cholestatic pattern, that is, a preferential increase in alkaline phosphatase.

Physiological increases in serum alkaline phosphatase activity can also occur in pregnancy, as a result of release of the placental isoenzyme, and during periods of growth in children and adolescents when the bone isoenzyme is released.

Pathological increases in serum alkaline phosphatase of bone origin may arise in disorders such as osteomalacia and rickets, Paget's disease of bone, bone tumours, renal bone disease, osteomyelitis and healing fractures. Alkaline phosphatase is also raised as part of the acute-phase response; for example, intestinal alkaline phosphatase may be raised in active inflammatory bowel disease. If in doubt, the origin of the enzyme can be indicated by assessment of γ-glutamyl transpeptidase or electrophoresis to separate alkaline phosphatase isoenzymes.

γ-Glutamyl transpeptidase

γ-Glutamyl transpeptidase (gamma GT), also known as γ-glutamyl transferase, is present in high concentrations in the liver, kidney and pancreas, where it is found within the endoplasmic reticulum of cells. It is a sensitive indicator of hepatobiliary disease but does not differentiate a cholestatic disorder from hepatocellular disease. It can also be elevated in alcoholic liver disease, hepatitis, cirrhosis and non-hepatic disease such as pancreatitis, heart failure, chronic obstructive pulmonary disease and renal failure.

Serum levels of γ-glutamyl transpeptidase activity can be raised by enzyme induction by certain drugs, such as phenytoin, phenobarbital, rifampicin and oral contraceptives.

Serum γ-glutamyl transpeptidase activity is usually raised in an individual with alcoholic liver disease. However, it can also be raised in heavy drinkers of alcohol who do not have liver damage, as a result of enzyme induction. Its activity can remain elevated for up to 4 weeks after stopping alcohol intake.

Although it lacks specificity, it has a high sensitivity for liver disease and is thus useful for identifying the cause of a raised alkaline phosphatase level.

Albumin

Albumin is quantitatively the most important protein synthesised in the liver, with 10–15 g/day being produced in a healthy man. About 60% is located in the interstitial compartment of the ECF, with the remainder in the smaller, but relatively impermeable, serum compartment where it is present at a higher concentration. The concentration in the serum is important in maintaining its volume because it accounts for approximately 80% of serum colloid osmotic pressure. A reduction in serum albumin concentration often results in oedema as a result of fluid redistribution into the extravascular compartment.

Many molecules bind to albumin including calcium, bilirubin and many drugs (e.g. warfarin and phenytoin), and assays of these may need adjusting as a result. A reduction in serum albumin will increase free levels of agents which are normally bound, and adverse effects can result if the 'free' entity is not rapidly cleared from the body.

The serum concentration of albumin depends on its rate of synthesis, volume of distribution and rate of catabolism. Synthesis falls in parallel with increasing severity of liver disease or in malnutrition states where there is an inadequate supply of amino acids to maintain albumin production. Synthesis also decreases in response to inflammatory mediators such as interleukin. A low serum albumin concentration will occur when the volume of distribution of albumin increases, as happens, for example, in cirrhosis with ascites, in fluid-retention states such as pregnancy or where a shift of albumin from serum to interstitial fluid causes dilutional hypoalbuminaemia after parenteral infusion of excess protein-free fluid. The movement of albumin from serum into interstitial fluid is often associated with increased capillary permeability in postoperative patients or those with septicaemia.

Other causes of hypoalbuminaemia include catabolic states associated with a variety of illnesses and increased loss of albumin, either in urine from damaged kidneys, as occurs in the nephrotic syndrome, or via the skin following burns or a skin disorder such as psoriasis, or from the intestinal wall in a protein-losing enteropathy. The finding of hypoalbuminaemia and no other alteration in liver tests virtually rules out hepatic origin of this abnormality.

Albumin's serum half-life of approximately 20 days precludes its use as an indicator of acute change in liver function, but levels are of prognostic value in chronic disease.

An increase in serum albumin is rare and can be iatrogenic, for example, inappropriate infusion of albumin, or the result of dehydration or shock.

A shift of protein is known to occur physiologically when moving from lying down to the upright position. This can account for an increase in the serum albumin level of up to 10 g/L and can contribute to the variation in serum concentration of highly bound drugs which are therapeutically monitored.

Table 6.8 Normal values for calcium and phosphate

Laboratory test	Reference range
Calcium (total adjusted)	2.12–2.60 mmol/L
Calcium (ionised)	1.19–1.37 mmol/L
Phosphate	0.80–1.44 mmol/L

Amylase

The pancreas and salivary glands are the main producers of the digestive enzyme amylase. The serum amylase concentration rises within the first 24 hours of an attack of pancreatitis and then declines to normal over the following week. Although a number of abdominal and extra-abdominal conditions, including loss of bowel integrity through infarction or perforation, chronic alcoholism, postoperative states and renal failure, can result in a high amylase activity, in patients with the clinical picture of severe upper abdominal symptoms the specificity and sensitivity of an amylase level over 1000 U/L in the diagnosis of pancreatitis is more than 90%. There is a lack of prognostic significance of absolute values of amylase because values are directly related to the degree of pancreatic duct obstruction and inversely related to the severity of pancreatic disease.

Ammonia

The concentration of free ammonia in the blood is very tightly regulated and is exceeded by two orders of magnitude by its derivative, urea. The normal capacity for urea production far exceeds the rate of free ammonia production by protein catabolism under normal circumstances, such that any increase in free blood ammonia concentration is a reflection of either biochemical or pharmacological impairment of urea cycle function or fairly extensive hepatic damage. Clinical signs of hyperammonaemia occur at concentrations greater than 60 mmol/L and include anorexia, irritability, vomiting, somnolence, disorientation, asterixis, seizures, cerebral oedema, coma and death; the appearance of these findings is generally proportional to free ammonia concentration. Causes of hyperammonaemia include genetic defects in the urea cycle and disorders resulting in significant hepatic dysfunction. Ammonia plays an important role in the increase in brain water, which occurs in acute liver failure. Measurement of the blood ammonia concentration in the evaluation of patients with known or suspected hepatic encephalopathy can help in diagnosis and assessing the effect of treatment. Valproic acid can induce hyperammonaemic encephalopathy as one of its adverse neurological effects.

Calcium and phosphate

Calcium

Calcium distribution

The regulation of calcium and regulation of phosphate levels, whilst measured independently (Table 6.8), are undoubtedly interrelated. An adult contains around 1000 g of calcium, and

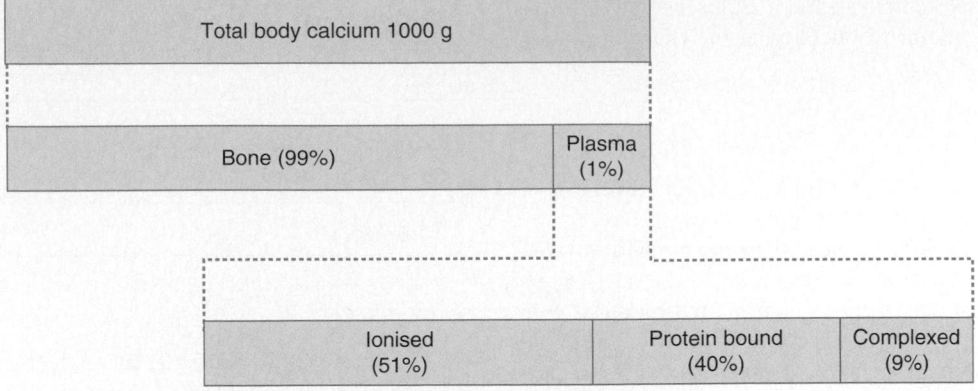

Fig. 6.5 Approximate distribution of calcium in a 70-kg adult.

Box 6.6	Formula for correction of total serum calcium concentration for changes in albumin concentration

For albumin < 40 g/L
$$\text{Corrected calcium} = [Ca] + 0.02 \times (40 - (alb)) \text{ mmol/L}$$

Albumin concentration = [alb] (albumin units = g/L);
calcium concentration = [Ca] (total calcium units = mmol/L)

Box 6.7	Drugs that are known to cause hypercalcaemia

- Thiazide diuretics
- Lithium
- Theophylline
- Tamoxifen
- Calcium supplements

more than 99% of this is bound within bone. Total calcium in the plasma is made up of ionised (which is free and biologically active), protein bound (predominantly to albumin but also to globulin) and complexed to anions like phosphates, sulphates, lactate and citrate (Fig. 6.5).

Calcium regulation

Calcium metabolism is regulated by parathyroid hormone (PTH), secreted by the parathyroid glands in response to a fall in serum calcium. PTH acts on the kidneys to increase tubular calcium reabsorption and bone resorption by activation of osteoclasts. PTH also stimulates the release of dihydroxycholecalciferol (vitamin D), which promotes gastro-intestinal absorption of calcium from the duodenum. PTH is under negative feedback control: as calcium increases, PTH decreases.

The serum calcium level is often determined by measuring total calcium, that is, both free and bound calcium. Normal values can be seen in Table 6.8. Changes in albumin can result in changes of the total calcium concentration while the ionised calcium remains unchanged. Therefore, measurement of free ionised calcium is important. Decreased total calcium with normal ionised calcium is referred to as pseudohypocalcaemia. Various equations are available to estimate the calcium concentration, and many laboratories report total and adjusted calcium routinely. A commonly used formula is shown in Box 6.6. Caution must be taken when using such a formula in the presence of disturbed blood hydrogen ion concentrations.

Acid–base balance plays a role in ionised calcium levels; alkalosis decreases ionised calcium levels, as hydrogen ions dissociate from albumin, and calcium binding to albumin increases, together with an increase in complex formation. If the concentration of ionised calcium falls sufficiently, clinical symptoms of hypocalcaemia may occur despite the total serum calcium concentration being unchanged. The reverse effect, that is, increased ionised calcium, occurs in acidosis.

Hypercalcaemia

Hypercalcaemia may be caused by a variety of disorders, the most common being primary hyperparathyroidism, often a single adenoma secreting excess PTH. Hypercalcaemia can also be as a result of malignancy, for example, in multiple myeloma or boney metastases as a result of increased osteoclast activity leading to increased bone resorption. However, in squamous carcinoma of the bronchus, hypercalcaemia occurs as a result of a peptide with PTH-like activity that is released by the tumour. Hypercalcaemia is also observed in thyrotoxicosis, vitamin A, vitamin D intoxication and sarcoidosis. PTH measurement can be pivotal in the establishment of the cause of hypercalcaemia. Drugs that can cause hypercalcaemia are shown in Box 6.7.

An artefactual increase in total serum calcium may sometimes be seen as a result of a tourniquet being applied during venous sampling. The resulting venous stasis may cause redistribution of fluid from the vein into the extravascular space, and the temporary haemoconcentration will affect albumin levels.

Clinical features and management. Hypercalcaemia can present with symptoms of general malaise, depression, bone pain, abdominal pain and renal stones and is classically described by 'moans, stones, groans and bones'. Mild hypercalcaemia (Ca^{2+} < 3 mmol/L) is often asymptomatic.

Management of acute hypercalcaemia involves correction of any dehydration with intravenous fluid (sodium chloride 0.9%). Following rehydration intravenous bisphosphonates, for example, zoledronic acid or pamidronate, are given to inhibit bone

Box 6.8   Drugs that are known to cause hypocalcaemia

- Aminoglycosides
- Bisphosphonates
- Calcitonin
- Caspofungin
- Cisplatin
- Denosumab
- Furosemide
- Phenobarbital
- Phenytoin

Table 6.9   Standard values of inflammatory markers

Laboratory test	Reference range
Erythrocyte sedimentation rate (ESR)	Younger adults <15 mm/h Male over 50 <20 mm/h Female over 50 <30 mm/h
C-reactive protein (CRP)	<5 mg/L
Procalcitonin	<0.05 ng/mL

turnover. Further treatment options include glucocorticoids (inhibit 1,25-$[OH]_2D_3$ production) or calcitonin.

Hypocalcaemia

Hypocalcaemia occurs mainly as a result of disorders of PTH or vitamin D. Inadequate intake of oral calcium is rarely the cause, whereas absorptive hypocalcaemia can occur as a result of dietary insufficiency of vitamin D or impaired production of vitamin D as seen in chronic kidney disease. Hypoparathyroidism, as a result of surgery or autoimmune conditions, results in decreased PTH production, which can be a cause of hypocalcaemia. Other causes include pancreatitis, reduced exposure to sunlight, acid–base disturbance and hypoalbuminaemia. Drugs that have been implicated as causing hypocalcaemia are shown in Box 6.8.

Clinical features. Hypocalcaemia results in increased excitability of nerves. It can present with numbness, commonly around the mouth and in the peripheries; later signs include cramps, tetany, convulsions and death.

Phosphate

Phosphate distribution

An adult contains around 700 g of phosphate, and 85% is in bone, where it is complexed with calcium. Phosphate is an intracellular anion, and its concentration is 100-fold higher than in the plasma.

Phosphate regulation

Phosphorus is an essential element and has roles in cell structure, cellular metabolism (ATP generation), cellular signalling, bone mineralisation and acid–base balance. Serum levels are regulated by absorption from the diet (both passive and active uptake). Vitamin D increases active absorption from the gut and bone, whereas PTH controls excretion by the kidneys and resorption from bone. Fibroblast growth factor 23, a phosphatonin, is released in response to hyperphosphatemia and reduces renal reabsorption of phosphate.

Hyperphosphataemia

Hyperphosphataemia occurs in chronic renal failure and is reduced by dietary phosphate binders. Less common causes are secondary to rhabdomyolysis, tumour lysis or severe haemolysis. Hyperphosphataemia can cause hypocalcaemia as a result of binding of calcium to phosphate. Treatment of hyperphosphataemia requires identification and correction of the underlying cause.

Hypophosphataemia

Severe hypophosphataemia can cause general debility, anorexia, anaemia, muscle weakness and wasting and some bone pain and skeletal wasting. Because phosphorus is ubiquitous in various foods, inadequate dietary phosphorus intake requires near starvation. Refeeding of those recovering from energy depletion, as a result of alcoholic bouts or diabetic ketoacidosis without adequate provision of phosphorus, can precipitate hypophosphataemia.

Inflammatory markers

The inflammatory process can be measured using a number of biochemical markers, including erythrocyte sedimentation rate, C-reactive protein and procalcitonin (Table 6.9).

Erythrocyte sedimentation rate

The erythrocyte sedimentation rate (ESR) is a measure of the settling rate of RBCs in a sample of anticoagulated blood, over a period of 1 hour, in a cylindrical tube. The ESR strongly correlates with the ability of RBCs to aggregate into orderly stacks or rouleaux. In disease, the most common cause of a high ESR is an increased protein level in the blood, such as the increase in acute-phase proteins seen in inflammatory diseases. Proteins are thought to affect the repellent surface charges on RBCs and cause them to aggregate into rouleaux, and hence the sedimentation rate increases.

In children, the normal value is often less than 10 mm/h, but normal values do rise with age. A normal ESR for men and women over 50 years old is 20 mm/h and 30 mm/h, respectively. The Westergren method, performed under standardised conditions, is commonly used. Although some conditions may cause a low ESR, the test is principally used to monitor inflammatory diseases such as rheumatoid arthritis, inflammatory bowel disease, malignancy and infection. The ESR is non-specific and, therefore, of little diagnostic value, but serial tests can be helpful in following the progress of disease and its response to treatment

C-reactive protein

C-reactive protein (CRP) is an acute-phase protein and named for its capacity to precipitate the somatic C-polysaccharide of *Streptococcus pneumoniae*. This nonspecific acute-phase response is instigated by tissue damage, infection, inflammation and malignancy. Production of CRP is rapidly and sensitively upregulated in hepatocytes under the control of cytokine (IL-6) originating at the site of pathology. CRP is recognised by, and subsequently activates, the complement system whilst also generating proinflammatory cytokines and aiding in the activation of the adaptive immune system.

Serum concentrations rise by about 6 hours, peaking around 48 hours. The serum half-life is around 19 hours, so serum level is determined by synthesis rate, which therefore reflects the intensity of the pathological process stimulating this, and falls rapidly when this ceases. CRP values are not diagnostic and can only be interpreted with the knowledge of all other clinical and pathological results. In most diseases, the circulating value of CRP reflects ongoing inflammation or tissue damage more accurately than other acute-phase parameters, such as serum viscosity or ESR. Drugs including HMG-CoA reductase inhibitors ('statins') have been shown to reduce CRP values potentially by affecting the underlying pathology providing the acute-phase stimulus.

Procalcitonin

Procalcitonin, a polypeptide, is one of many bloodstream biomarkers investigated as an early predictor of sepsis. It is produced rapidly in response to bacterial stimulus but not in systemic inflammatory response syndrome of noninfectious origin. Diagnostic thresholds for a positive procalcitonin, indicative of sepsis, have been proposed between 1.0 and 2.0 ng/mL. Although this approach has been demonstrated to change clinical practice in the diagnosis and treatment of sepsis, it is not yet embedded in routine practice.

Special tests

Several standalone tests are not routinely included in the various profiles discussed so far but are essential to the diagnosis and monitoring of certain conditions (Table 6.10).

Glucose

The serum glucose concentration is largely determined by the balance of glucose moving into, and leaving, the extracellular compartment. In a healthy adult, this movement and cellular metabolism are capable of maintaining serum levels below 10 mmol/L, regardless of the intake of meals of varying carbohydrate content.

The renal tubules have the capacity to reabsorb glucose from the glomerular filtrate via sodium glucose cotransporters (SGLT2), and minimal glucose is normally lost from the body. Glucose in the urine (glycosuria) is normally only present when the concentration in serum exceeds 10 mmol/L, the renal threshold for total reabsorption.

Table 6.10 Standard values of specialist tests

Laboratory test	Reference range
Glucose (fasting)	3.3–6.0 mmol/L
HbA$_{1C}$ (DCCT)	4–6%
HbA$_{1C}$ (IFCC)	20–42 mmol/mol
Glycosylated haemoglobin (HbA$_{1c}$)	4–5.9%
Troponin I (99th percentile of upper reference limit)	<0.04 microgram/L
Lactate dehydrogenase (LDH)	240–480 U/L
Beta-D-glucan (BDG)	<6 pg/mL
D-dimer	<0.5 microgram/mL
Creatine kinase (CK)	Male: 30–200 U/L Female: 20–170 U/L
Uric acid	180–420 mmol/L

DCCT, Diabetes Control and Complications Trial; IFFC, International Federation for Clinical Chemistry.

Capillary blood glucose testing using a finger-tip sample is the mainstay of routine serum glucose monitoring. Serum glucose concentrations are also displayed routinely on arterial blood gas reports.

Normal ranges for serum glucose concentrations are often quoted as non-fasting (<11.1 mmol/L) or fasting (3.3–6.0 mmol/L) concentration ranges. Fasting serum glucose levels between 6.1 and 7.0 mmol/L indicate impaired glucose tolerance. When symptoms are typical of diabetes, a fasting level above 7.0 mmol/L or a 2-hour post-glucose or random serum glucose level ≥11.1 mmol/L is consistent with a diagnosis of diabetes. Other signs and symptoms, if present, are notably those attributable to an osmotic diuresis and will suggest clinically the diagnosis of diabetes mellitus.

Glycated haemoglobin

Glucose binds to a part of the haemoglobin molecule to form a small glycated fraction. Normally, about 5% of haemoglobin is glycated, but this amount is dependent on the average blood glucose concentration over the lifespan of the RBCs (about 120 days), and where RBC lifespan is reduced, this leads to low glycated haemoglobin levels. The major component of the glycated fraction is referred to as HbA$_{1C}$.

Measurement of HbA$_{1C}$ is well established as an indicator of chronic glycaemic control in patients with diabetes. Guidelines for the diagnosis and monitoring of diabetes now stipulate that methods for measuring HbA$_{1c}$ must have been calibrated to the International Federation for Clinical Chemistry (IFCC) standardisation. These newer laboratory methods have a higher specificity for HbA$_{1c}$, and so results cannot be directly compared with the old Diabetes Control and Complications Trial (DCCT) method (National Institute for Health and Care

Excellence [NICE], 2015). One method adopted for preventing direct comparison is by moving to standard units of mmol/mol. Some reports will also report a percentage, comparable to the older assay, which is by a conversion calculation rather than performing both tests.

Cardiac markers

Troponins

Cardiac troponin I (cTnI) and cardiac troponin T (cTnT) are regulatory proteins that control the calcium-mediated interaction between actin and myosin in cardiac muscle. Both are comparable in diagnostic and prognostic efficacy, and the local decision may be a balance between cost and specific assay performance. Troponins offer extremely high cardiac tissue specificity and clinical sensitivity for myocardial necrosis but do not discriminate between ischaemic and non-ischaemic mechanisms, including myocarditis, cardiac surgery and sepsis.

Conventional approved cTn assays display a coefficient of variance of less than 20%. The major international cardiac societies (Daubert and Jeremias, 2010) define myocardial infarction through the detection of a 20% rise or fall with respect to the 99th percentile of the upper reference limit plus one of the following:

1. Symptoms of ischaemia
2. ECG evidence of ischaemia (e.g. ST-elevation or left bundle branch block)
3. Cardiac imaging findings consistent with ischaemia
4. Identification of an intracoronary thrombus by angiography

Sampling of cTn at two time points, usually admission and 12 hours from the worst pain, is usually needed, although if it is entirely clear that there has been a myocardial infarction, particularly in a late presentation, a second sample may not be needed. Newer high-sensitivity tests have much lower variance (≤10%) and, unlike conventional assays, can detect baseline cTn in healthy individuals. High sensitivity tests require careful interpretation through sex-specific reference ranges but potentially reduce the time to diagnosis through shorter sampling intervals (3–6 hours between the first and second test).

Lactate dehydrogenase

Lactate dehydrogenase (LDH) has five isoenzymes (LD1–LD5). Total LDH activity is rarely measured because of the lack of tissue specificity. Levels of activity are elevated following damage to the liver, skeletal muscle and kidneys, in both megaloblastic and immune haemolytic anaemias, and in intravascular haemolysis as seen in thrombotic thrombocytopenic purpura and paroxysmal nocturnal haemoglobinuria. In lymphoma, a high LDH activity indicates a poor prognosis. Elevation of LD1 and LD2 occurs after myocardial infarction, renal infarction or megaloblastic anaemia; LD2 and LD3 are elevated in acute leukaemia; LD3 is often elevated in some malignancies; and LD5 is elevated after damage to liver or skeletal muscle.

Beta-D-glucan

Beta-D-glucan (BDG) is a cell wall component released by most fungi and as such can be used as a serum marker of invasive fungal infection. BDG has been shown to have good diagnostic accuracy for identifying invasive fungal infections, particularly those attributable to *Candida* or *Aspergillus* species.

D-dimers

D-dimers are degradation products of fibrin clots, formed by the sequential action of three enzymes, thrombin, factor XIIIa and plasmin, which degrades cross-linked fibrin to release fibrin degradation products and expose the D-dimer antigen. D-dimer assays measure an epitope on fibrin degradation products using monoclonal antibodies. Because each has its own unique specificity, there is no standard unit of measurement or performance. Levels of D-dimers in the blood are raised in conditions associated with coagulation and are used to detect venous thromboembolism, although they are influenced by the presence of comorbid conditions such as cancer, surgery and infectious diseases. D-dimer measurement has been most comprehensively validated in the exclusion of venous thromboembolism in certain patient populations and in the diagnosis and monitoring of coagulation activation in disseminated intravascular coagulation. Diagnosis of deep vein thrombosis (DVT) or pulmonary embolism (PE) should include a clinical probability assessment as well as D-dimer measurements. In patients with a low clinical probability of pulmonary embolism, a negative quantitative D-dimer test result effectively excludes PE. In suspected DVTs, D-dimer measurements combined with a clinical prediction score and compression ultrasonography study have a high predictive value. More recently, assays are being used in the prediction of the risk of venous thromboembolism (VTE) recurrence.

Xanthochromia

Xanthochromia is a yellow discolouration of cerebrospinal fluid caused by haemoglobin catabolism. It is thought to arise within several hours of subarachnoid haemorrhage (SAH) and can help to distinguish the elevated RBC count observed after traumatic lumbar puncture from that observed following SAH, particularly if few RBCs are present. Spectrophotometry is used to detect the presence of both oxyhaemoglobin and bilirubin, both of which contribute to xanthochromia following SAH, although some hospitals rely on visual inspection.

Creatine kinase

Creatine kinase (CK) is an enzyme present in relatively high concentrations in the heart muscle, skeletal muscle and brain, in addition to being present in smooth muscle. Levels are markedly increased following shock and circulatory failure, myocardial infarction and muscular dystrophies. Less marked increases have been reported following muscle injury, surgery,

Table 6.11 Medications and toxic substances that increase the risk of rhabdomyolysis

Direct myotoxicity	Indirect muscle damage
HMG-CoA reductase inhibitors, especially in combination with fibrate-derived lipid-lowering agents such as niacin (nicotinic acid)	Alcohol
	Central nervous system depressants
	Cocaine
Ciclosporin	Amphetamine
Itraconazole	Ecstasy (MDMA)
Erythromycin	LSD
Colchicine	Neuromuscular blocking agents
Zidovudine	
Corticosteroids	

HMG-CoA, 3-Hydroxy-3-methylglutaryl coenzyme A; LSD, lysergic acid diethylamide; MDMA, methylene dioxymethamphetamine.

Table 6.12 Standard values in iron, B$_{12}$ and folate

Laboratory test	Reference range
Iron studies	
Iron	11–29 mmol/L
Ferritin	15–300 micrograms/L
Transferrin	1.7–3.4 g/L
Transferrin saturation	20–50%
Associated tests	
Folate	2.7–21.0 ng/mL
B$_{12}$	0.13–0.68 nmol/L

physical exercise, muscle cramp, an epileptic fit, intramuscular injection and hypothyroidism. The most important adverse effects associated with statins are myopathy and an increase in hepatic transaminases, both of which occur infrequently. Statin-associated myopathy represents a broad clinical spectrum of disorders, from mild muscle aches to severe pain and restriction in mobility, with grossly elevated CK levels. In rhabdomyolysis, a potentially life-threatening syndrome resulting from the breakdown of skeletal muscle fibres as a result of, for example, ischaemic crush injury where large quantities of CK are measurable in the blood with the level of CK predicting the developments of acute renal failure. Medications and toxic substances that increase the risk of rhabdomyolysis are shown in Table 6.11.

CK has two protein subunits, M and B, which combine to form three isoenzymes, BB, MM and MB. BB is found in high concentrations in the brain, thyroid and some smooth muscle tissue. Little of this enzyme is present in the serum, even following damage to the brain. The enzyme found in serum of normal subjects is the MM isoenzyme, which originates from skeletal muscle.

Cardiac tissue contains more of the MB isoenzyme than skeletal muscle. Following a myocardial infarction there is a characteristic increase in serum CK activity. Although measurement of activity of the MB isoenzyme was used in the past to detect myocardial damage, cardiac troponin measurement is now the preferred biomarker.

In some diseases, such as chronic lymphatic leukaemia, lymphoma and multiple myeloma, a discrete, densely staining band (paraprotein) can be seen in the γ region. In multiple myeloma, abnormal fragments of immunoglobulins are produced (Bence–Jones protein), which clear the glomerulus and are found in the urine.

Uric acid

The production of uric acid, the end product of purine metabolism, is catalysed by xanthine oxidase, an enzyme linked to oxidative stress, endothelial dysfunction and heart failure. The purines, which are used for nucleic acid synthesis, are produced by the breakdown of nucleic acid from ingested meat or synthesised within the body.

Monosodium urate is the form in which uric acid usually exists at the normal pH of body fluids. The term *urate* is used to represent any salt of uric acid.

Two main factors contribute to elevated serum uric acid levels: an increased rate of formation or a reduced excretion. Uric acid is poorly soluble, and an elevation in serum concentration can readily result in deposition, as monosodium urate in tissues or joints. Deposition usually precipitates an acute attack of gouty arthritis. The aim of treatment is to reduce the concentration of uric acid and prevent further attacks of gout. It has been hypothesised that measurement of urate could serve as a marker of cardiovascular risk because the serum uric acid level is an independent predictor of all causes of mortality in patients at high risk of cardiovascular disease, independent of diuretic use.

Immunoglobulins

Immunoglobulins are antibodies which are produced by B lymphocytes. They are detected by electrophoresis as bands in three regions: α, β and γ, with most occurring in the γ region. Hypergammaglobulinaemia may result from stimulation of B cells and produces an increased staining of bands in the γ region on electrophoresis. This occurs in infections, chronic liver disease and autoimmune disease.

Iron, transferrin and iron binding

Iron

Iron (Table 6.12) is a trace element and required for numerous cellular functions, but it is particularly important in cells producing haemoglobin and myoglobin. The adult body contains 3–4 g of iron, around 70% in heme compounds (e.g. haemoglobin). Iron circulates in the blood bound to transferrin, which transports it to the bone marrow, where it is incorporated into haemoglobin in developing RBCs. Iron intake from the diet is around 1–2 mg/day, whereas 40–60 mg/day is derived from the reticuloendothelial system from senescent red blood cells.

Serum iron levels are extremely labile and fluctuate throughout the day and, therefore, provide little useful information about iron status.

Iron balance is regulated by hepcidin, a circulating peptide hormone, which aims to provide iron as needed whilst avoiding excess iron promoting the formation of toxic oxygen radicals. Genetic iron overload results from mutations in molecules which regulate hepcidin production or activity.

Ferritin

Ferritin is an iron storage protein found in cell cytosol. It acts as a depot, accepting excess iron and allowing for mobilisation of iron when needed. Serum ferritin measurement is the test of choice in patients suspected of having iron-deficiency anaemia.

In normal individuals, the serum ferritin concentration is directly related to the available storage iron in the body. The serum ferritin level falls below the normal range in iron-deficiency anaemia, and its measurement can provide a useful monitor for repletion of iron stores after iron therapy. Raised ferritin can occur as a result of raised iron stores, but ferritin is an acute-phase protein and is released from damaged hepatocytes. Levels therefore can be raised in inflammatory disorders, liver disease or malignancy.

Transferrin

Transferrin, a simple polypeptide chain with two iron binding sites, is the plasma iron binding protein which facilitates its delivery to cells bearing transferrin receptors. Measurement of total iron binding capacity (TIBC), from which the percentage of transferrin saturation with iron may be calculated, gives more information. Saturation of 20% or lower is usually taken to indicate an iron deficiency, as is a raised TIBC of greater than 70 mmol/L.

Vitamin B$_{12}$ and folate

In the haematology literature, B$_{12}$ refers not only to cyanocobalamin but also to several other cobalamins with identical nutritional properties. Folic acid, which can designate a specific compound, pteroylglutamic acid, is also more commonly used as a general term for the folates. Deficiency of cobalamin can result both in macrocytic anaemia and neurological disease, including neuropathies, dementia and psychosis. Folate deficiency produces macrocytic anaemia, depression, dementia and neural tube defects.

Liver disease tends to increase B$_{12}$ levels, and they may be reduced in folate-deficient patients; malabsorption of B$_{12}$ may result from long-term ingestion of antacids, proton-pump inhibitors and H$_2$-receptor antagonists, or biguanides (e.g. metformin). Serum folate levels tend to increase in B$_{12}$ deficiency, and alcohol can reduce levels. RBC folate is a better measure of folate tissue stores.

Table 6.13 Tumour markers and their clinical application

Tumour marker	Primary malignancy	Clinical application
Prostate-specific antigen (PSA)	Prostate	Primary screening, determining prognosis and monitoring therapy
CA 125	Ovarian	Primary screening, determining prognosis and monitoring therapy
CA 19-9	Pancreatic	Monitoring therapy
CA 15-3	Breast	Monitoring therapy
Human chorionic gonadotropin (HCG)	Trophoblastic	Primary screening, determining prognosis and monitoring therapy
Human epidermal growth factor receptor 2 (HER-2)	Breast	Predicting response to therapy
Alpha-fetoprotein (AFP)	Hepatocellular	Primary screening and monitoring therapy
Pepsinogen	Gastric	Primary screening

Tumour markers

Tumour markers are defined as a qualitative or quantitative alteration or deviation from normal of a molecule, substance or process that can be detected by some form of assay above and beyond routine clinical and pathological evaluation. They may be detected within malignant cells, in surrounding stroma or metastases, or as soluble products in blood, secretions or excretions. In order to be useful clinically, the precise use of the marker in altering clinical management should have been defined by data based on a reliable assay and a validated clinical outcome trial.

Tumour markers could potentially be used in the diagnosis of cancers in asymptomatic individuals; however, they are more commonly used in contributing to the diagnosis in symptomatic patients. Tumour markers may be used to differentiate between benign and malignant disease (e.g. prostate-specific antigen), predicting response to therapeutic agents (e.g. human epidermal growth factor receptor-2 for trastuzumab therapy) and assessing prognosis following surgical removal (Table 6.13).

Arterial blood gases

Arterial blood gas analysis provides a rapid and accurate assessment of oxygenation, alveolar ventilation and acid–base status (Table 6.14), the three processes which maintain pH homeostasis.

Table 6.14 Standard values for arterial blood gases

Laboratory test	Reference range
Arterial blood gas	
pH	7.35–7.45
$PaCO_2$	4.6–6.1 kPa
PaO_2	10.6–13.3 kPa
HCO_3^-	22–28 mmol/L
BE	±2 mmol/L

BE, Base excess; HCO_3^- bicarbonate; $PaCO_2$, arterial partial pressure of carbon dioxide; PaO_2, arterial partial pressure of oxygen.

Box 6.9 Henderson–Hasselbalch equation

$$pH = pK_a + \log\frac{A^-}{HA}$$

A^-, molar concentration of this acid's conjugate base (HCO_3^-); HA, molar concentration of the dissociated weak acid (H_2CO_3); pH, plasma pH; pK_a, cologarithm of the dissociation constant of carbonic acid.

pH

A normal physiological pH (7.4) is required for many physiological functions, from enzymatic function to influencing oxygen release from haemoglobin. An acidosis is indicated by a pH less than 7.35; an alkalosis by a pH greater than 7.45. Two compensatory mechanisms exist to maintain the optimum physiological pH: the regulation of carbon dioxide concentration in the blood by the lungs (respiratory) and the excretion of hydrogen ions or reabsorption of bicarbonate by the kidneys (metabolic). Bicarbonate in the blood acts as an intermediary buffer, which is best represented by the Henderson–Hasselbalch equation (Box 6.9).

Carbon dioxide

The maintenance of arterial CO_2 tension ($PaCO_2$) depends on the quantity of CO_2 produced in the body and its removal through alveolar ventilation. High $PaCO_2$ (>6.1 kPa) indicates alveolar hypoventilation and without compensation would result in a respiratory acidosis. Low $PaCO_2$ (<4.5 kPa) implies alveolar hyperventilation and would in isolation result in a respiratory alkalosis.

Oxygenation

The adequate delivery of oxygen to the tissues depends on the cardiopulmonary system, PaO_2, oxygen fraction in inspired air (FiO_2) and haemoglobin content and its affinity for oxygen. Oxygen saturation is measured by pulse oximetry or by arterial blood gas analysis. Hypoxaemia is defined as a PaO_2 of less than 12 kPa at sea level in an adult patient breathing room air ($FiO_2 = 0.21$).

Table 6.15 Arterial blood gas interpretation

Step 1: Acidosis/ alkalosis	Acidosis (pH < 7.35)		Alkalosis (pH > 7.4)	
Step 2: Primary cause	Respiratory pCO_2 > 6.1 kPa	Metabolic HCO_3^- < 22 mmol/L	Respiratory pCO_2 < 4.6 kPa	Metabolic HCO_3^- > 28 mmol/L
Examples	COPD Guillain– Barre	DKA Sepsis Aspirin overdose	PE Anxiety	Diuretic use Severe vomiting
Step 3: Compen- sation	Metabolic HCO_3^- > 28 mmol/L	Respiratory pCO_2 < 4.6 kPa	Metabolic HCO_3^- < 22 mmol/L	Respiratory pCO_2 > 6.1 kPa

COPD, Chronic obstructive pulmonary disease; DKA, diabetic ketoacidosis; HCO_3^-, bicarbonate; $PaCO_2$, arterial partial pressure of carbon dioxide; PE, pulmonary embolus.

Bicarbonate

A raised bicarbonate on its own would cause metabolic alkalosis; a reduced bicarbonate metabolic acidosis. Bicarbonate is not the only base in the system, and the base deficit quantifies the amount of bicarbonate that theoretically must be added (or taken away) to achieve physiological pH. The base excess (BE) describes this explanation in reverse or the negative base deficit (BE = –[BD]).

Interpreting arterial blood gases

Arterial blood gases should always be interpreted in clinical context and not in isolation. The configuration of various parameters in the arterial blood gases can lead to a high suspicion of certain diagnoses combined with relevant signs and symptoms (Table 6.15).

The respiratory system can compensate for a metabolic abnormality and vice versa. This may not be seen immediately because whilst modification of the respiratory rate can occur within minutes, the renal response may take several days.

Case studies

Case 6.1

A 78-year-old man, Mr KB, with a history of atrial fibrillation on digoxin and apixaban is admitted with a 2-day history of vomiting, headache, dizziness and palpitations. He was recently started on furosemide for worsening leg oedema which was particularly troubling him. The results of his admission blood tests are as follows:

Sodium	135 mmol/L	(135–145 mmol/L)
Potassium	2.5 mmol/L	(3.4–5.0 mmol/L)
Creatinine	140 mmol/L	(75–155 mmol/L)
Urea	12 mmol/L	(3.1–7.9 mmol/L)

Questions

1. What is a possible diagnosis?
2. What additional tests might you perform to confirm your diagnosis?
3. Why has this occurred?
4. Mr KB is given 1 L of sodium chloride 0.9% with 40 mmol of potassium. A further sample shows a sodium of 152 mmol/L and potassium of 5.7 mmol/L. What has caused this?

Answers

1. Digoxin toxicity precipitated by hypokalaemia
2. Serum digoxin levels would be useful in confirming this diagnosis. The timing since the last dose should be confirmed if possible to ensure that the result is relevant. Other features of toxicity could include bradycardia, diarrhoea, yellow vision and rash. An ECG may display down-sloping ST-segment depression also known as the 'reverse tick'.
3. The initiation of furosemide has increased potassium excretion, which has not been sufficiently replaced. The resulting hypokalaemia has precipitated digoxin toxicity.
4. Beware of sudden changes in consecutive samples; always ask if they have been taken appropriately. The follow-up sample was taken from the line being used to infuse the fluid, giving an artificially high value of both electrolytes.

Case 6.2

A 23-year-old woman, Miss CB, is bought to the emergency department by ambulance late on a Friday night. Her respiratory rate is 10 breaths/min, and she is unconscious. Her arterial blood gas shows the following:

pH	7.25	(7.35–7.45)
PaCO$_2$	8.2 kPa	(4.6–6.1 kPa)
PaO$_2$	8.6 kPa	(10.6–13.3 kPa)
Bicarbonate	26 mmol/L	(22–28 mmol/L)

Questions

1. Describe Miss CB's acid–base status.
2. When trying to place an intravenous cannula, you notice injection marks on the inside of the arms and groin. On further examination, Miss CB has pinpoint pupils. What is the most likely diagnosis?
3. What treatment would you consider?

Answers

1. Respiratory acidosis with no metabolic compensation
2. Opiate overdose produces a respiratory acidosis by depressing respiratory drive. Hypoventilation causes accumulation of carbon dioxide, which tips the balance towards acidosis. The lack of compensation by the renal mechanism demonstrates the acute nature of this presentation.
3. A trial dose of naloxone, a competitive and specific opioid antagonist, would be expected to improve respiration if the intoxication was caused by an opiate overdose alone. Repeated doses or an infusion may be necessary because of the short half-life of the antidote.

Case 6.3

A 35-year-old obese information technology (IT) worker, Mr JC, complains of general aches and pains over the past few months. His friend has said that he has not been himself for the past few weeks and appears 'under the weather'. A blood sample was taken and a bone profile requested; the results are as follows:

Ca^{2+}	4.01 mmol/L	
Ca^{2+} (corrected)	4.09 mmol/L	(2.12–2.60 mmol/L)
Phosphate	0.41 mmol/L	(0.80–144 mmol/L)
Albumin	41 g/L	(34–50 g/L)

Questions

1. What is the cause of Mr JC's symptoms?
2. What further test would you request?
3. If that test returns high, what is the diagnosis?
4. How would you treat the patient?

Answers

1. Mr JC has hypercalcaemia. Patients with a high calcium often present with 'bones, stones and moans'.
2. Parathyroid releasing hormone (PTH)
3. A raised PTH would suggest a primary hyperparathyroidism, although a normal PTH would still be abnormal because PTH is under a negative feedback control from calcium. This is suggestive of a parathyroid adenoma that is producing PTH.
4. Management of hypercalcaemia includes i.v. rehydration with sodium chloride 0.9% and, following rehydration, the addition of an i.v. bisphosphonate. Ultimately, surgical removal of the parathyroid adenoma would be indicated.

Case 6.4

A 34-year-old aid worker, Miss AS, has just returned from Africa, having become increasingly unwell over the last month. She has been feverish on and off for the last 4 weeks with a worsening headache and abdominal pain, and she has noticed a yellow discolouration to her eyes. Miss AS's initial blood test shows the following:

Haemoglobin	8.5 g/L	(115–165 g/L)
Platelets	60 × 10^9/L	(150–450 × 10^9/L)
WBC	11.5 × 10^9/L	(4.0–11.0 × 10^9/L)
MCV	90 fL	(83–101 fL)
MCH	30 pg	(27–34 pg)

Questions

1. Describe this haematology profile.
2. What additional tests should be requested?
3. Given the clinical picture, what would you expect to see in these tests?

Answers

1. This profile shows a normocytic normochromic anemia with thrombocytopenia.
2. Liver function tests would be useful given Miss AS's possible jaundice and nonspecific abdominal pain. Given her recent travel, consideration must be given to various tropical diseases.
3. The clinical picture of jaundice would suggest a bilirubin of more than 50 mmol/L, over which it is usually detectable. Combined with her normocytic normochromic anaemia, Miss AS has a high probability of malaria where jaundice in adults can be attributable to a cholestatic picture. It is likely that the ALP and gamma-GT would also be raised whilst transaminases may be normal. Further specific investigations would be needed to confirm a diagnosis of malaria.

Acknowledgement

The authors acknowledge the contribution of H. A. Wynne and C. Edwards to versions of this chapter which appeared in previous editions.

References

Bahuleyan, B., 2015. Hemostasis: a cell based model. J. Phys. Pharm. Adv. 5 (5), 638–642.

Daubert, M.A., Jeremias, A., 2010. The utility of troponin measurement to detect myocardial infarction: review of the current findings Vasc. Health. Risk. Manag. 6, 691–699.

Hoffman, M., Monroe, D.M., 2001. A cell-based model of haemostasis. Thromb. Haemost. 85 (6), 958–965.

Jones, G.R.D., 2011. Estimating renal function for drug dosing decisions. Clin. Biochem. Rev. 32 (2), 81–88.

National Institute for Health and Care Excellence (NICE), 2015. Type 2 diabetes in adults: management. Available at: https://www.nice.org.uk/guidance/ng28.

Further reading

Benes, J., Zatloukal, J., Kletecka, J., 2015. Viscoelastic methods of blood clotting assessment – a multidisciplinary review. Front. Med. 14 (2), 62. https://doi.org/10.3389/fmed.2015.00062.

Broomhead, R.H., Mallett, S.V., 2013. Clinical aspects of coagulation and haemorrhage. Anaesth. Intensive Care Med. 14 (2), 57–62.

Hoffbrand, A.V., Moss, P.A.H. (Eds.), 2015. Hoffbrand's Essential Haematology, seventh ed. Wiley-Blackwell, Oxford.

Marshall, W.J., Lapsley, M., Day, A. (Eds.), 2016. Clinica Chemistry, eighth ed. Elsevier, Amsterdam.

Useful websites

LiverTox: Clinical and research information on drug-induced liver injury. Available at: https://livertox.nih.gov/

Acid–Base Tutorial. Available at: https://www.acid-base.com/

7 Parenteral Nutrition

Susanna J. Harwood and Alan G. Cosslett

Key points

- Parenteral nutrition is indicated in people who are malnourished or at risk of malnutrition as a result of a nonfunctional, inaccessible or perforated gastro-intestinal tract or who have inadequate or unsafe enteral nutritional intake.
- Combinations of oral diet, enteral feeding and parenteral nutrition, either peripherally or centrally, may be appropriate.
- Parenteral nutrition regimens should be tailored to the nutritional needs of the patient and should contain a balance of seven essential components: water, L-amino acids, glucose, lipids with essential fatty acids, vitamins, trace elements and electrolytes.
- Advances in technology alongside expertise in pharmaceutical stability often permit the required nutrients to be administered from a single container. Increasingly, standard formulations are used, including licensed preparations.
- Parenteral nutrition must be compounded under validated aseptic conditions by trained specialists.
- Prescriptions are guided by baseline nutritional assessment, calculation of requirements, knowledge of the patient's disease status and ongoing monitoring.
- The incidence of complications with parenteral nutrition is reducing; knowledge of management is improving.
- Many patients on parenteral nutrition are now being cared for successfully in the home environment.

Introduction

Malnutrition

Malnutrition can be described as a deficiency, excess, or imbalance of energy, protein, and other nutrients that causes measurable adverse effects on body tissue, size, shape, composition, function and clinical outcome.

In UK hospitals, most malnutrition appears to be a general undernutrition of all nutrients (protein, energy and micronutrients) rather than marasmus (insufficient energy provision) or kwashiorkor (insufficient protein provision). Alternatively, there may be a specific deficiency, such as thiamine in severe hepatic disease.

Multiple causes may contribute to malnutrition. They may include inadequate or unbalanced food intake, increased demand as a result of clinical disease status, defects in food digestion or absorption or a compromise in nutritional metabolic pathways. Onset may be acute or insidious. Even mild malnutrition can result in problems with adverse effects on clinical, physical and psychosocial status. Symptoms may include impaired immune response, reduced skeletal muscle strength and fatigue, reduced respiratory muscle strength, impaired thermoregulation and impaired skin barrier and wound healing. In turn, these predispose the patient to a wide range of problems including infection, delayed clinical recovery, increased clinical complications, inactivity, psychological decline and reduced quality of life. Because symptoms may be nonspecific, the underlying malnutrition may be left undiagnosed. Early nutritional intervention is associated with reduced average length of hospital stay and linked cost savings.

Nutrition screening

Routine screening is recommended by the Malnutrition Advisory Group of the British Association of Parenteral and Enteral Nutrition (BAPEN). This group has worked to promote awareness of the clinical significance of malnutrition and has produced guidelines to monitor and manage malnutrition. Screening criteria and tools have been developed and refined to assess nutritional status. Examples include the relatively simple and reproducible body mass index (BMI) tool with consideration of other key factors (Table 7.1). Body weight should not be used in isolation; significant weight fluctuations may reflect fluid disturbances, and muscle wasting may be a result of immobility rather than undernutrition. BAPEN has developed a new web-based nutritional care tool. This tool enables BAPEN to monitor the effectiveness of nutritional care plans.

Incidence of undernutrition

The incidence of undernutrition in hospitalised patients is not accurately known, although it is estimated as being between 20% and 40%.

Table 7.1 Body mass index as a screening tool	
BMI (kg/m²)	BMI category
<18.5	Underweight
18.5–25	Ideal BMI
25–29.9	Overweight
>30	Obese

BMI, Body mass index. BMI = weight (kg)/height (m²).

Indications for parenteral nutrition

Parenteral nutrition (PN) is a nutritionally balanced aseptically prepared or sterile physicochemically stable solution or emulsion for intravenous administration. It is indicated whenever the gastro-intestinal tract is inaccessible, perforated or nonfunctional or when enteral nutrition is inadequate or unsafe. PN should be considered if the enteral route is not likely to be possible for more than 5 days. PN may fulfil the total nutritional requirements or may be supplemental to an enteral feed or diet.

The simplest way to correct or prevent undernutrition is through conventional balanced food; however, this is not always possible. Nutritional support may then require oral supplements or enteral tube feeding. Assuming the gut is functioning normally, the patient will be able to digest and absorb their required nutrients. These include water, protein, carbohydrate, fat, vitamins, minerals and electrolytes; however, if the gut is not accessible or functioning adequately, or if gut rest is indicated, then PN may be used. Although the enteral route is the first choice, this may still fail to provide sufficient nutrient intake in a number of patients. Complications and limitations of enteral nutrition need to be recognised.

A decision pathway can be followed to guide initial and ongoing nutritional support. Although many are published, a locally tailored and regularly updated pathway is favoured. A useful starting point may be found in Fig. 7.1.

Close monitoring should ensure the patient's needs are met; a combination of nutrition routes is sometimes the best course. Where possible, patients receiving PN should also receive enteral intake; even minor gut stimulation has been linked with a reduction in the incidence of bacterial translocation through maintaining gut integrity and preventing overgrowth and cholestatic complications. PN should not be stopped abruptly but should be gradually reduced in line with the increasing enteral diet.

Nutrition support teams

A report published by the Kings Fund Report (1992) highlighted the issue of malnutrition both in the hospital and home setting. The findings led to the development of the BAPEN and nutrition support teams throughout the UK. These multidisciplinary nutrition support teams comprise a doctor, nurse, pharmacist and dietitian. They function in a variety of ways, depending on the patient populations and resources. In general, they adopt either a consultative or an authoritative role in nutrition management. Many studies have shown their positive contribution to the total nutritional care of the patient through efficient and appropriate selection and monitoring of feed and route (Gales and Gales, 1994).

Components of a parenteral nutrition regimen

In addition to water, six main groups of nutrients need to be incorporated in a PN regimen (Table 7.2).

Water volume

Water is the principal component of the body and accounts for approximately 60% and 55% of total body weight in men and women, respectively. Usually, homeostasis maintains appropriate fluid levels and electrolyte balance, and thirst drives the healthy person to drink; however, some patients are not able physically to respond by drinking, and so this homeostasis is ineffective. There is risk of over- or underhydration if the range of factors affecting fluid and electrolyte balance is not fully understood and monitored. In general, an adult patient will require 20–40 mL/kg/day fluid; however, Table 7.3 describes other factors that should be considered in tailoring input to needs.

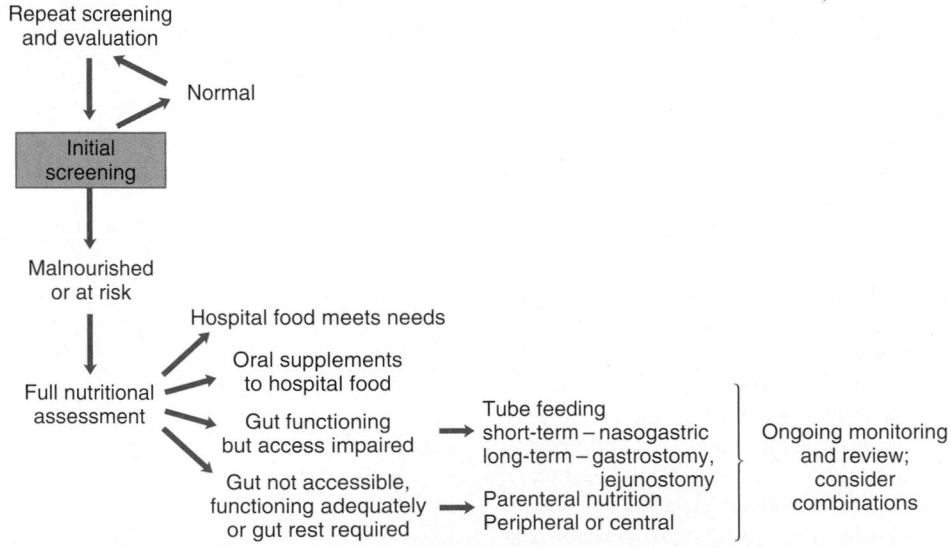

Fig. 7.1 Decision pathway to guide initial and ongoing nutritional support.

Table 7.2 Oral and equivalent parenteral nutrition source

Oral diet	Parenteral nutrition source
Water	Water
Protein	L-Amino acid mixture
Carbohydrate	Glucose
Fat with essential fatty acids	Lipid emulsions with essential fatty acids
Vitamins	Vitamins
Minerals	Trace elements
Electrolytes	Electrolytes

Table 7.3 Factors affecting fluid requirements

Consider increasing fluid input	Consider reducing fluid input
Signs/symptoms of dehydration	Signs/symptoms of fluid overload
Fever: increased insensible losses from lungs in hyperventilation and from skin in sweating; allow 10–15% extra water per 10 °C above normal	High humidity: reduced rate of evaporation
Acute anabolic state: increased water required for increased cell generation	Blood transfusion: volume input
High environmental temperature or low humidity: increased rate of evaporation	Cardiac failure: may limit tolerated blood volume
	Drug therapy: assess volume and electrolyte content of infused drug
Abnormal gastro-intestinal loss (vomiting, wounds, ostomies, diarrhoea): consider both volume loss and electrolyte content	
Burns or open wound(s): increased water evaporation	
	Renal failure: fluid may accumulate, so reduce input accordingly or provide artificial renal support
Blood loss: assess volume lost and whether replaced by transfusion, colloid, crystalloid	

Amino acids

Twenty L-amino acids are required for protein synthesis and metabolism, and the majority of these can be synthesised endogenously. Eight are called 'essential' amino acids because they cannot be synthesised (isoleucine, leucine, lysine, methionine, phenylalanine, threonine, tryptophan and valine). A further group of 'conditionally essential' amino acids (arginine, choline, glutamine, taurine and S-adenosyl-L-methionine) are defined as the patient's needs exceed synthesis in clinically stressed conditions. Also, because of the immature metabolic pathways of neonates, infants and children, some other amino acids are essential in the young patient; these include histidine, proline, cysteine, tyrosine and taurine. Immature neonatal metabolism does not fully metabolise glycine, methionine, phenylalanine and threonine, and so requirements are reduced.

To balance the patient's amino acid requirements and the chemical characteristics of the amino acids (solubility, stability and compatibility), commercially available licensed solutions have been formulated that contain a range of amino acid profiles (Table 7.4). Aminoplasmal, Aminoven, Synthamin and Vamin are

Table 7.4 Examples of amino acid and consequential nitrogen content of licensed amino acid solutions available in the UK

Name	Nitrogen content (g/L)	Electrolytes present
Aminoplasmal 5% E	8	Potassium, magnesium, sodium and phosphate
Aminoplasmal 10%	16	
Aminoplasmal 15%	24	
Aminoven 25	25.7	
Glamin	22.4	
Primene 10%	15	
Synthamin 9	9.1	Potassium, magnesium, sodium and phosphate
Synthamin 9 EF	9.1	
Synthamin 14	14	Potassium, magnesium, sodium and phosphate
Synthamin 14 EF	14	
Synthamin 17	17	Potassium, magnesium, sodium and phosphate
Synthamin 17 EF	17	
Vamin 14	13.5	Potassium, magnesium, sodium and calcium
Vamin 14EF	13.5	
Vamin 18EF	18	

designed for adult patients. The amino acid profiles of Primene, Vaminolact and Aminoplasmal Paediatric are specifically tailored to neonates, infants and children (reflecting the amino acid profile of maternal cord blood and breast milk, respectively).

L-Glutamine was initially excluded from formulations because of its low solubility and relatively poor stability in the aqueous environment; however, it is recognised that there is a clinical need for this amino acid in catabolic stress, and it is now available as an additive (Dipeptiven) and as an amino acid solution containing a dipeptide form of glutamine (Glamin) in which the peptide bond cleaves in the blood, releasing free L-glutamine.

Assuming adequate energy is supplied, most adult patients achieve nitrogen balance with approximately 0.2 g nitrogen/kg/day, although care should be taken with overweight patients. A 24-hour urine collection can be used as an indicator of nitrogen loss, assuming all urine is collected and urea or volume output is not compromised by renal failure; however, a true nitrogen output determination requires measurement of nitrogen output from all body fluids, including urine, sweat, faeces, skin and wounds. Nitrogen balance studies can indicate the metabolic state of the patient (positive balance in net protein synthesis, negative balance in protein catabolism). Urinary urea constitutes approximately 80% of the urinary nitrogen. The universally accepted conversion factor for nitrogen to protein is 1 g nitrogen per 6.25 g of protein.

Amino acid solutions are hypertonic to blood and should not be administered alone into the peripheral circulation.

Energy

Many factors affect the energy requirement of individual patients, and these include age, activity and illness (both severity and stage). Predictive formulae can be applied to estimate the energy requirement, for example, the Harris–Benedict equation or the more commonly used Henry equation, which is shown in Table 7.5 (Henry, 2005).

Alternatively, calorimetry techniques can be used; however, no single method is ideal or suits all scenarios. Often it is found that two methods result in different recommendations. The majority of adults can be appropriately maintained on 25–35 non-protein

kcal/kg/day. There is debate over whether to include amino acids as a source of calories because it is simplistic to assume they are either all spared for protein synthesis or fed into the metabolic pathways (Krebs cycle) and contribute to the release of energy-rich molecules. In general, the term to 'non-protein energy' is used, and sufficient lipid and glucose energy is supplied to spare the amino acids. As a rough guide, the ratio of non-protein energy to nitrogen is approximately 150:1, although an ideal ratio for all patients has not been absolutely defined. A lower ratio is considered for critically ill patients, whereas higher ratios are considered for less catabolic patients.

Dual energy

In general, energy should be sourced from a balanced combination of lipid and glucose; this is termed 'dual energy' and is more physiological than an exclusive glucose source. Typically, the fat-to-glucose ratio remains close to the 60:40–40:60 ranges.

Dual energy can minimise the risk of giving too much lipid or glucose because complications increase if the metabolic capacity of either is exceeded. A higher incidence of acute adverse effects is noted with faster infusion rates and higher total daily doses, especially in patients with existing metabolic stress. It is, therefore, essential that the administered dose complements the energy requirements and the infusion rate does not exceed the metabolic capacity. While effectively maintaining nitrogen balance, lipid inclusion is seen to confer a number of advantages (Box 7.1). Some patients, notably long-term home patients, do not tolerate daily lipid infusions and need to be managed on an individual basis. Depending on the enteral intake and nutritional needs, lipids are prescribed for a proportion of the days. A trial with the newer-generation lipid emulsions may be appropriate.

Glucose

Glucose is the recommended source of carbohydrate (1 g anhydrous glucose provides 4 kcal). Table 7.6 indicates the energy provision and tonicity for a range of concentrations. Glucose 5% is regarded as isotonic with blood. The higher concentrations

Table 7.5 Henry equation

	Age (years)	Kcal (day) (W = weight)
Male	10–18	18.4W + 581
	18–30	16.0W + 545
	30–60	14.2W + 593
	60–70	13.0W + 567
	70+	13.7W + 481
Female	10–18	11.1W + 761
	18–30	13.1W + 558
	30–60	9.74W + 694
	60–70	10.2W + 572
	70+	10.0W + 577

Adapted from Henry (2005).

Box 7.1 Examples of the advantages of dual-energy systems over glucose-only energy systems

- Minimise risk of hyperglycaemia and related complications
- Prevent and reverse fatty liver (steatosis)
- Reduce carbon dioxide production and respiratory distress
- Meet higher calorie requirements of septic and trauma patients when glucose oxidation reduced and lipid oxidation increased
- Reduce metabolic stress
- Support immune function
- Improve lean body mass and reduce water retention
- Permit peripheral administration, through reduced tonicity
- Facilitate fluid restriction, as lipid is a concentrated source of energy
- Are a source of essential fatty acids, preventing and correcting deficiency

Table 7.6 Energy provision and tonicity of glucose solutions

Concentration (w/v)	Energy content (kcal/L)	Osmolarity (mOsmol/L)
5%	200	278
10%	400	555
20%	800	1110
50%	2000	2775
70%	2800	3885

Table 7.7 Examples of licensed lipid emulsions available in the UK

Lipid emulsion type	Details of products
Soybean oil	Intralipid 10%, 20%, 30%
Purified olive oil/soybean oil	ClinOleic 20%
Medium chain triglycerides/ soybean oil	Lipofundin MCT/LCT 10%, 20%
Omega-3-acid triglycerides/ soybean oil/medium-chain triglycerides	Lipidem
Fish oil/olive oil/soybean oil/medium-chain triglycerides	SMOFLipid

cause phlebitis if administered directly to peripheral veins and should, therefore, be given by a central vein or in combination with compatible solutions to reduce the tonicity.

The glucose infusion rate should generally be between 2 and 4 mg/kg/min. An infusion of 2 mg/kg/min (equating to approximately 200 g [800 kcal] per day for a 70-kg adult) represents the basal glucose requirement, whereas 4 mg/kg/day is regarded as the physiologically optimal rate. Higher levels are tolerated by some patients, especially those at home on PN, but monitoring of blood glucose is required at least initially. Care needs to be taken because glucose oxidation occurs where there is an increased conversion to glycogen and fat. If excess glucose is infused and the glycogen storage capacity exceeded, the circulating glucose level rises, de novo lipogenesis occurs (production of fat from glucose) and there is an increased incidence of metabolic complications.

Lipid emulsions

Lipid emulsions are used as a source of energy and for the provision of the essential fatty acids, linoleic and alpha-linolenic acid. Supplying 10 kcal energy per gram of lipid, they are energy rich and can be infused directly into the peripheral veins because they are relatively isotonic with blood.

Typically, patients receive up to 2.5 g lipid/kg/day. Details of lipid emulsions available within the UK can be found in Table 7.7.

Lipid emulsions are oil-in-water formulations. Fig. 7.2 shows the structure of triglycerides (three fatty acids on a glycerol backbone) and a lipid globule, stabilised at the interface by phospholipids. Ionisation of the polar phosphate group of the phospholipid results in a net negative charge of the lipid globule and an electromechanically stable formulation. The lipid globule size distribution is similar to that of the naturally occurring chylomicrons (80–500 nm), as indicated in Fig. 7.3.

The first-generation lipid emulsions have been in use since the 1970s and utilise soybean oil as the source of long-chain fatty acids. More recent research on lipid metabolic pathways and clinical outcomes has indicated that the fatty acid profile of soybean oil alone is not ideal (Klek, 2016). For example, it is now recognised that these lipid emulsions contain excess essential polyunsaturated fatty acids, resulting in a qualitative and quantitative compromise to the eicosanoid metabolites that have important

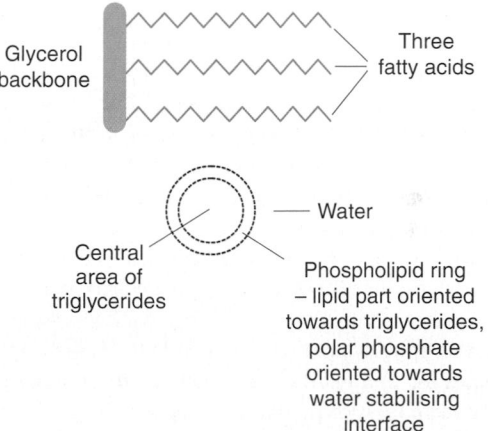

Fig. 7.2 Triglyceride structure and composition of lipid emulsion globule.

roles in cell structure, haemodynamics, platelet function, inflammatory response and immune response.

The molecular structure of the fatty acids has an important impact on the patient's oxidative stress. Two strategies have been applied to overcome this: a reduction in the polyunsaturated fatty acid content through an improved balance of fatty acids or the inclusion of medium chain fatty acids. This has resulted in the development of lipid emulsions that include olive oil (rich in monounsaturated oleic acid and antioxidant α-tocopherol with an appropriate level of essential polyunsaturated fatty acids), fish oil (rich in omega-3 fatty acids) and medium-chain triglycerides (reduced long-chain fatty acid content). Clinical application of these newer lipid emulsions depends on good clinical studies within the relevant patient population. Such studies should evaluate the efficacy of energy provision and clinical tolerance and report improvements in the eicosanoid-dependent functions or oxidative stress.

Both egg and soybean phospholipids include a phosphate moiety. There is a debate as to whether this is bioavailable. Therefore, some manufacturers include the phosphate content in their stability calculations, whereas others do not.

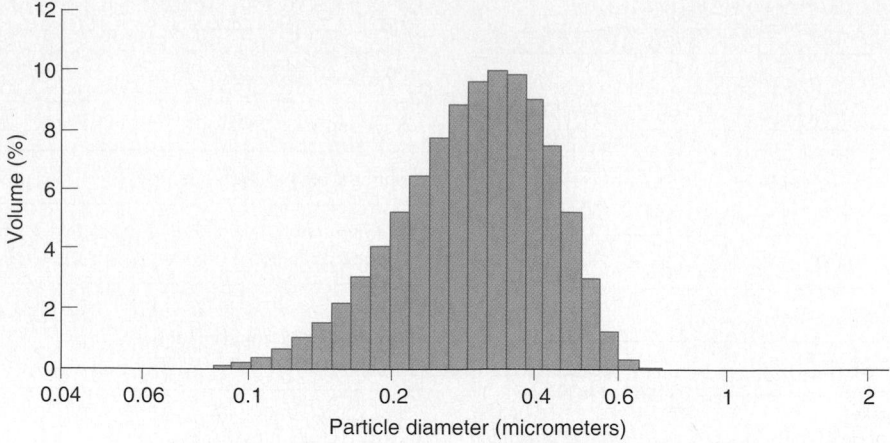

Fig. 7.3 Lipid-globule size-distribution curve of Ivelip 20%.

Micronutrients

Micronutrients naturally fall into two groups, the trace elements and vitamins, and they have a key role in intermediary metabolism, as both cofactors and coenzymes. For example, zinc is required by more than 200 enzyme systems and affects many diverse body functions, including acid–base balance, immune function and nucleic acid synthesis. It is evident, therefore, that the availability of micronutrients can affect enzyme activity and total metabolism. When disease increases the metabolism of the major substrates, the requirement for micronutrients is increased. Some of the micronutrients also play an essential role in the free-radical scavenging system. These include the following:

- Copper, zinc and manganese, in the form of superoxide dismutase, dispose of superoxide radicals.
- Selenium, in the form of glutathione peroxidase, removes hydroperoxyl compounds.
- Vitamin C is a strong reducing agent.
- Vitamins A and E and β-carotene react directly with free radicals.

By the time a patient starts PN, he or she may have already developed a deficiency of one or more essential nutrients. By the time a specific clinical deficiency is observed, for example, depigmentation of hair in copper deficiency or skin lesions in zinc deficiency, the patient will already have tried to compensate to maintain levels, compromised intracellular enzyme activity and antioxidant systems and expressed nonspecific symptoms such as fatigue and impaired immune response. A summary of factors that affect micronutrient needs is presented in Box 7.2. Measuring blood levels of vitamins and trace elements in acutely ill patients is of limited value. It is recommended that these are measured every 1–6 months, depending on levels, and in patients at home on PN (National Institute for Health and Care Excellence [NICE], 2006). Deficiency states are clinically significant, but with nonspecific symptoms, they are often difficult to diagnose.

Micronutrients should be included daily from the start of the PN. The requirements are increased during critical illness and in chronically depleted patients. Their supplementation may influence the outcome of the disease. Even if the patient has reasonable levels and reserves initially, they can

---

Box 7.2 Factors affecting micronutrient requirements

Baseline nutritional state on starting parenteral nutrition
- Acute or chronic onset of illness
- Dietary history
- Duration and severity of inadequate nutritional intake

Increased loss
- Small bowel fistulae/aspirate: rich in zinc
- Biliary fluid loss: rich in copper
- Burn fluid loss: rich in zinc, copper, selenium

Increased requirement
- Increased metabolism: acute in anabolic phase following catabolic phase of critically ill
- Active growth

Organ function
- Liver failure: copper and manganese clearance reduced
- Renal failure: aluminium, chromium, zinc and nickel clearance reduced

---

quickly become depleted if they are not supported by daily administration. Additional oral or enteral supplements may be considered if there is some intestinal absorption. However, copper deficiency can increase iron absorption and zinc intake can decrease copper absorption. Micronutrient preparations have been developed to provide more than basal amounts of all micronutrients. They should, therefore, meet the requirements of most patients, given they are administered intravenously. Micronutrients should be added to all PN infusions under appropriate, controlled environmental conditions prior to administration (NICE, 2006).

Trace elements

Trace elements are generally maintained at a relatively constant tissue concentration and are present to a level of less than 1 mg/kg body weight. They are essential; deficiency results in structural and physiological disorders which, if identified early enough, can be resolved by re-administration. Ten essential trace elements are known: iron, copper, zinc,

Table 7.8 UK reference nutritional intake (RNI) for trace elements in adults

	RNI (males)	RNI (females)
Iron (milligrams/day)	8.7	8.7
Zinc (milligrams/day)	9.5	7.0
Copper (milligrams/day)	1.2	1.2
Selenium (micrograms/day)	75	60
Iodine (micrograms/day)	140	140

RNI, reference nutritional intake.
Adapted from Department of Health HMSO (1991). SACN vitamin D and Health (2016).

Table 7.9 UK reference nutritional intake (RNI) for vitamins in adults

	RNI (males)	RNI (females)
Vitamin A (micrograms/day)	700	600
Vitamin C (milligrams/day)	40	40
Vitamin D (micrograms/day)	10	10
Vitamin B1 (Thiamin) (milligrams/day)	0.9	0.8
Vitamin B2 (Riboflavin) (milligrams/day)	1.3	1.1
Vitamin B6 (milligrams/day)	1.4	1.2
Vitamin B12 (micrograms/day)	1.5	1.5
Niacin (milligrams/day)	16	12
Folate (micrograms/day)	200	200

RNI, reference nutritional intake.
Adapted from Department of Health HMSO (1991). SACN vitamin D and Health (2016).

fluorine, manganese, iodine, cobalt, selenium, molybdenum and chromium.

Because the controversy which exists around the amount of trace elements to administer, the American Society of Enteral and Parenteral Nutrition (ASPEN) established a task force to consider this issue. The task force published guidelines for the trace element requirements during PN (Vanek et al., 2012). UK adult reference nutritional intake and ASPEN trace element requirements during PN can be found in Table 7.8. The differences in the advised amounts reflect the efficiency of the gut to absorb the various micronutrients.

Currently, three preparations are commercially available for adults (Tracutil, Additrace, Nutryelt), together with a single paediatric preparation (Peditrace).

Vitamins

There are two groups of vitamins: the water-soluble vitamins and the fat-soluble vitamins. Fat-soluble vitamins are stored in the body fat, whereas excess water-soluble vitamins are renally cleared; therefore, if there is inadequate provision, deficiency states for the water-soluble vitamins reveal themselves first. UK adult reference nutritional intake and ASPEN vitamin requirements during PN can be found in Table 7.9. Commercially available preparations are Solivito N (water soluble), Vitlipid N Adult/Infant (fat soluble) and Cernevit (water and fat soluble, except vitamin K).

In an attempt to reduce the risk of osteoporosis, especially in home PN patients, vitamin D is essential. Patients on long-term PN should have vitamin D levels measured every 6 months. If low, this should be supplemented to help protect against osteoporosis, which is a well-recognised complication of home PN. Although oral vitamin D is of benefit, patients should be encouraged to allow sunlight exposure to the skin. By doing so, not only can the skin generate large amounts of vitamin D, but also this is not affected by intestinal absorption of oral vitamin D. The recommended dietary vitamin D intakes for patients at risk of vitamin D deficiency 600 IU/day for those 19–70 years of age and 800 IU/day for more than 7 years (Holick et al., 2011).

Electrolytes

Electrolytes are included to meet the patient's needs. Typical daily parenteral requirements are:
- sodium (1–1.5 mmol/kg),
- potassium (1–1.5 mmol/kg),
- calcium (0.1–0.15 mmol/kg),
- magnesium (0.1–0.2 mmol/kg),
- phosphate (0.5–0.7 mmol/kg).

Depending on the stability of the patient's clinical state, they are kept relatively constant or adjusted on a near daily basis, reflecting changes in blood biochemistry. Hypophosphataemia and hypomagnesaemia should be corrected before starting parenteral or enteral nutrition to avoid the refeeding syndrome. Varying amounts of electrolytes are lost from the different gastro-intestinal secretions. Table 7.10 gives an indication of the content of various gastro-intestinal secretions. This should be taken into account when formulating PN for a patient who may have such losses.

Administration of parenteral nutrition

Routes of administration

PN can be administered peripherally or centrally.

Peripheral route

Administration of PN via a peripheral venous catheter should be considered for patients who are likely to need short-term feeding

Table 7.10 Electrolyte content of gastro-intestinal secretions

Intestinal tract locality	Volume (mL)	Sodium (mmol/L)	Potassium (mmol/L)	Chloride (mmol/L)	Bicarbonate (mmol/L)
Saliva	1500	10	25	10	30
Gastric juice (fasting)	1500	60	15	90	15
Pancreatic fistula	700	140	5	75	120
Biliary fistula	500	145	5	100	40
Jejunostomy	2000–3000	110	5	100	30
Ileostomy	500	115	8	45	30
Proximal colostomy	300	80	20	45	30
Diarrhoea	500–1500	120	25	90	45

(<14 days) and who have no other need for central venous access. Peripheral lines are less costly than central lines, and they may be inserted at the bedside providing the patient has good venous access. Ultrasound machines may be used to aid placement. There is no need for a chest X-ray to confirm placement because the line does not reach the central circulation. Mid-lines should be considered, which are usually about 20 cm long. Care should be taken when formulating PN to be administered via a peripheral catheter with regard to the tonicity of the solution. Some indications and contraindications to the use of the peripheral route are summarised in Box 7.3.

Peripheral administration is sometimes complicated or delayed by phlebitis, where an insult to the endothelial vessel wall causes inflammation, redness, pain and possible extravasation. Hot and cold compresses have been used to treat this. A 5 mg glyceryl trinitrate patch placed where the line tip is estimated to be may cause some local vasodilation, which is believed to prevent thrombophlebitis (Khawaja and Williams, 1991). Peripheral tolerance can be influenced by a range of factors (Box 7.4).

Many consider that the tonicity of the infused solution or emulsion is a key factor defining peripheral infusion tolerance. The total number of osmotically active particles in the intracellular and extracellular fluids is essentially the same, approximately 290–310 mOsmol/L. When a lipid emulsion is included, infusions of approximately three times this osmolarity are generally well tolerated via the peripheral route, and there are reports of success with higher levels. However, other factors should also be considered. Patient factors, such as vein fragility and blood flow, may mean that some infusion episodes are better tolerated than others. The osmolarity of a PN formulation can be estimated by applying the following equation:

$$= \frac{\sum [\text{osmolarity}_n\,(\text{mOsmol/L}) \times \text{volume}_n\,(\text{L})]}{\text{Total volume (L)}},$$

where n indicates the component.

By considering the macronutrients included in the regimen, that is, the amino acids, glucose and lipid, an estimation of the osmolarity can be made. The value will be increased by

Box 7.3 Indications and contraindications for the use of peripheral parenteral nutrition

Indications
- Duration of feed likely to be short-term
- Supplemental feeding
- Compromised access to central circulation, e.g. local trauma, surgery or thrombosis
- No immediate facilities or trained staff to insert central catheter
- High risk of fungal or bacterial sepsis, e.g. patients with purulent tracheostomy secretions, immune deficiency state, history of repeated sepsis
- Contraindication to central venous catheterisation

Contraindications
- Inadequate or inaccessible peripheral veins
- Large volumes of administration
- High calorie/nitrogen requirements alongside fluid restrictions (admixture osmolarity too high)

Box 7.4 Factors that improve tolerance to peripheral lines

- Aseptic insertion and line care
- Selection of large vessel with good blood flow and direct path, e.g. cephalic vein
- Fine-bore catheter (22G) for minimal trauma on insertion and disturbance of blood flow
- Fine polyurethane catheter
- Secured catheter to minimise physical trauma
- Glyceryl trinitrate patch placed distal to insertion site, over tip, to vasodilate vein
- Flushing of lines not in use
- Low-tonicity infusions
- Inclusion of lipid emulsion; venoprotective and isotonic with blood

electrolyte or micronutrient additions; however, because the peripheral tolerance is affected by so many factors, including tonicity, and because the limit is only an estimate, the effect of these additions is relatively low unless high levels of monovalent ions are included.

Central route

The central venous route is indicated when longer-term feeding is anticipated, high-tonicity or large-volume formulations are required, or the peripheral route is inaccessible. The rapid and turbulent blood flow in the central circulation and the constant movement of the heart ensure rapid mixing and reduce the risk of osmotically induced injury to the endothelium.

Single-, double-, triple- and quadruple-lumen central lines are available, and one lumen must be dedicated for the intravenous nutrition. These lines require skilful insertion, usually into the jugular or subclavian vein, and confirmation of their position by X-ray. This relatively invasive and costly procedure is performed by trained medical staff. Tunnelling of the line to an appropriate exit site facilitates line care and may reduce the incidence of line sepsis. The femoral route is not favoured because of a higher incidence of sepsis. If cared for well, a tunnelled central line placed in a patient receiving home PN may last for many years.

Peripherally inserted central catheters

Peripherally inserted central catheters (PICCs) are typically inserted into a peripheral vein, usually the cephalic or basilic in the upper arm, with the exit tip in the superior vena cava just above the right atrium. As the name suggests, they are used for the central administration of infusions. Single- and double-lumen versions are available; some also have a one-way valve to prevent backflow. Insertion is less invasive than for conventional central lines and can be undertaken by trained nurse practitioners at the bedside. A chest X-ray is necessary to confirm placement.

Infusion control

Pumps

PN must always be administered under the control of an infusion pump. Acute overload of fluid, nutrition and electrolytes can have morbid consequences.

Infusion pumps should be used with an appropriate infusion or giving set which is compatible with both the infusion pump and the PN admixture. For home patients, small, simple battery-powered ambulatory pumps are favoured.

Temperature

PN should be at room temperature when it is infused. It must, therefore, be removed from the refrigerator in which it is stored approximately 2 hours before connection. No external heat should be applied, although intermittent inversion of the bag may help.

If a cold admixture is infused, the patient may experience infusion discomfort, and the acute release of gas from where it was dissolved in the admixture may cause the pump to alarm 'air in line'.

Compounded formulations

Historically, PN was administered from a series of separate bottles, where healthcare staff had to accurately and safely manage a combination of giving sets, infusion rates and total infusion times. Patients now receive their complete nutrition from a single daily bag of a pharmaceutically stable PN formulation.

Various terms are used to describe the PN formulation, depending on whether lipid is included. If it contains lipid, it is called a 3-in-1, ternary or all-in-one admixture; if no lipid is present, the terms 2-in-1, binary or aqueous admixture are used. Various methods now exist for compounding PN. These range from high-tech, computer-run compounding machines through to basic-principle techniques such as gravity filling.

Formulations

Depending on the type (size and specialty) of the hospital, various formulations are used. The range is specifically selected to meet the needs of the patients managed by the hospital and will typically include a low-tonicity regimen suitable for peripheral administration, a higher calorie and nitrogen regimen for central administration to catabolic patients and a high-tonicity regimen for fluid-restricted patients. Baseline electrolytes will generally be included, although the flexibility for reduced levels is usually offered.

Licensed, ready-to-use products

Various licensed, ready-to-use preparations are available and should have micronutrients added prior to infusing. For convenience, baseline electrolyte levels are included in many formulations and meet the needs of most patients, and additional electrolytes may be added up to the limits set by the manufacturer. Electrolyte-free options are also available. Some are licensed for use in paediatrics and/or for peripheral use. Manufacturers advise on stability and shelf-life for electrolyte and micronutrient additions. The range of ready-to-use products includes the following:

- Triple-chamber bags (Triomel, Kabiven, SmofKabiven and Nutriflex Lipid ranges): chambers separately prefilled with lipid, amino acid and glucose and terminally sterilised. These are activated by applying external pressure so that weak seals peel open, mixing the contents to form a 3-in-1 formulation.
- Dual-chamber bags (Clinimix and Nutriflex ranges): chambers separately prefilled with amino acid and glucose and terminally sterilised. These are activated to form a 2-in-1 formulation. They provide the flexibility to allow staff to omit or add a compatible lipid.

The range of commercially available PN formulations is continually expanding. For hospital pharmacies without compounding facilities, this offers an opportunity to ensure the correct formulation is given to meet individual patient needs. PN formulations are now available with micronutrients added and with extended shelf-lives when stored in a refrigerator.

Cyclic infusions

Cyclic PN is when the daily requirements are administered over a short period. A classic example is stable home patients who administer their feed overnight, freeing themselves from the constraints of an infusion during the day. This enables them to have more physical freedom and improves their quality of life. Some patients, however, prefer to administer their PN during the day

Shelf-life and temperature control

The manufacturer may be able to provide physical and chemical stability data to support a formulation for a shelf-life of up to 90 days at 2–8°C followed by 24 hours at room temperature for infusion; this assumes that a strict aseptic technique is used during compounding. Units holding a manufacturing license covering aseptic compounding of PN are potentially able to assign this full shelf-life (if stability data are available), whereas unlicensed units are limited to a maximum shelf-life of 7 days.

PN must be stored and transported within the defined temperature limits and should not be exposed to temperature cycling (e.g. the formulations must not freeze); for this reason, a validated cold-chain must be employed, especially when delivering formulations to home care patients. Pharmaceutical-grade fridges should be used and monitored to ensure appropriate air cycling and temperature maintenance. The temperature during the infusion period should be known. Because neonatal units and their patient incubators are classically maintained at higher temperatures, formulations used for this environment must have been stability-validated at these temperatures.

Drug stability

The addition of drugs to PN admixtures, or Y-site coadministration, is actively discouraged unless the compatibility has been formally confirmed. Wherever possible, the PN should be administered through a dedicated line. Multilumen catheters can be used to infuse PN separately from other infusion(s); however, extreme competition for intravenous access may prompt consideration of drug and PN combinations. Many factors need to be considered: the physical and chemical stability of the PN, the physical and chemical stability of the drug, the bioavailability of the drug (especially when a lipid emulsion is present) and the effect of stopping and starting Y-site infusions on the actual administration rates. It is not possible to reliably extrapolate data from a specific PN composition, between brands of solutions and salt forms or between brands or doses of drugs. Various studies have been performed and published; however, these should be used with caution.

In practice, drugs should only be infused with PN when all other possibilities have been exhausted. These may include gaining further intravenous access and changing the drug(s) to clinically acceptable non-intravenous alternatives. The relative risks of stopping and starting the PN infusion and repeatedly breaking the infusion circuit should be fully considered before sharing a line for separate infusions of PN and drug. In most cases, the risks outweigh the benefits; however, if this option is adopted, the line must be flushed before and after with an appropriate volume of solution known to be stable with both the PN and the drug. Strict aseptic technique should be adopted to minimise the risk of contaminating the line and infusions.

Filtration

All intravenous fluids pass through the delicate lung microvasculature with its capillary diameter of 8–12 micrometers. The presence of particulate matter has been demonstrated to cause direct embolisation, direct damage to the endothelia, formation of granulomata and formation of foreign body giant cells and to have a thrombogenic effect. In addition, the presence of microbial and fungal matter can cause a serious infection or inflammatory response.

Precautions taken to minimise the particulate load of the compounded admixture must include:

- use of filter needles or straws (5 micrometers) during compounding to catch larger particles, such as cored rubber from bottles and glass shards from ampoules;
- air particle levels kept within defined limits in aseptic rooms by the use of air filters and non-shedding clothing and wipes;
- use of quality raw materials with minimal particulate presence, including empty bags and leads;
- confirmation of physical and chemical stability of the formulation prior to aseptic compounding applying approved mixing order (stability for the required shelf-life time and conditions).

Guidelines have been published that endorse the use of filters, especially for patients requiring intensive or prolonged parenteral therapy, including home patients, the immunocompromised, neonates and children (Bethune et al., 2001). The filter should be placed as close to the patient as possible and validated for the PN to be used. For 2-in-1 formulations, 0.2-micrometers filters may be used; for 3-in-1 formulations, validated 1.2-micrometers filters may be used.

Light protection

It is widely recognised that exposure to light, notably phototherapy light and intense sunlight, may increase the degradation rate of certain constituents such as vitamins A and E. It is recommended that all regimens should be protected from light both during storage and during infusion for the following reasons:

- The presence of a lipid emulsion does not totally protect against vitamin photodegradation.
- The Maillard reaction is influenced by light exposure.
- Ongoing research suggests lipid peroxidation is accelerated by a range of factors, including exposure to certain wavelengths of light.

Additionally, only validated bag and delivery set covers should be used.

Nutritional assessment and monitoring

Initial assessment

Once screening has identified that a patient is in need of nutritional intervention, a more detailed assessment is performed. This will include an evaluation of nutritional requirements, the expected course of the underlying disease, consideration of the enteral route and, where appropriate, identification of access routes for PN. This will be supported by a clinical assessment that will include:

- clinical history;
- dietary history;
- physical examination;
- anthropometry including muscle function tests;
- biochemical, haematological and immunological review.

Monitoring

PN monitoring has a number of objectives:

- evaluate ongoing nutritional requirements, including fluid and electrolytes;
- determine the effectiveness of the nutritional intervention;
- facilitate early recognition of complications;
- identify any deficiency, overload or toxicity to individual nutrients;
- determine discrepancies between prescribed, delivered and received dose.

Regular monitoring contributes to the success of the PN, and a monitoring protocol should be in place for each individual patient. Baseline data should be recorded so that deviations can be recognised and interpreted. In the early stages, while the patient is in the acute stage of the illness and the nutritional requirements are being established, the frequency of monitoring will be greatest. As the patient's status stabilises, the frequency of monitoring will reduce, although the range of parameters monitored is likely to increase. NICE (2006) has issued a comprehensive guideline for laboratory monitoring of nutrition support. Examples of parameters monitored can be found in Table 7.13.

Complications

Complications of PN fall into two main categories: catheter related and metabolic (Box 7.5). Overall, the incidence of such complications has reduced because of increased knowledge and

Table 7.13   Examples of parameters monitored during parenteral nutrition therapy

Parameter	Additional information
Clinical symptoms at presentation	May be specific (e.g. thrombophlebitis) or nonspecific (e.g. confusion)
Temperature, blood pressure and pulse	Vigilance for the risk of sepsis
Fluid balance and weight	Acute weight changes reflect fluid gain or loss and prompt review of the volume of the PN. Slow, progressive changes are more likely to reflect nutritional status.
Nitrogen balance	An assessment of urine urea and insensible loss and their relation to nitrogen input. It is difficult to obtain accurate figures.
Visceral proteins	Albumin levels may indicate malnutrition, but its long half-life limits sensitivity to detect acute changes in nutritional status. Other markers with a shorter half-life may be more useful, e.g. transferrin.
Haematology	Platelet counts and clotting studies for thrombocytopenia
C-reactive protein	Monitor the inflammatory process.
Blood glucose	Hyperglycaemia is a relatively frequent complication. Management includes either a reduction in the infused dose of glucose or lengthening of the infusion period. If these measures fail, insulin may be used. Hyperglycaemia may also indicate sepsis. Rebound hypoglycaemia can occur when an infusion is stopped. If this is a problem, the infusion should be tapered off during the last hour or two of the infusion. Some infusion pumps are programmed to do this automatically.
Lipid tolerance	Turbidity, cholesterol and triglyceride profiles are required.
Electrolyte profile	Indicates appropriate provision or complicating clinical disorder. In the first few days, low potassium, magnesium and/or phosphate with or without clinical symptoms may reflect the refeeding syndrome.
Liver function tests	An abnormal liver profile may be observed, and it is often difficult to identify a single cause. PN and other factors, such as sepsis, drug therapy and underlying disease, may all interplay. In adults, PN-induced abnormalities tend to be mild, reversible and self-limiting. In the early stages, fatty liver (steatosis) is seen. In longer-term patients, a cholestatic picture tends to present. Varying the type of lipid used and removing lipid from some formulations may be of benefit.
Anthropometry	Assesses longer-term status
Acid–base profile	Indicative of respiratory or metabolic compromise and may require review of PN formulation
Vitamin and trace element screen	A range of single compounds or markers to consider tolerance and identify deficiencies, although of limited value because some tests are nonspecific and inaccurate
Catheter entry site	Vigilance for phlebitis, erythema, extravasation, infection, misplacement

PN, Parenteral nutrition.

Box 7.5   Examples of complications during parenteral nutrition

Catheter related
- Thrombophlebitis (peripheral)
- Catheter-related infection, local or systemic
- Venous thrombosis
- Line occlusion (lipid, thrombus, particulate, mechanical)
- Pneumothorax, catheter malposition, vessel laceration, embolism, hydrothorax, dysrhythmias, incorrect placement (central)

Metabolic
- Hyperglycaemia or hypoglycaemia
- Electrolyte imbalance
- Lipid intolerance
- Refeeding syndrome
- Dehydration or fluid overload
- Specific nutritional deficiency or overload
- Liver disease or biliary disease
- Gastrointestinal atrophy
- Metabolic bone dysfunction (in long-term)
- Thrombocytopenia
- Adverse events with parenteral nutrition components
- Essential fatty acid deficiency

Table 7.14   Risk factors for developing refeeding syndrome (NICE, 2006)

One or more of the following	Two or more of the following
BMI <16 kg/m²	BMI <18.5 kg/m²
Unintentional weight loss greater than 15% within the last 3–6 months	Unintentional weight loss greater than 10% within the last 3–6 months
Little or no nutritional intake for more than 10 days	Little or no nutritional intake for more than 5 days
Low levels of potassium, phosphate or magnesium prior to feeding	A history of alcohol abuse or drugs including insulin, chemotherapy, antacids or diuretics

BMI, Body mass index.

skills together with more successful management (Maroulis and Kalfarentzos, 2000).

Line sepsis

Line sepsis is a serious and potentially life-threatening condition. Monitoring protocols should ensure that signs of infection are identified early, and a local decision pathway should be in place to guide efficient diagnosis and management. Management will depend on the type of line and the source of infection. Alternative sources of sepsis should be considered. Initially, the PN is usually stopped.

Line occlusion

Line occlusion may be caused by a number of factors, including:
- fibrin sheath forming around the line, or a thrombosis blocking the tip;
- internal blockage of lipid, blood clot or salt and drug precipitates;
- line kinking;
- particulate blockage of a protective inline filter.

Management will depend on the cause of the occlusion; in general, the aim is to save the line and resume feeding with minimum risk of the patient. The use of locks and flushes with alteplase (for fibrin and thrombosis), ethanol (for lipid deposits) and dilute hydrochloric acid (for salt and drug precipitates) may be considered. In some cases, the lines may need to be replaced. These complications can be minimised by having a dedicated line for PN and flushing the line well with sodium chloride 0.9% before and after use; a regular slow flush of ethanol 20% may be used to prevent lipid deposition.

Refeeding syndrome

Patients should be assessed as to their risk of developing refeeding syndrome (see Table 7.14). Refeeding syndrome can be defined as 'the potentially fatal shifts in fluids and electrolytes that may occur in malnourished patients receiving nutrition' (Mehanna et al., 2008). Undernourished patients are catabolic, and their major sources of energy are fat and muscle. As the PN infusion (which contains glucose) starts, this catabolic state is pushed to anabolic, which in turn causes a surge of insulin. As the insulin levels increase, there is an intracellular shift of magnesium, potassium and phosphate, and acute hypomanganesaemia, hypokalaemia and hypophosphataemia result. This can cause cardiac and neurological dysfunction and may be fatal. PN should be gradually increased over a period of 2–7 days, depending on the patient's BMI and risk of developing refeeding syndrome. Thiamine is an essential coenzyme in carbohydrate metabolism and deficiency results in Wernicke's encephalopathy (ocular abnormalities, ataxia, confusional state, hypothermia, coma) or Korsakoff's syndrome (retrograde and anterograde amnesia, confabulation). For these reasons, oral thiamine and vitamin B compound strong or full-dose intravenous vitamin B preparation may be administered before PN is started and for the first few days of infusion.

Specific disease states
Liver

Abnormal liver function tests associated with short-term PN are usually benign and transient. However, liver dysfunction in long-term PN patients is one of the most prevalent and severe complications. The underlying pathophysiology largely remains to be elucidated. The content of PN should be examined, and care should be taken not to overfeed with glucose and/or lipid. Various lipid preparations are now available, including preparations containing fish oils, which have been reported to be beneficial in reversing liver disease (De Meijer et al., 2009). Lipid emulsions containing a mix of medium- and long-chain triglycerides are also available and have an improved liver tolerability. Because of the complexity of liver function, the range of potential disorders and the liver's role in metabolism, the use of PN in liver disease can cause problems. Consensus guidelines for the use of PN in liver disease have been published (Plauth et al., 2009). Nutritional intervention may be essential for recovery, although care must be exercised with amino acid input and the risk of encephalopathy, calorie input and metabolic capacity, and the reduced clearance of trace elements such as copper and manganese (Maroulis and Kalfarentzos, 2000). Low-sodium, low-volume feeds are indicated if there is ascites. Cyclic feeding appears useful, especially in steatosis.

Renal failure

Fluid and electrolyte balance demand close attention, and guidelines for nutrition in adult renal failure are available (Cano et al., 2009). A low-volume and poor-quality urine output may necessitate a concentrated PN formulation with a reduction in electrolyte content, particularly a reduction in potassium and phosphate. In the polyuric phase or the nephrotic syndrome, a higher-volume formulation may be required. If there is fluid retention, ideal body weight should be used for calculating requirements rather than the actual body weight.

The metabolic stress of acute renal failure and the malnutrition of chronic renal failure may initially demand relatively high nutritional requirements; however, nitrogen restriction may be necessary to control uraemia in the absence of dialysis or filtration and to avoid uraemia-related impaired glucose tolerance, because of peripheral insulin resistance, and lipid clearance. Micronutrient requirements may also change in renal disease. For example, renal clearance of zinc, selenium, fluoride and chromium is reduced, and there is less renal 1α-hydroxylation of vitamin D.

Intradialytic PN (IDPN) may be administered at the same time as dialysis; however, this is not without complications. High blood sugars and fluid overload can be a problem, and there is uncertainty as to how much of the PN is retained by the body and how much is removed by dialysis. Administration requires local guidelines and monitoring to be in place (Dukkipati et al., 2010; Lazarus, 1999).

Pancreatitis

Acute pancreatitis is a metabolic stress that requires high-level nutritional support and pancreatic rest to recover. Guidelines for nutrition in acute pancreatitis are available (Gianotti et al., 2009). Whereas enteral nutrition stimulates the pancreas, PN does not appear to. Hyperglycaemia may occur and require exogenous insulin.

Sepsis and injury

Significant fluctuations in macronutrient metabolism are seen during sepsis and injury. There are two metabolic phases: the 'ebb' phase of 24–48 hours and the following 'flow' phase. The initial hyperglycaemia, reflecting a reduced utilisation of glucose, is followed by a longer catabolic state with increased utilisation of lipid and amino acids. The effect of the different lipid emulsions on immune function is the subject of much research. It is important not to overfeed and also to consider the reduced glucose tolerance during the critical days. This is a result of increased insulin resistance and incomplete glucose oxidation. Exogenous insulin may be required.

Respiratory

Whereas underfeeding and malnutrition can compromise respiratory effort and muscle function, overfeeding can equally compromise respiratory function as a result of increased carbon dioxide and lipid effects on the circulation. Although chronic respiratory disease may be linked with a long-standing malnutrition, the patient with acute disease will generally be hypermetabolic.

Heart failure

Heart failure and multiple-drug therapy may limit the volume of PN that can be infused. Concentrated formulations are used and, as a consequence of the high tonicity, administered via the central route. Close electrolyte monitoring and adjustment are required. Cardiac drugs may affect electrolyte clearance. Although central lines may already be in use for other drugs or cardiac monitoring, it is essential to maintain a dedicated lumen or line for the feed.

Diabetes mellitus

Diabetic patients can generally be maintained with standard dual-energy regimens. It is important to use insulin to manage blood glucose rather than reduce the nutritional provision of the feed. Close glucose monitoring will guide exogenous insulin administration. This should be given as a separate infusion (sliding scale) or, if the patient is stable, in bolus doses. Insulin should not be included within the PN formulation because of stability problems and variable adsorption to the equipment. Y-site infusion with the PN should be avoided because changes in insulin rates will be delayed, and changes in feed rates will result in significant fluctuations in insulin administration. Long-term PN patients may need differing insulin regimens, depending on the glucose load (aqueous/lipid) in the formulation. Although using oral antihypoglycaemic agents with PN may be considered, care should be taken as to the potentially erratic absorption and thus varying blood glucose levels.

Cancer and palliative care

The worldwide debate over the use of artificial nutrition and hydration in cancer and palliative care remains controversial. Nutritional support in cancer and palliative care is guided by the potential risks and benefits of the intervention, alongside the wishes of the patient and carers. Further research is required to evaluate the effects of PN on length and quality of life. Guidelines have been developed on ethical aspects of artificial nutrition (Druml et al., 2016). PN may be useful during prolonged periods of gastro-intestinal toxicity, as in bone marrow transplant patients.

Pre- and postsurgery

Only a minority of patients require pre- and postsurgical PN, as most are eating normal food within 1–3 days. In patients with severe undernutrition and who cannot be fed adequately enterally, 7–10 days preoperative PN improves postoperative outcome. Postoperative PN is recommended in patients who cannot meet their calorie requirements enterally within 7–10 days following surgery.

Short bowel syndrome

The small intestine is defined as 'short' if it is less than 100 cm. Treatment options depend on which part of the gut has been removed and the functional state of the remaining organ. The surface area for absorption of nutrition and reabsorption of fluid and electrolytes is significantly compromised. Fluid and electrolyte balance needs to be managed closely because of the high-volume losses. High-volume PN formulations with raised electrolyte content (notably sodium and magnesium) may be required. Vitamin and trace element provision is very important.

Long-term parenteral nutrition

Comprehensive guidelines have been developed for adult patients with chronic intestinal failure (Pironi et al., 2016). Chronic intestinal failure is described as 'the long lasting reduction of gut function below the minimum necessary for the absorption of macronutrients with or without water and electrolytes, such that intravenous supplementation is required to maintain health with or without growth' (Pironi et al., 2016).

Home care is well established in the UK, with some patients successfully supported for over 20 years. There are an increasing number of patients receiving long-term PN at home. In these patients, total or supplemental PN may be appropriate. Trace elements, notably selenium, should be managed closely because a patient's requirements may be increased.

Many patients are trained to connect and disconnect their PN and to care for their central lines. Patients are encouraged to lead as active and normal a life as possible. Foreign travel is now possible for patients on home PN, as are most other normal daily activities and sports (Staun et al., 2009). Most patients are extremely well informed about their underlying disease and their PN; many also benefit from the support group Patients on Intravenous and Nasogastric Nutrition Therapy (PINNT) and from Looking into the Requirements for Equipment (LITRE), a standing committee of BAPEN which looks at equipment issues.

Before patients are discharged home on PN, medication should be optimised to reduce the amount of PN they require. Medication therapy is used to reduce gut transit time, so loperamide is frequently prescribed. In practice, the dose of loperamide often exceeds the maximum dose recommended by the manufacturer. Opioids such as codeine phosphate may also be used to reduce gut transit time. However, loperamide is preferred to opiate drugs because it is not addictive or sedative. Proton pump inhibitors are also used to reduce gastric secretion and thereby reduce the amount of fluid lost through high-output stomas.

Paediatric parenteral nutrition

Nutritional requirements

Early nutritional intervention is required in paediatric patients because of their low reserve, especially in neonates. Where possible, premature neonates should commence feeding from day 1. In addition to requirements for the maintenance of body tissue, function and repair, it is also important to support growth and development.

Typical guidelines for average daily requirements of fluid, energy and nitrogen are shown in Table 7.15. The dual-energy approach is favoured in paediatrics. Most centres gradually increase the lipid provision from day 1 from 1 g/kg/day to 2 g/kg/day and then 3 g/kg/day, monitoring lipid clearance through the serum triglyceride level. This ensures the essential fatty acid requirements of premature neonates are met.

Formulation and stability issues

Many centres use PN formulations that include specific paediatric amino acid solutions (Primene, Vaminolact or Aminoplasmal Paediatric). Prescriptions and formulations are tailored to reflect clinical status, biochemistry and nutritional requirements. Micronutrients are included daily. Paediatric licensed preparations are available and are included on a mL/kg basis up to a maximum total volume (Peditrace, Solivito N and Vitlipid N Infant). Electrolytes are also monitored and included in all formulations on a mmol/kg basis. Acid–base balance should be considered. Potassium and sodium acetate salt forms are used in balance with the chloride salt forms in neonatal formulae to avoid excessive chloride input contributing to acidosis (acetate is metabolised to bicarbonate, an alkali). In the initial stages, neonates tend to be hypernatraemia as a result of relatively poor renal clearance; this should be reflected in the standard formulae used. If calcium gluconate is used, it must be from plastic containers because of the concerns over contamination with aluminium.

As a result of the balance of nutritional requirements, a relatively high glucose requirement with high calcium and phosphate provision, the neonatal and paediatric prescription may be supplied by a 2-in-1 formulation and separate lipid infusion. These are generally given concurrently, joining at a Y-site. Older children can sometimes be managed with 3-in-1 formulations. A single infusion is particularly useful in the home care environment. Some ready-to-use formulations are licensed for use in paediatrics.

Improved stability profiles with the new lipid emulsions, and increasing stability data, may support 3-in-1 formulations that meet the nutritional requirements of younger children.

Heparin

Historically, low concentrations of heparin were included in 2-in-1 formulations in an attempt to improve fat clearance through enhanced triglyceride hydrolysis, prevent the formation of fibrin around the infusion line, reduce thrombosis and reduce thrombophlebitis during peripheral infusion. However, this is no longer recommended because it was recognised that when the 2-in-1 formulation comes into contact with the lipid phase, calcium-heparin bridges form between these lipid globules, destabilising the formulation. Also, there is limited evidence of clinical benefit of the heparin inclusion.

Route of administration

Peripheral administration is less common in neonates and children because of the risk of thrombophlebitis; however, it is useful when low-concentration, short-term PN is required and there is

Table 7.15 Suggested paediatric daily parenteral nutrition requirements

		Day 1	Day 2	Day 3	Day 4	Na⁺	K⁺	Ca²⁺	Mg²⁺
			>1 month but <10 kg				mmol/kg/day		
Fluid requirement	100 mL/kg								
						3	2.5	0.6	0.1
Nitrogen	g/kg	0.15	0.2	0.3	0.4				
Glucose	g/kg	10	12	14	16				
Lipid	g/kg	1	2	2	3				
Phosphate[a]	mmol/kg/day	0.5	0.58	0.58	0.6				
			10–15 kg						
Fluid requirement	1000 mL + 50 mL/kg for each kg above 10 kg								
						3	2.5	0.2	0.07
Nitrogen	g/kg	0.15	0.2	0.3	0.3				
Glucose	g/kg	6	8	10	12				
Lipid	g/kg	1.5	2	2.5	2.5				
Phosphate[a]	mmol/kg/day	0.23	0.27	0.3	0.3				
			16–20 kg						
Fluid requirement	1000 mL + 50 mL/kg for each kg above 10 kg								
						3	2	0.2	0.07
Nitrogen	g/kg	0.15	0.2	0.3	0.3				
Glucose	g/kg	4	6	8	10				
Lipid	g/kg	1.5	2	2	2				
Phosphate[a]	mmol/kg/day	0.22	0.26	0.26	0.26				
			21–30 kg						
Fluid requirement	1500 mL + 20 mL/kg for each kg above 20 kg								
						3	2	0.2	0.07
Nitrogen	g/kg	0.2	0.3	0.3					
Glucose	g/kg	4	6	8					
Lipid	g/kg	1	2	2					
Phosphate[a]	mmol/kg/day	0.18	0.26	0.26					
			>30 kg						
Fluid requirement	1500 mL + 20 mL/kg for each kg above 20 kg								
						3	2	0.2	0.07
Nitrogen	g/kg	0.15	0.2						
Glucose	g/kg	3	5						
Lipid	g/kg	1	2						
Phosphate[a]	mmol/kg/day	0.18	0.25						

[a]Includes phosphate from lipid emulsion and Vitlipid preparations.
Adapted from Koletzko et al., (2005).

good peripheral access. The maximum glucose concentration for peripheral administration in paediatrics is generally regarded to be 12%. However, considering all the other factors that can affect the tonicity of a regimen and peripheral tolerance, it is clear that this is a relatively simplistic perspective. Many centres favour a limit of 10% with close clinical observation. Tonicity of the formulation should also be used when reviewing the route of administration.

Central administration is via a PICC a long-term tunnelled central line or a jugular or subclavian line. Femoral lines are a less preferred option because of their location and, therefore, high risk of becoming infected.

Case studies

Case 7.1

Mrs AB is 40-year-old and has been admitted to hospital for an elective bowel resection. She has suffered from Crohn's disease for 20 years and has had many previous episodes of surgery. Over the last 3 months Mrs AB has lost 6 kg body weight. Her current weight is 45 kg, and she is 1.6 m tall. Mrs AB is admitted 2 weeks prior to surgery for elective preoperative intravenous feeding to maximise the success of surgery.

Post-operatively, Mrs AB is left with an ileostomy, and her surgical notes inform you she has just 90 cm of small bowel remaining. There is no plan for further surgery.

Questions

1. Calculate Mrs AB's fluid requirements and nutritional requirements using the Henry equation.
2. What sort of intravenous access would be appropriate for Mrs AB's preoperative PN?
3. What electrolytes and vitamins may need to be supplemented as PN starts, and why?
4. What sort of access should be considered for postoperative PN?
5. What changes would you expect to see in Mrs AB's PN formulation?
6. What long-term care plan would you expect to see for Mrs AB?

Answers

1. The provision of 20–40 mL/kg fluid gives a requirement of between 900 mL and 1800 mL/day. Using the Henry equation Mrs AB's nutritional requirements are 1132 kcal/day ([9.74 × 45] + 694 = 1132 kcal/day).
2. Given Mrs AB's current weight of 45 kg and having calculated her fluid and nutritional requirements, it can be seen that they are not excessively high. Providing Mrs AB has good peripheral access, a long peripheral line would be suitable. This can be inserted at the bedside and is good for short-term feeding. PN suitable for peripheral infusion should be formulated.
3. Mrs AB is at risk of refeeding syndrome given that her BMI is 17.6 (BMI = weight [kg]/height [m^2]) and she has lost more than 10% of her body weight in the last 6 months. With this in mind potassium, magnesium and phosphate should be monitored closely and supplemented where necessary. Vitamin B compound strong or intravenous vitamin B should be given.
4. Given that Mrs AB now has a 'short bowel' (i.e. <100 cm), it is likely she will require long-term parenteral nutrition. For this reason, a more permanent central line should be considered, such as a tunnelled central line.

5. With only 90 cm of short bowel, Mrs AB will have a high-output ileostomy, likely greater than 1000 mL/day output. This means the volume of PN will need to be increased to prevent dehydration and to replace losses. Ileostomy secretions are rich in sodium, and therefore sodium will need to be increased. Magnesium loss will also mean an increased requirement in the PN.
6. It is likely Mrs AB will need to go home on PN. Prior to this, medication to slow gut transit time should be optimised. Her prescription may look like the following:

   Codeine phosphate 60 mg four times a day
   Loperamide 6 mg four times a day
   Omeprazole 40 mg once a day

   Once medication has been optimised, PN formulation should be stabilised—namely, electrolytes and fluid. Mrs AB may not need PN every day. The multidisciplinary nutrition team should then work to train Mrs AB to connect and disconnect her own PN and to care for her central line. A home care package and PN equipment installation will then be required before Mrs AB is discharged into the community. There will be close follow-up and regular outpatient clinic appointments.

Case 7.2

You arrive at work on a Monday morning to find the nutrition support pharmacist has phoned in sick and you have been asked to cover PN. During the course of the morning, you receive a referral for a patient who needs to start PN. You and the rest of the nutrition support team go to review the patient and find the following clinical details:
- The patient, Mrs T, is 40-year-old and weighs 70 kg.
- Mrs T has been diagnosed with a postoperative ileus following elective surgery. She is now 7 days post-op.
- Mrs T has no history of weight loss or malnutrition. Preoperatively, she was well, with a good healthy diet.
- Mrs T has a triple-lumen central line in situ, which was placed during surgery. One lumen has been used for intravenous fluids, another for intravenous antibiotics. The third lumen has not been used.
- Mrs T has no gastro-intestinal losses. Unfortunately, the last set of blood biochemistry taken was 3 days ago. The results that are available are all within normal limits.

Questions

1. Describe what course of action you would take to initiate PN, paying particular attention to the following:
   a. Nutritional requirements
   b. Fluid requirements
   c. Electrolyte requirements
   d. Intravenous access
2. Back in the pharmacy, you check which ready-to-use products are stocked. You find the following products on the shelf:

	Product 1	Product 2	Product 3
Volume (mL)	1500	2000	2500
Kcal	900	1720	2200
Nitrogen (g)	6.0	10.4	13.6
Sodium (mmol)	31.5	70	100
Potassium (mmol)	24	60	70
Magnesium (mmol)	3.3	8	8
Calcium (mmol)	3.0	7	8
Phosphate (mmol)	12.7	30	30

2. Describe which product is most suitable for Mrs T, and suggest any additions to be made.

The next day, the PN pharmacist is still off sick. You join the rest of the nutrition support team to review Mrs T. Her blood biochemistry results from yesterday are now available:

Sodium	130 mmol/L	(135–145 mmol/L)
Potassium	4.5 mmol/L	(3.4–5 mmol/L)
Magnesium	0.58 mmol/L	(0.7–1.0 mmol/L)
Corrected calcium	2.25 mmol/L	(2.12–2.6 mmol/L)
Phosphate	1.3 mmol/L	(0.8–1.44 mmol/L)

You find Mrs T to be apyrexial but in a positive fluid balance of 800 mL. On examination you observe mild ankle oedema.

3. Comment on the biochemistry and clinical findings, and describe what course of action you would take from a PN-formulation point of view.

4. Mrs T asks you if she is able to have some time not connected to the PN to take a walk on the ward. What is your response?

5. It is now Friday, and the PN pharmacist is still off sick. Mrs T has started to eat and drink and is progressing well. Describe what PN formulations you would compound for her for the weekend.

· ·

Answers

1. a. In discussion with the dietician, you estimate energy requirements to be 25–35 kcal/kg = 1750–2450 kcal/kg and protein to be 0.2 gN/kg/day = 14g.
   b. Given that there are no gastro-intestinal losses which need replacing, Mrs T's fluid requirements can be estimated as 20–40 mL/kg/day = 1400–2800 mL/day.
   c. Given that there is no recent blood biochemistry, basal requirements should be calculated and a set of blood taken for analysis. These results will then be available to aid compounding the next day.

Sodium 1–1.5 mmol/kg	= 70–105 mmol
Potassium 1–1.5 mmol/kg	= 70–105 mmol
Calcium 0.1–0.15 mmol/kg	= 7–10.5 mmol
Magnesium 0.1–0.2 mmol/kg	= 7–14 mmol
Phosphate 0.5–0.7 mmol/kg	= 35–49 mmol

   d. Given that Mrs T has a central line in situ, one port should be dedicated to PN. The central line should be examined to ensure the site is clean and well dressed.

2. The most suitable formulation is product 3. This formulation more or less meets all Mrs T's requirements. Only vitamins and trace elements need to be added to the bag prior to infusing.

3. Sodium abnormalities always warrant careful management. Given that Mrs T has no gastro-intestinal losses, she is in a positive fluid balance and she has ankle oedema, the low sodium is likely to be a result of fluid overload rather than sodium deficiency. Therefore fluid restriction is the correct course of action rather than administering a greater amount of sodium. The formulation should be changed to product 2. This means a reduction in volume to 2000 mL. Note also the reduced amount of sodium in this bag compared with product 3. However, even the 70 mmol sodium in product 2 meets Mrs T's basal requirements, and so there would be no need to increase further in the PN. Sodium level should come up with fluid restriction alone. The low magnesium is likely to be attributable to the fact that Mrs T has not received any magnesium supplementation postoperatively, and this is, therefore, a genuinely low level. The product literature for the chosen formulation should be checked to elucidate the maximum amount of magnesium that may be added to the bag. This should then be added as a manual addition in the pharmacy aseptic unit. Some other parameters in product 2 are slightly lower than the calculated requirements; however, these differences are negligible and are of secondary importance to the correction of sodium and fluid balance. Monitoring will continue during the course of treatment.

4. The first infusion should always be over 24 hours. Providing blood sugar levels are stable and within normal limits, the infusion time may then be reduced. You could suggest a 4-hour rest period on day 2 of PN, then a 6-hour rest period on day 3 of PN.

5. Given the good prognosis, it is likely Mrs T will no longer require PN by Monday. PN should, therefore, be tapered off over the weekend as oral diet increases. One possible way of doing this is to give just half the PN infusion over a 12-hour overnight period. Any remaining solution must be discarded once the PN is disconnected. This could be given Friday and Saturday nights and then no PN on Sunday. Mrs T should then be reviewed again on Monday morning with the intention of stopping PN and removing the central line, providing oral nutritional intake is deemed adequate.

Acknowledgement

This chapter is based on the contribution by S. J. Dunnett that first appeared in the fourth edition of this textbook.

References

Bethune, K., Allwood, M., Grainger, C., et al., 2001. Use of filters during the preparation and administration of parenteral nutrition: position paper and guidelines prepared by a British Pharmaceutical Nutrition Group Working Party. Nutrition 17, 403–408.

Cano, N.J.M., Aparicio, M., Brunori, G., et al., 2009. European Society for Parenteral and Enteral Nutrition (ESPEN) guidelines on parenteral nutrition: acute renal failure. Clin. Nutr. 28, 401–414.

De Meijer, V.E., Gura, K.M., Le, H.D., 2009. Fish oil-based emulsions prevent and reverse parenteral nutrition associated liver disease. The Boston experience. J. Parenter. Enteral Nutr. 33, 541–547.

Department of Health, 1991. Dietary reference values for food energy and nutrients for the United Kingdom. Report of the panel on dietary reference values of the committee on medical aspects of food policy. Department of Health, London.

Druml, C., Ballmer, P., Druml, W., et al., 2016. European Society for Parenteral and Enteral Nutrition (ESPEN) guideline on ethical aspects of artificial nutrition and hydration. Clin. Nutr. 35 (3), 545–556.

Dukkipati, R., Kalantar-Zaden, K., Kopple, J.D., 2010. Is there a role for intradialytic parenteral nutrition? A review of the evidence. Am. J. Kidney Dis. 55 (2), 352–364.

Gales, B.J., Gales, M.J., 1994. Nutritional support teams: a review of comparative trials. Ann. Pharmacother. 28 (2), 227–235.

Gianotti, L., Meier, R., Lobo, D., et al., 2009. European Society for Parenteral and Enteral Nutrition (ESPEN) guidelines on nutrition in pancreatitis. Clin. Nutr. 28, 428–435.

Henry, C.J.K., 2005. Basal metabolic rate studies in humans: measurement and development of new equations. Public Health Nutr. 8 (7a), 1133–1152.

Holick, M., Binkley, N., Bischoff-Ferrari, H., et al., 2011. Evaluation, treatment and prevention of vitamin D deficiency. An endocrine society clinical practice guideline. J. Clin. Endocrinol. Metab. 96 (7), 1911–1930.

Khawaja, H.T., Williams, J.D., 1991. Transdermal glyceryl trinitrate to allow peripheral total parenteral nutrition: a double blind placebo controlled feasibility study. J. R. Soc. Med. 84, 69–72.

Kings Fund Report, 1992. A Positive Approach to Nutrition as Treatment. Kings Fund, London.

Klek, S., 2016. Omega-3 fatty acids in modern parenteral nutrition: a review of the current evidence. J. Clin. Med. 5, 34. https://doi.org/10.3390/jcm5030034.

Koletzko, B., Goulet, O., Hunt, J., 2005. Guidelines on paediatric parenteral nutrition of the European Society of Paediatric Gastroenterology, Hepatology and Nutrition (ESPGHAN) and the European Society for Enteral and Parenteral Nutrition (ESPEN), supported by the European Society of Paediatric Research (ESPR). J. Parenter. Enteral Nutr. 41 (Suppl. 2), S1–S87. Available at http://espghan.med.up.pt/joomla/position_papers/con_22.pdf.

Lazarus, J.M., 1999. Recommended criteria for initiating and discontinuing intradialytic parenteral nutrition. Am. J. Kidney Dis. 33, 211–216.

Maroulis, J., Kalfarentzos, F., 2000. Complications of parenteral nutrition at the end of the century. Clin. Nutr. 19, 299–304.

Mehanna, H.M., Moledina, J., Travis, J., 2008. Refeeding syndrome: what it is, and how to prevent and treat it. BMJ 336 (7659), 1495–1498.

National Institute for Health and Care Excellence (NICE), 2006. Nutrition support in adults CG32. NICE, London. Available at: http://www.nice.org.uk/guidance/CG32.

Pironi, L., Arends, J., Bozzetti, F., et al., 2016. The home artificial nutrition and chronic intestinal failure special interest group of European Society of Parenteral and Enteral Nutrition (ESPEN) guidelines on chronic intestinal failure in adults. Clin. Nutr. 35, 247–307.

Plauth, M., Cabre, E., Canpillo, B., et al., 2009. European Society of Parenteral and Enteral Nutrition (ESPEN) guidelines on parenteral nutrition: hepatology. Clin. Nutr. 28, 436–444.

Staun, M., Pironi, L., Bozzetti, F., et al., 2009. European Society of Parenteral and Enteral Nutrition (ESPEN) guidelines on parenteral nutrition: home parenteral nutrition (HPN) in adult patients. Clin. Nutr. 28, 467–479.

The Scientific Advisory Committee on Nutrition (SACN) Vitamin D and Health, 2016.

Vanek, V.W., Borum, P., Buchman, A., et al., 2012. American Society for Parenteral and Enteral Nutrition (ASPEN) position paper: recommendations for the changes in commercially available parenteral multivitamin and multi-trace element products. Nutr. Clin. Pract. 27, 440–491.

Further reading

Austin, P., Stroud, M., 2007. Prescribing Adult Intravenous Nutrition. Pharmaceutical Press, London.

Bozzetti, F., Staun, M., Van Gossum, A., 2015. Home Parenteral Nutrition, second ed. Cabi, Wallingford.

Useful websites

British Pharmaceutical Nutrition Group. Available at: http://www.bpng.co.uk
European Society of Parenteral and Enteral Nutrition. Available at: http://www.espen.orgBritish

Association of Parenteral and Enteral Nutrition. Available at: http://www.bapen.org

8 Pharmacoeconomics

Jonathan Cooke

Key points

- Expenditure on medicines is increasing at a greater rate than other healthcare costs.
- Increasingly, governments are employing health economics to help prioritise between different medicines and other health technologies.
- In health economics, the consequences of a treatment can be expressed in monetary terms (cost–benefit), natural units of effectiveness (cost-effectiveness) and in terms of patient preference or utility (cost–utility).
- Head-to-head studies offer the best way of determining overall effectiveness and cost-effectiveness.
- Sensitivity analysis can be used to address areas of uncertainty.
- Medication non-adherence, medication errors and unwanted drug effects place a considerable burden on societal healthcare costs.
- Decision analysis techniques offer a powerful tool for comparing alternative treatment options.

The demand for and the cost of health care are growing in all countries. Many governments are focusing their activities on promoting the effective and economic use of resources allocated to health care. The increased use of evidence-based programmes not only concentrates on optimising health outcomes but also utilises health economic evaluations. Spending on health across the Organisation for Economic Co-operation and Development (OECD) edged up slightly in 2013, with preliminary estimates pointing to a continuation of this trend in 2014. The slow rise comes after health spending growth ground to a halt in 2010 in the wake of the global financial and economic crisis (OECD, 2016).

Although there have been marked gains in life expectancy in those countries which make up the OECD, health costs have also risen in all of them. The USA spent 16.4% of its national income (gross domestic product [GDP]) on health in 2013, a value considerably greater than many other OECD countries and almost twice that of the UK (Fig. 8.1).

Medicines form a small but significant proportion of total healthcare costs; this has been increasing consistently as new medicines are marketed. For example, the overall National Health Service (NHS) expenditure on medicines in 2014–15 was £15.5 billion, an increase of 7.8% from £14.4 billion in 2013–14 and an increase of 19.4% from £13.0 billion in 2010–11. In 2014–15 hospital use accounted for 42.9% of the total cost, up from 40.1% in 2013–14 and up from 32.1% in 2010/11. Expenditure on medicines rose by 7.8% overall and by 15.4% in hospitals from 2013–14 to 2014–15. The expenditure on medicines in hospitals has risen by 59.8% since 2010–11 (Health and Social Care Information Centre, 2015).

There are a number of reasons why prescribing costs are increasing:

- Demographic changes have resulted in an ageing population, with individuals living longer and with greater needs for therapeutic interventions. This patient group is more susceptible to unwanted effects of medicines which in turn consume more resources.
- More patients have complex clinical problems and comorbidities that have a higher dependency on medicines.
- Health screening programmes and improved diagnostic and imaging techniques are uncovering previously nonidentified diseases, which subsequently require treatment.
- New medicines that offer more effective and less toxic alternatives to existing agents are being marketed. Invariably these are more expensive, especially biotechnology medicines, such as monoclonal antibodies, which can cost in excess of £30,000 per patient per year.
- The use of existing agents is becoming more widespread as additional indications for their use are found.
- Increasing numbers of standards in guidelines for care are being set by national bodies, such as the National Institute for Health and Care Excellence (NICE).
- The public and patients have a higher expectation of their rights to access high-cost health care.
- Higher acquisition costs are also a result of inflation and currency fluctuations.

In the UK, health reforms over the past two decades have addressed the quality of care through the promotion of quality and safety standards. The formation of NICE in 1998 'to improve standards of patient care and to reduce inequities in access to innovative treatment' has formalised this process. NICE undertakes appraisals of medicines and other treatments (health technologies) and addresses the clinical and cost-effectiveness of therapies and compares outcomes with alternative use of NHS funds. The increased use of evidence-based programmes not only concentrates on optimising health outcomes but also utilises health economic evaluations. Formalised health technology assessments provide an in-depth and evidence-based approach to this process.

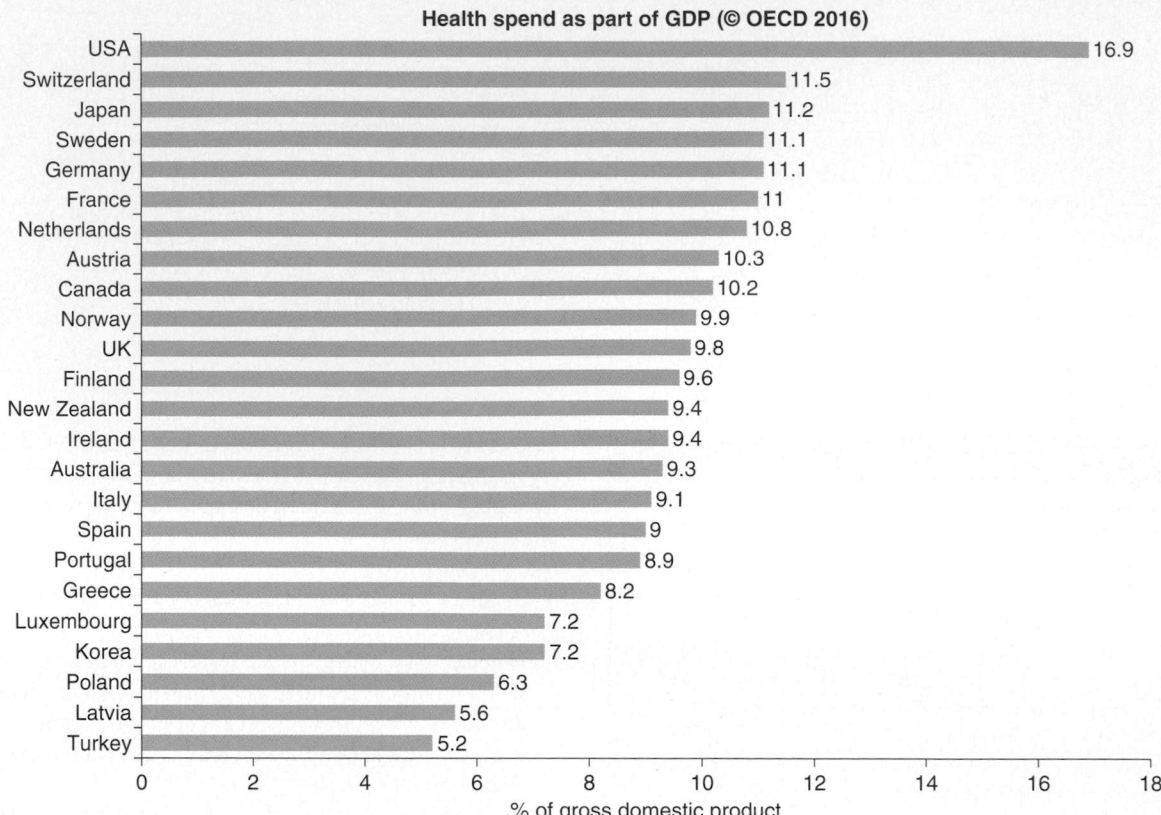

Fig. 8.1 Comparison of health spending as a percentage of gross domestic product in different countries in 2015. (© Organisation for Economic Co-operation and Development, 2016.)

Terms used in health economics

Pharmacoeconomics can be defined as the measurement of both the costs and consequences of therapeutic decision making. Pharmacoeconomics provides a guide for decision makers on resource allocation but does not offer a basis on which decisions should be made. Pharmacoeconomics can assist in the planning process and help assign priorities where, for example, medicines with a worse outcome may be available at a lower cost, and medicines with better outcome and higher cost can be compared.

When economic evaluations are conducted, it is important to categorise various costs. Costs can be direct to the organisation – physicians' salaries, the acquisition costs of medicines, consumables associated with drug administration, staff time in preparation and administration of medicines, laboratory charges for monitoring effectiveness and adverse drug reactions. Indirect costs include lost productivity from a disease, which can manifest itself as a cost to the economy or taxation system, as well as economic costs to the patient and the patient's family. All aspects of the use of medicines may be allocated costs, both direct, such as acquisition and administration costs, and indirect, such as the cost of a given patient's time off work because of illness, in terms of lost output and social security payments. The consequences of drug therapy include benefits for both the individual patient and society at large and may be quantified in terms of health outcome and quality of life, in addition to the purely economic impact.

It is worthwhile here to describe a number of definitions that further qualify costs in a healthcare setting. The concept of 'opportunity cost' is at the centre of economics and identifies the value of opportunities which have been lost by utilising resources in a particular service or health technology. This can be valued as the benefits that have been forsaken by investing the resources in the best alternative fashion. Opportunity cost recognises that there are limited resources available for utilising every treatment, and therefore the rationing of health care is implicit in such a system.

Average costs are the simplest way of valuing the consumption of healthcare resources. Quite simply, they represent the total costs (i.e. all the costs incurred in the delivery of a service) of a healthcare system divided by the units of production. For example, a hospital might treat 75,000 patients a year (defined as finished consultant episodes [FCEs]) and have a total annual revenue cost of £150 million. The average cost per FCE is therefore £2000.

Fixed costs are those that are independent of the number of units of production and include heating, lighting and fixed staffing costs.

Variable costs, on the other hand, are dependent on the numbers of units of productivity. The cost of the consumption of medicines is a good example of variable costs.

The inevitable increases in the medicines budget in a particular institution which is treating more patients, or treating those with a more complex pathology, have often been erroneously interpreted by financial managers as a failure to effectively manage the budget. To better describe the costs associated with a healthcare intervention, economists employ the term *marginal costs* to describe the costs of producing an extra unit of a particular service. The term *incremental cost* is employed to define the difference between the costs of alternative interventions.

Choice of comparator

Sometimes a claim is made that a treatment is cost-effective. But cost-effective against what? As in any good clinical trial, a treatment has to be compared against a reasonable comparator. The choice of comparator is crucial to this process. A comparator that is no longer in common use or in a dose that is not optimal will result in the evaluated treatment being seen as more effective than it actually is. Sadly, many evaluations of medicines fall into this trap, as sponsors seldom wish to undertake head-to-head studies against competitors. Again, the reader has to be careful when interpreting economic evaluations from settings which are different from those in local practice. A common error can be made when viewing international studies that have different healthcare costs and ways of treating patients and translating them directly into 'one's own practice'. This is sometimes referred as *generalisability* or *external validity*.

In addition, hospital charges, including those for hotel services such as heating and lighting overheads, meals and accommodation, which may constitute a major cost, should be considered. These are frequently included in an average cost per patient day.

Types of health economic evaluations
Cost–benefit analysis

In cost–benefit analysis (CBA), consequences are measured in terms of the total cost associated with a programme, where both costs and consequences are measured in monetary terms. Although this type of analysis is preferred by economists, its use in health care is problematic because it is frequently difficult to ascribe monetary values to clinical outcomes such as pain relief, avoidance of stroke or improvements in quality of life.

Methods are available for determining cost–benefit for individual groups of patients that centre around a concept known as *contingent valuation*. Specific techniques include 'willingness to pay', where patients are asked to state how much they would be prepared to pay to avoid a particular event or symptom, for example, pain or nausea following day-care surgery. Willingness to pay can be fraught with difficulties of interpretation in countries with socialised healthcare systems, which are invariably funded out of general taxation. 'Willingness to accept' is a similar concept but is based on the minimum amount an individual person or population would receive in order to be prepared to lose or reduce a service.

CBA can be usefully employed at a macro level for strategic decisions on healthcare programmes. For example, a countrywide immunisation programme can be fully costed in terms of resource utilisation consumed in running the programme. This can then be valued against the reduced mortality and morbidity that occur as a result of the programme.

CBA can be useful in examining the value of services – for example, centralised intravenous additive services where a comparison between a pharmacy-based intravenous additive service and ward-based preparation by doctors and nurses may demonstrate the value of the centralised pharmacy service, or a clinical pharmacokinetics service where the staffing and equipment costs can be offset against the benefits of reduced morbidity and mortality.

Cost-effectiveness analysis

Cost-effectiveness analysis (CEA) can be described as an examination of the costs of two or more programmes which have the same clinical outcome as measured in physical units (e.g. lives saved or reduced morbidity). Treatments with dissimilar outcomes can also be analysed by this technique. Where two or more interventions have been shown to be or are assumed to be similar, then if all other factors are equal, for example, convenience, side effects, availability, and so forth, selection can be made on the basis of cost. This type of analysis is called *cost-minimisation analysis* (CMA). CMA is frequently employed in formulary decision making where often the available evidence for a new product appears to be no better than that for existing products. This is invariably what happens in practice because clinical trials on new medicines are statistically powered for equivalence as a requirement for licensing submission.

As previously described, CEA examines the costs associated with achieving a defined health outcome. Although these outcomes can be relief of symptoms such as nausea and vomiting avoided, pain relieved, and so forth, CEA frequently employs years of life gained as a measure of the success of a particular programme. This can then offer a method of incrementally comparing the costs associated with two or more interventions. For example, consider a hypothetical case of the comparison of two drug treatments for the management of malignant disease.

Treatment 1 represents a 1-year course of treatment for a particular malignant disease. Assume that this is the current standard form of treatment and that the average total direct costs associated with this programme are £A per year. This will include the costs of the medicines, antiemetics, in-patient stay, radiology and pathology. Treatment 2 is a new drug treatment for the malignancy which has demonstrated, through comparative controlled clinical trials, an improvement in the average life expectancy for this group of patients from 3.5 years for treatment 1 to 4.5 years for treatment 2. The average annual total costs for treatment 2 are £B. A comparative table can now be constructed.

Strategy	Treatment costs	Effectiveness
Treatment 1	£A	3.5 years
Treatment 2	£B	4.5 years

Incremental cost-effectiveness ratio: = £B – £A/(4.5 – 3.5) per life-year gained.

Cost–utility analysis

An alternative measurement of the consequences of a healthcare intervention is the concept of utility. Utility provides a method

Table 8.1 Parameters for economic evaluation of infections due to surgical site infection in patients undergoing colorectal surgery (Information from NHS Payment by Results [PBR] Tariff 2012–13 [Classen et al., 1992; Frampton, 2010])

Description	
Probability of SSI in patients receiving antibiotic prophylaxis on time	0.0059
Probability of SSI in patients receiving antibiotic prophylaxis too early or late	0.03
Average cost of colorectal surgery	£5,901
Average additional cost of SSI in patients undergoing colorectal surgery	£10,366

SSI, Surgical site infection.

for estimating patient preference for a particular intervention in terms of the patient's state of well-being. Utility is described by an index which ranges between 0 (representing death) and 1 (perfect health). The product of utility and life years gained provides the term *quality-adjusted life-year* (QALY).

There are a number of methods for the calculation of utilities:

- The 'Rosser–Kind matrix' relies on preferences from population samples from certain disease groups.
- The 'visual analogue scale' method seeks to obtain patient preferences for their perceived disease state by scoring themselves on a line scaled between 0 and 1 as previously described.
- The 'standard gamble' method requires individuals to choose between living the rest of their lives in their current state of health or making a gamble on an intervention which will restore them to perfect health. Failure of the gamble will result in instant death. The probabilities of the gamble are varied until there is indifference between the two events.
- The 'time trade-off' method requires individuals to decide how many of their remaining years of life expectancy they would be prepared to exchange for complete health.

Using the previous model, if treatment 1 provides on average an increase of 3.5 years of life expectancy, but this is valued at a utility of 0.9, then the health gain for this intervention is $0.9 \times 3.5 = 3.15$ QALYs. Similarly, if the increase in life expectancy with treatment 2 only has a utility of 0.8 (perhaps because it produces more nausea), then the health gain for this option becomes $0.8 \times 4.5 = 3.6$ QALYs. An incremental CUA can be undertaken as follows:

Strategy	Treatment costs	Effectiveness	Utility
Treatment 1	£A	3.5 years	0.9
Treatment 2	£B	4.5 years	0.8

Incremental cost–utility ratio: $= (£B - £A)/[(4.5 \times 0.8) - (3.5 \times 0.9)]$ per QALY gained.

The calculation of QALYs provides a method which enables decision makers to compare different health interventions and assign priorities for decisions on resource allocation. However, the use of QALY league tables has provided much debate amongst stakeholders of health care as to their value and use.

According to NICE, there is no empirical basis for assigning a particular value (or values) to the cutoff between cost-effectiveness and cost-ineffectiveness. The general view is that those interventions with an incremental cost-effectiveness ratio

of less than £20,000 per QALY should be supported and that there should be increasingly strong reasons for accepting cost-effective interventions with an incremental cost-effectiveness ratio of over £30,000 per QALY.

Costs and consequences

Discounting

Discounting is an economic term which is based mainly on a time preference that assumes individuals prefer to forego a part of the benefits of a programme if they can have those benefits now rather than fully in an uncertain future. The value of this preference is expressed by the discount rate. There is intense debate amongst health economists regarding the value for this annual discount level and whether both costs and consequences should be subjected to discounting. If a programme does not exceed 1 year, then discounting is felt to be unnecessary. The current rate that is proposed by NICE is 3.5% per annum, although lower rates may be accepted in certain circumstances (NICE, 2013).

Decision analysis

Decision analysis offers a method of pictorial representation of treatment decisions. If the results from clinical trials are available, probabilities can be placed within the arms of a decision tree, and outcomes can be assessed in either monetary or quality units. An example of this can be found in the assessment of the timing of antibiotics used as prophylaxis to prevent surgical site infections (Classen et al., 1992). A pivotal large prospective study monitored the timing of antibiotic prophylaxis and studied the occurrence of surgical-wound infections. To populate a decision tree, it is necessary to obtain information from the literature on the probabilities for the clinical benefits and risks of each time frame (Table 8.1). The costs of the various procedures, consumables and bed stay are then calculated or taken from the literature. From these a decision tree can be constructed that determines the cost-effectiveness of one intervention over another (Fig. 8.2).

If there is uncertainty about the robustness of the values of the variables within the tree, they can be varied within defined ranges to see if the overall direction of the tree changes. This is referred to as *sensitivity analysis* and is one of the most powerful tools available in an economic evaluation.

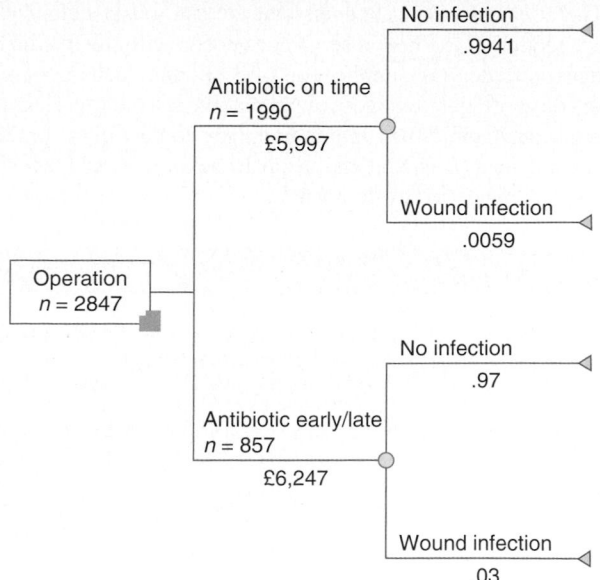

No infection
.9941

Antibiotic on time
n = 1990
£5,997

Wound infection
.0059

Operation
n = 2847

No infection
.97

Antibiotic early/late
n = 857
£6,247

Wound infection
.03

Fig 8.2   Decision tree for costs and outcomes on the effects of timing of antibiotic prophylaxis on surgical site infections. (Data from Classen et al., 1992.)

Economic evaluation of medicines

A number of countries have introduced explicit guidelines for the conduct of economic evaluations of medicines. Others require economic evaluations before allowing a medicine onto an approved list or formulary. Guidelines have been published which aim to provide researchers and peer reviewers with background guidance on how to conduct an economic evaluation and how to check its quality (Husereau et al., 2013), whereas others have set out how they incorporate health economics in the evaluation of medicines (NICE, 2014).

Risk management of unwanted drug effects

Avoiding the adverse effects of medicines has become a desirable goal of therapeutic decision makers as well as those who promote quality assurance and risk management. Not only can there be significant sequelae in terms of increased morbidity associated with adverse drug effects; the economic consequences can be considerable. For example, gentamicin is often regarded as a relatively inexpensive antibiotic, but in the USA, each case of nephrotoxicity has been reported to cost several thousands of pounds in terms of additional resources consumed even without any assessment of the reduction in a patient's quality of life. The increasingly litigious nature of society has resulted in the economic valuation of perceived negligence, for example, with irreversible vestibular toxicity associated with prolonged unmonitored aminoglycoside therapy. As a result, many healthcare systems have targeted a significant reduction in the number of serious errors in the use of prescribed medicines.

Medication non-adherence

The costs of non-adherence with medicines are considerable. In the USA, it has been calculated that 11% of all admissions to hospital are directly associated with some form of non-adherence.

Box 8.1   Ten examples of the application of pharmacoeconomics in practice

- The value of one treatment over another in terms of the cost for each unit of health gained
- Avoidance of costs associated with the failure to use an appropriate medicine, e.g. antimicrobial surgical prophylaxis
- Avoidance of the costs of the side effects or adverse effects of a medicine
- Financial planning and horizon scanning for new medicines
- Prioritisation of healthcare resources
- Health gain, quality-of-life issues and patient preferences
- Duration of care and balance between in-patient, day care and outpatient care
- Changes in legislative controls, e.g. reclassification of medicines from prescription-only to pharmacy status
- Costs of concordance and non-concordance
- Economics of health service delivery

This equates to 2 million hospital admissions a year in the USA resulting from medication non-adherence, at a total cost of over £5 billion. In addition, lost work productivity through non-adherence has been estimated to cost in excess of a further £3 billion per year. The scale of the problem in the UK is probably similar.

In the UK, between a half and one-third of all medicines prescribed for long-term conditions are not taken as recommended (Horne et al., 2005), and the estimated drug cost of unused or unwanted medicines in the NHS in England is around £300 million a year (Trueman et al., 2010). National guidance on medication adherence has been issued (NICE, 2009).

Incentives and disincentives

There are good examples of both incentives and disincentives being used in the NHS to save money. In England, the contract for hospitals penalises those organisations that fail to achieve their targets for reducing *Clostridium difficile* infections. Good antimicrobial stewardship is essential for addressing this, as each case of *C. difficile* infection can cost at least £4000. Reduction in prescribing of both fluoroquinolones and second- and third-generation cephalosporins is associated with a reduction in *C. difficile* infection (Department of Health and the Health Protection Agency, 2008). It follows from this that reducing the use of these agents can reduce acquisition costs of the medicines.

Examples of incentives to reduce expenditure can be seen within the NHS commissioning processes in England. A typical example involves a scheme where commissioners must make 1.5% of contract value (or equivalent non-contract activity value) available for each provider's quality and innovation scheme, and these include prescribing targets (NHS England 2015).

Conclusion

A fundamental element of the use of pharmacoeconomics in practice is the viewpoint from which the analysis is conducted. Ideally this should be from a societal perspective, but frequently it is from a government or Department of Health viewpoint.

Purchasers of health care may also have a different perspective from provider units, and the viewpoint of clinicians may differ from that of the patient. The pharmaceutical industry will probably have another viewpoint that will be focused on its particular products. As a consequence, with all economic evaluations, the perspective from which they have been analysed should be clear.

The effect of having budgets that are rigorously defended in every section of the health service, as occurs with the medicines budget, is to deny the application of economic decision making in the most efficient way for the population served. It is clear that pharmacoeconomics has an important part to play in the practice of therapeutics (Box 8.1) and needs to be an integral part of all planned therapeutic developments.

References

Classen, D.C., Evans, R.S., Pestotnik, S.L., et al., 1992. The timing of prophylactic administration of antibiotics and the risk of surgical-wound infection. N. Engl. J. Med. 326, 281–286.

Department of Health and the Health Protection Agency, 2008. *Clostridium difficile* infection: how to deal with the problem. Department of Health, London.

Frampton, L., 2010. Calculating the cost of surgical site infection. Microbiology update. The Biomedical Scientist 866–869.

Health and Social Care Information Centre, 2015. Prescribing costs in hospitals and the community. England 2014–15. Available at: http://digital.nhs.uk/article/2021/Website-Search?productid=19276&q=Prescribing+Costs+in+Hospitals+and+the+Community&sort=Relevance&size=10&page=1&area=both#top.

Horne, R., Weinman, J., Barber, N., et al., 2005. Concordance, adherence and compliance in medicine taking. National Co-ordinating Centre for NHS Service Delivery and Organisation R & D. Available at: https://www.researchgate.net/profile/Ian_Kellar/publication/271443859_Concordance_Adherence_and_Compliance_in_Medicine_Taking/links/54cfdb790cf298d65665b4d4.pdf.

Husereau, D., Drummond, M., Petrou, S., et al. on behalf of the CHEERS Task Force, 2013. Consolidated Health Economic Evaluation Reporting Standards (CHEERS) statement. BMC Medicine 11, 80. Available at: http://www.biomedcentral.com/1741-7015/11/80.

National Institute for Health and Care Excellence (NICE), 2009. Medicines adherence: involving patients in decisions about prescribed medicines and supporting adherence NICE guidelines [CG76]. Available at: http://www.nice.org.uk/guidance/cg76.

National Institute for Health and Care Excellence (NICE), 2013. Guide to the methods of technology appraisal 2013. Available at: https://www.nice.org.uk/process/pmg9/chapter/foreword.

National Institute for Health and Care Excellence (NICE), 2014. Developing NICE guidelines: the manual. Available at: https://www.nice.org.uk/process/pmg20/chapter/introduction-and-overview.

NHS England, 2015. Commissioning for quality and innovation guidance 2015–16. Available at: https://www.england.nhs.uk/wp-content/uploads/2015/03/9-cquin-guid-2015-16.pdf.

Organisation for Economic Co-Operation and Development (OECD), 2016. OECD health statistics 2016. Available at: http://www.oecd.org/health/health-data.htm.

Trueman, P., Taylor, D.G., Lowson, K., et al., 2010. Evaluation of the scale, causes and costs of waste medicine. Report of DH funded National Project York Health Economics Health Consortium and the School of Pharmacy. University of London, York and London. Available at: http://discovery.ucl.ac.uk/i350234/.

Further reading

Drummond, M., Sculpher, S., Claxton, K., et al., 2015. Methods for the Economic Evaluation of Health Care Programmes, fourth ed. Oxford University Press, Oxford.

Useful websites

National Institute for Health and Care Excellence (NICE), Assessing cost-effectiveness. https://www.nice.org.uk/process/pmg6/chapter/assessing-cost-effectiveness.

SECTION **2**

LIFE STAGES

9 Neonates

Martin P. Ward-Platt

Key points

- The survival of very premature babies has been greatly increased through the use of antenatal glucocorticoids and neonatal surfactant treatment to prevent and treat surfactant deficiency.
- The feto-placental unit creates a unique route for drug delivery.
- Drug disposition and metabolism in the neonate are very different from those at any other time of life.
- Preterm babies grow very fast, so doses have to be re-calculated at regular intervals.
- Drug elimination in the neonate can be much slower than in children, especially in the first week, so dose intervals have to be longer initially but may shorten as babies grow and mature.

The earliest in pregnancy at which newborn babies can sometimes survive is around 23 weeks' gestation, when survival, which used to be about 10%, is now more than 50% for live-born babies. In contrast, very few babies born at 22 weeks survive. Conventionally, any baby born at less than 32 weeks is regarded as being at relatively high risk of death or disability. About 7.5% of all births in the UK are technically 'premature' (<37 weeks), but only 1.4% of births take place before 32 weeks of gestation. Likewise, 7% of all babies are low birth weight (LBW), for example, less than 2500 g, and 1.4% are very low birth weight (VLBW). However, it is the gestation at birth rather than the birth weight which is of more practical and prognostic value. Over three-quarters of babies born at 25 weeks' gestation now survive to discharge home. The definitions of selected terms used for babies are given in Table 9.1.

Because mothers with high-risk pregnancies will often be transferred for delivery to a hospital capable of providing neonatal intensive care, the proportion of preterm and LBW babies cared for in such units is greater than that in smaller maternity units in peripheral hospitals. In the population as a whole, between 1% and 2% of all babies will receive intensive care, and the most common reason for this among preterm babies is the need for respiratory support of some kind.

Babies in between 28 and 32 weeks' gestation invariably need some degree of special or intensive care and generally go home when they are feeding adequately, somewhere between 35 and 40 weeks of postmenstrual age. Babies born at 23–25 weeks, however, need prolonged intensive care and may well go home some weeks after their due date. So although in epidemiological terms the neonatal period is defined as up to 28 postnatal days, babies may be 'neonatal' in-patients for as long as 4 or 5 months; during this time their weight may triple or quadruple, and their physiology and metabolism change dramatically.

Drug disposition

Absorption

An important and unique source of drug absorption, available until birth, is the placenta. Maternal drugs pass to the fetus and back again during pregnancy, but from delivery, any drugs present in the neonatal circulation can no longer be eliminated by that route and must be dealt with by the baby's own systems. Important examples of maternal drugs which may adversely affect the newborn baby include opiates given for pain relief during labour and β-adrenergic blockers given for pregnancy-induced hypertension, such as labetalol.

The placental route may also be used deliberately to give a mother drugs with the intention of treating not her but her fetus. There are two important and quite common examples of this. The first is the use of corticosteroids to promote fetal lung maturation when preterm delivery is planned or expected. In this situation, betametasone or dexamethasone are normally the drugs of choice because prednisolone is metabolised in the placenta and does not reach the fetus. The second example is the administration of magnesium sulfate to mothers in, or at high risk of preterm labour; the magnesium sulfate protects against subsequent cerebral palsy in their babies. Rarely, mothers may be given anti-arrhythmic drugs, such as flecainide, to control tachyarrhythmias in the fetus.

Enteral drug absorption is potentially erratic in any newborn baby and may be unavailable in the ill baby because the stomach does not always empty effectively. Therefore, most drugs are given intravenously to ensure maximum bioavailability. Some drugs, such as paraldehyde and diazepam (for neonatal seizures) and paracetamol (for simple analgesia), can be given rectally. The trachea may be used as the preferred route of administration when surfactant administration is required or where adrenaline (epinephrine) is given during resuscitation. The buccal route may be used to administer glucose gel in the treatment of hypoglycaemia, or for midazolam to control seizures. Intramuscular injection is generally avoided because of pain and low muscle bulk, although the widespread use of intramuscular vitamin K, to prevent bleeding caused by vitamin K deficiency, flies in the face of this precept.

Table 9.1 Definitions of terms

Normal length of human pregnancy (term)	40 weeks (280 days), range 37 up to 42 completed weeks of gestation
Preterm	<37 weeks of gestation at birth
Post-term	42 completed weeks onwards
Neonatal period	Up to the 28th postnatal day
Low birth weight (LBW)	<2500 g
Very low birth weight (VLBW)	<1500 g
Extremely low birth weight (ELBW)	<1000 g
Extremely low gestational age (ELGAN)	<28 weeks

In the very preterm baby of 28 weeks' gestation or less, the keratin layer of the skin is extremely thin and a poor barrier to water loss; consequently, it is also permeable to substances in contact with it. This is harmful to the baby if there is prolonged skin contact with alcohol, as in chlorhexidine in 70% methylated spirit, because it causes a severe chemical burn and can lead to systemic methyl alcohol poisoning.

Distribution

Drugs are distributed within a baby's body as a function of their lipid and aqueous solubility, as at any other time of life. The main difference in the neonate is that the size of the body water pool under renal control is related not to the baby's surface area but to body weight. Furthermore, the absolute glomerular filtration rate increases logarithmically with postmenstrual age irrespective of the length of a baby's gestation. This has implications for predicting the behaviour of water-soluble drugs such as gentamicin.

The amount of adipose tissue can vary substantially between different babies. Any baby born more than 10 weeks early, and babies of any gestation who have suffered intrauterine growth restriction, may have little body fat. Conversely, the infant of a diabetic mother may have a particularly large fat layer, and this affects the retention of predominantly lipid-soluble drugs.

Protein binding in the plasma is influenced by the amount of albumin available, and this in turn is related to gestation, with albumin values found 12 weeks before term being only two-thirds of adult concentrations.

Metabolism

The metabolic fate of drugs in the newborn is not qualitatively different from that in the older child, for example, hydroxylation, oxidation and conjugation to sulphate or glucuronate. It is the efficiency with which these processes are carried out that distinguishes the baby from the older person. In addition to the immaturity of the metabolic pathways for drug disposal, drug metabolism is also affected by the physiological hyperbilirubinaemia common in the newborn. The bilirubin can compete both for enzyme-binding sites and for glucuronate and may thus affect drug metabolism for as long as unconjugated hyperbilirubinaemia persists.

Elimination

The relative immaturity of hepatic and renal function results in correspondingly slow elimination of most drugs from the neonate. This is not necessarily a problem, so long as due account is taken of the slow elimination and dose intervals are modified accordingly. It may even be a useful property, as with phenobarbital, which when given as a loading dose (usually 20 mg/kg) will remain in circulation for days in useful therapeutic quantities, often avoiding the need for further doses. On the other hand, drugs such as gentamicin and vancomycin, which have a relatively narrow therapeutic index, must be given far less frequently than in children or adults, and serum drug levels must be assayed to avoid toxicity.

There has been little study of pharmacodynamics in the term or preterm neonate. Most clinicians work on the assumption that the kinetics of drug behaviour are so different in this group of patients that the pharmacodynamic properties must follow the same pattern. In practice, the most important pharmacodynamic effect is probably that of the behaviour of opiates derived from the mother in labour. Pethidine and diamorphine are the opiates most likely to cause significant respiratory depression in the neonate. Such respiratory depression can be treated with naloxone, and a special neonatal preparation (20 micrograms/mL) is available. However, after birth, the opiates and their metabolites have a long serum half-life in the baby, whereas the naloxone is rapidly eliminated. The initial dramatic effect of naloxone can give a false sense of security because the baby may become narcosed after a few hours after transfer to the postnatal ward. To try to prevent this late-onset narcosis, adult naloxone (400 micrograms/mL) may be given intramuscularly to ensure it remains active over several hours. Even when the respiratory effects have disappeared, opiates may have prolonged behavioural effects on both mother and baby.

Major clinical disorders
Respiratory distress syndrome

Classical respiratory distress syndrome (RDS), caused by lung immaturity as defined by surfactant insufficiency at the time of birth, is now relatively uncommon for several reasons: It is prevented by the use of antenatal glucocorticoids in the mother; most very preterm babies are given early postnatal surfactant; and the very early use of continuous positive airway pressure in these babies can achieve lung distension without respiratory distress. However, there is not always time to administer corticosteroids if delivery occurs rapidly and unexpectedly, so variants of RDS related to surfactant deficiency still occur. The condition is rare in babies born at or near term and becomes increasingly likely the more preterm a birth takes place. Alternative terminology is shown in Box 9.1.

Box 9.1 Respiratory distress syndrome: alternative terminology

Respiratory distress syndrome (RDS): The clinical appearance of a baby with increased work of breathing, nasal flaring, rib recession, tachypnoea, a requirement for oxygen therapy and/or retention of carbon dioxide on blood gas analysis. There are many causes for this clinical picture in addition to surfactant deficiency.

Surfactant-deficiency lung disease: A more precise term describing the most common underlying cause of respiratory distress in preterm babies.

Hyaline membrane disease (HMD): The histological appearance of lungs affected by lack of surfactant, first described in babies who had died of the condition without ever having been ventilated. Much of the alveolar air space is taken up with homogeneous pink-staining 'hyaline membranes' of proteinaceous exudate, and there is an accompanying inflammatory response.

Antenatal glucocorticoids given to the mother reduce the incidence, severity and mortality of RDS caused by surfactant deficiency. It is also better in terms of surfactant production for a baby to undergo labour rather than be delivered by caesarean section without labour. Babies of less than 32 weeks' gestation gain most benefit from antenatal corticosteroids because they are at greatest risk of death and disability from RDS, but net benefit continues up to 38 weeks for babies born by elective caesarean section. Optimum treatment is four oral doses of 6 mg betamethasone, each given 12-hourly, or two doses of 12 mg intramuscularly 24 hours apart.

A relatively big baby born around 32–34 weeks of gestation with mild RDS is usually treated with continuous positive airway pressure and some extra oxygen, delivered via the nose by a flow driver. In contrast, smaller, more premature or more severely affected babies often need artificial ventilation using an endotracheal tube. A few babies require high inspired concentrations of oxygen (up to 100%) for several days. Fortunately, pulmonary oxygen toxicity is not as much a problem for the neonate as it is for the adult, although it may have a causal role in the development of bronchopulmonary dysplasia (neonatal chronic lung disease; see later section). Oxygen therapy has to balance the concern about increasing the chance of retinopathy of prematurity with the knowledge from recent studies that targeting oxygen saturations more than 90% conveys a lower overall mortality.

Many sick, ventilated babies develop a degree of hypotension. In addition to volume expansion with boluses of normal saline, some of these babies are given inotropes to support their blood pressure. Adrenaline, dopamine, or dobutamine infusions are widely used in neonatal care, but there are no randomised controlled trials to guide either the first choice of inotrope or the exact indications for using it.

Paralysing agents such as pancuronium are sometimes given to ventilated neonates, but these only prevent the baby from moving and are not sedative. Pancuronium is widely used, partly because it wears off slowly so that the baby is not suddenly destabilised; vecuronium infusions are sometimes used. Shorter-acting agents such as atracurium are often given for temporary paralysis for intubation. Whether or not the baby is paralysed, morphine is commonly given, either as intermittent doses or as an infusion, to provide narcosis and analgesia to reduce the distress of neonatal intensive care.

Persistent pulmonary hypertension commonly complicates early-onset septicaemia and meconium aspiration syndrome. Inhaled nitric oxide, which is added to the ventilator circuit, dilates the pulmonary arterioles and lowers the excessive pulmonary blood pressure, and it is both more effective than the previously used drug therapies and much less likely to lead to systemic hypotension. For some babies of at least 34 weeks of gestation and at least 2 kg birth weight, extracorporeal membrane oxygenation (ECMO), in which a baby is, in effect, put on partial heart–lung bypass for a few days, may be life-saving if ventilation and nitric oxide fail to reverse hypoxaemia.

Patent ductus arteriosus

Patent ductus arteriosus (PDA) can be a problem in the recovery phase of respiratory distress syndrome in very preterm babies and usually shows itself as a secondary increase in respiratory distress and/or ventilatory requirement, an increasing oxygen requirement, wide pulse pressure and a characteristic heart murmur. The reason that an open duct becomes a problem is that as pressure in the pulmonary artery falls, the duct allows blood from the aorta to flow into the pulmonary artery, which is the opposite of what was happening in the fetus. This elevated pulmonary flow engorges the lungs and reduces their compliance while putting strain on the heart. Echocardiography is used to confirm the clinical suspicion. About one-third of all babies with birth weights less than 1000 g will develop signs of PDA, but treatment is mostly given when the baby is haemodynamically compromised. However, the optimum timing and selection of babies for treatment of the open duct remain controversial and have not yet been resolved in spite of years of research. When treatment is needed, the options are either medical treatment (with indometacin or ibuprofen) or surgical ligation.

Ibuprofen has largely replaced indometacin because it is equally efficacious and better tolerated. Potential serious side effects of both drugs include renal impairment, gastric haemorrhage and gut perforation. Surgery to ligate the duct is generally considered when one or more courses of medical treatment fail to close it, or if drugs are contraindicated.

Bronchopulmonary dysplasia

Bronchopulmonary dysplasia (BPD), also sometimes generically known as chronic lung disease of prematurity, most frequently occurs in very premature babies who have undergone prolonged respiratory support. The factors predisposing to BPD are the degree of prematurity, the severity of RDS, infection, the occurrence of PDA, oxygen toxicity and probably intrinsic genetic factors. BPD is diagnosed from the chest X-ray appearances of a baby who remains either on respiratory support or on oxygen, but who no longer has an acute respiratory illness.

Established BPD that is not severe enough to need continuing mechanical ventilation is either treated with nasal continuous positive airway pressure with or without oxygen supplementation or, if less severe, may be treated with supplemental high-flow or low-flow oxygen through nasal cannulae.

BPD leads to increases in both pulmonary artery pressure and lung water content. The consequent strain on the heart can lead to heart failure, with excessive weight gain, increasing oxygen requirements and clinical signs such as oedema, enlarged liver and a cardiac 'gallop' rhythm. The first-line treatment for heart failure is with diuretics. Diuretics improve pulmonary mechanics and treat heart failure. Sometimes furosemide is used, but its side effects are significant and include urinary loss of potassium and calcium and renal calcification. An alternative is to combine a thiazide diuretic with spironolactone, which causes less calcium and potassium loss. By reducing lung water content, diuretics can also improve lung compliance and reduce the work of breathing. However, BPD is not routinely treated with diuretics because many babies do well without specific treatment beyond oxygen supplementation.

A chronic inflammatory process is part of the pathology of BPD, and for this reason, much attention has been given to the role of glucocorticoids (generally dexamethasone) in treating it. Steroid use generally results in a rapid fall in oxygen requirements but has not yet been shown to improve mortality. Trials have shown that when dexamethasone is used early, within the first 1 or 2 postnatal weeks, there is an increased rate of cerebral palsy, so one of the principal indications for steroid use is when a baby remains ventilator dependent at the age of 4 weeks or more. Widely varying treatment regimens have been used in trials, and there is no standard approach; the initial dose (usually between 50 and 250 micrograms/kg/day) is dependent on physician preference and experience, whereas the rate of reduction of dose is generally individualised to the baby. Side effects such as hypertension and glucose intolerance are common but seldom require modification of the steroid dose or other treatment, but the effects on linear growth can be significant if steroids are given for a long time.

For some babies with severe BPD, in whom echocardiography demonstrates pulmonary arterial pressures close to, or greater than, systemic pressure, many neonatologists try sildenafil because there has been considerable experience using this drug off-label to prevent pulmonary hypertensive crises in babies after cardiac surgery. There are no randomised controlled trials of sildenafil in BPD. Systemic hypertension sometimes occurs among babies with BPD even without steroid exposure and may need treatment with antihypertensive drugs such as nifedipine.

Significantly preterm babies still in oxygen at 36 weeks' postmenstrual age are almost certain to need oxygen at home after discharge, and home oxygen programmes for ex-premature babies with BPD are now widespread. Most babies manage to wean off supplementary oxygen in a few months, but a very few may need it for up to 2 years.

Bacterial infection

Important pathogens in the first 2 or 3 days after birth are group B β-haemolytic streptococci and a variety of Gram-negative organisms, especially *Escherichia coli*. Coagulase-negative staphylococci and *Staphylococcus aureus* are more important subsequently. In line with good antimicrobial stewardship, it is

Table 9.2 Serious neonatal infections and common pathogens

Septicaemia	*Staphylococcus epidermidis*, group B streptococci, *Escherichia coli*
Systemic fungal infection	*Candida* spp.
Necrotizing enterocolitis	No single causal pathogen
Osteomyelitis	*Staphylococcus aureus*
Meningitis	Group B streptococci, *E. coli*

wise to use narrow-spectrum antibiotics when possible, to give them in short courses, and to discontinue treatment quickly if the blood culture is negative. The most serious neonatal infections are listed in Table 9.2.

Superficial candida infection is common in all babies, but systemic candida infection is a particular risk in very preterm babies, especially those receiving prolonged courses of broad-spectrum antibiotics, with central venous access or receiving intravenous feeding. Routine use of either enteral nystatin or systemic fluconazole is highly effective at preventing systemic candidiasis.

It is usual to give babies antibiotics prophylactically when preterm labour is unexplained, where there has been prolonged rupture of the fetal membranes before delivery, when a mother is known to carry group B streptococci but did not get intrapartum penicillin, and when a baby is ventilated from birth. A standard combination for such early treatment, now enshrined in National Institute of Health and Care Excellence (NICE, 2012) guidance is penicillin G and an aminoglycoside, to cover group B streptococci and the common Gram-negative pathogens. Treatment can be stopped after 36 or 48 hours (depending on local laboratory techniques) if cultures prove negative. The treatment of suspected infection that starts when a baby is more than 48 hours old has to take account of the expected local pathogens but will always include cover for *S. aureus*.

Meticillin-resistant *S. aureus* (MRSA) has emerged as a real problem in hospitals in recent years, but there is little evidence that neonatal units have any more problems than other intensive care areas. *Clostridium difficile* is not a problem pathogen in neonatal care.

Viral infections

The most important viral infection in neonates is cytomegalovirus (CMV). It may present as a congenital infection with a seriously ill baby or be a cause of later respiratory illness. CMV is a common cause of non-hereditary sensorineural hearing loss among term babies, for whom prolonged treatment with oral valganciclovir can greatly improve auditory outcome.

For HIV, the goal of management is to prevent 'vertical' transmission from mother to baby. The main strategy is to use aggressive maternal treatment throughout pregnancy to suppress the maternal viral load. After delivery, if the mother has a low viral load, the baby is given zidovudine as a single agent for 4 weeks. If the maternal load is high, the baby gets conventional triple therapy.

Ex-preterm babies often contract respiratory syncytial virus (RSV)–positive bronchiolitis once at home, especially if they are on home oxygen and have been discharged during the winter when bronchiolitis is epidemic. Palivizumab, an anti-RSV immunoglobulin, is recommended for prophylaxis and has to be given to the infant as monthly intramuscular injections for the duration of the annual epidemic. It is also good practice to ensure that oxygen-dependent babies and their families receive the seasonal flu immunisation.

The major emergent virus which may infect the fetus and has implications for the newborn is Zika virus (ZIKV). This flavivirus is unusual in that it is transmitted by *Aedes* mosquitos, but it behaves clinically much like rubella in the pre-immunisation days, causing a mild exanthematous illness in adults and children but being capable of infecting pregnant mothers and their fetuses. Fetal infection can damage the brain and give rise to neonatal microcephaly. Unlike rubella, there is no vaccine as yet, but as ZIKV continues to spread into densely populated areas of Central and North America, it is likely that there will be a concerted effort to produce a vaccine as soon as possible.

Necrotizing enterocolitis

Necrotising enterocolitis (NEC) can arise in any baby, but it is most common, and generally most lethal, in babies less than 27 weeks' gestation. There is general agreement that the pathophysiology is related to damage to the gut mucosa, which may occur because of hypotension or hypoxia, coupled with the presence of certain organisms in the gastro-intestinal tract that invade the gut wall to give rise to the clinical condition. Early 'trophic' feeding, feeding with the mother's expressed breast milk and enteral probiotics appear to be protective.

A baby who becomes ill with NEC is often septicaemic and may present acutely with a major collapse, respiratory failure and shock or more slowly with abdominal distension, intolerance of feeds with discoloured gastric aspirates and sometimes blood in the stool. The medical treatment is respiratory and circulatory support if necessary, broad-spectrum antibiotics and switching to intravenous feeding for a period of time, usually 7–10 days. The antibiotic strategy for NEC is to cover Gram-positive, Gram-negative and anaerobic bacteria. Metronidazole is used to cover anaerobes in the UK, but clindamycin is still used in some other countries. One of the most difficult surgical judgements is deciding whether and when to operate to remove necrotic areas of gut or deal with a perforation.

Apnoea

Apnoea is the absence of breathing. Babies (and adults) normally have respiratory pauses, but preterm babies in particular are prone to prolonged pauses in respiration of longer than 20 seconds which can be associated with significant falls in arterial oxygenation. Apnoea usually has both central and obstructive components, is often accompanied by bradycardia and requires treatment to prevent life-threatening episodes of arterial desaturation.

The main goal of medical treatment is to reduce the number and severity of the apnoeic episodes without having to resort to

> **Box 9.2** Grading of neonatal hypoxic-ischaemic encephalopathy
>
> **Grade 1:** Short-lived (<24 h) increase in tone; often high-pitched cry; sometimes difficult to feed. No seizures.
> **Grade 2:** More prolonged but usually <1 week; lethargy and reduced tone; usually needs tube feeding for some time; may have seizures.
> **Grade 3:** Comatose, floppy, often apnoeic and needing ventilation; seizures not always present clinically but if present, often difficult to control; highly abnormal cerebral function monitor trace, usually very suppressed initially.

artificial ventilation, so using either nasal continuous positive airway pressure, or caffeine or both is the first-line treatment. Caffeine both reduces apnoea in the short-term and improves neurodevelopmental outcome. Doxapram is occasionally given in addition to caffeine to avoid resorting to mechanical ventilation. Most clinicians stop giving caffeine when the baby is around 34 weeks' postmenstrual age, by which time most babies will have achieved an adequate degree of cardiorespiratory stability.

Hypoxic–ischaemic encephalopathy

Hypoxic–ischaemic encephalopathy (HIE) usually results either from intrapartum asphyxia or from an antepartum insult such as placental abruption. It is conventionally graded into three divisions (see Box 9.2). However, it is important to remember that although hypoxia-ischaemia is by far the most common cause of a neonatal encephalopathy, it is not the only one: metabolic disease, cerebral infarction and infection need to be considered as possibilities too.

No drug has been shown to improve outcome when given after a hypoxic-ischaemic insult has occurred, but cooling a baby to between 33 and 34 °C for 72 hours reduces the degree of neurodisability among survivors and is now standard therapy. In the trials of cooling therapy, it was babies with a grade 3 encephalopathy in whom benefit was shown, but currently, many babies at the worse end of grade 2 encephalopathy are cooled too. Cooling is a benign and well-tolerated therapy, so the tendency is to use it rather than not in borderline cases.

Assessing cerebral electrical activity using the cerebral function monitor (CFM) is now standard practice and helps in the decision making as to whether a particular baby should be offered cooling therapy. HIE of grades 2 and 3 may give rise to clinical seizures, or subclinical seizures may show up on the CFM. In the neonate, the first-choice anticonvulsant for the acute treatment of seizures in HIE is usually phenobarbital because it seldom causes respiratory depression and is active for many hours or days because of its long elimination half-life. Diazepam is best avoided because it upsets temperature control, causes unpredictable respiratory depression, and is very sedating compared with phenobarbital. Paraldehyde is occasionally used because it is easy to give rectally, is relatively non-sedating and is short acting. It is excreted by exhalation, and the smell can make the working environment quite unpleasant for staff. Phenytoin is often used when fits remain uncontrolled after two loading doses of phenobarbital (total 40 mg/kg) but is not usually given long-term because of its narrow therapeutic index, and its anti-inotropic effect can be a problem if there is ischaemic cardiomyopathy. When seizures are difficult to control, further options include clonazepam, midazolam or lidocaine; the last two can be given as infusions. There is little experience with intravenous sodium valproate in the neonate, but increasingly levetiracetam is being prescribed and appears to be very effective.

A therapeutic dilemma lies in the degree of aggression with which seizures should be treated because no anticonvulsant is reliably effective in reducing electrocerebral seizure activity, even when the clinical manifestations of seizures are abolished. In any case, seizures tend naturally to cease after a few days. However, seizures that compromise respiratory function need to be treated to prevent serious falls in arterial oxygen tension and possible secondary neurological damage. Also, babies with frequent or continuous seizure activity are difficult to nurse and cause great distress to their parents. Therefore, in practice, it is usual to try to suppress the clinical manifestation of seizure activity, and phenobarbital remains the most commonly used first-line treatment. Where a decision is taken to keep a baby on anticonvulsant medication, therapeutic drug monitoring can provide helpful information and may need to be repeated from time to time during follow-up.

Seizures may occur as isolated events in term or near-term babies in whom there is neurological normality between seizure episodes; this is sometimes seen in perinatal strokes. Seizures seldom complicate the course of very premature babies because cerebral injury in these babies is now a rare event. Investigations in term babies with seizures are directed to finding an underlying cause, but in about half of those having fits without an encephalopathy, no underlying cause can be found.

Haemorrhagic disease of the newborn

Haemorrhagic disease of the newborn, better described as vitamin K–dependent bleeding, is very rare but it may cause death or disability if it presents with an intracranial bleed. Except in the case of malabsorption, it affects only breastfed babies because they get very little vitamin K in maternal milk, and their gut bacteria do not synthesise it. Formula-fed infants get sufficient vitamin K in their milk, and only in the very rare situation of fat malabsorption do they need supplementing.

There are several possible strategies for giving vitamin K with a view to preventing haemorrhagic disease. An intramuscular injection of phytomenadione 1 mg (0.5 mL) can be given either to every newborn baby or selectively to babies who have certain risk factors such as instrumental delivery or preterm birth. Vitamin K can be given orally, so long as an adequate number of doses is given, and this has been shown to be effective in preventing disease. Intramuscular injections are an invasive and unpleasant intervention for the baby because muscle bulk is small in the newborn, and particularly the preterm, and other structures such as the sciatic nerve can be damaged even if the intention is to give the injection into the lateral thigh. Intramuscular injections can be reserved for those babies with doubtful oral absorption, for example, all those admitted for special care, or at high risk because of enzyme-inducing maternal drugs such as anticonvulsants.

Principles and goals of therapy

The ultimate aim of neonatal care at all levels is to maximise disability-free survival and identify treatable conditions that would otherwise compromise growth or development. It follows that potential problems should be anticipated, and the complexities of intensive care should be avoided if at all possible.

Many of the drugs used in neonatal care are not licensed for such use or are used off-label. There is a high potential for errors because of the small doses used, which sometimes calls for unusual levels of dilution when drawing up drugs. Constant vigilance and the use of specialised neonatal formularies are important in preventing harm; interestingly, there is at present little evidence of added safety from electronic prescribing.

Rapid growth

Once the need for intensive care has passed, the growth of a premature baby can be very rapid if the child is being fed with a high-calorie formula modified for use with preterm infants. Indeed, most babies born at 27 weeks and weighing around 1 kg can be expected to double their birth weight by the time they are 8 weeks old, and babies born at 23 or 24 weeks may triple or quadruple their weight before discharge home. Because the dose of all medications is calculated on the basis of body weight, constant review of the dose is necessary to maintain efficacy, particularly for drugs that may be given for several weeks, such as respiratory stimulants and diuretics. Conversely, all that is necessary to gradually wean a baby from a medication is to hold the dose constant so that the baby gradually 'grows out' of the drug. This practice is frequently used with diuretic medication in BPD, the need for which becomes less as the baby's somatic growth reduces the proportion of damaged lung in favour of healthy tissue.

Therapeutic drug monitoring

The assay of serum concentrations of various drugs has a place in neonatal medicine, particularly where the therapeutic index of a drug is narrow. It is routine to assay trough levels of certain antibiotics: for aminoglycosides, accumulation must be avoided, and for vancomycin, both avoiding accumulation and demonstrating adequate trough levels are desirable. Only rarely is it necessary to assay minimal inhibitory or bactericidal concentrations of antibiotics in blood or cerebrospinal fluid if serious infections are being treated, and constraints on sampling limit the frequency with which this may be undertaken.

Where phenobarbital or other anticonvulsants are given long-term intermittent measurement of serum levels can be a useful guide to increasing the dose. All these drugs have a long half-life, so it is most important that drug concentrations are not measured too early, or too frequently, to prevent inappropriate changes in dose being made before a steady state is reached.

Avoiding harm

Intramuscular injections are considered potentially harmful because of the small muscle bulk of babies. However, it is not always easy to establish venous access, and occasionally it may be necessary to use the intramuscular route instead. For vaccines, the intramuscular route is unavoidable.

For sick preterm infants ventilated for respiratory failure, handling of any kind is a destabilising influence, so the minimal necessary intervention should be the rule. Merely opening the doors of an incubator can destabilise a fragile baby. It is, therefore, a good practice to minimise the frequency of drug administration and to try to coordinate the doses of different medications.

Medication errors in neonatal care have been the subject of extensive study, but it is sufficient to say here that the root causes of error are most commonly one or more human factors relating to dose calculation, distraction, urgency, poor team function, and other factors commonly found in intensive care environments. Encouraging a culture of reporting, investigating, understanding and learning from errors and near misses remains the keystone of improving safety and minimising harm.

Time scale of clinical changes

In babies, the time scale for starting drug treatments is very short because the clinical condition of any baby can change with great rapidity. For example, where a surfactant is required it should be given as soon as possible after birth to premature babies who are intubated and ventilated. Similarly, infection can be rapidly progressive, so starting antibiotics is a priority when the index of suspicion is high or where congenital bacterial infection is likely. The same applies for antiretroviral drugs when a baby is born to a mother positive for HIV, especially if the maternal viral load is high.

For the sick preterm infant, this model applies to a wide range of interventions. It is seldom possible to wait a few hours for a given drug, and this has obvious implications for the level of support required by a neonatal service.

Early urgent immunisation with hepatitis B vaccine and the administration of anti-hepatitis B immunoglobulin are very important in preventing vertical transmission of hepatitis B when the mother is e-antigen positive. Of less urgency, but considerable importance, is making sure that premature babies who are still on the neonatal unit 8 weeks after birth get their routine immunisations because these should be given according to chronological age irrespective of prematurity.

Patient and parent care

It is all too easy to take a mechanistic approach to neonatal medicine, on the grounds that premature infants cannot communicate their needs. Such an approach to therapy is inappropriate. Even when receiving intensive care, any infant who is not either paralysed or very heavily sedated does in fact respond with a wealth of cues and nonverbal communication in relation to their needs. Monitors, therefore, do not replace clinical skills but provide supplementary information and potentially advance warning of problems. Even the most premature babies show individual characteristics, which emphasises that individualised care is as important in this age group as in any other. In particular, neonatal pain and distress have effects on nociception and behaviour well into childhood.

It has become increasingly apparent in recent years that involvement of parents in every aspect of care is a necessary goal with clear advantages to the baby in relation to developmental outcome. Not only is care increasingly regarded as a partnership between professionals and parents rather than the province of professionals alone, but it makes sense to involve parents in as many aspects of care with which they feel comfortable. For babies who have special rather than intensive care needs, provision of single rooms with parent facilities, as is standard in paediatric care, has many advantages. In the traditional model, parents only visit until a day or two before discharge when they are encouraged to room-in with their baby for the first time, but this increasingly looks out of touch with the way parents and babies should be kept together. Routine administration of oral medication is thus an act in which parents may be expected to participate, and for those whose baby has to be discharged home still requiring continuous oxygen, the parent will rapidly obtain complete control, with support from the hospital and the primary healthcare team. The growing number of babies who survive very premature birth but whose respiratory state requires continued support after discharge presents an increasing therapeutic challenge for the future.

Case studies

Case 9.1

Ms A went into labour as a result of an antepartum haemorrhage at 28 weeks of gestation. There was no time to give her steroids when she arrived at the maternity unit, and her son, J, was born by vaginal delivery in good condition. However, he required intubation and ventilation at the age of 10 minutes to sustain his breathing; surfactant was immediately given down the endotracheal tube. He was not weighed at the time but was given intramuscular vitamin K and then taken to the special care unit. On arrival in the unit, baby J was weighed (1270 g) and placed in an incubator for warmth. He was connected to a ventilator. Blood was taken for culture and basic haematology, and he was prescribed antibiotics. A radiograph showed well-aerated lungs.

Questions

1. Which antibiotic(s) would be appropriate initially for baby J?
   After 12 hours, baby J was extubated onto continuous positive airway pressure and remained on antibiotics. Parenteral feeding was commenced on day 1 as per unit policy, and simultaneously very slow continuous milk feeding into his stomach was started. Blood cultures were negative at 48 hours, and the antibiotics were stopped.
   On day 5, baby J looked unwell, with a rising oxygen requirement, increased work of breathing and poor peripheral perfusion. Examination revealed little else except that his liver was enlarged and a little firm, his pulses rather full and easy to feel and there was a moderate systolic heart murmur. One possibility was infection.
2. Which antibiotics would be appropriate for baby J on day 5?
   Another possibility was a patent arterial duct leading to heart failure.
3. How could his heart failure and patent ductus arteriosus be treated?
   After appropriate treatment he looked progressively better, and when the blood culture was negative after 2 days, the antibiotics

were stopped. By the age of 10 days, baby J was on full milk feeds, and the duct had closed. He was in air. However, he began to have increasingly frequent episodes of spontaneous bradycardia, sometimes after apnoeic spells in excess of 20 seconds in duration. Examination between episodes showed a healthy, stable baby. Investigations such as haematocrit, serum sodium and an infection screen were normal.

4. At 2 weeks, which drug of choice could be used to treat his apnoea and bradycardia? What would be the expected duration of treatment with this drug?

Answers

1. Antibiotic cover is usually started without knowledge of any organism until negative blood cultures are received. Penicillin and gentamicin provide good cover for streptococci and Gram-negative organisms, which are the most likely potential pathogens at this stage, and is the combination recommended by NICE (2012). If cultures were negative at 48 hours, antibiotics could be stopped provided that there were no clinical indications to continue.

2. At day 5, antibiotic therapy should take account of the likely pathogens such as *S. aureus* and others causing nosocomial infections. A suitable choice for the former would be flucloxacillin, if there was no concern about MRSA, or vancomycin if there was. The addition of another agent with good Gram-negative activity such as gentamicin or a third-generation cephalosporin would provide appropriate broad-spectrum cover.

3. Intravenous indometacin or ibuprofen would be suitable for the treatment of patent ductus arteriosus. Furosemide is the drug of choice for acute heart failure.

4. Caffeine is now the drug of choice. A suitable dose of caffeine for baby J would be a loading dose of 20 mg/kg with maintenance dose of 5 mg/kg/day, increasing to 10 mg/kg/day if necessary. The frequency of episodes of apnoea and bradycardia should decline immediately. The treatment is likely to continue until he is about 34 weeks of postmenstrual age, when his control of breathing should be mature enough to maintain good respiratory function. In some units, a loading dose of caffeine is given routinely just before extubation.

Case 9.2

Baby B was born at 25 weeks' gestation and was ventilated for 5 days before being extubated onto continuous positive airway pressure. On extubation she was initially in air, but now at the age of 4 weeks, she is mostly in about 30% oxygen, fully fed on milk, and growing well. Her chest X-ray showed the pattern typical of chronic lung disease. One morning she is noticed to be in 45% oxygen. She has had a large weight gain, and she looks quite oedematous all over.

Questions

1. What do these symptoms suggest?
   After careful evaluation, baby B is given an oral dose of furosemide 1 mg/kg, after which the oedema settles, her weight falls and her oxygen requirement returns to 30%.
2. What are the disadvantages of giving regular furosemide in this situation?
   A thiazide diuretic and spironolactone are prescribed. Four days later, routine biochemistry tests show a sodium of 125 mmol/L.
3. What is the choice the attending team has to make?

Answers

1. The symptoms suggest heart failure. Medical examination would probably have revealed an enlarged liver, and the heart might also have had a 'gallop' rhythm. In babies, the symptoms and signs commonly suggest both left and right ventricular failure.
2. Regular treatment with furosemide causes hypercalciuria, as well as excessive loss of sodium and potassium. Chronic hypercalciuria can lead to nephrocalcinosis. For this reason, a combination of thiazide diuretics and spironolactone is commonly used.
3. The sodium is low. The normal range in preterm babies is 130–140 mmol/L, lower than in children and adults. That it is low is probably an effect of the diuretics. The choice is between carrying on with the diuretics and supplementing the sodium intake or stopping the diuretics and observing the baby for any recurrence of heart failure.

Reference

National Institute for Health and Care Excellence (NICE), 2012. Neonatal infection (early onset): antibiotics for prevention and treatment. Clinical Guideline CG149. NICE, London. Available at: https://nice.org.uk/Guidance/cg149.

Further reading

Ainsworth, S.B., 2014. Neonatal Formulary: Drug Use in Pregnancy and the First Year of Life, seventh ed. Wiley-Blackwell, Oxford.

Holmes, A.P., 2016. NICU Primer for Pharmacists. American Society of Health-System Pharmacists, Bethesda.

Lissauer, T., Fanaroff, A.A., Miall, L., et al., 2015. Neonatology at a Glance, third ed. Wiley-Blackwell, Oxford.

Rennie, J.M., Kendall, G.S., 2013. A Manual of Neonatal Intensive Care, fifth ed. Routledge, London.

10 Paediatrics

Catrin Barker and Octavio Aragon Cuevas

Key points

- Children are not small adults.
- Patient details such as age, weight and surface area need to be accurate to ensure appropriate dosing of medicines.
- Weight and surface area may change in a relatively short time period and necessitate dose adjustment.
- Pharmacokinetic changes in childhood are important and have a significant influence on drug handling and need to be considered when choosing an appropriate dosing regimen for a child.
- The ability of the child to use different dosage forms changes with age, so a range of formulations should be available, for example, oral liquid, dispersible tablets and capsules.
- The availability of a medicinal product does not mean it is appropriate for use in children.
- The use of an unlicensed medicine in children is not illegal, although it must be ensured that the choice of drug and dose is appropriate.

Paediatrics is the branch of medicine dealing with the development, diseases and disorders of children. Infancy and childhood are periods of rapid growth and development. The various organs, body systems and enzymes that handle drugs develop at different rates; hence, drug dosage, formulation, response to drugs and adverse reactions vary throughout childhood. Compared with adult medicine, drug use in children is not extensively researched, and the range of licensed medicines in appropriate dosage forms is limited.

For many purposes, it has been common to subdivide childhood into the following periods:
- neonate: the first 4 weeks of life,
- infant: from 4 weeks to 1 year,
- child: from 1 to 12 years.

For the purpose of drug dosing, children older than 12 years are often classified as adults. This is inappropriate because many 12-year-olds have not been through puberty and have not reached adult height and weight. The International Committee on Harmonization (European Medicines Agency [EMA], 2001) suggested that childhood be divided into the following age ranges for the purposes of clinical trials and licensing of medicines:
- preterm newborn infants,
- term newborn infants (0–27 days),
- infants and toddlers (28 days to 23 months),
- children (2–11 years),
- adolescents (12–16/18 years).

These age ranges are intended to reflect biological changes: the newborn (birth to 4 weeks) covers the climacteric changes after birth, 4 weeks to 2 years covers the early growth spurt, 2–11 years covers the gradual growth phase and 12–18 years covers puberty and the adolescent growth spurt to final adult height. Manufacturers of medicines and regulatory authorities are still working towards standardising the age groups quoted in each product's Summary of Product Characteristics.

Demography

The population of the UK in 2016 was reported to be 65.6 million, of which 12 million were children younger than 16 years (Office of National Statistics, 2017a). But figures published by the Office for National Statistics in 2017 indicate that over the last 25 years the percentage of the population aged 16 years and younger has decreased from 21% to 19%. This trend is predicted to continue, and by 2036 the percentage of the population younger than 16 years is predicted to be 18%.

Children make substantial use of hospital-based services. In 2016 there were 23.57 million attendances at England's accident and emergency (A&E), and on average, one-quarter of these were for patients aged 19 or younger (Baker, 2017).

Congenital anomalies

Congenital anomalies remain an important cause of infant and child mortality. A congenital anomaly is an abnormality of structure, function or metabolism present at birth that results in physical or mental disability or is fatal. Congenital anomalies may be inherited or sporadic, and some may result from environmental causes, including diet, drugs, toxins, radiation or infection. Up to 1 in 20 babies are born with problems such as cleft palate, spina bifida or Down's syndrome. Screening during pregnancy can detect some congenital anomalies, whereas some are found at birth. Others become obvious only as a baby grows older.

Rare diseases affect a small number of people compared with the general population and, because they are rare, can be difficult to diagnose, treat and/or prevent. A disease is considered to be rare when it affects 1 person in 2000 or fewer (Genetic Alliance UK, 2016). The National Congenital Anomaly and Rare Disease Registration Service (NCARDRS) was established by Public Health England in 2013–14 and records those people with congenital abnormalities and rare diseases across the whole of England.

Cancer

Cancer is very rare in childhood. The most common cancers diagnosed in childhood are leukaemias and malignant neoplasms of the brain. As a consequence of the technical advances in treatment and the centralisation of services in specialist centres, much greater numbers of childhood cancer sufferers are surviving into adulthood. For all childhood cancers combined, the trend for children (0–14 years) diagnosed between 1990 and 2014 is of an increasing 5-year survival; 5-year survival is predicted to be 83.9% for children diagnosed in 2015 (Office of National Statistics, 2017b).

Asthma, eczema and allergy

Asthma, eczema and hay fever (allergic rhinitis) are among the most common chronic diseases of childhood, and most of the affected children are managed in primary care. During the 1970s and 1980s there was considerable expansion of epidemiological research into these disorders, prompted mainly by concern about the increase in hospital admissions for childhood asthma despite the availability of effective anti-asthma medication. These studies failed to identify any demographic, perinatal or environmental factor that could explain more than a small proportion of the large changes in prevalence of asthma, hay fever or eczema. Asthma continues to be an important childhood illness placing a burden on the health service. One in 11 children is reported to have asthma, and it is the most common long-term medical condition (Asthma UK, 2017). Asthma prevalence is thought to have plateaued since the late 1990s, although the UK still has some of the highest prevalence rates in Europe.

Prevalence rates for food allergy have also increased, with peanut allergy now affecting 1 in 70 children in the UK (Grundy et al., 2002). This is reflected in a documented increase in admission rates of children with very severe (anaphylactic) reactions (Turner et al., 2015).

Allergic diseases are not static. The distribution and pattern of disease change as the child matures. Infants are more likely to present with atopic eczema, food allergy, gastro-intestinal symptoms and wheezing, whilst older children typically present with asthma and allergic rhinoconjunctivitis. These observed differences are frequently referred to as the allergic march, which recognises the association between these diseases and the tendency for children to 'outgrow' certain aspects of their allergic disease (e.g. eczema or milk allergy).

Infections

Despite a dramatic decline in the incidence of childhood infectious diseases during the 20th century, they remain an important cause of ill health in childhood. Major advances in the prevention of infections have been achieved through the national childhood vaccination programme (information available at https://www.gov.uk/government/publications/the-complete-rou tine-immunisation-schedule).

The importance of maintaining high vaccine uptake has been demonstrated by the resurgence of vaccine-preventable diseases where children have not been vaccinated. Adverse publicity surrounding the measles, mumps and rubella (MMR) vaccine, involving a possible association with Crohn's disease and autism, resulted in a loss of public confidence in the vaccine and a decrease in MMR coverage. However, evidence does not support an association between measles vaccine and bowel disease (Davis and Bohlke, 2001) or autism (Jain et al., 2015).

Meningococcal disease occurs as a result of a systemic bacterial infection by *Neisseria meningitidis*. Meningococci colonise the nasopharynx of humans and are frequently harmless commensals. It is not fully understood why disease develops in some individuals but not in others. Meningococcal infection most commonly presents as either meningitis or septicaemia, or a combination of both. Early symptoms and signs are usually malaise, pyrexia and vomiting. Headache, neck stiffness, photophobia, drowsiness or confusion and joint pains may variably occur. In meningococcal septicaemia, a rash may develop, along with signs of advancing shock and isolated limb and/or joint pain. The rash may be nonspecific early on, but as the disease progresses, the rash may become petechial or purpuric and may not blanch. This can readily be confirmed by gentle pressure with a glass (the 'glass test') when the rash can be seen to persist. In young infants particularly, the onset may be insidious, and the signs may be nonspecific, without 'classical' features of meningitis, including the rash.

In January 2013, a four-component meningococcal B (4CMenB) protein vaccine was authorised for use by the European Medicines Agency. In 2015 4CMenB was added to the routine UK immunisation schedule, and the MenC conjugate vaccine provided at around 14 years of age was replaced with MenACWY conjugate vaccine.

Respiratory syncytial virus (RSV) is the most important cause of lower respiratory tract infection in infants and young children in the UK, in whom it causes bronchiolitis, tracheobronchitis and pneumonia. It is responsible for seasonal outbreaks of respiratory tract infection most commonly between October and April. The main burden of disease is borne by children younger than 2 years, and on average in England each year there are 30,000 RSV-associated hospital admissions in children younger than 5 years (Reeves et al., 2017). During the winter months, RSV is the single greatest cause of admission to hospital in children. Palivizumab provides passive immunity against RSV. The objective of the passive immunisation is to protect at-risk infants, for example, babies born with heart and lung disorders and premature babies, for whom RSV infection is likely to cause serious illness or death, and all children less than 24 months of age with severe combined immunodeficiency syndrome (SCID).

Mental health disorders

The emotional well-being of children is just as important as their physical health. Good mental health allows children and young people to develop resilience and grow into well-rounded, healthy adults. However, mental health disorders are another emerging concern in the child health arena. Mental health problems affect about 1 in 10 children and young people (Green et al., 2005). They include depression, anxiety and conduct disorder and are often a direct response to what is happening in children's lives. Alarmingly, however, 70% of children and young people who experience a mental health problem have not had appropriate interventions at a sufficiently early age (Children's Society, 2008). Groups at particularly high risk of psychiatric disorder include children in the care system, young people who are homeless and young offenders. Biological, psychological and social factors all seem likely to contribute to the risk of psychiatric disorders and may act in combination.

Drugs, smoking and alcohol

The harm that drugs, smoking and drinking can do to the health of children and young people is recognised, and a number of targets have been set in an attempt to reduce prevalence. In 2014–15, 1% of school children aged 8–15 in England reported that they smoked regularly (at least once a week) (Scholes and Mindell, 2016). Similar proportions of boys and girls had tried smoking and smoked regularly, and the prevalence increased with age. The proportion of children who had ever smoked cigarettes declined from 19% in 1997 to 4% in 2015. In 2007, the minimum age for buying tobacco was increased from 16 years old to 18 years old.

The proportion of 11- to 15-year-old children in England who have tried alcohol has been decreasing since 2003 (NHS Digital, 2017). In a survey in 2014, 38% of 11- to 15-year-olds had tried alcohol at least once, the lowest proportion since the survey began. There was little difference between the prevalence of drinking between girls and boys; the prevalence of drinking alcohol also increased with age.

In England, between 2001 and 2010, the prevalence of drug use among 11- to 15-year-olds declined (Agalioti-Sgompou, 2015); since 2010, the decline has slowed. In 2014, 15% of pupils had ever taken drugs, 10% had taken drugs in the last year and 6% had taken drugs in the last month.

Nutrition and exercise

Health during childhood can affect well-being in later life. Good nutrition and physical exercise are vital both for growth and development and for preventing health complications in later life. In addition, dietary patterns in childhood and adolescence have an influence on dietary preferences and eating patterns in adulthood. The World Health Organization (WHO) regards childhood obesity as one of the most serious global public health challenges for the 21st century. Obese children and adolescents are at an increased risk of developing various health problems and are also more likely to become obese adults with an increased risk of developing diseases such as diabetes, heart disease, stroke and certain types of cancers.

The National Child Measurement Programme (NCMP) measures the height and weight of around 1 million school children in England every year, providing a detailed picture of the prevalence of child obesity. In England, 28% of children aged 2–15 were classified as overweight or obese (14% overweight, 14% obese) (Conolly and NatCen Social Research, 2016), with a slightly higher percentage of boys in the obese category compared with girls (15% vs. 13%). Childhood obesity increased with age, with 11% of children between 2 and 4 years of age being obese compared with 16% of those aged 13–15.

Obese children have a higher percentage of fat mass and a lower percentage of lean mass compared with normal-weight children. Drug-dose calculation and pharmacokinetics in obese children are poorly understood. The harmful consequences of inadvertent overdosing of obese children are of increasing concern to clinicians prescribing drugs with serious side effects, such as morphine and paracetamol. Ideal body weight (IBW) and lean body mass (LBM) are, depending on the drug, often recommended as safer alternatives to total body weight during weight-based dose calculation.

The normal child

Growth and development are important indicators of a child's general well-being, and paediatric practitioners should be aware of the normal developmental milestones in childhood. In the UK, development surveillance and screening of babies and children is well established through child health clinics and more recently the introduction of the NCMP, where children are weighed and measured by trained staff at school.

Weight is one of the most widely used and obvious indicators of growth, and progress is assessed by recording weights on a percentile chart. A weight curve for a child which deviates from the usual pattern requires further investigation. Separate recording charts are used for boys, girls and children with Down's syndrome, and because percentile charts are usually based on observations of the white British population, adjustments may be necessary for some ethnic groups. WHO has challenged the widely used growth charts, based on growth rates of infants fed on formula milk. In 2006, it published new growth standards based on a study of more than 8000 breast-fed babies from six countries around the world. The optimum size is now that of a breast-fed baby. Recently, new growth charts have been introduced for children from birth to 4 years of age, although specific 'neonatal and infant close monitoring charts' for infants from 0 to 2 years of age and 'childhood and puberty close monitoring charts' for children 2–20 years of age are also available. These combine the UK and WHO data. Copies are available from the Royal College of Paediatrics and Child Health (RCPCH) website (http://www.rcpch.ac.uk/Research/UK-WHO-Growth-Charts).

Height (or length in children <2 years of age) is another important tool in developmental assessment. In a similar way to weight, height or length should follow a percentile line. If this is not the case, or if growth stops completely, then further investigation is required. The normal rate of growth is taken to be 5 cm or more per year, and any alteration in this growth velocity should be investigated. In secondary care, height is not always measured routinely in practice, and this can lead to difficulties in assessing important factors such as body mass index (BMI), adjusted body weight and renal function.

Obesity is a growing concern in the paediatric population in the UK, as described previously. Available equations for adults may not give relevant BMI values in children; thus, BMI charts have been developed. These charts should be used rather than the popular BMI equation for adults to get accurate results. They are available from the RCPCH website. NHS Choices offers a useful online 'healthy weight calculator' (http://www.nhs.uk/tools/page s/healthyweightcalculator.aspx) and offers advice and signposting to parents/carers and healthcare professionals dealing with an overweight or obese child.

For infants up to 2 years of age, head circumference is also a useful parameter to monitor. In addition to the previously described evaluations, assessments of hearing, vision, motor development and speech are undertaken at the child health clinics. A summary of age-related development is shown in Fig. 10.1.

Child health clinics play a vital role in the national childhood immunisation programme, which commences at 2 months of age. Immunisation is a major success story for preventive medicine, preventing diseases that have the potential to cause serious damage to a child's health or even death. An example of the impact that immunisation can have on the profile of infectious diseases is demonstrated by the meningitis C immunisation campaign, which began in November 1999. The UK was the first country to introduce the meningitis C conjugate (MenC) vaccine, and uptake levels have been close to 90%. The programme was targeted at under-20-year-olds and has been a huge success, with a 90% reduction in cases in that age group. A vaccine for the serotype B of the meningococcal microbe was developed in June 2013. Initially, the Joint Committee on Vaccination and Immunisation (JCVI) deemed the vaccine not cost-effective. However, after months of pressure from parents, health professionals and charity groups, the JCVI reviewed the decision in 2014, and the vaccine is now available for infants younger than 1 year as part of the routine immunisation schedule.

The human papilloma virus vaccine has also recently been introduced to the immunisation programme in the UK for females aged 12–13 years of age, to reduce the risk of cervical cancer. More recently, the Rotavirus vaccine, an oral live attenuated vaccine, has been added to the UK immunisation schedule with the aim of reducing the number of annual deaths in young infants due to this viral infection and also of reducing the burden and spread of the disease in A&E or walk-in centres.

Advice on the current immunisation schedule can be found in the current online edition of the British National Formulary for Children and the government website https://www.gov.uk/government/publica tions/the-complete-routine-immunisation-schedule.

Drug disposition

Pharmacokinetic factors

An understanding of the variability in drug disposition is essential if children are to receive rational and appropriate drug therapy. However, when treating a patient, all the factors have a dynamic relationship, and none should be considered in isolation.

Absorption

Oral absorption. The absorption process of oral preparations may be influenced by factors such as gastric and intestinal transit time, gastric and intestinal pH and gastro-intestinal contents. Posture, disease state and therapeutic interventions such as naso-gastric aspiration or drug therapy can also affect the absorption process. It is not until the second year of life that gastric acid output increases and is comparable on a per-kilogram basis with that observed in adults. In addition, gastric emptying time only approaches adult values at about 6 months of age.

The bioavailability of sulfonamides, digoxin and phenobarbital has been studied in infants and children of a wide age distribution. Despite the different physicochemical properties of the drugs, a similar bioavailability pattern was observed in each case. The rate of absorption was correlated with age, being much slower in neonates than in older infants and children. However, few studies have specifically reported on the absorption process in older infants or children. The available data suggest that in older infants and children, orally administered drugs will be absorbed at a rate and extent similar to those in healthy adults. Changes in the absorption rate would appear to be of minor importance when compared with the age-related differences of drug distribution and excretion.

Intramuscular absorption. Absorption in infants and children after intramuscular (i.m.) injection is noticeably faster than in the neonatal period because muscle blood flow is increased. On a practical note, intramuscular administration is very painful and should, where possible, be avoided. The route should not be used for the convenience of staff if alternative routes of administration are available.

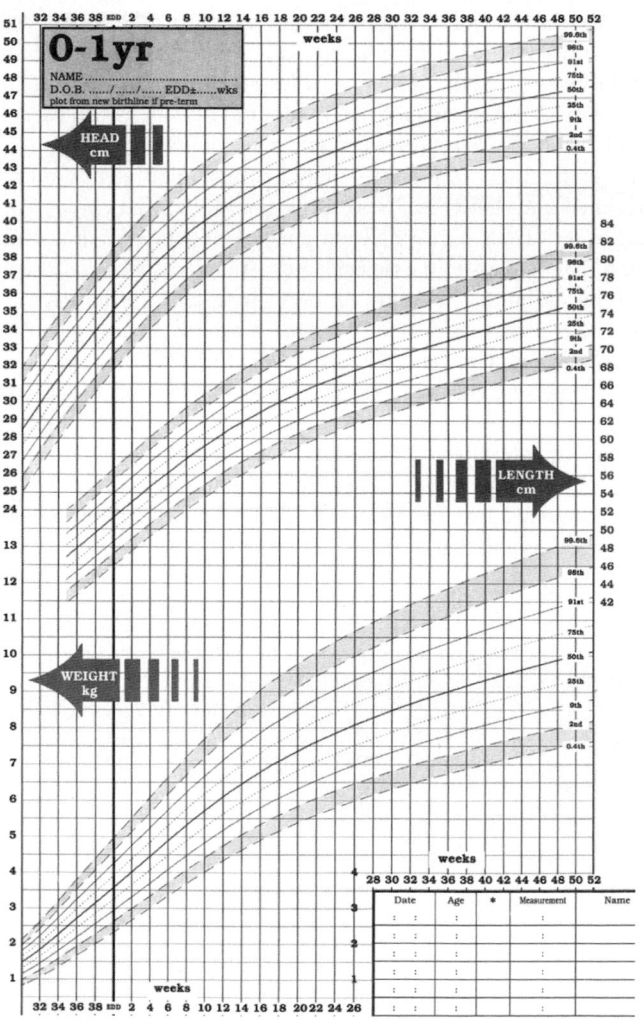

Fig. 10.1 A summary of the various stages of development.

Intraosseous absorption. Intraosseous absorption is a useful route of administration in patients in whom intravenous access cannot be obtained. It is especially useful in paediatric cardio-respiratory arrests where rapid access is required. A specially designed needle is usually inserted into the flat tibial shaft until the marrow space is reached. This route is considered equivalent to the intravenous route for rate of drug absorption, and most drugs can be given by this route.

Topical absorption. Advances in transdermal drug delivery systems have led to an increased use of this route of administration. For example, patch formulations of hyoscine hydrobromide have been found to be very useful to dry up secretions in children with excess drooling; likewise, fentanyl patches can be useful in pain management. Percutaneous absorption, which is inversely related to the thickness of the stratum corneum and directly related to skin hydration, is generally much greater in the premature and term newborn than in the adult. This can lead to adverse drug reactions (ADRs). For example, the topical application of a preparation containing prilocaine and lidocaine (EMLA) should not be used in preterm infants (<37 weeks) because of concerns about significant absorption of prilocaine in this age group, which may lead to methaemoglobinaemia (Aspen, 2016). Another route of topical absorption is the ophthalmic route. Significant amounts of drugs may be absorbed from ophthalmic preparations through ophthalmic or nasolacrimal duct absorption; for example, administration of phenylephrine eye drops can lead to hypertensive episodes in children (Apt and Gaffney, 2016).

Subcutaneous absorption. The development of needle-free subcutaneous jet injection systems appears to bring many benefits as a method of drug administration. They have been shown to give comparable levels to standard subcutaneous injections and overcome the problems of needle phobia, with less pain on administration. This system has been used with growth hormone, insulin and sedative medicines given before procedures and vaccination in children. However, it should be borne in mind that the system is not completely painless, and it can be quite frightening to young children because it is very noisy.

Rectal absorption. The mechanism of rectal absorption is probably similar to that of the upper part of the gastro-intestinal tract, despite differences in pH, surface area and fluid content. Although some products are erratically absorbed from the rectum, the rapid onset of action can be invaluable.

Buccal absorption. The buccal cavity is a potentially useful route of administration in patients who cannot tolerate medications via the oral route, for example, postoperative patients or those with severe nausea. Highly lipophilic drugs such as fentanyl can rapidly cross the buccal mucosa.

There are a number of 'melt' and 'wafer' formulations available, such as ondansetron. These preparations have the advantage of palatability; however, they are not absorbed via the buccal mucosa but require swallowing and enteral absorption of the active constituent. Desmopressin melts, on the other hand, are designed for buccal absorption, and thus the buccal dose is smaller than the enteral dose.

Intranasal absorption. The intranasal route is another useful route of administration. Medicines can be administered intranasally for their local action, for example, sympathomimetics, or for their systemic effects, for example, desmopressin in the treatment of diabetes insipidus. Highly lipophilic analgesics such as fentanyl and diamorphine are used via this route for the treatment of acute pain, particularly in situations where intravenous access is difficult, for example, reduction of fractures in the emergency department. Significant systemic absorption of medicines given intranasally for their local effect can also occur. For example, corticosteroids used in the treatment of allergic rhinitis could lead to cushingoid symptoms (Raveendran, 2014). Furthermore, administration may be difficult in the uncooperative child, and drugs administered may irritate the mucosa or be painful and unpleasant.

Distribution

Some of the factors that determine drug distribution within the body are subject to change with age. These include vascular perfusion, body composition, tissue-binding characteristics, and the extent of plasma protein binding.

As a percentage of total body weight, the total body water and extracellular fluid volume decrease with age (Table 10.1). Thus, for water-soluble drugs such as aminoglycosides, larger doses on the basis of a milligram per kilogram of body weight are required in the neonate than in the older child to achieve similar plasma concentrations.

Protein binding. Despite normal blood pH, free fatty acid and bilirubin levels in infants, binding to plasma proteins is reduced as a result of low concentrations of both globulins and albumin. It has been suggested that binding values comparable with those seen in adults are reached within the third year of life for acidic drugs, whereas for basic drugs, adult values are not reached until between 7 and 12 years of life. The clinical significance of this reduction in infants and older children is minimal. The influence of disease states, such as renal impairment, on plasma protein binding is more important. In the neonatal period these issues are complicated further by high circulating levels of endogenous agents such as bilirubin and immaturity of transporting proteins such as albumin. In this age range, care should be exercised when using drugs with an albumin binding affinity greater than 90% because they could displace bilirubin from its binding sites and lead to kernicterus. Ceftriaxone and phenytoin are two examples of drugs where use needs careful consideration in these situations.

Table 10.1 Extracellular fluid volume and total body water as a percentage of body weight at different life stages

Age	Total body water (%)	Extracellular fluid (%)
Preterm neonate	85	50
Term neonate	75	45
3 months	75	30
1 year	60	25
Adult	60	20

Drug metabolism

At birth, the majority of the enzyme systems responsible for drug metabolism are either absent or present in considerably reduced amounts compared with adult values, and evidence indicates that the various systems do not mature at the same time. This reduced capacity for metabolic degradation at birth is followed by a dramatic increase in the metabolic rate in the older infant and young child. In the age group of 1–9 years in particular, metabolic clearance of drugs is shown to be greater than in adults, as exemplified by theophylline, phenytoin and carbamazepine. Thus, to achieve plasma concentrations similar to those observed in adults, children in this age group may require a higher dosage than adults on a milligram-per-kilogram basis (Table 10.2).

Metabolic pathways that play only a minor role in adults may play a more significant role in children and compensate for any deficiencies in the normal adult metabolic pathway. For example, glucuronidation accounts for up to 70% of the metabolic pathway of paracetamol in adulthood; however, in the early newborn period, glucuronidation is deficient, accounting for less than 20% of paracetamol metabolism. This is compensated for by a more pronounced sulphate conjugation, and this leads to an apparently normal half-life in newborns. Paracetamol appears to be less toxic in children than in adults, and this may be in part explained by the compensatory routes of metabolism.

Metabolic differences may be further complicated by genetic polymorphism. The contribution of genetic factors to explain heterogeneity of drug response in infants and children is another important issue, with the ultimate goal for better treatment of children based on the individual genetic makeup. CYP2D6, the enzyme responsible for converting the prodrug codeine into the active compound morphine, is one example of an enzyme that displays genetic polymorphism. The enzyme production changes as the child grows (it is very low in the first weeks of life and in the teenage years, but it is highly available during infancy and childhood), and it has four genetic subtypes; a number of deaths in patients with the ultra-rapid metaboliser subtype led to the discontinuation of codeine use in infants and children.

Renal excretion

The anatomical and functional immaturity of the kidneys at birth limits renal excretory capacity. Younger than 3–6 months, the glomerular filtration rate is lower than that of adults but may be partially compensated for by a relatively greater reduction in tubular reabsorption. Tubular function matures later than the filtration process.

Generally, the complete maturation of glomerular and tubular function is reached only towards 12–18 months of age. After 18 months, the renal excretion of drugs is comparable with that observed in older children and adults. Changes in renal clearance of gentamicin provide a good example of the maturation of renal function (Table 10.3).

Other factors

In addition to age-related changes in drug disposition, nutritional status and disease states can influence drug handling. High plasma clearance of antibiotics such as penicillins and aminoglycosides has been demonstrated in children with cystic fibrosis, increased elimination of furosemide has been reported in children with nephrotic syndrome and prolonged elimination of furosemide has been reported in infants with heart failure. Altered protein binding has been demonstrated in hepatic disease, nephrotic syndrome, malnutrition and heart failure.

Drug therapy in children
Dosage

Doses of medicines in children should be obtained from a paediatric dosage handbook and should not be extrapolated from the adult dose. There are a number of such texts available internationally. The information within them may be based on evidence from clinical studies in children or reflect the clinical experience of the contributors. In the UK, the British National Formulary for Children (BNFC) is a national formulary that includes prescribing guidelines and drug monographs. It contains information on licensed, unlicensed and off-label use of medicines. When consulting any dosage reference resource, care should be taken to identify the dosage convention being used. Most formularies use a single-dose convention and indicate the number of times the dose should be repeated in a 24-hour period. Other formularies indicate the total daily dose and the number of doses this is divided into. Some formularies combine both conventions. Confusing the total daily dose with the single dose to be repeated may have catastrophic consequences, and the single-dose convention has become the preferred convention.

Table 10.2	Theophylline dosage in children older than 1 year
Age	Dosage (mg/kg/day)
1–9 years	24
9–12 years	20
12–16 years	18
Adult	13

Table 10.3	Renal clearance of gentamicin
	Plasma half-life (h)
Small premature infants weighing less than 1.5 kg	11.5
Small premature infants weighing 1.5–2 kg	8
Term infants and large premature infants less than 1 week of age	5.5
Infants 1 week to 6 months	3–3.5
Infants more than 6 months to adulthood	2–3

Although age, weight and height are the easiest parameters to measure, the changing requirement for drug dosage during childhood corresponds most closely with changes in body surface area (BSA). Nomograms which allow the surface area to be easily derived are available. There are practical problems in using the surface area method for prescribing; accurate height and weight may be difficult to obtain in a sick child, and manufacturers rarely provide dosage information on a surface-area basis. The surface-area formula for children has been used to produce the percentage method, giving the percentage of adult dose required at various ages and weights, although use should be reserved for exceptional circumstances (Table 10.4).

In selecting a method of dosage calculation, the therapeutic index of the drug should be considered. For agents with a narrow therapeutic index, such as cytotoxic agents, where recommendations are quoted per square metre, dosing must be based on the calculated surface area. However, there may be exceptions, for example, in children less than 1 year of age who have a proportionally larger surface area than other age groups, and where dosages of chemotherapeutic agents are often based on weight rather than surface area to prevent overestimation of the dose in this age group.

For drugs with a wide therapeutic index, such as penicillin, single doses may be quoted for a wide age range. Between these two extremes, doses are quoted in milligrams per kilogram, and this is the most widely used method of calculation. Whichever method is used, the resulting dosage should be rounded sensibly to facilitate dose measurement and administration and subsequently modified according to response or adverse effects.

It is important to note that none of the available methods of dosage calculation accounts for the change in dosage interval that may be required because of age-related changes in drug clearance. Where possible, the use of therapeutic drug monitoring to confirm the appropriateness of a dose is recommended.

Table 10.4   Percentage of adult dose required at various ages and body weights

	Mean weight for age (kg)	Percentage of adult dose
Newborn (full term)	3.5	12.5
2 months	4.5	15
4 months	6.5	20
1 year	10	25
3 years	15	33.3
7 years	23	50
10 years	30	60
12 years	39	75
14 years	50	80
16 years	58	90
Adult	68	100

Choice of preparation

The choice of preparation and its formulation will be influenced by the intended route of administration, the age of the child, availability of preparations, other concomitant therapy and, possibly, underlying disease states. The acceptability of a drug will vary with the type of formulation and age of the child. The problems of administering medicines to children were reviewed by the EMA, and guidelines on developing medicines for paediatric use were produced (EMA, 2005, 2013). It is common for healthcare professionals to manipulate medicines to try to provide the required dose for children. Guidance on this is available at http://www.medsiq.org/tool/manipulation-drugs-required-children-modric-%E2%80%93-guide-health-professionals.

Buccal route

Drugs may be absorbed rapidly from the buccal cavity (the cheek pouch), or they may dissolve when administered and be swallowed and absorbed from the stomach. 'Melt' technology, in which the drug and flavourings are freeze-dried into a rapidly dissolving pellet, can be very useful. The 'melt' dissolves instantly into a very small volume which is difficult for the child to reject. Gels, sprays and liquids can also be administered into the buccal cavity, an example being midazolam to treat seizures.

Oral route

The oral route is usually the most convenient, but in an uncooperative child, it can be the least reliable. Safe and effective drug therapy requires accurate administration, yet the 5 mL spoon is a difficult means of administering liquid medicines. Use of an oral syringe can provide controlled administration and ensure accurate measurement of the calculated dose, and it avoids the need for dilution of preparations with syrup. Use of oral syringes (which will not fit an intravenous Luer connector) is mandatory in UK practice. Concentrated formulations may be administered as oral drops in a very small volume. Although convenient, there could be significant dosage errors if drops are not delivered accurately.

In general, liquid preparations are often considered to be more suitable for children younger than 7 years. However, there is a wide variability in the age at which children can swallow tablets and capsules, and some quite young children can cope with solid dose formulations, especially mini-tablets. Some commercially available products contain excipients such as alcohol, propylene glycol and dyes that may cause adverse effects or be inappropriate for use in children with particular disease states. The osmolality and tonicity of preparations may be important; necrotising enterocolitis (a disorder seen in the neonatal period) has been associated with many different factors, including high-osmolality infant feeding formulae and pharmaceutical preparations, although a causal relationship has not been established. Oral liquids with high-osmolality or extremes of pH may irritate the stomach and should be diluted for administration. Sugar-free preparations may be necessary for the diabetic child or be desirable in other children for the prevention of dental caries. It is, however, important to be aware of the potential problems associated with substitutes for sucrose. The artificial sweetening agent aspartame, used in some preparations, should be used with caution in children with phenylketonuria because of its phenylalanine content. Other substitutes such as sorbitol and glycerol may not contribute to dental caries but produce diarrhoea if large doses are given. In these instances, a specially formulated preparation containing a higher amount of the active drug in a smaller volume may be preferable.

Injection solutions can sometimes be administered orally, although their concentration and pH must be considered together with the presence of unsuitable excipients. Powders or small capsules may be prepared and used as an alternative. However, lactose is a common diluent in powders and caution must be exercised in children with lactose intolerance.

Parents/carers are often discouraged from adding the dose of medicine to an infant's feed. On top of potential interactions which may arise with milk feeds, if the entire feed is not taken, a proportion of the dose will be lost. It is also important to advise parents/carers when it is not appropriate to crush solid dosage forms (e.g. sustained-release preparations). However, it should be recognised that addition of a medicine to a food or liquid may be the only way of rendering an unpalatable medicine acceptable. Whenever possible, evidence that this is pharmaceutically acceptable should be sought.

Manufacturers are increasingly recognising the difficulties associated with administration of medicines to children and are responding with novel formulations.

Mini tablets of just a few millimetres diameter may be useful to ease administration and allow flexibility of dosage. They may be presented in capsules or counted from bulk and can be individually coated for modified or sustained release. Increased surface area may present larger quantities of excipients to the child and requires careful control.

If an age-appropriate formulation is not available, for example, for a medicine used off-label, a liquid oral preparation may be prepared extemporaneously, often by crushing the 'adult' tablets and suspending the powder in commercial or locally produced suspending agents. Alternatively, the 'adult' dosage form may be manipulated, for example, by splitting tablets or dispersing it in water to take a proportion of the solution. Due consideration must be given to safety, solubility, accuracy and stability when modifying dosage forms.

Nasogastric, gastrostomy and jejunostomy administration

Medicines may be administered into the stomach via a nasogastric tube in the unconscious child or when swallowing is difficult. A gastrostomy tube may be placed into the stomach transcutaneously if the problem is long-term, for example, in some children with cerebral palsy. Enteral nutrition may also be administered through such tubes. Jejunostomies may be used when reflux persists despite use of a gastrostomy and or fundoplication surgery. Drugs such as phenytoin may adsorb to the plastic of the tubes and interact with enteral feeds, requiring special administration techniques to ensure bioavailability. Crushed tablets may block thin-bore nasogastric tubes. Some drugs may be absorbed early in the duodenum, making administration via a jejunostomy inappropriate. Furthermore, the jejunum lacks the secretions to buffer drugs with certain pH or high osmolality, making the dilution of these drugs with water or choosing a different formulation necessary. Suitability of drugs for nasogastric, gastrostomy and jejunostomy tube administration should always be checked.

Rectal route

The rectal route of administration is generally less favoured in the UK than in other European countries. It can be useful in patients who are vomiting or in infants or children reluctant or unable to take oral medication, but it is limited by the range of products available and the dosage inflexibility associated with rectal preparations. Some oral liquid preparations such as chloral hydrate and carbamazepine can be administered rectally. The route is useful in the unconscious child in the operating theatre or intensive care unit, and it is not uncommon to administer perioperative analgesics such as diclofenac and paracetamol and the antiemetic ondansetron using suppository formulations. Parents/carers and teachers may express concerns about using this route, fearing accusations of child abuse, but it is an important route of administration for diazepam or paraldehyde in the fitting child, although increasingly, buccal administration of midazolam may be preferred in this situation.

Parenteral route

When oral and rectal routes are inappropriate, the parenteral route may be necessary.

The problems associated with the administration of intramuscular injections in infants and children have been described earlier in this chapter. The route has a limited role in paediatric drug therapy and should not be used routinely. The intravenous route of administration is more widely used, but it is still associated with a number of potential problems that are outlined in the following sections.

Intravenous access. The practical difficulties of accessing small veins in the paediatric patient do not require explanation. However, these difficulties can often explain the sites of access that are chosen. Scalp veins, commonly used in newborn infants, are often very prominent in this age group, allowing easy access. It is also more difficult for the infant to dislodge a cannula from this site than from a site on the arm or foot. Likewise, the umbilical artery offers a useful route for monitoring the patient but can also be used for drug administration in some circumstances. Vasoconstrictive drugs, such as adrenaline (epinephrine), dopamine and isoprenaline, should not be given via this route.

Fluid overload. In infants and children, the direct administration of intravenous fluids from the main infusion container is associated with the risk of inadvertent fluid overload. This problem can be avoided by the use of a paediatric administration set and/or a volumetric infusion device to control the flow rate. A paediatric administration set incorporates a graduated volumetric chamber with a maximum capacity of 150 mL. Although this system is intended primarily as a safety device, the volume within the burette chamber can be readily adjusted, allowing its use for intermittent drug administration and avoiding the need for the 'piggyback system' commonly used in adult intravenous administration.

Dilution of parenteral preparations for infusion may also cause inadvertent fluid overload in children. In fluid-restricted or very young infants, it is possible that the volume of diluted drug can exceed the daily fluid requirement. To appreciate this problem, the paediatric practitioner should become familiar with the fluid volumes that children can tolerate. As a guide, these volumes can be calculated using the following formula: 100 mL/kg for the first 10 kg, plus 50 mL/kg for the next 10 kg, plus 20 mL/kg thereafter. Worked examples are given in Table 10.5. It is important to remember that these volumes do not account for losses such as those caused by dehydration, diarrhoea or artificial ventilation. Although the use of more concentrated infusion solutions may overcome the problem of fluid overload, stability data on concentrated solutions are often lacking. It may, therefore, be necessary to manipulate other therapy to accommodate the treatment or even to consider alternative treatment options. Fluid overload may also result from excessive volumes of flushing solutions and is described later. Guidance on selecting appropriate intravenous fluids for administration to children to avoid fluid induced hyponatraemia was published by the National Patient Safety Agency (NPSA, 2007a). Additional guidance on intravenous fluid therapy in children and young people in hospital was published by the National Institute for Health and Care Excellence (NICE) in December 2015 (NICE, 2015).

Lack of suitable paediatric formulations. Many parenteral products are only available in adult dose sizes. The concentrations of these products can make it difficult to measure the small doses required in paediatrics. Dilution to achieve measurable concentrations, miscalculations and misinterpretation of decimal points may lead to errors. 'Ten times' errors are common particularly when drawing the dose from a single ampoule or vial that contains sufficient quantity for an adult patient.

Displacement volume. Reconstitution of powder injections in accordance with manufacturers' directions usually makes no allowance for the displacement volume of the powder itself. Hence, the final volume may be greater than expected, and the concentration will, therefore, be less than expected. This can result in the paediatric patient receiving an underdose, which becomes even more significant in younger patients receiving smaller doses or more concentrated preparations. Paediatric units usually make available modified reconstitution directions which take account of displacement volumes.

Rates of infusion. The slow infusion rates often necessary in paediatrics may influence drug therapy. The greater the distance between the administration port and the distal end of the delivery system, and the slower the flow rate, the longer the time required for the drug to be delivered to the patient. In very young infants and children, it may take several hours for the drug to reach the patient, depending on the point of injection. This is an important consideration if dosage adjustments are being made in response to plasma level monitoring. Bolus injections should always be given as close to the patient as possible.

Dead space. After administration via an injection port, a residual amount of drug solution can remain trapped at the port. If dose volumes are small, the trapped fluid may represent a considerable proportion of the intended dose. Similarly, the volume of solution required to prime the intravenous lines or the inline filters (i.e. the dead space) can be a significant proportion of the intended dose. This problem can be minimised by ensuring that drugs are flushed at an appropriate rate into the main infusion line after administration via an injection port or through a filter and by priming the lines initially with a compatible solution. The small volumes required to prime filters and tubing specifically designed for infants and children can be used to minimise the dead space. Modern filter materials can produce less adsorption of drugs so that more of the drug is delivered to the patient.

It is important to remember that flushing volumes can add a significant amount to the daily fluid and sodium intake, and it may be important to record the volume of flushing solutions used in patients susceptible to fluid overload.

Excipients. Analogous to oral preparations, excipients may be present in parenteral formulations and can be associated with adverse effects. Benzyl alcohol, polysorbates and propylene glycol are commonly used agents which may induce a range of adverse effects in children, including metabolic acidosis, altered plasma osmolality, central nervous system depression, respiratory depression, cardiac arrhythmias and seizures. Knowledge of the products that contain these ingredients may influence drug selection.

The National Patient Safety Agency highlighted the risks associated with the preparation of injectable preparations in 2007 (NPSA, 2007b). Many hospitals have established centralised intravenous additive services (CIVAS) that prepare single intravenous doses under aseptic conditions, thus avoiding the need for preparation at ward level. Such services have not only significantly decreased the risks associated with intravenous therapy, particularly in the paediatric population, but can also produce considerable cost savings because more than one dose may be drawn up from the one vial.

Pulmonary route

The use of aerosol inhalers for the prevention and treatment of asthma presents particular problems for children because of the coordination required. The availability of breath-activated devices and spacer devices and large-volume holding chambers has greatly improved the situation. Guidance has been published on the use of inhaler devices in children less than 5 years of age (NICE, 2000) and older children (NICE, 2002) and was updated in 2014 (British Thoracic Society and Scottish Intercollegiate Guidelines Network, 2014). Recent experience has shown that different types of large-volume holding chambers alter drug delivery and absorption and should not be considered as interchangeable.

Table 10.5 Calculation of standard daily fluid requirements in paediatric patients

15-kg patient	35-kg patient
100 mL/kg × 10 kg = 1000 mL	100 mL/kg × 10 kg = 1000 mL
Plus 50 mL/kg × 5 kg = 250 mL	Plus 50 mL/kg × 10 kg = 500 mL
Total = 1250 mL/day	Plus 20 mL/kg × 15 kg = 300 mL
	Total = 1800 mL/day

It must be remembered that drugs can be absorbed into the systemic circulation after pulmonary administration or may be absorbed via the enteral route when excess drug is swallowed. High-dose corticosteroid inhalation may suppress the adrenal cortical axis and growth by this mechanism.

Dose regimen selection

A summary of the factors to be considered when selecting a drug dosage regimen or route of administration for a paediatric patient is shown in Table 10.6.

Medicines optimisation

Medicines optimisation is about ensuring that the right patients get the right choice of medicine, at the right time. By focusing on patients and their experiences, the goal is to help patients improve their outcomes, take their medicines correctly, avoid taking unnecessary medicines, reduce wastage of medicines and improve medicine safety. Ultimately, medicines optimisation can help encourage patients to take ownership of their treatment.

Parents or carers are often responsible for the administration of medicines to their children, and, therefore, basic principles of medicines optimisation such as concordance and adherence of both parties must be considered. The literature on nonadherence and concordance in children is limited, but the problem is considered to be widespread and similar to that reported in adults.

Nonadherence may be caused by several factors, such as patient resistance to taking the medicine, complicated dosage regimens, misunderstanding of instructions and apparent ineffectiveness or side effects of treatment. In older children and adolescents who may be responsible for their own medication, different factors may be responsible for nonadherence; for example, they may be unwilling to use their medication because of peer pressure.

Several general principles should be considered in an attempt to improve adherence. Adherence is usually better when fewer medicines are prescribed. Attention should be given to the formulation, taste, appearance and ease of administration of treatment. The regimen should be simple and tailored to the child's waking day. If possible, the child should be involved in choosing a suitable preparation when choice is available.

Many health professionals often counsel the parents/carers only, rather than involving the child in the counselling process. Where possible, treatment goals should be set in collaboration with the child.

Table 10.6 Factors to be considered when selecting a drug dosage regimen or route of administration for a paediatric patient

Factor	Comment
1. Age/weight/surface area	Is the weight appropriate for the stated age? If it is not, confirm the difference. Can the discrepancy be explained by the patient's underlying disease (e.g. patients with neurological disorders such as cerebral palsy may be significantly underweight for their age)? Is there a need to calculate dosage based on surface area, e.g. cytotoxic therapy? Remember heights and weights may change significantly in children in a very short space of time. It is essential to recheck the surface area at each treatment cycle using recent heights and weights.
2. Assess the appropriate dose	The age/weight of the child may have a significant influence on the pharmacokinetic profile of the drug and the manner in which it is handled. In addition, the underlying disease state may influence the dosage or dosage interval.
3. Assess the most appropriate interval	In addition to the influence of disease states and organ maturity on dosage interval, the significance of the child's waking day is often overlooked. A child's waking day is generally much shorter than that of an adult and may be as little as 12 h. Instructions given to parents particularly should take account of this; e.g. the instruction 'three times a day' will bear no resemblance to 'every 8 h' in a child's normal waking day. If a preparation must be administered at regular intervals, then the need to wake the child should be discussed with the parents, or preferably an alternative formulation, such as a sustained-release preparation, should be considered.
4. Assess the route of administration in the light of the disease state and the preparations and formulations available	Some preparations may require manipulation to ensure their suitability for administration by a specific route. Even preparations which appear to be available in a particular form may contain undesirable excipients that require alternatives to be found; e.g. patients with the inherited metabolic disorder phenylketonuria should avoid oral preparations containing the artificial sweetener aspartame because of its phenylalanine content.
5. Consider the expected response and monitoring parameters	Is the normal pharmacokinetic profile altered in children? Are there any age-specific or long-term adverse effects, such as on growth, that should be monitored?
6. Interactions	Drug interactions remain as important in reviewing paediatric prescriptions as they are in adult practice. However, drug–food interactions may be more significant, particularly drug–milk interactions in babies having 5–6 milk feeds per day.
7. Legal considerations	Is the drug licensed? If an unlicensed drug is to be used, the pharmacist should have sufficient information to support its use.

Parents consider the age group of 8–10 years the most appropriate at which to start including the child in the counselling process. As well as verbal instruction, parents often want written information. However, current patient information leaflets (PILs) must reflect the Summary of Product Characteristics and so are often inappropriate. If a drug is used in an 'off-label' manner, statements such as 'not recommended for use in children' may cause confusion and distress. Care needs to be taken, therefore, to ensure that the information provided, whether written or spoken, is appropriate for both the parents/carers and the child.

Information provided with medicines is often complex and may not always be relevant to children. The Royal College of Paediatrics and Child Health in conjunction with other bodies has launched a range of information leaflets on medicines for parents and carers. The leaflets cover off-label use of specific drugs and aim to provide appropriate, accurate and easily understandable information on dosage and side effects to those administering medicines to children. The leaflets can be downloaded from the website http://www.medicinesforchildren.org.uk.

Medicines in schools

Children with medical conditions should be properly supported at school so that they have full access to education, including school trips and physical education. Children who are acutely ill will be treated with medicines at home or in hospital, although it may be possible to return to school during their recovery phase. Children with chronic illness, such as asthma or epilepsy, and children recovering from acute illnesses may require medicines to be administered whilst at school. In addition, there are some medical emergencies that may occur at school or on school trips that require prompt drug administration before the arrival of the emergency services. These emergencies include anaphylaxis (associated with food allergy or insect stings), severe asthma attacks and seizures.

Policies and guidance

There is considerable controversy over the administration of medicines in schools. Whilst governing bodies must ensure that arrangements are in place to support pupils at school with medical conditions, there is no legal or contractual duty on school staff to administer medicine or supervise a pupil taking it. This is a voluntary role. Some support staff may have specific duties to provide medical assistance as part of their contract. Policies and procedures are required to ensure that prescribed medicines are labelled, stored and administered safely and appropriately and that teachers and care assistants are adequately trained and understand their responsibilities.

Advice has been provided for schools and their employers on how to manage medicines in schools in "Supporting pupils at school with medical conditions: Statutory guidance for governing bodies of maintained schools and proprietors of academies in England" (Department for Education, 2015). The roles and responsibilities of employers, parents and carers, governing bodies, head teachers, teachers and other staff and of local health services are all explained. The advice considers staffing issues such as employment of staff, insurance and training. Other issues covered include drawing up a healthcare plan for a pupil; confidentiality; record keeping; the storage, access and disposal of medicines; home-to-school transport; and on-site and off-site activities. It also provides general information on four common conditions that may require management at school: asthma, diabetes, epilepsy and anaphylaxis.

Responsibility for common medicines

Responsible pupils should be allowed to administer their own medication. Children with asthma should carry their 'reliever' inhaler (e.g. salbutamol or terbutaline); a spare inhaler should be available in school, and easy access to it before and during sports should be assured. There should be no need to have 'preventer' inhalers at school because administration schedules of two or three times daily are appropriate and can avoid school hours. Medicines with an administration schedule of two or three times a day should be supplied wherever possible so that dosing during school hours is avoided. Sustained-release preparations or drugs with intrinsically long half-lives may be more expensive but avoid the difficulties of administration at school. Sustained-release methylphenidate and atomoxetine, both used in the management of attention-deficit/hyperactivity disorder (ADHD), are examples. When administration at school is unavoidable, the school time doses can be provided in a separate, labelled container.

Special schools

Some children with severe, chronic illness will go to special rather than mainstream schools where their condition can receive attention from teachers and carers who have undergone appropriate training. Some special schools will be residential. Pupils may also attend another institution for respite care. Particular attention to communication of changes to drug treatment between parents/carers, primary care doctors, hospital doctors and school staff is required if medication errors are to be avoided.

Monitoring parameters

Paediatric vital signs as specified in the Advanced Paediatric Life Support (APLS) guidelines are described in Table 10.7. The figures presented in the tables are given as examples and may vary from hospital to hospital.

For standard paediatric haematological and biochemical parameters, local laboratory reference ranges should be consulted because these change throughout childhood.

Assessment of renal function

There are a number of methods of measuring renal function in children. These include the use of exogenous markers such as ^{51}Cr-EDTA, ^{99m}Tc-DTPA and using endogenous serum and urine creatinine concentrations measured over a timed period. Exogenous markers methods are used when an exact determination of renal function is needed, for example, before commencing

Table 10.7 Paediatric vital signs (Advanced Life Support Group, 2016)

Age	Respiration rate at rest (breaths/min) 5th–95th centile	Heart rate (beats/min) 5th–95th centile	Blood pressure systolic		
			5th centile	50th centile	95th centile
Birth	25-50	120-170	65-75	80-90	105
1 month					
3 months	25-45	115-160			
6 months	20-40	110-160			
12 months			70-75	85-95	
18 months	20-35	100-155			
2 years	20-30	100-150	70-80	85-100	110
3 years		90-140			
4 years		80-135			
5 years			80-90	90-110	111-120
6 years		80-130			
7 years					
8 years	15-25	70-120			
9 years					
10 years					
11 years					
12 years	12-24	65-115	90-105	100-120	125-140
14 years		60-110			
Adult					

complex chemotherapy. Despite some limitations, serum creatinine and estimated creatinine clearance are the most frequently used and most practical methods for 'bedside' assessment of renal function.

In adults, several formulae and nomograms are available for calculating and estimating renal function. However, these cannot be extrapolated to the paediatric population; the Cockcroft and Gault equation and the modification of diet in renal disease (MDRD) are validated only for patients aged 18 years and older.

Specific validated models are available for use in children. These equations use combinations of serum creatinine, height, weight, BSA, age and sex and, more recently, cystatin C (Cys-C) and blood urea nitrogen (BUN) to provide an estimate of creatinine clearance. Some of these equations have been further modified to better predict creatinine clearance; however, the advantage of simplicity is thereby lost. Several examples with their validated age ranges are shown here. The equations retain the limitations of the adult equations and tend to underperform in children with extreme weights or

rapidly changing creatinine levels, and they are affected by gender, ethnicity and concurrent illness and should be interpreted with care. Furthermore, the equations have been determined using different assays to measure parameters such as creatinine or Cys-C. An awareness of the method used by the local laboratory is needed to choose one equation or the other. Examples include the following:

- The most commonly used bedside equation (although more accurate ones are now available) is the original Schwartz equation:
  - GFR (mL/min/1.73 m^2) = K × height/serum creatinine (SCr)
    - Height in cm
    - SCr in mmol/L
    - Age range validation: 1–21 years
    - GFR range validation: 3–220 mL/min
    - Jaffe assay method for creatinine determination
    - K is a constant dependent on analytical method used to measure SCr, body composition, age and gender

- $K = 40$; however, different K values are available for different ages/genders:
  - $K = 29$ in low-birth-weight (<2.5 kg) infants
  - $K = 49$ in girls 2–16 and boys 2–13 years old
  - $K = 62$ in boys 13–16 years old
- The most reliable paediatric equation using endogenous markers to date is the improved Schwartz equation from 2009 eGFR-CKiD2. This equation is complex but can be used if the BUN and Cys-C values are available; it will perform exceedingly well (close to exogenous methods) if the patient's GFR is 15–75 mL/min.
  - $eGFR = 39.8 \times [ht(m)/Scr]^{0.456} \times [1.8/\ Cys\text{-}C]^{0.418} \times [30/BUN]^{0.079} \times [ht(m)/1.4]^{0.179}$
    - SCr in mg/dL
    - Height in metres
    - SCys in mg/L
    - BUN in mg/dL
    - × 1.076 if male
    - Age range: 1–17 years
    - Enzymatic method for creatinine determination
    - PENIA assay for cystatin C determination
    - NB: different units
- If Cys-C or BUN is not available, the most accurate endogenous markers equation is the 2008 Schwartz-Lyon equation:
  - GFR (mL/min/1.73 m^2) = K × height/SCr
    - SCr in mmol/L
    - Height in cm
    - Age range: 1–18 years
    - GFR range: 18–150 mL/min
    - Jaffe method for creatinine, but converted to enzymatic result.
    - Calculates different K values for age and gender:
      - K in all girls and boys <13 years = 32.5
      - K in boys ≥13 years = 36.5
- If height is not available:
  - Use Schwartz-Lyon with average height.

Adverse drug reactions

Drug safety is an important issue in all medical disciplines, but in paediatrics, this is compounded by the fact that medicines are often not tested in children, and therefore at the time of licensing there is no indication for use in children. This leads to off-label and/or unlicensed (OLUL) prescribing, estimated to occur in 25% of paediatric in-patient prescriptions. It is clear that extrapolation of efficacy, dosing regimens and adverse drug reactions (ADRs) from adult data to children is inappropriate owing to size differences, developmental changes in physiology and drug handling. Taken together with the fact that the pattern of diseases in children is different from that in adults, this puts them at high risk of serious and unpredictable ADRs.

Studies have shown an incidence of ADRs in paediatric patients of between 0.4% and 17% of patients (Smyth et al., 2012), with the incidence of adverse drug reactions causing admission to hospital as 2.9%. The wide range reflects the limited number of formal prospective and retrospective studies examining the incidence and characteristics of ADRs in the paediatric age group and the variations in study setting, patient group and definition of ADR used. Data can also be skewed by vaccination campaigns because adverse effects are common, and reporting is encouraged. One consistent finding is that the greater the number of medications the child is exposed to, the greater the risk of ADRs (Smyth et al., 2012).

ADRs in infants and older children typically occur at lower doses than in adults, and symptoms may be atypical. Examples include:

- enamel hypoplasia and permanent discolouration of the teeth with tetracyclines;
- growth suppression with long-term corticosteroids in prepubertal children;
- paradoxical hyperactivity in children treated with phenobarbital;
- hepatotoxicity associated with the use of sodium valproate; there are three major risk factors:
  - age under 3 years,
  - child receiving other anticonvulsants,
  - developmental delay;
- increased risk of Reye's syndrome with the use of salicylates in children with mild viral infection. Reye's syndrome is a life-threatening illness associated with drowsiness, coma, hypoglycaemia, seizures and liver failure. The mechanism of this toxicity remains unknown, but aspirin should generally be avoided in children younger than 16 years.

Many ADRs occur less frequently in the paediatric population, for example, gastro-intestinal bleeds with non-steroidal anti-inflammatory drugs (NSAIDs), hepatotoxicity with flucloxacillin and severe skin reactions with trimethoprim/sulfamethoxazole.

The reporting of ADRs is particularly important because the current system of drug development and authorisation not only deprives children of useful drugs because of the lack of clinical trials in children but may also exclude them from epidemiological studies of ADRs to prescribed drugs. The Medicines and Healthcare products Regulatory Agency (MHRA) and the Commission on Human Medicines (CHM) strongly encourage the reporting of serious ADRs in children, including those relating to unlicensed or off-label use of medicines, even if the intensive monitoring symbol (an inverted black triangle) has been removed. This reporting scheme has been extended in recent years to allow pharmacists, nurses and patients/carers to report suspected ADRs.

Medication errors

In contrast to ADRs, medication errors occur as a result of human mistakes or system flaws. Medication errors are now recognised as an important cause of adverse drug events in paediatric practice and should always be considered as a possible causative factor in any unexplained situation. They can produce a variety of problems ranging from minor discomfort to death. The National Patient Safety Agency (now the Patient Safety Agency within NHS England) reported that children aged up to 4 years were involved in 10% of medication incident reports where age was stated (NPSA, 2009). Further review of these reports highlighted issues with dose calculation, including 10-fold errors, and particular medicines (e.g. gentamicin).

Again, different reporting systems and criteria for errors make direct comparisons between studies difficult.

The incidence of medication errors and the risk of serious errors occurring in children are significantly greater than in adults. The causes are many and include:

- heterogeneous nature of the paediatric population and the corresponding lack of standard dosage;
- calculation errors by the prescriber, pharmacist, nurse or caregiver;
- lack of available dosage forms and concentrations appropriate for administration to children, necessitating additional calculations and manipulations of commercially available products or preparation of extemporaneous formulations from raw materials;
- lack of familiarity with paediatric dosing guidelines;
- confusion between adult and paediatric preparations;
- limited published information;
- need for precise dose measurement and appropriate drug delivery systems, the absence of which leads to administration errors and use of inappropriate measuring devices;
- 10-fold dosing errors, which are particularly important and potentially catastrophic, with reports still appearing regularly in the published literature.

The reporting and prevention of medication errors are important. The causes of medication errors are usually multifactorial, and it is essential that when investigating medication errors, particular focus should be placed on system changes and human factors.

Licensing medicines for children

Medicines licensing process

All medicines marketed in the UK must have been granted a product licence (PL) under the terms of the Medicines Act 1968 or a marketing authorisation (MA) following more recent European legislation on the authorisation of medicines. The aim of licensing is to ensure that medicines have been assessed for safety, quality and efficacy. In the UK, evidence submitted by a pharmaceutical company is assessed by the MHRA with independent advice from the CHM and its paediatric medicines expert group.

The licensed indications for a drug are published in the summary of product characteristics. Many medicines granted a product license or MA for adult use have not been scrutinised by the licensing authorities for use in children. This is reflected by contraindications or cautionary wording in the summary of product characteristics. There has been a lack of commercial incentive to develop medicines for the relatively small paediatric market and perceived difficulties in carrying out clinical trials in this group. It is not illegal to use medicines for indications or ages not specified in the summary of product characteristics, but to ensure safe and effective treatment, health professionals should have adequate supporting information about the intended use before proceeding. Failure to ensure that the use of a medicine is reasonable could result in a suit for negligence if the patient comes to harm.

Unlicensed and 'off-label' medicines

Several reports on drug prescribing in the paediatric setting show that the use of 'off-label' (use of a medicine outside the terms of the licence) or unlicensed medicines is extensive both within hospital and in outpatient settings. In hospital and neonatal care studies the proportion of 'off-label' use varied between 10% and 65%. In outpatient settings the proportion of off-label use varied between 11% and 31% (Kimland and Odlind, 2012). Many 'off-label' medicines will have to be produced by using an 'adult' dose forms, such as tablets, and preparing an extemporaneous liquid preparation suitable for the child. This may be made from the licensed dose form, for example, by crushing tablets and adding suitable excipients, or from chemical ingredients. An appropriate formula with a validated expiry period and ingredients to approved standards should be used. Care must be taken to ensure accurate preparation, particularly when using formulae or ingredients which are unfamiliar.

On some occasions the drug to be used has no product licence or MA, perhaps because it is only just undergoing clinical trials in adults, has been imported from another country, has been prepared under a 'specials' manufacturing licence or is being used for a rare condition for which it has not previously been employed. As with 'off-label' use, there must always be information to support the quality, efficacy and safety of the medicine, as well as information on the intended use. There is always a risk in using such a medicine, which must be balanced against the seriousness of the child's illness and discussed with the parents/carers if practicable.

Many authorities require that the patient should always be informed if the medicine prescribed is unlicensed or 'off-label' and even that written informed consent be obtained before treatment begins. In many situations in paediatrics, this would be impractical, but if parents/carers are not informed, the PIL included with many medicines may cause confusion because it may state that it is 'not for use in children'. Patient or parent/carer information specific to the situation should be prepared and provided.

Legislation on medicines for children

The Paediatric Regulation came into force in the European Union (EU) in January 2007. Its objective was to improve the health of children in Europe by facilitating the development and availability of medicines for children aged 0–17 years. The regulation aims to ensure that medicines for use in children are of high quality, ethically researched and authorised appropriately and also improve the availability of information on the use of medicines for children. It aims to achieve this without subjecting children to unnecessary trials or delaying the authorisation of medicines for use in adults.

The regulation dramatically changed the regulatory environment for paediatric medicines in Europe. Its main impact was the establishment of the Paediatric Committee (PDCO) of the EMA, which is responsible for coordinating the agency's work on medicines for children. The PDCO's main role is to determine the studies that companies must carry out on children as part of paediatric investigation plans (PIPs). In return for such development, the company receives an additional 6 months of market exclusivity for its product.

In July 2012, the EMA published a report for the European Commission on the first 5 years of the regulation (EMA, 2012). This report concludes that paediatric development has become a more integral part of the overall development of medicinal products in the EU, with the regulation working as a major catalyst to improve the situation for young patients. The EMA and its PDOC have agreed to more than 600 PIPs with pharmaceutical companies, to provide data on the efficacy and safety of medicines for diseases of children. More paediatric clinical trials were done, around 350–400 clinical trials per year, that included children (0–18 years), and the proportion of clinical trials including children has increased in the last 6 years, to approximately 10%. Neonates are the most neglected group when it comes to medicines development, but medicines very often need to be used without any proper data on efficacy and safety. The EMA requested the inclusion of more neonates and infants in clinical trials to obtain these data in a safe way; currently 30% of the PIPs include studies with neonates, and more neonates and infants (26%) have been included in trials in recent years. The report also identifies some areas for improvement, such as the low uptake of paediatric-use marketing authorisations (PUMAs) by companies.

Several European governments have funded paediatric clinical trials networks to stimulate research and help undertake studies resulting from the paediatric medicines regulations. In the UK, the Clinical Research Network (Children Specialty) is part of the UK National Institute for Health Research (https://www.crn.nihr.ac.uk/children/).

WHO has a 'Make medicines child size' programme to stimulate the development of age-appropriate formulations of medicines for children, particularly for those which appear in the List of Essential Medicines for Children: http://www.who.int/medicines/publications/essentialmedicines/en/.

Case studies

Case 10.1

Name: PT
Age: 7 years old
Sex: Male
Weight: 16 kg

Presenting condition:	Presented in the emergency department with a 2-day history of worsening groin and hip pain. Could not bear weight. Patient was febrile with a temperature of 39.2 °C, vomiting and dehydrated. There was no history of injury.
Previous medical history:	Nil of note
Allergies:	No known drug allergies
Drug history:	Nil of note
Differential diagnosis:	Septic arthritis, osteomyelitis

Tests:	Urea and electrolytes
	Full blood count
	C-reactive protein (CRP), erythrocyte sedimentation rate (ESR)
	Blood culture and sensitivities
	X-ray (hips and abdomen)
	Bone scan
Results:	Bone scan revealed right pubic osteomyelitis
	CRP = 56 mg/L (normal range 0–10 mg/L)
	ESR = 34 mm/h (normal range 1–10 mm/h)
	Blood culture revealed *Staphylococcus aureus* sensitive to flucloxacillin
Prescribed:	Flucloxacillin i.v. 800 mg four times a day for 2 weeks, to be followed by oral flucloxacillin 800 mg four times a day for 4 weeks
Progress:	Temperature settled and ESR/CRP decreased after initiation of antibiotic therapy

On the third day of treatment the patient developed a raised red rash which was suspected of being an allergic reaction to flucloxacillin. Treatment was changed to i.v. clindamycin 160 mg three times a day (10 mg/kg/dose) for 2 weeks followed by oral clindamycin 160 mg three times a day for a further 4 weeks.

Question

Comment on the drug therapy and any monitoring required.

Answer

There are a number of points to consider for PT:
- Body weight appears low for age; therefore, there is a need to check if the weight is correct (expected weight for a 7-year-old is approximately 23 kg). If incorrect, doses of medication will need to be recalculated.
- Recommended i.v. dose of flucloxacillin of 50 mg/kg/dose is correct. However, the usual maximum oral dose of flucloxacillin is 25 mg/kg/dose. This is because of the increased risk of gastric side effects with high oral doses of flucloxacillin.
- There is a need to consider adherence with oral flucloxacillin therapy due to poor palatability of the suspension formulation (if PT would not take capsules) and the frequent dosing regimen.
- Whilst the risk of flucloxacillin-induced hepatotoxicity is low in children, there is a need to consider measuring baseline and repeat liver function tests because of the prolonged course (>2 weeks) of flucloxacillin therapy.
- Clindamycin has good oral bioavailability, so i.v. therapy may be unnecessary. However, guidelines on the treatment of osteomyelitis suggest 1–2 weeks of i.v. therapy before switching to oral therapy.
- The recommended dose of clindamycin by i.v. infusion is up to 10 mg/kg dose 6 hourly in severe infection. The infusion should be diluted to 6 mg/mL with sodium chloride 0.9% or dextrose 5% (or a combination) and administered over 30–60 minutes at a maximum rate of 20 mg/kg/h. Consider 160 mg in 27 mL sodium chloride 0.9% over 30 minutes.
- The recommended standard oral dose of clindamycin is 3–6 mg/kg/dose four times a day. This may contribute to problems with adherence to long-term therapy. A three-times-daily dosing

regimen is to be preferred, particularly because PT may return to school, and four-times-daily dosing would require a dose to be administered at school, which may be problematic.

- Consideration should be given to how to administer clindamycin. Clindamycin palmitate suspension, which was palatable, is no longer available as a licensed preparation in the UK. Whilst extemporaneous formulations are available that use clindamycin hydrochloride capsules, the palatability of the resultant suspension is a major concern, particularly given the prolonged course of therapy. A 75 mg/5 mL suspension, licensed in Belgium, can be imported. From a safety and efficacy perspective, it is preferable to use such a product, which has been through a regulatory process similar to that of the UK, than to compound an extemporaneous preparation, which has not undergone appropriate pharmaceutical/pharmacokinetic evaluation.
- Consideration could be given to decreasing the dose of clindamycin to 150 mg three times a day to accommodate capsules, although PT may have difficulty taking these.
- The most serious adverse effect of clindamycin is antibiotic-associated colitis; however, this is often asymptomatic in children due to lack of receptors to the enterotoxin produced by *Clostridium difficile*. It is important to monitor for diarrhoea. If this arises, treatment should be discontinued.

Case 10.2

Name: CS
Age: 18 months old
Sex: Female
Weight: 10 kg

Presenting condition:	**Severe right-sided abdominal pain**
	Vomiting and loss of appetite
	Increased temperature 38.2°C
Previous medical history:	Nil of note
Allergies:	No known allergies
Drug history:	Nil of note
Tests:	Ultrasound
Provisional diagnosis:	Appendicitis

CS went to theatre where an appendicectomy was performed. The appendix was noted to be perforated.

The prescription reads:	Morphine i.v. 50 mg in 50 mL to run at 1–4 mL/h (10–40 micrograms/kg/h)
	Paracetamol 200 mg four times a day as required orally or per rectum
	Diclofenac 12.5 mg twice a day as required per rectum
	or
	Ibuprofen 100 mg four times a day as required orally when tolerating milk
	Five days of i.v. antibiotic therapy with:
	• Gentamicin 70 mg once daily
	• Cefotaxime 500 mg four times a day
	• Metronidazole 75 mg three times a day

Question

Comment on CS's drug therapy.

Answer

- Consideration must be taken of the fact that CS is small for her age. Investigate if the weight has been recorded accurately in the drug chart.
- The morphine dose is incorrect. If the infusion is prepared as directed, 1 mL/h will actually provide 100 micrograms/kg/h (the dose of morphine is between 10 and 40 micrograms/kg/h). This is a 10-fold overdose, which is a medication error frequently seen in children.
- There is a need to consider how to administer the appropriate rectal dose of paracetamol to CS. Often, post-appendicectomy patients will need to be nil by mouth for a few days. Rectal bioavailability is lower than oral bioavailability, and there may be a need to consider giving a larger rather than smaller paracetamol dose, that is, possibly 250 mg/rectum 8 hourly rather than 125 mg 6 hourly, for up to 48 hours, but not exceeding 90 mg/kg/day.
- Regarding the use of the rectal route, i.v. paracetamol might be a better option for CS. The i.v. preparation is cost-effective compared with the suppositories, is more acceptable (in most cases) for the parents/carers and the child and is fast and effective. It has been shown to be morphine sparing postoperatively. This patient already has an i.v. cannula in situ, so i.v. paracetamol would be the drug of choice rather than rectal.
- Suggest that paracetamol and NSAID are administered regularly in addition to the morphine for at least the first few days post-surgery. Multimodal analgesic therapy is recommended. The NSAID should not be administered, even rectally, until CS is feeding. The gastro-intestinal side effects caused by NSAIDs are systemic, by affecting the prostaglandin pathways, not topical.
- There will be a need to monitor CS for side effects. Nausea, vomiting and pruritus all occur frequently with morphine but can be treated/prevented. It might be a good idea to get a laxative, anti-emetic and antihistamine prescribed so that the medication can be given in a timely manner should the need arise.
- Young children are particularly susceptible to developing myoclonic jerks with morphine. These are often worrying for parents/carers but resolve on withdrawal of the morphine.
- NSAIDs are well tolerated by children, and the risk of adverse events is much lower in children than the adult population. However, it is important to ensure adequate hydration status postoperatively, particularly when using NSAIDs. Acute renal failure has been reported in children who have been treated with NSAIDs and not adequately hydrated, especially bearing in mind that a second nephrotoxic agent, gentamicin, has been prescribed.
- The choice of antibiotics for CS offers adequate cover; however, it could be rationalised. High-dose (7 mg/kg) once-daily aminoglycoside (gentamicin/tobramycin) therapy is now routinely used in children. It is administered by short infusion over 20 minutes. Plasma drug levels should be monitored to achieve an 18- to 24-hour trough level of less than 1 mg/L to avoid toxicity. Monitor urea and electrolytes and serum creatinine. Cefotaxime can be given as a bolus injection over 3–5 minutes. Metronidazole can be given as a short bolus or as a short infusion over 20 minutes. Current practice is to use a broad-spectrum antibiotic such as co-amoxiclav that will offer cover against the most likely causative organisms, Gram-negative enterobacteria, anaerobes and Gram-positive bacteria potentially from surgical equipment. It will also avoid using three antibiotics, accessing the line multiple times, using cefotaxime (there is an increase of microorganisms showing resistances to cephalosporins) and using gentamicin (which is nephrotoxic and best avoided in the peri-operative period).

References

Advanced Life Support Group, 2016. Advanced Paediatric Life Support: The Practical Approach, 6th ed. Wiley Blackwell, London.

Agalioti-Sgompou, V., Christie, S., Fiorini, P., et al., 2015. Smoking, drinking and drug use among young people in England in 2014. Available at: http://content.digital.nhs.uk/catalogue/PUB17879/smok-drin-drug-youn-peop-eng-2014-rep.pdf.

Apt, L., Gaffney, W.L., 2016. Adverse effects of topical eye medication in infants and children. Available at: https://entokey.com/adverse-effects-of-topical-eye-medication-in-infants-and-children/.

Aspen, 2016. EMLA cream 5%. Summary of product characteristics. Available at: https://www.medicines.org.uk/emc/medicine/171.

Asthma, U.K., 2017. Asthma facts and statistics. Available at: https://www.asthma.org.uk/about/media/facts-and-statistics/.

Baker, C., 2017. Accident and emergency statistics: demand, performance and pressure. Briefing Paper No. 6964. House of Commons Library Search. Available at: http://researchbriefings.files.parliament.uk/documents/SN06964/SN06964.pdf.

British Thoracic Society and Scottish Intercollegiate Guidelines Network, 2014. SIGN 141 British guideline on the management of asthma. Available at: https://www.brit-thoracic.org.uk/document-library/clinical-information/asthma/btssign-asthma-guideline-2014/.

Children's Society, 2008. The Good Childhood Inquiry: Health Research Evidence. Children's Society, London.

Conolly, A., NatCen Social Research, 2016. Health survey for England 2015. Children's body mass index, overweight and obesity. Available at: http://www.content.digital.nhs.uk/catalogue/PUB22610/HSE2015-Child-obe.pdf.

Davis, R.L., Bohlke, K., 2001. Measles vaccination and inflammatory bowel disease: controversy laid to rest? Drug Saf. 24, 939–946.

Department for Education, 2015. Supporting pupils at school with medical conditions. Statutory guidance for governing bodies of maintained schools and proprietors of academies in England. Available at: https://www.gov.uk/government/uploads/system/uploads/attachment_data/file/484418/supporting-pupils-at-school-with-medical-conditions.pdf.

European Medicines Agency, 2001. International Committee on Harmonization, Topic E11 on clinical investigation of medicinal products in the paediatric population Step 5. Note for guidance on clinical investigation of medicinal products in the paediatric population. European Medicines Agency, London. Available at: http://www.ema.europa.eu/docs/en_GB/document_library/Scientific_guideline/2009/09/WC500002926.pdf.

European Medicines Agency, 2005. Reflection paper: formulations of choice for the paediatric population. Available at: http://www.ema.europa.eu/docs/en_GB/document_library/Scientific_guideline/2009/09/WC500003782.pdf.

European Medicines Agency, 2012. 5-year report to the European Commission. General report on the experience acquired as a result of the application of the paediatric regulation. Available at: https://ec.europa.eu/health/sites/health/files/files/paediatrics/2012-09_pediatric_report-annex1-2_en.pdf.

European Medicines Agency, 2013. Guideline on pharmaceutical development of medicines for paediatric use. Available at: http://www.ema.europa.eu/docs/en_GB/document_library/Scientific_guideline/2013/07/WC500147002.pdf.

Genetic Alliance, U.K., 2016. What is a rare disease? Available at: http://www.raredisease.org.uk/what-is-a-rare-disease/.

Green, H., McGinnity, A., Meltzer, H., et al., 2005. Mental health of children and young people in Great Britain: 2004. Office for National Statistics.

Available at: http://content.digital.nhs.uk/catalogue/PUB06116/ment-heal-chil-youn-peop-gb-2004-rep2.pdf.

Grundy, J., Matthews, S., Bateman, B., et al., 2002. Rising prevalence of allergy to peanut in children: Data from 2 sequential cohorts. J. Allergy Clin. Immunol. 110, 784–789.

Jain, A., Marshall, J., Buikema, A., et al., 2015. Autism occurrence by MMR vaccine status among US children with older siblings with and without autism. JAMA 313, 1534–1540.

Kimland, E., Odlind, V., 2012. Off-label drug use in paediatric patients. Clin. Pharm. Therapeut. 91, 796–801. http://www.ema.europa.eu/docs/en_GB/document_library/Other/2013/06/WC500143984.pdf.

National Institute for Health and Care Excellence (NICE), 2000. Guidance on the use of inhaler systems (devices) in children under the age of 5 years with chronic asthma. Technical appraisal guidance [TA10]. Available at: https://www.nice.org.uk/guidance/ta10.

National Institute for Health and Care Excellence (NICE), 2002. Inhaler devices for routine treatment of chronic asthma in older children (aged 5–15 years). Technical appraisal guidance [TA38]. Available at: https://www.nice.org.uk/guidance/ta38.

National Institute for Health and Care Excellence (NICE), 2015. Intravenous fluid therapy in children and young people in hospital. NICE guideline [NG29]. Available at: https://www.nice.org.uk/guidance/ng29.

National Patient Safety Agency, 2007a. Reducing the risk of hyponatraemia when administering intravenous infusions to children. Patient Safety Alert 22. NPSA, London.

National Patient Safety Agency, 2007b. Promoting safer use of injectable medicines. Patient Safety Alert 20. NPSA, London.

National Patient Safety Agency, 2009. Review of patient safety for children and young people. NPSA, London.

NHS Digital, 2017. Statistics on alcohol England, 2017. Available at: https://digital.nhs.uk/media/30886/Statistics-on-Alcohol...2017.../alc-eng-2017-rep.

Office of National Statistics, 2017a. Overview of the UK population: July 2017. Available at: https://www.ons.gov.uk/peoplepopulationandcommunity/populationandmigration/populationestimates/articles/overviewoftheukpopulation/july2017.

Office of National Statistics, 2017b. Childhood cancer survival in England: children diagnosed from 1990 to 2014 and followed up to 2015. Available at: https://www.ons.gov.uk/peoplepopulationandcommunity/healthandsocialcare/conditionsanddiseases/bulletins/childhoodcancersurvivalinengland/childrendiagnosedfrom1990to2014andfollowedupto2015.

Raveendran, A.V., 2014. Inhalational steroids and iatrogenic Cushing's syndrome. Open Respir. Med. J. 8, 74–84.

Reeves, R.M., Hardelid, P., Gilbert, R., et al., 2017. Estimating the burden of respiratory syncytial virus (RSV) on respiratory hospital admissions in children less than five years of age in England, 2007-2012. Influenza Other Respir. Viruses 11, 122–129.

Scholes, S., Mindell, J., 2016. Health survey for England 2015. Children's smoking and exposure to other people's smoke. Available at: http://www.content.digital.nhs.uk/catalogue/PUB22610/HSE2015-Child-smo.pdf.

Smyth, R.M.D., Gargon, E., Kirkham, J., et al., 2012. Adverse drug reactions in children – a systematic review. PLoS One 7, e24061.

Turner, P.J., Gowland, M.H., Sharma, V., et al., 2015. Increase in anaphylaxis-related hospitalizations but no increase in fatalities: an analysis of United Kingdom national anaphylaxis data, 1992–2012. J. Allergy Clin. Immunol 135, 956–963.

Further reading

Kliegman, R.M., Stanton, B., St. Geme, J., et al., 2015. Nelson Textbook of Pediatrics, twentyth ed. Elsevier, Philadelphia.

Lewisham and North Southwark Health Authority, 2012. Guy's, St Thomas's and Lewisham Hospitals Paediatric Formulary, nineth ed. Lewisham and North Southwark Health Authority, London.

NHS Education for Scotland, 2014. An introduction to paediatric pharmaceutical care. Available at: http://www.nes.scot.nhs.uk/media/3068550/paeds_december_2014.pdf.

Phelps, S.J., Hagemann, T.M., Lee, K.R., et al., 2013. Teddy Bear Book: Pediatric Injectable Drugs, tenth ed. American Society of Health System Pharmacists, Bethesda.

Taketomo, C.K., 2016–17. Pediatric and neonatal dosage handbook, twenty third ed. Wolters Kluwer, Alphen aan den Rijn.

Useful websites

UK WHO growth charts: http://www.rcpch.ac.uk/Research/UK-WHO-Growth-Charts.

Contact a Family (for families with disabled children): http://www.cafamily.org.uk/.

Immunization against infectious diseases: https://www.gov.uk/government/collections/immunisation-against-infectious-disease-the-green-book.

Information leaflets on medicines for parents and carers: http://www.medicinesforchildren.org.uk.

Manipulation of drugs required in children (MODRIC) – A guide for health professionals: http://www.medsiq.org/tool/manipulation-drugs-required-children-modric-%E2%80%93-guide-health-professionals.

Neonatal and Paediatric Pharmacists Neonatal and Paediatric Pharmacists Group (NPPG): http://www.nppg.org.uk/.

NHS Choice BMI healthy weight calculator: http://www.nhs.uk/tools/pages/healthyweightcalculator.aspx.

Royal College of Paediatrics and Child Health: http://www.rcpch.ac.uk/.

UK Immunization schedule: https://www.gov.uk/government/publications/the-complete-routine-immunisation-schedule.

UK National Institute for Health Research: https://www.crn.nihr.ac.uk/children/.

WHO list of essential medicines for children: http://www.who.int/medicines/publications/essentialmedicines/en/.

11 Geriatrics

Hamsaraj Shetty and Ken Woodhouse

Key points

- Older people form about 18% of the population and receive about one-third of health service prescriptions in the UK.
- Ageing results in physiological changes that affect the absorption, metabolism, distribution and elimination of drugs.
- Alzheimer's disease and vascular dementia are the most important diseases of cognitive dysfunction in the elderly. Donepezil, rivastigmine and galantamine are inhibitors of acetylcholinesterase and improve cognitive function in Alzheimer's disease.
- The elderly patient with Parkinson's disease is more susceptible to the adverse effects of levodopa such as postural hypotension, ventricular dysrhythmias and psychiatric effects.
- Aspirin, clopidogrel and anticoagulants (in patients with atrial fibrillation) reduce the reoccurrence of non-fatal strokes in the elderly.
- Calcium channel blockers (CCBs) are the first-line drugs for the treatment of hypertension in older people. In those intolerant to CCBs and in those who have contraindications, thiazide diuretics should be offered.
- Urinary incontinence can be classified as stress incontinence, overflow incontinence or due to detrusor instability. Commonly used drugs used in detrusor instability include oxybutynin, solifenacin, trospium and tolterodine.
- Non-steroidal anti-inflammatory drugs (NSAIDs) are more likely to cause gastroduodenal ulceration and bleeding in the elderly.

There has been a steady increase in the number of older people since the beginning of the 20th century. In addition, the 'oldest of the old' are getting older. People older than 65 years formed only 4.8% of the population in 1901, increasing to about 18% in 2014. Among people older than 65 years, those in their 80s accounted for 19% and those older than 90 years accounted for 2% in 1984. In 2014, 22% of those older than 65 years were in their 80s and 5% were older than 90 years. The number of centenarians has gone up by 6030, a 72% increase, over the past decade. It was estimated that there were 14,450 centenarians (aged older than 100 years) living in the UK in 2014 (Office for National Statistics, 2015). The number of centenarians is projected to increase to 80,000 in 2033. The significant increase in the number of very elderly people will have important social, financial and healthcare planning implications.

The elderly have multiple and often chronic diseases. It is not surprising, therefore, that they are the major consumers of drugs. Elderly people receive about one-third of National Health Service (NHS) prescriptions in the UK. In most developed countries, the elderly now account for 25–40% of drug expenditures.

A UK survey of drug usage in elderly people aged 65 and older identified that the prevalence of medication use was 75% in those aged 65–74 years and 84% in those aged 75 and older. The commonly used drugs were cardiovascular, followed by central nervous system (which included non-narcotic analgesics). A usage rate higher than 9% was identified in both age groups for gastro-intestinal, musculoskeletal, haematological, dietetic, endocrine and respiratory medicines (Chen et al., 2001).

Institutionalised patients tend to be on larger numbers of drugs compared with patients in the community. Patients in long-term care facilities are likely to be receiving, on average, seven to eight drugs (Centre for Policy on Ageing, 2012). Many of nursing and residential home residents are prescribed psychotropic drugs for conditions including dementia and depression and therefore may be at risk of drug interactions and adverse drug reactions (ADRs). Much work is being undertaken in such homes on reducing the prescribing of inappropriate medicines, and the role of the pharmacist in undertaking such medication reviews has been highlighted (Royal Pharmaceutical Society Wales, 2016).

For optimal drug therapy in the elderly, a knowledge of age-related physiological and pathological changes that might affect the handling of and response to drugs is essential. This chapter discusses the age-related pharmacokinetic and pharmacodynamic changes (Mangoni and Jackson, 2003) which might affect drug therapy and the general principles of drug use in the elderly.

Pharmacokinetics

Ageing results in many physiological changes that could theoretically affect absorption, first-pass metabolism, protein binding, distribution and elimination of drugs. Age-related changes in the gastro-intestinal tract, liver and kidneys are:
- reduced gastric acid secretion
- decreased gastro-intestinal motility
- reduced total surface area of absorption
- reduced splanchnic blood flow
- reduced liver size
- reduced liver blood flow
- reduced glomerular filtration
- reduced renal tubular filtration

Absorption

There is a delay in gastric emptying and reduction in gastric acid output and splanchnic blood flow with ageing. These changes do not significantly affect the absorption of the majority of drugs. Although the absorption of some drugs such as digoxin may be slower, the overall absorption is similar to that in the young.

First-pass metabolism

After absorption, drugs are transported via the portal circulation to the liver, where many lipid-soluble agents are metabolised extensively (>90–95%). This results in a marked reduction in systemic bioavailability. Obviously, even minor reductions in first-pass metabolism can result in a significant increase in the bioavailability of such drugs.

Impaired first-pass metabolism has been demonstrated in the elderly for several drugs, including clomethiazole, labetalol, nifedipine, nitrates, propranolol and verapamil. The clinical effects of some of these, such as the hypotensive effect of nifedipine, may be significantly enhanced in the elderly. In frail hospitalised elderly patients, that is, those with chronic debilitating disease, the reduction in pre-systemic elimination is even more marked.

Distribution

The age-related physiological changes which may affect drug distribution are:
- reduced lean body mass
- reduced total body water
- increased total body fat
- lower serum albumin level
- α_1-Acid glycoprotein level unchanged or slightly raised

Increased body fat in the elderly results in an increased volume of distribution for fat-soluble compounds such as clomethiazole, diazepam, desmethyl-diazepam and thiopental. On the other hand, reduction in body water results in a decrease in the distribution volume of water-soluble drugs such as cimetidine, digoxin and ethanol.

Acidic drugs tend to bind to plasma albumin, whereas basic drugs bind to α_1-acid glycoprotein. Plasma albumin levels decrease with age, and therefore the free fraction of acidic drugs such as cimetidine, furosemide and warfarin will increase. Plasma α_1-acid glycoprotein levels may remain unchanged or may rise slightly with ageing, and this may result in minimal reductions in free fractions of basic drugs such as lidocaine. Disease-related changes in the level of this glycoprotein are probably more important than age *per se*.

The age-related changes in distribution and protein binding are probably of significance only in the acute administration of drugs because, at steady state, the plasma concentration of a drug is determined primarily by free drug clearance by the liver and kidneys rather than by distribution volume or protein binding.

Renal clearance

Although there is a considerable interindividual variability in renal function in the elderly, in general the glomerular filtration rate declines, as do the effective renal plasma flow and renal tubular function. Because of the marked variability in renal function in the elderly, the dosages of predominantly renally excreted drugs such as dabigatran should be individualised. Reduction in dosages of drugs with a low therapeutic index, such as digoxin and aminoglycosides, may be necessary. Dosage adjustments may not be necessary for drugs with a wide therapeutic index, for example, penicillins.

Hepatic clearance

The hepatic clearance (Cl_H) of a drug is dependent on hepatic blood flow (Q) and the steady-state extraction ratio (E), as can be seen in the following formula:

$$Cl_H = Q \times \frac{C_a - C_v}{C_a}$$
$$= Q \times E$$

where C_a and C_v are arterial and venous concentrations of the drug, respectively. It is obvious from this formula that when E approaches unity, Cl_H will be proportional to and limited by Q. Drugs which are cleared by this mechanism have a rapid rate of metabolism, and the rate of extraction by the liver is very high. The rate-limiting step, as mentioned earlier, is hepatic blood flow, and therefore drugs cleared by this mechanism are called 'flow limited'. On the other hand, when E is small, Cl_H will vary according to the hepatic uptake and enzyme activity and will be relatively independent of hepatic blood flow. The drugs which are cleared by this mechanism are termed 'capacity limited'.

Hepatic extraction is dependent upon liver size, liver blood flow, uptake into hepatocytes, and the affinity and activity of hepatic enzymes. Liver size falls with ageing, and there is a 20–40% decrease in hepatic mass between the 3rd and 10th decade. Hepatic blood flow falls equally with declining liver size. Although it is recognised that the microsomal mono-oxygenase enzyme systems are significantly reduced in ageing male rodents, evidence suggests that this is not the case in ageing humans. Conjugation reactions have been reported to be unaffected in the elderly by some investigators, but a small decline with increasing age has been described by others.

Impaired clearance of many hepatically eliminated, particularly lipid-soluble, drugs has been demonstrated in the elderly. Morphological changes rather than impaired enzymatic activity appear to be the main cause of impaired elimination of these drugs. In frail debilitated elderly patients, however, the activities of drug-metabolising enzymes such as plasma esterases and hepatic glucuronyltransferases may well be impaired.

Pharmacodynamics

Molecular and cellular changes that occur with ageing may alter the response to drugs in the elderly. There is, however, limited information about these alterations because of the technical difficulties and ethical problems involved in measuring them. It is not surprising, therefore, that there is relatively little information about the effect of age on pharmacodynamics.

Changes in pharmacodynamics in the elderly may be considered under two headings:

- those due to a reduction in homeostatic reserve,
- those that are secondary to changes in specific receptor and target sites.

Reduced homeostatic reserve

Orthostatic circulatory responses

In normal elderly subjects, there is blunting of the reflex tachycardia that occurs in young subjects on standing or in response to vasodilatation. Structural changes in the vascular tree that occur with ageing are believed to contribute to this observation, although the exact mechanism is unclear. Antihypertensive drugs, drugs with α-receptor blocking effects (e.g. tricyclic antidepressants, phenothiazines and some butyrophenones), drugs which decrease sympathetic outflow from the central nervous system (e.g. barbiturates, benzodiazepines, antihistamines and morphine) and antiparkinsonian drugs (e.g. levodopa and pramipexole) are, therefore, more likely to produce hypotension in the elderly.

Postural control

Postural stability is normally achieved by static reflexes, which involve sustained contraction of the musculature, and phasic reflexes, which are dynamic, short-term and involve transient corrective movements. With ageing, the frequency and amplitude of corrective movements increase and an age-related reduction in dopamine (D_2) receptors in the striatum has been suggested as the probable cause. Drugs which increase postural sway, for example, hypnotics and tranquillisers, have been shown to be associated with the occurrence of falls in the elderly.

Thermoregulation

There is an increased prevalence of impaired thermoregulatory mechanisms in the elderly, although it is not universal. Accidental hypothermia can occur in the elderly with drugs that produce sedation, impaired subjective awareness of temperature, decreased mobility and muscular activity, and vasodilatation. Commonly implicated drugs include phenothiazines, benzodiazepines, tricyclic antidepressants, opioids and alcohol, either on their own or with other drugs.

Cognitive function

Ageing is associated with marked structural and neurochemical changes in the central nervous system. Cholinergic transmission is linked with normal cognitive function, and in the elderly the activity of choline acetyltransferase, a marker enzyme for acetylcholine, is reduced in some areas of the cortex and limbic system. Several drugs cause confusion in the elderly. Anticholinergics, hypnotics, H_2 antagonists and β-blockers are common examples.

Visceral muscle function

Constipation is a common problem in the elderly because there is a decline in gastro-intestinal motility with ageing. Anticholinergic drugs, opiates, tricyclic antidepressants and antihistamines are more likely to cause constipation or ileus in the elderly. Anticholinergic drugs may cause urinary retention in elderly men, especially those who have prostatic hypertrophy. Bladder instability is common in the elderly, and urethral dysfunction more prevalent in elderly women. Loop diuretics may cause incontinence in such patients.

Age-related changes in specific receptors and target sites

Many drugs exert their effect via specific receptors. Response to such drugs may be altered by the number (density) of receptors, the affinity of the receptor, postreceptor events within cells resulting in impaired enzyme activation and signal amplification, or altered response of the target tissue itself. Ageing is associated with some of these changes.

α-Adrenoceptors

α_2-Adrenoceptor responsiveness appears to be reduced with ageing, whereas α_1-adrenoceptor responsiveness appears to be unaffected.

β-Adrenoceptors

β-Adrenoceptor function declines with age. It is recognised that the chronotropic response to isoprenaline infusion is less marked in the elderly. Propranolol therapy in the elderly produces less β-adrenoceptor blocking effect than in the young. In isolated lymphocytes, studies of cyclic adenosine monophosphate (AMP) production have shown that on β-adrenoceptor stimulation, the dose–response curve is shifted to the right, and the maximal response is blunted.

An age-related reduction in β-adrenoceptor density has been shown in animal adipocytes, erythrocytes and brain, and also in human lymphocytes in one study, although this has not been confirmed by other investigators. Because maximal response occurs on stimulation of only 0.2% of β-adrenoceptors, a reduction in the number by itself is unlikely to account for age-related changes. Some studies have shown a reduction in high-affinity binding sites with ageing, in the absence of change in total receptor numbers, and others have suggested that there may be impairment of postreceptor transduction mechanisms with ageing that may account for reduced β-adrenoceptor function.

Cholinergic system

The effect of ageing on cholinergic mechanisms is less well known. Atropine produces less tachycardia in elderly humans than in the young. It has been shown in ageing rats that the hippocampal pyramidal cell sensitivity to acetylcholine is reduced. The clinical significance of this observation is unclear.

Benzodiazepines

The elderly are more sensitive to benzodiazepines than the young, and the mechanism of this increased sensitivity is not known. No difference in the affinity or number of benzodiazepine-binding sites has been observed in animal studies. Habituation to benzodiazepines occurs to the same extent in the elderly as in the young. A prospective population-based study did not support a causal association between benzodiazepine use and dementia (Gray et al., 2016).

Warfarin

The elderly are more sensitive to warfarin. This phenomenon may be due to age-related changes in pharmacodynamic factors. The exact mechanism is unknown.

Digoxin

The elderly appear to be more sensitive to the adverse effects of digoxin, but not to the cardiac effects.

Common clinical disorders

This section deals in detail only with the most important diseases affecting older people. Other conditions are mentioned primarily to highlight areas where the elderly differ from the young or where modifications of drug therapy are necessary.

Dementia

Dementia is an important cause of disability and dependence and is estimated to affect around 150 million people worldwide by 2050 (Public Health England, 2016). Caring for dementia is estimated to cost $1 trillion by 2030.

Dementia is characterised by a gradual deterioration of intellectual capacity. Alzheimer's disease (AD), vascular dementia (VaD), dementia with Lewy bodies and frontotemporal dementia are the most important diseases of cognitive dysfunction in the elderly. The term mild cognitive impairment (MCI) is used to describe a decline in cognitive function without an associated difficulty in performing complex functional tasks such as shopping or social and occupational activities. Around 50% of patients with MCI develop AD within 4 years of diagnosis. AD has a gradual onset, and it progresses slowly. Forgetfulness is the major initial symptom followed by difficulty with occupational activities and the activities of daily living such as dressing and bathing. The individual with AD tends to get lost in his or her own environment. Eventually, the social graces are lost. Pathological examination of the brain characteristically reveals neuritic plaques containing amyloid beta (Aβ), neurofibrillary tangles which are composed of hyperphosphorylated tau filaments and accumulation of Aβ in cerebral blood vessel walls.

VaD is the second most important cause of dementia. It usually occurs in patients in their 60s and 70s and is more common in those with a previous history of hypertension or stroke. It is

---

Box 11.1 Drugs causing confusion in the elderly

Antiparkinsonian drugs
Barbiturates
Benzodiazepines
Diuretics
Hypoglycaemic agents
Monoamine oxidase inhibitors
Opioids
Steroids
Tricyclic antidepressants

commonly associated with mood changes and emotional lability. Gait disorders, difficulties with executive function, dysarthria, dysphagia and incontinence become evident with advancing disease. Physical examination may reveal focal neurological deficits. A number of drugs and other conditions cause confusion in the elderly, and their effects may be mistaken for dementia. These are listed in Box 11.1.

In patients with AD, damage to the cholinergic neurones connecting subcortical nuclei to the cerebral cortex has been consistently observed. Postsynaptic muscarinic cholinergic receptors are usually not affected, but ascending noradrenergic and serotonergic pathways are damaged, especially in younger patients. Based on those abnormalities, several drugs have been investigated for the treatment of AD. Lecithin, which increases acetylcholine concentrations in the brain, 4-aminopyridine, piracetam, oxiracetam and pramiracetam, all of which stimulate acetylcholine release, have been tried but have produced no, or unimpressive, improvements in cognitive function. Anticholinesterases block the breakdown of acetylcholine and enhance cholinergic transmission. Donepezil, galantamine and rivastigmine are recommended for treatment of patients with AD of moderate severity only – that is, those with a Mini-Mental State Examination (MMSE) score of between 10 and 20 points (National Institute for Health and Care Excellence [NICE], 2016). Donepezil is a piperidine-based acetylcholinesterase inhibitor. It has been shown to improve cognitive function in patients with mild to moderately severe AD. However, it does not improve day-to-day functioning, quality-of-life measures or rating scores of overall dementia. Rivastigmine is a non-competitive cholinesterase inhibitor. It has been shown to slow the rate of decline in cognitive and global functioning in AD. Galantamine, a reversible and competitive inhibitor of acetylcholinesterase, has also been shown to improve cognitive function significantly and is well tolerated. Adverse effects of cholinesterase inhibitors include nausea, vomiting, diarrhoea, weight loss, agitation, confusion, insomnia, abnormal dreams, muscle cramps, bradycardia, syncope and fatigue. Treatment with these drugs should only be continued in people with dementia who show an improvement or no deterioration in their MMSE score, together with evidence of global (functional and behavioural) improvement after the first few months of treatment. The treatment effect should then be reviewed critically every 6 months, before a decision to continue drug therapy is made.

Memantine, an *N*-methyl-D-aspartate (NMDA) antagonist, has also been used for the treatment of moderate to severe AD. It acts mainly on subtypes of glutamate receptors related to memory (i.e. NMDA), resulting in improvements in cognition. It has also been shown to have some beneficial effects on behaviour, and its use is recommended in patients with moderate to severe AD as part of well-designed clinical studies (NICE, 2016).

Deposition of amyloid (in particular, the peptide β/A4) derived from the Alzheimer amyloid precursor protein (APP) is an important pathological feature of the familial form of AD that accounts for about 20% of patients. Point mutation of the gene coding for APP (located in the long arm of chromosome 21) is thought to be associated with familial AD. So far, the anti-amyloid treatment strategy in AD has been disappointing. Vaccination against $A\beta_{42}$, which was very effective in clearing and accumulation brain amyloid in mouse models, was associated with serious adverse effects in human beings. Bapineuzumab, a monoclonal antibody that targets the N-terminus of Aβ, and solanezumab, a monoclonal antibody that binds to soluble Aβ, were both found to be ineffective in clinical trials. Tarenflurbil, avagacestat and semagacestat, all γ-secretase inhibitors which reduce $A\beta_{42}$ production, were found be ineffective in placebo-controlled human trials, and the latter drug was associated with faster cognitive decline. β-Secretase inhibitors are also currently being investigated in phase 2 and 3 clinical trials for early AD. Tau neurofibrillary tangles found in AD patients are noted to be associated with synaptic loss and cognitive decline. Tau antibodies and drugs that modify Tau phosphorylation and aggregation are currently being investigated. Insulin signalling is thought to play a role in the pathogenesis of AD, and the benefit of insulin in mild AD is undergoing investigation (Scheltens et al., 2016).

A formulation containing caprylic triglyceride, fractionated coconut oil (Axona), is approved for treatment of AD in the USA. Souvenaid, which contains vitamins and supplements, is approved for early AD in some European countries, Australia, and China.

Depression is common in AD patients and is usually treated with a selective serotonin reuptake inhibitor (SSRI) drug. Agitation is also common, and whilst risperidone is the only antipsychotic licensed in the UK for treatment of severe aggression in AD, antipsychotic drugs such as quetiapine and olanzapine are now preferred in practice.

In some studies, donepezil and galantamine have been shown to improve cognition, behaviour and activities of daily living in patients with VaD, and in those with AD and coexistent cerebrovascular disease. Memantine has been reported to stabilise progression of VaD compared with placebo. However, acetylcholinesterase inhibitors and memantine should not be prescribed for the treatment of cognitive decline in patients with VaD, except as part of properly constructed clinical studies. Aspirin therapy has also been reported to slow the progression of VaD. The incidence of VaD is likely to decrease with other stroke-prevention strategies, such as smoking cessation, anticoagulation for atrial fibrillation and control of hypertension and hyperlipidemia.

Parkinsonism

Parkinsonism is a relatively common disease of the elderly, with a prevalence between 50 and 150 per 100,000. It is characterised by resting tremors, muscular rigidity and bradykinesia (slowness of initiating and carrying out voluntary movements). The patient has a mask-like face and monotonous voice and walks with a stoop and a slow, shuffling gait.

The elderly are more susceptible than younger patients to some of the adverse effects of antiparkinsonian drugs. Age-related decline in orthostatic circulatory responses means that postural hypotension is more likely to occur in elderly patients with levodopa therapy. The elderly are more likely to have severe cardiac disease, and levodopa preparations should be used with caution in such patients because of the risk of serious ventricular dysrhythmias. Psychiatric adverse effects such as confusion, depression, hallucinations and paranoia occur with dopamine agonists and levodopa preparations. These adverse effects may persist for several months after discontinuation of the offending drug and may result in misdiagnosis (e.g. of AD) in the elderly. Bromocriptine and other ergot derivatives should be avoided in elderly patients with severe peripheral arterial disease because they may cause peripheral ischaemia. Antiparkinsonian drugs should be commenced in low doses and the dose increased gradually. 'Drug holidays', which involve discontinuation of drugs, for example, for 2 days per week, may reduce the incidence of adverse effects of antiparkinsonian drugs, but their role is questionable.

Stroke

In 2010, stroke was the second most common cause of death and the third most common cause of lost disability-adjusted life years (DALYs), with an estimated incidence of 16.9 million strokes worldwide. There were 33.0 million prevalent stroke cases, 5.9 million stroke deaths and 102.2 million DALYs lost. Over 38% of new strokes, 30% of prevalent strokes, 55% of stroke deaths and 28% of DALYs lost were in people aged older than 75 years. In developed countries, about 85% of strokes are ischaemic and 15% are due to haemorrhages. However, most stroke burden worldwide is due to haemorrhagic stroke.

Treatment of acute stroke

Thrombolytic agents. Intravenous alteplase increases the odds of a good stroke outcome if given within 4.5 hours of onset. The benefit is time dependent (odds ratio [OR] 1.75 if given within 3 hours and 1.26 if given between 3 and 4.5 hours). Odds of improved outcome are highest if it is given within 90 minutes, and it is not effective beyond 4.5 hours. The benefit occurs irrespective of stroke severity and age of patients. Alteplase compared with placebo significantly increased the odds of symptomatic intracranial haemorrhage (OR 5.55) and of fatal intracranial haemorrhage within 7 days (OR 7.140). Alteplase therapy was associated with higher 90-day mortality (hazard ratio 1.11). Although there was an absolute increase of about 2% in the risk of early death from intracranial haemorrhage, by 3–6 months, the risk was offset by absolute increase in disability-free survival of about 10% for patients treated in less than 3.0 hours and about 5% for patients treated after 3.0 hours, up to 4.5 hours (Emberson et al., 2014). Thrombolysis is a potentially dangerous treatment, especially in older people. Therefore, it should only be given to carefully selected patients after excluding patients who have contraindications and those who are at very high risk of bleeding. Older people should not be denied this very effective treatment purely on the basis of chronological age. Careful adherence to thrombolysis protocol has been shown to reduce the risk of haemorrhagic complications after treatment with alteplase. Currently, alteplase is the only thrombolytic agent that is licensed for use in acute ischaemic stroke. Other thrombolytic agents such as tenecteplase are currently undergoing clinical trials. Endovascular therapy, especially with stent-based clot retrievers, in combination with alteplase therapy has been shown to be highly effective and is likely to become the standard therapy for acute stroke (NICE, 2016).

Antiplatelet therapy. Aspirin in doses of 150–300 mg commenced within 48 hours of onset of ischaemic stroke has been shown to reduce the relative risk of death or dependency by 2.7% up to 6 months after the event in two large studies (Chen et al., 2000).

Anticoagulation. Use of intravenous unfractionated heparin and low-molecular-weight heparin has not been shown to be beneficial and is associated with an increased risk of intracranial haemorrhage.

Neuroprotective agents. Many neuroprotective agents have been used for the treatment of acute ischaemic stroke, but none has been shown to have long-term beneficial effects.

Secondary prevention

Patients with ischaemic stroke, if they are in sinus rhythm, should receive aspirin 300 mg as soon as possible after the diagnosis. Aspirin should be discontinued after 2 weeks, and clopidogrel 75 mg daily should be started for secondary stroke prevention. If there is a history of allergy or intolerance to clopidogrel, the combination of aspirin 75 mg daily plus modified-release dipyridamole 200 mg twice daily or the latter drug on its own if the patient is allergic to aspirin, should be prescribed (NICE, 2010). Clopidogrel plus aspirin (75 mg each daily) compared with aspirin alone is associated with an absolute increase in the risk of life-threatening bleeding by 1.3%, and therefore this combination is not recommended for secondary stroke prevention (Diener et al., 2004).

In patients with atrial fibrillation who have had a previous stroke or transient ischaemic attack, anticoagulation with warfarin (international normalised ratio [INR] 1.5–2.7) has been shown to be significantly better than aspirin for secondary prevention (Hart et al., 2007). Anticoagulation has not been shown to be effective for secondary prevention in patients with sinus rhythm. The oral anti-factor Xa drugs apixaban, edoxaban and rivaroxaban and the antithrombin drug dabigatran are also approved by NICE for stroke prevention in patients who have had a transient ischaemic attack (TIA) or stroke if they are in atrial fibrillation. Compared with warfarin, they significantly reduce the risk of stroke or systemic embolism by 19% and significantly reduce all-cause mortality. They are associated with significantly lower risk of intracerebral haemorrhage, similar risk of major bleeding as warfarin, but slightly higher incidence of gastro-intestinal haemorrhage (Verheugt and Granger, 2015). They are very convenient to use because they are given once or twice daily and do not require routine monitoring. Because they have very short half-lives (between 9 and 17 hours), adherence to treatment is absolutely essential if they are to be effective. Dabigatran is predominantly renally excreted and should be avoided in patients with severe renal impairment (creatinine clearance <30 mL/min). As with warfarin, older patients should be carefully counselled before commencing treatment with the direct oral anticoagulants (DOACs), and their full blood count, renal and liver function should be monitored at regular intervals.

Adequate control of hypertension (aiming for a blood pressure of <140/80 mmHg), hyperlipidaemia (ideally with a statin) and diabetes; stopping smoking; losing weight and reducing alcohol consumption are also important in secondary stroke prevention.

Primary prevention

Randomised controlled trials have shown that anticoagulation with warfarin compared with placebo reduces the risk of stroke in patients with atrial fibrillation (Hart et al., 2007). Control of risk factors such as hypertension, hyperlipidaemia, diabetes and smoking is likely to play an important role in primary prevention.

Osteoporosis

Osteoporosis is a progressive disease characterised by low bone mass and micro-architectural deterioration of bone tissue resulting in increased bone fragility and susceptibility to fracture. It is an important cause of morbidity in postmenopausal women. The most important complication of osteoporosis is fracture of the hip. Fractures of wrist, vertebrae and humerus also occur. Increasing age is associated with higher risk of fractures, which occur mostly in those aged older than 75 years. In the UK, more than 200,000 fractures occur each year, costing the NHS £1.8 billion per year, of which 87% is spent on hip fractures. In Europe, more than 3.7 million osteoporotic fractures occur annually, costing £22.5bn.

Prevention

Because complications of osteoporosis have enormous economic implications, preventive measures are extremely important. Regular exercise has been shown to halve the risk of hip fractures. Stopping smoking before menopause reduces the risk of hip fractures by 25%.

Treatment

Vitamin D and calcium. Vitamin D deficiency is common in elderly people. Treatment for 12–18 months with 800 IU of vitamin D plus 1.2 g of calcium given daily has been shown to reduce hip and non-vertebral fractures in elderly women (mean age 84 years) living in sheltered accommodation. Clinical trials have shown that vitamin D supplementation without co-administration of calcium do not prevent fracture. Recent evidence from clinical trials indicates that it is inappropriate to use vitamin D for osteoporosis prevention in community-dwelling adults who do not have specific risk factors for vitamin D deficiency. Calcium supplementation on its own also does not reduce fracture incidence and is no longer recommended for treatment of osteoporosis (Black and Rosen, 2016).

Calcitriol and alfacalcidol. Calcitriol (1,25-dihydroxyvitamin D), the active metabolite of vitamin D, and alfacalcidol, a synthetic analogue of calcitriol, reduce bone loss and have been shown to reduce vertebral fractures, but not consistently. Serum calcium should be monitored regularly in patients receiving these drugs.

Bisphosphonates. Bisphosphonates, synthetic analogues of pyrophosphate, bind strongly to the bone surface and inhibit bone resorption. Currently, five bisphosphonates are available for the prevention and treatment of osteoporosis: alendronate, etidronate, risedronate, ibandronate and zoledronate. Compared with placebo, alendronate, zoledronate and risedronate significantly reduce the risk of hip and vertebral fractures. Ibandronate significantly reduces the risk of vertebral fractures but not that of nonvertebral fractures. Ibandronate by intravenous route is approved only for treatment, but not the prevention, of postmenopausal osteoporosis. Alendronate, risedronate and zoledronate are approved for treatment of osteoporosis in men and steroid-induced osteoporosis. Risedronate and zoledronate are also approved for prevention of steroid-induced osteoporosis.

Alendronate can be given either daily (10 mg) or weekly (70 mg) with equal efficacy. It is effective in reducing vertebral fractures, wrist and hip fractures by about 50%. Etidronate is given cyclically with calcium supplements to reduce the risk of bone mineralisation defects. It reduces the risk of vertebral fractures by 50% in postmenopausal women. There is no evidence to support its effectiveness in preventing hip fractures. It is used less commonly now and is not approved for treatment of osteoporosis in the USA.

Risedronate can be administered once daily (5 mg), weekly (35 mg) or monthly (150 mg). It reduces vertebral fractures by 41% and non-vertebral fractures by 39%. It has been shown to reduce the risk of hip fractures by 40% in postmenopausal women.

Ibandronate can be given intravenously at a dose of 3 mg once every 3 months and by oral route either 150 mg once monthly or 2.5 mg daily. It reduces the incidence of clinical vertebral fractures by about 50% compared with placebo but does not reduce the risk of non-vertebral fractures.

Zoledronic acid significantly reduces the incidence of clinical vertebral fractures by 70%, hip fractures by 41% and non-vertebral fractures by 25% in patients with osteoporosis. It is administered intravenously at a dose of 5 mg, once a year.

All oral bisphosphonates cause gastro-intestinal side effects. Alendronate and risedronate are associated with severe oesophageal reactions including oesophageal stricture. Patients should not take these tablets at bedtime and should be advised to stay upright for at least 30 min after taking them. They should avoid food for at least 2 hours before and after taking etidronate. Alendronate and risedronate should be taken 30 min before the first food or drink of the day. Bisphosphonates should be avoided in patients with renal impairment. Serum calcium and vitamin D levels should be checked before commencing treatment with bisphosphonates because hypocalcemia can occur, especially with zoledronate. Patients with vitamin D deficiency may develop severe and prolonged hypocalcemia.

Rarely, atypical sub-trochanteric and femoral shaft fractures have been associated with prolonged (especially beyond 5 years) bisphosphonate therapy. The evidence for benefit with bisphosphonate therapy beyond 5 years is limited, and therefore the decision about long-term therapy should be carefully reviewed and individualised.

Osteonecrosis of the jaw can occur rarely (annual incidence: 0.067%) with bisphosphonate therapy, and it appears to depend on the potency of the drug used (highest risk with zoledronate), the indication for its use (more likely to occur when used for treatment of skeletal metastases than for osteoporosis or Paget's disease), the duration of therapy (more likely to occur with treatment beyond 3 years) and the route of administration (significantly higher with intravenous route). The risk factors for osteonecrosis include recent dental procedure with exposure of bone, dental disease, ill-fitting dental appliances, diabetes, smoking, concomitant treatment with steroids and comorbid conditions. Patients on bisphosphonates should be advised to maintain good dental hygiene and have regular dental checkups.

Strontium ranelate. Strontium ranelate, which both increases bone formation and reduces bone resorption, reduces vertebral (by 37%) and non-vertebral (including hip) fractures (by 14%) in postmenopausal women with osteoporosis. It is well tolerated. It can be used in those who are unable to tolerate bisphosphonates. It should be avoided in patients with severe renal disease (creatinine clearance less than 30 mL/min). It has been reported to cause severe drug rash with eosinophilia and systemic symptoms (DRESS), which causes skin rash, fever, lymphadenopathy and raised white cell count. It can involve the liver, kidneys and lungs and can cause death. Analysis of pooled data from randomised studies in around 7500 postmenopausal women with osteoporosis showed an increased risk of myocardial infarction with strontium ranelate compared with placebo, with a relative risk of 1.6 (95% confidence interval [CI], 1.07–2.38), and an increased risk of venous thrombotic and embolic events with a relative risk of 1.5 (95% CI, 1.04–2.19). Strontium ranelate is now restricted to the treatment of severe osteoporosis in postmenopausal women and adult men at high risk of fracture who cannot use other osteoporosis treatments.

Hormone replacement therapy. Oestrogens increase bone formation and reduce bone resorption. They also increase calcium absorption and decrease renal calcium loss. Hormone replacement therapy (HRT), if started soon after menopause, is effective in preventing vertebral fractures but has to be continued lifelong if protection against fractures is to be maintained. It is associated with increased risk of endometrial cancer, breast cancer and venous thromboembolism. One study has shown that HRT may increase the risk of death due to myocardial disease in elderly women with pre-existing ischaemic heart disease. It should be avoided in older patients.

Raloxifene. Raloxifene is an oral selective oestrogen receptor modulator (SERM) that has oestrogenic actions on bone and anti-oestrogenic actions on the uterus and breast. It reduces the risk of vertebral fractures, but not those at other sites. Adverse effects include hot flushes, leg cramps and risk of venous thromboembolism. It also protects against breast cancer. Its use is restricted, as a second-line drug, to younger postmenopausal women with vertebral osteoporosis.

Parathyroid hormone peptides. Teriparatide is the recombinant portion of human parathyroid hormone, amino acid sequence 1–34, of the complete molecule (which has 84 amino acids). It reduces vertebral and non-vertebral fractures in postmenopausal women. It does not reduce hip fractures. It is given subcutaneously at a dose of 20 micrograms daily. The recombinant (full 1–84 amino acid sequence) parathyroid hormone peptide (Preotact) can also be used at a dose of 100 micrograms daily. It has similar efficacy as teriparatide. Both these drugs are expensive, and teriparatide is associated with an increased risk of osteosarcoma in animal studies. Teriparatide is recommended for secondary prevention of osteoporotic fractures in postmenopausal women who are unable to tolerate or have a contraindication for treatment with bisphosphonates or strontium.

Calcitonin. Calcitonin inhibits osteoclasts and decreases the rate of bone resorption, reduces bone blood flow and may have central analgesic actions. It is effective in all age groups in preventing vertebral bone loss. It is costly and has to be given parenterally or intranasally. Antibodies do develop against calcitonin, but they do not affect its efficacy. Calcitonin is useful in treating acute pain associated with osteoporotic vertebral fractures but is no longer recommended for treatment of osteoporosis because it is associated with malignancy with long-term use.

Denosumab. Denosumab is a fully human monoclonal antibody to RANKL (receptor activator of nuclear factor-κβ ligand). It acts as an antiresorptive agent by inhibiting the formation of mature osteoclasts by binding to RANKL, which regulates osteoclast formation, activity and survival. It reduces vertebral fractures by 68%, hip fractures by 40% and nonvertebral fractures by 20%. It has been approved for treatment of postmenopausal osteoporosis and also for osteoporosis in men. Atypical femoral fractures and osteonecrosis of the jaw have both been associated with denosumab. Atypical femoral fractures occur rarely after treatment for more than 2.5 years. Osteonecrosis of the jaw has mainly been reported in cancer patients receiving 120 mg of denosumab subcutaneously every 4 weeks. For treatment of postmenopausal osteoporosis, the dose used is 60 mg subcutaneously every 6 months. Risk factors for osteonecrosis and precautions for its prevention, discussed under bisphosphonates, should be considered in all patients before starting denosumab therapy. Severe hypocalcemia has been reported, usually in the first week of treatment with denosumab, especially in patients with renal impairment. Serum calcium level should be checked before starting, within 2 weeks of the first dose and in patients experiencing symptoms of hypocalcemia, such as muscle spasms, cramps or tingling of fingers/perioral region.

Arthritis

Osteoarthrosis (also known as osteoarthritis), gout, pseudogout, rheumatoid arthritis and septic arthritis are the important joint diseases in the elderly. Treatment of these conditions is similar to that in the young. If possible, NSAIDs should be avoided in patients with osteoarthrosis. Total hip and knee replacements should be considered in patients with severe arthritis affecting these joints.

Hypertension

Hypertension is an important risk factor for cardiovascular and cerebrovascular disease in the elderly. The incidence of myocardial infarction is 2.5 times higher, and that of cerebrovascular accidents is twice as high, in elderly hypertensive patients compared with non-hypertensive subjects. Elevated systolic blood pressure is the single most important risk factor for cardiovascular disease and more predictive of stroke than diastolic blood pressure.

Blood pressure lowering has been shown to be beneficial in those patients younger and older than 65 years with no substantial variation in the reduction of major vascular events with different drug classes (Blood Pressure Lowering Treatment Trialists' Collaboration, 2008). There is evidence that treatment of both systolic and diastolic blood pressure in the elderly is beneficial. One large study has shown reductions in cardiovascular events, and mortality associated with cerebrovascular accidents in treated elderly patients with hypertension (Amery et al., 1986). The treatment did not reduce the total mortality significantly. Another study (SHEP, 1991), which used low-dose chlorthalidone to treat isolated systolic hypertension (systolic blood pressure 160 mmHg or more with diastolic blood pressure less than 95 mmHg), showed a 36% reduction in the incidence of stroke, with a 5-year benefit of 30 events per 1000 patients. It also showed a reduction in the incidence of major cardiovascular events, with a 5-year absolute benefit of 55 events per 1000 patients. In addition, this study reported that antihypertensive therapy was beneficial even in patients older than 80 years. Subgroup meta-analysis of seven randomised controlled trials, which included 1670 patients older than 80 years, showed that antihypertensive therapy for about 3.5 years reduces the risk of heart failure by 39%, strokes by 34% and major cardiovascular events by 22% (Gueyffier, 1999). In one placebo-controlled study which included 3845 patients who were 80 years of age or older and had a sustained systolic blood pressure of 160 mmHg or more, treatment with the diuretic indapamide (sustained release, 1.5 mg) plus perindopril (2 or 4 mg) to achieve the target blood pressure of 150/80 mmHg resulted in a 30% reduction in the rate of fatal or non-fatal stroke, a 39% reduction in the rate of death from stroke, a 21% reduction in the rate of death from any cause, a 23% reduction in the rate of death from cardiovascular causes and a 64% reduction in the rate of heart failure (Beckett et al., 2008). These studies demonstrate the increasing evidence that antihypertensive therapy in patients older than 80 years is beneficial.

Treatment of hypertension

Non-pharmacological. In patients with asymptomatic mild hypertension, non-pharmacological treatment is the method of choice. Weight reduction to within 15% of desirable weight, restriction of salt intake to 4–6 g/day, regular aerobic exercise such as walking, restriction of alcohol consumption and stopping smoking are the recommended modes of therapy.

Pharmacological. The current NICE guidance on the management of hypertension (NICE, 2011) states that for patients older than 55 years, calcium channel blockers (CCBs) are the first line. Step 2 adds an angiotensin-converting enzyme (ACE) inhibitor or an angiotensin II receptor blocker to the CCB, whilst step 3 adds a thiazide-like diuretic.

Thiazide diuretics. Thiazides lower peripheral resistance and do not significantly affect cardiac output or renal blood flow.

They are effective, cheap and well tolerated and have also been shown to reduce the risk of hip fracture in elderly women. They can be used in combination with other antihypertensive drugs. Adverse effects include mild elevation of creatinine, glucose, uric acid and serum cholesterol levels, as well as hypokalaemia. They should be used in low doses because higher doses only increase the incidence of adverse effects without increasing their efficacy.

Calcium channel blockers. CCBs act as vasodilators. Amlodipine is the recommended first-line drug for treatment of hypertension in older people. It does not have significant negative inotropic or chronotropic effect and is generally well tolerated. Leg oedema is a common side effect. Verapamil and, to some extent, diltiazem decrease cardiac output and are generally not used first line. These drugs do not have a significant effect on lipids or the central nervous system. They may be more effective in the elderly, particularly in the treatment of isolated systolic hypertension. Adverse effects include headache, oedema and postural hypotension. Short-acting dihydropyridine, for example, nifedipine, should be avoided. Some studies indicate adverse outcomes with these agents, particularly in those patients with angina or myocardial infarction.

ACE inhibitors and angiotensin receptor blockers. ACE inhibitors and angiotensin receptor blockers (ARBs) used for the treatment of hypertension are discussed elsewhere (see Chapter 19). These drugs should be used with care in the elderly, who are more likely to have underlying atherosclerotic renovascular disease that could result in renal failure. Excessive hypotension is also more likely to occur in the elderly.

β-Adrenoceptor blockers. Although theoretically the β-blockers are expected to be less effective in the elderly, they have been shown to be as effective as diuretics in clinical studies. Water-soluble β-blockers such as atenolol may cause fewer adverse effects in the elderly. With the availability of better-tolerated and more effective alternative drugs, β-blockers are now mainly used in patients with coexistent ischaemic heart disease.

Myocardial infarction

The diagnosis of myocardial infarction in the elderly may be difficult in some patients because of an atypical presentation (Bayer et al., 1986). In the majority of patients, chest pain and dyspnoea are the common presenting symptoms. Confusion may be a presenting factor in up to 20% of patients older than 85 years. The diagnosis is made on the basis of history, serial electrocardiograms and cardiac enzyme estimations.

The principles of management of myocardial infarction in the elderly are similar to those in the young. Thrombolytic therapy has been shown to be safe and effective in elderly patients.

Cardiac failure

In addition to the typical features of cardiac failure, that is, exertional dyspnoea, oedema, orthopnoea and paroxysmal nocturnal dyspnoea (PND), elderly patients may present with atypical symptoms. These include confusion due to poor cerebral circulation, vomiting and abdominal pain due to gastro-intestinal and hepatic congestion, or insomnia due to PND.

Dyspnoea may not be a predominant symptom in an elderly patient with arthritis and immobility. Treatment of cardiac failure depends on the underlying cause and is similar to that in the young. Loop diuretics, ACE inhibitors, and β-blockers are the important drugs used in the treatment of cardiac failure in the elderly.

Leg ulcers

Leg ulcers are common in the elderly. They are mainly of two types: venous or ischaemic. Other causes of leg ulcers are blood diseases, trauma, malignancy and infections (Cornwall et al., 1986), but these are less common in the elderly. Venous ulcers occur in patients with varicose veins who have valvular incompetence in deep veins due to venous hypertension (Alavi et al., 2016). They are usually located near the medial malleolus and are associated with varicose eczema and oedema. These ulcers are painless unless there is gross oedema or infection. Ischaemic ulcers, on the other hand, are due to poor peripheral circulation and occur on the toes, heels, foot and lateral aspect of the leg. They are painful and are associated with signs of lower limb ischaemia, such as absent pulse or cold lower limb. There may be a history of smoking, diabetes or hypertension.

Venous ulcers respond well to treatment, and more than 75% heal within 3 months. Elevation of the lower limbs, exercise, compression bandage, local antiseptic creams when there is evidence of infection, with or without steroid cream, are usually effective. Advanced wound dressings are needed for management of large, chronic, exudative ulcers. Hydrogels donate fluid, hydrocolloids maintain hydration, alginates and foams absorb the exudate present in wounds. Hydrogel, hydrocolloid and medical-grade honey dressings are useful to deslough wounds. Sterile maggots can also be used for removal of wound debris. Antiseptics should not be used when there is granulation tissue. Cotton or viscose tulle dressings impregnated with soft paraffin are useful as low-adherence dressings on granulating wounds and those with minimal exudation. They prevent the wound bed from coming into direct contact with secondary dressings. The type of dressing chosen should depend on the type of leg ulcer and comorbid conditions of the patient. Skin grafting may be necessary for large ulcers. Ischaemic ulcers do not respond well to medical treatment, and such patients should be assessed by vascular surgeons.

Urinary incontinence

Urinary incontinence in the elderly may be of three main types: stress incontinence, overflow incontinence and detrusor instability.

Stress incontinence

Stress incontinence is due to urethral sphincter incompetence. It occurs almost exclusively in women and is associated with weakening of pelvic musculature. It can occur in men after prostatic surgery. Involuntary loss of small amounts of urine occurs on performing activities which increase intra-abdominal pressure – for example, coughing, sneezing, bending and lifting. It does not cause significant nocturnal symptoms.

Overflow incontinence

Overflow incontinence is characterised by constant involuntary loss of urine in small amounts. Prostatic hypertrophy is a common cause and is often associated with symptoms of poor stream and incomplete emptying. Increased frequency of micturition at night is often a feature. Use of anticholinergic drugs and diabetic autonomic neuropathy are other causes.

Detrusor instability

This condition, also called overactive bladder (OAB), causes urge incontinence, where a strong desire to pass urine is followed by involuntary loss of large amounts of urine either during the day or night. It is often associated with neurological lesions or urinary outflow obstruction, for example, prostatic hypertrophy, but in many cases the cause is unknown. The prevalence of OAB has been reported to be around 11.8%. Around 19.1% of men and 18.3% of women older than 60 years were noted to have urgency of micturition in a multinational cross-sectional survey (Irwin et al., 2006).

Stress incontinence is not amenable to drug therapy. However, duloxetine is licensed for the treatment of moderate to severe stress incontinence in women along with pelvic floor exercises. In patients with prostatic hypertrophy α_1-blockers such as prazosin, indoramin, alfuzosin, terazosin, and tamsulosin have all been shown to increase peak urine flow rate and improve symptoms in about 60% of patients. They reduce outflow obstruction by blocking α_1-receptors and thereby relaxing prostate smooth muscle. Postural hypotension is an important adverse effect and occurs in between 2% and 5% of patients.

5α-Reductase converts testosterone to dihydrotesterone (DHT), which plays an important role in the growth of the prostate. The 5α-reductase inhibitor finasteride reduces the prostate volume by 20% and improves peak urine flow rate. The clinical effects, however, might not become apparent until after 3–6 months of treatment. The main adverse effects are reductions in libido and erectile dysfunction in 3–5% of patients.

Several antimuscarinic drugs, including darifenacin, fesoterodine fumarate, oral and transdermal oxybutynin hydrochloride, modified-release propiverine hydrochloride, solifenacin succinate, trospium chloride, and modified-release tolterodine, have all been licensed for OAB (Wagg, 2012). The antimuscarinic drugs decrease detrusor contractions by inhibiting the M2 and M3 subtypes of muscarinic receptors in the urinary bladder. All these drugs are similar in efficacy and cause antimuscarinic side effects such as dry mouth, blurred vision and constipation. Transdermal and modified-release preparations are better tolerated but are more expensive.

Mirabegron, a β_3-adrenoceptor agonist which relaxes the bladder, has been approved by NICE (2013) for the treatment of OAB, 'only for people in whom antimuscarinic drugs are contraindicated or clinically ineffective, or have unacceptable side effects'. The recommended dose is 50 mg daily. The lower dose of 25 mg daily should be used in patients with mild hepatic impairment or mild to moderate renal impairment if they are on strong inhibitors of cytochrome P450 3A, such as itraconazole, ketoconazole, ritonavir, or clarithromycin.

Mirabegron should not be used in patients with blood pressure higher than 160/100 mmHg and also in those with severe renal impairment. It is also contraindicated in in those with moderate hepatic impairment, who are concurrently on strong inhibitors of cytochrome P450 3A.

A double-blind, double-placebo–controlled, randomised trial compared solifenacin, 5 mg initially (with possible escalation to 10 mg and, if necessary, subsequent switch to trospium XR, 60 mg) plus one intradetrusor injection of saline or one intradetrusor injection of 100 U of onabotulinum toxin A plus daily oral placebo showed that both interventions reduced the urge incontinence to a similar degree. Dry mouth was less common with onabotulinum toxin A, but it was more likely to result in complete resolution of urge incontinence. It was also associated with higher rates of transient urinary retention and urinary tract infections. A meta-analysis has concluded that onabotulinum toxin A is an effective treatment for idiopathic OAB symptoms, with side effects mainly confined to the urinary tract (Cui et al., 2015).

Drug therapy for OAB should be combined with pelvic floor exercises and bladder training. The need for continued drug therapy should be critically reviewed at regular intervals, and patients should be monitored for adverse effects.

Constipation

Chronic constipation accounts for around 8 million visits to doctors annually in the USA. The age-related decline in gastro-intestinal motility and treatment with drugs (e.g. opiates, antimuscarinics, calcium-channel blockers, antidepressants) which decrease gastro-intestinal motility predispose the elderly to constipation. Decreased mobility, wasting of pelvic muscles and a low intake of solids and liquids are other contributory factors. Faecal impaction may occur with severe constipation, which in turn may cause subacute intestinal obstruction, abdominal pain, spurious diarrhoea and faecal incontinence. Adequate intake of dietary fibre, regular bowel habit and use of bulking agents such as bran or ispaghula husk may help prevent constipation. When constipation is associated with a loaded rectum, a stimulant laxative such as senna or bisacodyl may be given. Frail, ill elderly patients with a full rectum may have atonic bowels that will not respond to bulking agents or softening agents, and in such cases, a stimulant is more effective. A stool-softening agent such as docusate sodium is effective when stools are hard and dry. For severe faecal impaction, a phosphate enema may be needed. Long-term use of stimulant laxatives may lead to abuse and atonic bowel musculature.

Linaclotide acts on guanylate cyclase C receptor to increase intestinal fluid secretion and transit. It is licenced for use in moderate to severe irritable bowel syndrome associated with constipation. Lubiprostone, a bicyclic fatty acid derived from prostaglandin E, which activates chloride channel, increases intestinal water secretion and motility. It has been approved for use in chronic severe constipation and irritable bowel syndrome. Prucalopride, a prokinetic agent, which is a selective 5 HT4-receptor agonist, is licensed for chronic severe constipation in women. However, because of its comparable efficacy with less expensive laxatives, further studies are probably needed to establish the cost effectiveness this drug.

Gastro-intestinal ulceration and bleeding

Gastro-intestinal bleeding associated with peptic ulcer is less well tolerated by the elderly. The clinical presentation may sometimes be atypical, with, for example, patients presenting with confusion. *Helicobacter pylori* infection is common, and its treatment is similar to that in younger patients. NSAIDs are more likely to cause gastroduodenal ulceration and bleeding in the elderly.

Principles and goals of drug therapy in older people

A thorough knowledge of the pharmacokinetic and pharmacodynamic factors discussed is essential for optimal drug therapy in older people. In addition, some general principles based on common sense, if followed, may result in even better use of drugs.

Avoid unnecessary drug therapy

Before commencing drug therapy, it is important to ask the following questions:
- Is it really necessary?
- Is there an alternative method of treatment?

In patients with mild hypertension, non-drug therapies which are of proven efficacy should be considered in the first instance. Similarly, unnecessary use of hypnotics should be avoided. Simple measures such as emptying the bladder before going to bed to avoid having to get up, avoidance of stimulant drugs in the evenings or at night or moving the patient to a dark, quiet room may be all that is needed.

Effect of treatment on quality of life

The aim of treatment in elderly patients is not just to prolong life but also to improve the quality of life. To achieve this, the correct choice of treatment is essential. In a 70-year-old lady with severe osteoarthrosis of the hip, for example, total hip replacement is the treatment of choice rather than prescribing NSAIDs with all their associated adverse effects.

Treat the cause rather than the symptom

Symptomatic treatment without specific diagnosis is not only bad practice but can also be potentially dangerous. A patient presenting with 'indigestion' may in fact be suffering from angina, and therefore treatment with proton pump inhibitors or antacids is clearly inappropriate. When a patient presents with a symptom, every attempt should be made to establish the cause of the symptom and specific treatment, if available, should then be given.

Drug history

A drug history should be obtained in all elderly patients. This will ensure that patients are not prescribed a drug or drugs to which they may be allergic or the same drug or group of drugs to which they have previously not responded. It will also help avoid potentially serious drug interactions.

Concomitant medical illness

Concurrent medical disorders must always be taken into account. Cardiac failure, renal impairment and hepatic dysfunction are particularly common in the elderly and may increase the risk of adverse effects of drugs.

Choosing the drug

Once it is decided that a patient requires drug therapy, it is important to choose the drug likely to be the most efficacious and least likely to produce adverse effects. It is also necessary to take into consideration coexisting medical conditions. For example, it is inappropriate to commence diuretic therapy to treat mild hypertension in an elderly male with prostatic hypertrophy.

Dose titration

In general, older people require relatively smaller doses of all drugs compared with young adults. It is recognised that the majority of adverse drug reactions occurring in them are dose related and potentially preventable. It is, therefore, rational to start with the smallest possible dose of a given drug in the least number of doses and then gradually increase both, if necessary. Dose titration should obviously take into consideration age-related pharmacokinetic and pharmacodynamic alterations that may affect the response to the chosen drug.

Choosing the right dosage form

Many older people find it easy to swallow syrups, suspensions or effervescent tablets rather than large tablets or capsules.

Packaging and labelling

Many elderly patients with arthritis find it difficult to open child-resistant containers and blister packs. Medicines should be dispensed in easy-to-open containers that are clearly labelled using large print.

Good record keeping

Information about a patient's current and previous drug therapy, alcohol consumption, smoking and driving habits may help in choosing appropriate drug therapy and when the treatment needs to be altered. It will help reduce costly duplications and will also identify and help avoid dangerous drug interactions.

Regular supervision and review of treatment

A UK survey showed that 59% of prescriptions to the elderly had been given for more than 2 years, 32% for more than 5 years and 16% for more than 10 years. Of all prescriptions given to the elderly, 88% were repeat prescriptions; 40% had not been discussed with the doctor for at least 6 months, especially prescriptions for hypnotics and anxiolytics. It also showed that 31% of prescriptions were considered pharmacologically questionable, and 4% showed duplication of drugs.

It is obvious that there is a need for regular and critical review of all prescriptions, especially when long-term therapy is required.

Adverse drug reactions

It is recognised that ADRs occur more frequently in the elderly. A UK multicentre study in the UK showed that ADRs were the only cause of admission in 2.8% of 1998 admissions to 42 units of geriatric medicine (Williamson and Chopin, 1980). It also showed that ADRs were contributory to a further 7.7% of admissions. On the basis of this study, it was estimated that up to 15,000 geriatric admissions per annum in the UK are at least partly due to an ADR. Obviously, this has enormous economic implications.

The elderly are more susceptible to ADRs for a number of reasons. They are usually on multiple drugs, which in itself can account for the increased incidence of ADRs. It is, however, recognised that ADRs tend to be more severe in the elderly, and gastrointestinal and haematological ADRs are more common than would be expected from prescribing figures alone. Age-related pharmacokinetic and pharmacodynamic alterations and impaired homeostatic mechanisms are the other factors which predispose the elderly to ADRs, by making them more sensitive to the pharmacological effects of the drugs. Not surprisingly, up to 80% of ADRs in the elderly are dose-dependent and therefore predictable.

Adherence

Although it is commonly believed that the elderly have poor adherence with their drug therapy, there is no clear evidence to support this. Studies in Northern Ireland and continental Europe have shown that the elderly are as adherent with their drug therapy as the young, provided that they do not have confounding disease. Cognitive impairment, which is common in old age, multiple drug therapy and complicated drug regimens may impair adherence in the elderly. Poor adherence may result in treatment failure. The degree of adherence required varies depending on the disease being treated. For treatment of a simple urinary tract infection, a single dose of an antibiotic may be all that is required, and therefore adherence is not important. On the other hand, adherence of 90% or more is required for successful treatment of epilepsy or difficult hypertension. Various methods have been used to improve adherence. These include prescription diaries, special packaging, training by pharmacists and counselling.

Conclusion

The number of elderly patients, especially those older than 75 years, is steadily increasing, and they are accounting for an ever-increasing proportion of healthcare expenditure in the West. Understanding age-related changes in pharmacodynamic factors, avoiding polypharmacy and regular and critical review of all drug treatments will help in the rationalisation of drug prescribing, reduction in drug-related morbidity and cost of drug therapy for this important subgroup of patients.

Case studies

Case 11.1

An 80-year-old man with Parkinson's disease, Mr JB, was admitted to hospital with increasing confusion and recurrent falls. He had a past history of ischaemic heart disease. Mr JB's primary care doctor had recently commenced him on antihypertensive therapy. His drug therapy included co-careldopa 12.5/50 mg three times a day, amlodipine 10 mg once a day, simvastatin 40 mg once a day, clopidogrel 75 mg once a day and isosorbide mononitrate 10 mg twice a day.

Question

Which drugs could have contributed to Mr JB's symptoms?

Answer

Co-careldopa, amlodipine and isosorbide mononitrate all cause postural hypotension. Recent addition of amlodipine is likely to have caused symptomatic postural hypotension. Significant postural hypotension could lead to falls and decreased cerebral blood flow, which in turn may cause confusion.

Case 11.2

An 85-year-old lady, Mrs FW, presented to hospital with sudden onset of right-sided weakness and loss of speech. She had a previous history of hypertension, ischemic heart disease, hyperlipidemia and atrial fibrillation (AF). Mrs FW was on bisoprolol 2.5 mg once a day, rivaroxaban 15 mg once a day, simvastatin 20 mg once a day and amlodipine 5 mg once a day. A computed tomography (CT) head scan revealed an intracerebral haemorrhage involving the left frontal lobe.

Question

How should Mrs FW be managed?

Answer

It is very likely that rivaroxaban, a DOAC, has contributed to the intracerebral haemorrhage. Patients who develop intracerebral haemorrhage whilst on anticoagulants (both warfarin and DOACs) continue to bleed as long as they are anticoagulated. The larger the haematoma, the worse is the outcome. Therefore, the priority is to reverse the anticoagulation with a specific antidote (in this case, an anti-Xa antidote) as soon as possible. Surgical evacuation of the haematoma is not routinely performed at present because there is no evidence for its efficacy.

Case 11.3

An 80-year-old woman with a previous history of hypothyroidism presented with a history of abdominal pain and vomiting. She had not moved her bowels for the previous 7 days. Two weeks earlier her primary care doctor had prescribed a combination of paracetamol and codeine to control pain in her osteoarthritic hips.

Question

What are the likely underlying causes of this patient's bowel dysfunction?

Answer

This patient developed severe constipation after taking a codeine-containing analgesic. Ageing is associated with decreased gastro-intestinal motility. Hypothyroidism, which is common in the elderly, is also associated with reduced gastro-intestinal motility. Whenever possible, drugs that are known to reduce gastro-intestinal motility should be avoided in the elderly.

Case 11.4

A 75-year-old lady who suffered from osteoarthrosis of the hip and knee joints presented with a history of passing black stools. Her drug therapy included naproxen 500 mg twice daily and paracetamol 1 g as required.

Question

What is the likely cause of this patient's symptoms?

Answer

The likely cause is upper gastro-intestinal bleeding due to naproxen, which is an NSAID. Elderly people are more prone to develop ulceration in the stomach and duodenum with NSAIDs compared with young patients. Pain in osteoarthrosis is not inflammatory in origin. If at all possible, NSAIDs should be avoided in such patients. If a mild NSAID is indicated, ibuprofen is preferred in older people because it is better tolerated. A yellow card should be submitted to the Medicines and Healthcare Products Regulatory Agency (MHRA) if a serious adverse event occurs with NSAID treatment. The MHRA is particularly interested in receiving reports of ADRs in patients older than 65 years.

Case 11.5

A 75-year-old man, Mr AJ, presented to his primary care physician with exertional dyspnoea and increasing leg oedema for 4 weeks. He had a previous history of hypertension, ischaemic heart disease and hyperlipidemia. Mr AJ smoked 30 cigarettes per day. He was on amlodipine 10 mg once a day, atorvastatin 40 mg once a day and clopidogrel 75 mg once a day. The primary care doctor diagnosed heart failure and commenced him on ramipril 2.5 mg once a day. Four weeks later, Mr AJ returned to his primary care doctor with anorexia, nausea and vomiting.

Question

What may have caused Mr AJ's new symptoms?

Answer

Mr AJ has probably gone into renal failure causing anorexia, nausea and vomiting due to the resultant uraemia. Patients with atherosclerotic vascular disease, which Mr AJ is likely to have, sometimes develop bilateral renal artery stenosis (as a result of atherosclerosis). Prescribing ACE inhibitors in such patients may result in acute renal failure due to the significant reduction in renal blood flow.

References

Alavi, A., Sibbald, R.G., Phillips, T.J., et al., 2016. What's new: management of venous leg ulcers: approach to venous leg ulcers. J. Am. Acad. Dermatol. 74, 627–640.

Amery, A., Birkenhager, W., Brixko, P., et al., 1986. Efficacy of antihypertensive drug treatment according to age, sex, blood pressure, and previous cardiovascular disease in patients over the age of 60. Lancet 2, 589–592.

Bayer, A.J., Chadha, J.S., Farag, R.R., et al., 1986. Changing presentation of myocardial infarction with increasing old age. J. Am. Geriatr. Soc. 34, 263–266.

Beckett, N.S., Peters, R., Fletcher, A.E., for the HYVET Study Group, 2008. Treatment of hypertension in patients 80 years of age or older. N. Engl. J. Med. 358, 1887–1898.

Black, D.M., Rosen, C.J., 2016. Postmenopausal osteoporosis. N. Engl. J. Med. 374, 254–262.

Blood Pressure Lowering Treatment Trialists' Collaboration, 2008. Effects of different regimens to lower blood pressure on major cardiovascular events in older and younger adults: meta-analysis of randomised trials. Br. Med. J. 336, 1121–1123.

Centre for Policy on Ageing, 2012. Managing and administering medication in care homes for older people. A report for the project: 'Working together to develop practical solutions: an integrated approach to medication in care homes'. Available at: http://www.cpa.org.uk/information/reviews/Managing_and_Administering_Medication_in_Care_Homes.pdf.

Chen, Y.-F., Dewey, M.E., Avery, A.J., the Analysis Group of the MRCCFA Study, 2001. The Medical Research Council Cognitive Function Ageing Study (MRC CFAS) 2001: Self-reported medication use for older people in England and Wales. J. Clin. Pharm. Therap. 26, 129–140.

Chen, Z.M., Sandercock, P., Pan, H.C., et al., 2000. Indications for early aspirin use in acute ischaemic stroke: a combined analysis of 40,000 randomised patients from the Chinese acute stroke trial and the international stroke trial. On behalf of the CAST and IST collaborative groups. Stroke 31, 1240–1249.

Cornwall, J.V., Dore, C.J., Lewis, J.D., 1986. Leg ulcers: epidemiology and aetiology. Br. J. Surg. 73, 693–696.

Cui, Y., Zhou, X., Zong, H., Yan, H., et al., 2015. The efficacy and safety of onabotulinumtoxin A in treating idiopathic OAB: a systematic review and meta-analysis. Neurourol. Urodynam. 34, 413–419.

Diener, H.C., Bogousslavsky, J., Brass, L.M., et al., 2004. Aspirin and clopidogrel compared with clopidogrel alone after recent ischaemic stroke or transient ischaemic attack in high-risk patients (MATCH): randomised, double-blind, placebo-controlled trial. Lancet 364, 331–337.

Emberson, J., Lees, K.R., Lyden, P., 2014. Effect of treatment delay, age, and stroke severity on the effects of intravenous thrombolysis with alteplase for acute ischaemic stroke: a meta-analysis of individual patient data from randomised trials. Lancet 384, 1929–1935.

Gray, S.L., Dublin, S., Yu, O., et al., 2016. Benzodiazepine use and risk of incident dementia or cognitive decline: prospective population based study. BMJ. 352, i90. https://doi.org/10.1136/bmj.i90.

Gueyffier, F., Bulpitt, C., Boissel, J.P., et al., 1999. Antihypertensive drugs in very old people: a subgroup meta-analysis of randomised controlled trials. Lancet 353, 793–796.

Hart, R.G., Pearce, L.A., Aguilar, M.I., 2007. Meta-analysis antithrombotic therapy to prevent stroke in patients who have nonvalvular atrial fibrillation. Ann. Intern. Med. 146, 857–867.

Irwin, D.E., Milsom, I., Hunskaar, S., et al., 2006. Population-based survey of urinary incontinence, overactive bladder, and other lower urinary tract symptoms in five countries: results of the EPIC study. Eur. Urol. 50 (6), 1306–1314.

Mangoni, A.A., Jackson, S.H.D., 2003. Age-related changes in pharmacokinetics and pharmacodynamics: basic principles and practical applications. Br. J. Clin. Pharmacol. 57, 6–14.

National Institute for Health and Care Excellence (NICE), 2010. Clopidogrel and modified-release dipyridamole for the prevention of occlusive vascular events. Available at: https://www.nice.org.uk/guidance/ta210.

National Institute for Health and Care Excellence (NICE), 2011. Hypertension in adults: diagnosis and management. Available at: https://www.nice.org.uk/guidance/cg127.

National Institute for Health and Care Excellence (NICE), 2013. Mirabegron for treating symptoms of overactive bladder. Technology appraisal guidance. Available at: https://www.nice.org.uk/guidance/ta290.

National Institute for Health and Care Excellence (NICE), 2016. Mechanical clot retrieval for treating acute ischaemic stroke. Interventional procedure guidance. Available at: https://www.nice.org.uk/guidance/ipg548.

Office for National Statistics, 2015. Statistical bulletin: estimates of the very old (including centenarians): England and Wales, and United Kingdom, 2002 to 2014. Available at: http://www.ons.gov.uk/peoplepopulationandcommunity/birthsdeathsandmarriages/ageing/bulletins/estimatesoftheveryoldincludingcentenarians/2015-09-30.

Public Health England, 2016. Health matters: midlife approaches to reduce dementia risk. Available at: https://www.gov.uk/government/publications/health-matters-midlife-approaches-to-reduce-dementia-risk/health-matters-midlife-approaches-to-reduce-dementia-risk.

Royal Pharmaceutical Society Wales, 2016. Improving medicines use for care home residents. Royal Pharmaceutical Society Wales, Cardiff. Available at: https://www.rpharms.com/Portals/0/RPS%20document%20library/Open%20access/Publications/Improving%20medicines%20use%20for%20care%20home%20residents.pdf.

Scheltens, P., Blennow, K., Monique, M.B., et al., 2016. Alzheimer's disease. Lancet. 388(10043), 505–517. Available at: http://www.thelancet.com/pdfs/journals/lancet/PIIS0140-6736(15)01124-1.pdf.

SHEP Cooperative Research Group, 1991. Prevention of stroke by antihypertensive drug treatment in older persons with isolated systolic hypertension: final results of the systolic hypertension in the elderly programme (SHEP). J. Am. Med. Assoc. 265, 3255–3264.

Verheugt, F.W.A., Granger, C.W., 2015. Oral anticoagulants for stroke prevention in atrial fibrillation: current status, special situations, and unmet needs. Lancet 386 (9990), 303–310.

Wagg, A.S.A., 2012. Antimuscarinic treatment in overactive bladder: special considerations in elderly patients. Drugs Aging 29 (7), 539–548.

Williamson, J., Chopin, J.M., 1980. Adverse reactions to prescribed drugs in the elderly: a multicentre investigation. Age Ageing 9, 73–80.

Further reading

Alhawassi, T.M., Krass, I., Bajorek, B.V., et al., 2014. A systematic review of the prevalence and risk factors for adverse drug reactions in the elderly in the acute care setting. Clin. Interventions Aging 9, 2079–2086.

Ettehad, D., Emdin, C.A., Kiran, A., et al., 2016. Blood pressure lowering for prevention of cardiovascular disease and death: a systematic review and meta-analysis. Lancet 387 (10022), 957–967.

Kalia, L.V., Lang, A.E., 2015. Parkinson's disease. Lancet 386 (9996), 896–912.

Kernan, W.N., Ovbiagele, B., Black, H.R., et al., 2014. Guidelines for the prevention of stroke in patients with stroke and transient ischemic attack: a guideline for healthcare professionals from the American Heart Association/American Stroke Association. Stroke 45, 2160–2236.

Maraka, S., Kennel, K.A., 2015. Bisphosphonates for the prevention and treatment of osteoporosis. BMJ 351, h3783. https://doi.org/10.1136/bmj.h3783.

National Collaborating Centre for Chronic Conditions, 2008. Stroke. National clinical guideline for diagnosis and initial management of acute stroke and transient ischaemic attack (TIA). Royal College of Physicians, London.

Robinson, L., Tang, E., Taylor, J.-P., 2015. Dementia: timely diagnosis and early intervention. BMJ 350, h3029. https://doi.org/10.1136/bmj.h3029.

Scientific Committee of the First International Consultation on Incontinence, 2000. Assessment and treatment of urinary incontinence. Lancet 355, 2153–2158.

Wald, A., 2016. Constipation: advances in diagnosis and treatment. JAMA 315, 185–191.

SECTION **3**

THERAPEUTICS

12 Dyspepsia, Peptic Ulcer Disease and Gastro-Oesophageal Reflux Disease

Dan Greer

Key points

- Symptoms of dyspepsia lack specificity and are poor predictors of underlying causes; therefore, undiagnosed dyspepsia without ALARM symptoms should be treated empirically without an endoscopic diagnosis.

- For patients without ALARM symptoms, lifestyle advice on healthy eating, weight reduction and smoking cessation should be offered together with a review of medication for potential causes of dyspepsia. If these fail to control symptoms, treatment options are 1 month of proton pump inhibitor (PPI) or to test and treat for Helicobacter pylori (H. pylori).

- A diagnosis of peptic ulcer disease, gastro-oesophageal reflux disease (GORD) or functional dyspepsia can only be confirmed by endoscopy.

- Treatment of peptic ulcer disease centres on removal of the underlying cause, most commonly non-steroidal anti-inflammatory drugs (NSAIDs) or H. pylori. In some cases further acid suppression is required for 1–2 months.

- For H. pylori eradication, a 1-week course of twice-daily triple therapy with a PPI, clarithromycin and amoxicillin or metronidazole remains first-line therapy, but a recent history of antibiotic exposure may affect choice because resistance to clarithromycin and metronidazole is increasingly common.

- Gastroprotection should be offered to all patients on chronic NSAID therapy to reduce the risk of ulcer disease. The highest-risk groups are older people and those with previous ulcer disease or gastro-intestinal bleeding, and NSAIDs should be avoided where possible in these groups.

- Dual antiplatelet therapy carries a similar risk of gastro-intestinal bleeding to NSAIDs, and therefore gastroprotection is warranted.

- Treatment for endoscopically confirmed GORD consists of 1–2 months of PPI therapy. Some patients with recurrent symptoms may require maintenance therapy; those with severe oesophagitis should remain on full dose PPI. There is no role for H. pylori eradication therapy in GORD.

- Functional dyspepsia is difficult to treat; initial treatment options are to eradicate H. pylori if present or to offer 1 month of low-dose PPI or an H_2 antagonist.

- The association of long-term PPI treatment with Clostridium difficile and osteoporosis means that PPIs should only be continued where there is a clear indication. Long-term PPI treatment is indicated for NSAID gastroprotection and severe oesophagitis only. Patients receiving PPIs for other indications should receive short courses of 1–2 months, with maintenance offered at the lowest effective dose only for those with resistant or recurrent symptoms.

Dyspepsia is an umbrella term used to describe a range of symptoms associated with the upper gastro-intestinal tract and includes upper abdominal pain or discomfort, heartburn, acid reflux, nausea and vomiting. The underlying causes of dyspepsia symptoms include gastric and duodenal ulcers, gastro-oesophageal reflux disease (GORD) and oesophageal or gastric cancers; however, the cause is often unknown, which is classified as functional dyspepsia. The key challenge in managing dyspepsia is to differentiate the majority of patients who can be managed symptomatically from those who may have more serious underlying pathology that requires further investigation before treatment.

Epidemiology

In the UK, dyspepsia occurs in 40% of the population annually and leads to a primary care doctor consultation in 5% and referral for endoscopy in 1%. In those patients with signs or symptoms severe enough to merit endoscopy, 40% have functional dyspepsia, 40% have GORD and 13% have peptic ulcer disease, whereas gastric and oesophageal cancers are very rare, occurring in only 3% of endoscopies (National Institute for Health and Care Excellence [NICE], 2014a).

The incidence of peptic ulcer disease in the Western world is declining, probably driven by the declining prevalence of Helicobacter pylori (H. pylori) infection, reduction in non-steroidal anti-inflammatory drugs (NSAIDs) use and increased use of gastroprotective agents.

Pathophysiology

The pathophysiology of dyspepsia depends on the underlying cause.

Peptic ulcer disease

An ulcer is defined as a breach in the gastric or duodenal mucosa down to the submucosa (Fig. 12.1). The two main causes of peptic ulcer disease are H. pylori infection and the use of aspirin and NSAIDs. Less common is ulcer disease associated with massive hypersecretion of acid, which occurs in the rare gastrinoma

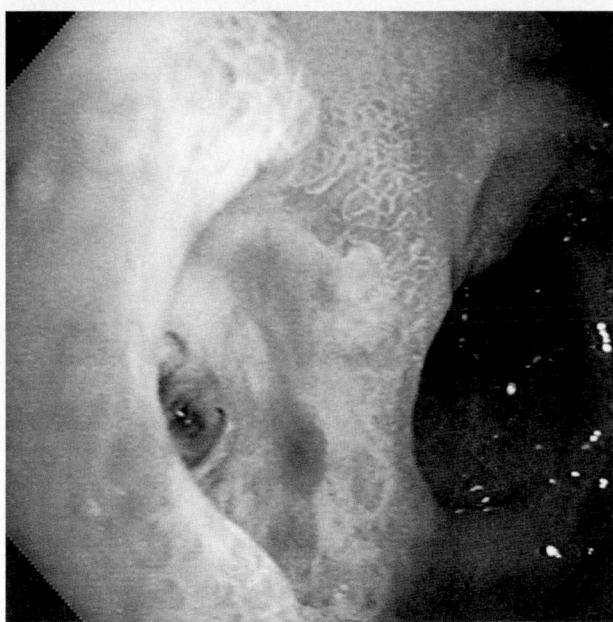

Fig. 12.1 Duodenal ulcer seen at endoscopy. Note also a visible blood vessel that is a stigma of recent haemorrhage.

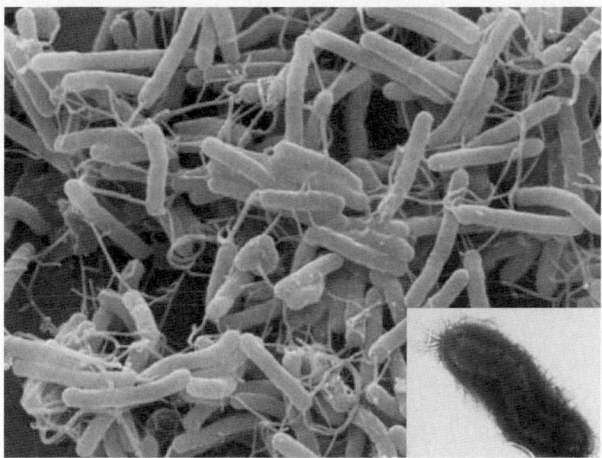

Fig. 12.2 *Helicobacter pylori*. The Gram-negative spiral bacterium *H. pylori*, formerly known as *Campylobacter pylori*, was isolated serendipitously from patients with gastritis by Barry Marshall and Robin Warren in 1982. Seven years later, it was conceded that *H. pylori* is responsible for most cases of gastric and duodenal ulcer.

(Zollinger–Ellison) syndrome. Stress ulcers are ulcers that form due severe physiological stress, such as head injury, spinal cord injury, burns, multiple trauma or sepsis. Mechanical ventilation and the presence of coagulopathies place patients at particular risk of stress-related mucosal bleeding and may warrant prophylactic treatment (Quenot et al., 2009).

Helicobacter pylori

H. pylori is a Gram-negative microaerophilic bacterium found primarily in the gastric antrum of the human stomach (Fig. 12.2). Ninety-five percent or more of duodenal ulcers and 80–85% of gastric ulcers are associated with *H. pylori*. *H. pylori* infection is thought to occur in infancy or early childhood, and infection is associated with poor socioeconomic conditions. Transmission most likely occurs via the oral-oral and faeco-oral route. In developed countries, the prevalence among middle-aged adults is falling, whereas in many developing countries, the prevalence in the same age group is much greater. Only about 15% of infected individuals develop ulcers (Kuipers, 1997). This is likely to be due to variation in virulence between strains of *H. pylori*, differences in host response to infection and other environmental factors.

The underlying pathophysiology associated with *H. pylori* infection involves the production of cytotoxin-associated gene A (*CagA*) proteins and vacuolating cytotoxins, such as vac A, which activate the inflammatory cascade. *CagA* status and one genotype of the vac A gene are also predictors of the ulcerogenic capacity of a strain. In addition, a number of enzymes produced by *H. pylori* may be involved in causing tissue damage and include urease, haemolysins, neuraminidase and fucosidase.

There appear to be two patterns of infection with *H. pylori*. Infection in infancy is thought to lead to pan gastritis and gastric ulcers, whereas acquisition in later childhood may lead to a predominantly antral gastritis only, causing duodenal ulcers.

In antral gastritis, a bacterially mediated decrease of antral D cells that normally secrete somatostatin leads to a loss of the negative-feedback action of somatostatin on gastrin, which is the main hormone involved in stimulating gastric acid secretion. The resulting hypergastrinaemia and high acid content in the proximal duodenum leads to metaplastic gastric-type mucosa, which provides a niche for *H. pylori* infection followed by inflammation and ulcer formation.

In pan gastritis, there is a more generalised inflammatory response to infection in the gastric mucosa, leading to mucosal damage and ulceration.

Non-steroidal anti-inflammatory drugs

The major systemic action of NSAIDs that contributes to the formation of ulcers is the reduction of mucosal prostaglandin production via COX-1 (Fig. 12.3). This leads to a reduction in the mucosal protective mechanisms of mucous, bicarbonate production and mucosal repair. Patients taking NSAIDs have a fourfold increase in the risk of ulcer complications compared with nonusers (Hernandez-Diaz and Rodriguez, 2000). The absolute risk of ulcer complications in patients on NSAIDs is approximately 1% per year.

Ulcers have been found to be more common in patients who have taken NSAIDs for less than 3 months, with the highest risk observed during the first month of treatment. The risk of ulcer complications (Box 12.1) is progressive depending on the number of risk factors present (Lanza et al., 2009). The most important risk factors are a history of ulcer complications and advancing age, particularly older than 75 years. Corticosteroids alone are an insignificant ulcer risk but potentiate the ulcer risk when added to NSAIDs, particularly in daily doses of at least 10 mg of prednisolone (Lanza et al., 2009).

Low-dose aspirin (75 mg/day) alone increases the risk of ulcer bleeding by approximately twofold, and dual antiplatelet use increases this risk to fourfold. This effect may be due to the antiplatelet action, independent of other risk factors. Concomitant use of aspirin with NSAIDs further increases the risk. There is no evidence that anticoagulants increase the risk of NSAID ulcers,

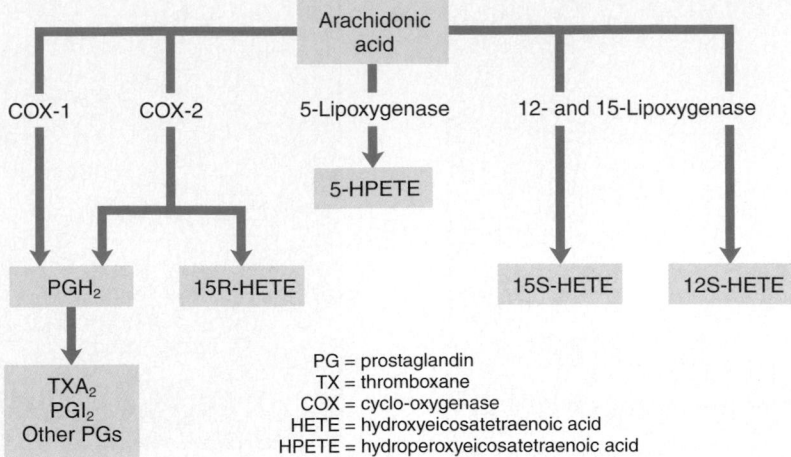

Fig. 12.3 Arachidonic acid pathway.

PG = prostaglandin
TX = thromboxane
COX = cyclo-oxygenase
HETE = hydroxyeicosatetraenoic acid
HPETE = hydroperoxyeicosatetraenoic acid

Box 12.1 Risk factors for non-steroidal anti-inflammatory drug ulcers

- Age >65 years
- Previous peptic ulceration/bleeding
- High dose of NSAID or more than one NSAID (including aspirin)
- Short-term history of NSAID use (<1 month)
- Concomitant corticosteroid or anticoagulant use
- Cardiovascular disease

NSAID, Non-steroidal anti-inflammatory drug.

Box 12.2 Odds ratio of peptic ulcer bleeding with different non-steroidal anti-inflammatory drugs (Langman et al., 1994)

Ibuprofen	2.0
Diclofenac	4.2
Naproxen	9.1
Indometacin	11.3
Piroxicam	13.7
Ketoprofen	23.7
Azapropazone	31.5

---

but they are associated with an increase in the risk of haemorrhage (García Rodríguez et al., 2011). Use of selective serotonin reuptake inhibitors (SSRIs) also increases the risk of bleeding, due to the antiplatelet effect of serotonin. The presence of cardiovascular disease is also considered as an independent risk factor.

NSAIDs differ in their propensity to cause ulceration (Box 12.2), with ibuprofen and diclofenac considered lowest risk, and ketoprofen and azapropazone considered highest. The risk also increases with higher doses of NSAIDs (García Rodríguez and Jick, 1994).

Selective cyclo-oxygenase-2 inhibitors

The gastro-intestinal side effects of conventional NSAIDs are mediated through the inhibition of COX-1 (see Fig. 12.3). COX-1 stimulates synthesis of homeostatic prostaglandins, whereas COX-2 is predominantly induced in response to inflammation. Selective COX-2 inhibitors tend not to reduce the mucosal production of protective prostaglandins to the same extent as NSAIDs. COX-2 inhibitors are, therefore, considered to be safer than nonselective NSAIDs in patients at high risk of developing gastro-intestinal mucosal damage. Although studies have confirmed the reduction of endoscopic and symptomatic ulcers (Hooper et al., 2004), an increase in cardiovascular risk, including heart attack and stroke, has resulted in the withdrawal of some COX-2 inhibitors from the market. Additional contraindications are now in place for those COX-2 inhibitors that remain; these include the recommendation that they should not be taken by patients with established heart or cerebrovascular disease or taken in combination with low-dose aspirin because this negates any gastro-intestinal protective effects. More recently, a European safety review concluded that diclofenac also has a similar thrombotic risk to COX-2 inhibitors (European Medicines Agency [EMA], 2013). The need for and choice of anti-inflammatory agent should therefore take into account gastro-intestinal, cardiovascular and other risks such as potential cardio-renal effects. For all agents, the lowest effective dose should be used for the shortest duration.

Gastro-oesophageal reflux disease

Gastro-oesophageal reflux disease (GORD) is caused by reflux of acid or bile from the stomach into the oesophagus, or beyond, causing symptoms and/or complications (Katz et al., 2013). The pathophysiology of reflux is multifactorial and involves increased transient lower oesophageal sphincter relaxations, reduced tone of the lower oesophageal sphincter, hiatus hernia, abnormal oesophageal acid clearance and delayed gastric emptying. Risk factors include obesity, pregnancy and certain medications.

Drug-related causes of gastro-oesophageal reflux disease

Some drug classes cause relaxation of the lower oesophageal sphincter, increasing the risk of GORD. These include calcium channel blockers, nitrates and theophylline. Bisphosphonates are

---

Box 12.3 ALARM features

- Dysphagia
- Unintentional weight loss
- Melaena or haematemesis
- Anaemia
- Persistent vomiting
- Epigastric mass

Box 12.4 Drugs causing dyspepsia

- Antibiotics
- Bisphosphonates
- Calcium channel blockers
- Corticosteroids
- Drugs with antimuscarinic effects (e.g. tricyclic antidepressants)
- Iron
- Nitrates
- Non-steroidal anti-inflammatory drugs, including aspirin
- Potassium chloride
- Theophylline

---

thought to be directly toxic to oesophageal mucosa, hence the need to swallow with a glass of water and remain upright after administration. Smoking is also thought to reduce oesophageal sphincter pressure, although a direct association has not been proven.

Functional dyspepsia

The pathophysiology of functional dyspepsia is unclear and likely to be multifactorial. Dysmotility and visceral hypersensitivity have been proposed as possible causes, and there are also changes in brain activity, suggesting that central processing may be altered (Ford and Moayyedi, 2013). *H. pylori* may be implicated, as eradication results in symptom improvement in some patients.

Patient assessment and clinical manifestations

Typical symptoms for the underlying causes of dyspepsia are described herein; however, it should be emphasised that symptoms lack specificity and, alone, are poor indicators of the underlying cause. It is for this reason that UK guidelines (NICE, 2014a) recommend a single treatment pathway for those with 'undiagnosed' dyspepsia, with the emphasis on assessing patients at any age for ALARM features (Box 12.3) and referring them for endoscopic investigation. These groups of patients are at a higher risk of underlying serious disease, such as cancer, peptic ulcer disease or severe oesophagitis. Referral is also recommended for patients over the age of 55 if symptoms are unexplained or persistent despite initial management (NICE, 2014a). Malignant disease is rare in young people and in those without ALARM features. Medication should also be reviewed for potential causes of dyspepsia (Box 12.4). The possibility of cardiac or biliary disease should be considered as part of the differential diagnosis.

Peptic ulcer disease

Peptic ulcers classically present with epigastric pain, described as a gnawing or burning sensation, although some ulcers (particularly NSAID-induced ulcers) are asymptomatic. Duodenal ulcers typically cause pain occurring 1–3 hours after meals, which is relieved by food, whereas gastric ulcer pain is typically triggered by food. Complications of peptic ulcer disease may occur with or without previous dyspeptic symptoms. These are haemorrhage (haematemesis or melaena), chronic iron-deficiency anaemia,

pyloric stenosis and perforation. In the setting of acute gastro-intestinal bleeding with significant blood loss, patients may present with tachycardia and hypotension.

Gastro-oesophageal reflux disease

Classical symptoms of GORD are heartburn, regurgitation, volume reflux, odynophagia (painful swallowing) or dysphagia. Complications include oesophageal stricture, oesophageal ulceration and Barrett's oesophagus, a metaplasia where squamous cells are replaced by columnar epithelium. Barrett's oesophagus can be a precursor to oesophageal cancer, with 0.5–1% of patients progressing to cancer per year (Shaheen and Richter, 2009).

Investigations

Endoscopy

Endoscopy is generally the investigation of choice for diagnosing the underlying cause of dyspepsia, although the investigation is invasive and expensive. Routine endoscopy in patients presenting with dyspepsia without ALARM features (see Box 12.3) is not necessary but should be undertaken in patients with ALARM features and in those patients older than 55 years who present with unexplained or persistent symptoms of dyspepsia. Biopsies may be taken to exclude malignancy and uncommon lesions such as in Crohn's disease.

Patients presenting with severe upper gastro-intestinal bleeding should undergo endoscopy immediately after resuscitation, whereas others should undergo endoscopy within 24 hours (NICE, 2012). Risk assessment scores such as the Blatchford score (Blatchford et al., 2000) pre-endoscopy can be used to identify low-risk patients who can be managed safely without endoscopy or admission to hospital (Table 12.1). The Rockall score (Rockall et al., 1996) post-endoscopy includes endoscopic findings to predict those with high mortality (Table 12.2). Where gastric ulcer is found, endoscopy should be repeated to confirm ulcer healing because gastric ulcers can be malignant.

Patients with iron-deficiency anaemia who have a normal endoscopy are likely to undergo a colonoscopy to look for a lower gastro-intestinal source of blood loss. In such cases iron therapy should be withheld until after this investigation because the dark stools resultant from iron therapy can impair views of the mucosa despite bowel preparation.

Radiology

Double-contrast barium radiography should detect 80% of peptic ulcers but is only done where endoscopy has failed or the patient declines endoscopy. Endoscopy is preferred because of the ability to take biopsies and administer endoscopic therapy if required for bleeding lesions.

Table 12.1 Blatchford score (Blatchford et al., 2000)

Risk factor	Score[a]
Urea (mmol/L)	
6.5–8.0	2
8.0–10.0	3
10.0–25	4
>25	6
Haemoglobin (g/L), men	
12.0–12.9	1
10.0–11.9	3
<10.0	6
Haemoglobin (g/L), women	
10.0–11.9	1
<10.0	6
Systolic blood pressure (mmHg)	
100–109	1
90–99	2
<90	3
Other markers	
Pulse ≥100/min	1
Presentation with melaena	1
Presentation with syncope	2
Hepatic disease	2
Cardiac failure	2

[a]Add scores for each risk factor to give a total score. A score of zero is associated with a low risk of the need for endoscopic intervention, whereas scores of 6 or more are associated with a greater than 50% risk of needing an endoscopic intervention.

Helicobacter pylori detection

There are several methods of detecting *H. pylori* infection. They include noninvasive tests such as serological tests to detect antibodies, [13C] urea breath tests and stool antigen tests. Urea breath tests have a sensitivity and specificity over 90% and are accurate for both initial diagnosis and confirmation of eradication. The breath test is based on the principle that urease activity in the stomach of infected individuals hydrolyses urea to form ammonia and carbon dioxide. The test contains carbon-labelled urea which, when hydrolysed, results in the production of labelled carbon dioxide that appears in the patient's breath. The stool antigen test uses an enzyme immuno-assay to detect *H. pylori* antigen in stool. This test also has a sensitivity and specificity over 90% and can be used in the initial diagnosis and also to confirm eradication. However, the breath test is preferred for confirming eradication because there is currently insufficient evidence for the stool test as a test of eradication. Serological tests are based on the detection of anti–*H. pylori* immunoglobulin G (IgG) antibodies but are not able to distinguish between active or previous exposure to infection. Near-patient serology tests are not recommended because they are inaccurate (NICE, 2014a).

Invasive tests requiring gastric antral biopsies include urease tests, histology and culture. Of these, the biopsy urease test is widely used. Agar-based biopsy urease tests are designed to be read at 24 hours, whereas the strip-based biopsy urease tests can be read at 2 hours following incubation with the biopsy material. Increasing the number of biopsy samples increases the sensitivity of the test because infection can be patchy. The accuracy of the urea breath test, biopsy urease test and stool test can be reduced by drug therapy; therefore, it is recommended patients discontinue PPIs at least 2 weeks before testing and discontinue antibiotics at least 4 weeks before testing to reduce the risk of false-negative results.

Treatment

Undiagnosed dyspepsia

National guidelines (NICE, 2014a) provide algorithms to guide practitioners through the management of patients presenting

Table 12.2 Rockall score (Rockall et al., 1996)

Variable[a]	Score 0	Score 1	Score 2	Score 3
Age (years)	<60	60–79	>80	
Shock	No shock	Pulse >100 beats/min Blood pressure >100 systolic mmHg	SBP <100 mmHg	
Comorbidity	Nil major		CHF, IHD, major morbidity	Renal failure, liver failure, metastatic cancer
Diagnosis	Mallory–Weiss tear	All other diagnoses	GI malignancy	
Evidence of bleeding	None		Blood, adherent clot, spurting vessel	

[a]Add score for each risk factor to give total score.
CHF, Chronic heart failure; GI, gastro-intestinal; IHD, ischaemic heart disease; SBP, systolic blood pressure.

with dyspepsia (Fig. 12.4) who do not need referral for endoscopy. Medicines should be reviewed for potential causes of dyspepsia (see Box 12.4), and lifestyle advice should be offered on healthy eating, weight reduction and smoking cessation. Patients should be advised to avoid known precipitants where possible, such as smoking, alcohol, coffee, chocolate, fatty foods and being overweight. Raising the head of the bed and having a main meal well before going to bed may help some.

There is, however, little evidence that these measures improve symptoms.

If these initial steps fail, options are either to test and treat for *H. pylori* or to offer 1 month of full-dose PPI. No difference has been found between efficacy or costs of the two options (Ford et al., 2008), but if the prevalence of *H. pylori* in the population being considered is known to be low, it probably makes more sense to give acid suppression first line. Retesting

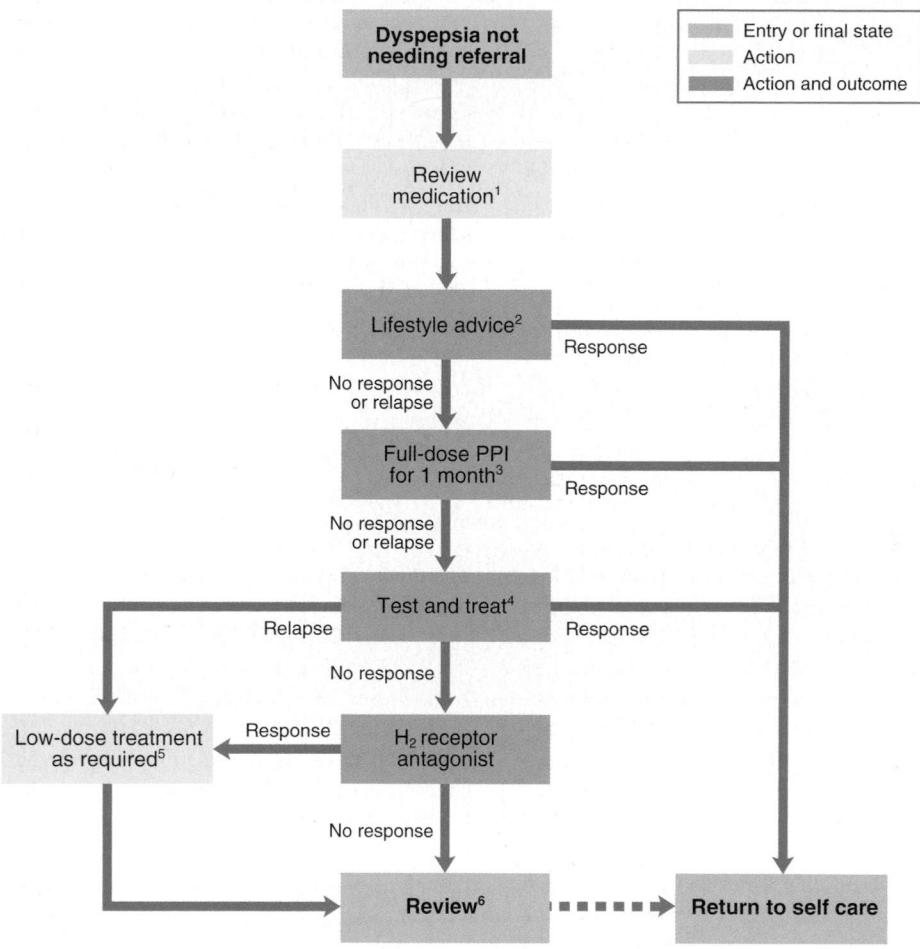

Fig. 12.4 Decision algorithm for management of uninvestigated dyspepsia. (With permission from NICE.)

1 Review medications for possible causes of dyspepsia, for example, calcium antagonists, nitrates, theophyllines, bisphosphonates, steroids and NSAIDs.

2 Offer lifestyle advice, including advice on healthy eating, weight reduction and smoking cessation, promoting continued use of antacid/alginates.

3 There is currently inadequate evidence to guide whether full-dose PPI (proton pump inhibitor) for 1 month or *H. pylori* test and treat should be offered first. Either treatment may be tried first with the other offered if symptoms persist or return.

4 Detection: use carbon-13 urea breath test, stool antigen test or, when performance has been validated, laboratory-based serology.

5 Offer low-dose treatment with a limited number of repeat prescriptions. Discuss the use of treatment on an as-required basis to help patients manage their own symptoms.

6 In some patients with an inadequate response to therapy it may become appropriate to refer to a specialist for a second opinion. Emphasise the benign nature of dyspepsia. Review long-term patient care at least annually to discuss medication and symptoms.

for *H. pylori* to confirm eradication is not considered worthwhile in this scenario. H_2 receptor antagonists are considered second line because they are less effective. If symptoms recur, PPI therapy should be tailored to the lowest dose needed to control symptoms, including discussing with patients the possibility of using them on an 'as-needed' basis to manage their own symptoms.

Peptic ulcer disease

Acute bleeding peptic ulcer

Peptic ulcer is the most common cause of nonvariceal upper gastro-intestinal bleeding. In major bleeding, the priority is to resuscitate initially with fluids, with or without blood, to stabilise before endoscopy. NSAIDs should be stopped, and if patients are actively bleeding, anticoagulants should be reversed. For warfarin this should be with a combination of prothrombin complex concentrate (PCC) and 5 mg vitamin K. Vitamin K alone in this scenario is insufficient because it can take up to 12 hours for full reversal (Keeling et al., 2011). Endoscopy allows identification of the severity of disease as well as endoscopic haemostatic therapy, which is successful in reducing mortality. Endoscopic therapy is necessary only in patients who exhibit high-risk stigmata (active bleeding, nonbleeding visible vessel, adherent clot) on endoscopy.

Pharmacological agents used for endoscopic injection therapy include 1:10,000 adrenaline (epinephrine), human thrombin and fibrin glue. Mechanical endoscopic treatment options include thermocoagulation using a heater probe or endoscopic clipping. Combination therapies are superior to monotherapy and so are recommended (Barkun et al., 2010; NICE, 2012). The need for surgery, re-bleeding rates and mortality are reduced with endoscopic therapy, but bleeding recurs in about 10% of patients and can cause death (Hearnshaw et al., 2011). Patients with uncontrolled bleeding should receive repeat endoscopic treatment, arterial embolisation or surgery.

The use of intravenous PPI therapy before endoscopy in patients with upper gastro-intestinal bleeding may reduce the need for endoscopic therapy but does not affect relevant clinical outcomes such as re-bleeding, need for surgery or mortality (Sreedharan et al., 2010). Therefore, it is not recommended before endoscopy (NICE, 2012).

Acid suppression reduces the re-bleeding rate and should be given to those patients at high risk of re-bleeding following endoscopic haemostatic therapy. The rationale for this is that gastric acid inhibits clot formation, and if intragastric pH is maintained above 6 during the first 3 days after the initial bleed, there is opportunity for clot stabilisation and haemostasis. Results from a meta-analysis suggest that PPIs significantly reduce re-bleeding rates compared with H_2-receptor antagonists and are the preferred choice of treatment (Leontiadis et al., 2010). In similar dosage regimens, there are no data to suggest any PPI is more efficacious than another. The optimal dose and route of PPI are unknown in this indication, although reduction in mortality is observed in high-risk patients when high-dose PPI therapy is given (e.g. 80 mg bolus omeprazole, pantoprazole or esomeprazole followed by 8 mg/h for 72 hours) following endoscopic haemostasis (Barkun

et al., 2010; Scottish Intercollegiate Guidelines Network [SIGN], 2008).

Successful eradication of *H. pylori* reduces the rate of re-bleeding to a greater extent than antisecretory non-eradicating therapy (Gisbert et al., 2004). Following successful *H. pylori* eradication and healing of the ulcer, there is no need to continue maintenance antisecretory therapy beyond 4 weeks unless required for prophylaxis of ulcer complications in those continuing to take aspirin or NSAIDs (SIGN, 2008).

Patients receiving aspirin monotherapy for secondary prevention of vascular events should continue aspirin once bleeding is controlled because although the risk of rebleeding is increased by restarting aspirin early, the overall risk of mortality is lower (Sung et al., 2010), and the addition of a PPI is of benefit in the prevention of recurrent bleeding (Lai et al., 2002). If aspirin is being taken for primary prevention, the risk of bleeding may outweigh benefits, and stopping aspirin permanently should be considered. Clopidogrel alone is not a safer alternative than aspirin and PPI in terms of prevention of recurrent ulcer bleeding. For patients on other antiplatelets or dual antiplatelet therapy, the balance of risk and benefit is less clear and is likely to depend on the indication (e.g. acute coronary syndrome or for cardiac stent) and how long ago the procedure or event occurred. Generally, non-aspirin antiplatelets are stopped acutely, and then advice should be taken from the appropriate specialist.

Uncomplicated peptic ulcer disease

Treatment of endoscopically proven uncomplicated peptic ulcer disease centres on removal of the principal underlying causes, namely, eradication of *H. pylori* infection and discontinuation of NSAIDs. Algorithms for treatment are available from the National Institute for Health and Care Excellence (NICE, 2014a) (Fig. 12.5A and B).

***Helicobacter pylori* eradication.** Eradication of *H. pylori* speeds healing of ulcers, but the major benefit is in reduction of recurrence and avoidance of the need for long-term acid-suppression therapy. Eradication reduces recurrence from 64 per 100 patients to 13 per 100 patients in duodenal ulcer, and from 52 per 100 patients to 16 in 100 patients for gastric ulcer (Ford et al., 2016). Antibiotics alone, or acid-suppressing agents alone, do not eradicate *H. pylori*. Both therapies act synergistically because growth of the organism occurs at elevated pH, and antibiotic efficacy is enhanced during growth. Additionally, increasing intragastric pH may enhance antibiotic absorption.

The standard regimen is a triple therapy consisting of a PPI, clarithromycin and amoxicillin or metronidazole in a twice-daily simultaneous course. However, there are concerns that this regimen is losing efficacy in some areas of the world, principally driven by an increase in *H. pylori* resistance to clarithromycin. In Central, Western and Southern Europe resistance is now greater than 20%, though in Northern Europe resistance rates are still less than 10%, so clarithromycin-based therapies are still considered appropriate (Megraud et al., 2013). The current NICE (2014a) recommendation is 1 week of therapy, whereas more recent European guidelines recommend 2 weeks of therapy, which is thought to increase eradication by approximately 10% (Malfertheiner et al., 2017). A significant factor in driving resistance is individual exposure to antibiotics; therefore, previous exposure to clarithromycin and metronidazole or quinolone should be checked. Amoxicillin resistance is rare. Data reflecting current recommendations by NICE (2014a) are shown in Tables 12.3 and 12.4. However, the discontinued manufacture of the bismuth containing tripotassium dicitratobismuthate in early 2016 in the UK means that bismuth-based therapies may be difficult to source. An unlicensed alternative is to use bismuth subsalicylate (Pepto-Bismol) (Public Health England, 2016). *H. pylori* eradication for peptic ulcer disease should be confirmed 6–8 weeks after beginning treatment by retesting. If first- and second-line regimens fail, gastric biopsy and sensitivity testing are recommended.

Successful eradication relies on patient adherence to the medication regimen. It is, therefore, important to educate patients about the principles of eradication therapy and also about coping with common adverse effects associated with the regimen. Diarrhoea is the most common adverse effect and should subside after treatment is complete. In rare cases, this can be severe and continue after treatment. If this happens, patients should be advised to return to their doctor because rare cases of antibiotic-associated colitis have been reported. If drugs are not taken as intended, then nonadherence may result in antibiotic resistance. If eradication is successful, uncomplicated active peptic ulcers heal without the need to continue ulcer-healing drugs beyond the duration of eradication therapy (Gisbert et al., 2004).

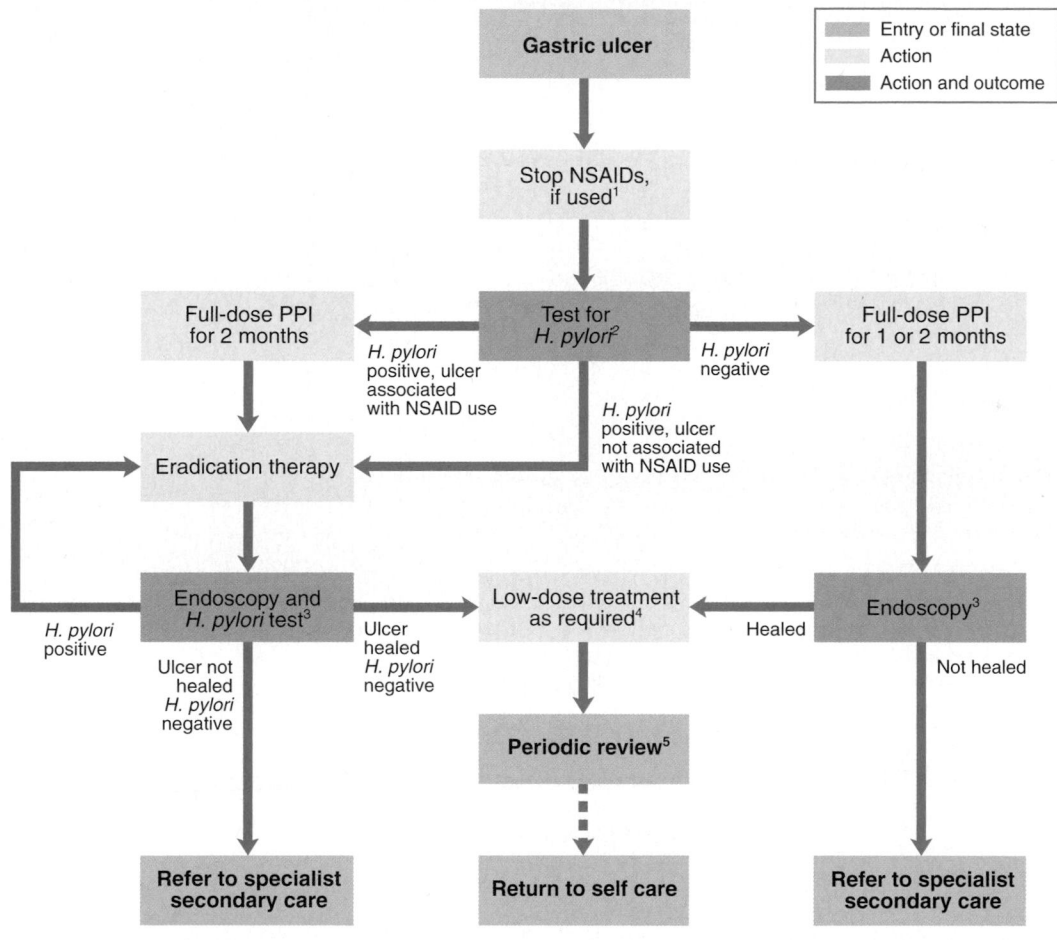

A

1. If NSAID continuation is necessary, after ulcer healing offer long-term gastric protection or consider substitution to a newer COX-2-selective NSAID.
2. Use a carbon-13 urea breath test, stool antigen test or, when performance has been validated, laboratory-based serology.
3. Perform endoscopy 6 to 8 weeks after treatment. If re-testing for *H. pylori* use a carbon-13 urea breath test.
4. Offer low-dose treatment, possibly used on an as-required basis, with a limited number of repeat prescriptions.
5. Review care annually, to discuss symptoms, promote stepwise withdrawal of therapy when appropriate and provide lifestyle advice. In some patients with an inadequate response to therapy it may become appropriate to refer to a specialist.

Fig. 12.5 (A) Management algorithm for gastric ulcer. (B) Management algorithm for duodenal ulcer (NICE, 2014a.). (With permission from NICE.) NSAID, Non-steroidal anti-inflammatory drug.

(Continued)

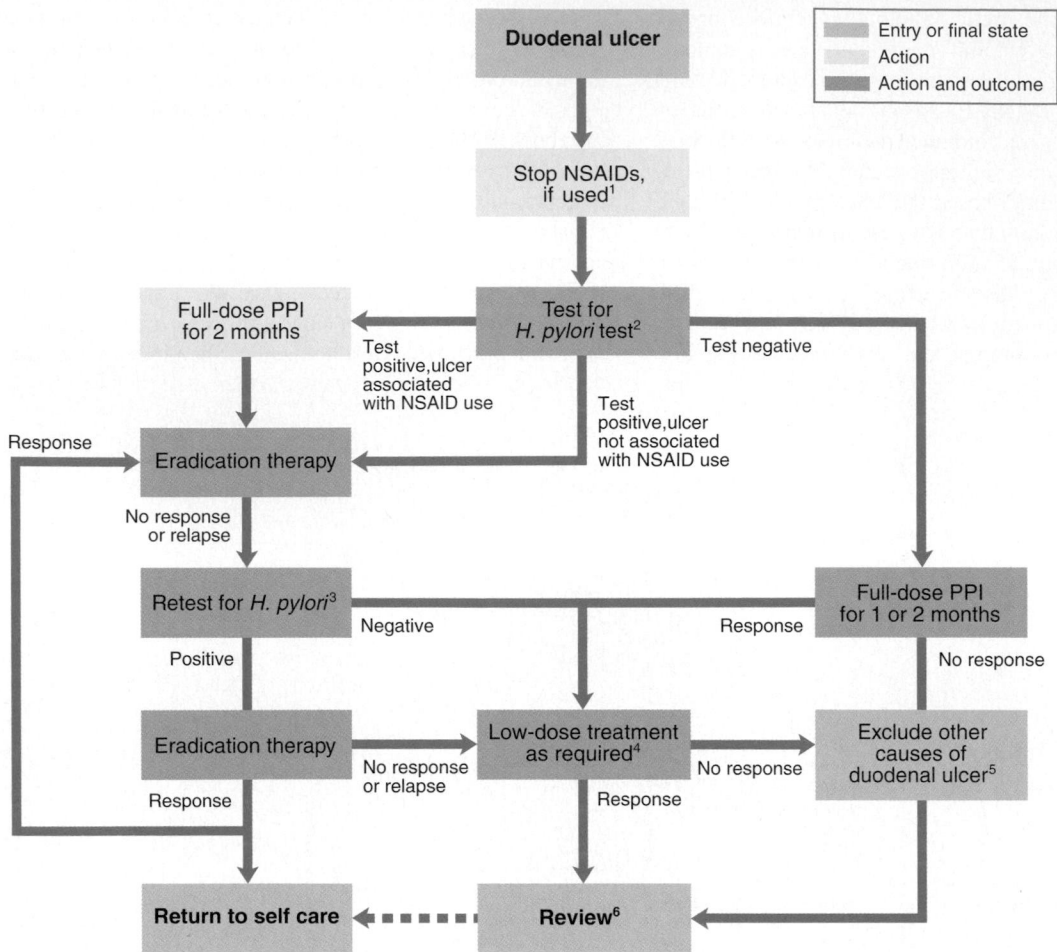

B

1 If NSAID continuation is necessary, after ulcer healing offer long-term gastric protection or consider substitution to a newer COX-2-selective NSAID.

2 Use a carbon-13 urea breath test, stool antigen test or, when performance has been validated, laboratory-based serology.

3 Use a carbon-13 urea breath test.

4 Offer low-dose treatment, possibly used on an as required basis, with a limited number of repeat prescriptions.

5 Consider: non-adherence with treatment, possible malignancy, failure to detect *H. pylori* infection due to recent PPI or antibiotic ingestion, inadequate testing or simple misclassification; surreptitious or inadvertent NSAID or asprin use; ulceration due to ingestion of other drugs; Zollinger-Ellison syndrome, Crohn's disease.

6 Review care annually, to discuss symptoms, promote stepwise withdrawal of therapy when appropriate and provide lifestyle advice.

Fig. 12.5, cont'd.

Table 12.3 *Helicobacter pylori* eradication first-line regimens	
Standard (7 days)	PPI twice a day, amoxicillin 1 g twice a day, clarithromycin 500 mg twice a day Or PPI twice a day, amoxicillin 1 g twice a day metronidazole 400 mg twice a day
Penicillin allergy (7 days)	PPI twice a day, clarithromycin 250 mg twice a day, metronidazole 400 mg twice a day
Penicillin allergy and previous clarithromycin exposure	PPI twice a day, tripotassium dicitratobismuthate (De-nol) 240 mg four times a day[a] tetracycline 500 mg four times a day, metronidazole 400 mg twice a day

[a]Alternatively, bismuth subsalicylate 525 mg four times a day (Pepto-Bismol).
PPI doses for *H. pylori* eradication: esomeprazole 20 mg, lansoprazole 30 mg, omeprazole 20–40 mg, pantoprazole 40 mg, rabeprazole 20 mg.
PPI, Proton pump inhibitor.
See also NICE (2014a).

Table 12.4 *Helicobacter pylori* eradication second-line regimens

Standard (use whichever was not used first line)	PPI twice a day, amoxicillin 1 g twice a day, clarithromycin 500 mg twice a day Or PPI twice a day. amoxicillin 1g twice a day, metronidazole 400 mg twice a day
Previous clarithromycin and metronidazole exposure	PPI twice a day, quinolone twice a day, tetracycline 500 mg twice a day
Penicillin allergy with no previous quinolone exposure	PPI twice a day, metronidazole 400 mg twice a day, levofloxacin 500 mg twice a day
Penicillin allergy with previous quinolone exposure	PPI twice a day, tripotassium dicitratobismuthate (De-nol) 240 mg four times a day,[a] tetracycline 500 mg four times a day, metronidazole 400 mg twice a day

[a]Alternatively, bismuth subsalicylate 525 mg four times a day (Pepto-Bismol).
PPI, Proton pump inhibitor.
PPI doses for *H. pylori* eradication: esomeprazole 20 mg, lansoprazole 30 mg, omeprazole 20–40 mg, pantoprazole 40 mg, rabeprazole 20 mg.
See also NICE (2014a).

Other accepted indications for *H. pylori* eradication include mucosal-associated lymphoid tissue (MALT) lymphoma of the stomach, severe gastritis, and in patients with a high risk of gastric cancer, such as those with a family history of the disease.

Treatment of non-steroidal anti-inflammatory drug-associated ulcers

When NSAIDs are discontinued, most uncomplicated ulcers heal using standard doses of a PPI, H$_2$-receptor antagonist, misoprostol or sucralfate, although in practice, PPIs are used first line. Healing is impaired if NSAID use is continued. Studies have demonstrated conflicting results for comparative healing rates between PPIs and H$_2$-receptor antagonists in this situation (Goldstein et al., 2007; Yeomans et al., 2006). PPIs demonstrate higher healing rates at 4 weeks but similar healing rates to H$_2$-receptor antagonists at 8 weeks. There is no evidence that high-dose PPI is better than treatment with the standard dose. Although effective, misoprostol use is limited by treatment-related adverse events, principally diarrhoea.

Patients should be advised to avoid over-the-counter aspirin and NSAIDs and to use paracetamol-based products. This is probably best facilitated by advising patients to seek pharmacy advice when purchasing over-the-counter analgesic preparations.

Prophylaxis of non-steroidal anti-inflammatory drug ulceration

The most effective way to reduce NSAID-related ulcers is to avoid their use in patients who are at highest risk of gastro-intestinal toxicity (see Box 12.1). However, some patients with chronic rheumatological conditions may require long-term NSAID treatment, in which case the lowest effective dose should be used.

Treatment for ulcer prophylaxis is now considered cost-effective for all patients who require NSAIDs for any period of time, not just in those at high risk (NICE, 2014b). Options include co-therapy with acid-suppressing agents or a synthetic prostaglandin analogue, or substitution of a selective COX-2 inhibitor for

Table 12.5 Drugs for prophylaxis for non-steroidal anti-inflammatory drug-induced ulceration

Drug	Licensed indication	Prophylaxis dose
Omeprazole	Prophylaxis of further DU or GU	20 mg every day
Esomeprazole	Prophylaxis of DU or GU	20 mg every day
Lansoprazole	Prophylaxis of DU or GU	15–30 mg every day
Pantoprazole	Prophylaxis of DU or GU	20 mg daily
Misoprostol	Prophylaxis of DU or GU	200 micrograms 2–4 times a day
Ranitidine	Prophylaxis of DU	150 mg twice a day
Ranitidine	Prophylaxis of DU (unlicensed)	300 mg twice day

DU, Duodenal ulcer; GU, gastric ulcer.

a nonselective NSAID. The prostaglandin analogue misoprostol at a dose of 800 micrograms daily has the strongest evidence of being effective at reducing NSAID-associated ulcer complications and symptomatic ulcers (Rostom et al., 2002). However, it is rarely used in practice because adverse effects, primarily diarrhoea, abdominal pain and nausea, limit its use, and lower doses are less effective. PPIs are effective in reducing endoscopically diagnosed ulcers and symptomatic ulcers. Studies have not demonstrated any advantage in using higher-than-standard doses of PPIs to reduce the risk of ulcers. Standard doses of H$_2$-receptor antagonists (e.g. ranitidine 150 mg twice a day) are effective in reducing the risk of endoscopic duodenal ulcers. However, reduction in the risk of gastric ulcers requires double this dose, and therefore standard-dose ranitidine is not recommended. Gastroprotective agents licensed for prophylaxis of NSAID ulceration are listed in Table 12.5.

In patients with no history of peptic ulcer bleeding but with risk factors, a combination of COX-2 inhibitor with a PPI was found to be similar in efficacy to a combination of nonselective NSAID with a PPI (Scheiman et al., 2006). In patients with a history of ulcer bleeding, a combination of selective COX-2 inhibitor with a PPI reduced recurrent ulcer bleeding compared with COX-2 inhibitor alone (Chan et al., 2007); however, this was not compared with a combination of a nonselective NSAID and a PPI. An earlier study suggested COX-2 inhibitors alone offered similar protection to that offered by a combination of nonselective NSAID with PPI (Lai et al., 2005). However, overall results suggest that in high-risk patients with a history of gastro-intestinal bleeding in whom an NSAID is indicated where alternative analgesic therapies have failed and in whom there are no contraindications to selective COX-2 inhibitors, a combination of PPI with a selective COX-2 inhibitor may be the safest strategy.

Helicobacter pylori and prevention of non-steroidal anti-inflammatory drug–related ulcers

Trials on eradication of *H. pylori* for prevention of NSAID-related ulcers are not consistent in their outcomes, with benefits shown in those patients about to start NSAIDs but not in those already receiving long-term NSAIDs (Malfertheiner et al., 2017). The value of eradication of *H. pylori* in chronic NSAID users is, therefore, unclear. It would be considered mandatory in patients with a prior history of peptic ulcer disease, but the cost-effectiveness of such a strategy is unknown in those patients at low risk of peptic ulcer.

Prophylaxis of gastro-intestinal bleeding during anti-platelet therapy

In low-dose aspirin users, standard-dose PPIs are more effective than high dose H_2-receptor antagonists in preventing recurrent ulcer bleeding following ulcer healing and eradication of *H. pylori* (Ng et al., 2010). However, in those patients who do not have a history of peptic ulcer bleeding, high-dose H_2-receptor antagonists might be an alternative to PPIs (Taha et al., 2009). When the combination of aspirin and clopidogrel is indicated, concomitant PPI therapy has been shown to reduce the risk of ulcer complications (Bhatt et al., 2010).

There is no UK guidance available regarding who should receive prophylaxis with antiplatelet therapy. However, American guidelines suggest a pragmatic approach (Fig. 12.6) by offering prophylaxis to those at highest risk, which includes those on single antiplatelet therapy with a history of gastro-intestinal bleeding or peptic ulcer disease, and all patients with either dual antiplatelet therapy or antiplatelet and anticoagulant (Bhatt et al., 2008).

Helicobacter pylori–negative, non-steroidal anti-inflammatory drug–negative ulcers

Ulceration in the absence of *H. pylori* infection or NSAID or aspirin use is rare, and validation of a negative medication history and *H. pylori* status should be confirmed using biopsy samples and a careful medication history that includes over-the-counter preparations. Many analgesics contain aspirin or NSAIDs, and some patients purchase low-dose aspirin. If both of these are excluded, standard therapy is 4 weeks of a PPI.

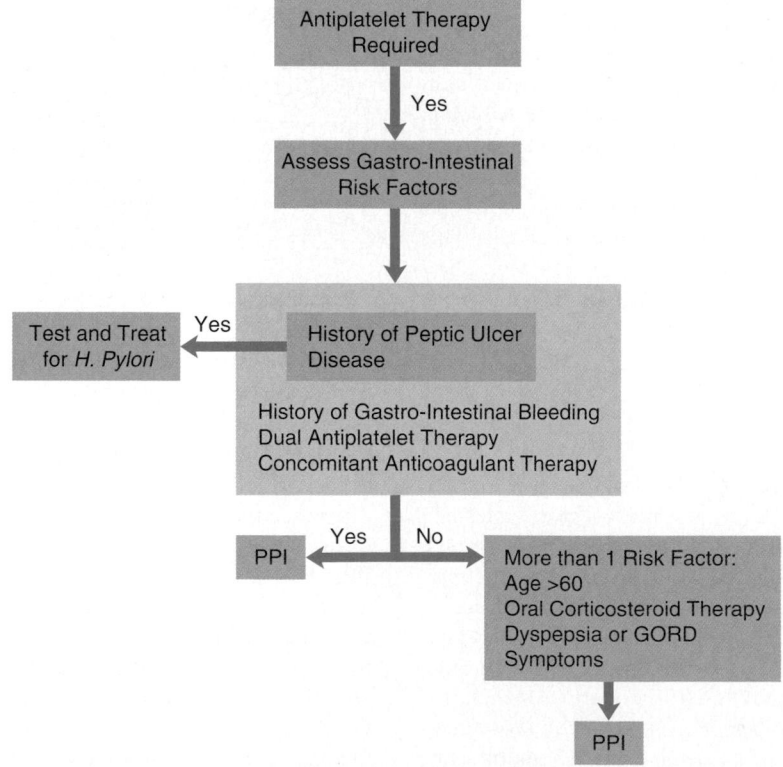

Fig. 12.6 Decision algorithm for gastroprophylaxis with antiplatelet therapy. (Adapted from Bhatt et al., 2008.)

Table 12.6	The Los Angles classification of severity of reflux oesophagitis (Lundell et al., 1999)
Grade A	One or more mucosal breaks <5 mm in maximal length
Grade B	One or more mucosal breaks >5 mm but without continuity across mucosal folds
Grade C	Mucosal breaks continuous between >2 mucosal folds but involving <75% of the oesophageal circumference
Grade D	Mucosal breaks involving >75% of oesophageal circumference

Gastro-oesophageal reflux disease

Table 12.6 describes the classification of oesophagitis severity (Lundell et al., 1999). Reflux disease should be diagnosed on the basis of endoscopy, classifying into those with oesophagitis and those with endoscopy-negative reflux disease (ENRD), no oesophagitis but predominant reflux-like symptoms. A treatment algorithm as described by NICE (2014a) is shown in Fig.12.7. Patients with predominant reflux symptoms but with no prior endoscopy should be managed as undiagnosed dyspepsia. NICE (2014a) defines standard- and high-dose PPI differently when treating severe oesophagitis. Definitions of standard, high and maintenance doses of PPIs are given in Tables 12.7 and 12.8.

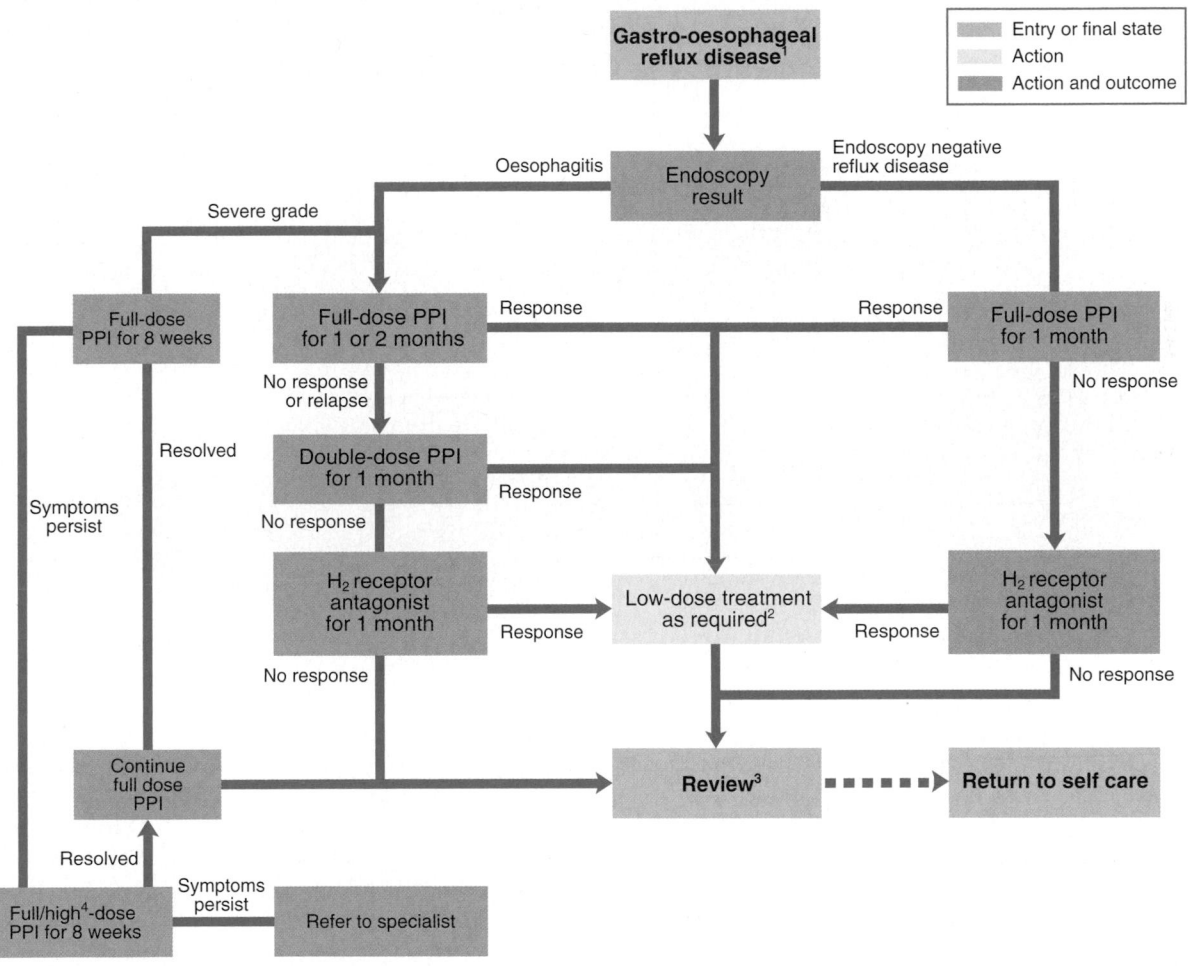

1 GORD refers to endoscopically determined oesophagitis or endoscopy-negative reflux disease. Patients with uninvestigated 'reflux-like' symptoms should be managed as patients with uninvestigated dyspepsia.
There is currently no evidence that *H. pylori* should be investigated in patients with GORD.

2 Offer low-dose treatment, possibly used on an as-required basis, with a limited number of repeat prescriptions.

3 Review long-term patient care at least annually to discuss medication and symptoms.
In some patients with an inadequate response to therapy or new emergent symptoms it may become appropriate to refer to a specialist for a second opinion.

A minority of patients have persistent symptoms despite PPI therapy and this group remains a challenge to treat.
Therapeutic options include adding an H_2 receptor antagonist at bedtime.

4 Consider a high dose of the initial PP, switching to another full-dose PPI or switching to another high-dose PPI.

Fig. 12.7 Management algorithm for gastro-oesophageal reflux disease (NICE, 2014a). (With permission from NICE.)
GORD, Gastro-oesophageal reflux disease; PPI, proton pump inhibitor.

Table 12.7 Definitions of maintenance-, standard- and high-dose proton pump inhibitors for dyspepsia, peptic ulcer disease and gastro-oesophageal reflux disease

PPI	Full/standard dose	Low dose (on-demand dose)	Double dose
Esomeprazole	20 mg[a] once a day	Not available	40 mg[c] once a day
Lansoprazole	30 mg once a day	15 mg once a day	30 mg[b] twice a day
Omeprazole	20 mg once a day	10 mg[b] once a day	40 mg once a day
Pantoprazole	40 mg once a day	20 mg once a day	40 mg[b] twice a day
Rabeprazole	20 mg once a day	10 mg once a day	20 mg[b] twice a day

[a]Lower than the licensed starting dose for esomeprazole in gastro-oesophageal reflux disease (GORD), which is 40 mg, but considered to be dose-equivalent to other proton pump inhibitors (PPIs). When undertaking meta-analysis of dose-related effects, NICE (2014a) classed esomeprazole 20 mg as a full-dose equivalent to omeprazole 20 mg.
[b]Off-label dose for GORD.
[c]40 mg is recommended as a double dose of esomeprazole because the 20 mg dose is considered equivalent to omeprazole 20 mg.
See also NICE, 2014a.

Table 12.8 Definitions of maintenance-, standard- and high-dose proton pump inhibitors for dyspepsia, peptic ulcer disease and gastro-oesophageal reflux disease – severe oesophagitis only

PPI	Full/standard dose	Low dose (on-demand dose)	High/double dose
Esomeprazole	40 mg[a] once a day	20 mg[a] once a day	40 mg[a] twice a day
Lansoprazole	30 mg once a day	15 mg once a day	30 mg[b] twice a day
Omeprazole	40 mg[a] once a day	20 mg[a] once a day	40 mg[a] twice a day
Pantoprazole	40 mg once a day	20 mg once a day	40 mg[b] twice a day
Rabeprazole	20 mg once a day	10 mg once a day	20 mg[b] twice a day

[a]Change from the NICE 2004 dose, specifically for severe oesophagitis, agreed by the guideline development group during the NICE 2014 update.
[b]Off-label dose for gastro-oesophageal reflux disease (GORD).
See also NICE, 2014a.

A 4- to 8-week course of standard-dose PPI therapy is most effective for healing of oesophagitis and in ENRD, being more effective than H$_2$ antagonists (Moayyedi et al., 2011; Sigterman et al., 2013). Extending the course from 4 to 8 weeks increases healing by 14% (NICE, 2014a), and therefore an 8-week course is recommended for endoscopically severe oesophagitis (Los Angeles class C or D; Lundell et al., 1999). If initial courses fail, high-dose PPI, switching PPI, or adding an H$_2$ antagonist at night are options.

For maintenance therapy if symptoms return, intermittent courses can be given or, alternatively, on-demand single doses can be taken immediately as symptoms occur. Patients who relapse frequently may require continuous maintenance therapy using the lowest dose that provides effective symptom relief, although in milder disease, on-demand therapy has been shown to be as effective and as acceptable to patients as continuous maintenance therapy (Pace et al., 2007).

An exception to this is patients with endoscopically severe oesophagitis (Los Angeles class C or D) or oesophageal stricture, who should remain on standard-dose PPI as maintenance. Because uncontrolled acid reflux is thought to be an underlying cause of progression of Barrett's oesophagus to oesophageal adenocarcinoma, patients with Barrett's oesophagus should also continue on standard-dose PPI. *H. pylori* eradication is not recommended in the management of GORD (Malfertheiner et al., 2017).

Prokinetics are no longer licensed for GORD because their evidence of efficacy is poor, and following a safety review, licensed use of domperidone and metoclopramide is now restricted to short-term use in nausea and vomiting only (Medicines and Healthcare Products Regulatory Agency [MHRA], 2013, 2014a). If patients have severe symptoms that are uncontrolled by medical therapy or if there are refractory complications such as recurrent strictures, anti-reflux surgery can be performed after appropriate confirmatory pH and manometry tests.

Functional dyspepsia

Patients with dyspeptic symptoms but with a normal endoscopy are classified as having functional dyspepsia. A treatment algorithm is given in Fig. 12.8. Eradication of *H. pylori*, if present, may improve symptoms and is recommended as

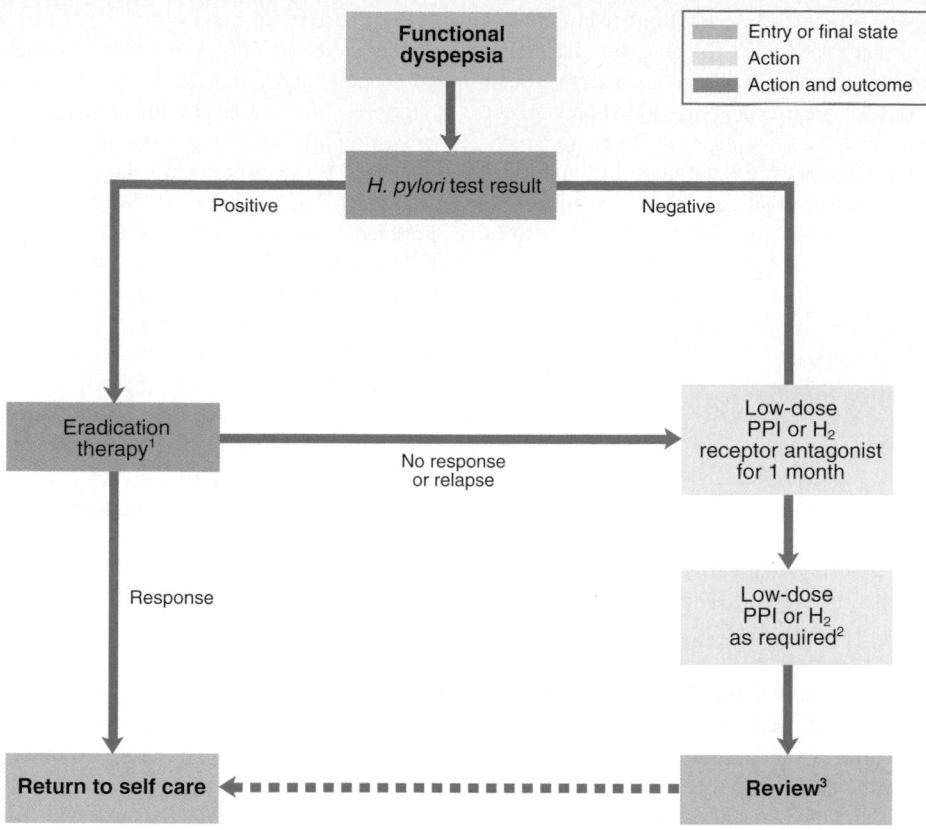

Fig. 12.8 Decision algorithm for management of functional dyspepsia. (With permission from NICE.)

first-line therapy by NICE (2014a). Second-line therapy is low-dose PPI or an H_2 antagonist for 4 weeks, for which there is little difference in efficacy for this indication. As for undiagnosed dyspepsia, if symptoms recur therapy should be tailored to the lowest dose needed to control symptoms. This should include discussing with patients the possibility of using therapy on an 'as-needed' basis to manage their own symptoms.

Pyloric stenosis

Malignancy is the most common cause of gastric outlet obstruction. Peptic ulcer disease is the underlying cause in about 10% of cases. There is limited anecdotal evidence that incomplete gastric outlet obstruction may improve within several months of successful *H. pylori* eradication. Conventional treatment with acid-suppressive therapy may also help. If medical therapy fails to relieve the obstruction, endoscopic balloon dilation or surgery may be required.

Zollinger–Ellison syndrome

Zollinger–Ellison syndrome is a rare syndrome that consists of a triad of non-β islet cell tumours of the pancreas that contain and release gastrin, leading to gastric acid hypersecretion and severe ulcer disease. Extrapancreatic gastrinomas are also common and may be found frequently in the duodenal wall. A proportion of these patients have tumours of the pituitary gland and parathyroid gland (multiple endocrine neoplasia type I). Surgical resection of the gastrinoma may be curative. Medical management consists of greater-than-standard doses of PPIs. The somatostatin analogue octreotide inhibits secretion of gastrin and can be used as a second-line agent.

Stress ulcers

Histamine H_2-receptor antagonists, PPIs, and sucralfate (4–6 g daily in divided doses) have been used to prevent stress ulceration in the intensive care unit until the patient tolerates enteral feeding. UK guidelines recommend the use of either H_2 antagonists or PPIs (orally or intravenously) for acutely ill patients admitted to critical care (NICE, 2012). These agents have been shown to reduce the risk of gastro-intestinal bleeding but not mortality. It is important that the ongoing need for these agents is reviewed when patients recover or are discharged from critical care. Sucralfate is rarely used in practice because of the risk of bezoar formation and the need to administer at different times from other medicines.

Drugs for dyspepsia

Proton pump inhibitors

The PPIs are all benzimidazole derivatives that control gastric acid secretion by inhibition of gastric H^+, K^+-ATPase, the enzyme responsible for the final step in gastric acid secretion from the parietal cell (Fig. 12.9).

The PPIs are inactive prodrugs that are carried in the bloodstream to the parietal cells in the gastric mucosa. The prodrugs readily cross the parietal cell membrane into the cytosol. These drugs are weak bases and therefore have a high affinity for acidic environments. They diffuse across the secretory membrane of the parietal cell into the extracellular secretory canaliculus, the site of the active proton pump (see Fig. 12.9). Under these acidic conditions the prodrugs are converted to their active form, which irreversibly binds the proton pump, inhibiting acid secretion. Because the 'active principle' forms at a low pH, it concentrates selectively in the acidic environment of the proton pump and results in extremely effective inhibition of acid secretion. The different PPIs (omeprazole, esomeprazole, lansoprazole, pantoprazole and rabeprazole) bind to different sites on the proton pump, which may explain their differences in potency on a milligram-per-milligram basis.

PPIs require an enteric coating to protect them from degradation in the acidic environment of the stomach. This delays absorption, and a maximum plasma concentration is reached after 2–3 hours. Because these drugs irreversibly bind to the proton pump, they have a sustained duration of acid inhibition that does not correlate with the plasma elimination half-life of 1–2 hours. The apparent half-life is approximately 48 hours. This prolonged duration of action allows once-daily dosing of PPIs, although twice-daily dosing is recommended in some cases of severe oesophagitis or in *H. pylori* eradication. All PPIs are most effective if taken about 30 minutes before a meal because they inhibit only actively secreting proton pumps, and meals are the main stimulus for proton pump activity.

Intravenous PPIs are most frequently used to prevent recurrent ulcer bleeding in high-risk patients. Intravenous preparations are therapeutically equivalent to oral preparations. In the UK, omeprazole, pantoprazole and esomeprazole can be given intravenously.

PPIs are metabolised in the liver to various sulphate conjugates that are extensively eliminated by the kidneys (80%). With the exception of severe hepatic dysfunction, no dose adjustments are necessary in liver disease or in renal disease. The clinical effect of PPIs is similar among all agents when administered chronically in equivalent standard doses. Their efficacy and relative safety has led them to be first-line agents for treating dyspepsia, GORD and peptic ulcer disease.

Adverse drug reactions

Experience suggests that PPIs are a remarkably safe group of drugs. The most commonly reported side effects are diarrhoea, headaches, abdominal pain, nausea, fatigue and dizziness which resolve on drug discontinuation (Table 12.9). Possible mechanisms for diarrhoea include bacterial overgrowth, changes in intestinal pH and bile salt abnormalities. Some cases of persistent chronic watery diarrhoea associated with lansoprazole have been diagnosed as microscopic colitis, although this may be a class effect.

Although PPIs are very safe on an individual patient basis, the extensive use of PPIs on a population basis has led to some public health concerns. PPIs are associated with an approximately twofold increased risk of *Clostridium difficile*. The absolute risk is low in the general population, with a number needed to harm (NNH) of 3900 at 1 year, but is much greater in high-risk patients such as hospitalised patients receiving antibiotics, where

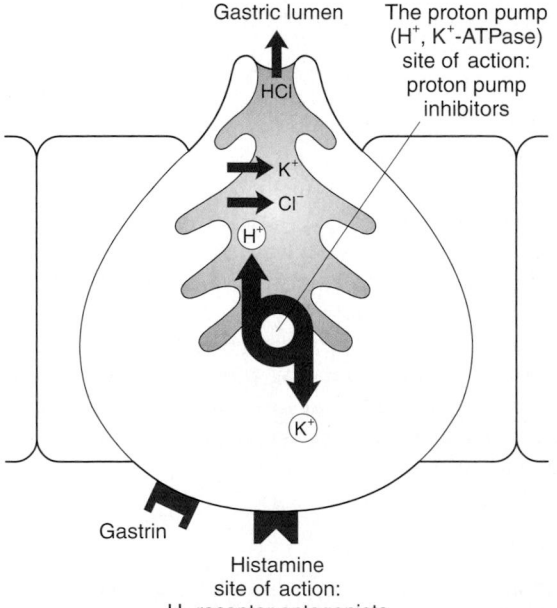

Gastric lumen

The proton pump (H^+, K^+-ATPase) site of action: proton pump inhibitors

HCl

K^+

Cl^-

H^+

K^+

Gastrin

Histamine site of action: H_2 receptor antagonists

Fig. 12.9 Receptor stimulation of acid secretion.

Table 12.9 Common adverse reactions to ulcer-healing drugs

Proton pump inhibitors	H_2-receptor antagonists	Sucralfate
Diarrhoea	Diarrhoea	Constipation
Headache	Headache	
Abdominal pain	Abdominal pain	
Nausea	Confusion	
Fatigue		
Dizziness		

the NNH may be as high as 50 at 2 weeks (Tleyjeh et al., 2012). Long-term use is also associated with an increased risk of hip fractures, although the association is not strong (hazard ratio of fracture 1.28 at 1 year), and the absolute risk is also low, with an NNH of 2000 at 1 year (Khalili et al., 2012).

Drug interactions

The cytochrome P450 isoenzyme CYP2C19 is the main route of metabolism of esomeprazole, lansoprazole, omeprazole and pantoprazole and is also involved in the metabolism of rabeprazole. Omeprazole and esomeprazole are potent inhibitors of CYP2C19, and therefore they may increase the levels of drugs that are metabolised by this isoenzyme. There are, however, relatively few drug interactions of clinical significance. Omeprazole partially inhibits the metabolism of R-warfarin via CYP2C19, and there are isolated case reports of increases in INR with other PPIs.

Omeprazole and esomeprazole at a dose of 40 mg may inhibit the metabolism of phenytoin, but this is unlikely to be clinically relevant.

Absorption of ketoconazole, posaconazole and itraconazole is reduced by omeprazole due to a reduction in acidity required for absorption. This is likely to be a class effect of PPIs, and concomitant use should be avoided. A similar interaction with PPIs reduces absorption of the HIV-protease inhibitors indinavir, nelfinavir and atazanavir, and so concomitant use should be avoided. Conversely, exposure to saquinavir appears to be increased, although the mechanism for this is unknown.

The conversion of clopidogrel to its active form is reliant on CYP2C19, and the inhibition of this activity by omeprazole and esomeprazole may be of concern, although the clinical relevance of this is unclear. The most recent MHRA guidance advises avoidance of concurrent use of esomeprazole and omeprazole, but not other PPIs, acknowledging the lack of clear evidence to support an interaction and the potential benefits of concurrent use in reducing the risk of gastro-intestinal bleeding (MHRA, 2010).

H$_2$-receptor antagonists

The H$_2$-antagonists are all structural analogues of histamine. They competitively block the histamine receptors in gastric parietal cells, thereby preventing acid secretion. Pepsinogen requires acid for conversion to pepsin, and so when acid output is reduced, pepsin generation is, in turn, also reduced.

All the available drugs (cimetidine, ranitidine, famotidine, nizatidine) have similar properties. Maximum plasma concentration is reached within 1–3 hours after administration. First-pass hepatic metabolism varies; ranitidine is most extensively metabolised, which explains the difference between the intravenous and oral dose. All H$_2$-antagonists are eliminated to a variable and significant extent via the kidneys, and all require dosage reduction in moderate to severe renal impairment. They are equally effective at suppressing daytime and nocturnal acid secretion, and they do not cause total achlorhydria. The evening dose of an H$_2$-antagonist is particularly important because during the daytime, gastric acid is buffered for long periods by food; however, during the night this does not occur, and the intragastric pH may fall below 2.0 for several hours. For healing oesophagitis, intragastric pH must

remain above 4.0 for 18 hours or more per day. H$_2$-receptor antagonists are, therefore, less effective in healing oesophagitis. Adding a bedtime dose of H$_2$-receptor antagonist to PPI therapy may enhance nocturnal gastric pH control in patients in whom nocturnal gastric acid breakthrough is problematic.

The role of H$_2$-receptor antagonists in the management of dyspepsia has diminished because PPIs are more effective and generally recommended as first line. They do provide an alternative or addition in those unresponsive to PPIs, and their availability for purchase means they still have a role to play in self-management of dyspepsia.

Adverse drug reactions

H$_2$-receptor antagonists are a safe group of drugs. The risk of any adverse reaction is below 3%, and serious adverse reactions account for less than 1%. Diarrhoea and headache are the most common, and occasionally mental confusion and rashes have been reported (see Table 12.9). Hepatotoxicity is a rare adverse effect. Cimetidine, due to its antiandrogenic effects, has been associated with gynaecomastia and impotence when used in high doses.

Drug interactions

Cimetidine is a nonspecific, weak inhibitor of a number of the cytochrome P450 isoenzymes and therefore inhibits the metabolism of many drugs, which is potentially important for drugs with a narrow therapeutic index. Clinically relevant interactions are established for theophylline, warfarin, and phenytoin. The other H$_2$ antagonists do not inhibit cytochrome P450 to a clinically relevant extent, and for this reason, cimetidine is now rarely used in practice.

The absorption of some drugs may be affected by the changes in gastric pH that can be produced by any of the H$_2$-receptor antagonists. Clinically relevant examples include reduction of posaconazole and atazanavir absorption.

Bismuth chelate

Bismuth has been included in antacid mixtures for many decades but fell from favour because of its neurotoxicity. Bismuth chelate is a relatively safe form of bismuth that has ulcer-healing properties comparable to those of H$_2$-antagonists. Its mode of action is not clearly understood, but it is thought to have cytoprotective properties. Bismuth is toxic to *H. pylori* and was one of the first agents to be used to eradicate the organism and reduce ulcer recurrence. Tripotassium dicitratobismuthate in combination with tetracycline, metronidazole and a PPI has been used in quadruple-therapy regimens in patients resistant to triple therapy, although manufacture of this agent in the UK ceased in early 2016. An alternative is to use bismuth subsalicylate (Pepto-Bismol) (Public Health England, 2016).

Adverse drug reactions

Small amounts of bismuth are absorbed from bismuth chelate, and urinary bismuth excretion may be raised for several weeks after a course of treatment. The risk of bismuth intoxication is small if these products are used at the recommended dose and for short courses of treatment. Bismuth may accumulate in patients with impaired renal function. The most commonly reported events are nausea, vomiting, blackened tongue and dark faeces.

Sucralfate

Sucralfate is the aluminium salt of sucrose octasulphate. Although it is a weak antacid, this is not its principal mode of action in peptic ulcer disease. It has mucosal protective effects, including stimulation of bicarbonate and mucus secretion and stimulation of mucosal prostanoids. At a pH less than 4.0, it forms a sticky, viscid gel that adheres to the ulcer surface and may afford some physical protection. It is capable of adsorbing bile salts. These activities appear to reside in the entire molecular complex and are not due to the aluminium ions alone. Sucralfate has no acid-suppressing activity. Sucralfate is now less commonly used in practice due to the practicalities of managing other medicines and because of the risk of bezoar formation (an undigested mass trapped in the gastro-intestinal tract). When prescribed, the liquid formulation is often used because the tablets are large and difficult to swallow.

Adverse drug reactions

Constipation appears to be the most common problem with sucralfate, and this is thought to be related to the aluminium content (see Table 12.9). About 3–5% of a dose is absorbed, and therefore there is a risk of aluminium toxicity with long-term treatment. This risk is correspondingly greater in patients with renal impairment. Caution is required to avoid oesophageal bezoar formation around a nasogastric tube in patients managed in the intensive care unit.

Drug interactions

Sucralfate may bind to other agents in the gastro-intestinal tract and reduce the absorption of other drugs. Therefore, it should be taken at least 2 hours following other medicines.

Antacids

Antacids have a place in symptomatic relief of dyspepsia, in particular, self-management. The choice of antacid lies between aluminium-based and magnesium-based products, although many proprietary products combine both. Calcium-based products are less suitable because calcium stimulates acid secretion. Antacids containing sodium bicarbonate are unsuitable for regular use because they deliver a high sodium load and generate large quantities of carbon dioxide. It should be noted that magnesium trisilicate mixtures contain a large amount of sodium bicarbonate. Some products contain other agents, such as dimethicone or alginates. Products containing sodium alginate with a mixture of antacids are effective in relief of symptoms in GORD but are not particularly effective antacids.

Antacids provide immediate symptom relief, and a more rapid response is achieved with liquid preparations. They have a limited duration of action and need to be taken several times a day, usually after meals (to coincide with peak acid production) and at bedtime.

Adverse drug reactions

Aluminium-based antacids cause constipation, and magnesium-based products cause diarrhoea. When combination products are used, diarrhoea tends to predominate as a side effect. Although these are termed 'non-absorbable', a proportion of aluminium and magnesium is absorbed and the potential for toxicity exists, particularly with coexistent renal failure.

Drug interactions

Administration should be separate from drugs with potential for chelation, such as tetracycline and ciprofloxacin, and also pH-dependent controlled-release products.

Case studies

Case 12.1

A 62-year-old man, Mr BD, presented to the emergency department following haematemesis and melaena. He was suffering no pain. His past medical history included non-ST-elevated myocardial infarction (NSTEMI) for which he had undergone percutaneous coronary intervention (PCI) and bare metal stent insertion 4 months previously. Mr BD stopped smoking 2 years ago, drinks alcohol in moderation and is not obese. He is prescribed the following prescribed medicines:

- aspirin (dispersible) 75 mg daily,
- clopidogrel 75 mg daily,
- ramipril 2.5 mg twice daily,
- atorvastatin 80 mg daily,
- bisoprolol 5 mg daily,
- GTN spray prn.

On investigation, Mr BD's blood pressure was 98/60 mmHg with a heart rate of 120 beats/min and respiratory rate of 20 beats/min. There was no jaundice or stigmata of liver disease. Mr BD's blood results were as follows:

	Value	Reference range
Urea	18 mmol/L	3.1–7.9 mmol/L
Creatinine	87 mmol/L	75–155 mmol/L
INR	1.0	
Sodium	142 mmol/L	135–145 mmol/L
Potassium	4.3 mmol/L	3.4–5.0 mmol/L
Haemoglobin	8 g/dL	13.5–18 g/dL
MCV	90 fL	78–100 fL

Endoscopy revealed an actively bleeding gastric ulcer.

Questions

1. What immediate treatment should Mr BD have received before endoscopy?
2. What treatment should he receive at the time of endoscopy?
3. Why should biopsies be taken at the time of endoscopy?
4. What pharmacological treatment should be given to Mr BD to reduce the risk of re-bleeding following endoscopic haemostatic therapy?

5. What was the likely cause of Mr BD's bleeding ulcer?
6. When should antiplatelet therapy be restarted, and which agent(s) should be prescribed?
7. Should Mr BD receive gastroprotection following ulcer healing?
8. Identify what aspects of Mr BD's medicines you would want to discuss with him.

· ·

Answers

1. Mr BD's age, comorbidity and clinical signs of shock place him at risk of death and in need of emergency hospital admission for aggressive resuscitation with intravenous fluids and red blood cell transfusion. Crystalloid solutions should be used for volume restoration before administering blood products. Sodium chloride 0.9% is appropriate fluid replacement. There is no evidence to support the use of intravenous PPIs before diagnosis by endoscopy.

2. Patients who are in shock and have active peptic ulcer bleeding are at high risk of continuing to bleed and should receive haemostatic endoscopic therapy. Endoscopic treatment is indicated only for those with high-risk lesions (active bleeding, nonbleeding visible vessels or adherent blood clot). Endoscopic injection of large volume (at least 13 mL) 1:10,000 adrenaline achieves haemostasis through vasoconstriction, and haemostasis is sustained if this is combined with thermal coagulation or mechanical endoscopic clipping. The patient should receive combination endoscopic therapy.

3. The presence of *H. pylori* should be sought at the time of endoscopy. Biopsies should be taken from the antrum and the body of the stomach. Samples are sent for testing for the presence of malignant cells, and samples are used for the rapid urease test for *H. pylori*. The presence of bleeding may reduce the sensitivity of the rapid urease test, and if negative results are obtained, a urea breath test or stool sample can be undertaken once oral intake is established.

4. In patients who have received endoscopic haemostatic therapy, high-dose intravenous PPI therapy reduces the risk of re-bleeding. The optimum dose and route are unclear, but improved mortality is observed in high-risk patients when a dose of 80 mg bolus followed by 8 mg/h infusion for 72 hours is given. Maintaining intragastric pH above 6 is considered to stabilise clot formation and prevent re-bleeding. Because a positive test for *H. pylori* was obtained, oral eradication therapy should be given, although there is no evidence to suggest this must be given in the acute phase; therefore, the usual practice is to wait until oral intake is established. *H. pylori* eradication therapy is effective in the prevention of re-bleeding from peptic ulcer. Ulcer healing can be achieved with an additional 3-week treatment with standard-dose PPI.

5. Mr BD was taking dual antiplatelet therapy to reduce the risk of myocardial infarction and cardiovascular death. Both of these agents carry an increased risk of bleeding events, the risk being additive with dual therapy. Mr BD did not have any additional risk factors for peptic ulcer disease, but it is important to take a careful medication history to identify if he had been taking NSAID analgesics and ensure he avoids such medicines in the future. The bleeding peptic ulcer was likely caused by the combination of aspirin and clopidogrel.

6. In patients with NSTEMI, most benefit is gained from the addition of clopidogrel to aspirin therapy in the first 3 months (CURE Study Investigators, 2001). Prolonged treatment for 12 months is indicated if a drug-eluting stent is inserted, but because this patient had a bare metal stent inserted 4 months previously, the benefit from the addition of clopidogrel probably does not outweigh the gastro-intestinal bleeding risk, and consideration should be given to discontinuation of clopidogrel. Aspirin should be continued at a dose of 75 mg daily. There is no evidence to suggest enteric coating

is of any benefit, so the dispersible formulation should be continued. It is suggested that aspirin should be restarted within 7 days of discontinuation to maintain cardiovascular secondary prevention.

7. Mr BD should be prescribed the standard dose of PPI as maintenance therapy to reduce the risk of further aspirin-induced gastro-intestinal bleeding.

8. Mr BD needs to be aware of both his cardiovascular and gastro-intestinal risks. He does need to continue aspirin, but he should be aware of the need to discontinue clopidogrel now because it is 4 months following his NSTEMI, and the benefit does not outweigh the risk. He should be advised not to take any other aspirin or NSAID-containing medicines. If the test for *H. pylori* is positive, Mr BD should be prescribed 7 days of treatment with a twice-daily PPI, such as omeprazole 20 mg, amoxicillin 1 g and clarithromycin 500 mg, after ascertaining he is not penicillin sensitive and checking for recent antibiotic use. The importance of this treatment in prevention of re-bleeding should be emphasised to encourage adherence to the prescribed course, which he may complete after discharge from hospital. Aspirin will be restarted, and the dose of omeprazole will be reduced to 20 mg daily long-term for gastroprotection after any *H. pylori* eradication.

Case 12.2

A 68-year-old male, Mr MF, presents with melaena. He has a past medical history of atrial fibrillation and hypertension. On examination, Mr MF is pale and clammy, with a blood pressure of 95/60 mmHg and a pulse of 110 beats/min with a Blatchford score of 11. His drug history is recorded as follows:
- warfarin 4 mg daily,
- amlodipine 5 mg daily,
- simvastatin 40 mg daily.

Mr MF's blood results were as follows:

	Value	Reference range
Sodium	140 mmol/L	135–145 mmol/L
Potassium	3.9 mmol/L	3.4–5.0 mmol/L
Urea	11.5 mmol/L	3.1–7.9 mmol/L
Creatinine	90 mmol/L	75–155 mmol/L
WCC	7.6×10^9/L	$3.5–11 \times 10^9$/L
MCV	90 fL	78–100 fL
INR	2.8	
Haemoglobin	10.5 g/dL	13.5–18 g/dL

The impression is that Mr MF has had an upper gastro-intestinal bleed. The plan is for Mr MF to undergo reversal of anticoagulation, resuscitation with intravenous fluids and then an urgent endoscopy.

· ·

Questions

1. If you were confirming Mr MF's medication history, what particular aspects should be checked?
2. How should warfarin be reversed?
3. An endoscopy reveals Mr MF has a bleeding duodenal ulcer for which he receives a 72-hour PPI infusion. A *H. pylori* test is negative. How should Mr MF's anticoagulation be managed?

· ·

Answers

1. Mr MF should be asked about potential over-the-counter use of aspirin or NSAIDs; this is often missed because they have not been prescribed. If Mr MF has been using these medicines, then he should be advised to avoid future use.

2. For active bleeding, warfarin should be reversed even though Mr MF'S INR is within the therapeutic range. This is undertaken by administration of 5 mg intravenous vitamin K and prothrombin complex 25–50 units/kg.

3. As the risk of re-bleeding is highest within the first 72 hours following endoscopy, in this case, it would be advisable to withhold anticoagulation at least until this point. When the risk of thrombus is higher, for example, in metallic valve or recent pulmonary embolism (PE), anticoagulation may be restarted once the patient is stable using heparin or low-molecular-weight heparin. With regard to restarting warfarin in this patient with atrial fibrillation, the risk of stroke can be calculated using the CHA2DS2-VASC score, and the risk of bleeding can be calculated using the HAS-BLED score. These figures can be used to help Mr MF make an informed decision about his preferences for restarting anticoagulation. If warfarin is to be restarted, it would be reasonable to continue a PPI long-term for gastroprotection.

Case 12.3

A 57-year-old woman, Mrs MG, presents to her primary care doctor with symptoms of epigastric pain that have interfered with her normal activities over the previous few weeks. Medication history reveals that Mrs MG takes no prescribed medicines and only occasional paracetamol as an analgesic for minor ailments. Although she has occasional heartburn, this is not the predominant symptom. Mrs MG has not vomited and does not have difficulty or pain on swallowing. She has not lost weight recently and has normal stools with no evidence of bleeding. The pain is not precipitated by exercise and does not radiate to the arms and neck. Mrs MG is a nonsmoker and only drinks a small quantity of alcohol on social occasions. She is not overweight. She has an allergy to penicillin.

....

Questions

1. How should Mrs MG be treated?
2. Which *H. pylori* test should be used in primary care?

....

Answers

1. It is important to ascertain if Mrs MG has ALARM features (see Box 12.3), which should be investigated particularly because her age places her at higher risk of gastro-intestinal cancer. It is also important to consider differential diagnoses such as cardiac pain, although the lack of radiation and lack of link with exertion suggests a cardiac cause is unlikely. Because she has no ALARM features, she can be treated following the pathway for uninvestigated dyspepsia. Because there are no obvious medication-related causes or lifestyle-related factors to address, an initial strategy of testing and treating for *H. pylori* or a month of PPI would be appropriate. If her *H. pylori* test is positive, a 7-day course of twice-daily eradication therapy of omeprazole 20 mg, metronidazole 400 mg and clarithromycin 250 or 500 mg can be prescribed. Mrs MG should be advised to complete the course of therapy to avoid eradication failure and/or resistance to antibiotics. The potential interaction between metronidazole and alcohol should be explained to the patient in terms of the risk of nausea, vomiting, flushing and breathlessness, which may occur during and for a few days after discontinuing metronidazole. Mrs MG should also be alerted to the common adverse effect of diarrhoea associated with triple therapy. Patients should be encouraged to cope with the inconvenience but report symptoms to their doctor if they continue after the course of treatment is finished. If neither *H. pylori*

eradication nor a month of PPI is successful, Mrs MG should be offered H$_2$ antagonist therapy.

2. The most accurate noninvasive *H. pylori* test is the carbon-13 urea breath test. Alternative tests are the stool antigen test and a laboratory-based serology test. Local facilities and costs determine the choice of tests. Serology tests based on measurement of serum antibody are commonly used for initial detection of *H. pylori* but cannot be used to confirm eradication because circulating antibody remains after removal of the antigen.

Case 12.4

A 68-year-old woman, Ms WR, presents for review of her medication. Her medical history includes hypertension and osteoarthritis of the knees. Ms WR receives a regular prescription for the following:
- bendroflumethiazide 2.5 mg daily,
- naproxen 500 mg twice daily.

Ms WR stopped smoking 4 years ago and drinks no more than 10 units of alcohol per week. She is overweight, with a body mass index (BMI) of 30 kg/m^2. Ms WR occasionally purchases an antacid to treat symptoms of heartburn if she's eaten a large meal at night. Her blood pressure is 148/92 mmHg with a pulse of 82 beats/min. The results of Ms WR's routine blood tests are as follows:

	Value	Reference range
Sodium	138 mmol/L	135–145 mmol/L
Potassium	3.9 mmol/L	3.4–5.0 mmol/L
Creatinine	110 mmol/L	75–155 mmol/L
Blood glucose	6.8 mmol/L	<11.1 mmol/L
Total cholesterol	4.5 mmol/L	<4.0 mmol/L
Haemoglobin	12.0 g/dL	11.5–16.5 g/dL

....

Questions

1. What is the mechanism for NSAID-induced peptic ulcer disease?
2. What are the risks associated with NSAID use in this patient?
3. What are the options for treating Ms WR's pain and minimising the risk of peptic ulceration?

....

Answers

1. NSAIDs cause superficial erosions, but the main mechanism for causing ulcers is through their systemic inhibition of mucosal prostaglandin production. COX-1 is the enzyme responsible for the synthesis of prostaglandins responsible for gastro-intestinal mucosal protection through maintenance of blood flow and production of mucus and bicarbonate. Another isoform of COX, COX-2 is involved in the inflammatory response, and the prostaglandins produced are associated with pain and inflammation. The anti-inflammatory action of NSAIDs is thought to be as a result of inhibition of COX-2. Inhibition of COX-1 is thought to be responsible for the gastro-intestinal and renal adverse effects of NSAIDs.

2. Patients older than 60 years of age are at higher risk of peptic ulcer complications than their younger counterparts, and the risk is much higher in those above 75 years of age (Hernandez-Diaz and Rodriguez, 2000). Other risk factors include a previous history of peptic ulcer disease, in particular, peptic ulcer bleeding. Dyspepsia symptoms do not correlate with those who develop peptic ulcer disease and are, therefore, not a risk factor and can be treated symptomatically. Concomitant drug therapy, such as aspirin, corticosteroids and anticoagulants, increases the risk of peptic ulcer complications. In this case, the patient's age places Ms WR

at risk, and therefore the benefits of the NSAID should be weighed against the risks and potential options for risk management considered. Age is also a risk factor for NSAID-induced decrease in renal perfusion caused by inhibition of prostaglandin-stimulated renal blood flow, a compensatory mechanism that is activated when renal perfusion is impaired. Withdrawal of NSAID therapy can improve renal perfusion and associated haemodynamic effects such as hypertension.

3. The safest option for Ms WR is to manage the pain with regular use of a paracetamol-based product and to withdraw the NSAID, thus removing the risk of peptic ulcer disease but also removing the potential detrimental effect the NSAID may have on blood pressure because the patient is just above the target for blood pressure control. Weight loss may also help reduce the burden on her knees and may also have some positive effect on Ms WR's blood pressure. The relative risk of ulcer complications has been compared among groups of NSAIDs, with naproxen being of intermediate risk (García Rodríguez and Jick, 1994). Different NSAIDs vary in their selectivity for COX isoenzymes and may account for the relative toxicities observed. Selective COX-2 inhibitors are associated with low risk but are contraindicated in patients with cardiovascular disease because they have been associated with an increased incidence of myocardial infarction. However, some other nonselective NSAIDs have also been associated with thrombotic risk, although naproxen seems to have the lowest risk and so is an appropriate choice of NSAID if indicated in this patient (Trelle et al., 2011). There is no clear evidence to test for and eradicate *H. pylori* in chronic NSAID users. An assessment of Ms WR's pain should be undertaken, and the risks associated with naproxen use should be explained. Ms WR may be willing to change to regular paracetamol with the addition of codeine if necessary. Otherwise adding a standard dose of PPI to naproxen reduces the gastrointestinal risks but not the renal risks.

Case 12.5

Mr LP, aged 64 years, is attending a medication review clinic. While discussing any concerns Mr LP has about his medication, he mentions that he suffers from heartburn. On further questioning, Mr LP explains that his heartburn has been recently getting worse, and that food occasionally "gets stuck" when he is eating. Mr LP has a past medical history of hypertension, angina and heart failure. He lives alone and smokes 30–40 cigarettes per day. Mr LP's medication history is as follows:

- aspirin 75 mg daily,
- ramipril 5 mg twice a day,
- furosemide 40 mg each morning,
- amlodipine 5 mg each morning,
- isosorbide mononitrate MR 30 mg each morning,
- simvastatin 40 mg at night,
- GTN spray 1–2 sprays when required.

Despite changing his angina medication to a β-blocker, Mr LP's symptoms did not resolve, and in view of his dysphagia, he was admitted for endoscopy. It has been 4 weeks since Mr LP's hospital admission (2 months since you last saw him). His current medication is as follows:

- bisoprolol 5 mg each morning,
- furosemide 40 mg each morning,
- ramipril 5 mg twice a day,
- lansoprazole 30 mg each morning.

The interim discharge note states that the endoscopy found a grade B oesophagitis. However, there is no information as to the course length required for Mr LP's PPI.

Questions

1. What nonmedication advice can you offer Mr LP?
2. What recommendations could you make regarding Mr LP's drug therapy?
3. Does Mr LP require any further investigation at this stage?
4. How long should the PPI be continued at the treatment dose?
5. Will Mr LP require any further treatment once he has finished the course of treatment-dose PPI?

Answers

1. Lifestyle advice can be offered. Smoking cessation may help symptoms of dyspepsia. If Mr LP is overweight, weight reduction may also help. Other options include exploring dietary intake for potential triggers. Avoiding eating late at night and using extra pillows to prop up his head at night may potentially help Mr LP's reflux-like symptoms, although there is no evidence to support this strategy.
2. Calcium channel blockers and nitrates can lower oesophageal sphincter pressure and could, therefore, be contributing to his heartburn. Alternatives, such as a β-blocker, for his angina could be explored.
3. Mr LP describes symptoms of dysphagia, which is an ALARM symptom. Therefore, although the previous options could be explored, he should be referred as soon as possible for an endoscopy. Dysphagia could represent an underlying oesophageal stricture or tumour.
4. Because Mr LP has confirmed oesophagitis, 1–2 months of treatment-dose PPI should be offered. Because Mr LP has now had a month of treatment, you should discuss with him whether he has any continuing symptoms. If he does, it would be appropriate for the PPI to be continued at the treatment dose for a further month.
5. Initially, treatment could be stopped, although GORD is a chronic disease, with approximately two-thirds of patients requiring further treatment. If Mr LP's symptoms recur, treatment should be offered at the lowest dose that controls symptoms. The option of Mr LP taking the PPI on an on-demand basis (i.e. taking PPI only when symptoms occur) could be considered.

Acknowledgment

The author acknowledges the contribution of M. Kinnear to versions of this chapter that appeared in previous editions.

References

Barkun, A.N., Bardou, M., Kuipers, E.J., et al., 2010. International consensus recommendations on the management of patients with nonvariceal upper gastro-intestinal bleeding. Ann. Intern. Med. 152, 101–113.

Bhatt, D., Scheiman, J., Abraham, N., et al., 2008. ACCF/ACG/AHA 2008 Expert consensus document on reducing the gastrointestinal risks of antiplatelet therapy and NSAID use a report of the American College of Cardiology Foundation Task Force on clinical expert consensus documents. J. Am. Coll. Cardiol. 52, 1502–1517.

Bhatt, D.L., Cryer, B.L., Contant, C.F., et al., 2010. Clopidogrel with or without omeprazole in coronary artery disease. N. Engl. J. Med. 36, 1909–1917.

Blatchford, O., Murray, W.R., Blatchford, M., 2000. A risk score to predict need for treatment for upper-gastrointestinal haemorrhage. Lancet 356, 1318–1321.

Chan, F.K.L., Wong, V.W.S., Suen, B.Y., et al., 2007. Combination of a cyclo-oxygenase-2 inhibitor and a proton-pump inhibitor for prevention of recurrent ulcer bleeding in patients at very high risk: a double-blind, randomised trial. Lancet 369, 1621–1626.

CURE Study Investigators, 2001. Effects of Clopidogrel in addition to aspirin in patients with acute coronary syndromes without ST-segment elevation. N. Engl. J. Med. 345, 494–502.

European Medicines Agency (EMA), 2013. PRAC recommends the same cardiovascular precautions for diclofenac as for selective COX-2 inhibitors. Available at: http://www.ema.europa.eu/docs/en_GB/document_library/Referrals_document/Diclofenac-containing_medicinal_products/Recommendation_provided_by_Pharmacovigilance_Risk_Assessment_Committee/WC500144452.pdf.

Ford, A.C., Gurusamy, K., Delaney, B., Forman, D., et al., 2016. Eradication therapy for peptic ulcer disease in Helicobacter pylori positive patients. Cochrane DB Syst. Rev. 2016 (4), Art. No. CD003840.

Ford, A.C., Moayyedi, P., 2013. Dyspepsia. BMJ 347, f5059.

Ford, A.C., Moayyedi, P., Jarbol, D.E., et al., 2008. Meta-analysis: Helicobacter pylori 'test and treat' compared with empirical acid suppression for managing dyspepsia. Aliment Pharmacol. Ther. 28, 534–544.

García Rodríguez, L.A., Jick, H., 1994. Risk of upper gastrointestinal bleeding and perforation associated with individual non-steroidal anti-inflammatory drugs. Lancet 343, 769–772.

García Rodríguez, L.A., Lin, J.K., Hernandez-Diaz, S., et al., 2011. Risk of upper gastrointestinal bleeding with low-dose acetylsalicylic acid alone and in combination with clopidogrel and other medications. Circulation 123, 1108–1115.

Gisbert, J.P., Khorrami, S., Carballo, F., et al., 2004. Helicobacter pylori eradication therapy vs. antisecretory non-eradication therapy (with or without long-term maintenance antisecretory therapy) for the prevention of recurrent bleeding from peptic ulcer. Cochrane DB Syst. Rev. 2004 (2), Art No. CD004062. https://doi.org/10.1002/14651858.CD004062.pub2.

Goldstein, J.L., Johanson, J.F., Hawkey, C.J., et al., 2007. Clinical trial: healing of NSAID-associated gastric ulcers in patients continuing NSAID therapy – a randomised study comparing ranitidine with esomeprazole. Aliment. Pharmacol. Ther. 26, 1101–1111.

Hearnshaw, S.A., Logan, R.F., Lowe, D., et al., 2011. Acute upper gastrointestinal bleeding in the UK: patient characteristics, diagnoses and outcomes in the 2007 UK audit. Gut 60, 1327–1335.

Hernandez-Diaz, S., Rodriguez, L.A., 2000. Association between non-steroidal anti-inflammatory drugs and upper gastro intestinal tract bleeding/perforation: an overview of epidemiologic studies published in the 1990s. Arch. Intern. Med. 160 (14), 2093–2099.

Hooper, L., Brown, T.J., Elliott, R.A., et al., 2004. The effectiveness of five strategies for the prevention of gastro-intestinal toxicity induced by non-steroidal anti-inflammatory drugs: systematic review. BMJ 329, 948–952.

Katz, P., Gerson, L., Vela, M., 2013. Guidelines for the diagnosis and management of gastroesophageal reflux disease. Am J Gastroenterol. 108, 308–328.

Keeling, D., Baglin, T., Tait, C., et al., 2011. Guidelines on oral anticoagulation with warfarin (4th ed.). Br. J. Haematol. 154 (3), 311–324.

Khalili, H., Huang, E., Jacobson, B., et al., 2012. Use of proton pump inhibitors and risk of hip fracture in relation to dietary and lifestyle factors: a prospective cohort study. BMJ 344, e372.

Kuipers, E.J., 1997. Helicobacter pylori and the risk and management of associated diseases: gastritis, ulcer disease, atrophic gastritis and gastric cancer. Aliment Pharmacol. Ther. 11 (Suppl. 1), 71–88.

Lai, K.C., Chu, K.M., Hui, W.M., et al., 2005. Celecoxib compared with lansoprazole and naproxen to prevent gastro-intestinal ulcer complications. Am. J. Med. 118, 1271–1278.

Lai, K.C., Lam, S.K., Chu, K.M., et al., 2002. Lansoprazole for the prevention of recurrences of ulcer complications from long-term low dose aspirin use. N. Engl. J. Med. 346, 2033–2038.

Langman, M.J., Weil, J., Wainwright, P., et al., 1994. Risks of bleeding peptic ulcer associated with individual non-steroidal anti-inflammatory drugs. Lancet 343 (8905), 1075–1078.

Lanza, F.L., Chan, F.K., Quigley, E.M., 2009. Practice parameters Committee of the American College of Gastroenterology 2009 guidelines for prevention of NSAID-related ulcer complications. Am. J. Gastroenterol. 104, 728–738.

Leontiadis, G.I., Sharma, V.K., Howden, C.W., 2010. Proton pump inhibitor treatment for acute peptic ulcer bleeding. Cochrane Database Syst. Rev. 2010 (5), Art. No. CD002094.

Lundell, L., Dent, J., Bennett, J., et al., 1999. Endoscopic assessment of esophagitis: clinical and functional correlates and further validation of Los Angeles classification. Gut 45, 172–180.

Malfertheiner, P., Megraud, F., O'Morain, C., et al., 2017. Management of Helicobacter pylori infection – the Maastricht V/Florence Consensus Report. Gut 66, 6–30.

Megraud, F., Coenen, S., Versporten, A., et al., 2013. Helicobacter pylori resistance to antibiotics in Europe and its relationship to antibiotic consumption. Gut 62 (1), 34–42.

Medicines and Healthcare Products Regulatory Agency (MHRA), 2010. Clopidogrel and proton pump inhibitors: interaction – updated advice. Drug Safety Update 3 (9), 4.

Medicines and Healthcare Products Regulatory Agency (MHRA), 2013. Metoclopramide: risk of neurological adverse effects. Drug Safety Update 7 (1), S2.

Medicines and Healthcare Products Regulatory Agency, 2014. Domperidone: risks of cardiac side effects. Drug Safety Update 7 (10), A1.

Moayyedi, P., Santana, J., Khan, M., et al., 2011. Medical treatments in the short-term management of reflux oesophagitis. Cochrane DB Syst. Rev. 2011 (2), Art. No. CD003244. Available at: http://cochranelibrary-wiley.com/doi/10.1002/14651858.CD003244.pub2/abstract;jsessionid=B241148ABB585A493C36E758353DAEE6.f01t02.

National Institute for Health and Care Excellence (NICE), 2012. Acute upper gastrointestinal bleeding in over 16s: management. NICE, London. Available at: http://www.nice.org.uk/guidance/cg141.

National Institute for Health and Care Excellence (NICE), 2014a. Gastro-oesophageal reflux disease and dyspepsia in adults: investigation and management. NICE, London. Available at: http://www.nice.org.uk/guidance/cg184.

National Institute for Health and Care Excellence (NICE), 2014b. Osteoarthritis: care and management. NICE, London. Available at: http://www.nice.org.uk/guidance/cg177.

Ng, F.H., Wong, S.Y., Lam, K.F., et al., 2010. Famotidine is inferior to pantoprazole in preventing recurrence of aspirin-related peptic ulcers or erosions. Gastroenterology 138, 82–88.

Pace, F., Tonini, M., Pallotta, S., et al., 2007. Systematic review: maintenance treatment of gastro-oesophageal reflux disease with proton pump inhibitors taken 'on-demand'. Alimentary Pharmacol. Therap. 26, 195–204.

Public Health England, 2016. Test and treat for Helicobacter pylori (HP) in dyspepsia. Quick reference guide for primary care. For consultation and local adaptation. Available at: https://www.gov.uk/government/uploads/system/uploads/attachment_data/file/560852/Hellicobacter_pylori_quick_reference_guide.pdf.

Quenot, J.P., Theiry, N., Barbar, S., 2009. When should stress ulcer prophylaxis be used in the ICU? Curr. Opin. Crit. Care 15, 139–143.

Rockall, T.A., Logan, R.F., Devlin, H.B., et al., 1996. Risk assessment after acute upper gastrointestinal haemorrhage. Gut 38, 316–321.

Rostom, A., Dube, C., Wells, G.A., et al., 2002. Prevention of NSAID-induced gastroduodenal ulcers. Cochrane DB Syst. Rev. 2002 (4), Art. No. CD002296. https://doi.org/10.1002/14651858.CD002296.

Scheiman, J.M., Yeomans, N.D., Talley, N.J., et al., 2006. Prevention of ulcers by esomeprazole in at-risk patients using non-selective NSAIDs and COX-2 inhibitors. Am. J. Gastroenterol. 101, 701–710.

Scottish Intercollegiate Guidelines Network, 2008. Management of acute upper and lower gastro-intestinal bleeding (Guideline 105). Scottish Intercollegiate Guideline Network, Edinburgh. Available at: http://www.sign.ac.uk/sign-105-management-of-acute-upper-and-lower-gastrointestinal-bleeding.html.

Shaheen, N.J., Richter, J.E., 2009. Barrett's oesophagus. Lancet 373, 850–861.

Sigterman, K.E., van Pinxteren, B., Bonis, P.A., et al., 2013. Short-term treatment with proton pump inhibitors, H2-receptor antagonists and prokinetics for gastro-oesophageal reflux disease-like symptoms and endoscopy negative reflux disease. Cochrane DB Syst. Rev. 2013 (5), Art. No. CD002095. https://doi.org/10.1002/14651858.CD002095.pub5.

Sreedharan, A., Martin, J., Leontiadis, G.I., et al., 2010. Proton pump inhibitor treatment initiated prior to endoscopic diagnosis in upper gastrointestinal bleeding. Cochrane DB Syst. Rev. 2010 (7), Art. No. CD005415. https://doi.org/10.1002/14651858.CD005415.pub3.

Sung, J.J., Lau, J.Y., Ching, J.Y., et al., 2010. Continuation of low-dose aspirin therapy in peptic ulcer bleeding: a randomized trial. Ann. Intern. Med. 152 (1), 1–9.

Taha, A.S., McCloskey, C., Prasad, R., et al., 2009. Famotidine for the prevention of peptic ulcers and oesophagitis in patients taking low dose aspirin (FAMOUS): a phase III, randomised, double-blind, placebo-controlled trial. Lancet 374, 119–125.

Tleyjeh, I.M., Bin Abdulhak, A.A., Riaz, M., et al., 2012. Association between proton pump inhibitor therapy and *Clostridium difficile* infection: a contemporary systematic review and meta-analysis. PLoS One 7 (12), e50836.

Trelle, S., Reichenbach, S., Wandel, S., et al., 2011. Cardiovascular safety of non-steroidal anti-inflammatory drugs: network meta-analysis. BMJ 342, c7086.

Yeomans, N.D., Svedberg, L.E., Naesdal, J., 2006. Is ranitidine therapy sufficient for healing peptic ulcers associated with non-steroidal anti-inflammatory drug use? Int. J. Clin. Pract. 60, 1401–1407.

Further reading

Braden, B., 2012. Diagnosis of *Helicobacter pylori* infection. BMJ 344, e828. Available at: http://www.bmj.com/content/344/bmj.e828.

Ford, A.C., Moayyedi, P., 2013. Dyspepsia. BMJ 347 (47), 29–33. Available at: http://www.bmj.com/content/347/bmj.f5059.

Marks, D.J.B., 2016. Time to halt the overprescribing of proton pump inhibitors. Clin. Pharm. 8 (8). Available at: http://www.pharmaceutical-journal.com/opinion/insight/time-to-halt-the-overprescribing-of-proton-pump-inhibitors/20201548.fullarticle.

National Institute for Health and Care Excellence, 2015. Clinical knowledge summaries: dyspepsia-proven peptic ulcer. NICE, London. Available at: http://cks.nice.org.uk/dyspepsia-proven-peptic-ulcer.

Scottish Intercollegiate Guidelines Network, 2008. Management of acute upper and lower gastrointestinal bleeding 105. SIGN, Edinburgh. Available at: hhttp://www.sign.ac.uk/sign-105-management-of-acute-upper-and-lower-gastrointestinal-bleeding.html..

Useful website

NHS Choices, 2016. Indigestion. http://www.nhs.uk/Conditions/Indigestion/Pages/Introduction.aspx.

13 Inflammatory Bowel Disease

Sarah Cripps

Key points

- Ulcerative colitis and Crohn's disease are the two most common types of inflammatory bowel disease (IBD) of the gut. Both are chronic relapsing conditions with a high ongoing morbidity and remain largely incurable.
- Ulcerative colitis and Crohn's disease are related diseases, but there are contrasting features which relate to the clinical presentation, the site of involvement and extent of inflammation across the bowel wall. Ulcerative colitis is limited to the large bowel and the mucosa, whereas Crohn's disease frequently involves the small intestine, with inflammation extending through the bowel wall to the serosal surface.
- The aims of treatment are to control acute attacks promptly and effectively and to induce and maintain remission. Successful treatment also aims to prevent inflammatory damage and/or dysplasia which leads to surgical intervention.
- Choice and route of therapy will depend on the site and the extent and severity of the disease, together with knowledge of current or previous treatment.
- A reduction in inflammation with corticosteroids and aminosalicylates is the mainstay of treatment, with immunosuppressants (e.g. azathioprine, methotrexate, ciclosporin) and biologic agents (e.g. infliximab, adalimumab and vedolizumab) reserved for more severe and refractory cases.
- The management of IBD poses a challenge to the multidisciplinary team both clinically and economically.
- The biggest cost for commissioners relates to hospital care and biological treatments.
- National standards and management guidelines for IBD aim to ensure patients receive consistent, high-quality, evidence-based care and IBD services throughout the UK.

Introduction

Inflammatory bowel disease (IBD) can be divided into two chronic inflammatory disorders of the gastro-intestinal tract, namely, Crohn's disease and ulcerative colitis. Crohn's disease can affect any part of the gastro-intestinal tract, whereas ulcerative colitis affects only the large bowel.

IBD follows a relapsing and remitting course that is unpredictable and causes disruption to a patient's lifestyle and places a burden on the workplace and healthcare setting.

The management of IBD patients poses a challenge to the multidisciplinary team both clinically and economically. Current available treatment for IBD is not curative. In practice, complex cases

and those prescribed biologics are increasingly managed by specialist hospital centres. Patients whose disease is less severe are still managed predominantly by gastroenterologists and IBD specialist nurses with support from primary care doctors. Situations when primary care doctors should refer patients to secondary care include failure to respond to oral treatment for acute exacerbations and toxicity to immunomodulators. It is essential that primary care doctors and pharmacists recognise signs of an acute severe exacerbation and refer patients to hospital promptly for intensive treatment. National standards and management guidelines for IBD aim to ensure patients receive consistent, high-quality care and IBD services throughout the UK that are evidence based; engaged in local, national and international networking; and meet specific minimum standards.

Epidemiology

The incidence of IBD is greater in North America, Europe, Australia and New Zealand, although the incidence in Africa, Asia and South America is rising steadily. This increase in developing countries may be due to improved sanitation and vaccination programmes along with a decreased exposure to enteric infections. Jewish and Asian people living in USA and UK are more commonly affected by IBD than those living in Israel and Asia. There appears to be no association between IBD and social class.

Up to 260,000 people are affected by IBD in the UK (National Institute for Health and Care Excellence [NICE], 2012). Around 146,000 of these have a diagnosis of ulcerative colitis compared with 115,000 who are diagnosed with Crohn's disease. These figures differ from those published by the National IBD Standards Group (2013), which estimated around 620,000 people had IBD in 2012. The incidence of ulcerative colitis is stable, whereas the incidence of Crohn's disease appears to be increasing.

The peak incidence of IBD occurs between 10 and 40 years, although it can occur at any age, with 15% of cases diagnosed in individuals over the age of 60 years. Up to one-third of patients with Crohn's disease are diagnosed before the age of 21 (NICE, 2012). The incidence appears equal between males and females, although some studies in Crohn's disease suggest it is more common in females. The incidence of new cases of ulcerative colitis in Europe and USA is 2–8 per 100,000 per year with a prevalence of 40–80 per 100,000 per year. The incidence has remained fairly static over the last 40 years. In the UK, Crohn's disease occurs with a similar frequency to ulcerative colitis, with around 4 per 100,000 per year and a prevalence of 50 per 100,000. The rates in Central and Southern Europe are lower. In South America, Asia and Africa, Crohn's disease is uncommon but appears to be on the rise (Mpofu and Ireland, 2006).

Aetiology

The precise aetiology of IBD is unclear, although its development and progression are multifactorial.

Environmental

Diet

Evidence that dietary intake is involved in the aetiology of IBD is inconclusive. Breastfeeding may reduce the risk of developing IBD (Mpofu and Ireland, 2006). Some other dietary factors have been associated with IBD, including fat intake, fast-food ingestion, milk and fibre consumption and total protein and energy intake. A large number of case-control studies have reported a causal link between the intake of refined carbohydrates and Crohn's disease (Gibson and Shepherd, 2005). The mechanism for diet as a trigger is poorly understood but is likely to involve dietary effects on the microbiome.

There is limited evidence that altering diet reduces inflammation or the risk of flare-ups. Patients with Crohn's disease may improve if they take an exclusive elemental (amino acid based), oligomeric (peptides) and polymeric (whole protein) feeds, although symptoms typically return when their normal diet is reintroduced. Other dietary modifications have not been proved to be effective, although patients are often able to identify foods that aggravate or exacerbate their coexistent irritable bowel syndrome (IBS).

Smoking

There is a higher rate of smoking amongst patients with Crohn's disease than in the general population, with up to 40% of patients with the disease being smokers. Smoking worsens the clinical course of the disease and increases the risk of relapse and the need for surgery. Fewer patients with ulcerative colitis smoke (approximately 10%). Former smokers are at the highest risk of developing ulcerative colitis, whereas current smokers have the lowest risk. Stopping smoking can provoke the emergence of ulcerative colitis, indicating that smoking may help to prevent the onset of the disease. In part this effect may be caused by nicotine (Guslandi, 1999).

Infection

Exposure to *Mycobacterium paratuberculosis* has been considered a causative agent of Crohn's disease, although current evidence indicates it is not an aetiological factor.

Ulcerative colitis may present after an episode of infective diarrhoea, but overall, there is little evidence to support the role of a single infective agent.

Enteric microflora

Enteric microflora plays an important role in the pathogenesis of IBD because the gut acts as a sensitising organ that contributes to the systemic immune response. Patients with IBD show a loss of immunological tolerance to intestinal microflora, and consequently, antibiotics often play a role in the treatment of IBD, particularly Crohn's disease. Although there is inconclusive evidence for a specific pathogen causing IBD, evidence suggests that there is a reduced diversity of luminal microbiota in IBD, with a decrease in *Firmicutes* such as bifidobacteria, lactobacillus and *Faecalibacterium prausnitzii* and an increase in mucosal-adherent bacteria.

Manipulating the intestinal flora using probiotics, prebiotics and symbiotics is an attractive therapeutic aim, but there is currently limited evidence of efficacy or clinical use. Probiotics such as *Bifidobacteria* and *Lactobacilli* favourably alter the intestinal microflora balance. More trials are needed to support the use of probiotics as therapy in IBD.

Drugs

Non-steroidal anti-inflammatory drugs (NSAIDs) such as diclofenac have been reported to exacerbate IBD (Felder et al., 2000). It is thought this may result from direct inhibition of the synthesis of cytoprotective prostaglandins. Antibiotics may also precipitate a relapse in disease due to a change in the enteric microflora. The risk of developing Crohn's disease is marginally increased in women taking the oral contraceptive pill, possibly caused by vascular changes.

Measles, mumps and rubella vaccine. There has been much debate about the link between bowel disease and measles, measles vaccine or combined measles, mumps and rubella (MMR) immunisation. However, current evidence has indicated no proven correlation.

Appendicectomy

Appendicectomy has an inverted association with Crohn's disease and ulcerative colitis. For ulcerative colitis, it is protective against disease development, whereas appendicectomy for appendicitis appears to marginally increase one's risk of Crohn's disease (Radford-Smith et al., 2002). It is unclear whether this protective effect is immunologically based or whether individuals who develop appendicitis and consequently have an appendicectomy are physiologically, genetically or immunologically distinct from the general population.

Stress

Some patients find that stress triggers a relapse in their IBD, and this has been reproduced in animal models. It is thought that stress activates inflammatory mediators at enteric nerve endings in the gut wall. In addition to stress as a trigger factor, living with IBD can also be stressful. Its chronic nature, lack of curative treatment, distressing symptoms and impact on lifestyle can make it difficult for patients to cope.

Genetic

A genetic predisposition to IBD is well established. Evidence for this predominantly comes from an observed high concordance rate for Crohn's disease amongst monozygotic twins and a 3- to 20-fold increased risk of IBD in first-degree relatives. Disease location (e.g. colonic versus ileal) and type of clinical presentation (e.g. fibrostenotic) appear to have a heritable pattern, and an earlier onset and increased severity at presentation also appear to occur in the offspring of affected parents in subsequent generations. Studies have implicated over 200 distinct susceptibility loci for IBD. Variants within these loci further increase the overall genetic variation associated with IBD risk. Genetic studies have enabled us to identify specific pathways that are important in the pathogenesis of the disease. The colitis phenotype results from interactions among multiple genetic loci, but actual disease is more likely to be dependent upon enteric microflora (Snapper and Podolsky, 2016).

Ethnic and familial

Jews are more prone to IBD than non-Jews, with Ashkenazi Jews having a higher risk than Sephardic Jews. In North America, IBD is more common in whites than blacks.

Pathophysiology

In individuals with IBD, trigger factors typically cause a severe, prolonged and inappropriate inflammatory response in the gastrointestinal tract, and the ongoing inflammatory reaction leads to an alteration in the normal architecture of the digestive tract. Genetically susceptible individuals seem unable to downregulate immune or antigen-nonspecific inflammatory responses. It is thought that chronic inflammation is characterised by increased activity of effector lymphocytes and proinflammatory cytokines that override normal control mechanisms. Others, however, have suggested that IBD may result from a primary failure of regulatory lymphocytes and cytokines, such as interleukin-10 and transforming growth factor-β, to control inflammation and effector pathways. In Crohn's disease, it is also thought that T cells are resistant to apoptosis after inactivation. The presence of non-pathogenic bowel flora appears to be an essential factor.

Disease location

The character and distribution, both macroscopic and microscopic, of chronic inflammation define and distinguish ulcerative colitis and Crohn's disease. Table 13.1 shows the differences in location and distribution of ulcerative colitis and Crohn's disease. Fig. 13.1 details the histological differences.

Table 13.1	Location and distribution of ulcerative colitis and Crohn's disease	
	Ulcerative colitis	Crohn's disease
Location	Colon and rectum 40% proctitis 20% pancolitis 10–15% backwash ileitis	Entire gut (mouth to anus, rectal sparing) 45% ileocaecal disease 25% colitis only 20% terminal ileal disease 5% small bowel disease 5% anorectal, gastroduodenal, oral disease
Distribution	Continuous, diffuse	Often discontinuous and segmental 'skip lesions' Full thickness (transmural)
	No granulomas	Granulomatous inflammation
	Inflammation of mucosa	
	Ulceration is fine and superficial	Deep ulceration with mucosal extension
Fissures, fistulae and stricture	Absent	Common
Perianal disease	Absent	Present

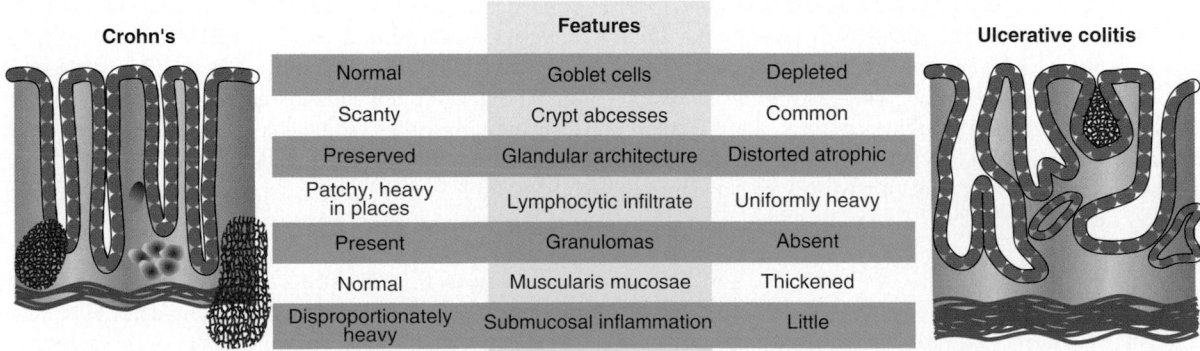

Crohn's	Features	Ulcerative colitis
Normal	Goblet cells	Depleted
Scanty	Crypt abcesses	Common
Preserved	Glandular architecture	Distorted atrophic
Patchy, heavy in places	Lymphocytic infiltrate	Uniformly heavy
Present	Granulomas	Absent
Normal	Muscularis mucosae	Thickened
Disproportionately heavy	Submucosal inflammation	Little

Fig. 13.1 Histological features in the rectal biopsy that help to distinguish between ulcerative colitis and Crohn's disease. (From Misiewicz et al., 1994, with kind permission from Blackwell Scientific Publications, Oxford.)

Crohn's disease

Crohn's disease can affect any part of the gut from the mouth to the anus. Approximately 45% of patients have ileocaecal disease, 25% colitis only, 20% terminal ileal disease, 5% small bowel disease and 5% anorectal, gastroduodenal or oral disease. Crohn's disease can involve one area of the gut or multiple areas, with unaffected areas in between being known as 'skip lesions'. The areas of the small bowel affected are typically thickened and narrow. A 'red ring' is often the first visible abnormality seen on colonoscopy. This is a lymphoid follicular enlargement with a surrounding ring of erythema, which develops into aphthoid ulceration and may progress to deep fissuring ulcers with a cobblestone appearance, fibrosis and strictures. Intestinal strictures arise from chronic and extensive inflammation and fibrosis, and bowel obstruction may arise. Local gut perforation may cause abscesses, which may also lead to fistulae.

Microscopically, inflammation and ulceration are transmural (i.e. extend through all layers of the bowel wall). Inflammatory cells are seen throughout, resulting in ulceration and microabscess formation. Non-caseating epithelioid cells, sometimes with Langhans's giant cells, are seen in about 25% of colonic biopsies and in 60% of surgically resected bowels. Chronic inflammation in the small intestine, colon, rectum and anus leads to an increased risk of carcinoma.

Ulcerative colitis

At first presentation, ulcerative colitis is confined to the rectum (proctitis) in 40% of cases, the sigmoid and descending colon (left-sided colitis) in 40% and the whole colon (total ulcerative colitis or pancolitis) in 20% of cases. Proctitis extends to involve more of the colon in a minority, with 15–30% of patients developing more extensive disease over 10 years. Fig. 13.2 highlights the location of colonic disease. The reason why some patients have extensive disease and some have limited disease is unknown. In severe total ulcerative colitis, there may also be inflammation of the terminal ileum. This is known as 'backwash ileitis' but is not clinically significant. The colon appears mucopurulent, erythematous and granular with superficial ulceration that in severe cases leads to ulceration. As the colon heals by granulation, postinflammatory polyps may form.

Microscopically, superficial inflammation is seen with inflammatory cells infiltrating the lamina propria and crypts. Crypt abscesses occur, the crypt structure is lost and goblet cell depletion arises as mucin is lost. Dysplasia, which can potentially progress to carcinoma, may be seen in biopsies taken from patients with long-standing total colitis.

Colitis not yet classified

Colitis not yet classified (sometimes referred to indeterminate colitis) is when the clinical, biochemical, endoscopic and histologic features of the disease do not allow a distinction between Crohn's colitis or ulcerative colitis. This occurs in approximately 10% of IBD colitis.

Other types of colitis

Another type of chronic colitis is microscopic colitis (which can be differentiated into lymphocytic colitis or collagenous colitis). The main feature is watery diarrhoea in the presence of a normal colonoscopy and chronic inflammation in the absence of crypt architectural distortion on mucosal biopsies. Drugs such as NSAIDs and proton pump inhibitors (PPIs) are implicated as the cause in up to 50% of cases of microscopic colitis. Diversion colitis is when inflammation occurs in the defunctioned colon, causing a mucous discharge. Pseudomembranous colitis is caused by *Clostridium difficile*, usually after prolonged or multiple antibiotics. The use of PPIs predisposes patients to *C. difficile* infection. It is diagnosed by sigmoidoscopy and detection of *C. difficile* toxin in the stool.

Clinical manifestation

The clinical differences between Crohn's disease and ulcerative colitis are described in Table 13.2.

Crohn's disease

The clinical features of Crohn's disease depend in part on the site of the bowel affected, the extent, severity and the pathological process in each patient. Crohn's disease tends to be more disabling than ulcerative colitis, with 25% of patients unable to work 1 year after diagnosis. The predominant symptoms in Crohn's disease are diarrhoea (which may contain some blood and mucus), abdominal pain and weight loss. Weight loss occurs in most patients, irrespective of disease location. Ten to twenty

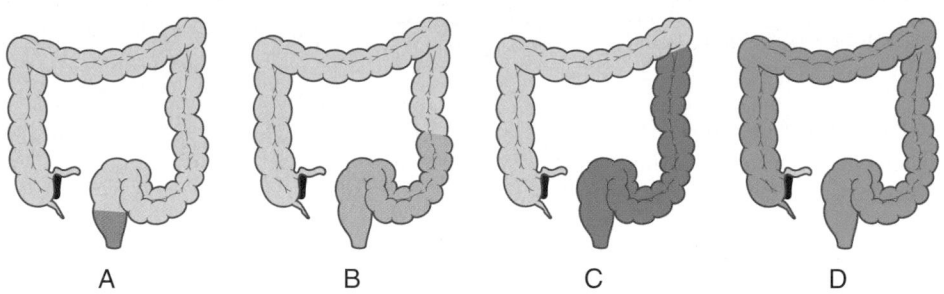

Fig. 13.2 Location of colonic disease in ulcerative colitis. (A) Proctitis involves only the rectum. (B) Proctosigmoiditis involves the rectum and sigmoid colon. (C) Distal colitis involves only the left side of the colon. (D) Pancolitis involves the entire colon.

Table 13.2 Clinical differences between ulcerative colitis and Crohn's disease

	Ulcerative colitis	Crohn's disease
Symptoms of active disease		
Prominent symptom	Bloody diarrhoea, urgency to pass stool	Diarrhoea, abdominal pain, weight loss 30% no gross bleeding
Fever	Implies acute severe colitis or infection	Common
Abdominal pain	Varies	Common
Diarrhoea	Very common	Fairly common
Rectal bleeding	Very common	Fairly common
Weight loss	Fairly common	Common
Signs of malnutrition	Fairly common	Common
Abdominal mass	Absent	Common
Dehydration	Very common	Common
Autoantibodies	Common	Rare
Electrolyte disturbances, iron deficiency anaemia raised inflammatory markers (CRP/ESR), hypoalbuminaemia	Common	Common
Pattern of disease	Both characterised by unpredictable periods of remission and relapse	
Occurrence	Occurs more in people of Caucasian and Ashkenazic Jewish origin than in other racial and ethnic subgroups Incidence fairly static 146,000 patients in UK	Occurs more in people of Caucasian and Ashkenazic Jewish origin than in other racial and ethnic subgroups 5-fold increase in incidence at all ages since 1950s 115,000 patients in UK Can occur at any age – up to one-third diagnosed before 21 years old peak 20–40 years
Occurrence in smokers	Uncommon in smokers	3–4 times more common in smokers
Occurrence in breastfeeding and appendectomy	Breastfeeding and appendectomy protective	Breastfeeding protective Appendectomy may increase risk
Fissures, fistulae and strictures	Absent	Common
Perianal disease	Absent	Present
Extra-intestinal manifestations	Present	Present

CRP, C-reactive protein; ESR, erythrocyte sedimentation rate.

percent of patients will have weight loss greater than 20%. The main cause is decreased oral intake, although malnutrition is also common. As a result, patients sometimes have a low body mass index (BMI). Growth retardation is common in young Crohn's patients. There is a slight increase in mortality in patients with extensive Crohn's disease.

It is estimated that only 10% patients have prolonged remission, with 20% requiring hospital admission each year and 50% requiring surgery within 10 years of diagnosis. This is unlike ulcerative colitis, where mortality appears to be slightly increased compared with the general population.

Small bowel, ileocaecal and terminal ileal disease

Patients present with pain and/or a tender palpable mass in the right iliac fossa with weight loss and diarrhoea, which usually contains no blood. Diarrhoea is caused by mucosal inflammation, bile salt malabsorption or bacterial overgrowth proximal to a stricture. Small bowel obstruction may also occur as a consequence of inflammation, fibrosis and stricture formation. Patients often describe a more generalised intermittent pain which is colicky, with loud gurgling bowel sounds (borborygmi), abdominal distension, vomiting and constipation. When inflammation or abscesses are the predominant pathology, patients then present with constant pain and fever. Enteric fistulae occur and may involve the skin, bladder or vagina. Although rare, perforation of the gut may present with an acute abdomen and peritonitis. Vitamin B_{12} and iron deficiencies are common, predisposing patients to anaemia, while bile acid malabsorption also occurs in such patients and predisposes them to cholesterol gallstones and oxalate renal stones.

Crohn's colitis

The main symptoms are abdominal pain, profuse and frequent diarrhoea usually without blood, and weight loss. Patients also complain of lethargy, anorexia and nausea and may appear thin, tachycardic, anaemic, malnourished and febrile. Colitis may present insidiously with minimal discomfort. Patients with severe involvement of the colon or the terminal ileum often have electrolyte abnormalities, hypoalbuminaemia and iron-deficiency anaemia. Extra-intestinal complications are more common in those patients with large bowel disease.

Perianal disease

Patients may present with an anal fissure, fistula or a perirectal abscess. These symptoms can have a significant impact on the patient's lifestyle. Fistulae are abnormal channels lined with granulation tissue that can form between the intestine and the skin as well as organs such as the bladder, vagina, or other parts of the intestine.

Gastroduodenal and oral disease

Gastroduodenal and oral disease are both rare manifestations. Gastroduodenal Crohn's disease presents as dyspepsia, pain, weight loss, anorexia, nausea and vomiting. Oral disease is very painful and may cause chronic ulceration, resulting in anorexia.

Stricturing Crohn's disease

Strictures, narrowed segments of bowel, are common and can lead to blockages, acute dilatation and perforation if not surgically treated. Patients usually present with pain, vomiting and constipation (see Fig. 13.3).

Ulcerative colitis

Typical symptoms of ulcerative colitis include bloody diarrhoea (the most predominant symptom) with mucus, urgency and frequency. Abdominal pain usually is of cramps associated with (and relieved by) the urge to defaecate. Weight loss occurs in severe cases. Frank blood loss is more common in ulcerative colitis than Crohn's disease. Approximately 50% of patients with ulcerative colitis have some form of relapse each year,

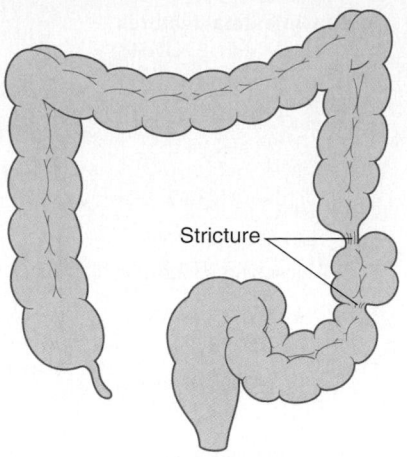

Fig. 13.3 Stricture formation in Crohn's disease.

and severe attacks can be life-threatening. Up until the 1960s, one-third of ulcerative colitis patients died from the condition; with advances in medical and surgical treatment, death is now extremely rare.

Most patients diagnosed with ulcerative colitis will have mild disease at first presentation, and only 10% will have severe disease. Up to 30% will undergo colectomy within 10 years of diagnosis (Mowat et al., 2011).

Acute severe disease

In addition to the typical symptoms of ulcerative colitis, patients with acute severe disease present with more than six bloody stools per day (10–20 liquid stools per day is not unusual), with one or more of the following: a fever (>37.8 °C), tachycardia (>90 bpm), anaemia (Hb <10.5 g/dL) or elevated inflammatory markers (erythrocyte sedimentation rate [ESR] >30 mm/h; C-reactive protein [CRP] >8 mg/L). Severity is commonly assessed using the Truelove and Witts's criteria (see investigations).

Moderately active disease

Stool frequency is less than six motions each day with diarrhoea, mucus and rectal bleeding. Moderately active disease is more common in 'left-sided' disease. Toxic megacolon is rare in patients with rectosigmoidal involvement, and the incidence of colon cancer is much lower in these patients than those with total colitis.

Proctitis

The manifestations of active proctitis are less severe. These are tenesmus, pruritus ani, rectal bleeding and mucous discharge. Patients are often constipated and may require an osmotic laxative such as a macrogol.

Toxic dilatation

This can occur in untreated severe ulcerative colitis. There is a high risk of perforation, with a historical mortality of 50%.

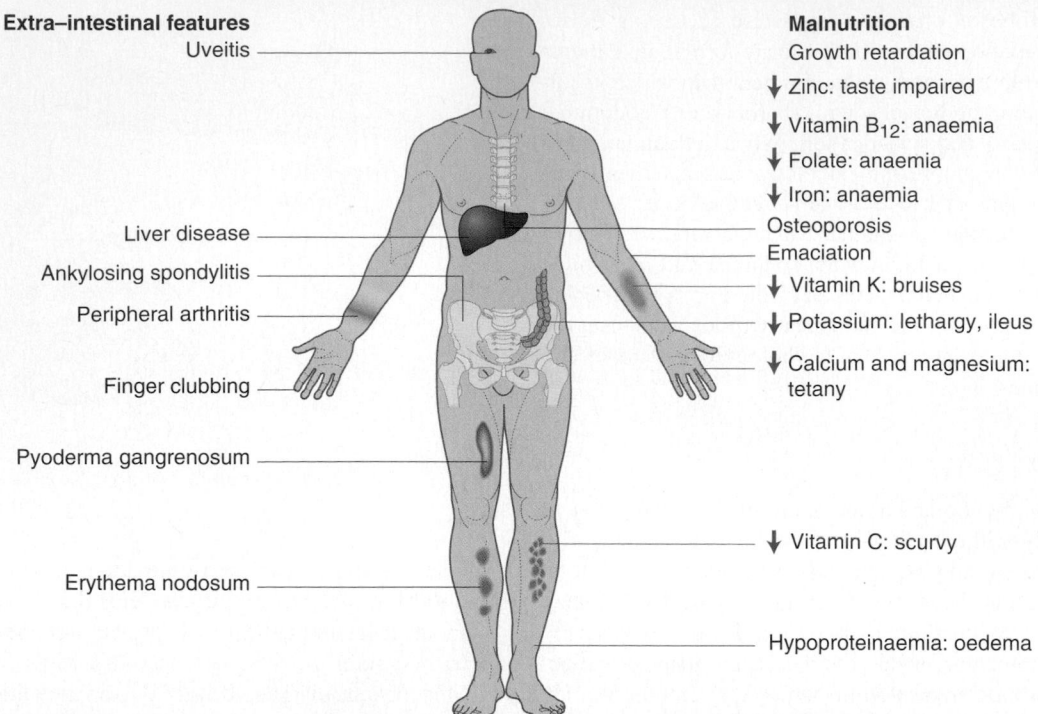

Extra-intestinal features
Uveitis

Liver disease
Ankylosing spondylitis
Peripheral arthritis

Finger clubbing

Pyoderma gangrenosum

Erythema nodosum

Malnutrition
Growth retardation
↓ Zinc: taste impaired
↓ Vitamin B$_{12}$: anaemia
↓ Folate: anaemia
↓ Iron: anaemia
Osteoporosis
Emaciation
↓ Vitamin K: bruises
↓ Potassium: lethargy, ileus
↓ Calcium and magnesium: tetany

↓ Vitamin C: scurvy

Hypoproteinaemia: oedema

Fig. 13.4   Some of the extra-intestinal illnesses and features of malnutrition found in patients with inflammatory bowel disease. (From Misiewicz et al., 1994, with kind permission from Blackwell Scientific Publications, Oxford.)

Extra-intestinal complications

Around 20–30% of patients with IBD will present with extra-intestinal manifestations. They are more commonly seen in patients when IBD affects the colon. Complications affect the joints, skin, bone, eyes, liver and biliary tree and are mostly (but not exclusively) associated with active disease. Fig. 13.4 highlights some of the extra-intestinal features of IBD.

Joints and bones

Arthropathies occur in 10% of patients with IBD, are more common in women and are a well-recognised complication of IBD. Patients with pauciarticular disease, characterised by arthritis limited to five or fewer joints, often experience a flare in the arthropathy when there is an exacerbation of the IBD symptoms. When the IBD relapse is treated, the arthropathy improves. This is in contrast to polyarticular arthropathy, a chronic condition which affects more than five joints; a flare of the IBD appears not to be temporally related to the activity of the arthropathy. About 5% of patients with IBD also have ankylosing spondylitis. This is thought to be immunologically mediated and not associated with IBD activity. Osteopenia, potentially leading to osteoporosis, is often seen in patients with IBD because of chronic steroid use (particularly when the cumulative dose of prednisolone exceeds 10 g) and/or malabsorption.

Skin

Both erythema nodosum and pyoderma gangrenosum are associated with IBD. Erythema nodosum appears as tender, hot, red nodules usually on the shins that subside over a few days to leave a brown skin discolouration. The onset is normally directly related to IBD activity in the 8% of patients affected.

Pyoderma gangrenosum presents as a discrete pustule that develops into an ulcer. In the 2% of patients affected, IBD activity does not appear to be directly related to the pyoderma gangrenosum, which may begin or worsen when the IBD is quiescent.

Sweet's syndrome (an acute febrile neutrophilic dermatosis), which has some similarity to erythema nodosum, may also be associated with IBD.

Eye

Ocular complications are infrequent, occurring in less than 10% of cases. Episcleritis (intense burning and itching with localised area of blood vessels) is the most common complication of IBD. Scleritis may impair vision. Uveitis (headache, burning red eye, blurred vision) is often associated with joint and skin manifestations of IBD. Conjunctivitis is frequently seen in IBD patients but is not specific, and no true association has been demonstrated.

Hepatobiliary

Biliary complications of IBD are gallstones and primary sclerosing cholangitis (PSC). The latter occurs in 5% of patients with ulcerative colitis but less frequently in those with Crohn's disease. Conversely, the prevalence of IBD (mostly ulcerative colitis) in patients with PSC is 70–80%. PSC, found predominantly in males, is a chronic cholestatic condition characterised by inflammation and fibrosis of the intrahepatic and extrahepatic bile ducts. Patients present with obstructive jaundice, cholangitis and raised cholestatic liver enzymes. Magnetic resonance chol-angiopancreatography (MRCP) is the diagnostic test of choice, with endoscopic retrograde cholangiopancreatography (ERCP) restricted to when intervention is required (e.g. for removal of obstructing gallstones). There is an increased risk of cholangio-carcinoma, cirrhosis and hepatocellular carcinoma (HCC) with a liver transplant being the only effective treatment.

Thromboembolic

Thromboembolic complications occur in around 1–2% of IBD patients. The most common cause of death in hospitalised IBD patients was once pulmonary embolism (Solem et al., 2004). However, the risk of this is now reduced because of the routine use of venous thromboembolism prophylaxis in hospitalised patients.

Anaemia

Anaemia is the most common systemic complication of IBD. In the majority of cases, IBD-associated anaemia is a unique example of the combination of chronic iron deficiency and anaemia of chronic disease (ACD). Other causes of anaemia in IBD include vitamin B_{12} and folate deficiency and the toxic effects of medications such as azathioprine and methotrexate.

All patients with IBD should be regularly assessed for the presence of anaemia because of its impact on quality of life and comorbidity. About two-thirds of IBD patients have anaemia at diagnosis.

The cause of iron-deficiency anaemia includes continuous blood loss from the ulcerated surface of the bowel or malnutrition with reduced iron intake. Diagnostic criteria depend on the level of inflammation. In patients without clinical, endoscopic or biochemical evidence of active disease, serum ferritin less than 30 micrograms/L is indicative. However, in the presence of inflammation, a serum ferritin up to 100 micrograms/L may still be consistent with iron deficiency and warrant active treatment. In comparison the diagnostic criteria for ACD in the presence of biochemical or clinical evidence of inflammation are a serum ferritin greater than 100 micrograms/L and transferrin saturation less than 20%. If the serum ferritin level is between 30 and 100 micrograms/L, a combination of true iron deficiency and ACD is likely.

Patients with IBD should be monitored for recurrent iron deficiency every 3 months for at least a year after correction and between 6 and 12 months thereafter. After effective iron replenishment, anaemia recurs rapidly, and patients with IBD should be monitored for iron deficiency every 3 months using a combination of haemoglobin, ferritin, transferrin saturation, and CRP (Dignass et al., 2015).

Other complications of inflammatory bowel disease

Complications of ulcerative colitis include toxic dilatation of the colon (>5.5 cm identified by abdominal X-ray) and the risk of perforation. Repeated resections can lead to short bowel in Crohn's disease and the need for lifelong total parenteral nutrition and medication to control a high-output stoma. There is a risk of colorectal cancer in patients with colonic disease,

and routine colonoscopic surveillance is recommended for patients at increased risk (NICE, 2011).

Investigations

A full patient history should include recent travel, medication (such as recent use of antibiotics or NSAIDs), sexual and vaccination history as appropriate and identifying potential risk factors such as smoking, family history and recent infection, such as gastroenteritis. A combination of clinical signs and symptoms and endoscopic, radiological, histological and haematological investigations will help to confirm diagnosis, disease recurrence and response to treatment (Dignass et al., 2015). Differential diagnoses of IBD include carcinoma, infection, drug-induced colitis, ischaemia, radiation damage, irritable bowel syndrome and diverticulitis.

Endoscopy

The key diagnostic investigation in IBD is lower gastro-intestinal tract endoscopy (sigmoidoscopy and colonoscopy), which allows direct visualisation of the large bowel and histopathological assessment from biopsies. Treatment response to biologics can be assessed via mucosal healing seen at colonoscopy. In patients with severe symptoms, it is sometimes necessary to delay a full colonoscopy because of the increased risk of perforation.

To enable a good view of the mucosa, bowel-cleansing agents (e.g. Citramag, Picolax or Moviprep) are taken prior to the procedure. Phosphate enemas are given prior to sigmoidoscopy and are considered safe in acute severe colitis provided there is no colonic dilatation.

The Ulcerative Colitis Endoscopic Index of Severity (UCEIS) predicts overall assessment of endoscopic severity of disease (Travis et al., 2012). Three descriptors are graded as vascular pattern, bleeding and ulceration to give a score out of 8. A higher score is more predictive of likely colectomy. The use of the UCEIS has reduced variance in endoscopic reporting from 73% to 14% (Travis et al., 2012).

Wireless capsule endoscopy allows the small bowel to be viewed and can be useful in patients with non-stricturing Crohn's disease. The patient swallows a small single-use capsule, usually after an overnight fast. This capsule consists of a camera, a light source and a wireless circuit for the acquisition and transmission of signals. As the capsule moves through the gastro-intestinal tract, images are transmitted to a data recorder, worn on a belt outside the body. These data are transferred to a computer for interpretation. The capsule is then passed in the patient's stool (NICE, 2004).

Radiology

Radiological imaging is used in the initial evaluation or diagnosis, preoperative review, to highlight the presence of complications during exacerbations and to evaluate extra-intestinal manifestations. Radiological examination still plays a key role in IBD affecting the small bowel, although endoscopy has generally replaced conventional X-ray examinations of the colon. There are various types of radiological tests, and the most appropriate imaging technique is ideally discussed with a radiologist to minimise unnecessary ionising radiation.

Abdominal X-ray is essential in severe indeterminate colitis to exclude colonic dilatation and may help assess disease extent of ulcerative colitis or identify proximal constipation. In Crohn's disease, abdominal radiography may identify a potential mass in the right iliac fossa or highlight evidence of small bowel dilatation.

Computed tomography (CT scan) and magnetic resonance imaging (MRI) are the best radiological methods for locating and defining fistulae and abscesses in active Crohn's disease. MRI has the advantage over CT in that there is no radiation, which is advantageous in a young population, and with Crohn's disease, where repeat imaging is likely.

Radiolabelled leucocyte scans that utilise autologous leucocytes labelled with ^{99}technetium-hexamethylenamine oxime are very rarely used because modern imaging provides superior information about disease severity and complications.

Laboratory findings

Although not diagnostic, active disease is suggested in patients with raised inflammatory markers that include erythrocyte sedimentation rate (ESR) and C-reactive protein (CRP) in addition to a low haemoglobin, raised ferritin and raised platelet count. Vitamin B_{12} may be low in patients with chronic terminal ileal disease. Low red cell folate and serum albumin, magnesium, calcium, zinc and essential fatty acids also indicate chronic inflammation and malabsorption. Anti-*Saccharomyces cerevisiae* antibodies (ASCAs) are more likely to be present in Crohn's disease. Serology is used by some clinicians but is not sensitive or specific enough to be a commonly used diagnostic tool.

Malabsorption, indicated by low serum trace elements (e.g. magnesium and zinc), is not seen in ulcerative colitis. Low albumin may indicate relapse in active disease. Patients with sclerosing cholangitis often present with altered liver function tests (LFTs).

Cytomegalovirus (CMV) should be considered in severe or refractory colitis, particularly in the presence of high fevers and/or deranged LFTs. Reactivation is common in patients taking immunosuppressants.

Stool tests

Stool tests do not diagnose IBD but contribute to excluding alternative diagnoses, such as infection and identifying a potential precipitant for a flare in symptoms. Red and white blood cells can be seen on microscopic examination of fresh stools. Microscopic identification of infective cells such as amoeba may also be visualised. *C. difficile* toxin can be assessed through culture and toxin assay. *C. difficile* has a higher prevalence in IBD patients and is associated with increased mortality.

Faecal calprotectin is often used as indicator for IBD. It is a useful diagnostic marker for predicting relapses or flares and can help assess the efficacy of treatment. Increased levels of faecal calprotectin correlate with endoscopic disease activity and can

Table 13.3 Truelove and Witts's criteria for assessing severity of ulcerative colitis (NICE, 2013)

Feature	Mild	Moderate	Severe
Motions per day	<4	4–6	>6
Rectal bleeding	Little	Moderate	Large amounts
Temperature	Apyrexial	Intermediate	>37.8 °C on 2 of 4 days
Pulse rate	Normal	Intermediate	>90 bpm
Haemoglobin	Normal	Intermediate	<10.5 g/dL
ESR	Normal	Intermediate	>30 mm/h

bpm, Beats per minute; ESR, erythrocyte sedimentation rate.

help distinguish between a diagnosis of IBD and irritable bowel syndrome (IBS) in which faecal calprotectin levels are normal. Proton pump inhibitors (e.g. omeprazole) may be associated with elevated calprotectin values so this should be taken into account when interpreting results.

Clinical assessment tools

The Crohn's Disease Activity Index (CDAI) (Best et al., 1976) or the Harvey–Bradshaw Index (HBI) (Harvey and Bradshaw, 1980) are used in most clinical trials to define remission in Crohn's disease. However, in clinical practice the CDAI is rarely used because it needs to be measured prospectively and is complex. The HBI is a simple measure of stool frequency, pain and other clinical features that is increasingly used to document selection for and response to biologic therapy. A CDAI of <150 or an HBI of 3 or below suggests the patient is in remission (NICE, 2010). When using these scores, consideration should be made for any physical, sensory or learning disabilities or communication difficulties that could affect the scores and make any adjustments as appropriate. The Truelove and Witts's criteria (NICE, 2013) comprise a useful tool in defining the severity of ulcerative colitis in adults (see Table 13.3). A severe attack is defined as more than six bloody stools a day plus one or more of the following: pulse greater than 90 beats/min, temperature greater than 37.8 °C, haemoglobin less than 10.5 g/dL or ESR greater than 30 mm/h. In this case, the patient should be admitted to hospital. The Paediatric Ulcerative Colitis Activity Index (PUCAI) is used with children (Turner et al., 2007a).

The Simple Clinical Colitis Activity Index (SCCAI) (Walmsley et al., 1998) allows initial evaluation of exacerbations of ulcerative colitis using scores for five clinical criteria. These are ESR, bowel frequency per day and at night/day, urgency of defaecation, presence of blood in stool, general well-being and extracolonic features.

Predicting the outcome of severe ulcerative colitis (resistance to steroids and likelihood of requiring colectomy) should be assessed on day 3 of intensive treatment with intravenous corticosteroids. Those patients with frequent stools (>8/day) or raised CRP (>45 mg/L) predicts the need for surgery in 85% cases (Travis et al., 1996). Remission in ulcerative colitis is defined

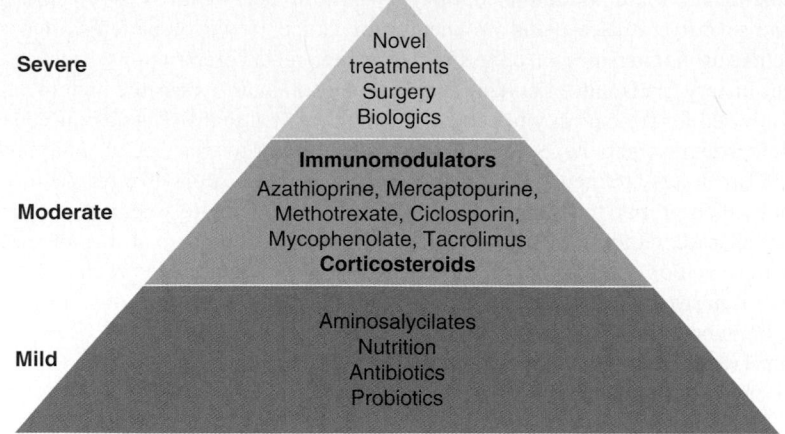

Fig. 13.5 Treatment options in inflammatory bowel disease from mild to moderate and severe disease.

as complete resolution of symptoms with a normal bowel pattern (<3 stools/day), no urgency and no visible bleeding. Mucosal healing is confirmed by endoscopy.

Treatment of inflammatory bowel disease

At present there is no cure for IBD because the exact cause of the condition is unknown. Widely ranging drugs and nutritional supplements are available to maintain the patient in long periods of remission in both Crohn's disease and ulcerative colitis. However, surgical intervention often becomes necessary if a complication occurs or if the patient fails to respond to medical therapy. Because the majority of people with IBD are diagnosed under the age of 30, effective treatment and avoidance of relapses are of paramount importance in this chronic, long-term condition. Steroid-free remission remains one of the main goals of therapy.

The available treatments for inflammatory bowel disease are not curative. They are largely aimed at:
- treating acute attacks promptly and inducing remission,
- maintenance of remission,
- minimising toxicity related to drug treatment,
- optimising nutrition and/or growth,
- encouraging smoking cessation in patients with Crohn's disease,
- minimising psychological concerns,
- detecting cases of colorectal cancer,
- managing disease complications,
- maintaining or improving quality of life.

In addition, identification and selection of patients who would benefit from surgery and/or endoscopic treatment are also undertaken.

Nutritional therapy

Nutritional therapy can be considered as an adjunctive or primary treatment. Although a potential problem for all patients with IBD, patients with Crohn's disease are at particular risk of becoming malnourished and developing a variety of nutritional deficiencies.

Although of benefit in Crohn's disease, there is no indication for enteral feeding in the treatment of ulcerative colitis. In Crohn's disease, there is evidence that enteral liquid feed favourably alters the inflammatory response and may be useful in inducing remission. However, there is little evidence to support its use as maintenance treatment. Exclusive enteral nutrition for 3–6 weeks is an alternative to corticosteroids to induce remission. This is commonly used in paediatrics, where avoidance of corticosteroids because of their side effects, such as growth retardation, is desirable. Up to 80% of paediatric patients achieve remission with exclusive elemental nutrition. The efficacy in adults is lower, primarily as a result of tolerability and adherence. There does not appear to be a difference in efficacy between elemental and polymeric diets (Mowat et al., 2011).

Patients who have extensive small bowel resection may experience many nutritional deficiencies because of malabsorption. Iron depletion, hypoproteinaemia, deficiencies in water- and fat-soluble vitamins, trace elements and electrolytes may all occur and must be corrected using a suitable replacement regimen.

Where appropriate, and when enteral nutrition is not indicated or adequate, a total parenteral nutrition (TPN) regimen may be prescribed. Some patients receive concurrent enteral and parenteral feeding.

Drug treatment

Drug treatments are often required for many years, and patient preference, acceptability and potential side effects affect both choice and potential medication adherence. A therapeutic strategy and consistency in the management of patients with IBD are essential. Strategies for the management of induction of remission and maintenance of remission for both conditions are set out in the respective NICE (2012, 2013) management guidelines and other international guidelines such as those from the European Crohn's and Colitis Organisation (Dignass et al., 2012a, 2012b; Gionchetti et al., 2016; Gomollon et al., 2016). Patients are likely to receive several different treatments during the course of their illness as a result of intolerance or lack of response, and medicine optimisation is key to ensure patients get the most out of their medicines.

The mainstays of drugs used in the treatment of IBD are corticosteroids, aminosalicylates, immunomodulators and biologics. Fig. 13.5 illustrates the stepwise approach to drug treatment options.

The choice of drug treatment and route of administration depends on the site, extent and severity of disease and whether it is being used for the induction or maintenance of remission. Consideration of the treatment history is also an important factor. Maintenance treatment is advised for the majority of patients (except those ulcerative colitis patients who have undergone colectomy). The majority of IBD patients are managed successfully as hospital outpatients or by their primary care doctor. Only severe extensive or fulminant disease requires hospitalisation and the use of parenteral therapy and/or surgical intervention. Oral medication can be given to most patients for maintenance of mild to moderate disease. Immunomodulators and biologics, which are reserved for more severe disease, should only be initiated by/on the advice of a specialist gastroenterologist. The use of immunomodulators, biologics or surgery is invariably required if steroid treatment alone fails to induce remission or cannot be withdrawn. An algorithm for drug treatment in IBD is shown in Fig. 13.6.

Although commonly used and accepted practice in the UK, many of the drugs recommended in the treatment of IBD, such as the immunomodulators (azathioprine, mercaptopurine, methotrexate, ciclosporin, and tacrolimus), are used outside of their UK marketing authorisation. In addition, many drugs do not have a UK licence for use in children. This includes some oral and topical aminosalicylates, and therefore reference should be made to the British National Formulary for Children (BNFC). Informed consent for the use of these drugs should therefore be obtained and documented because the prescriber must take full responsibility for their use.

The route of administration is a particularly important factor in IBD. In contrast to most other conditions, minimal systemic absorption and maximal intestinal wall drug levels are required with oral therapy. Several delivery strategies have been used to achieve this, including the chemical modification of drug molecules, delayed and controlled-release formulations and the use of bioadhesive particles.

Rectal route

Disease confined to the anus, rectum or left side of the colon is more appropriately treated with rectally administered topical preparations where the drug is applied directly to the site of inflammation (Table 13.4). Rectally administered topical preparations of aminosalicylates and corticosteroids are recommended in mild to moderate ulcerative colitis (NICE, 2013).

Drugs administered rectally have reduced systemic absorption and fewer side effects than those administered orally or intravenously. The choice of formulation (suppository, foam or liquid enema) depends on the site of inflammation, product presentation, acceptability, patient preference and cost. Adherence to topical therapy is generally poor, and good patient education is required for effective benefit. Patients with poor dexterity may find the use of rectal products difficult, and these preparations may therefore be poorly tolerated and consequently have a limited advantage.

Proctitis is best treated with suppositories. Where inflammation affects the rectum and sigmoid colon (up to 15–20 cm), foam enemas are preferred. In more extensive disease extending to the splenic flexure (30–60 cm), liquid enemas are the agents of choice. However, patients often require a combination of different rectal preparations because, for example, over 90% of liquid enemas bypass the rectum and thereby exert no therapeutic benefit at that site. As a consequence, a suppository may also be required to treat rectal inflammation. The propellant action of foam applicators also results in some preparations bypassing the rectal mucosa. Enemas or suppositories should be administered just before bedtime in a supine position because this allows a much longer retention time. Liquid enemas can be warmed and should be inserted while lying in the left lateral position.

Corticosteroids

The glucocorticoid properties of hydrocortisone and prednisolone are the mainstay of treatment in active ulcerative colitis and Crohn's disease to induce remission. Prednisolone administered orally or rectally (if colonic or rectal disease) is the steroid of choice, although in emergency situations, hydrocortisone or methylprednisolone is used when the parenteral route is required. Corticosteroids have direct anti-inflammatory and immunosuppressive actions which rapidly control symptoms. They can be used either alone or in combination, with a suitable mesalazine (5-aminosalicylic acid, 5-ASA) formulation or immunosuppressant, to induce remission. Rectal corticosteroids are recommended for use in mild to moderate proctitis/sigmoiditis but are not as effective as rectal aminosalicylates.

Corticosteroids are ineffective in preventing relapse once remission has occurred. If disease symptoms recur during the withdrawal period, the dose should be increased and a slower taper schedule commenced. The addition of an immunomodulator should be considered. Oral corticosteroids should not be used for maintenance treatment because of serious long-term side effects, such as osteoporosis, and abrupt withdrawal should be avoided. Patients should be maintained on aminosalicylates, immunosuppressants or biologics or a combination of these, as appropriate, or referred for surgery.

Oral corticosteroids. Oral prednisolone will control mild and moderate IBD, and 70% of patients improve after 2–4 weeks of 40 mg/day. This is gradually reduced over the next 4–6 weeks to prevent acute adrenal insufficiency and early relapse. Prednisolone at doses higher than 40 mg/day increases the incidence of adverse effects and has little therapeutic advantage. Initial doses below 20 mg/day, faster reduction regimens or short pulses of corticosteroids are generally ineffective in active disease (St Clair Jones, 2014). An example of a reducing oral prednisolone regimen is detailed in Box 13.1.

Oral corticosteroids should be taken in the morning to mimic the diurnal rhythm of the body's cortisol secretion and prevent sleep disturbance. Uncoated steroid tablets are suitable for most patients, whereas enteric-coated preparations do not offer any proven advantage and should be avoided in patients with short bowel or strictures because of poor absorption and bolus release at stricture sites.

Short-term side effects of corticosteroids include moon face, acne, sleep and mood disturbance, dyspepsia, hypokalaemia,

Ulcerative colitis
Induction of remission

Mild to moderate proctitis/proctosigmoiditis
1. Offer topical aminosalicylate (enema/suppository) <u>OR</u>
2. Consider <u>adding</u> an oral aminosalicylate (combination more efficacious) <u>OR</u>
3. Consider oral aminosalicylate alone

If aminosalicylate declined/not tolerated/contra-indicated
1. Consider topical corticosteroid <u>OR</u> oral prednisolone

Left-sided and extensive ulcerative colitis
1. Offer high induction dose of oral aminosalicylate
2. Consider <u>adding</u> topical aminosalicylate OR beclometasone dipropionate

If aminosalicylate declined/not tolerated/contra-indicated OR clinical features of sub-acute ulcerative colitis
1. Offer oral prednisolone

Sub-acute
1. Infliximab (NICE, 2008) or vedolizumab (NICE, 2015a)

All extents of disease
If no improvement after 4 weeks of starting step one
1. Consider adding oral prednisolone to aminosalicylate. Stop beclometasone dipropionate if used

If inadequate response to prednisolone
1. Consider adding oral tacrolimus to oral prednisolone (treatment usually up to 3/12)

Acute severe ulcerative colitis: all extents of disease – first presentation or inflammatory exacerbation

Management should involve gastroenterologist and colorectal surgeon. If pregnant, obstetric and gynaecology team should also be included.
1. Offer IV corticosteroids AND assess likely need for surgery

If no improvement or deterioration after 72 hours of IV corticosteroids OR IV corticosteroids not tolerated OR IV corticosteroids contra-indicated
2. Consider adding ciclosporin or surgery
3. Consider adding infliximab if ciclosporin contra-indicated or inappropriate (refer to NICE, 2008)

Ulcerative colitis – maintenance of remission

Mild to moderate proctitis/proctosigmoiditis
1. Consider topical aminosalicylate (enema/suppository) and/or oral low dose oral aminosalicylate (combination more efficacious)

Left-sided and extensive ulcerative colitis
1. Offer low dose of oral aminosalicylate
Consider patient preference, side effects and cost in choice of aminosalicylate
Once daily aminosalicylate

All extents
If two or more exacerbations in 12 months that require systemic corticosteroids OR remission not maintained with aminosalicylate OR to maintain remission after a single episode of acute severe colitis
1. Consider azathioprine or mercaptopurine
2. Consider anti-TNF or vedolizumab

After a single episode of acute severe ulcerative colitis
1. Consider azathioprine or mercaptopurine
2. Consider low dose aminosalictlyate (if azathioprine/mercaptopurine contra-indicated/not tolerated)

Crohn's disease
Induction of remission

Monotherapy
First presentation/single inflammatory exacerbation in 12 month period
1. Conventional glucocorticosteroid, e.g. prednisolone, IV hydrocortisone
2. Enteral nutrition (if child/young person and concerns about growth or side effects)
3. Budesonide (if conventional glucocorticosteroid contra-indicated and distal ileal, ileocaecal or right sided colonic disease). Less effective but may have fewer side effects
4. Aminosalicylate (if glucocorticosteroid declined, contra-indicated, not tolerated). Less effective than conventional glucocorticosteroid or budesonide

Add-on therapy
If 2 or more inflammatory exacerbations in a 12 month period or the dose of glucocorticosteroid cannot be tapered
1. Azathioprine or mercaptopurine (TPMT activity to be assessed prior to initiating treatment)
2. Methotrexate (if azathioprine/mercaptopurine not tolerated or TPMT activity deficient)

Anti-TNF (infliximab, adalimumab)
If fulfils NICE (2010) criteria anti-TNF agent must only be prescribed by a Gastroenterology specialist

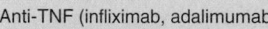

Crohns – maintenance of remission

Patients may or may not be on maintenance treatment. They should be made aware of risk of inflammatory exacerbations (on/off treatment), potential side effects of medication, follow up plan, access to healthcare if experiences a relapse
All extents
1. Azathioprine or mercaptopurine (if previously used with conventional glucocorticosteroid or budesonide to induce remission or if poor prognostic factors e.g. early age onset, perianal disease, glucocorticosteroid use at presentation)
2. Methotrexate (if azathioprine/mercaptopurine not tolerated, contra-indicated e.g. pancreatitis, TPMT deficient)
3. Do not offer a conventional glucocorticosteroid or budesonide to maintain remission
4. Anti-TNF or ustekinumab
5. Stop smoking

Maintenance of remission post surgery

Maintenance treatment post- surgery
1. Azathioprine or mercaptopurine (if adverse prognostic factors e.g. more than one resection; previously complicated or debilitating disease such as abscess, fistulae, penetrating disease)
2. Aminosalictlyate (if Azathioprine or mercaptopurine not tolerated or contra-indicated).
3. Do not offer budesonide or enteral nutrition
4, Anti-TNF

Anti-TNF = anti-tumour necrosis factor (e.g. infliximab, adalimumab)
TPMT = thiopurine methyltransferase
IV = intravenous

Fig. 13.6 Drug treatment algorithm for inflammatory bowel disease. (Adapted from NICE, 2012, 2013.)

Table 13.4 Comparison of commercially available preparations for rectal administration in inflammatory bowel disease

Generic name (proprietary name)	Formulation	Site of release
Budesonide (Entocort)	Retention enema	Rectum and rectosigmoid colon
Budesonide (Budenofalk)	Foam enema	Rectum and rectosigmoid colon
Hydrocortisone acetate (Colifoam)	Foam enema	Rectum and rectosigmoid colon
Mesalazine (Pentasa, Salofalk)	Retention enema	Transverse and descending colon and rectum
Mesalazine (Asacol, Salofalk)	Foam enema	Rectum and rectosigmoid colon
Mesalazine (Asacol, Pentasa, Salofalk)	Suppositories	Rectum
Prednisolone sodium metasulfobenzoate (nonproprietary)	Foam enema	Rectum and rectosigmoid colon
Prednisolone sodium phosphate (Predsol)	Retention enema	Transverse and descending colon
Prednisolone sodium phosphate (nonproprietary)	Suppositories	Rectum
Sulfasalazine (Salazopyrin)	Suppositories	Rectum

Box 13.1 An example of a reducing regimen for oral steroids (prednisolone)

40 mg/day for 1 week
30 mg/day for 1 week
20 mg/day for 4 weeks
15 mg/day for 1 week
10 mg/day for 1 week
5 mg/day for 1 week then stop

Local regimen used at the Oxford University Hospitals NHS Foundation Trust.

---

hypernatraemia and glucose intolerance. Prolonged use can cause cataracts, osteoporosis and increased risk of infection. All patients taking corticosteroids must be issued with a steroid card and counselled on potential side effects.

Rectal corticosteroids. The distribution and absorption characteristics of rectally administered steroids vary greatly. Hydrocortisone (e.g. Colifoam) is readily absorbed from the rectal mucosa, with high peak concentrations compared with prednisolone sodium metasulphobenzoate. Topical preparations may play a role either alone or in combination with oral steroids.

Intravenous corticosteroids. Intravenous corticosteroids remain the mainstay of therapy in severe ulcerative colitis. The landmark article by Truelove and Witts (1955) showed a reduction in mortality from 24% in the placebo group to 7% in the steroid-treated group. Severe extensive or fulminant disease (often referred to as acute severe colitis [ASC]) or disease that is not responding to oral corticosteroids requires hospital admission with parenteral corticosteroids. Patients are given either hydrocortisone sodium succinate, administered intramuscularly or intravenously at doses of 100 mg three or four times a day, or methylprednisolone 15–20 mg three or four times a day, for 5 days. No additional benefit is gained after 7–10 days.

Additional therapy used in severe disease (ulcerative colitis or Crohn's) may include intravenous fluid and electrolyte replacement (especially potassium), blood transfusion and/or intravenous iron replacement, topical therapy for rectal and/or colonic involvement, thromboprophylaxis with prophylactic heparin (IBD is associated with increased coagulopathy), antibiotics and nutritional support. Aminosalicylates should be stopped during an acute severe exacerbation because of poor absorption and the side effect of diarrhoea, which could exacerbate or be misleading. Care should also be taken with the use of anti-motility drugs such as codeine and loperamide and antispasmodic drugs in an acute exacerbation of colitis because they can precipitate a paralytic ileus and toxic megacolon in active disease. Treatment with corticosteroids should not be delayed whilst awaiting microbiological results for possible infective causes.

If improvement is seen with intravenous corticosteroids, oral prednisolone treatment is normally introduced as soon as possible and withdrawn over the following 6–8 weeks. Too-rapid reduction is associated with relapse. Corticosteroids are ineffective in preventing relapse once remission has occurred. The use of immunomodulators or biologics should be considered to induce and maintain remission as the steroids are withdrawn. The use of these drugs (plus surgery) is invariably required if steroid treatment alone fails to induce remission or cannot be withdrawn.

A typical treatment algorithm for the management of an acute attack of ulcerative colitis is presented in Fig. 13.7.

Other steroids. In the UK, oral budesonide (Budenofalk or Entocort) is licensed for the induction of remission in patients with mild to moderate active Crohn's disease affecting the ileum and/or the ascending colon. Budenofalk is also licensed for microscopic colitis. Cortiment is licensed for induction of remission in adults with mild to moderate active ulcerative colitis where aminosalicylates are not sufficient. Rectal budesonide (Entocort enemas) are licensed for ulcerative colitis.

Budesonide is less effective than conventional corticosteroids in inducing remission in active disease, but it has fewer side effects than prednisolone because of its rapid and extensive first-pass metabolism. However, the absorbed drug has a higher affinity for glucocorticoid receptors, 50–100 times that of prednisolone, and so long-term or maintenance treatment is not advocated. Budesonide is useful for moderate terminal ileal Crohn's disease or for patients intolerant to prednisolone, as it is more expensive. A standard dose for induction of remission would be 9 mg/day orally for up to 8 weeks reducing the dose for the last 2 weeks of treatment. Budesonide should not be used in severe active disease.

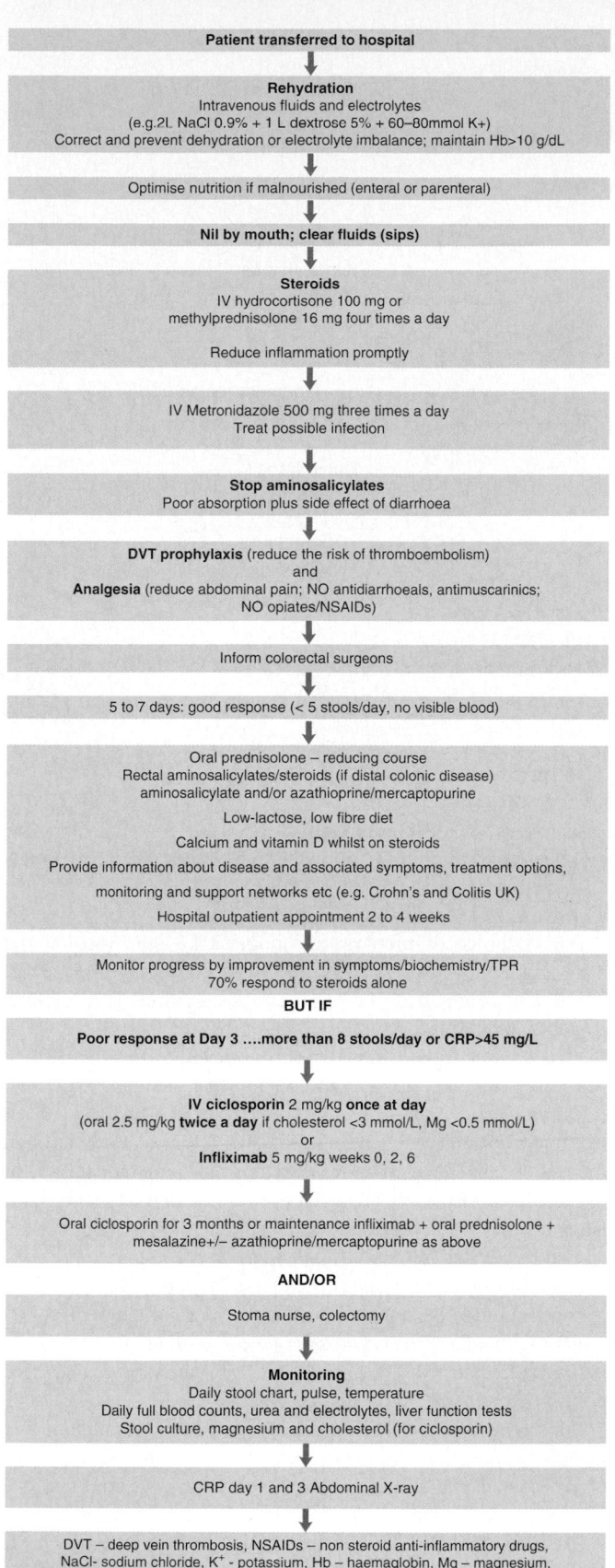

Patient transferred to hospital

↓

Rehydration
Intravenous fluids and electrolytes
(e.g.2L NaCl 0.9% + 1 L dextrose 5% + 60–80mmol K+)
Correct and prevent dehydration or electrolyte imbalance; maintain Hb>10 g/dL

↓

Optimise nutrition if malnourished (enteral or parenteral)

↓

Nil by mouth; clear fluids (sips)

↓

Steroids
IV hydrocortisone 100 mg or
methylprednisolone 16 mg four times a day

Reduce inflammation promptly

↓

IV Metronidazole 500 mg three times a day
Treat possible infection

↓

Stop aminosalicylates
Poor absorption plus side effect of diarrhoea

↓

DVT prophylaxis (reduce the risk of thromboembolism)
and
Analgesia (reduce abdominal pain; NO antidiarrhoeals, antimuscarinics;
NO opiates/NSAIDs)

↓

Inform colorectal surgeons

↓

5 to 7 days: good response (< 5 stools/day, no visible blood)

↓

Oral prednisolone – reducing course
Rectal aminosalicylates/steroids (if distal colonic disease)
aminosalicylate and/or azathioprine/mercaptopurine

Low-lactose, low fibre diet

Calcium and vitamin D whilst on steroids

Provide information about disease and associated symptoms, treatment options,
monitoring and support networks etc (e.g. Crohn's and Colitis UK)

Hospital outpatient appointment 2 to 4 weeks

↓

Monitor progress by improvement in symptoms/biochemistry/TPR
70% respond to steroids alone

BUT IF

Poor response at Day 3 ....more than 8 stools/day or CRP>45 mg/L

↓

IV ciclosporin 2 mg/kg **once at day**
(oral 2.5 mg/kg **twice a day** if cholesterol <3 mmol/L, Mg <0.5 mmol/L)
or
Infliximab 5 mg/kg weeks 0, 2, 6

↓

Oral ciclosporin for 3 months or maintenance infliximab + oral prednisolone +
mesalazine+/– azathioprine/mercaptopurine as above

AND/OR

↓

Stoma nurse, colectomy

↓

Monitoring
Daily stool chart, pulse, temperature
Daily full blood counts, urea and electrolytes, liver function tests
Stool culture, magnesium and cholesterol (for ciclosporin)

↓

CRP day 1 and 3 Abdominal X-ray

↓

DVT – deep vein thrombosis, NSAIDs – non steroid anti-inflammatory drugs,
NaCl- sodium chloride, K$^+$ - potassium, Hb – haemaglobin, Mg – magnesium,
CRP – C-reactive protein, IV – intravenous, TPR – temperature, pulse and respiration, L - litre

Fig. 13.7 Treatment algorithm for an acute severe attack of ulcerative colitis.

Oral beclometasone dipropionate (Clipper) is licensed as adjunct therapy with aminosalicylates for a maximum duration of 4 weeks in ulcerative colitis. It should not be used with other corticosteroids.

Aminosalicylates

The aminosalicylates currently licensed for the treatment of IBD include sulfasalazine, mesalazine, olsalazine and balsalazide. Their mode of action is unclear, but a local effect on epithelial cells by a variety of mechanisms to moderate the release of lipid mediators, cytokines and reactive oxygen species is proposed. Different formulations deliver variable amounts of the active component, mesalazine (5-ASA), to the gut lumen, where it exerts a predominantly local action independent of blood levels. The dissolution profile and site of ulceration determine the effectiveness of different preparations. Diagnosis, disease location, activity, side-effect profile, efficacy and cost all affect the choice of aminosalicylate. Available as oral or rectal preparations, aminosalicylates can be used in combination with steroids to induce and maintain remission in mild to moderate ulcerative colitis. Sulfasalazine is cheaper, but the newer aminosalicylates are generally used in practice. Mesalazine also reduces the risk of colorectal cancer by 75% (St Clair Jones, 2014).

The use of aminosalicylates in Crohn's disease is less well established. They should only be considered for the induction of remission in patients who decline or cannot tolerate glucocorticosteroids and/or for maintenance postoperatively (dose >2 g/day) if an immunosuppressant or biologic is unsuitable (NICE, 2012). Fig. 13.6 highlights the place in therapy of aminosalicylates in the management of ulcerative colitis.

Sulfasalazine consists of sulfapyridine diazotised to mesalazine. It is broken down by bacterial azoreductase in the colon to mesalazine and sulfapyridine. Sulfapyridine is absorbed in the colon, metabolised by hepatic acetylation or hydroxylation followed by glucuronidation and excreted in urine. Mesalazine is partly absorbed, metabolised by the liver and excreted via the kidneys as *n*-acetyl 5-ASA. However, the majority is acetylated as it passes through the intestinal mucosa. Sulfasalazine itself is poorly absorbed, and that which is absorbed is recycled back into the gut, via the bile, either unchanged or as the *n*-acetyl metabolite.

Elimination of sulfapyridine depends on the patient's acetylator phenotype. Those who inherit the 'slow' acetylator phenotype experience more side effects. The dissolution profile of the drug and the site of ulceration determine effectiveness (Fig. 13.8). The optimal dose of sulfasalazine to achieve and maintain remission is usually in the range of 2–4 g/day in 2–4 divided doses. Acute attacks require 4–8 g/day in divided doses until remission occurs, but at these doses, associated side effects are often observed.

About 30% of patients taking sulfasalazine experience adverse effects, which are either dose related and dependent on acetylate phenotype or idiosyncratic and not dose related. Dose-related side effects include nausea, vomiting, abdominal pain, diarrhoea, headache, metallic taste, haemolytic anaemia, reticulocytosis and methaemoglobinaemia. Side effects which are not dose related include rashes, aplastic anaemia, agranulocytosis,

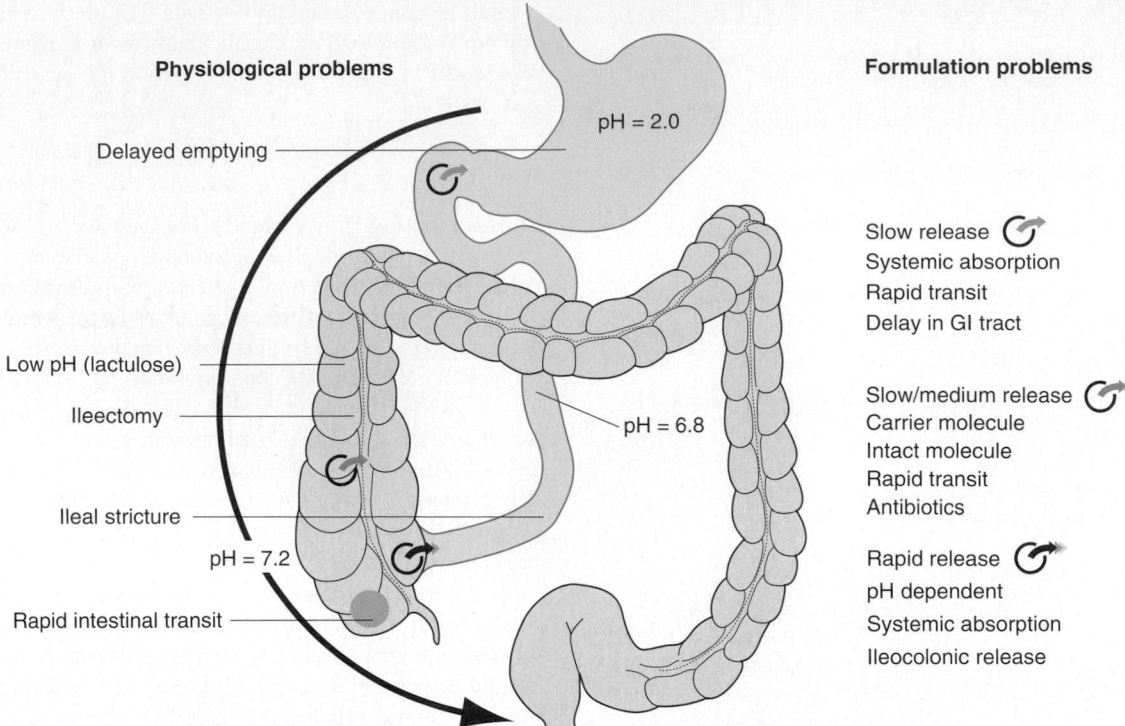

Physiological problems

Delayed emptying

Low pH (lactulose)

Ileectomy

Ileal stricture

pH = 7.2

Rapid intestinal transit

pH = 2.0

pH = 6.8

Formulation problems

Slow release
Systemic absorption
Rapid transit
Delay in GI tract

Slow/medium release
Carrier molecule
Intact molecule
Rapid transit
Antibiotics

Rapid release
pH dependent
Systemic absorption
Ileocolonic release

Fig. 13.8 Physiological and formulation problems encountered with mesalazine and delivery systems.

pancreatitis, hepatic and pulmonary dysfunction, renal impairment, peripheral neuropathy and oligospermia. In 3% of patients, acute intolerance may be seen. The most frequent manifestation is diarrhoea. Adverse effects usually occur during the first 2 weeks of therapy, the majority being related to plasma sulfapyridine levels. Sulfasalazine metabolites are responsible for the yellow colouration of bodily fluids and staining of soft contact lenses.

Sulfasalazine is now only used in favour of mesalazine in those patients who have enteropathy (colitis-associated arthropathy). Mesalazine is tolerated by 80% of patients who are intolerant of sulfasalazine. Many of the sulfonamide-related adverse effects of sulfasalazine are avoided by using one of the newer aminosalicylate formulations. However, mesalazine alone can still cause side effects, including blood disorders, pancreatitis, renal dysfunction and lupoid phenomenon. Patients should be counselled on how to recognise and report blood dyscrasias, and if they occur, treatment should be stopped. Olsalazine-induced diarrhoea may help patients with distal disease and proximal constipation, and in these cases, olslazine is often the 5-ASA of choice.

Formulations of mesalazine. Mesalazine is unstable in acid medium and rapidly absorbed from the gastro-intestinal tract. To increase the stability and/or alter the site of release of active drug in oral formulations, 5-ASA is modified by different delivery systems:

- acrylic resin-coat that releases 5-ASA pH-dependently (Asacol, Salofalk, Octasa);
- ethyl cellulose mesalazine granules that release 5-ASA in a timely manner throughout the gastro-intestinal tract irrespective of pH (Pentasa);

- diazotisation of mesalazine to itself or inert carrier with release of drug in colon by splitting by bacterial enzymes (sulfasalazine, olsalazine, balsalazide);
- multimatrix (Mezavant XL).

Initial choice of preparation should take into account the dose frequency, cost, availability and patient preference. Table 13.5 compares the oral aminosalicylate preparations currently available.

Although once considered not interchangeable, the British National Formulary (BNF) now advises that patients prescribed oral mesalazine should be closely monitored if the preparation needs to be changed (e.g. because of a local formulary). Although there is no evidence to show that any one oral preparation of mesalazine is more effective than the other, delivery characteristics do vary, so patients who are switched to a different brand should be advised to report any changes in their symptoms.

High dose oral aminosalicylate (≥4 g/day) should be given for the induction of remission in mild-moderate ulcerative colitis with or without a rectal aminosalicylate and often in combination with a corticosteroid. For maintenance of remission in ulcerative colitis, doses of ≥2 g/day should be used.

For remission doses, NICE (2013) guidance recommends that a once-daily dosing regimen of aminosalicylate should be considered based on evidence that it can be more effective than multiple dosing and may even be superior. However, it may result in more side effects. It should be noted that not all oral aminosalicylates currently have a UK licence for once-daily dosing, and therefore the prescriber should follow relevant professional guidance and take full responsibility for the decision. Informed consent should be obtained and documented.

Table 13.5 Comparison of available oral aminosalicylate preparations for patients with inflammatory bowel disorder

Drug	Formulation	Optimal drug release pH	Site of drug release
Mesalazine			
Asacol MR	Tablets: 400 mg: Enteric coated with Eudragit S 800 mg: Enteric coated with layer of Eudragit S followed by Eudragit S+L	pH-dependent Delayed release (pH >7)	Terminal ileum and large bowel (colon and rectum)
Octasa MR	Tablets: Enteric coated with Eudragit S	pH >7	Terminal ileum and colon
Mezavant XL	Tablets: Film coated with methacrylate copolymers Type A, Type B	Gastroresistant coating with lipophilic and hydrophilic matrix (pH >7)	Terminal ileum and colon
Pentasa	Tablets and granules: Ethylcellulose-coated microgranules to allow slow, continuous release	Diffusion through semipermeable membrane (any enteral pH[a])	Duodenum to rectum
Salofalk	Tablets: Enteric coated with Eudragit L Granules: Eudragit L and matrix granule structure (slow, continuous release)	pH-dependent Delayed release (pH >6) and matrix	Terminal ileum and colon
Azo-bonded preparations			
Salazopyrin (Sulfasalazine) Colazide (Balsalazide) Dipentum (Olsalazine)	5-ASA + SA Prodrug Dimer	Cleavage by intestinal bacteria azoreductase (pH >7)	Colon

[a]Released at all gastro-intestinal tract pH conditions.
5-ASA, 5-Aminosalicylic acid; SA, sulfasalazine.

Renal function should be monitored before starting an oral aminosalicylate, at 3 months of treatment and then annually during treatment (more frequently in renal impairment), Blood disorders can also occur, and patients should be advised to report any unexplained bruising, bleeding, purpura, sore throat, fever or malaise. The drug should be stopped if there is a suspicion of blood dyscrasias.

In the UK, all mesalazine preparations are licensed for ulcerative colitis; however, only Octasa MR and Asacol MR are licensed for Crohn's disease. Mesalazine has limited efficacy for the treatment of Crohn's disease and in general is not recommended. Mesalazine enemas (1 g), foam enemas (1 g per application) or suppositories (250 mg, 500 mg and 1 g) are effective alternatives for treating distal ulcerative colitis and proctitis. The optimum rectal dose is 1 g. Rectal administrations of 5-ASA formulations are significantly better than rectal corticosteroids in inducing remission in ulcerative colitis, but steroids are cheaper, although availability is now limited. In severe ulcerative colitis, oral and topical formulations should be combined to give prompt symptom relief. Topical and oral 5-ASA is better than either alone (NICE, 2013).

Immunosuppressants

Azathioprine, 6-mercaptopurine, methotrexate, ciclosporin and mycophenolate are immunosuppressants used in patients unresponsive to steroids and aminosalicylates or who relapse when steroids are withdrawn. They are used to induce and maintain remission. They can take several weeks to work and require regular monitoring. They are often referred to as steroid-sparing agents or immunomodulators.

Thiopurines (azathioprine, mercaptopurine). The thiopurines remain the first-line immunomodulators used for the treatment of IBD. Azathioprine is metabolised to 6-mercaptopurine by the liver. Mercaptopurine is further metabolised to pharmacologically active 6-thioguanine nucleotides (TGN). Mercaptopurine is also metabolised by the enzyme thiopurine methyltransferase (TPMT), which produces methylmercaptopurine (MeMP), and xanthine oxidase (XO), which produces thiouric acid. Neither of these metabolites are pharmacologically active. Patients who have high levels of TPMT can produce high levels of MeMP, which can cause hepatotoxicity. High levels of TGN can cause dose-related adverse effects, such as myelosuppression. Fig. 13.9 shows the metabolic pathway of azathioprine. Competing pathways result in inactivation by TPMT or XO or incorporation of cytotoxic nucleotides into DNA.

TPMT activity should be assessed before initiating azathioprine or mercaptopurine to inform the initial starting dose and identify patients at increased risk of myelosuppression or liver dysfunction. TPMT measurements are not used in dose optimisation. In patients where the TPMT activity is deficient (very low or absent), azathioprine or mercaptopurine should not be used. Lower treatment doses (half recommended initiation doses) can be considered if TPMT activity is below normal but not deficient.

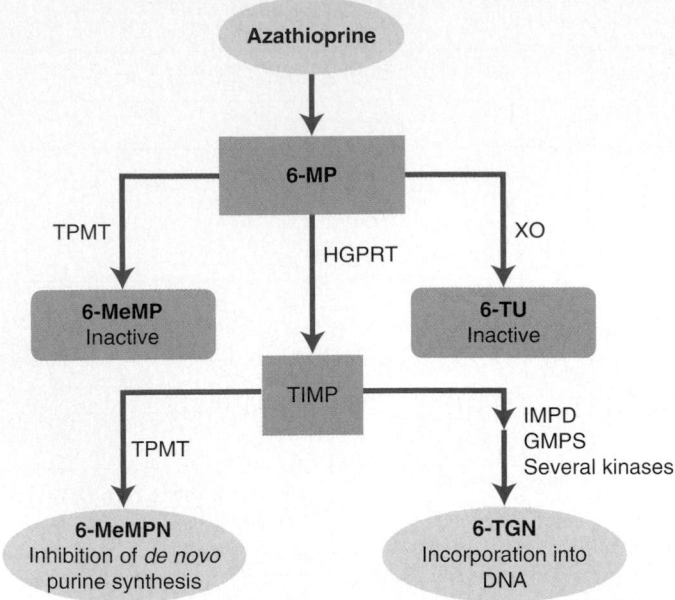

6-MP = mercaptopurine; TPMT = thiopurine methyltransferase; 6-MeMP = methylmercaptopurine; XO = xanthine oxidase; TIMP = thioiosinic acid; 6-TGN = thioguanine nucleotides; 6-MeMPN = methylmercaptopurine nucleotide; 6-TU = thiouric acid; GMPS = guanosine monophosphate synthetase; HGPRT = hypoxanthine-guanosine-phosphoribosyl-transferase; IMPD = inosine monophosphate dehydrogenase

Fig. 13.9 Metabolic pathway of azathioprine. (Adapted from Dervieux et al., 2001; McLeod and Siva, 2002.)

Box 13.2	Thiopurine methyltransferase levels
<10 mU/L	Deficient
20–67 mU/L	Low
68–150 mU/L	Normal
>150 mU/L	High

One in 300 people have no functional TPMT activity, and most patients who develop leucopenia will have a normal TPMT. TPMT levels are used for predicting early events rather than long-term control (see Box 13.2).

Both azathioprine and 6-mercaptopurine have steroid-sparing properties. Although the action in IBD is unclear, their active metabolites inhibit purine ribonucleotide synthesis, which may in turn inhibit lymphocyte function, primarily T cells.

Azathioprine and mercaptopurine are recommended for the induction and maintenance of remission in IBD, although they have a much slower onset of action than steroids in active disease. They should be considered in patients who:

- require two or more steroid courses in 1 year;
- continue to have chronic active disease when prednisolone is reduced below 15 mg/day or within 6 weeks of stopping;
- are intolerant of aminosalicylate therapy;
- are post-op for prophylaxis of complex Crohn's disease (fistulising/extensive disease);
- fail to maintain remission with 5-ASA in ulcerative colitis;
- have suffered a single episode of acute severe ulcerative colitis;
- require thiopurine to maintain remission in Crohn's disease if used to induce remission with steroids and/or have poor prognostic signs.

Oral maintenance doses for azathioprine are usually 2–2.5 mg/kg/day (typically 100–250 mg/day) and for mercaptopurine, 1–1.5 mg/kg/day (typically 50–150 mg/day). Doses are adjusted to patient response, tolerance, white blood cell and platelet counts and 6-thioguanine levels. Patients are usually prescribed a reducing dose of corticosteroid, in addition, to induce remission because mercaptopurine and azathioprine can take several weeks to show a therapeutic benefit.

Seventy percent of patients will tolerate azathioprine. Of the remaining 30%, a further 70% will tolerate mercaptopurine. The most common side effects occur within 2–3 weeks of starting treatment and rapidly stop on withdrawal. These include flu-like symptoms (myalgia, headache), nausea and diarrhoea. Nausea is reduced by taking the medicine with food. Although rare (<3%), leucopenia can develop suddenly and unpredictably. Hepatotoxicity and pancreatitis have also been reported in less than 5% of patients. Thioguanine has been used but is associated with a greater risk of hepatotoxicity.

There is ongoing debate as to how long thiopurines can safely be used for, particularly because the patient is likely to be young when treatment is initiated. One of the main concerns is the increased risk of developing lymphoproliferative disorders (lymphoma, non-melanoma skin cancers and cervical dysplasia) (Gomollon et al., 2016). This risk remains very small (<1%) after 10 years of use (Mowat et al., 2011). There is currently insufficient data to suggest that anti-tumour necrosis factor (anti-TNF) agents alone increase the risk of lymphoproliferative disorders

Table 13.6 Therapeutic drug monitoring of thiopurines and actions required

Metabolite level	Reason	Action
MeMP and TGN low/absent	Not adhering to treatment	Patient education
TGN and MeMP low/absent but adhering to treatment	Subtherapeutic dosing	Increase dose. Recheck levels after 4 weeks (when reach steady state).
TGN low, MeMP high	May be unresponsive to treatment and at risk of hepatotoxicity	Consider co-prescribing allopurinol, which, by inhibiting XO and possibly methylating pathways, results in higher ratio of thiopurine converted to TGN. In this case, the dose of azathioprine needs to be reduced to 25–50% of the standard dose to avoid excessive TGN levels.
TGN and MeMP high with patient not responding to treatment	Nonresponder to treatment	Stop thiopurine and consider alternative treatment.

The recommended range is 200–400 pmol/8x10^8 red blood cells for TGN and <5700 pmol/8x10^8 red blood cells for MeMP.
MeMP, methylmercaptopurine; TGN, thioguanine nucleotides; XO, xanthine oxidase.

or solid tumors. In contrast, their combination with thiopurines significantly increases the risk of lymphoproliferative disorders, and there have been rare cases of fatal hepatosplenic T-cell lymphoma reported. Cases have been predominantly young males (≤35 years) (NICE, 2012). Although the absolute risk of malignancy is low, the risks should always be balanced carefully against the substantial benefits associated with these treatments and discussed with the patient.

Therapeutic drug monitoring of thiopurine metabolites (TGN and MeMP) is increasingly used to assess adherence and dose optimisation and to allow patients who were previously considered intolerant of or not responding to thiopurines to remain on this treatment. The recommended therapeutic range is of TGN is 200–400 pmol/8 × 10^8 red blood cells and <5700 pmol/8 × 10^8 red blood cells for MeMP. Table 13.6 highlights how these results should be interpreted and action to take. Low white blood cell counts or abnormal LFTs may be caused by high TGN or MeMP levels, respectively.

Methotrexate. A low-dose regimen of methotrexate is effective in inducing and maintaining remission in patients with chronically active Crohn's disease. The evidence for use in ulcerative colitis is less convincing, although use is common in practice.

Patients receive once-weekly doses of methotrexate ranging from 15 to 25 mg on the same day each week. These can be given orally or by subcutaneous or intramuscular injection. Oral medication is more practical, although parenteral administration may be more effective and better tolerated. Methotrexate is reserved for patients intolerant or unresponsive to thiopurines. Methotrexate can take between 6 weeks to 3 months to have a full effect.

Methotrexate metabolites inhibit dihydrofolate reductase, although this cytotoxic action does not explain the drug's anti-inflammatory effect. Inhibition of cytokine and eicosanoid synthesis and modification of adenosine levels probably contribute.

Adverse effects associated with methotrexate are essentially gastro-intestinal (nausea, vomiting, diarrhoea and stomatitis). These may also be reduced by prescribing weekly doses of folic acid 5 mg. Folic acid should not be taken on the same day as the methotrexate. Monitoring is undertaken because of the serious side effects of hepatotoxicity, bone marrow suppression and pneumonitis.

Methotrexate is teratogenic, and all male and female patients should be counselled about using contraception while taking the medication and also for 3 months after therapy is withdrawn. Guidance to improve the safety of methotrexate use and minimise the potential risk of overdose has been issued (National Patient Safety Agency [NPSA], 2007). Measures include the issue of patient handheld monitoring cards detailing dose and blood test results, comprehensive written and verbal medication information, dispensing one strength of tablet (2.5 mg) and ensuring in-patient medication charts clearly state once-weekly dosing and the number and strength of tablets routinely used. A memory aid commonly recommended to patients to remember dose frequency is to take methotrexate on Mondays and folic acid on Fridays. Tablets disperse in water, which may help adherence because there are typically large numbers of tablets per dose.

Calcineurin inhibitors (ciclosporin, tacrolimus). Ciclosporin is a calcineurin inhibitor that acts at an early stage on precursors of helper T cells by interfering with the release of interleukin-2. This inhibits the formation of the cytotoxic lymphocytes which cause tissue damage. Both controlled and uncontrolled studies suggest that ciclosporin is effective rescue therapy for severe ulcerative colitis failing to respond to intravenous steroids (Campbell et al., 2005). Its use in Crohn's disease is unproven.

Doses of 2–5 mg/kg/day in treating acute severe colitis have been shown to be effective. A dose of 2 mg/kg/day intravenously has been shown to be as effective as 4 mg/kg/day, and because of dose-related toxicity, 2 mg/kg/day should be used. Patient response to ciclosporin has varied, with adverse effects causing withdrawal of treatment in some cases. However, some patients have stopped concurrent steroid therapy and have remained in remission for some time.

When patients with severe colitis fail to show little or no improvement within 72 hours of starting parenteral steroids, or their symptoms worsen at any time despite corticosteroid treatment, then ciclosporin at an intravenous dose of 2 mg/kg/day/i.v. is indicated.

If patients respond to parenteral ciclosporin, they can subsequently be maintained on an oral dose (5 mg/kg in two divided doses) for 3–6 months. If patients have a low plasma magnesium (<0.5 mmol/L) or low cholesterol (<3 mmol/L), they are at an increased risk of ciclosporin-induced seizures when given intravenously. In these circumstances, treatment with an oral ciclosporin preparation from the outset at a dose of 5 mg/kg/day in two divided doses (to account for variation in bioavailability), is preferred. Ciclosporin therapy is used for many patients but normally as a bridge to colectomy or starting maintenance treatment with azathioprine or mercaptopurine. When used to bridge to azathioprine maintenance therapy, it is estimated that 30–50% of patients with steroid-refractory ulcerative colitis remain in clinical remission at the end of 1 year (Turner et al., 2007b). Treatment with ciclosporin should not be longer than 3–6 months because significant toxicity precludes long-term use.

Infliximab is an alternative 'rescue therapy' for acute severe colitis (NICE, 2008) if ciclosporin is contraindicated or clinically inappropriate. The result of a multi-centre randomised controlled trial (CONSTRUCT) that compared the clinical and cost-effectiveness of infliximab and ciclosporin in the treatment of steroid-resistant acute severe colitis showed similar efficacy in prevention of short- and long-term colectomy rates (Duijvis et al., 2016). Forty percent of patients who receive ciclosporin develop minor side effects, such as tremor, paraesthesia, headache, gum hyperplasia, burning sensations of the hands and feet and hirsutism. Major complications include nephrotoxicity, neurotoxicity, hepatotoxicity and hypertension with low mortality reported. In severe proctitis, refractory to standard treatments, ciclosporin enemas have been used with some success at a dose of 250 mg at night for 1 month. No commercial preparation is available, which prohibits routine use in practice.

Tacrolimus is an alternative calcineurin inhibitor to ciclosporin that has shown some benefit in inducing remission in ulcerative colitis. It can be considered as a treatment option if there is an inadequate response to oral prednisolone after 2–4 weeks in mild to moderate ulcerative colitis (NICE, 2013) at a dose of 0.025 mg/kg twice daily. Tacrolimus has limited value in Crohn's disease.

Tacrolimus is also associated with bone marrow suppression, hypertension and renal dysfunction. It may also induce diabetes.

The main concern with calcineurin inhibitors is opportunistic infection, such as *Pneumocystis carinii* pneumonia (PCP) and *Aspergillus fumigatus* pneumonia. Routine use of PCP prophylaxis may be considered, particularly if patients are on dual or triple immunosuppression.

Trough drug levels, taken before a dose, should be monitored for both ciclosporin and tacrolimus. For ciclosporin, the target level is within the range of 100–200 ng/mL; for tacrolimus, the target level is within the range of 5–15 ng/mL. Both drugs take 2–3 days to reach steady state. Grapefruit juice, macrolide antibiotics (mainly erythromycin and clarithromycin), ketoconazole, fluconazole, itraconazole, diltiazem, verapamil, oral contraceptives and protease inhibitors are just some of the drugs that increase both ciclosporin and tacrolimus levels and can cause toxicity. Both ciclosporin and tacrolimus should be prescribed by brand because of variations in absorption and subsequent effects on efficacy and toxicity.

Mycophenolate. Mycophenolate (MMF) has shown to be of some benefit in the management of IBD in patients intolerant to thiopurines. It appears to be safe, well tolerated and efficacious for both short- and long-term therapy, without the need for dose escalation. Further evaluation of mycophenolate comparing it to conventional immunosuppressants is required (Gomollon et al., 2016).

Monitoring of aminosalicylates and immunosuppressants. It is essential that patients who are receiving aminosalicylates and immunomodulators have regular blood monitoring to ensure they avoid toxicity associated with these drugs as a result of bone marrow suppression and hepatotoxicity. The effects of these drugs should be monitored as advised. Documented local safety monitoring policies and procedures (including audit) for people receiving drugs that need monitoring is strongly recommended. Shared care policies are developed where care of a patient is the joint responsibility of both secondary and primary care doctors. These policies should clearly highlight the responsibilities of primary and secondary care healthcare staff and the patient with ulcerative colitis or Crohn's disease or the patient's parent/carer as appropriate. A member of the staff within the multidisciplinary team should be nominated to act on abnormal results and communicate with primary care or secondary care doctors and patients with ulcerative colitis and/or their parents or carers, as appropriate.

Blood tests should include full blood counts and LFTs, including plasma bilirubin and alkaline phosphatase. These should be undertaken weekly for the first month and then every 2 to 3 months unless there is a dose change, when bloods should be repeated more frequently. Although often advised, there is no evidence that more frequent monitoring is more effective. Patients should be taught to recognise the signs of bone marrow suppression and liver toxicity (e.g. jaundice) and educated about the need for earlier blood tests and the increased risk of infection because of immunosuppression. It is recommended that all patients initiated or maintained on immunosuppressants are provided with a record card detailing current dose and blood test results. Guidance on appropriate action following abnormal blood results is provided in Box 13.3.

All patients taking immunomodulators should be vaccinated against seasonal influenza and pneumococcal pneumonia. Patients should be advised to avoid live vaccines such as polio and yellow fever while taking immunosuppressants, including corticosteroids. Sunscreens and protective covering should be encouraged to reduce sunlight exposure to patients taking immunosuppressants to reduce the risk of skin cancers.

Biologic agents

Monoclonal antibodies are a significant treatment development in recent years for IBD. They are used to induce and maintain remission in severe disease. If effective, they can reduce corticosteroid requirements, help to drain fistulae, achieve mucosal healing and reduce the need for major abdominal surgery or hospitalisation. The main licensed monoclonal antibodies currently used are anti-tumour necrosis factor α (anti-TNF-α) antagonists (infliximab, adalimumab, golimumab), the α4β7 integrin antagonist (vedolizumab) and the IL-12, IL-23 antagonist (utekinumab).

Biologics should only be started by doctors with experience in their use in IBD, and their clinical benefit should be reviewed regularly. They are generally indicated for patients who have

Box 13.3 Guidance on dealing with abnormal blood results for patients on immunosuppressant therapy

Baseline U & Es, LFTs and FBC should be carried out prior to initiation of therapy. These should be repeated weekly for 4 weeks then every 2–3 months. If there is a dose change, blood should be rechecked after 2 weeks.

Methotrexate should be withheld and the relevant expert advice obtained if any of the following occur:

WBC	$<3.5 \times 10^9$/L
Neutrophils	$<2 \times 10^9$/L
Platelets	$<150 \times 10^9$/L
AST/ALT	$>3 \times$ normal range

- Unexplained respiratory symptoms, e.g. dyspnoea, dry cough, especially if accompanied by fever and sweats
- Renal impairment
- Mouth or throat ulceration/rash/unexplained bleeding/fever/alopecia/recurrent sore throats, infections, fever or chills/nausea/vomiting/diarrhoea

Azathioprine or **mercaptopurine** should be withheld and the relevant expert advice obtained if any of the following occur:

WBC	$<3.5 \times 10^9$/L
Neutrophils	$<2 \times 10^9$/L
Platelets	$<150 \times 10^9$/L
AST/ALT	$>3 \times$ normal range

- Significant reduction in renal function
- Mouth or throat ulceration/rash/unexplained bleeding/fever/upper abdominal or back pain/alopecia/recurrent sore throats, infections, fever or chills/nausea/vomiting/diarrhoea
- Nausea may be relieved by taking the dose with/after food or in divided doses

Ciclosporin should be withheld and the relevant expert advice obtained if any of the following occur:
- High blood levels (will require dose adjustment)
- Significant reduction in renal function
- Uncontrolled hypertension
  Drug blood levels should be done at similar intervals to FBC. A 12-h trough level should be taken (i.e. before a dose). Target level within the range of 100–200 ng/mL. It takes 2–3 days to reach steady state after dose change.

ALT, Alanine transaminase; AST, aspartate transaminase; FBC, full blood count; LFTs, liver function tests; U & Es, urea and electrolytes; WBC, white blood cell.

The use of biosimilars has made a significant impact on the financial costs of treating IBD with these agents; costs are now up to 40% cheaper than the originator biologic. The licence of the biosimilar was based on extrapolated data from a rheumatology population. However, studies in the IBD population have demonstrated comparable efficacy and safety in patients who were switched to an infliximab biosimilar compared to naïve anti-TNF-α users and also patients who had been previously exposed to one or more biologics (Fiorino et al., 2016). Table 13.7 summarises the biological agents currently used in IBD. The choice should take into account drug licensing, funding, access and cost.

There is currently no specific guidance regarding how long biologics should be continued. Many patients in clinical remission for greater than 1 year, with a normal CRP and complete mucosal healing on endoscopy, will remain in remission during the following year after stopping treatment with an anti-TNF agent. All biologics should be reviewed regularly to assess appropriate use. If patients clinically respond to induction doses, maintenance should be given until treatment failure (including the need for surgery) or until 12 months after initiation of treatment, whichever is shorter. Patients should then have their disease reassessed and continue treatment if there is clear evidence of ongoing active disease and treatment is still clinically appropriate. Treatment can be restarted if patients subsequently relapse. The STORI trial (Louis et al., 2012) identified that infliximab withdrawal was associated with a high risk of relapse. Patients in the study were on combination therapy with infliximab and thiopurine. Treatment was stopped after 6 months of remission (clinical and endoscopic). The average relapse rate was 58% at 1 year, which suggested that if well tolerated, treatment should not be interrupted. Patients with two or fewer identified risk factors had a relapse risk of only 14–16%. Risk factors were identified as male sex, no previous surgical resection, WCC $>6 \times 10^9$/L, haemoglobin <145 g/L, CRP >5 mg/L, faecal calprotectin >300 micrograms/g. The study also found that restarting treatment with infliximab following symptoms relapse was successful in 98% of patients if restarted within 6 months of stopping treatment.

Monoclonal antibodies are contraindicated in patients with tuberculosis (TB); therefore, all patients should have a chest X-ray prior to administration to exclude active or latent TB. Other contraindications include moderate to severe cardiac failure, history of malignancy (excluding non-melanoma skin cancer), sepsis (including pelvic or perianal) and optic neuritis. Intestinal stricturing is a relative contraindication because obstruction may be exacerbated through rapid healing at the stricture site. Chronic hepatitis B/C carriers, primary failure or absence of inflammatory activity (normal CRP) are also contraindications.

Infliximab and vedolizumab are given via an intravenous infusion, whereas adalimumab, golimumab, certolizumab and ustekinumab can be given subcutaneously, enabling patients to self-administer at home. Infliximab must be administered in a setting where there are adequate resuscitation facilities available and patients can be closely monitored because of the potential risk of an acute infusion-related reaction, including anaphylactic shock, and delayed hypersensitivity reactions. As yet, there have been no reported anaphylactic or severe infusion reactions reported for vedolizumab.

Infection is the main concern with all anti-TNF agents. Patients self-administering adalimumab, golimumab or certolizumab at

failed, are intolerant or have contraindications to conventional therapy including corticosteroids and immunomodulators.

Study design and patient populations are sufficiently different between studies of different biological agents used in IBD. Therefore, direct comparisons of efficacy should be viewed with caution.

In Crohn's disease, those patients with a high disease activity and features indicating a poor prognosis may derive greater benefit from earlier use – for example, patients diagnosed younger than 40 years old and patients with stricturing disease, steroid dependency, perianal disease, greater than 5 kg weight loss and complex fistulae (Gomollon et al., 2016).

Not all patients will require biological therapy, which is expensive. Currently, only infliximab is commercially available as a biosimilar, with a biosimilar of adalimumab anticipated in 2018.

Table 13.7 Summary of biological agents used in inflammatory bowel disease (adults only)

Agent	Mode of action	Indication	Criteria	Licensed in UK	Standard dose	UK National funding/ access decisions NICE TA
Infliximab	Anti-TNF-α antagonist	Crohn's disease	Moderately to severely active disease in patients who have not responded despite a full and adequate course of therapy with a corticosteroid and/or an immunosuppressant or who are intolerant to or have medical contraindications for such therapies	Yes	5 mg/kg at weeks 0, 2 and 6; if responds, maintenance 5 mg/kg every 8 weeks	TA187 (NICE, 2010) Infliximab and adalimumab for the treatment of Crohn's disease
			Fistulising active disease, in patients who have not responded despite a full and adequate course of therapy with conventional treatment (including antibiotics, drainage and immunosuppressive therapy)	Yes	5 mg/kg at weeks 0, 2 and 6, then refer to product literature	TA187 (NICE, 2010) Infliximab and adalimumab for the treatment of Crohn's disease
		Ulcerative colitis	Induction and maintenance of remission of moderate to severe active disease in patients who have had an inadequate response to conventional therapy including corticosteroids and or who are intolerant to or have medical contraindications for such therapies	Yes	5 mg/kg at weeks 0, 2 and 6; if responds, maintenance 5 mg/kg every 8 weeks	TA329 (NICE, 2015b) Infliximab, adalimumab and golimumab for treating moderately to severely active ulcerative colitis after the failure of conventional therapy
			Option for treatment of acute exacerbation of severe ulcerative colitis when treatment with ciclosporin is contraindicated or inappropriate	Yes	5 mg/kg at weeks 0, 2 and 6; if responds maintenance 5 mg/kg every 8 weeks	TA163 (NICE, 2008) Infliximab for acute exacerbation of ulcerative colitis
Adalimumab	Anti-TNF-α antagonist	Crohn's disease	Moderately to severely active disease unresponsive to full and adequate course of therapy with a corticosteroid and/or an immunosuppressant or who are intolerant to or have medical contraindications for such therapies	Yes	160 mg subcutaneously on week 1, 80 mg week 2 then 40 mg subcutaneously on alternate weeks; can increase to weekly if loss of response. Review treatment if no response within 12 weeks of initial dose.	TA187 (NICE, 2010) Infliximab and adalimumab for the treatment of Crohn's disease
		Ulcerative colitis	Moderately to severely active disease unresponsive to full and adequate course of therapy with a corticosteroid and/or an immunosuppressant or who are intolerant to or have medical contraindications for such therapies	Yes	160 mg subcutaneously on week 1, 80 mg week 2 then 40 mg subcutaneously on alternate weeks	TA329 (NICE, 2015b) Infliximab, adalimumab and golimumab for treating moderately to severely active ulcerative colitis after the failure of conventional therapy
Golimumab	Anti-TNF-α antagonist	Ulcerative colitis	Moderate to severely active disease who have not responded adequately to conventional therapy or who are intolerant to it	Yes	200 mg week 0, 100 mg week 2, then 50 mg every 4 weeks (100 mg if >90 kg)	TA329 (NICE, 2015b) Infliximab, adalimumab and golimumab for treating moderately to severely active ulcerative colitis after the failure of conventional therapy

Table 13.7 Summary of biological agents used in inflammatory bowel disease (adults only)—cont'd

Agent	Mode of action	Indication	Criteria	Licensed in UK	Standard dose	UK National funding/access decisions NICE TA
Certolizumab pegol	Anti-TNF-α antagonist	Crohn's disease	Moderate to severely active disease when patients have lost response to or are intolerant of alternative licensed anti-TNF antagonist	No	400 mg subcutaneously at weeks 0, 2, 4 and then 400 mg every 4 weeks	No NICE TA undertaken Individual funding request required
Vedolizumab	α4β7 antagonist	Crohn's disease	Moderately to severely active disease who have had an inadequate response with, lost response to or were intolerant to either conventional therapy or a TNF-α antagonist	Yes	300 mg intravenously at weeks 0, 2, 6 and then maintenance every 8 weeks. Review treatment if no response after 10 weeks. Can increase to every 4 weeks if loss of response.	TA352 (NICE, 2015c) Vedolizumab for treating moderately to severely active Crohn's disease after prior therapy
Vedolizumab	α4β7 antagonist	Ulcerative colitis	Moderately to severely active disease who have had an inadequate response with, lost response to, or were intolerant to either conventional therapy or a TNF-α antagonist	Yes	300 mg at weeks 0, 2, 6 and then maintenance every 8 weeks. Review treatment if no response after 10 weeks. Can increase to every 4 weeks if loss of response.	TA342 (NICE, 2015a) Vedolizumab for treating moderately to severely active ulcerative colitis
Ustekinumab	IL-12, IL-23 antagonist	Crohn's disease	Moderately to severely active Crohn's disease who have had an inadequate response with, lost response to or were intolerant to either conventional therapy or a TNF-α antagonist or have medical contraindications to such therapies	Yes	Intravenous induction treatment (dose depends on body weight and is approximately 6 mg/kg). Maintenance subcutaneous treatment at week 8 (90 mg), then every 12 weeks	TA456 (NICE, 2017) Ustekinumab for moderately to severely active Crohn's disease after previous treatment

6-MP, 6-Mercaptopurine; AZA, azathioprine; IL, interleukin; TA, technology appraisal; TNF, tumour necrosis factor.

home should be educated on how to recognise signs of infection, for example, fever, productive cough, toothache, stinging on passing urine or if neurological symptoms develop and therefore delay their dose.

Anti-TNF-α antagonists (infliximab, adalimumab, golimumab, certolizumab) are monoclonal antibodies which inhibit the functional activity of the proinflammatory cytokine TNF-α, which damages cells lining the gut, causing pain, cramping and diarrhoea. Colonic biopsies post-treatment with these agents show a substantial reduction in TNF-α and a reduction in the commonly elevated plasma inflammatory marker CRP.

Around 40% of patients with Crohn's disease do not respond to treatment with anti-TNF agents, 30% to 50% achieve complete remission after 6 months and 30% of patients maintain the response for 12 months with continual treatment (Mowat et al., 2011).

Infliximab. Infliximab is a chimeric human murine monoclonal antibody licensed for treating patients who have moderate to severely active Crohn's disease (with or without fistulae) or ulcerative colitis, who are unresponsive/intolerant or who have contraindications to conventional therapy such as corticosteroids and/or immunosuppressants or antibiotics. NICE (2010) defines appropriate use of infliximab in Crohn's disease as a CDAI score of 300 or more or a Harvey–Bradshaw score of 8 or 9 or above. For ulcerative colitis, moderate disease is defined as more than 4 daily bowel movements but the patient is not systemically ill; and severe ulcerative colitis as more than 6 bowel movements daily and the patient is also systemically unwell (with tachycardia, fever, anaemia or a raised ESR) (NICE, 2015b).

Infliximab is administered by intravenous infusion at a standard dose of 5 mg/kg, which in practice is often rounded up or down to the nearest 100 mg vial. The induction dosing is at weeks 0 and 2 and if a clinical response is seen, and then a maintenance dose of 5 mg/kg every 8 weeks should be given. Fixed dosing is superior to intermittent dosing because of the reduced risk of immunogenicity (NICE, 2010). The effectiveness of infliximab for maintenance of Crohn's disease was demonstrated in the ACCENT 1 study (Hanauer et al., 2002) and, the ACCENT II for fistulising disease (Sands et al., 2004) and confirmed in the SONIC study (Colombel et al., 2010). The effectiveness of infliximab in maintaining clinical remission and mucosal healing in ulcerative colitis was observed in ACT 1 and 2 studies (Gomollon et al., 2016).

In some patients, infliximab has been associated with either infusion (during or shortly after infusion) or delayed hypersensitivity reactions. It may also affect the normal body immune responses in a significant number of patients. Anaphylactic reactions have been reported. All doses should be preceded with intravenous corticosteroid (hydrocortisone 100 mg) unless the patient has been taking an immunosuppressant for more than 3 months, to reduce the risk of a hypersensitivity reaction. Other side effects include headache, dizziness, nausea, rash, raised LFTs, abdominal pain and fatigue.

Adalimumab. Adalimumab is a fully humanised anti-TNF monoclonal antibody which is licensed for the treatment of moderate to severely active Crohn's disease and ulcerative colitis where patients are refractory or intolerant to corticosteroids and/or conventional immunomodulators. It may also be used in those patients who have primary or secondary nonresponse to infliximab or developed a hypersensitivity reaction. Because adalimumab is fully humanised, it is less immunogenic than infliximab. It also has the advantage of being given as a subcutaneous injection, which enables patients to self-administer at home, therefore reducing nursing time and hospital bed occupancy. This also lends itself to being supplied by home delivery services. The licensed dose is an initial induction of 80 mg followed by 40 mg at week 2 and then 40 mg on alternate weeks thereafter as maintenance. An accelerated dose of 160 mg followed by 80 mg and then 40 mg on alternate weeks maintenance is more commonly used in practice, particularly in those patients who have previously been on infliximab. The maintenance dose can be increased to 40 mg weekly if a diminished or suboptimal response is seen, Treatment should be stopped if no response is seen within 12 weeks of the initial dose in Crohn's disease or within 8 weeks in ulcerative colitis.

Adalimumab effectiveness in maintaining clinical remission in Crohn's disease was proven in the CHARM study (Colombel et al., 2007). The ULTRA 2 study supported the benefit versus placebo for maintaining remission in ulcerative colitis (Sandborn et al., 2012).

Certolizumab. Certolizumab is a PEGylated monoclonal antibody fragment TNF-α antibody. It was given a negative opinion by the European Medicines Agency Committee for Medicinal Products for Human use in IBD and is not approved by NICE. It is therefore rarely used and only in difficult cases where a TNF antagonist may be justified but other drugs within the class have exhibited secondary loss of response or are not tolerated. It is administered by subcutaneous injection.

Golimumab. Golimumab is only licensed for ulcerative colitis. It is administered by subcutaneous injection. Efficacy was demonstrated in the PUSUIT studies (Sandborn et al., 2014). The standard dosing regimen is 200 mg at initial induction, 100 mg at week 2, then 50 mg every 4 weeks (100 mg if >90 kg); treatment should be reviewed if no response after 4 doses.

Vedolizumab. Vedolizumab is a humanised monoclonal antibody and is a highly gut-selective immunosuppressive biologic. It works by exclusively binding to α4β7 integrin, which is a protein preferentially expressed on a subset of lymphocytes. These lymphocytes migrate to the gastro-intestinal tract and cause inflammation characteristic of IBD. Vedolizumab binds to the α4β7 integrin and subsequently inhibits the ability of the lymphocytes to interact with gut endothelial cells (via the mucosal address in cell adhesion molecule-1 [MAdCAM-1]) and thus inhibits their ability to cross the endothelium and cause inflammation.

Clinical studies suggest it is more effective in ulcerative colitis than Crohn's disease. Efficacy in achieving significant rates of clinical remission compared to placebo was demonstrated in the GEMINI 1 and II studies (Feagan et al., 2013; Sandborn et al., 2013).

Vedolizumab can take up to 10 weeks to show clinical benefit. This relatively slow onset of action makes it inappropriate for acute severe colitis. If no therapeutic benefit is observed by week 10, treatment should be stopped. Longer-term remission data appear to be more favourable compared to anti-TNF-α antagonists. The standard dosing regimen is 300 mg at initiation, weeks 2 and 6 and then every 8 weeks. Vedolizumab is administered by intravenous infusion over 30 minutes. Current advice states it should only be used during pregnancy if the benefits clearly outweigh any potential risk to both the mother and foetus.

The gut-specific mode of action appears to result in minimal systemic immunosuppressive effects when compared with anti-TNF-α antagonists. The most common reported side effects are nasopharyngitis, headache and arthralgia. Malignancy has been reported in less than 1% of cases (colon cancer and melanoma). This safety profile suggests vedolizumab can be prescribed long-term to young and elderly patents (Bryant et al., 2015).

Ustekinumab. Ustekinumab is a human monoclonal antibody that targets the p40 subunit of the interleukins (IL)-12 and IL-23, thereby preventing their binding to receptors of T-cells and natural killer cells. It was licensed in early 2017 for patients with moderately to severely active Crohn's disease who have had an inadequate response with, lost response to, or are intolerant of either conventional therapy or a TNF-α antagonist or who have medical contraindications to such therapies. Maintenance dosing is administered subcutaneously every 8–12 weeks. Clinical efficacy has been demonstrated in the UNITI-1, UNITI-2 and IM-UNITI studies (Feagan et al., 2016).

Other biologics. There are several trials in IBD looking at other biologics which target different molecules in the inflammatory process to modulate the immune response. These include Janus kinase (JAK) inhibitors.

Combination of biologics with immunomodulators. Concomitant immunosuppressant therapy (e.g. thiopurines, methotrexate) with anti-TNF agents is not associated with better clinical efficacy in patients who have already failed these drugs. However, in the SONIC study, a combination of infliximab plus azathioprine was shown to be more efficacious in achieving and maintaining steroid-free remission than infliximab monotherapy or azathioprine monotherapy in patients naïve to both therapies (Colombel et al., 2010). The rate of infusion-related infliximab reactions was also less with combination treatment, with no significant difference in the rate of serious infection. Immunomodulators are thought to reduce the risk of anti-drug antibody formation and potentiate efficacy. In practice, the results of this study have been extrapolated to other biologics and immunomodulator combinations. At present there is no clear evidence that this is required for vedolizumab, but theoretically, anti-drug antibodies could lead to loss of response. This is counterbalanced by one of the benefits of vedolizumab monotherapy, which is the avoidance of systemic immunosuppression. Until further evidence is available, it is usually recommended by most gastro-enterologists that immunomodulators do not need to be routinely started alongside vedolizumab. However, if a patient is already on and tolerating an immunomodulator, it is reasonable to continue this pending further information.

A recent review of the clinical management of Crohn's disease by NICE states that there is uncertainty regarding the comparative effectiveness and long-term adverse effects of immuno-suppressants when combined with biologics (infliximab and adalimumab), and the use of monotherapy or combination therapy should be discussed with patients when initiating treatment with an anti-TNF antagonist and regularly throughout treatment (NICE, 2016).

Medication optimisation of biologics. Current strategies to overcome a loss of response or concerns regarding adherence of biologics include increasing the dose, decreasing the interval between administrations or switching to a different agent (same class or one with a different mode of action). Optimising the use of a concurrent immunomodulator may also be indicated.

The ability to measure drug levels (trough) and anti-drug antibodies for infliximab and adalimumab provides an alternative strategy to optimise the use of these treatment options. Assays to measure levels of other biologics are under development. The benefit of therapeutic drug monitoring was highlighted in the TAXIT trial, which investigated the value of optimising infliximab by measuring trough levels and anti-drug antibodies in patients in clinical remission (Vande Casteele et al., 2012).

The main indications for requesting trough anti-TNF and antibody levels in IBD are if there is a loss of response, annual review of stable disease and following dose alteration. Assessment of levels and anti-drug antibodies serum concentrations after induction may also be a predictive tool for estimating the long-term clinical response to biological therapy.

The timing of testing is important. Levels must be taken just prior to a dose (up to maximum of 24–48 hours). The results must be considered in context with symptoms, disease activity (e.g. C-reactive protein [CRP], full blood count [FBC], ferritin, Harvey–Bradshaw index), patient history (e.g. previous surgery, disease severity, current life events) and endoscopic, histological and radiological findings before dose adjustments are made. NICE has developed guidance on the use of therapeutic drug monitoring of anti-TNF inhibitors in Crohn's disease (NICE, 2016).

Antibiotics

The gut microbiota plays a role in promoting and maintaining inflammation in inflammatory bowel diseases, hence the rationale for the use of antibiotics in the treatment of those disorders. Antibiotics, however, may induce undesirable side effects and resistance, especially during long-term therapy. Most of the evidence for benefit is in Crohn's disease associated with perianal disease, sepsis associated with abscesses, fistulae, perforation and bacterial overgrowth in the small bowel. There is little benefit demonstrated for their use in ulcerative colitis, except for in pouchitis.

Different antibiotics, including ciprofloxacin, metronidazole, and the combination of both rifaximin and anti-tuberculous regimens, have been evaluated in clinical trials for the treatment of inflammatory bowel disease, although more studies are needed to define their exact role. Rifaximin is virtually unabsorbed after oral administration and is devoid of systemic side effects. Rifaximin has provided promising results in inducing remission of Crohn's disease and ulcerative colitis. It may also have a role in maintaining remission of ulcerative colitis and pouchitis. The potential therapeutic activity of rifaximin in IBD requires further research.

Pseudomembranous colitis caused by *C. difficile* usually occurs after prolonged or multiple antibiotics. This can be distinguished from other causes of colitis by biopsy and stool culture. If it is unclear whether a patient has pseudomembranous or acute colitis, empirical treatment with metronidazole or vancomycin and steroids is advised. A colonoscopy can be performed once symptoms resolve.

Cytomegalovirus (CMV) affects more than 40% of the population. When it occurs, CMV colitis usually affects IBD patients who are significantly immunosuppressed. It occurs more frequently with ulcerative colitis than with Crohn's disease. The most common clinical presentation mimics a flare or relapse, with bloody diarrhoea, fever and abdominal pain. Poor response to corticosteroids should prompt investigation of CMV as a cause for symptoms. There is a high mortality associated with CMV (up to 30%), and therefore prompt treatment with ganciclovir or valganciclovir is indicated (Filizzola et al., 2004).

Other treatments

Thalidomide. Thalidomide has been used, under specialist supervision, in refractory cases of Crohn's disease. Thalidomide acts as a TNF-α inhibitor and probably stabilises lysosomal membranes. At therapeutic doses, it also inhibits the formation of superoxide and hydroxyl radicals, both potent oxidants capable of causing tissue damage. Daily doses in the range of 50–400 mg have proved beneficial when used for periods of 1 week to several months. Side effects during treatment include sedation, dry skin and reduced libido. Thalidomide is teratogenic and should never be used in women of childbearing age.

Antidiarrhoeals. Codeine and loperamide should be used with caution to treat diarrhoea and abdominal cramping in IBD. Their use may mask inflammation, infection, obstruction or colonic dilation, thereby delaying correct diagnosis.

Bile salt sequestrants. Diarrhoea resulting from the loss of bile salt absorption such as bowel resection of terminal ileal disease, may improve with a bile sequestrant such as cholestyramine. Doses of up to 4 g three times a day inhibit the secretion of water and electrolytes stimulated by bile acids. Colestipol and colesevelam are alternatives. Patients may undergo a ^{75}Se tauroselcholic acid (SeHCAT) scan to formally diagnose bile salt malabsorption.

Fish oils (omega-3 fatty acids). Fish liver oils containing eicosapentaenoic and docosahexaenoic acids have been used with some success in the treatment of both ulcerative colitis and Crohn's disease. These products cause unpleasant regurgitation, which renders them unpalatable in long-term use. Enteric-coated preparations have reduced this problem. It is thought that fish oils work by diverting fatty acid metabolism from leukotriene B4 to the formation of the less inflammatory leukotriene B5.

Miscellaneous treatments. There are many limited trials, studies and case series in the literature evaluating other therapies for ulcerative colitis and Crohn's disease. These include sodium cromoglicate, bismuth and arsenic salts, sucralfate, nicotine, oxygen-derived free radical scavengers, somatostatin analogues, lidocaine, chloroquine, D-penicillamine, carbomers, antituberculous agents, heparin, aloe vera and worm therapy (helminths). In general, these treatments are not recommended, although the variety illustrates the limitations of current therapy. When a patient is not responding to conventional agents, consideration should be given to referral to a specialist centre for a review of current therapy and a plan for future management. Complementary treatments, for example, acupuncture and aromatherapy, may have a role in improving quality of life, but if used, this use should be concomitant with standard medical and surgical care.

Leukapheresis has been shown to have some benefit in patients with IBD. It involves removal of leucocytes from the blood, either through an adsorptive system or by centrifugation. In each system, venous blood is removed in a continuous flow, anticoagulated, processed to deplete the leucocytes and returned to the circulation (NICE, 2005).

There is some evidence that faecal microbiota transplantation (FMT) may have a therapeutic role in IBD (Lopez and Grinspan, 2016). FMT is the administration of a solution of faecal matter from a donor into the intestinal tract of a recipient to directly change the recipient's gut microbial composition and confer a health benefit. Faecal microbiota transplantation has the potential to be an effective and safe treatment for IBD, although well-designed randomised controlled trials are required in this area (Anderson et al., 2012). FMT has been used to successfully treat recurrent *C. difficile* infection (NICE, 2014).

Autologous hematopoietic stem cell transplantation has been used in a small number of patients with severe refractory Crohn's disease, with encouraging results (Gomollen et al., 2016). Further studies are required to define its place in therapy

VSL♯3, a probiotic, has efficacy in the maintenance treatment of pouchitis, although real-world remission rates, palatability, availability and cost all limit its use. Another probiotic, Mutaflor (*Escherichia coli* Nissle), is as effective as 5-ASA in the maintenance of ulcerative colitis and is utilised in occasional cases. Prebiotics stimulate the growth of specific, beneficial microorganisms in the colon, whilst symbiotics are a combination of both prebiotics and probiotics.

Surgical treatment

Of Crohn's disease patients, 50–80% will require surgery within 5–10 years of diagnosis. In contrast, 20–30% of ulcerative colitis patients will usually undergo colectomy over long-term follow-up (20 years).

In ulcerative colitis, proctocolectomy is curative. Most patients elect to subsequently have an ileoanal pouch formed, although this is a quality-of-life decision, and some decide to continue with a permanent ileostomy. Up to 30% of patients will ultimately require surgical intervention. In those who undergo ileal pouch surgery, half will suffer from pouchitis, in which antibiotics are commonly required to treat and prevent symptoms.

All patients admitted to hospital with acute severe colitis should be assessed daily for the likelihood of requiring surgery. Acute severe colitis is typically defined using the Truelove and Witts's criteria. These are met if the patient is passing 6 or more bloody stools in 24 hours plus has at least one of the following: a tachycardia (pulse >90 bpm), a fever (>37.8 °C), raised ESR >30 mm/h (CRP often used as a surrogate), and/or anaemia (Hb <10.5g/dL). The severity of the colitis is related to the additional number of Truelove and Witts's criteria met, with other markers including endoscopic severity (as defined by the ulcerative colitis endoscopic index of severity), a low albumin and adverse features on an abdominal X-ray (colonic dilatation, mucosal oedema, mucosal islands). The need for rescue therapy (failure of i.v. steroids) is usually determined by stool frequency of >8 on day 3 or a CRP >45 mg/L on day 3 of steroid treatment. Ciclosporin or infliximab can be used as rescue therapy (NICE, 2013).

Curative surgery is not possible in Crohn's disease because recurrence is normal. Complications (stenosis, abscess, fistula) in the course of their illness result in about 70% of patients with Crohn's disease requiring at least one surgical procedure. Surgical techniques vary and include resection and anastomosis, and strictureplasty. The choice of surgical procedure will depend on type and extent of disease, presence of complications and previous response to medical treatment. If a significant length of gut is removed, this can result in short gut syndrome, which may require long-term parenteral nutrition and medication to control a high-output stoma.

Control of a high-output stoma either because of short gut or following colectomy should be carefully managed to prevent dehydration and metabolic disturbance, for example, hyponatraemia and hypomagnesaemia. Drinking more non-isotonic solutions can make the situation worse because this flushes the contents of the small intestine through and exacerbates dehydration. Food and drink can promote secretion and increase volume. The causes of high-output stomas need to be considered and may include high lactose intake, partial obstruction, intraabdominal sepsis, gastric hypersecretion, inappropriate diet, laxatives and diuretics. Treatment options should include a high-dose proton pump inhibitor (PPI) to reduce gastric acid hypersecretion and codeine phosphate (180–240 mg/day) and/or loperamide (doses up to 100 mg/day are common) to reduce gut motility. In the absence of a colon, a dose of loperamide that exceeds 16 mg/day can be used without adverse effect. Octreotide has been used as an alternative to the antimotility drugs but would appear to offer limited benefit and is best reserved for when other measures have been tried. Intake of isotonic fluids with a sodium concentration greater than 90 mmol/L, to allow the jejunum to absorb water, is also indicated. Care should be taken with medication that could be affected by rapid transit through the gastro-intestinal tract, leading to reduced or erratic absorption (e.g. modified-release preparations) or medication that could alter fluid and electrolytes or be affected by changes caused by dehydration (e.g. digoxin).

Prophylactic treatment should be considered to maintain remission after surgery for Crohn's disease. The choice of therapy will depend on the presence of adverse prognostic factors for disease recurrence, the most reliable of which are active smoking and perforating disease. Smoking cessation in patients who smoke significantly reduces postoperative relapse (Gionchetti et al., 2016). Other factors such as disease location, previous response to therapy, and disease recurrence after previous operations should be considered. The choice of postoperative therapy is currently as for standard maintenance (immunomodulators and/or anti-TNF therapy). The role of vedolizumab has yet to be established. Whatever strategy is initially used, it is now good practice to reassess disease activity at colonoscopy with or without small bowel imaging at 6–12 months postoperatively and adjust management accordingly. Because ulcerative colitis is confined to the colon, prophylactic treatment in ulcerative colitis is unnecessary following colectomy.

Patient care

The impact of a diagnosis of IBD should not be underestimated. In general, most patients are diagnosed when they are relatively young, and the disease can have a significant effect on the rest of their lives. In addition to managing symptoms, the condition can result in loss of education and difficulty in gaining employment or insurance. In young patients, it can cause psychological problems and growth failure or retarded sexual development. Anxiety and loss of self-esteem are commonly described. In addition to pharmacological treatments, psychological support is also important. It is important to counsel patients on the importance of medication adherence during periods of remission. Medical treatment with corticosteroids and immunosuppressants may cause secondary health problems such as infection, and surgery may result in complications such as intestinal failure. The care of patients with IBD is therefore a challenge for the multidisciplinary team.

NICE management guidelines for ulcerative colitis (NICE, 2013) and Crohn's disease (NICE, 2016) highlighted patient information and support as key priorities for implementation (i.e. having the biggest impact on patient care and outcomes) in the management of induction and maintenance of remission. All information and advice should be appropriate for the patient's age, cognitive/literacy levels and cultural/linguistic needs and in an understandable format. Discussions with patients should include treatment options, monitoring, side effects, diet and nutrition, fertility, prognosis and cancer risk. Patients and/or their parents or carers should be informed of contact details for support groups (e.g. Crohn's and Colitis UK), which can provide leaflets on such issues as the disease itself, treatments, insurance, employment and pregnancy. Patients and/or parents and carers should be aware of whom to contact when symptoms of active disease develop. Primary care doctors and community pharmacists should be aware of the contact details for their local IBD nurse specialist, if available, and how to get rapid access to secondary care services when necessary. As with any condition, patients should be warned about unreliable information sources. Pharmacists have a key role in providing information to patients about their medication and have an integral role within the multidisciplinary team in caring for this patient group.

All patients should be educated about their illness and medication and reminded that even in periods of remission, it is important to continue taking prescribed therapy. This should take the form of verbal and written information. Drug use is invariably lifelong, and patients are likely to receive several different treatments during the course of their illness as a result of intolerance or lack of response. Certain patients, such as females or newly diagnosed patients, may require more tailored information about the condition or treatment. Patients with poor dexterity may find the use of rectal preparations difficult, and these preparations may therefore be poorly tolerated.

Patients and primary care doctors may require additional reassurance because several of the treatments used, for example, azathioprine, are unlicensed for IBD. Regular blood monitoring of aminosalicylates and immunosuppressants is essential to ensure patients avoid the toxicity associated with these drugs. All patients taking steroids must be issued a steroid card. Shared care policies between primary care doctors, gastroenterologists and patients should be in place.

Optimising pharmacological treatments in inflammatory bowel disease

Table 13.8 summarises the pharmacological profile of drugs used in adults with IBD. Medicine optimisation is important in IBD patients to maximise the beneficial clinical outcomes, particularly because medication is associated with toxic side effects and in the case of biologics, high financial costs. Adherence to medication, even in periods of remission, is very important. Treatments can be optimised by the following strategies:

- Provide tailored information on the condition, its complications and the medication used to individuals and/or their carers.
- Ensure good communication within the multidisciplinary team and across primary and secondary care interfaces.
- Encourage adherence even during periods of remission; studies have shown non-adherence to be one of the main factors contributing to relapse (Robinson et al., 2013).
- Provide good education for patients on how to take medication, especially administration of topical therapy, which is essential to ensure effectiveness and adherence.
- Use an appropriate dose and reduction regimen of corticosteroids during an acute flare.
- Advise patients taking aminosalicylates on how to increase their dose during a flare and how to reduce to an appropriate maintenance dose when in remission.
- Prescribe the most appropriate rectal formulation therapy for the site of disease (e.g. enema for descending colon, foam for sigmoid colon, suppositories for rectum), with the patient's dexterity and the cost of the formulation also taken into account.
- Review medication choice in patients who are in clinical remission.
- Develop rescue strategies in patients who have stopped treatment and subsequently relapsed.
- Use therapeutic drug monitoring to optimise treatment with thiopurines and biologics.

Table 13.8 Pharmacological profile of drugs used in adults with inflammatory bowel disease

Pharmacological group	Daily dose	t½	Metabolism
Steroids			
Hydrocortisone	125–250 mg as foam enema	1.5 h	Hepatic metabolism 70% and 30% unchanged
	100–400 mg in 0.9% w/v in sodium chloride intravenous injection	1.5 h	Hepatic metabolism 70% and 30% unchanged
Prednisolone	20–40 mg orally	3 h	Hepatic metabolism 70% and 30% unchanged
	20 mg as foam or liquid enema	3 h	Hepatic metabolism 70% and 30% unchanged
	5–10 mg as suppositories	3 h	Hepatic metabolism 70% and 30% unchanged
Budesonide	3–9 mg orally 2mg/dose as foam or liquid enema	2.8 h	90% Hepatic metabolism
Aminosalicylates			
Mesalazine	500 mg to 1.5 g as suppositories	0.7–2.4 h	Local and systemic hepatic acetylation, glucuronidation
	1 g as enema	0.7–2.4 h	Local and systemic hepatic acetylation, glucuronidation
	1.2–4.8 g orally	0.7–2.4 h	Local and systemic hepatic acetylation, glucuronidation
Olsalazine	1–3 g orally	1.0 h	Local and systemic hepatic acetylation, glucuronidation
Sulfasalazine	3 g as enema	5–8 h	Colonic azo-reduction Local and systemic acetylation Hepatic glucuronidation
	1–2 g as suppositories	5–8 h	Colonic azo-reduction Local and systemic acetylation Hepatic glucuronidation
	4–8 g orally	5–8 h	Colonic azo-reduction Local and systemic acetylation Hepatic glucuronidation
Balsalazide	3–6.75 g orally	1.0 h	Local and systemic hepatic acetylation
Antibiotics			
Metronidazole	600 mg–1.2 g orally	6–24 h	Hepatic metabolism
	1.5 g intravenously	6–24 h	Hepatic metabolism
Immunosuppressants			
Azathioprine	2–2.5 mg/kg/day orally	3 h	Hepatic metabolism to 6-mercaptopurine
Mercaptopurine	1–1.5 mg/kg/day orally	1.5 h	Hepatic metabolism to inactive metabolite
Methotrexate	15–25 mg orally/intramuscular/subcutaneous injection once weekly	3–10 h	Insignificant metabolism at low doses
Ciclosporin	2 mg/kg intravenously 2.5 mg/kg twice daily orally	19–27 h	Mainly hepatic metabolism Mainly hepatic metabolism
Mycophenolate	1–2 g/day orally	11–24 h	Hepatic metabolism
Tacrolimus	0.025 mg/kg twice daily orally	43 h	Hepatic metabolism

Table 13.8 Pharmacological profile of drugs used in adults with inflammatory bowel disease—cont'd

Pharmacological group	Daily dose	t½	Metabolism
Monoclonal antibodies			
Infliximab	5 mg/kg intravenous infusion every 8 weeks (maintenance)	8–9 days	Unknown
Adalimumab	40 mg subcutaneous injection every 2 weeks (maintenance)	10–19 days	Unknown
Certolizumab	400 mg subcutaneous injection every 4 weeks (maintenance)	14 days	Unknown
Golimumab	50 mg subcutaneous injection every 4 weeks (maintenance)	9–15 days	Unknown
Vedolizumab	300 mg intravenous infusion every 8 weeks (maintenance)	25 days	Unknown
Ustekinumab	90 mg subcutaneous injection every 8–12 weeks (maintenance)	3 weeks	unknown
Miscellaneous			
Arsenic salts	250 mg to 1 g rectally	72 h	Tissue deposition excreted unchanged
Bismuth salts	200 mg to 1.2 g rectally	60–80 h	Tissue deposition excreted unchanged
Fish oils	3–4 g	None	Used in the arachidonic acid cycle
Sodium cromoglicate	200–800 mg orally 100–400 mg rectally	Unknown	Poorly absorbed, excreted unchanged in urine and bile
Nicotine	5–15 mg transdermally	0.5–2.0 h	Hepatic oxidation to cotinine 5% excreted unchanged
Lidocaine	200–800 mg rectally	1–2 h	Hepatic de-ethylation and hydrolysis 3% excreted unchanged Largely excreted unchanged
Human growth hormone	1.5–5 mg daily by subcutaneous injection	0.5–4 h	Unknown
Thalidomide	100–400 mg orally	7–16 h	Hydrolysis
Cholestyramine	4–12 g orally		Not absorbed
Probiotics, e.g. VSL#3	1–2 sachets daily orally		Poorly absorbed

Pregnancy

IBD affects young adults, so pregnancy is not uncommon. Patients are strongly advised to discuss any plans for pregnancy with their gastroenterologist. Information should be provided on the effects of disease on pregnancy and the potential risks and benefits of medical treatment. There needs to be good communication across specialties involved in the joint care of pregnant women (e.g. primary care doctors, obstetrics, gastroenterology and colorectal surgeons). Good nutrition, stopping smoking and adherence to medication are important.

Most women with IBD have a normal pregnancy and deliver a healthy baby. Active disease is more of a risk to a normal pregnancy than medication. Disease control prior to conception and throughout the pregnancy is associated with the best outcomes for both mother and baby. Conception occurring at a time of active disease increases the risk of persistent activity during pregnancy. Women who continue maintenance treatment throughout pregnancy reduce the risk of a flare in the postpartum period, when the risk is more likely.

There is no evidence that inactive Crohn's disease and ulcerative colitis affect fertility, although active Crohn's disease or previous pelvic or pouch surgery can reduce it. There is no evidence that medication affects fertility in females. In males, sulfasalazine causes reversible oligospermia. In such cases, an alternative aminosalicylate should be used as appropriate.

Children of parents with IBD have an increased risk of developing IBD, although the overall risk remains low. The risk is higher for Crohn's disease and also if both parents are affected. Although most babies born are normal and healthy, caesarean delivery is more frequent in women with IBD. There is also an increased risk of low birthweight and preterm birth, which is linked to disease activity at conception or during the pregnancy (van der Woude et al., 2015).

With the exception of methotrexate, mycophenolate and thalidomide, which are contraindicated in pregnancy, most drugs used in the treatment of IBD do not present a significant hazard. There is currently little information for the use in vedolizumab in pregnancy. Despite most patient information leaflets cautioning use in pregnancy or breastfeeding, most specialists agree that maintenance treatment should continue to keep disease under control (van der Woude et al., 2015). The risk of infection with anti-TNF agents alone or in combination with immunomodulators is controversial.

Infliximab and adalimumab are generally considered low risk. Because both drugs cross the placenta and can stay in the circulation of the baby for several months, consideration to discontinue at around 32 weeks of pregnancy should be discussed. Because these drugs remain in the baby's circulation, live vaccines such as the rotavirus vaccine and Bacillus Calmette–Guérin vaccine (BCG) should be avoided in the first 6 months after birth. Table 13.9 summarises the risks associated with the use of IBD medications during pregnancy and lactation.

Vaginal delivery or caesarean section should be discussed because the pelvic floor muscles used to deliver naturally are also important for bowel function. This is particularly important if surgery (such as a pouch formation) may be required in the future. A caesarean section is almost always recommended when there is active perianal Crohn's disease or when there is an ileo-anal pouch or ileorectal anastomosis. It is worth considering a caesarian section in those with ulcerative colitis who have higher risk factors for future surgery, such as those with more than one admission for acute severe ulcerative colitis.

Smoking

Encouraging patients to stop smoking, especially those with Crohn's disease, can have a significant impact on the course of the disease as well as other health benefits. Smoking increases the risk of flare and postoperative relapse and increases the risk of blood clots. In pregnant women with IBD who smoke, there is a higher chance of a low-birth-weight baby and a higher risk of deformity and miscarriage.

Osteoporosis

Long-term steroid use and underlying IBD both contribute to a higher risk of developing osteoporosis. This is prevalent in up to 50% of the patient population with IBD. Patients with Crohn's disease appear more susceptible to osteoporosis than those with ulcerative colitis. Regular DEXA-scanning should be considered, and preventive treatment with bisphosphonate and/or calcium and vitamin D supplements may be necessary.

Table 13.9 Risks of inflammatory bowel disease medications used during pregnancy and lactation

Drug	During pregnancy	During lactation
Mesalazine	Low risk	Low risk
Sulfasalazine	Low risk	Low risk
Corticosteroids	Low risk	Low risk, 4 h delay before breastfeeding is advised
Azathioprine, mercaptopurine	Low risk	Low risk
Anti-TNF agents	Low risk; consider stopping around third trimester in patients with sustained remission	Probably low risk, limited data
Vedolizumab	Limited data	Avoid
Methotrexate	Contraindicated	Contraindicated
Thalidomide	Contraindicated	Contraindicated
Ciclosporin, tacrolimus	Low risk	Avoid
Mycophenolate	Contraindicated	Avoid
Metronidazole	Avoid first trimester	Avoid
Ciprofloxacin	Avoid first trimester	Avoid

TNF, Tumour necrosis factor.

Guidance for the treatment of osteoporosis in IBD has been published by NICE (2013).

Anaemia

Iron supplementation is recommended in all IBD patients with iron-deficiency anaemia. Although there is evidence of benefit in treating iron deficiency without anaemia in other conditions, such as chronic fatigue and heart failure, such evidence is not yet available in the context of IBD.

The aim of iron supplementation is to normalise haemoglobin levels and iron stores. An increase in haemoglobin of at least 2 g/dL within 4 weeks of treatment is an acceptable speed of response.

Intravenous iron should be considered as first-line treatment in patients with clinically active IBD, with previous intolerance to oral iron, with haemoglobin below 10 g/dL, and in patients who need erythropoiesis-stimulating agents. The usual treatment of iron-deficiency anaemia with oral iron has relevant limitations in IBD patients such as malabsorption and gastro-intestinal irritation. Intravenous iron is more effective, shows a faster response and is better tolerated than oral iron. It is, however, more expensive. There is no difference in efficacy between the available licensed intravenous preparations.

Opportunistic infections and vaccination

IBD patients at most risk of opportunistic infections are those treated with immunomodulators and biologics, especially in combination, and those with malnutrition. The European Crohn's and Colitis Organisation has published evidence-based consensus guidelines on the prevention, diagnosis and management of opportunistic infections in IBD (Rahier et al., 2014). UK practice currently recommends influenza (annually), pneumococcal and human papilloma virus (HPV) (female) vaccinations if age appropriate. Hepatitis B vaccinations should be considered prior to starting immunosuppressants (including steroids and biologics) in the non-immune high-risk patient. Patients taking immunosuppressants, including biologics, should avoid live vaccines such as MMR, oral polio, yellow fever, live typhoid, varicella and BCG.

Immunosuppressants should be withheld and specialists informed in those patients suffering from chickenpox or active skin lesions in shingles. For those with exposure to chickenpox or shingles and no history of infection/vaccination, passive immunisation with varicella zoster immune globulin (VZIG) should be carried out.

Colonoscopic surveillance

Adults with IBD may have a higher risk of developing colorectal cancer than the general population. The increased risk is typically associated with the extent, severity and longevity of inflammation and other factors, such as the presence of coexistent primary sclerosing cholangitis (PSC), an inflammatory disease of the bile ducts. Colorectal cancer is the third most common cancer in the UK. Colonoscopic surveillance in people with IBD can detect any problems early and potentially prevent progression to colorectal cancer. In the UK, for people who are not already in surveillance programmes, the NHS Bowel Cancer Screening Programme offers screening using faecal occult blood testing every 2 years to all men and women aged 60–74 years. People undergoing colonoscopic surveillance are not generally offered screening as part of the Bowel Cancer Screening Programme. Colonoscopic surveillance in the UK should be offered in line with NICE (2011) guidelines.

Since the original Quality Care: Service Standards for the Healthcare of People Who Have Inflammatory Bowel Disease (IBD) was published (IBD Standards Group UK, 2009), there have been marked improvements in the delivery of IBD services, as shown by the findings of the UK-wide IBD audits. Care should be delivered by a multidisciplinary team comprising a medical gastroenterologist, nurse specialist, pharmacist, dietician, psychologist, colorectal surgeon, primary care doctor, radiologist and histopathologist. The aim of these standards is to ensure patients receive consistent, high-quality care and that IBD services throughout the UK are evidence based, engaged in local and national networking, based on modern information technology (IT) and audited to meet specific minimum standards. A quality standard for IBD was published by NICE (2015d) to improve services across the UK. There are several published guidelines for the management of IBD (Mowat et al., 2011; Dignass et al., 2012a, 2012b; NICE, 2012, 2013; Gomollen et al., 2016) that aim to provide a consistent, evidence-based and cost-effective strategy for treating this challenging group of patients.

Case studies

Case 13.1

Miss AT presents with weight loss, fluctuating symptoms of abdominal pain and occasional blood in stool. On examination she appears thin and pale and complains of angular stomatitis and mouth ulcers causing problems with eating. Her abdomen is tender. On imagining and colonoscopy there is ileocaecal and perianal distribution of Crohn's disease. She is a social drinker and smokes 10 cigarettes/day.

Miss AT has been on adalimumab (40 mg on alternate weeks) for the last 6 months, and a recent serum trough level came back as 1.2 micrograms/mL (reference range of assay 4.9–6.5 micrograms/mL). She started a reducing course of steroids 2 weeks ago.

Other blood results included Hb 8.9 g/dL, CRP 21 mg/L, platelets 400×10^9/L, temperature 37 °C.

Questions

1. What action should be taken with a subtherapeutic level of adalimumab?
2. What advice, if any, would you give regarding Miss AT smoking?

Answers

1. The reason for a suboptimal therapeutic level may be poor adherence, suboptimal dosing or the presence of anti-drug antibodies. Adherence should be questioned, but if Miss AT is taking her adalimumab as prescribed, the dose should be increased to 40 mg weekly. Another trough level should be performed after a couple of months.

   If there were high levels of anti-drug antibodies detected, then it would be appropriate to switch to a different anti-TNF agent, such as infliximab. If Miss AT has previously had infliximab, and had secondary loss of response or it was not tolerated, then consider different target, for example, usteknumab.

   Miss AT is not currently on an immunomodulator. Provided there are no contraindications or previous reports of intolerance, azathioprine should be added at a dose of 2–2.5 mg/kg/day. The TPMT level should be checked prior to starting azathioprine. If the TPMT activity is deficient (very low or absent), azathioprine should not be used. Lower treatment doses (half recommended initiation doses) can be considered if TPMT activity is below normal but not deficient. Alternatively, methotrexate could be considered.
2. Encouraging patients to stop smoking, especially those with Crohn's disease, can have a significant impact on the course of the disease as well as other health benefits. Smoking increases the risk of disease flare and postoperative relapse and increases the risk of blood clots.

Case 13.2

Mr BG is newly diagnosed with mild ulcerative colitis. His abdominal X-ray suggests predominantly disease of the rectum and sigmoid colon. His past medical history includes joint stiffness as a result of rheumatoid arthritis. He presents at the pharmacy with a prescription for Asacol MR tablets 800 mg three times a day and Salofalk 1 g rectal foam enemas, two administrations at bedtime.

Questions

1. What advice would you give Mr BG about the administration of Salofalk enemas?
2. The community pharmacist substitutes Asacol MR tablets for Octasa MR tablets 800 mg three times a day. Does the change of mesalazine brand matter?
3. Can Octasa MR be taken in a single daily dose?
4. What are the side effects of 5-ASA treatments?

Answers

1. Rectal therapy is appropriate for mild left-sided disease. Enemas are best administered just before bedtime when the supine position allows longer retention times. Salofalk rectal foam comes in a canister that is first fitted with an applicator and then shaken for about 20 seconds before the applicator is inserted into the rectum as far as is comfortable. To administer a dose of Salofalk, the pump dome is fully pushed down and released. The spray will only work properly when held with the pump dome pointing down. Following the first or second activation, depending on need, the applicator should be held in position for 10–15 seconds before being withdrawn from the rectum. If the patient has difficulty in holding this amount of foam, the foam can also be administered in divided doses: one at bedtime and one in the morning. The best results are obtained after the bowels have been emptied. A new applicator is used for each dose. Patients with rheumatoid arthritis may have difficulty in using enemas, and this may affect adherence and treatment success. Mr BG should be shown how to use the product. The aerosol canister is flammable, and care should be taken in sunlight and temperatures over 30 °C.

2. To increase the stability and/or alter the site of release of active drug in oral formulations, 5-ASA is modified by different delivery systems. Both Asacol MR and Octasa MR tablets have an acrylic resin-coat that releases 5-ASA pH-dependently. Although once considered not interchangeable, the British National Formulary (BNF) now advises that patients prescribed oral mesalazine should be closely monitored if the preparation needs to be changed (e.g., because of the local drug formulary). Although there is no evidence to show that any one oral preparation of mesalazine is more effective than the other, patients who are switched to a different brand should be advised to report any changes in their symptom control. The dose, frequency and patient acceptability are more important than the product.

3. For maintenance of remission NICE (2013) recommends that a once-daily dosing regimen of aminosalicylate should be considered based on evidence that it can be more effective than multiple dosing and may even be superior. However, it may result in more side effects.
The licensed dose of Octasa MR tablets for induction of remission of mild acute ulcerative colitis is 2.4 g (three tablets) once daily or in divided doses. For moderate disease, this can be increased to six tablets. Maintenance doses are in the range of 1.6 g to 2.4 g (two to three tablets) taken once daily or in divided doses. The maximum adult dose should not exceed six tablets a day and not exceed three tablets taken together at any one time.

4. The side effects of aminosalicylates include diarrhoea, nausea, vomiting, abdominal pain, headache, exacerbation of colitis. Renal function should be monitored before starting an oral aminosalicylate, at 3 months of treatment and then annually during treatment. More frequent monitoring is required for patients with renal impairment. Blood disorders can also occur, and patients should be advised to report any unexplained bruising, bleeding, purpura, sore throat, fever or malaise. The drug should be stopped if there is a suspicion of blood dyscrasias. Aminosalicylates should be avoided in patients with salicylate hypersensitivity.

Case 13.3

Miss CP presents with a 3-week history of acute, foul-smelling, bloody diarrhoea accompanied by mild to severe lower abdominal discomfort. Frequency of bowel movements is eight per day for the last week. She has had two previous attacks in the past year requiring steroids. On examination Miss CP is thin and pale, tender in left iliac fossa, abdomen distended, active bowel sounds. She is currently taking Pentasa 2 g twice a day.

Her ulcerative colitis endoscopic index score (UCEIS) on colonoscopy is 7/8, in keeping with acute severe colitis. On admission, her results were Hb 10.7 g/dL, CRP 84 mg/L, albumin 29 g/dL, platelets 624 × 10⁹/L, potassium 3.0 mmol/L, creatinine 79 mmol/L, pulse >90 beats/min, temperature >37.8 °C.

Intravenous corticosteroids, fluid and electrolyte replacement and subcutaneous unfractionated heparin are prescribed. However, at day 3, her CRP is still elevated at 70 mg/L, and bowel frequency remains at more than 6 motions/day.

Questions

1. What action should be taken if there is little response to intravenous corticosteroids at day 3 in the management of acute severe colitis?
2. What assessments should be done before and during treatment with intravenous ciclosporin?
3. If Miss CP responds to i.v. ciclosporin, on what maintenance treatment should she be discharged?
4. What counselling would you offer Miss CP about her ciclosporin treatment?

Answers

1. Predicting the outcome of acute severe colitis (resistance to steroids and likelihood of requiring colectomy) should be assessed on day 3 of intensive treatment with intravenous corticosteroids. Those patients with frequent stools (>8/day), or stool frequency of 3–8 and raised CRP (>45 mg/L) should have treatment escalation with the addition of ciclosporin or infliximab because they are most likely to require colectomy. After 7 days of treatment, patients with >3 stools/day with visible blood have a 60% chance of continuous symptoms and 40% chance of colectomy in the following months (Travis et al., 1996).

2. The use of ciclosporin for acute severe colitis is an unlicensed indication but approved by NICE (2013). The i.v. dose is 2 mg/kg/day. Provided cholesterol >3.0 mmol/L, then i.v. route is safe. There is an increased risk of fitting if the patient has low cholesterol. Hypomagnesia can also lead to an increase risk of fitting, so this should be corrected if necessary. Ensure there is no infection, and if so, consider antibiotics. The patient should also be informed of potential need for a colectomy if medical treatment fails. The patient could also have an appointment with a stoma nurse specialist and surgeon in case of emergency surgery, in which the risks and benefits of surgery are discussed.
Signs of ciclosporin toxicity include hypertension, renal dysfunction and tremor. A trough level should be done after 48 hours of treatment, aiming for therapeutic range of 100–200 ng/mL.

3. The hydrocortisone should be switched to oral steroids (prednisolone) and tapered over 8 weeks because steroids are not indicated for long-term maintenance treatment.
Intravenous ciclosporin should be converted to oral at a dose of 2.5 mg/kg twice a day for 3–6 months.
As Miss CP has experienced a severe acute exacerbation, then 5-ASA may no longer be sufficient for maintenance treatment. Therefore, Miss CP should be considered for azathioprine when

the dose of prednisolone is reduced. NICE (2013) states that after a single episode of acute severe colitis or if two or more exacerbations have occurred within 12 months that require systemic corticosteroids, or remission is not maintained with aminosalicylate, then azathioprine or mercaptopurine can be considered.

Miss CP should start calcium/vitamin D supplements when on oral steroids. Miss CP should have a DEXA scan to see if bisphosphonate therapy is required because she has had several steroid courses over the last year. Miss CP should be encouraged to get mild exercise. Her bone mineral density should be monitored, particularly because of her low body mass index (BMI) and steroid use.

4. Miss CP should be counselled on the importance of remaining on the same brand of ciclosporin because there are different release characteristics between brands. She should have bloods tests (FBC, renal, ciclosporin trough levels) weekly for the first month, then every month or after a change in dose. Miss CP should be educated on how to recognise signs of over immunosuppression, such as a sore throat, fever or bruising. Miss CP should avoid grapefruit juice. In the UK, there should be a shared care protocol in place if primary care doctors are to continue prescribing and monitoring the ciclosporin.

Case 13.4

Mr DS has been admitted for his first dose of vedolizumab. He was diagnosed with ulcerative colitis 5 years ago and recently received infliximab for an acute exacerbation of this disease. Unfortunately, Mr DS experienced an adverse reaction to infliximab. He is currently taking azathioprine 100 mg once a day.

Questions

1. Is vedolizumab an appropriate treatment option for Mr DS?
2. What dose would you recommend?
3. What are the potential side effects which Mr DS might develop?
4. Because Mr DS is already prescribed azathioprine, should this be continued if he is prescribed vedolizumab as maintenance treatment?

Answers

1. Vedolizumab is licensed for patients with moderately or severely active inflammatory bowel disease (ulcerative colitis or Crohn's disease) who have had an inadequate response with, lost response to or become intolerant of either standard therapy for these conditions or a TNF-α inhibitor (e.g., infliximab or adalimumab). Mr DS has had a reaction to infliximab, so vedolizumab is appropriate.
2. The licensed dose of vedolizumab in moderate/severe ulcerative colitis is 300 mg by i.v. infusion to be given at initiation and then weeks 2 and 6. Further doses can be given every 8 weeks, following a review of continued therapeutic benefit at week 10. Patients established on therapy who begin to lose response may benefit from a 4-week interval between doses.
3. Vedolizumab is given as an infusion over 30 minutes. Mr DS should be observed continuously throughout and after his infusion for signs of acute hypersensitivity reactions. If a severe anaphylactic reaction occurs during the infusion, it should be immediately

stopped. If Mr DS has a mild or moderate infusion-related reaction, then a slower infusion rate or temporary interruption of therapy may be considered. Pre-treatment with hydrocortisone can be useful. The most common reported side effects are nasopharyngitis, headache and arthralgia.

4. Immunomodulators are thought to reduce the risk of anti-drug antibody formation and potentiate efficacy (Colombel et al., 2010). In practice, the results of this study on infliximab and azathioprine are extrapolated to other biologics and immunomodulator combinations. Currently, there is no clear evidence that this is required for vedolizumab, but theoretically, anti-drug antibodies could lead to loss of response, so until additional evidence is available, it is common practice to continue immunomodulators in those patients already taking and tolerating them.

Case 13.5

Mrs EW was diagnosed with Crohn's disease 4 years ago and is prescribed mercaptopurine 75 mg once a day and infliximab every 8 weeks as maintenance therapy. She would like to become pregnant and wants to know if she should stop her mercaptopurine and infliximab treatment to avoid any congenital defects.

Questions

1. What advice would you give Mrs EW?
2. What advice should Mrs EW be given regarding vaccinations both for herself and her baby?

Answers

1. Most women with IBD have a normal pregnancy and deliver a healthy baby. Active disease is more of a risk to a normal pregnancy than medication. Mrs EW therefore needs to keep well and continue current treatment to ensure her disease is well controlled prior to conception and throughout the pregnancy. Mercaptopurine and infliximab are considered safe during pregnancy and breastfeeding. However, because infliximab crosses the placenta and can stay in the circulation of the baby for several months, consideration to discontinue at around 32 weeks of pregnancy should be discussed with Mrs EW.

   There needs to be good communication across specialties involved in the joint care of Mrs EW (e.g., primary care, obstetrics, gastroenterology and colorectal surgeons).

   Mrs EW should be advised on nutrition and the avoidance of smoking and alcohol consumption. A higher dose of folic acid (5 mg/day) is recommend in IBD patients such as Mrs EW to prevent neural tube defects.

2. Patients taking immunosuppressants, including biologics, should avoid live vaccines. The seasonal flu jab and pneumococcal vaccine is safe during pregnancy and should be given to anyone prescribed an immunosuppressant.

   Because infliximab remains in the baby's circulation, live vaccines such as the MMR vaccine, rotavirus or BCG against tuberculosis should be avoided in the first 6 months after birth.

Acknowledgments

The author would like to thank Dr Oliver Brain, Consultant Gastroenterologist, Oxford University Hospitals NHS Foundation Trust, for his support and contribution to this chapter.

References

Anderson, J.L., Edney, R.J., Whelan, K., 2012. Systematic review: faecal microbiota transplantation in the management of inflammatory bowel disease. Aliment Pharmacol. Ther. 36 (6), 503–516.

Best, W.R., Becktel, J.M., Singleton, J.W., et al., 1976. Development of a Crohn's disease activity index. National Cooperative Crohn's disease study. Gastroenterology 70 (3), 439–444.

Bryant, R.V., Sandborn, W.J., Travis, S.P.L., 2015. Introducing vedolizumab to clinical practice: who, when and how? J. Crohn's Colitis 9 (4), 356–366.

Campbell, S., Travis, S., Jewell, D., 2005. Ciclosporin use in acute ulcerative colitis: a long-term experience. Eur. J. Gastroenterol. Hepatol. 17, 79–84.

Colombel, J.F., Sandborn, W.J., Reinisch, W., et al., 2010. Infliximab, azathioprine, or combination therapy for Crohn's disease. N. Engl. J. Med. 362, 1383–1395.

Colombel, J.F., Sandborn, W.J., Rutgeerts, P., et al., 2007. Adalimumab for maintenance of clinical response and remission in patients with Crohn's disease. The CHARM trial Gastroenterology 132 (1), 52–65.

Dervieux, T., Blanco, J.G., Krynetski, E.Y., et al., 2001. Differing contribution of thiopurine methyltransferase to mercaptopurine versus thioguanine effects in human leukemic cells. Cancer Res. 61, 5810–5816.

Dignass, A., Eliakim, R., Magro, F., et al., 2012a. Second European evidence-based consensus on the diagnosis and management of ulcerative colitis 2012. Part 1: definitions and diagnosis. J. Crohn's Colitis 6 (10), 965–990.

Dignass, A., Lindsay, J., Sturm, A., et al., 2012b. Second European evidence-based consensus on the diagnosis and management of ulcerative colitis 2012. Part 2: current management. J. Crohn's Colitis 6 (10), 991–1030.

Dignass, A.U., Gasche, C., Bettenworth, D., et al., 2015. European consensus on the diagnosis and management of iron deficiency and anaemia in inflammatory bowel disease. J. Crohn's Colitis 9 (3), 211–222.

Duijvis, N.W., ten Hove, A.S., Ponsioen, C.I.J., et al., 2016. Similar short- and long-term colectomy rates with ciclosporin and infliximab treatment in hospitalised ulcerative colitis patients. J. Crohn's Colitis 10 (7), 821–827.

Feagan, B.G., Rutgeerts, P., Sands, B., et al., 2013. Vedolizumab as induction and maintenance therapy for ulcerative colitis. N. Engl. J. Med. 369, 699–710.

Feagan, B.G., Sanhborn, W.J., Gasink, C., et al., 2016. Ustekinumab as induction and maintenance therapy for Crohn's disease. N. Engl. J. Med. 375, 1946–1960.

Felder, J.B., Burton, I.K., Rajapakse, R., 2000. Effects of nonsteroidal anti-inflammatory drugs on inflammatory bowel disease: a case–control study. Am. J. Gastroenterol. 95, 1949–1954.

Filizzola, M.J., Gill, S., Martinez, F., et al., 2004. Cytomegalovirus infection exacerbating inflammatory bowel disease. Infect. Med. 21 (11), 567–570.

Fiorino, G., Manetti, N., Variola, A., 2016. Prospective observational study on safety and efficacy of infliximab biosimilar in patients with inflammatory bowel disease: preliminary results of the PROSIT-BIO cohort. Abstract ECCO conference 2016. Available at: https://www.ecco-ibd.eu/publications/congress-abstract-s/abstracts-2016/item/p544-prospective-observational-study-on-inflammatory-bowel-disease-patients-treated-with-infliximab-biosimilars-preliminary-results-of-the-prosit-bio-cohort-of-thex00a0ig-ibd.html.

Gibson, P.R., Shepherd, S.J., 2005. Personal view: food for thought – Western lifestyle andsusceptibility to Crohn's disease. The FODMAP hypothesis. Aliment. Pharmacol. Ther. 21, 1399–1409.

Gionchetti, P., Dignass, A., Danese, S., et al., 2016. Third European evidence-based consensus on the diagnosis and management of Crohn's disease 2016: part 2: surgical management and special situations. J. Crohn's Colitis 11 (2), 135–149.

Gomollon, F., Dignass, A., Annese, V., et al., 2016. Third European evidence-based consensus on the diagnosis and management of Crohn's disease 2016: part 1: diagnosis and current management. J. Crohn's Colitis 11 (1), 3–25.

Guslandi, M., 1999. Nicotine treatment for ulcerative colitis. Br. J. Clin. Pharmacol. 48, 481–484.

Hanauer, S.B., Feagan, B.G., Lichtenstein, G.R., et al., 2002. Maintenance infliximab for Crohn's disease: the ACCENT I randomised trial. Lancet 359 (9317), 1541–1549.

Harvey, R., Bradshaw, J., 1980. A simple index of Crohn's-disease activity. Lancet 315 (8167), 514.

IBD Standards Group UK, 2009. Quality Care: Service Standards for the Healthcare of People Who Have Inflammatory Bowel Disease (IBD). Oyster Healthcare Communications, London.

Lopez, J., Grinspan, A., 2016. Fecal microbiota transplantation for inflammatory bowel disease Gastroenterol. Hepatol. (NY) 12 (6), 374–379.

Louis, E., Mary, J.Y., Vernier-Massouille, G., et al., 2012. Maintenance of remission among patients with Crohn's disease on antimetabolite therapy after infliximab therapy is stopped. Gastroenterology 142, 63–70.

McLeod, H.L., Siva, C., 2002. The thiopurine S-methyltransferase gene locus – implications for clinical pharmacogenomics. Pharmacogenomics 3 (1), 89–98.

Misiewicz, J., Pounder, R.E., Venables, C.W. (Eds.), 1994. Diseases of the Gut and Pancreas, second ed. Blackwell Scientific Publications, Oxford.

Mowat, C., Cole, A., Windsor, A., et al., 2011. British Society of Gastroenterology Guidelines for the management of inflammatory bowel disease in adults. Gut 60, 571–607.

Mpofu, C., Ireland, A., 2006. Inflammatory bowel disease – the disease and its diagnosis. Hosp. Pharm. 13, 153–158.

National IBD Standards Group, 2013. Standards for the healthcare of people who have inflammatory bowel disease (IBD). IBD Standards 2013 update. Available at: http://www.ibdstandards.org.uk.

National Institute for Health and Care Excellence (NICE), 2004. Wireless capsule endoscopy for investigation of the small bowel. Interventional Procedures Guidance IPG101. Available at: https://www.nice.org.uk/guidance/ipg101.

National Institute for Health and Care Excellence (NICE), 2005. Leukapheresis for inflammatory bowel disease. Available at: https://www.nice.org.uk/guidance/ipg126.

National Institute for Health and Care Excellence (NICE), 2008. Infliximab for acute exacerbations of ulcerative colitis. Technology Appraisal No. 163. Available at: https://www.nice.org.uk/guidance/ta163.

National Institute for Health and Care Excellence (NICE), 2010. Infliximab (review) and adalimumab for the treatment of Crohn's disease (includes a review of Technology Appraisal Guidance 40). Technology Appraisal No. 187. Available at: https://www.nice.org.uk/guidance/ta187.

National Institute for Health and Care Excellence (NICE), 2011. Colorectal cancer prevention: colonoscopic surveillance in adults with ulcerative colitis, Crohn's disease or adenomas. Clinical Guideline No. 118. Available at: https://www.nice.org.uk/guidance/cg118.

National Institute for Health and Care Excellence (NICE), 2012. Crohn's disease: Management in adults, children and young people. Clinical Guideline No. 152. Available at: https://www.nice.org.uk/guidance/cg152.

National Institute for Health and Care Excellence (NICE), 2013. Ulcerative colitis: management in adults, children and young people. Clinical Guideline No. 166. Available at: https://www.nice.org.uk/guidance/cg166.

National Institute for Health and Care Excellence (NICE), 2014. Faecal microbiota transplant for recurrent Clostridium difficile infection 2014. Interventional procedures guidance [IPG485]. Available at: https://www.nice.org.uk/guidance/ipg485.

National Institute for Health and Care Excellence (NICE), 2015a. Vedolizumab for treating moderately to severely active ulcerative colitis. Technology Appraisal No. 342. Available at: https://www.nice.org.uk/guidance/ta342.

National Institute for Health and Care Excellence (NICE), 2015b. Infliximab, adalimumab, golimumab for treating moderately to severely active ulcerative colitis after the failure of conventional therapy. Technology Appraisal 329. Available at: https://www.nice.org.uk/guidance/ta329.

National Institute for Health and Care Excellence (NICE), 2015c. Vedolizumab for treating moderately to severely active Crohn's disease after prior therapy. Technology Appraisal No. 352. Available at https://www.nice.org.uk/guidance/ta352.

National Institute for Health and Care Excellence (NICE), 2015d. Inflammatory bowel disease QS81. Available at: https://www.nice.org.uk/guidance/q81.

National Institute for Health and Care Excellence (NICE), 2016. Therapeutic monitoring of TNF-alpha inhibitors in Crohn's disease (LISA-TRACKER ELISA kits, IDK monitor ELISA kits, and Promonitor ELISA kits). Diagnostics Guidance DG22. Available at: https://www.nice.org.uk/guidance/dg22.

National Institute for Health Care Excellence (NICE), 2017. Ustekinumab for moderately to severely active Crohn's disease after previous treatment. Available at: https://www.nice.org.uk/guidance/ta456.

National Patient Safety Agency (NPSA), 2007. Patient safety alert 13. Improving compliance with oral methotrexate guidelines. NPSA, London. Available at: http://www.nrls.npsa.nhs.uk/resources/?entryid45=59800.

Radford-Smith, G.L., Edwards, J.E., Purdie, D.M., 2002. Protective role of appendicectomy on onset and severity of ulcerative colitis and Crohn's disease. Gut 51, 808–813.

Rahier, J.F., Ben-Horin, S., Chowers, Y., et al., 2014. The second European evidence based consensus on the prevention, diagnosis and management of opportunistic infections in inflammatory bowel disease. J. Crohn's Colitis 8 (6), 443–468.

Robinson, A., Hanins, M., Wiseman, G., et al., 2013. Maintaining stable symptom control in inflammatory bowel disease: a retrospective analysis of adherence, medication switches and risk of relapse. Aliment Pharmacol. Ther. 38, 531–538.

Sandborn, W.J., Feagan, B.G., Marano, C., et al., 2014. Subcutaneous golimumab maintains clinical response in patients with moderate-to-severe ulcerative colitis. Gastroenterology 146 (1), 96–109.

Sandborn, W.J., Feagan, B.G., Rutgeerts, P., et al., 2013. Vedolizumab as induction and maintenance therapy for Crohn's disease. N. Engl. J. Med. 369, 711–721.

Sandborn, W.J., van Assche, G., Reinisch, N., et al., 2012. Adalimumab induces and maintains clinical remission in patients with moderate-to-severe ulcerative colitis. Gastroenterology 142 (2) 275–265.

Sands, B.E., Blank, M.A., Patel, K., et al., 2004. Long-term treatment of rectovaginal fistulas in Crohn's disease: response to infliximab in the ACCENT II study Clin. Gastroenterol. Hepatol 2 (10), 912–920.

Snapper, S.B., McGovern, D.P.B., 2016. Genetic factors in inflammatory bowel disease. https://www.uptodate.com/contents/genetic-factors-in-inflammatory-bowel-disease.

Solem, C.A., Loftus, E.V., Tremaine, W.J., et al., 2004. Venous thromboembolism in inflammatory bowel disease. Am. J. Gastroenterol. 99, 97–101.

St Clair Jones, A., 2014. Optimising therapy for inflammatory bowel disease. Clinical Pharmacist 6 (9). https://doi.org/10.1211/CP.2014.20067117.

Travis, S.P.L., Farrant, J.M., Ricketts, C., et al., 1996. Predicting outcome in severe ulcerative colitis. Gut 38 (6), 905–910.

Travis, S.P.L., Schnell, D., Krzeski, P., et al., 2012. Developing an instrument to assess the endoscopic severity of ulcerative colitis: the Ulcerative Colitis Endoscopic Index of Severity (UCEIS). Gut 61, 535–542.

Truelove, S.C., Witts, L.J., 1955. Cortisone in ulcerative colitis: final report on a therapeutic trial. BMJ 2 (4947), 1041–1048.

Turner, D., Otley, A.R., Mack, D., et al., 2007a. Development, validation, and evaluation of a pediatric ulcerative colitis activity index: a prospective multicentre study. Gastroenterology 133 (2), 423–432.

Turner, D., Walsh, C.M., Steinhart, A.M., et al., 2007b. Response to corticosteroids in severe ulcerative colitis: a systematic review of the literature and a meta-regression. Clin. Gastroenterol. Hepatol. 5 (1), 103–110.

van der Woude, C.J., Ardizzone, S., Bengton, M.B., et al., 2015. The second European-based consensus on reproduction and pregnancy in inflammatory bowel disease. J. Crohn's Colitis 9 (2), 107–124.

Vande Casteele, N., Comperolle, G., Ballet, V., et al., 2012. Individualised infliximab treatment using therapeutic drug monitoring: a prospective controlled trough level adapted infliximab treatment (TAXIT) trial. European Crohn's and Colitis Organisation oral presentation. Available at: https://www.ecco-ibd.eu/index.php/publications/congress-abstracts/abstracts-2012/item/op11-indivi-2.html.

Walmsley, P.S., Ayres, R.C.S., Pounder, R.E., et al., 1998. A simple clinical colitis activity index Gut 43 (1), 29–32.

Further reading

Silva, S., 2011. Inflammatory bowel disease – clinical features and diagnosis. Clinical Pharmacist 3, 73–76.

St Clair Jones, A., Kelly, M., 2011. Inflammatory bowel disease – management. Clinical Pharmacist 3, 78–84.

Useful websites

British Society of Gastroenterology (BSG): http://www.bsg.org.uk
European Crohn's and Colitis Organisation: https://www.ecco-ibd.eu
Crohn's and Colitis UK: https://www.crohnsandcolitis.org.uk

14 Constipation and Diarrhoea

Ian Smith and Jonathan Berry

Key points

Constipation
- Constipation is most commonly considered as less frequent evacuation of the bowels with difficulty in passing a stool.
- Constipation can affect all age groups.
- When assessing the patient, it is important to understand what they mean by the term constipation and why they believe they are constipated.
- The evidence for the safety and efficacy of laxatives is limited, which means the process of managing constipation is based more on expert opinion than on evidence.

Diarrhoea
- Diarrhoea is a symptom and can be due to many causes and conditions.
- Diarrhoea can be considered to be acute (<14 days), persistent (>14 days but <4 months) or chronic (>4 months).
- Hydration and nutrition are the interventions with the greatest impact on the course of acute diarrhoea.

Constipation and diarrhoea are two of the most common disorders of the gastro-intestinal (GI) tract. They can both be considered to be either a symptom or a disorder, usually depending on how long they last. The majority of cases of both constipation and diarrhoea are not life-threatening but will cause varying degrees of morbidity. When assessing patients with these conditions, it should be considered that they may be a symptom of another, more serious disorder. For example, constipation may be secondary to hypothyroidism, hypokalaemia, diabetes, multiple sclerosis or GI obstruction. Likewise, diarrhoea may be secondary to ulcerative colitis, Crohn's disease, malabsorption or bowel carcinoma. Both constipation and diarrhoea can also be drug-induced which should also be considered when assessing a patient.

Constipation

Constipation is most commonly considered as less frequent evacuation of the bowels with difficulty in passing a stool. Abnormal, in terms of frequency, would be considered to be fewer than three bowel actions a week (Connell et al., 1965), and this has been incorporated into the Rome III diagnostic criteria for functional constipation (Longstreth et al., 2006). As well as frequency, other criteria can be added into the definition of constipation,

such as stool hardness, straining and the feeling of incomplete evacuation. This all leads to the subjectivity of a true definition. Constipation, it can be said, is defined by the sufferer. If, after a discussion with a patient when normal and abnormal bowel habits are described, the patient says he or she is constipated, then the patient should be considered to require help with his or her constipation (National Institute of Health and Care Excellence [NICE], 2015a).

Incidence

Constipation can affect all age groups. The prevalence of the condition is difficult to measure due to the subjectivity of the definition, but a review article indicated that the prevalence rate worldwide ranged from 2.5% to 79% in adults and from 0.7% to 29.6% in children. The prevalence of self-reported constipation was stated to be about 20% (Mugie et al., 2011). This review indicted that constipation is more common in women than in men, and that the incidence increases with age, particularly after 65 years. There is a higher incidence in elderly patients in nursing homes (Rao and Go, 2010). In the elderly, contributing factors have been identified such as poor diet, insufficient intake of fluids, lack of exercise, concurrent disease states and the use of medicines that can cause constipation. Increased prevalence has also been found in people of high body mass index and low socioeconomic status.

Changes in hormones and mechanical factors during pregnancy lead to an increase in prevalence of constipation compared with the general population. The prevalence rate is higher during the second trimester, and about 40% are affected at some stage during pregnancy (Cullen and O'Donoghue, 2007).

Aetiology

The digestive system can be divided into the upper and lower GI tracts. The upper GI tract starts at the mouth, includes the oesophagus and stomach, and is responsible for the ingestion and digestion of food. The lower GI tract consists of the small intestine, large intestine (colon), rectum and anus (Fig. 14.1), and is responsible for the absorption of nutrients, conserving body water and electrolytes, drying the faeces and elimination. Normally there is a net absorption of water during transit to the rectum. If too much water is reabsorbed, this will, generally, lead to constipation, whereas too much water in the faeces will result in diarrhoea.

The contents of the intestine are swept along the GI tract by waves of muscular contractions called peristalsis. These

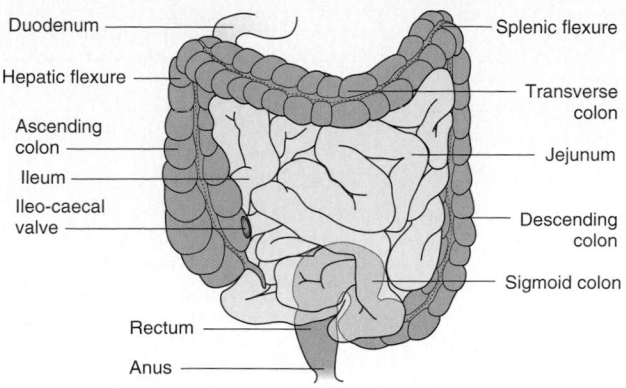

Fig. 14.1 The lower gastro-intestinal tract.

peristaltic waves eventually move the faeces from the colon to the rectum, and this then induces the urge to defaecate. This process is under the influence of the autonomic nervous system (sympathetic and parasympathetic).

Agents that alter intestinal motility, either directly or by acting on the autonomic nervous system, affect the transit time of substances along the GI tract. Because the extent of absorption and secretion of fluid from the GI tract generally parallels transit time, a slower transit time will lead to the formation of hard stools and constipation. Transit times are faster in males than in females (Degen and Phillips, 1996) and can be affected by the type of food that is ingested and the amount of fluid that is drunk.

Motility is largely under parasympathetic (cholinergic) control, with stimulation bringing about an increase in motility, whereas antagonists such as antimuscarinics, or drugs with antimuscarinic side effects, decrease motility and induce constipation. This mechanism is distinct from that of the other major group of drugs that induce constipation, the opioids. Opioids cause constipation by maintaining or increasing the tone of smooth muscle, suppressing forward peristalsis, raising sphincter tone at the ileocaecal valve and anal sphincter, and reducing sensitivity to rectal distension. This delays the passage of faeces through the gut, with a resultant increase in absorption of electrolytes and water in the small intestine and colon.

Constipation can be classed as primary or secondary (Rao and Meduri, 2011). Chronic primary constipation can be subclassified into five categories:

- normal transit
- slow transit
- dyssynergic defecation, which is the difficulty in expelling stools
- slow transit–dyssynergic combination
- irritable bowel syndrome (IBS) with constipation

Secondary constipation can be caused by many different factors including diet, drugs and behaviour. These and other factors are highlighted in Table 14.1.

Differential diagnosis

When assessing patients, it is important to understand what patients mean by the term constipation and why they believe they are constipated. The onset, duration and severity of the condition will need to be assessed. This will require information about the frequency and consistency of their stools and any other issues which affect defaecation, such as straining or incomplete evacuation. An assessment of the action the person has taken to manage his or her condition and how effective it has been will be required. Predisposing factors will also require investigation to identify any possible causes. Current medication will need investigation with particular regard to medicines known to cause constipation (Table 14.2). In the UK, more than 700 medicinal products, including ophthalmic preparations, have constipation listed as a possible side effect.

The Rome III diagnostic criteria identify patients with functional constipation when 25% of bowel movements are associated with at least two of the following symptoms: straining; hard or lumpy stools; a sense of incomplete evacuation; a sense of anorectal obstruction; the need for manual manoeuvres; or fewer than three defaecations per week in the previous 3 months with an onset of symptoms longer than 6 months (Longstreth et al., 2006). The Bristol Stool Chart (see Useful Websites) provides practitioners and patients with a practical guide to stool consistency (Lewis and Heaton, 1997).

Patients will require referral and further investigation if they are passing blood or mucus in their stools, have unintentional and unexplained weight loss, experience fever or have nocturnal symptoms which disturb their sleep. The longer the constipation has lasted the more likely it is to need further investigation, in particular if it is unresponsive to treatment. A person older than 50 years who has started to complain about constipation without a previous history may require referral. Recurrent abdominal pain or discomfort with constipation is more associated with IBS (Lui, 2011).

Rao and Meduri (2011) gave an outline of the methods which can be used to investigate chronic constipation. These include clinical evaluation and diagnostic tests. The diagnostic tests are further broken down as follows:

- radiographic studies including plain abdominal radiography, barium enema, magnetic resonance imaging (MRI), endoscopy, and defecography;
- tests for colonic function including colonic transit study, colonic transit scintigraphy, wireless motility capsule and colonic manometry;
- tests for anorectal function including anorectal manometry, high-resolution manometry, balloon expulsion test and rectal barostat test.

General management

The aim, when managing constipation, should be to restore normal bowel function. This aim may not be realistic in some patients. The general approach to treating constipation is first to clear faecal loading or impaction before starting to treat chronic constipation. When treating the condition it is recommended that individual preference and the response to treatment are considered. A stepped approach is recommended, which will involve adjusting the dose, frequency and combination of laxatives (NICE, 2015a). Little evidence is available about the most effective treatments for constipation, and what evidence does exist concentrates on the treatment of chronic constipation. Non-drug advice is widely accepted as the first-line treatment,

Table 14.1 Causes of constipation

Cause	Comments
Poor diet	Diets high in animal fats (e.g. meats, dairy products, eggs) and refined sugar (e.g. sweets), but low in fibre predispose to constipation
Irritable bowel syndrome	Spasm of colon delays transit of intestinal contents; patients have a history of alternating constipation and diarrhoea
Poor bowel habit	Ignoring and suppressing the urge to have a bowel movement will contribute to constipation
Laxative abuse	Habitual consumption of laxatives necessitates increase in dose over time until intestine becomes atonic and unable to function without laxative stimulation
Travel	Changes in lifestyle, daily routine, diet and drinking water may all contribute to constipation
Hormone disturbances	For example, hypothyroidism and diabetes
Pregnancy	Mechanical pressure of womb on intestine and hormonal changes (e.g. high levels of progesterone)
Fissures and haemorrhoids	Painful disorders of the anus often lead patients to suppress defaecation, leading to constipation
Diseases	Many disease states may have constipation as a symptom (e.g. scleroderma, lupus, multiple sclerosis, Parkinson's disease, stroke and dementia)
Mechanical compression	Scarring, inflammation around diverticula and tumours can produce mechanical compression of intestine
Nerve damage	Spinal cord injuries and tumours pressing on the spinal cord affect nerves that lead to intestine
Colonic motility disorders	Peristaltic activity of intestine may be ineffective, resulting in colonic inertia
Medication	See Table 14.2
Dehydration	Insufficient fluid intake or excessive fluid loss; water and other fluids add bulk to stools, making bowel movements soft and easier to pass
Immobility	Prolonged bedrest after an accident, during an illness or general lack of exercise
Electrolyte abnormalities	Hypercalcaemia or hypokalaemia
Anxiety and depression	The psychological symptoms can be a result of the distress associated with constipation, or constipation can be an expression of the depressive or anxiety disorder

although there is a lack of evidence that it is effective (Lui, 2011). Laxatives can be used if the patient does not respond to non-drug advice or if they need relief while the non-drug advice is taking effect. If there is a medicine which is causing or contributing to the problem, this should be withdrawn or adjusted if possible.

Patients with opioid-induced constipation will require treatment with an osmotic or stimulant laxative alone or in combination. Methylnaltrexone bromide injection can also be added to their treatment if required. This is an opioid-receptor antagonist which does not alter the central analgesic effect of opioids.

Non-drug advice

Non-drug advice is advocated for all patient groups, except those who are terminally ill. Education and discussion about their current bowel habits may be required because some people believe that if they do not have a bowel movement each day they are constipated, and this may lead to laxative overuse. All advice given should incorporate any of the predisposing factors identified. General advice about the patient not ignoring the urge to have a bowel movement, as well as increasing fluid intake, dietary fibre and activity, may help the patient, particularly if any of these have been identified as a possible predisposing factor. This will require understanding the fluid intake, exercise activity and diet of the patient, to give effective advice.

It is generally recommended that fibre intake in the form of fruit, vegetables, cereals, grain foods, wholemeal bread and so on be increased to between 18 and 30 g/day. Studies have shown that low-fibre diets can lead to constipation. High-fibre diets can lead to a decrease in transit time and an increase in stool weight (Rao and Go, 2010). Fibre intake should be increased gradually to prevent flatulence and bloating. The effect of increasing fibre could be seen within a few days but may take up to 4 weeks to have an effect (NICE, 2015a). Advice on adequate fluid intake could be appropriate, and this will be important in patients who are consuming a high-fibre diet. A high-fibre diet is not recommended in those with megacolon or hypotonic colon/rectum because they do

Table 14.2 Examples of medicines known to cause constipation [frequency defined as very common (>10%) or common (1–10%)]

Class	Examples
α-Blocker	Prazosin
Antacid	Aluminium and calcium salts
Antimuscarinic	Trihexyphenidyl, hyoscine, oxybutynin, procyclidine, tolterodine
Antidepressant	Tricyclics, selective serotonin reuptake inhibitors, reboxetine, venlafaxine, duloxetine, mirtazapine
Antiemetic	Palonosetron, dolasetron, aprepitant
Antiepileptic	Carbamazepine, oxcarbazepine
Antipsychotic	Phenothiazines, haloperidol, pimozide and atypical antipsychotics such as amisulpride, aripiprazole, olanzapine, quetiapine, risperidone, zotepine, clozapine
Antiviral	Foscarnet
β-Blocker	Oxprenolol, bisoprolol, nebivolol; other β-blockers cause constipation more rarely
Bisphosphonate	Alendronic acid
Central nervous system stimulant	Atomoxetine
Calcium channel blocker	Diltiazem, verapamil
Cytotoxic	Bortezomib, buserelin, cladribine, docetaxel, doxorubicin, exemestane, gemcitabine, irinotecan, mitoxantrone, pentostatin, temozolomide, topotecan, vinblastine, vincristine, vindesine, vinorelbine
Dopaminergic	Amantadine, bromocriptine, carbegolide, entacapone, tolcapone, levodopa, pergolide, pramipexole, quinagolide
Growth hormone antagonist	Pegvisomant
Immunosuppressant	Basiliximab, mycophenolate, tacrolimus
Lipid-lowering agent	Colestyramine, colestipol, rosuvastatin, atorvastatin (other statins uncommon), gemfibrozil
Iron	Ferrous sulphate
Metabolic disorder	Miglustat
Muscle relaxant	Baclofen
NSAID	Meloxicam; other NSAIDs, e.g. aceclofenac, and cyclo-oxygenase-2 inhibitors reported as uncommon
Smoking cessation	Bupropion
Opioid analgesic	All opioid analgesics and derivatives
Ulcer healing	All proton pump inhibitors, sucralfate

NSAID, Non-steroidal anti-inflammatory drug.

not respond to bulk in the colon. Similarly, a high-fibre diet may not be appropriate in those with opioid-induced constipation.

An increased level of exercise could also be advised. Although it has not been associated with improvement in constipation, it has been associated with an increase in quality of life and deceased bowel symptoms (Rao and Meduri, 2011).

Drug treatment

Evidence for the safety and efficacy of laxatives is limited, which means the process of managing constipation is based more upon expert opinion than on evidence. If non-drug advice is unsuccessful, or there is a clinical need, a short course of treatment with laxatives would be appropriate. Bulk-forming agents are seen as the first-line treatment. Osmotic and stimulant laxatives are used as second-line treatments. Where the constipation is believed to be due to opioid medication, the recommendation is not to use a bulk-forming agent but to use an osmotic or stimulant laxative instead.

In pregnancy there is very little evidence to support the use of laxatives. It is generally accepted that a bulk-forming laxative would be the first choice if non-drug advice is unsuccessful followed by lactulose (Rungsiprakarn et al., 2015).

Laxatives are subcategorised into groups related to their mechanism of action; however, some laxatives have more than one mechanism of action; that is, bulk-forming agents also have softening properties. Docusate sodium can be considered as a stimulant laxative and faecal softener. Glycerol suppositories have a lubricant effect, in additional to a stimulant effect.

Bulk-forming agents. Ispaghula formulated as powder, granules and effervescent granules, methylcellulose tablets and sterculia granules are all bulk-forming agents. Their use is most appropriate in situations where the patient has small, hard stools and the dietary intake of fibre cannot be increased.

The mechanism of action for bulk-forming agents is that they are polysaccharides which are not digested. There is some evidence to indicate that ispaghula can cause an increase in frequency, weight and consistency of stools (Ashraf et al., 1995). Following ingestion it usually takes 12–36 hours before any effect is seen but may be longer. An adequate volume of fluid should be ingested to avoid intestinal obstruction. Bulk-forming agents can be used safely long-term during pregnancy or when breast-feeding, but many users will experience problems with flatulence and distension. The use of bulk-forming agents is not recommended in patients with colonic atony, intestinal obstruction or faecal impaction. They are less effective, or may even exacerbate constipation, in those who lack mobility.

Stimulant laxatives. Medicines in the stimulant laxative group include bisacodyl, sodium picosulfate, senna and dantron. They directly stimulate colonic nerves that cause movement of the faecal mass, reduce transit time and result in the passage of stool within 6–12 hours. As a consequence of their time to onset, oral dosing at bedtime is generally recommended. Suppositories that contain laxatives have a more immediate effect, causing defaecation within 20–60 minutes. Abdominal cramps are a common side effect of stimulant laxatives. Chronic use of stimulant laxatives should be avoided and discouraged because this can lead to electrolyte disturbances and an atonic colon. In the elderly atonic colon is of less concern, and prolonged use may be required in a few cases. Stimulant laxatives should be avoided in patients with intestinal obstruction.

Co-danthramer and co-danthrusate are stimulant laxatives with limited use. Their carcinogenic effects, identified from rodent studies, have limited their use to those patients who are terminally ill.

Osmotic laxatives. Osmotic laxatives include magnesium salts, phosphate enemas, sodium citrate enemas, lactulose and macrogols. These agents retain fluid in the bowel by osmosis and change the water distribution in faeces to produce a softer, bulkier stool. Their ingestion should be accompanied by an appropriate fluid intake. Bowel-cleansing preparations of phosphates and sodium citrate in the form of enemas are mainly used before bowel surgery, colonoscopy or radiological examination.

Lactulose is a semisynthetic disaccharide, which is not absorbed from the gut. It may take 48 hours or longer to work. It is also useful in the treatment of hepatic encephalopathy because it produces an osmotic diarrhoea of low faecal pH that discourages the growth of ammonia-producing organisms.

Macrogols are inert polymers of ethylene oxide. They are formulated in enemas, powders or liquid with salts such as sodium chloride and potassium chloride. Macrogol-containing enemas are mainly used as bowel-cleansing preparations. Macrogol powders and liquid are used for chronic constipation or faecal impaction.

Faecal softeners. Docusate sodium is a non-ionic surfactant that has stool-softening properties. It reduces surface tension, increases the penetration of intestinal fluids into the faecal mass and has weak stimulant properties. Oral preparations, like lactulose, can take up to 48 hours to act. Enemas have a rapid onset of action (within 20 minutes) but should not be used in individuals with haemorrhoids or an anal fissure.

Liquid paraffin, a traditionally used laxative, has very limited use because of the problems it may cause, including anal irritation and seepage, granulomatous reactions and lipoid pneumonia. It can also reduce the absorption of fat-soluble vitamins.

Other drugs used in constipation. Linaclotide, lubiprostone and prucalopride have very limited use. For example, within the UK, linaclotide is licensed for the treatment of moderate-to-severe IBS associated with constipation; lubiprostone is licensed for the treatment of chronic idiopathic constipation in adults whose condition has not responded adequately to lifestyle changes; prucalopride is licensed for the treatment of chronic constipation in women, when other laxatives have failed to provide an adequate response.

Diarrhoea

Diarrhoea, as a symptom, can be due to many causes and conditions. A definition of diarrhoea is the abnormal passing of loose or liquid stools, with increased frequency and/or increased volume (NICE, 2013). Increased frequency is defined as the presence of three or more abnormally loose or watery stools in the preceding 24 hours (World Gastroenterology Organisation, 2012).

Diarrhoea can be considered acute (<14 days), persistent (>14 days but <4 months) or chronic (>4 months). The usual cause of acute diarrhoea, in all age groups, is viral or bacterial infection (Tam et al., 2012). Other causes of acute diarrhoea include food allergies, anxiety or alcohol misuse. Chronic diarrhoea can be associated with conditions such as IBS, inflammatory bowel disease, colorectal cancer and malabsorption syndromes. Certain medicines can also cause diarrhoea as a side effect. This section will consider acute diarrhoea caused by infection or drugs.

Incidence

As with constipation, prevalence rates of diarrhoea are difficult to estimate. Worldwide there are an estimated 1.7 billion cases

Table 14.3 Types of diarrhoea

Type	Cause
Osmotic diarrhoea	Solutes in the intestinal lumen increasing the osmotic gradient
Secretory diarrhoea	Water being secreted in the intestinal lumen
Inflammatory and infectious diarrhoea	Infection or inflammation affecting the lining of the intestine
Accelerated transit time diarrhoea	An increase in transit time through the intestine, which is then too fast to allow absorption of enough water

of diarrhoeal disease every year. Each year 760,000 children younger than 5 years die of diarrhoea, mostly in developing countries (World Health Organisation [WHO], 2013a). This means that more than 2000 children are dying every day as a result of diarrhoeal diseases. Chronic diarrhoea in the Western population is said to be about 4–5% (Thomas et al., 2003). The incidence of diarrhoea among adults in Great Britain is stated as, on average, just under one episode per person each year (Feldman and Banatvala, 1994). It has been estimated that there are just less than 17 million cases per year of infectious intestinal disease (IID), and this leads to just greater than 1 million primary care doctor consultations per year in the UK (Tam et al., 2012). Of these cases, viral causes are more common than bacterial causes. Norovirus is the most common cause, being responsible for nearly 3 million cases. The most common bacterial cause is *Campylobacter*, with just more than half a million cases. Since the mid-1990s it would appear that the incidence of IID has increased by about 40%. Over the same period the number of primary care doctor consultations for IID has halved, which is believed to be because of changes in healthcare usage. *Clostridium difficile*, which is an important cause of IID in hospital and other healthcare settings, appears to be a rare cause of community IID. Worldwide, rotavirus is the most common cause of severe debilitating diarrhoea in children younger than 5 years (WHO, 2013b).

Aetiology

There are four types of diarrhoea. These are described in Table 14.3. Pathogens produce secretory diarrhoea and inflammatory and infectious diarrhoea via a number of methods.

They can cause a secretory diarrhoea by producing enterotoxins which have a dual action of activating adenylyl cyclase and directly acting on the nerves in the intestine to release water (e.g. *Vibrio cholerae*, *Staphylococcus aureus* and *Clostridium* species).

Inflammatory and infectious diarrhoea is caused by the pathogen disrupting or destroying the epithelium of the intestine. Bacteria such as *Salmonella*, *Escherichia coli* O157, *Shigella* and *Campylobacter* and protozoa such as *Cryptosporidium* and *Giardia* cause this type of infectious diarrhoea. Norovirus and rotavirus also cause this type of diarrhoea, although the mechanism of action may be more complicated (Shetty and Tang, 2009).

Many medicines (Table 14.4), particularly broad-spectrum antibiotics such as ampicillin, erythromycin and neomycin, induce diarrhoea secondary to therapy. With antibiotics, the mechanism involves the overgrowth of antibiotic-resistant bacteria and fungi in the large bowel after several days of therapy. The diarrhoea is generally self-limiting; however, when the overgrowth involves *C. difficile*, it can be life-threatening. *C. difficile*–associated diarrhoea is a major concern in the hospital setting. Pathogenic strains produce two enterotoxins: toxin A, which causes fluid accumulation in the lumen of the large intestine; and toxin B, which is responsible for ulceration of the bowel wall. These are responsible for the severe diarrhoea, and consequential pseudomembranous colitis and toxic megacolon which characterise the *C. difficile* infection (Shetty, 2009).

Signs and symptoms

Diarrhoea, like constipation, is a change from the normal bowel function. In diarrhoea there is an increase in frequency or an increase in weight of the stools, or both. Acute diarrhoea is associated with loose or watery stools that may be accompanied by anorexia, nausea, vomiting, abdominal cramps, flatulence or bloating.

Getting a complete history of the patient is important. The duration of the diarrhoea, along with its severity and symptoms, will need to be ascertained to establish whether referral is warranted. Warning signs that warrant further investigation include blood in the stools, persistent vomiting, unintentional and unexplained weight loss, or nocturnal symptoms which disturb sleep.

Patients should be questioned about whether other members of the family or other people they have been in contact with are ill. They should also be questioned about the food they have eaten, any medicines they have taken and if they have recently travelled abroad, because all of these factors are important in assessing the condition.

Dehydration can be a consequence of diarrhoea, and this can be exacerbated if the patient is also vomiting. Signs and symptoms of dehydration should be reviewed when assessing a patient, and particularly if the patient is very young or very old.

In mild dehydration there are usually no signs, but symptoms such as lassitude, anorexia, nausea, light-headedness and postural hypotension may be described. Symptoms such as apathy, tiredness, dizziness, headache and muscles cramps together with signs such as pinched face, dry tongue or sunken eyes, reduced skin elasticity, postural hypotension, tachycardia and oliguria could indicate moderate dehydration. In severe dehydration, the above symptoms are more marked and may also include profound apathy, weakness and confusion, leading to coma with signs of shock, tachycardia, marked peripheral vasoconstriction, systolic blood pressure less than 90 mmHg uraemia, oliguria or anuria (NICE, 2015b).

Investigations

Before any investigations are undertaken, a medication history is required to eliminate drug-induced diarrhoea. Testing for *C. difficile*–induced pseudomembranous colitis is indicated in those with severe symptoms or where hospitalisation or antibiotic

Table 14.4 Examples of medicines known to cause diarrhoea (defined as very common [>10%] or common [1–10%])

Class	Examples
α-Blocker	Prazosin
Angiotensin-converting enzyme inhibitor	Lisinopril, perindopril
Angiotensin receptor blocker	Telmisartan
Acetylcholinesterase inhibitor	Donepezil, galantamine, rivastigmine
Antacid	Magnesium salts
Antibacterial	All
Antidiabetic	Metformin, acarbose
Antidepressant	Selective serotonin reuptake inhibitors, clomipramine, venlafaxine
Antiemetic	Aprepitant, dolasetron
Antiepileptic	Carbamazepine, oxcarbazepine, tiagabine, zonisamide, pregabalin, levetiracetam
Antifungal	Caspofungin, fluconazole, flucytosine, nystatin (in large doses), terbinafine, voriconazole
Antimalarial	Mefloquine
Antiprotozoal	Metronidazole, sodium stibogluconate
Antipsychotic	Aripiprazole
Antiviral	Abacavir, emtricitabine, stavudine, tenofovir, zalcitabine, zidovudine, atazanavir, indinavir, lopinavir, nelfinavir, saquinavir, efavirenz, ganciclovir, valganciclovir, adefovir, oseltamivir, ribavirin, fosamprenavir
β-Blocker	Bisoprolol, carvedilol, nebivolol
Bisphosphonate	Alendronic acid, disodium etidronate, ibandronic acid, risedronate, sodium clodronate, disodium pamidronate, tiludronic acid
Cytokine inhibitor	Adalimumab, infliximab
Cytotoxic	All classes of cytotoxics
Dopaminergic	Levodopa, entacapone
Growth hormone antagonist	Pegvisomant
Immunosuppressant	Ciclosporin, mycophenolate, leflunomide
Non-steroidal anti-inflammatory drug	All
Ulcer healing	All proton pump inhibitors
Vaccine	Pediacel (5 vaccines in 1), haemophilus, meningococcal
Miscellaneous	Calcitonin, strontium ranelate, colchicine, dantrolene, olsalazine, anagrelide, nicotinic acid, pancreatin, eplerenone, acamprosate

therapy with lincomycin, broad-spectrum β-lactams or cephalosporins has occurred within the preceding 6 weeks.

In general, stool culture is required in patients who are unwell (fever or dehydration), immunocompromised, with blood or pus in the stool, or where there is no improvement within a week. Stool culture is also required when there is a history of recent overseas travel other than to Europe, North America, Australia or New Zealand.

Further tests that may be required in chronic diarrhoea are listed in Table 14.5.

Treatment

Acute infective diarrhoea, including traveller's diarrhoea, is usually a self-limiting disorder. However, depending on the causative agent, a number of complications may have to be addressed. Dehydration and electrolyte disturbance can be readily treated but may, if severe, progress to acidosis and circulatory failure with hypoperfusion of vital organs, renal failure and death.

General measures

Patients should be advised on handwashing and other hygiene-related issues to prevent transmission to other family members.

Table 14.5 Blood tests in patients with chronic diarrhoea

Test	Comments
Full blood count	Detection of anaemia or raised platelet count suggesting inflammation
Liver function tests	Including albumin level
Tests for malabsorption	Calcium; vitamin B_{12} and red blood cell folate; iron status (ferritin)
Thyroid function test	Reduced thyroid-stimulating hormone and elevated free T_3 and T_4 levels would be suggestive of overt hyperthyroidism
Erythrocyte sedimentation rate and C-reactive protein	Elevated levels may indicate inflammatory bowel disease
Antibody testing for coeliac disease	IgA tissue transglutaminase antibody or IgA endomysial antibody

IgA, Immunoglobulin A.

The promotion of handwashing may reduce the incidence of diarrhoea by approximately one-third (Ejemot-Nwadiaro et al., 2015). Exclusion from work or school until the patient is free of diarrhoea is advised. In acute, self-limiting diarrhoea, children, healthcare workers and food handlers should be symptom free for 48 hours before returning to school or work. More exacting criteria for return to work, such as testing for negative stool samples, are rarely required.

Patients, either adults or children, should be advised to commence eating as soon as they want. In babies, breast-feeding and bottle-feeding should be continued, although there is some evidence that moving bottle-fed babies to lactose-free milk may be beneficial (MacGillivray et al., 2013). The BRAT diet (bananas, rice, applesauce and toast) has long been recommended by healthcare workers. However, there is little evidence to promote this diet, and it is believed to be too restrictive (Churgay and Aftab, 2012). In weaned and non-weaned children with gastroenteritis, early feeding after rehydration has been shown to result in higher weight gain, no deterioration or prolongation of the diarrhoea and no increase in vomiting or lactose intolerance (Conway and Ireson, 1989).

Dehydration treatment

The interventions of greatest impact on acute diarrhea are hydration and nutrition (Brandt et al., 2015). Because diarrhoea results in fluid and electrolyte loss, it is important to prevent or reverse any fluid and electrolyte depletion. Most patients can be advised to increase their intake of fluids.

Young children and the frail and elderly are prone to diarrhoea-induced dehydration, and the use of an oral rehydration solution (ORS) is recommended. The formula recommended by the WHO contains glucose, sodium, potassium, chloride and bicarbonate and is almost isotonic with body fluid. A number of similar preparations are available commercially in the form of sachets that require reconstitution in clean water before use (Table 14.6). The reasoning behind the ingredients within ORS are that the glucose facilitates the absorption of sodium (and hence water) on a 1:1 molar basis in the small intestine. Some preparations replace glucose with rice powder. Sodium and potassium are needed to replace the body losses of these essential ions during diarrhoea (and vomiting), and the citrate corrects the acidosis that occurs as a result of diarrhoea and dehydration (WHO, 2006). Previously the WHO ORS contained 90 mmol/L sodium, because cholera is more common in developing countries and is associated with rapid loss of sodium and potassium. However, a systematic

Table 14.6 Composition of oral rehydration solutions

	Osmolarity (mOsm/L)	Glucose (mmol/L)	Sodium (mmol/L)	Chloride (mmol/L)	Potassium (mmol/L)	Base (mmol/L)
Dioralyte	240	90	60	60	20	Citrate 10
Electrolade	251	111	50	40	20	Bicarbonate 30
World Health Organisation oral rehydration solution	245	75	75	65	20	Citrate 10

review of trials using a reduced osmolarity ORS concluded that solutions with a reduced osmolarity compared with the standard WHO formula were associated with 33% fewer unscheduled intravenous infusions, a trend towards reduced stool output and less vomiting in children with mild-to-moderate diarrhoea (Hahn et al., 2001). Based on this and other findings, the WHO ORS now has a reduced osmolarity of 245 mOsm/L and contains 75 mmol of sodium.

ORS should be routinely used in both primary and secondary care settings. For healthy adults, an appropriate substitute for a rehydration sachet is 2.5 mL of table salt plus 30 mL of sugar in 1 L of drinking water. The volume of ORS to be taken in treating mild-to-moderate diarrhoea is dependent on age. In adults, 2 L of oral rehydration fluid should be given in the first 24 hours, followed by unrestricted normal fluids with 200 mL of rehydration solution per loose stool or vomit. For children, 30–50 mL/kg of an ORS should be given over 3–4 hours. This can be followed with unrestricted fluids, either with normal fluids alternating with ORS or normal fluids with 10 mL/kg rehydration solution after each loose stool or vomit. The solution is best sipped every 5–10 minutes rather than drunk in large quantities less frequently. However, care is required in patients with diabetes because they may need to monitor blood glucose levels more carefully. They should also be advised not to stop taking insulin.

Drug treatment

Antimotility agents. In uncomplicated acute diarrhoea, antimotility agents such as loperamide, diphenoxylate and codeine are occasionally useful for symptomatic control in adults. They act by binding to opiate receptors in the gut wall, reducing propulsive peristalsis, increasing intestinal transit time and enhancing the reabsorption of water and electrolytes. Antimotility agents are not recommended for use in children because trial results appear contradictory and any benefits are small with unacceptable levels of side effects observed. Antimotility agents should be avoided in severe gastroenteritis or dysentery.

Loperamide. Loperamide is a synthetic opioid analogue. It should have an effect within 1 hour of oral administration. For acute diarrhoea in adults, 4 mg of loperamide is taken initially followed by 2 mg after every loose stool, up to a maximum of 16 mg each day for 5 days. It is relatively free of central nervous system (CNS) effects at therapeutic doses because it does not readily cross the blood–brain barrier, although CNS depression may be seen in overdose, particularly in children. Because it undergoes hepatic metabolism it should be used with caution in patients with hepatic dysfunction. It is also of use in patients with high-output stomas; the tablet rather than the capsule formulation should be dispensed to avoid the formulation passing unchanged into an ostomy bag.

Diphenoxylate. Diphenoxylate is a synthetic opioid available as co-phenotrope in combination with a subtherapeutic dose of atropine. The atropine is present to discourage abuse but may cause atropinic effects in susceptible individuals. Administration of co-phenotrope at the recommended dosage carries minimal risk of dependence. However, prolonged use or administration of high doses may produce a morphine-type dependence. It has a similar adverse effect profile to that of morphine. If an overdose is taken, the symptoms can be delayed for a considerable period and respiratory depression may not be seen for up to 30 hours. Young children are particularly susceptible to diphenoxylate overdose, whereas few as 10 tablets of co-phenotrope may be fatal. Concurrent use of diphenoxylate with monoamine oxidase inhibitors can precipitate a hypertensive crisis, while the action of CNS depressants such as barbiturates, tranquilisers and alcohol is enhanced.

Codeine and morphine. The constipating side effect of the opioid analgesics codeine and morphine may be used to treat diarrhoea. Both are susceptible to misuse and, given in large doses, may induce tolerance and psychological and physical dependence. Morphine may still be obtained in combination with the adsorbent kaolin, but this combination is no longer recommended for the treatment of acute diarrhoea.

Absorbants. Kaolin, used as an absorbant, is not recommended for the treatment of acute diarrhoea.

Antimicrobials. Antibiotics are generally not recommended in diarrhoea associated with acute infective gastroenteritis. This is because the cause is more commonly viral, and the symptoms tend to resolve quickly on their own. Inappropriate treatment of diarrhoea with antibiotics will only further contribute to the problem of resistant organisms. Antibiotics should be reserved for patients who produce a positive stool culture for bacteria and where the symptoms are not receding or for traveller's diarrhoea (De Bruyn et al., 2000). Rifaximin, a rifamycin antibiotic which is not absorbed when administered orally, is licensed in the UK to treat traveller's diarrhoea without fever, blood in the stools and where there have been less than eight unformed stools in the past 24 hours.

C. difficile is a facultative anaerobe and as such will normally respond to a 10-day course of metronidazole. Other effective antibiotics include oral vancomycin and fidaxomicin. Infections which are resistant to antibiotic treatment have been treated with immunoglobulins. More recently attention has focused on faecal transplantation (intestinal microbiota transplantation) as a novel mode of treatment. This involves infusing intestinal microorganisms from a healthy donor into the bowel of an affected patient, most commonly via an enema. A systematic review showed a 92% success rate (Gough et al., 2011).

Enkephalinase inhibitors. Racecadotril is a pro-drug of thiorphan. Thiorphan, an enkephalinase inhibitor, inhibits the breakdown of endogenous opioids, thereby reducing intestinal secretions. It does not change intestinal transit time. Racecadotril can be used as an adjunct to rehydration for the symptomatic treatment of acute uncomplicated diarrhoea.

Probiotics. Probiotics have been defined as components of microbial cells or microbial cell preparations that have a beneficial effect on health. Well-known probiotics include lactic acid bacteria and the yeast *Saccharomyces*. The rationale for their use in infectious diarrhoea is that they act against enteric pathogens in a number of ways and increase the immune responses within the body. A Cochrane review identified a reduction on duration and severity of diarrhoea when probiotics were administered with rehydration therapy. Probiotics were not associated with adverse effects. The use of probiotics is therefore recommended as an adjunct to ORS; however, there was insufficient evidence to develop an evidence-based treatment guideline for probiotics (Allen et al., 2010).

Zinc. The use of zinc has been reviewed in the treatment of diarrhoea in children in developing countries (Lazzerini and Wanzira, 2016). In this context, zinc has been beneficial in children older than 6 months, probably because they have a prior underlying zinc deficiency. The WHO (2011) has recommended both ORS and zinc supplementation for the clinical management of diarrhoea.

Rotavirus vaccine. The monovalent rotavirus vaccine Rotarix was introduced to the standard UK childhood immunisation programme in September 2013. It is administered at 2 and 3 months of age. Reported cases of rotavirus have declined by 74% in 2015/2016 season when compared with the 10-year average (Public Health England, 2016). Considering that Tam et al. (2012) estimated that there were 147 community cases and 10 primary care doctor consultations for every reported case of rotavirus within the UK, this would represent a 220,000 reduction in clinical cases of rotavirus.

Some of the common therapeutic problems in the management of individuals with constipation and diarrhoea are outlined in Table 14.7.

Case studies

Case 14.1

Mrs CB, a woman in her 40s, asks to speak to the pharmacist. She has had constipation on and off for the last 2 months. She is a busy working mother, 5′4″ tall (1.63 m) and weighs 13 stone (82.6 kg). She states that she has put on weight over the last 12 months.

Question

What further information do you need to obtain to be in a position to help Mrs CB?

Answer

Constipation can be a common problem in someone of Mrs CB's age. A full medical and social history is required to establish the root cause. Ignoring the need to defecate which could be combined with a diet low in fibre, inadequate fluid intake and inadequate exercise may all be contributory factors. The nature of the condition should be established alongside the duration of the problem and whether there are any other symptoms such as blood in the stools, pain and bloating. Her normal bowel habits could be discussed, and she should be asked to explain why she thinks she is constipated. It would be important to establish if there has been any change which may have precipitated the constipation. These may include physical and social factors such as life changes. Particularly, in this case, one should further probe the weight gain over the past 12 months. If the patient eats a healthy diet and has been exercising on a regular basis, then hypothyroidism could be suspected. If other symptoms of hypothyroidism, such as lethargy, tiredness, malaise and feeling cold are present, then it may be prudent to refer to the primary care doctor for thyroid function tests.

If her replies to the questions raise no suspicion of underlying medical problems, then non-drug advice only may be needed. If the patient would benefit from an increase in exercise, fluid intake or increase in fibre, then this can be recommended. Often patients will request a

Table 14.7 Common therapeutic problems in constipation and diarrhoea

Problem	Comments
Constipation	
Bulk laxative (e.g. ispaghula) taken at bedtime	Drugs such as ispaghula should not be taken before going to bed because of risk of oesophageal blockage.
Urine changes colour	Anthraquinone glycosides (e.g. senna) are excreted by the kidney and may colour urine yellowish brown to red, depending on pH.
Patient claims dietary and fluid advice ineffective in resolving constipation	May find high-fibre diet difficult to adhere to, socially unacceptable, and expect result in less than 4 weeks.
Patient who is taking docusate reports unpleasant aftertaste or burning sensation	Advise to take with plenty of fluid after ingestion.
Sterculia as Normacol and Normacol Plus granules or sachets	The granules should be placed dry on the tongue and swallowed immediately with plenty of water or a cool drink. They can also be sprinkled onto and taken with soft food such as yogurt.
Methylcellulose (Celevac)	Each tablet should be taken with at least 300 mL of liquid.
Diarrhoea	
Antimotility agent requested for a young child	Antimotility agents must be avoided in young children or patients with severe gastroenteritis or dysentery.
Antimotility agent requested by patient with persistent diarrhoea (>10 days)	Antimotility agent inappropriate. Stool culture required to exclude parasitic infection, such as Giardia, Entamoeba and Cryptosporidium.
Adult with diarrhoea stops eating and drinking to allow diarrhoea to settle	Patient should eat and drink as normally as possible. Plenty of fluids are required to prevent dehydration. Fruit juice (glucose and potassium), soup (salt), bread and pasta (carbohydrate) are of particular benefit.
Reconstitution of oral rehydration solution	Each sachet of Dioralyte and Electrolade; requires 200 mL of water. They should be discarded after 1 h after preparation unless stored in a fridge when they may be kept for 24 h.

particular product. Mrs CB should be recommended a bulk-forming laxative as first-line treatment. It is important to counsel the patient about how long the laxative will take to work (12–36 hours), because patients often have misconceptions about the onset of therapeutic benefit.

Case 14.2

Mr RJ is an 82-year-old man who was admitted to hospital following a fall at home. On admission he was confused and spiking a temperature of 38.7 °C. Urine analysis was strongly positive for nitrites and white blood cells. He was commenced on co-amoxiclav 1.2 g three times a day i.v. for a urinary tract infection. Two days later his temperature was normal and he was eating and drinking well. The decision was made to convert i.v. co-amoxiclav to oral for a further 5 days to ensure resolution of his infection. Three days later you are asked as the ward pharmacist if there is anything you can recommend because Mr RJ has diarrhoea. This morning his temperature is 39.2 °C and his C-reactive protein (CRP) is 45 mg/L. His regular medicines are furosemide 40 mg, lansoprazole 30 mg, atenolol 50 mg and aspirin 75 mg. All these medicines are taken once a day.

Answer

Broad-spectrum antibiotics are often used to treat infections empirically in the hospital setting. In elderly patients this is a potential risk. In addition to treating the infection they will also kill many of the normal gut microflora, which can allow pathogenic organisms to colonise the large intestine. Mr RJ shows two signs of an acute infection with a raised temperature and CRP. New-onset diarrhoea following a course of broad-spectrum antibiotic should always raise the possibility of *C. difficile*–associated diarrhoea. Proton pump inhibitors have been associated with an increased prevalence of *C. difficile* because by raising the pH of the stomach they remove a natural barrier to infection. Because Mr RJ is elderly this also increases the risk of *C. difficile* infection. Stool samples should be sent to the laboratory for culture and enterotoxin testing. Immediate action would involve isolating the patient and stopping any unnecessary treatment with broad-spectrum antibiotics. The lansoprazole should also be stopped to prevent colonisation from further pathogenic species. Antibiotic treatment to eradicate *C. difficile* should be commenced immediately. This normally involves a 10-day course of metronidazole in treatment-naive patients. However, increasingly resistant strains of *C. difficile* are being reported from UK hospitals. As a result local policies may recommend oral vancomycin or fidaxomicin as first-line treatment options. Treatment-resistant cases may be treated with a second antibiotic. In severe cases immunoglobulins or intestinal microflora transplants may be considered before total colectomy which can be lifesaving.

Case 14.3

Mr BT is a busy 45-year-old executive who works for a large, multi-national company. He complains of constipation. He has also noticed blood in his stools over the past 2 weeks, and for 3 days he has had continuous abdominal discomfort. He has discussed his symptoms with his wife, and they suspect haemorrhoids are the cause. Mr BT regularly travels to Africa with work and is due to go again in 6 days. He would like your advice on a suitable treatment.

Question

What advice should be given to Mr BT?

Answer

Blood in the stool is not necessarily serious. If the blood appears fresh and can only be seen on the surface of the stool it is likely the source is the anus or distal colon. It is probably caused by straining when defaecating, leading to bleeding from haemorrhoids or an anal fissure. Similarly, if the blood appears as specks or as a smear on the toilet paper after defaecation, this is also likely to indicate haemorrhoids, particularly if such a diagnosis has been made previously following clinical examination. Larger amounts of fresh blood in the stool may indicate diverticulitis in older people, or if combined with other infective symptoms such as fever or rash may indicate infection with an enteroinvasive species such as *Shigella*, *E. coli* O157 or typhoid.

If the blood is mixed with the faeces and has a dark or 'tarry' appearance and a particularly offensive smell, then a more serious underlying cause is possible. The darker the faeces, the more suggestive that there has been an upper GI bleed or a substantial loss of blood from the large bowel. If this is the case the patient should be referred to have a full clinical examination, alongside a full blood count and urea and electrolyte tests. Iron tablets or bismuth preparations can cause darkened stools, so it is important to take a medication history from the patient.

However, given Mr BT's age, recent onset of symptoms, travel plans and the presence of continuous abdominal pain accompanying the constipation, referral for further investigation would be appropriate.

Case 14.4

Miss LS, the 15-year-old daughter of one of your regular patients, makes a request for stimulant laxative for herself for constipation. She is normally healthy, if a little thin, and seems a little nervous today.

Questions

What questions would you ask Miss LS in response to her over-the-counter medication request for a laxative?

Answers

Laxative abuse should be a consideration when receiving such a request from a person of this age. For individuals suffering from an eating disorder such as anorexia or bulimia nervosa, the prevalence of laxative abuse has been reported to range from approximately 10% to 60% (Roerig et al., 2010). As a result, although this request should be treated with suspicion, it should always be dealt with professionally and tactfully. Abuse should not be assumed without supporting evidence. Questions, regarding the length and duration of symptoms, any other medication, current diet and exercise patterns and her current social situation, will help to build up a more complete picture of the patient, and possibly help her reveal any underlying issues. It is important to investigate why she wants this product, as well as if she has used stimulant laxatives before and how often to eliminate abuse and chronic use. Stimulant laxatives are more prone to abuse because they are seen as a weight-reduction aid, because of their fast onset of action. Whatever the outcome of the consultation with Miss LS, healthy eating habits should be encouraged. This may include five portions of fruit and vegetables per day, 8 cups of water per day and regular exercise. It may also be useful to measure her weight and height to calculate her body mass index to show her that she does not need to lose weight.

Her age also complicates the issues in this case. Within the UK, Fraser guidelines and Gillick competence can be used to assess whether Miss LS is competent to make decisions about her own care (National Society for the Prevention of Cruelty to Children, 2017). Parents should not be informed as routine practice. If Miss LS has been chronically using stimulant laxatives, referral to her primary care doctor may be advised; however, she should not be forced to go.

Case 14.5

Mr GH is planning to travel to Mexico on business. He was last there 6 months ago but was incapacitated with diarrhoea for 3 of 6 days during a busy work schedule. He does not want a repeat experience on his forthcoming visit and is seeking advice about taking a course of antibiotics with him to use as empirical treatment, should the need arise.

Questions

1. Is there any evidence that antibiotics are of benefit in traveller's diarrhoea?
2. Are there any problems associated with empirical use of antibiotics in traveller's diarrhoea?

Answers

1. The empirical use of antibiotics has been shown to increase the cure rate in individuals suffering from traveller's diarrhoea.

Studies in travellers, including students, package tourists, military personnel and volunteers, have compared antibiotic use against placebo (De Bruyn et al., 2000). The antibiotics studied have included aztreonam, ciprofloxacin, co-trimoxazole, norfloxacin, ofloxacin and trimethoprim given for durations varying from a single dose to a 5-day treatment course. Overall, antibiotics increased the cure rate at 72 hours (defined as cessation of unformed stools or less than one unformed stool/24 hours) without additional symptoms. There has been an increase in reports of fluoroquinolone resistance from South East Asia; macrolides such as azithromycin are a useful treatment in these cases (Tribble et al., 2007).

2. The use of antibiotics in the treatment of traveller's diarrhoea does have problems. Adverse effects in up to 18% of recipients have been reported, with GI (cramp, nausea, or anorexia), dermatological (rash) and respiratory (cough and/or sore throat) symptoms the most frequently reported. Antibiotic-resistant isolates have also been reported following the use of ciprofloxacin, co-trimoxazole and norfloxacin. Rifaximin is licensed for the treatment of traveller's diarrhoea.

Acknowledgement

The authors would like to acknowledge the contribution of Paul Rutter to previous versions of this chapter which appeared in fourth and fifth editions of this book.

References

Allen, S.J., Martinez, E.G., Gregorio, G.V., Dans, L.F., 2010. Probiotics for treating acute infectious diarrhoea. Cochrane Database Syst. Rev. 2010 (11), CD003048. https://doi.org/10.1002/14651858.CD003048.pub3.

Ashraf, W., Park, F., Lof, J., Quigley, E.M., 1995. Effects of psyllium therapy on stool characteristics, colon transit and anorectal function in chronic idiopathic constipation. Aliment. Pharmacol. Ther. 9, 639–647.

Brandt, K.G., Castro Antunes, M.M., Silva, G.A., 2015. Acute diarrhea: evidence-based management. J. Pediatr. (Rio J.) 91 (6 Suppl. 1), S36–S43.

Churgay, C.A., Aftab, Z., 2012. Gastroenteritis in children: part II. Prevention and management. Am. Fam. Physician 85 (11), 1066–1070.

Connell, A.M., Hilton, C., Irvine, G., et al., 1965. Variation of bowel habit in two population samples. BMJ 1965, 1095–1099.

Conway, S.P., Ireson, A., 1989. Acute gastroenteritis in well nourished infants: comparison of four feeding regimens. Arch. Dis. Child. 64, 87–91.

Cullen, G., O'Donoghue, D., 2007. Constipation and pregnancy. Best Pract. Res. Clin. Gastroenterol. 21 (5), 807–818.

De Bruyn, G., Hahn, S., Borwick, A., 2000. Antibiotic treatment for travellers' diarrhoea. Cochrane Database Syst. Rev. 2000 (3), CD002242. https://doi.org/10.1002/14651858.CD002242.

Degen, L.P., Phillips, S.F., 1996. Variability of gastrointestinal transit in healthy women and men. Gut 39, 299–305.

Ejemot-Nwadiaro, R.I., Ehiri, J.E., Arikpo, D., Meremikwu, M.M., Critchley, J.A., 2015. Hand washing promotion for preventing diarrhoea. Cochrane Database Syst. Rev. 2015 (9), CD004265. https://doi.org/10.1002/14651858.CD004265.pub3.

Feldman, R.A., Banatvala, N., 1994. The frequency of culturing stools from adults with diarrhoea in Great Britain. Epidemiol. Infect. 113 (1), 41–44.

Gough, E., Shaikh, H., Manges, A.R., 2011. Systematic review of intestinal microbiota transplantation (fecal bacteriotherapy) for recurrent *Clostridium difficile* infection. Clin. Infect. Dis. 53 (10), 994–1002.

Hahn, S., Kim, Y., Garner, P., 2001. Reduced osmolarity oral rehydration solution for treating dehydration due to diarrhoea in children: systematic review. BMJ 323 (73404), 81–85.

Lazzerini, M., Wanzira, H., 2016. Oral zinc for treating diarrhoea in children. Cochrane Database Syst. Rev. 2016 (12), CD005436. https://doi.org/10.1002/14651858.CD005436.pub5.

Lewis, S.J., Heaton, K.W., 1997. Stool form scale as a useful guide to intestinal transit time. Scand. J. Gastroenterol. 32 (9), 920–924.

Liu, L.W., 2011. Chronic constipation: current treatment options. Can. J. Gastroenterol. 25 (Suppl. B), 22B–28B.

Longstreth, G.F., Thompson, W.G., Chey, W.D., et al., 2006. Functional bowel disorders. Gastroenterology 130, 1480–1491.

MacGillivray, S., Fahey, T., McGuire, W., 2013. Lactose avoidance for young children with acute diarrhoea. Cochrane Database Syst. Rev. 2013 (10), CD005433. https://doi.org/10.1002/14651858.CD005433.pub2.

Mugie, S.M., Benninga, M.A., Di Lorenzo, C., 2011. Epidemiology of constipation in children and adults: a systematic review. Best Pract. Res. Clin. Gastroenterol. 25 (1), 3–18.

National Institute of Health and Care Excellence (NICE), 2013. CKS: diarrhoea adult's assessment. Available at: https://cks.nice.org.uk/diarrhoea-adults-assessment.

National Institute of Health and Care Excellence (NICE), 2015a. CKS: constipation. Available at: http://cks.nice.org.uk/constipation.

National Institute of Health and Care Excellence (NICE), 2015b. CKS: gastroenteritis. Available at: http://cks.nice.org.uk/gastroenteritis.

National Society for the Prevention of Cruelty to Children, 2017. A child's legal rights Gillick competency and Fraser guidelines. Available at: https://www.nspcc.org.uk/preventing-abuse/child-protection-system/legal-definition-child-rights-law/gillick-competency-fraser-guidelines.

Public Health England, 2016. Winter health watch summary. 17 March 2016. Available at: https://www.gov.uk/government/publications/winter-health-watch-summary-17-march-2016/winter-health-watch-summary-17-march-2016.

Rao, S.S.C., Go, J.T., 2010. Update on the management of constipation in the elderly: new treatment options. Clin. Interv. Aging. 5, 163–171.

Rao, S.S.C., Meduri, K., 2011. What is necessary to diagnose constipation? Best Pract. Res. Clin. Gastroenterol. 25 (1), 127–140.

Roerig, J.L., Steffen, K.J., Mitchell, J.E., et al., 2010. Laxative abuse: epidemiology, diagnosis and management. Drugs 70 (12), 1487–1503.

Rungsiprakarn, P., Laopaiboon, M., Sangkomkamhang, U.S., et al., 2015. Interventions for treating constipation in pregnancy. Cochrane Database Syst. Rev. 2015 (9), CD011448. https://doi.org/10.1002/14651858.CD011448.pub2.

Shetty, N., 2009. Healthcare associated infections. In: Shetty, N., Tang, J.W., Andrews, J. (Eds.), Infectious Disease: Pathogenesis, Prevention and Case Studies. Wiley-Blackwell, Chichester, UK.

Shetty, N., Tang, J.W., 2009. Gastroenteritis. In: Shetty, N., Tang, J.W., Andrews, J. (Eds.), Infectious Disease: Pathogenesis, Prevention and Case Studies. Wiley-Blackwell, Chichester, UK.

Tam, C.C., Rodrigues, L.C., Viviani, L., et al., 2012. Longitudinal study of infectious intestinal disease in the UK (IID2 study): incidence in the community and presenting to general practice. Gut 61, 69–77.

Thomas, P.D., Forbes, A., Green, J., et al., 2003. Guidelines for the investigation of chronic diarrhoea, 2nd edition. Gut 52 (Suppl. V), v1–v15.

Tribble, D.R., Saunders, J.W., Pang, L.W., et al., 2007. Traveler's diarrhea in Thailand: randomized, double-blind trial comparing single-dose and 3-day azithromycin-based regimens with a 3-day levofloxacin regimen. Clin. Infect. Dis. 44, 338–346.

World Gastroenterology Organisation, 2012. Acute diarrhea in adults and children: a global perspective. Available at: http://www.worldgastroenterology.org/guidelines/global-guidelines/acute-diarrhea/acute-diarrhea-english.

World Health Organisation (WHO), 2006. Oral rehydration salts: production of the new ORS. Available to download from: http://www.who.int/maternal_child_adolescent/documents/fch_cah_06_1/en.

World Health Organisation (WHO), 2011. Zinc supplementation in the management of diarrhea. Available at: http://www.who.int/elena/titles/bbc/zinc_diarrhoea/en.

World Health Organisation (WHO), 2013a. Diarrhoeal disease Fact Sheet. Available at: http://www.who.int/mediacentre/factsheets/fs330/en.

World Health Organisation (WHO), 2013b. Weekly epidemiological paper. 88(5), 49–64. Available at: www.who.int/wer/en

Further reading

National Institute of Health and Care Excellence, 2016. CKS: palliative care – constipation. Available at: https://cks.nice.org.uk/palliative-care-constipation.

National Institute of Health and Care Excellence, 2015. CKS: constipation in children. Available at: https://cks.nice.org.uk/constipation-in-children.

National Institute of Health and Care Excellence, 2015. CKS: gastroenteritis. Available at: https://cks.nice.org.uk/gastroenteritis.

National Institute of Health and Care Excellence, 2013. CKS: diarrhoea-prevention and advice for travellers. Available at: https://cks.nice.org.uk/diarrhoea-prevention-and-advice-for-travellers.

National Institute of Health and Care Excellence, 2013. CKS: diarrhoea-antibiotic associated. Available at: https://cks.nice.org.uk/diarrhoea-antibiotic-associated.

Pinto Sanchez, M.I., Bercik, P., 2011. Epidemiology and burden of chronic constipation. Can. J. Gastroenterol. 25 (Suppl. B), 11B–15B.

Schuster, B.G., Kosar, L., Kamrul, R., 2015. Constipation in older adults: stepwise approach to keep things moving. Can. Fam. Physician 61 (2), 152–158.

Trottier, M., Erebara, A., Bozzo, P., 2012. Treating constipation during pregnancy. Can. Fam. Physician 58 (8), 836–838.

Useful websites

Bristol Stool Chart is available through the NICE website: https://www.nice.org.uk/guidance/cg99/resources/bristol-stool-chart-pdf-245459773

15 Adverse Effects of Drugs on the Liver

Sara Sawieres

Key points

- Approximately 20–30% of acute liver failure cases are attributed to drugs.
- The risk of drug-induced liver disorders increases with age and is generally more common in women.
- Generally, drug-induced liver damage is either dose-related or idiosyncratic.
- Drugs can cause all types of liver disorder and should always be considered in patients presenting with liver-related problems.
- The clinical features of drug-induced hepatotoxicity vary widely, depending on the type of liver damage caused.
- Treatment of drug-induced hepatotoxicity relies on correct diagnosis, prompt withdrawal of the causative agent and supportive therapy.
- Patients given potentially hepatotoxic drugs should be monitored regularly and taught how to recognise signs of liver dysfunction and advised to report symptoms immediately.
- Drugs causing dose-related hepatic toxicity may do so at lower doses in patients with liver disease than in patients with normal liver function, and idiosyncratic reactions may occur more frequently in patients with existing liver disease.
- Any new drug has the potential to cause hepatotoxicity. Post-marketing surveillance is important to highlight new potential hepatotoxic effects.

Traditionally, the definition of an adverse drug reaction (ADR) is an effect that is unintentional, noxious and occurs at doses used for diagnosis, prophylaxis and treatment (World Health Organization [WHO], 1972). In 2014 the European Medicines Evaluation Agency (EMEA) defined an ADR as

a response to a medicinal product which is noxious and unintended.
[...]
Adverse reactions may arise from use of the product within or outside the terms of the marketing authorisation or from occupational exposure. Use outside the marketing authorisation includes off-label use, overdose, misuse, abuse and medication errors (EMEA, 2014).

A hepatic drug reaction is an ADR that predominantly affects the liver.

Drugs can induce almost all forms of acute or chronic liver disease, with some drugs producing more than one type of hepatic reaction. Although not a particularly common form of ADR, drugs should always be considered as a possible cause of liver disease.

Drug-induced liver injury (DILI) is termed as either intrinsic or idiosyncratic DILI. Intrinsic DILI, which can also be termed as type A DILI, includes drugs that have the potential to affect all individuals with varying degrees. The reaction tends to be predictable and is often dose dependent; an example is paracetamol. Idiosyncratic DILI, which can also be termed type B DILI, occurs in susceptible individuals. The reaction is not predictable, so it is not dose dependent (Chalasani et al., 2014). The latency period for the manifestation of idiosyncratic reactions is variable, ranging from 5 to 90 days from the initial ingestion of the drug. This type of reaction may be due to either drug hypersensitivity or a metabolic abnormality. Examples of drugs that induce idiosyncratic reactions are chlorpromazine, halothane and isoniazid (Leise et al., 2014).

Epidemiology

WHO has been tracking ADRs since 1968 and has issued a report indicating that since the 1990s, the number of incidences of DILI has continued to increase (Bjornsson and Olsson, 2006). However, the incidence of idiosyncratic reactions occurring at therapeutic doses for most drugs remains low, from 1 in every 1000 patients to 1 in every 100,000 patients. DILI is not usually life-threatening; however, for the small number of patients who develop drug-induced acute liver failure (ALF), the prognosis is poor. Ten percent of those who develop hepatocellular damage and jaundice will either need a liver transplant or die. It is estimated that 15–40% of ALF cases may be attributable to drugs (Chalasani et al., 2014). Table 15.1 presents the suggested classification of ALF: hyperacute, acute and subacute (Richardson and O'Grady, 2002).

Hepatotoxicity induced by such drugs as halothane, the antituberculous agents isoniazid and rifampicin, psychotropics, antibiotics and cytotoxic drugs still continues to cause concern. ALF induced by paracetamol has become an important indication for liver transplantation. A trial carried out between 2002 and 2007 using six English hospitals and the National Registry of deliberate self-harm identified that there were 10,208 presentations to hospitals for paracetamol overdose in the UK and 9057 in Ireland (Hawton et al., 2011).

Many drugs cause elevated liver enzymes with apparently no clinically significant adverse effect, although in a few patients there may be significant hepatotoxicity. For

Table 15.1 Characteristics of the different types of acute liver failure (Richardson and O'Grady, 2002)

Characteristic	Hyperacute	Acute	Subacute
Transition time from jaundice to encephalopathy	0–7 days	8–28 days	29–84 days
Cerebral oedema	Common	Common	Rare
Renal failure	Early	Late	Late
Ascites	Rare	Rare	Common
Coagulation disorder	Marked	Marked	Modest
Prognosis	Moderate	Poor	Poor

example, isoniazid causes elevated liver enzymes in 10–36% of patients taking the drug as a single agent. However, only 1% suffer significant hepatotoxicity, with the liver function tests (LFTs) of the majority returning to normal if therapy is discontinued.

Although it is not possible to identify patients who will suffer ADRs manifesting in hepatic toxicity, a number of risk factors have been identified.

Risk factors

There are three types of risk factors that need to be considered: patient factors, drug factors and disease factors.

Patient factors

Age

Age as a risk factor for DILI only applies to some medications. For example, younger age puts people at risk of Reye's syndrome associated with aspirin. Agents such as erythromycin, halothane, isoniazid, nitrofurantoin and flucloxacillin are considered to have a greater risk of hepatotoxicity as age increases (Chalasani and Bjornsson, 2010). The US tuberculosis study showed an incidence of isoniazid hepatotoxicity of 4.4 per 1000 patients aged 25–34 years but 20–83 per 1000 patients aged 50 years or older (Fountain et al., 2005). Younger individuals commonly develop hepatocellular DILI, whereas cholestatic DILI is more common in the elderly. The reason for age as a risk factor in DILI or the type of injury is unclear. The clearance of certain CYP3A substrates is altered by older age; however, the activity of phase I or II drug metabolising enzymes is not significantly affected by age. Elderly patients tend to be on multiple medications that may increase the risk of DILI; however, there is conflicting evidence around this (Chalasani and Bjornsson, 2010).

Sex

Traditionally, it was believed that the frequency of drug-induced hepatotoxicity was higher in females than males. However, Lucena et al. (2009) carried out a prospective study and showed 51% of patients with DILI were male, and 49% were female. Specific medications have shown differences between genders. Halothane, isoniazid, nitrofurantoin, chlorpromazine and erythromycin have been shown to cause DILI more frequently in women, whereas men are more susceptible to azathioprine DILI. Medication causing hepatocellular patterns of damage, that is, damage to the cells in the liver, is seen more frequently in women and is associated with a poorer outcome, whereas cholestatic jaundice associated with co-amoxiclav has been reported to be more common in males than females (Chalasani and Bjornsson, 2010).

Genetics

The rarity and unpredictable nature of idiosyncratic DILI suggest that there is a strong genetic component. Significant connections have been made between certain genetic traits and DILI. This has only been shown for a few compounds. It is difficult to isolate genetic traits from environmental risk factors. There are different suggestions and studies that have considered mitochondrial DNA mutations and their effect on DILI, genetic changes involved in the glycoproteins used to transport drug metabolites and genetic changes affecting immune response. It is thought that toxic metabolites formed by cytochrome P450 isoenzymes in phase I metabolism are involved in the pathogenesis of DILI. The evidence for this is weak except for in a few compounds where there are some case reports. There is some evidence showing that CYP2E1 mutant genotypes can reduce the risk of isoniazid-induced hepatotoxicity.

N-Acetylation involved in phase II metabolism is also thought to be involved in DILI. The enzyme involved is N-acetyltransferase 2 (NAT2); polymorphs of this enzyme have different enzymatic activity, with NAT2*4 having the fastest rate of acetylation. Studies have shown that the polymorphs associated with slower rates of acetylation are linked to hepatotoxicity associated with isoniazid and sulfonamides. Slow acetylators do not detoxify acetyl-hydrazine quickly and so promote oxidation by CYP2E1 into toxic metabolites.

It is thought that a genetic predisposition to allergic forms of drug hypersensitivity could be a factor in some types of liver disease. Flucloxacillin liver injury has been associated with the human leukocyte antigen B*5701. Having this HLA haplotype confers an 80-fold increase in susceptibility to liver injury with flucloxacillin (Chalasani and Bjornsson, 2010).

Enzyme induction and metabolism

A study carried out in the US looked at the metabolism of 207 of the most commonly prescribed medications and their association with DILI. Drugs that were significantly metabolised by the liver, greater than 50% hepatic metabolism, had a significantly increased incidence of raised alanine aminotransferase, liver failure and fatal DILI. The study looked at four common cytochrome P450 pathways. The different pathways were associated with different indicators of liver injury. CYP2C9 and CYP2C19 were found to have the stronger association with DILI (Lammert et al., 2010).

Alcohol, rifampicin and other drugs that induce cytochrome P450 isoenzyme 2El potentiate the risk of hepatotoxicity with other drugs such as paracetamol, isoniazid and halothane. The role of alcohol as a risk factor for DILI is, however, not clear-cut, and acute and chronic alcohol consumption may have different effects.

Concomitant therapy with other anticonvulsants, particularly phenytoin and phenobarbital, is a risk factor for toxicity with sodium valproate, where 90% of cases of liver injury are associated with combination therapy (Chalasani and Bjornsson, 2010).

Drug factors

Daily dose

It has already been mentioned that idiosyncratic DILI cannot be predicted by the dose of a medication. However, co-amoxiclav, flucloxacillin and diclofenac are examples of medications that can cause idiosyncratic DILI that have shown a dose effect. Idiosyncratic DILI can occur at lower doses of these agents; however, an increase in dose has shown a worsening of DILI. Conversely, some agents, such as duloxetine, have caused DILI only on increasing the dose. These patients had previously not suffered from any underlying liver impairment at the lower doses (de Abajo et al., 2004).

Polypharmacy

A typical example of this is seen with non-steroidal anti-inflammatory drugs (NSAIDs). The risk of liver disease with NSAIDs is normally extremely low but is increased when NSAIDs are used with other hepatotoxic drugs. As mentioned previously, there is an association between drugs metabolised by CYP450 isoenzymes and DILI. Co-commitment use of drugs that interact by inducing CYP450 are thought to act as predisposing factors to DILI. CYP inducers include rifampicin, phenytoin, isoniazid, smoking and alcohol. A meta-analysis carried out looking at hepatotoxicity associated with taking isoniazid and rifampicin together or alone showed significantly greater incidences of hepatotoxicity when taken together than alone (Steele et al., 1991).

Disease factors

Pre-existing liver disease

Pharmacodynamics can be altered in pre-existing liver disease, making side effects more pronounced. For example, caution is needed when using anticoagulants in patients with impaired coagulopathy. It is also important to measure the risks of not using a specific agent versus the risks of using it. Patients with pre-existing liver damage should not be excluded from using agents that may cause liver injury. However, there are some agents where greater caution should be exhibited in patients with pre-existing liver disease. Examples include methotrexate, cytotoxic agents, aspirin and sodium valproate. A past medical history of DILI from any medication has been shown to be a predictor of future DILI from other drugs (Chalasani and Bjornsson, 2010).

Table 15.2 Examples of host factors that predispose to drug hepatotoxicity

Risk Factor	Drugs
Female sex	Nitrofurantoin, sulfonamides
Male sex	Azathioprine, amoxicillin/clavulanate
Advanced age	Isoniazid, amoxicillin/clavulanate
Young age	Valproic acid
Chronic alcohol abuse	Paracetamol, isoniazid, methotrexate
Malnutrition or fasting	Paracetamol
Pregnancy	Isoniazid
Diabetes	Methotrexate
Chronic liver disease	Methotrexate, niacin (vitamin B_3)
Chronic kidney disease	Allopurinol
HIV infection	Dapsone, trimethoprim/sulfamethoxazole
Hepatitis B or C infection	Antiretroviral agents, antituberculosis agents
Genetic predisposition	Phenytoin, sulfonamides, isoniazid, antiepileptics

Adapted from Kim and Phongsamran (2009).

Concurrent diseases and pregnancy

Pre-existing renal disease, diabetes, poor nutrition and pregnancy may all affect the ability of the liver to metabolise drugs effectively and may put the patient at risk of developing liver damage. Table 15.2 summarises the host factors that may predispose a patient to drug hepatotoxicity.

Aetiology/pathophysiology/clinical manifestation

Drug-induced hepatotoxicity may present as an acute insult that may or may not progress to chronic disease, or it can present as an insidious development of chronic disease. The type of lesion may be cytotoxic (cellular destruction) or cholestatic (impaired bile flow). Cytotoxic damage may be further classified as necrotic (cell death) or steatic (fatty degeneration). The liver damage resulting from drug toxicity often presents as a mixed picture of cytotoxic and cholestatic injury. The mechanisms of drug-induced hepatic damage can be divided into intrinsic (type A) and idiosyncratic (type B) hepatotoxicity (Table 15.3). Intrinsic hepatotoxicity is predictable, is dose-dependent and usually has a short latency period ranging from hours to weeks. The majority

Table 15.3 Characteristics of intrinsic and idiosyncratic hepatotoxic reactions

Intrinsic drug-induced liver injury	Idiosyncratic drug-induced liver injury
Dose related reaction (usually at the same dose)	Attacks only susceptible individuals (unclear relationship with dose)
Predictable time frame for onset of symptoms	Variable onset relative to exposure
Distinctive liver lesion	Variable liver pathology
Predictable using routine animal testing	Not predictable using routine animal tests

Adapted from Roth and Ganey (2010).

Table 15.4 Examples of adverse drug reactions on the liver (Leise et al., 2014)

Adverse reaction	Drugs associated with reaction
Hepatocellular necrosis	Paracetamol, propylthiouracil, salicylates, iron salts, allopurinol, dantrolene, halothane, ketoconazole, isoniazid, mitomycin, cocaine, 'ecstasy' (methylenedioxymethamphetamine [MDMA])
Fatty liver	Amiodarone, tetracyclines, steroids, sodium valproate, l-asparaginase, methotrexate
Cholestasis	Oral contraceptives, carbimazole, anabolic steroids, ciclosporin
Cholestasis with hepatitis	Chlorpromazine, tricyclic antidepressants, erythromycin, flucloxacillin, co-amoxiclav, angiotensin-converting enzyme (ACE) inhibitors, sulfonamides, sulfonylureas, phenytoin, non-steroidal anti-inflammatory drugs (NSAIDs), cimetidine, ranitidine, trazodone
Granulomatous hepatitis	Phenytoin, allopurinol, carbamazepine, clofibrate, hydralazine, sulfonamides, sulfonylureas
Acute hepatitis	Dantrolene, isoniazid, phenytoin
Chronic active hepatitis	Methyldopa, nitrofurantoin, isoniazid
Fibrosis and cirrhosis	Methotrexate, methyldopa, vitamin A (dose-related)
Vascular disorders	Azathioprine, dactinomycin, dacarbazine

of individuals who take a toxic dose are affected and exhibit the same type of injury. Examples are paracetamol, salicylates, methotrexate and tetracycline. Toxicity may be avoided by ensuring the recommended doses are not exceeded.

Idiosyncratic reactions occur at a low frequency. The latency period is variable, ranging from 5 to 90 days from the initial ingestion of the drug. The type of injury is less predictable and not dose-related. This type of reaction may be due to either drug hypersensitivity or a metabolic abnormality. Examples of drugs that induce idiosyncratic reactions are chlorpromazine, halothane and isoniazid.

The precise mechanisms resulting in DILI are often not completely understood, although injury to the hepatocytes may result directly from interference with intracellular function or membrane integrity or indirectly by immune-mediated damage to cells.

The range of DILIs is illustrated in Table 15.4. An increased serum level of hepatobiliary enzymes without clinical liver disease occurs with variable frequency between drugs, but for some agents, it may occur in up to half of the patients who receive a drug. This may reflect subclinical liver injury.

Cholestasis

Cholestasis is defined as the stagnated movement of bile throughout the bile ducts. This can occur in the intrahepatic ductiles in conditions such as primary biliary cirrhosis or can be extrahepatic due to disruption by gallstones (North-Lewis, 2008).

Aetiology

Some drugs injure bile ducts and cause partial or complete obstruction of the common bile duct, resulting in retention of bile acids. Cholestasis caused by anabolic and contraceptive steroids is due to inhibition of bilirubin excretion from the hepatocyte into the bile.

The penicillins, although commonly associated with allergic drug reactions, are a very rare cause of liver disease. The isoxazolyl group present in the synthetic β-lactamase-resistant oxypenicillins has been implicated as a cause of liver injury. Acute cholestatic hepatitis has increasingly been reported during treatment with flucloxacillin, and in some countries this has become the most important cause of drug-induced cholestatic hepatitis. The incidence

appears to be about twice that of the related isoxazolyl penicillins cloxacillin and dicloxacillin. Moreover, there is likely to be underreporting due to a delay in onset of up to 42 days after stopping treatment. Female sex, age over 55 years, longer courses and high daily doses also seem to be associated with a higher risk of liver injury associated with flucloxacillin (Farrell, 1997).

Rifampicin causes hyperbilirubinaemia by inhibiting uptake of bilirubin by the hepatocyte and inhibiting bilirubin excretion into bile. This is generally not an indication for interrupting rifampicin therapy, although liver function will need to be closely monitored. Other therapeutic agents affect sinusoidal or endothelial cells and may result in veno-occlusive disease or fibrosis. Vitamin A affects the fat-storing cells, causing toxicity that leads to fibrosis.

Pathophysiology

Cholestasis without hepatitis is associated with a raised bilirubin and a normal or minimally raised alanine aminotransferase level. No inflammation or hepatocellular necrosis is seen. In contrast, cholestasis associated with hepatitis presents with raised bilirubin, alanine aminotransferase and alkaline phosphatase levels and a certain amount of liver damage.

Clinical manifestation

The main clinical feature of pure cholestasis is severe pruritus, with or without other features, according to the severity, such as dark urine, pale stools and jaundice.

Drug-induced cholestatic hepatitis usually presents with gastro-intestinal symptoms after an influenza-like illness. Abdominal pain with typical features of cholestasis then occurs. The pruritus is generally less severe than with pure cholestasis (Leise et al., 2014; North-Lewis, 2008).

Steatosis

The liver is the main organ involved in fat metabolism. Damage to the hepatocytes disrupts this process and leads to steatosis. Steatosis is the accumulation of fat within the hepatocytes. It can also be termed fatty liver. The size of the droplets can be small (micro-vesicular) or large (macro-vesicular).

Aetiology

As mentioned previously, the cause of steatosis is the accumulation of fat in the hepatocytes. Tetracyclines are thought to cause steatosis by interfering with the synthesis of lipoproteins that normally remove triglycerides from the liver.

Pathophysiology

Steatosis is associated with abnormal LFTs, although the elevation of alanine aminotransferase is not as high as that seen in acute hepatocellular necrosis. Hyperammonia, hypoglycaemia, acidosis and clotting factor deficiency may also be present. Histologically, the liver damage resembles the acute fatty liver of pregnancy. Micro-vesicular droplets occur with tetracycline, aspirin and sodium valproate, and macro-vesicular droplets occur with steroids, methotrexate, alcohol and amiodarone.

A less severe, more chronic form of fatty liver, steatohepatitis, also occurs. Steatohepatitis differs from diffuse fatty change. Notably, the clinical symptoms and biochemistry resemble chronic parenchymal disease, and the histology is similar to that seen in alcoholic hepatitis. Amiodarone is an example of a drug that can cause chronic steatohepatitis associated with phospholipidosis (North-Lewis, 2008).

Clinical manifestation

A patient presenting with steatosis generally shows fatigue, nausea, vomiting, hypoglycaemia and confusion. Jaundice is present in severe cases.

Hepatitis

When hepatocytes are damaged or die, an inflammatory response is triggered. The inflammatory response is characterised by inflammatory cells, oedema and congestion surrounding the hepatocytes. Inflammation can be acute or chronic and can present differently depending on the degree of damage.

Aetiology

Hepatitis can occur from any number of insulting agents, such as medication or viruses, or can be autoimmune regulated.

Acute hepatitis

Pathophysiology

Acute hepatitis resembles viral hepatitis, with LFTs raised in proportion to the severity of the hepatocellular damage. The best indicator of severity is the prothrombin time. Histologically, necrosis and cellular degeneration are seen in combination with an inflammatory infiltrate.

Clinical manifestation

Acute hepatitis may present with a prodromal illness with non-specific symptoms or include features of drug allergy followed by anorexia, nausea and vomiting, dark urine, pale stools and jaundice. Jaundice tends to be present in severe cases. Weight loss may also be a feature of acute hepatitis. Fatalities occur in 5–30% of jaundiced patients. Acute hepatitis is second only to paracetamol self-poisoning as a cause of DILI.

Chronic active hepatitis

Pathophysiology

Chronic active hepatitis may present as an acute injury or progress to cirrhosis. Serum transaminases are usually raised, and albumin is low. The histology resembles that of autoimmune chronic active hepatitis and is associated with circulating auto-antibodies. Methyldopa is an example of a drug that can cause chronic active hepatitis (North-Lewis, 2008).

Clinical manifestation

Drug-induced chronic active hepatitis may present with tiredness, lethargy and malaise, in a manner similar to other types of chronic liver disease. The symptoms may evolve over many months. Gastro-intestinal symptoms are usually present, and patients may show one or more complications of severe liver disease, including ascites, bleeding oesophageal varices or hepatic encephalopathy. If the ADR has an allergic component, a skin rash and other extrahepatic features of a drug allergy, such as lymphadenopathy, evidence of bone marrow suppression (particularly petechial haemorrhages) may be present.

Fibrosis

Fibrosis of the liver occurs from excessive accumulation of scar tissue as a result of ongoing inflammation of hepatocytes.

Aetiology

A fibrotic liver is characterised by collagen deposits in response to continuous insult to hepatocytes. This then develops into scar tissue. The scarred tissue disrupts the blood flow through the liver and disrupts the passage of substrates from the blood to the hepatocytes.

Pathophysiology

In patients with fibrosis, the serum transaminase levels may be only slightly raised and are not good predictors of hepatic damage. Microscopy shows deposition of fibrous tissues. Fibrosis may proceed to cirrhosis. Such damage may be seen with long-term methotrexate use (North-Lewis, 2008).

Clinical manifestations

Clinical manifestations can vary depending on the severity of fibrosis. Some patients may not have any symptoms at all, and some can present with general symptoms such as abdominal pain, fatigue and malaise (North-Lewis, 2008).

Tumours

Tumours that originate in the liver are termed hepatocellular carcinomas (HCCs).

Aetiology

Of patients who develop an HCC, 90–95% have an underlying cirrhosis; the rest will have a non-cirrhotic HCC. Cirrhosis can be caused by hepatitis B or C, alcoholism, primary biliary cirrhosis, diabetes or smoking and, on rare occasions, medications (Forn et al., 2012).

Pathophysiology

Drugs have been associated with a variety of hepatic tumours. The drugs most commonly linked to malignancy are the oral contraceptives, anabolic steroids and danazol (North-Lewis, 2008).

Clinical manifestation

Patients with small tumours tend to be asymptomatic. However, when clinical manifestations occur, symptoms can be very general to liver impairment. Abdominal pain may or may not be reported, together with a feeling of fullness after eating. Weight loss, fatigue, anorexia, nausea and, occasionally, vomiting can occur, especially in advanced cases (North-Lewis, 2008).

Necrosis

The course of liver necrosis is similar to acute toxic liver injury with a sudden onset.

Aetiology

Necrosis is characterised by cytotoxic cellular breakdown (hepatocellular destruction) and is generally associated with a poor prognosis. Drugs commonly associated with DILI have a variable propensity to cause hepatic necrosis. For example, hepatic necrosis has been reported in 3% of cases with co-amoxiclav DILI compared with 89% in individuals with halothane-induced liver injury cases (North-Lewis, 2008).

Paracetamol causes hepatic necrosis when its normal metabolic pathway is saturated. Subsequent metabolism occurs by an alternative pathway that produces a toxic metabolite that covalently binds to liver cell proteins and causes necrosis (Heard, 2008).

Pathophysiology

In severe cases, acute hepatocellular necrosis presents with jaundice and LFT abnormalities, including a modestly raised alkaline phosphatase and a markedly elevated alanine aminotransferase level of up to 200 times the upper limit of the reference range. Prolongation of the prothrombin time occurs but depends on the severity of the injury, increasing dramatically in severe cases. Microscopy reveals necrosis of the hepatocytes in a characteristic pattern.

Clinical manifestation

In acute hepatocellular necrosis caused by paracetamol, early symptoms include anorexia, nausea and vomiting, malaise and lethargy. Abdominal pain may be the first indication of liver damage but is not usually apparent for 24–48 hours. A period of apparent recovery precedes the development of jaundice and production of dark urine. If the liver injury is severe, deterioration follows, with repeated vomiting, hypoglycaemia, metabolic acidosis, bruising and bleeding, drowsiness and hepatic encephalopathy. Oliguria (diminished urine output) and anuria (complete cessation of urine production) may result from acute tubular necrosis. Renal failure may occur even in the absence of severe liver disease. In addition to acute renal failure, myocardial injury and pancreatitis have also been reported. In fatal cases, death from acute liver failure occurs between 4 and 18 days after ingestion.

Vascular disorders

A variety of drugs can cause veno-occlusive disease, which is characterised by non-thrombotic narrowing of small centrilobular veins and is typically caused by cytotoxic agents and some herbal remedies. The use of oral contraceptives or cytotoxic agents may exacerbate an underlying thrombotic disorder and increase the risk of Budd–Chiari syndrome (obstruction of the large veins) developing. Veno-occlusive disease may present with painful hepatomegaly, ascites and jaundice, along with other features of liver insufficiency. It has been reported after chemotherapy with drugs such as cyclophosphamide, doxorubicin and dacarbazine. It has also been reported as a common complication of bone marrow transplantation (Leise et al., 2014; North-Lewis, 2008).

Investigations

Various types of investigation are used in the diagnosis of drug-induced hepatotoxicity, with the number and type of tests depending on the clinical presentation. Unfortunately, available laboratory tests do not provide ideal markers for DILI, and the diagnosis is generally one of exclusion.

Biochemical tests

Routine LFTs are measured, which generally include total bilirubin, alanine transaminase (ALT) and alkaline phosphatase (ALP). Impairment of the synthetic function of the liver is detected by total protein, albumin and the prothrombin time. Other biochemical tests may include measurement of γ-glutamyl transpeptidase (GGT), which may be elevated in all forms of liver disease, including drug-induced disease. α-Fetoprotein (AFP) may be measured to exclude malignancy. Conjugated bilirubin may be measured to establish if there is biliary obstruction.

Serological markers

Serological markers for hepatitis A, B and C and other viruses such as the Epstein–Barr virus should be determined in patients with symptoms of hepatitis with appropriate risk factors to exclude an infective cause.

Radiological investigations

Radiological investigations, such as ultrasound, computed tomography (CT), percutaneous cholangiograms and endoscopic retrograde cholangiopancreatography (ERCP), are used to look for physical obstruction of bile ducts by gallstones, masses or strictures.

Liver biopsy

Liver biopsy is seldom helpful for diagnosis of DILI, but certain drugs can cause characteristic lesions, such as the distribution of micro-vesicular fat droplets seen with tetracyclines. Specific diagnostic tests for drug-induced disease exist for few drugs.

Other causes of liver dysfunction, such as autoimmune chronic active hepatitis, acute severe cholestasis, ischemic hepatic necrosis, pregnancy-related liver disease, the Budd–Chiari syndrome, rare metabolic disorders or liver disease related to alcohol abuse, must also be excluded.

Treatment

The aim of treatment for drug-induced hepatotoxicity is a complete recovery. This relies on correct diagnosis, withdrawal of any and all suspected drugs, and supportive therapy, which may include liver transplantation where appropriate.

Diagnosis

Drug-induced hepatic injury should be considered in every patient with jaundice alongside all other causes of liver disease by the clinical history and the results of investigations (Chalasani et al., 2014). The typical process in screening

patients presenting with jaundice is outlined in Fig. 15.1, and the general approach to the differential diagnosis of acute hepatitis is set out in Fig. 15.2.

Identifying the causative agent and stopping it is important in reducing the morbidity and mortality associated with DILI. Agents such as nitrofurantoin, minocycline and statins tend to cause DILI after prolonged use. Agents such as antibiotics and antiepileptics are more common agents known to cause more than 60% of DILI. Antihypertensive and diabetic medications are known to cause DILI; however, their incidence is much less.

A detailed and thorough drug history, including the use of oral contraceptives, over-the-counter medicines, vitamins, herbal preparations and illicit drug use, should be obtained. Examples of herbal and dietary preparations implicated in causing liver damage are listed in Box 15.1. Attention to the duration of treatment with a specific drug and the relationship to the onset of symptoms is important. The likelihood of a drug-related disease is greatest when the abnormality begins between 5 and 90 days after taking the first dose and within 15 days of taking the last dose. The latent period, that is, the time between starting therapy and the appearance of symptoms, may vary but for many drugs is sufficiently reproducible to be of some diagnostic value (Chalasani et al., 2014).

Recovery normally follows discontinuation of a hepatotoxic drug. Serious toxicity or ALF may result if the drug is continued after symptoms appear or the serum transaminases rise significantly. Failure to discontinue the drug may give grounds for claims of negligence.

Predisposing factors for liver toxicity should also be noted. If the liver injury is accompanied by fever, rash and eosinophilia, the likelihood of drug-induced disease increases, although lack of these features does not exclude it. Unequivocal diagnosis cannot be made in most circumstances, and improvement on withdrawal of the implicated drug may provide the strongest evidence for drug-induced disease. Time for resolution of the abnormalities is dependent on the individual drug and type of liver disease. In some cases, several months may elapse.

Idiosyncratic reactions may also need to be considered and the literature consulted for previous reports. A key component of secondary prevention is the reporting of all suspected hepatic drug reactions to the appropriate monitoring agency.

Practice points for diagnosing DILI are shown in Box 15.2, and examples of drugs associated with chronic liver injury are shown in Box 15.3.

Withdrawal

Once drug-induced hepatotoxicity has been recognised as a possibility, therapy should be stopped. If the patient is receiving more than one potentially hepatotoxic drug, all drugs should be stopped. Withdrawal of the agent usually results in recovery that begins within a few days. However, LFTs may take many months or even years to return to normal. Co-amoxiclav and phenytoin are examples of drugs that have been associated with a worsening of the patient's condition for several weeks after withdrawal and a protracted recovery period of several months.

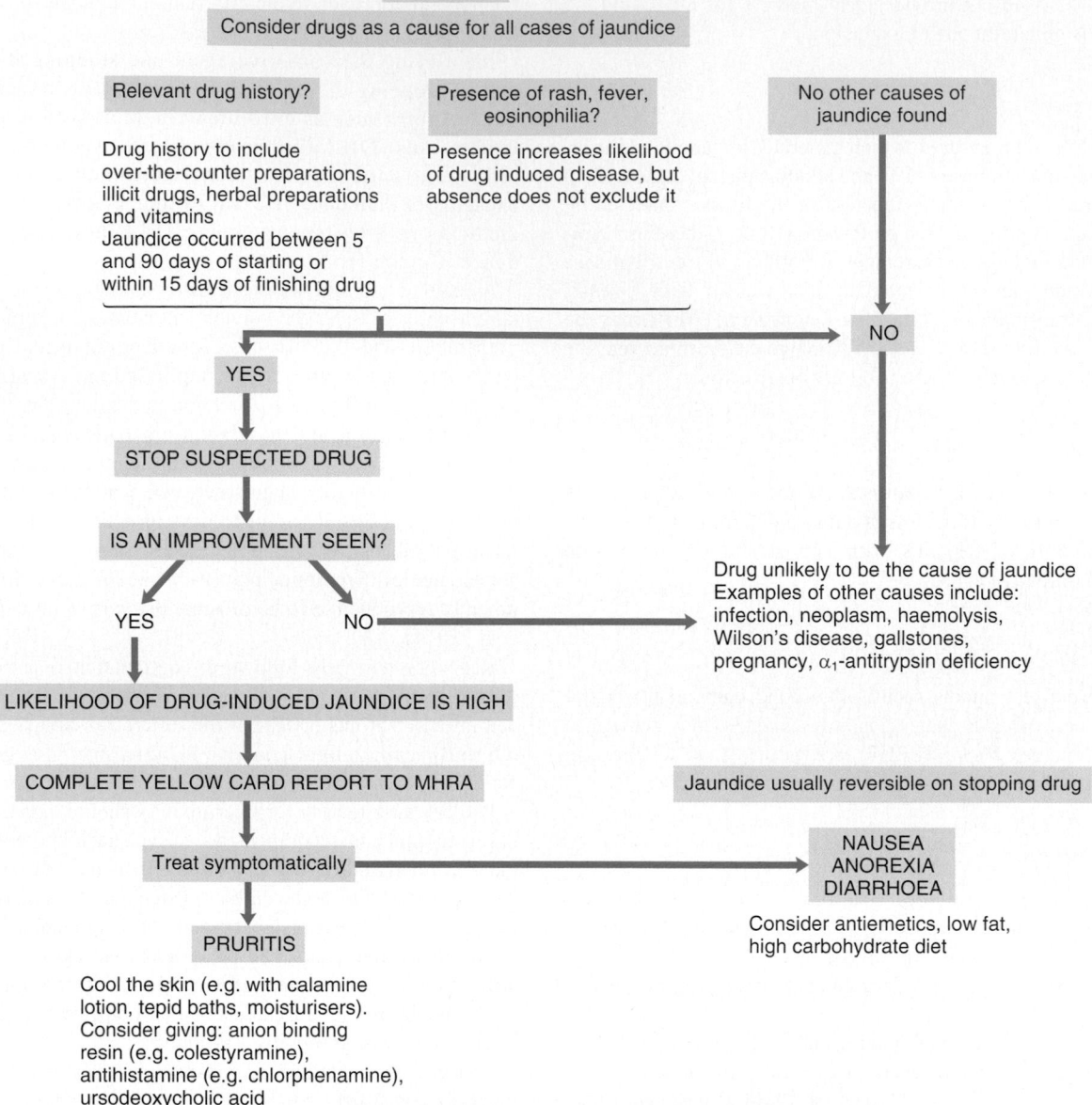

Fig. 15.1 General approach to the diagnosis and management of drug-induced jaundice.
MHRA, Medicines and Healthcare Products Regulatory Agency.

Rechallenge

When drug-induced hepatotoxicity has been confirmed by improvement on drug withdrawal, subsequent use in the patient is generally contraindicated. Rechallenge is not normally justified because this is potentially dangerous for the patient, although a positive rechallenge is the most definitive confirmation of drug-induced disease. Inadvertent rechallenge may occur. If the rechallenge is negative, this is usually taken to indicate that the patient may resume using the drug. Another adverse reaction on re-exposure to the drug precludes any further use (Chalasani et al., 2014).

Management

If clinical or laboratory signs of hepatic failure appear, hospitalisation is mandatory. After withdrawal of the drug, attempts to remove it from the body are only relevant for acute hepatotoxins such as paracetamol, metals or toxic mushrooms such as *Amanita phalloides* (death cap). If patients present a few hours post-ingestion, any unabsorbed drug may best be removed by gastric lavage, rather than by use of emetics.

Antidotes

Specific antidotes are acetylcysteine and methionine for paracetamol, and desferrioxamine for iron overdose. Desferrioxamine is administered orally as soon as possible after ingestion for acute iron poisoning. Parenteral desferrioxamine is indicated in addition to oral administration, to chelate absorbed iron where the plasma levels exceed 89.5 mmol/L, where the plasma levels exceed 62.6 mmol/L and there is evidence of free iron, and in patients with signs and symptoms of acute iron poisoning.

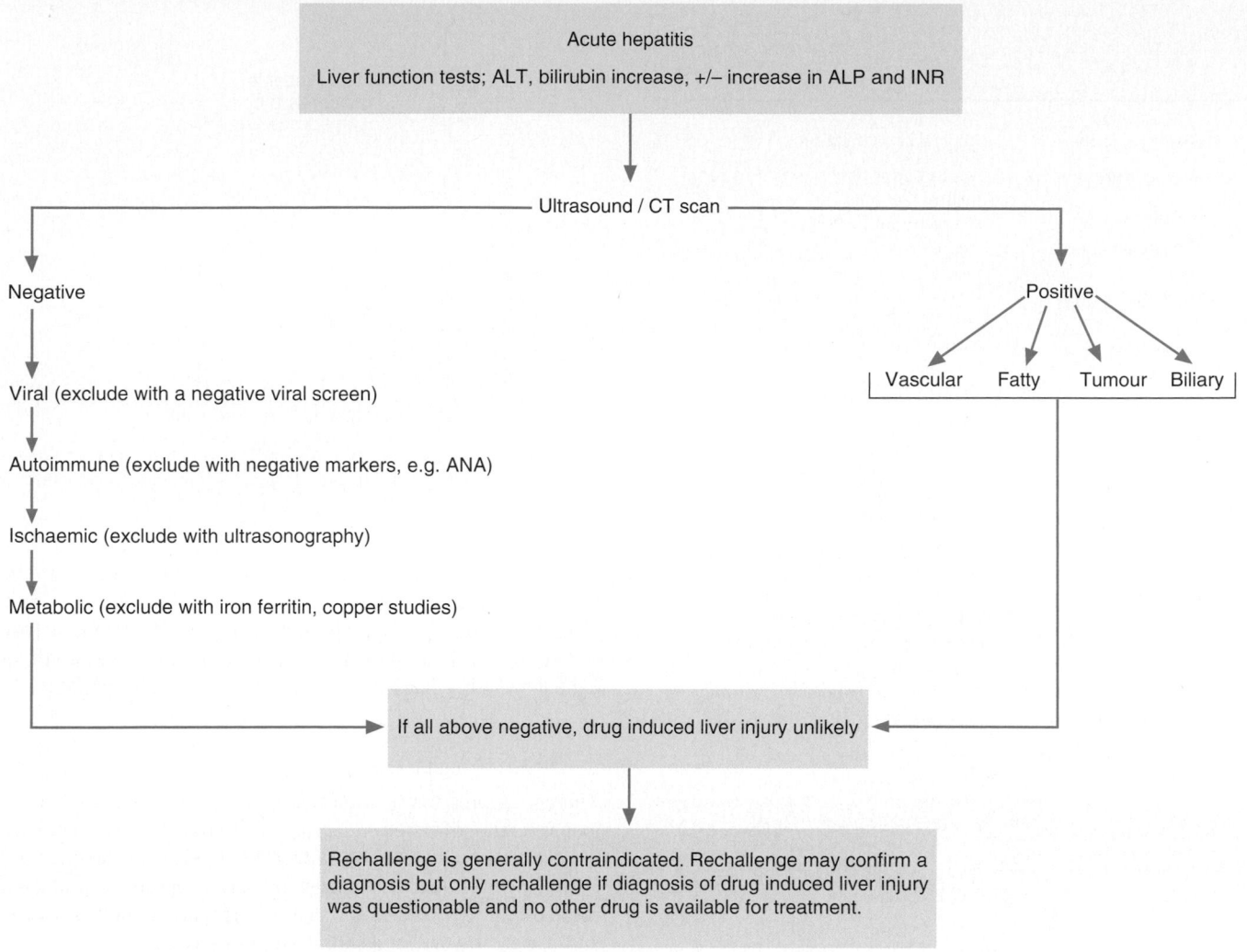

Fig. 15.2 General approach to the differential diagnosis of acute hepatitis.
ALP, Alkaline phosphatase; ALT, alanine transferase; ANA, antinuclear antibodies; CT, computed tomography; INR, international normalised ratio.

Paracetamol-induced hepatotoxicity. Paracetamol causes a dose-related toxicity resulting in centrilobular necrosis. It normally undergoes the phase II reactions of glucuronidation and sulphation. However, paracetamol is metabolised by cytochrome P450 2E1 to *N*-acetyl-*p*-benzoquinoneimine (NABQI) if the capacity of the phase II reactions is exceeded or if cytochrome P450 2E1 is induced. After normal doses of paracetamol, NABQI is detoxified by conjugation with glutathione to produce mercaptopurine and cysteine conjugates. After overdose, tissue stores of glutathione are depleted, allowing NABQI to accumulate and cause cell damage. Illness, starvation and alcohol deplete glutathione stores and increase the predisposition to paracetamol toxicity, while acetylcysteine and methionine provide a specific antidote by replenishing glutathione stores.

Ingestion of doses as low as 10–15 g of paracetamol has been reported to cause severe hepatocellular necrosis. Activated charcoal may be administered to reduce further absorption of paracetamol and facilitate removal of un-metabolised paracetamol from extracellular fluids if presenting early after ingestion. A plasma paracetamol concentration should be taken as soon as possible but not within 4 hours of ingestion due to the fact that a misleading and low level may be obtained because of continuing absorption and distribution of the drug. The plasma concentration measured should be compared with a standard nomogram reference line of a plot of plasma paracetamol concentration against time in hours after ingestion. This may be a semilogarithmic plot (Fig. 15.3).

Generally, administration of intravenous acetylcysteine is the treatment of choice for paracetamol overdose when the blood paracetamol level is in the range predictive of possible or probable liver injury (Fig. 15.3). Patients allergic to acetylcysteine may receive oral methionine.

Acetylcysteine is most effective within 8 hours of overdose. However, late administration in patients who present more than

Box 15.1 Examples of herbal remedies and food supplements implicated in hepatotoxicity (Kim and Phongsamran, 2009)

Dietary supplement	Clinical presentation
Atractylis gummifera	Acute hepatitis, fulminant hepatic failure
Black cohosh	Acute hepatitis
Callilepis laureola	Acute hepatitis, fulminant hepatic failure
Camellia sinensis	Acute hepatitis, fulminant hepatic failure
Chaparral	Cholestasis, acute and chronic hepatitis
Chinese herbal medicines (Sho-saiko-to, Dai-saiko-to)	Acute hepatitis, cholestasis, autoimmune hepatitis
Germander	Acute and chronic hepatitis, hepatic fibrosis
Hydroxycut	Acute hepatitis
Jin Bu Huan	Acute hepatitis, chronic cholestatic hepatitis, hepatic fibrosis
Kava	Acute hepatitis, cholestasis, fulminant hepatic failure
Ma Huang	Acute hepatitis, autoimmune hepatitis
Pyrrolizidine alkaloids	Veno-occlusive disease
Valerian	Mild hepatitis

Box 15.2 Practice points for the diagnosis of drug-induced liver disease

- Consider drugs as a cause for all cases of liver damage in patients presenting with liver disease.
- Take a careful drug history, including prescription, over-the-counter, herbal and alternative medicines and illicit drugs.
- Has the drug implicated been previously reported to cause drug-induced liver disease?
- Does the patient have risk factors for drug-induced liver disease?
- Consider the temporal relationship (onset of symptoms between 5 and 90 days after initial exposure?).
- Is there improvement on discontinuation of the suspected agent?
- Rechallenge with the suspected drug is not recommended; however, a positive rechallenge is the most definite evidence of drug-induced disease.

Box 15.3 Examples of drugs associated with the development of chronic liver disease

- Amiodarone
- Flucloxacillin
- Isoniazid
- Methotrexate
- Nitrofurantoin
- Non-steroidal anti-inflammatory drugs
- Pyrazinamide
- Rifampicin

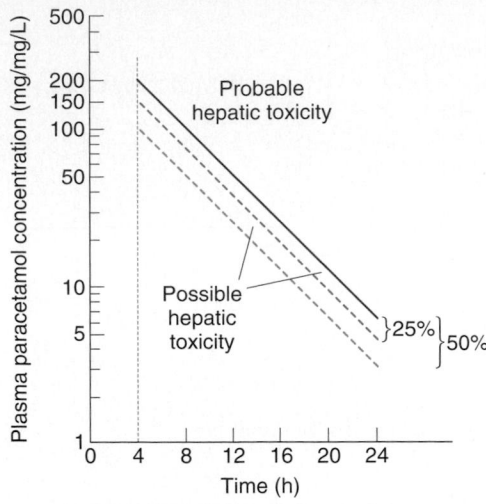

Fig. 15.3 Semilogarithmic plot of plasma paracetamol concentration versus time in hours after ingestion.

16–24 hours post-ingestion may be appropriate. Acetylcysteine administered at this stage will not counteract the oxidative effects of paracetamol, but it may have a cytoprotective role in hepatic failure and has been shown to reduce morbidity and mortality in patients who have already developed ALF (Brok et al., 2006).

Corticosteroids

Immunosuppression with corticosteroids has been used in the management of drug-induced hepatotoxicity, but evidence indicates their use does not affect the survival of patients with ALF. However, there have been anecdotal reports of impressive responses to corticosteroids that are persuasive, and it may be appropriate to conduct a short trial in rare types of drug-induced disease (Chalasani et al., 2014).

Supportive treatment

For most patients there is no specific treatment available. General supportive treatment is necessary in liver failure, with appropriate attention to fluid and electrolyte balance. Nutritional support should be along conventional medical lines for those suffering from malnourishment as a result of chronic injury.

Pruritus

The main symptom of drug-induced cholestasis is pruritus due to high systemic concentrations of bile acids deposited in tissues. General measures include light clothing (avoid wool), cooling the skin with tepid baths or calamine lotion and use of a general moisturising agent such as aqueous cream. The management of liver-induced pruritus is discussed in Chapter 16.

Coagulation disorders

Coagulation disorders should be treated by correcting vitamin K deficiency with intravenous phytomenadione injection. This should correct the prothrombin time within 3–5 days. Oral phytomenadione is ineffective in cholestasis. Menadiol sodium phosphate, the water-soluble vitamin K analogue, may be effective in an oral dose of 10 mg daily. If bleeding occurs, infusion of fresh frozen plasma or clotting factor concentrates will be indicated. The administration of other fat-soluble vitamins may also be necessary (North-Lewis, 2008).

Long-term treatment

When the DILI is under control, consideration will have to be given to the treatment of the original condition for which the implicated drug was prescribed. In many cases, drug therapy will still be required, and caution must therefore be exercised because drugs with similar chemical structures may cause similar hepatotoxicity.

Hepatotoxicity may occur with different derivatives of a drug. Erythromycin-induced cholestatic hepatitis has been more frequently reported with the estolate preparation than with other erythromycin esters (ethylsuccinate, stearate, propionate and lactobionate). It is not clear which part of the drug is responsible for hypersensitivity.

Patient counselling

Patients who recover from drug-induced hepatotoxicity should be informed of the causative agent, warned to avoid it in the future, and advised to inform their doctor, dentist, nurse and pharmacist about the occurrence of such an event.

Patients who purchase preparations containing paracetamol should be made aware of the danger of overdosing, which may occur if other preparations containing paracetamol are taken simultaneously. Since 1994 the European guidelines on package labelling have required products containing paracetamol to warn patients of the need to avoid other products containing paracetamol. The pack size of paracetamol sold from general sales outlets has been limited to 16 tablets or capsules (32 where paracetamol is sold under the supervision of a pharmacist) with the aim of limiting availability and reducing residual stocks in the home. This appears to have reduced the incidence of ALF secondary to paracetamol overdose (Hawton et al., 2011).

All patients should be advised of potential side effects. This information needs to be reinforced with the use of patient information leaflets. For medications known to cause liver injury, patients and their carers should be helped to recognise signs of liver disorder and know to report immediately symptoms such as malaise, nausea, fever and abdominal discomfort that may be significant. If these are accompanied by elevated LFTs, the drug needs to be assessed for its safety.

Parents of children commenced on sodium valproate should be warned to report side effects that may be suggestive of liver injury, such as the onset of anorexia, abdominal discomfort, nausea and vomiting. Early features include drowsiness and disturbed consciousness. DILI associated with sodium valproate usually occurs within 6 months. The maximum risk period is between 2 and 12 weeks of starting.

The challenge for all members of the healthcare team is to alert patients to the potentially toxic effects of drugs without creating so much concern that they fail to comply with vital medication. For the limited number of drugs presented in Table 15.5,

careful monitoring of LFTs during the first 6 months of treatment is advisable, although not always practical. Thereafter, regular monitoring of LFTs is appropriate in patients who are at greater risk of hepatotoxicity. Such patients would include those with known liver disease, those taking other hepatotoxic drugs, those older than 40 years, and heavy alcohol consumers. Surveillance should be particularly frequent in the first 2 months of treatment. In patients with no risk factors and normal pretreatment liver function, LFTs need only be repeated if fever, malaise, vomiting, jaundice or unexplained deterioration during treatment occurs.

Because many drugs cause elevation of LFTs, there may be difficulty in assessing when to stop a drug, particularly when treating an individual for tuberculosis or epilepsy. An empirical guideline is that the drug should be stopped if the levels of alanine transaminase exceed three times the upper limit of the reference range (Joshi et al., 2015). Any clinical features of liver disease or drug allergy would require immediate discontinuation of the drug. Conversely, a raised γ-glutamyl transpeptidase level and elevated alanine transaminase level in the absence of symptoms often reflect microsomal induction and would not indicate drug-induced injury.

It should be noted that monitoring of LFTs is not a complete safeguard against hepatotoxicity because some drug reactions develop very quickly, and the liver enzymes are an unreliable indicator of fibrosis.

Minimising the risk of drug-induced liver injury

The risk of acute liver injury with co-amoxiclav is higher than that of amoxicillin and increases with treatment courses longer than 14 days. Hence, the indications for co-amoxiclav have been restricted to cover infections caused by amoxicillin-resistant β-lactam-producing infections.

Patients admitted for procedures requiring a general anesthetic should be questioned about past exposure and any previous reactions to halothane. Halothane is well known to be associated with hepatotoxicity, particularly if patients are re-exposed. Repeated exposure to halothane within a period of less than 3 months should be avoided, and some increase in risk persists regardless of the time interval since last exposure. Unexplained jaundice or delayed-onset postoperative fever in a patient who has received halothane is an absolute contraindication to future use in that individual. Patients with a family history of halothane-related liver injury should also be treated with caution.

Although hepatic ADRs are rare for most drugs, when they do occur they can cause significant morbidity and mortality. More than 600 drugs have been associated with hepatotoxicity, and any new drug released to the market may have the potential to cause hepatotoxicity. Pemoline and troglitazone are examples of drugs withdrawn from the market due to reports of serious hepatic reactions. These examples help highlight the importance of postmarketing surveillance and yellow card reporting.

Appropriate selection of drugs, an awareness of predisposing factors and avoidance of toxic dose thresholds and potentially hepatotoxic drug–drug interactions will minimise the risk to patients.

Practice points for patient care and minimising the risk of DILI are outlined in Box 15.4.

Table 15.5 Examples of drugs where regular monitoring of liver function is recommended

Drug	Baseline measurement[a]	Frequency of monitoring
Anti-TB therapy (isoniazid, rifampicin, pyrazinamide)	Yes	Patients with pre-existing chronic liver disease: check LFTs regularly, every week for the first 2 weeks, then twice a week for the first 2 months. Patients with normal liver function tests and no evidence of pre-existing liver disease: regular monitoring is not necessary, but LFTs repeated if signs of liver dysfunction develop, e.g. fever, malaise, vomiting or jaundice. Patients with raised pretreatment hepatic transaminases: two or more times normal: check LFTs weekly for 2 weeks, then twice a week until normal. Less than two times normal: check LFTs at 2 weeks. If these transaminases have fallen, further tests are only needed if symptoms occur.
Amiodarone	Yes	Check LFTs every 6 months.
Cyproterone	Yes	Recheck if any symptoms.
Dantrolene	Yes	Repeat LFTs after first 6 weeks of therapy.
Itraconazole	Yes	Monitor LFTs if therapy continues for more than 1 month. Recheck if any symptoms.
Ketoconazole	Yes	LFTs checked on weeks 2 and 4 of therapy and then every month.
Methotrexate	Yes	LFTs checked every 2 weeks for the first 2 months, then monthly for 4 months, then every 3 months.
Methyldopa	Yes	Check LFTs at intervals during the first 6–12 weeks of treatment.
Micafungin	Yes	Periodic monitoring of LFTs recommended. Recheck if any symptoms.
Nevirapine	Yes	Check LFTs every 2 weeks for the first 2 months, then at month 3 and then regularly.
Pioglitazone	Yes	Periodic monitoring of LFTs recommended. Recheck if any symptoms.
Sodium valproate	Yes	Check LFTs regularly during the first 6 months of therapy.
Statins	Yes	LFTs checked 12 weeks after initiation or after a dose increase and periodically thereafter.
Sulfasalazine	Yes	LFTs checked every 2 weeks for the first 2 months, then monthly for 4 months then every 3 months
Tipranavir	Yes	Check LFTs on weeks 2, 4 and 8 of treatment and then every 2–3 months.
Vildagliptin	Yes	LFTs checked every 3 months for the first year and then periodically.

[a]Baseline and subsequent LFTs difficult to interpret in critically ill patients because LFTs will be affected by multiple factors.
LFT, Liver function test; TB, tuberculosis.

Box 15.4 Practice points for minimising the risk of drug-induced liver injury

- Minimise DILI by ensuring appropriate monitoring of drugs associated with hepatotoxicity.
- Minimise DILI by following recommendations – e.g. use co-amoxiclav for penicillin β-lactam-resistant infections only; counsel all patients on paracetamol not to exceed 4 g/day and to be alert to other preparations containing paracetamol.
- Counsel all patients (or carers of patients) on potentially hepatotoxic medicines to recognise and report signs of liver damage.
- Inform all patients who have DILI of the causative agent and the importance of avoiding this in the future.

DILI, Drug-induced liver injury.

Case studies

Case 15.1

Mrs RS, a 42-year-old female, presented to her local hospital after a paracetamol overdose. She had recently separated from her husband, went on an alcohol binge and then on impulse had taken approximately 90 paracetamol tablets. She presented to her local hospital 30 hours after the overdose. At presentation she was feeling nauseous and had right subcostal pain. Her results at this time were as follows:

	Actual value (normal range)
Paracetamol	18 mg/mL
Albumin	24 g/dL (30–50 g/L)
Alanine transaminase	6543 units/L (0–50 units/L)
Bilirubin	70 mmol/L (<17 mmol/L)
Alkaline phosphatase	66 units/L (30–135 units/L)
Prothrombin time	58 s (9.8–12.6 s)
Creatinine	200 mmol/L (35–125 mmol/L)
Urea	5.6 mmol/L (0–7.5 mmol/L)

Other test results:

Hepatitis screen negative
Autoantibody screen negative

At this stage, supportive treatment was given. However, she deteriorated, with worsening test results and the development of encephalopathy. She was then transferred to a specialist intensive care unit, with a diagnosis of ALF secondary to paracetamol overdose. Her test results on admission to the intensive care unit were as follows:

	Actual value (normal range)
Albumin	22 g/dL (30–50 g/L)
Alanine transaminase	10,000 units/L (0–50 units/L)
Bilirubin	150 mmol/L (<17 mmol/L)
Alkaline phosphatase	80 units/L (30–135 units/L)
Prothrombin time	90.8 s (9.8–12.6 s)
Arterial pH	7.226 (7.350–7.450)
Lactate	8 mmol/L (0.4–2.2 mmol/L)
Creatinine	420 mmol/L (35–125 mmol/L)
Urea	7.4 mmol/L (0–7.5 mmol/L)

She was discussed by a liver transplant multidisciplinary team and was identified as needing a liver transplant extremely urgently. Within 2 days of the overdose, she was transplanted.

Questions

1. What risk factors does Mrs RS have that suggest a worse prognosis?
2. On initial presentation, what treatment should have been initiated?
3. What is the significance of the high creatinine result?
4. Can Mrs RS be prescribed paracetamol for pain relief?

Answers

1. The progression of paracetamol toxicity can be categorised into four stages: preclinical, hepatic injury, hepatic failure and recovery. The prognosis varies depending on the stage at presentation. Mrs RS's late presentation to hospital also increases her risk of a worse prognosis. She presented to hospital 30 hours after the overdose, with raised ALT and some symptoms of liver injury, indicating that she was in the hepatic injury stage and progressed to the liver failure stage with the development of encephalopathy. Patients presenting with liver injury have a variable prognosis, but patients who present with hepatic failure have a mortality rate of 20–40%. Had she presented in the preclinical stage, she would have been expected to make a full recovery with treatment. Although Mrs RS had acutely ingested alcohol at the time of paracetamol overdose, this is not a risk factor for a worse prognosis. Theoretically, acute alcohol ingestion competes with paracetamol for CYP2E1 metabolism, resulting in lower formation of NAPQI and thus less toxicity. Chronic alcohol consumption induces the CYP2E1 isoenzyme, resulting in increased NAPQI production and increased risk of hepatotoxicity. Mrs RS developed hepatorenal syndrome; this is a poor prognostic indicator and has an associated mortality of 50–100%.

   A poor prognosis is also associated with the following:

Prothrombin time	>36 s
Creatinine	>200 mmol/L
pH	<7.3
Encephalopathy	Present
Cerebral oedema	Present
Time from onset of jaundice to encephalopathy	0–7 days

2. A plasma paracetamol level needs to be taken as soon as possible, although not within the first 4 hours after paracetamol overdose. A toxic screen should be performed to exclude other drug overdoses. Supportive therapy with intravenous fluids and oxygen, if necessary, should be given. This patient should also have been treated with N-acetylcysteine. Treatment with N-acetylcysteine is particularly beneficial when administered within 8 hours of paracetamol overdose when the blood paracetamol level is in the range predictive of possible or probable liver injury (see Fig. 15.3). However, late administration in patients who present more than 16–24 hours post-ingestion is also appropriate. Acetylcysteine administered at this stage will not counteract the oxidative effects of paracetamol, but it may have a cytoprotective role in hepatic failure, improving hemodynamics and oxygen use. Late administration of N-acetylcysteine has been shown to reduce morbidity and mortality in patients who have already developed hepatic failure. Available data for the use of N-acetylcysteine after paracetamol overdose suggests that although the evidence for benefit is limited, it should be given to patients with overdose (Brok et al., 2006).

3. Mrs RS developed renal impairment secondary to the liver damage, which is known as the hepato-renal syndrome (HRS). Other causes of renal impairment should be excluded. Where necessary, drug doses should be adjusted for renal impairment. Once the liver recovers, or transplantation of the liver occurs, the kidneys are likely to recover.
4. Paracetamol should be avoided in the acute phase after an overdose. However, if the patient needs either an analgesic or antipyretic after the acute phase, then paracetamol in small doses may be used. After a liver transplant, standard paracetamol doses can be used as long as the patient is adequately nourished and does not have any psychological issues with the use of paracetamol.

Case 15.2

Mr SS is a 43-year-old man with type 2 diabetes who was commenced on simvastatin 40 mg at night 3 months ago. He has no other relevant past medical history. He does not drink alcohol and does not consume grapefruit. He also takes metformin 1g twice a day. A routine blood test revealed an increase in ALT from baseline (pre-simvastatin) of 21–197 units/L (0–50 units/L) at 3 months.

Questions

1. What are the likely causes of the increase in ALT?
2. Should liver function tests be routinely monitored in patients on a statin?
3. What action, if any, should be taken in this case?
4. Can statins be used in patients with pre-existing liver disease?

Answers

1. The most likely cause of the increase in ALT is the introduction of simvastatin 3 months previously. All statins are reported to cause elevations in transaminases, which may be transient or persistent. The incidence of transaminitis with statins is low, being reported to occur between 1 in 1000 and 1 in 10,000 patients. Other causes of liver disease should also be considered in this case, for example, non-alcoholic steatohepatitis (NASH) associated with diabetes.
2. Monitoring of liver function tests in patients taking a statin is recommended in the Summary of Product Characteristics and hence should be monitored for medico-legal reasons (McKenney et al., 2006). It is recommended to monitor liver function tests at baseline and then at 12 weeks or after a dose increase. However, the true value for monitoring liver function test is not clear as it does not identify those at risk of liver damage, is expensive and may lead to patient anxiety and unnecessary cessation of statin therapy. Moreover, hepatic function does not appear to be compromised by statin use, and there is no apparent link between an elevation in liver function tests and the development of toxicity (McKenney et al., 2006).
3. Mr SS had a single high ALT result. The general recommendation is that if the patient is asymptomatic and the transaminase levels are greater than three times the upper limit of normal, the test should be repeated. If transaminases are still more than three times the upper limit of normal, the patient should have a full liver investigation. In this case, the simvastatin was switched to atorvastatin before a repeat liver function test. Follow-up liver function tests showed that the ALT had returned to within the normal range. It is highly probable that this rise in ALT on simvastatin would have been transient, and had the patient continued with simvastatin, the ALT would have normalised. However, the patient was anxious, did not want to risk any progression of liver toxicity and was keen to switch to an alternative statin.

4. Statins are contraindicated in ALF and decompensated chronic liver disease. However, they can probably be used safely in liver disease where there is no, or mild, synthetic dysfunction. Statin use may actually improve elevations in transaminases in patients with fatty liver disease (Gomez-Dominguez et al., 2006).

Case 15.3

Mr CB, a 66-year-old who has been recently diagnosed with tuberculosis (TB), was started on Rifater (rifampicin, isoniazid and pyrazinamide) 5 tablets a day and ethambutol 800 mg daily. He takes no other medication; however, he has told his doctor he drinks about 30 units of alcohol a week. He presents to his doctor with a 2-week history of fever, malaise and vomiting. Before starting his treatment, his liver function tests were as follows:

	Actual value (normal range)
Albumin	40 g/dL (30–50 g/L)
Alanine transaminase	30 units/L (0–50 units/L)
Bilirubin	6 mmol/L (<17 mmol/L)
Aspartate aminotransferase	20 units/L (10-50 units/L)

His doctor repeated his liver function tests, kidney function test and full blood count and tested for viruses such as cytomegalovirus (CMV) and hepatitis A, B, C, D and E. His viral screens all came back as negative. His liver and kidney function tests were as follows:

	Actual value (normal range)
Albumin	32 g/dL (30–50 g/L)
Alanine transaminase	500 units/L (0–50 units/L)
Bilirubin	120 mmol/L (<17 mmol/L)
Aspartate aminotransferase	600 units/L (10–50units/L)
Creatinine	89 mmol/L (35–125 mmol/L)
Urea	6 mmol/L (0–7.5 mmol/L)

He was admitted to hospital.

Questions

1. For which drug(s) would Mr CB be having routine liver function tests?
2. Does Mr CB have any risk factors for developing drug-associated hepatotoxicity?
3. What actions should be taken in relation to Mr CB's TB medication?

Answers

1. Rifampicin, isoniazid and pyrazinamide
   Each of these drugs has been associated with liver dysfunction. LFTs should be carried out for all patients receiving these agents pre-treatment. This includes baseline hepatic enzymes and bilirubin, as well as serum creatinine and a full blood count including platelets. Patients should be seen monthly throughout the duration of treatment and questioned about symptoms associated with adverse reactions.
   Mr CB would be considered to have normal LFTs pre-treatment. In addition to his LFTs, he would need to be monitored for symptoms of vomiting, jaundice or other signs of deterioration. He should be advised to see his doctor should he develop any of these symptoms.

2. Age increases the risk associated with DILI caused by iso-niazid, as well as large amounts of alcohol (Kumar et al., 2014). Patients older than 35 years have a higher frequency of isoniazid-associated hepatitis. A transaminase measurement should be obtained at baseline and at least monthly during the duration of treatment in this age group. Other risk factors that will increase the risk of hepatitis include daily use of alcohol, chronic liver disease, intravenous drug use and being a black or Hispanic woman. Mr CB only has alcohol as an additional risk factor.

3. In general, Rifater should be discontinued in hepatotoxicity after a discussion with the chest physicians. Mr CB shows signs of clinical hepatitis, with symptoms of general malaise and vomiting, in conjunction with raised LFTs. On discontinuation, his liver function should be monitored closely. Once his liver function has settled, individual agents could be cautiously reintroduced with close monitoring. This is as per guidance from the British Thoracic Society (BTS) and the American Thoracic Society (ATS). Because rifampicin has been shown to be the least toxic of the three agents, it should be started first. Subsequent agents should only be reintroduced if the liver function remains stable. If hepatotoxicity continues, the causative agent should be stopped and an alternative started (Kumar et al., 2014).

Acknowledgment

The author acknowledges the contribution of B. E. Featherstone to versions of this chapter which appeared in previous editions.

References

Bjornsson, E., Olsson, R., 2006. Suspected drug induced liver fatalities reported to the WHO database. Digest. Liver Dis. 38, 33–38.

Brok, J., Buckley, N., Gluud, C., 2006. Interventions for paracetamol (aceta-minophen) overdose. Cochrane Database Syst. Rev. 2006 (2) Art No. CD003328. doi:10.1002/14651858.CD003328.pub2.

Chalasani, N., Bjornsson, E., 2010. Risk factors for idiosyncratic drug-induced liver injury. Gastroenterol. 138, 2246–2259.

Chalasani, N., Hayashi, P., Bonkovsley, H., 2014. Diagnosis and manage-ment of idiosyncratic drug induced liver injury. Am. Coll. Gastroent. 109, 950–966.

de Abajo, F.J., Montero, D., Madurga, M., et al., 2004. Acute and clinically relevant drug induced liver injury: A population based case control study. Brit. J. Clin. Pharmaco. 58, 71–80.

European Medicines Evaluation Agency, 2014. Guidelines on good pharmacovigilance practices (GVP). Annex I – Definitions (Rev. 4). EMA/87633/2011 Rev 4. EMA, London. Available at: http://www.ema.europa.eu/docs/en_GB/document_library/Scientific_guideline/2013/05/WC500143294.pdf.

Farrell, G., 1997. Drug-induced hepatic injury. J. Gastroent. Hepatol. 12, 5242–5250.

Forn, A., Llove, J.M., Bruix, J., 2012. Hepatocellular carcinoma. Lancet 379, 1245–1255.

Fountain, F.F., Tolley, E., Chrisman, C.R., et al., 2005. Isoniazid hepatotox-icity associated with treatment of latent tuberculosis infection: a 7 year evaluation from a public health tuberculosis clinic. Chest 128, 116–123.

Gomez-Dominguez, E., Gisbert, J., Moreno-Monteagudo, J., et al., 2006. A pilot study of atorvastatin treatment in dyslipemid, non-alcoholic fatty liver patients. Am. J. Cardiol. 97, 131–136.

Hawton, K., Burgen, H., Simkin, S., et al., 2011. Impact of different sizes of paracetamol in the United Kingdom and Ireland on intentional overdose: a comparative study. BioMed Central Pub. Health 11 (1), 460.

Heard, K.J., 2008. Acetylcysteine for acetaminophen poisoning. New Engl. J. Med 359, 285–292.

Joshi, D., Keane, G., Brind, A., 2015. Drug-induced liver injury. In: Hepatology at a Glance. Wiley-Blackwell, Hoboken.

Kim, J., Phongsamran, P., 2009. Drug-induced liver disease and drug use considerations in liver disease. J. Pharm. Pract. 22, 278–289.

Kumar, N., Kedarisetty, C.K., Kumar, S., et al., 2014. Antitubercular therapy in patients with cirrhosis: Challenges and options. World J. Gastroent 20, 5760–5772.

Lammert, C., Niklasson, A., Bjornsson, E., et al., 2010. Oral medicines with significant hepatic metabolism are at higher risk of hepatic adverse events. Hepatology 51, 615–620.

Leise, M.D., Poterucha, J.J., Talwalkar, J.A., 2014. Drug-induced liver injury. Mayo Clin. Proc. 89 (1), 95–106.

Lucena, H., Andrade, R.J., Kaplowitz, N., et al., 2009. Phenotypic characterization of idiosyncratic drug induced liver injury: the influence of age and gender. Hepatology 49, 2001–2009.

McKenney, J., Davidson, M.H., Jacobson, T.A., et al., 2006. Final conclusions and recommendations of the National Lipid Association Statin Safety Assessment Task Force. Am. J. Cardiol. 97, 89C–94C.

North-Lewis, P. (Ed.), 2008. Drugs and the Liver. Pharmaceutical Press, London.

Richardson, P., O'Grady, J., 2002. Acute liver disease. Hospital Pharm. J. 9, 131–136.

Roth, R., Ganey, P., 2010. Intrinsic versus idiosyncratic drug induced hepa-totoxicity – two villains or one? J. Pharmacol. Exp. Ther. 332, 692–967.

Steele, M.A., Burk, R.F., DesPrez, R.M., 1991. Toxic hepatitis with isonia-zid and rifampin. A meta-analysis. Chest 99, 465–471.

World Health Organization (WHO), 1972. International drug monitoring: the role of national centres. Technical Report Series No. 498. WHO, Geneva.

Further reading

Bell, L.N., Chalasani, N., 2009. Epidemiology of idiosyncratic drug-induced liver injury. Semin. Liver Dis. 29, 337–347.

Bjornsson, E., 2007. long-term follow up of patients with mild to moderate drug induced liver injury. Aliment. Pharm. Ther. 26, 79–85.

Bjornsson, E., 2009. The natural history of drug-induced liver injury. Semin. Liver Dis 24, 357–363.

Lee, W.L., 2003. Drug induced hepatotoxicity. New Engl. J. Med. 349, 474–485.

Suzuki, A., Andrade, R.J., Bjornsson, E., et al., 2010. Drugs associated with hepatotoxicity and their reporting frequency of liver adverse events in VigiBase: unified list based on international collaborative work. Drug. Saf. 33, 503–522.

Watkins, P., 2009. Biomarkers for the diagnosis and management of drug induced liver injury. Semin. Liver Dis. 24, 393–399.

16 Liver Disease

Apostolos Koffas and Patrick Kennedy

Key points

- The liver is a complex organ central to the maintenance of homeostasis.
- The liver is notable for its capacity to regenerate unless cirrhosis has developed. However, now some evidence suggests that cirrhosis can, in fact, be reversible in selected cases (e.g. treated hepatitis B virus).
- The spectrum of liver disease extends from mild, self-limiting conditions to serious illnesses which may carry significant morbidity and mortality.
- Liver disease is defined as acute or chronic on the basis of whether the history of disease is less than or greater than 6 months, respectively.
- Viral infections and paracetamol overdose are leading causes of acute liver disease, but a significant number of patients have no defined cause (seronegative hepatitis).
- Alcohol abuse and chronic viral hepatitis (B and C) are the major causes of chronic liver disease.
- Cirrhosis may be asymptomatic for considerable periods.
- Ascites, encephalopathy, varices and hepatorenal failure are the main serious complications of cirrhosis.
- A careful assessment is required before the use of any drug in a patient with liver disease because of unpredictable effects on drug handling.

The liver weighs up to 1500 g in adults and as such is one of the largest organs in the body. The main functions of the liver include protein synthesis, storage and metabolism of fats and carbohydrates, detoxification of drugs and other toxins, excretion of bilirubin and metabolism of hormones, as summarised in Fig. 16.1. The liver has considerable reserve capacity, reflected in its ability to function normally despite surgical removal of 70–80% of the organ or the presence of significant disease. It is noted for its capacity to regenerate rapidly. However, once it has been critically damaged, multiple complications develop involving many body systems. The distinction between acute and chronic liver disease is conventionally based on whether the history is less than or greater than 6 months, respectively.

The hepatocyte is the functioning unit of the liver. Hepatocytes are arranged in lobules and within a lobule hepatocytes perform different functions depending on how close they are to the portal tract. The portal tract is the 'service network' of the liver and contains an artery and a portal vein delivering blood to the liver and bile duct which forms part of the biliary drainage system (Fig. 16.2). The blood supply to the liver is 30% arterial, and the remainder is from the portal system which drains most of the abdominal viscera. Blood passes from the portal tract through sinusoids that facilitate exposure to the hepatocytes before the blood is drained away by the hepatic venules and veins. There are a number of other cell populations in the liver, but two of the most important are Kupffer cells, fixed monocytes that phagocytose bacteria and particulate matter, and stellate cells responsible for the fibrotic reaction that ultimately leads to cirrhosis.

Acute liver disease

Acute liver disease is a self-limiting episode of hepatocyte damage which in most cases resolves spontaneously without clinical sequelae, but acute liver failure (ALF) can develop. This is a rare condition in which there is a rapid deterioration in liver function with associated encephalopathy (altered mentation) and coagulopathy. ALF carries a significant morbidity and mortality and may require emergency liver transplantation.

Chronic liver disease

Chronic liver disease occurs when permanent structural changes within the liver develop secondary to longstanding cell damage, with the consequent loss of normal liver architecture. In many cases this progresses to cirrhosis, where fibrous scars divide the liver cells into areas of regenerative tissue called nodules (Fig. 16.3). Conventional wisdom is that this process is irreversible, but therapeutic intervention in hepatitis B (and even hepatitis C virus) in addition to haemochromatosis has demonstrated the ability to reverse cirrhosis (Sohrabpour et al., 2012). Once chronic liver disease progresses, patients are at risk of development of liver failure, portal hypertension or hepatocellular carcinoma (HCC). Cirrhosis is a sequel of chronic liver disease of any aetiology and it develops over a variable time frame from 5 to ≥20 years.

Causes of liver disease
Viral infections

Viruses commonly affect the liver and can result in a transient and an innocuous hepatitis. Viruses which target the liver primarily are described as hepatotropic viruses, and each of these can lead to clinically significant hepatitis and in some cases to the development of chronic viral hepatitis with viral persistence. Five human viruses have been well described to date: hepatitis A (HAV), B (HBV), C (HCV), D (HDV) and E (HEV). Each type of viral hepatitis causes a similar pathology with acute inflammation of the liver. HAV and HEV are classically associated with an acute and sometimes severe hepatitis which is invariably self-limited, but occasionally fatal. HBV causes acute hepatitis in the majority of adults; only 5% of patients become chronic carriers, whereas 95% of those infected in the neonatal period or early childhood

experience chronic infection. HCV rarely causes an acute hepatitis, but up to 85% of patients become chronic carriers. Both viruses cause chronic liver inflammation or hepatitis, cirrhosis and HCC.

Hepatitis A

HAV is a non-enveloped RNA virus and a major cause of acute hepatitis worldwide, accounting for up to 25% of clinical hepatitis in the developed world (Brook et al., 2016). HAV is an enteric virus and the faecal–oral route is the main mechanism of transmission. The virus is particularly contagious and constitutes a public health problem throughout the world. The virus may go unnoticed by the patient in the absence of an icteric episode, particularly in children. However, HAV can cause ALF in less than 1% of patients (Brook et al., 2016); this is typically seen in older adults. The virus is particularly prevalent in areas of poor sanitation and is often associated with water- and food-borne epidemics. HAV has a relatively short incubation period (2–7 weeks), during which time the virus replicates and abnormalities in liver function tests (LFTs) can be detected.

Hepatitis B

Up to 500 million people worldwide are chronically infected with HBV. Chronic hepatitis B (CHB) is characterised by the presence of hepatitis B surface antigen (HBsAg) for a period of more than 6 months. In endemic areas of Africa and the Far East, up to

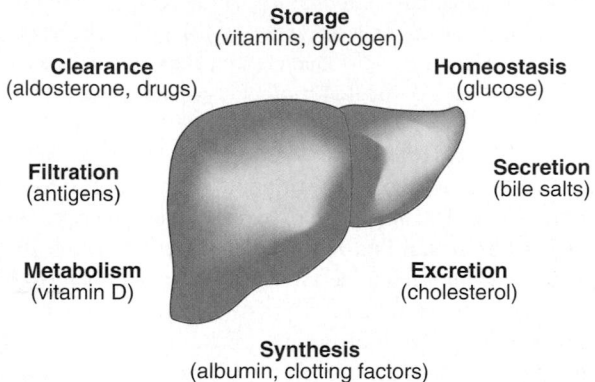

Fig. 16.1 Normal physiological functions of the liver, with examples of each.

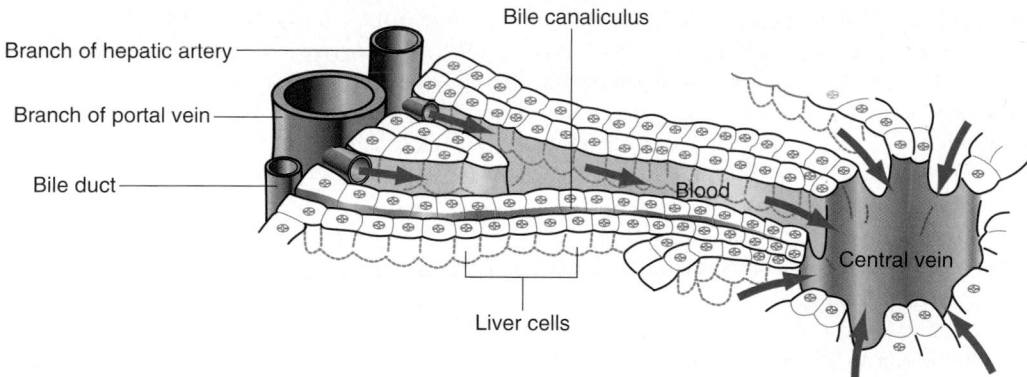

Fig. 16.2 Illustration of the relationship among the three structures that comprise the portal tract, with blood from both the hepatic artery and portal vein perfusing the hepatocytes before draining away towards the hepatic veins (central veins). Each hepatocyte is also able to secrete bile via the network of bile ducts. (Reproduced with permission of McGraw-Hill from Vander, 1980.)

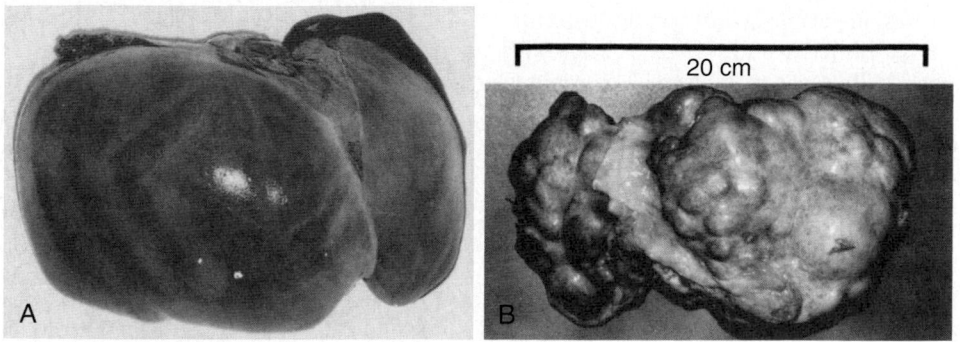

Fig. 16.3 The gross postmortem appearance of (A) a normal and (B) a cirrhotic liver demonstrating scarring and nodule formation in B.

20% of the population are chronic carriers of HBV (Brook et al., 2016), and exposure to HBV at birth (vertical or perinatal transmission) is the single most important risk factor for the development of CHB infection. Acquisition of HBV in adulthood is often via sexual transmission and is usually associated with a discrete episode of hepatitis. HBV can also be transmitted parenterally, by the transfusion of blood or blood products from contaminated stocks and by intravenous drug use or needle sharing.

Many factors determine the outcome of HBV infection, ranging from age at the time of exposure and genetic factors of the host to virus characteristics. Acute HBV infection by definition resolves within a 6-month time frame. It is generally self-limiting, and antiviral therapy is not indicated in the majority of patients. Most patients recover within 1–2 months of the onset of jaundice. The protracted incubation period of HBV and the ability of the virus to escape the host immune response contribute to the development of CHB. CHB is associated with varying levels of viraemia and hepatic inflammation. The level of viraemia, and thus infectivity, is determined by the presence of the hepatitis B e antigen (HBeAg); thus, HBeAg loss and the development of anti-HBe antibody (HBeAg seroconversion) results in a significant reduction in replicating virus and the potential to transmit the virus. Low levels of HBV DNA and normal transaminases are associated with a more favourable disease outcome. However, HBeAg-negative chronic hepatitis can progress with the development of significantly elevated levels of HBV DNA and associated biochemical activity; a disease profile with a poorer prognosis is now recognised as a growing healthcare challenge globally. HBeAg-negative CHB results as a consequence of the emergence of escape mutants from the core promoter or pre-core regions of the virus. It is estimated that 10–50% of HBV carriers will develop serious sequelae during their lifetime (Brook et al., 2016), namely, liver cirrhosis and/or HCC, which may even develop in CHB in the absence of cirrhosis. Perinatal or childhood infection is synonymous with a higher percentage of patients developing CHB, characterised by a protracted disease phase often referred to as immune-tolerant CHB. Because of this protracted phase of disease and long-term exposure to the virus, a higher proportion of those infected at birth or in early childhood (up to 25%) are at risk of development of cirrhosis and/or HCC.

Hepatitis D

Hepatitis D (HDV) is an incomplete virus that can establish infection only in patients simultaneously infected by HBV. It is estimated that 5% of HBV carriers worldwide are infected with HDV. It is endemic in the Mediterranean Basin and is transmitted permucosally, percutaneously or sexually. In other geographical areas, it is confined to intravenous drug users.

Hepatitis C

An estimated 185 million people worldwide are chronically infected with HCV (Brook et al., 2016). HCV is a hepatotropic, non-cytopathic, predominantly blood-borne virus with greater infectivity than the human immunodeficiency virus (HIV). It is estimated that more than 2.7 million people in the USA are chronically infected with HCV (Centers for Disease Control and Prevention, 2017), where it is the leading cause of death from liver disease. An estimated 214,000 people are chronically infected with hepatitis C in the UK (Public Health England, 2015), although a considerable proportion of individuals have not yet been diagnosed. HCV is transmitted parenterally, most commonly through intravenous drug use and the sharing of contaminated needles. Before its identification in 1990, HCV (previously known as non-A, non-B viral hepatitis) was also contracted through contaminated blood and blood products. The introduction of widespread screening of blood donors and pooled blood products has largely consigned blood transfusion as a mode of transmission to history. There remains a small risk of HCV infection associated with tattooing, electrolysis, ear piercing, acupuncture and sexual contact. The vertical transmission rate from HCV-infected mother to child is less than 3% (Tosone et al., 2014).

HCV infection is associated with the development of a recognised episode of acute hepatitis in only a small percentage of individuals. The majority of patients remain asymptomatic and so are often unaware of the infection or the timing at which they contracted the virus. Symptoms associated with HCV infection tend to be mild constitutional upset, with malaise, weakness and anorexia being most commonly reported. Up to 85% of subjects exposed to HCV experience development of chronic disease (Brook et al., 2016), which can lead to progressive liver damage, cirrhosis and HCC. Unlike HBV, the risk of development of HCC is almost totally linked to the presence of cirrhosis. Up to 30% of patients with chronic HCV infection progress to end-stage liver disease within 14–30 years (Brook et al., 2016), and alcohol consumption is a recognised co-factor that accelerates disease progression. HCV infection is the leading indication for liver transplantation worldwide and accounts for approximately 400,000 deaths per year (World Health Organization, 2017).

Hepatitis E

HEV is endemic in India, Asia, the Middle East and parts of Latin America. It is an RNA virus which is transmitted enterically and leads to acute hepatitis. It has an average incubation period of 42 days. The symptoms of HEV are no different from other causes of viral hepatitis. It is believed that the risk of death is increased in pregnancy, especially in the final trimester (World Health Organization, 2016).

Alcohol

Alcohol is the single most significant cause of liver disease throughout the Western world, accounting for between 40% and 60% of cases of cirrhosis in different countries. In general, deaths from alcoholic liver disease (ALD) in each country correlate with the consumption of alcohol per head of population, although additional factors can influence this trend. Liver disease related to recent alcohol consumption can present as a broad spectrum of conditions, ranging from the relatively benign fatty liver disease or hepatic steatosis to the development of alcoholic hepatitis (AH). An estimated 20% of alcohol abusers develop progressive liver fibrosis, which can eventually lead to alcoholic cirrhosis, typically after a period of 10–20 years of alcohol misuse (Mueller et al., 2009).

The central event in the development of hepatic fibrosis is the transformation of hepatic stellate cells into matrix-secreting cells producing pericellular fibrosis. This network of collagen fibres develops around the liver cells and gradually leads to hepatocyte cell death. The extent of fibrosis progresses and micronodular fibrotic bands develop characterising alcoholic cirrhosis. The anatomical changes within the liver increase resistance to blood flow from the portal system, causing an increase in pressure within this system resulting in portal hypertension. As the number of normally functioning liver cells reduces further, because of continued liver cell failure and death, the clinical condition is characterised by a progressive deterioration and ultimately liver failure. The rate of disease progression, and indeed regression, is strongly linked to whether patients continue to consume alcohol.

Non-alcoholic fatty liver disease

Non-alcoholic fatty liver disease (NAFLD) refers to a spectrum of disease ranging from simple hepatic steatosis to liver fibrosis and cirrhosis. Hepatic steatosis, which is the most common entity of NAFLD, refers to the infiltration of more than 5% of the liver with fat and is now the most common liver disorder in the developed world; it is estimated that at least one in five people (20%) in the UK are affected. Non-alcoholic steatohepatitis (NASH) is characterised by inflammation of the liver and hepatocellular injury which may progress to fibrosis or cirrhosis. The majority of cases previously reported as cryptogenic cirrhosis probably reflect the end stage of the NAFLD/NASH disease process, even though by this advanced stage the characteristic fatty infiltrate has disappeared. By definition, alcohol consumption of more than 20 g/day (about 25 mL/day net ethanol) excludes the condition. People who are more at risk of development of NAFLD are overweight or obese individuals, smokers, those who have a poor diet and lack of physical exercise, in addition to those with the metabolic syndrome. Its prevalence is increasing worldwide, and in the USA, NASH is reported to be the second leading cause of liver disease among adults awaiting liver transplantation (Wong et al., 2015). Different theories regarding the pathogenesis of NAFLD exist, but insulin resistance plays a key role in the development of the disorder.

Immune disorders

Autoimmune disease can affect the hepatocyte or bile duct and is characterised by the presence of auto-antibodies and raised serum immunoglobulin levels.

Autoimmune hepatitis

Autoimmune hepatitis (AIH) is an unresolving inflammation of the liver characterised by the presence of auto-antibodies (anti–smooth muscle ([type 1] or anti-kidney, liver microsomal [type 2]), hypergammaglobulinemia and an interface hepatitis on liver histology. It is usually a chronic, progressive disease which can occasionally present acutely with a severe hepatitis.

AIH typically occurs in young women, between 20 and 40 years, and a history or family history of autoimmune disorders is often present.

Primary biliary cholangitis

Primary biliary cholangitis (PBC) is an autoimmune disease of the liver which predominantly affects middle-aged women (95% of cases are female). It is characterised by the presence of anti-mitochondrial antibodies and a granulomatous destruction of the interlobular bile ducts leading to progressive ductopenia, fibrosis and cirrhosis. The disease is progressive, albeit over a period of 20 years or longer if diagnosed at an early age; liver transplantation is often the only effective treatment.

Primary sclerosing cholangitis

Primary sclerosing cholangitis (PSC) is an idiopathic chronic inflammatory disease resulting in intrahepatic and extrahepatic biliary strictures, cholestasis and eventually cirrhosis. There is a strong association with inflammatory bowel disease, particularly ulcerative colitis (UC); 75% of patients with PSC have UC and 5% of patients with UC develop PSC (Lee and Kaplan, 1995; Loftus et al., 2005). It has a predilection for young Caucasian males (mean age at presentation 39 years), but it can occur in infancy or childhood and can affect any race. Cholangiocarcinoma develops in up to 10% of patients with PSC.

Vascular abnormalities

Budd–Chiari syndrome is a rare, heterogeneous and potentially fatal condition related to the obstruction of the hepatic venous outflow tract. The prevalence of underlying thrombophilias is markedly increased in patients with Budd–Chiari syndrome. Affected patients are commonly women with an average age at presentation of 35 years. Early recognition and immediate use of anticoagulation has vastly improved outcome. More advanced disease can be treated in a number of ways including venoplasty, transjugular intrahepatic portosystemic shunt (TIPSS), surgical shunts or liver transplantation.

Metabolic and genetic disorders

Various inherited metabolic disorders can affect the functioning of the liver.

Haemochromatosis

Hereditary haemochromatosis is the most commonly identified genetic disorder in the Caucasian population. It is associated with increased absorption of dietary iron resulting in deposition within the liver, heart, pancreas, joints, pituitary gland and other organs. This can lead to cirrhosis and HCC.

Wilson's disease

Wilson's disease is an autosomal recessive disorder of copper metabolism. The disorder leads to excessive absorption and deposition of dietary copper within the liver, brain, kidneys and other tissues. Presentation can vary widely from chronic hepatitis, asymptomatic cirrhosis, ALF to neuropsychiatric symptoms with cognitive impairment.

α₁-Antitrypsin deficiency

α_1-Antitrypsin deficiency is an autosomal recessively inherited disease and is the most common genetic metabolic liver disease. The disease results in a reduction in α_1-antitrypsin which is protective against a variety of proteases including trypsin, chymotrypsin, elastase and proteases present in neutrophils. The homozygous form of the disease (ZZ phenotype) is associated with the development of liver disease and cirrhosis in 15–30% of both adult and paediatric patients.

Glycogen storage disease

Glycogen storage disease is a rare disease that occurs in 1 in 100,000 births. Enzymatic deficiencies at specific steps in the pathway of glycogen metabolism cause impaired glucose production and accumulation of abnormal glycogen in the liver.

Gilbert's syndrome

Gilbert's syndrome is characterised by persistent mild unconjugated hyperbilirubinaemia. It is most frequently recognised in adolescents and young adults with an incidence rate between 2% and 7% in the general population. Serum bilirubin levels fluctuate but can increase to 80–100 mmol/L during periods of stress, sleep deprivation, prolonged fasting, menstruation and intercurrent infections. Gilbert's syndrome is an asymptomatic condition that requires no therapy. However, patients may inappropriately associate being jaundiced with the symptoms of the condition that triggered the increased bilirubin levels.

Drugs

Drugs are particularly important causes of abnormal LFTs and acute liver injury, including ALF. DILI (drug-induced liver injury) is an acronym for any drug toxin that causes abnormal liver enzymes. Drugs can also be relevant to a number of chronic liver diseases including steatosis, fibrosis/cirrhosis, autoimmune and vascular disease. In most situations the drug is implicated because of an appropriate temporal relationship between the disease and drug exposure.

Clinical manifestations of liver disease

Symptoms of liver disease

In patients who have liver disease, weakness, increased fatigue and general malaise are common but non-specific symptoms. Weight loss and anorexia are more commonly seen in chronic liver disease, and loss of muscle bulk is a characteristic of advanced disease. Abdominal discomfort may be described by patients with an enlarged liver or spleen, whereas abdominal distension with the accumulation of ascites is usually the cause in more advanced disease. Abdominal pain is common in hepatobiliary disease, frequently localised to the right upper quadrant. This is often a feature of rapid or gross enlargement of the liver when the pain is thought to be a consequence of capsular stretching. Tenderness over the liver is a symptom of acute hepatitis, hepatic abscess or hepatic malignancy.

Jaundice is the most striking symptom of liver disease and can present with or without pain, depending on the underlying aetiology of disease. Pruritus can be a distressing symptom in cholestatic liver disease, and patients usually report that it is worse at night. Patients with acute and chronic liver disease can develop bleeding complications because of defective hepatic synthesis of coagulation factors and low platelet counts.

Signs of liver disease

Table 16.1 presents physical signs of chronic liver disease.

Cutaneous signs

Hyperpigmentation is common in chronic liver disease and results from increased deposition of melanin. It is particularly associated with PBC and haemachromatosis. Scratch marks on the skin suggest pruritus, which is a common feature of cholestatic liver disease. Vascular 'spiders', referred to as spider naevi, are small vascular malformations in the skin and are found in the drainage area of the superior vena cava, commonly seen on the face, neck, hands and arms. Examination of the limbs can reveal several signs, none of which are specific to liver disease. Palmar erythema, a mottled reddening of the palms of the hands, can be associated with both acute and chronic liver disease. Dupuytren's contracture, thickening and shortening of the palmar fascia of the

Table 16.1 Physical signs of chronic liver disease	
Common findings	**End-stage findings**
Jaundice	Ascites
Gynaecomastia and loss of body hair	Dilated abdominal blood vessels
Hand changes:	Fetor hepaticus
Palmar erythema	Hepatic flap
Clubbing	Neurological changes:
Dupuytren's contracture	Hepatic encephalopathy
Leukonychia	Disorientation
Liver mass reduced or increased	Changes in consciousness
Parotid enlargement	Peripheral oedema
Scratch marks on skin	Pigmented skin
Purpura	Muscle wasting
Spider naevi	
Splenomegaly	
Testicular atrophy	
Xanthelasma	
Hair loss	

hands causing flexion deformities of the fingers, was traditionally associated with alcoholic cirrhosis. It is now considered to be multifactorial and not to reflect primary liver disease. Nail changes, highly polished nails or white nails (leukonychia) can be seen in up to 80% of patients with chronic liver disease. Leukonychia is a consequence of low serum albumin. Finger clubbing is most commonly seen in hypoxaemia related to hepato-pulmonary syndrome, but it is also a feature of chronic liver disease.

Abdominal signs

Abdominal distension, notably of the flanks, is suggestive of ascites which can develop in both acute (less commonly) and chronic liver disease. An enlarged liver (hepatomegaly) is a common finding in acute liver disease. In cirrhotic patients the liver may be large, but alternatively it may be small and shrunken, reflecting end-stage chronic disease. An enlarged spleen (splenomegaly) in the presence of chronic liver disease is the most important sign of portal hypertension. Dilated abdominal wall veins are a notable finding in chronic liver disease with the detection of umbilical and para-umbilical veins a feature of portal hypertension.

Jaundice

Jaundice is the physical sign regarded as synonymous with liver disease and is most easily detected in the sclerae. It reflects impaired liver cell function (hepatocellular pathology), or it can be cholestatic (biliary) in origin. Hepatocellular jaundice is commonly seen in acute liver disease, but may be absent in chronic disease until the terminal stages of cirrhosis are reached. The causes of jaundice are shown in Fig. 16.4.

Portal hypertension

The increased pressure in the portal venous system leads to collateral vein formation and shunting of blood to the systemic circulation. Portal hypertension is an important contributory factor to the formation of ascites and the development of encephalopathy due to bypassing of blood from the liver to the systemic circulation. The major, potentially life-threatening complication of portal hypertension is a variceal bleed (torrential venous haemorrhage) from the thin-walled veins in the oesophagus and upper stomach. Patients with portal hypertension are often asymptomatic, whereas others may present with bleeding varices, ascites and/or encephalopathy.

Ascites

Ascites is the accumulation of fluid within the abdominal cavity. The precise mechanism by which ascites develops in chronic liver disease remains unclear, but the following factors are all thought to contribute:

- Activation of the renin–angiotensin–aldosterone axis as a consequence of central hypovolaemia, leading to a reduction in sodium excretion by the kidney and fluid retention. Reduced aldosterone metabolism caused by reduced liver function may also contribute to increased fluid retention.

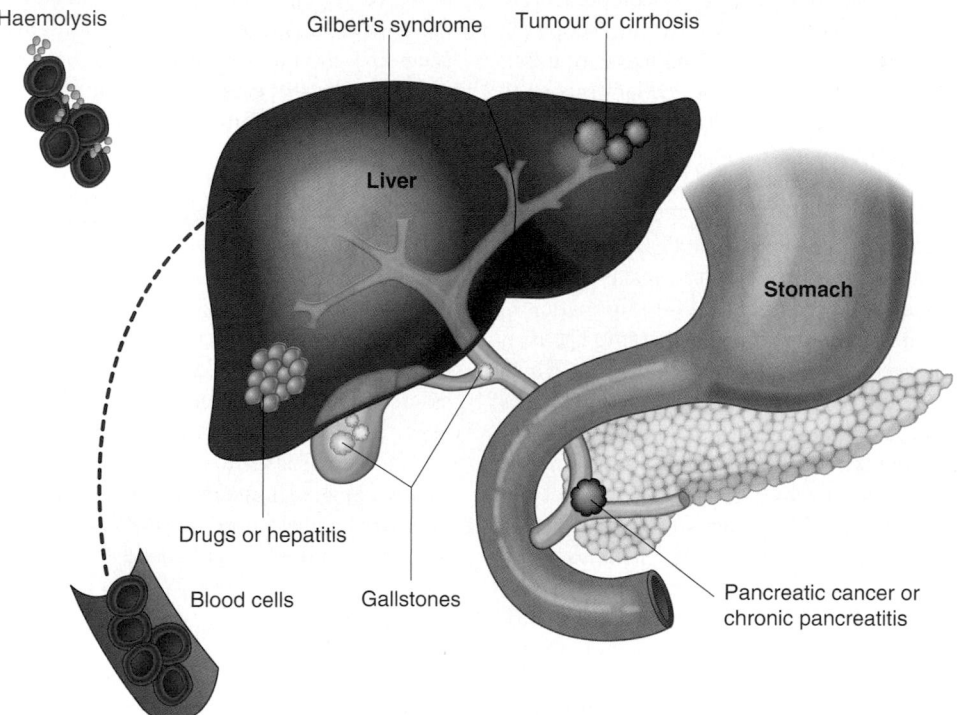

Fig. 16.4 Common causes of jaundice: obstructive, due to blockage of the bile ducts; hepatocellular, due to drugs, hepatitis, chronic liver disease or tumour formation; and prehepatic, due to increased blood breakdown such as occurs in haemolysis.

- A reduction in serum albumin and reduced oncotic pressure is thought to contribute to the collection of fluid in the third space. Peripheral oedema (swollen lower limbs) occurs through this mechanism in a manner similar to the development of ascites.
- Portal hypertension and splanchnic arterial vasodilation alter intestinal capillary pressure and permeability, and thus facilitate the accumulation of retained fluid in the abdominal cavity.

Sexual characteristics

Endocrine changes are well documented in chronic liver disease and tend to be more common in ALD. Hypogonadism is common in patients with cirrhosis. In males, hypogonadism results in testicular atrophy, female body hair distribution and gynaecomastia. This is thought in part to occur because the cirrhotic liver cannot metabolise oestrogen, leading to feminisation in males. Gynaecomastia is found particularly in alcoholics but is also seen in those who are taking spironolactone, when there is usually associated tenderness of the nipples. In women with chronic liver disease, menstrual irregularity, amenorrhoea and reduced fertility are common findings in females of reproductive age, but few detectable physical signs are seen as a result of gonadal atrophy.

Investigation of liver disease

All patients with liver disease must undergo a comprehensive and thorough assessment to ascertain the underlying aetiology. Although causes of acute and chronic liver disease may differ, a similar approach is used to investigate both patient groups to ensure no primary cause or co-factor is overlooked.

Biochemical liver function tests

Biochemical LFTs are simple, inexpensive and easy to perform, but they usually cannot be used in isolation to make a diagnosis. Biochemical parameters provide very useful information in monitoring disease progression or response to therapy. The liver enzymes usually measured are the aminotransferases, which reflect hepatocellular pathology and the cholestatic liver enzymes serum alkaline phosphatase (AST) and γ-glutamyl transpeptidase. Serum aspartate transaminase and alanine transaminase (ALT) are two intracellular enzymes present in hepatocytes which are released into the blood of patients as a consequence of hepatocyte damage. Extremely high values, where transaminases are recorded in the thousands, occur in acute liver disease (e.g. viral hepatitis or paracetamol overdose). In chronic hepatitis serum transaminases are rarely more than five to eight times the upper limit of normal. Alkaline phosphatase is present in the canalicular and sinusoidal membranes of the liver but is also present in some other sites, especially bone. Concomitant elevation of the enzyme γ-glutamyl transpeptidase confirms the hepatic origin of an elevated alkaline phosphatase. The serum alkaline phosphatase activity may be raised by up to four to six times the normal limit in intrahepatic or extrahepatic cholestasis. It can also be raised in conditions associated with liver infiltration, such as metastases.

Bilirubin is commonly elevated in hepatocellular pathology and especially in acute hepatitis and end-stage chronic liver disease. An increase in bilirubin concentration results in jaundice and is usually clinically apparent when the serum bilirubin level exceeds 50 mmol/L. In acute liver disease the serum bilirubin reflects severity of disease but is of little prognostic value. In chronic liver disease a gradual increase for no apparent reason usually reflects serious disease progression. Hepatocellular damage, cholestasis and haemolysis can all cause elevations in the serum bilirubin concentration.

Synthetic function capacity is very important in assessing liver disease. Prothrombin time (PT), international normalised ratio (INR) and other coagulation studies are useful short-term markers of the synthetic function, especially in acute liver insults, where they reflect the severity of the liver injury. PT or INR are also important indicators of chronic liver disease when combined with serum albumin levels. Albumin is synthesised in the liver and serum albumin levels reflect liver function over the preceding months rather than days as with coagulation studies. Alternative causes of hypoalbuminaemia need to be considered, especially proteinuria.

Laboratory investigation of aetiology

All individuals presenting with derangement of liver function should be tested for HAV, HBV, HCV and HEV as part of a routine liver disease screen. Auto-antibodies and immunoglobulins to screen for autoimmune disease are also relevant to both acute and chronic liver disease. Serum ferritin, caeruloplasmin (in patients <40 years old), α_1-antitrypsin phenotype and lipid profile are standard investigations in patients with evidence of chronic liver disease.

Imaging techniques

Ultrasound is a non-invasive, low-risk procedure that is pivotal in the preliminary assessment of liver disease because it assesses the size, shape and echotexture of the liver and screens for dilatation of the biliary tract. In patients with chronic liver disease it assesses patency of the portal vein and may detect signs of portal hypertension (e.g. increased spleen size, ascites). It is also routinely used to screen for HCC and other hepatobiliary malignancies. Computed tomography and magnetic resonance imaging scans are regularly used for further characterisation of any abnormalities identified on ultrasound.

Liver biopsy and Fibroscan

Liver biopsy is an invasive procedure with an associated morbidity and mortality, albeit extremely low. Nevertheless, it remains the gold standard in establishing a diagnosis and assessing the severity of chronic liver disease. Significant progress has being made in developing non-invasive techniques for the assessment of liver fibrosis, and elastography (Fibroscan) is now widely used in clinical practice. Although Fibroscan is considered the first-line investigation for the assessment of liver fibrosis, in some instances liver histology can still contribute to the diagnostic and management process (e.g. whether to initiate antiviral therapy for HBV or less commonly HCV). In acute hepatic dysfunction, a liver biopsy is usually unnecessary, especially if the condition is self-limiting.

Patient care

Pruritus

Pruritus is a prominent and sometimes distressing symptom of chronic liver disease and tends to be most debilitating in the context of cholestatic conditions. The pathogenesis of pruritus in liver disease is poorly understood, but the deposition of bile salts within the skin is considered to be central to its development. However, the concentration of bile salts in the skin does not appear to correlate with the intensity of pruritus. Management of pruritus is variable. Relief of biliary obstruction by endoscopic, radiological or surgical means is indicated in patients with obstructed biliary systems. In other cases pharmacological agents are used initially, but in some cases plasmapheresis, molecular absorbants recirculating system or even liver transplantation may be needed.

Anion exchange resins

Colestyramine and colestipol act by binding bile acids and preventing their reabsorption. These anion exchange resins are the first line of therapy in the treatment of pruritus. Colestyramine is usually initiated at a dosage of 4 g once or twice daily, and the dosage is then titrated to optimise relief without causing side effects, which are predominantly gastro-intestinal. Such adverse effects are common and include constipation, diarrhoea, fat and vitamin malabsorption. Palatability is variable, and consequently adherence is often a problem. To enhance adherence, patients should be advised that the benefits of therapy may take time to become apparent, often up to a week. Anion exchange resins can reduce the absorption of concomitant therapy, and such drugs should be taken 1 hour before or 4–6 hours after colestyramine or colestipol ingestion. Drugs which are susceptible to this interaction include digoxin, levothyroxine, ursodeoxycholic acid (UDCA), thiazide diuretics, lomitapide, tetracycline, sodium valproate, mycophenolate, raloxifene, calcitriol and paracetamol.

Antihistamines

Although frequently used, antihistamines are usually ineffective in the management of the pruritus caused by cholestasis and should not be considered first-line therapy. A non-sedating antihistamine such as cetirizine (10 mg once daily) or loratadine (10 mg once daily) is preferred because these avoid precipitating or masking encephalopathy. Antihistamines such as chlorphenamine or hydroxyzine provide little more than sedative properties,

although they may be useful at night if the severity of pruritus is sufficient to prevent a patient from sleeping.

Ursodeoxycholic acid

The bile acid UDCA (13–15 mg/kg daily in two divided doses) has been used frequently in cholestatic liver disease. However, its effect on pruritus is uncertain; for instance, two large trials in PBC and PSC demonstrated no improvement in pruritus when used at the above dose (Heathcote et al., 1994; Lindor, 1997). In comparison, in a different report it was shown that ursodeoxycholic at a higher dosage (30 mg/kg/day in three divided doses) led to relief of itching within 1 month (Matsuzaki et al., 1990).

Rifampicin

Rifampicin induces hepatic microsomal enzymes, which may benefit some patients, possibly by improving bile flow. Rifampicin, administered at a dosage of up to 600 mg/day, may be effective in the treatment of pruritus, albeit over a more prolonged period (1–3 weeks). It is most commonly used in patients with primary biliary cirrhosis (PBC). Its use is restricted by its potential hepatotoxicity and drug interactions with other agents.

Opioid antagonists

A growing spectrum of opioid antagonists have been used to treat pruritus because it is believed that endogenous opioids in the central nervous system are potent mediators of itch. As a consequence the centrally acting opioid antagonists naloxone, naltrexone and nalmefene are thought to reverse the actions of these endogenous opioids. The use of such agents is limited by their route of administration. Naloxone is given by subcutaneous, intramuscular or intravenous injection, whereas naltrexone and nalmefene are reported to be more substantially bioavailable after oral administration.

Topical preparations

Topical therapy may benefit some patients. Calamine lotion or menthol 2% in aqueous cream are standard preparations, but improvement of pruritus with such agents is variable.

A summary of drugs used in the management of pruritus is shown in Table 16.2.

Clotting abnormalities

The relationship of liver disease to clotting abnormalities is shown diagrammatically in Fig. 16.5. Haemostatic abnormalities develop in approximately 75% of patients with chronic liver disease and 100% of patients with ALF. The majority of clotting factors (with the exception of factor V) are dependent on vitamin K. Patients with liver disease who experience deranged blood clotting should receive intravenous doses of phytomenadione (vitamin K), usually 10 mg daily for 3 days. Administration of vitamin K to patients with significant liver disease does not usually improve the PT because the liver is unable to utilise the

Table 16.2 Drugs commonly used in the management of pruritus

Drug	Indications	Daily dose	Advantages	Disadvantages
Colestyramine	Cholestatic jaundice Itching (first line)	4–16 g (in two or three divided doses)	Reduce systemic bile salt levels	Poor patient adherence because of unpalatability Diarrhoea/constipation Increased flatulence Abdomin discomfort
Ursodeoxycholic acid	Cholestatic jaundice Itching	13–15 mg/kg (in two divided doses)		Variable response
Menthol 2% in aqueous cream	Itching	As required	Local cooling effect	Variable response
Chlorphenamine	Itching	4–16 mg (in three or four divided doses)	Sedative effects may be useful for nighttime itching	May precipitate/aggravate encephalopathy
Hydroxyzine	Itching	25–100 mg (in three or four divided doses)	Sedative effects may be useful for nighttime itching	May precipitate/aggravate encephalopathy
Cetirizine	Itching	10 mg (once daily)	Antihistamine with low incidence of sedation	Variable response
Naltrexone	Itching	50 mg/day	Shown to be beneficial in primary biliary cirrhosis	Opiate withdrawal symptoms, usually transient

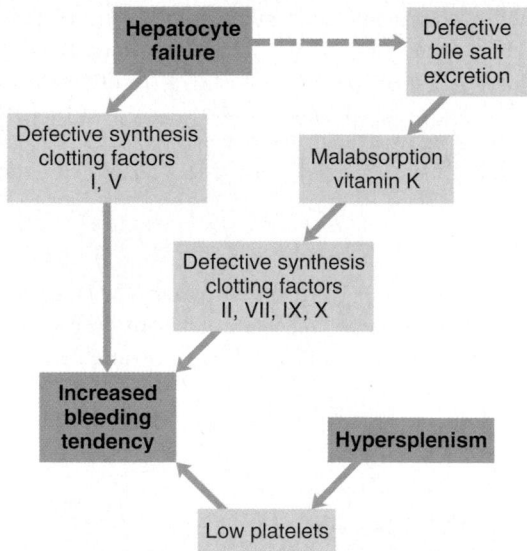

Fig. 16.5 Mechanisms of deranged clotting in chronic liver disease.

vitamin to synthetize clotting factors. Oral vitamin K is less effective than the parenteral form, and thus has little or no place in the management of clotting abnormalities and bleeding secondary to liver disease.

Aspirin, non-steroidal anti-inflammatory drugs (NSAIDs) and anticoagulants should be avoided in all patients with liver disease because of the risk of altering platelet function, causing gastric ulceration and bleeding. NSAIDs have also been implicated in precipitating renal dysfunction and variceal bleeding in patients with end-stage liver disease. Although cyclo-oxygenase-2 inhibitors may cause a lower incidence of bleeding complications, currently they are avoided in patients with liver disease because their use still poses a risk.

Ascites

The aim in the treatment of ascites is to mobilise the collection of third space fluid (intra-abdominal fluid), and this can be achieved by simple measures such as reduced sodium intake. A low-salt diet (60–90 mEq/day) may be enough to facilitate the elimination of ascites and delay reaccumulation of fluid. Salt reduction combined with fluid restriction (approximately 1–1.5 L/day) are practical measures taken to mobilise fluid and provide weight reduction and symptomatic relief.

Aggressive weight reduction in the absence of peripheral oedema should be avoided because it is likely to lead to intravascular fluid depletion and renal failure. To prevent renal failure, weight loss should not exceed 300–500 g/day in the absence of peripheral oedema and 800–1000 g/day in those with peripheral oedema. However, diuretics and/or paracentesis are the cornerstone in the management of moderate- to large-volume ascites. Box 16.1 outlines a sequential approach to the management of ascites.

Diuretics

The aldosterone antagonist spironolactone is usually used as a first-line agent in the treatment of ascites. In most instances a negative sodium balance and loss of ascitic fluid can be achieved with low doses of diuretics. Spironolactone can be used alone or in combination with a more potent loop diuretic. The specific agents and dosages used are outlined in Table 16.3. Spironolactone acts by blocking sodium reabsorption in the collecting tubules of the kidney. It is usually commenced at 50–100 mg/day, but this varies, depending on the patient's clinical status, electrolyte levels and concomitant drug therapies. It can take many days to have a therapeutic effect, so dose augmentation should be conducted with caution and with strict monitoring of renal parameters. The addition of a loop diuretic, furosemide 40 mg/day, enhances the natriuretic activity of spironolactone and should be used when ascites is severe or when spironolactone alone fails to produce acceptable diuresis.

The use of more potent diuretic combinations may result in excessive diuresis which can lead to renal failure of pre-renal origin. The initiation and augmentation of diuretic therapy should ideally be carried out in hospital. This allows strict urea and electrolyte monitoring to detect impending hyperkalaemia and/ or hyponatraemia, which commonly occur with diuretic therapy. It also allows the baseline measurement of urinary sodium excretion; subsequent changes in diuretic dose should be titrated against urinary sodium excretion. Aggressive and unchecked diuresis will precipitate the hepatorenal syndrome, which has a very poor prognosis. Generally if the serum sodium level decreases to less than 130 mmol/L or if serum creatinine levels rise to greater than 130 mmol/L, then the diuretic regimen should be reviewed and stopped if indicated. Diuretic therapy can be complicated by hepatic encephalopathy, hyperkalaemia, hyponatraemia and azotaemia. Gynaecomastia and muscle cramps are side effects of diuretic therapy.

Refractory ascites, which occurs in 5–10% of patients with ascites, is associated with a 6-month to 1-year survival rate of as low as 50% (Arroyo et al., 1996; Guardiola et al., 2002). Therapeutic strategies include repeated large-volume paracentesis combined with the administration of plasma expanders, or alternatively, TIPSS, and in some cases the Alfapump. In some patients liver transplantation may be indicated. Ascites is considered to be refractory or diuretic resistant if there is no response with once-daily doses of 400 mg spironolactone and 160 mg furosemide. Again, urinary sodium excretion provides important information in terms of the response to or viability of dose augmentation with diuretic therapy. Patients on lower doses of diuretics are also considered to have refractory ascites if side effects are a problem (e.g. hepatic encephalopathy, hyperkalaemia, hyponatraemia or azotemia).

Paracentesis

Repeated large-volume paracentesis in combination with albumin administration is the most widely accepted therapy for refractory ascites. Patients generally require paracentesis every 2–4 weeks, and the procedure is often performed in the outpatient setting. Paracentesis, however, does not affect the mechanism responsible for ascitic fluid accumulation, and thus early recurrence is common. Intravenous colloid replacement or plasma expanders are used to prevent adverse effects on the renal and systemic circulation. Colloid replacement in the form of 6–8 g albumin per litre of ascites removed – equivalent to 100 mL of 20% human albumin solution (1 unit) for every 2.5 L of ascitic fluid removed – is a standard regimen.

Transjugular intrahepatic portosystemic shunting

TIPSS is an invasive procedure, used to manage refractory ascites or control refractory variceal bleeding. It is carried out under radiological

---

Box 16.1 Sequential approach to the management of cirrhotic ascites

Bed rest and sodium restriction (60–90 mEq/day, equivalent to 1500–2000 mg of salt/day)
▼
Spironolactone (or other potassium-sparing diuretic)
▼
Spironolactone and loop diuretic
▼
Large-volume paracentesis and colloid replacement

Other measures
Alfapump
Transjugular intrahepatic portosystemic shunt (TIPSS)
Peritoneovenous shunt
Consider orthotopic liver transplantation

Table 16.3 Diuretics used in the management of ascites

Drug	Indication	Daily dose	Advantage	Disadvantage
Spironolactone	Fluid retention	50–400 mg	Aldosterone antagonist Slow diuresis	Painful gynaecomastia Variable bioavailability Hyperkalaemia
Furosemide	Fluid retention	40–160 mg	Rapid diuresis Sodium excretion	Nephrotoxic Hypovolaemia Hypokalaemia Hyponatraemia Caution in pre-renal uraemia
Amiloride	Mild fluid retention	5–10 mg	As K$^+$-sparing agent or weak diuretic if spironolactone contraindicated	Lacks potency

guidance. An expandable intrahepatic stent is placed between the hepatic vein and the portal vein by a transjugular approach (Fig. 16.6). In contrast with paracentesis, the use of TIPSS is effective in preventing recurrence in patients with refractory ascites. It reduces the activity of sodium-retaining mechanisms and improves the renal response to diuretics. However, a disadvantage of this procedure is the high rate of shunt stenosis (up to 30% after 6–12 months), which leads to recurrence of ascites. TIPSS can also induce or exacerbate hepatic encephalopathy (Zervos and Rosemurgy, 2001).

Automated low-flow pump system (Alfapump)

The Alfapump is a device recently introduced for the management of refractory ascites. It consists of an intra-peritoneal catheter connected to a subcutaneously implanted, battery-powered device that moves fluid from the peritoneal cavity, with a second catheter that connects the subcutaneous pump to the urinary bladder, resulting in patients directly urinating the ascites. Implantation of the Alfapump requires a minor surgical procedure usually performed under general anaesthesia. Post-implant, the need for paracentesis is markedly reduced and in some instances is not required at all (Stirnimann et al., 2017). The most frequently encountered complications in clinical practice relate to the surgery, development of infections, catheter dysfunction and renal insufficiency.

Spontaneous bacterial peritonitis

Patients with ascites should be closely observed for spontaneous bacterial peritonitis (SBP) because it develops in 10–30% of patients and has a high mortality rate. Hepatorenal syndrome can complicate SBP in up to 30% of patients and also carries a high mortality rate. Conventional signs and symptoms of peritonitis are rarely present in such patients and if suspected, treatment with appropriate antibiotics should be started immediately after a diagnostic ascitic tap has been taken. A polymorphonuclear leucocyte count of greater than 250 cells/mm^3 is diagnostic of this condition. The causative organism is of enteric origin in approximately

three-fourths of infections, and originates from the skin in the remaining one-fourth. Cefotaxime (2 g, 8 hourly) is effective in 85% of patients with SBP and is commonly used as first-line antimicrobial therapy. Other antibiotic regimens have been used including co-amoxiclav, but third-generation cephalosporins are the treatment of choice. The quinolone norfloxacin (400 mg/day) has a role in the prevention of recurrence of SBP, estimated as 70% at 1 year, and is recommended for long-term antibiotic prophylaxis (Moore and Aithal, 2006). However, the emergence of quinolone-resistant bacteria is a growing problem in the management of SBP.

Hepatic encephalopathy

Hepatic encephalopathy is a reversible neuropsychiatric complication that occurs with significant liver dysfunction. The precise cause of encephalopathy remains unclear, but three factors are known to be implicated, namely, portosystemic shunting, metabolic dysfunction and an alteration of the blood–brain barrier. It is thought that intestinally derived neuroactive and neurotoxic substances such as ammonia pass through the diseased liver or bypass the liver through shunts and go directly to the brain. This results in cerebral dysfunction. Ammonia is thought to increase the permeability of the blood–brain barrier, enabling other neurotoxins to enter the brain and indirectly alter neurotransmission. Other substances implicated in causing hepatic encephalopathy include free fatty acids, γ-aminobutyric acid and glutamate.

Clinical features of hepatic encephalopathy range from trivial lack of awareness, altered mental state to asterixis (liver flap) through to gross disorientation and coma. During low-grade encephalopathy, the altered mental state may present as impaired judgement, altered personality, euphoria or anxiety. Reversal of day/night sleep patterns is typical of encephalopathy. Somnolence, semistupor, confusion and finally coma can ensue (Table 16.4).

Encephalopathy associated with cirrhosis and/or portal systemic shunts may develop as a result of specific precipitating factors (Box 16.2) or can occur spontaneously. Common precipitating factors include gastro-intestinal bleeding, SBP, constipation, dehydration, electrolyte abnormalities and certain drugs (including narcotics and sedatives). Identification and removal of such precipitating

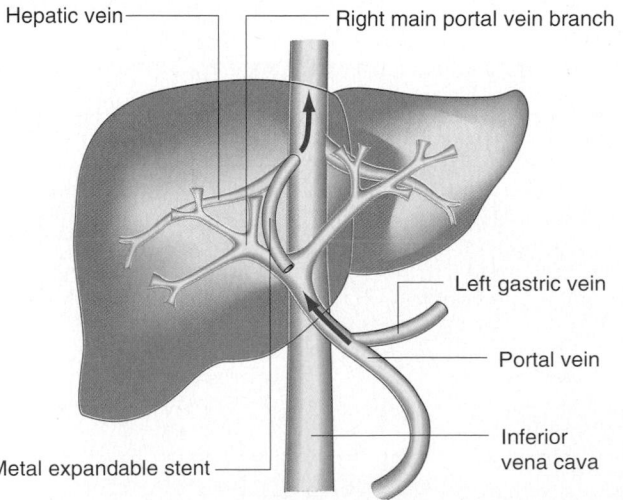

Fig. 16.6 Intrahepatic stent shunt links the hepatic vein with the intrahepatic portal vein.

Labels: Hepatic vein · Right main portal vein branch · Left gastric vein · Portal vein · Inferior vena cava · Metal expandable stent

Table 16.4	Grading of hepatic encephalopathy
Grade 0	Normal
Subclinical	Abnormal psychometric tests for encephalopathy (e.g. number correction test)
Grade 1	Mood disturbance, abnormal sleep pattern, impaired handwriting with or without asterixis
Grade 2	Drowsiness, grossly impaired calculation ability, asterixis
Grade 3	Confusion, disorientation, somnolent but arousable, asterixis
Grade 4	Stupor to deep coma, unresponsive to painful stimuli

factors are mandatory. Therapeutic management is then aimed at reducing the amount of ammonia or nitrogenous products in the circulatory system. Treatment with laxatives increases the throughput of bowel contents, by reducing transit time, and also increases soluble nitrogen output in the faeces. Drug therapies for encephalopathy are summarised in Table 16.5.

Lactulose, a non-absorbable disaccharide, decreases ammonia production in the gut. It is widely used because it is broken down by gastro-intestinal bacteria to form lactic, acetic and formic acids. The effect of lactulose is to acidify the colonic contents which leads to the ionisation of nitrogenous products within the bowel, with a consequent reduction in their absorption from the gastro-intestinal tract. Lactulose is commenced in doses of 30–40 mL/day and titrated to result in two to three bowel motions each day. Patients unable to take oral medication or those with worsening encephalopathy are treated with phosphate enemas.

The non-absorbable antibiotic rifaximin has emerged as a key therapeutic strategy in the management of hepatic encephalopathy. Rifaximin is concentrated in the gastro-intestinal tract, has broad-spectrum in vitro activity against Gram-positive and Gram-negative aerobic and anaerobic enteric bacteria, and appears to carry a low risk of inducing bacterial resistance. A potential mechanism for the activity of rifaximin is its effects on the metabolic function of the gut microbiota, rather than a change in the relative bacterial abundance. Rifaximin is administered in dosages of 550 mg twice daily. Peripheral oedema and nausea are reported by patients. Metronidazole or neomycin may also be used to reduce ammonia production from gastro-intestinal

bacteria, but both of these options have largely been abandoned with the emergence of rifaximin. Other therapies investigated for the treatment of encephalopathy include L-ornithine-L-aspartate, sodium benzoate, L-dopa, bromocriptine and the benzodiazepine receptor antagonist flumazenil.

Oesophageal varices

Variceal bleeding is the most feared complication of portal hypertension in patients with cirrhosis, and there is a 30% lifetime risk of at least one bleeding episode among patients with cirrhosis and varices. Treatment of variceal bleeding includes endoscopic band ligation (EBL), or rarely sclerotherapy, of oesophageal varices in parallel with splanchnic vasoconstrictors and intensive medical care. Patients with variceal bleeding refractory to endoscopic intervention or patients bleeding from ectopic or uncontrolled gastric varices will need TIPSS or surgical decompressive shunts. Refractory variceal bleeding should therefore be managed in centres with an appropriate level of expertise.

Initial treatment is aimed at stopping or reducing the immediate blood loss, treating hypovolaemic shock, if present, and subsequent prevention of recurrent bleeding. Immediate and prompt resuscitation is an essential part of treatment. Only when medical treatment has been initiated and optimised should endoscopy be performed. Endoscopy confirms the diagnosis and allows therapeutic intervention. Fluid replacement is invariably required and should be in the form of colloid or packed red cells and administered centrally. Sodium chloride 0.9% should generally be avoided in all patients with cirrhosis. Fluid replacement must be administered with caution because over-zealous expansion of the circulating volume may precipitate further bleeding by raising portal pressure, thereby exacerbating the clinical situation. A flow chart for the management of bleeding oesophageal varices is shown in Fig. 16.7.

Endoscopic management

Variceal band ligation uses prestretched rubber bands applied to the base of a varix which has been sucked into the banding chamber attached to the front of an endoscope. Endoscopic balloon ligation controls bleeding in the majority of cases. It is at

---

Box 16.2 Precipitating causes of hepatic encephalopathy

Gastro-intestinal bleeding
Infection (spontaneous bacterial peritonitis [SBP], other sites of sepsis)
Hypokalaemia, metabolic alkalosis
High-protein diet
Constipation
Drugs, opioids and benzodiazepines
Deterioration of liver function
Postsurgical portosystemic shunt or transjugular intrahepatic portosystemic shunt

---

Table 16.5 Drugs commonly used in the management of encephalopathy

Drug	Dosage	Comment	Side effects
Lactulose	15–30 mL orally 2–4 times daily	Aim for two to three soft stools daily	Bloating, diarrhoea
Metronidazole	400–800 mg orally daily in divided doses	Metabolism impaired in liver disease	Gastro-intestinal disturbance and neurotoxicity (especially when administered prolongedly)
Neomycin	2–4 g orally daily in divided doses	Maximum duration of 6 days, used less frequently now	Potential for nephrotoxicity and ototoxicity
Rifaximin	550 mg twice daily	Unclear whether long-term treatment could induce microbial resistance	Potential for nausea, peripheral oedema, and *Clostridium difficile* infection

least as effective as sclerotherapy, which it has largely superseded, and is associated with fewer side effects. Balloon tamponade with a Sengstaken–Blakemore balloon or Linton balloon may be used to stabilise a patient with actively bleeding varices by direct compression, until more definitive therapy can be undertaken. Balloon tamponade can control bleeding in up to 80% of cases, but 50% re-bleed when the balloon is deflated (Avgerinos and Armonis, 1994). Gastric varices develop in approximately 20% of patients with portal hypertension (Chang et al., 2013). The risk of gastric variceal bleeding is lower than that of oesophageal variceal bleeding, but bleeding from fundal varices is notoriously more difficult to manage and is associated with a higher mortality. The most effective treatment strategy for fundal varices is now considered to be variceal obturation with tissue adhesives or 'glue injection'. The use of cyanoacrylate injection in the treatment of fundal varices is associated with less re-bleeding and is now the treatment of choice in the hands of experienced endoscopists (National Institute for Health and Care Excellence, 2012).

Pharmacological therapy

Several pharmacological agents are available for the emergency control of variceal bleeding (Table 16.6). Most act by lowering portal venous pressure. They are generally used to control bleeding in addition to balloon tamponade and emergency endoscopic techniques. Vasopressin was the first vasoconstrictor used to reduce portal pressure in patients with actively bleeding varices. However, its associated systemic vasoconstrictive adverse effects limited its use. The synthetic vasopressin analogue, terlipressin, is highly effective in controlling bleeding and in reducing mortality. It can be administered in bolus doses every 4–6 hours and has a longer biological activity and a more favourable side effect profile. Once a diagnosis of variceal bleeding has been established, a vasoactive drug infusion (usually terlipressin) should be started without further delay and continued for 2–5 days. Somatostatin and the somatostatin analogue, octreotide, are reported to cause selective splanchnic vasoconstriction and reduce portal pressure. Although they are reported to cause less adverse effects on the systemic circulation, terlipressin remains the agent of choice.

Self-expanding metallic stents

Current treatment strategies of variceal bleeding are highlighted earlier in this section; however, up to 10% of bleeding events remain refractory to standard therapy and are associated with high mortality. Implantation of a self-expanding metallic stent appears to sufficiently result in immediate haemostasis and stopping of bleeding in refractory variceal bleeding. Additionally it appears to be associated with fewer adverse effects compared with conventional therapeutic strategies and decreased incidence of bleeding recurrence. The Danis stent system is an example of a self-expanding stent which offers effective haemostasis through direct compression of the bleeding oesophageal varices. It does not require image guidance, allows post-procedure endoscopic investigations and patients can also resume oral intake of food. The main clinically significant adverse outcomes reported to date are stent migration and oesophageal ulceration; the former does not appear to be associated with increased incidence of re-bleeding, and the latter occurs in approximately 6% (Kumbhari et al., 2013).

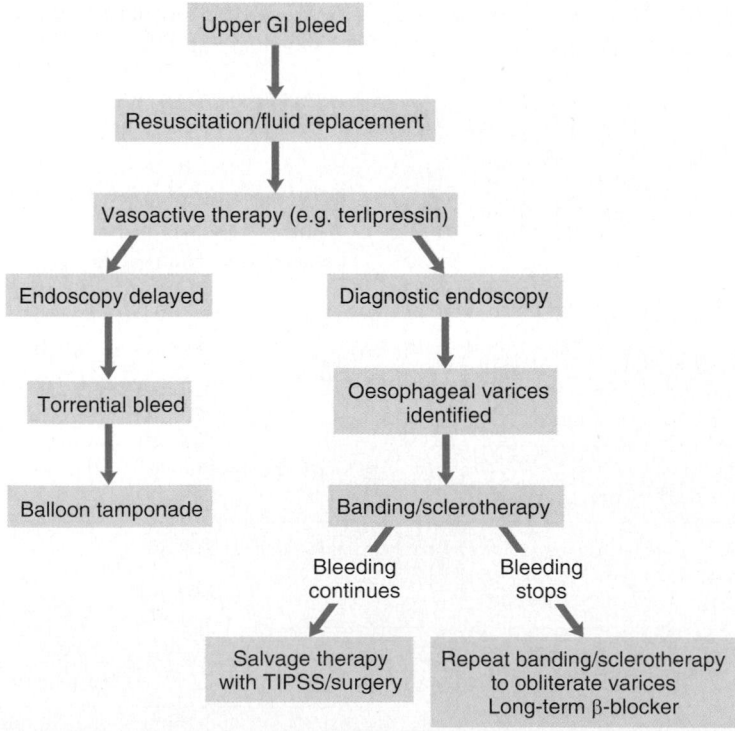

Fig. 16.7 Management of oesophageal variceal haemorrhage.
GI, Gastro-intestinal; TIPSS, transjugular intrahepatic portosystemic shunt.

Transjugular intrahepatic portosystemic stent shunt

TIPSS stent is now established as the preferred rescue therapy in cases where endoscopic intervention has failed to control bleeding (see Fig. 16.7). Recent data suggest the use of early TIPSS within the first 48 hours may be lifesaving in patients with advanced liver failure (Lopera, 2005).

Prevention of re-bleeding

EBL is performed at regular intervals (1–2 weeks) as part of an eradication programme to obliterate the varices. Once varices have been eradicated, endoscopic follow-up can be performed less frequently (3 monthly) for the first year, and then twice yearly thereafter. If varices reappear they should be banded regularly until eradicated again. Non-selective β-blockers, such as propranolol, are the medication of choice to prevent re-bleeding and can also be used as primary prophylaxis against variceal bleeding in patients with known varices. The mechanism of action is complex, but they reduce portal hypertension by causing splanchnic vasoconstriction and reduced portal blood flow. At higher doses they can have a more marked negative effect on cardiac output and thus must be titrated accordingly.

Acute liver failure

ALF occurs when there is a rapid deterioration in liver function in previously healthy individuals, resulting in encephalopathy and a coagulopathy. ALF is a multisystem disorder, with cerebral oedema and renal impairment being particularly important complications. In the past, viral hepatitis was a major consideration in the cause of ALF. However, the development of a commercial vaccine for hepatitis B has seen a dramatic decline in the contribution of HBV to ALF in Western countries. The most common cause of ALF in the UK and USA is paracetamol (acetaminophen) toxicity. Seronegative hepatitis is the other common aetiological group. Management of ALF is complicated, involving supporting the central nervous, cardiovascular and renal systems. All patients with ALF are at risk of infection, and prophylactic administration of broad-spectrum antibiotics and antifungal agents is standard practice. Coagulopathy and bleeding resulting from liver failure are well-recognised life-threatening complications which require specialised monitoring and early correction.

Liver transplantation

Liver transplantation is the established treatment for selected patients with ALF, decompensated chronic liver disease, inherited metabolic disorders and primary liver cancer. HCV and alcohol-related end-stage liver disease are the commonest indications for liver transplantation in Europe and the USA. Typical 1-year survival rates are around 90% for elective transplants. Remarkably few transplants fail because of rejection and, nowadays, technical problems, infection and multisystem failure account for most deaths in the first year. Recurrence of the primary disease, malignancy and death with a functioning graft account for most late deaths.

An increasing number of immunosuppressive agents are now available, and this has enabled clinicians to tailor immunosuppression to achieve a balance of good graft function and an acceptable side effect profile. The calcineurin inhibitors, tacrolimus and ciclosporin, remain the mainstay of immunosuppressive therapy. Corticosteroids are still commonly used, at least during the first 3 months after transplantation. The other drugs used regularly for long-term immunosuppression include azathioprine, mycophenolate, sirolimus and everolimus. Therapy is monitored closely and increasingly tailored to individual patients, with a particular emphasis on preserving renal function and reducing the risk of cardiovascular disease.

Disease-specific therapies
Hepatitis B

The primary goal in the management of CHB infection is to prevent cirrhosis, hepatic failure and HCC. The ideal treatment endpoint is HBsAg loss, which is considered a functional cure. However, the eradication of HBV at this juncture is considered impossible because of integration of HBV into the host genome and the presence of an intracellular conversion pathway which replenishes the pool of transcriptional templates in the hepatocyte nucleus without the need for reinfection. For this reason, current treatment strategies revolve around continuous viral suppression to reduce immune-mediated liver damage and prevent the development of fibrosis and cirrhosis. Although viral suppression can significantly reduce the risk of HCC, it does not necessarily prevent it.

It is the persistence of covalently closed circular DNA (cccDNA) which is considered to preclude eradication of HBV. Thus, therapies currently available for the treatment of CHB are measured in terms of HBeAg seroconversion (in eAg-positive disease), viral suppression, ALT normalisation and improvement in liver histopathology. There has been increased focus on HBsAg quantification, with HBsAg levels considered a surrogate of cccDNA levels (Martinot-Peignoux et al., 2013). Thus, all new therapies for the treatment of HBV should be benchmarked against their ability to achieve HBsAg loss, which is associated with reduced risk of disease progression and the development of HCC.

Recommended first-line therapies vary in different guidelines. Both the international guidelines from the European Association for the Study of the Liver (EASL) and the American Association for the Study of Liver Diseases (AASLD) offer flexibility in treatment selection, with the choice of first-line agent being left to physician's discretion along with an element of patient choice in making a joint decision (EASL, 2017; Terrault et al., 2016). Treatment strategies have broadened and include the potent oral antiviral agents tenofovir and entecavir, as well as pegylated

Table 16.6	Drugs used in the treatment of acute bleeding varices
Drug	Dosage and administration
Terlipressin	1–2 mg bolus 4–6 hourly for 2–5 days
Octreotide	50 micrograms/h i.v. infusion for ≥48 h

interferon (peginterferon) alfa-2a. Tenofovir and entecavir have emerged as the leading oral antivirals, and agents with a low genetic barrier to resistance, such as telbivudine, lamivudine and adefovir, should not be used as first-line antivirals. The use of lamivudine or adefovir as a monotherapy is no longer recommended and should be avoided if at all possible, owing to high rates of resistance with these drugs. Peginterferon alfa-2a is also used in the treatment of CHB. This is due primarily to its potent immunomodulatory effects which give it a clear advantage over oral antivirals. Significant rates of HBsAg loss have been reported in both eAg- positive and -negative disease, and the inclusion of quantitative HBsAg levels provides an objective 'stopping rule' to terminate treatment early where the response is deemed suboptimal. The advantages of interferon therapy, such as a finite treatment course and good rates of HBsAg loss in selected patients, must be weighed against the disadvantages associated with an injection-based therapy and the inherent side effect profile associated with interferons. Therefore, a careful and rational approach must be followed when considering treatment of CHB. The treatment landscape for CHB has changed dramatically from the high rates of resistance previously seen with lamivudine and adefovir to the extremely low rates of resistance reported for entecavir and tenofovir. However, when commencing oral antiviral agents, the patient and treating prescriber must be aware that they are potentially embarking on a lifelong course of treatment.

An issue which must be considered nonetheless is the potential side effect profile of these relatively new drugs, notwithstanding their potency and documented efficacy. More recently, reports of renal toxicity have emerged in some patients treated with tenofovir (glomerular and tubular dysfunction); as a consequence, tenofovir alafenamide (TAF), a prodrug of tenofovir, has emerged as an alternative antiviral agent with non-inferior efficacy but a better safety profile (Kayaaslan and Guner, 2017; Scott and Chan, 2017). TAF is now considered a first-line treatment for the management of CHB, owing to its high genetic barrier to resistance, but distinguished by its better safety profile. Access to TAF in clinical practice is likely to be determined by cost, while the existing antivirals (tenofovir and entecavir) come off patent and relatively cheap generics will be available. However, prescribers will need to remain vigilant for the emergence of resistant virus (and the development of side effects), even with these newer more potent agents, because the treatment landscape in CHB is set to change dramatically over the coming years.

Hepatitis C

The primary aim of treating patients with chronic HCV is viral clearance with sustained virologic response (SVR). SVR is defined as the absence of viraemia, that is, undetectable HCV RNA in a sensitive assay (≤15 IU/mL), 12 weeks (SVR 12) and 24 weeks (SVR 24) after antiviral therapy has been completed. The goal of therapy is ultimately to eradicate HCV and prevent the development of liver cirrhosis, decompensated liver disease, HCC and death.

The backbone of hepatitis C treatment had been for many years an interferon-based regimen with the addition of ribavirin

in 1998 and pegylation of interferon in 2001. This antiviral regimen was characterised by suboptimal response rates, that is, 55% for genotypes 1 and 4 and 80–85% for genotypes 2 and 3. The main limitation of interferon-based treatment was the side effect profile, complications of therapy and poor patient tolerability. Common side effects of therapy included influenza-like symptoms, decrease in haematological parameters (haemoglobin, neutrophils, white blood cell count and platelets), gastrointestinal complaints, psychiatric disturbances (anxiety and depression), and hypothyroidism or hyperthyroidism. Hence HCV management was characterised more by toxicity than treatment success.

The landscape changed significantly with the emergence of the first direct-acting antiviral (DAA) agents boceprevir and telaprevir in 2011. More recently, second-generation DAAs, approved in 2013, have revolutionised treatment of HCV, and they are now considered the standard of care in HCV management. DAAs are molecules that target specific non-structural proteins of the virus that results in disruption of viral replication and infection. There are four classes of DAAs, which are defined by their mechanism of action and therapeutic target. The four classes are non-structural proteins 3/4A (NS3/4A), protease inhibitors, NS5B nucleoside polymerase inhibitors, NS5B non-nucleoside polymerase inhibitors and NS5A inhibitors.

In 2013 the U.S. Food and Drug Administration approved sofosbuvir and simeprevir as the first all-oral therapies to be used in clinical practice and were subsequently followed by the approval of daclatasvir, ledipasvir, ombitasvir, paritaprevir, ritonavir and dasabuvir. DAAs are used with or without the addition of ribavirin and/or peginterferon-alfa. Selection of a combination of drugs and duration of treatment (either a 12- or 24-week course) is considered primarily on the basis of whether the patient has cirrhosis; other factors which may determine the treatment regimen and duration include prior treatment failure and HCV genotype. SVR is achievable in more than 90% of all patients irrespective of the presence/absence of cirrhosis, varying between 82% and 100% (Solbach and Wedemeyer, 2015). DAAs are well tolerated with few individuals reporting side effects and even fewer, if any, discontinuing treatment because of adverse effects. The most common side effects reported are fatigue, headache, rash and pruritus, nausea, insomnia and asthenia.

A recognised episode of acute hepatitis in individuals with HCV develops only in a small percentage of individuals. Based on recently published guidelines, patients with acute hepatitis C should be treated with a combination of DAAs, in order to prevent progression to chronic hepatitis C. High SVR rates (>90%) have been reported with sofosbuvir-based, interferon-free regimens (EASL, 2016).

DAAs should also be used in patients with an indication for liver transplantation because antiviral treatment prevents graft rejection, and similarly they should be considered in patients with HCC who are being considered for transplantation. The tolerability of the DAAs means there are few cases where their use is precluded, and drug cost is often the main barrier to their wider use. Treatment with DAAs in transplanted patients with post-transplant HCV recurrence is now considered routine, and the debate about the use of DAAs in the transplant setting now revolves around the most appropriate timing of treatment, be that pretransplantation or restriction to the post-transplant setting. Special groups such as individuals with HIV co-infection, HBV co-infection, individuals with bleeding disorders, active drug addicts and patients on stable maintenance substitution have all shown excellent treatment outcomes with DAAs. More challenging subgroups, such as individuals with renal failure (creatinine clearance <30 mL/min and/or on renal replacement therapy), should be considered for treatment with DAAs; however, there remains a paucity of data, mainly on pharmacokinetics, safety and efficacy, in these patients which mandates further research to establish the best treatment strategy.

It is clear that the emergence of the DAAs marked the dawn of a new era in the management of patients with HCV infection. The challenges faced in a real-world setting with restricted access to DAAs, because of drug cost, have resulted in patients with the greatest clinical need being treated first. Even in this setting, treating those with the most advanced disease has reinforced the potency of the DAAs and the potential to achieve HCV cure in these difficult-to-treat patients without jeopardizing patients' health.

Alcoholic liver disease

The backbone of managing ALD and more specifically alcoholic cirrhosis is abstinence from alcohol which reduces the risks of complications and associated mortality. Additionally, cofactors which include obesity, insulin resistance, smoking, malnutrition, iron overload and viral hepatitis should be identified and managed. Liver transplantation was shown to be beneficial in patients with a Child-Pugh C ALD and/or a Model for End-Stage Liver Disease score ≥15. All the major liver disease organisations concur that a 6-month period of abstinence is necessitated to assess patient progress and the potential to avoid liver transplantation in those with spontaneous improvement.

AH is a clinical syndrome characterised by jaundice and/or ascites of recent onset in a patient with ongoing alcohol misuse. The recommended first-line treatment of choice in patients with AH is corticosteroids. In the recent STOPAH study conducted in the UK (Thursz et al., 2015), it was suggested that the administration of 40 mg prednisolone daily for 1 month may have a beneficial effect on short-term mortality, but not on the medium-term or long-term outcome of AH. Early non-response to steroids should be identified, and cessation of therapy should be considered. Until recently, pentoxifylline was considered an alternative first-line treatment to steroids in patients with AH and ongoing sepsis; however, the STOPAH trial did not show improvement of outcomes in patients with AH treated with pentoxifylline.

N-acetylcysteine, an antioxidant substance that replenishes glutathione stores in hepatocytes, could also be considered in addition to steroids because it was suggested that the combination regimen has a better 1-month survival (Nguyen-Khac et al., 2011).

Non-alcoholic fatty liver disease

Epidemiological evidence suggests a strong relationship between an unhealthy lifestyle and NAFLD; therefore, all patients with NAFLD should receive counselling for lifestyle intervention, namely, a more healthy diet and increased physical activity. A target 7–10% weight loss should be set for patients because this has been correlated with improvement of liver enzymes and histology.

Pharmacotherapy should be reserved for those with evidence of NASH and stage 2 or higher fibrosis and/or those with the potential for disease progression. Although further studies are necessitated, pioglitazone appears to improve all histological features (except for fibrosis) and additionally improves ALT and insulin resistance (Shyangdan et al., 2011); resolution of the clinical features of NASH was achieved more often (when compared with placebo). Vitamin E at a dosage of 800 IU/day also appears to improve steatosis, inflammation and ballooning and could induce resolution of NASH in a third of patients with NASH based on recent studies; vitamin E demonstrated better safety and tolerability in the short-term in comparison with pioglitazone (Sanyal et al., 2010). A combination of the above could also be used. The role of statins is more clear; they can be used with confidence to reduce cardiovascular risk without having any benefits (or conversely causing harm) to the liver.

As a strategy to tackle obesity and diabetes, bariatric surgery has a role in the management of NAFLD because it reduces fat in the liver and therefore is thought to reduce NASH progression; prospective data showed improvement of all histological lesions of NASH, including fibrosis (Nostedt et al., 2016). Finally, liver transplantation may be the only therapeutic option for some patients with end-stage NAFLD; in this cohort overall survival is comparable with other indications for transplantation.

Autoimmune hepatitis

Corticosteroids and/or azathioprine are the standard therapies for AIH. Prednisone or prednisolone are administered at dosages of 40–60 mg/day (0.5–1 mg/kg/day) alone or at lower dosages when combined with azathioprine. The steroid dosage is reduced over a 6-week to 3-month period to a target maintenance dosage of ≤7.5 mg/day. The disturbance in aminotransferases usually normalises within 6–12 weeks, but histological remission tends to lag by 6–12 months. Azathioprine at a dosage of 1–2 mg/kg/day is used as an adjunct to corticosteroid therapy. Azathioprine used alone is ineffective in treating the acute phase of AIH, and therefore is usually added in once the steroid therapy has improved the biochemical abnormality. In patients intolerant of azathioprine, or in cases of proven treatment failure, other immunosuppressive agents have been used (e.g. tacrolimus and mycophenolate). Newer corticosteroids such as budesonide, which is associated with fewer systemic side effects, have also been used effectively, but this is not recommended in patients with established cirrhosis. Budesonide is likely to have a greater role in the treatment of AIH in the future.

Primary biliary cholangitis

Several therapies have been associated with short-term improvements in LFTs. UDCA 13–15 mg/kg/day is the medication of choice and is widely used to treat PBC by reducing the retention of bile acids and increasing their hepatic excretion; therefore, it is effective in protecting against the cytotoxic effects of dihydroxy bile acids which accumulate in PBC. UDCA has been demonstrated to markedly decrease serum bilirubin, alkaline phosphatase (ALP), gamma-glutamyl transpeptidase (γGT), cholesterol and immunoglobulin M levels and also to ameliorate histological features in patients with PBC when compared with placebo (Pares et al., 2000). However, no significant effect on symptoms such as fatigue or pruritus were observed. Additionally, it was shown that long-term treatment with UDCA delayed the histological progression of the disease, especially in patients in whom treatment was started at an early stage (Angulo et al., 1999). With respect to the effect of UDCA on survival, most large studies do not show a significant beneficial effect, although, in a combined analysis of raw data from the French, Canadian and Mayo cohorts, treatment was associated with a significant reduction in the likelihood of liver transplantation or death (Tsochatzis et al., 2009).

There is currently no consensus on how to treat patients with a suboptimal biochemical response to UDCA; one approach could be the combination of UDCA and budesonide (6–9 mg/day) in non-cirrhotic patients, although further studies are required. Development of portal vein thrombosis, probably related to short-term budesonide administration, was reported in stage 4 patients with portal hypertension; therefore, budesonide should not be administered to patients with cirrhosis.

Liver transplantation remains the only effective option in patients with end-stage disease. Survival rates above 90% and 80–85% at 1 and 5 years, respectively, have been reported by many centers. After orthotopic liver transplantation, most patients' antimitochondrial antibody status does not change, but they have no signs of liver disease. PBC has a calculated weighted disease recurrence rate of 18%. However, recurrence is rarely associated with graft failure.

Immunosuppressive agents such as ciclosporin, azathioprine and methotrexate have also been assessed for the treatment of PBC, but clinically significant adverse events outweigh the potential benefits. Other medications, including antifibrotic agents such as D-penicillamine and colchicine or antiretroviral agents, were also studied, but outcomes were shown to be inferior or non-superior to UDCA or reported adverse events outweighed the benefits (Angulo et al., 1999).

Recent results on the use of obeticholic acid show promise for its role in the treatment of PBC (Bowlus, 2016). Obeticholic acid binds to the farnesoid X receptor; a key regulator of bile acid metabolic pathways found in the nucleus of cells in the liver and intestine. Obeticholic acid, given orally, appears to increase bile flow from the liver and to suppress bile acid production in the liver, thus reducing exposure of the liver to toxic levels of bile acids. It is indicated in combination with UDCA in adults with an inadequate response to UDCA, or as monotherapy in adults unable to tolerate UDCA. Most common side effects (>5%) include, amongst others, pruritus, fatigue and gastro-intestinal disturbances.

Primary sclerosing cholangitis

Effective treatment for PSC does not exist to date. Although paucity of data does not allow a specific recommendation for the general use of UDCA in the management of PSC, it appears that UDCA at a higher dosage (>15 mg/kg/day) can be used to manage associated cholestasis. This has been shown to improve serum liver enzymes and surrogate markers of prognosis, but it has not been shown to have proven benefit on survival. Studies with various immunosuppressive agents have been disappointing, and transplantation remains the only effective treatment option in patients with advanced disease.

Wilson's disease

Wilson's disease, a rare autosomal recessive condition, is usually managed with chelation therapy. Penicillamine is the agent of choice in Wilson's disease because it promotes urinary copper excretion in affected patients and prevents copper accumulation in presymptomatic individuals. Initial treatment of 1.5–2 g/day is given in divided doses. Initially neurological symptoms may worsen because of deposition of mobilised copper in the basal ganglia, but symptomatic patients tend to improve over a period of several weeks. Other therapy-related adverse effects include renal dysfunction, haematological abnormalities and disseminated lupus erythematosus. Therefore, regular monitoring of full blood count and electrolytes is required, as well as small doses of pyridoxine (25 mg), to counteract the antipyridoxine effect of penicillamine and the associated neurological toxicity. Patients unable to tolerate penicillamine may respond to trientine. This chelating agent is less potent than penicillamine but has fewer adverse effects. Oral zinc is also used, but again is limited by its lack of potency when compared with penicillamine.

Case studies

Case 16.1

Mr AD, a 56-year-old man, is admitted to hospital following haematemesis and melaena. He has a known history of ALD (stopped drinking alcohol 1 year ago) with marked ascites. A provisional diagnosis of bleeding oesophageal varices is made. A Sengstaken–Blakemore tube is inserted and the balloon inflated as a temporary measure to arrest bleeding. The patient is transferred 8 hours later to a specialist regional centre for further management.

Laboratory data on admission are:

		Reference range
Na+	124	133–143 mmol/L
K+	3.0	3.5–5.0 mmol/L
Creatinine	131	80–124 mmol/L
Urea	14.3	2.7–7.7 mmol/L
Bilirubin	167	3–17 mmol/L
ALT	24	0–35 IU/L
PT	18.9	13 seconds
Albumin	24	35–50 g/dL
Haemoglobin	8.9	13.5–18 g/dL

Drugs on admission:

spironolactone 200 mg one each morning.

Questions

1. What other action would you have recommended before Mr AD was transferred to the regional centre?
2. What options (drug and/or non-drug) are likely to be available at the regional centre for managing the patient's bleeding varices?
3. What further long-term measures would you recommend for Mr AD?

Answers

1. Initial restoration of circulating blood volume with colloid, followed by cross-matched blood. Fluid replacement is necessary to protect renal perfusion. In view of Mr AD's ascites, sodium chloride 0.9% should be avoided. Dextrose 5% with added potassium (hypokalaemia present) would be a reasonable choice. A pharmacological agent to reduce portal pressure, such as terlipressin 1–2 mg every 4–6 hours or octreotide 50 micrograms/h, should be started (Abid et al., 2009). Broad-spectrum intravenous antibiotics such as a fluoroquinolone (including ciprofloxacin and norfloxacin) for short-term use (7 days) are recommended in most expert guidelines (Lee et al., 2014). Intravenous cephalosporin (especially ceftriaxone), given in a hospital setting with prevalent quinolone-resistant organisms, has also been shown to be beneficial, particularly in high-risk patients with advanced cirrhosis. There is no evidence that gastric acid suppression is beneficial, and routine commencement of a proton pump inhibitor (PPI) is not recommended; if the bleeding is caused by a gastric mucosal lesion, a PPI such as lansoprazole or omeprazole, or a histamine type 2 receptor antagonist such as ranitidine can be administered. Spironolactone is likely to be either causing or exacerbating the low sodium and should be discontinued. Vitamin K, 10 mg intravenously once daily for 3 days, should be administered in an attempt to correct the raised PT. Because the patient has severe liver disease with varices and ascites there is a possibility he may experience development of encephalopathy. It would be advisable to start lactulose or, if the patient is unable to take medicines orally, administer an enema such as a phosphate enema.

2. Banding/ligation: This is considered superior to sclerotherapy with fewer postendoscopic complications. It involves mechanical strangulation of variceal channels by small elastic plastic rings mounted on the tip of the endoscope.
   TIPSS: This can be used to reduce portal pressure, but there is a risk of precipitating encephalopathy.
   Banding is the first-line option for managing bleeding oesophageal varices. Balloon tamponade with a Sengstaken–Blakemore balloon or Linton balloon may be used to stabilise a patient with active bleeding varices by direct compression, until more definitive therapy can be undertaken. Implantation of a self-expanding metal stent (SEMS) can also result in immediate haemostasis and bleeding control in refractory variceal bleeding. Patients who continue to bleed after two endoscopic treatments should be considered for TIPSS. Surgery involving portal-systemic shunts or devascularisation are possible options if the above alternative modalities fail. Extrahepatic portal-systemic shunts are situated outside the liver and divert portal blood flow into the systemic circulation bypassing the liver. Devascularisation involves obliteration of the collateral vessels supplying blood to the varices.

3. Banding/ligation can be performed on Mr AD at regular intervals of 1–2 weeks to obliterate bleeding varices. Once varices have been eradicated, endoscopic follow-up should be undertaken every 3 months for the first year, then every 6–12 months thereafter. If varices reappear they should be banded regularly until endoscopic eradication. Non-selective β-blockers, such as propranolol, are used in the prophylaxis of further bleeds, with the

dose adjusted until the heart rate is reduced by 25%, but to not less than 55 beats/min.

Case 16.2

Mrs AL, a 68-year-old woman with a long-standing history of ALD, is admitted to hospital with a 2-week history of vomiting, confusion, increased abdominal distension and worsening jaundice.

On admission laboratory data are as follows:

		Reference range
Na	116	133–143 mmol/L
K	3.8	3.5–5.0 mmol/L
Urea	8.5	2.7–7.7 mmol/L
Creatinine	119	80–124 mmol/L
Bilirubin	459	3–17 mmol/L
Albumin	23	35–50 g/L
ALT	23	0–35 IU/L
Alkaline phosphatase	524	70–300 IU/L
PT	18.6	13 seconds

Drugs on admission are as follows:

spironolactone 300 mg each morning
temazepam 10 mg at night
lactulose 10 mL twice daily

Questions

Discuss Mrs AL's initial treatment plan for the management of:
1. ascites
2. nausea and vomiting
3. confusion

Answers

From the presenting features and LFTs on admission it is apparent that Mrs AL's liver disease is getting progressively worse, probably as a result of continued alcohol intake. She is confused on admission and this suggests encephalopathy, a common complication of chronic liver disease.

1. Ascites management: Mrs AL has increased abdominal distension on admission suggestive of worsening ascites. This might be due to poor adherence with spironolactone, or alternatively her ascites may have become diuretic resistant. The patient should be sodium restricted and confined to bed. Spironolactone therapy should be stopped in view of the low sodium and confusion, because overuse of diuretics can precipitate encephalopathy. Fluid restriction is necessary to reduce the ascites, but sufficient fluid is required to rehydrate the patient following vomiting. Paracentesis should be used to manage the ascites. Every litre of ascitic fluid removed should be replaced with 6–8 g of albumin. A diagnostic ascitic tap should be undertaken to exclude the presence of spontaneous bacterial peritonitis (or infection in the ascites).

2. Nausea/vomiting management: Mrs AL's urea is slightly raised, indicating possible dehydration as a result of vomiting. Given the low serum sodium, Mrs AL should be rehydrated with 20% human albumin solution until formal assessment of the total body sodium status; 5% dextrose in this instance may further exacerbate the hyponatraemia. Additional potassium should be given to correct the low serum potassium. Note that if Mrs AL has been taking spironolactone, there would normally be an increase in potassium, but in this case the vomiting has probably reduced this. Mrs AL's nausea can be managed

with a suitable antiemetic such as domperidone 10 mg four times a day initially and then titrated according to the response.

3. Confusion: Confusion may be an early sign of encephalopathy in Mrs AL. Temazepam should be stopped. The patient is on an inadequate dose of lactulose for the management of encephalopathy, so this should be increased to produce two to three loose motions per day. A typical dose would be 20 mL three or four times daily. In view of Mrs AL's confusion it may be worth considering other agents in the management of the encephalopathy, such as rifaximin 550 mg twice daily. Precipitating factors should be identified and treated appropriately, such as the profound hyponatraemia.

Case 16.3

Mrs PB, a 54-year-old woman with PBC, has been complaining of increasing backache over the last 3 months. Her general condition has deteriorated over the past year during which she has suffered from ascites and encephalopathy. Her main complaint is of continuous back pain, which disturbs her sleep.

Question

How would you manage Mrs PB's back pain?

Answer

Back pain secondary to osteoporosis-related vertebral fractures is common in patients with chronic liver disease, such as PBC. This is due to the fact that most patients with PBC are postmenopausal women in their late fifties on whom loss of bone density is likely, secondary to both menopause and chronic liver disease. Once the diagnosis has been confirmed, the patient should be counselled that the bone pain is chronic, tends to be intermittent, and may take several months to settle depending on the presence and extent of fractures. Bed rest is useful in the acute situation, but prolonged bed rest can accelerate bone loss; adequate exercise is therefore recommended. The patient should be advised to take adequate calcium supplementation of 1–1.5 g/day in addition to her normal diet. Vitamin D deficiency is common in chronic liver disease and should be corrected; it is advisable to administer 800 IU daily or alternatively 25,000 IU once or twice per week. Oral bisphosphonates have been found to be safe, especially in patients with PBC, and can improve bone mineral density. Hormone replacement therapy remains contentious because of potential carcinogenic properties and the increased risk of thromboembolism; thus, it is not considered a first-line therapy. In patients with chronic liver disease, transdermal oestradiol is considered a safer option.

For symptomatic management of the pain, a variety of analgesics are available. The choice of drug is influenced by both the severity of the pain and the degree of liver impairment. For mild pain, paracetamol is the mainstay of treatment and may be used in standard doses in the majority of patients with liver dysfunction. Patients pretreated with cytochrome P450–inducing drugs or patients with a history of alcohol abuse are at increased risk of paracetamol-induced liver injury and should receive only short courses at low doses (maximum of 2 g/day for an adult). Opioid analgesics should usually be avoided in liver disease because of their sedative properties and the risks of precipitating or masking encephalopathy. If a patient has stable mild-to-moderate liver disease, then short-term use of opioids can be considered. Moderate potency opioids, such as dihydrocodeine and codeine, are eliminated almost entirely by hepatic metabolism. Therapy should be initiated at a low dose, and the dosage interval titrated according to the response of the patient. Despite their low potency, these preparations may still precipitate encephalopathy.

In severe pain, the use of potent opioids is usually unavoidable. They undergo hepatic metabolism and are therefore likely to accumulate in liver disease. To compensate for this, it is important to increase the dosage interval when using these drugs. Morphine, pethidine or diamorphine should be administered at doses at the lower end of the dosage range at intervals of 6–8 hours. The patient should be regularly observed and the dose titrated according to patient response. In any patient with liver disease who is receiving an opioid it is advisable to co-prescribe a laxative because constipation can increase the possibility of development of encephalopathy. NSAIDs should be avoided in patients with liver disease. All NSAIDs can prolong bleeding time via their effects on platelet function. Impaired liver function itself can lead to a reduced synthesis of clotting factors and an increased bleeding tendency. NSAIDs may also be dangerous because of the increased risk of gastro-intestinal haemorrhage and potential to precipitate renal dysfunction.

References

Abid, S., Jafri, W., Hamid, S., et al., 2009. Terlipressin vs. octreotide in bleeding esophageal varices as an adjuvant therapy with endoscopic band ligation: a randomized double-blind placebo-controlled trial. Am. J. Gastroenterol. 104, 617–623.

Angulo, P., Batts, K.P., Therneau, T.M., et al., 1999. Long-term ursodeoxycholic acid delays histological progression in primary biliary cirrhosis. Hepatology 29, 644–647.

Arroyo, V., Gines, P., Gerbes, A.L., et al., 1996. Definition and diagnostic criteria of refractory ascites and hepatorenal syndrome in cirrhosis. International Ascites Club. Hepatology 23, 164–176.

Avgerinos, A., Armonis, A., 1994. Balloon tamponade technique and efficacy in variceal haemorrhage. Scand. J. Gastroenterol. 207, 11–16.

Bowlus, C.L., 2016. Obeticholic acid for the treatment of primary biliary cholangitis in adult patients: clinical utility and patient selection. Hepat. Med. 8, 89–95.

Brook, G., Bhagani, S., Kulasegaram, R., et al., 2016. United Kingdom national guidelines on the management of the viral hepatitides A, B and C 2015. Int. J. STD AIDS 27, 501–525.

Centers for Disease Control and Prevention, 2017. Hepatitis C FAQs for health professionals. Available at: https://www.cdc.gov/hepatitis/hcv/hcvfaq.htm.

Chang, C.J., Hou, M.C., Liao, W.C., et al., 2013. Management of acute gastric varices bleeding. J. Chin. Med. Assoc. 76, 539–546.

European Association for the Study of Liver Disease (EASL), 2016. EASL recommendations on treatment of Hepatitis C. J. Hepatol. 66, 153–194.

European Association for the Study of the Liver (EASL), 2017. Clinical Practice Guidelines on the management of hepatitis B virus infection. J. Hepatol. 67, 370–398.

Guardiola, J., Baliellas, C., Xiol, X., et al., 2002. External validation of a prognostic model for predicting survival of cirrhotic patients with refractory ascites. Am. J. Gastroenterol. 97, 2374–2378.

Heathcote, E.J., Cauch-Dudek, K., Walker, V., et al., 1994. The Canadian multicenter double-blind randomized controlled trial of ursodeoxycholic acid in primary biliary cirrhosis. Hepatology 19, 1149–1156.

Kayaaslan, B., Guner, R., 2017. Adverse effects of oral antiviral therapy in chronic hepatitis B. World J. Hepatol. 9, 227–241.

Kumbhari, V., Saxena, P., Khashab, M.A., 2013. Self-expandable metallic stents for bleeding esophageal varices. Saudi J. Gastroenterol. 19, 141–143.

Lee, Y.M., Kaplan, M.M., 1995. Primary sclerosing cholangitis. N. Engl. J. Med. 332, 924–933.

Lee, Y.Y., Tee, H.P., Mahadeva, S., 2014. Role of prophylactic antibiotics in cirrhotic patients with variceal bleeding. World J. Gastroenterol. 20, 1790–1796.

Lindor, K.D., 1997. Ursodiol for primary sclerosing cholangitis. Mayo Primary Sclerosing Cholangitis-Ursodeoxycholic Acid Study Group. N. Engl. J. Med. 336, 691–695.

Loftus, E.V., Harewood, G.C., Loftus, C.G., et al., 2005. PSC-IBD: a unique form of inflammatory bowel disease associated with primary sclerosing cholangitis. Gut 54, 91–96.

Lopera, J.E., 2005. Role of emergency transjugular intrahepatic portosystemic shunts. Semin. Interv. Radiol. 22, 253–265.

Martinot-Peignoux, M., Lapalus, M., Asselah, T., et al., 2013. The role of HBsAg quantification for monitoring natural history and treatment outcome. Liver Int. 33 (Suppl. 1), 125–132.

Matsuzaki, Y., Tanaka, N., Osuga, T., et al., 1990. Improvement of biliary enzyme levels and itching as a result of long-term administration of ursodeoxycholic acid in primary biliary cirrhosis. Am. J. Gastroenterol. 85, 15–23.

Moore, K.P., Aithal, G.P., 2006. Guidelines on the management of ascites in cirrhosis. Gut 55 (Suppl. 6), vi1–vi12.

Mueller, S., Millonig, G., Seitz, H.K., 2009. Alcoholic liver disease and hepatitis C: a frequently underestimated combination. World J. Gastroenterol. 15, 3462–3471.

National Institute for Health and Care Excellence, 2012. Acute upper gastrointestinal bleeding in over 16s: management CG141. NICE, London. Available at: https://www.nice.org.uk/guidance/cg141/chapter/guidance#gastric-varices.

Nguyen-Khac, E., Thevenot, T., Piquet, M.A., for the AAH-NAC Study Group, et al., 2011. Glucocorticoids plus N-acetylcysteine in severe alcoholic hepatitis. N. Engl. J. Med. 365, 1781–1789.

Nostedt, J.J., Switzer, N.J., Gill, R.S., et al., 2016. The effect of bariatric surgery on the spectrum of fatty liver disease. Can. J. Gastroenterol. Hepatol. 2016 2059245.

Pares, A., Caballeria, L., Rodes, J., et al., 2000. Long-term effects of ursodeoxycholic acid in primary biliary cirrhosis results of a double-blind controlled muticentric trial. J. Hepatol. 32, 561–566.

Public Health England, 2015. Hepatitis C in the UK: 2015 report. Available at: https://www.gov.uk/government/uploads/system/uploads/attachment_data/file/448710/NEW_FINAL_HCV_2015_IN_THE-_UK_REPORT_28072015_v2.pdf.

Sanyal, A.J., Chalasani, N., Kowdley, K.V., et al., for the NASH CRN, 2010. Pioglitazone, vitamin E, or placebo for nonalcoholic steatohepatitis. N. Engl. J. Med. 362, 1675–1685.

Scott, L.J., Chan, H.L.Y., 2017. Tenofovir alafenamide: a review in chronic hepatitis B. Drugs 77, 1017–1028.

Shyangdan, D., Clar, C., Ghouri, N., et al., 2011. Insulin sensitisers in the treatment of non-alcoholic fatty liver disease: a systematic review. Health Technol. Assess. 15, 1–110.

Sohrabpour, A.A., Mohamadnejad, M., Malekzadeh, M., 2012. The reversibility of cirrhosis. Aliment. Pharmacol. Ther. 36, 824–832.

Solbach, P., Wedemeyer, H., 2015. The new era of interferon-free treatment of chronic hepatitis C. Viszeralmedizin 31, 290–296.

Stirnimann, G., Banz, V., Storni, V., De Gottardi, A., 2017. Automated low-flow ascites pump for the treatment of cirrhotic patients with refractory ascites. Therap. Adv. Gastroenterol. 10, 283–292.

Terrault, N.A., Bzowej, N.H., Chang, K.M., et al., 2016. American Association for the Study of Liver Diseases. AASLD guidelines for treatment of chronic hepatitis B. Hepatology 63, 261–283.

Thursz, M.R., Richardson, P., Allison, M., et al., 2015. Prednisolone or pentoxifylline for alcoholic hepatitis. N. Engl. J. Med. 372, 1619–1628.

Tosone, G., Maraolo, A.E., Mascolo, S., et al., 2014. Vertical hepatitis C virus transmission: main questions and answers. World J. Hepatol. 6, 538–548.

Tsochatzis, E.A., Gurusamy, K.S., Gluud, C., et al., 2009. Ursodeoxycholic acid and primary biliary cirrhosis: EASL and AASLD guidelines. J. Hepatol. 51, 1084–1085 author reply 1085–1086.

Wong, R.J., Aguilar, M., Cheung, R., et al., 2015. Nonalcoholic steatohepatitis is the second leading etiology of liver disease among adults awaiting liver transplantation in the United States. Gastroenterology 148, 547–555.

World Health Organization (WHO), 2016. Hepatitis E. Available at: http://www.who.int/mediacentre/factsheets/fs280/en/.

World Health Organization, 2017. Hepatitis C. Available at: http://www.who.int/mediacentre/factsheets/fs164/en/.

Zervos, E.E., Rosemurgy, A.S., 2001. Management of medically refractory ascites. Am. J. Surg. 181, 256–264.

Further reading

North-Lewis, P. (Ed.), 2008. Drugs and the Liver. Pharmaceutical Press, London.

Friedman, L.S., Martin, P., 2017. Handbook of Liver Disease, fourth ed. Elsevier, London.

Greenburger, N., Blumberg, R., Burakoff, R., 2016. CURRENT Diagnosis & Treatment: Gastroenterology, Hepatology, and Endoscopy, third ed. McGraw Hill Education, New York.

Hauser, S.C., 2015. Mayo Clinic Gastroenterology and Hepatology Board Review, fifth ed. Mayo Clinic Scientific Press–Oxford University Press, New York.

Mahl, T.E., O'Grady, J., 2014. Fast Facts: Liver Disorders (Fast Facts series), second ed. Health Press Limited, Oxford.

Useful websites

European Association for the Study of the Liver (EASL): https://www.easl.eu/research/our-contributions/clinical-practice-guidelines

American Association for the Study of Liver Diseases (AASLD). https://www.aasld.org/publications/practice-guidelines-0

17 Acute Kidney Injury

Paul Cockwell, Stephanie Stringer and John Marriott

Key points

- Acute kidney injury (AKI) is diagnosed when the excretory function of the kidney declines rapidly over a period of hours or days and is usually associated with the accumulation of metabolic waste products and water.
- A wide range of factors can precipitate AKI, including trauma, obstruction of urine flow or any event that causes a reduction in renal blood flow, including surgery and medical conditions, for example, sepsis, diabetes, acute liver disease and rapidly progressive glomerulonephritis.
- Drug involvement in the development of AKI is common.
- There are no specific signs and symptoms of AKI. The condition is typically indicated by raised blood levels of creatinine and/or a low urine output.
- The clinical priorities in AKI are to manage life-threatening complications, correct intravascular fluid balance and establish the cause, reversing factors causing damage where possible.
- The aim of medical treatment is to remove causative factors and maintain patient well-being so that the kidneys have a chance to recover.
- Treatment of AKI is essentially supportive, although there are conditions that cause AKI that are reversible with specific treatment.
- AKI is a serious condition with mortality rates up to 70%, varying according to cause and at its highest with concurrent failure of other organs.

Table 17.1 Kidney Disease Improving Global Outcomes (KDIGO) classification criteria for acute kidney injury staging (only one criterion is required to fulfil stage)

Stage	Serum creatinine criteria	Urine output criteria
Stage 1	Rise by ≥0.3 mg/dL (≥26.4 mmol/L) or ≥1.5–2 times from baseline	<0.5 mL/kg/h for ≥6 h
Stage 2	Rise to ≥2–2.9 times from baseline	<0.5 mL/kg/h for ≥12 h
Stage 3	Rise to ≥3 times from baseline or ≥4.0 mg/dL (≥352 mmol/L) or receiving renal replacement therapy	<0.3 mL/kg/h for ≥24 h or anuria for ≥12 h

these cases sustain AKI, and this increases to ≥30% in those who are critically ill. Most cases are caused by pre-renal AKI and are reversed with appropriate intervention. However, severe AKI, which may include a requirement for dialysis treatment, is often associated with failure of one or more non-renal organs (this is called *multi-organ failure*); in this setting there is a mortality rate of 70% in patients with sepsis and AKI and 45% in patients without sepsis. AKI that occurs in the community is responsible for around 1% of all hospital admissions.

Definition and incidence

Acute kidney injury (AKI) is a common and serious problem in clinical medicine. It is characterised by an abrupt reduction (usually within a 48-hour period) in kidney function. This results in an accumulation of nitrogenous waste products and other toxins. Many patients become oliguric (low urine output) with subsequent salt and water retention. In patients with pre-existing chronic kidney disease (CKD), a rapid decline in renal function is termed *acute on chronic*. The nomenclature of AKI has recently entered clinical practice and has replaced the previously used term *acute renal failure*.

The diagnostic and classification criteria for AKI are based on an increase in serum creatinine or the presence of oliguria (Table 17.1 and Fig. 17.1).

The large majority of cases of AKI occur in patients who are already hospitalised for other medical conditions; up to 7% of

Classification and causes

AKI is not a single disease state with a uniform aetiology, but a consequence of a range of different diseases and conditions. The most useful practical classification comprises three main groupings: (1) pre-renal, (2) renal or (3) post-renal. More than one category may be present in an individual patient. Common causes of each type of AKI are outlined in Table 17.2.

The kidneys are predisposed to haemodynamic injury owing to hypovolaemia or hypoperfusion. This relates to the high blood flow through the kidneys in normal function; the organs represent 5% of total body weight but receive 25% of blood flow. Furthermore, the renal microvascular bed is unique. Firstly, the glomerular capillary bed is on the arterial side of the circulation. Secondly, the

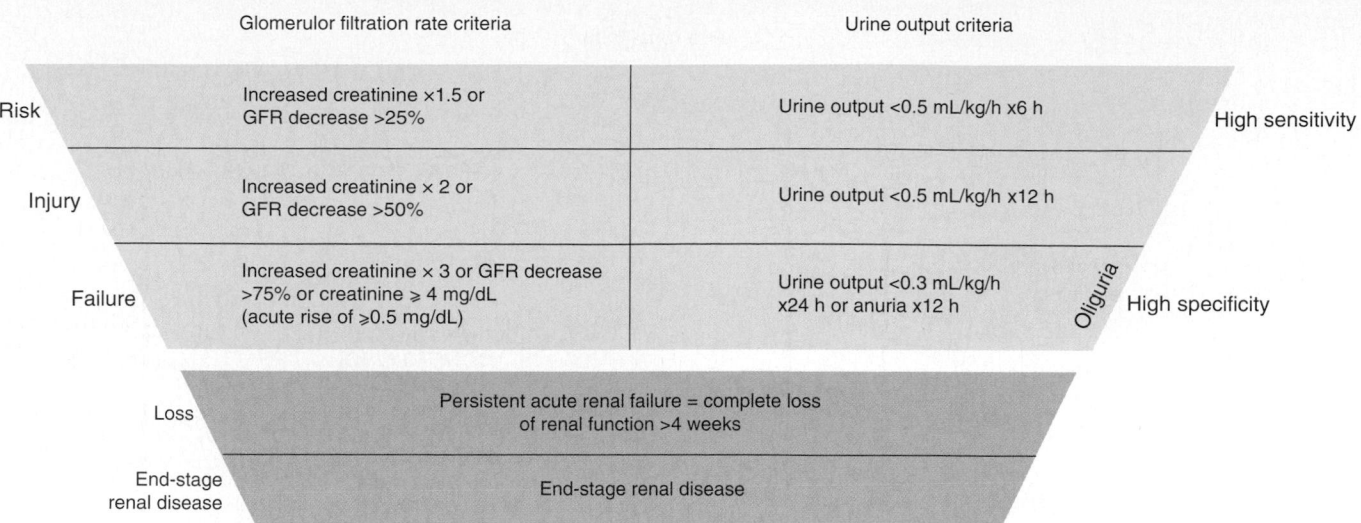

Fig. 17.1   The RIFLE (risk, injury, failure, loss, end-stage renal disease) criteria for the definition and staging of acute renal disease.

Table 17.2   Common causes of the categories of acute kidney injury

Pre-renal	Renal	Post-renal
Sepsis	Prolonged pre-renal AKI	Tumours (pelvic or retroperitoneal)
Hypovolaemia	Rapidly progressive glomerulonephritis	Prostate disease (in men)
Vaso-active drugs[a] (e.g. NSAIDs and ACEi/ARBs)	Acute interstitial nephritis	Renal calculi (obstructing the ureter)

[a]More common in patients with chronic kidney disease; drugs that are usually protective (e.g. ACEi/ARBs) can increase the risk of if a patient has an acute intercurrent illness (e.g. sepsis, diarrhea, acute heart failure).
ACEi, angiotensin-converting enzyme inhibitors; AKI, acute kidney injury; ARB, angiotensin receptor blocker; NSAIDs, non-steroidal anti-inflammatory drugs.

peri-tubular capillaries are downstream of the glomerular capillary bed. Finally, renal cells are highly specialised and are, therefore, predisposed to ischaemic and inflammatory injury.

Pre-renal acute kidney injury

Pre-renal AKI is caused by impaired perfusion of the kidneys with blood and is usually a consequence of decreased intravascular volumes (hypovolaemia) and/or decreased intravascular pressures. Some of the commonest causes of pre-renal AKI are summarised in Fig. 17.2. Perfusion of the kidneys at the level of the microvascular beds (glomerular and tubulo-interstitial) is usually maintained through wide systemic variations in pressure and flow through highly efficient auto-regulatory pathways, including the renin–angiotensin–aldosterone system (RAAS) and regulated prostaglandin synthesis. However, when the systolic blood pressure (BP) drops below 80 mmHg, AKI

may develop. In individuals with CKD or in the elderly, AKI may occur at higher levels of systolic BP. Drugs that inhibit the RAAS, such as angiotensin-converting enzyme (ACE) inhibitors and angiotensin receptor blockers (ARBs), or block the production of prostaglandins, such as non-steroidal anti-inflammatory drugs (NSAIDs), can predispose to the development of pre-renal AKI. These drugs are discussed in more detail in the following sections.

Hypovolaemia

Hypovolaemia results from any condition that causes intravascular fluid depletion, either directly by haemorrhage or indirectly to compensate for extravascular loss. Examples of this include diarrhoea and vomiting, burns and excessive use of diuretics. Hypotension is a secondary effect of significant hypovolaemia.

Hypotension

In addition to hypovolaemia, hypotension can result from pump (cardiac) failure, of which there are a number of causes, the most common of which is ischaemic heart disease. Another important cause is septic shock, where there is peripheral vasodilatation and low peripheral resistance which leads to profound hypotension despite a high cardiac output.

Intra-renal acute kidney injury

Intra-renal acute kidney injury has a variety of causes (see Tables 17.2 and 17.3), most commonly (in >80% of cases) acute tubular necrosis (ATN). ATN usually occurs in patients with sustained pre-renal AKI leading to tubular injury; this is caused by hypotension and hypovolaemia, often in the setting of sepsis and nephrotoxic agents including drugs. Other endogenous sources can cause direct tubular damage, including myoglobin, haemoglobin and immunoglobulin light chains in multiple myeloma.

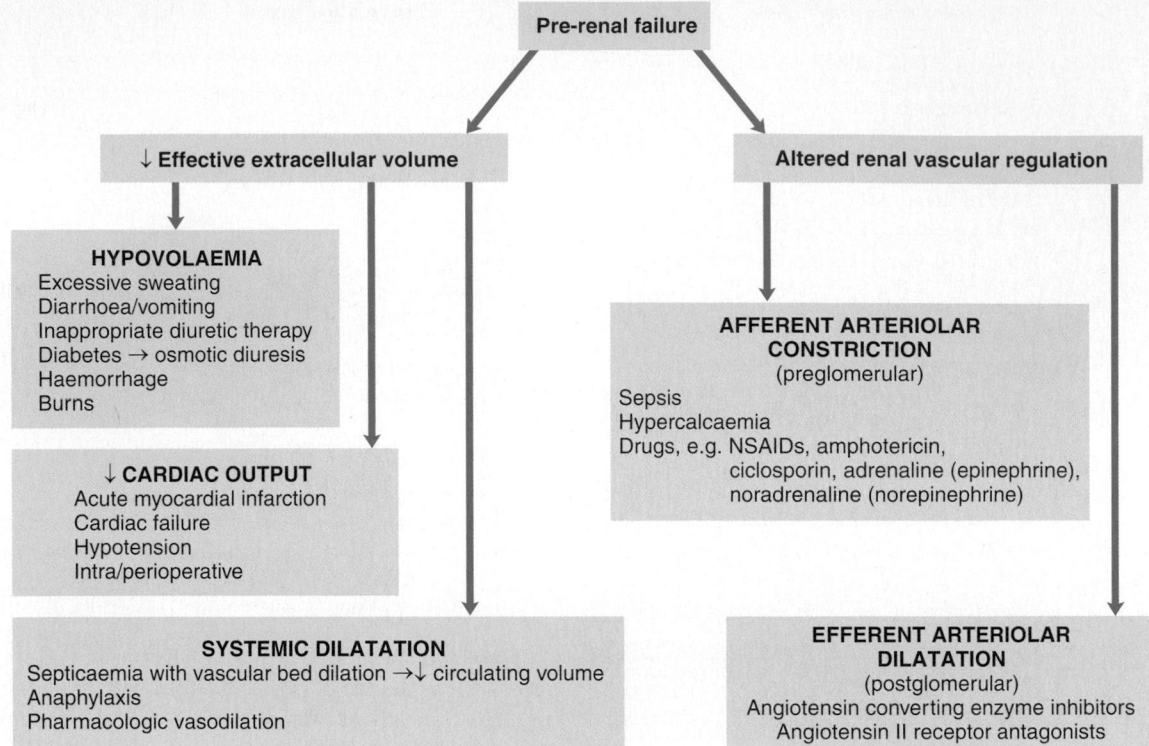

Fig. 17.2 Causes of pre-renal failure.

Acute tubular necrosis

ATN is a diagnosis made by renal biopsy; the findings can include damage to the proximal tubule and the ascending limb of the loop of Henle, interstitial oedema and sparse infiltrating inflammatory cells. Although severe and sustained hypoperfusion can lead to ATN, it usually develops when there is a combination of factors including the presence of one or more of a range of nephrotoxins. These may arise exogenously from drugs or chemical poisons, or from endogenous sources such as haemoglobin, myoglobin, crystals (uric acid, phosphate), immunoglobulin light chains and toxic products from sepsis or tumours (see Table 17.3). Some endogenous toxins may be released as a direct consequence of drug exposure. For example, myoglobin may be released (rhabdomyolysis) following muscle injury or necrosis, hypoxia, infection or after drug treatment, for example, with fibrates and statins, particularly when both are used in combination. The mechanism of the subsequent damage to renal tissue is not fully understood but probably results from a combination of factors including hypoperfusion, haem-catalysed free radical tubular cytotoxicity and haem cast formation and precipitation leading to tubular injury.

Vascular bed and development of acute tubular necrosis. Regional blood flow within the kidney varies, resulting in relatively hypoxic regions such as the outer medulla. This area is also the site of highly metabolically active parts of the nephron. Owing to the relatively poor oxygen supply and high metabolic demands, the outer medulla is at risk of ischaemia, even under normal conditions. The regulation of regional blood flow, and therefore the oxygen supply to these areas, relies upon vasomotor

mechanisms mediated in part by adenosine. Adenosine appears to exert either vasoconstrictor or vasodilator effects within the kidney depending upon the relative distribution of A_1 and A_2 receptors.

Clearly any circumstance that interferes with the delicate balance of blood flow and, therefore, oxygen supply within the kidney can result in ATN because of ischaemia and a greater vulnerability to nephrotoxins. The likelihood of ATN is increased by underlying conditions that predispose to ischaemia such as pre-existing CKD of any cause, atheromatous renovascular disease and cholesterol embolisation from upstream atheromatous plaque rupture.

Common causes of acute tubular necrosis. Table 17.3 shows a summary of some of the common factors encountered clinically that may cause ATN.

Immune and inflammatory renal disease

The kidney is vulnerable to a range of immunological processes that can cause AKI. These are divided into glomerular causes (glomerulonephritis) and interstitial causes (interstitial nephritis). Rarely acute pyelonephritis, which is an infection of renal parenchyma, usually as a consequence of ascending infection, can cause AKI.

Rapidly progressive glomerulonephritis. Glomerulonephritis refers to an inflammatory process within the glomerulus. If that process causes AKI it is called rapidly progressive glomerulonephritis (RPGN). Most cases of RPGN are caused by a small-vessel vasculitis (SVV); this gives a pattern of injury in the glomerulus that is called a focal segmental necrotising glomerulonephritis

Table 17.3 Common clinical factors known to cause acute tubular necrosis

Clinical factor	Mechanism
Hypoperfusion	Reduced oxygen/nutrient supply
Radiocontrast media	Medullary ischaemia may result from contrast media–induced renal vasoconstriction. The high ionic load of contrast media may produce ischaemia, particularly in patients with diabetes and those with myeloma (who produce large quantities of light chain immunoglobulins)
Sepsis	Infection produces endotoxaemia and systemic inflammation in combination with a pre-renal state and nephrotoxins. The immunological response to sepsis involves release of vasoconstrictors and vasodilators (e.g. eicosanoids, nitric oxide) and damage to vascular endothelium with resultant thrombosis
Rhabdomyolysis	Damaged muscles release myoglobin, which can cause ATN through direct nephrotoxicity and by a reduction in blood flow in the outer medulla
Renal transplantation	The procedures and conditions encountered during renal transplantation can induce ischaemic ATN, which can be difficult to distinguish from the nephrotoxic effects of immunosuppressive drug therapy used in these circumstances and rejection
Hepato-renal syndrome	Renal vasoconstriction is frequently seen in patients with end-stage liver disease. Progression to ATN is common
Nephrotoxins	
Aminoglycosides	Aminoglycosides are transported into tubular cells, where they exert a direct nephrotoxic effect. Current dosage regimens recommend once-daily doses, with frequent monitoring of drug levels, to minimise total uptake of aminoglycoside
Amphotericin	Amphotericin appears to cause direct nephrotoxicity by disturbing the permeability of tubular cells. The nephrotoxic effect is dose dependent and minimised by limiting total dose used, by limiting rate of infusion, and by volume loading. These precautions also apply to newer liposomal formulations
Immunosuppressants	Ciclosporin and tacrolimus cause intra-renal vasoconstriction that may result in ischaemic AIN. The mechanism is unclear but enhanced by hypovolaemia and other nephrotoxic drugs
NSAIDs	Vasodilator prostaglandins, mainly E_2, D_2 and I_2 (prostacyclin), produce an increase in blood flow to the glomerulus and medulla. In normal circumstances they play no part in the maintenance of the renal circulation. However, increased amounts of vasoconstrictor substances arise in a variety of clinical conditions such as volume depletion, congestive cardiac failure or hepatic cirrhosis associated with ascites. Maintenance of renal blood flow then becomes more reliant on the release of vasodilatory prostaglandins. Inhibition of prostaglandin synthesis by NSAIDs may cause unopposed arteriolar vasoconstriction, leading to renal hypoperfusion
Cytotoxic chemotherapy	For example, cisplatin
Anaesthetic agents	Methoxyflurane, enflurane
Chemical poisons/naturally occurring poisons	Insecticides, herbicides, alkaloids from plants and fungi, reptile venoms

ATN, Acute tubular necrosis; NSAIDs, non-steroidal anti-inflammatory drugs.

(FSNGN) with crescent proliferation; crescents are the presence of cells and extracellular matrix in Bowman's space. Most cases of FSNGN are caused by anti-neutrophil cytoplasmic antibody (ANCA)-associated SVV. ANCAs refer to the presence of circulating antibodies that are targeted against primary neutrophil cytoplasmic antigens (proteins including proteinase 3 and myeloperoxidase).

The two main types of ANCA-associated SVV are granulomatosis with polyangiitis, previously known as Wegener's granulomatosis, and microscopic polyangiitis. Other important causes of RPGN include Goodpasture's disease, which is caused by antibodies against glomerular basement membrane (anti-GBM antibodies). Systemic lupus erythematosus, which usually affects young women and is more common with black ethnicity, and secondary vasculitis are triggered by drugs, infection and tumours. There are many drug triggers for secondary vasculitis; the commonest clinical presentation is a cutaneous vasculitis, secondary to immune complex deposition. Kidney involvement can occur and has been reported with a range of drugs.

Interstitial nephritis. Interstitial nephritis is thought to be a nephrotoxin-induced hypersensitivity reaction associated with infiltration of inflammatory cells into the interstitium with secondary involvement of the tubules. The nephrotoxins involved

Table 17.4 Differentiating pre-renal from renal acute kidney injury

Laboratory test	Pre-renal	Renal
Urine osmolality (mOsm/kg)	>500	<400
Urine sodium (mEq/L)	<20	>40
Urine/serum creatinine (mmol/L)	>40	<20
Urine/serum urea (mmol/L)	>8	<3
Fractional excretion of sodium (%)	<1	>2

Table 17.5 Factors associated with acute kidney injury

	Volume depletion	Volume overload
History	Thirst Excessive fluid loss (vomiting or diarrhoea) Oliguria	Weight increase Orthopnoea/ nocturnal dyspnea
Physical examination	Dry mucosae ↓ Skin elasticity Tachycardia ↓ Blood pressure ↓ Jugular venous pressure	Ankle swelling Oedema Jugular venous distension Pulmonary crackles Pleural effusion

are usually drugs and/or the toxic products of infection. Drugs that have been most commonly shown to be responsible include NSAIDs, antibiotics (especially penicillins, cephalosporins and quinolones), proton pump inhibitors such as omeprazole, furosemide, allopurinol and azathioprine, although many other drugs have been implicated.

Differentiating pre-renal from renal acute kidney injury

It is sometimes possible to distinguish between cases of pre-renal and renal AKI through examination of biochemical markers (Table 17.4). In renal AKI, the kidneys are generally unable to retain Na$^+$ because of tubular damage. This can be demonstrated by calculating the fractional excretion of sodium (FENa); in practice this is not often done because it lacks sensitivity and specificity, and may be difficult to interpret in the elderly who may have pre-existing concentrating defects.

$$FENa = sodium\ clearance/creatinine\ clearance$$

$$FENa = \frac{urine\ sodium \times serum\ creatinine}{serum\ sodium \times urine\ creatinine}$$

If FENa is less than 1%, this indicates pre-renal AKI with preserved tubular function; if FENa is greater than 1%, this is indicative of ATN. This relationship is less robust if a patient with renal AKI has glycosuria, pre-existing renal disease, has been treated with diuretics or has other drug-related alterations in renal haemodynamics, for example, through use of ACE inhibitors or NSAIDs. One potential use of urinary electrolytes is in the patient with liver disease and AKI, where the diagnosis of hepato-renal syndrome is being considered; one of the diagnostic criteria is a urinary sodium concentration less than 10 mmol/L.

Post-renal acute kidney injury

Post-renal AKI results from obstruction of the urinary tract by a variety of mechanisms. Any mechanical obstruction from the renal pelvis to the urethral orifice can cause post-renal AKI; these can be divided into causes within the ureters (e.g. calculi or clots), a problem within the wall of the ureter (e.g. malignancies or benign strictures) and external compression (e.g. retroperitoneal tumours). It is extremely unusual for drugs to be responsible for post-renal AKI. Practolol-induced retroperitoneal fibrosis resulting in bilateral ureteric obstruction is a rare example.

Clinical manifestations

The signs and symptoms of AKI are often non-specific, and the diagnosis can be confounded by co-existing clinical conditions. The patient may exhibit signs and symptoms of volume depletion or overload, depending upon the precipitating conditions, course of the disease and prior treatment.

Acute kidney injury with volume depletion

In those patients with volume depletion, a classic pathophysiological picture is likely to be present, with tachycardia, postural hypotension, reduced skin turgor and cold extremities (Table 17.5). The most common sign in AKI is oliguria, where urine production declines to <0.5 mL/kg/h for several hours. This is less than the volume of urine required to effectively excrete products of metabolism to maintain a physiological steady state. Therefore, the serum concentration of those substances normally excreted by the kidney will rise and differentially applies to all molecules up to a molecular mass of around 50 kDa. This includes serum creatinine, which at a molecular mass of 113 Da is normally freely filtered by the kidneys, but with loss of kidney function the serum level climbs. Although the term uraemia is still in widespread use, it merely describes a surrogate for the overall metabolic disturbances that accompany AKI; these include excess potassium, hydrogen ions (acidosis) and phosphate in blood. Most cases of AKI are first identified by an abnormal blood test, although some patients may have symptoms that are specifically attributable to AKI; these include nausea, vomiting, diarrhoea, gastro-intestinal haemorrhage, muscle cramps and a declining level of consciousness.

Acute kidney injury with volume overload

In those patients with AKI who have maintained a normal or increased fluid intake as a result of oral or intravenous administration, there may be clinical signs and symptoms of fluid overload (see Table 17.5).

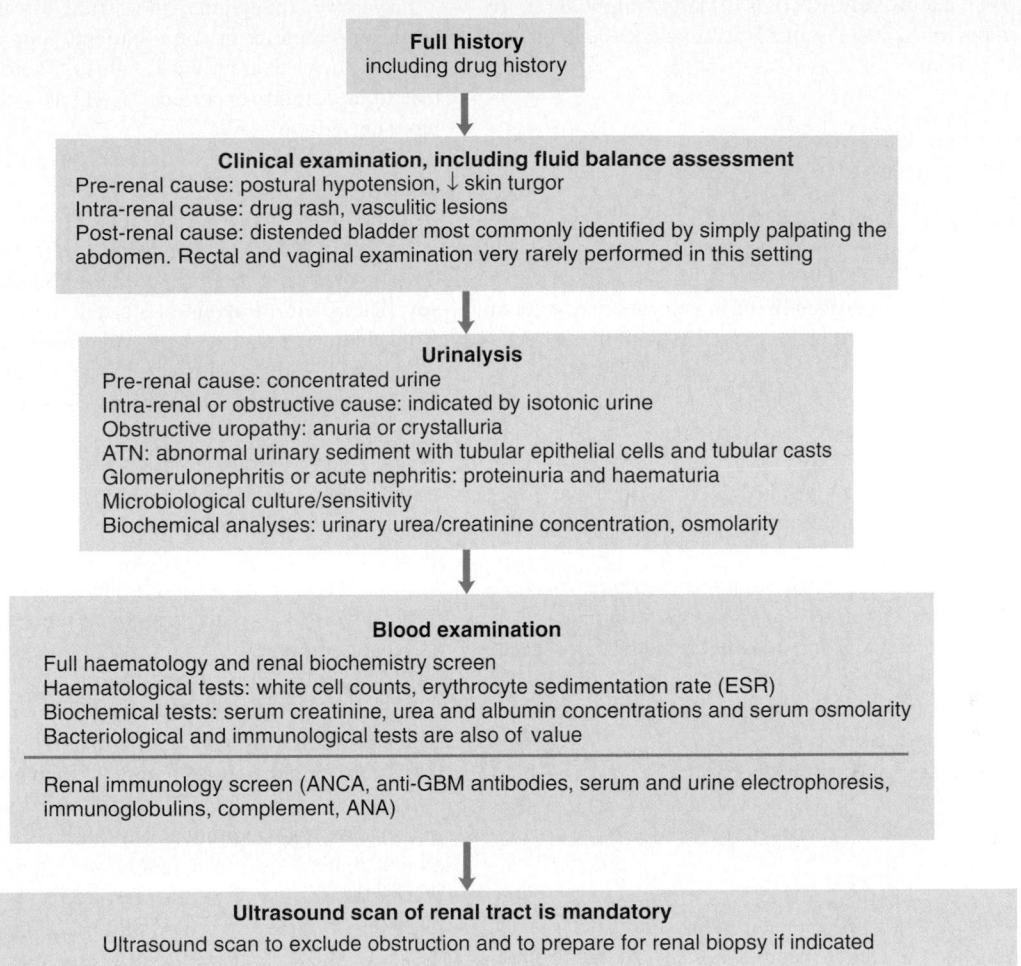

Full history
including drug history

Clinical examination, including fluid balance assessment
Pre-renal cause: postural hypotension, ↓ skin turgor
Intra-renal cause: drug rash, vasculitic lesions
Post-renal cause: distended bladder most commonly identified by simply palpating the abdomen. Rectal and vaginal examination very rarely performed in this setting

Urinalysis
Pre-renal cause: concentrated urine
Intra-renal or obstructive cause: indicated by isotonic urine
Obstructive uropathy: anuria or crystalluria
ATN: abnormal urinary sediment with tubular epithelial cells and tubular casts
Glomerulonephritis or acute nephritis: proteinuria and haematuria
Microbiological culture/sensitivity
Biochemical analyses: urinary urea/creatinine concentration, osmolarity

Blood examination
Full haematology and renal biochemistry screen
Haematological tests: white cell counts, erythrocyte sedimentation rate (ESR)
Biochemical tests: serum creatinine, urea and albumin concentrations and serum osmolarity
Bacteriological and immunological tests are also of value

Renal immunology screen (ANCA, anti-GBM antibodies, serum and urine electrophoresis, immunoglobulins, complement, ANA)

Ultrasound scan of renal tract is mandatory
Ultrasound scan to exclude obstruction and to prepare for renal biopsy if indicated

Fig. 17.3 Investigations of acute kidney injury.
ANA, Anti-nuclear antibody; ANCA, Anti-neutrophil cytoplasmic antibodies; GBM, glomerular basement membrane.

Diagnosis and clinical evaluation

In hospitalised patients, AKI is usually diagnosed incidentally by the detection of increasing serum creatinine and/or a reduction in urine output.

The assessment of renal function is described in detail in Chapter 18. However, unless a patient is at steady state, measurement of serum creatinine does not provide a reliable guide to renal function. For example, serum creatinine levels will usually rise by only 50–100 mmol/L/day following complete loss of renal function in a previously normal patient. Thus changes in serum creatinine are not sufficiently responsive to serve as a practical indicator of a rapidly changing glomerular filtration rate (GFR), particularly in AKI in critical care scenarios.

In the hospital situation, when AKI is detected incidentally, the cause(s) of the condition, such as fluid depletion (hypovolaemia), infection or the use of nephrotoxic drugs, are often apparent on close examination of the clinical history. The development of AKI in this setting is more likely to occur in people with pre-existing CKD. People with normal baseline kidney function usually need to sustain at least two separate triggers for the development of AKI; for example, hypovolaemia will rarely cause AKI in this setting, but when hypovolaemia occurs in the presence of nephrotoxic drugs, then AKI may occur. In patients with pre-existing CKD, AKI (i.e. acute on chronic renal failure) can occur in patients with one trigger. By definition, the worse the baseline kidney function, the smaller the trigger required for the development of AKI.

Irrespective of the presentation of AKI, it is wise to consider the complete differential diagnosis in all people; active exclusion of post-renal AKI and immune and inflammatory AKI should be considered in all cases. In AKI without an obvious precipitating pre- or post-renal cause, there is a greater need to consider these causes. Although the majority of patients have ATN, other causes such as RPGN, interstitial nephritis, multiple myeloma or urinary tract obstruction must be screened for and systematically excluded. In addition to supportive care that is generic for all causes of AKI, disease-specific treatment may also be required. The investigation of AKI is outlined in Fig. 17.3.

Various other parameters should be monitored through the course of AKI. Fluid balance charts may be inaccurate and should not be relied upon exclusively. Records of daily weight are more reliable indicators of volume status but are dependent on the mobility of the patient.

Monitoring fluid balance in acute kidney disease

Maintaining appropriate fluid balance in AKI is a critical component of the clinical management of the patient. Detailed clinical assessment includes:

1. measurement of BP, which needs to be interpreted in respect of the baseline for the affected patient together with the patient's heart rate;
2. auscultation of the heart for the presence of third (and fourth) heart sounds, the presence of which indicate cardiac strain associated with fluid overload;
3. presence of added sounds in the chest, in particular fine inspiratory crackles that are found in some patients with pulmonary oedema;
4. a chest X-ray for the presence of pulmonary oedema;
5. pulse oximetry to assess arterial oxygen saturation;
6. although the presence of pitting oedema of the legs or sacrum indicates longer-term fluid overload, it may also be a useful marker of overall endothelial function and the potential for extravascular fluid accumulation;
7. evaluation for decreased skin turgor, which is a sign of fluid loss.

Intravascular monitoring

Central venous pressure (CVP) can be measured following insertion of a central venous catheter and is a measure of the pressure in the large systemic veins and the right atrium produced by venous return. CVP assesses circulating volume and, therefore, the degree of fluid deficit, and reduces the risk of pulmonary oedema following over-rapid transfusion. CVP should usually be maintained within the normal range of 5–12 cm H_2O.

Most patients with AKI do not require invasive monitoring to the extent described earlier and recover with supportive care based on careful clinical observations.

Monitoring key parameters in acute kidney disease

Serum electrolytes, including potassium, bicarbonate, calcium, phosphate and acid–base balance, should be measured on a daily basis. In patients with severe AKI, acid–base balance may need to be assessed every few hours because this may direct fluid replacement, respiratory support and dialysis treatment. Patients should be weighed daily as this is an important measure of fluid balance.

Course and prognosis
Pre-renal acute kidney injury

The majority of cases will recover within days of onset following prompt correction of the underlying causes. The urine output improves and waste products of metabolism are cleared by the kidneys. Even though the kidney function usually stabilises to the pre-event baseline, in some patients long-term kidney function resets to lower than previous values. There is excellent evidence that some patients experience CKD as a consequence of one or more episodes of AKI.

ATN may be divided into three phases. The first is the oliguric phase (<400 mL/day of urine produced), where patients have sustained pre-renal AKI and move from the potential for early reversibility to a situation where uraemia and hyperkalaemia develop and the patient may die unless renal replacement therapy (RRT) with dialysis is started. The oliguric phase is usually no longer than 7–14 days but may last for up to 6 weeks. This is followed by a diuretic phase, which is characterised by a urine output that rises over a few days to several litres per day. This phase lasts for up to 7 days and corresponds to the recommencement of tubular function. The onset of this phase is associated with an improving prognosis unless the patient sustains an intercurrent infection or a vascular event. Finally, the patient enters a recovery phase, where tubular cells regenerate slowly over several months, although the GFR often does not return to initial levels. The elderly recover renal function more slowly and less completely.

The mortality rate of AKI varies according to the cause but increases when AKI occurs in patients with multi-organ failure, where mortality rates of up to 70% are seen. Higher mortality rates are seen in patients aged more than 60 years.

Death resulting from uraemia and hyperkalaemia is very uncommon. Consequently, the major causes of death associated with AKI are septicaemia and intercurrent acute vascular events such as myocardial infarction and stroke. High circulating levels of uraemic toxins that occur in AKI result in general debility. These, together with the significant number of invasive procedures such as bladder catheterisation and intravascular cannulation, which are necessary in the management of AKI, leave such patients prone to infection and septicaemia. Uraemic gastro-intestinal haemorrhage is a recognised consequence of AKI, probably as a result of reduced mucosal cell turnover.

Post-renal acute kidney injury

Prompt identification and relief of the obstruction is important. The prognosis is then dependent on the underlying cause of the obstruction of the renal tract and the baseline to which the kidney function returns after the obstruction has been relieved. If the underlying problem is benign, then there may be no long-term adverse consequences. However, if the cause of the obstruction is due to an underlying malignancy, then long-term survival is dependent on whether this can be cured.

Angiotensin-converting enzyme inhibitors and angiotensin receptor blockers in acute kidney injury

ACE inhibitors and ARBs are not directly nephrotoxic and can be used in most patients with kidney disease. However, profound hypotension can occur if they are initiated in susceptible patients such as those who are receiving high-dose diuretics as treatment for fluid overload. This might result in the development of pre-renal AKI. It is, therefore, wise to monitor BP and carefully titrate dosages whilst monitoring renal function in such patients. Nonetheless, it is common to see increases in serum creatinine levels of up to 25% on initiation of an ACE inhibitor or ARB, and this is not necessarily a cause for discontinuing therapy with these agents.

ACE inhibitor use is, however, absolutely contraindicated when a patient has bilateral renal artery stenosis, or renal artery stenosis in a patient with a single functioning kidney. If an ACE inhibitor or ARB is initiated under these circumstances, then pre-renal AKI may ensue. This may occur because the renin–angiotensin system is stimulated by low renal perfusion resulting from stenotic lesions in the arteries supplying the kidneys, most often at the origin of the renal artery from the abdominal aorta. Angiotensin II is produced which causes renal vasoconstriction, in part, through increased efferent arteriolar tone. This creates a 'back pressure' which paradoxically maintains glomerular filtration pressure in an otherwise poorly perfused kidney. If angiotensin II production is inhibited by an ACE inhibitor, or the effect is blocked by an ARB, then efferent arteriole dilatation will result. Because increased efferent vascular tone maintains filtration in such patients, then the overall result of ACE inhibitor or ARB therapy will be to reduce or shut down filtration at the glomerulus and put the patient at risk of pre-renal AKI (Fig. 17.4).

Importantly, many patients with renal artery stenosis have not been identified. Consequently this is one of the reasons why patients should have kidney function testing before commencing an ACE inhibitor or ARB, and a repeat kidney function test 7–14 days after starting the drug or after a dose increase. In patients with an increase in creatinine level of more than 25%, the drug should be stopped and referral to a nephrologist considered for further investigation and management.

Management

The aim of the medical management of a patient with AKI is to stabilise the patient to allow recovery of kidney function. Effective management of AKI depends upon a rapid diagnosis. If the underlying acute deterioration in renal function is detected early enough, it is often possible to prevent progression. If the condition is advanced, however, management consists mainly of supportive strategies, with close monitoring and appropriate correction of metabolic, fluid and electrolyte disturbances. Patients with severe AKI often require RRT with dialysis. Specific therapies that promote recovery of ischaemic renal damage remain under investigation. Patients with immune-mediated causes of AKI should be treated with appropriate immunosuppressant regimens to treat the underlying cause of the AKI. Post-renal AKI is treated by relieving the obstruction.

Early preventive and supportive strategies

Identification of patients at risk

Any patient who has concurrent or pre-existing conditions that increase the risk of development and progression of AKI must be identified, and this includes those with pre-existing CKD, diabetes, jaundice, myeloma and the elderly. These patients either have baseline impaired renal function (CKD) or are sensitised to the development of AKI by the comorbid condition. Meticulous attention to fluid balance, assessment of infection and the use of drugs are crucial to minimise the risk of development of AKI.

Withdrawal and avoidance of nephrotoxic agents

Irrespective of whether the aetiology of the AKI directly involves nephrotoxic drugs, the drug and treatment regimens should be examined so that potential nephrotoxins are withdrawn. Particular care

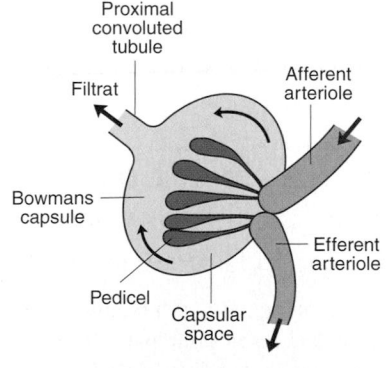
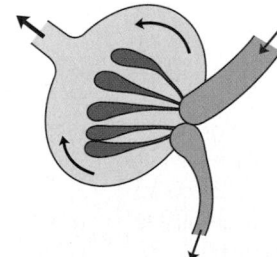
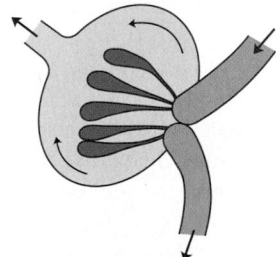

A. Normal glomerulus with efferent arteriolar tone (narrowed outflow of blood) causing a 'back pressure' producing filtration with water and solutes progressing through the capsular space to the proximal convoluted tubule.

B. Glomerulus in an untreated patient with renal artery stenosis. There is increased efferent arteriolar tone caused by the vasoconstrictive actions of angiotensin II. The efferent arteriole is narrowed more than normal promoting filtration.

C. Glomerulus in a patient with renal artery stenosis but treated with an ACE inhibitor or angiotensin receptor blocker. Blockade of the vasoconstrictive effects of angiotensin II has produced dilation of the efferent arteriole resulting in failure of the back pressure promoting filtration.

Fig. 17.4 Actions of angiotensin-converting enzyme (ACE) inhibition and angiotensin receptor blockade in patients with renal artery stenosis.

should be taken with ACE inhibitors, NSAIDs, radiological contrast media and aminoglycosides. The doses should be adjusted of any drugs or their active metabolites that are excreted by the kidneys.

Optimisation of renal perfusion

Initial treatment should include rapid correction of fluid and electrolyte balance to maximise renal perfusion. In patients for whom it is difficult to assess fluid balance by use of clinical examination, a urinary catheter may be placed in order that fluid losses may be easily measured. With the recent focus on the prevention of catheter-related bacteraemia, central lines are seldom used outside specialist renal and intensive care units, but they should be considered in patients with multi-organ failure.

A diagnosis of pre-renal AKI caused by renal underperfusion secondary to hypovolaemia and/or hypotension implies that restoration of renal perfusion would reverse impairment by improving renal blood flow, reducing renal vasoconstriction and flushing nephrotoxins from the kidney. The use of crystalloids in the form of 0.9% sodium chloride is an appropriate initial choice of intravenous fluid because it replaces both water and sodium ions in a concentration approximately equal to serum. The usual approach to fluid replacement is to use 250–500 mL bolus fluids up to a maximum initial volume of 2 L. If the patient does not respond to this, then senior medical review is required. In the patient with sustained hypotension that does not respond to a fluid challenge, the patient may need to move to an intensive care unit and be commenced on vasoconstrictor and inotropic drugs (e.g. noradrenaline) to improve BP.

The effect of fluid replacement on urine flow and intravascular pressures should be carefully monitored. Over-hydration of sick patients is very common and associated with an increased mortality risk. There is no evidence that colloids such as gelofusine or albumin provide any additional benefit for volume expansion and renal recovery over the use of crystalloids. A National Institute of Health and Care Excellence (NICE, 2013) intravenous fluid guideline provides detailed guidance.

The use of inotropes such as noradrenaline and cardiac doses of dopamine should be restricted to non-renal indications.

Establishing and maintaining an adequate diuresis

Although loop diuretics (most commonly furosemide) may facilitate the management of fluid overload and hyperkalaemia in early or established AKI, there is no evidence that these agents are effective for the prevention of, or early recovery from, AKI. It is reasonable to use these agents whilst the urine output is maintained because this provides space for intravenous drugs and parenteral feeding including oral supplements. In experimental settings loop diuretics decrease renal tubular cell metabolic demands and increase renal blood flow by stimulating the release of renal prostaglandins, a haemodynamic effect inhibited by NSAIDs. However, there is no demonstrable impact on clinical outcomes. Indeed, diuretic therapy should only be initiated in the context of fluid overload. If not, any diuresis might produce a negative fluid balance and precipitate or exacerbate a pre-renal state.

Doses of up to 100 mg/h of furosemide can be given as bolus injections or as an infusion. Higher infusion rates may cause transient deafness. There is probably little practical difference between using bolus intravenous doses of furosemide or a continuous infusion.

The addition of small oral doses of metolazone has been used for diuretic purposes in patients with renal impairment and volume overload. Metolazone is a weak thiazide diuretic alone but produces a synergistic action with loop diuretics. It should be used with great care because it may initiate a profound diuresis and the patient can rapidly experience intravascular depletion and worsen renal failure.

Mannitol. Mannitol has historically been recommended for the treatment of AKI. The rationale for using mannitol in AKI arises from the concept that tubular debris may contribute to oliguria. There is no evidence for mannitol-producing benefit in AKI over and above aggressive hydration. Indeed, mannitol can cause volume overload. Consequently, mannitol is now not recommended for patients with AKI.

Dopamine. Historically, dopamine has been recommended at low dose to improve renal blood flow and urine output. Dopamine at low dose acts as a renal vasodilator in normal kidneys, but in renal failure it is a renal vasoconstrictor even at a low dose. This translates into no demonstrable clinical benefit and it should no longer be used. Dopamine has α- and β-adrenergic effects. Fenoldopam, a pure dopaminergic D_1 agonist, has been investigated in a range of clinical trials; the results have not currently demonstrated a trend towards benefit in recovery of renal function from AKI (Gillies et al., 2015).

Drug therapy and renal auto-regulation

Intra-renal blood flow is controlled by an auto-regulatory mechanism unique to the kidney called tubuloglomerular feedback. This mechanism produces arteriolar constriction in response to an increased solute load to the distal nephrons. GFR and kidney workload are thus reduced. It has been proposed that oliguria is an adaptive response to renal ischaemia, and therapy designed to improve GFR would increase solute load to the nephrons and might increase kidney workload and worsen AKI. Clearly, reversal of a pre-renal state with fluids is a logical therapeutic aim.

Non-dialysis treatment of established acute kidney injury

Uraemia and intravascular volume overload

In AKI (and CKD) the symptoms of uraemia include nausea, vomiting and anorexia, and result principally from accumulation of toxic products of protein metabolism including urea.

Unfortunately, because uraemia causes anorexia, nausea and vomiting, many severely ill patients are unable to tolerate any kind of diet. In these patients and those who are catabolic, the use of enteral or parenteral nutrition should be considered at an early stage.

Intravascular fluid overload must be managed by restricting NaCl intake to about 1–2 g/day if the patient is not hyponatraemic and total fluid intake to less than 1 L/day plus the volume of urine and/or loss from dialysis. Care should be taken with the so-called low-salt products, because these usually contain KCl, which will exacerbate hyperkalaemia.

Hyperkalaemia

Hyperkalaemia is a particular problem in AKI not only because urinary excretion is reduced but also because intracellular potassium may be released. Rapid rises in extracellular potassium are to be expected when there is tissue damage, as in burns, crush injuries and sepsis. Acidosis also aggravates hyperkalaemia by provoking potassium leakage from healthy cells. The condition may be life-threatening, causing cardiac arrhythmias, and, if untreated, can result in asystolic cardiac arrest.

Dietary potassium should be restricted to less than 40 mmol/day, and potassium supplements and potassium-sparing diuretics removed from the treatment schedule. Emergency treatment is necessary if the serum potassium level reaches 7.0 mmol/L (reference range 3.5–5.5 mmol/L) or if there are the progressive changes in the electrocardiogram (ECG) associated with hyperkalaemia. These include tall, peaked T waves, reduced P waves with increased QRS complexes or the 'sine wave' appearance that often presages cardiac arrest (see Chapter 18, Fig. 18.11).

Emergency treatment of hyperkalaemia consists of the following:
1. 10–30 mL (2.25–6.75 mmol) of calcium gluconate 10% intravenously over 5–10 minutes: This improves myocardial stability but has no effect on the serum potassium levels. The protective effect begins in minutes but is short-lived (<1 hour), although the dose can be repeated.
2. 50 mL of 50% glucose together with 8–12 units of soluble insulin over 10 minutes: Endogenous insulin, stimulated by a glucose load or administered intravenously, stimulates intracellular potassium uptake, thus removing it from the serum. The effect becomes apparent after 15–30 minutes, peaks after about 1 hour, and lasts for 2–3 hours and will decrease serum potassium levels by around 1 mmol/L.
3. Nebulised salbutamol has also been used to lower potassium; however, this is not effective for all patients and does not permanently lower potassium. If used it is seen as a temporary emergency measure.

Acidosis

The inability of the kidney to excrete hydrogen ions may result in a metabolic acidosis. This may contribute to hyperkalaemia. It may be treated orally with sodium bicarbonate 1–6 g/day in divided doses (although this is not appropriate for acute metabolic acidosis seen in AKI), or 50–100 mmol of bicarbonate ions (preferably as isotonic sodium bicarbonate 1.4% or 1.26%, 250–500 mL over 15–60 minutes) intravenously may be used. The administration of bicarbonate in acidotic patients will also tend to reduce serum potassium concentrations. Bicarbonate will cause an increase in intracellular Na^+ through activation of the cell membrane Na^+/H^+ exchanger, which promotes increased activity of Na/K ATPase producing increased intracellular sequestration of K^+.

If calcium gluconate is used to treat hyperkalaemia, care should be taken not to mix it with sodium bicarbonate (by giving this through the same intravenous access site) because the resulting calcium bicarbonate forms an insoluble precipitate. If elevation of serum sodium or fluid overload precludes the use of sodium bicarbonate, extreme acidosis (serum bicarbonate of <10 mmol/L) is best treated by dialysis.

Hypocalcaemia

Calcium malabsorption, probably secondary to disordered vitamin D metabolism, can occur in AKI. Hypocalcaemia usually remains asymptomatic, as tetany of skeletal muscles or convulsions does not normally occur until serum concentrations are as low as 1.6–1.7 mmol/L (reference range 2.20–2.55 mmol/L). Should it become necessary, oral calcium supplementation with calcium carbonate is usually adequate, and although vitamin D may be used to treat the hypocalcaemia of AKI, it rarely has to be added. Effervescent calcium tablets should be avoided because they contain a high sodium or potassium load.

Hyperphosphataemia

Because phosphate is normally excreted by the kidney, hyperphosphataemia can occur in AKI but rarely requires treatment. Should it become necessary to treat, phosphate-binding agents may be used to retain phosphate ions in the gut. The most commonly used agents are calcium containing, such as calcium carbonate or calcium acetate, and are given with food. For further information, see Chapter 18.

Infection

Patients with AKI are prone to infection and septicaemia, which can ultimately cause death. Bladder catheters, central catheters and even peripheral intravenous lines should be used with care to reduce the chance of bacterial invasion. Leucocytosis is sometimes seen in AKI and does not necessarily imply infection. However, pyrexia must be immediately investigated and treated with appropriate antibiotic therapy if accompanied by toxic symptoms such as disorientation or hypotensive episodes. Samples from blood, urine and any other material such as catheter tips should be sent for culture before antibiotics are started. Antibiotic therapy should be broad spectrum until a causative organism is identified.

Other problems

Uraemic gastro-intestinal erosions

Uraemic gastro-intestinal erosions are a recognised consequence of AKI, probably as a result of reduced mucosal cell turnover owing to high circulating levels of uraemic toxins. Proton pump inhibitors and H_2 antagonists are effective. However, proton pump inhibitors should be used with caution in hospitals where there are significant rates of *Clostridium difficile* diarrhoea, because they may predispose to the development of this organism. H_2 antagonists are an appropriate alternative. In addition, there is increasing epidemiological evidence linking proton pump inhibitors with kidney disease (Lazarus et al., 2016).

Nutrition

There are two major constraints concerning the nutrition of patients with AKI:
- patients may be anorexic, vomiting and too ill to eat;
- oliguria associated with renal failure limits the volume of enteral or parenteral nutrition that can be safely given.

The introduction of dialysis or haemofiltration allows fluid to be removed easily and, therefore, makes parenteral nutrition possible. Large volumes of fluid may then be administered without producing fluid overload. A requirement for parenteral nutrition is rare, but where needed the factors to be considered include fluid balance, calorie/protein requirements, electrolyte balance/requirements, and vitamin and mineral requirements.

The basic calorie requirements are similar in patients with AKI irrespective of whether they require dialysis, although the need for protein may occasionally be increased in haemodialysis and haemofiltration because of amino acid loss. In all situations, protein is usually supplied as 12–20 g/day of an essential amino acid formulation, although individual requirements may vary.

Electrolyte-free amino acid solutions should be used in parenteral nutrition formulations for patients with AKI because they allow the addition of electrolytes as appropriate. Potassium and sodium requirements can be calculated on an individual basis depending on serum levels. There is usually no need to try to normalise serum calcium and phosphate levels because they will stabilise with the appropriate therapy or, if necessary, with haemofiltration or dialysis. Water-soluble vitamins are removed by dialysis and haemofiltration, but the standard daily doses normally included in parenteral nutrition fluids more than compensate for this loss. Magnesium and zinc supplementation may be required, not only because tissue repair often increases requirements but also because they may be lost during dialysis or haemofiltration.

It is necessary to monitor the serum urea, creatinine and electrolyte levels daily to make the appropriate alterations in the required nutritional support. The glucose concentration should also be checked daily because patients in renal failure sometimes develop insulin resistance. The plasma pH should be checked initially to determine whether addition of amino acid solutions is causing or aggravating metabolic acidosis. It is also valuable to check calcium, phosphate and albumin levels regularly, and when practical, daily weighing gives a useful guide to fluid balance.

Renal replacement therapy

RRT is indicated in a patient with AKI when kidney function is so poor that life is at risk. However, it is desirable to introduce RRT early in AKI, because complications and mortality are reduced if the serum urea level is kept to less than 35 mmol/L. Generally, RRT is urgently indicated in AKI to:

1. remove uraemic toxins when severe symptoms are apparent, for example, impaired consciousness, seizures, pericarditis and rapidly developing peripheral neuropathy;
2. remove fluid resistant to diuretics, for example, pulmonary oedema;
3. correct electrolyte and acid–base imbalances, for example, hyperkalaemia greater than 6.5 or 5.5–6.5 mmol/L where there are ECG changes, increasing acidosis (pH < 7.1 or serum bicarbonate < 10 mmol/L) despite bicarbonate therapy, or where bicarbonate is not tolerated because of fluid overload.

Forms of renal replacement therapy

The types of RRTs used in clinical practice for AKI (and with the addition of kidney transplantation for end-stage renal failure secondary to CKD) are:
- haemodialysis
- haemofiltration
- haemodiafiltration
- peritoneal dialysis

Although the basic principles of these replacement therapies are similar, clearance rates, that is, the extent of solute removal, vary.

In all types of dialysis, blood is presented to a dialysis solution across some form of semi-permeable membrane that allows free movement of low molecular weight compounds. The processes by which movement of substances occur are:
- *Diffusion:* Diffusion depends upon concentration differences between blood and dialysate and molecule size. Water and low molecular weight solutes (up to a molecular weight of about 10,000) move through pores in the semi-permeable membrane to establish equilibrium. Smaller molecules can be cleared from blood more effectively as they move more easily through pores in the membrane.
- *Ultrafiltration:* A pressure gradient (either +ve or −ve) across a semi-permeable membrane will produce a net directional movement of fluid from relative high- to low-pressure regions. The quantity of fluid dialysed is the ultrafiltration volume.
- *Convection:* Any molecule carried by ultrafiltrate may move passively with the flow by convection. Larger molecules are cleared more effectively by convection.

Haemodialysis

In haemodialysis, the form of vascular access used in AKI is a dialysis line. This is placed in a vein (the jugular, femoral or subclavian), which has an arterial lumen through which the blood is removed from the patient and a venous lumen by which it is returned to the patient after passing through a dialyser. The terms arterial and venous lumen can be misleading because both lumens are situated in the same vein. They are part of the same line which bifurcates and has two lumens: the longer lumen is the 'arterial' lumen, and the shorter the 'venous' lumen.

Heparin is added to the blood as it leaves the body to prevent the dialyser clotting. Blood is then actively pumped through the artificial kidney before being returned to the patient (Fig. 17.5). In those patients at high risk of haemorrhage, the amount of heparin used can be reduced or even avoided altogether. The dialyser consists of a cartridge comprising a bundle of hollow tubes (hollow fibre dialyser) made of a synthetic semi-permeable membrane. Dialysis fluid flows around the membrane countercurrent (opposite) to the flow of blood to maximise diffusion gradients. The dialysis solution is essentially a mixture of electrolytes in water with a composition approximating to extracellular fluid into which solutes diffuse. The ionic concentration of the dialysis fluid can be manipulated to control the rate and extent of electrolyte transfer. Calcium and bicarbonate concentrations can also be increased in dialysis fluid to promote diffusion into blood as replacement therapy. By manipulating the hydrostatic pressure of the dialysate and blood circuits, the extent and rate of water removal by ultrafiltration can be controlled.

Haemodialysis can be performed in either intermittent or continuous schedules. The latter regimen is preferable in the critical care situation, providing 24-hour control and minimising swings in blood volume and electrolyte composition that are found using intermittent regimens. The haemodialysis described in this section is indistinguishable from that used as maintenance therapy for many patients with end-stage renal failure; the method of access in this group is often via an arterio-venous fistula (see Chapter 18).

The capital cost of haemodialysis is considerable, requires specially trained staff and is seldom undertaken outside a renal unit. It does, however, rapidly treat renal failure and is, therefore, essential in hypercatabolic renal failure where urea is produced faster than, for example, it could be removed by peritoneal dialysis. Haemodialysis can also be used in patients who have recently undergone abdominal surgery in whom peritoneal dialysis would be ill advised.

Haemofiltration

Haemofiltration is an alternative technique to dialysis where simplicity of use, fine fluid balance control and low cost have ensured its widespread application in the treatment of AKI.

A similar arrangement to haemodialysis is employed, but dialysis fluid is not used. The hydrostatic pressure of the blood drives a filtrate, similar to interstitial fluid, across a high-permeability dialyser (passes substances of molecular weight up to 30,000) by ultrafiltration. Solute clearance occurs by convection. Commercially prepared haemofiltration fluid may then be introduced into the filtered blood in quantities sufficient to maintain optimal fluid balance. As with haemodialysis, haemofiltration can be intermittent or continuous. In continuous arterio-venous haemofiltration, blood is diverted, usually from the femoral artery, and returned to the femoral vein; this is now very seldom used.

In continuous venovenous haemofiltration, a dual-lumen vascular catheter is inserted into a vein (as described earlier). Blood is removed from the body via the distal lumen (the one farthest from the right side of the heart) in a process assisted by a blood pump, passed through a haemofilter and returned to the body via the proximal lumen. In slow, continuous ultrafiltration, the process is performed so slowly that no fluid substitution is necessary.

In addition to avoiding the expense and complexity of haemodialysis, this system enables continuous but gradual removal of fluid, thereby allowing very fine control of fluid balance in addition to electrolyte control and removal of metabolites. This control of fluid balance often facilitates the use of parenteral nutrition. Because of the advantages of haemofiltration over peritoneal dialysis and haemodialysis, continuous haemofiltration is currently the most common type of RRT used in patients in intensive care units.

Haemodiafiltration

Haemodiafiltration is a technique that combines the ability to clear small molecules, as in haemodialysis, with the large-molecule clearance of haemofiltration. It is more expensive than traditional haemodialysis, but does offer potential benefits. Although some studies suggest that haemodiafiltration may provide a clinical benefit compared with haemofiltration or haemodialysis, this is controversial (Borthwick et al., 2017). However, the enhanced combined control of fluid and solute removal provided by this technique means that it is being increasingly used in clinical practice. However, the evidence base for the optimum haemodialysis, haemofiltration or haemodiafiltration approach in patients with AKI is of poor quality, and further clinical trials are required to identify the best treatment (Borthwick et al., 2017).

Acute peritoneal dialysis

Acute peritoneal dialysis is rarely used now for AKI except in circumstances where haemodialysis is unavailable. A semi-rigid catheter is inserted into the abdominal cavity. Warmed sterile peritoneal dialysis fluid (typically 1–2 L) is instilled into the abdomen, left for a period of about 30 minutes (dwell time) and then drained into a collecting bag (Fig. 17.6). This procedure may be performed manually or by semi-automatic equipment. The process may be repeated up to 20 times a day, depending on the condition of the patient.

Acute peritoneal dialysis is relatively cheap and simple, and does not require specially trained staff or the facilities of a renal unit. It does, however, have the disadvantages of being

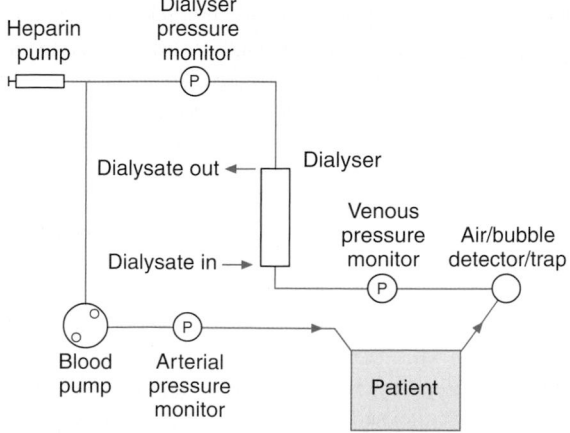

Fig. 17.5 A typical dialysis circuit representing emergency dialysis via a dialysis catheter.

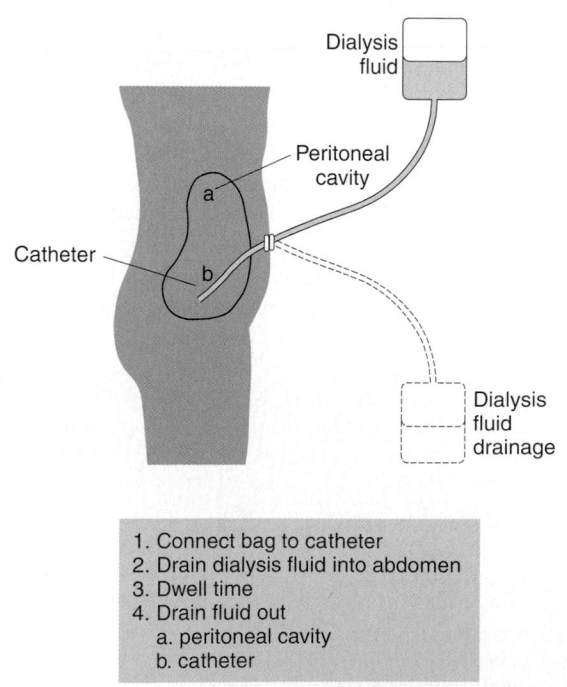

Fig. 17.6 Procedure for peritoneal dialysis.

uncomfortable and tiring for the patient. It is associated with a high incidence of peritonitis and permits protein loss, because albumin crosses the peritoneal membrane.

Drug dosage in renal replacement therapy

Whether a drug is significantly removed by dialysis or haemofiltration is an important clinical issue. Drugs that are not removed may well require dose reduction to avoid accumulation and minimise toxic effects. Alternatively, drug removal may be significant and require a dosage supplement to ensure an adequate therapeutic effect is maintained. In general, because haemodialysis, peritoneal dialysis and haemofiltration depend on filtration, the process of drug removal can be considered analogous to glomerular filtration. Table 17.6 gives an indication of approximate clearances of common renal replacement therapies, which for continuous regimens provide an estimate for the creatinine clearance of the system.

Drug characteristics that favour clearance by the glomerulus are similar to those that favour clearance by dialysis or haemofiltration. These include:
- low molecular weight
- high water solubility
- low protein binding
- small volume of distribution
- low metabolic clearance

Unfortunately, a number of other factors inherent in the dialysis process affect clearance; they include:
- duration of dialysis procedure,
- rate of blood flow to dialyser,
- surface area and porosity of dialyser,
- composition and flow rate of dialysate.

For peritoneal dialysis other factors come into play and include:
- rate of peritoneal exchange,
- concentration gradient between plasma and dialysate.

In view of the above, it is usually possible to predict whether a drug will be removed by dialysis, but it is very difficult to quantify the process except by direct measurement, which is rarely practical. Consequently, a definitive, comprehensive guide to drug dosage in dialysis does not exist. However, limited data for specific drugs are available in the literature, whereas many drug manufacturers have information on the dialysability of their products and some include dosage recommendations in their summaries of product characteristics. The most practical method for treating patients undergoing dialysis is to assemble appropriate dosage guidelines for a range of drugs likely to be used in patients with renal impairment and attempt to restrict use to these.

Because drug clearance by haemofiltration is more predictable than in dialysis, it is possible that standardised guidelines on drug elimination may become available. In the interim, a set of individual drug dosage guidelines similar to those described earlier would be useful in practice.

Factors affecting drug use

How the drug to be used is absorbed, distributed, metabolised and excreted, and whether it is intrinsically nephrotoxic are all factors that must be considered. The pharmacokinetic behaviour of many drugs may be altered in renal failure.

Absorption

Oral absorption in AKI may be reduced by vomiting or diarrhoea, although this is frequently of limited clinical significance.

Metabolism

The main hepatic pathways of drug metabolism appear unaffected in renal impairment. The kidney is also a site of metabolism in the body, but the effect of renal impairment is clinically important in only two situations. The first involves the conversion of 25-hydroxycholecalciferol to 1,25-dihydroxycholecalciferol (the active form of vitamin D) in the kidney, a process that is impaired in renal failure. Patients with AKI occasionally require vitamin D replacement therapy, and this should be in the form of 1α-hydroxycholecalciferol (alfacalcidol) or 1,25-dihydroxycholecalciferol (calcitriol). The latter is the drug of choice in the presence of concomitant hepatic impairment. The second situation involves the metabolism of insulin. The kidney is the major site of insulin metabolism, and the insulin requirements of patients with diabetes with AKI are often reduced.

Distribution

Changes in drug distribution may be altered by fluctuations in the degree of hydration or by alterations in tissue or serum protein binding. The presence of oedema or ascites increases the volume of distribution, whereas dehydration reduces it. In practice these changes will be significant only if the volume of distribution of the drug is small, that is, less than 50 L. Serum protein binding may be reduced because of either protein loss or alteration in binding caused by uraemia. For certain highly bound drugs the net result of reduced protein binding is an increase in free drug, and care is therefore required when interpreting serum concentrations. Most analyses measure the total serum concentration, that is, free plus bound drug. A drug level may, therefore, fall within the accepted concentration range but still result in toxicity because of the increased proportion of free drug. However, this is usually only a temporary effect. Because the unbound drug is now available for elimination, its concentration will eventually return to the original value, albeit with a lower total bound and unbound level. The total drug concentration may, therefore, fall below the therapeutic range while therapeutic effectiveness is maintained.

The time required for the new equilibrium to be established is about four or five elimination half-lives of the drug, and this may be altered itself in renal failure. Some drugs that show reduced serum protein binding include diazepam, morphine, phenytoin, levothyroxine,

Table 17.6	Approximate clearances of common renal replacement therapies	
Renal replacement therapy	**Clearance rate (mL/min)**
Intermittent haemodialysis	150–200
Intermittent haemofiltration	100–150
Acute intermittent dialysis	10–20
Continuous haemofiltration	5–15

theophylline and warfarin. Tissue binding may also be affected; for example, the displacement of digoxin from skeletal muscle binding sites by metabolic waste products that accumulate in renal failure result in a significant reduction in digoxin's volume of distribution.

Excretion

Alteration in renal clearance of drugs in renal impairment is the most important parameter to consider when considering dosage. Generally a decline in renal drug clearance indicates a decline in the number of functioning nephrons. The GFR can be used as an estimate of the number of functioning nephrons. Thus, a 50% reduction in the GFR will suggest a 50% decline in renal clearance.

Renal impairment, therefore, often necessitates drug dosage adjustments. Loading doses of renally excreted drugs are often necessary in renal failure because of the prolonged elimination half-life which leads to an increased time to reach steady state. The equation for a loading dose is the same in renal disease as in normal patients, thus:

$$\text{loading dose (mg)} = \text{target concentration (mg/L)} \times \text{volume of distribution (L)}$$

The volume of distribution may be altered but generally remains unchanged.

It is possible to derive other formulae for dosage adjustment in renal impairment. One of the most useful is:

$$DR_{rf} = DR_{n} \times [(1 - F_{eu}) + (F_{eu} \times RF)]$$

where DR_{rf} is the dosing rate in renal failure, DR_{n} is the normal dosing rate, RF is the extent of renal impairment = patient's creatinine clearance (mL/min)/ideal creatinine clearance (120 mL/min) and F_{eu} is the fraction of drug normally excreted unchanged in the urine. For example, when RF = 0.2 and F_{eu} = 0.5, 60% of the normal dosing rate should be given.

An alteration in dosing rate can be achieved by altering either the dose itself or the dosage interval, or a combination of both as appropriate. Unfortunately, it is not always possible to obtain the fraction of drug excreted unchanged in the urine. In practice it is simpler to use the guidelines for prescribing in renal impairment found in the British National Formulary. These are adequate for most cases, although the specialist may need to refer to other texts.

Nephrotoxicity

The list of potentially nephrotoxic drugs is long. Although the most common serious forms of renal damage are interstitial nephritis and glomerulonephritis, the majority of drugs only cause damage by hypersensitivity reactions and are safe in many patients. Some drugs, however, are directly nephrotoxic, and their effects on the kidney are more predictable. Such drugs include aminoglycosides, amphotericin, colistin, the polymyxins and ciclosporin. The use of any drug with recognised nephrotoxic potential should be avoided where possible. This is particularly true in patients with pre-existing CKD. Fig. 17.7 summarises the most important and common adverse effects of drugs on renal function, indicating the likely regions of the nephron in which damage occurs. Additional information on adverse effects can be found in Hems and Currie (2005).

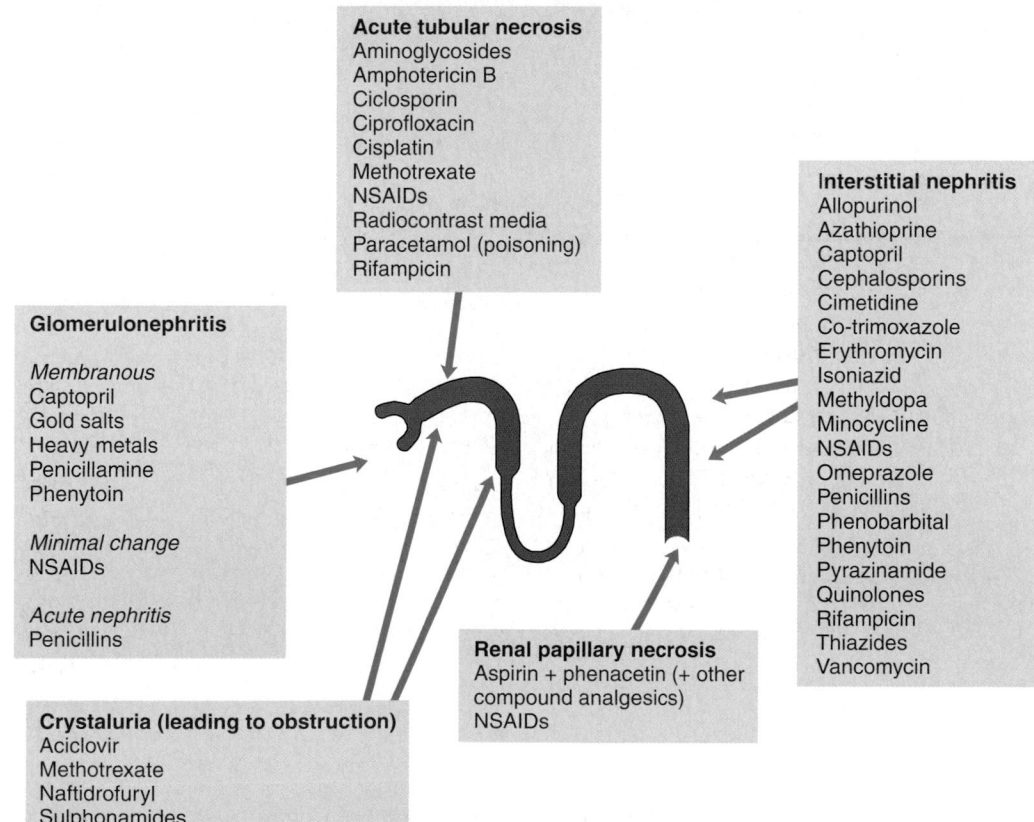

Acute tubular necrosis
Aminoglycosides
Amphotericin B
Ciclosporin
Ciprofloxacin
Cisplatin
Methotrexate
NSAIDs
Radiocontrast media
Paracetamol (poisoning)
Rifampicin

Interstitial nephritis
Allopurinol
Azathioprine
Captopril
Cephalosporins
Cimetidine
Co-trimoxazole
Erythromycin
Isoniazid
Methyldopa
Minocycline
NSAIDs
Omeprazole
Penicillins
Phenobarbital
Phenytoin
Pyrazinamide
Quinolones
Rifampicin
Thiazides
Vancomycin

Glomerulonephritis

Membranous
Captopril
Gold salts
Heavy metals
Penicillamine
Phenytoin

Minimal change
NSAIDs

Acute nephritis
Penicillins

Renal papillary necrosis
Aspirin + phenacetin (+ other compound analgesics)
NSAIDs

Crystaluria (leading to obstruction)
Aciclovir
Methotrexate
Naftidrofuryl
Sulphonamides

Fig. 17.7 Common adverse effects of drugs on the kidney. The likely sites of damage to the nephron (stylised) are indicated.
NSAID, Non-steroidal anti-inflammatory drug.

Box 17.1 Characteristics of the ideal drug for use in a patient with renal failure

- No active metabolites
- Disposition unaffected by fluid balance changes
- Disposition unaffected by protein binding changes
- Response unaffected by altered tissue sensitivity
- Wide therapeutic margin
- Not nephrotoxic

Inevitably, occasions will arise when the use of potentially nephrotoxic drugs becomes necessary, and on these occasions constant monitoring of renal function is essential. In conclusion, when selecting a drug for a patient with renal failure, an agent should be chosen that approaches the ideal characteristics listed in Box 17.1.

Case studies

Case 17.1

Mrs J, a 60-year-old widow, had long-standing hypertension that was unsatisfactorily controlled on a variety of agents. Her drug therapy included furosemide 40 mg once a day, amlodipine 10 mg daily and a salt-restricted diet. Following a routine review of her therapy, ramipril 2.5 mg once daily was added to her treatment regimen in an attempt to improve BP control.

Mrs J was recently diagnosed with gastroenteritis. A week after her diagnosis she presented to her local hospital accident and emergency unit with ongoing diarrhoea. Her BP was found to be 100/60 mmHg and serum biochemistry revealed creatinine levels of 225 mmol/L (50–120 mmol/L), Na^+ 125 mmol/L (135–145 mmol/L) and K^+ 5.2 mmol/L (3.5–5.0 mmol/L).

Questions

1. What was the likely cause and underlying mechanism to this patient's problem?
2. What treatment should be given?

Answers

1. ACE inhibitors reduce angiotensin II production and, thus, attenuate angiotensin II–mediated vasoconstriction of the efferent arterioles that contributes to the high-pressure gradient across the glomerulus necessary for filtration. It is not usually a problem in the majority of individuals; however, in patients with pre-existing compromised renal blood flow, such as renal artery stenoses, the kidney relies more heavily on angiotensin-mediated vasoconstriction of the postglomerular arterioles to maintain renal function. Hypovolaemia caused, for example, by diuretic use and a diarrhoeal illness would tend to exacerbate this problem. Moreover, it is likely that sodium depletion would render the kidney even more dependent upon vasoconstriction of efferent arterioles through activation of the tubuloglomerular feedback system, further sensitising the kidney to the effects of ACE inhibitors.

Mrs J might well have been suffering from incipient renal failure, but remained asymptomatic until her renal reserve diminished.

2. The inappropriate use of an ACE inhibitor should be stopped, as should the diuretic temporarily. Mrs J should be rehydrated using sodium chloride 0.9% and kidney function markers monitored in the hope that recovery will occur. Investigations should be arranged to determine whether Mrs J has renal artery stenosis as a cause of her AKI after initiation of the ACE inhibitor (see Chapter 18).

Case 17.2

Mr B, a known intermittent heroin and cocaine abuser, was discovered comatose in his room early in the morning. He was admitted to hospital as an emergency. An indirect history from an acquaintance indicated that Mr B had been drinking very heavily prior to the incident (probably more than a bottle of whisky in a 24-hour period) and had smoked both heroin and cocaine of unknown source and purity.

On examination he was found to be dehydrated and serum biochemistry revealed the following:

		Reference range
Sodium	147 mmol/L	135–145 mmol/L
Potassium	6.1 mmol/L	3.5–5.0 mmol/L
Calcium	1.72 mmol/L	2.20–2.55 mmol/L
Phosphate	2.0 mmol/L	0.9–1.5 mmol/L
Creatinine	485 mmol/L	50–120 mmol/L
Creatinine kinase	120,000 IU/L	<200 IU/L

Urine dipstick reacted positive for blood with no signs of red blood cells on microscopy. The urine was faintly reddish brown.

Question

What is likely to have occurred, and how should Mr B be treated?

Answer

Cocaine, heroin or alcohol abuse sometimes causes muscle damage resulting in rhabdomyolysis. The mechanism is unclear, but includes vasoconstriction and an increase in muscle activity, possibly because of seizures, self-injury, adulterants in the drug (e.g. arsenic, strychnine, amphetamine, phencyclidine, quinine) or compression (associated with long periods of inactivity). ATN may ensue from a direct nephrotoxic effect of the myoglobin released from damaged muscle cells, microprecipitation of myoglobin in renal tubules (as casts) or a reduction in medullary blood flow. The presence of myoglobin is suggested by the urine dipstick test, which reacts not only to red cells but also to free haemoglobin and myoglobin. Extremely high levels of myoglobinuria may result in urine the colour of black tea. High serum creatinine kinase levels are indicative of rhabdomyolysis together with the presence of free myoglobin in serum and urine. Serum levels of potassium and phosphate are elevated partly by the effects of incipient renal failure but also through tissue breakdown and intracellular release. Creatinine levels are often higher than expected because of muscle damage.

Treatment should involve fluid replacement with normal saline to reverse dehydration. Furosemide and other loop diuretics should be avoided because these decrease intra-tubular pH which may be a co-factor for cast precipitation. Indeed, in cases where urine pH is less than 6, administration of intravenous isotonic sodium bicarbonate may be of use. The patient's ECG should be monitored because of the risks involved with rapid elevation in serum potassium. Timely, appropriate corrective therapy must be instigated where necessary. In 50–70% of cases with rhabdomyolysis, dialysis is required to support recovery.

Case 17.3

Mr D is a patient who has been admitted to an intensive care unit with AKI, which developed following a routine cholecystectomy. His electrolyte results are as follows:

		Reference range
Sodium	138 mmol/L	135–145 mmol/L
Potassium	7.2 mmol/L	3.5–5.0 mmol/L
Bicarbonate	19 mmol/L	22–31 mmol/L
Urea	32.1 mmol/L	3.0–6.5 mmol/L
Creatinine	572 mmol/L	50–120 mmol/L
pH	7.28	7.36–7.44

The patient was connected to an ECG monitor, and the resultant trace indicated absent P waves and a broad QRS complex.

Question

Explain the biochemistry and ECG abnormalities, and indicate what therapeutic measures must be implemented?

Answer

Hyperkalaemia is one of the principal problems encountered in patients with renal failure. The increased levels of potassium arise from failure of the excretory pathway and also from intracellular release of potassium. Attention should also be paid to pharmacological or pharmaceutical processes that might lead to potassium elevation (e.g. inappropriate potassium supplements, ACE inhibitors). The acidosis noted in this patient, which is common in AKI, also aggravates hyperkalaemia by promoting leakage of potassium from cells. A serum potassium level greater than 7.0 mmol/L indicates that emergency treatment is required because the patient risks life-threatening ventricular arrhythmias and asystolic cardiac arrest. If ECG changes are present, as in this case, emergency treatment should be initiated when serum potassium concentration rises to more than 6.5 mmol/L. The emergency treatment should include:

1. Stabilisation of the myocardium is achieved by intravenous administration of 10–30 mL of calcium gluconate 10% over 5–10 minutes. The effect is temporary, but the dose can be repeated.
2. Intravenous administration of 10–20 units of soluble insulin with 50 mL of 50% glucose stimulates cellular potassium uptake. The dose may be repeated. The blood glucose should be monitored for at least 6 hours to avoid hypoglycaemia.
3. Acidosis may be corrected with an intravenous dose of sodium bicarbonate, preferably as an isotonic solution. Correction of acidosis stimulates cellular potassium reuptake.
4. Intravenous salbutamol 0.5 mg in 100 mL 5% dextrose administered over 15 minutes has been used to stimulate the cellular Na/K ATPase pump and thus drive potassium into cells. This may cause disturbing muscle tremors at the doses required to reduce serum potassium levels.

References

Borthwick, E.M.J., Hill, C.J., Rabindranath, K.S., et al., 2017. High-volume haemofiltration for sepsis in adults. Cochrane Database Syst. Rev. 2017 (1), CD008075. https://doi.org/10.1002/14651858.CD008075.pub3.

Gillies, M.A., Kalkar, V., Parker, R.J., et al., 2015. Fenoldapam to prevent acute kidney injury after major surgery – a systematic review and meta-analysis. Crit. Care 19, 449–458.

Hems, S., Currie, A., 2005. Renal disorders. In: Lee, A. (Ed.), Adverse Drug Reactions, second ed. Pharmaceutical Press, London.

Lazarus, B., Chen, Y., Wilson, F.P., et al., 2016. Proton pump inhibitor use and the risk of chronic kidney disease. JAMA Intern. Med. 176 (2), 238–246. https://doi.org/10.1001/jamainternmed.2015.7193.

National Institute for Health and Care Excellence (NICE), 2013. Intravenous fluid therapy in adults in hospital. Clinical Guideline 174. NICE, London. Available at: https://www.nice.org.uk/guidance/cg174.

Further reading

National Institute for Health and Care Excellence, 2013. Acute kidney injury: prevention, detection and management. Clinical Guideline 169. NICE, London. Available at: https://www.nice.org.uk/guidance/cg169.

Plant, L., Short, A., 2011. ABC of intensive care: renal failure, second ed. BMJ Books, Wiley-Blackwell, Oxford.

Steddon, S., Chesser, A., Cunningham, J., et al., 2014. Oxford Handbook of Nephrology and Hypertension. Oxford University Press, Oxford.

Useful websites

'Think Kidneys' website includes case histories and information targeted for different healthcare professionals, patients and the general public: https://www.thinkkidneys.nhs.uk/aki

UK Renal Registry website has a wide range of information including links to renal, patient, academic and healthcare organisations: https://www.renalreg.org

18 Chronic Kidney Disease and End-Stage Renal Disease

John Marriott, Paul Cockwell and Stephanie Stringer

Key points

- The prevalence of chronic kidney disease (CKD) increases with age and is greater in females and some ethnic populations.

- CKD is classified according to severity from G1 to G5, where G5 is the most advanced and G1 the least.

- Stage G1–G3 CKD is common and may not cause symptoms. It is unusual for stage G1–G3 CKD to progress to end-stage renal disease (ESRD) requiring renal replacement therapy (dialysis and/or transplantation).

- CKD is an important risk factor for cardiovascular disease (CVD).

- As CKD becomes more advanced (stage G4 and G5), virtually all body systems are adversely affected.

- Clinical symptoms and signs of advanced CKD include oedema, nocturia, hypertension, anaemia, bone pain, neurological changes and disordered muscle function.

- The aims of treatment are to slow or halt the progression of CKD, relieve symptoms and reduce CVD morbidity and mortality.

- Adequate control of blood pressure and reduction of proteinuria are essential to slow progression of CKD.

- Renal anaemia is common when the glomerular filtration rate (GFR) falls to lower than 30 mL/min but can be corrected by iron supplementation and erythropoiesis-stimulating agents (ESAs) in 90–95% of cases.

- ESRD is the point at which life can only be sustained by dialysis or transplantation. Some patients present with ESRD, but the large majority have been previously identified as having less severe CKD which has subsequently progressed to ESRD.

- The need for dialysis therapy is increasing at about 2% per annum with attendant resource implications.

- There are two principal types of dialysis: haemodialysis and peritoneal dialysis. In both, waste products and metabolites are transferred from the patient's blood across a semi-permeable membrane to a dialysis solution.

- Renal transplantation remains the treatment of choice for many patients with ESRD. However, up to 60% of patients on dialysis programmes are not fit enough to be put on the transplant list.

Chronic kidney disease (CKD) is defined by a reduction in the glomerular filtration rate (GFR) and/or urinary abnormalities or structural abnormalities of the renal tract. The severity of CKD is classified from G1 to G5 depending upon the level of GFR (Table 18.1). CKD is additionally classified by the degree of proteinuria, measured in clinical practice as albumin/creatinine ratio (ACR), from normal range (A1) to very heavy (A3). Stages G1 and G2, in a person with A1, will classify that individual as having CKD only if there is persistent haematuria of renal origin and/or if there is a structural abnormality of the renal tract, for example, renal cysts and/or a hereditary renal disease or a history of kidney transplantation.

It is a common condition that affects up to 15% of the population in Western societies and is more common in some ethnic minority populations and in females. The incidence increases with age such that many people older than 80 years of age have CKD. Social deprivation is also associated with a higher prevalence of CKD. The scale of CKD and the consequences for the health service have been appreciated only in the last few years.

Estimates for the prevalence of the stages of CKD are shown in Table 18.1 and have been derived from population-based studies, including from the UK. In the past, patients with CKD were often unrecognised because kidney function tests were not routinely performed in many individuals who were at high risk of CKD. However, individuals at higher risk of CKD are now routinely screened and monitored by kidney function testing. The accuracy of CKD assessment has improved over the past two decades; this is a consequence of utilising equations to estimate kidney function by incorporating serum creatinine into equations that correct for confounders of creatinine that are independent of kidney function, including age, gender and ethnicity. National guidance on the management of CKD has been published and includes management in primary and secondary care (National Institute for Health and Care Excellence [NICE], 2014).

CKD differs from acute kidney injury (AKI) in terms of cause, speed of onset and occurring in the community, rather than in hospitalised patients. However, AKI and CKD are not mutually exclusive; patients with AKI may not recover renal function to their baseline and may be left with residual CKD. In addition, patients with CKD are at increased risk of AKI.

Renin–angiotensin–aldosterone system

The renin–angiotensin–aldosterone system (RAAS) has a critical role in the progression of CKD, and an awareness of this system is important for understanding the pathophysiology of CKD and the targets for therapeutic intervention. Most of the renal effects of this system are through regulating intraglomerular pressures and salt and water balance. Renin is an enzyme which is formed and stored in the juxtaglomerular apparatus and released in response to decreased afferent intra-arterial pressures, decreased glomerular ultrafiltrate sodium levels and sympathetic nervous system activation. In patients with CKD, intra-renal pressures are often low, and sympathetic overactivity is common; these factors lead to increased renin secretion. This can occur with both normal and elevated systemic blood pressure (BP).

Renin cleaves the protein angiotensinogen, which is produced by the liver, to produce angiotensin I (ATI). ATI is converted to angiotensin II (ATII) by angiotensin-converting enzyme (ACE). ATII has two major physiological effects. First, it acts on the zona glomerulosa of the adrenal cortex to promote production of the mineralocorticoid hormone aldosterone, with resultant increased distal tubular salt and water reabsorption. Furthermore, ATII promotes antidiuretic hormone (ADH) release, which increases proximal tubular sodium reabsorption and promotes thirst. In combination, these cause salt and fluid retention, high intravascular volumes, hypertension and oedema. Second, ATII is a direct vasoconstrictor and promotes systemic and (preferential) renal hypertension. The renal effects are predominantly on the efferent glomerular arteriole. Vasoconstriction at this site is mediated by a high density of ATII receptors. When these receptors are ligated by ATII, there is increased intra-glomerular pressure. Although this leads to an overall increase in GFR in the short-term over a longer period glomerular hypertension promotes accelerated glomerular scarring and worsening CKD. In addition to the vascular and endocrine effects of the RAAS, it is now recognised that there is a local immune-modulatory role for this system. Both resident (e.g. tubular epithelial) and inflammatory (monocytes and macrophages) cells synthesise components of the RAAS and are themselves targeted by the system. For example, monocytes and macrophages express the ATII receptor, and activation through this receptor leads to an enhanced inflammatory and fibrotic phenotype of the cell. This raises the intriguing concept that some of the effects of blocking the RAAS are due to direct anti-inflammatory and antifibrotic effects. Fig. 18.1 shows this pathway and identifies the points at which pharmacological interventions targeted for a biological effect translate into improved clinical outcomes.

Measurement of renal function

The scale of CKD has only been recognised in recent years because detection is dependent upon an accurate estimation of the GFR. The GFR is defined as the volume of filtrate produced by the glomeruli of both kidneys each minute and is a reliable indicator of renal function.

It is laborious and expensive to measure GFR by gold standard tests such as inulin or radiolabelled isotope clearance. These tests are used only when extremely accurate assessment of kidney function is required. An example of this is measurement of kidney function in a potential living kidney donor where an individual is proposing to donate a kidney to a family member or close friend.

As a consequence, a number of equations have been validated for use in the routine clinical setting. These equations provide an estimate of glomerular filtration rate (eGFR) based on the combination of serum or plasma creatinine and a number of variables, which add precision to the estimation of kidney function. The equation that is currently recommended for clinical practice is the CKD epidemiology (EPI) equation; this has generally taken over from the four-variable MDRD (Modification of Diet in Renal Disease Study) equation. The biochemical variable that the eGFR equations utilise is serum creatinine.

Table 18.1 Classification of chronic kidney disease

Glomerular filtration rate stage[a]	Global prevalence[b] (%)	eGFR (mL/min/1.73 m^2)	Description
G1	3.5	≥90	Normal or high
G2	3.9	60–89	Normal or mildly decreased
G3a	7.6 (stage 3 total)	45–59	Mild to moderately decreased
G3b		30–44	Moderate to severely decreased
G4	0.4	15–29	Severely decreased
G5	0.1	<15 (or dialysis)	Kidney failure
Albuminuria stage (by ACR)	ACR (mg/mmol) (urine dip test)		Description
A1	<3 (–ve to trace)		Normal to high normal
A2	3–30 (trace to 1+)		High
A3	>30 (>1+)		Very high

[a]Use the suffix p- to denote the presence of proteinuria when staging chronic kidney disease. Clinically important proteinuria is defined by an ACR ≥3 mg/mmol.
[b]Data are from Hill et al. (2016).
ACR, Albumin/creatinine ratio.

Serum creatinine

Although serum creatinine concentration is related to renal function, it is also dependent upon the rate of production of creatinine by the patient. Creatinine is a by-product of normal muscle metabolism and is formed at a rate proportional to muscle mass (20 g of muscle equates to approximately 1 mg of creatinine production), and therefore is related to age, sex and ethnicity.

Creatinine is freely filtered by the glomerulus, so when muscle mass is stable any change in serum creatinine levels reflects a change in renal clearance. Consequently, measurement of serum creatinine can be utilised to give an estimate of the kidney function. It is important to note, however, that creatinine also undergoes significant tubular secretion (~10–20%). This becomes important in advanced CKD (stages G4 and G5) and limits the value of measuring serum creatinine to determine renal function in stage G4–G5 CKD.

Chronic kidney disease epidemiology estimate of glomerular filtration rate equation

The CKD EPI equation was first published in 2009 and is now recommended in the UK and elsewhere for reporting eGFR. It uses creatinine, age, gender and ethnicity (black or other ethnic groups) to report an eGFR (Fig. 18.2).

This equation is the most accurate equation for estimating kidney function where the patient has kidney function that is either in or close to the normal range. However, caution is needed because the equation performs differently in different populations of patients. The CKD classification system is based on the eGFR.

Previously the four variable MDRD equation (Fig. 18.3) was recommended for eGFR. Some laboratories are still reporting this equation.

Other estimates of kidney function

Creatinine clearance

Creatinine clearance (Cl_{Cr}) is similar to the GFR because nearly all the filtered creatinine appears in the urine. It is a measurement of the volume of blood that is cleared of creatinine with time. Measurements of Cl_{Cr} require accurate collection of 24-hour urine samples with a serum creatinine sample midway through this period. This is time-consuming, inconvenient, prone to inaccuracy and now is rarely used in clinical practice. Fig. 18.4 shows the equation for measuring Cl_{Cr}.

Cockroft–Gault equation

The Cockroft–Gault equation uses weight, sex and age to estimate Cl_{Cr} and was derived using average population data (Cockroft and Gault, 1976). The equation is shown in Fig. 18.5.

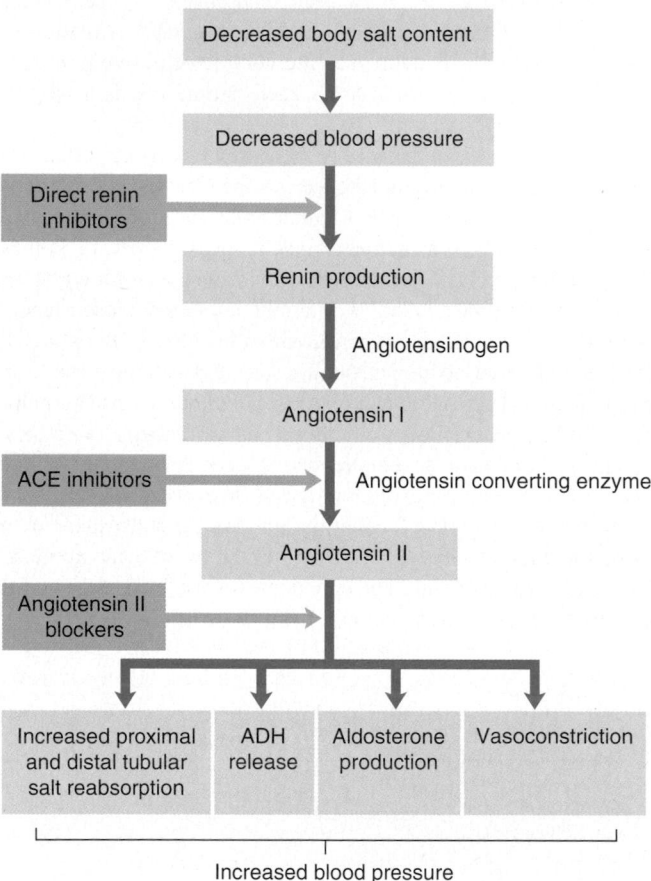

Fig. 18.1 The renin–angiotensin–aldosterone system and targets for pharmaceutical intervention.
ACE, Angiotensin-converting enzyme; ADH, antidiuretic hormone.

GFR = $141 \times \min(S_{cr} < /k, 1)^{\alpha} \times \max(S_{cr}/k, 1)^{-1.209} \times 0.993^{Age} \times 1.018\ [\text{if female}] \times 1.159\ [\text{if black}]$

where:
S_{cr} is serum creatinine in mmol/L,
k is 61.9 for females and 79.6 for males,
α is −0.329 for females and −0.411 for males,
min indicates the minimum of S_{cr}/k or 1,
and max indicates the maximum of S_{cr}/k or 1.

The equation does not require weight because the results are reported normalised to 1.73 m² body surface area, which is an accepted average adult surface area.

Fig. 18.2 The chronic kidney disease epidemiology (EPI) estimate of glomerular filtration rate (eGFR) equation.

MDRD eGFR (mL/min/1.73m²) = $186 \times [\text{serum creatinine (mmol/L)}/88.4]^{-1.154} \times [\text{age}]^{-0.203} \times [0.742\ \text{if } \textbf{female}] \times [1.212\ \text{if } \textbf{African-American}]$

Fig. 18.3 Four-variable MDRD (Modification of Diet in Renal Disease Study) equation used to calculate estimate of glomerular filtration rate (eGFR).

Estimates of glomerular filtration rate in paediatric patients

Estimates of GFRs in paediatric patients can be made using the Schwartz formula (Schwartz, 1985) or the Counahan–Barratt method (Counahan et al., 1976), which both rely upon inclusion of the height of the child in estimating Cl_{Cr}, because height correlates with muscle mass.

Urea

Serum urea is also used in the assessment of renal function despite a variable production rate and diurnal fluctuation in response to the protein content of the diet. Urea may also be elevated by dehydration or an increase in protein catabolism such as that accompanying gastro-intestinal haemorrhage, severe infection, trauma (including surgery) and high-dose steroid therapy. Serum urea levels are, therefore, an unreliable measure of renal function, but they can be used as an indicator of the patient's general condition and state of hydration. A rapid elevation of serum urea, before any rise in corresponding creatinine levels, is often a sign of an impending deterioration in renal function or a marker for pre-renal failure associated with intravascular volume depletion.

Significance of chronic kidney disease

CKD is significant because it indicates the possibility of progression to end-stage renal disease (ESRD) and a strong association with accelerated cardiovascular disease (CVD) similar in magnitude to that observed in individuals with diabetes. The CVD risk increases with the severity of CKD but is detectable at all levels. Thus, it is important to pay particular attention to traditional CVD risk factors such as smoking, cholesterol and BP in patients with CKD. However, these risk factors contribute only around 50% of the total CVD risk, and there is great interest in the identification of novel risk factors to explain the remainder of the risk.

$$Cr_{Cl} = \frac{(U \times V)}{S}$$

where **U** is the urine creatinine concentration (mmol/L), **V** is the urine flow rate (mL/min) and **S** is the serum creatinine concentration (mmol/L)

Fig. 18.4 Creatinine clearance (Cr_{Cl}) calculation.

$$Cr_{Cl} = \frac{F(140 \text{ age (years)}) \times \text{weight (kg)}}{\text{Serum creatinine (mmol/L)}}$$

where **F** = 1.04 (females) or 1.23 (males)

Fig. 18.5 The Cockroft–Gault formula. Cr_{Cl}, creatinine clearance.

It is important to make a distinction between CVD related to macrovascular atherosclerosis and arteriosclerosis which causes vascular stiffness and which contributes also to microvascular changes associated with endothelial dysfunction. In patients with more severe CKD, arteriosclerosis becomes the dominant lesion. As a consequence, cardiac disease in patients with CKD can represent a spectrum from left ventricular hypertrophy associated with hypertension, through to classical myocardial ischaemia, both irreversible (as in myocardial infarction) and reversible, and progressing to fibrotic myocardial disease with a high risk of sudden death, which is very common in patients with ESRD.

Progression to more advanced stages of CKD may occur, particularly if the BP is high and there is significant proteinuria. With good BP control, many patients with CKD can have stable kidney function for years or even decades. These patients need to be followed up with regular blood and urine tests to monitor for progression. Most patients with stage G1–G3 CKD do not require long-term follow-up by a kidney specialist, and their monitoring and management of risk factors are carried out in primary care.

Patients with stage G1–G3 CKD (see Table 18.1) are frequently asymptomatic. The reduction of GFR does not cause uraemic symptoms, and the presence in the urine of protein (proteinuria) or blood (haematuria) is usually not noticed by the patient and is only detectable on monitoring by specialist tests. There is a frequent association with high BP, which may be the cause or a consequence of renal damage. Recognition of these patients is important because it allows early modification of traditional cardiovascular risk factors. These patients should be investigated to determine whether there is a treatable cause for their CKD and followed up to identify those individuals with progressive disease.

Patients with stage G4 and G5 CKD and/or A3 level albuminuria (see Table 18.1) should usually be followed up in a nephrology clinic because they may require specialist management of the complications of CKD such as anaemia and bone disease, whilst many will also be undergoing preparation for renal replacement therapy (RRT).

Causes of chronic kidney disease

The reduction in renal function observed in CKD is often a patchy process, resulting from damage to the infrastructure of the kidney in discrete areas rather than throughout the kidney. The functional unit of the kidney is the nephron; there are 1 million nephrons in each kidney. Although the mechanism of damage depends on the underlying cause of renal disease, as individual nephrons become damaged and fail, remaining nephrons compensate for loss of function through hyperfiltration secondary to raised intra-glomerular pressure. This causes 'bystander' damage with secondary nephron loss. This vicious cycle is illustrated in Fig. 18.6. The patient remains well until so many nephrons are lost that the GFR can no longer be maintained despite activation of compensatory mechanisms. As a consequence, there is a progressive decline in kidney function.

CKD arises from a variety of causes (Table 18.2), although by the time a patient has established CKD it may not be possible to identify the exact cause. However, attempting to establish the cause is useful in the identification and elimination of reversible factors, to plan for likely outcomes and treatment needs, and for appropriate counselling when a genetic basis is established. The causes of CKD listed in Table 18.2 are ordered according to prevalence. It is important to note that the prevalence of these factors is different in CKD and ESRD. In ESRD some diseases (e.g. adult polycystic kidney disease [APKD]) are overrepresented and some (e.g. ischaemic/hypertensive nephropathy) are underrepresented. The reasons for this are that individuals with APKD are likely to survive to reach ESRD, whereas those with ischaemic renal damage are more likely to die of CVD before ESRD is reached.

Ischaemic/hypertensive renal disease

Ischaemic nephropathy was traditionally referred to as under-perfusion of the kidneys caused by renal artery stenosis. This explanation fell from favour and this term is now used for impairment of renal function caused by vascular disease distal to occlusion

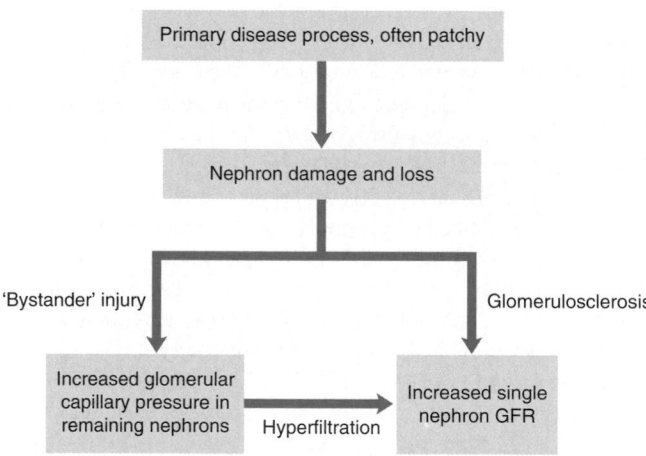

Fig. 18.6 Mechanism of progressive renal damage. GFR, Glomerular filtration rate.

of the main renal arteries. Hypertension results in atherosclerosis and arteriosclerosis which can cause occlusive renovascular disease and small-vessel damage. In patients with significant large-vessel occlusive disease, arteriolar nephrosclerosis, interstitial fibrosis and glomerular collapse may be present (Lerman and Textor, 2001). These diagnoses account for around 30% of CKD and a smaller proportion of ESRD. The effective management of hypertension is crucial to reduce renal damage.

Metabolic diseases

Diabetes mellitus is the most common metabolic disease that causes CKD. The predominant lesion is glomerular and is referred to as diabetic nephropathy or diabetic kidney disease when diabetic nephropathy is likely but the patient has not had a kidney biopsy performed to confirm the diagnosis. Around 95% of all diabetes cases are type 2 diabetes. Diabetes is present in up to one-third of patients with CKD (see Table 18.2), but in many of these patients processes other than diabetic nephropathy cause kidney disease. Diabetic nephropathy is associated with a faster decline in kidney function than other pathologies; these patients are also at high risk of CVD as a consequence of CKD and diabetes functioning as independent risk factors for CVD. Both type 1 and type 2 diabetes can result in diabetic nephropathy. Patients with type 1 diabetes usually present with CKD at a younger age, and if they progress to ESRD may benefit from combined kidney and pancreas transplantation. Patients with diabetes usually have high levels of protein in the urine (proteinuria); high levels of proteinuria are associated with an increased risk of progression of CKD to ESRD.

Chronic glomerulonephritis

Glomerulonephritis is a term that is used to describe the process of inflammation of the glomerulus. Chronic glomerulonephritis causes around 15% of cases of advanced CKD. The commonest

Table 18.2 Primary diagnosis in patients receiving renal replacement therapy by age and gender (UK Renal Registry, 2008)

Primary diagnosis	% All patients	Inter-centre range (%)	Age<65 years (%)	Age>65 years (%)	Male/female ratio
Aetiology uncertain/glomerulonephritis (not biopsy proven)	21.6	2.1–84.3	19.2	26.6	1.6
Glomerulonephritis (biopsy proven)	15.3	2.3–22.4	17.8	10.0	2.2
Pyelonephritis	11.9	3.2–19.4	13.6	8.3	1.1
Diabetes	13.2	2.8–26.0	12.3	15.1	1.6
Polycystic kidney	9.2	2.0–15.8	9.6	8.3	1.1
Hypertension	5.4	1.0–16.0	4.6	6.9	2.4
Renal vascular disease	3.5	0.3–16.1	1.1	8.2	2.0
Other	14.5	1.9–36.1	16.0	11.3	1.3
Not sent	5.5	0.1–46.2	5.7	5.2	1.5

cause of chronic glomerulonephritis is IgA nephropathy; this is characterised by deposition of polymeric IgA in the glomerulus with subsequent immune activation. Other patterns of glomerulonephritis include membranous nephropathy, where there is granular deposition of immunoglobulin on the glomerular capillary basement membrane. Systemic autoimmune diseases such as systemic lupus erythematosus can cause a variety of types of glomerulonephritis. Finally, some chronic forms of glomerulonephritis are pauci-immune; that is, they have no immune deposition. An example of this type is focal and segmental glomerulosclerosis.

Lower urinary tract disease

A variety of differing pathologies make up this group and together they represent 5–10% of all cases of CKD. They include the following conditions: reflux disease, renal stone disease, chronic pyelonephritis and extrinsic renal tract obstruction.

Reflux disease

Reflux disease results from reflux of urine back up the renal tract towards the kidneys. This can result in recurrent infections and subsequent scarring.

Renal stone disease

Kidney stones are primarily formed of calcium oxalate and calcium phosphate. They can cause urinary tract obstruction and infection.

Chronic pyelonephritis

Recurrent urinary tract infections which ascend to involve the kidneys can cause renal scarring; this is often associated with reflux disease but may occur without it.

Extrinsic renal tract obstruction

In males the commonest cause of extrinsic renal tract obstruction is prostatic hypertrophy. There are many other causes.

Hereditary/congenital diseases

There are many inherited renal diseases and together they represent 5% of CKD cases. It is, however, important to remember that they make up a higher proportion of cases of ESRD. The commoner inherited conditions are APKD and Alport's syndrome. Autosomal dominant polycystic kidney disease is an inherited condition which results in the formation of multiple cysts in both kidneys throughout life. The kidneys become enlarged and frequently fail in middle age. Alport's syndrome is a disorder of glomerular basement membranes caused by a mutation affecting type IV collagen; X-linked, autosomal dominant and autosomal recessive forms of inheritance are all seen. The clinical manifestations include progressive nephritis with haematuria, proteinuria and sensorineural deafness.

Unknown cause

The cause of CKD is unknown in around 30% of patients, who typically present with small kidneys and unremarkable immunological investigations. When the kidneys are small it is often not possible to carry out a renal biopsy to determine the underlying cause.

Clinical manifestations

Symptoms of advanced kidney disease are known as uraemic symptoms. Although uraemic symptoms are rare in stage G4 CKD, they become more apparent as the patient enters stage G5 CKD and approaches ESRD. In some patients symptoms only develop when ESRD develops, and as a consequence some patients are admitted to hospital as an emergency and require immediate dialysis at their first contact with the medical professional.

ESRD is characterised by the requirement of RRT to sustain life. It is usually accompanied by symptoms of uraemia and variably, anaemia, acidosis, osteodystrophy, and neuropathy. Most patients have hypertension and fluid retention. There is an increased susceptibility to infections (Fig. 18.7). These clinical features result from the major reduction in excretory, homeostatic, metabolic and endocrine functions of the kidney that have usually occurred over many years.

In the following sections the clinical features of CKD are described, along with the underlying pathogenesis.

Polyuria and nocturia

Polyuria, where the patient frequently voids high volumes of urine, is often seen in CKD and results from medullary damage and insensitivity to ADH. In people with advanced CKD it can also be related to the osmotic effect of a high serum urea level (>40 mmol/L). The ability to concentrate urine is also accompanied by physiological nocturnal antidiuresis, which when modified in CKD invariably results in nocturia, where the patient will wake overnight needing to pass urine.

Proteinuria and albuminuria

A small amount of protein is detectable in normal urine. However, when protein levels in the urine climb above a threshold level the patient is classified as having proteinuria. Around 70% of all proteinuria is albuminuria, and it is albuminuria that is used to contribute to the classification of CKD (see Table 18.1). Albuminuria is measured in clinical practice by using single urine samples to determine the ACR or (in some laboratories) the protein/creatinine ratio. These spot methods have almost entirely replaced the previously used 24-hour urine collection which was inconvenient and often unreliable. An ACR of 3–30 mg/mmol is classified as high albuminuria (previously micro-albuminuria) and an ACR greater than 30 mg/mmol as very high albuminuria (previously macroalbuminuria). In nephrotic-range proteinuria the ACR is greater than 250 mg/mmol.

Around 5% of adults have albuminuria/proteinuria. There are two reasons why this is measured. Firstly, it helps in making the diagnosis of the underlying cause of CKD. Albuminuria suggests glomerular pathology (e.g. diabetic nephropathy) in a patient with diabetes mellitus or a newly diagnosed glomerulonephritis. Secondly, albuminuria is a major risk factor for CKD

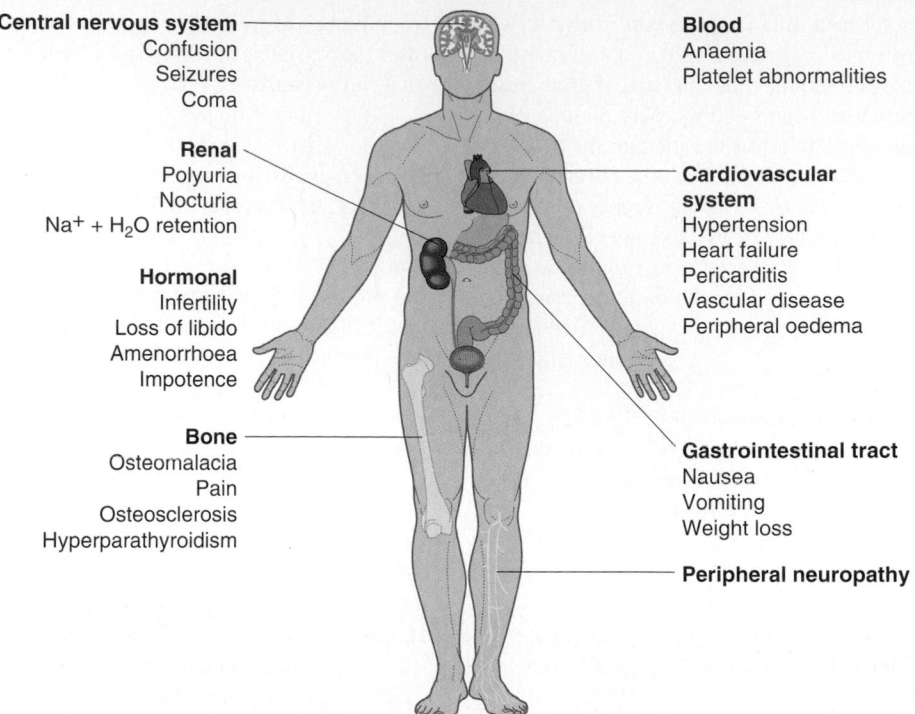

Central nervous system
Confusion
Seizures
Coma

Renal
Polyuria
Nocturia
$Na^+ + H_2O$ retention

Hormonal
Infertility
Loss of libido
Amenorrhoea
Impotence

Bone
Osteomalacia
Pain
Osteosclerosis
Hyperparathyroidism

Blood
Anaemia
Platelet abnormalities

**Cardiovascular
system**
Hypertension
Heart failure
Pericarditis
Vascular disease
Peripheral oedema

Gastrointestinal tract
Nausea
Vomiting
Weight loss

Peripheral neuropathy

Fig. 18.7 Typical signs and symptoms of chronic kidney disease.

progression; therefore, it identifies patients who require additional attention for management of risk factors and counselling about the long-term impact of CKD.

Haematuria

Haematuria refers to the presence of blood in the urine and can be caused by either renal or lower urinary tract pathology. The presence of blood and/or protein in the urine is described as an active urinary sediment. Whenever blood in the urine is detected, an infection should be considered and excluded by quantification of white cells (by microscopy or flow cytometry) and culture for organisms.

Haematuria can be either invisible (microscopic) or visible (macroscopic). The best way to test for haematuria is with a urinary dip test. This is a near-patient test, carried out when the patient provides the sample. If there is a delay in testing, the sample red cells in urine can lyse so microscopy may miss the presence of haematuria. Microscopy, however, does have a role in identifying the presence of casts, which are also seen in glomerular diseases and allow the discrimination of the course of haematuria.

Hypertension and fluid overload

Most patients with CKD will have hypertension, and this may be a cause or a consequence (or a combination of both) of their kidney disease. Furthermore, raised BP may exacerbate renal damage and lead to accelerated deterioration of CKD.

CKD leads to sodium retention, which in turn produces circulatory volume expansion with consequent hypertension. Volume-dependent hypertension occurs in about 80% of patients with CKD, and this is more prevalent with more advanced CKD. This form of hypertension is often termed 'salt-sensitive' because it may be exacerbated by salt intake. Lesser degrees of renal impairment reduce kidney perfusion, which activates RAAS. Treatment of BP, irrespective of choice of therapy, generally slows the rate of deterioration of kidney function in patients with CKD. As the eGFR falls to very low levels the kidneys are unable to excrete salt and water adequately, resulting in the retention of extravascular fluid. All patients with fluid overload will by definition also have salt retention; this does not show itself as an increase in serum sodium levels, but reflects the fact that extracellular fluid including excess extravascular fluid is sodium rich.

Clinical findings

Hypertension can lead to cardiac disease (left ventricular hypertrophy, ischaemic heart disease and heart failure), peripheral vascular disease, and cerebrovascular disease (including strokes). Fluid retention can manifest as peripheral and pulmonary oedema and ascites. Oedema may be seen around the eyes on waking, the sacral region in supine patients and from the feet upwards in ambulatory patients.

Uraemia

Many small molecules including urea, creatinine and water are normally excreted by the kidney and accumulate as renal function decreases. Uraemia refers to the clinical manifestation of the accumulation of small molecules in CKD. In patients with ESRD, some of the molecules responsible for the toxicity of uraemia are intermediate in size between small, readily dialysed molecules and large, non-dialysable proteins. These are described as 'middle molecules' and include phosphate, guanidines, phenols and organic acids. There are a wide range of uraemic toxins, but it is the blood level of urea that is still used to estimate the degree of toxin accumulation in CKD. True symptomatic uraemia occurs only in very advanced CKD.

Clinical findings

The symptoms of uraemia include anorexia, nausea, vomiting, constipation, foul taste and skin discolouration that is presumed to be due to pigment deposition compounded by the pallor of anaemia. The characteristic complexion is often described as 'muddy' and can be associated with severe pruritus without an underlying rash. In severe cases crystalline urea is deposited on the skin (uraemic frost).

In uraemia, there is also an increased tendency to bleed, which can exacerbate pre-existing anaemia because of impaired platelet adhesion including modified interactions between platelets and blood vessels resulting from altered blood rheology.

Anaemia

Anaemia affects most people with stages G4 and G5 CKD. The decrease in haemoglobin level is a slow, insidious process accompanying the decline in renal function. A normochromic, normocytic pattern is usually seen with haemoglobin levels declining to around 80 g/L by ESRD.

Several factors contribute to the pathogenesis of anaemia in CKD, including shortened red cell survival, marrow suppression by uraemic toxins and iron or folate deficiency associated with poor dietary intake or increased loss, for example, from gastro-intestinal bleeding. However, the principal cause results from damage of peritubular cells leading to inadequate secretion of erythropoietin. This hormone, which is produced mainly, although not exclusively, in the kidney, is the main regulator of red cell proliferation and differentiation in bone marrow. Hyperparathyroidism also reduces erythropoiesis by damaging bone marrow and, therefore, exacerbates anaemia associated with CKD. The RAAS is also involved in erythropoiesis; ACE inhibitors can cause small reductions in haemoglobin through reducing ATII production; ATII can also function as a stimulator of erythropoiesis.

Clinical findings

Anaemia in CKD is a major cause of fatigue, breathlessness at rest and on exertion, and lethargy. Patients may also complain of feeling cold, poor concentration and reduced appetite and libido. Compensatory haemodynamic changes include an increase in cardiac output to improve oxygen delivery to tissues, although this may result in tachycardia and palpitations. The anaemia of CKD usually responds to treatment with erythropoietin-stimulating agents (ESAs).

Bone disease (renal osteodystrophy)

Renal osteodystrophy describes the four types of bone disease associated with CKD:
- secondary hyperparathyroidism
- osteomalacia (reduced mineralisation)
- mixed renal osteodystrophy (both hyperparathyroidism and osteomalacia)

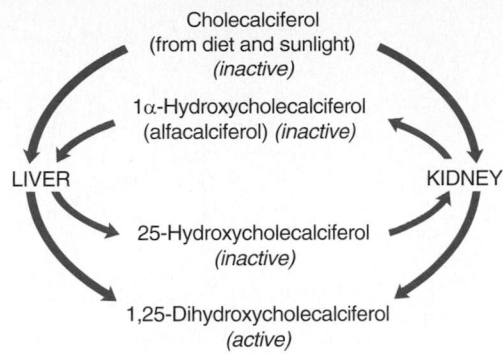

Fig. 18.8   Renal and hepatic involvement in vitamin D metabolism.

- adynamic bone disease (reduced bone formation and resorption)

Cholecalciferol, the precursor of active vitamin D, is both absorbed from the gastro-intestinal tract and produced in the skin by the action of sunlight. Production of active vitamin D, 1,25-dihydroxycholecalciferol (calcitriol) requires the hydroxylation of the colecalciferol molecule at both the 1α and the 25 position (Fig. 18.8).

Hydroxylation at the 25 position occurs in the liver, whereas hydroxylation of the 1α position occurs in the kidney; this latter process is impaired in CKD. The resulting deficiency in active vitamin D leads to defective mineralisation of bone and subsequent osteomalacia, which occurs in patients with stage G3–G5 CKD.

The deficiency in vitamin D with the consequent reduced calcium absorption from the gut in combination with the reduced renal tubular reabsorption results in hypocalcaemia (Fig. 18.9).

These disturbances are compounded by hyperphosphataemia caused by reduced phosphate excretion, which in turn reduces the concentration of ionised serum calcium by sequestering calcium phosphate in bone and in soft tissue. Hypocalcaemia, hyperphosphataemia and a reduction in the direct suppressive action of 1,25-dihydroxycholecalciferol on the parathyroid glands result in an increased secretion of parathyroid hormone (PTH).

Because the failing kidney is unable to respond to PTH by increasing renal calcium reabsorption, serum PTH levels remain persistently elevated, and hyperplasia of the parathyroid glands occurs. The resulting secondary hyperparathyroidism produces a disturbance in the normal architecture of bone, and this is termed osteosclerosis (hardening of the bone). A further possible consequence of secondary hyperparathyroidism produced in response to hypocalcaemia is that bone reabsorption is increased to maintain adequate calcium levels. This, in combination with hyperphosphataemia, may result in soft tissue calcification caused by calcium phosphate deposition.

Clinical findings

Bone pain is the main symptom, and distinctive appearances on radiography may be observed, such as 'rugger-jersey' spine, where there are alternate bands of excessive and defective mineralisation in the vertebrae (Fig. 18.10).

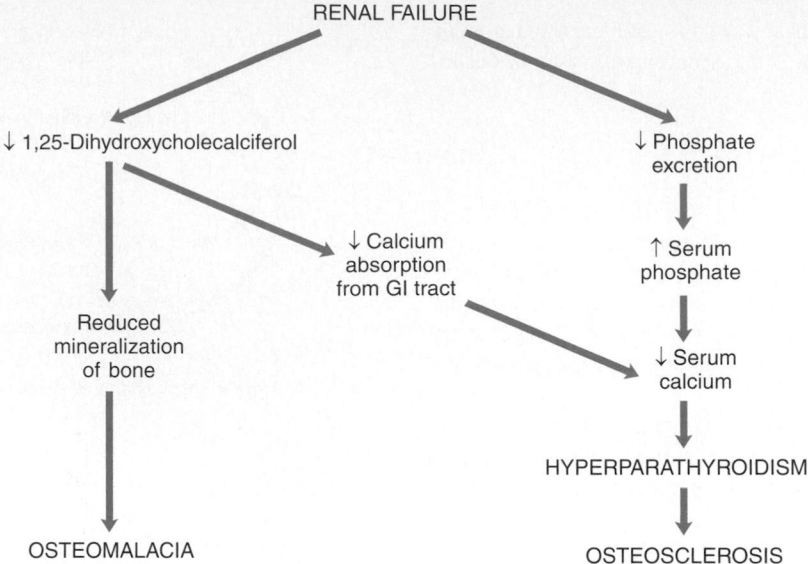

RENAL FAILURE

↓ 1,25-Dihydroxycholecalciferol

↓ Phosphate excretion

↓ Calcium absorption from GI tract

↑ Serum phosphate

Reduced mineralization of bone

↓ Serum calcium

HYPERPARATHYROIDISM

OSTEOMALACIA

OSTEOSCLEROSIS

Fig. 18.9 Disturbance of calcium and phosphate balance in chronic renal failure. GI, Gastro-intestinal.

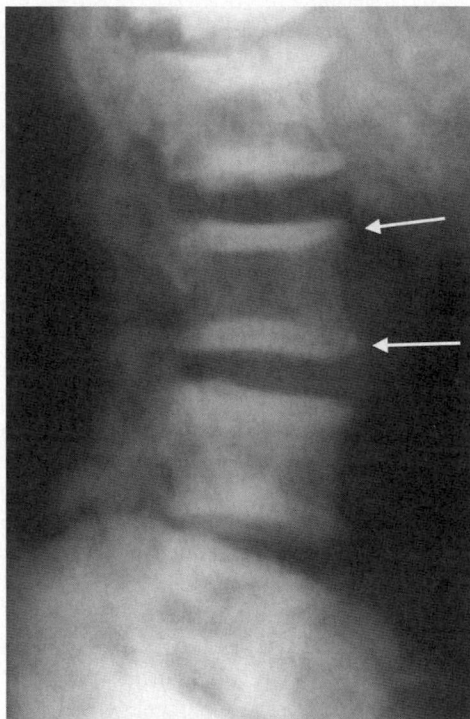

Fig. 18.10 Lateral radiograph of the spine in a patient with chronic renal failure. Characteristic endplate sclerosis (arrows) is referred to as 'rugger-jersey spine'. (Reproduced by kind permission of Dr M. J. Kline, Department of Diagnostic Radiology, Cleveland Clinic Foundation.)

Neurological changes

The most common neurological changes are non-specific and probably caused by uraemic toxins; they include poor concentration, memory impairment, irritability and stupor.

Clinical features

Fits caused by cerebral oedema or hypertension may occur. A 'glove and stocking' peripheral neuropathy and/or a mono-neuritis multiplex can occur.

Muscle function

Muscle symptoms are probably caused by general nutritional deficiencies and electrolyte disturbances, notably of divalent cations and especially by hypocalcaemia.

Clinical findings

Muscle cramps and restless legs are common and may be major symptoms causing distress to patients, particularly at night. Rarely a proximal myopathy of shoulder and pelvic girdle muscles may develop.

Electrolyte disturbances

Because the kidneys play such a crucial role in the maintenance of volume, extracellular fluid composition and acid–base balance, disturbances of electrolyte levels are common in CKD.

Sodium

Serum sodium levels are usually normal, even when the GFR is very low. However, patients may have hyponatraemia or hypernatraemia depending upon the condition and therapies (Table 18.3).

Potassium

Potassium levels can be elevated (hyperkalaemia) in CKD; this is a potentially catastrophic complication because the first indication of elevated potassium levels may be a cardiac arrest. Serum potassium levels greater than 7.0 mmol/L are life-threatening and should be treated as an emergency. Hyperkalaemia may be exacerbated in acidosis as potassium shifts from within cells.

Electrocardiogram (ECG) changes occur with an increase in serum potassium and become more pronounced as levels increase. The progressive changes comprise: T wave peak ('tenting'), reduction in P wave size, increase in the PR interval and widening of the QRS complex. P waves eventually disappear

Table 18.3 Causes and mechanism of serum sodium abnormalities in chronic kidney disease

	Mechanism	Cause/effect
Hypernatraemia	Sodium overload	Drugs, e.g. antibiotic sodium salts
	Hypotonic fluid loss	Osmotic diuresis Sweating
	↓ Water intake	Unconsciousness
Hyponatraemia	Dilution by intracellular water movement	Mannitol
Hyperglycaemia	Water overload	Acute dilution by intravenous fluids, e.g. 5% dextrose infusion Excessive intake Congestive cardiac failure Nephrotic syndrome

A. Normal serum potassium (3.5–5.0) mmol/L

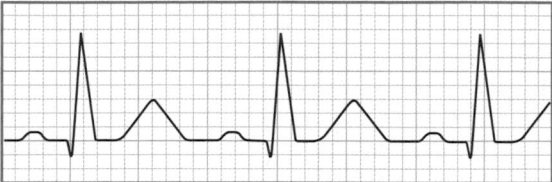

B. Serum potassium approximately 7.0 mmol/L

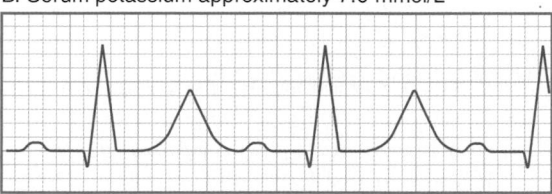

C. Serum potassium approximately 8.0–9.0 mmol/L

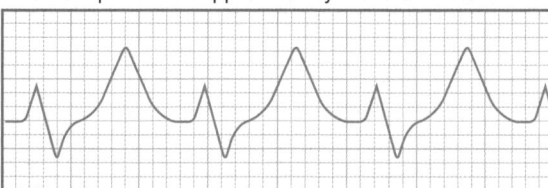

D. Serum potassium greater than 10.0 mmol/L

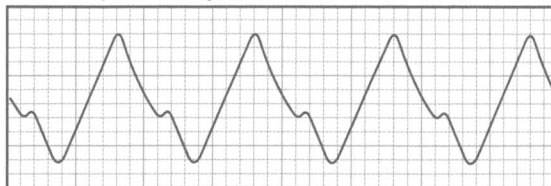

Fig. 18.11 Typical electrocardiogram changes in hyperkalaemia.

and the QRS complex becomes even wider. Ultimately, the ECG assumes a sinusoidal appearance prior to a cardiac arrest (Fig. 18.11).

Hydrogen ions

Hydrogen ions (H^+) are a common end-product of many metabolic processes, and about 40–80 mmol is normally excreted by the kidneys each day. In CKD, H^+ is retained, causing acidosis; the H^+ combines with bicarbonate (HCO_3^-), resulting in removal of some hydrogen as water, elimination of carbon dioxide via the lungs and reduction in serum bicarbonate level.

Diagnosis, investigations and monitoring

Although the diagnosis of CKD may be suspected because of signs and symptoms of renal disease, it is usually discovered on a routine blood test. In some patients no cause of CKD can be identified, often because they have two small kidneys which are not safe to biopsy. This appearance results from damage at some unspecified time in the past.

Family, drug and social histories are all important in elucidating the causes of CKD, because genetics or exposure to toxins, including prescription, over-the-counter and herbal drugs, might be implicated.

Physical examination may be helpful. Signs of anaemia and skin pigmentation, excoriations from scratching and whitening of the skin with crystalline urea ('uraemic frost') may indicate severe CKD. Palpable or audible bruits over the femoral arteries are strongly associated with extensive atherosclerosis and are commonly found in patients with co-incident renal vascular disease. Ankle oedema and a raised jugular venous pressure suggest fluid retention. In severe CKD a fishy smell on the breath known as 'uraemic foetor' is characteristic. In some patients the kidneys may be palpable. Large, irregular kidneys are indicative of polycystic kidney disease, whereas smooth, tender enlarged kidneys are likely to be infected or obstructed. However, in the large majority the kidneys are not palpable. A palpable bladder suggests outflow tract obstruction which is often due to prostatic hypertrophy in men.

Functional assessment of the kidney may be performed by testing serum and urine. The serum creatinine level, incorporated into an eGFR equation, is the measurement of choice for estimating excretory kidney function. Hyperkalaemia, acidosis with a correspondingly low serum bicarbonate level, hypocalcaemia and hyperphosphataemia are frequently present and can help to differentiate a new presentation of CKD from AKI.

The patient may report a change in urine colour, which might result from blood staining by whole cells or haemoglobin, drugs or metabolic breakdown products. Urine may also appear milky after connection with lymphatics; cloudy following infection; contain solid material such as stones, crystals and casts; or froth excessively in proteinuria. Urine should be examined visually, by dipstick test, microscopically if indicated, and with a spot urine assessment for ACR.

Dipstick tests enable simple, rapid estimation of a wide range of urinary parameters including pH, specific gravity, leucocytes, nitrites, glucose, blood and protein. Positive results should, however, be quantified by more specific methods.

Structural assessments of the kidney may be performed using a number of imaging procedures, including:

- ultrasonography;
- intravenous urography (IVU);
- plain abdominal radiography;
- computed tomography (CT), magnetic resonance imaging (MRI) and magnetic resonance angiography.

Ultrasonography

Ultrasonography produces two-dimensional images using sound waves and is used as the first-line investigational tool in many hospitals. The technique is harmless, non-invasive, quick, inexpensive, enables measurements to be made and produces images in real time. The latter feature allows accurate and safe positioning of biopsy needles for patients who undergo a kidney biopsy. Ultrasonography is particularly useful in the differentiation of renal tumours from cysts and in the assessment of renal tract obstruction. Doppler ultrasonography enables measurement of flow rate and direction of the intra-renal and extra-renal blood supply.

Computed tomography, magnetic resonance imaging and intravenous urography

Recently introduced cross-sectional imaging techniques have transformed the assessment of kidney disease. Both CT and MRI can produce very detailed images that include an assessment of the blood supply into the kidney and the drainage of the kidneys. IVU is now rarely used because it uses high doses of radiation and contrast media, and provides less information. For example, a CT urogram is now used as an investigation of choice for patients with obstruction of the renal tract by renal imaging. MRI scans provide enhanced soft tissue assessment and also avoid the use of contrast media that can cause kidney damage. However, the use of gadolinium as a contrast medium for MRI has been associated, in patients with stage G4 and G5 CKD, with nephrogenic systemic fibrosis which results in death in a proportion of patients. Although the use of gadolinium is not contraindicated in this group, it must be used with great care, and protocols will vary from unit to unit.

Cross-sectional imaging with CT or MRI can provide information that includes:

- the presence, length and position of the kidneys; in CKD the kidneys generally shrink in proportion to nephron loss, the exception being the enlarged kidneys seen in polycystic disease;
- the presence or absence of renal scarring and the shape of the calices and renal pelvis; renal cortical scarring and caliceal distortion indicate chronic pyelonephritis;

- obstruction to the ureters, for example, by a stone, tumour or retroperitoneal fibrosis; these may require surgical intervention;
- the presence of a cyst or solid mass in the kidneys and the features of this;
- detailed information on the blood supply into and out of the kidneys.

Nuclear medicine investigations

There are two commonly used nuclear medicine investigations. The first uses mercapto acetyl triglycerine. This is used for assessment of renal perfusion and the identification of outflow obstruction. The other is a dimercaptosuccinic acid scan, the purpose of which is to ascertain the percentage that each kidney contributes to overall function.

Renal biopsy

If imaging techniques fail to give a cause for the reduction in renal function, then a renal biopsy may be performed, although in advanced disease extensive scarring of the renal tissue may obscure the original (primary) diagnosis. Also, it is difficult to perform a biopsy of the small shrunken kidneys often seen in CKD and they may subsequently bleed. Most clinicians do not perform biopsies in this setting.

Rate of progression of chronic kidney disease

All patients with CKD should be monitored regularly. The recommendations for monitoring frequency can be found in the NICE guideline for assessment and management of CKD (NICE, 2014). In some patients with CKD the decline in renal function progresses at a constant rate and may be monitored by plotting the eGFR against time (see Fig. 18.11). The intercept with the x-axis indicates the time at which renal function will fall to zero and can be used to predict when the GFR will reach approximately 10 mL/min, that is, the level at which RRT should be initiated (Fig. 18.12A). If an abrupt decline in the slope of the reciprocal plot is noted (see Fig. 18.12B), this indicates a worsening of the condition or the presence of an additional renal insult.

It is, however, increasingly recognised that most patients with CKD do not sustain a predictable decline. Many stabilise or follow a path of episodes of accelerated decline followed by months or years of stability. These observations are of great interest and are an increasing focus of clinical research.

Prognosis

When the GFR has declined to about 20 mL/min, a continuing deterioration in renal function to ESRD is common even when the initial cause of the kidney damage has been removed and appropriate treatment instigated. The mechanisms for this decline in renal function include uncontrolled hypertension, proteinuria and damage resulting from hyperfiltration through the remaining intact nephrons. Serial GFR measurements should be monitored in conjunction with the patient's clinical condition to ensure the

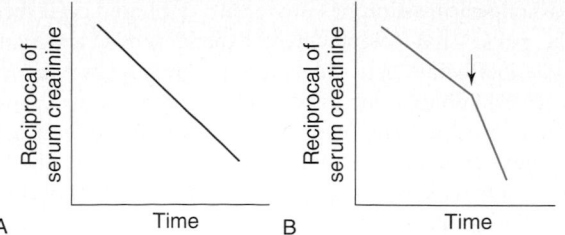

Fig. 18.12 Stylised reciprocal creatinine plots. (A) Linear, uniform progression in the decline in renal function. (B) Sudden decline in renal function (arrow).

Box 18.1 Factors that might exacerbate established chronic renal failure

Reduced renal blood flow
Hypotension
Hypertension
Nephrotoxins including drugs
Renal artery disease
Obstruction, e.g. prostatic hypertrophy

---

detection of the most appropriate point at which to commence RRT. Patients with an eGFR less than 20 mL/min should be supported to ensure that decisions have been made about the preferred modality of dialysis if ESRD is reached, suitability for and timing of transplantation, and for those patients who do not wish to receive dialysis or transplantation supportive care for symptom management if they reach ESRD.

There is now an accurate online tool for assessing the risk of progression of CKD to ESRD at the level of the individual patient (the Kidney Failure Risk Equation, see Useful Websites).

Treatment

The following are the aims of the treatment of CKD:
- halt or slow the process causing the renal damage (this may not be possible);
- avoid conditions that might worsen renal failure (Box 18.1);
- treat the secondary complications of CKD (renal anaemia and bone disease);
- relieve symptoms;
- implement treatment for ESRD in a controlled and timely manner.

Reversal or arrest of primary disease

By definition, CKD rarely has a readily reversible component, in contrast with acute renal failure. However, it is sometimes possible to identify a disease-specific factor that is contributing to declining renal function and remove it. Glomerulonephritis may respond to immunosuppressants and/or steroids. When drug-induced renal disease is suspected, the offending agent should be stopped. A post-renal lesion such as a ureter obstructed by a stone or a ureteric tumour may be successfully treated.

Hypertension

Optimum control of BP is usually the most important therapeutic measure. There is a cycle of events whereby hypertension causes damage to the intrarenal vasculature resulting in thickening and hyalinisation of the walls of arterioles and small vessels. This damage effectively reduces renal perfusion, contributing to stimulation of the RAAS. Arteriolar vasoconstriction, sodium and water retention result, which in turn exacerbates the hypertension.

Antihypertensive therapy with certain agents might produce a transient reduction in eGFR over the first 3 months of treatment as the systemic and glomerular BP drop; this is mainly seen with ACE inhibitors/angiotensin receptor blockers (ARBs). However, this is not an indication to stop the drugs unless the decline in eGFR is greater than 25%, because in the long-term the improvement in BP will slow the decline in renal function.

The drugs used to treat hypertension in CKD are generally the same as those used in other forms of hypertension, although allowance must be made for the effect of renal failure on drug disposition (NICE, 2014).

Calcium channel blockers

For patients without proteinuria, calcium channel blockers (CCBs) are the agents of choice. They produce vasodilatation principally by reducing Ca^{2+} influx into vascular muscle cells. CCBs also appear to promote sodium excretion in hypertension associated with fluid overload. The mechanism of this is unclear but may relate to the finding that high sodium levels can cause vasoconstriction by interfering with calcium transport.

Both verapamil and diltiazem (non-dihydropyridine CCBs) block conduction across the atrioventricular node and should not be used in conjunction with β-blockers. They are also negative cardiac inotropes. By contrast, dihydropyridine CCBs such as nifedipine and amlodipine produce less cardiac depression and differentially dilate afferent arterioles in the kidney.

CCBs can produce headache, facial flushing and oedema. The latter can be confused with the symptoms of volume overload but is resistant to diuretics. These effects occur because of changes in pre-capillary hydrostatic pressure, which forces fluid into the interstitial compartment. The oedema is not related to salt or water retention; hence the lack of response to diuretic therapy.

Angiotensin-converting enzyme inhibitors and angiotensin receptor blockers

The role of ACE inhibitors and ARBs in the management of CKD is now firmly established. In some patients the drugs have a protective effect over and above their impact on BP control. For example, patients with diabetes and albuminuria should be treated with ACE inhibitors or ARBs regardless of BP. In patients with CKD, but not with diabetes, the evidence indicates the use of these drugs as first-line treatment in patients with very heavy proteinuria.

ACE inhibitors reduce circulating ATII, and ARBs block binding to the ATII receptor; these actions result in vasodilatation and reduced sodium retention. ACE inhibitors and ARBs preferentially protect the glomerulus over and above their effect as systemic hypertensive agents, through decreasing efferent glomerular arteriolar vasoconstriction and therefore intra-glomerular hypertension and hyperfiltration. In the short-term they can cause a reduction in GFR by preventing the ATII-mediated vasoconstriction of the efferent glomerular arteriole. However, this decline is offset in the long-term by the protective effect of the agents in clinical practice.

Although the evidence for use of these drugs in patients with diabetic renal disease and proteinuric non-diabetic CKD is clear, care must be exercised in the following settings:

- Patients who sustain an early decline (in the first 7–10 days after ACE inhibitors/ARBs commencement) in kidney function of more than 25%: The drug should be stopped and potential renal artery stenosis investigated.
- Patients with non-proteinuric, non-diabetic CKD: These agents may be overused in this setting. There is no evidence that they provide a real renal benefit over other antihypertensive drugs.
- Patients with an accelerated decline in kidney function in the months to years after commencement of ACE inhibitors/ARBs: This is increasingly described and may reflect a resetting of the intra-renal perfusion to a level that potentiates chronic renal ischaemia present in most cases of CKD irrespective of cause.
- Patients with an intercurrent acute illness, particularly those admitted to hospital: Hypotension or infection will put patients at an increased risk of AKI.

For long-term management, it is usually preferable to use an agent with a duration of action that permits once-daily dosing. There is little to choose clinically between the ACE inhibitors currently on the market; however, consideration should be given to the cost benefits of choosing an agent that does not require dose adjustment in renal failure.

It has been reported that ACE inhibitors may reduce thirst, which may be useful in those patients who have a tendency to fluid overload as a result of excessive drinking. ACE inhibitors are potassium sparing; therefore, serum potassium should be monitored. If the potassium level is greater than 5.5 mmol/L on an ACE inhibitor or ARB, then a loop diuretic can be added because this will increase renal potassium clearance and lower serum potassium. A low-potassium diet may be necessary.

ARBs have properties similar to ACE inhibitors; however, because they do not inhibit the breakdown of kinins such as bradykinin, they do not cause the dry cough associated with the ACE inhibitors. There was interest in the potential use of dual blockade of the RAAS using ACE inhibitors and ARBs to produce more complete blockade of ATII. However, a number of studies have shown no added benefit and some evidence of worse outcomes, and this combination of drugs should be avoided (Mann and Böhm, 2015). Recently renin inhibitors have also been evaluated in clinical practice; however, this group of drugs was associated with a higher complication rate when used in combination with an ACE inhibitor and should not be used.

Diuretics

Diuretics are of use in patients with salt and volume overload, which is usually indicated clinically by the presence of oedema. This type of hypertension may be particularly difficult to treat. The choice of agent is generally limited to a loop diuretic.

Potassium-sparing diuretics are usually contraindicated because of the risks for development of hyperkalaemia, and thiazides become ineffective as renal failure progresses. In combination with ACE inhibitors, the mineralocorticoid receptor antagonists spironolactone and eplerenone can significantly reduce proteinuria; however, the combination of these agents raises the risk of significant hyperkalaemia, and care must be taken (Bianchi et al., 2005). The combination should be avoided when the eGFR falls to less than 30 mL/min. Studies are currently in progress assessing a role for spironolactone in patients with stage G1–G3 CKD.

Because loop diuretics need to be filtered to exert an action, progressively higher dosages are required as CKD worsens. Dosages of more than 250 mg/day furosemide may be required in advanced renal failure. Patients who do not respond to oral loop diuretic therapy alone may benefit from concomitant administration of metolazone, which acts synergistically to produce a profound diuresis. Alternatively, the loop diuretic may be given intravenously (i.v.). Care must be taken to avoid hypovolaemia (by monitoring body weight) and electrolyte disturbances such as hypokalaemia and hyponatraemia.

Thiazide diuretics, with the notable exception of metolazone, are ineffective at an eGFR less than 30 mL/min and may accumulate, causing an increased incidence of side effects.

β-Blockers

β-Blockers are commonly used in the treatment of hypertension in CKD. They exhibit a range of actions including a reduction of renin production. Consequently, β-blockers have a particular role in the rational therapy of hypertension without fluid overload. However, β-blockers can reduce cardiac output, cause peripheral vasoconstriction and exacerbate peripheral vascular disease.

It is advisable to use the more cardioselective β-blockers atenolol or metoprolol. Atenolol is excreted renally and consequently should require dosage adjustment in renal failure. In practice, however, atenolol is effective and tolerated well by renal patients at standard doses. Metoprolol is theoretically a better choice because it is cleared by the liver and needs no dosage adjustment, although small initial doses are advised in renal failure because there may be increased sensitivity to its hypotensive effects.

Selective α₁-blockers

These vasodilators produce a variety of actions that may be of benefit in hypertension associated with CKD. Sympathetic adrenergic activity can lead to sodium retention. Selective α₁-blockers have also been shown to produce improvements in insulin sensitivity, adverse lipid profiles and obstruction caused by hypertrophy of the prostate, all of which might be associated with some forms of CKD. These agents are used less commonly because there is some evidence that, in comparison with other antihypertensives, use is associated with adverse cardiovascular outcomes, especially the development of heart failure.

Vasodilators

The vasodilators hydralazine and minoxidil have been used to treat hypertension in CKD with varying degrees of success but are usually only used when other measures inadequately control BP. The sensitivity of patients to these drugs is often increased in renal failure, so, if used, therapy should be initiated with small doses. These agents cause direct peripheral vasodilation with resultant reflex tachycardia, which may require suppression by co-prescription of a β-blocker.

Centrally acting drugs

Methyldopa and clonidine are not commonly used as antihypertensives in CKD because of their adverse side effect profiles. If they are used in renal failure, initial doses should be small because of increased sensitivity to their effects.

Management of symptoms

Gastro-intestinal

Nausea and vomiting may persist after starting a low-protein diet. Metoclopramide is useful to treat this, but sometimes accumulation of the drug and its metabolites may occur, leading to extrapyramidal side effects. Patients should be started on a low dose, which should then be increased slowly. Prochlorperazine or cyclizine may also be useful. The 5-HT$_3$ antagonists such as ondansetron have also been shown to be effective. The patient with anaemia often becomes less nauseated when treated with an ESA.

Constipation is a common problem in patients with renal disease, partly as a result of fluid restriction and anorexia, and partly as a consequence of drug therapy with agents such as phosphate binders. It is particularly important that patients managed with peritoneal dialysis do not become constipated because this can reduce the efficacy of dialysis. Conventional laxative therapy may be used, such as bulk-forming laxatives or increased dietary fibre for less severe constipation. Alternatively, a stimulant such as senna with enemas or glycerine suppositories may be used for severe constipation. Higher doses of senna, typically two to four tablets at night, may be required. It should be noted that certain brands of laxatives that contain ispaghula husk may also contain significant quantities of potassium, and should be avoided in renal failure because of the risk of hyperkalaemia. Sterculia preparations are an effective alternative.

Pruritus

Pruritus (itching) associated with advanced CKD can be extremely severe, distressing and difficult to treat. It can also be disfiguring as a result of scratching. The exact mechanism responsible for the itching is not clear; the possibilities include one or more of xerosis (dry skin), skin micro-precipitation of divalent ions, elevated PTH levels and increased dermal mast cell activity.

Sometimes correction of serum phosphate or calcium levels improves itching, as does parathyroidectomy in patients with severe secondary or tertiary hyperparathyroidism. Conventionally, oral antihistamines have been used to treat pruritus; however, topical versions should not be used because of the risk of allergy. Non-sedating antihistamines such as loratadine are generally less effective than sedating antihistamines such as chlorphenamine or alimemazine, which may be useful, particularly at night. Topical crotamiton lotion and creams may also be useful in some patients. Other non-drug therapies include either warming or cooling the skin using baths, three times weekly ultraviolet B phototherapy and modified electrical acupuncture.

Recently, there is increasing evidence for the use of gabapentin, a drug which affects the neurotransmitter γ-aminobutyric acid and is usually used for epilepsy and neuropathic pain. Although gabapentin can be extremely effective for the itch associated with CKD (Rayner et al., 2012), dosing adjustments are required as it accumulates in CKD. There is less experience with the related drug, pregabalin, which can also be effective because it has a similar mechanism of action.

Dietary modifications

Historically, low-protein diets were used for patients with CKD; however, it is now accepted that this modification has limited evidence and is not used in mainstream clinical practice. The dietary modifications currently used include sodium and fluid restriction to reduce the risk of fluid overload, potassium restriction to reduce the risk of hyperkalaemia, and phosphate restriction. The dietary restrictions for patients with CKD can be arduous and difficult to follow.

Fluid retention

Oedema may occur as a result of sodium retention and the resultant associated water retention. Patients with CKD may also have hypoalbuminaemia secondary to very heavy proteinuria, and this can contribute to extravascular fluid retention (oedema) both through further activation of the RAAS and osmotic extravasation of fluid and its retention in tissues. The daily fluid intake for patients with CKD should be individualised, based on their predisposition to develop oedema. There is no clear evidence for a target fluid input (e.g. 3 L/day); however, it may be important to avoid dehydration because this may increase the risk of AKI.

For patients with ESRD, pulmonary and peripheral oedema is treated or avoided by using dialysis; however, the loop diuretic furosemide (often used at a very large dose) is used in patients who have a residual urine output because it can maintain urine output. In patients with ESRD, who have little (oliguria) or no (anuria) urine output, fluid restriction is critical. The fluid restriction for patients with ESRD can be limited to as little as 750 mL/day. This fluid allowance can be very difficult to maintain because it must include fluids ingested in any form, including sauces, medicines and fruits, in addition to drinks. Sucking ice cubes may relieve an unpleasant dry mouth, but patients should be encouraged not to swallow the melted water.

Sodium restriction. Sodium intake can be limited to 80 mmol/day by avoiding convenience foods and snacks or the addition of salt to food at the table. This is usually tolerable to patients. It is important to be aware of the potential contribution of sodium-containing medication to sodium loading, including some antibiotics, soluble or effervescent preparations, magnesium trisilicate mixture, Gaviscon, sodium bicarbonate and the plasma expanders hetastarch and gelatin.

Potassium restriction. Hyperkalaemia often occurs in CKD and may cause life-threatening cardiac arrhythmias. If untreated, asystolic cardiac arrest and death may result. Patients are often put on a potassium-restricted diet by avoiding potassium-rich foods such as fruit and fruit drinks, vegetables, chocolate, beer, instant coffee and ice cream. Many medicines have a high potassium content, for example, potassium citrate mixture, some antibiotics and ispaghula husk sachets. Emergency treatment is necessary if the serum potassium level is greater than 7.0 mmol/L or if there are ECG changes. The most effective treatment is dialysis, but if this is not available other measures may be tried (see Chapter 17).

The rationale and necessity for a renal diet and fluid restriction can be difficult for a patient to understand, and adherence may be a problem. A renal dietician is highly important in the management of patients with advanced CKD and is an established member of the multidisciplinary team of healthcare professionals required for a specialist renal service.

Anaemia

The anaemia of CKD is normochromic, normocytic and does not respond to iron or folic acid unless there is a coexisting deficiency. Functional iron deficiency in patients with CKD can occur at levels of serum ferritin that are in the normal range for patients with normal kidney function; consequently, there is a lower threshold for iron supplementation in patients with CKD. In addition, oral iron supplements are not well absorbed and/or tolerated in many patients with CKD, and therefore i.v. iron supplementation is commonly used.

Historically, the only treatment available for severe anaemia was red blood cell transfusions; however, this approach was a blood-borne infection risk, led to iron overload and promoted alloantibody formation, which decreased the likelihood of and increased the risk of subsequent kidney transplantation. The introduction of ESAs, initially as recombinant human erythropoietins (epoetin alfa and beta), into clinical practice in the early 1990s transformed the management of renal anaemia. Epoetin alfa and beta were thought to be indistinguishable in practical terms, as well as being immunologically and biologically indistinguishable from physiological erythropoietin. However, it has now been recognised that epoetins can be associated with the production of anti-erythropoietin antibodies leading to a severe anaemia which is unresponsive to exogenous epoetin. This is known as pure red cell aplasia and is more commonly associated with epoetin alfa when given by the subcutaneous route. The subcutaneous route is preferred because it provides equally effective clinical results while using similar or smaller doses (up to 30% less) than i.v. Most patients report a dramatically improved quality of life after starting epoetin therapy.

Epoetin alfa and beta have a short half-life and require dosing up to three times a week. Darbepoetin alfa is a novel erythropoiesis-stimulating protein that is a recombinant hyperglycosylated analogue of epoetin which stimulates red blood cell production by the same mechanism as the endogenous hormone. The terminal half-life in human is three times longer than that of epoetin and consequently requires a once-weekly or alternate weekly dosing schedule. A longer acting ESA has been introduced (methoxy polyethylene glycol-epoetin beta, pegzerepoetin alfa). This is a continuous erythropoietin receptor activator, which can be used in a once-monthly dosing schedule.

Iron and folate deficiencies must be corrected before therapy is initiated; patients receiving ESAs generally require concurrent iron supplements because of increased marrow requirements. Supplemental iron is usually given i.v. Maintaining iron stores ensures the effect of ESA is optimised for minimum cost, because with insufficient iron stores a patient will not respond to treatment with epoetin.

ESA therapy should aim to achieve a slow rise in the haemoglobin concentration to avoid cardiovascular side effects associated with a rapidly increasing red cell mass, such as hypertension, increased blood viscosity/volume, seizures and clotting of vascular accesses. BP should be closely monitored.

An initial subcutaneous or i.v. epoetin dosage of 50 units/kg body weight three times weekly, increased as necessary in steps of 25 U/kg every 4 weeks, should be given to produce a haemoglobin increase of not more than 2 g/dL per month. The target haemoglobin concentration is 10–12 g/dL, with most aiming for a target around 11.5 g/dL. Once this has been reached, a maintenance dosage of epoetin in the region of 33–100 U/kg three times a week or 50–150 U/kg twice weekly should maintain this level. Dosing adjustment and equivalence calculations are available for all currently used ESAs.

Several studies of ESAs have shown an increased risk of cardiovascular morbidity and overall mortality in people treated to a target greater than 12.5 g/dL (Phrommintikul et al., 2007). As a consequence, a discontinuation or reduction of dose is required in patients with a haemoglobin level greater than 12.5 g/dL.

Correcting anaemia usually helps control the symptoms of lethargy and myopathy, and often greatly reduces nausea. Improved appetite while receiving ESA therapy can, however, increase potassium intake and may necessitate additional dietary adjustment.

Acidosis

Because the kidney is the main route for excreting H^+ ions, CKD may result in a metabolic acidosis. This will cause a reduction in serum bicarbonate that may be treated readily with oral doses of sodium bicarbonate of 1–6 g/day. Because the dose of bicarbonate is not critical, it is easy to experiment with different dosage forms and strengths to suit individual patients. If acidosis is severe and persistent, then dialysis may be required. There is some evidence that correcting acidosis may slow the decline in renal function.

Neurological problems

Neurological changes are generally caused by uraemic toxins and improve on the treatment of uraemia by dialysis or diet. Muscle cramps are common and are often treated with quinine sulphate. Restless legs may respond to low doses of clonazepam or co-careldopa. In addition to their use for itching, gabapentin and pregabalin can also be used for restless legs.

Osteodystrophy

The osteodystrophy of renal failure is associated with three factors: hyperphosphataemia, vitamin D deficiency and hyperparathyroidism.

Hyperphosphataemia

The management of hyperphosphataemia depends initially upon restricting dietary phosphate. This can be difficult to achieve effectively, even with the aid of a specialist dietician, because phosphate is found in many palatable foods such as dairy products, eggs, chocolate and nuts. Phosphate-binding agents, when taken a few minutes before or with meals, can be used to reduce the absorption of orally ingested phosphate in the gut, by forming insoluble, non-absorbable complexes. Traditionally, phosphate-binders were usually salts of a di- or trivalent metallic ion, such as aluminium, calcium or occasionally magnesium. Although calcium-containing phosphate binders remain in widespread use, sevelamer and lanthanum-based binders are increasingly used.

Calcium carbonate has been used as a phosphate binder but is less effective as a phosphate binder than aluminium, and sometimes has been used in dosages of up to 10 g daily. However, this is no longer mainstream clinical practice and many clinicians advocate limiting elemental calcium dosing to ≤2 g/day because there is increasing evidence in patients with ESRD showing a relationship between calcium load and an increased risk of CVD events and early mortality (West et al., 2010). Calcium acetate is widely used as a phosphate binder. The capacity of calcium acetate and calcium carbonate to control serum phosphate appears to be similar. However, phosphate control is achieved using between half and a quarter of the dose of elemental calcium when calcium acetate is used.

Sevelamer, a hydrophilic but insoluble polymeric compound, is used increasingly as a phosphate binder. Sevelamer binds phosphate with an efficacy similar to calcium acetate but with no risk of hypercalcaemia. Mean levels of total and low-density cholesterol are also reduced with sevelamer use. This compound does not appear to present any risk of toxicity but may cause bowel obstruction and is relatively expensive when compared with other phosphate binders.

Lanthanum, like sevelamer, is a non-calcium-containing phosphate binder; there is therefore no resultant risk of hypercalcaemia, but there are gastro-intestinal side effects and these drugs are significantly more expensive than the alternatives. Although both of the non-calcium-containing phosphate binders available have been shown to reduce phosphate levels and keep calcium within acceptable levels, there is limited evidence to date for improvements in cardiovascular endpoints.

Historically, aluminium hydroxide was widely used as a phosphate binder because of the avid binding capacity of aluminium ions. However, a small amount of aluminium may be absorbed by patients with CKD owing to poor clearance of this ion, which can produce toxic effects including encephalopathy, osteomalacia, proximal myopathy and anaemia. Dialysis dementia was a disease observed among haemodialysis patients associated with aluminium deposition in the brain and exacerbated by aluminium in the water supply and the use of aluminium cooking pans.

Desferrioxamine (4–6 g in 500 mL of saline 0.9% per week) has been used to treat this condition by removing aluminium from tissues by chelation. The tendency of aluminium to cause constipation is an added disadvantage. Therefore, aluminium as a phosphate binder in CKD is controversial, and most clinicians advocate that it should only be used in shorter courses (e.g. months).

Vitamin D deficiency and hyperparathyroidism

Vitamin D deficiency may be treated with the synthetic vitamin D analogue 1α-hydroxycholecalciferol (alfacalcidol) at 0.25–1 microgram/day or 1,25-dihydroxycholecalciferol (calcitriol) at 1–2 micrograms/day. The serum calcium level should be monitored, and the dose of alfacalcidol or calcitriol adjusted accordingly. Hyperphosphataemia should be controlled before starting vitamin D therapy because the resulting increase in the serum calcium concentration on commencing vitamin D treatment may result in soft tissue calcification.

Paricalcitol is a synthetic, biologically active vitamin D analogue that selectively upregulates the vitamin D receptor in the parathyroid glands, reducing PTH synthesis and secretion. It also upregulates the calcium-sensing receptor in the parathyroids and reduces PTH by inhibiting parathyroid proliferation, PTH synthesis and secretion without affecting calcium or phosphorus levels. Paricalcitol is expensive, and the clinical evidence for the use of the drug is not strong enough at present for routine clinical practice.

The rise in 1,25-dihydroxycholecalciferol and calcium levels that result from starting vitamin D therapy usually suppresses the production of PTH by the parathyroids. If vitamin D therapy does not correct PTH levels, then parathyroidectomy, to remove part or most of the parathyroid glands, may be needed. This surgical procedure was once commonly performed on patients with CKD, but is now less frequent because of effective vitamin D supplementation and the introduction of cinacalcet.

Cinacalcet is a calcimimetic which increases the sensitivity of calcium-sensing receptors to extracellular calcium ion; this results in reduced PTH production. The benefit of this treatment is the suppression of PTH without resultant hypercalcaemia. It is recommended for use as an alternative to parathyroidectomy for patients who are not fit enough to undergo this procedure (NICE, 2007).

Common therapeutic problems in CKD are summarised in Table 18.4.

Renal transplantation

Renal transplantation has transformed the outlook for many patients with ESRD. The clinical outcomes of renal transplantation are now excellent. One-year patient and graft survival rates are 98% and 90–95%, respectively, and most patients who receive a transplant will never need to return to dialysis treatment. A renal transplant performed today in the developed world will continue to function, on average, in excess of

Table 18.4 Common therapeutic problems in chronic renal failure

Problem	Comment
Drug choice	Care with choice/dose of all drugs. Care to avoid renotoxic agents pre-dialysis to preserve function. Beware of herbal therapies because some contain immune system boosters (reverse immunosuppressant effects) and some are nephrotoxic.
Drug excretion	Chronic kidney disease will lead to accumulation of drugs and their active metabolites if they are normally excreted by the kidney.
Dietary restrictions	Restrictions on patient are often severe. Fluid allowance includes foods with high water content, e.g. gravy, custard, and fruit.
Hypertension	Frequently requires complex multiple-drug regimens. Calcium channel blockers can cause oedema that might be confused with fluid overload.
Analgesia	Side effects are increased. Initiate with low doses and gradually increase. Avoid pethidine as metabolites accumulate. Avoid non-steroidal anti-inflammatory drugs unless specialist advice is available.
Anaemia	Epoetin requires sufficient iron stores to be effective. Absorption from oral iron supplements may be poor, and intravenous iron supplementation might be required. Care is required to make sure that epoetin use does not produce hypertension.
Immunosuppression	Use of live vaccines should be avoided (i.e. bacille Calmette–Guérin, MMR [measles, mumps, rubella], mumps, oral polio, oral typhoid, smallpox, yellow fever).
Pruritus (itching)	Symptoms can be severe. Treat with chlorphenamine; less sedating antihistamines are often less effective. Some relief given with topical agents, e.g. crotamiton.
Restless legs	Involuntary jerks can prevent sleep. Clonazepam 0.5–1 mg at night may help.

15 years. However, an important consideration is that renal transplantation is the treatment of choice for patients with ESRD who are fit to receive a renal transplant; this recognises that many patients with advanced kidney disease are frail and elderly and/or have a number of co-existing medical problems such that they are not fit to undergo a major operation (implantation of the kidney) or to tolerate the immunosuppressive drugs that are required to prevent transplant rejection. This means that at any given time the majority of patients with ESRD are not actually on a national waiting list for a renal transplant.

For those patients who are fit enough to receive a renal transplant and are successfully transplanted, there is a profound survival benefit compared with remaining on dialysis treatment. The average transplant recipient lives two or three times as long as a matched dialysis patient who does not receive a renal transplant but remains on dialysis treatment. In addition, a transplant patient is less likely to be hospitalised and has a better quality of life than a dialysis patient. The secondary complications of CKD such as anaemia and bone disease resolve in many patients who are successfully transplanted. Furthermore, there are major health economic benefits to renal transplantation compared with dialysis. Transplantation is a far less expensive treatment than dialysis, particularly after the first year, when the large majority of the costs are limited to payment for the immunosuppressive drugs.

One of the major challenges for renal transplantation is the identification of a sufficient number of donor kidneys to fulfil demand. This is reflected in the increasing number of people who are waiting for a kidney; in the UK the average time on the waiting list before transplantation is around 3 years. Kidneys donated for the national waiting list are harvested from deceased donors. At the time of donation, donors are classified as dead as a consequence of either brainstem or cardiac death; these are also called heart beating and non–heart beating donors, respectively.

There is a shortage in the numbers of deceased donor kidneys available for transplantation; therefore, living donor transplantation has become increasingly common. In addition to addressing the scarcity of donor organs, patients who receive kidney transplants from living donors have better outcomes than patients who receive deceased donor kidneys. This is due to a number of factors, including the quality of the organs; living donors undergo a detailed health screening and if there is any indication that they have significant medical problems they are excluded from donation.

One of the major factors responsible for excellent outcomes for kidney transplant recipients is the use of immunosuppressive drugs to control the response as the immune system of the recipient mounts against the donor kidney. This is called an alloresponse. Alloimmunity refers to an immune response against tissue derived from an individual of the same species as the recipient of the tissue.

The major disadvantage of all immunosuppressive agents is their relative non-specificity, in that they cause a general depression of the immune system. This exposes the patient to an increased risk of malignancy and infection, which is an important cause of morbidity and mortality.

Table 18.5 Mechanism of action of immunosuppressants commonly used following renal transplantation

Drug	Mechanism	Comment
Steroids	Bind to steroid receptors and inhibit gene transcription and function of T cells, macrophages and neutrophils	Prophylaxis against and reversal of rejection
Ciclosporin	Forms complex with intracellular protein cyclophilin → inhibits calcineurin; ultimately inhibits interleukin-2 synthesis and T cell activation	Long-term maintenance therapy against rejection
Tacrolimus	Forms complex with an intracellular protein → inhibits calcineurin	Long-term maintenance therapy against rejection. Rescue therapy in severe or refractory rejection
Sirolimus	Inhibits interleukin-2 cell signalling → blocks T cell cycling and inhibits B cells	Usually used in combination with ciclosporin ± steroids
Mycophenolate	Inhibits inosine monophosphate dehydrogenase → reduces nucleic acid synthesis → inhibits T and B cell function	Usually used in combination with ciclosporin/ tacrolimus ± steroids
Azathioprine	Incorporated as a purine in DNA → inhibits lymphocyte and neutrophil proliferation	Usually used in combination with ciclosporin/ tacrolimus ± steroids
Muromonab (OKT3, mouse monoclonal anti-CD3)	Binds to CD3 complex → blocks, inactivates or kills T cell; short $t_{1/2}$	Prophylaxis against rejection. Reversal of severe rejection
Polyclonal horse/rabbit antithymocyte or antilymphocyte globulin	Antibodies against lymphocyte proteins → alter T and B cell activity	Prophylaxis against rejection. Reversal of severe rejection
Humanised or chimeric anti-CD25 (basiliximab and daclizumab)	Monoclonal antibodies that bind CD25 in interleukin-2 complex → prevent T cell proliferation	Prophylaxis against acute rejection in combination with ciclosporin and steroids

Immunosuppressants

The major pharmacological groups of immunosuppressive agents are summarised in Table 18.5.

Transplant recipients receive a high load of immunosuppression at the time of transplantation; this is known as induction immunosuppression. Induction immunosuppression is to protect the transplant from the high immunological risk that is present in the first few weeks after surgery. In the months following the transplant, the immunosuppression load is then incrementally reduced. Most patients will reach long-term low-dose maintenance immunosuppression sometime between 6 and 12 months after the transplant. However, whilst the transplant remains in the recipient it continues to represent an immunological risk; although overt, late rejection is uncommon, it can occur at any time if the patient stops taking his or her immunosuppressants. For a transplant to last many years, sustained day-to-day adherence with treatment is essential.

The most common combination used at induction is the calcineurin inhibitor (CNI) tacrolimus, the antiproliferative agent mycophenolate mofetil (MMF) and corticosteroids. Most patients also receive antibody induction. The antibody that is most commonly used is a monoclonal anti-CD25 antibody for people at low or medium immunological risk and anti–T cell polyclonal antibodies (thymoglobulin or ATG) for people at high immunological risk. There is also increasing use of alemtuzumab, a humanised CD52-specific complement-fixing (lymphocyte-depleting)

antibody. Patients at high immunological risk include those who have lost a previous transplant because of rejection, the presence of preformed circulating anti-human leucocyte antigen (HLA) antibodies at the time of transplantation (sensitisation), and major HLA mismatches (particularly at HLA-DR) between donor and recipient. Guidelines for the use of immunosuppressive therapy in kidney transplant patients have been issued and are currently being revised (NICE, 2004). International consensus guidelines now recommend use of newer agents such as MMF and emphasise the use of tacrolimus (rather than ciclosporin) as the CNI of choice (Kasiske et al., 2009). Tacrolimus is associated with less acute rejection than ciclosporin and may be associated with better graft function at 1 year and less graft loss (Knoll and Bell, 1999). It should be noted that generic/proprietary formulations of some drugs (e.g. tacrolimus and ciclosporin) are not interchangeable.

Calcineurin inhibitors (ciclosporin and tacrolimus)

The discovery and development of ciclosporin and latterly tacrolimus has led to a step improvement in 1-year renal transplant survival rate from 50–70% to 85–95%.

In T cells that have been exposed to T cell receptor ligation (signal 1) and co-stimulation (signal 2), there is activation of intra-cytoplasmic signalling pathways that include mobilisation of a molecule called calcineurin. Calcineurin contributes to the activation of a molecule called nuclear factor of activated T cells.

This factor then migrates to the nucleus and initiates transcription of interleukin-2 (IL-2) and other proinflammatory cytokines which are involved in driving an activated T cell into a proliferative phase, so that it makes multiple copies of itself. Ciclosporin and tacrolimus affect calcineurin through blocking binding proteins (cyclophilin and tacrolimus-binding protein, respectively) that are important for calcineurin activity.

The action of CNIs is partially selective in that they predominantly target T cells and have no direct effect on B cells; as a consequence, CNIs are associated with infections seen in people with deficiencies in the cellular limb of the immune response. These are predominantly intracellular infections such as viral, fungal, protozoal and mycobacterial infections.

Both ciclosporin and tacrolimus are critical dose drugs. That is, there is a narrow therapeutic window between underdosing and toxicity. Both drugs, therefore, require monitoring by serum levels. Trough levels are usually taken 12 hours after the previous dose and immediately before the next dose.

Ciclosporin

Ciclosporin causes a wide range of side effects, including nephrotoxicity, hypertension, fine muscle tremor, gingival hyperplasia, nausea and hirsutism. Hyperkalaemia, hyperuricaemia, hypomagnesaemia and hypercholesterolaemia may also occur. Nephrotoxicity is a particularly serious side effect and occasionally necessitates the withdrawal of ciclosporin. There is major inter-patient and intra-patient variation in absorption of ciclosporin. Blood level monitoring is required to achieve maximum protection against rejection and minimise the risk of side effects. The range regarded as acceptable varies between centres, but for ciclosporin it is commonly around 100–200 ng/mL in the first 6 months after transplantation and 80–150 ng/mL from 6 months onwards.

Ciclosporin interacts with a number of drugs that either lead to a reduction in ciclosporin levels, increase the risk of rejection or cause an elevation in ciclosporin levels leading to increased toxicity. Some drugs enhance the nephrotoxicity of ciclosporin (Box 18.2).

Ciclosporin should not be administered with grapefruit juice, which should also be avoided for at least an hour pre-dose, because this can result in marked increases in blood concentrations. This effect appears to be due to inhibition of enzyme systems in the gut wall resulting in transiently reduced ciclosporin metabolism.

Tacrolimus

Tacrolimus is not chemically related to ciclosporin, but acts by a similar mechanism. The side effect profile is similar to that of ciclosporin with some subtle differences. Disturbances of glucose metabolism leading to impaired glucose tolerance and new-onset diabetes after transplantation occurs in around 10–15% of patients who receive tacrolimus; this is twice as common as the incidence seen in patients who receive ciclosporin. In contrast, hirsutism is less of a problem in patients who receive tacrolimus than those who receive ciclosporin. In patients who are commenced on ciclosporin and then experience an episode of acute rejection, conversion to tacrolimus lowers the risk of recurrent rejection. Tacrolimus is an easier drug to use than ciclosporin. Careful monitoring is required with a target level of 8 ng/mL in the first weeks following transplantation, which is usually decreased in patients who follow an uncomplicated course to 5 ng/mL from 6 months.

> **Box 18.2** Examples of drug interactions involving ciclosporin
>
> - Reduce ciclosporin serum levels (hepatic enzyme inducers): phenytoin, phenobarbital, rifampicin, isoniazid
> - Increase ciclosporin serum levels (hepatic enzyme inhibitors): diltiazem, erythromycin, corticosteroids, ketoconazole
> - Enhance ciclosporin nephrotoxicity: aminoglycosides, amphotericin, co-trimoxazole, melphalan

---

Steroids

Prednisolone is the oral agent commonly used for immunosuppression after renal transplantation, whereas high-dose i.v. methylprednisolone is given as a single dose at induction with further use limited for cases of acute rejection. The maintenance dose of prednisolone to minimise adrenal suppression is around 0.1 mg/kg/day given as a single dose in the morning. The use of steroid therapy often leads to complications, particularly if high doses are given for long periods. In addition to a cushingoid state, the use of steroids may cause gastro-intestinal bleeding, hypertension, dyslipidaemia, diabetes, osteoporosis and mental disturbances. Patients who are temporarily unable to take oral prednisolone should be given an equivalent dose of hydrocortisone i.v.

Developments in therapy have led to an increasing use of steroid avoidance regimens. This term is misleading because patients still receive steroids, but use is restricted to the first week of transplantation. Currently, there is no long-term evidence to show this approach provides equivalence to a continuous steroid dosing regimen, but 1-year outcomes are comparable (Haller et al., 2016). If steroids are subsequently withdrawn months after the transplant, then outcomes with steroid avoidance regimens are worse.

Azathioprine

Azathioprine is derived from 6-mercaptopurine and is, therefore, an antimetabolite which reduces DNA and RNA synthesis-producing immunosuppression.

Azathioprine is given orally in a dosage of up to 2 mg/kg/day. There is no advantage in giving it in divided doses. Because azathioprine interferes with nucleic acid synthesis, it may be mutagenic, and pharmacy and nursing staff should avoid handling the tablets. Azathioprine has a significant drug interaction with allopurinol, causing fatal marrow suppression, and this combination should be avoided.

Mycophenolate mofetil

MMF is a prodrug of mycophenolic acid. It inhibits the enzyme inosine monophosphate dehydrogenase needed for guanosine synthesis which leads to reduced B cell and T cell proliferation. However, other rapidly dividing cells are less affected, as guanosine is produced in other cells. Consequently, mycophenolate has a more selective mode of action than azathioprine.

The drug is given in combination with tacrolimus at a dosage of 1 g twice a day which can subsequently be reduced after 6 weeks to 750 mg twice a day. A dose of 1.5 g twice a day is prescribed when used in combination with ciclosporin because the ciclosporin interferes with enterohepatic recirculation of mycophenolate metabolites with consequent lower exposure at a similar dose.

Compared with azathioprine, MMF reduces the risk of acute rejection episodes and improves long-term graft survival. However, it is a more potent immunosuppressant than azathioprine and is associated with a significantly increased risk of opportunistic infections.

Sirolimus

Sirolimus is a macrolide antibiotic that binds to the FKBP-25 cellular receptor. This complex initiates a sequence that produces modulation of regulatory kinases that ultimately interfere with the proliferative effects of IL-2 on lymphocytes. The progression of T cells from the G_1 to S phase is blocked, thus inhibiting cell division and therefore cell proliferation.

Adverse effects include hyperkalaemia, hypomagnesaemia, hyperlipidaemia, hypertriglyceridaemia, leukopenia, anaemia, impaired wound healing and joint pain. Sirolimus should not be used in the first few weeks after transplantation because it inhibits would healing through an antiproliferative effect. In combination with CNIs, it produces additive nephrotoxicity; when used with MMF it increases the risk of marrow suppression and mucosal side effects. Most experts currently limit the use of sirolimus to patients who have declining kidney function as a consequence of CNIs, but where graft function is still maintained to a GFR greater than 40 mL/min without significant proteinuria. Sirolimus may improve the outcomes of patients with skin cancer, and switching from a CNI to sirolimus in patients in this setting is increasingly utilised in clinical practice.

Monoclonal antibodies

The humanised or chimeric anti-CD25 monoclonal antibodies basiliximab and daclizumab are clinically similar and bind to CD25 in the IL-2 complex of activated T lymphocytes. This renders all T cells resistant to IL-2, and therefore prevents T cell proliferation. They are used as prophylaxis against acute rejection in combination with CNIs and steroids (NICE, 2004). Daclizumab is currently not available in the UK.

Polyclonal antibodies

Polyclonal antibodies were the first antibodies used as immunosuppressants and contain antibodies with a number of different antigen-combining sites. Polyclonal antibodies are used perioperatively as prophylaxis against rejection and in some cases to reverse episodes of severe rejection. The main preparations are antithymocyte globulin (ATG) or antilymphocyte globulin (ALG).

ATG is produced from rabbit or equine serum immunised with human T cells. It contains antibodies to human T cells, which on injection will attach to, neutralise and eliminate most T cells, thereby weakening the immune response. ALG is similar to ATG, is of equine origin, but is not specific to T cells as it also acts on B cells.

Polyclonal antibodies may act to inhibit T cell–mediated immune responses through a variety of mechanisms, including depletion of circulating T cells, modulation of cell surface receptor molecules, induction of anergy and apoptosis of activated T cells.

The main drawback to the use of anti–T cell sera is the relatively high incidence of side effects, notably anaphylactic reactions including hypotension, fever and urticaria. These reactions are more frequently observed with the first dose and may require supportive therapy with steroids and antihistamines. Severe reactions may necessitate stopping treatment. Steroids and antihistamines may be given prophylactically to prevent or minimise allergic reactions. Pyrexia often occurs on the first day of treatment but usually subsides without requiring treatment. Tolerance testing by administration of a test dose is advisable, particularly in patients such as asthmatics who commonly experience allergic reactions. In the event of adverse reactions, ALG and ATG can be substituted for each other.

Other precautions

Transplant patients are given prophylactic antibiotic therapy for varying periods postoperatively because of the risks of infection associated with immunosuppression. Treatment with co-trimoxazole to prevent *Pneumocystis carinii*, isoniazid and pyridoxine in high-risk patients to prevent tuberculosis, valganciclovir to prevent cytomegalovirus, and nystatin or amphotericin to prevent oral candidiasis are commonly used. Vaccination with live organisms (e.g. bacille Calmette–Guérin, MMR [measles, mumps, rubella], oral poliomyelitis, oral typhoid) must be avoided in the immunosuppressed patient.

Implementation of regular dialysis treatment

End-stage renal failure is the point at which the patient will die without the institution of renal replacement by dialysis or transplantation.

The principle of dialysis is simple. The patient's blood and a dialysis solution are positioned on opposing sides of a semi-permeable membrane across which exchange of metabolites occurs. The two main types of dialysis used in CKD are haemodialysis and peritoneal dialysis. Neither has been shown to be superior to the other in any particular group of patients, and so the personal preference of the patient is important when selecting dialysis modality. Haemodialysis and acute peritoneal dialysis are discussed in Chapter 17.

Because patients with ESRD may require dialysis treatment for many years, adaptations to the process of peritoneal dialysis have been made that enable the patient to follow a lifestyle as near normal as possible. Continuous ambulatory peritoneal dialysis involves a flexible non-irritant silicone rubber catheter (Tenckhoff catheter) that is surgically inserted into the abdominal cavity. Dacron cuffs on the body of the catheter become infiltrated with scar tissue during the healing process, causing the catheter to be firmly anchored in place. Such catheters may remain viable for many years. During the dialysis process thereafter, a bag typically containing 2.5 L of warmed dialysate and a drainage bag are connected to the catheter using aseptic techniques. Used dialysate is drained from the abdomen under gravity into the drainage bag, fresh dialysate is run into the peritoneal cavity and the giving set is disconnected. The patient continues his or her activities until the next exchange some hours later. The procedure is repeated regularly so that dialysate is kept in the abdomen 24 hours a day. This is usually achieved by repeating the process four times a day with an average dwell time of 6–8 hours. A number of different dialysis solutions are available of which the majority are glucose based.

Another form of peritoneal dialysis is known as automated peritoneal dialysis in which exchanges are carried out overnight while the patient sleeps. Dialysis fluid is exchanged, three to five times over a 10-hour period with volumes of 1.5–3 L each time. During the daytime the patient usually has a dwell of fluid within the abdominal cavity.

Because peritoneal dialysis is continuous and corrects fluid and electrolyte levels constantly, dietary and fluid restrictions are less stringent than required for patients treated with haemodialysis. Blood loss is also avoided, meaning that ESA requirements may be less. Unfortunately, peritoneal dialysis is not an efficient process; it only just manages to facilitate excretion of the substances required and, as albumin crosses the peritoneal membrane, up to 10 g of protein a day may be lost in the dialysate. It is also uncomfortable and tiring for the patient, and is contraindicated in patients who have recently undergone abdominal surgery.

Peritonitis is the most frequently encountered complication of peritoneal dialysis. Its diagnosis usually depends on a combination of abdominal pain, cloudy dialysate or positive microbiological culture. Empirical antibiotic therapy should, therefore, be commenced as soon as peritonitis is clinically diagnosed. Gram-positive cocci (particularly *Staphylococcus aureus*) and Enterobacteriaceae are the causative organisms in the majority of cases, while infection with Gram-negative species and *Pseudomonas* species are well recognised. Fungal infections are also seen, albeit less commonly.

Most centres have their own local protocol for antibiotic treatment of peritonitis. In one example, levofloxacin, a quinolone with good Gram-negative activity, is given orally, in combination with vancomycin, which has excellent activity against Gram-positive bacteria, being administered via the intraperitoneal route. As in all situations, the antibiotic regimen should be adjusted appropriately after the results of microbiological culture and sensitivity have been obtained.

Haemodialysis is particularly suitable for patients producing large amounts of metabolites, such as those with high nutritional demands or a large muscle mass, where these substances are produced faster than peritoneal dialysis can remove them. It also provides a backup for those patients in whom peritoneal dialysis has failed.

The various techniques of haemofiltration, a technique related to haemodialysis, are also discussed in detail in Chapter 17.

Case studies

Case 18.1

Mr D, a 19-year-old undergraduate student, visited his university health centre describing a 3-month history of fatigue, weakness, nausea and vomiting that he had attributed to 'examination stress'. His medical history indicated an ongoing history of bed wetting from an early age. Laboratory results from a routine blood screen showed the following:

		Reference range
Sodium	137 mmol/L	135–145 mmol/L
Potassium	4.8 mmol/L	3.5–5.0 mmol/L
Phosphate	2.5 mmol/L	0.9–1.5 mmol/L
Calcium	1.6 mmol/L	2.20–2.55 mmol/L
Urea	52 mmol/L	3.0–6.5 mmol/L
Creatinine	620 µmol/L	50–120 µmol/L
Haemoglobin	7.5 g/dL	13.5–18.0 g/dL

Subsequent referral to a specialist hospital centre established a diagnosis of CKD secondary to reflux nephropathy.

Question

Explain the signs and symptoms experienced by Mr D and the likely course of his disease?

Answer

Mr D is suffering from the signs and symptoms of uraemia resulting from CKD. Mechanical reflux damage to his kidneys has compromised renal function and resulted in an accumulation of toxins, including urea and creatinine, that, in turn, have contributed to his nausea, vomiting and general malaise. His biochemical results indicate other features typical of uraemic syndrome associated with chronic renal failure. The low haemoglobin is indicative of reduced erythropoietin production following progressive kidney damage. Renal osteodystrophy is also present, because inadequate vitamin D production and the raised serum phosphate have contributed to the hypocalcaemia.

This patient is likely to have remained symptom free for a period of years despite progressively worsening renal function. The kidneys operate with a substantial functional reserve under normal conditions. Patients generally remain asymptomatic as their renal reserve diminishes. Eventually there is a failure in the ability of the damaged kidney to compensate and symptoms appear late in the condition.

Case 18.2

Mr K, a 43-year-old man with established CKD, had been maintained for 3 years on continuous ambulatory peritoneal dialysis. He was admitted to hospital for cadaveric renal transplantation. On examination he was found to have slight ankle oedema. He weighed 60 kg, his BP was 135/90 mmHg and pulse rate 77 beats/min. He was administered the following immunosuppressants preoperatively: an anti-CD25 antibody, tacrolimus, mycophenolate and prednisolone.

Question

How should the immunosuppressants be administered to Mr K, and how should immunosuppression be managed postoperatively?

Answer

Anti-CD25 antibodies and high-dose methylprednisolone are given i.v. at the time of the operation. Typically tacrolimus at 200–300 micrograms/kg/day is given as two split doses, although once-daily formulations are also available. Specific tacrolimus preparations are not interchangeable, and as a result they must be prescribed by brand name; changes between preparations must only be made by a transplant specialist. Mycophenolate mofetil (MMF) at 1 g twice a day and prednisolone at 10 mg twice a day are given as oral doses to continue in the days and weeks following transplantation. These are commenced within 12 hours of the operation. In living kidney donation where the transplant operation is planned, patients are preloaded for several days before the transplant. i.v. tacrolimus is available, but should only be used in exceptional circumstances, usually when the gut is not working and all drugs and nutrition need to be given by the parenteral route.

Early dose adjustments in tacrolimus following transplantation are common and directed by drug levels. These are checked daily for the first week following transplantation; by 6 months they will be checked on alternate weeks. In the long-term the median dose of tacrolimus is around 2 mg twice a day and the dosage of mycophenolate mofetil can be reduced to 500–750 mg twice a day in the large majority of patients. The dosage of prednisolone is titrated down so that by 3 months it is 5–10 mg/day. Acute rejection episodes, diagnosed on a renal biopsy performed for a decline in graft function, are treated with high-dose steroids. For antibody-mediated (severe) rejection, plasma exchange and i.v. immunoglobulin are used.

Case 18.3

Mr A is a patient with CKD secondary to chronic interstitial nephritis. He reports chronic fatigue, lethargy and breathlessness on exertion, palpitations and poor concentration. His recent haematological results were found to be:

		Reference range
Haemoglobin	7.6 g/dL	13.5–17.5 g/dL
Red cell count	2.92×10^9 L^{-1}	4.5–6.5×10^9 L^{-1}
Haematocrit	0.208	0.40–0.54
Serum ferritin	88.0 micrograms/L	15–300 micrograms/L

Question

Explain Mr A's symptoms and haematological results, and outline the optimal treatment.

Answer

Mr A's symptoms are most likely a result of a normochromic, normocytic anaemia caused by CKD. Levels of erythropoietin produced by the kidney are reduced in renal failure. Production of erythropoietin from extra-renal sites (e.g. liver) are not sufficient to maintain erythropoiesis, which is also inhibited by uraemic toxins and hyperparathyroidism. The anaemia associated with renal failure is further compounded by a reduction in red cell survival through low-grade haemolysis, bleeding from the gastro-intestinal tract, and blood loss through dialysis, aluminum toxicity which interferes with haem synthesis, and iron deficiency, usually through poor dietary intake.

Therapy with erythropoietin-stimulating agent is the treatment of choice. However, iron and folate deficiencies should be corrected if epoetin therapy is to be successful. Iron demands are generally raised during epoetin treatment, and iron status should be regularly monitored. If serum ferritin declines to less than 200 micrograms/L, then iron supplementation should be started. Often i.v. iron is required to provide an adequate supply.

References

Bianchi, S., Bigazzi, R., Campese, V.M., 2005. Antagonists of aldosterone and proteinuria in patients with chronic kidney disease: a controlled pilot study. Am. J. Kidney Dis. 46, 45–51.

Cockroft, D., Gault, M., 1976. Predication of creatinine clearance from serum creatinine. Nephron 16, 31–34.

Counahan, R., Chantler, C., Ghazali, S., et al., 1976. Estimation of glomerular filtration from plasma creatinine concentration in children. Arch. Dis. Childhood. 51, 875–878.

Haller, M.C., Royuela, A., Nagler, E.V., Pascual, J., Webster, A.C., 2016. Steroid avoidance or withdrawal for kidney transplant recipients. Cochrane Database Syst. Rev. 2016 (8), CD005632. https://doi.org/10.1002/14651858.CD005632.pub3.

Hill, N.R., Fatoba, S.T., Oke, J.L., et al., 2016. Global prevalence of chronic kidney disease: a systematic review and meta-analysis. PLoS One 11 (7), e0158765. https://doi.org/10.1371/journal.pone.0158765.

Kasiske, B.L., Zeier, M.G., Chapman, J.R., et al., 2009. KDIGO Clinical Practice Guideline for the care of kidney transplant recipients. Am. J. Transplant. 9 (Suppl. 3), S10–S13.

Knoll, G.A., Bell, R.C., 1999. Tacrolimus versus ciclosporin for immunosuppression in renal transplant: meta-analysis of randomized trials. Br. Med. J. 318, 1104–1107.

Lerman, L., Textor, S.C., 2001. Pathophysiology of ischaemic nephropathy. Urol. Clin. North Am. 28, 793–803.

Mann, J.F., Böhm, M., 2015. Dual renin-angiotensin system blockade and outcome benefits in hypertension: a narrative review. Curr. Opin. Cardiol. 30, 373–377.

National Institute for Health and Care Excellence (NICE), 2004. Immunosuppressive therapy for renal transplantation in adults. Technology Appraisal 85. NICE, London. Available at: https://www.nice.org.uk/guidance/ta85.

National Institute for Health and Care Excellence (NICE), 2007. Cinacalcet for the treatment of secondary hyperparathyroidism in patients with end stage renal disease on maintenance dialysis therapy. Technology Appraisal 117. NICE, London. Available at: https://www.nice.org.uk/guidance/ta117.

National Institute for Health and Care Excellence (NICE), 2014. Chronic kidney disease in adults: assessment and management. Clinical Guideline 182. NICE, London. Available at: https://www.nice.org.uk/guidance/cg182.

Phrommintikul, A., Haas, S.J., Elsik, M., et al., 2007. Mortality and target haemoglobin concentrations in anaemic patients with chronic kidney disease treated with erythropoietin: a meta-analysis. Lancet 369, 381–388.

Rayner, H., Baharani, J., Smith, S., et al., 2012. Uraemic pruritus: relief of itching by gabapentin and pregabalin. Nephron Clin. Pract. 122 (3–4), 75–79.

Schwartz, G.J., 1985. A simple estimate of glomerular filtration rate in adolescent boys. J. Pediatr. 106, 522–526.

UK Renal Registry, 2008. The 11th Annual Report. Renal Association, Bristol.

West, S.L., Swan, V.J.D., Jamal, S.A., 2010. Effects of calcium on cardiovascular events in patients with kidney disease and in a healthy population. Clin. J. Am. Soc. Nephrol. 5, S41–S47.

Further reading

Daugirdas, J.T., Blake, P.G., Ing, S.T., 2014. Handbook of Dialysis, fifth ed. Lippincott Williams & Wilkins, Philadelphia.

Go, A.S., Chertow, G.M., Fan, D., et al., 2004. Chronic kidney disease and the risks of death, cardiovascular events and hospitalisation. N. Engl. J. Med. 351, 1296–1305.

Johnson, R.J., Feehally, J., Floege, J., 2015. Comprehensive Clinical Nephrology, fifth ed. Elsevier, Philadelphia.

National Institute for Health and Care Excellence, 2011. Chronic kidney disease (stage 5): peritoneal dialysis. Clinical Guideline 125. NICE, London. Available at: https://www.nice.org.uk/guidance/cg125.

National Institute for Health and Care Excellence, 2013. Chronic kidney disease (stage 4 or 5): management of hyperphosphataemia. Clinical Guideline 157. NICE, London. Available at: https://www.nice.org.uk/guidance/cg157.

National Institute for Health and Care Excellence, 2015. Chronic kidney disease: managing anaemia. Clinical Guideline 8. NICE, London. Available at: https://www.nice.org.uk/guidance/ng8.

ONTARGET Investigators, 2008. Telmisartan, ramipril, or both in patients at high risk of vascular events. N. Engl. J. Med. 358, 1547–1559.

Steddon, S., Chesser, A., Cunningham, J., et al., 2014. Oxford Handbook of Nephrology and Hypertension. Oxford University Press, Oxford.

Useful websites

National Institute of Diabetes and Digestive and Kidney Diseases. U.S. site with useful glomerular filtration rate calculators including those with SI units: https://www.niddk.nih.gov/health-information/health-communication-programs/nkdep/lab-evaluation/gfr-calculators/Pages/gfr-calculators.aspx

The Kidney Failure Risk Equation. Find out your real risk of kidney failure at: http://www.kidneyfailurerisk.com

19 Hypertension

Helen Williams

Key points

- Hypertension can be defined as a condition in which blood pressure (BP) is elevated to a level likely to lead to adverse consequences. There is no clear-cut blood pressure threshold separating normal blood pressure from high blood pressure, with hypertension arbitrarily defined as a systolic blood pressure equal to or greater than 140 mmHg and/or diastolic blood pressure equal to or greater than 90 mmHg. The risk of complications is related to the degree to which blood pressure is elevated.

- The World Health Organization has identified hypertension as the leading risk factor for death worldwide. The complications of hypertension include stroke, myocardial infarction, heart failure, renal failure and dissecting aortic aneurysm. Modest reductions in blood pressure result in substantial reductions in the relative risks of these complications.

- Hypertension should not be seen as a risk factor in isolation, and decisions on management should not focus on blood pressure alone but on the total cardiovascular risk present for an individual, which, in the absence of established cardiovascular (CV) disease, should be calculated using a validated CV risk calculator such as QRisk2.

- The diagnosis of hypertension should be based on the results of ambulatory blood pressure monitoring or home blood pressure monitoring, not on clinic blood pressure readings.

- Non-pharmacological interventions are important and include weight reduction, avoidance of excessive salt and alcohol, increased intake of fruit and vegetables and regular physical activity. Other cardiovascular risk factors, such as smoking, dyslipidaemia and diabetes, should be addressed.

- Different antihypertensive drugs are available. Drug choice should aim to maximise blood-pressure-lowering effectiveness and minimise patient side effects.

- The most appropriate choice of initial drug therapy depends on the age and racial origin of the patient, as well as the presence of other medical conditions. For patients younger than 55 years, an angiotensin-converting enzyme (ACE) inhibitor is recommended as first-line treatment. For older patients and people of black African or Caribbean origin of any age, a calcium channel blocker is an appropriate initial choice. Most people need a combination of drugs to achieve adequate blood pressure control.

Hypertension (high blood pressure) is an important risk factor for the future development of cardiovascular disease. It can be defined as a condition in which blood pressure (BP) is elevated to a level likely to lead to adverse consequences and where clinical benefit will be obtained from BP lowering. BP

measurement includes systolic and diastolic components, and both are important in determining an individual's cardiovascular risk.

Blood pressure is continuously distributed in the population, and there is no clear cut-off point between hypertensive and normotensive subjects, although a figure of systolic/diastolic blood pressure of 140/90 mmHg is considered the upper limit of 'normal'. Hypertension has therefore been arbitrarily defined as a systolic blood pressure above 140 mmHg or a diastolic blood pressure above 90 mmHg, or both. Hypertension is largely a condition affecting older individuals. Whereas diastolic pressure peaks at age 50, systolic pressure continues to increase with advancing age, and hence isolated systolic hypertension is a common feature of older age. Generally, the risk of cardiovascular disease doubles for every 20/10-mmHg rise in blood pressure.

The cardiovascular complications associated with hypertension are shown in Box 19.1. The most common and important of these are stroke and myocardial infarction. The risk associated with increasing blood pressure is continuous, with each 2-mmHg rise in systolic blood pressure associated with a 7% increased risk of mortality from ischemic heart disease and a 10% increased risk of mortality from stroke (National Institute for Health and Care Excellence [NICE], 2011). The risk of heart failure is increased sixfold in hypertensive subjects. Meta-analysis of clinical trials has indicated that these risks are reversible, with relatively modest reductions in blood pressure of 10/6 mmHg associated with a 38% reduction in stroke and 16% reduction in coronary events (Collins et al., 1990), whereas a 5-mmHg reduction in blood pressure is associated with a 25% reduction in risk of renal failure. There is considerable evidence

---

Box 19.1 Complications of hypertension

- Myocardial infarction
- Stroke
  - Cerebral/brainstem infarction
  - Cerebral haemorrhage
  - Lacunar syndromes
  - Multi-infarct disease
- Hypertensive encephalopathy/malignant hypertension
- Dissecting aortic aneurysm
- Hypertensive nephrosclerosis
- Peripheral vascular disease

from clinical trials to demonstrate that the treatment of subjects with blood pressures above the threshold (BP >140/90 mmHg) currently used in clinical practice results in important clinical benefits.

The absolute benefits of blood pressure lowering achieved as a result of these relative risk reductions depend on the underlying level of cardiovascular risk present for an individual. High-risk subjects gain more benefit in terms of events saved per year of therapy. Absolute risk is highest in those who already have evidence of cardiovascular disease, such as previous myocardial infarction, transient ischaemic attack or stroke, or who have other evidence of cardiovascular dysfunction such as electrocardiogram (ECG) or echocardiograph abnormality. Risk is also increased in the elderly and in people with diabetes or renal failure and is further enhanced by other risk factors, such as smoking, dyslipidaemia, obesity and sedentary lifestyle. In those under the age of 75, men are at greater risk than women. Cardiovascular risk of an individual with no known cardiovascular disease can be estimated using cardiovascular risk calculators, such as QRisk (UK) (https://www.qrisk.org/), SCORE (Europe) (https://www.escardio.org/Education/Practice-Tools/CVD-prevention-toolbox/SCORE-Risk-Charts#) and ASSIGN (Scotland) (http://assign-score.com).

Epidemiology

Hypertension is a very common condition. It is estimated that approximately 25% of the adult population has hypertension, rising to above 50% of people over the age of 60 years old (NICE, 2011), although much of this remains undiagnosed.

In 90–95% of cases of hypertension, there is no underlying medical illness to cause high blood pressure. This is termed 'essential' hypertension, so named because at one time it was erroneously believed to be an 'essential' compensation mechanism to maintain adequate circulation. The precise aetiology of essential hypertension is currently unknown. Genetic factors clearly play a part because the condition clusters in families, with hypertension being twice as common in subjects who have a hypertensive parent. Genetic factors account for about one-third of the blood pressure variation between individuals, although no single gene appears to be responsible except in some rare conditions such as polycystic kidney disease and other metabolic conditions such as Liddle's syndrome (Beevers et al., 2001). The remaining 5–10% of cases are secondary to some other disease process (Box 19.2).

Hypertension is more common in black people of African or Caribbean family origin, who are also at particular risk of stroke and renal failure. Hypertension is exacerbated by other factors, for example, high salt or alcohol intake or obesity.

Regulation of blood pressure

The mean blood pressure is the product of cardiac output and total peripheral resistance. In most hypertensive individuals, cardiac output is not increased, and high blood pressure arises as a

---

Box 19.2 Causes of hypertension

Primary hypertension (90–95%)
- Essential hypertension

Secondary hypertension (5–10%)
- Renal diseases
- Endocrine diseases
  - Steroid excess: hyperaldosteronism (Conn's syndrome); hyperglucocorticoidism (Cushing's syndrome)
  - Growth hormone excess: acromegaly
  - Catecholamine excess: phaeochromocytoma
  - Others: pre-eclampsia
- Vascular causes
- Renal artery stenosis: fibromuscular hyperplasia; renal artery atheroma; coarctation of the aorta
- Drugs
  - Sympathomimetic amines
  - Oestrogens (e.g. combined oral contraceptive pills)
  - Ciclosporin
  - Erythropoietin
  - Non-steroidal anti-inflammatory drugs
  - Steroids

---

result of increased total peripheral resistance caused by constriction of small arterioles.

Control of blood pressure is important in evolutionary terms, and homeostatic reflexes have evolved to provide blood pressure homeostasis. Minute-to-minute changes in blood pressure are regulated by the baroreceptor reflex, whereas the renin–angiotensin–aldosterone system is important for longer-term salt, water and blood pressure control. Long-term increases in shear stress can cause vascular remodelling of the endothelium, which leads to the formation of a procoagulant rather than anticoagulant surface. At the same time, systems that lead to vascular relaxation, for example, nitric oxide, are overcome by increased sensitivity to vasoconstrictor substances such as endothelin, which predispose to vascular disease and further increases in peripheral resistance, which lead to a vicious cycle that increases blood pressure further due to the increase in vascular resistance. Other substances with a role in controlling blood pressure include atrial natriuretic peptide, bradykinin and antidiuretic hormone.

Clinical presentation

Hypertension is asymptomatic in most cases and is often, therefore, an incidental finding when subjects present with unrelated conditions or may be identified during a cardiovascular risk assessment. Severe cases may present with headache, visual disturbances or evidence of target organ damage (including stroke, ischaemic heart disease, renal failure or retinopathy). In the UK, adults, particularly those over 40 years of age, should have their blood pressure checked at least every 5 years, with an annual review for those with high normal values in the range 135–139 mmHg systolic or 85–89 mmHg diastolic.

Malignant (accelerated) hypertension

Malignant or accelerated hypertension is an uncommon condition characterised by greatly elevated blood pressure (usually BP >220/120 mmHg) associated with evidence of ongoing small vessel damage. Fundoscopy may reveal papilloedema, haemorrhages and/or exudates, and renal damage can manifest as haematuria, proteinuria and impaired renal function. The condition may be associated with hypertensive encephalopathy, which is caused by small vessel changes in the cerebral circulation associated with cerebral oedema. The clinical features are confusion, headache, visual loss, seizures and coma. Brain imaging, particularly magnetic resonance imaging (MRI), usually demonstrates extensive white matter changes. Malignant hypertension is a medical emergency that requires hospital admission and rapid control of blood pressure over 12–24 hours towards normal levels.

Urgent specialist care is recommended for patients with accelerated hypertension, defined as BP usually higher than 180/110 mmHg with signs of papilloedema and/or retinal haemorrhage or suspected phaeochromocytoma (labile or postural hypotension, headache, palpitations, pallor and diaphoresis) (NICE, 2011).

Management of hypertension

In the UK, the management of hypertension is guided by guidelines produced by NICE (2011). Joint guidelines from the European Society of Hypertension and European Society of Cardiology were published in 2013 (Mancia et al., 2013).

Diagnosis of hypertension

Blood pressure should be measured using a validated manual or automated sphygmomanometer, which should be well maintained and regularly calibrated. Blood pressure should initially be measured in both arms, and if there is a difference of more than 20 mmHg sustained after repeat measurement, the arm with the highest value should be used for subsequent monitoring readings. Differences of more than 15 mmHg between arms may indicate risk of underlying vascular disease and an increased risk of all-cause and cardiovascular (CV) mortality (Clark et al., 2012).

The subject should be relaxed, and at least at the first presentation, blood pressure should be measured in both the sitting and the standing positions to identify any postural changes. An appropriate-sized cuff should be used because one that is too small will result in an overestimation of the patient's blood pressure. The arm should be supported level with the heart. Where blood pressure is measured manually, the Korotkov sounds appear (the first phase) and disappear (the fifth phase) over the brachial artery as pressure in the cuff is released. Cuff deflation should occur at approximately 2 mmHg per second to allow accurate measurement of the systolic and diastolic blood pressures. The fourth Korotkov phase (muffling of sound) has previously been used for diastolic blood pressure measurement but is not currently recommended unless Korotkov V cannot

be defined. Where blood pressure is measured using an automated device, it is important to palpate the radial or brachial pulse before measuring blood pressure to identify if there is a pulse irregularity, for example, atrial fibrillation. In such situations the automated device may not measure blood pressure accurately, and therefore blood pressure should be measured manually.

If the manual or automated blood pressure reading is 140/90 mmHg or higher, a second measurement should be taken, and if the result is substantially different from the first, a third measurement should be taken. The lower of the last two measurements should be recorded as the clinic blood pressure.

Having established that the blood pressure in the clinic setting is 140/90 mmHg or greater, a diagnosis of hypertension should be confirmed by ambulatory blood pressure monitoring (ABPM) or home blood pressure monitoring (HBPM), except in the case of severe hypertension (systolic blood pressure equal to or greater than 180 mmHg and diastolic blood pressure equal to or great than 110 mmHg), when the treatment should be initiated immediately.

Ambulatory or home blood pressure measurements

NICE (2011) recommended that ambulatory or home blood pressure monitoring should be used to confirm the diagnosis of blood pressure because some people develop excessive and unrepresentative blood pressure rises when in the clinic setting, so-called 'white-coat' hypertension. White-coat hypertension can be largely excluded by 24-hour ABPM or by the patients checking their blood pressure at home away from the clinic setting. A systematic review of the relative effectiveness of clinic BP monitoring and HBPM compared with ABPM in diagnosis of hypertension concluded that ABPM was the most accurate strategy based on the evidence available at the time (Hodgkinson et al., 2011). ABPM over 24 hours is also useful for patients who have unusual variability in blood pressure, resistant hypertension or symptoms suggesting hypotension. Home blood pressure measurement is inexpensive, but it is important to have a machine of validated accuracy that the patient can use properly. Because ambulatory and home blood pressure measurements are usually lower than clinic recordings, NICE (2011) recommended that the diagnostic threshold for hypertension using these strategies should be systolic BP equal to or greater than 135 mmHg and/or diastolic BP equal to or greater than 85 mmHg.

Hypertension classification

The NICE (2011) guidance classifies hypertension as follows:
- Stage 1 hypertension: Clinic blood pressure is 140/90 mmHg or higher, and subsequent ABPM daytime average or HBPM average blood pressure is 135/85 mmHg or higher.
- Stage 2 hypertension: Clinic blood pressure is 160/100 mmHg or higher, and subsequent ABPM daytime average or HBPM average blood pressure is 150/95 mmHg or higher.
- Severe hypertension: Clinic systolic blood pressure is 180 mmHg or higher or clinic diastolic blood pressure is 110 mmHg or higher.

Assessment of the hypertensive patient

Secondary causes

Although most cases of hypertension are essential or primary, it is important to take a careful history, checking for features that might suggest a possible secondary cause of hypertension. Examples would be symptoms of renal disease, such as haematuria or polyuria, or the paroxysmal symptoms that suggest the rare diagnosis of phaeochromocytoma and include headache, postural dizziness and syncope. A careful physical examination should be performed for abdominal bruits, which suggests possible renal artery stenosis; radiofemoral delay, which suggests coarctation of the aorta; and palpable kidneys, which suggests polycystic kidney disease. Laboratory analysis should include a full blood count, electrolytes, urea, creatinine and urinalysis, checking the albumin/creatinine ratio (ACR) as well as for glucosuria. In some patients, further investigations may be appropriate, for example, ultrasound of the abdomen or isotope renogram where renal disease is suspected. A renin/angiotensin ratio is a useful screening test to investigate for possible hyperaldosteronism, and serum metanephrine and urinary catecholamines may detect underlying phaeochromocytoma.

A low serum potassium may alert to the presence of hyperaldosteronism, but it should be remembered that renin levels are suppressed by β-blockers and aldosterone by ACE inhibitors and receptor antagonists. A very high aldosterone/renin ratio may suggest Conn's syndrome or primary hyperaldosteronism. This is usually caused by a benign adenoma or simple hyperplasia within the zona glomerulosa of the adrenal gland, the presence of which may be demonstrated by computed tomography (CT) or magnetic resonance imaging (MRI) scanning. The tumours may be surgically resected, but where there is a suggestion of hyperaldosteronism and no obvious tumour on imaging, patients may still respond to spironolactone, an aldosterone antagonist, while remaining relatively resistant to other antihypertensives.

Contributing factors

The patient should also be assessed for possible contributory factors to the development of hypertension, such as obesity, excess alcohol or salt intake and lack of exercise. Occasionally, hypertension may be provoked by the use of drugs (see Box 19.2), including over-the-counter medicines used as cold and flu remedies. Other risk factors should also be documented and addressed, for example, smoking, diabetes and hyperlipidaemia. It is important to establish whether there is a family history of cardiovascular disease.

Evidence of end-organ damage

The patient should also be examined carefully for evidence of end-organ damage from hypertension. This should include examination of the optic fundi to detect retinal changes. An ECG should be performed to detect left ventricular hypertrophy or subclinical ischaemic heart disease. It is advisable to check the renal function and test the urine for signs of microalbuminuria, which may be an indicator of a higher risk of future end-stage renal disease and overall vascular risk. The presence of end-organ damage indicates the need for early intervention with drug therapy to control blood pressure in patients with stage 1 hypertension.

Determination of cardiovascular risk

An accurate assessment of cardiovascular disease risk is essential before recommending appropriate management in hypertension. Patients with documented atheromatous vascular disease, for example, previous myocardial infarction or stroke, angina or peripheral vascular disease are at high risk of recurrent events. Similarly, patients with evidence of target organ damage are at higher risk. For patients without established vascular disease, it is necessary to estimate cardiovascular risk (see Chapter 24). A 10-year cardiovascular disease (CVD) risk of 20% is regarded as an appropriate threshold for antihypertensive therapy in patients with stage 1 hypertension, with lipid-lowering therapy to be considered in patients with 10-year CVD risk of 10% or more. Treatment decisions based on these calculations will favour treatment in older patients. Although a younger patient with stage 1 hypertension may be at lower absolute risk over 10 years and may not meet the criteria for antihypertensive drug therapy and lipid treatment, the younger patient may be at higher lifetime and longer-term risk of premature death and vascular disease and, thus, still merit risk factor intervention.

Other factors to consider include microalbuminuria, which increases cardiovascular risk by a factor of 2–3, and the combination of reduced glomerular filtration rate (GFR) and microalbuminuria, which may increase risk by as much as sixfold (Cirillo et al., 2008; Sehestedt et al., 2009).

Treatment

Non-pharmacological approaches

Non-pharmacological management of hypertension is an important aspect of treatment for all people with hypertension and is the first-line strategy in people with stage 1 hypertension at low risk of cardiovascular events. Lifestyle advice should include discussion of weight loss, diet and physical activity, as well as salt and alcohol intake and smoking cessation, with signposting to relevant local services to support the patient's efforts to address these issues. The impact of common lifestyle interventions on systolic blood pressure is summarised in Table 19.1. In order to maximise potential benefit, patients should receive clear and unambiguous advice, including written information they can digest in their own time. Written advice for patients can be downloaded from the British Heart Foundation website (http://www.bhf.org.uk) and the Blood Pressure UK website (http://www.bloodpressureuk.org/Home).

In patients who are overweight, reductions in systolic blood pressure of 0.5–2 mmHg per kg weight loss can be achieved. The Dietary Approaches to Stop Hypertension (DASH) diet was evaluated in a clinical trial and found to lower blood pressure significantly (4.5/2.7 mmHg) compared with a typical US diet. This diet emphasises fruit, vegetables and low-fat dairy produce in addition to fish, low-fat poultry and whole grains while

Table 19.1 Impact of lifestyle modifications on blood pressure (DiPiro et al., 2014)

Modification	Recommendation	Approximate systolic blood pressure reduction (mmHg)[a]
Weight loss	Maintain normal body weight	5–20 per 10-kg weight loss
DASH-type diet	Consume a diet rich in fruits, vegetables and low-fat dairy products with reduced saturated and total fat	8–14
Reduced salt intake	Reduce daily dietary sodium intake	2–8
Physical activity	Regular aerobic physical activity (at least 30 min/day, most days of the week)	4–9
Moderation of alcohol intake	Limit consumption to 2 drinks/day in men and 1 drink/day in women and lighter-weight persons	2–4

[a]Effects of implementing these modifications are time and dose dependent and could be greater for some patients.
DASH, Dietary approaches to stop hypertension.

minimising red meat, confectionaries and sweetened drinks (Appel et al., 1997). Subjects should reduce their salt intake, for example, by not adding salt to food when cooking, using spices to add flavour and not adding additional salt to food on the plate. A daily sodium intake of less than 100 mmol (i.e. 6 g sodium chloride or 2.4 g elemental sodium) should be the aim. There is a significant amount of hidden salt in processed meat, ready meals, cheese and even bread. A dietary assessment may be required to accurately quantify a patient's salt intake and advise on how reductions might be made. Most subjects will need to limit their calorie and saturated fat intake. Regular physical activity should be encouraged, at a level appropriate to the individual subject, aiming for a total of 150 minutes of moderate-intensity exercise per week or 75 minutes of high-intensity activity per week. This results in improved physical fitness and a reduction in blood pressure. Alcohol intake should be restricted to a maximum of 14 units per week, with 2 consecutive days alcohol-free. Although smoking does not have a direct effect on blood pressure, it increases cardiovascular risk, and patients should stop or, if this is not possible, reduce their cigarette consumption.

For low-risk stage 1 hypertension, lifestyle approaches are currently the only recommended intervention. However, if there is a more urgent need for drug treatment, for example, in stage 2 and severe hypertension, non-pharmacological interventions should occur in parallel with the initiation of drug therapy.

Drug treatment

Treatment thresholds

Treatment thresholds are summarised in Table 19.2. Patients with severe hypertension (>180/110 mmHg confirmed on several readings on the same occasion) should be treated immediately, and some guidance suggests that dual therapy should be commenced immediately in patients at high risk or with markedly high baseline blood pressure because monotherapy is unlikely to be effective (Mancia et al., 2013). People with stage 2 hypertension should have drug treatment initiated, alongside

Table 19.2 Threshold blood pressures for intervention

Category	Intervention
Stage 1 hypertension with no additional risk factors	Lifestyle advice and support If under 40 years old, consider referral for specialist assessment of secondary causes and possible target organ damage
Stage 1 hypertension with ≥1 of the following: • established CVD • target organ damage (left ventricular hypertrophy, chronic kidney disease, hypertensive retinopathy), • renal disease, • diabetes, • a 10-year CVD risk ≥20%.	Lifestyle advice and support Drug treatment for all ages
Stage 2 hypertension	Lifestyle advice and support Drug treatment for all ages
Severe hypertension	Lifestyle advice and support Drug treatment for all ages Refer to specialist care the same day if patient has: • accelerated hypertension, • blood pressure usually higher than 180/110 mmHg with signs of papilloedema, • suspected phaeochromocytoma (labile or postural hypotension, headache, palpitations, pallor and diaphoresis).

CVD, Cardiovascular disease.

lifestyle advice. People below the age of 80 with stage 1 hypertension and the presence of other complications, such as evidence of target organ damage, cardiovascular complications, diabetes, renal disease or a calculated cardiovascular risk more than 20% over 10 years, should also have drug treatment initiated alongside lifestyle advice. Patients with blood pressure in the high normal range (systolic BP 135–139 and/or diastolic BP 85–89 mmHg) should be reassessed annually, whereas those with blood pressure lower than this can be rechecked every 5 years.

Target blood pressures

The optimal blood pressure treatment target has not been established. Current guidance in the UK (NICE, 2011) suggests that for uncomplicated hypertension, patients should be treated to achieve a clinic blood pressure less than 140/90 mmHg, except those older than 80 years, for whom a clinic blood pressure target of 150/90 mmHg is recommended (Table 19.3). More aggressive targets for patients with comorbidities are summarised in Table 19.4.

Studies that have sought to establish optimal blood pressure treatment targets include the following:

- In the Hypertension Optimal Treatment (HOT) study (Hansson et al., 1998), patients were allocated diastolic target blood pressures of less than 90, 85 and 80 mmHg. The study struggled to stratify patients effectively into these treatment groups, but analysis suggested that the optimum target blood pressure was less than 140/85 mmHg, with little benefit in lowering to lower levels of 120/70 mmHg but also little evidence of harm.
- The UK Prospective Diabetes Study Group (1998a, 1998b) suggested 'tight' blood pressure control was better than less tight in patients with non-insulin-dependent diabetes (type II

diabetes). The targets in the UK Prospective Diabetes Study were 'tight' less than 150/85 mmHg and 'less tight' less than 180/105 mmHg, but the actually achieved blood pressures were lower, for example, 154/87 mmHg versus 144/82 mmHg.
- The Cardio-Sis study randomised non-diabetic subjects with systolic blood pressure greater than 150 mmHg to target systolic blood pressure of less than 140 or less than 130 mmHg (Verdecchia et al., 2009). The primary end point was left ventricular hypertrophy, although the secondary end point of a composite cardiovascular end point was reduced (as well as the primary end point) in the 130-mmHg group, with no increase in adverse events. This, however, is not robust enough evidence to recommend a reduction in blood pressure target levels and would require a larger study of hard clinical end points to confirm these findings.
- Most recently, the SPRINT study (SPRINT Research Group, 2015) sought to compare the impact of intensive blood pressure (target systolic <120 mmHg) versus standard treatment (target systolic <140 mmHg). The trial was stopped early due to a significant reduction in fatal and nonfatal major cardiovascular events and death from any cause in the intensive-treatment group. Higher rates of some adverse events were observed in this group, including hypotension, syncope, electrolyte abnormalities, and acute kidney injury or failure, but not injurious falls.

A recent systematic review was designed to assess the association of mean achieved systolic blood pressure levels with the risk of cardiovascular disease and all-cause mortality in adults with hypertension treated with antihypertensive therapy. It concluded that reducing systolic blood pressure to levels below currently recommended targets significantly reduces the risk of cardiovascular disease and all-cause mortality, with a mean achieved systolic BP of 120–124 mmHg being associated with the lowest CV risk (Bundy et al., 2017). Although the authors concluded that these data support more intensive control of systolic blood pressure among adults with hypertension, the study did not assess the potential adverse effects of such intensive blood-pressure-lowering therapy.

Table 19.3	Target blood pressures in uncomplicated hypertension (NICE, 2011)	
	Clinic BP target	ABPM/HBPM target (average daytime BP)
People younger than 80 years	<140/90 mmHg	<135/85 mmHg
People older than 80 years	<150/90 mmHg	<145/85 mmHg

ABPM, Ambulatory blood pressure monitoring; BP, blood pressure; HBPM, home blood pressure monitoring.

Table 19.4	Target clinic blood pressures in the presence of comorbidities (NICE, 2014a, 2015a, 2015b)	
	Clinic BP target without complications	Clinic BP target with complications
People with type 1 diabetes mellitus	135/85 mmHg	130/80 mmHg
People with type 2 diabetes mellitus	140/80 mmHg	130/80 mmHg
People with chronic kidney disease	140/90 mmHg	130/80 mmHg

BP, Blood pressure.

Antihypertensive drug classes

Renin–angiotensin system antagonists

Angiotensin converting enzyme (ACE) inhibitors block the conversion of angiotensin I to angiotensin II, whereas angiotensin receptor blockers (ARBs) block the action of angiotensin II at the angiotensin II type 2_1 receptor. Because angiotensin II is a vasoconstrictor and stimulates the release of aldosterone, antagonism results in vasodilation and potassium retention, as well as inhibition of salt and water retention. ACE inhibitors also block kininase production and, thus, prevent the breakdown of bradykinin. This appears to be important in the aetiology of ACE-inhibitor-induced cough, which is a troublesome side effect in 10–20% of users. ARBs do not inhibit kininase and are an appropriate choice for patients who are intolerant of ACE inhibitors because of cough. ACE inhibitors are also associated with a significant incidence of angioedema, which can in severe cases cause dangerous swelling of the pharyngolaryngeal area leading to stridor, threatening the patient's airway. This adverse reaction is more common in black subjects; as a result, ARBs are preferred to ACE inhibitors in people of black African or Caribbean family origin.

Calcium channel blockers

These agents block slow calcium channels in the peripheral blood vessels and/or the heart. The dihydropyridine group work almost exclusively on L-type calcium channels in the peripheral arterioles and reduce blood pressure by reducing total peripheral resistance. In contrast, the effect of verapamil and diltiazem are primarily on the heart, reducing heart rate and cardiac output. Long-acting dihydropyridines are preferred because they are more convenient for patients and avoid large fluctuations in plasma drug concentrations that may be associated with adverse effects.

Although effective for lowering blood pressure and preventing cardiovascular events, adverse effects are common, for example, oedema and flushing. Gum hypertrophy may occur with dihydropyridines and constipation with verapamil. Concerns have previously been raised by observational studies (Psaty et al., 1995) and meta-analysis (Furberg et al., 1995) that there may be an increased risk of coronary heart disease in recipients of dihydropyridine calcium channel blockers, although this was likely associated with use of short-acting preparations causing large fluctuations in blood pressure. Randomised clinical trials utilising long-acting dihydropyridines have not confirmed these observations (Gong et al., 1996; Staessen et al., 1997) and have indicated that dihydropyridines have similar efficacy to thiazide diuretics in preventing cardiovascular events (Brown et al., 2000).

Diuretics

There is substantial clinical trial evidence that benefit is obtained from the use of thiazide diuretics in hypertension. Examples of drugs include bendroflumethiazide and hydrochlorothiazide, or thiazide-like diuretics, for example, chlortalidone and indapamide. These drugs are both inexpensive and well tolerated by most patients. Their diuretic action is achieved by blockade of distal renal tubular sodium reabsorption. Initially, they reduce blood pressure by reducing circulating blood volume, but in the longer-term, they reduce total peripheral resistance, suggesting a direct vasodilatory action. Although generally well tolerated, thiazide and thiazide-like diuretics may cause hypokalaemia, small increases in low-density lipoprotein (LDL) cholesterol and triglycerides, and gout associated with impaired urate excretion. Erectile dysfunction is also common.

Until recently bendroflumethiazide and hydrochlorothiazide were the most commonly prescribed agents at low doses to minimise adverse effects; however, evidence of reduced CV events with these low doses is lacking. NICE (2011) recommended the preferred agents were thiazide-like diuretics, indapamide (1.5 mg modified release or 2.5 mg daily) or chlortalidone (12.5–25 mg daily, due to the greater evidence of reduced CV events at lower doses.

Many studies of diuretics have also incorporated β-blockers, and this combination can have adverse metabolic consequences that may lead to new-onset diabetes. Within the Antihypertensive and Lipid Lowering Treatment to Prevent Heart Attack Trial (ALLHAT), the absolute risk of developing diabetes was 3.5% higher in the chlortalidone group than the lisinopril group (ALLHAT Collaborative Research Group, 2002). It remains an issue of contention as to whether this diabetic tendency is clinically significant. There was no reduction in efficacy associated with thiazide use in ALLHAT, and indeed, there was less heart failure in the diuretic-treated patients compared with those receiving calcium channel blockers or ACE inhibitors.

Loop diuretics are no more effective at lowering blood pressure than thiazides unless renal function is significantly impaired or the patient is receiving agents that inhibit the renin–angiotensin system. They are also a suitable choice if heart failure is present.

Spironolactone, an aldosterone antagonist, is not suitable for first-line therapy but is an increasingly important treatment option at low dose (25 mg daily) for patients with resistant hypertension. Where hyperaldosteronism is suspected, spironolactone may prove to be effective. Spironolactone is a potassium-sparing diuretic and should be used with caution, especially if used in combination with ACE inhibitors or ARBs, and should almost always be avoided with other potassium-sparing diuretics, for example, amiloride.

α-Adrenoreceptor blockers

α-Adrenoreceptor blockers antagonise α-adrenoceptors in the blood vessel wall and, thus, prevent noradrenaline (norepinephrine)-induced vasoconstriction. As a result, they reduce total peripheral resistance and blood pressure. Prazosin was originally used but had the disadvantage of being short-acting and causing first-dose hypotension. Newer agents such as doxazosin and terazosin have a longer duration of action. There are concerns about the first-line use of α-blockers because the ALLHAT study has indicated that doxazosin is more often associated with heart failure and stroke than thiazide diuretics (ALLHAT Collaborative Research Group, 2000). However, they may be considered as add-in therapy for patients with resistant hypertension inadequately controlled using other agents. They can frequently cause postural hypotension but may alleviate symptoms in men with prostatic hypertrophy.

Centrally acting agents

Methyldopa and moxonidine inhibit sympathetic outflow from the brain, resulting in a reduction in total peripheral resistance. Methyldopa is not widely used because it has pronounced central adverse effects, including tiredness and depression. It continues to be used in pregnancy because it does not cause fetal abnormalities. It is also occasionally used in patients with resistant hypertension. Moxonidine blocks central imidazoline and α_2-adrenoceptors found within the medulla oblongata of the brain. It can cause side effects of dry mouth, headache, fatigue and dizziness, although it appears to have fewer central adverse effects than methyldopa. Other centrally acting agents such as clonidine and reserpine are almost never used in modern practice because of their pronounced adverse effects.

β-Adrenoreceptor antagonists

The mode of action of β-adrenoreceptor antagonists in hypertension is uncertain. The β-adrenoreceptor blockade reduces cardiac output in the short-term and during exercise. It also reduces renin secretion by antagonising β-receptors in the juxtaglomerular apparatus. Central actions may also be important for some agents. Non-selective β-blockers may give rise to adverse effects as a result of antagonism of β_2-adrenoceptors, that is, asthma and worsened intermittent claudication. However, the so-called 'cardioselective' (β_1-selective) β-blockers are not entirely free of these adverse effects. Patients who develop very marked bradycardia and tiredness may tolerate a drug with partial agonist activity such as pindolol.

β-Adrenoreceptor antagonists also have substantial clinical trial evidence of benefit over placebo in hypertension and are relatively inexpensive. However, their use is declining, and they have been relegated to use as one of a number of options in resistant hypertension in the UK according to NICE (2011) guidance (Fig. 19.1). This recommendation largely stems from the evidence that they may be less effective at preventing stroke in conjunction with their diabetogenic effects. The Losartan for Endpoint Reduction in Hypertension (LIFE) study compared an atenolol/thiazide-based regimen with a losartan-based regimen and demonstrated equivalent levels of blood pressure reduction but with a small excess incidence of stroke in the atenolol arm (Dahlöf et al., 2002). In the Anglo Scandinavian Cardiac Outcomes Trial (ASCOT) study, the risk of diabetes was 2.5% higher in the atenolol arm compared with the amlodipine arm, with similar increased risk of diabetes found within the atenolol arm of the LIFE study (Dahlöf et al., 2005). A Cochrane review warned of the excess risk in developing diabetes in patients prescribed combinations of thiazide diuretics and β-blockers. This would equate to one new case per 500 treated (Mason et al., 2005). The combination of thiazide and a β-blocker should, therefore, be avoided if possible, particularly in those who are at risk of developing diabetes (e.g. obese, strong family history of diabetes, South Asian origin).

To complicate matters, however, a long-term 20-year follow-up study of the UK Prospective Diabetes Study (UKPDS) found similar cardiovascular outcomes between patients on β-blockers and ACE inhibitors, with a reduction in all causes of mortality that actually favoured β-blockers (Holman et al., 2008). β-Blockers do remain suitable for younger hypertensives who have another indication for β-blockade, such as coronary heart disease. β-Blockers are also effective in suppressing atrial fibrillation, and this may be one group of patients where first-line therapy with β-blockers is still merited. Additionally, where anxiety is a significant driver of hypertension, β-blockers may have a role.

Other agents

Several other drugs are available for use for people with more resistant hypertension. Minoxidil is a powerful antihypertensive drug, but its use is associated with severe peripheral oedema and reflex tachycardia. It should be restricted to patients with severe hypertension who are also taking β-blockers and diuretics. It

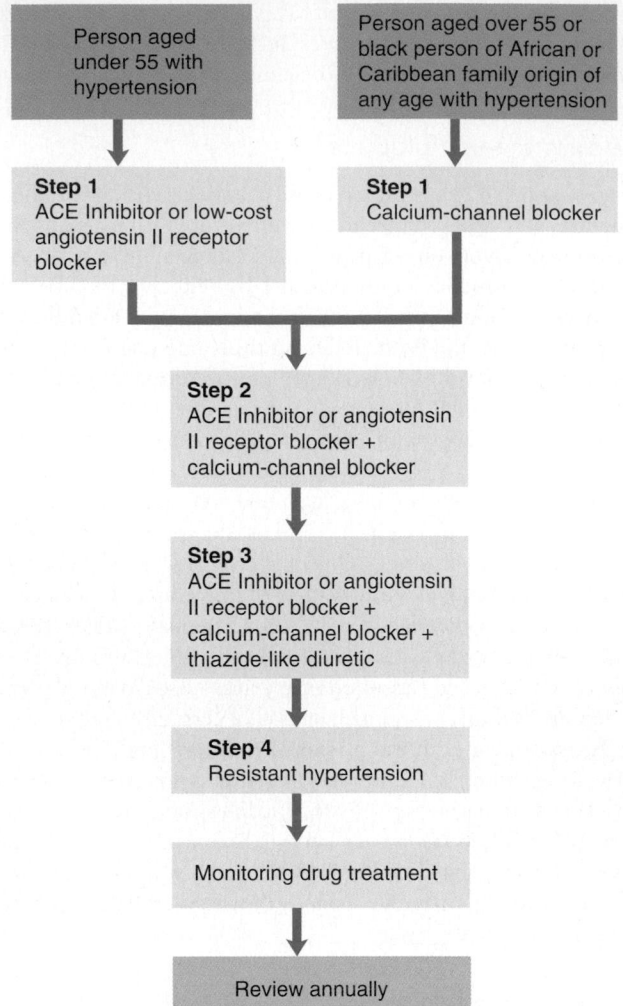

Fig. 19.1   Summary of antihypertensive drug treatment (NICE, 2017). ACE, Angiotensin converting enzyme.

causes pronounced hirsutism and is not a suitable treatment for women. Hydralazine can be used as add-on therapy for patients with resistant hypertension but is not well tolerated because it is a profound vasodilator and may occasionally be associated with drug-induced systemic lupus erythematosus. Sodium nitroprusside is a direct-acting arterial and venous dilator that is administered as an intravenous infusion for treating hypertensive emergencies and for the acute control of blood pressure during anaesthesia. Hypertension has previously been treated with ganglion blockers such as guanethidine, but these drugs are now of historical interest only.

There is evidence that the renin antagonist aliskiren may have a blood-pressure-lowering effect similar to that of other agents and may be safely added to other inhibitors of the renin–angiotensin–aldosterone system to provide a greater level of inhibition (O'Brien et al., 2007). Due to its cost and a lack of outcome data, it can only be suggested as an add-on therapy where other, more established treatment options have failed to control blood pressure. It is generally well tolerated but may cause diarrhoea at higher doses.

Drug selection

Drugs should be chosen on the basis of efficacy, safety, convenience to the patient and cost. For assessing efficacy, it is essential to use evidence from large-scale clinical trials that demonstrate measurable effects on hard end points such as the incidence of stroke and other cardiovascular events or death. Smaller-scale studies looking at the effects of drugs on blood pressure and surrogate markers such as left ventricular hypertrophy or carotid artery stenosis may generate a hypothesis of a future treatment strategy but should not be used to change current strategies. When considering safety, it is important to recognise that these drugs will be taken long-term, and there are advantages to using drugs that have long-established safety records. It is also important to recognise the importance of symptomatic adverse effects because these may reduce adherence. Patient convenience is another important factor, and use of once-daily preparations will result in better adherence than more frequent regimens. Because the hypertensive population is very large, it is necessary to be conscious of the cost of individual preparations. Combinations of low doses of antihypertensive drugs are often better tolerated than single drugs taken in high dose. The choice of drugs available for treating hypertension is shown in Table 19.5, and common therapeutic problems are noted.

Clinical trial evidence

Initial evidence of benefit in placebo-controlled clinical trials came from studies that primarily involved thiazide diuretics or β-blockers. However, there is increasing evidence of clinical benefit from newer drug classes, including ACE inhibitors and calcium channel blockers.

The Blood Pressure Lowering Treatment Trialists Collaboration (2000) carried out a meta-analysis of old against new treatments. They concluded that newer treatments were no more effective than older therapies. Since this study was done, several landmark comparative clinical trials have been published.

The Captopril Prevention Project (CAPPP) demonstrated that captopril was as effective as diuretics or β-blockers for preventing cardiovascular morbidity (Hansson et al., 1999a). However, captopril was associated with a 25% higher stroke risk, perhaps because it did not reduce blood pressure as effectively as conventional therapy in this particular study.

The LIFE study demonstrated that losartan was more effective at preventing vascular events, especially stroke, than atenolol in just over 9000 hypertensive patients with left ventricular hypertrophy, although reductions in blood pressure were similar. Losartan was also better tolerated (Dahlöf et al., 2002).

The ALLHAT study (ALLHAT Collaborative Research Group, 2002) involved over 40,000 older, high-risk hypertensive patients with the aim of determining whether the occurrence of fatal coronary heart disease or non-fatal myocardial infarction was lower in those treated with newer agents (amlodipine, lisinopril or doxazosin) compared with a thiazide-like diuretic (chlortalidone). The doxazosin arm was discontinued early because of a higher rate of events, especially heart failure, compared with the diuretic. For the remaining three drugs, there was no difference in the occurrence of the primary end point. Chlortalidone was more effective than amlodipine and lisinopril in lowering blood pressure and

preventing heart failure and was also marginally more effective than lisinopril in preventing stroke.

The second Australian National Blood Pressure Study Group (Wing et al., 2003) compared enalapril with hydrochlorothiazide

Table 19.5 Summary of oral antihypertensive drugs and common therapeutic problems

Class	Examples	Major adverse effects
Angiotensin-converting enzyme inhibitor	Ramipril, Lisinopril, Perindopril, Enalapril	Cough, Rash, Taste disturbance, Renal dysfunction, Angioedema
Angiotensin receptor blockers	Candesartan, Irbesartan, Losartan, Valsartan	Headache, Rash, Renal failure
Calcium channel blocker	*Dihydropyridine:* Amlodipine, Felodipine, Lacidipine, Lercanidipine	Flushing, Ankle swelling, Headache
	Non-dihydropyridine: Diltiazem, Verapamil	Bradycardia/heart block, Constipation (verapamil only)
Diuretics	*Thiazide-type:* Indapamide, Chlortalidone; *Thiazide:* Bendroflumethiazide, Hydrochlorothiazide; *Loop:* Furosemide, Bumetanide	Hypokalaemia, Gout, Glucose intolerance, Hyperlipidaemia, Impotence, Uraemia, Dehydration
Aldosterone antagonists	Spironolactone, Eplerenone	Hyperkalaemia, Renal dysfunction, Gynaecomastia (spironolactone only), Dehydration, Hyponatraemia
Beta-blockers	Bisoprolol, Atenolol, Metoprolol, Nebivolol, Labetalol	Tiredness/fatigue, Reduced exercise tolerance, Bradycardia, Cold peripheries, Claudication, Wheezing, Impotence
α-Blockers	Doxazosin, Prazosin	Postural hypotension, Headache, Rash
Centrally acting vasodilator	Methyldopa, Moxonidine	Tiredness, Depression

in just over 6000 hypertensive subjects recruited in primary care. The primary end point was any cardiovascular event or death from any cause. In this relatively small study, there was a trend in favour of the ACE inhibitor that was of borderline statistical significance.

The VALUE study (Julius et al., 2004) compared amlodipine and valsartan in high-risk hypertensive subjects. No differences in the primary composite cardiac end point were observed, although non-fatal myocardial infarction was less common with amlodipine, which also lowered blood pressure to a greater extent. Conversely, onset of diabetes was less common with valsartan.

The ASCOT study (Dahlöf et al., 2005) compared a modern treatment regimen based on amlodipine and perindopril with a traditional regimen based on atenolol and bendroflumethiazide. The study involved over 20,000 high-risk hypertensives. The amlodipine-based therapy was associated with better blood pressure reduction and reductions in the occurrence of cardiovascular events, total mortality and diabetes, although the primary composite end point was not significantly affected. It is uncertain how much of the benefit can be attributed to the better blood pressure control achieved in the amlodipine-based arm and how specific these findings are to the drug doses and sequencing specified in the trial protocol for each arm of the study.

These various trials have provided results that are conflicting, in part because of differences in trial design and quality. However, there is increasing evidence that β-blockers may be less effective at preventing cardiovascular end points, as suggested by LIFE and ASCOT studies. In a meta-analysis (Lindholm et al., 2005), β-blockers were less effective than other antihypertensives at preventing stroke, although no significant differences were observed in effects on myocardial infarction or death. There is no consistent evidence that thiazides or thiazide-like drugs are less effective than newer agents in preventing cardiovascular events.

Recommendations for drug sequencing

In England and Wales, the NICE (2011) guidelines include an algorithm for the use of antihypertensive therapies based on the age and ethnicity of the individual being treated (Fig. 19.1).

At step 1, these recommend an initial choice of an ACE inhibitor or ARB as first-line therapy in younger (<55 years) non-black patients. The rationale for this is that these patients often have hypertension associated with high concentrations of circulating renin. It is, therefore, logical to treat these patients with drugs that antagonise the renin–angiotensin system. For patients older than 55 years and patients of black African or Caribbean family origin of any age, who tend to have hypertension associated with low renin concentrations, calcium channel blockers (CCBs) are advocated as the preferred first-line option. Diuretic therapy, in the form of a thiazide-type diuretic, is recommended as an alternative if a CCB is not suitable, for example, because of oedema or intolerance, or if there is evidence of heart failure or a high risk of heart failure.

If initial monotherapy at step 1 fails to control blood pressure, a combination of an ACE inhibitor or ARB and a CCB is recommended at step 2 for both groups of patients, although the addition of an ARB is preferred in patients of black African or Caribbean family origin due to the higher risk of angioedema with ACE inhibitor seen in this group.

Step 3 recommends a combination of ACE inhibitor/ARB plus CCB plus a thiazide-type diuretic.

Step 4, defined as resistant hypertension, recommends the addition of spironolactone or a higher dose of thiazide-like diuretic, although the evidence for any option at this stage is limited, and other possible additions include β-blockers or α-blockers. β-Blockers may be used in those patients with a high sympathetic drive. European guidance (Table 19.6) has eschewed a formal ranking of treatments and instead suggests a table of drugs and indications where they might be most appropriately indicated (Mancia et al., 2013).

Timing of dosing

There remains uncertainty about the optimal timing for the dosing of antihypertensive drug therapy, with one Cochrane review (Zhao et al., 2011) concluding that evening dosing was associated with a small, but significant reduction in blood pressure compared with morning dosing. However, the quality of the studies included in this meta-analysis was poor, and therefore more research is required in this area.

Special patient groups

Race

People of African Caribbean origin have an increased prevalence of hypertension and left ventricular hypertrophy and are at high risk of stroke and renal failure. They obtain particular benefit from reduced salt intake and are also sensitive to diuretic and calcium channel blockers, whereas β-blockers appear less effective, at least when used as monotherapy. People of black African or Caribbean origin have reduced plasma renin activity, and as a result, ACE inhibitors and ARBs are also less effective. This was illustrated in the ALLHAT study (ALLHAT, 2000, 2002) where stroke and coronary events were more common in black patients randomised to lisinopril compared with those receiving chlortalidone. In this group NICE recommends CCBs as the first line with the addition of an ARB at step 2.

British Asians also have an increased prevalence of hypertension, diabetes and insulin resistance and a particularly high risk of coronary heart disease and stroke. There is currently no evidence of a difference in drug response when compared with white Europeans. However, combinations of β-blockers and thiazides should be avoided when possible because of the higher risk of diabetes.

Elderly

The elderly have a high prevalence of hypertension, with over 70% having blood pressures greater than 140/90 mmHg. Because they are at high absolute risk of cardiovascular events, the absolute benefits of blood pressure treatment are particularly large in this group. Antihypertensive therapy may also reduce the risk of heart failure and dementia. The Study of Cognition and Prognosis

Table 19.6 European Society of Cardiology: Drugs to be preferred in specific conditions (Mancia et al., 2013)

Condition	Drug
Asymptomatic organ damage	
Left ventricular hypertrophy	ACE inhibitor, CCB, ARB
Asymptomatic atherosclerosis	CCB, ACE inhibitor
Microalbuminuria	ACE inhibitor, ARB
Renal dysfunction	ACE inhibitor, ARB
Clinical cardiovascular event	
Previous stroke	Any agent effectively lowering blood pressure
Previous myocardial infarction	β-Blocker, ACE inhibitor, ARB
Angina pectoris	β-Blocker, CCB
Heart failure	Diuretic, β-blocker, ACE inhibitor, ARB, aldosterone antagonist
Aortic aneurysm	β-Blocker
Atrial fibrillation, prevention	Consider ARB, ACE inhibitor, β-blocker or aldosterone antagonist
Atrial fibrillation, ventricular rate control	β-Blocker, non-dihydropyridine CCB
End-stage renal disease/proteinuria	ACE inhibitor, ARB
Peripheral artery disease	ACE inhibitor, CCB
Other	
Isolated systolic hypertension (elderly)	Diuretic, CCB
Metabolic syndrome	ACE inhibitor, ARB, CCB
Diabetes mellitus	ACE inhibitor, ARB
Pregnancy	Methyldopa, β-blocker, CCB
Blacks	Diuretic, CCB

ACE, Angiotensin-converting enzyme; ARB, angiotensin receptor blocker; CCB, calcium channel blocker.

in the Elderly (SCOPE) study (Lithell et al., 2003) was designed to investigate the effects of candesartan on the occurrence of cognitive decline or dementia but revealed no benefit, probably because of the lack of difference in blood pressure between the two arms of the study.

The elderly are at particular risk of certain adverse effects of treatment such as postural hypotension, and it is important that both sitting and standing blood pressure are monitored. Nevertheless, the benefits of therapy are so great that blood-pressure-lowering strategies should be employed at all ages, in the form of lifestyle modification with or without drug therapy (NICE, 2011), unless the patient is very frail or the patient's life expectancy is very short. Isolated systolic hypertension (systolic >160 mmHg, diastolic <90 mmHg) is common in the elderly, and there is irrefutable evidence that drug treatment is beneficial in this group (Staessen et al., 1997; Systolic Hypertension in the Elderly Programme [SHEP] Co-operative Research Group, 1991). The elderly have more variable blood pressure, and larger numbers of measurements may be required to confirm hypertension; hence, ABPM is preferred to confirm a diagnosis.

Calcium channel blockers and low-dose thiazide diuretics are safe and effective treatments for elderly hypertensive people, and their use is endorsed by large-scale clinical trials. β-Blockers are less effective at reducing blood pressure and preventing clinical end points. The Swedish Trial in Old Patients with hypertension-2 (STOP-2) compared the effects of conventional (β-blocker or thiazide) and newer drugs (ACE inhibitors or calcium channel blockers) on cardiovascular morbidity in older subjects and did not detect significant differences (Hansson et al., 1999b).

In the Hypertension in the Very Elderly Trial (HYVET) (Beckett et al., 2008), 4000 patients with a mean age of 84 and blood pressure of 160–199 mmHg systolic at entry were treated to a target of systolic 150 mmHg for 1.8 years with indapamide (a thiazide-like diuretic) and, if required, the ACE inhibitor perindopril. There was a 30% reduction in fatal and non-fatal stroke, 21% reduction in death from all causes, and fewer adverse events in the actively treated group (Beckett et al., 2008).

The elderly certainly benefit from treatment of hypertension, but the threshold and target for treatment have not been fully elucidated. Most studies in the elderly recruited patients with relatively high baseline targets (>160–190 mmHg systolic) achieving blood pressure on treatment of between 150 and 170 mmHg, and only one achieved target blood pressure lower than 140 mmHg, and in this study outcome was poorer in the treated group (JATOS Study Group 2008).

The HYVET study (Beckett et al., 2008) was the first to confirm the safety and efficacy of lowering systolic blood pressure to less than 150 mmHg, and therefore this has been established as the treatment target for people older than 80 years.

Diabetes

In type 1 diabetes, the presence of hypertension often indicates the presence of diabetic nephropathy. In this group, blood pressure reduction and ACE inhibition slow the rate of decline in renal function. To achieve adequate blood pressure control, combinations of drugs will be needed. Thiazides, β-blockers, calcium channel blockers and α-blockers are all suitable as add-on treatments to ACE inhibitors, which should be first-line therapy.

Target blood pressure should be less than 135/85 mmHg or less than 130/80 mmHg if there is albuminuria or two or more signs of metabolic syndrome present; however, achieving these targets in clinical practice is challenging (NICE, 2015a).

In type 2 (non-insulin-dependent) diabetes, hypertension is particularly common, affecting 70% of people in this group. It is strongly associated with obesity and insulin resistance, and control of blood pressure is more important for preventing complications than tight glycaemic control. There is no evidence that one group of drugs is more or less effective than any other in terms of lowering blood pressure. The ADVANCE trial treated diabetics with indapamide and perindopril in addition to prestudy antihypertensive agents. The active group was found to have a further reduction in blood pressure and a significant reduction in adverse renal outcomes (21%) (Patel et al., 2007). It remains a subject of debate whether ACE inhibitors and ARBs have specific renoprotective benefits over and above their effects on blood pressure. In 2015, the guideline development group for the NICE diabetes type II guidelines concluded that the best evidence for prevention of renal disease and limitation of metabolic worsening related to the renin–angiotensin–system-blockers (RAS-blockers) (ACEI and ARB) as a class. Hence, NICE (2015b) guidance for England and Wales now recommends an ACE inhibitor as the first line in everyone except those of black African or Caribbean family origin where initial dual therapy with an ACE inhibitor plus diuretic therapy or CCB is recommended. If further antihypertensive therapy is required, ACEI plus CCB with the addition of a diuretic if necessary is endorsed. Many people with diabetes require four or even five antihypertensive agents to approach target levels. After triple therapy, there is little evidence to support the choice of one drug class over another, and any α-blocker, β-blocker or potassium-sparing diuretic can be added at this stage.

Renal disease

In patients with chronic renal impairment, good blood pressure control slows the progression of renal dysfunction. Renin–angiotensin system antagonists, including ACE inhibitors, ARBs and direct renin inhibitors, reduce the incidence of end-stage renal failure, but it is not clear if this is a specific effect or nonspecific action as a result of blood pressure lowering. The drugs also reduce protein loss and should be used in patients with hypertension and an albumin/creatinine ratio (ACR) of 30 mg/mmol or more or rapidly progressive renal dysfunction. Renin–angiotensin–aldosterone system antagonists may worsen renal impairment in patients with renal vascular disease, and careful monitoring of electrolytes and creatinine is mandatory. Salt restriction is particularly important in managing hypertension in renal disease. Thiazide diuretics are ineffective in patients with significant renal dysfunction (eGFR <30 mL/min/1.73 m²), and loop diuretics should be used when a diuretic is needed.

A further note of caution regarding overtreatment of blood pressure to overaggressive targets comes from the ONTARGET study, which randomised patients with vascular disease or high-risk diabetics to high-dose ramipril, telmisartan or both. Many patients were already taking polypharmacy for hypertension, and blood pressures at entry were approximately 142/82 mmHg

in all groups. Treatment reduced blood pressure by 6.4/4.3 mmHg in the ramipril group, 7.4/5.0 mmHg in the telmisartan group and 9.8/6.3 mmHg in the combination group. This would give the combination group a post-treatment blood pressure of 132/76 mmHg. This combination group was associated with adverse renal outcomes, for example, renal failure and high potassium with no improvement in other cardiovascular outcomes (Yusuf et al., 2008). The Medicines and Healthcare Regulatory Agency in the UK issued a warning in 2014 to avoid combining medicines from two classes of RAS-blocking agents (ACE inhibitors, ARBs, or aliskiren) for the treatment of hypertension (Medicines and Healthcare Regulatory Authority [MHRA], 2014).

Stroke

Hypertension is the most important risk factor for stroke in patients with or without previous stroke. There is increasing evidence that in those with a previous stroke, blood pressure reduction reduces the risk of stroke recurrence as well as other cardiovascular events. The PROGRESS study, although clearly demonstrating a benefit of lowering blood pressure in patients with cerebrovascular disease, only demonstrated benefit in those whose blood pressure was greater than 140 mmHg on entry or who were already on antihypertensives. The size of benefit was proportional to the size of the blood pressure reduction. The combination of perindopril and indapamide lowered systolic blood pressure by 12.3 mmHg and stroke incidence by an impressive 43%, whereas perindopril alone was associated with a small drop in systolic blood pressure and no reduction in stroke risk (PROGRESS Collaborative Group, 2001). On treatment, blood pressure in the actively treated group was 132 mmHg systolic.

In the Secondary Prevention of Small Subcortical Strokes (SPS3) trial, targeting a systolic blood pressure of below 130 mmHg in patients with recent lacunar stroke, reductions in the rate of all stroke, disabling or fatal stroke and the composite outcome of myocardial infarction or vascular death were not significant, but the rate of cerebral haemorrhage was reduced, and the lower target was well tolerated (SPS Study Group, 2013). A meta-analysis of 123 studies and 613,815 subjects found that blood-pressure-lowering treatment significantly reduced cardiovascular events and death in proportion to the magnitude of blood pressure reduction achieved, with no differences in the proportional benefits between trials with lower (below 130 mmHg) or higher systolic BP at baseline (Ettehad et al., 2016). Overall, a 10-mmHg reduction in systolic BP reduced the risk of cardiovascular disease by 20% and stroke by 27%.

The UK Royal College of Physicians national clinical guideline for stroke (Intercollegiate Stroke Working Party, 2016) recommends that patients post-stroke should be treated to achieve a clinic systolic blood pressure below 130 mmHg, except for people with severe bilateral carotid artery stenosis, for whom a systolic blood pressure target of 140–150 mmHg is appropriate.

Treatment of hypertension in the setting of acute stroke has been a subject of much debate. Blood pressure naturally rises then falls in the days and hours following acute stroke, and some have argued that elevated levels are necessary to maintain brain circulation due to the failure of cerebral autoregulatory mechanisms around the time of stroke. The theory that lowering blood pressure could reduce cerebral perfusion due to a lack of the usual autoregulatory mechanisms is counterweighted by the potential for further damage due to cerebral oedema. There are no large-scale clinical trials to guide treatment, and national guidance from the UK (Intercollegiate Stroke Working Party, 2016) currently only recommends lowering blood pressure in the setting of acute ischaemic stroke if there is an indication for emergency treatment, such as:

- systolic blood pressure above 185 mmHg or diastolic blood pressure above 110 mmHg when the patient is otherwise eligible for thrombolysis,
- hypertensive encephalopathy,
- hypertensive nephropathy,
- hypertensive cardiac failure or myocardial infarction,
- aortic dissection,
- pre-eclampsia or eclampsia.

In patients with intracerebral haemorrhage, acute reduction of blood pressure has also been demonstrated to be feasible and probably safe, with reduced haematoma growth in the actively treated group (Anderson et al., 2008).

Following the acute phase of treatment, patients with acute stroke admitted on antihypertensive medication should resume oral treatment once they are medically stable and as soon as they can swallow medication safely. For newly identified hypertension, blood-pressure-lowering treatment for people with stroke should be initiated before the transfer of care out of hospital or at 2 weeks, whichever is the soonest.

Pregnancy

An increased blood pressure before 20 weeks of gestation usually indicates pre-existing chronic hypertension that may not have been previously diagnosed. As in all younger hypertensive patients, a careful assessment is needed to exclude possible secondary causes, although radiological and radionuclide investigations should usually be deferred until after pregnancy. Hypertension diagnosed after 20 weeks of gestation may also indicate chronic hypertension, which may have been masked during early pregnancy by the fall in blood pressure that occurs at that time. Patients with elevated blood pressure in pregnancy are at increased risk of pre-eclampsia and intrauterine growth retardation. They need frequent checks of their blood pressure, urinalysis and fetal growth. Pre-eclampsia is diagnosed when the blood pressure increases by 30/15 mmHg from measurements obtained in early pregnancy or if the diastolic blood pressure exceeds 110 mmHg and proteinuria is present. There is general consensus that blood pressure should be treated with drugs if it exceeds 150/100 mmHg (NICE, 2010), although some clinicians use a lower threshold, for example, 140/90 mmHg. Methyldopa is the most suitable drug choice for use in pregnancy because of its long-term safety record. Calcium channel blockers, hydralazine and labetalol are also used. β-Blockers, particularly atenolol, are used less often because they are associated with intrauterine growth retardation. Although diuretics reduce the incidence of pre-eclampsia, they are little used in pregnancy because of

concerns about decreasing maternal blood volume. ACE inhibitors and ARBs are contraindicated because they are associated with oligohydramnios, renal failure and intrauterine death.

Meta-analysis of trials suggests that antihypertensive drugs reduce the risk of progression to severe hypertension and reduce hospital admissions, although excessive blood pressure reduction may reduce fetal growth.

Oral contraceptives

Use of combined oral contraceptives results, on average, in an increase of 5/3 mmHg in blood pressure. However, severe hypertension can occur in a small proportion of recipients months or years into treatment. Progesterone-only preparations do not cause hypertension very often but are less effective for contraception, especially in younger women. Combined oral contraceptives are not absolutely contraindicated in hypertension unless other risk factors for cardiovascular disease, such as smoking, are present.

Hormone replacement therapy

There is little evidence that hormone replacement therapy is associated with an increase in blood pressure, and women with hypertension should not be denied access to these agents if there is an appropriate indication. Controversy remains regarding whether hormone replacement therapy reduces or increases the risk of CV events overall. Large increases in blood pressure have occasionally been reported in individuals, and it is important to monitor blood pressure during the first few weeks of therapy and every 6 months thereafter. In women with resistant hypertension, during treatment with hormone replacement therapy, the effectiveness of discontinuing hormone replacement should be assessed.

A list of the indications and contraindications to the various antihypertensive agents can be found in Table 19.7.

Ancillary drug treatment

Aspirin

The use of aspirin reduces cardiovascular events at the expense of an increase in gastro-intestinal complications, and it is no longer recommended for primary prevention of cardiovascular events. Its use in hypertensive patients should be restricted to those who have evidence of established vascular disease.

Lipid-lowering therapy

Guidelines clearly support the use of statins in all patients requiring secondary prevention of CVD. In the absence of established CV disease, the decision to initiate statin therapy should be based on the results of a cardiovascular risk assessment using an approved risk calculator, such as QRisk. NICE guidance recommends that statins should be considered in patients with a CV risk greater than 10% over 10 years, after other modifiable risk factors have been addressed (NICE, 2014b, 2014c).

Table 19.7 Use of antihypertensive drugs adapted from British Hypertension Society guidelines

Class	Indications	Contraindications
Diuretics	Elderly ISH Heart failure Secondary stroke prevention	Gout
β-Blockers	Myocardial infarction Angina (Heart failure)	Asthma/chronic obstructive pulmonary disease Heart block (Heart failure) (Dyslipidaemia) (Peripheral vascular disease) (Diabetes, except with coronary heart disease)
Calcium antagonists: dihydropyridine	Elderly ISH (Elderly) (Angina)	
Calcium antagonists (rate limiting)	Angina (Myocardial infarction)	Combination with β-blocker (Heart block) (Heart failure)
ACE inhibitors	Heart failure Left ventricular dysfunction Type 1 diabetic nephropathy Secondary stroke prevention (Chronic renal disease) (Type 2 diabetic nephropathy) (Proteinuric renal disease)	Pregnancy Renovascular disease (Renal impairment) (Peripheral vascular disease)
α-Blockers	Benign prostatic hypertrophy (Dyslipidaemia)	Urinary incontinence (Postural hypotension) (Heart failure)
Angiotensin receptor blockers	ACE inhibitor intolerance Type 2 diabetic nephropathy Hypertension with LVH Heart failure in ACE inhibitor-intolerant subjects Post-MI (LV dysfunction post-MI) (Intolerance of other antihypertensive drugs) (Proteinuric renal disease) (Chronic renal failure) (Heart failure)	As ACE inhibitors
Centrally acting vasodilators	Pregnancy (methyldopa only) Resistant hypertension unresponsive to first-line therapy	
Direct-acting vasodilators	Resistant hypertension, unresponsive to first-line therapy	

Note: Strong indications and contraindications are shown. Text in parentheses indicates weak/possible indications or contraindications.
ACE, Angiotensin-converting enzyme; ISH, isolated systolic hypertension; LV, left ventricular; LVH, left ventricular hypertrophy; MI, myocardial infarction.

Case studies

Case 19.1

Mrs PP, a 55-year-old woman of African Caribbean origin, is found to have consistently elevated blood pressure over several weeks; her lowest reading was 155/98 mmHg. She is overweight and has diabetes and is being treated with metformin. Her renal function and urinalysis are both normal.

Questions

1. Should Mrs PP be initiated on drug therapy for her hypertension?
2. If her hypertension was treated with drugs, which agents should be offered and in what order?

Answers

1. Provided Mrs PP's blood pressure has been measured accurately over several weeks, it demonstrates stage 1 hypertension. It is important to ensure that an appropriately sized blood pressure cuff is being used, in view of her obesity. She should be treated with both lifestyle advice and drug therapy because she also has diabetes. Restriction of salt intake may be particularly helpful in people of black African or Caribbean family origin, and weight reduction would benefit her hypertension and diabetes.

2. NICE (2015b) guidance recommends that first-line antihypertensive drug treatment for a person of African or Caribbean family origin should be an ACE inhibitor plus either a diuretic or a calcium channel blocker. This conflicts with the recommendation in the 2011 NICE guideline, which suggests that ARBs are preferred to ACE inhibitors in people of black African or Caribbean family origin, but the recommendation is based on the greater wealth of clinical trial data to support ACE inhibitors in people with diabetes. Calcium channel blockers do not have adverse metabolic effects and are effective in people of this origin and would, therefore, be an appropriate choice. If blood pressure remains uncontrolled, the addition of either diuretic or CCB should be considered (whichever was not initiated at step 1). Tight blood pressure control is important, and if blood pressure is not controlled with three agents, an α-blocker, β-blocker or potassium-sparing diuretic could be considered for addition at this stage.

Case 19.2

Mr PT, a 35-year-old man, is overweight and has a blood pressure of 178/108 mmHg. He smokes 25 cigarettes daily and drinks 28 units of alcohol per week. He has a sedentary occupation. He eats excessive quantities of saturated fat and salt.

Mr PT subsequently stopped smoking and lost some weight but remained hypertensive. He was treated with atenolol 50 mg daily. His blood pressure fell to 136/84 mmHg, but he developed tiredness and bradycardia and complained of erectile impotence.

Questions

1. How should Mr PT be managed?
2. What are the treatment options for Mr PT?

Answers

1. Since Mr PT is a young man, his absolute risk of cardiovascular events is likely to be low, at least for the time being; however, this should be confirmed using QRisk. His total cholesterol and high-density lipoprotein (HDL) cholesterol levels, as well as height and weight, will be needed to accurately access his risk. Mr PT has several cardiovascular risk factors that need to be addressed, including his sedentary lifestyle and his smoking. Non-pharmacological methods have the potential of reducing his blood pressure considerably, including dietary modification, weight loss, and reduced salt intake. He is unlikely to qualify for lipid-lowering therapy at this point because of his young age and presumed low cardiovascular risk. Because he has stage 2 hypertension, drug treatment should be initiated in parallel with lifestyle advice.

2. β-Blockers are no longer recommended for the first-line treatment of hypertension, and Mr PT is complaining of significant adverse effects, which may affect adherence. In line with guidance and to address his adverse effects, he should be changed to a drug of a different class such as an ACE inhibitor, in view of his age (NICE, 2011). This is likely to be more effective for blood pressure lowering than

a calcium channel blocker or diuretic. Other drugs could be added or substituted if Mr PT was intolerant to initial therapy or it did not reduce his blood pressure to target levels; with calcium channel blocker recommended at step 2 and the addition of a thiazide type diuretic at step 3 (although these can also cause impotence).

Case 19.3

A 24-year-old woman, Ms SR, with a family history of hypertension is prescribed an oral contraceptive. Six months after starting this, she is noted to have a blood pressure of 148/96 mmHg.

Question

How should Ms SR be managed?

Answer

If Ms SR's blood pressure is consistently raised, she may have either essential hypertension or hypertension induced by the oral contraceptive (secondary hypertension) or a combination. Her blood pressure may fall if her oral contraceptive is discontinued. Ms SR will, however, need advice on adequate contraceptive methods. A progesterone-only preparation would be one possibility. She would need careful counselling about the methods available and how successful they are. If her blood pressure remained elevated after discontinuing her oral contraception, she is likely to have underlying hypertension. This may be essential in nature, in view of the family history; however, because of her age, Ms SR should undergo some investigations to exclude possible secondary causes of hypertension. She is at low risk of complications, and there is no urgency to consider drug treatment. If there is a strong wish to use combined oral contraception, it would be important to control other risk factors as far as possible and to consider drug treatment for her hypertension.

Case 19.4

Mrs GJ, a 73-year-old woman, has a long-standing history of hypertension and intolerance to antihypertensive drugs. Bendroflumethiazide was associated with acute attacks of gout, she developed breathlessness and wheezing while taking bisoprolol, amlodipine caused flushing and headache and doxazosin was associated with intolerable postural hypotension. Four weeks earlier she had been started on enalapril but then complained of a dry, persistent cough. Her blood chemistry has remained normal.

Questions

1. Is Mrs GJ's cough likely to be an adverse effect of enalapril?
2. What other options are available for controlling her blood pressure?

Answers

1. Yes, a dry cough is a common adverse effect of ACE inhibitors. It affects approximately 10–20% of recipients and is more common in women. Some patients are able to tolerate the symptom, but in many, the drug has to be discontinued.

2. Angiotensin receptor blockers can be used in patients intolerant of ACE inhibitors due to cough. They are unlikely to produce this symptom because they do not inhibit the metabolism of

pulmonary bradykinin. Centrally acting agents such as methyldopa or moxonidine could also be considered. However, these are not well tolerated, and side effects are quite likely in this patient. A non-dihydropyridine calcium channel blocker such as diltiazem or verapamil is another alternative. Measurement of plasma uric acid could also be considered followed by prophylactic treatment with allopurinol before introducing a diuretic. Alternatively, a trial of spironolactone could be considered, although renal function will need careful monitoring.

Case 19.5

Mrs KB, a 23-year-old woman, has a normal blood pressure (118/82 mmHg) when reviewed at 8 weeks of pregnancy. In the 24th week of pregnancy, she is reviewed by her midwife and found to have a blood pressure of 148/96 mmHg. Urinalysis is normal.

Questions

1. What is the likely diagnosis?
2. What complications does Mrs KB's high blood pressure place her at increased risk of?
3. Should she receive drug treatment? If so, with which drug, and if not, how should she be managed?

Answers

1. Mrs KB may have gestation-induced hypertension or chronic hypertension that had previously been masked by the fall in blood pressure that happens in early pregnancy.
2. She is at increased risk of pre-eclampsia and intrauterine growth retardation.
3. There are differences of opinion between specialists as to whether blood pressure should be treated at this level during pregnancy. In favour of treatment is the substantial rise over the earlier blood pressure recording. Some specialists would not treat unless the blood pressure was greater than 170/110 mmHg or other complications were present, but NICE (2010) recommends intervention if the BP is greater than 150/100 mmHg. If Mrs KB was treated, methyldopa would be a suitable choice. In any event, Mrs KB requires close monitoring of her blood pressure, urinalysis and fetal growth.

Case 19.6

An elderly patient, Mr GD, comes to the pharmacy with a prescription for the following medications: salbutamol inhaler 200 micrograms as required, beclometasone inhaler 200 micrograms twice daily, bendroflumethiazide 2.5 mg daily, modified release diltiazem 180 mg once daily and atenolol 50 mg daily. The atenolol was being started by Mr GD's primary care doctor, apparently because of inadequate blood pressure control.

Question

What action should the pharmacist take?

Answer

There are three reasons to be concerned about the addition of atenolol to Mr GD's drug regimen. First, there is a potentially hazardous interaction with diltiazem, which may result in severe bradycardia or heart block. Second, Mr GD is receiving treatment for obstructive

airways disease, and this may be worsened by the atenolol. Third, there is increasing evidence to demonstrate that the combination of a thiazide and a β-blocker increases the risk of developing diabetes. The prescription should be discussed with the prescriber. The addition of an ACE inhibitor or ARB would be a suitable alternative in line with NICE (2011) guidance.

Case 19.7

A patient, Mr AG, is admitted to hospital with a stroke. A CT scan of the brain shows a cerebral infarct. The patient's blood pressure is 178/102 mmHg and remains at this level over the first 6 hours after admission to the ward.

Question

Should Mr AG be prescribed antihypertensive medication?

Answer

There is no good evidence that antihypertensive drug treatment is beneficial in the early stages of acute stroke, and there is a risk that lowering blood pressure may compromise cerebral perfusion further. However, in the longer-term, blood pressure reduction is valuable for preventing further strokes and other cardiovascular events. It would be appropriate to monitor Mr AG's blood pressure and start treatment after a few days if it remains persistently elevated. A thiazide diuretic and/or ACE inhibitor are commonly used under these circumstances, following the demonstration of benefit in the PROGRESS study (PROGRESS Collaborative Group, 2001).

Case 19.8

Mr TH, a 67-year-old man, has been treated for hypertension with atenolol 50 mg daily for several years. He feels well, and his blood pressure is controlled. Mr TH has read an article in the paper that suggests atenolol is not considered the most suitable drug for treating high blood pressure and enquires about changing his prescription.

Question

Should an alteration to Mr TH's treatment be recommended?

Answer

There is increasing evidence that β-blockers, including atenolol, may be less effective at preventing cardiovascular events, especially stroke, than other drugs and are associated with a higher risk of development of diabetes, especially if used in combination with thiazide diuretics. They are also less effective at reducing blood pressure in older people. However, if Mr TH's blood pressure is well controlled and the treatment suits him, there is no strong reason to change his medication unless he is at particular risk of diabetes.

Case 19.9

Mr AB, a 58-year-old man, is noted to have high blood pressure by his primary care doctor. There is no evidence of end-organ damage, and he has no other cardiovascular risk factors. The blood pressure remains greater than 160/100 mmHg each time it is checked in the surgery over several weeks, in spite of salt and alcohol reduction. Mr AB buys a wrist blood pressure monitor at a pharmacy and takes several readings at home. These are all below 130/75 mmHg.

Question

What advice should Mr AB be given about the need for drug treatment?

Answer

Mr AB may have 'white-coat' hypertension. Because this is associated with a lower risk than sustained hypertension, he may not need drug treatment. However, before making this judgment, it is important to check that his machine is accurate. This can be done by comparing readings with a validated machine or by checking to see if the make of the blood pressure monitor has been verified as accurate by the British Hypertension Society.

References

ALLHAT Collaborative Research Group, 2000. Major cardiovascular events in hypertensive patients randomised to doxazosin vs. chlorthalidone. Antihypertensive and lipid lowering treatment to prevent heart attack trial (ALLHAT). J. Am. Med. Assoc. 283, 1967–1975.

ALLHAT Collaborative Research Group, 2002. Major outcomes in high-risk hypertensive patients randomized to angiotensin-converting enzyme inhibitor or calcium channel blocker vs. diuretic: the antihypertensive and lipid lowering treatment to prevent heart attack trial (ALLHAT). J. Am. Med. Assoc. 288, 2981–2997.

Anderson, C.S., Yining, H., Wang, J.G., et al., 2008. Intensive blood pressure reduction in acute cerebral haemorrhage trial (INTERACT): a randomised pilot trial. Lancet Neurol. 7, 391–399.

Appel, L.J., Moore, T.J., Obarzanek, E., et al., 1997. A clinical trial of the effects of dietary patterns on blood pressure. N. Engl. J. Med. 336, 1117–1124.

Beckett, N.S., Peters, R., Fletcher, A.E., et al., 2008. Treatment of hypertension in patients 80 years of age or older. N. Engl. J. Med. 358, 1887–1898.

Beevers, G., Lip, G.Y.H., O'Brien, E., 2001. The pathophysiology of hypertension. Br. Med. J. 322, 912–916.

Blood Pressure Lowering Treatment Trialists Collaboration, 2000. Effects of ACE inhibitors, calcium antagonists, and other blood pressure lowering drugs: results of prospectively designed overviews of randomized trials. Lancet 356, 1955–1964.

Brown, M.J., Palmer, C.R., Castaigne, A., et al., 2000. Morbidity and mortality in patients randomised to double blind treatment with a long acting calcium channel blocker or diuretic in the international nifedipine GITS study (INSIGHT). Lancet 356, 366–372.

Bundy, J.D., Li, C., Stuchlik, P., et al., 2017. Systolic blood pressure reduction and risk of cardiovascular disease and mortality A systematic review and network meta-analysis. JAMA Cardiol. https://doi.org/10.1001/jamacardio.2017.1421.

Cirillo, M., Lanti, M.P., Menotti, A., et al., 2008. Definition of kidney dysfunction as a cardiovascular risk factor: use of urinary albumin excretion and estimated glomerular filtration rate. Arch. Int. Med. 168, 617–624.

Clark, C.E., Taylor, R.S., Shine, A.C., et al., 2012. Association of a difference in systolic blood pressure between arms with vascular disease and mortality: a systematic review and meta-analysis. Lancet 379, 905–914.

Collins, R., Petro, R., MacMahon, S., et al., 1990. Blood pressure, stroke and coronary heart disease. Part 2. Short-term reductions in blood pressure: overview of randomised drugs trials in their epidemiological context. Lancet 335, 827–838.

Dahlöf, B., Devereux, R., Kjeldsen, S.E., et al., 2002. Cardiovascular morbidity and mortality in the Losartan for Endpoint reduction in hypertension study (LIFE): a randomised trial against atenolol. Lancet 359, 995–1003.

Dahlöf, B., Sever, P.S., Poulter, N.R., ASCOT Investigators, 2005. Prevention of cardiovascular events with an antihypertensive regimen of amlodipine adding perindopril as required versus atenolol adding bendroflumethiazide as required, in the Anglo Scandinavian Cardiac Outcomes Trial – Blood Pressure Lowering Arm (ASCOT–BPLA). Lancet 366, 895–906.

DiPiro, J.T., Talbert, R.L., Yee, G.C., et al., 2014. Pharmacotherapy: a Pathophysiologic Approach, ninth ed. McGraw-Hill Education, New York.

Ettehad, D., Emdin, C.A., Kiran, A., et al., 2016. Blood pressure lowering for prevention of cardiovascular disease and death: a systematic review and meta-analysis. Lancet 387, 957–967.

Furberg, C.D., Psaty, B.M., Meyer, J.V., 1995. Nifedipine: dose-related increase in mortality in patients with coronary heart disease. Circulation 92, 1326–1331.

Gong, L., Zhang, W., Zhu, Y., et al., 1996. Shanghai trial of nifedipine in the elderly (STONE). J. Hypertens. 14, 1237–1245.

Hansson, L., Lindholm, L.H., Niskanen, L., et al., 1999a. Effect of angiotensin-converting-enzyme inhibition compared with conventional therapy on cardiovascular morbidity and mortality in hypertension. The Captopril Prevention Project (CAPPP). Lancet 353, 611–616.

Hansson, L., Lindholm, L.H., Ekbom, T., et al., 1999b. Randomised trial of old and new antihypertensive drugs in elderly patients: cardiovascular mortality and morbidity in the Swedish Trial in Old Patients with hypertension-2 study. Lancet 354, 1751–1756.

Hansson, L., Zanchetti, A., Carruthers, S.G., for the HOT Study Group, 1998. Effects of intensive blood-pressure lowering and low-dose aspirin in patients with hypertension: principal results of the hypertension optimal treatment (HOT) randomised trial. Lancet 351, 1755–1762.

Hodgkinson, J., Mant, J., Martin, U., et al., 2011. Relative effectiveness of clinic and home blood pressure monitoring compared with ambulatory blood pressure monitoring in diagnosis of hypertension: systematic review. Br. Med. J. 342, d3621.

Holman, R.R., Paul, S.K., Bethel, M.A., et al., 2008. Long-term follow-up after tight control of blood pressure in type 2 diabetes. N. Engl. J. Med. 359, 1565–1576.

Intercollegiate Stroke Working Party, 2016. Royal College of Physicians National Clinical Guideline for Stroke, fifth ed. Available at: https://www.strokeaudit.org/SupportFiles/Documents/Guidelines/2016-National-Clinical-Guideline-for-Stroke-5t-(1).aspx.

JATOS Study Group, 2008. Principal results of the Japanese trial to assess optimal systolic blood pressure in elderly hypertensive patients. Hypertens. Res. 31, 2115–2127.

Julius, S., Kjeldsen, S.E., Weber, M., et al., 2004. Outcomes in hypertensive patients at high cardiovascular risk treated with regimens based on valsartan or amlodipine: the VALUE randomised trial. Lancet 363, 2022–2031.

Lindholm, L.H., Carlberg, B., Samuelsson, O., 2005. Should beta blockers remain first choice in the treatment of primary hypertension? A meta-analysis. Lancet 366, 1545–1553.

Lithell, H., Hansson, L., Skoog, I., SCOPE Study Group, 2003. The Study of Cognition and Prognosis in the Elderly (SCOPE): principal results of a randomised double-blind intervention trial. J. Hypertens. 21, 875–1866.

Mancia, G., Fagard, R., Narkiewicz, K., et al., 2013. ESH/ESC Guidelines for the management of arterial hypertension. Eur. Heart J. 34, 2159–2219.

Mason, J., Dickinson, H., Nicolson, D., et al., 2005. The diabetogenic potential of thiazide diuretics and beta-blocker combinations in the management of hypertension. J. Hypertens. 23, 1777–1781.

Medicines and Healthcare Regulatory Authority, 2014. Combination use of medicines from different classes of renin-angiotensin system blocking agents: risk of hyperkalaemia, hypotension, and impaired renal function – new warnings. Available at: https://www.gov.uk/drug-safety-update/combination-use-of-medicines-from-different-classes-of-renin-angiotensin-system-blocking-agents-risk-of-hyperkalaemia-hypotension-and-impaired-renal-function-new-warnings.

National Institute for Health and Care Excellence (NICE), 2010. CG 107: Hypertension in pregnancy: diagnosis and management. Available at: https://www.nice.org.uk/guidance/cg107.

National Institute for Health and Care Excellence (NICE), 2011. CG127: hypertension in adults: diagnosis and management. Available at: https://www.nice.org.uk/guidance/cg127.

National Institute for Health and Care Excellence (NICE), 2014a. CG182: Chronic kidney disease in adults: assessment and management. Available at: https://www.nice.org.uk/guidance/cg182.

National Institute for Health and Care Excellence (NICE), 2014b. Clinical knowledge summaries: CVD risk assessment and management. Available at: https://cks.nice.org.uk/cvd-risk-assessment-and-management.

National Institute for Health and Care Excellence (NICE), 2014c. CG181: Cardiovascular disease: risk assessment and reduction, including lipid modification. Available at https://www.nice.org.uk/guidance/cg181.

National Institute for Health and Care Excellence (NICE), 2015a. Type 1 diabetes in adults: diagnosis and management. Available at: https://www.nice.org.uk/guidance/ng17.

National Institute for Health and Care Excellence (NICE), 2015b. Type 2 diabetes in adults: management. Available at: https://www.nice.org.uk/guidance/ng28.

National Institute for Health and Care Excellence (NICE), 2017. Treatment steps for hypertension. Available at: https://pathways.nice.org.uk/pathways/hypertension#path=view%3A/pathways/hypertension/treatment-steps-for-hypertension.xml&content=view-index.

O'Brien, E., Barton, J., Nussberger, J., et al., 2007. Aliskiren reduces blood pressure and suppresses plasma renin activity in combination with a thiazide diuretic, an angiotensin-converting enzyme inhibitor, or an angiotensin receptor blocker. Hypertension 49, 276–284.

Patel, A., MacMahon, S., Chalmers, J., et al., 2007. Effects of a fixed combination of perindopril and indapamide on macrovascular and microvascular outcomes in patients with type 2 diabetes mellitus (the ADVANCE trial): a randomised controlled trial. Lancet 370, 829–840.

PROGRESS Collaborative Group, 2001. Randomised trial of a perindopril-based blood pressure lowering regimen among 6105 individuals with previous stroke or transient ischaemic attack. Lancet 358, 1033–1041.

Psaty, B.M., Heckbert, S.R., Kocpsell, T.D., et al., 1995. The risk of myocardial infarction associated with antihypertensive drug therapies. J. Am. Med. Assoc. 274, 620–625.

Sehestedt, T., Jeppesen, J., Hansen, T.W., et al., 2009. Which markers of subclinical organ damage to measure in individuals with high normal blood pressure? J. Hypertens. 27, 1165–1171.

SPRINT Research Group, 2015. A randomized trial of intensive versus standard blood-pressure control. N. Engl. J. Med. 373, 2103–2116.

SPS Study Group, 2013. Blood-pressure targets in patients with recent lacunar stroke: the SPS3 randomised trial. Lancet 382 (9891), 507–515.

Staessen, J.A., Fagard, R., Thijs, L., for the Systolic Hypertension in Europe (Syst-Eur) Trial Investigators, 1997. Randomised double-blind comparison of placebo and active treatment for older patients with isolated systolic hypertension. Lancet 350, 757–764.

Systolic Hypertension in the Elderly Programme (SHEP) Co-operative Research Group, 1991. Prevention of stroke by antihypertensive drug treatment in older persons with isolated systolic hypertension: final results of the Systolic Hypertension in the Elderly Program (SHEP). J. Am. Med. Assoc. 265, 3255–3264.

UK Prospective Diabetes Study Group, 1998a. Tight blood pressure control and risk of macrovascular and microvascular complications in type 2 diabetes: UKPDS 38. Br. Med. J. 317, 703–713.

UK Prospective Diabetes Study Group, 1998b. Efficacy of atenolol and captopril in reducing risk of macrovascular and microvascular complications in type 2 diabetes: UKPDS 39. Br. Med. J. 317, 713–726.

Verdecchia, P., Staessen, J.A., Angeli, F., on behalf of the Cardio-Sis investigators, 2009. Usual versus tight control of systolic blood pressure in non-diabetic patients with hypertension (Cardio-Sis): an open-label randomised trial. Lancet 374, 525–533.

Wing, L.M.H., Reid, C.M., Ryan, P., et al., 2003. A comparison of outcomes with angiotensin-converting-enzyme inhibitors and diuretics for hypertension in the elderly. N. Engl. J. Med. 348, 583–592.

Yusuf, S., Teo, K.K., Pogue, J., ONTARGET investigators, et al., 2008. Telmisartan, ramipril, or both in patients at high risk for vascular events. N. Engl. J. Med. 358, 1547–1559.

Zhao, P., Xu, P., Wan, C., et al., 2011. Evening versus morning dosing regimen drug therapy for hypertension. Cochrane DB Syst. Rev. (10), 2011. https://doi.org/10.1002/14651858.CD004184.pub2. Art. No. CD004184.

Further reading

Messerli, F., Williams, B., Ritz, E., 2007. Essential hypertension. Lancet 370, 591–603.

Taddei, S., 2015. Combination therapy in hypertension: what are the best options according to clinical pharmacology principles and controlled clinical trial evidence? Am. J. Cardiovasc. Drugs 15, 185–194.

Williams, H., 2015. Hypertension: management. Clinical Pharmacist. Available at: http://www.pharmaceutical-journal.com/learning/cpd-article/hypertension-management/20067719.cpdarticle.

Williams, H., 2015. Hypertension: pathophysiology and diagnosis. Clinical Pharmacist. Available at http://www.pharmaceutical-journal.com/learning/cpd-article/hypertension-pathophysiology-and-diagnosis/20067718.cpdarticle.

Useful websites

British Heart Foundation: http://www.bhf.org.uk
British Hypertension Society: http://bhsoc.org/
Blood Pressure UK: http://www.bloodpressureuk.org/Home
Cardiovascular risk calculators:
    ASSIGN: http://assign-score.com

SCORE: https://www.escardio.org/Education/Practice-Tools/CVD-prevention-toolbox/SCORE-Risk-Charts#
QRISK: https://www.qrisk.org

20 Coronary Heart Disease

Duncan McRobbie and Imran Hafiz

Key points

- Coronary heart disease (CHD) is common, often fatal and frequently preventable.
- High dietary fat, smoking and sedentary lifestyle are risk factors for CHD and require modification if present.
- Hypertension, hypercholesterolaemia, diabetes mellitus, obesity and personal stress are also risk factors and require optimal management.
- Stable angina should be managed with nitrates for pain relief and β-blockers, unless contraindicated, for long-term prophylaxis. Where β-blockers are inappropriate, the use of calcium channel blockers and/or nitrates may be considered.
- Acute coronary syndromes arise from unstable atheromatous plaques and may be classified as to whether there is ST-elevation myocardial infarction (STEMI) or non-ST-elevation myocardial infarction (NSTEMI).
- ST elevation on the electrocardiogram (ECG) indicates an occluded coronary artery and is used to determine treatment with fibrinolysis or primary angioplasty.
- Patients with NSTEMI may have experienced myocardial damage, are at increased risk of death and may benefit from a glycoprotein IIb/IIIa inhibitor.

Coronary heart disease (CHD), sometimes described as coronary artery disease (CAD) or ischaemic heart disease (IHD), is a condition in which the vascular supply to the heart is impeded by atheroma, thrombosis or spasm of coronary arteries. This may impair the supply of oxygenated blood to cardiac tissue sufficiently to cause myocardial ischaemia which, if severe or prolonged, may cause the death of cardiac muscle cells. Similarities in the development of atheromatous plaques in other vasculature, in particular the carotid arteries, with the resultant cerebral ischaemia has resulted in the term cardiovascular disease (CVD) being adopted to incorporate CHD, cerebrovascular disease and peripheral vascular disease.

Myocardial ischaemia occurs when the oxygen demand exceeds myocardial oxygen supply. The resultant ischaemic myocardium releases adenosine, the main mediator of chest pain, by stimulating the A1 receptors located on the cardiac nerve endings. Myocardial ischaemia may be 'silent' if the duration is of insufficient length, the afferent cardiac nerves are damaged (as with diabetics) or there is inhibition of the pain at the spinal or supraspinal level.

Factors increasing myocardial oxygen demand often precipitate ischaemic episodes and are commonly associated with increased work rate (heart rate) and increased workload (force of contractility). Less commonly, myocardial ischaemia can also arise if oxygen demand is abnormally increased, as may occur in patients with thyrotoxicosis or severe ventricular hypertrophy due to hypertension. Myocardial oxygen supply is dependent on the luminal cross-sectional area of the coronary artery and coronary arteriolar tone. Atheromatous plaques decrease the lumen diameter and, when extensive, reduce the ability of the coronary artery to dilate in response to increased myocardial oxygen demand. Ischaemia may also occur when the oxygen-carrying capacity of blood is impaired, as in iron-deficiency anaemia, or when the circulatory volume is depleted.

Epidemiology

An estimated 17.5 million people die from CVD worldwide each year, accounting for almost one-third of all deaths (World Health Organization, 2017). In the UK, just more than 150,000 people die from CVD each year, with CHD accounting for almost a half of these (British Heart Foundation, 2017). About 25% of premature deaths (<75 years old) in men and 17% of premature deaths in women result from CVD.

The epidemiology of CHD has been studied extensively, and risk factors for developing CHD are now well described. The absence of established risk factors does not guarantee freedom from CHD for any individual, and some individuals with several major risk factors seem perversely healthy. Nonetheless, there is evidence that in developed countries, education and publicity about the major risk factors have led to changes in social habits, particularly with respect to a reduction in smoking and fat consumption, and this has contributed to a decrease in the incidence of CHD.

The UK has seen a steady decline in deaths from CVD. Since the early 1960s the number of deaths has more than halved (British Heart Foundation, 2017). A study has indicated that both reductions in major risk factors and improvements in treatment have contributed to this reduction (Unal et al., 2004).

The improvement in deaths from CHD has been chiefly among those with higher incomes; however, the less prosperous social classes continue to have almost unchanged levels of CHD.

Better treatment has also contributed to a decrease in cardiac mortality, although CHD still accounts for some 70,000 deaths in the UK each year (British Heart Foundation, 2017), including 70% of sudden natural deaths, 14% of male deaths and 9% of female deaths. In the UK, CHD is the leading cause of death in men between 50 and 79 years old (second to lung cancer in women) (Office of National Statistics, 2015). In the over-80s, Alzheimer's disease and dementia are the leading causes of death in both men and women, followed by CHD in both groups. In the UK, in comparison with Caucasians, people of South Asian descent have a higher death rate from CHD, potentially due to a combination of genetic and environmental factors, including increased prevalence of metabolic syndrome and abdominal obesity, which increase the risk of diabetes and premature atherosclerosis. African Caribbeans and West Africans in the UK have a lower rate of CHD mortality, potentially explained by low levels of very low-density lipoprotein (VLDL), small dense LDL, and triglycerides.

Prevalence

In the UK, 2.3 million people have CHD, more than 60% of whom are male (British Heart Foundation, 2017). It has a prevalence of 5% in men and 3% in women. A quarter of men aged 55–74 years have evidence of CHD, and this proportion increases with age. Every year nearly 200,000 people suffer a myocardial infarction in the UK, of whom 70% survive. There are currently 915,000 people who have survived a myocardial infarction.

Mortality increases with age and is probably not due to a particular age-related factor but to the cumulative effect of risk factors that lead to atheroma and thrombosis and hence to CHD. Whilst the death rates for CHD in the UK have fallen (British Heart Foundation, 2017), the number of people living with CHD is increasing because of the ageing population.

Women appear less susceptible to CHD than men, although they seem to lose this protection after menopause, presumably because of hormonal changes. Race has not proved to be a clear risk factor because the prevalence of CHD seems to depend much more strongly on location and lifestyle than on ethnic origin or place of birth. It has been shown that lower social or economic class is associated with increased obesity, poor cholesterol indicators, higher blood pressure and higher C-reactive protein (CRP) measurements (an indicator of inflammatory activity).

Risk factors

Traditionally, the main potentially modifiable risk factors for CHD have been considered to be hypertension, cigarette smoking, raised serum cholesterol and diabetes. More recently psychological stress and abdominal obesity have gained increased prominence (Box 20.1). Patients with a combination of all these risk factors are at risk of suffering a myocardial infarction some 500 times greater than individuals without any of the risk factors. Stopping smoking, moderating alcohol intake, regular exercise and consumption of fresh fruit and vegetables were associated independently and additively with a reduction in the risk of having a myocardial infarction.

Box 20.1 Factors that increase or decrease the risk of developing coronary heart disease

Factors that increase the risk of CHD
- Cigarette smoking
- Raised serum cholesterol
- Hypertension
- Diabetes
- Abdominal obesity
- Increased personal stress

Factors that decrease the risk of CHD
- Regular consumption of fresh fruit and vegetables
- Regular exercise
- Moderate alcohol consumption
- Modification of factors that increase the risk of CHD

CHD, Coronary heart disease.

Diabetes mellitus is a positive risk factor for CHD in developed countries with high levels of CHD. Insulin resistance, as defined by high fasting insulin concentrations, is an independent risk factor for CHD in men. In the UK, the mortality rates from CHD is higher for people with diabetes.

Although unusual physical exertion is associated with an increased risk of infarction, an active lifestyle that includes regular, moderate exercise is beneficial; however, the optimum level has not been determined, and its beneficial effect appears to be readily overwhelmed by the presence of other risk factors. A family history of CHD is a positive risk factor, independent of diet and other risk factors. Hostility, anxiety and depression are associated with increased CHD and death, especially after a myocardial infarction.

Epidemiological studies have shown associations between CHD and prior infections with several common micro-organisms, including *Chlamydia pneumoniae* and *Helicobacter pylori*, but a causal connection has not been found. The influence of fetal and infant growth conditions, and their interaction with social conditions in childhood and adult life, has been debated strongly for decades, but it is clear that lower socioeconomic status and being underweight in very early life are linked to higher incidences of CHD.

Aetiology

The vast majority of CHD occurs in patients with atherosclerosis of the coronary arteries (Fig. 20.1) that starts before adulthood. The cause of spontaneous atherosclerosis is unclear, although it is thought that in the presence of hypercholesterolaemia, a non-denuding form of injury occurs to the endothelial lining of coronary arteries and other vessels. This injury is followed by subendothelial migration of monocytes and the accumulation of fatty streaks containing lipid-rich macrophages and T-cells. Almost all adults, and 50% of children aged 11–14 years, have fatty streaks in their coronary arteries. Thereafter, there is migration and proliferation of smooth muscle cells into the intima, with further lipid deposition. The smooth muscle cells, together with fibroblasts, synthesise and secrete collagen, proteoglycans, elastin and glycoproteins that make up a fibrous cap surrounding cells

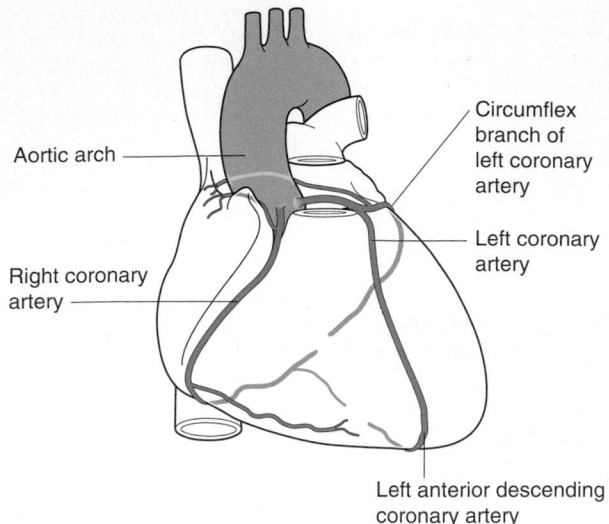

Fig. 20.1 Main coronary arteries.

Labels: Aortic arch; Right coronary artery; Circumflex branch of left coronary artery; Left coronary artery; Left anterior descending coronary artery

Table 20.1 Effect of interventions on risk of myocardial infarction

Intervention	Control	Benefit of intervention
Stopping smoking for ≥5 years	Current smokers	50–70% lower risk
Reducing serum cholesterol		2% lower risk of each 1% reduction in cholesterol
Treatment of hypertension		2–3% lower risk of each 1-mmHg decrease in diastolic pressure
Active lifestyle	Sedentary lifestyle	45% lower risk
Mild to moderate alcohol consumption (approx. 1 unit/day)	Total abstainers	25–45% lower risk
Low-dose aspirin	Non-users	33% lower risk in men
Postmenopausal oestrogen replacement	Non-users	44% lower risk

The quality of data associated with these interventions varies greatly, and figures may not apply to all patient groups.

and necrotic tissue, together called a plaque. The presence of atherosclerotic plaques results in narrowing of vessels, reduction in blood flow and a decrease in the ability of the coronary vasculature to dilate. This may manifest as angina. Associated with the plaque rupture is a loss of endothelium. This can serve as a stimulus for the formation of a thrombus and result in more acute manifestations of CHD, including unstable angina (UA) and myocardial infarction. Plaque rupture caused by physical stresses or plaque erosion may precipitate an acute reaction. Other pathological processes are probably involved, including endothelial dysfunction, which alters the fibrin–fibrinolysis balance and the vasoconstriction–vasodilation balance. There is interest in the role of statins and angiotensin-converting enzyme (ACE) inhibitors in modifying endothelial function.

There is also great interest in the role of inflammation, especially in acute episodes. At postmortem, many plaques are found to contain inflammatory cells, and inflammatory damage is found at the sites of plaque rupture.

Measurement of acute phase inflammatory reactions, such as fibrinogen and CRP, has a predictive association with coronary events. High-sensitivity CRP assays have been used in populations without acute illness to stratify individuals into high-, medium- and low-risk groups. In patients with other risk factors, however, CRP adds little prognostic information. CRP is produced by atheroma, in addition to the major producer, which is the liver, and is an inflammatory agent as well as a marker of inflammation. Evidence is emerging that drug therapy that reduces CRP in otherwise healthy individuals reduces the incidence of major cardiac events (Ridker et al., 2008).

Oxidative stress that involves the uncontrolled production of reactive oxygen species (ROS) or a reduction in antioxidant species has been linked in the laboratory to several aspects of cardiovascular pathogenesis including endothelial malfunction, lipid metabolism, atheroma formation and plaque rupture, but the clinical importance is unclear. The use of antioxidants has been disappointingly unsuccessful, but there is interest in peroxisome proliferator-activated receptor (PPAR) agonists that modify ROS production; some of these are already in use for treating diabetes

and are associated with favourable changes in many metabolic markers for CVD. Other agents that reduce ROS production include statins and drugs that reduce angiotensin production.

Modification of risk factors

Common to all stages of CHD treatment is the need to reduce risk factors (Table 20.1). The patient needs to appreciate the value of the proposed strategy and to be committed to a plan for changing their lifestyle and habits, which may not be easy to achieve after years of smoking or eating a particular diet. Preventing CHD is important but neither instant nor spectacular. It may require many sessions of counselling over several years to initiate and maintain healthy habits. It may also involve persuasion of patients to continue taking medication for asymptomatic disorders such as hypertension or hypercholesterolaemia.

National campaigns to encourage healthy eating or exercise are expensive, as is the long-term medical treatment of hypertension or hypercholesterolaemia, and such strategies must have the backing of governments to succeed. It has been argued that community-wide campaigns on cholesterol reduction have had measurable benefits in Finland, the USA and elsewhere, at least in high-risk, well-educated and affluent groups. It follows that the next challenge is to extend that success to poorer, ethnically diverse groups and to those portions of the population with mild to moderate risk.

National campaigns to reduce smoking, either by raising public awareness of the risks or by legislation that prohibits smoking in enclosed public places and workplaces, on public transport and in vehicles used for work, have reduced the number of smokers in the UK to an all-time low (although 17% of adults still smoke).

For every individual there is a need to act against the causative factors of CHD. Thus, attempts should be made to control hypertension, heart failure, arrhythmias, hypercholesterolaemia, obesity, diabetes mellitus, thyroid disease, anaemia and cardiac valve disorders. Apart from medication, these will require careful attention to diet and exercise and will necessitate smoking cessation. Cardiac rehabilitation classes and exercise programmes improve many risk factors, including obesity, lipid indices, insulin resistance, psychological state and lifestyle. They also impact on morbidity and mortality.

The role of antioxidants and hormone replacement therapy in preventing and treating coronary disease has been debated. However, a randomised clinical trial of antioxidant vitamins and/or hormone replacement therapy suggested that these agents are not of benefit and may indeed result in higher rates of cardiovascular events (Waters et al., 2002).

Clinical syndromes

The primary clinical manifestation of CHD is chest pain. Chest pain arising from stable coronary atheromatous disease leads to stable angina and normally arises when narrowing of the coronary artery lumen exceeds 50% of the original luminal diameter. Stable angina is characterised by chest pain and breathlessness on exertion; symptoms are relieved promptly by rest.

A stable coronary atheromatous plaque may become unstable as a result of either plaque erosion or rupture. Exposure of the subendothelial lipid and collagen stimulates the formation of thrombus, which causes sudden narrowing of the vessel. The spectrum of clinical outcomes that results is grouped under the term acute coronary syndrome (ACS) and is characterised by chest pain of increasing severity either on minimal exertion or, more commonly, at rest. These patients are at high risk of myocardial infarction and death and require prompt hospitalisation. Many aspects of the treatment of stable angina and ACS are similar, but there is a much greater urgency and intensity in the management of ACS.

Stable angina

Stable angina is a clinical syndrome characterised by discomfort in the chest, jaw, shoulder, back, or arms, typically elicited by exertion or emotional stress and relieved by rest or nitroglycerin. Characteristically, the discomfort (it is often not described by the patient as a pain) occurs after a predictable level of exertion, classically when climbing hills or stairs, and resolves within a few minutes on resting. The Canadian Cardiovascular Society (1976) classification is often used to measure the severity of the angina (Table 20.2). Unfortunately, the clinical manifestations of angina are very variable. Many patients mistake the discomfort for indigestion. Some patients, particularly diabetics and the elderly, may not experience pain at all but present with breathlessness or fatigue; this is termed silent ischaemia.

Table 20.2	Classification of angina severity according to the Canadian Cardiovascular Society (1976)
Class I	Ordinary activity does not cause angina, such as walking and climbing stairs.
Class II	Slight limitation of ordinary activity
Class III	Marked limitation of ordinary physical activity
Class IV	Inability to carry on any physical activity without discomfort

Further investigations are needed to confirm the diagnosis and assess the need for intervention. The resting electrocardiogram (ECG) is normal in more than half of patients with angina. However, an abnormal ECG substantially increases the probability of coronary disease; in particular, it may show signs of previous myocardial infarction. Noninvasive testing is helpful. Exercise testing is useful both in confirming the diagnosis and in giving a guide to prognosis. Alternatives such as myocardial scintigraphy (isotope scanning) and stress echocardiography (ultrasound) provide similar information.

Coronary angiography is regarded as the gold standard for the assessment of CHD and involves the passage of a catheter through the arterial circulation and the injection of radio-opaque contrast media into the coronary arteries. The X-ray images obtained permit confirmation of the diagnosis, aid assessment of prognosis and guide therapy, particularly with regard to suitability for angioplasty and coronary artery bypass grafting.

Noninvasive techniques, including magnetic resonance imaging (MRI) and multi-slice computerised tomography (CT) scanning, are being developed and tested as alternatives to angiography.

Treatment of stable angina is based on two principles:
- improve prognosis by preventing myocardial infarction and death,
- relieve or prevent symptoms.

Pharmacological therapy can be considered a viable alternative to invasive strategies, providing similar results without the complications associated with percutaneous coronary intervention (PCI). An algorithm for addressing both of these principles is outlined in Fig. 20.2. In addition, diabetes, hypertension and Legislation under the Health Act 2006, which prohibits smoking in enclosed public places and workplaces, on public transport and in vehicles used for work in patients with stable angina should be well controlled. Smoking cessation, without or with pharmacological support, and weight loss should be attempted.

Treatment to reduce risk

One of the major complications arising from atheromatous plaque is thrombus formation. This causes an increase in plaque size and may result in myocardial infarction. Antiplatelet agents, in particular aspirin, are effective in preventing platelet activation and thus thrombus formation. Aspirin is of proven benefit in all forms of established CHD, although the risk/benefit ratio in people at risk of CHD is less clear.

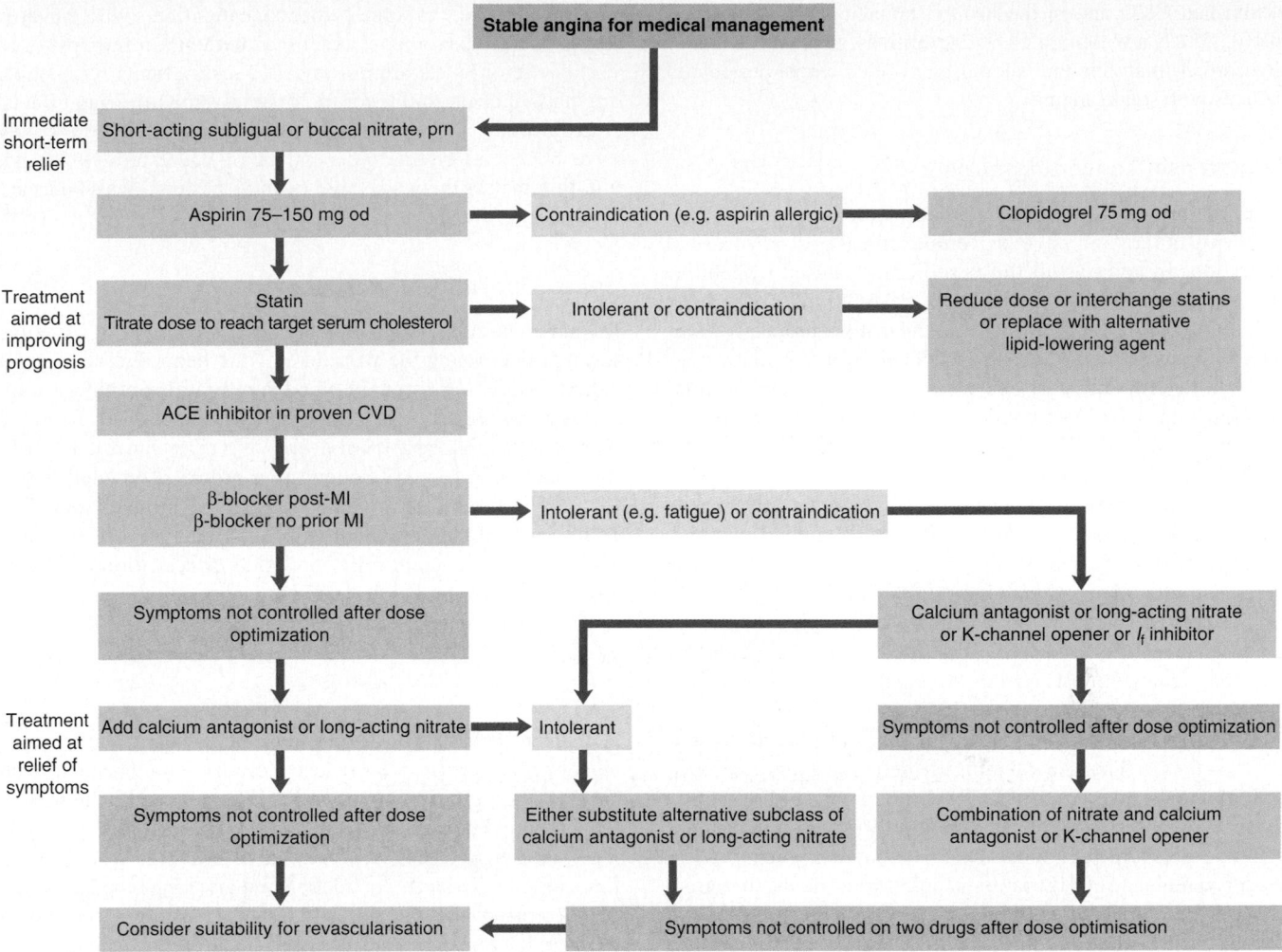

Fig. 20.2 Algorithm for the medical management of stable angina.
CVD, Cardiovascular disease; MI, myocardial infarction; od, once a day; prn, when required. (Adapted from Fox et al., 2006.)

Aspirin. Aspirin acts via irreversible inhibition of platelet cyclooxygenase 1 (COX-1) and thus thromboxane production, which is normally complete with chronic dosing of 75 mg/day. This antiplatelet action is apparent within an hour of taking a dose of 300 mg. The effect on platelets lasts for the lifetime of the platelet, around 8–10 days.

The optimal maintenance dose seems to be 75–150 mg/day, with lower doses having limited cardiac risk protection and higher doses increasing the risk of gastro-intestinal side effects. Dyspepsia is relatively common in patients taking aspirin, and patients should be advised to take the medicine with or immediately after food. Enteric-coated preparations are no safer, and patients with ongoing symptoms of dyspepsia may require concomitant acid suppression with a proton pump inhibitor or should be switched to clopidogrel. Adverse reactions to aspirin include allergy, including bronchospasm. The benefits and risks of using aspirin in patients with asthma or a previous history of gastro-intestinal bleeding need to be carefully considered.

Clopidogrel. Clopidogrel inhibits adenosine diphosphate (ADP) activation of platelets and is useful as an alternative to

aspirin in patients who are allergic or cannot tolerate aspirin. Data from one major trial (CAPRIE Steering Committee, 1996) indicate that clopidogrel is at least as effective as aspirin in patients with stable coronary disease. The usual dose is 300 mg once, then 75 mg daily. Although less likely to cause gastric erosion and ulceration, gastro-intestinal bleeding is still a major complication of clopidogrel therapy. There is evidence that the combination of a proton pump inhibitor and aspirin is as effective as using clopidogrel alone in patients with a history of upper gastro-intestinal bleeding.

COX-2 inhibitors. The analgesic and anti-inflammatory action of non-steroidal anti-inflammatory drugs (NSAIDs) is believed to depend mainly on their inhibition of COX-2, and the unwanted gastro-intestinal effects of NSAIDs on their inhibition of COX-1. COX-2 inhibition reduces the production of prostacyclin, which has vasodilatory and platelet-inhibiting effects. Studies have raised concern about the cardiovascular safety of NSAIDs. Initially, the concern was focussed on the selective cyclo-oxygenase-2 inhibitors and a link to an increased cardiovascular risk. Evidence has shown the more traditional nonselective NSAIDs increase cardiovascular risk in both patients with established CVD and in the healthy population (Fosbøl et al., 2010). NSAIDs with high COX-2 specificity increase the risk of myocardial infarction and should be avoided where possible in patients with stable angina.

Angiotensin-converting enzyme inhibitors

ACE inhibitors are established treatments for hypertension and heart failure and have proven beneficial post–myocardial infarction. In addition to the vasodilation caused by inhibiting the production of angiotensin II, ACE inhibitors have anti-inflammatory, antithrombotic and antiproliferative properties. Some of these effects are mediated by actions on vascular endothelium and might be expected to be of benefit in all patients with CHD. ACE inhibitors also reduce the production of ROS.

The use of ACE inhibitors in patients without myocardial infarction or left ventricular damage is based on two trials: the HOPE study (Yusuf et al., 2000), which studied ramipril, and the EUROPA (2003) study, which used perindopril. These trials also identified an incidental delay in the onset of diabetes mellitus in susceptible individuals, which may be of long-term benefit to them. The HOPE study (Yusuf et al., 2000), a secondary prevention trial, investigated the effect of an ACE inhibitor on patients older than 55 years who had known atherosclerotic disease or diabetes plus one other cardiovascular risk factor. The use of ramipril decreased the combined endpoint of stroke, myocardial infarction or cardiovascular death by approximately 22%. The benefits were independent of blood pressure reduction. This has major implications for the management of CHD patients, both for the decision to treat all and the choice of treatment. At present the use of ACE inhibitors in patients with coronary disease and at least one additional risk factor, but without myocardial infarction, has general acceptance and is recommended in European guidelines (Montalescot et al., 2013).

Statins

Studies have repeatedly demonstrated the benefit of reducing cholesterol, especially low-density lipoprotein-cholesterol (LDL-C), in patients with CHD.

Earlier studies focused on patients with 'elevated' cholesterol, but all patients with coronary risk factors benefit from reduction of their serum cholesterol level. It is now clear that there is no 'safe' level of cholesterol for patients with CHD and that there is a continuum of risk down to very low cholesterol levels. Levels of LDL-C of less than 1.8 mmol/L used to be recommended for patients with established CVD, but a 40% reduction in non-HDL cholesterol from baseline is now recommended (National Institute for Health and Care Excellence [NICE], 2014a). Statins should be prescribed alongside lifestyle advice for both primary prevention of CVD and in those with established CVD (see Chapter 24 for more detail).

In addition to cholesterol-lowering properties, statins also have antithrombotic, anti-inflammatory and antiproliferative properties. They are also important in restoring normal endothelial function and inhibit the production of ROS in the vessel wall. There is some evidence that patients with elevated levels of CRP have better outcomes with statin therapy, even if cholesterol levels are not raised. Most patients with stable angina will be on statins for their cholesterol-lowering effects. It is important, however, to recognise that these drugs may have beneficial effects independent of cholesterol lowering, and this makes them valuable even in patients with 'normal' cholesterol levels.

Symptom relief and prevention

In stable angina, much of the drug treatment is directed towards decreasing the workload of the heart and, to a lesser extent, improving coronary blood supply; this provides symptomatic relief and improves prognosis. Therapy to decrease workload is targeted at both decreasing afterload and controlling heart rate. Evidence suggests a prognostic benefit when the resting heart rate is controlled below 70 beats/min (Fox et al., 2008). Drug treatment is initiated in a stepwise fashion according to symptom relief and side effects. Some patients will require a number of anti-anginal medicines to control their angina symptoms.

β-Blockers

β-Blockers are now considered first-line agents in the management of angina. β-Blockers reduce mortality in both patients who have suffered a previous myocardial infarction and in those with heart failure. They reduce myocardial oxygen demand by blocking β-adrenergic receptors, thereby decreasing the heart rate and force of left ventricular contraction and lowering blood pressure. The decreased heart rate not only reduces the energy demand on the heart but also permits better perfusion of the subendocardium by the coronary circulation. β-Blockers may also reduce energy-demanding supraventricular or atrial arrhythmias and counteract the cardiac effects of hyperthyroidism or pheochromocytoma.

β-Blockers are particularly useful in exertional angina. Patients treated optimally should have a resting heart rate of around 60 beats/min. Although many patients may dislike the side effects of β-blockers, they should be urged to continue wherever reasonable. β-Blockers should be used with caution in patients with diabetes because the production of insulin is under adrenergic system control, and thus their concomitant use may worsen glucose control. β-Blockers can also mask the symptoms of hypoglycaemia and patients in whom the combination is considered of value should be warned of this; however, most clinicians now believe that the benefits of taking β-blockers, even in diabetics, outweigh the risks, and they are frequently prescribed.

Although β-blockers are widely used, their tendency to cause bronchospasm and peripheral vascular spasm means that they are contraindicated in patients with asthma and used with caution in chronic obstructive pulmonary disease and peripheral vascular disease as well as in acute heart failure and bradycardia.

Cardioselective agents such as atenolol, bisoprolol and metoprolol are preferred because of their reduced tendency to cause bronchoconstriction, but no β-blocker is completely specific for the heart. Agents with low lipophilicity, for example, atenolol, penetrate the central nervous system (CNS) to a lesser extent

Table 20.3 Properties and pharmacokinetics of β-blockers

	Blockade	Lipophilicity	ISA	Oral absorption	Elimination
Acebutolol	β₁ (some β2)	+	+	90%[a]	Active metabolite ($t_{1/2}$ 11–13 h, renal)
					Gut 50%, $t_{1/2}$ 3–4 h
Atenolol	β₁	–	–	50%	Renal $t_{1/2}$ 5–7 h
Betaxolol	β₁	+	–	100%	Hepatic + renal $t_{1/2}$ 15 h
Bisoprolol	β₁	+	–	90%	Hepatic + renal $t_{1/2}$ 10–12 h
Carteolol	β₁ β₂	–	++	80%	Hepatic + renal $t_{1/2}$ 3–7 h
Carvedilol	β₁β₂α₁	+	–	80%[a]	Hepatic + renal $t_{1/2}$ 4–8 h
Celiprolol	β₁α₂	–	β₂+	30–70%	Renal + gut $t_{1/2}$ 5–6 h
Esmolol	β₁	–	–	i.v.	Blood enzymes $t_{1/2}$ 9 min
Labetalol	β₁β₂α₁	–	–	100%[a]	Hepatic $t_{1/2}$ 6–8 h
Metoprolol	β₁	+	–	95%[a]	Hepatic $t_{1/2}$ 3–4 h
Nadolol	β₁β₂	–	–	30%	Renal $t_{1/2}$ 16–18 h
Nebivolol	β₁	+	–	12–96%[b]	Hepatic $t_{1/2}$ 8–27 h[b]
Oxprenolol	β₁β₂	+	++	90%[a]	Hepatic + $t_{1/2}$ 1–2 h
Pindolol	β₁β₂	+	+++	90%	Hepatic + renal $t_{1/2}$ 3–4 h
Propranolol	β₁β₂	+	–	90%[a]	Hepatic $t_{1/2}$ 3–6 h
Sotalol	β₁β₂	–	–	70%	Renal $t_{1/2}$ 15–17 h
Timolol	β₁β₂	+	–	90%[a]	Hepatic + renal $t_{1/2}$ 3–4 h

[a]Extensive first-pass metabolism may result in a significant decrease in bioavailability.
[b]Genetically determined groups of slow and fast metabolisers have been identified.
All figures are approximate and subject to interpatient variability. Therapeutic ranges are not well defined.
ISA, Intrinsic sympathomimetic activity; i.v., intravenous; $t_{1/2}$, elimination half-life.

than others, and do not so readily cause the nightmares, hallucinations and depression that are sometimes found with lipophilic agents, for example, propranolol and metoprolol, which should not be used in patients with psychiatric disorders. CNS-mediated fatigue or lethargy is found in some patients with all β-blockers, although it must be distinguished from that of myocardial suppression. β-Blockers should not be stopped abruptly for fear of precipitating angina through rebound receptor hypersensitivity. They should be avoided in the rare Prinzmetal's angina where coronary spasm is a major factor.

All β-blockers tend to reduce renal blood flow, but this is only important in renal impairment. Drugs eliminated by the kidney (Table 20.3) may need to be given at lower doses in the renally impaired or in the elderly, who are particularly susceptible to the CNS-mediated lassitude. Drugs eliminated by the liver have a number of theoretical interactions with other agents that affect liver blood flow or metabolic rate, but these are rarely of clinical significance because the dose should be titrated to the effect.

Likewise, although there is theoretical support for the use of agents with high intrinsic sympathomimetic activity (ISA) to reduce the incidence or severity of drug-induced heart failure, there is no β-blocker that is free from this problem, and clinical trials of drugs with ISA have generally failed to show any extra benefit.

Calcium channel blockers

Calcium channel blockers (CCBs) act on a variety of smooth muscle and cardiac tissues, and there are a large number of agents that have differing specificities for different body tissues.

Although short-acting dihydropyridine CCBs have been implicated in the exacerbation of angina due to the phenomenon of 'coronary steal', longer-acting dihydropyridines, for example, amlodipine and felodipine, or longer-acting formulations, for example, nifedipine LA, have demonstrated symptom-relieving potential similar to β-blockers. Dihydropyridines have no effect on the conducting tissues and are effective arterial dilators, decreasing afterload and improving coronary perfusion but also causing flushing, headaches and reflex tachycardia. This may be overcome by combination with a β-blocker. The use of dihydropyridines in angina is based on efficacy in trials that have used surrogate markers such as exercise tolerance rather than mortality as the endpoint.

CCBs with myocardial rate control as well as vasodilatory properties, for example, diltiazem, and those with predominantly rate-controlling effects, for example, verapamil, have also been shown to improve symptom control, reduce the frequency of anginal attacks and increase exercise tolerance. They should be avoided in patients with compromised left ventricular function and conduction abnormalities. Verapamil and diltiazem are suitable for rate-control patients in whom β-blockers are contraindicated on the grounds of respiratory or peripheral vascular disease. They should be used with caution in patients already receiving β-blockers because bradycardia and heart block have been reported with this combination.

CCBs have a particular role in the management of Prinzmetal's (variant) angina, which is thought to be due to coronary artery spasm.

Nitrates

Organic nitrates are valuable in angina because they dilate veins and thereby decrease preload, dilate arteries to a lesser extent, thereby decreasing afterload, and promote flow in collateral coronary vessels, diverting blood from the epicardium to the endocardium. They are available in many forms, but all relax vascular smooth muscle by releasing nitric oxide (formerly known as endothelium-derived relaxing factor), which acts via cyclic GMP. The production of nitric oxide from nitrates is probably mediated by intracellular thiols, and it has been observed that when tolerance to the action of nitrates occurs, a thiol donor (such as N-acetylcysteine) may partially restore the effectiveness of the nitrate. Antioxidants such as vitamin C have also been used. Although clinical trials have not established any mortality gain from the use of oral nitrate preparations, their role in providing symptom relief is well established.

Tolerance is one of the main limitations to the use of nitrates. This develops rapidly, and a 'nitrate-free' period of a few hours in each 24-hour period is beneficial in maintaining the effectiveness of treatment. The nitrate-free period should coincide with the period of lowest risk of infarction, usually night time, and not early morning, the period with the highest risk. Many patients receiving short-acting nitrates two or three times a day would do well to have their doses between 7 a.m. and 6 p.m. (say, 8 a.m. and 2 p.m. for isosorbide mononitrate). This is generally not practised in unstable angina where there is no low-risk period; continuous dosing is used, with doses increased if tolerance develops.

There are many nitrate preparations available, including intravenous infusions, conventional or slow-release tablets and capsules, transdermal patches, sublingual tablets and sprays and adhesive buccal tablets. Slow-release preparations and transdermal patches are expensive and do not generally offer such flexible dosing regimens as short-acting tablets. Sustained-release tablets do not release the drug over the whole 24-hour period, producing a 'nitrate free period', whereas patches need to be removed for a few hours each day. Buccal tablets are expensive and offer no real therapeutic advantage in regular therapy. Like sublingual sprays and tablets, however, they have a rapid onset of action, and the drug bypasses the liver, which has an extensive first-pass metabolic effect on oral nitrates. The sublingual preparations, whether sprays or suckable or chewable tablets, are used for the prevention or relief of acute attacks of pain but may elicit the two principal side effects of nitrates: hypotension with dizziness and fainting, and a throbbing headache. To minimise these effects, patients should be advised to sit down, rather than lie or stand, when taking short-acting nitrates, and to spit out or swallow the tablet once the angina is relieved. Sublingual glyceryl trinitrate (GTN) tablets have a very short shelf-life on exposure to air and need to be stored carefully and replaced frequently. As a consequence, they are now little used. All nitrates may induce tachycardia.

Three main nitrates are used: GTN (mainly for sublingual, buccal, transdermal and intravenous routes), isosorbide dinitrate and isosorbide mononitrate. All are effective if given in appropriate doses at suitable dose intervals (Table 20.4). Because isosorbide dinitrate is metabolised to the mononitrate, there is a preference for using the more predictable mononitrate, but this is not a significant clinical factor. A more relevant feature may be that whereas the dinitrate is usually given three or four times a day, the mononitrate is given once or twice a day. Slow-release preparations exist for both drugs.

Nicorandil

Nicorandil is a compound that exhibits the properties of a nitrate but which also activates adenosine triphosphate (ATP)-dependent potassium channels. The IONA Study Group (2002) compared nicorandil with placebo as 'add-on' treatment in 5126 high-risk patients with stable angina. The main benefit for patients in the nicorandil group was a reduction in unplanned admission to hospital with chest pain. The study did not discuss when to add nicorandil to combinations of antianginals such as β-blockers, CCBs and long-acting nitrates. There is a theoretical benefit from these agents in their action to promote ischaemic preconditioning. This phenomenon is seen when myocardial tissue is exposed to a period of ischaemia before sustained coronary artery occlusion. Prior exposure to ischaemia renders the myocardial tissue more resistant to permanent damage. This mechanism is mimicked by the action of nicorandil.

Ivabradine

Ivabradine represents a class of antianginal agents which block the I_f current. I_f is a mixed Na^+–K^+ inward current activated by hyperpolarisation and modulated by the autonomic nervous system. This regulates pacemaker activity in the sinoatrial node and controls heart rate. Inhibition, therefore, reduces heart rate without affecting the force of contraction. Ivabradine is similar in efficacy to atenolol and CCBs and may be of particular use in patients in whom β-blockers are contraindicated. The most frequent adverse drug reactions are dose-dependent transient visual symptoms that manifest as enhanced brightness commonly associated with abrupt changes in light intensity. They may be related to the action of ivabradine at hyperpolarisation-activated, cyclic

Table 20.4 Properties of commonly used nitrates

Drug	Speed of onset	Duration of action	Notes
GTN			
Intravenous	Immediate	Duration of infusion	
Transdermal	30 min	Designed to release drug steadily for 24 h	Tolerance develops if applied continuously
SR tablets and capsules	Slow	8–12 h	
Sublingual tablets	Rapid (1–4 min)	<30 min	Inactivated if swallowed Less effective if dry mouth
Spray	Rapid (1–4 min)	<30 min	
Buccal tablets	Rapid (1–4 min)	4–8 h	Nearly as rapid in onset as sublingual tablets
Isosorbide dinitrate			
SR tablets	Similar to GTN		
Intravenous	Similar to GTN		
Sublingual	Slightly slower than GTN	As for GTN	
Chewable tablets	2–5 min	2–4 h	Less prone to cause headaches than sublingual tablets
Oral tablets	30–40 min	4–8 h	
Isosorbide mononitrate			
Oral tablets	30–40 min	6–12 h	
SR tablets or capsules	Slow	12–24 h	Some brands claim a nitrate-free period if given once daily

GTN, Glyceryl trinitrate; SR, sustained-release.

nucleotide-gated cation current channels present in the retina. Visual symptoms may resolve spontaneously during therapy or after drug discontinuation.

Ranolazine

Ranolazine, a selective inhibitor of late sodium influx, attenuates the abnormalities of ventricular repolarisation and contractility associated with ischaemia. It has been shown to increase exercise tolerance, reduce anginal episodes and reduce the use of GTN. Side effects include dizziness, constipation, nausea, and the potential for prolongation of the QTc interval. Ranolazine seems to be a safe addition to current traditional drugs for chronic stable angina, especially in aggressive multidrug regimens.

Acute coronary syndrome

Definition and cause

The group of conditions referred to as ACS often present with similar symptoms of chest pain which is not, or only partially, relieved by GTN. These conditions include acute myocardial infarction (AMI), unstable angina (UA) and non-ST-elevation myocardial infarction (NSTEMI). AMI with persistent ST-segment elevation on the ECG usually develops Q waves, indicating transmural infarction. UA and NSTEMI present without persistent ST-segment elevation and are managed differently, although a similar early diagnostic and therapeutic approach is employed. All patients with ACS should be admitted to hospital for evaluation, risk stratification and treatment. The spectrum of ACS is described in Fig. 20.3.

ACS arises from the rupture of an unstable atheromatous plaque. This exposes the cholesterol-rich plaque in the intima to the blood, initiating platelet activation and eventual thrombus formation. The volume of the eventual thrombus and the time the vessel is occluded determine the degree of myocardial necrosis that occurs. The major difference in approach to these patients arises from whether the coronary artery involved is felt to be occluded or open.

Patients with an occluded coronary artery suffer myocardial damage, the extent of which is determined by the duration and site of the occlusion. The primary strategy for these patients is the restoration of coronary flow with either a fibrinolytic agent or primary angioplasty. If the coronary artery is

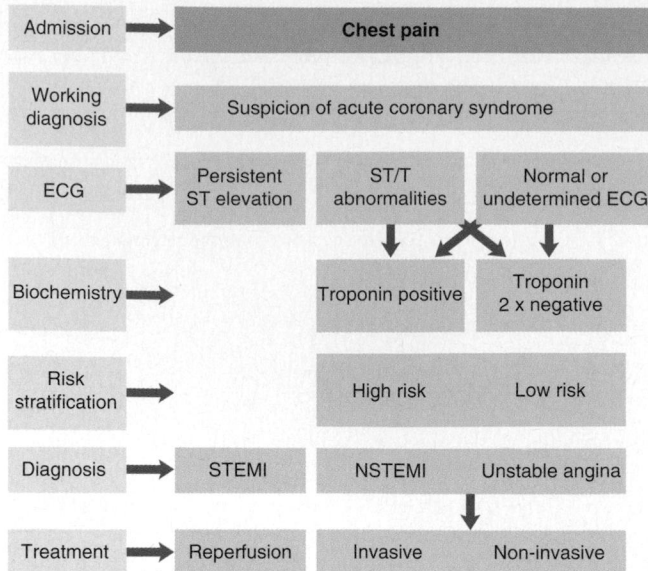

Fig. 20.3 The spectrum of acute coronary syndrome (Thygesen et al., 2007).
ECG, Electrocardiogram; NSTEMI, non-ST-elevation myocardial infarction; STEMI, ST elevation myocardial infarction.

patent, then fibrinolysis is unnecessary and probably harmful, although angioplasty may still be appropriate. When the vessel is open, for both groups, patient management focuses on the unstable coronary plaque and is, therefore, fundamentally similar.

Troponins (troponin I or troponin T) are cardiac muscle proteins that are released after myocardial cell damage and are highly sensitive and specific for myocardial infarction. They are useful in diagnosing patients with ACS and for predicting response to drug therapy; they are now key to the management of these patients and have replaced cardiac enzymes such as creatinine kinase (CK), aspartate transaminase (AST) and lactate dehydrogenase (LDH).

Diagnostic criteria for AMI have changed to incorporate the increasing availability of new diagnostic techniques with traditional symptoms and ECG changes. The following criteria for AMI, agreed by the European Society of Cardiology (Steg et al., 2012) rely on the rise of cardiac biomarkers (preferably troponin) with at least one value above the 99th percentile of the upper reference limit, together with evidence of myocardial ischaemia characterised by at least one of the following symptoms:

- ECG changes indicative of new ischaemia: new ST changes (STEMI or new left bundle branch block [LBBB]),
- development of pathological Q waves in the ECG,
- image evidence of new loss of viable myocardium or new regional wall motion abnormality.

Mortality rates of patients with presumed myocardial infarction or ACS in the first month is approximately 30%, and of these deaths, about half occur within the first 2 hours. The prognosis of an individual who has suffered a STEMI and receives hospital treatment has improved since the widespread use of thrombolytic therapy and primary percutaneous intervention.

The most dangerous time after a myocardial infarction is the first few hours when ventricular fibrillation (VF) is most likely to occur.

Patients without persistent ST elevation on the ECG may still have experienced myocardial damage due to the temporary occlusion of the vessel or emboli from the plaque-related thrombus blocking smaller distal vessels and will have raised levels of troponin. These patients have had a NSTEMI. The long-term prognosis in NSTEMI is similar to that of STEMI. The early adverse event rate is lower, but these patients are more likely to suffer death, recurrent myocardial infarction or recurrent ischaemia after hospital discharge than patients with STEMI. More emphasis is now placed on improving the treatment of patients with NSTEMI than was previously the case. Patients without ST elevation and without a rise in troponin or cardiac enzymes are defined as having UA.

The Global Registry of Acute Coronary Events (GRACE; available at http://www.gracescore.org) is an international registry which has enrolled patients with ACS (UA, NSTEMI and STEMI) since 1999. The registry indicates a similar incidence of UA, NSTEMI and STEMI. The GRACE 2.0 risk calculator (available via http://www.gracescore.org) provides a direct estimation of mortality while in hospital, at 6 months, 1 year and at 3 years. The combined risk of death or myocardial infarction at 1 year is also provided. Variables used in the GRACE 2.0 risk calculation include age, systolic blood pressure, pulse rate, serum creatinine, Killip class at presentation, cardiac arrest at admission, elevated cardiac biomarkers and ST deviation (Roffi et al., 2016).

The classification of ACS based on ECG findings and measurement of troponin is shown in Fig. 20.4.

Treatment of ST-elevation myocardial infarction

Treatment of STEMI may be divided into four categories:

- provide immediate care to alleviate pain, prevent deterioration and improve cardiac function;
- restore coronary flow and myocardial tissue perfusion;
- manage complications, notably heart failure and arrhythmias;
- prevent further infarction or death (secondary prophylaxis).

The management of heart failure and arrhythmias is covered more extensively in Chapters 21 and 22, respectively, and will not be discussed here. The remaining therapeutic aims are to relieve pain, return patency to the coronary arteries, minimise infarct size, provide prophylaxis to arrhythmias and institute secondary prevention.

Immediate care to alleviate pain, prevent deterioration and improve cardiac function

Pain relief. Patients with suspected STEMI should receive sublingual GTN under the tongue, and intravenous access should be established immediately. If sublingual GTN fails to relieve the chest pain, intravenous morphine may be administered together with an antiemetic such as prochlorperazine or metoclopramide. There is no benefit in leaving a patient in pain while the diagnosis is considered. Pain is associated

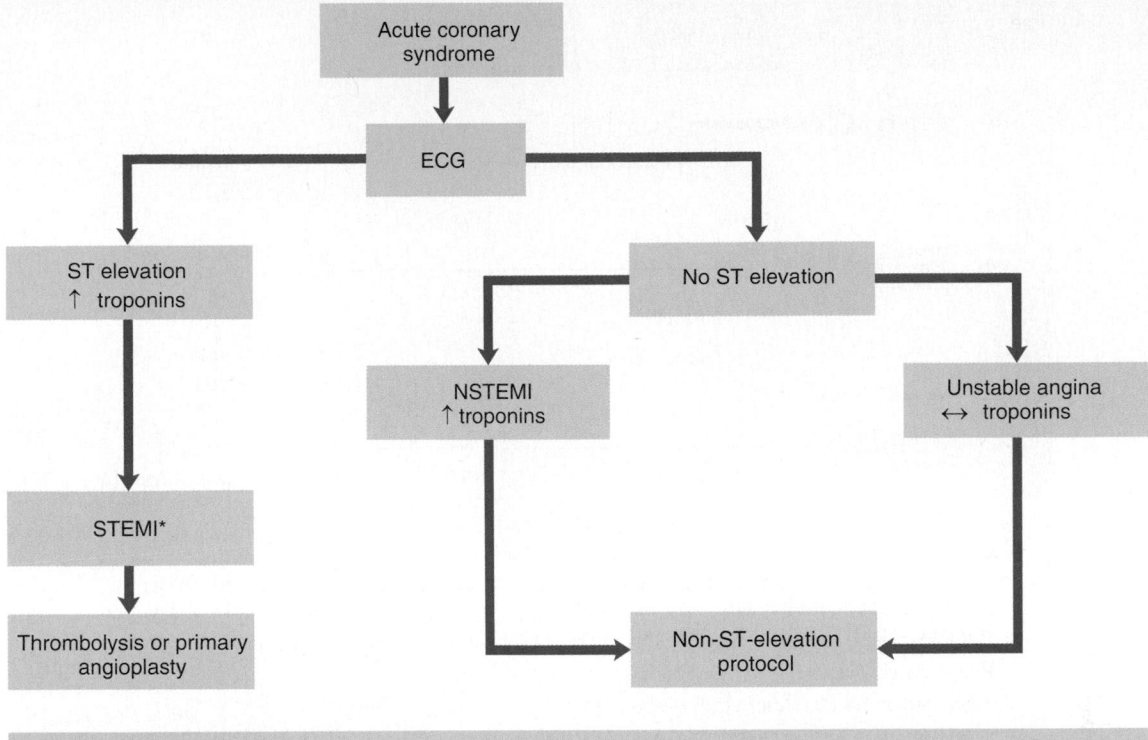

* A small number of patients have ST elevation without infarction, these may represent aborted myocardial infarction or cornary artery spasm.
STEMI, ST elevation myocardial infarction   NSTEMI, Non-ST- elevation myocardial infarction

Fig. 20.4 Classification of acute coronary syndrome based on electrocardiogram (ECG) and measurement of troponins.

with sympathetic activation, which causes vasoconstriction, increases the workload of the heart and can exacerbate the underlying condition. Oxygen should only be administered in cases of hypoxaemia or respiratory distress; a recent trial has demonstrated the potential of harm if used in normoxaemic patients (Stub et al., 2015).

Antiplatelet therapy. An aspirin tablet (300–325 mg) chewed as soon as possible after the infarct and followed by a daily dose of 75 mg for at least 1 month has been shown to reduce mortality and morbidity. The reduction in mortality is additional to that obtained from thrombolytic therapy (Table 20.5). Current recommendations state aspirin should be taken indefinitely (Ibanez et al., 2018). Clopidogrel, a $P2Y_{12}$ inhibitor given in addition to aspirin, can further improve coronary artery blood flow, but the additional absolute reduction in mortality is small, at approximately 0.4% (Sabatine et al., 2005). Clopidogrel is a prodrug that undergoes a two-step metabolic activation process within the body. This alongside its variable absorption results in a delayed response and increases inter-patient variability. The newer $P2Y_{12}$ inhibitors, prasugrel (another thienopyridine) and ticagrelor (an acyclopentyl-triazolo-pyrimidine), offer a quicker onset of action and less interpatient variability, with an absolute risk reduction of 2% (Lindholm et al., 2014; Montalescot et al., 2009). Cangrelor, an intravenous $P2Y_{12}$ inhibitor, has most recently been licensed in the UK, but its role in therapy is still to be ascertained.

Table 20.5 Vascular deaths at 35 days in the ISIS-2 (1990) study	
Placebo	13.2%
Aspirin	10.7%
Streptokinase	10.4%
Aspirin + streptokinase	8.0%

Restoring coronary flow and myocardial tissue perfusion

In patients with STEMI, early restoration of coronary artery patency results in an improved outcome. The timing of treatment is vital because myocardial damage after the onset of an acute ischaemic episode is progressive, and there are pathological data to suggest it is irreversible beyond 6 hours. Hospitals need to maintain fast-track systems to ensure maximum benefit, although there is still some worthwhile benefit up to 12 hours after infarction.

Treatment within 1 hour has been found to be particularly advantageous, although difficult to achieve, for logistical reasons, in anyone who has an infarct outside hospital. Prioritisation of ambulances to emergency calls for chest pain and appropriately equipped paramedics or primary care doctors administering fibrinolytics out of hospital have all helped reduce delay

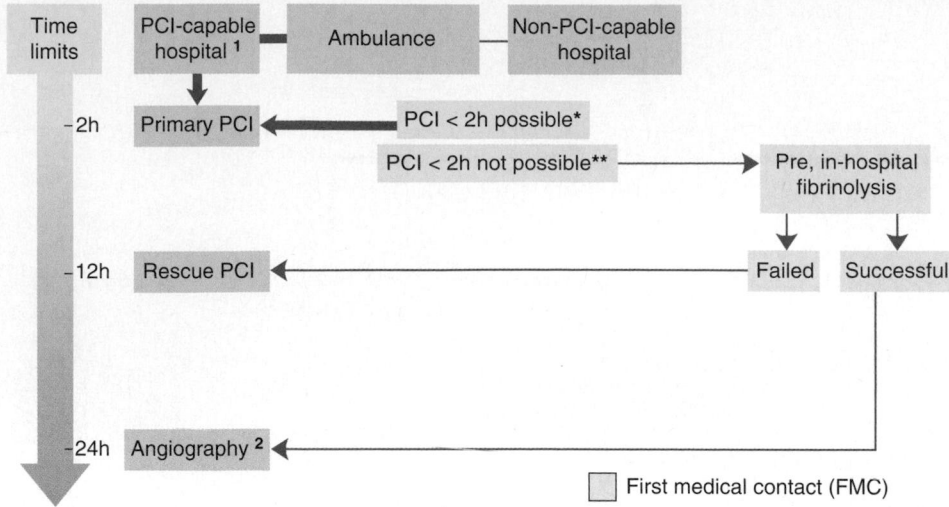

* Time FMC to first balloon inflation must be shorter than 90 min in patients presenting early
(<2 h after symptom onset), with large amount of viable myocardium and low risk of bleeding
** If PCI is not possible <2 h of FMC, start fibrinolytic therapy as soon as possible
[1] 24/7 service
[2] Not earlier than 3 h after starting fibrinolysis
PCI, Percutaneous coronary intervention

Fig. 20.5 Reperfusion strategies. The thick arrow (dark blue) indicates the preferred strategy (Van de Werf, 2008).

Table 20.6 Fibrinolytic agents (thrombolytics)

	Fibrin specificity	Elimination	Half-life (minute)	Dosing	Antigenic	Mode of action
Streptokinase		Hepatic	18–23	1 h infusion	Yes	Activator complex
Alteplase	++	Hepatic	3–8	Bolus + 90 min infusion	No	Direct
Reteplase	+	Renal	15–18	Two boluses	No	Direct
Tenecteplase	+++	Hepatic	20–28	One bolus	No	Direct

in fibrinolysis administration. Increased numbers of and direct access to hospitals offering primary angioplasty sites have further reduced the time to myocardial tissue reperfusion. Current reperfusion strategies are outlined in Fig. 20.5.

Fibrinolytics. Fibrinolytic agents (Table 20.6) have transformed the management of these patients by substantially improving coronary artery patency rates, which has translated into a 25% relative reduction in mortality. The risk of haemorrhagic stroke (around 1%) (Ibanez et al., 2018) and a failure to adequately reperfuse the affected myocardium have remained despite advances in fibrinolytics.

Percutaneous coronary intervention. Percutaneous coronary intervention (PCI) involves the passing of a catheter via the femoral or radial artery and aorta into the coronary vasculature under radio-contrast guidance. Inflation of a balloon at the end of the catheter in the area of the atheromatous plaques opens the lumen of the artery. For patients undergoing PCI, there is a small risk of death, myocardial infarction and long-term restenosis. This is reduced by insertion of a coronary artery stent and the use of pre- and peri-procedural antiplatelet therapy. Over the last 10 years the proportion of patients undergoing PCI and stent insertion has accounted for more than 95% of all PCI procedures.

The introduction of primary PCI (angioplasty and/or stent insertion without prior or concomitant fibrinolytic therapy) has demonstrated superiority to fibrinolysis when it can be performed expeditiously by an experienced team in a hospital with an established 24-hour-a-day interventional programme. In this context, primary angioplasty is better than fibrinolysis at reducing the overall short-term death, non-fatal reinfarction and stroke. The target for time from first medical contact to first balloon inflation should be less than 2 hours. If the delay to angioplasty is likely to be longer than 2 hours, facilitated PCI can be undertaken.

Table 20.7 Key features and differences of the oral P2Y$_{12}$ Inhibitors

	Clopidogrel	Prasugrel	Ticagrelor
Class	Thienopyridine	Thienopyridine	Acyclopentyl-triazolo-pyrimidine
Loading dose	300–600 mg	60 mg	180 mg
Maintenance dose	75 mg daily	5–10 mg daily	90 mg twice daily
Activation	Prodrug with variable metabolic activation	Prodrug with predictable metabolic activation	Active drug
Binding	Irreversible	Irreversible	Reversible
Onset	2–6 h	30 min	30 min
Duration of effect	3–10 days	7–10 days	3–5 days

Facilitated PCI involves the use of a fibrinolytic to achieve reperfusion before a planned PCI. This approach allows the clinical team to bridge an anticipated delay in undertaking a PCI.

Rescue PCI is performed on coronary arteries which remain occluded despite attempts at fibrinolysis. It has better outcomes than repeated fibrinolytic therapy or conservative management.

PCIs encompass various invasive procedures to improve myocardial blood delivery by opening up the blood vessels. PCIs open stenosed coronary vessels and are less invasive than coronary bypass surgery, where the coronary vessels are replaced.

A percutaneous (through the skin) transluminal (through the lumen of the blood vessels) coronary (into the heart) angioplasty (surgery or repair of the blood vessels) (PTCA) was first carried out on a conscious patient in 1977. Now more than 2 million people a year undergo PCIs. The procedure is less invasive than coronary artery bypass graft (CABG) surgery.

Antiplatelet and anticoagulant therapy. After stent insertion, there is a short-term risk of thrombus formation until the endothelial lining of the blood vessel has been re-established. The combination of aspirin and a P2Y$_{12}$ inhibitor has been shown to reduce the risk of myocardial infarction and need for reperfusion therapy and decrease the length of hospital stay. Patients undergoing primary PCI should receive aspirin and an oral P2Y$_{12}$ inhibitor as early as possible. In comparison to clopidogrel, prasugrel has less metabolic activation steps and a faster and more reliable onset of antiplatelet action. In combination with aspirin, in the UK it is recommended as an option for preventing atherothrombotic events in adults with acute coronary syndrome having primary or delayed percutaneous coronary intervention (NICE, 2014b). Ticagrelor does not require metabolic activation and has a faster and more reliable onset of antiplatelet action. In combination with aspirin, in the UK it is recommended (NICE, 2011) in the following individuals:

• those with STEMI who are to be treated with percutaneous coronary intervention,
• those with NSTEMI or unstable angina.

Most centres are now using the newer P2Y$_{12}$ inhibitors due to their favourable properties (Table 20.7).

Heparin is routinely administered during the PCI procedure and is titrated to maintain an activated clotting time (ACT) of 250–350 seconds. Glycoprotein IIb/IIIa receptor antagonists, particularly abciximab, have been shown to reduce mortality if used during the procedure. These are used in combination with heparin, and a lower ACT (200–250 seconds) is targeted to reduce bleeding complications. Bivalirudin, a direct thrombin inhibitor, has demonstrated less bleeding compared with abciximab and may be useful in those at risk of increased bleeding.

Much of the evidence for the use of glycoprotein IIb/IIIa receptor antagonists was accumulated before high-dose clopidogrel or more potent antiplatelets were in routine practice. Current recommendations are that in the setting of dual-antiplatelet therapy with unfractionated heparin or bivalirudin as the anticoagulant, glycoprotein IIb/IIIa receptor antagonists can be useful at the time of primary PCI for bailout (intraprocedure thrombus formation, slow flow, threatened vessel closure) but cannot be recommended as routine therapy (Ibanez et al., 2018).

Intracoronary administration of vasodilators such as adenosine, verapamil, nicorandil, papaverine, and nitroprusside during and after primary PCI has been shown to improve flow in the infarct-related coronary artery and myocardial perfusion, and/or to reduce infarct size, but large prospective randomised trials with hard clinical outcomes are missing.

Fibrinolytics. Fibrinolytic agents fall into two categories: fibrin specific (alteplase, tenecteplase and reteplase) and fibrin nonspecific (streptokinase). There are theoretical advantages for the fibrin-specific agents, which are superior in terms of achieving coronary artery patency in angiographic studies, and these are therefore recommended in current guidance (Ibanez et al., 2018). Fast injection of fibrin-specific agents is better than slower infusion of streptokinase, especially in younger patients with anterior infarcts. Tenecteplase and reteplase have the advantage that they can be administered by bolus injection, which facilitates pre-hospital administration and reduces errors.

Patients receiving alteplase also receive a 5000-unit heparin bolus followed by a 48-hour infusion adjusted to maintain the activated partial thromboplastin time (APTT) in the therapeutic range. Intravenous enoxaparin followed by subcutaneous injections may be an alternative. Heparin has not been compared with a placebo in trials of tenecteplase or reteplase, but it is standard practice to use heparin with these agents. Heparin has no advantage in addition to streptokinase, which has a longer-lasting and less specific fibrinolytic action.

A low dose of fondaparinux, a synthetic, indirect anti-Xa agent, has been found to be superior to placebo or heparin in preventing death and reinfarction in patients who received fibrinolytic therapy (OASIS-6 Trial Group, 2006).

Bivalirudin, a direct thrombin inhibitor, reduces reinfarction rates compared with heparin when given with streptokinase but has not been studied with fibrin-specific agents. This combination resulted in a nonsignificant increase in noncerebral bleeding complications (HERO-2 Trial Investigators, 2001).

Trials using various dosing combinations of glycoprotein IIb/IIIa inhibitors with newer fibrinolytic agents have not found a regimen that increases overall survival (Menon et al., 2004).

All fibrinolytics cause haemorrhage, which may present as a stroke or a gastro-intestinal bleed, and there is an increased risk with regimens that use intravenous heparin. Recent strokes, bleeds, pregnancy and surgery are contraindications to fibrinolysis. Streptokinase induces cross-reacting antibodies which reduce its potency and may cause an anaphylactoid response. Patients with exposure to streptokinase, or with a history of rheumatic fever or recent streptococcal infection, should not receive the drug. The use of hydrocortisone to reduce allergic responses has fallen out of favour, but patients should be carefully observed for hypotension during the administration of streptokinase.

Old age is no longer considered to be a contraindication to fibrinolysis. Although the risks are greater, the benefit is also greater, but the doses of alteplase and tenecteplase need to be adjusted for body weight.

All the major trials have used specific ECG criteria for entry, usually ST elevation in adjacent leads or LBBB, and eliminated patients with major contraindications to fibrinolysis (Box 20.2). Confusion often arises about the term 'relative contraindication'. For example, systolic hypertension is common in AMI, so most protocols recommend lowering the blood pressure with either a β-blocker or intravenous nitrates before commencing fibrinolysis. An increasing number of patients are on warfarin, and this again is regarded as a relative contraindication to fibrinolysis; thresholds for the use of fibrinolysis in patients on warfarin vary from an international normalised ratio (INR) of 2 to 2.4. The use of fibrinolytic therapy in patients with relative contraindications should take into account both the site and size of the myocardial infarction. For example, in patients with a large anterior myocardial infarction the benefits of fibrinolysis may outweigh its risk. In patients in whom there is a serious concern regarding bleeding after fibrinolysis, primary angioplasty should be considered.

Management of complications

Heart failure. Heart failure during the acute phase of STEMI is associated with a poor short- and long-term prognosis. It should be managed with oxygen, intravenous furosemide and nitrates.

> **Box 20.2** Contraindications to fibrinolysis (Van de Werf et al., 2008)
>
> Absolute contraindications
> - Haemorrhagic stroke of unknown origin at any time
> - Ischaemic stroke in preceding 6 months
> - Central nervous system damage or neoplasms
> - Recent major trauma/surgery/head injury (within preceding 3 weeks)
> - Gastro-intestinal bleed within the last month
> - Known bleeding disorder
> - Non-compressible punctures
> - Aortic dissection
>
> Relative contraindications
> - Transient ischaemic attack in preceding 6 months
> - Oral anticoagulant therapy
> - Pregnancy or within 1 week postpartum
> - Advanced liver disease
> - Active peptic ulcer
> - Infective endocarditis
> - Traumatic resuscitation
> - Refractory hypertension (systolic blood pressure >180 mmHg)

More severe failure or cardiogenic shock (tissue hypoperfusion resulting from cardiac failure with symptoms of hypotension, peripheral vasoconstriction, diminished pulses, decreased urine output and decreased mental status) should be treated with inotropes and/or intra-aortic balloon pumps to maintain the systolic blood pressure greater than 90 mmHg. Invasive monitoring may be required.

Arrhythmias. Life-threatening arrhythmias such as ventricular tachycardia, sustained VF or atrio-ventricular block occur in about one-fifth of patients presenting with a STEMI, although this is decreasing due to early reperfusion therapy. β-Blockers have been the subject of many studies because of their anti-arrhythmic potential and because they permit increased subendocardial perfusion. In studies undertaken before the widespread use of fibrinolytics, the early administration of an intravenous β-blocker was shown to limit infarct size and reduce mortality from early cardiac events. A post hoc analysis of the use of atenolol in the GUSTO-I trial and a systematic review (Freemantle et al., 1999) did not support the routine, early intravenous use of β-blockers; therefore, oral β-blockers are started within 24 hours of the event. If a β-blocker is contraindicated because of respiratory or vascular disorders, verapamil may be used because it has been shown to reduce late mortality and reinfarction in patients without heart failure, although it shows no benefit when given immediately after an infarct. Diltiazem is less effective but may be used as an alternative. This is clearly not a class effect; other calcium channel blockers have produced different results, and nifedipine increases mortality in patients after a myocardial infarction.

Initially, magnesium infusions looked promising when given early after infarction. However, in large trials (ISIS-4, 1995), no reductions in mortality were found, making the routine use of magnesium inappropriate. Magnesium infusions are used, however, to correct low serum magnesium levels if cardiac arrhythmias are present.

Sinus bradycardia and heart block may also occur after a myocardial infarction, and patients may require temporary or permanent pacemaker insertion.

Blood glucose. Patients with a myocardial infarction are often found to have high serum and urinary glucose levels, usually described as a stress response. The CREATE-ECLA trial (Mehta et al., 2005) studied more than 20,000 patients and showed a neutral effect of insulin on mortality, cardiac arrest and cardiogenic shock. Current guidelines do not support the routine use of insulin in STEMI in patients not previously known to be diabetic.

Up to 20% of patients who have a myocardial infarction have diabetes. Moreover, diabetic patients are known to do poorly after infarction, with almost double the mortality rate of non-diabetics. In these patients, an intensive insulin regimen, both during admission and for 3 months after, was found to save lives (Malmberg, 1997). However, the follow-up study (Malmberg et al., 2005) did not show any mortality benefit from intensive insulin therapy compared with standard therapy. In patients with diabetes, it appears reasonable, however, to continue to control blood glucose levels within the normal range immediately post-infarct.

Prevention of further infarction or death (secondary prophylaxis)

Lipid-lowering agents. Reduction of cholesterol through diet and use of lipid-lowering agents is effective at reducing subsequent mortality and morbidity in patients with established CHD. Levels of LDL-C of less than 1.8 mmol/L used to be recommended for patients with established CVD, but a 40% reduction in non-HDL cholesterol from baseline is now recommended (NICE, 2014a). In patients with AMI or high-risk NSTEMI, there was a reduction in the combination end point of death, myocardial infarction, or documented UA requiring hospitalisation, revascularisation or stroke when patients were treated with high-intensity statin therapy (atorvastatin 80 mg daily) compared with standard statin therapy (Cannon et al., 2004). A meta-analysis of studies (Josan et al., 2008) reaffirmed the benefit of high-intensity statin therapy especially in those patients with ACS. An additional finding of particular interest was that the results were significant for the high-intensity treatment arms despite approximately half of patients not achieving LDL-C of less than 2 mmol/L.

β-Blockers. Long-term use of a β-blocker is recommended to decrease mortality in patients in whom there is no contraindication (Ibanez et al., 2018). β-Blockade should be avoided in individuals with heart block, bradycardia and asthma and used with caution in individuals with chronic obstructive pulmonary disease or peripheral vascular disease. One large cohort study compared low and high doses of β-blockers with no therapy and found benefit in all treated patients, with similar survival rates but a lower heart failure rate in the low-dose group (Rochon et al., 2000).

Angiotensin-converting enzyme inhibitors. Various doses and durations of ACE inhibitors have proved beneficial in reducing the incidence of heart failure and mortality. In all but the earliest trials, patients were given an ACE inhibitor for 4–6 weeks,

Table 20.8	Relative benefits of treating 1000 patients for myocardial infarction
Intervention	**Events prevented**
Intravenous β-adrenoceptor blocker	6 deaths
ACE inhibitor	6 deaths
Aspirin	20–25 deaths
Streptokinase (in hospital)	20–25 deaths
Alteplase (in hospital)	35 deaths
Streptokinase (before hospital)	35–40 deaths
Fibrinolysis 4½–1 h earlier	15 deaths
Long-term aspirin	16 deaths/MI/strokes
Long-term β-blockade	18 deaths/MI
Long-term ACE inhibitor	21–45 deaths/MI
10% reduction in serum cholesterol	7 deaths/MI
Stopping smoking	27 deaths

ACE, Angiotensin-converting enzyme; MI, myocardial infarction.
Adapted from McMurray and Rankin (1994).

and treatment continued in patients with signs or symptoms of heart failure or left ventricular dysfunction. The HOPE study (Yusuf et al., 2000) found that ramipril improved survival in all groups of patients with CHD, and this has led clinicians to continue ACE inhibitors in all patients with a myocardial infarction older than 55 years and in younger patients with evidence of left ventricular dysfunction. Contraindications to their use include hypotension and intractable cough.

There is considerable interest in focusing on the possible benefits of combining ACE inhibition with angiotensin II receptor blockers. Angiotensin receptor blockade alone does not cause the accumulation of bradykinins which may be part of the benefit of using ACE inhibitors. Clinical trials (OPTIMAAL Study Group, 2002; VALIANT Investigators, 2003) have failed to find a benefit over ACE inhibition. Nonetheless, angiotensin receptor blockers are probably suitable in patients who cannot tolerate an ACE inhibitor. The relative benefits of ACE inhibitors and other treatments are shown in Table 20.8.

Eplerenone. In patients with heart failure post-AMI, in the EPHESUS Trial (Pitt et al., 2003) an improvement in survival and decreased cardiovascular mortality and hospitalisation was seen in those taking the aldosterone antagonist eplerenone. Serious hyperkalemia occurred more frequently in the eplerenone arm, and monitoring of serum potassium is warranted when used in practice.

Antidepressants. Anxiety is almost inevitable, and a quarter of patients who have suffered a myocardial infarction subsequently experience marked depression. Post–myocardial infarction depression is associated with poor medication compliance, a lower quality-of-life score and a fourfold increase in mortality (Januzzi et al., 2000). Antidepressant treatments have not been subjected to formal trials, but it seems reasonable to try to reduce the depression. There is concern about the potential for older antidepressants, such as tricyclic antidepressants, to increase the QT interval and cause arrhythmias. Newer antidepressants are less prone to cause these arrhythmias, and selective serotonin receptor inhibitors (SSRIs) are preferred.

Rehabilitation programmes which include some measure of social interaction, physical activity and education are also of proven benefit. Although psychological stress clearly worsens outcomes, stress reduction interventions have not been tested and proven to work independently of other measures.

Nitrates. Studies on nitrates in myocardial infarction were mostly completed before fibrinolysis was widely used. Nitrates improve collateral blood flow and aid reperfusion, thus limiting infarct size and preserving functional tissue. ISIS-4 (1995) and GISSI-3 (1994) demonstrated that nitrates did not confer a survival advantage in patients receiving fibrinolysis. Sublingual nitrates may be given for immediate pain relief, and the use of intravenous or buccal nitrates can be considered in patients whose infarction pain does not resolve rapidly or who develop ventricular failure.

Anticoagulants and antiplatelets. Anticoagulation with warfarin is not generally recommended after a myocardial infarction, despite promising results in trials that have practised exceptionally good anticoagulant monitoring. This is partly because of the success of antiplatelet therapy with aspirin. Aspirin does not have the same need for expensive and time-consuming follow-up and monitoring as warfarin and is associated with fewer drug interactions. The $P2Y_{12}$ inhibitors (clopidogrel, prasugrel and ticagrelor) have been shown to be beneficial, when combined with aspirin, in patients who have had a myocardial infarction. As the number of patients who receive a stent increases, dual antiplatelet therapy (DAPT) with aspirin and a $P2Y_{12}$ inhibitor is more common. The duration of DAPT therapy has been the topic of much debate, with most guidelines recommending 12-month therapy, but this is reduced in patients at a high risk of bleeding and increased in those with a heightened risk of reinfarction. A lower dose of ticagrelor (60 mg twice daily) given after the initial year of DAPT has demonstrated a reduction in CVD-associated death (Bonaca et al., 2015).

A low dose of the direct acting oral anticoagulant (DOAC) rivaroxaban (2.5 mg twice daily) combined with aspirin and clopidogrel or aspirin alone has demonstrated a reduction in atherothrombotic events in individuals post-ACS (Mega et al., 2012). Higher doses were found to increase the risk of bleeding.

For patients who require long-term oral anticoagulation, either with warfarin or a DOAC, for other therapeutic indications (e.g., stroke prevention in atrial fibrillation or treatment of venous thromboembolism) in addition to dual antiplatelet therapy, a combination which minimises bleeding risk should be considered. Evidence currently favours DAPT (with aspirin and clopidogrel) for a shorter period (followed by clopidogrel alone for up to 12 months) with the lowest recommended therapeutic dose of oral anticoagulant. The use of prasugrel or ticagrelor as part of triple therapy should be avoided unless there is a clear need for these agents (Kirchhof et al., 2016).

Treatment of non-ST-elevation acute coronary syndromes

ACS without ST elevation is classified as either UA or NSTEMI. UA is defined as angina that occurs at rest or with minimal exertion, new (within 1 month) onset of severe angina, or worsening of previously stable angina. NSTEMI (or non-Q wave MI) is the more severe manifestation of ACS.

Patients with NSTEMI may be treated either with an interventional strategy, where all patients undergo angiography and PCI after admission, or conservatively, where they undergo angiography and intervention only if they remain unstable or have a positive exercise test. Initial trials of early intervention did not demonstrate any benefit, but with the advent of advanced angioplasty techniques using stents and adjuvant drug therapies including clopidogrel and glycoprotein IIb/IIIa antagonists, there appears to be a clear advantage for an interventional strategy in high-risk patients (Fox et al., 2005).

Patients presenting with UA/NSTEMI can be classified into three categories of risk (low, intermediate and high), depending on their risk of death or likelihood of developing an AMI. High-risk patients (those with ST-segment changes during chest pain, chest pain within 48 hours, troponin T-positive patients and those presenting already on intensive anti-anginal therapy) can be effectively managed with aggressive medical and interventional therapy. This results in fewer individuals progressing to AMI.

Various pharmacological agents such as antithrombin and antiplatelet drugs, and coronary revascularisation (particularly PCI) have been shown to improve the outcome of patients with UA or NSTEMI. These interventions are known to be associated with some treatment hazards, particularly bleeding complications. The risks must be balanced against potential treatment benefits for each individual patient. This balance is influenced by the patient's estimated risk of an adverse cardiovascular outcome as a consequence of the ACS. The absolute magnitude of benefit from an intervention is generally greatest in those at highest risk. A confounding issue is that treatment hazards, such as bleeding complications, are often also greatest in those at highest risk of an ischaemic event.

Measures of risk can be derived from the clinical assessment of a patient and the use of a formal risk scoring system, such as the GRACE, PURSUIT, PREDICT or TIMI scores. Scores based on clinical trial data generally exclude patients who are at high risk of an adverse cardiovascular outcome such as the elderly, or those with renal or heart failure. As a consequence, the evidence for clinical and cost-effectiveness of therapeutic interventions is confined to patients at lower to intermediate levels of risk. Risk score based on registry data (e.g. GRACE) may provide a more realistic estimation of risk.

In patients with NSTEMI, the immediate administration of 300 mg aspirin can reduce mortality or subsequent myocardial infarction by 50%. Risk stratification according to a recognised tool should be used to guide the subsequent choice of pharmacological and/or surgical intervention. The exclusion of STEMI and

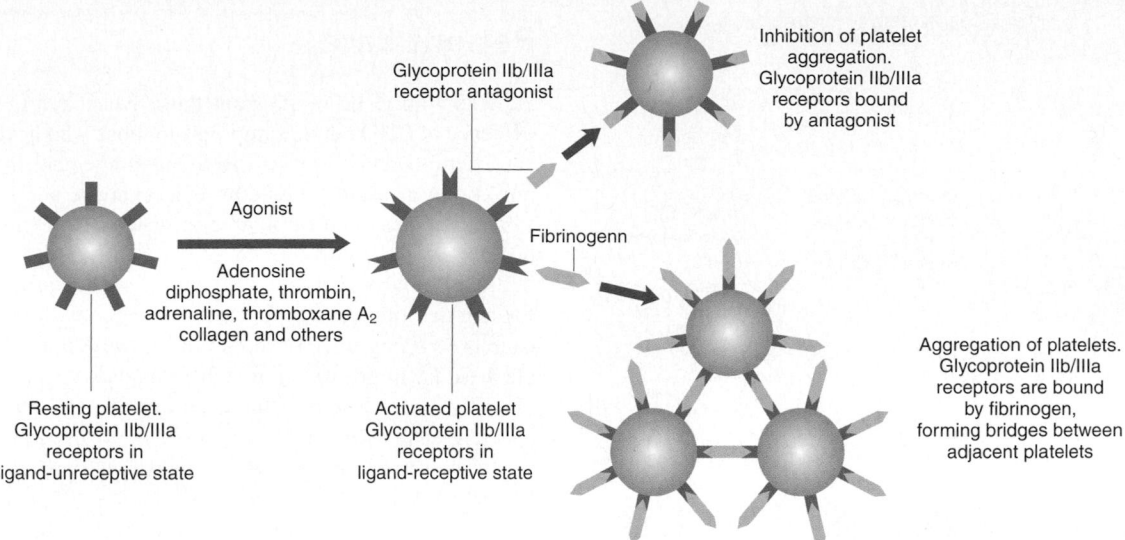

Fig. 20.6 Schematic representation of mechanism of action of glycoprotein IIb/IIIa inhibitors.

confirmation of NSTEMI is important, as the use of fibrinolysis in NSTEMI confers no benefit and merely increases the risk of bleeding. In patients with NSTEMI, the preferred treatment normally involves a combination of antiplatelet agents to reduce the formation of a thrombus.

Antiplatelet and anticoagulant drugs

The current range of antiplatelet and anticoagulant drugs available for the reduction of thrombotic events in ACS leads to the potential for a large number of combinations. In all cases, the benefit of reducing thrombotic events must be balanced against the potential for an increased risk of bleeding.

In the early 1990s, unfractionated heparin combined with aspirin showed a reduction in death and subsequent myocardial infarction compared with aspirin alone. The use of the low-molecular-weight heparin (LMWH), enoxaparin, subsequently demonstrated superiority over unfractionated heparin, with both usually continued for 48 hours, or until chest pain resolves or patient is discharged. Both groups of drugs were tested in the era before PCI became part of routine practice.

The CURE study (2001) showed that clopidogrel, given as a loading dose of 300 mg followed by 75 mg daily in combination with aspirin and heparin, reduced the combined end point of death, myocardial infarction and revascularisation in all patients with NSTEMI. Clopidogrel needs to be continued for 12 months but should be stopped 5–7 days before any major surgery to reduce the risk of bleeding.

Because PCI has become more routine as part of the management of high-risk NSTEMI patients, more aggressive antiplatelet treatment has been required to reduce both peri-procedural and post-procedural thromboembolic complications.

Expression of glycoprotein IIb/IIIa is one of the final steps in the platelet aggregation cascade. Inhibiting these receptors has been a strategy before, and during, PCI for some time. Glycoprotein IIb/IIIa inhibitors bind to the IIb/IIIa receptors on platelets (Fig. 20.6)

and prevent cross-linking of platelets by fibrinogen. There are three classes of these agents: murine-human chimeric antibodies, (e.g. abciximab); synthetic peptides (e.g. eptifibatide); and non-peptide synthetics (e.g. tirofiban). Oral agents are ineffective, and the murine-human chimeric antibodies appear to be effective only in the context of PCI.

In high-risk patients undergoing PCI and receiving background heparin, triple antiplatelet therapy (aspirin, clopidogrel and a glycoprotein IIb/IIIa inhibitors) has been shown to be superior to standard dose dual-antiplatelet therapy (aspirin and clopidogrel), particularly in troponin-positive individuals (Kastrati et al., 2006). However, much of this evidence was generated before the introduction of higher doses of clopidogrel or the newer, more potent oral antiplatelet agents.

There is no clear benefit to giving glycoprotein IIb/IIIa inhibitors more than 4 hours before PCI ('upstream') compared with waiting until immediately before or during the procedure ('deferred' or 'downstream') (Stone et al., 2007).

Currently, all patients with a likely or definite diagnosis of NSTEMI should receive a loading dose of aspirin 300 mg (see Fig. 20.7). Patients undergoing PCI intervention should have a higher loading dose of 600 mg of clopidogrel or 60 mg of prasugrel, unless contraindicated, to reduce events during and after PCI. Clopidogrel is often given as 300 mg on admission and a further 300 mg when the decision to intervene is made. Patients who are not planned for intervention should receive a lower loading dose of clopidogrel 300 mg. Prasugrel, with its faster time to maximum effect, has demonstrated some benefit but routine use is not recommended (NICE, 2014b). Ticagrelor is a suitable alternative, and a loading dose of 180 mg can be given in those already loaded on clopidogrel.

All patients should receive heparin; bivalirudin or fondaparinux are suitable alternatives in combination with aspirin and clopidogrel. Unfractionated heparin is preferred for patients with compromised renal function. Fondaparinux, a synthetic pentasaccharide factor Xa inhibitor which has predictable and

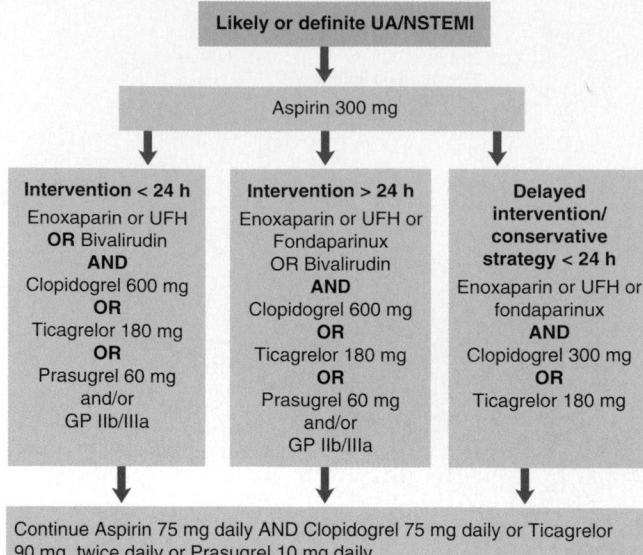

Fig. 20.7 Treatment options for patients with likely or definite unstable angina (UA) or non-ST-elevation myocardial infarction (NSTEMI) in relation to time of percutaneous coronary intervention (PCI) intervention. UFH, Unfractionated heparin.

sustained anticoagulation with fixed dose, once-a-day subcutaneous administration, causes less bleeding than enoxaparin, an LMWH. Concerns over catheter-related thrombus mean it should not be considered if patients are planned for PCI within 24 hours of chest pain. Bivalirudin is a synthetic analogue of hirudin that binds reversibly to thrombin and inhibits clot-bound thrombin.

The decision to use glycoprotein IIb/IIIa inhibitors is dependent on the centre and operator and whether the planned intervention for the patient is to be surgical or pharmacological. The introduction of higher loading doses of clopidogrel and more potent oral agents, as well as an increased focus on the bleeding risks associated with combination therapy, has reduced the use of these agents in many centres.

The recommendation of an anticoagulant regimen has become more complicated by a number of new choices suggested by contemporary trials, some of which do not provide adequate comparative information for common practice settings (see section in previous STEMI discussion).

Anti-ischaemic drugs

The use of both β-blockers and nitrates in the management of patients with NSTEMI is based on studies of their use in stable angina and AMI. Their use is, however, well established and based on a firm pathophysiological and pharmacological rationale.

Statins

High-intensity statins have been shown to benefit patients when given early in ACS. They are usually started on admission if the diagnosis of CHD is definite, independent of the patient's cholesterol level. Treatment should aim to achieve a 40% reduction in non-HDL cholesterol from baseline.

Patient care

Patients with CHD range from those who have investigational evidence of CHD but no symptoms to those who have major pain and exercise limitation. All need encouragement in adhering to preventive measures, including diet, exercise and smoking cessation. Patients need to be able to discuss concerns about their health.

Exercise must be tailored according to the patient's threshold for angina, aiming for moderate- to vigorous-intensity aerobic exercise training three or more times a week and for 30 minutes per session. In general, although some patients are too cavalier, most are likely to err on the cautious side and may need to be encouraged to do more. Many centres now run cardiac rehabilitation classes to encourage patients to exercise and adopt a suitable lifestyle.

There are simple treatments and important lifestyle changes that can reduce cardiovascular risk and slow or even reverse the progression of established coronary disease. The most important of these to address is smoking cessation. The risk of CHD is two to four times higher in heavy smokers (those who smoke at least 20 cigarettes/day) than in those who do not smoke. Other reports estimate the age-adjusted risk of smokers of more than 25 cigarettes/day is 5–21 times that of non-smokers. Smokers should be encouraged to quit. Within months of stopping smoking, CHD risk begins to decline. Within 5 years of smoking cessation, the risk decreases to approximately the level found in people who have never smoked, regardless of the amount smoked, duration of the habit and the age at cessation. The use of nicotine replacement therapy almost doubles a smokers' chance of successfully stopping smoking (18% vs. 11%). All patients who smoke should be offered advice on cessation and encouraged to attend specialist smokers' clinics to further improve their chance of quitting.

Patient beliefs about medicines and medication-taking behaviour (and therefore adherence) are also important determinants of outcome and are influenced by many factors. These can largely be divided into beliefs about the importance of the medicine and concerns about the medicine's harmful effects. To ensure the patient's concordance with medication regimens, it is necessary to address each individual patient's beliefs and concerns. One approach to counselling patients with CHD may be to divide the medication prescribed into those used to reduce the risk of heart attacks and death and those for symptom control. Key points to be discussed will relate to side effects and what to do if they occur, the need to continue medication until told otherwise and ensuring they do not run out of medication. Patients should be encouraged to identify their concerns, and these should be addressed as openly and honestly as possible.

Patients also need up-to-date advice when faced with difficult choices regarding medical treatment, angiographic procedures or surgery. Patients have good reason to be anxious at times, but some patients restrict their activities unnecessarily out of fear of angina and infarction.

Some of the common therapeutic problems encountered in the management of CHD are described in Table 20.9.

Table 20.9 Common therapeutic problems in coronary heart disease

Problem	Comment
Used incorrectly, nitrates may cause hypotensive episodes or collapse.	Advise to sit down when using nitrate sprays or sublingual tablets.
A daily nitrate-free period is required to maintain efficacy of nitrates.	Avoid long-acting preparations and prescribe asymmetrically (e.g. 8 a.m. and 2 p.m.).
NSAIDs are associated with renal failure when given with ACE inhibitors.	Advise patients to use paracetamol as their analgesic of choice.
Speed is essential when patients need fibrinolytic drugs after infarction.	Arrange emergency admission to hospital where fast-track systems should exist.
Aspirin may cause gastro-intestinal bleeding.	Advise on taking with food and water. Consider use of prophylactic agents in high-risk patients.
β-Blockers are often considered unpleasant to take.	Encourage patient to use regularly. Change the time of day. Consider a vaso-dilator if cold extremities are a problem. Consider verapamil or diltiazem.
β-Blockers are contraindicated in asthma.	Consider verapamil or diltiazem. Pay strict attention to other treatments and removal of precipitating factors.
Patients often receive multiple drugs for prophylaxis and for treatment of co-existing disorders.	Use once-daily preparations, dosing aids and intensive social and educational support. Avoid all unnecessary drugs.
ACE inhibitors are contraindicated in pregnancy, especially the first trimester.	Advise women of child-bearing years to avoid conception or seek specialist advice first.

ACE, Angiotensin-converting enzyme; NSAID, non-steroidal anti-inflammatory drug.

Case studies

Case 20.1

A 55-year-old man, Mr HG, presents to his primary care doctor complaining of tightness in his chest when he digs the garden. It eases when he has a rest. On investigation, Mr HG has a raised serum glucose concentration and is considered to be a newly diagnosed non-insulin-dependent type II diabetic.

Question

What cardiovascular investigations and treatments should Mr HG receive?

Answer

Mr HG's blood pressure and ECG should be checked, and he should be examined for signs of hypertensive or diabetic target organ damage, including albuminuria. His serum lipid profile should be measured.

Mr HG should receive GTN spray or sublingual tablets for the chest symptoms that are almost certainly angina. He should take aspirin 75 mg daily. Prescribers would give a statin in almost all diabetic CHD patients and likewise an ACE inhibitor (unless there is a contraindication). Certainly, any hypertension should be treated aggressively so that the diastolic pressure is less than 80 mmHg. A β-blocker may also be useful to control blood pressure and prevent further episodes of angina, but many prescribers would wait until there was evidence of failure of the other therapies. In view of Mr HG's relatively young age, a referral to a cardiologist for possible angiography should be considered. Dietary advice and help stop smoking, if needed, should be given. Diabetic treatments should be given (see Chapter 45 diabetes).

Case 20.2

The following patients are admitted for treatment of myocardial infarction:
1. A patient with asthma
2. A man previously treated for infarction

Question

What considerations are there for standard treatment in these two patients?

Answers

Standard treatment for myocardial infarction includes the use of aspirin (or dual antiplatelet therapy if a PCI was performed), lipid lowering with a statin, rate control with a β-blocker and the prevention of cardiac remodeling with an ACE inhibitor. Treatment of further chest pain should be with GTN for acute chest pain and anti-anginals (long-acting nitrates or amlodipine) for ongoing chest pain.

1. A patient with asthma should not receive a β-blocker without careful consideration and supervision because of the risk of bronchoconstriction; there is also a small risk of bronchoconstriction with aspirin.
2. A previous infarct may have been treated with streptokinase, and a repeat dose within 12 months should be avoided because of the build-up of antibodies to the initial dose rendering subsequent doses ineffective. Tissue plasminogen activator should be used instead. Consideration of patient adherence to previously prescribed medicines should be assured.

Case 20.3

A patient, Mr TD, with rheumatoid disease, treated with naproxen, has CHD.

Question

Is there any benefit or harm in adding aspirin to Mr TD's treatment?

Answer

A recent meta-analysis of the major randomised controlled trials on the effect of NSAIDs has concluded that, except for naproxen, NSAIDs used commonly in clinical practice are associated with increased risk of AMI at high doses or in patients previously diagnosed with coronary heart disease. For diclofenac and rofecoxib, the risk is elevated for both low and high doses (Varas-Lorenzo, 2013).

Aspirin is more beneficial than any other non-steroidal anti-inflammatory agent in modifying platelet activity and reducing mortality and morbidity in CHD. There is an increased risk of gastro-intestinal bleeding if two agents are given, but this should not be a major consideration at low doses of aspirin. There is some evidence, however, that some NSAIDs interfere with the action of aspirin by blocking access to the active site on the COX-1 enzyme. Such agents should be avoided. Diclofenac does not block the receptor, and ibuprofen has a short action and is acceptable if given 2 hours after the daily dose of aspirin.

Case 20.4

A patient, Ms LV, who has recently been started on aspirin and ticagrelor post-PCI with a drug-eluting stent (after an ACS), has been diagnosed a left ventricular thrombus.

Question

What changes to her medication therapy are required?

Answer

Left ventricular thrombi commonly develop in patients with severe left ventricular dysfunction. Treatment will require full anticoagulation for at least 3–6 months to allow the clot to disperse. Although the combination of aspirin and ticagrelor produces better outcomes than aspirin and clopidogrel, there is a bleeding risk associated with adding full-dose anticoagulation. Recent European

Society of Cardiology (ESC) guidelines (Roffi et al., 2016) do not recommend using ticagrelor or prasugrel with full anticoagulation post-PCI.

The recommended option would be to commence warfarin (bridged with parenteral anticoagulation; e.g. LMWH) and switch ticagrelor to clopidogrel 75 mg once daily. The duration of triple therapy (i.e. aspirin, clopidogrel and warfarin) should be minimised based on several factors, balancing the risk of atherothrombosis and bleeding.

Case 20.5

A patient with angioedema, Ms MJ, who is allergic to aspirin, has suffered a STEMI.

Question

What antiplatelet therapy would you recommend for Ms MJ post-PCI?

Answer

Due to the lack of research in patients with aspirin allergy, there is currently no dual antiplatelet regimen recommended post-PCI without aspirin. Options include the following:

- Allergy desensitisation to aspirin – a rapid desensitisation protocol has been described in the literature and can be performed in the cardiac laboratory within 2 hours before/after PCI.
- Single antiplatelet agent – this is an option, with a greater preference for the newer agents (prasugrel or ticagrelor). There is no evidence to suggest the combination of prasugrel and ticagrelor would be beneficial because both act on the ADP-receptor, potentially competing for the same site.
- Anticoagulation with clopidogrel – if there is another reason to anticoagulate (e.g. the presence of atrial fibrillation), then the combination of warfarin or DOAC with clopidogrel is a treatment option.

Case 20.6

A patient with angina, Mr WF, has just been started on ranolazine.

Question

What drug interactions do you need to consider before starting therapy?

Answer

Before commencing any drug therapy, there are two types of effects that need to be considered: pharmacokinetic and pharmacodynamic interactions.

With respect to pharmacokinetic effects, ranolazine is metabolised by the cytochrome P450 3A4 isoenzyme (CYP3A4), resulting in a range of drug interactions. Plasma levels are increased by CYP3A4 inhibitors (e.g. diltiazem, verapamil, macrolide antibiotics, grapefruit juice). Ranolazine clearance is also reduced by renal and hepatic impairment; thus, dose adjustments may be required.

Pharmacodynamically, ranolazine may increase the risk of arrhythmias by prolonging the QTc. It should be avoided in patients with prolonged-QT and used with caution with other QT-prolonging medication (e.g. fluconazole and erythromycin).

References

Bonaca, M.P., Bhatt, D.L., Cohen, M., et al., 2015. Long-term use of tica-grelor in patients with prior myocardial infarction (PEGASUS-TIMI 54). New Engl. J. Med. 372, 1791–1800.

British Heart Foundation, 2017. CVD statistics – BHF UK factsheet. Available at: https://www.bhf.org.uk/research/heart-statistics.

Canadian Cardiovascular Society, 1976. Canadian Cardiovascular Society grading of angina pectoris. Available at: https://www.ccs.ca/images/Guide lines/Guidelines_POS_Library/Ang_Gui_1976.pdf.

Cannon, C.P., Braunwald, E., McCabe, C.H., et al., 2004. Intensive versus moderate lipid lowering with statins after acute coronary syndromes. New Engl. J. Med. 350, 1495–1504.

CAPRIE Steering Committee, 1996. A randomised, blinded, trial of clopi-dogrel versus aspirin in patients at risk of ischaemic events (CAPRIE). Lancet 348, 1329–1339.

CURE (Clopidogrel in Unstable Angina to Prevent Recurrent Events) Trial Investigators, 2001. Effects of clopidogrel in addition to aspirin in pa-tients with acute coronary syndromes without ST-segment elevation. New Engl. J. Med. 345, 494–502.

EUROPA Study Investigators, 2003. The European trial on reduction of cardiac events with perindopril in stable coronary artery disease investigators. Effi-cacy of perindopril in reduction of cardiovascular events among patients with stable coronary artery disease: randomised, double-blind, placebo-controlled, multicentre trial (the EUROPA study). Lancet 362, 782–788.

Fosbøl, E.L., Folke, F., Jacobsen, S., et al., 2010. Cause-specific cardiovas-cular risk associated with nonsteroidal anti-inflammatory drugs among healthy individuals. Circ. Cardiovasc. Qual. Outcomes 3, 395–405.

Fox, K., Ford, I., Steg, P.G., on behalf of the BEAUTIFUL Investigators, et al., 2008. Ivabradine for patients with stable coronary artery disease and left-ventricular systolic dysfunction (BEAUTIFUL): a randomised, double-blind, placebo-controlled trial. Lancet 372, 807–816.

Fox, K., Garcia, M.A.A., Ardissino, D., et al., 2006. The task force on the management of stable angina pectoris of the European Society of Cardiology. Guidelines on the management of stable angina pectoris. Eur. Heart J. 27, 1341–1381.

Fox, K.A.A., Poole-Wilson, P., Clayton, T., et al., 2005. Five-year outcome of an interventional strategy in non-ST-elevation acute coronary syndrome: the British Heart Foundation RITA 3 randomised trial. Lancet 366, 914–920.

Freemantle, N., Cleland, J., Young, P., et al., 1999. Beta blockade after myocardial infarction: systematic review and meta regression analysis. Br. Med. J. 318, 1730–1737.

GISSI-3 (Gruppo Italiano per lo Studio della Sopravvivenza nell'infarto Miocardico), 1994. Effects of lisinopril and transdermal glyceryl trinitrate singly and together on 6-week mortality and ventricular function after acute myocardial infarction. Lancet 343, 1115–1122.

HERO (Hirulog and Early Reperfusion or Occlusion)-2 Trial Investigators, 2001. Thrombin-specific anticoagulation with bivalirudin versus heparin in patients receiving fibrinolytic therapy for acute myocardial infarction: the HERO-2 randomised trial. Lancet 358, 1855–1863.

Ibanez, B., James, S., Agewall, S., et al., 2018. 2017 ESC Guidelines for the management of acute myocardial infarction in patients presenting with ST-segment elevation: The Task Force for the management of acute myocardial infarction in patients presenting with ST-segment elevation of the European Society of Cardiology (ESC). Eur. Heart J. 39, 119–177.

IONA Study Group, 2002. Effect of nicorandil on coronary events in patients with stable angina: the Impact of Nicorandil in Angina (IONA) randomised trial. Lancet 349, 1269–1275.

ISIS-2 (Second International Study of Infarct Survival) Collaborative Group, 1990. In-hospital mortality and clinical course of 20,891 patients with sus-pected acute myocardial infarction randomised between tissue plasminogen activator or streptokinase with or without heparin. Lancet 336, 71–75.

ISIS-4 (Fourth International Study of Infarct Survival) Collaborative Group, 1995. A randomised factorial trial assessing early oral captopril, oral mononitrate, and intravenous magnesium sulphate in 58,050 patients with suspected acute myocardial infarction. Lancet 345, 669–685.

Januzzi, J.L., Stern, T.A., Pasternak, R.C., et al., 2000. The influence of anxiety and depression on outcomes of patients with coronary artery disease. Arch. Int. Med. 160, 1913–1921.

Josan, K., Majumdar, S.R., McAlister, F.A., 2008. The efficacy and safety of intensive statin therapy: a meta-analysis of randomized trials. Can. Med. Assoc. J. 178, 576–584.

Kastrati, A., Mehilli, J., Neumann, F.J., et al., 2006. Abciximab in patients with acute coronary syndromes undergoing percutaneous coronary inter-vention after clopidogrel pretreatment: the ISAR-REACT 2 randomized trial. J. Am. Med. Assoc. 295, 1531–1538.

Kirchhof, P., Benussi, S., Kotecha, D., ESC Guidelines for the management of atrial fibrillation developed in collaboration with EACTS, et al., 2016. The task force for the management of atrial fibrillation of the European Society of Cardiology (ESC). Eur. Heart J. 37, 2893–2962.

Lindholm, D., Varenhorst, C., Cannon, C.P., et al., 2014. Ticagrelor vs. clopidogrel in patients with non-ST-elevation acute coronary syndrome with or without revascularization: results from the PLATO trial. Eur. Heart J. 35, 2083–2093.

Malmberg, K., for the DIGAMI (Diabetes Mellitus Insulin Glucose Infusion in Acute Myocardial Infarction) Study Group, 1997. Prospective randomised study of intensive insulin treatment on long-term survival after acute myocar-dial infarction in patients with diabetes mellitus. Br. Med. J. 314, 1512–1515.

Malmberg, K., Ryden, L., Wedel, H., et al., 2005. Intense metabolic control by means of insulin in patients with Diabetes Mellitus and Acute Myo-cardial Infarction (DIGAMI 2): effects on mortality and morbidity. Eur. Heart J. 26, 650–661.

McMurray, J.J.V., Rankin, A.C., 1994. Treatment of myocardial infarction, unstable angina and angina pectoris. Br. Med. J. 309, 1343–1350.

Mega, J.L., Braunwald, E., Wiviott, S.D., et al., 2012. Rivaroxaban in patients with a recent acute coronary syndrome. ATLASACS 2–TIMI 51 Investigators. New Engl. J. Med. 366, 9–19.

Mehta, S.R., Yusuf, S., Diaz, R., et al., 2005. Effect of glucose-insulin-potassium infusion on mortality in patients with acute ST-segment elevation myocardial infarction: the CREATE-ECLA randomized controlled trial. J. Am. Med. Assoc. 293, 437–446.

Menon, V., Harrington, R.A., Hochman, J.S., et al., 2004. Thrombolysis and adjunctive therapy in acute myocardial infarction. Chest 126, 549S–575S.

Montalescot, G., Sechtem, U., Achenbach, S., et al., 2013. ESC guidelines on the management of stable coronary artery disease. The task force on the management of stable coronary artery disease of the European Soci-ety of Cardiology. Eur. Heart J. 34, 2949–3003.

Montalescot, G., Wiviott, S.D., Braunwald, E., et al., 2009. Prasugrel compared with clopidogrel in patients undergoing percutaneous coronary intervention for ST-elevation myocardial infarction (TRITON-TIMI 38): double-blind, randomised controlled trial. Lancet 373, 723–731.

National Institute for Health and Care Excellence (NICE), 2011. Ticagrelor for the treatment of acute coronary syndromes. NICE, London. Available at http://www.nice.org.uk/guidance/ta236.

National Institute for Health and Care Excellence (NICE), 2014a. Cardiovas-cular disease: risk assessment and reduction, including lipid modification. NICE, London. Available at: http://www.nice.org.uk/guidance/cg181.

National Institute for Health and Care Excellence (NICE), 2014b. Prasugrel with percutaneous coronary intervention for treating acute coronary syndromes. NICE, London. Available at http://www.nice.org.uk/guidance/ta317.

OASIS-6 Trial Group, 2006. Effects of fondaparinux on mortality and reinfarction in patients with acute ST-segment elevation myocardial infarction. J. Am. Med. Assoc. 295, 1519–1530.

Office of National Statistics, 2015. Deaths registered in England and Wales (Series DR): 2015 registered deaths by age, sex, selected underlying causes of death and the leading causes of death for both males and females. Available at: https://www.ons.gov.uk/peoplepopulationandcomm unity/birthsdeathsandmarriages/deaths/bulletins/deathsregisteredinenglan dandwalesseriesdr/2015.

OPTIMAAL Study Group, 2002. Effect of losartan and captopril on mortal-ity and morbidity in high-risk patients after acute myocardial infarction: the OPTIMAAL randomized trial. Lancet 360, 752–780.

Pitt, B., Remme, W., Zannad, F., for the Eplerenone Post-Acute Myocardial Infarction Heart Failure Efficacy and Survival Study Investigators, et al., 2003. Eplerenone, a selective aldosterone blocker, in patients with left ventricular dysfunction after myocardial infarction. New Engl. J. Med. 348, 1309–1321.

Ridker, P.M., Danielson, E., Fonseca, F.A.H., for the JUPITER Study Group, et al., 2008. Rosuvastatin to prevent vascular events in men and women with elevated C-reactive protein. New Engl. J. Med. 359, 2195–2207.

Rochon, P.A., Tu, J.V., Anderson, G.M., et al., 2000. Rate of heart failure and 1-year survival for older people receiving low-dose β-blocker therapy after myocardial infarction. Lancet 356, 639–644.

Roffi, M., Patrono, C., Collet, J.-P., et al., 2016. ESC Guidelines for the management of acute coronary syndromes in patients presenting without persistent ST-segment elevation. Eur. Heart J. 37, 267–315 [including web addenda].

Sabatine, M.S., Cannon, C.P., Gibson, C.M., for the CLARITY-TIMI 28 Investigators, et al., 2005. Addition of clopidogrel to aspirin and fibrinolytic therapy for myocardial infarction with ST-segment elevation. New Engl. J. Med. 352, 1179–1189.

Steg, G., James, S.K., Atar, D., et al., 2012. ESC guidelines for the management of acute myocardial infarction in patients presenting with ST-segment elevation. The task force on the management of ST-segment elevation acute myocardial infarction of the European Society of Cardiology (ESC). Eur. Heart J. 33, 2569–2619.

Stone, G.W., Bertrand, M.E., Moses, J.W., et al., 2007. Routine upstream initiation vs deferred selective use of glycoprotein IIb/IIIa inhibitors in acute coronary syndromes: the ACUITY Timing Trial. J. Am. Med. Assoc. 297, 591–602.

Stub, D., Smith, K., Bernard, S., et al., 2015. Air versus oxygen in ST-segment-elevation myocardial infarction. Circulation 131, 2143–2150.

Thygesen, K., Alpert, J.S., White, H.D., Joint ESC/ACCF/AHA/WHF Task Force for the redefinition of myocardial infarction, et al., 2007. Universal definition of myocardial infarction. Eur. Heart J. 28, 2525–2538.

Unal, B., Critchley, J.A., Capewell, S., 2004. Explaining the decline in coronary heart disease mortality in England and Wales between 1981 and 2000. Circulation 109, 1101–1107.

VALIANT (VALsartan In Acute myocardial iNfarction Trial) Investigators, 2003. Valsartan, captopril, or both in myocardial infarction complicated by heart failure, left ventricular dysfunction, or both. New Engl. J. Med. 349, 1893–1906.

Van de Werf, F., Bax, J., Betriu, A., et al., 2008. The task force on the management of ST-segment elevation acute myocardial infarction of the European Society of Cardiology. Management of acute myocardial infarction in patients presenting with persistent ST-segment elevation. Eur. Heart J. 29, 2909–2945.

Varas-Lorenzo, C., Riera-Guardia, N., Calingaert, B., et al., 2013. Myocardial infarction and individual nonsteroidal anti-inflammatory drugs meta-analysis of observational studies. Pharmaco. Drug Safety 22, 559–570.

Waters, D.D., Alderman, E.L., Hsia, J., et al., 2002. Effects of hormone replacement therapy and antioxidant vitamin supplements on coronary atherosclerosis in post-menopausal women: a randomized controlled trial. JAMA 288, 2432–2440.

World Health Organization, 2017. Cardiovascular disease. Fact sheet. Available at: http://www.who.int/mediacentre/factsheets/fs317/en/.

Yusuf, S., Sleight, P., Pogue, J., et al., 2000. Effects of an angiotensin-converting-enzyme inhibitor, ramipril, on cardiovascular events in high-risk patients. The Heart Outcomes Prevention Evaluation (HOPE) Study Investigators. New Engl. J. Med. 342, 145–153.

Further reading

Montalescot, G., Sechtem, U., Achenbach, S., et al., 2013. ESC guidelines on the management of stable coronary artery disease: the task force on the management of stable coronary artery disease of the European Society of Cardiology. Eur. Heart J. 34, 2949–3003.

National Institute for Health and Care Excellence, 2011. Unstable angina and NSTEMI. The early management of unstable angina and non-ST-segment-elevation myocardial infarction. NICE, London. Available at: http://www.nice.org.uk/guidance/cg94.

National Institute for Health and Care Excellence, 2013. Myocardial infarction with ST-segment elevation: acute management. NICE, London. Available at http://www.nice.org.uk/guidance/cg167.

Shahzad, A., Kemp, I., Christine, M., et al., 2014. Unfractionated Heparin versus Bivalirudin in Primary Percutaneous Coronary Intervention (HEAT-PPCI): an open-label, single centre, randomised controlled trial. Lancet 384 (9957), 1849–1858.

Steg, P.G., James, S.K., Atar, D., et al., 2012. ESC guidelines for the management of acute myocardial infarction in patients presenting with ST-segment elevation. Eur. Heart J. 33, 2569–2619.

Useful websites

GRACE risk score: http://www.gracescore.org
TIMI risk score: http://www.timi.org

British Heart Foundation: https://www.bhf.org.uk

21 Chronic Heart Failure

John McAnaw and Tobias Dreischulte

Key points

- Heart failure is a common condition that affects the quality of life, causing fatigue, breathlessness and oedema. It often has a poor prognosis.

- Heart failure is a maladaptive condition with haemodynamic and neurohormonal disturbances. Increased understanding of its pathophysiology and the strength of the evidence base allow a rational approach to therapeutic management.

- The aims of drug treatment are to control symptoms and improve survival. By slowing disease progression, the aim is to maintain quality of life.

- Angiotensin-converting enzyme (ACE) inhibitors, β-blockers and mineralocorticoid receptor antagonists are first-line options in treating patients with systolic dysfunction.

- Angiotensin II receptor blockers (ARBs) are an alternative choice in patients intolerant of or resistant to ACE inhibitors or mineralocorticoid receptor antagonist therapy.

- Diuretics are used for symptomatic management of heart failure and are combined with other agents in the treatment of systolic dysfunction.

- The use of sacubitril/valsartan should be considered under specialist advice in patients with systolic dysfunction who have ongoing symptoms of heart failure despite optimal therapy.

- Ivabradine should be considered under specialist advice in patients with systolic dysfunction who have had a hospital admission for heart failure in the preceding 12 months but have stabilised on standard therapy for at least 4 weeks.

- Digoxin may still have a role in improving symptoms and reducing the rate of hospitalisation for patients with heart failure in sinus rhythm, but it has not been demonstrated to affect mortality. The combination of hydralazine and nitrate may still have a place for specific patients on the advice of a specialist.

- Heart failure is a condition in which integration of pharmaceutical care within multidisciplinary models of patient care can improve clinical outcomes for patients and contribute to the continuity of care.

Chronic heart failure results from a deficiency in the heart's function as a pump, where the delivery of blood, and therefore oxygen and nutrients, becomes inadequate for the needs of the tissues. Chronic heart failure is a complex condition associated with a number of symptoms arising from defects in left ventricular filling and/or emptying, of which shortness of breath (exertional dyspnoea, orthopnoea and paroxysmal nocturnal dyspnoea), fatigue and ankle swelling are the most common. The symptoms of heart failure are due to inadequate tissue perfusion, venous congestion and disturbed water and electrolyte balance. Impairment of renal function, and the associated water retention, adds to the burden placed on the heart. In chronic heart failure, the physiological mechanisms that aim to maintain adequate tissue perfusion become counterproductive and contribute to the progressive nature of the condition.

Treatment is aimed at improving left ventricular function, controlling the secondary effects that lead to the occurrence of symptoms and delaying disease progression. Drug therapy is indicated in all patients with heart failure to control symptoms (where present), improve quality of life and prolong survival. Patients with heart failure usually have their functional status assessed and categorised using the New York Heart Association (NYHA) classification system shown in Table 21.1.

Epidemiology

Chronic heart failure is a common condition, affecting about 2% of the adult population (Metra and Teerlink, 2017). Prevalence increases with age; less than 2% of people younger than 60 years of age to greater than 10% in those aged 75 years or older. Heart failure accounts for 5% of adult emergency medical admissions to hospital (National Institute for Health and Care Excellence [NICE], 2010). There is a loss of cardiac reserve with age, and heart failure may often complicate the presence of other conditions in the elderly.

Heart failure is a progressive condition with complex possible causes, and mortality varies according to aetiology and severity. The variable prognosis is represented by a median survival of about 5 years after diagnosis. The prognosis can be predicted according to the severity of the disease, with an overall annual mortality rate for patients with stable heart failure estimated at 6–7%, up to 25% or more in patients admitted to hospital with acute heart failure (Metra and Teerlink, 2017). Main causes of death are progressive pump failure, sudden cardiac death and recurrent myocardial infarction (MI).

Aetiology

Heart failure may be a consequence of MI, but as a chronic condition, it is often gradual in onset with symptoms arising

Table 21.1 New York Heart Association classification of functional status of the patient with heart failure

I	No symptoms with ordinary physical activity (such as walking or climbing stairs)
II	Slight limitation with dyspnoea on moderate to severe exertion (climbing stairs or walking uphill)
III	Marked limitation of activity, less than ordinary activity causes dyspnoea (restricting walking distance and limiting climbing to one flight of stairs)
IV	Severe disability, dyspnoea at rest (unable to carry on physical activity without discomfort)

Adapted from the Criteria Committee of the New York Heart Association (1994).

insidiously and without any specific cause over a number of years. The common underlying aetiologies in patients with heart failure are coronary artery disease and hypertension. The appropriate management of these predisposing conditions is also an important consideration in controlling heart failure in the community. Identifiable causes of heart failure include aortic stenosis, cardiomyopathy, mechanical defects such as cardiac valvular dysfunction, hyperthyroidism and severe anaemia. Conditions that place increased demands on the heart can create a shortfall in cardiac output and lead to intermittent exacerbation of symptoms. Symptoms of heart failure may occur as a consequence of hyperthyroidism, where the tissues place a greater metabolic demand, or severe anaemia, where there is an increased circulatory demand on the heart. Cardiac output may also be compromised by bradycardia or tachycardia, or by a sustained arrhythmia such as that experienced by patients in atrial fibrillation.

Atrial fibrillation often accompanies hyperthyroidism and mitral valve disease, where a rapid and irregular ventricular response can compromise cardiac efficiency. Improved management of the underlying causes, where appropriate, may alleviate the symptoms of heart failure, whereas the presence of mechanical defects may require the surgical insertion of prosthetic valve(s). Although around 50% of patients with heart failure have significant left ventricular systolic dysfunction, the other half comprises patients who have either a normal or insignificantly reduced left ventricular ejection fraction (EF). However, there is no consensus on the threshold for compromised EF, and assessment of each patient relies mainly on clinical symptoms. These patients are referred to as having heart failure with preserved left ventricular ejection fraction (HFPEF). Most of the available evidence from clinical trials regarding the pharmacological treatment of heart failure to date relates to those patients with heart failure due to left ventricular systolic dysfunction. Clinical symptomatic description of chronic heart failure is mild, moderate or severe heart failure. 'Mild' is used for patients who are mobile with no important limitations of dyspnoea or fatigue, 'severe' for patients who are markedly symptomatic in terms of exercise intolerance and 'moderate' for those with restrictions in

between. Trials tend to formalise these categories into NYHA Categories I–IV (Table 21.1).

Pathophysiology

In health, cardiac output at rest is approximately 5 L/min with a mean heart rate of 70 beats/min and stroke volume of 70 mL. Because the filled ventricle has a normal volume of 130 mL, the fraction ejected is more than 50% of the ventricular contents, with the remaining (residual) volume being approximately 60 mL. In left ventricular systolic dysfunction, the EF is reduced to less than 45%, and symptoms are common when the fraction is less than 35%, although some patients with a low EF can remain asymptomatic. When the EF falls below 10%, patients have the added risk of thrombus formation within the left ventricle, and in most cases anticoagulation with warfarin is indicated.

Left ventricular systolic dysfunction can result from cardiac injury, such as MI, or by exposure of the heart muscle to mechanical stress, such as long-standing hypertension. This may result in defects in systolic contraction, diastolic relaxation or both. Systolic dysfunction arises from impaired contractility and is reflected in a low EF and cardiac dilation. Diastolic dysfunction arises from impairment of the filling process. Diastolic filling is affected by the rate of venous return, and normal filling requires active diastolic expansion of the ventricular volume. The tension on the ventricular wall at the end of diastole is called the preload and is related to the volume of blood available to be pumped. That tension contributes to the degree of stretch on the myocardium. In diastolic dysfunction, there is impaired relaxation or reduced compliance of the left ventricle during diastole, and therefore less additional blood is accommodated. In pure diastolic dysfunction, the EF can be normal, but cardiac dilation is absent. Sustained diastolic dysfunction, which is a feature in a minority of patients with heart failure, may lead to systolic dysfunction associated with disease progression and left ventricular remodelling (structural changes and/or deterioration).

During systolic contraction, the tension on the ventricular wall is determined by the degree of resistance to outflow at the exit valve and that within the arterial tree, that is, the systemic vascular resistance. Arterial hypertension, aortic narrowing and disorders of the aortic valve increase the afterload on the heart by increasing the resistance against which the contraction of the ventricle must work. The result is an increased residual volume and consequently an increased preload as the ventricle overfills and produces greater tension on the ventricular wall. In the normal heart, a compensatory increase in performance occurs as the stretched myocardium responds through an increased elastic recoil. In the failing heart, this property of cardiac muscle recoiling under stretch is diminished, with the consequence that the heart dilates abnormally to accommodate the increased ventricular load. With continued dilation of the heart, the elastic recoil property can become much reduced. Failure of the heart to handle the increasing ventricular load leads to pulmonary and systemic venous congestion. At the same time, the increased tension on the ventricular wall in heart failure raises myocardial oxygen requirements, which increases the risk of an episode of myocardial ischaemia or arrhythmias.

The failing heart may show cardiac enlargement due to dilation, which is reversible with successful treatment. An irreversible increase in cardiac muscle mass, cardiac hypertrophy, occurs with progression of heart failure and is a consequence of long-standing hypertension. Although hypertrophy may initially alleviate heart failure, the increased mass is pathologically significant because it ultimately increases the demands on the heart and oxygen consumption.

A reflex sympathetic discharge caused by the diminished tissue perfusion in heart failure exposes the heart to catecholamines where positive inotropic and chronotropic effects help sustain cardiac output and produce a tachycardia. Arterial constriction diverts blood to the organs from the skin and gastro-intestinal tract but overall raises systemic vascular resistance and increases the afterload on the heart.

Reduced renal perfusion due to heart failure leads to increased renin release from the glomerulus in the kidney. Circulating renin raises blood pressure through the formation of angiotensin I and angiotensin II, a potent vasoconstrictor, and renin also prompts adrenal aldosterone release. Aldosterone retains salt and water at the distal renal tubule and so expands blood volume and increases preload. Arginine vasopressin released from the posterior pituitary in response to hypoperfusion adds to the systemic vasoconstriction and has an antidiuretic effect by retaining water at the renal collecting duct.

These secondary effects become increasingly detrimental to cardiac function as heart failure progresses because the vasoconstriction adds to the afterload, and the expanded blood volume adds to the preload. The expanded blood volume promotes the atrial myocytes to release a natural vasodilator, atrial natriuretic peptide (ANP), to attenuate the increased preload.

The compensatory mechanisms for the maintenance of the circulation eventually become overwhelmed and are ultimately highly counterproductive, leading to the emergence and progression of clinical signs and symptoms of heart failure. The long-term consequences are that the myocardium of the failing heart undergoes biochemical and histological changes that lead to remodelling of the left ventricle, which further complicates disease progression. In those patients where the condition is severe and has progressed to an end stage, heart transplantation may be the only remaining treatment option.

Clinical manifestations

The reduced cardiac output, impaired oxygenation and diminished blood supply to muscles cause fatigue. Shortness of breath occurs on exertion (dyspnoea) or on lying (orthopnoea). When the patient lies down, the postural change causes abdominal pressure on the diaphragm which redistributes oedema to the lungs, leading to breathlessness. At night the pulmonary symptoms give rise to cough, and an increase in urine production prompts micturition (nocturia), which adds to the sleep

Table 21.2 Clinical manifestations of heart failure

Venous (congestion)	Cardiac (cardiomegaly)	Arterial (peripheral hypoperfusion)
Dyspnoea	Dilation	Fatigue
Oedema	Tachycardia	Pallor
Hypoxia	Regurgitation	Renal impairment
Hepatomegaly	Cardiomyopathy	Confusion
Raised venous pressure	Ischaemia, arrhythmia	Circulatory failure

disturbance. The patient can be inclined to waken at night as gradual accumulation of fluid in the lungs may eventually provoke regular attacks of gasping (paroxysmal nocturnal dyspnoea). Characteristically, the patient describes the need to sit or stand up to seek fresh air and often describes a need to be propped up by three or more pillows to remedy the sleep disturbances that are due to fluid accumulation.

Patients with heart failure may appear pale and their hands cold and sweaty. Reduced blood supply to the brain and kidney can cause confusion and contribute to renal failure, respectively. Hepatomegaly occurs from congestion of the gastro-intestinal tract, which is accompanied by abdominal distension, anorexia, nausea and abdominal pain. Oedema affects the lungs, ankles and abdomen. Signs of oedema in the lungs include crepitations heard at the lung bases. In acute heart failure, symptoms of pulmonary oedema are prominent and may be life-threatening. The sputum may be frothy and tinged red from the leakage of fluid and blood from the capillaries. Severe dyspnoea may be complicated by cyanosis and shock. Table 21.2 presents the clinical manifestations of heart failure.

Investigations

Patients with chronic heart failure are diagnosed and monitored on the basis of signs and symptoms from physical examination, history and an exercise tolerance test. On physical examination of the patient, a lateral and downwards displacement of the apex beat can be identified as evidence of cardiac enlargement. Additional third and/or fourth heart sounds are typical of heart failure and arise from valvular dysfunction. Venous congestion can be demonstrated in the jugular vein of the upright, reclining patient by an elevated jugular venous pressure (JVP), which reflects the central venous pressure. The JVP is measured by noting the visible distension above the sternum and may be accentuated in heart failure by the application of abdominal compression in the reclining patient. Confirmation of heart failure, however, should not be based on symptom assessment alone.

After clinical examination, patients should have their brain-type natriuretic peptide (BNP) and N-terminal (NT) proBNP (BNP/NT-proBNP) measured and then have an

Table 21.3 Investigations performed to confirm a diagnosis of heart failure

Investigation	Comment
Blood test	The following assessments are usually performed: • Urinalysis • Serum creatinine and urea to assess renal function • Full blood count to investigate possibility of anaemia • Thyroid function tests to investigate possibility of thyrotoxicosis • Serum BNP or NT pro-BNP to indicate whether echocardiography is necessary • Fasting blood glucose to investigate possibility of diabetes mellitus
12-Lead electrocardiogram	A normal ECG along with low BNP/NT-ProBNP levels usually excludes the presence of left ventricular systolic dysfunction. An abnormal ECG will require further investigation including echocardiography
Chest radiograph	A chest radiograph (X-ray) is performed to look for an enlarged cardiac shadow and consolidation in the lungs
Echocardiography	An echocardiogram is used to confirm the diagnosis of heart failure and any underlying causes, e.g. valvular heart disease

BNP or NT pro-BNP, brain-type natriuretic peptid6e (BNP) and N-terminal (NT) proBNP; ECG, electrocardiogram.

electrocardiogram (ECG) taken. If BNP/NT-proBNP level is found to be low and the ECG result is normal, it is unlikely that the patient has heart failure. Therefore, another underlying cause for the symptoms should be considered. If a raised BNP/NT-proBNP level is found or the patient's ECG is abnormal, then the patient should be referred for echocardiography. Echocardiography is important when investigating patients with a suspected diagnosis of heart failure. An echocardiogram allows visualisation of the heart in real time and will identify whether heart failure is due to systolic dysfunction, diastolic dysfunction or heart valve defects. Table 21.3 shows the investigations that are routinely performed in the assessment of heart failure symptoms.

Treatment of heart failure

Until the 1980s, pharmacotherapy was driven by the aim to control symptoms, when diuretics and digoxin were the mainstays of treatment. Although relieving the symptoms of heart failure remains decisive in improving a patient's quality of life, a better understanding of the underlying pathophysiology has led to major advances in the pharmacological treatment of heart failure. With the introduction of angiotensin-converting enzyme (ACE) inhibitors, β-blockers, angiotensin II receptor

blockers (ARBs) and mineralocorticoid receptor antagonists (MRAs), delaying disease progression and ultimately improving survival have become realistic goals of therapy. An outline of the site of action of the various drugs is schematically presented in Fig. 21.1.

In heart failure patients with comorbid conditions known to contribute to heart failure, such as hyperthyroidism, anaemia, atrial fibrillation and valvular heart disease, attention must be given to ensuring these underlying contributing factors are well controlled. Patients with atrial fibrillation may be candidates for electrocardioversion. Tachycardia from atrial fibrillation usually requires control of the ventricular rate through suppression of atrioventricular node conduction. In patients with heart failure, the use of β-blockers or digoxin are options in such circumstances. In these patients, the use of an anticoagulant may be necessary and should be based on an assessment of stroke risk.

In patients with heart failure and preserved EF, diuretics are commonly used for symptom control. However, the use of all other agents of proven benefit in treating heart failure due to left ventricular systolic dysfunction is currently not supported by an evidence base.

There is consensus that all patients with left ventricular systolic dysfunction should be treated with an ACE inhibitor in the absence of intolerance or contraindications (Scottish Intercollegiate Guidelines Network [SIGN], 2016). The evidence base for treatment clearly shows that use of an ACE inhibitor in patients with heart failure due to left ventricular systolic dysfunction leads to an improvement in symptoms and reduction in mortality. Beneficial effects on morbidity and mortality have also been shown for the use of ARBs, β-blockers, mineralocorticoid receptor antagonists and hydralazine/nitrate combinations when used in the treatment of chronic heart failure. Digoxin has been shown to improve morbidity and reduce the number of hospital admissions in patients with heart failure, although its effect on mortality has not been demonstrated. Table 21.4 describes the treatment of acute heart failure in the hospital setting, and Table 21.5 highlights the possible treatment options for patients with chronic heart failure due to left ventricular systolic dysfunction.

The selection of adjunctive therapy beyond the use of ACE inhibitor, β-blocker and mineralocorticoid receptor antagonist therapy is largely dependent on the nature of the patient and the preference of the heart failure specialist involved in the patient's care. It is accepted that there is a limit as to how many agents any one patient can tolerate; therefore, the selection of drug therapy will probably be tailored to each individual patient, meaning that treatment plans will vary.

Diuretics

In chronic heart failure, diuretics are used to relieve pulmonary and peripheral oedema by increasing sodium and chloride excretion through blockade of sodium re-absorption in the renal tubule. Normally, in the proximal tubule, about 70% of sodium is reabsorbed along with water. In mild heart failure, either a thiazide or more often a loop diuretic is chosen depending on the severity of the symptoms experienced by the patient

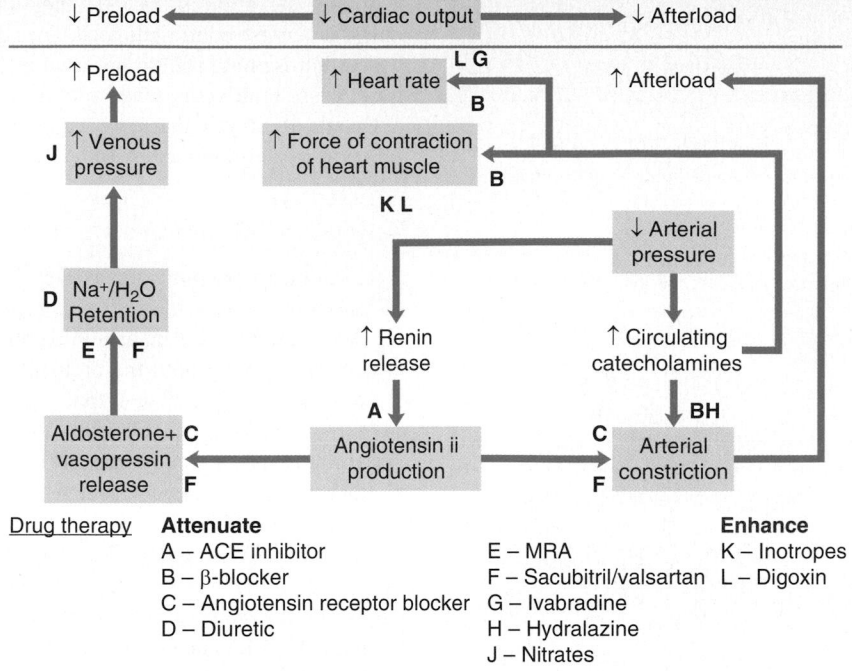

Fig. 21.1 Schematic representation of the physiological response to reduced cardiac output and arterial pressure, and where heart failure drugs act.

Table 21.4 Treatment of acute heart failure due to left ventricular systolic dysfunction in patients requiring hospitalisation

Problem	Drug therapy indicated
Anxiety	Use of opiates to reduce anxiety and reduce preload through venodilation might be considered for some patients, although routine use should be avoided due to a potentially increased risk of mortality.
Breathlessness	High-flow oxygen (60–100%) may be required in conjunction with i.v. furosemide as either direct injection or 24-h infusion (5–10 mg/h). GTN may be considered to help relieve pulmonary congestion.
Arrhythmia	Digoxin is useful in the control of atrial fibrillation. Amiodarone is the drug of choice in ventricular arrhythmias.
Expansion of blood volume after blood transfusion	An elevation in preload, such as can occur acutely by the expansion of blood volume after a transfusion, can exacerbate the degree of systolic dysfunction. Therefore, it is necessary to continue or increase diuretic dosage during this time.

GTN, glyceryl trinitrate; i.v., intravenous.

and the degree of diuresis required. Thiazides are described as 'low-ceiling agents' because maximum diuresis occurs at low doses, and they act mainly on the cortical diluting segment (the point of merger of the ascending limb with the distal renal tubule), at which 5–10% of sodium is normally removed. Although thiazides have some action at this site, they fail to produce a marked diuresis because a compensatory increase in sodium re-absorption occurs in the loop of Henle, and consequently thiazides are ineffective in patients with moderate to severe renal impairment (eGFR <30 mL/min/1.73 m^2) or persisting symptoms. Additionally, doses above the equivalent of bendroflumethiazide 5 mg have an increased risk of adverse metabolic effects with no additional symptomatic benefit. Thiazides are, therefore, now rarely used as sole diuretic therapy and are reserved for cases where the degree of fluid retention is very mild, renal function is not compromised or as an adjunct to loop diuretics.

Loop diuretics are indicated in the majority of symptomatic patients, and most patients will be prescribed one of either furosemide, bumetanide or torasemide in preference to a thiazide. These agents are known as 'high-ceiling agents' because their blockade of sodium re-absorption in the loop of Henle continues with increased dose. They have a shorter duration of action (average 4–6 hours) compared with thiazides (average 12–24 hours), and they produce less hypokalaemia. In high doses, however, their intensity of action may produce hypovolaemia with risk of postural hypotension, worsening of symptoms and renal failure. In practice, high doses of furosemide (up to 500 mg/day) may be required to control oedema in patients with poor renal function. In the acute situation, doses of loop diuretics are titrated to produce a weight loss of 0.5–1 kg/day.

Table 21.5 Outline of the treatment options for patients with chronic heart failure due to left ventricular systolic dysfunction

NYHA	Drug therapy options
I	Asymptomatic patients with a reduced ejection fraction Angiotensin-converting enzyme inhibitor (or ARB if intolerant)
II–IV	Patients with symptoms of heart failure and reduced ejection fraction ACE inhibitor (or ARB if intolerant) β-Blocker MRA (or ARB if NYHA II–III and intolerant of MRA) Diuretic (where dyspnoea and/or oedema present)
II–IV	Additional options where specialist advice required before use Angiotensin receptor/neprilysin inhibitor (only where ongoing symptoms despite optimal therapy; requires stopping both ACE inhibitor and/or ARB) Ivabradine (only if sinus rhythm heart rate ≥75 beats/min and maximum tolerated β-blocker dose reached) Digoxin (only in sinus rhythm if patient still symptomatic despite optimal therapy) Hydralazine/isosorbide dinitrate (only where ACE inhibitor or ARB intolerant due to renal dysfunction or raised potassium, or where the patient is African-American and NYHA III–IV)

ACE, angiotensiin-converting enzyme; ARB, angiotensin receptor blocker; MRA, mineralocorticoid receptor antagonist; NYHA, New York Heart Association.

In longer-term use, patients with heart failure frequently develop some resistance to the effects of loop diuretic due to a compensatory rebound in sodium retention. In this situation, a combination of thiazide and loop diuretics has been shown to have a synergistic effect, even in patients with reduced renal function. In the UK, metolazone is also used as an adjunct to augment the effects of loop diuretics. The potentially profound diuresis produced by such a combination poses serious risks, such as dehydration and hypotension, and patients who are prescribed metolazone in addition to an existing loop diuretic must be carefully monitored. In practice, patients with oedema treated with loop diuretics may best be treated using a degree of self-management. Some patients are instructed to make upwards adjustment of loop diuretic dose or to add metolazone therapy on particular days, for example, when they self-record a gain of 2 kg or more in their body weight over a short period of time.

Diuretics also have a mild vasodilator effect that helps improve cardiac function, and the intravenous use of loop diuretics reduces preload acutely by locally relieving pulmonary congestion before the onset of the diuretic effect. Effective diuretic therapy is demonstrated by the normalisation of filling pressure. Therefore,

continued elevation of the JVP suggests a need for more diuretic unless otherwise contraindicated. The administration rate of intravenous furosemide should not usually exceed 4 mg/min because it can cause ototoxicity when administered more rapidly.

Details of diuretic therapy used in left ventricular systolic dysfunction are summarised in Table 21.6.

Angiotensin-converting enzyme inhibitors

ACE inhibitors are indicated as first-line treatment for all grades of heart failure due to left ventricular systolic dysfunction, including those patients who are asymptomatic. These agents exert their effects by reducing both the preload and afterload on the heart, thereby increasing cardiac output.

ACE inhibitors act on the renin–angiotensin–aldosterone system, and they reduce afterload by reducing the formation of angiotensin II, a potent vasoconstrictor in the arterial system. These drugs also have an indirect effect on sodium and water retention by inhibiting the release of aldosterone and vasopressin, thereby reducing venous congestion and preload. The increase in cardiac output leads to an improvement in renal perfusion, which further helps alleviate oedema. ACE inhibitors also potentiate the vasodilator bradykinin and may intervene locally on ACE in cardiac and renal tissues.

ACE inhibitors are generally well tolerated by most patients and have been shown to improve the quality of life and survival in patients with mild-to-severe systolic dysfunction (CONSENSUS I, 1987; CONSENSUS II, 1992; SOLVD-P, 1992; SOLVD-T, 1991; V-HeFT II, 1991), including those patients who have experienced an MI (AIRE, 1993; SAVE, 1992; TRACE ,1995). When an ACE inhibitor is prescribed, it is important to ensure that the dose is started low and increased gradually, paying close attention to renal function and electrolyte balance. The dose should be titrated to achieve the target dose that has been associated with long-term benefits shown in clinical trials or (if not possible) the maximum tolerable dose. There is some evidence to suggest that high doses of ACE inhibitor are more effective than low doses in relation to reduction in mortality, although it is uncertain whether this is a general class effect (ATLAS, 1999). In clinical practice, it is possible that some patients may be treated with ACE inhibitors at doses lower than those used in clinical trials. As a consequence, actual outcomes in heart failure treatment may not be as good as expected from the trial findings.

The introduction of an ACE inhibitor may produce hypotension, which is most pronounced after the first dose and is sometimes severe. Patients at risk include those already on high doses of loop diuretics, where the diuretics cannot be stopped or reduced beforehand, and patients who may have a low-circulating fluid volume (due to dehydration) and an activated renin–angiotensin system. Hypotension can also occur where the ACE inhibitor has been initiated at too high a dose or where the dose has been increased too quickly after initiation. In the primary care setting, treatment must be started with a low dose, which is usually administered at bedtime. In patients at particular risk of hypotension, a test dose of the shorter-acting agent captopril can be given to assess suitability for treatment

Table 21.6 Diuretics and mineralocorticoid receptor antagonists used in the treatment of patients with heart failure with reduced ejection fraction

Class and agent	Onset and duration of effect		Comment
Thiazide and related	**Oral**		
Bendroflumethiazide	Onset 1–2 h Duration 12–18 h		Thiazides are effective in the treatment of sodium and water retention, although there is generally a loss of action in renal failure (GFR <30 mL/min). Metolazone has an intense action when added to a loop diuretic and is effective at low GFR.
Metolazone	Onset 1–2 h Duration 12–24 h		
Loop	**Oral**	**Parenteral**	
Furosemide	Onset 0.5–1 h Duration 4–6 h	Onset 5 min Duration 2 h	Loop diuretics are preferred in the treatment of sodium and water retention where renal dysfunction is evident or more severe grades of heart failure present. Agents can be given orally or by infusion, and all are effective at low GFR.
Bumetanide	As above	As above	
Torasemide	Onset <1 h Duration <8 h	Onset 10 min Duration <8 h	
Mineralocorticoid receptor antagonist	**Oral**		
Spironolactone	Onset 7 h Duration 24 h		Mineralocorticoid receptor antagonists can improve symptoms and survival when given as an adjunct to ACE inhibitor and β-blocker therapy. Spironolactone has a recommended starting dose of 25 mg daily (or on alternate days), with a target dose of 25–50 mg daily. With eplerenone, a starting dose of 25 mg daily is given, titrating up to a target dose of 50 mg daily.
Eplerenone	Steady-state within 2 days		

ACE, Angiotensin-converting enzyme; GFR, glomerular filtration rate.

before commencing long-term treatment with a preferred ACE inhibitor. Once it has been established that the ACE inhibitor can be initiated safely, the preferred option would be to switch to a longer-acting agent with once- or twice-daily dosing, starting with a low dose that would be gradually titrated upwards to the recommended target (Table 21.7). Monitoring of fluid balance, blood biochemistry and blood pressure is an essential safety check during initiation and titration of ACE inhibitor therapy.

One of the most common adverse effects seen with ACE inhibitors is a dry cough. However, because a cough can occur naturally in patients with heart failure, it is sometimes difficult to determine the true cause. ACE inhibitor therapy can also compromise renal function, although in patients in whom there is a reduction in renal perfusion due to worsening heart failure or hypovolaemia, renal dysfunction can also occur. Therefore, there are a number of instances where ACE inhibitor intolerance can be misdiagnosed in practice. Where ACE inhibitor intolerance is suspected, patients can usually be successfully rechallenged with an ACE inhibitor once their heart failure is more stable, although careful monitoring of the patient should be undertaken during initiation and subsequent dose titration. If the increase in the patient's serum creatinine is greater than 100% from baseline, the ACE inhibitor should be stopped, intolerance confirmed and specialist advice sought. Where the increase from baseline is 50–100%, the ACE inhibitor dose should be halved and serum creatinine concentration rechecked after 1–2 weeks. If renal function is stable and no cough or other adverse effects are reported, therapy should be continued. Where the problem persists, an alternative treatment option might be required. For example, an ARB will have similar benefits for morbidity and mortality, but there is a possibility of similar adverse effects on blood pressure and renal function. Alternatively, a mineralocorticoid receptor antagonist could be used.

ACE inhibitors are potentially hazardous in patients with pre-existing renal disease because blockade of the renin–angiotensin system may lead to reversible deterioration of renal function. In particular, ACE inhibitors are contraindicated in patients with bilateral renal artery stenosis, in whom the renin–angiotensin system is highly activated to maintain renal perfusion. Because most ACE inhibitors or their active metabolites rely on elimination via the kidney, the risk of other forms of dose-related toxicity is also increased in the presence of renal failure. Fosinopril, which is partially excreted by metabolism, may be the preferred agent in patients with renal failure. ACE inhibitors are also contraindicated in patients with severe aortic stenosis because their use can result in a markedly reduced cardiac output due to decreased filling pressure within the left ventricle. Table 21.7 summarises the activity and use of ACE inhibitors.

Table 21.7 Vasodilators used in the treatment of heart failure

	Dose	Frequency	Half-life (h)	Comment
ACE inhibitors				
Captopril	Target: 50 mg Start: 6.25 mg	Three times daily	8	First-dose hypotension may occur. May worsen renal failure. Adjust dose in renal failure. Hypokalaemia, cough, taste disturbance and hypersensitivity may occur, particularly with captopril. ACE inhibitors have been shown to improve survival, with starting and target dose for those agents used in clinical trials highlighted.
Enalapril	Target: 10-20 mg Start: 2.5 mg	Twice daily	11	
Fosinopril	Target: 40 mg Start: 10 mg	Once daily	11-14	
Lisinopril	Target: 20-35 mg Start: 2.5-5 mg	Once daily	12	
Perindopril	Target: 4 mg Start: 2 mg	Once daily	25	
Quinapril	Target: 10-20 mg Start: 2.5 mg	Once daily (or divided dose)	2-3	
Ramipril	Target: 10 mg Start: 2.5 mg	Once daily (or divided dose)	13-17	
Trandolapril	Target: 4 mg Start: 0.5 mg	Once daily	16-24	
B-Blocker				
Bisoprolol	Target: 10 mg Start: 1.25 mg	Once daily	10-12	May initially exacerbate symptoms, but if initiated at low dose and slowly titrated, can improve long-term survival, even in elderly patients with heart failure. Half-life of nebivolol can be 3-5 times longer in slow metabolisers.
Carvedilol	Target: 25-50 mg Start: 3.125 mg	Twice daily	6-10	
Nebivolol	Target: 10 mg Start: 1.25 mg	Once daily	10	
Angiotensin II receptor blocker				
Losartan	Target: up to 150 mg Start:12.5mg	Once daily	6-9	Comparable effectiveness to ACE inhibitor in patients with ACE inhibitor intolerance, although similar effect on renal function and blood pressure. Evidence suggests improved survival when ARB used as adjunctive therapy. However, increased potential for deterioration in renal function and/or hyperkalaemia
Candesartan	Target:32 mg Start:4-8 mg	Once daily	9	
Valsartan	Target:160 mg Start:40 mg	Twice daily	9	
Angiotensin II receptor/ Neprilysin inhibitors	**Oral**			
Sacubitril/Valsartan	Target: 96/104 mg Start:24/26 mg to 49/51 mg	Twice daily	1.4-10	Comparable effectiveness to ACE inhibitor regarding survival and hospitalisation for heart failure. If patient on an ACE inhibitor or ARB, this must be stopped 36h before initiation to minimise the risk of angioedema. During titration the dose should be doubled at 2-4 weekly intervals until target reached, with patients who have moderate renal impairment or systolic blood pressure ≥ 100-110mmHg starting on the lower starting dose.

Table 21.7 Vasodilators used in the treatment of heart failure—cont'd

	Dose	Frequency	Half-life (h)	Comment
Hydralazine				
	Target: 50-75mg Start: 25mg	Three to four times daily	2-3	Has a direct action on arteries. Tolerance occurs. May cause drug-induced lupus and sodium retention. Used in combination with oral nitrates.
Nitrates				
Isosorbide dinitrate	Target: 40-160mg	Daily in divided doses	1	High doses of Isosorbide dinitrate needed and may require up to 240mg daily in divided doses. With isosorbide mononitrate, up to 120mg daily in divided doses may be required. Tolerance can be prevented by nitrate-free period of >8 hours. Protective against cardiac ischaemia. Used in combination with hydralazine.
Isosorbide mononitrate	Target: variable Start:10mg	Twice daily	5	

ARB, angiotensin receptor blocker; ACE, angiotensin-converting enzyme.

Angiotensin II receptor blockers

Although comparisons of ACE inhibitors and ARBs have shown similar benefits on morbidity and heart failure mortality, only ACE inhibitors have been shown to have positive effects on all-cause mortality. ARBs should, therefore, not be used instead of ACE inhibitors, unless the patient experiences intolerable side effects.

The use of ARBs as an adjunct to ACE inhibitor and β-blocker therapy has been associated with significant reductions in cardiovascular events and hospitalisation rate (CHARM Added, 2003). Although this finding is encouraging, the impact on mortality alone remains inconsistent, and there is no clear consensus on when to use an ARB as adjunctive therapy. In studies involving patients unable to tolerate an ACE inhibitor, ARBs have been shown to be comparable to ACE inhibitors in reducing the risk of cardiovascular death and rate of hospitalisation and in the control of symptoms in heart failure patients (CHARM Alternative, 2003; Val-HeFT, 2002). Therefore, ARBs are recommended for use as an alternative to ACE inhibitor therapy where intolerance has been confirmed. It is important to note that in patients who have renal failure secondary to ACE inhibitors, switching to an ARB is of no theoretical or practical benefit because similar adverse effects are likely.

β-Blockers

Formerly, β-blockers have been contraindicated in patients with heart failure. However, the sympathetic neurohormonal overactivity that occurs in response to the failing heart has been identified as a decisive factor in the progression of ventricular dysfunction. Consequently, β-blockers have been tested in a number of clinical trials. There is now substantial evidence that β-blockers reduce mortality among patients with mild-to-moderate symptomatic heart failure (ANZ Carvedilol, 1997; CAPRICORN, 2001; CIBIS II, 1999; MERIT-HF, 1999; US Carvedilol, 1996;) and those with severe heart failure (COPERNICUS, 2001). This beneficial effect also extends to the elderly heart failure population (SENIORS, 2005).

The use of β-blockers is, therefore, recommended for all patients with symptoms of heart failure due to left ventricular systolic dysfunction, irrespective of age and the degree of dysfunction. However, due to their negative inotropic effects, β-blockers should only be initiated when the patient's condition is stable. There is insufficient evidence for a class effect to be assumed illustrated by the fact that in one trial, metoprolol tartrate was found to be inferior to carvedilol (COMET, 2003). Currently, nebivolol, bisoprolol and carvedilol are the only licensed β-blockers for the treatment of heart failure in the UK.

It is likely that patients will experience a worsening of symptoms during initiation of therapy, and therefore, patients are started on very low doses of β-blocker (e.g. carvedilol 3.125 mg daily), with careful titration occurring over a number of weeks or months with careful monitoring. The goal is to titrate the dose towards those used in clinical trials that have been associated with morbidity and mortality benefits (carvedilol 25–50 mg daily). Table 21.7 summarises the activity and use of β-blockers in heart failure.

Despite the demonstrated benefits, there is ongoing concern that certain subgroups of patients with heart failure continue to be undertreated with β-blockers. These groups include patients with chronic obstructive pulmonary disease (COPD), peripheral vascular disease, diabetes mellitus and erectile dysfunction and older adults. With the exception of patients with reversible pulmonary disease, who have typically been excluded from β-blocker trials (CIBIS II, 1999; MERIT-HF, 1999), there is now sufficient evidence to justify the use of β-blockers licensed for heart failure in these patients. In addition, a systematic review of trials on cardio-selective β-blockers found no clinically significant adverse respiratory effects in patients with reversible COPD, although it would be prudent to use these agents in such patients with caution and with appropriate monitoring in place (Salpeter et al. 2005).

Mineralocorticoid receptor antagonists

The use of MRAs as an adjunct to standard treatment has been shown to reduce morbidity and mortality in patients with heart failure. Spironolactone has been shown to reduce mortality and hospitalisation rates in patients with moderate to severe heart failure (RALES, 1999). The use of eplerenone has also been shown to be associated with similar benefits in early post-MI patients with symptomatic heart failure or early post-MI diabetic patients with asymptomatic heart failure (EMPHASIS-HF, 2011; EPHESUS, 2003).

Aldosterone can cause sodium and water retention, sympathetic activation and parasympathetic inhibition, all of which are associated with harmful effects in the patient with heart failure. Aldosterone antagonists counteract these effects by directly antagonising the activity of aldosterone, providing a more complete blockade of the renin–angiotensin–aldosterone system when used in conjunction with an ACE inhibitor. Although the combination of spironolactone (at a dose of 50 mg daily or more) and an ACE inhibitor is associated with an increased risk of developing hyperkalaemia, the use of a 25 mg daily dose has been shown to have little effect on serum potassium and provides a significant reduction in mortality. The use of spironolactone is, however, contraindicated in those patients with a serum potassium >5.5 mmol/L or serum creatinine >200 mmol/L. With eplerenone, similar contraindications exist, and therefore close monitoring of blood biochemistry and renal function must be undertaken for the use of either agent. The activity and use of spironolactone and eplerenone are summarised in Table 21.5.

Currently, there is no evidence available regarding the effectiveness and safety of combining an ACE inhibitor, ARB and a mineralocorticoid receptor antagonist, and therefore it is recommended that this combination is avoided until more information about this particular combination becomes available.

Sacubitril

Sacubitril is a neprilysin inhibitor, a new class of medicine with a unique mechanism of action. Neprilysin breaks down endogenous vasoactive peptides (e.g. natriuretic peptides, bradykinin), meaning that neprilysin inhibition elevates plasma levels of these peptides, which in turn offset the activation of the renin–angiotensin–aldosterone system and its negative consequences on symptom control and disease progression in heart failure (see Fig. 21.1).

Replacing ACE inhibitor therapy in suitable patients with the combination of the neprilysin inhibitor, sacubitril, and the ARB valsartan has been shown to reduce cardiovascular mortality and hospital admissions for heart failure in patients who are poorly controlled under treatment with an ACE inhibitor (or ARB), β-blockers and/or mineralocorticoid receptor antagonist (PARADIGM-HF, 2014). Patients shown to benefit are those with moderate to severe heart failure who have either markedly elevated plasma BNP levels or previous hospital admission for heart failure.

Because both ACE inhibitors and sacubitril inhibit the breakdown of bradykinin, there is an increased risk of angioedema with overlapping use of these agents, and therefore it is recommended that ACE inhibitor is stopped at least 36 hours before initiating sacubitril/valsartan. There is also a higher risk of symptomatic hypotension with sacubitril/valsartan than with ACE inhibitors or ARBs alone, and with limited post-marketing experience to date, it is currently recommended that specialist advice is sought before treatment with sacubitril/valsartan is initiated.

Ivabradine

Ivabradine is a new type of medicine that reduces the pacemaker activity of the sinoatrial node. As with β-blockers, ivabradine reduces the heart rate, but in contrast to β-blockers, it lacks negative inotropic effects, which has obvious advantages in patients with heart failure. However, a disadvantage is that it only slows the heart rate when the heart rhythm is driven by the sinoatrial node (sinus rhythm).

The use of ivabradine in heart failure is supported by trial evidence showing that it reduces heart failure deaths and hospitalisation due to heart failure when added to usual care of patients with moderate to severe heart failure (SHIFT, 2010). It is recommended for use in patients who have had a hospital admission for heart failure in the preceding 12 months but have stabilised on standard therapy for at least 4 weeks. Due to the risk of severe bradycardia with the combined use of β-blockers and ivabradine, it is recommended that patients have a sinus rhythm heart rate ≥75 beats/min despite maximum tolerated doses of β-blockers, and specialist advice should be sought before choosing to initiate ivabradine.

Digoxin

There is evidence to show that when digoxin has been used to treat heart failure in patients in sinus rhythm, as an adjunct to ACE inhibitor and diuretic therapy, worsening of symptoms occurs on withdrawal of digoxin (PROVED, 1993; RADIANCE, 1993). Although the use of digoxin in heart failure in patients in sinus rhythm has no measurable impact on mortality, it reduces the number of hospital admissions (DIG, 1997). Consequently, digoxin is currently recommended for use as add-on therapy at low doses in patients with moderate to severe heart failure who remain symptomatic despite adequate doses of ACE inhibitor, β-blocker and diuretic treatment. Due to the lack of effect on mortality, it is unlikely that digoxin would be considered before the other adjunctive therapies available.

Digoxin is a positive inotropic agent and acts by increasing the availability of calcium within the myocardial cell through an inhibition of sodium extrusion, thereby increasing sodium–calcium exchange and leading to enhanced contractility of cardiac muscle. Digoxin increases cardiac output in patients with co-existing atrial fibrillation by suppressing atrioventricular conduction and controlling the ventricular rate. In patients with atrial fibrillation, the serum digoxin concentration usually needs to be at the higher end of the reference range (0.8–2 micrograms/L) or beyond to control the arrhythmia. However, a high serum digoxin concentration is not necessarily required to achieve an inotropic effect in patients in sinus rhythm. Digoxin is also associated with both vagal stimulation and a reduction in sympathetic nerve activity, and these may play important roles in the symptomatic benefits experienced by those patients in sinus rhythm receiving lower doses. In practice, the dose prescribed will be judged appropriate by the clinical response expressed as relief of symptoms and control of ventricular rate. Routine monitoring of serum digoxin concentrations in the pharmaceutical care of the patient is not recommended, other than to confirm or exclude digoxin toxicity or investigate issues around patient adherence.

Digoxin treatment is potentially hazardous due to its low therapeutic index, and so all patients receiving this drug should be regularly reviewed to exclude clinical signs or symptoms of adverse effects. Digoxin may cause bradycardia and lead to potentially fatal cardiac arrhythmias. Other symptoms associated with digoxin toxicity include nausea, vomiting, confusion and visual disturbances. Digoxin toxicity is more pronounced in the presence of metabolic or electrolyte disturbances and in patients with cardiac ischaemia. Those patients who develop hypokalaemia, hypomagnesaemia, hypercalcaemia, alkalosis, hypothyroidism or hypoxia are at particular risk of toxicity. Treatment may be required to restore serum potassium, and in emergency situations, intravenous digoxin-specific antibody fragments can be used to treat life-threatening digoxin toxicity. Table 21.8 summarises the activity and use of digoxin.

Nitrates/hydralazine

Nitrates exert their effects in heart failure predominantly on the venous system, where they cause venodilation, thereby reducing the symptoms of pulmonary congestion. The preferred use of nitrates is in combination with an arterial vasodilator such as hydralazine, which reduces the afterload, to achieve a balanced effect on the venous and arterial circulation. The combined effects of these two drugs lead to an increase in cardiac output, and there is evidence to show the combination is effective and associated with a reduction in mortality in patients with heart failure (V-HeFT I, 1986). Although the combination can improve survival, the reduction in mortality is much smaller than that seen with ACE inhibitors (V-HeFT II, 1991), especially in the white population. The combination has been shown to reduce mortality, heart failure hospitalisation rates and quality of life in patients of African descent, when added as an adjunct to optimum medical therapy (A-HeFT, 2004), and this benefit is sustained (A-HeFT, 2007).

The evidence supports the use of hydralazine 300 mg daily with isosorbide dinitrate (ISDN) 160 mg daily (although in practice an equivalent dose of isosorbide mononitrate, ISMN, is often used). Since the emergence of ACE inhibitors, with their superior effects on morbidity and mortality, the combination has mainly been reserved for patients unable to tolerate or with a contraindication to ACE inhibitor therapy or for those patients of African descent.

Organic nitrate vasodilators work by interacting with sulphydryl groups found in the vascular tissue. Nitric oxide is released from the nitrate compound, and this in turn activates soluble guanylate cyclase in vascular smooth muscle, leading to the vasodilatory effect. Plasma nitric oxide concentrations are not clearly related to pharmacological effects because of their indirect action on the vasculature. Depletion of tissue sulphydryl groupings can occur during continued treatment with nitrates and is partly responsible for the development of tolerance in patients with sustained exposure to high nitrate doses. Restoration of sulphydryl groupings occurs within hours of treatment being interrupted; therefore, nitrate tolerance can be prevented by the use of an asymmetrical dosing regimen to ensure that the patient experiences a daily nitrate-free period of more than 8 hours.

In the acute setting, glyceryl trinitrate (GTN) might be administered intravenously, along with a loop diuretic, to patients with heart failure and concomitant myocardial ischaemia. When using

---

Table 21.8 Inotropic agents used in the treatment of heart failure

Class and agent	Pharmacological half-life	Comment
Cardiac glycosides		
Digoxin	39 h	In renal failure, half-life of digoxin is prolonged. Dosage individualisation required. Serum drug concentration monitoring used to confirm or exclude toxicity or effectiveness. Dose of digitoxin unaffected by renal failure. CNS, visual and GI symptoms linked to digoxin toxicity. No benefit in terms of mortality, but use associated with improved symptoms and reduced hospitalisation for heart failure. Beneficial in AF, although risk of arrhythmias with high doses. If given i.v., must be administered slowly (20 min) to avoid cardiac ischaemia.
Digitoxin	5–8 days	
Phosphodiesterase inhibitors		
Enoximone	4.2 h	Used only in severe heart failure as adjunctive therapy. Associated with arrhythmias and increased mortality with chronic use.
Milrinone	2.4 h	
Sympathomimetics		
Dopexamine	6–7 min	Continuous i.v. use only and should be used with caution in acute heart failure. Generally given in lower doses and titrated up with close monitoring in critical care setting. Dopamine and dobutamine may also be useful agents where appropriate.

AF, Atrial fibrillation; CNS, central nervous system; GI, gastro-intestinal; i.v., intravenous.

this route of administration, it is important that a Teflon-coated catheter is used to avoid adsorption of the GTN onto the intravenous line, and blood pressure is closely monitored.

ISDN can be given orally and is completely absorbed; however, only 25% of a given dose appears as ISDN in serum, with 60% of an oral dose being rapidly converted to ISMN. ISMN is longer acting, and therefore most of the accumulated effects of a dose of ISDN are attributable to the 5-isosorbide mononitrate metabolite. Consequently, a 20 mg dose of ISDN is approximately equivalent to a 10 mg dose of ISMN. In practice, nitrate preparations are usually given orally in the form of ISMN (see Table 21.7).

Hydralazine has a direct action on arteriolar smooth muscle to produce arterial vasodilation. Its use is associated with the risk of causing drug-induced systemic lupus erythematosus (SLE). SLE is an uncommon multisystem connective tissue disorder that is more likely to occur in patients classified as slow acetylators of hydralazine, which accounts for almost half the UK population.

Inotropic/Vasopressor agents

The use of inotropic/vasopressor agents (except digoxin) is almost exclusively limited to hospital practice, where acute heart failure with potentially reversible cardiogenic shock may require the use of agents such as the sympathomimetic dopexamine in an intravenous continuous infusion. They may be used to address persisting hypotension and hypoperfusion in the critical care setting. These agents have inotrope-vasodilator effects that differ according to their action on α, β_1, β_2 and dopamine receptors. Dopexamine acts on β_2 adrenoceptors in cardiac muscle with a lesser effect on peripheral dopamine receptors, which together produces a positive inotropic effect and an increase in renal perfusion (see Table 21.8). Generally, inotropes would only be used where there is hypotension or hypoperfusion. Tolerance to sympathomimetic inotropic agents may develop on prolonged administration, particularly in patients with underlying ischaemia, and is also associated with a risk of precipitating arrhythmias.

Noradrenaline (norepinephrine) is an α-adrenoreceptor agonist; its vasoconstrictor action limits its usefulness in severely hypotensive patients such as those in septic shock. Adrenaline (epinephrine) has β_1-, β_2- and α-adrenoreceptor agonist effects and is used in patients with low vascular resistance. However, it is more arrhythmogenic than dobutamine and should be used with caution.

Phosphodiesterase inhibitors are rarely used in clinical practice as a consequence of trials showing an increased risk of mortality (PROMISE, 1991) and there being little evidence to date to show they improve prognosis or survival (Tang et al, 2015).

Other agents

Direct-acting vasodilators such as sodium nitroprusside are rarely used.

Patients with coronary heart disease may be candidates for calcium-blocking antianginal vasodilators. However, some of these agents can exacerbate co-existing heart failure because their negative inotropic effects offset the potentially beneficial arterial vasodilation. Amlodipine and felodipine have a more selective action on vascular tissue and, therefore, a less pronounced effect on cardiac contractility than other calcium antagonists and should be the agents of choice where appropriate.

In hospitalised patients in whom compromised respiratory function remains despite medical management of heart failure, the treatment options include mechanical ventilation, continuous positive airway pressure ventilation and the use of intra-aortic balloon pumping.

Guidelines

Several groups have produced evidence-based consensus clinical guidelines for the management of chronic heart failure. The focus of the various guidelines tends to be on chronic medication use (European Society of Cardiology, 2016; NICE, 2010; ACC/AHA/HFSA, 2016; SIGN, 2016). All guidelines confirm that ACE inhibitors should be given to all patients with all grades of heart failure, whether symptomatic or asymptomatic, in the absence of contraindication or intolerance.

In patients intolerant of ACE inhibitors, the preferred alternative is an ARB. However, it should be remembered that where ACE inhibitor intolerance is due to renal dysfunction, hypotension or hyperkalaemia, similar effects could be expected with an ARB. For patients with symptomatic heart failure, a loop diuretic is usually recommended to treat oedema and control symptoms. In heart failure patients who are still symptomatic despite being on optimum therapy (ACE inhibitor, β-blocker, mineralocorticoid receptor antagonist with/without a diuretic), the use of adjunctive therapies is recommended, which can include sacubitril/valsartan, ivabradine, hydralazine/nitrate combination and digoxin where the patient is still in sinus rhythm.

There is also debate as to whether diastolic dysfunction is a true diagnosis. The cause of 'apparent' heart failure symptoms can in many cases be attributed to another disease/condition such as respiratory disease, obesity or ischaemic heart disease. However, there may also be some patients in whom the cause of heart failure symptoms remains uncertain. Therefore, specific recommendations for the drug treatment of diastolic heart failure are still lacking.

Patient care

Heart failure remains poorly understood by the general public, among whom only 3% were able to identify the condition when presented with a list of typical symptoms. Patients with heart failure are often elderly and often include patients with comorbidity such as coronary heart disease and hypertension. Other complications include renal impairment, polypharmacy and variable adherence to prescribed medication regimens. Where renal function is compromised, careful attention to dosage selection is required for drugs excreted largely unchanged in the urine. Patients with heart failure are at particular risk of fluid or electrolyte imbalance, adverse effects and drug interactions. Consequently, careful monitoring is indicated to help detect problems associated with suboptimal drug therapy, unwanted drug effects and poor patient adherence.

A number of therapeutic problems may be encountered by the patient with heart failure. Notably, heart failure often complicates other serious illness and is a common cause of hospital admission. In addition to monitoring clinical signs and symptoms in the acute setting, there should be monitoring of fluid and electrolyte balance, assessment of renal and hepatic function, and performance of chest radiograph, electrocardiograph and haemodynamic measurements where appropriate.

Patient education and self-monitoring

The patient must be in a position to understand the need for treatment and the benefits and risks offered by prescribed medication before concordance with a treatment plan can be achieved. Appropriate patient education is necessary to encourage an understanding of the condition and inform patients of the extent of the condition and how prescribed drug treatment will work and affect their daily lives. It is also important to encourage them to be an active participant in their care where appropriate. Specific advice should be given to reinforce the timing of doses and how each medication should be taken. Patients also need to be advised of potentially troublesome symptoms that may occur with the medication and whether such effects are avoidable, self-limiting or a cause for concern.

Patients should be made aware that diuretics will increase urine production and that doses are usually timed for the morning to avoid inconvenience during the rest of the day or overnight. However, there are cases where patients are advised that they can alter the timing of the dose(s) if required to suit their lifestyle or social commitments, with the agreement of their doctor. There are also some patients who use a flexible diuretic dosing regimen, where they can take an extra dose of diuretic in response to worsening signs or symptoms as part of an agreed self-management protocol. To use such a regimen, the patient has to monitor and record his or her weight on a daily basis, have clear instructions to take an extra dose of diuretic when a notable increase in weight is detected as a result of fluid retention and know when to seek medical attention.

Patients with heart failure are at an increased risk of acute kidney injury when experiencing intercurrent illness that can cause dehydration (e.g. diarrhoea, vomiting, bacterial or viral infections) as a result of their condition and the medicines they are taking. In dehydration, the reduced cardiac output is further exacerbated by a loss in circulating blood volume, leading to reduced renal perfusion. In this situation the renin–angiotensin–aldosterone system is normally activated to maintain renal blood flow, but the use of ACE inhibitors, ARBs and/or MRAs in patients with heart failure offsets this compensatory mechanism. It is therefore important that patients and carers are made aware of the potential harms of continuing to take these medicines when acutely ill. In Scotland, a 'Medicine Sick Day Rules' card has been introduced that lists those problematic medicines that patients should stop

for 24–48 hours when they experience a dehydrating illness (http://ihub.scot/spsp/primary-care/medicine-sick-day-rules-card/).

It is also important for patients to be aware of signs and symptoms of drug toxicity with medicines such as digoxin (e.g. anorexia, diarrhoea, nausea and vomiting), and to be aware of the action to be taken should these symptoms occur.

Timing of doses is also important. If a nitrate regimen is being used, then patients must be made aware that the last dose of the nitrate should be taken in mid- to late afternoon to ensure that a nitrate-free period occurs overnight, thus reducing the risk of nitrate tolerance. However, patients with prominent nocturnal symptoms require separate consideration. Where β-blockers are introduced, it is important that the patient is aware of the need for gradual dose titration due to the risk of the medication aggravating heart failure symptoms. Certain medicines for the treatment of minor ailments that are available for purchase over the counter without a prescription can aggravate heart failure, such as ibuprofen, antihistamines and effervescent formulations. It is important that patients know what action to take if their symptoms become progressively worse and whom to contact when necessary for advice. Table 21.9 provides a general patient education and self-monitoring checklist, highlighting the typical areas where advice should be given.

Monitoring effectiveness of drug treatment

Therapeutic effectiveness is confirmed by assessing the patient for improvements in reported symptoms, such as shortness of breath and oedema, and for noticeable changes in exercise tolerance. Oedema is often visible and remarked upon by patients, especially in the feet (ankles) and hands (wrists and fingers). Increased oedema may be reflected by an increase in the patient's body weight and can be more easily assessed if the patient routinely records his or her weight and reviews this on a daily basis. Questions about tolerance to exercise are also useful in identifying patients who may be experiencing difficulties with their condition or where the treatment plan is suboptimal. Onset or deterioration of symptoms is often slow, and patients are more inclined to adapt their lifestyle gradually by moderating daily activities to compensate. This should be borne in mind whenever a patient assessment is undertaken.

Identifying the symptoms of poor heart failure control can be complicated by many factors, such as the presence of conditions like arthritis and parkinsonism, which can also affect a patient's mobility. Poor control of respiratory disease, presenting as an increased shortness of breath or exacerbation of other respiratory symptoms, can also be mistaken for loss of control of heart failure. Therefore, consideration of these and other factors is necessary in the interpretation of presenting symptoms because a deterioration in symptoms may not be solely due to worsening heart failure or ineffective heart failure medication.

Dietary factors can lead to loss of symptom control, where failure to restrict sodium intake may contribute to an ongoing problem of fluid retention. Simple dietary advice to avoid

Table 21.9 Patient education and self-monitoring in the treatment of heart failure

Topic	Advice	Comment
Diuretics	• Will cause diuresis • Timing of dose • Flexible dosing (where indicated)	Monitor for incontinence, muscle weakness, confusion, dizziness, gout, unusual gain in weight within very short time period (few days). Use of diary to record and monitor daily weight can help identify when to take an agreed extra dose of diuretic. Patient also able to adjust time of dose to suit lifestyle where necessary.
Angiotensin-converting enzyme inhibitors and angiotensin II receptor blockers	• Improve symptoms • Avoid standing rapidly	Monitor for hypotension, dizziness, cough, taste disturbance, sore throat, rashes, tingling in hands, joint pain, signs of swelling under the skin (if the throat/tongue are involved and breathing is affected, urgent medical attention is required).
β-Blockers	• Symptoms worsen initially • Gradual increase in dose	Monitor for hypotension, dizziness, headache, fatigue, gastro-intestinal disturbances, bradycardia.
Sacubitril/valsartan	• Improve symptoms • Gradual increase in dose required	Monitor for dizziness, light-headedness, cough, diarrhoea, tiredness, signs of swelling under the skin (if the throat/tongue are involved and breathing is affected, urgent medical attention is required).
Cardiac glycosides	• Report toxic symptoms	Monitor for signs or symptoms of toxicity, such as anorexia, nausea, visual disturbances, diarrhoea, confusion, social withdrawal.
Nitrates	• Timing of dose • Postural hypotension • Avoid standing rapidly	Monitor for headache, hypotension, dizziness, flushing (face or neck), gastro-intestinal upset. Ensure asymmetrical dosing pattern for nitrates to provide nitrate-free period and reduce risk of tolerance developing.
Potassium salts	• Administration of dose (soluble + non-soluble)	Monitor for gastro-intestinal disturbances, swallowing difficulty, diarrhoea, tiredness, limb weakness. Ensure patient knows how to take the medication safely, e.g. swallow whole immediately after food, or soluble forms to be taken with appropriate amount of water/fruit juice after allowing fizzing to stop.
Purchased medicines	• Choice of medicines	Ensure patient is aware of need to seek advice when purchasing medicines for minor ailments. Ask pharmacist to confirm suitability when selecting.
Understanding the condition	• What heart failure is • Impact on lifestyle • Treatment goals	Ensure patient understands the condition, treatment goals and complications that may affect quality of life. Important to motivate the patient with respect to lifestyle modification and achievement of agreed treatment goals relative to the degree of heart failure present (asymptomatic, mild, moderate or severe symptoms).
Health issues	• Diet; sodium intake • Alcohol intake • Smoking • Exercise • Other risk factors	Issues related to diet, alcohol consumption, smoking habit, regular gentle exercise (walking). Other associated risk factors (e.g. hypertension, ischaemic heart disease) need to be addressed where appropriate.

processed foods and not to add salt to food should be reinforced. According to some manufacturers, the absorption of ACE inhibitors, for example, captopril and perindopril, may be slowed by food or antacids, and therefore patients should be advised to take the dose before food in the morning to ensure maximum effect.

Patients with heart failure may often receive suboptimal drug treatment, due to the fact that they are not prescribed first-line therapy, such as ACE inhibitors, β-blockers and mineralocorticoid receptor antagonists, and the dosage is less than the recommended target dose. All patients at risk of suboptimal treatment need to be routinely identified, and this will

Box 21.1 Criteria for the assessment of drug treatment in a patient with chronic heart failure (Scottish Intercollegiate Guidelines Network, 2016)

Need for drug therapy (all patients)
1. Is an ACE inhibitor prescribed?
If symptomatic (NYHA II or above)
2. Is a β-blocker prescribed?
3. Is a MRA prescribed?
4. If intolerant to ACE inhibitor or MRA, is an ARB prescribed?
5. Has patient received pneumococcal vaccination?
6. Has patient received influenza vaccination?

Need for drug therapy (as appropriate)
7. If symptomatic on optimised doses of ACE inhibitor, β-blocker and MRA, has specialist advice on use of sacubitril/valsartan been considered?
8. If symptomatic on optimised therapy with a β-blocker, has specialist advice on use of ivabradine been considered?
9. If symptomatic on optimised therapy including 7 and/or 8 above, has specialist advice on use of digoxin or H-ISDN been considered?
10. If post-MI, is an antiplatelet and statin prescribed?
11. In AF is thromboembolic prophylaxis prescribed?

Need for dose titration
12. If an ACE inhibitor is prescribed, is target dose achieved?
13. If an ARB is prescribed, is target dose achieved?

14. If a β-blocker is prescribed, is target dose achieved?
15. If an MRA is prescribed, is target dose achieved?
16. If warfarin is prescribed, is dose titrated to INR?

Medication safety
17. Aggravating drugs avoided (if possible):
 a. NSAIDs
 b. Tricyclic antidepressants
 c. Some antihistamines (e.g. diphenhydramine)
 d. Dihydropyridine calcium channel blockers (except amlodipine or felodipine)
 e. Diltiazem, verapamil
 f. Anti-diabetics (e.g. glitazones, gliptins)
 g. Minoxidil
 h. Itraconazole and other azole antifungals
 i. Macrolide antibiotics
 j. Corticosteroids
 k. Tadalafil
 l. Lithium

ACE, Angiotensin-converting enzyme; AF, atrial fibrillation; ARB, angiotensin receptor blocker; H-ISDN, hydralazine-isosorbide dinitrate; INR, international normalised ratio; MI, myocardial infarction; MRA, mineralocorticoid receptor antagonist; NSAID, non-steroidal anti-inflammatory drug.

require the involvement of healthcare professionals in the monitoring of symptoms and the individualisation of each patient's therapeutic plan.

In an effort to systematically identify whether a patient's therapeutic plan adheres to the current evidence base for treatment and whether any changes might be required to optimise therapy, the audit tool shown in Box 21.1 could be used in routine practice. The tool has been derived from published consensus-based clinical guidelines and could underpin a more comprehensive medication review.

Monitoring safety of drug treatment

A number of issues around the safe use of medication must be considered, especially in those patients with comorbidity and/or a high number of prescribed medicines. In these patients there is an increased risk of drug–drug and drug–disease interactions (Tables 21.10–21.12). It is important to be aware of clinically important interactions and to investigate potentially problematic combinations, as well as to regularly assess the patient for any signs or symptoms of drug therapy problems. Monitoring for problems such as negative inotropic effects, excessive blood pressure reduction and salt and fluid retention should be undertaken, and where appropriate, laboratory measurement of serum drug concentration (digoxin) or physiological markers (potassium, creatinine) should be performed to confirm or exclude adverse effects. Patients started on an ACE inhibitor should have renal function and serum electrolytes checked at 1 and 3 months after starting therapy, and every 6 months once a maintenance dose is reached.

Potential problems with diuretic therapy

The use of diuretic therapy for sodium and water retention is common in the treatment of heart failure, although there can be a number of problems for the patient to contend with. Elderly patients in particular are at risk from the unwanted effects of diuretics. The increase in urine volume can worsen incontinence or precipitate urinary retention in the presence of an enlarged prostate, whereas overuse can lead to a loss of control of heart failure and worsening of symptoms. Rapid diuresis with a loop diuretic leading to more than a 1 kg loss in body weight per day may exacerbate heart failure due to an acute reduction in blood volume, hypotension and diminished renal perfusion, with a consequent increase in renin release. Prolonged and excessive doses of diuretics can also contribute to symptoms of fatigue as a consequence of electrolyte disturbance and dehydration. The adverse biochemical effects of excessive diuresis include uraemia, hypokalaemia and alkalosis. Diuretic-induced glucose intolerance may affect diabetic control in type 2 diabetes, but more commonly diuretics reveal glucose intolerance in patients who are not diagnosed as being diabetic. Diuretics also increase serum urate, leading to hyperuricaemia, although this may not require a change in drug therapy if symptoms of gout are absent (estimated incidence of 2%).

Hyponatraemia may occur with diuretics and is usually due to water retention rather than sodium loss. Severe hyponatraemia (serum sodium concentration of less than 115 mmol/L) causes confusion and drowsiness. It commonly arises when potassium-sparing agents are used in diuretic combinations.

Table 21.10 Monitoring the effectiveness of drug treatment in patients with heart failure

Consider	Monitor for	Comment
Clinical markers	Poor symptom control Achievement of agreed treatment goals	Signs or symptoms of undertreatment or advancing disease need to be addressed (dyspnoea, breathlessness and/or fatigue). The aim is for good symptom control and either maintenance or improvement in quality of life. Persisting symptoms or hospitalisation may indicate a revision of drug therapy or the addition of other agents where appropriate.
Interactions	Drug–drug interactions	Some interactions may result in reduced effectiveness and require dosage adjustment or change in choice of drug.
Adherence	Formulation acceptability Dose timing and interval Unusual time interval between requests for prescription medication	Poor adherence can result from drug being ineffective (over- or underuse), experience of side effects, a complicated drug regimen or patient behaviour (intentional nonadherence or forgetfulness). Reasons need to be identified and addressed where possible, e.g. adjusting frequency and timing of doses, review choice of formulation, education. Initiation of devices to improve compliance should be considered where appropriate.
Evidence-based prescribing	Implementation of evidence-based guidelines Audit of prescribed treatment for heart failure	The drug of choice for a particular patient may not reflect the evidence base for treatment for patients with heart failure. It is important to ensure evidence-based treatments are considered for every patient, and choices of medication confirmed or changed where appropriate. Audit of guideline recommendations to help confirm that treatment plans are optimal can be systematically applied to help assess appropriateness of treatment (see Box 21.1).
Multidisciplinary working	Input from other healthcare professionals	It is important to be aware of what care has already been provided to minimise the risk of giving conflicting advice to the patient or duplicating work already done. It may also allow reinforcement of key information. There is an increasing evidence base for the benefits of multidisciplinary models of care for chronic heart failure patients.

Table 21.11 Common drug–drug interactions with prescribed heart failure medication

Drug	Interacts with	Result of interaction
Diuretic	NSAIDs Carbamazepine Lithium	Decreased effect of diuretic and increased risk of renal impairment Increased risk of hyponatraemia Excretion of lithium impaired (thiazides worse than loop diuretics)
ACE inhibitor or ARB	NSAIDs Ciclosporin Lithium Diuretics Sacubitril/valsartan	Antagonism of hypotensive effect; increased risk of renal impairment Increased risk of hyperkalaemia Excretion of lithium impaired Enhanced hypotensive effect; increased risk of hyperkalaemia with potassium-sparing drugs Increased risk of angioedema, hypotension, hyperkalaemia, renal impairment
Sacubitril/valsartan	ACE inhibitor or ARB Aliskiren Statins, e.g. atorvastatin Ciclosporin or rifampicin Cidofovir or tenofovir	Increased risk of angioedema, hypotension, hyperkalaemia, renal impairment Increased risk of hypotension, hyperkalaemia, renal impairment Increased risk of statin adverse effects Increased risk of hypotension Increased risk of hypotension
β-Blocker	Amiodarone Diltiazem Verapamil	Increased risk of bradycardia Increased risk of AV block and bradycardia Increased risk of hypotension, heart failure and asystole
Mineralocorticoid receptor antagonists	ACE inhibitor or ARB Digoxin Carbamazepine Antibacterials, e.g. clarithromycin Anticonvulsants, e.g. phenytoin Antifungals, e.g. ketoconazole St John's Wort	Increased risk of hyperkalaemia Increased plasma concentration of digoxin Decreased plasma concentration of eplerenone Increased plasma concentration of eplerenone Decreased plasma concentration of eplerenone Increased plasma concentration of eplerenone Decreased plasma concentration of eplerenone

Table 21.11 Common drug–drug interactions with prescribed heart failure medication—cont'd

Drug	Interacts with	Result of interaction
Digoxin	Amiodarone	Increased digoxin level (need to halve maintenance dose of digoxin)
	Propafenone	Increased digoxin level (need to halve maintenance dose of digoxin)
	Quinidine	Increased digoxin level (need to halve maintenance dose of digoxin)
	Verapamil	Increased risk of AV block
	Diuretics	Increased risk of hyperkalaemia and therefore toxicity
	Amphotericin	Increased cardiac toxicity if hypokalaemia present
Nitrates	Sildenafil	Increased hypotensive effect
	Heparin	Increased excretion of heparin

ACE, Angiotensin-converting enzyme; ARB, angiotensin receptor blocker; AV, atrioventricular; NSAIDs, non-steroidal anti-inflammatory drugs.

Table 21.12 Common drug–disease interactions with prescribed heart failure medication

Drug	Concurrent disease	Potential outcome
Diuretic	Prostatism	Urinary retention/incontinence
	Hyperuricaemia	Exacerbation of gout
	Liver cirrhosis	Encephalopathy
ACE inhibitor or ARB	Renal artery stenosis	Renal failure
	Severe aortic stenosis	Exacerbation of heart failure
	Renal impairment	Renal failure
	Hypotension	Further hypotension and cardiogenic shock
Sacubitril/valsartan	Renal artery stenosis	Renal failure
	Renal impairment	Renal failure
	Hepatic impairment	Hepatic failure
	Hypotension	Further hypotension and cardiogenic shock
β-Blocker	Asthma	Bronchoconstriction/respiratory arrest
	Bradyarrhythmias	Exacerbation of heart failure
	Hypotension	Further hypotension and cardiogenic shock
Mineralocorticoid receptor antagonists	Renal impairment	Hyperkalaemia
Digoxin	Bradyarrhythmias	Exacerbation of heart failure
	Renal impairment	Exacerbation of heart failure and digoxin toxicity leading to cardiac arrhythmias

ACE, Angiotensin-converting enzyme; ARB, angiotensin receptor blocker.

Diuretics may also lead to hypokalaemia as a result of urinary sodium increasing the rate of K^+/Na^+ exchange in the distal tubule. The occurrence of hypokalaemia is hazardous for patients receiving digoxin and also for those with ischaemic heart disease or conduction disorders. It is more commonly found with thiazide diuretics than loop agents and is more likely to occur when diuretics are used for heart failure than for hypertension. This is probably due to the fact that higher doses are used, and there is an associated activation of the renin–angiotensin system. Patients with a serum potassium level of less than 3.5 mmol/L require treatment with potassium supplements or the addition of a potassium-sparing diuretic. The use of a potassium-sparing diuretic is considered to be more effective at preventing hypokalaemia than using potassium supplements. Prevention of hypokalaemia requires at least 25 mmol of potassium, whereas treatment requires 60–120 mmol of potassium daily. Because proprietary diuretic-potassium combination products usually contain less than 12 mmol in each dose, their use is often inappropriate.

Potassium supplements are poorly tolerated at the high doses often needed to treat hypokalaemia, and a liquid formulation is more preferable to a solid form. This is mainly due to the fact that solid forms can produce local high concentrations of potassium salts in the gastro-intestinal tract, with the risk of damage to the tract in patients with swallowing difficulties or delayed gastro-intestinal transit. In patients with deteriorating renal function or renal failure, the use of potassium supplements or potassium-sparing diuretics might cause hyperkalaemia, and therefore careful monitoring of these agents is essential.

Potential problems with angiotensin-converting enzyme inhibitor, angiotensin II receptor blocker and mineralocorticoid receptor antagonist therapy

ACE inhibitors are the cornerstone of the treatment of heart failure, but there are also risks associated with their use. ARBs, which also act on the renin–angiotensin–aldosterone system, pose similar risks to those recognised for ACE inhibitors. Both agents can predispose patients to hyperkalaemia through a reduction in circulating aldosterone; therefore, potassium supplements or potassium-retaining agents should be used with care when co-prescribed, and careful monitoring of serum potassium should be mandatory. Although potassium retention can be a problem with ACE inhibitors and ARBs, it can also be an advantage by helping counteract the potassium loss that can result from the use of diuretic therapy. However, because this effect on potassium cannot be predicted, laboratory monitoring is still necessary to confirm that serum potassium concentration remains within safe limits.

The use of a mineralocorticoid receptor antagonist with an ACE inhibitor (or ARB if the patient is ACE inhibitor intolerant) can be safely undertaken with minimal effects on the serum potassium concentration, provided that recommended target doses for the mineralocorticoid receptor antagonist are not exceeded (see Table 21.6). Although this is usually the case, laboratory monitoring of potassium is mandatory to ensure patient safety. Heparin therapy has also been shown to increase the risk of hyperkalaemia when used alongside ACE inhibitor or ARB therapy, and therefore a similar approach to monitoring should be taken when co-prescribed.

When initiating ACE inhibitor or ARB therapy, volume depletion due to prior use of a diuretic increases the risk of a large drop in blood pressure occurring after the first dose. As a consequence, diuretic treatment is usually withheld during the initiation phase of therapy in an effort to minimise this effect.

A dry cough, which may be accompanied by a voice change, occurs in about 10% of patients receiving an ACE inhibitor. It is more common in women and is associated with a raised level of kinins. Rashes, loss or disturbances of taste, mouth ulcers and proteinuria may also occur with ACE inhibitor therapy, particularly with captopril. These unwanted effects tend to be more common in patients with connective tissue disorders.

A number of ACE inhibitors are administered as pro-drugs, so close monitoring is advised in patients with liver dysfunction, as this could reduce the benefits associated with their use. Most ACE inhibitors are dependent on the kidney for excretion and require careful dosage titration in patients with existing renal dysfunction. Differences in the pharmacokinetic characteristics do not fully explain the differences in duration of action seen with the ACE inhibitors because this is also related to ACE binding affinity. Throughout treatment, the dose must be individualised to obtain maximum benefit in relation to symptom relief and survival, with minimum side effects. When the experience of adverse effects requires a review of therapeutic alternatives, ARBs can be considered as an alternative treatment option. Although the side-effect profile of ARB therapy is very similar to that of ACE inhibitors, it is not identical.

Potential problems with β-blocker therapy

Previously, the use of β-blockers was contraindicated in patients with heart failure due to negative inotropic and chronotropic effects. However, β-blockers have clearly been shown to be safe and effective in patients with symptoms of heart failure and should be used in patients in the absence of contraindications or intolerance. Initiation of treatment and titration of dose must be done under close supervision, with very small dose increments used to minimise transient worsening of heart failure symptoms. Titration of the dose to target is normally performed over a number of weeks or months, and close patient monitoring is required to ensure safety is not compromised. The maximum tolerable dose for a patient may be less than the target dose and may limit further dose titration. Monitoring for excessive bradycardia or rapid deterioration of symptoms is necessary to ensure patient safety while also monitoring the patient's prescribed dose to ensure that dosage increments are gradual and that the patient is not subjected to an overall worsening of symptoms.

Potential problems with sacubitril/valsartan therapy

The sacubitril/valsartan combination is the most recent addition to the range of medicines to treat heart failure, and given that one of the agents is an ARB, there will be a need for a similar approach to monitoring patient safety as outlined previously. There is also a need to be alert to the possible development of angioedema, particularly where there is a family history. Any swelling of the face, lips, tongue and/or throat, which may cause difficulties in breathing or swallowing, require immediate medical attention. Careful monitoring should be undertaken when switching from an ACE inhibitor to this combination, and it is important to ensure an interval of at least 36 hours between stopping the ACE inhibitor and starting the new therapy.

Potential problems with digoxin therapy

Although digoxin has been shown to reduce hospitalisation rates for patients with heart failure, its use is associated with a range of adverse effects, including nonspecific signs and symptoms of toxicity such as nausea, anorexia, tiredness, weakness, diarrhoea, confusion and visual disturbances. Digoxin also has the potential to cause fatal arrhythmias. It slows atrioventricular conduction and produces bradycardia, but it may also cause various ventricular and supraventricular arrhythmias. Digoxin toxicity typically causes conduction disturbances, with enhanced automaticity leading to premature ventricular contractions. Patients at particular risk are those with myocardial ischaemia, hypoxia, acidosis or renal failure.

The appropriateness of digoxin dosage should be guided by assessment of the patient's renal function (from serum creatinine and creatinine clearance determinations) and from the patient's

Table 21.13 Monitoring the safety of drug treatment in patients with heart failure

Consider	Monitor	Comment
Clinical markers	Side effects Toxicity Adverse drug reactions	There is a need to monitor for signs/symptoms of overtreatment with prescribed medication, such as diuretics (dehydration) and digoxin (nausea and vomiting). Look for signs of patient intolerance, allergy, serious adverse effects or troublesome side effects. Document unexpected adverse drug reactions if reported.
Laboratory markers	Changes in organ function Biochemical changes Haematological changes Suspected digoxin toxicity	Renal function assessment and implications for drug choice and dosage individualisation required, especially in the elderly and for initiation or titration of ACE inhibitor therapy (creatinine, potassium, urea). Hypokalaemia can lead to digoxin toxicity, and serum drug concentration measurement may be performed to confirm or exclude toxicity. Haematological side effects with some drugs have been reported, e.g. ACE inhibitors; therefore, laboratory checks may be required in response to clinical signs/symptoms presented.
Interactions	Drug–drug interactions Drug–disease interactions	Some interactions may result in harm to the patient.
Comorbidity	Drug selection for concomitant conditions	The presence of heart failure may influence treatment choice for co-existing diseases or conditions, e.g. coronary artery disease, thyroid disease, respiratory disease. Where possible, ensure drugs known to worsen heart failure are avoided or used with caution, e.g. non-steroidal anti-inflammatory agents or corticosteroids in rheumatoid arthritis.

ACE, Angiotensin-converting enzyme.

pulse rate. Renal function may also be affected by drug therapy or loss of control of heart failure; therefore, any medicine that affects in digoxin clearance will have an impact on the serum digoxin concentration. The possibility of a high serum digoxin concentration should also be considered in any patient whose health deteriorates or who shows signs and symptoms of potential digoxin toxicity.

Potential problems with other cardiovascular drugs

There are a number of other cardiovascular drugs that may be prescribed for patients with diseases or conditions other than heart failure, with some agents capable of worsening or aggravating symptoms. Patients with coronary artery disease may be candidates for calcium-blocking antianginal vasodilators. However, some of these agents, for example, diltiazem and verapamil, can exacerbate co-existing heart failure because their negative inotropic effects offset the potentially beneficial arterial vasodilation. Second-generation dihydropyridines such as amlodipine and felodipine have a preferential action on the vasculature. They have less pronounced effects on cardiac contractility than other calcium antagonists, and this makes them the agents of choice where a limitation of the heart rate is not required.

Symptoms of fainting or dizziness on standing may indicate a need to review diuretic or vasodilator therapy. Patients should be reassured about mild postural effects and given advice to avoid standing from a chair too quickly. The patient and the healthcare team need to confirm the safety of the patient's treatment plan regularly and be vigilant for any signs or symptoms suggesting otherwise.

A summary of the monitoring activity required to ensure the safety of drug use is outlined in Table 21.13.

Potential problems with non-cardiovascular agents

A number of agents should be avoided or used with caution in patients with heart failure because of their known negative inotropic or pro-arrhythmic effects that may aggravate symptoms of heart failure (see Box 21.1). In particular, the use of non-steroidal anti-inflammatory drugs (NSAIDs) should be actively discouraged where possible. Not only do NSAIDs cause fluid retention and put patients at increased risk of bleeding, especially if they are already taking antiplatelets or anticoagulants, but there is also an increased risk of acute renal failure, particularly in those on long-term use and in the elderly, particularly when they experience intercurrent illness (diarrhoea, vomiting, severe infections) with dehydration. Recent articles have described the synergistic/cumulative adverse renal effects of combinations of ACE inhibitors or ARBs with diuretics and NSAIDs, which are particularly common in patients with heart failure.

Case studies

Case 21.1

Mr GF, a 57-year-old, suffered an MI 12 months ago and at that time was also found to have left ventricular systolic dysfunction on echocardiography. His functional status is currently classed as NYHA II. At your request, he has agreed to see you for a medication review regarding his drug therapy. He has a history of type 2 diabetes mellitus (8 years), and his current prescription includes enalapril 10 mg twice daily, gliclazide 80 mg twice daily, bisoprolol 5 mg daily, aspirin 75 mg daily, and a glyceryl trinitrate spray to use when required.

Question

Is the current treatment plan for heart failure optimal?

Answer

Mr GF has echocardiographic evidence of left ventricular systolic dysfunction, and some signs and symptoms of heart failure are present. The absence of diuretic therapy should be explored as part of the review, and monitoring for signs/symptoms of fluid retention would be included as part of ongoing patient monitoring activity. He is prescribed an ACE inhibitor at the recommended target dose (enalapril 10–20 mg twice daily). Treatment with this agent could be increased if required. The current dose of bisoprolol (5 mg daily) is less than the recommended target and could, therefore, be titrated to a dose of 10 mg daily or the maximum tolerable dose. Any titration should be implemented gradually over a period of weeks or months, with close monitoring of blood pressure and heart rate. Regular assessment of the patient for side effects or signs and symptoms of heart failure should also be undertaken because each incremental rise in β-blocker dose may be accompanied by a worsening of heart failure symptoms. When considering other potential changes to the treatment plan for heart failure, there may be an opportunity for the introduction of a mineralocorticoid receptor antagonist.

With Mr GF's history of MI and type 2 diabetes mellitus, his cardiovascular risk is high, and he should therefore also be prescribed lipid-lowering therapy (regardless of his serum cholesterol measurement), for example, a statin.

Case 21.2

Mrs JM, 66-year-old, presents with a new prescription for candesartan 4 mg daily. On checking her medication record, she has been prescribed lisinopril 20 mg daily, bisoprolol 10 mg daily and furosemide 40 mg daily for the last 6 months to treat her heart failure (NYHA II–III). Her blood pressure was measured 2 weeks ago and was 128/78 mmHg.

Question

How do you respond to the new prescription?

Answer

It is unclear from the information given whether candesartan is prescribed as an adjunct to ACE inhibitor therapy (provided the dose has been optimised) or as an alternative to ACE inhibitor due to intolerance. If being used as an adjunct, it is also unclear whether the patient has an intolerance to an MRA, which would be the preferred choice according to the available evidence. Therefore, it is important to confirm the intended use of candesartan in this case through speaking to the patient and/or prescriber. If candesartan is being used as an alternative to either the ACE inhibitor or MRA, it is important to establish the reason for intolerance and ensure the therapeutic choice is appropriate for the patient. Patients are usually found to be intolerant of ACE inhibitors for three main reasons: dry cough, hypotension or compromised renal function. Because heart failure can produce

symptoms of a dry cough, it can sometimes be difficult to ascertain whether the ACE inhibitor or the heart failure is responsible. Dry cough occurs secondary to the inhibition of bradykinin metabolism and is generally identified shortly after initiation of an ACE inhibitor or after a dose increase; therefore, inquiry into the timing of symptoms attributed to ACE inhibitor intolerance is important. If the reason is due to persistent dry cough, an ARB would be a suitable alternative. However, if the ACE inhibitor intolerance is related to hypotension or renal dysfunction, it is likely an ARB would induce similar adverse effects, and therefore other alternatives may need to be discussed with a heart failure specialist. In patients intolerant of an MRA, the main reasons tend to be related to hyperkalaemia or unacceptable side effects such as gynaecomastia in men, gastro-intestinal intolerance and renal dysfunction.

If candesartan is being used as adjunctive therapy, careful introduction and titration of dose must be undertaken due to the increased risk of hypotension, renal dysfunction and hyperkalaemia. ACE inhibitors and ARBs are both potassium conserving. The addition of candesartan would normally be under the guidance of a heart failure specialist and should be initiated at a low dose and gradually titrated up to the target (32 mg daily) or maximum tolerable dose. It is important to note that dose increases during the titration period should be at least 2 weeks apart. Although Mrs JM has a normal blood pressure measurement at present, it is unclear whether renal function or blood biochemistry has previously been checked, and it is important that this is confirmed before starting candesartan. The monitoring plan for Mrs JM should include regular checks of blood pressure, serum creatinine (and estimation of renal function) and serum potassium and clinical assessment for any signs/symptoms of adverse effects/intolerance. This should be done 7–14 days after initiation and final dose titration. Because the addition of candesartan should improve heart failure symptom control, regular patient monitoring will allow an assessment of the effectiveness of therapy.

Case 21.3

Mr HS, 72-year-old, is admitted to hospital with increasing shortness of breath at rest. He has a previous medical history of severe left ventricular systolic dysfunction, confirmed by echocardiography, and angina. Before admission he had been taking the following medication: lisinopril 10 mg daily, furosemide 80 mg each morning and 40 mg at 2 pm, digoxin 62.5 micrograms each morning, ISMN SR 60 mg daily, glyceryl trinitrate spray 1–2 doses as required, aspirin 75 mg dispersible each morning. His chest X-ray shows severe pulmonary oedema, his blood pressure is 110/70 mmHg and serum urea and electrolytes are within normal range. During the admission, carvedilol 3.125 mg twice daily is started.

Questions

1. What therapeutic options would you choose to treat the acute symptoms presented by Mr HS at the beginning of his admission?
2. Was the addition of carvedilol appropriate for this patient?
3. What other drug treatment options might be considered for this patient in the longer-term?

Answers

1. The administration of furosemide by the intravenous route is necessary because there is decreased absorption of oral furosemide secondary to gastro-intestinal oedema in acute heart failure. The administration of i.v. furosemide allows rapid serum levels to be

achieved, which has the benefit of producing venodilation (reducing the preload), which helps improve symptoms long before there is diuresis. Only after the oedema has resolved should the patient revert back to oral administration of diuretics. At this time, the dosage can be adjusted to maintain an appropriate fluid balance. Where diuresis is inadequate with an oral loop diuretic alone, the addition of a thiazide diuretic such as bendroflumethiazide or metolazone should be considered. Metolazone should be given initially at a low dose of 2.5 mg daily, or less often if required, to avoid rapid diuresis leading to hypotension and/or renal failure.

2. Although there is good evidence to show that β-blocker therapy is safe and effective for patients with NYHA stage IV heart failure, it is not currently recommended that it should be initiated in patients with acute symptoms of heart failure. Where β-blocker therapy is indicated, initiation should occur when the patient's heart failure has been stable for at least 2 weeks and started at a very low dose on specialist advice (i.e. carvedilol 3.125 mg twice daily). The dose should be titrated gradually over a period of months towards the recommended target dose where appropriate, provided the patient tolerates each increment. In Mr HS's case, however, there is evidence to suggest that β-blocker use at discharge can be done safely in patients with heart failure, with positive effects on survival for both heart failure and coronary heart disease.

3. There is also scope to increase the dose of lisinopril to 20–35 mg daily, provided the patient can tolerate the higher dose, because this is associated with greater benefits on morbidity and mortality. Based on his systolic blood pressure and assuming satisfactory renal function, there is no reason why this option cannot be explored, and it would be reasonable to delay any titration of dosage until the symptoms become more stable. This is important because the use of large doses of loop diuretics in acutely ill patients may predispose to ACE inhibitor–induced renal impairment. A mineralocorticoid receptor antagonist could be added to Mr HS's existing drug therapy if the patient is poorly controlled on optimised doses of ACE inhibitor and β-blocker. This would provide benefits to morbidity and mortality if added to the existing treatment plan. The decision to initiate further treatment options would usually lie with a heart failure specialist based on the individual patient, which may include replacing digoxin therapy with a more effective agent. As Mr HS approaches end-stage heart failure, there may be a need to focus solely on symptom relief.

Case 21.4

Mrs FM, a 70-year-old with chronic asthma and mild heart failure, has been prescribed naproxen 250 mg three times daily. On inspection of her medication record, it is discovered that she is also receiving:

- furosemide 40 mg each morning,
- ramipril 5 mg in the morning,
- prednisolone 5 mg daily,
- salbutamol inhaler two puffs four times daily when required,
- salmeterol 50 micrograms inhaler one puff twice daily,
- beclometasone 250 micrograms inhaler two puffs twice daily,
- omeprazole 10 mg daily.

When asked her about symptom control, she said she is still breathless at night, which, in addition to her painful knee, is keeping her awake.

Questions

1. Do you think Mrs FM should be taking naproxen?
2. What other aspects of this patient's medication regimen could be improved?

3. What is the likely effect of the prescribed therapy on serum potassium concentrations?

Answers

1. NSAIDs such as naproxen can exacerbate asthma and heart failure by inducing bronchospasm and by causing fluid retention, respectively. They can also lead to upper gastro-intestinal problems, particularly when co-prescribed with oral steroids. It would be worth checking what has been tried already. If the painful knee is responsive to a simple analgesic such as paracetamol, this would be the preferred option. Alternatively, if an NSAID is necessary and tolerated, the use of ibuprofen in low dosage would be slightly less likely to have an effect on respiratory and renal function, although it may still aggravate symptoms of heart failure. Further investigation into the persistence of respiratory symptoms is required because it is unclear whether the patient's breathlessness is due to an exacerbation of her asthma or a worsening of her heart failure, and therefore the interpretation of this symptom is difficult.

2. The clinical nature of the breathlessness is not easy to determine and therefore makes the solution to this case uncertain at this stage. A number of issues, which also include confirming both diagnoses, should be considered. It is important to establish whether the patient is receiving maximum benefit from the inhaled treatment. Inhaler technique must be checked and improved if necessary and the dose of beclometasone optimised. A regular regimen of salbutamol is not advisable because it may impair control of asthma by masking the onset of exacerbations. A review of the need for an oral steroid should be undertaken, and any reduction in the use of an oral steroid must be done gradually to avoid exacerbation of the asthma and ensure that the patient does not experience adrenal insufficiency. Reduction of the oral steroid dose may benefit the heart failure. Although the prednisolone dose is low, its impact on treated heart failure is probably low but nevertheless should be taken into account in the review of its use.

When considering the treatment of heart failure, application of the criteria set identified the following issues in Mrs FM's treatment:

- Target dose of ACE inhibitor not achieved
- Not prescribed any mineralocorticoid receptor antagonist
- Potentially aggravating drug prescribed (NSAID, naproxen)
- Has specialist advice on use of sacubitril/valsartan been sought?
- Has specialist advice on use of ivabradine been sought?

There is scope to increase the dose of ramipril to 5 mg twice daily if tolerated, which is the target dose in heart failure patients. However, because a β-blocker is contraindicated in this patient due to her asthma, consideration may be given to adjunctive therapy such as an MRA, for example, spironolactone. If the patient was known to be intolerant of an MRA, an ARB, for example, candesartan, could be added instead. The decision about which agent to select first may come down to personal choice if symptoms are moderate. An increase in the dose of furosemide could also be considered, provided the breathlessness is due to heart failure.

3. Mrs FM is receiving a number of medications with the potential to affect serum potassium. Diuretics, oral and inhaled steroids (high dose) and β-agonists can reduce potassium, whereas ACE inhibitors can increase potassium. It is impossible to predict the extent to which each agent will affect potassium, especially with inhaled treatments, because the dose normally needs to be high before there is any significant systemic absorption. Determination of serum potassium is necessary, and if it remains low under the current treatment plan or is at risk of being altered due to changes in drug dosage such as an increase in ramipril to 5 mg twice daily, then close observation will be required.

Case 21.5

Mr CH, a 78-year-old, regularly visits your pharmacy for his medication and has moderately symptomatic heart failure (NYHA III). During a recent review with his primary care doctor, Mr CH described worsening of his heart failure symptoms. His doctor has said he could take an extra dose of furosemide 40 mg if required, but Mr CH would need to be referred back to the hospital cardiology consultant before changing any other medication. He is currently prescribed ramipril 5 mg daily, nebivolol 2.5 mg daily and furosemide 40 mg daily. His blood pressure has been measured as 103/62 mmHg (heart rate 54 bpm), and he has an eGFR of 30 ml/min/1.73 m².

Questions

1. What is the rationale behind the decision to refer Mr CH to the cardiology consultant?
2. What other drug treatment options might be considered?

Answers

1. Mr CH is prescribed both ACE inhibitor and β-blocker therapy in accordance with the evidence base for treatment. As Mr CH has symptomatic heart failure (NYHA III), he is also prescribed furosemide in response to signs and symptoms of fluid retention. When Mr CH reports deterioration in the control of his heart failure symptoms, the prescriber must consider what treatment options are available for Mr CH and make any necessary changes. Neither the ACE inhibitor nor β-blocker is prescribed at the recommended target dose (see Table 21.7); therefore, there is scope to titrate the dose of either agent to the target dose, which should result in improvement of symptoms and a reduced need for diuretic therapy. However, there may be reluctance to increase the dose of ACE inhibitor, possibly due to the fact that Mr CH has a relatively low blood pressure and compromised renal function (eGFR of 30 ml/min/1.73 m²). However, it is unclear whether Mr CH is receiving maximally tolerated doses and whether his apparent hypotension is indeed symptomatic. Similarly, there may be reluctance to increase the dose of β-blocker due to a low blood pressure and heart rate (54 beats/min). Because both options may adversely affect the patient, the doctor has decided to treat the symptoms with additional diuretic when required as a short-term solution before Mr CH's appointment with the cardiology consultant for advice. In Mr CH's case, it is likely that specialist supervision is required in considering the addition of further agents and for the optimisation of therapy.

2. It is unlikely that there will be much scope to add further medication, and optimising either ACE inhibitor or β-blocker therapy will be limited due to their effects on blood pressure and/or renal function. There are some agents that could be added, although Mr CH may be a likely candidate for cardiac resynchronisation therapy (CRT) and should probably be assessed for this. An ECG would confirm his eligibility for therapy if his QRS duration was greater than 120 ms, and this would be likely to improve his symptoms and survival. It may also help increase his blood pressure and renal function to a point where further optimisation of ACE inhibitor and β-blocker dose or addition of other therapeutic options might become possible.

References

A-HeFT: Taylor, A.L., Ziesche, S., Yancy, C., et al., for the African-American Heart Failure Trial Investigators, 2004. Combination of isosorbide dinitrate and hydralazine in blacks with heart failure. New Eng. J. Med. 351, 2049–2057.

A-HeFT: Taylor, A.L., Ziesche, S., Yancy, C., et al., for the African-American Heart Failure Trial Investigators, 2007. Early and sustained benefit on event-free survival and heart failure hospitalization from fixed-dose combination of isosorbide dinitrate/hydralazine: consistency across subgroups in the African-American Heart Failure Trial. Circulation 115, 1747–1753.

ACC/AHA/HFSA: Yancy, C.W., Jessup, M., Bozkurt, B., et al., 2016. ACC/AHA/HFSA focused update on new pharmacological therapy for heart failure: an update of the 2013 ACCF/AHA guideline for the management of heart failure: a report of the American College of Cardiology Foundation/American Heart Association Task Force on Clinical Practice Guidelines and the Heart Failure Society of America. J. Am. Coll. Cardiol. 68, 1476–1488.

AIRE: Acute Infarction Ramipril Efficacy Study Investigators, 1993. Effect of ramipril on mortality and morbidity of survivors of acute myocardial infarction with clinical evidence of heart failure. Lancet 342, 821–828.

ANZ Carvedilol, 1997. Randomised, placebo-controlled trial of carvedilol in patients with congestive heart failure due to ischaemic heart disease. Australia/New Zealand Heart Failure Research Collaborative Group. Lancet 349, 375–380.

ATLAS: Packer, M., Poole-Wilson, P.A., Armstrong, P.W., et al., 1999. Comparative effects of low and high doses of the angiotensin-converting enzyme inhibitor, lisinopril, on morbidity and mortality in chronic heart failure. ATLAS Study Group. Circulation 100, 2312–2318.

CAPRICORN Investigators, 2001. Effect of carvedilol on outcome after myocardial infarction in patients with left-ventricular dysfunction: the CAPRICORN randomised trial. Lancet 357, 1385–1390.

CHARM Added: McMurray, J.J., Ostergren, J., Swedberg, K., et al., 2003. Effects of candesartan in patients with CHF and reduced left-ventricular systolic dysfunction taking angiotensin-converting-enzyme inhibitors: the CHARM Added trial. Lancet 362, 767–771.

CHARM Alternative: Granger, C.B., McMurray, J.J., Yusuf, S., et al., 2003. Effects of candesartan in patients with CHF and reduced left-ventricular systolic function intolerant to angiotensin-converting-enzyme inhibitors: the CHARM Alternative trial. Lancet 362, 772–776.

CIBIS II: Investigators Committees, 1999. The Cardiac Insufficiency Bisoprolol Study II (CIBIS II): a randomised trial. Lancet 353, 9–13.

COMET: Poole-Wilson, P.A., Swedberg, K., Cleland, J.G.F., et al., for the COMET Investigators, 2003. Comparison of carvedilol and metoprolol on clinical outcomes in patients with chronic heart failure in the Carvedilol Or Metoprolol European Trial (COMET): a randomised controlled trial. Lancet 362, 7–13.

CONSENSUS I: CONSENSUS Trial Study Group, 1987. Effects of enalapril on mortality in severe congestive heart failure. New Eng. J. Med. 316, 1429–1435.

CONSENSUS II: Swedberg, K., Held, P., Kjekshus, J., et al., 1992. Effects of the early administration of enalapril on the mortality in patients with acute myocardial infarction. Results from the co-operative new Scandinavian enalapril survival study II. New Eng. J. Med. 327, 678–684.

COPERNICUS: Packer, M., Coats, A.J., Fowler, M.B., for the Carvedilol Prospective Randomized Cumulative Survival Study Group, et al., 2001. Effect of carvedilol on survival in severe chronic heart failure. New Eng. J. Med. 334, 1651–1658.

Criteria Committee of the New York Heart Association, 1994. Nomenclature and Criteria for Diagnosis of Diseases of the Heart and Great Vessels, ninth ed. Little, Brown & Co, Boston.

DIG: Digitalis Investigation Group, 1997. The effect of digoxin on mortality and morbidity in patients with heart failure. New Eng. J. Med. 336, 525–533.

EMPHASIS-HF: Zannad, F., McMurray, J.J.V., Krum, H., et al., for the EMPHASIS-HF Study Group, 2011. Eplerenone in patients with systolic heart failure and mild symptoms. New Eng. J. Med. 364, 11–21.

EPHESUS: Pitt, B., Remme, W., Zannad, F., et al., 2003. Eplerenone, a selective aldosterone blocker, in 38 patients with left ventricular dysfunction after myocardial infarction. New Eng. J. Med. 348, 1309–1321.

European Society of Cardiology, 2016. ESC Guidelines for the diagnosis and treatment of acute and chronic heart failure. The Task Force for the diagnosis and treatment of acute and chronic heart failure of the European Society of Cardiology (ESC). Eu. Heart J. 37, 2129–2200.

MERIT-HF Study Group, 1999. Effect of metoprolol CR/XL in chronic heart failure: metoprolol CR/XL randomised intervention trial in congestive heart failure (MERIT-HF). Lancet 353, 2001–2007.

Metra, M., Teerlink, J.R., 2017. Heart failure. Lancet. Available at: https://doi.org/10.1016/S0140-6736(17)31071-1.

National Institute for Health and Care Excellence (NICE), 2010. Chronic heart failure in adults: management (Clinical Guideline CG108). NICE, London. Available at: https://www.nice.org.uk/guidance/cg108/

PARADIGM-HF: McMurray, J.J., Packer, M., Desai, A.S., et al., 2014. Angiotensin-neprilysin inhibition versus enalapril in heart failure. New Eng. J. Med. 371, 993–1004.

PROMISE: Packer, M., Carver, J.R., Rodeheffer, R.J., for the PROMISE Study Research Group, et al., 1991. Effect of oral milrinone on mortality in severe chronic heart failure. New Eng. J. Med. 325, 1468–1475.

PROVED: Uretsky, B.F., Young, J.B., Shahidi, F.E., for the PROVED Investigative Group, et al., 1993. Randomized study assessing the effect of digoxin withdrawal in patients with mild to moderate chronic congestive heart failure: results of the PROVED trial. J. Am. Coll. Cardiol. 22, 955–962.

RADIANCE: Packer, M., Gheorghiade, M., Young, J.B., et al., 1993. Withdrawal of digoxin from patients with chronic heart failure treated with angiotensin-converting-enzyme inhibitors. RADIANCE Study. New Eng. J. Med. 329, 1–7.

RALES Pitt, B., Zannad, F., Remme, W.J., et al., for the Randomized Aldactone Evaluation Study Investigators, 1999. The effect of spironolactone on morbidity and mortality in patients with severe heart failure. New Eng. J. Med. 341, 709–717.

Salpeter, S., Ormiston, T., Salpeter, E., 2005. Cardioselective beta-blockers for chronic obstructive pulmonary disease. Cochrane DB Syst. Rev. 2005 (4). https://doi.org/10.1002/14651858.CD003566.pub2. Art. No. CD003566.

SAVE Pfeffer, M.A., Braunwald, E., Moye, L.A., et al., 1992. Effect of captopril on mortality and morbidity in patients with left ventricular dysfunction after myocardial infarction. Results of the Survival and Ventricular Enlargement trial (SAVE). New Eng. J. Med. 327, 669–677.

Scottish Intercollegiate Guidelines Network, 2016. Management of chronic heart failure (Guideline 147). SIGN, Edinburgh. Available at: http://www.sign.ac.uk/assets/sign147.pdf

SENIORS: Flather, M.D., Shibata, M.C., Coats, A.J., et al., 2005. Randomized trial to determine the effect of nebivolol on mortality and cardiovascular hospital admission in elderly patients with heart failure (SENIORS). Eur. Heart J. 26, 215–225.

SHIFT: Swedberg, K., Komajda, M., Bohm, M., et al., 2010. Ivabradine and outcomes in chronic heart failure (SHIFT): A randomised placebo-controlled study. Lancet 376, 875–885.

SOLVD-P: SOLVD Investigators, 1992. Effect of enalapril on mortality and the development of heart failure in asymptomatic patients with reduced left ventricular ejection fractions. New Eng. J. Med. 327, 685–691.

SOLVD-T: SOLVD Investigators, 1991. Effect of enalapril on survival in patients with reduced left ventricular ejection fractions and congestive heart failure. New Eng. J. Med. 325, 293–302.

Tang, X, Liu, P, Runjun, L, et al., 2015. Milrinone for the treatment of acute heart failure after acute myocardial infarction: a systematic review and meta-analysis. Basic & Clinical Pharmacology & Toxicology 117, 186–194.

TRACE: Trandolapril Cardiac Evaluation Study Group, 1995. A clinical trial of the angiotensin-enzyme inhibitor trandolapril in patients with left ventricular dysfunction after myocardial infarction. New Eng. J. Med. 333, 1670–1676.

US Carvedilol: Packer, M., Bristow, M.R., Cohn, J.N., et al., 1996. The effect of carvedilol on morbidity and mortality in patients with chronic heart failure. US Carvedilol Heart Failure Study Group. New Eng. J. Med. 334, 1349–1355.

V-HeFT I: Cohn, J., Archibald, D., Ziesche, S., et al., 1986. Effect of vasodilator therapy on mortality in chronic congestive heart failure. Results of a Veterans Administration Cooperative Study. New Eng. J. Med. 314, 1547–1552.

V-HeFT II Cohn, J.N., Johnson, G., Ziesche, S., et al., for the V-HeFT II Study, 1991. A comparison of enalapril with hydralazine-isosorbide dinitrate in the treatment of chronic congestive heart failure. New Eng. J. Med. 325, 303–310.

Val-HeFT: Maggioni, A.P., Anand, I., Gottlieb, S.O., et al., 2002. Effects of valsartan on morbidity and mortality in patients with heart failure not receiving angiotensin-converting enzyme inhibitors. J. Am. Coll. Cardiol. 40, 1422–1424.

Further reading

Williams, H., 2014. Heart failure management. Clin. Pharm. 6, 123–128.

Useful websites

American College of Cardiology: http://www.acc.org
British Heart Foundation: http://www.bhf.org.uk
British Society for Heart Failure: http://www.bsh.org
European Society of Cardiology: http://www.escardio.org

Heart Failure Matters: http://www.heartfailurematters.org
National Institute for Health and Care Excellence: http://www.nice.org.uk
Scottish Intercollegiate Guidelines Network: http://www.sign.ac.uk

22 Arrhythmias

Simon Sporton and Sotiris Antoniou

Key points

- The heart functions most efficiently in sinus rhythm. Any arrhythmia compromises cardiac function.
- Although drugs have been the mainstay of arrhythmia treatment, they are often of limited efficacy and may be associated with significant toxicity.
- An understanding of the ionic basis of the cardiac action potential is important because antiarrhythmic drugs act predominantly by altering the function of transmembrane ion channels.
- Antiarrhythmic drugs are grouped by the Vaughan–Williams classification, based on their action upon specific transmembrane ion channels.
- Antiarrhythmic drugs may be proarrhythmic in certain circumstances.
- The use of non-pharmacological treatments for arrhythmias (catheter ablation and device therapy) is increasing.
- Atrial fibrillation is the most common arrhythmia and is associated with an increased risk of thromboembolic stroke. All patients with atrial fibrillation should undergo assessment of their stroke risk.

Normal cardiac electrophysiology

The normal cardiac rhythm, sinus rhythm, is characterised by contraction of first the atria and then the ventricles (systole) followed by relaxation (diastole), during which the heart refills with blood before the next cardiac cycle begins. This orderly sequence of contraction and relaxation is regulated by the heart's electrical activity. Heart muscle cells (myocytes) are electrically active and capable of generating action potentials, which initiate contraction of the myocyte through a process known as excitation–contraction coupling. Adjacent myocytes form electrical connections through protein channels called gap junctions. An action potential in one myocyte causes current flow between itself and adjacent myocytes, which in turn generate their own action potentials, and in this way an 'activation wavefront' spreads though the myocardium, resulting in a wave of contraction.

Cardiac action potential

An understanding of the ionic basis of the cardiac action potential is important because drugs used in the treatment of cardiac arrhythmias act by altering the function of transmembrane ion channels. Inherited abnormalities of ion channel function ('channelopathies') are an important cause of sudden cardiac death due to arrhythmia and are increasingly implicated in the pathogenesis of other arrhythmias including atrial fibrillation (AF).

The phospholipid membrane of cardiac myocytes is spanned by numerous proteins known as ion channels, whose permeability to specific ions varies during the cardiac cycle, resulting in a resting (diastolic) membrane potential, diastolic depolarisation in cells with pacemaker activity, and action potentials.

Resting membrane potential

The resting membrane potential of −60 to −90 mV occurs because the intracellular potassium (K^+) concentration is much higher than the extracellular K^+ concentration as a result of a transmembrane pump known as Na^+-K^+-ATPase, which pumps K^+ ions into the cell in exchange for sodium (Na^+) ions. K^+ ions diffuse out of the cell through selective K^+ channels (the inward rectifier current or I_{K1}) unaccompanied by anions, resulting in a net loss of charge and thus a negative resting, diastolic or phase 4, transmembrane potential (Fig. 22.1A).

Pacemaker activity

Certain specialised myocytes form the cardiac conduction system and these cells have pacemaker activity; that is, they are capable of generating their own action potentials because of gradual depolarisation of the transmembrane potential during diastole (phase 4), referred to as the pacemaker potential (see Fig. 22.1B). The pacemaker potential occurs as a result of: (1) a gradual reduction in an outward K^+ current called the delayed rectifier (I_{K1}) current, (2) a gradual reduction in an acetylcholine-activated outward K^+ current I_{KAch}, and (3) increasing dominance of an inward current of Na^+ and some K^+ ions known as I_f (f stands for 'funny').

As a result of the pacemaker potential, the transmembrane potential gradually becomes less negative until a threshold potential is reached at which an action potential is triggered. The rate of depolarisation of the pacemaker potential, and hence

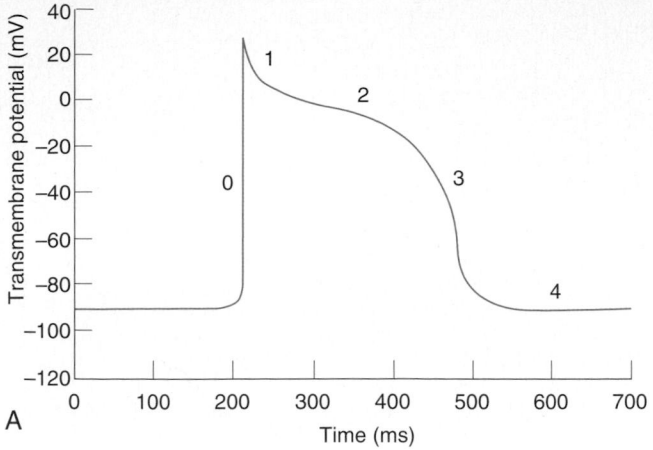

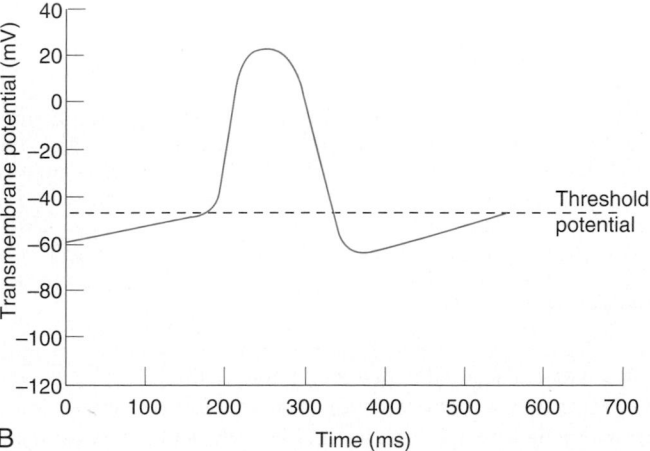

Fig. 22.1 Cardiac action potential. (A) An action potential from ventricular myocardium. During diastole (phase 4), the resting transmembrane potential is constant at −90 mV. The upstroke (phase 0) of the action potential is due to the rapid influx of Na^+ ions. The early phase of repolarisation (phase 1) is due to efflux of K^+ ions, followed by a plateau phase (phase 2) at about 0 mV during which influx of Ca^{2+} ions is balanced by efflux of K^+ ions. Towards the end of diastole, influx of Ca^{2+} ions diminishes and efflux of K^+ ions increases, resulting in repolarisation (phase 3) back to the negative resting membrane potential. (B) An action potential from the sinus node. During diastole (phase 4), there is progressive depolarisation towards a threshold potential at which an action potential is triggered. The upstroke (phase 0) of the action potential is less steep than in ventricular myocardial cells because the sinus node cells lack 'fast' Na^+ channels, and so depolarisation is dependent upon influx of Ca^{2+} ions.

the heart rate, is influenced by the autonomic nervous system. Sympathetic nervous system activation and circulating catecholamines increase the heart rate by binding to β_1-adrenoreceptors, leading to an increase in intracellular cyclic adenosine monophosphate (cAMP), which increases the pacemaker current I_f, leading to more rapid depolarisation of the sinus node and hence a faster heart rate. Parasympathetic nervous system activation, mediated by muscarinic cholinergic receptors, has the opposite effect: reduction of cAMP with inhibition of the pacemaker current I_f and an increase in the outward K^+ current I_{KAch}, reducing the rate of depolarisation of the sinus node and hence a slower heart rate.

Depolarisation

The rapid depolarisation of the cardiac action potential (see Fig. 22.1A, phase 0) occurs because of a rapid increase in the permeability of the cell membrane to Na^+ ions, which enter rapidly through 'fast' Na^+ channels in a current known as I_{Na}. The I_{Na} current is brief because the 'fast' Na^+ channels inactivate rapidly.

Repolarisation

The early phase of repolarisation (phase 1) is due to closure of the fast Na^+ channels, an outward K^+ current known as I_{to} (to – transient outward), and in atrial myocytes, a further K^+ current known as the ultra-rapid component of the delayed rectifier current, or I_{Kur}. The plateau phase (phase 2) of the cardiac action potential occurs because the inward movement of Ca^{2+} ions (I_{Ca}) is balanced by the outward movement of K^+ ions. Repolarisation (phase 3) is completed as I_{Ca} diminishes, and two further components of the delayed rectifier (I_K) current known as the rapid (I_{Kr}) and slow (I_{Ks}) components predominate, with an important contribution from I_{K1} and also I_{KAch}.

There is considerable variation in the expression of transmembrane ion channels in different parts of the heart, with corresponding variation in the morphology of the action potential. The most marked example is that myocytes in the sinus and AV nodes contain few Na^+ channels. The upstroke of the action potential in these cells is due, predominantly, to the influx of Ca^{2+} ions and, therefore, is considerably slower than the upstroke in other myocytes (see Fig. 22.1B). This results in slow propagation of the cardiac impulse in nodal tissue. The variation in ion channel expression throughout the heart is essential for normal cardiac function, helps explain the pathophysiology of many inherited and acquired diseases complicated by cardiac arrhythmia, and accounts for the relative selectivity of antiarrhythmic and other drugs for certain parts of the heart.

Refractoriness

The action potential of cardiac myocytes differs from that seen in nerve cells by the presence of a plateau phase during which the myocyte is electrically inexcitable (refractory), that is, incapable of generating another action potential. It is only towards the end of repolarisation (phase 3) that the myocyte regains excitability. The time interval between the onset of the action potential and the regaining of electrical excitability is known as the refractory period. Under most circumstances the refractory period of a cardiac myocyte corresponds closely to the duration of the cardiac action potential; therefore, drugs that prolong action potential duration (APD) prolong the refractory period.

Normal cardiac conduction

During sinus rhythm (Fig. 22.2), an activation wavefront begins in the sinus node, a group of cells with pacemaker activity on the upper free wall of the right atrium. The rate of diastolic depolarisation, and hence the rate of discharge of the sinus node, is increased

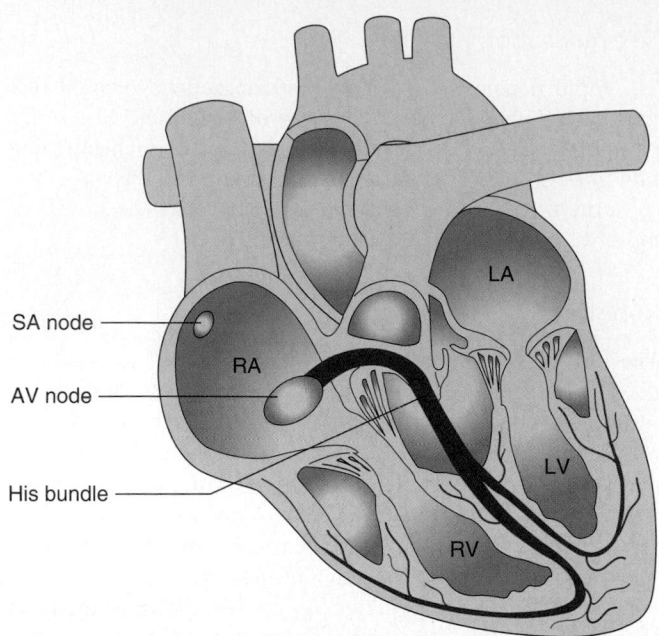

Fig. 22.2 Normal cardiac conduction system. During sinus rhythm, an activation wavefront spreads from the sinus (sinoatrial [SA]) node across the atrial myocardium before entering the atrioventricular (AV) node. The activation wavefront then enters the bundle of His, which penetrates the annulus fibrosus and forms the only electrical connection between the atria and ventricles. The bundle of His divides into right and left bundle branches, which ramify into a subendocardial network of Purkinje fibres that transmit the activation wavefront rapidly across the ventricles. Activation of the ventricles proceeds from endocardium to epicardium.
LA, Left atrium; LV, left ventricle; RA, right atrium; RV, right ventricle.

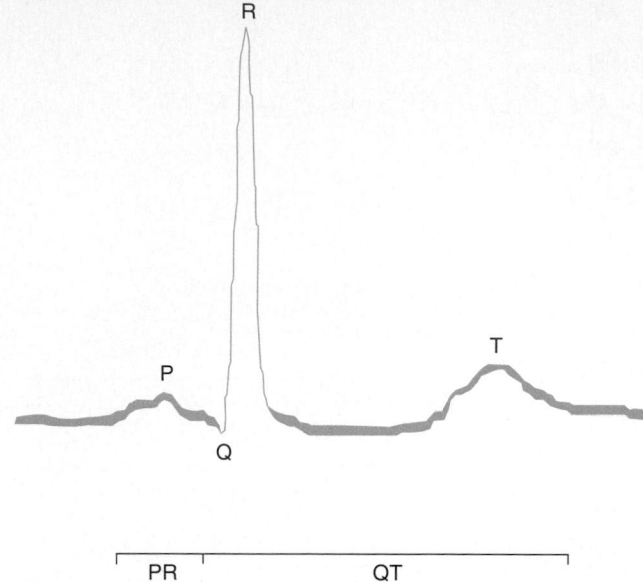

Fig. 22.3 Normal electrocardiogram (ECG). The P wave results from activation (depolarisation of the atria). The PR interval is isoelectric as the activation wavefront proceeds slowly through the atrioventricular node. The QRS complex reflects activation of the ventricles and is large compared with the P wave because of the much greater mass of the ventricular myocardium and brief, reflecting extremely rapid conduction in the His–Purkinje system. The T wave represents ventricular repolarisation.

by sympathetic nerve stimulation, circulating catecholamines or sympathomimetic drugs mediated by β_1-adrenoreceptors on the cell membranes of the sinus node myocytes. Parasympathetic (vagus) nerve stimulation exerts the opposite effect, mediated by muscarinic cholinergic receptors.

An activation wavefront spreads across the atrial myocardium, leading to atrial contraction and generating the P wave on the surface electrocardiogram (ECG; Fig. 22.3). The last part of the atria to be activated is the atrioventricular (AV) node, the electrical and structural properties of which result in a slow conduction velocity, allowing atrial emptying to be completed before ventricular contraction begins and reflected by the PR interval on the ECG. Conduction velocity in the AV node is increased by sympathetic nerve stimulation, circulating catecholamines or sympathomimetic drugs, mediated by β_1-adrenoreceptors, whereas parasympathetic (vagus) nerve stimulation exerts the opposite effect via muscarinic cholinergic receptors.

The atria and ventricles are electrically isolated from each other by the annulus fibrosus, the electrically non-conductive fibrous tissue forming the valve rings. In the normal heart, there is just one electrical connection between the atria and ventricles, the bundle of His, which conveys the activation wavefront from the AV node and penetrates the annulus fibrosus before dividing into the right and left bundle branches. The bundle branches ramify

into a sub-endocardial network of Purkinje fibres, which convey the activation wavefront rapidly across the ventricles ensuring near-simultaneous contraction of the ventricular myocardium, reflected by the narrow QRS complex of the ECG. Finally, the activation wavefront spreads from endocardium to epicardium. A wave of repolarisation then spreads across the ventricles resulting in the T wave. The QT interval on the ECG therefore represents the duration of ventricular depolarisation and repolarisation. There is an inverse relationship between the time to activation of different areas of the ventricular myocardium and APD such that the latest areas to be activated have the shortest APD. The purpose of this relationship is that repolarisation is rapid and uniform throughout the ventricular myocardium, which serves to maintain electrical stability.

Arrhythmia mechanisms

Cardiac arrhythmias occur because of abnormalities of impulse formation or propagation.

Abnormal impulse formation

Abnormal automaticity

Automaticity is another term for pacemaker activity, a characteristic possessed by all cells of the specialised cardiac conduction system during health and, potentially, by other cardiac

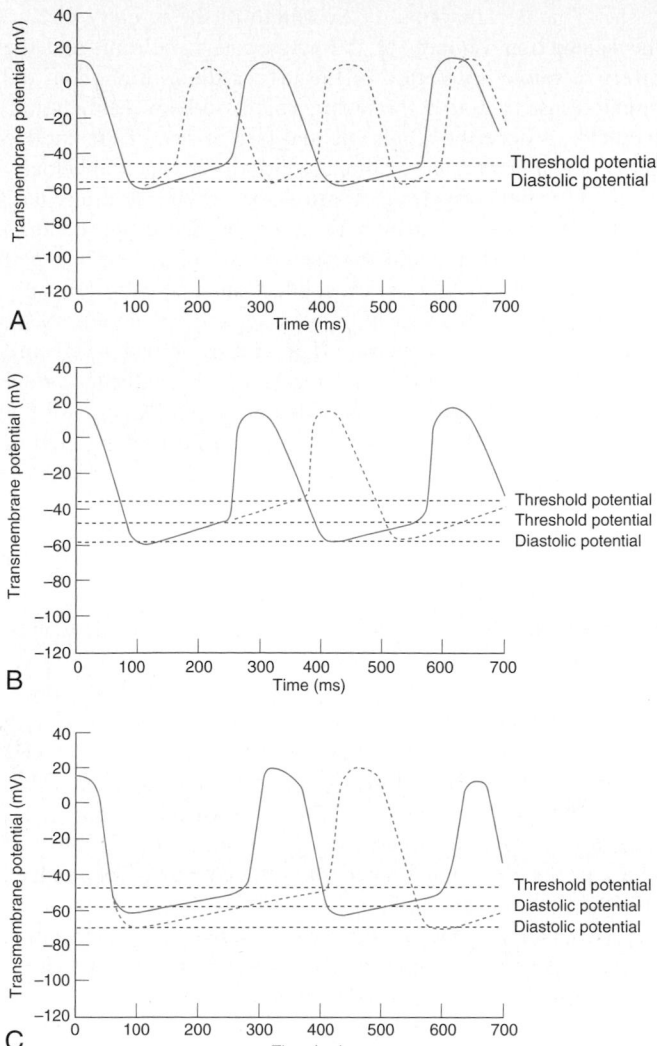

Fig. 22.4 Abnormal automaticity. A sinus node action potential is shown (in bold) with a characteristic slow upstroke. After repolarisation, gradual diastolic depolarisation occurs as a result of pacemaker currents. When the threshold potential is reached, a further action potential is generated. The rate of firing of the pacemaker cell is governed largely by the duration of the diastolic interval, which is in turn determined by (A) the slope of diastolic depolarisation, (B) the threshold potential, and (C) the maximum diastolic potential. Each of these (shown by dotted lines) may be altered by disease states leading to abnormal automaticity.

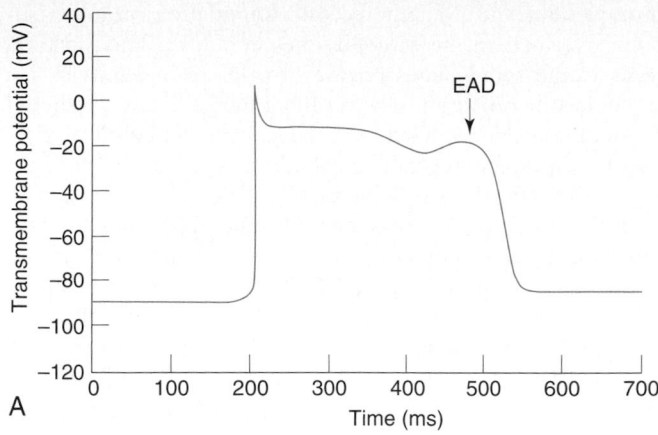

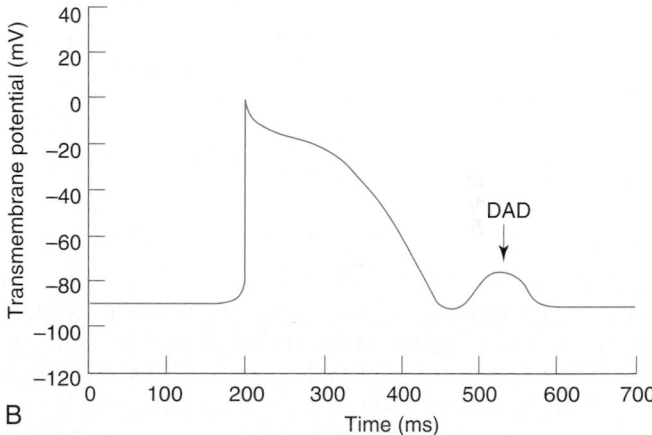

Fig. 22.5 Triggered activity. (A) An early afterdepolarisation (EAD) occurring at the start of phase 3 of the cardiac action potential. (B) A delayed afterdepolarisation (DAD) occurring after repolarisation, during phase 4. Either EADs or DADs may reach the threshold potential for generation of a further action potential.

myocytes during certain disease states. The rate of firing of a pacemaker cell is largely determined by the duration of the phase 4 diastolic interval (Fig. 22.4). This in turn is determined by: (1) the maximum diastolic potential following repolarisation of the preceding action potential, (2) the slope of diastolic depolarisation due to pacemaker currents, and (3) the threshold potential for generation of a new action potential. In the healthy state, there is a hierarchy of firing rates within the specialised conduction system, with the highest rate in the sinus node followed by the AV node and then the His–Purkinje system. The sinus node is, therefore, the dominant pacemaker and determines the heart rate, whereas the pacemaker activity in the distal conduction system is 'overdriven' by the sinus node. Abnormal automaticity describes either accelerated pacemaker activity in cells of the distal cardiac conduction system such that they escape from overdrive suppression by the sinus node, or the development of pacemaker activity in cells that do not form part of the cardiac conduction system.

Triggered activity

Triggered activity describes impulse formation dependent upon afterdepolarisations. Early afterdepolarisations (EADs) occur during phase 2 or 3 of the cardiac action potential, whereas delayed afterdepolarisations (DADs) occur during phase 4 (Fig. 22.5). In both cases, afterdepolarisation may reach the threshold potential required for generation of a new action potential.

EADs are characteristic of the congenital and acquired long QT syndromes. The prolonged APD promotes reactivation of the inward calcium current I_{Ca}, which may directly cause EADs during phase 2. Furthermore, action potential prolongation and β-adrenoreceptor stimulation promote calcium overload in the sarcoplasmic reticulum. This, in turn, leads to the spontaneous release of calcium in bursts by the sarcoplasmic reticulum. The resultant increase in intracellular calcium concentration activates the transmembrane Na^+/Ca^{2+} exchanger, which moves one calcium ion out of the myocyte in exchange for three sodium ions and, therefore, results in an EAD during phase 3. In the long QT syndromes, an EAD may initiate a form of polymorphic ventricular tachycardia (VT) known as Torsade de pointes. EADs are more prominent at slow heart rates.

DADs are seen during reperfusion following ischaemia, heart failure, digitalis toxicity, and in catecholaminergic polymorphic VT. They occur because of spontaneous release of calcium in bursts by the sarcoplasmic reticulum, activating the Na^+/Ca^{2+} exchanger as described for EADs and resulting in a DAD during phase 4. A DAD may result in a single extrastimulus ('ectopic beat') or in repetitive firing, that is, tachycardia. DADs are more prominent at rapid heart rates and during sympathetic nervous stimulation of β-adrenoreceptors.

Abnormal impulse propagation

Re-entry

Many clinically important arrhythmias are due to re-entry, in which an activation wavefront rotates continuously around a circuit. Re-entry depends upon a trigger in the form of a premature beat and a substrate, that is, the re-entry circuit itself. A precise set of electrophysiological conditions must be met for re-entry to occur (Fig. 22.6): (1) there must be a central non-conducting obstacle around which the re-entry circuit develops; (2) a premature beat must encounter unidirectional conduction block in one limb (a) of the re-entry circuit; (3) conduction must proceed slowly enough down the other limb (b) of the re-entry circuit that electrical excitability has returned in the original limb (a), allowing the activation wavefront to propagate in a retrograde direction along that limb; and (4) the circulating activation wavefront must continue to encounter electrically excitable

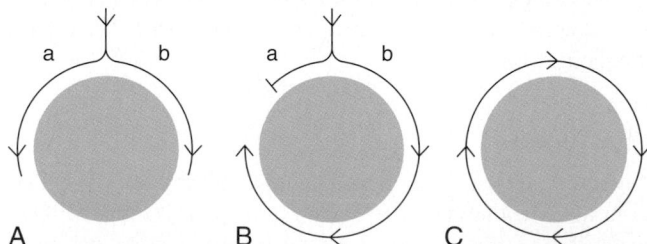

Fig. 22.6 Re-entry. During sinus rhythm, (A) an activation wavefront encounters a zone of fixed conduction block but can propagate anterogradely on either side of this zone, down limbs (a) and (b) of a potential re-entry circuit. A premature beat (B) encounters unidirectional conduction block in limb (a), but propagates anterogradely down limb (b) and re-enters limb (a) retrogradely. If limb (a) is now capable of retrograde conduction, the re-entry circuit is completed and re-entry continues (C) as long as the activation wavefront continually meets electrically excitable tissue.

tissue. This is a function of the length of the re-entry circuit, the conduction velocity of the activation wavefront, and the effective refractory period of the myocardium throughout the circuit. Class I antiarrhythmic drugs block sodium channels and, therefore, reduce the amplitude and rate of rise of the cardiac action potential and, in so doing, reduce the conduction velocity of an activation wavefront. Class I antiarrhythmic drugs may exert their major antiarrhythmic effect by abolishing conduction altogether in areas of diseased myocardium forming part of a re-entry circuit in which conduction is already critically depressed. Class III antiarrhythmic drugs prolong cardiac APD, and hence the refractory period. If previously activated cells in a re-entry circuit (the 'tail') remain refractory when the re-entrant wavefront (the 'head') returns to that area, conduction will fail and re-entry will be abolished. Drug-induced prolongation of the refractory period may, therefore, terminate and/or prevent re-entrant arrhythmias.

Clinical problems

Patients with a cardiac arrhythmia may present with a number of symptoms:

- The most common symptom is palpitation, an awareness of an abnormal heartbeat, although some patients with clearly documented arrhythmia have no palpitation. Arrhythmias start suddenly; therefore, if the patient clearly describes palpitation of sudden onset ('like flicking a switch'), this is a useful pointer to an arrhythmia rather than heightened awareness of sinus tachycardia, which has a less sudden onset.
- The heart is designed to work most efficiently in sinus rhythm. Any arrhythmia compromises cardiac function. Symptoms that arise due to reduced cardiac output and/or pulmonary venous congestion include reduced exercise capacity, breathlessness and fatigue.
- Angina may accompany tachycardia, even in the absence of coronary artery disease. Tachycardia increases the metabolic rate of cardiac muscle and hence its demand for blood flow. Myocardial perfusion occurs predominantly during diastole, and during tachycardia proportionately less time is spent in diastole and so myocardial demand for blood can exceed supply, resulting in angina.
- A sudden drop in cardiac output may accompany either bradycardia or tachycardia, causing episodes of dizziness (presyncope), loss of consciousness (syncope) or, in extreme cases, sudden death from cardiac arrest.
- Atrial tachyarrhythmias such as atrial flutter and AF may be complicated by the development of intracardiac thrombus, usually within the left atrial appendage (LAA). This thrombus may embolise to any part of the body, but the most common clinical presentation is with a transient ischaemic attack or stroke.
- Arrhythmias may aggravate heart failure in two ways: (1) the haemodynamic effect of the arrhythmia may precipitate heart failure or aggravate existing heart failure, and (2) prolonged tachycardia of any type may lead to tachycardia-induced cardiomyopathy.

Diagnosis

A detailed history should be obtained, covering all of the symptoms listed above. A characteristic of cardiac arrhythmias is their random onset. Symptoms that occur under specific circumstances are less likely to be due to arrhythmia, but there are exceptions including certain uncommon types of VT, some cases of supraventricular tachycardia (SVT) due to an accessory pathway, and vasovagal syncope (faints). Other key features of the history include:

- a history of cardiac disease;
- a family history of heart disease and of sudden unexpected death;
- other diagnosed medical conditions;
- a full drug history, including over-the-counter medicines and recreational drugs including alcohol.

Physical examination is essential but often normal between episodes of arrhythmia. Mandatory investigation includes a 12-lead ECG and an echocardiogram to detect structural heart disease. Other investigations for structural and ischaemic heart disease may be indicated at this stage with the aim of detecting any underlying structural heart disease. If the history does not include sinister features such as syncope or a family history of sudden unexpected death at a young age, and the resting 12-lead ECG and echocardiogram are normal, then the patient can be reassured that they are extremely unlikely to have a serious heart rhythm disturbance. The extent of further investigation will be dictated by how troublesome the symptoms are.

The most certain way of reaching a firm diagnosis is a 12-lead ECG recorded during the patient's symptoms demonstrating arrhythmia. Because many arrhythmias occur intermittently, some form of ECG monitoring is often necessary. This may include a continuous ambulatory ECG (Holter) recording for up to 7 days at a time if the symptoms occur frequently, or for less frequent symptoms an event recorder, which may store ECG strips automatically if it detects an arrhythmia or if activated by the patient during their symptoms. An insertable loop recorder may be implanted subcutaneously and is an ECG event recorder with a battery life of about 3 years, making it a useful tool for the diagnosis of infrequent arrhythmias. There are now attachments for mobile phones that turn them into single-lead ECG recorders, enabling patients with suspected or actual arrhythmia to make high-quality recordings of their heart rhythm at any time, although the onset of the arrhythmia is unlikely to be captured, which may limit their usefulness.

Management

Tachycardia

Tachycardia is conventionally defined as a resting heart rate greater than 100 beats/min and can be classified according to whether it arises in or involves the atria (supraventricular tachycardias [SVTs]) or the ventricle (ventricular tachyarrhythmias). Management of tachycardia may involve the use of drugs, direct current (DC) cardioversion, catheter ablation or implantable devices. DC cardioversion is performed under either anaesthesia or sedation and may be either 'external', where a shock is delivered across the chest wall via either handheld paddles or adhesive patches, or 'internal', where a shock is delivered using a catheter inserted into the heart via a vein. DC cardioversion converts most tachycardias promptly to sinus rhythm, but the recurrence rate is high. Catheter ablation may cure many types of tachycardia and involves the delivery of either radiofrequency or cryothermal energy via a catheter, resulting in the destruction of arrhythmogenic tissue by highly localised heating or freezing, respectively.

Supraventricular tachycardias

Supraventricular tachycardias are tachycardias that arise from or involve the atria.

Inappropriate sinus tachycardia

Although uncommon, inappropriate sinus tachycardia, that is, sinus tachycardia with no identifiable underlying cause, is one of the more difficult arrhythmias to treat. The presenting symptom is usually palpitation, and the typical patient is a young, predominantly female, adult with no history of heart disease or other physical illness. The 12-lead ECG shows sinus tachycardia and ambulatory ECG monitoring demonstrates sinus tachycardia, but with diurnal variation in heart rate. Echocardiography is required to exclude structural heart disease, and thyroid function and urinary catecholamine excretion should be measured to detect thyrotoxicosis and phaeochromocytoma, respectively, as rare underlying causes of sinus tachycardia. If treatment is required on symptomatic grounds, β-blockers or verapamil are first-line therapy. Ivabradine, a selective 'funny channel' blocker, has been used in resistant cases but is not currently licensed for this indication. These drugs are typically taken regularly in an attempt to control the heart rate and hence the symptoms. Catheter ablation of the sinus node has been performed in highly symptomatic, drug-resistant, inappropriate sinus tachycardia, but with limited success and risks including symptomatic sinus bradycardia and phrenic nerve palsy.

Atrial flutter

Atrial flutter is a right atrial tachycardia with a re-entry circuit around the tricuspid valve annulus. The atrial rate is typically 300 per minute. The long refractory period of the AV node protects the ventricles from 1:1 conduction: In the presence of a healthy AV node and the absence of AV node–modifying drugs, there is usually 2:1 AV conduction resulting in a regular narrow-complex tachycardia with a ventricular rate of 150 per minute.

Atrial flutter confers a risk of thromboembolism similar to that of AF, and this risk should be managed in the same way as for AF (see later). Emergency management of atrial flutter is dictated by the clinical presentation but may include DC cardioversion or ventricular rate control with drugs that increase the refractory period of the AV node such as β-blockers, verapamil, diltiazem, or digoxin. DC cardioversion would be appropriate in the case of significant haemodynamic compromise and might be considered in a chronically anticoagulated patient or where the onset of the arrhythmia is certain and is less than 48 hours. In other situations, ventricular rate control with drugs would be appropriate.

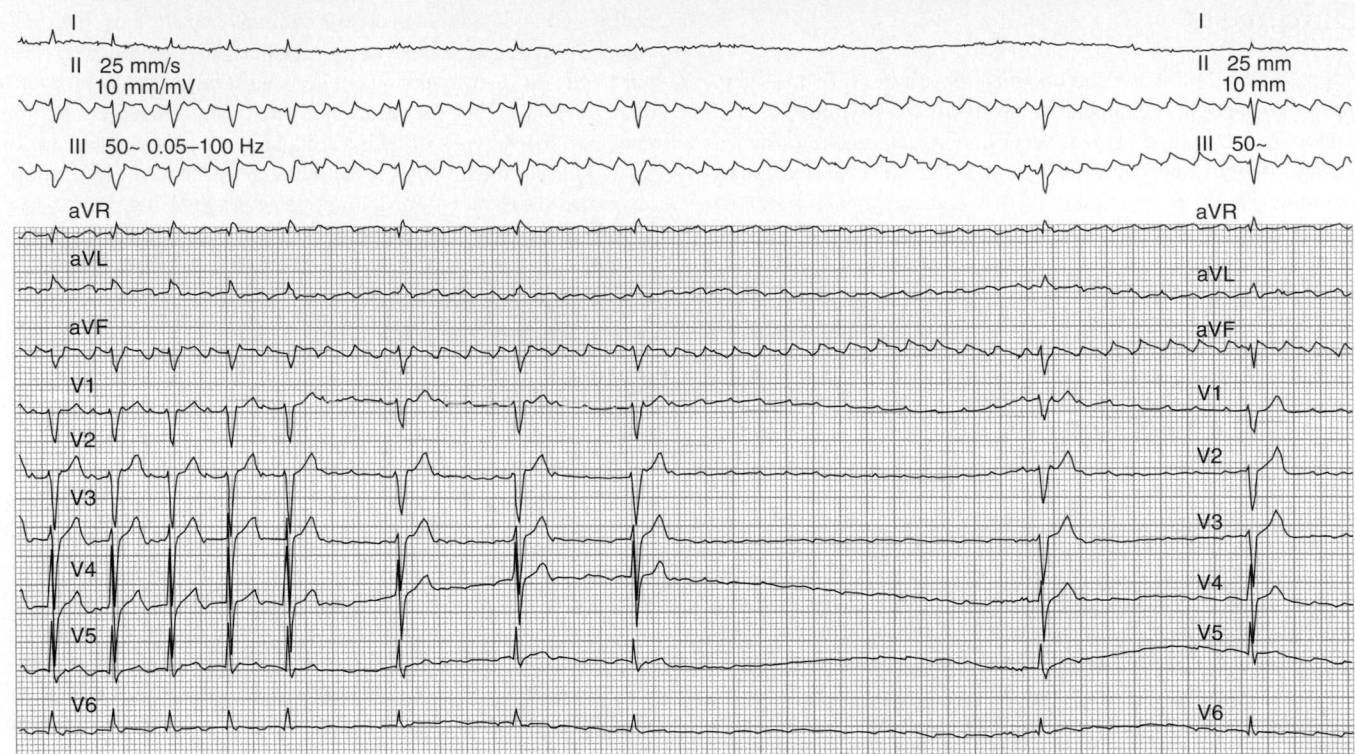

I

II 25 mm/s
10 mm/mV

III 50~ 0.05–100 Hz

aVR

aVL

aVF

V1

V2

V3

V4

V5

V6

I

II 25 mm
10 mm

III 50~

aVR

aVL

aVF

V1

V2

V3

V4

V5

V6

Fig. 22.7 A 12-lead electrocardiogram (ECG) recorded during the administration of intravenous adenosine. The initial rhythm is atrial flutter with 2:1 conduction from atria to ventricles. The QRS complexes obscure the atrial activity on the ECG. Adenosine does not terminate the atrial flutter but causes temporary atrioventricular block, revealing the characteristic 'sawtooth' ECG morphology of typical atrial flutter.

β-Blockers, verapamil, and digoxin may be given intravenously. β-Blockers or calcium channel blockers (CCBs) would usually be used as first-line treatment, whereas the delayed onset of action of digoxin makes it less useful for rapid heart rate control in an acute setting. Because the re-entry circuit is confined to the right atrium and does not involve the AV node, adenosine will not terminate atrial flutter but will produce transient AV block, allowing the characteristic flutter waves to be seen on the ECG (Fig. 22.7).

There is a limited role for antiarrhythmic drugs, whether used acutely to achieve chemical cardioversion or in the longer-term to maintain sinus rhythm. Class Ic antiarrhythmic drugs such as flecainide or propafenone should be used only in conjunction with AV node–modifying drugs such as β-blockers, verapamil, diltiazem, or digoxin because they may otherwise cause slowing of the atrial flutter circuit and 1:1 conduction though the AV node, which may be life-threatening. Sotalol and amiodarone have been used to restore and maintain sinus rhythm and have the advantage of helping to control the ventricular rate where rhythm control is incomplete. Catheter ablation of atrial flutter is highly effective, safe, and is increasingly used in preference to long-term drug treatment.

Focal atrial tachycardia

As its name implies, this relatively uncommon arrhythmia results from the repetitive discharge of a focal source within the atria or surrounding venous structures. The tachycardia mechanism may be caused by abnormal automaticity, triggered activity or microreentry. Management is as described for atrial flutter with three exceptions: (1) some focal atrial tachycardias terminate with adenosine; (2) the potential for class Ic antiarrhythmic drugs to slow tachycardia and result in 1:1 AV conduction is lower than for atrial flutter; and (3) catheter ablation of focal atrial tachycardia may be more challenging than that of atrial flutter, but it is curative in a majority of cases.

Junctional re-entry tachycardia

The term supraventricular tachycardias is widely used to describe junctional re-entry tachycardias, but it is a misnomer because it implies any tachycardia arising from the atria. Junctional re-entry tachycardia is a more specific term and may be preferable.

Two mechanisms account for most junctional re-entry tachycardias, and both involve a macroreentry circuit (Fig. 22.8). AV nodal re-entry tachycardia (AVNRT) rotates around a circuit including the AV node itself and the so-called AV nodal fast and slow pathways, which feed into the AV node. AV re-entry tachycardia (AVRT) comprises a re-entry circuit involving the atrial myocardium, the AV node, the ventricular myocardium and an accessory pathway, a congenital abnormality providing a second electrical connection between the atria and ventricles in addition to the His bundle, thus forming a potential re-entry circuit.

Many accessory pathways conduct only retrogradely from the ventricles to the atrium. In these cases, the ECG during sinus

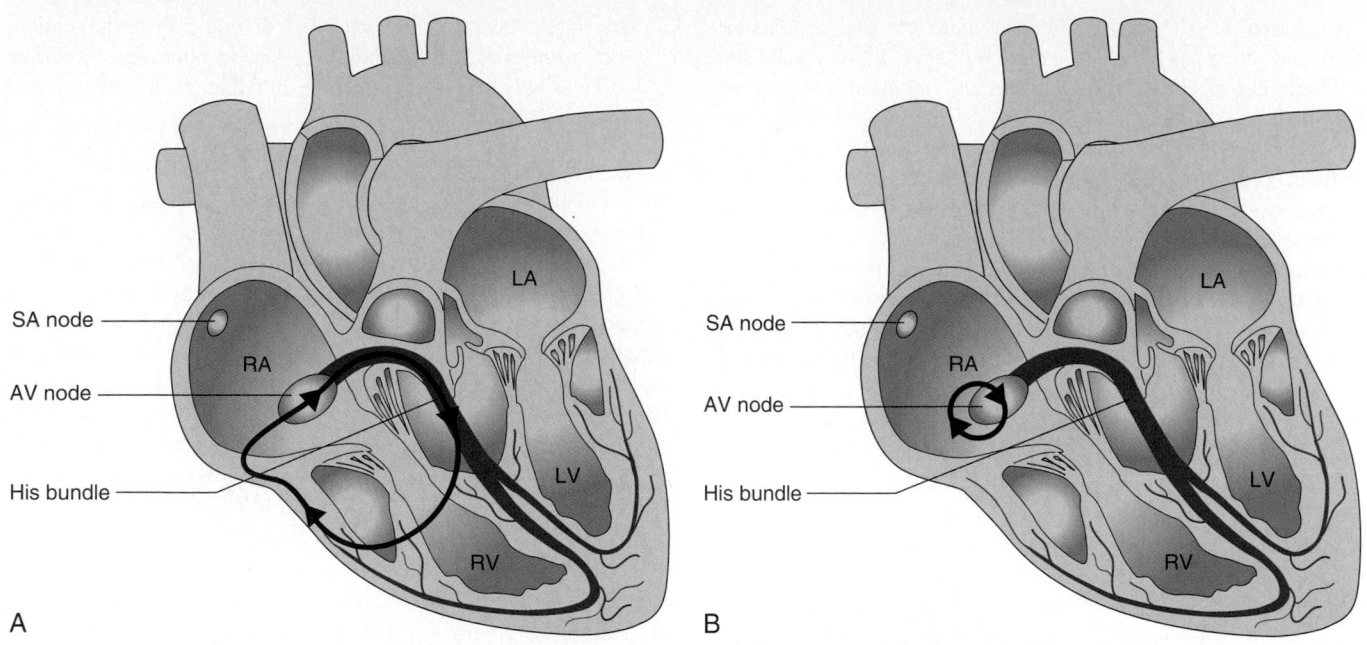

SA node
AV node
His bundle
RA
LA
LV
RV

A

SA node
AV node
His bundle
RA
LA
LV
RV

B

Fig. 22.8 The re-entry circuits of (A) atrioventricular (AV) re-entry tachycardia (AVRT) and (B) AV nodal re-entry tachycardia (AVNRT). (A) The AVRT circuit comprises atrial myocardium, the AV node and His bundle, ventricular myocardium and an accessory pathway, a small strand of muscle providing a second, abnormal, connection between atrium and ventricle, thus forming a potential re-entry circuit. The accessory pathway itself is the target of catheter ablation. (B) The AVNRT circuit comprises 'fast' and 'slow' pathways feeding into the AV node itself. The slow pathway is the target of catheter ablation. AV, Atrioventricular; LA, left atrium; LV, left ventricle; RA, right atrium; RV, right ventricle; SA, sinoatrial.

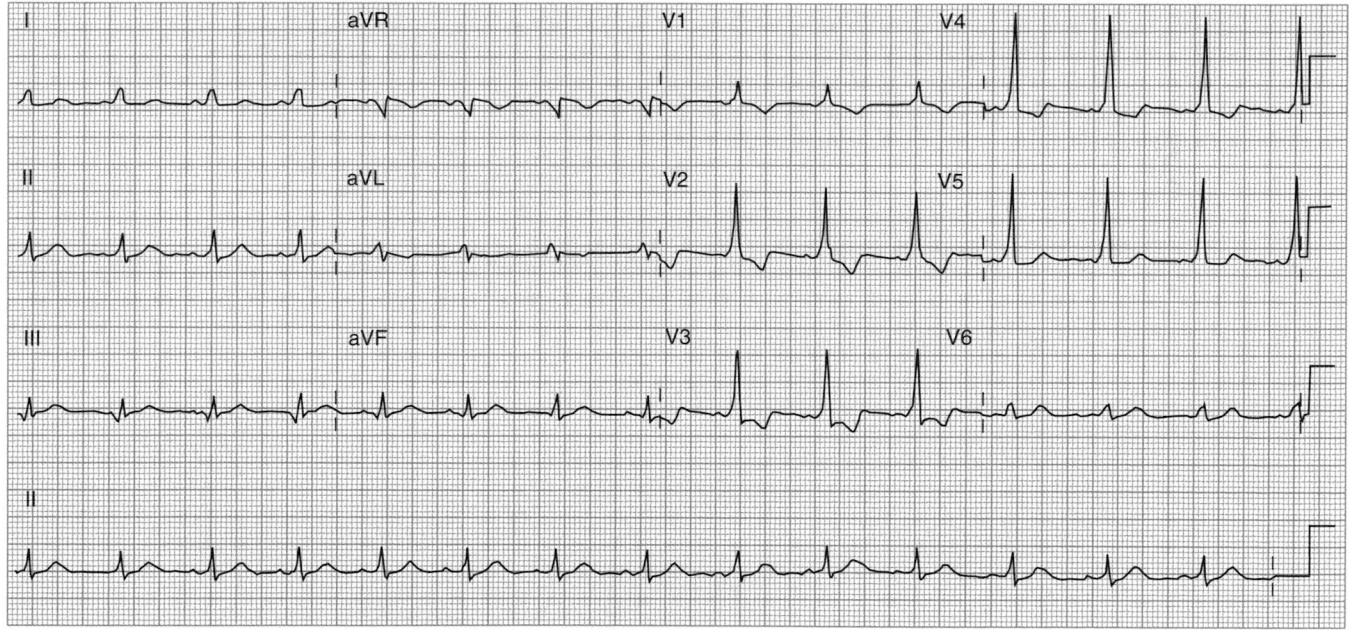

Fig. 22.9 Electrocardiogram showing a Wolff–Parkinson–White pattern. The PR interval is short and the QRS complex is abnormally broad, with a slurred upstroke or delta wave.

rhythm appears normal and the accessory pathway is described as 'concealed'. Other accessory pathways conduct anterogradely and retrogradely. In these cases, the ECG during sinus rhythm is abnormal and is described as having a Wolff–Parkinson–White pattern (Fig. 22.9). This abnormality is characterised by a short PR interval, because the conduction velocity of an accessory pathway is usually faster than that of the AV node, and a delta wave, a slurred onset to the QRS complex that occurs because an accessory pathway inserts into the ventricular myocardium which conducts more slowly than the His–Purkinje system.

Junctional re-entry tachycardias are characterised by a history of discrete episodes of rapid regular palpitation that start and stop suddenly and occur without warning and apparently at random. The peak age range at which symptoms begin is from the mid-teens to the mid-thirties, and the condition is more common in women. There are no symptoms between episodes, and cardiac examination and investigation at these times are usually normal. The diagnosis is usually made on the basis of the history, ideally confirmed by an ECG recorded during an episode showing a regular narrow-complex tachycardia with no discernible P waves or P waves occurring in a 1:1 relationship with the QRS complexes.

Acute treatment of junctional re-entry tachycardia aims to terminate the tachycardia by causing transient conduction block in the AV node, an obligatory part of the re-entry circuit. Vagotonic manoeuvres such as carotid sinus massage, a Valsalva manoeuvre or eliciting the diving reflex by immersion of the face in ice-cold water may all result in a brief vagal discharge sufficient to block conduction in the AV node, terminating tachycardia. The same effect may be achieved with intravenous adenosine given as a rapid bolus injection in doses up to 12 mg. Intravenous verapamil 5 mg as a rapid bolus injection is also a good alternative where adenosine is contraindicated, for example, in patients with asthma. However, verapamil should not be used if the patient has been recently treated with β-blockers.

Junctional re-entry tachycardia is often recurrent. There is a limited role for prophylactic drug treatment because this is generally not a dangerous condition affecting young and otherwise healthy people. Among other factors, the efficacy, toxicity, and acceptability of what may be long-term drug treatment requires careful consideration. Options for prophylactic drug treatment include β-blockers, verapamil, diltiazem, flecainide, and sotalol. Particular importance should be given to discussion about the management of junctional re-entry tachycardia during pregnancy. Catheter ablation is curative in one sitting in a majority of cases and is widely regarded as preferable to long-term drug therapy in this typically young and otherwise healthy group of patients.

Atrial fibrillation

AF is the most common sustained arrhythmia, affecting about 1% of the population. AF is rare before the age of 50 years, but its prevalence approximately doubles with each decade thereafter such that about 10% of those older than 80 years are affected. AF is characterised by extremely rapid and uncoordinated electrical activity in the atria and variable conduction through the AV node, resulting in irregular and usually rapid ventricular contraction.

The clinical importance of AF results from:
1. symptoms including palpitation, reduced exercise capacity, breathlessness and fatigue;
2. increased risk of thromboembolic stroke;
3. exacerbation of heart failure through its direct haemodynamic effect and by causing tachycardia-induced cardiomyopathy;
4. increased all-cause mortality (odds ratio 1.5 for men and 1.9 for women).

AF may be classified as:

Paroxysmal: self-limiting episodes of AF lasting no more than 7 days;

Persistent: AF lasting more than 7 days or requiring cardioversion; *Longstanding persistent*: continuous AF for more than 1 year; or *Permanent*: where a decision has been made not to attempt cure of persistent AF.

AF may also be classified as 'valvular' or 'nonvalvular'. The term valvular AF is used for AF in the context of rheumatic valvular disease (predominantly mitral stenosis) or prosthetic heart valves.

Stroke risk. Non-valvular AF is associated with a fivefold increase in the risk of stroke. Most strokes complicating AF are ischaemic, as a result of embolism of thrombus that forms predominantly within the left atrial appendage due, at least in part, to sluggish blood flow within the fibrillating atria. Oral anticoagulants reduce stroke risk in AF by between 60% and 70% (Hart et al., 2007), whereas antiplatelet drugs prescribed as monotherapy provide little or no protection against stroke in this population and confer a risk of intracranial bleeding similar to that seen with oral anticoagulants, especially in elderly patients.

Guidelines for stroke risk management. Stroke risk management in patients with atrial flutter and AF is the subject of national and international guidelines (Camm et al., 2012; National Institute for Health and Care Excellence [NICE], 2014). All patients presenting with AF (or atrial flutter) should undergo assessment of their stroke risk. The type of AF (paroxysmal, persistent, or permanent) does not appear substantially to influence stroke risk, but there is strong evidence that stroke risk in AF is determined by the entire stroke risk factor profile.

Patients with valvular AF (i.e. rheumatic mitral valve disease or a prosthetic heart valve) should be treated with a vitamin K antagonist (VKA) such as warfarin.

For patients with non-valvular AF, stroke risk is currently assessed by the CHA_2DS_2-VASc score (Table 22.1), which ranges from 0 to 9. The risk of thromboembolism is directly

Table 22.1 The CHA_2DS_2-VASc score for the assessment of stroke risk in non-valvular atrial fibrillation

Stroke risk factor	CHA_2DS_2-VASc score
Congestive cardiac failure and/or moderate-to-severely impaired left ventricular systolic function	1
Hypertension	1
Age ≥75 years (2 points)	2
Diabetes mellitus	1
History of stroke, transient ischaemic attack or other thromboembolism	2
Arterial vascular disease (history of myocardial infarction, aortic atheroma or peripheral vascular disease)	1
Age between 65 and 74 years	1
Sex category (female)	1
Adapted from Lip et al. (2010a).	

proportional to the CHA_2DS_2-VASc score (Fig. 22.10) (Olesen et al., 2011). Patients younger than 65 years with non-valvular AF and no other stroke risk factors (including female patients) are considered to have a low enough stroke risk that no stroke-preventative therapy is indicated. For all other patients, the CHA_2DS_2-VASc score should be calculated, and those with a CHA_2DS_2-VASc score ≥1 should be considered for treatment with either a VKA or a non-VKA oral anticoagulant (NOAC; also referred to as a direct oral anticoagulant [DOAC]): a direct thrombin inhibitor such as dabigatran or one of the factor Xa inhibitors apixaban, rivaroxaban and edoxaban.

Antiplatelet agents are no longer recommended for stroke prevention in patients with AF. Dual antiplatelet therapy with aspirin and clopidogrel has been shown to reduce stroke risk by comparison with aspirin alone in patients with AF with moderately high stroke risk considered unsuitable for treatment with an oral anticoagulant (ACTIVE Investigators et al., 2009), but is associated with a significantly increased risk of internal bleeding, and this combination is not recommended by current guidance.

Assessment of bleeding risk. The benefit of oral anticoagulants in terms of stroke risk reduction in patients with AF is partially offset by an increased risk of bleeding. Several bleeding risk scores have been proposed, among them the HAS-BLED score (Table 22.2), which has been validated in the AF population (Pisters et al., 2010) (Fig. 22.11).

The use of bleeding risk scores is not sufficiently refined to allow accurate assessment of the anticipated net clinical benefit of anticoagulation in individuals with AF according to their CHA_2DS_2-VASc score. However, it prompts consideration of the risk of bleeding, modification where possible of bleeding risk factors and perhaps intensified monitoring.

Choice of oral anticoagulant. VKAs, such as warfarin, which inhibit the synthesis of clotting factors II, VII, IX and X, have been the mainstay of oral anticoagulant treatment for AF. The beneficial effect of VKAs is seen with an international normalised ratio (INR) in the range 2.0–3.0. A sub-therapeutic INR increases substantially the risk of stroke or arterial thromboembolism. Conversely, a high INR increases the risk of bleeding (Fig. 22.12). The approximate annual frequency of major and minor bleeding with VKAs is 3% and 10%, respectively. It may be difficult to maintain an INR within the therapeutic range of 2.0–3.0, and indeed there is evidence from real-world studies that the INR may be outside of this range for much of the time. Patients' and doctors' concerns about the use of VKAs have resulted in their under-utilisation, particularly among elderly people, who are at the greatest risk of stroke. This concern has led to the development of the NOACs (also referred to as DOACs). The perceived advantages of the DOACs over VKAs include:

1. a predictable effect of the drugs upon coagulation such that a standard dose is taken without the need for blood tests to assess its effect,

Table 22.2	The HAS-BLED score for calculation of the risk of bleeding (Pisters et al., 2010)	
Hypertension (systolic blood pressure >160 mmHg)		1
Abnormal renal and/or liver function		1 or 2
Stroke		1
Bleeding tendency or predisposition		1
Labile international normalised ratios (if on warfarin, time in therapeutic range <60%)		1
Elderly (age >65 years, frail condition)		1
Drugs (antiplatelets, non-steroidal anti-inflammatories) or alcohol excess/abuse		1 or 2

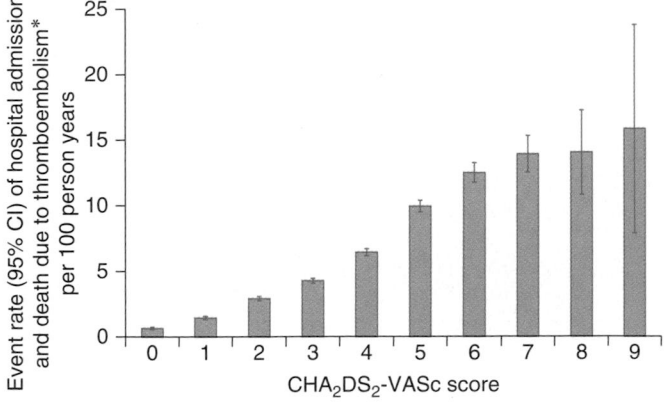

*Ischaemic stroke, peripheral artery embolism and pulmonary embolism, based upon 10 year follow-up.

Fig. 22.10 Hospital admission or death due to thromboembolism per 100 person-years as a function of CHA_2DS_2-VASc score, based upon 10-year follow-up. CI, Confidence interval. (Data from Olesen et al., 2011.)

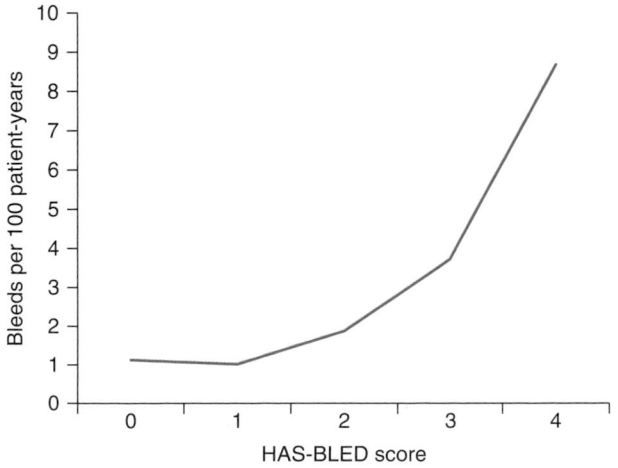

Fig. 22.11 Risk of major bleeding within 1 year as a function of the HAS-BLED score. (Data are from Pisters et al., 2010.)

2. lower potential for interaction with other drugs,
3. no dietary restrictions.

The following are potential disadvantages of DOACs by comparison with VKAs:

1. Assessing adherence may be problematic.
2. The DOACs are all to some extent renally excreted: Dose reduction is necessary in patients with impaired renal function, and the drugs are contraindicated in those with severely impaired renal function.
3. The ability to achieve rapid reversal of the anticoagulant effect of DOACs is a concern, although there is evidence that the intravenous administration of dried prothrombin complex (factors II, VII, IX and X) may reverse the anticoagulant of factor Xa inhibitors. Specific reversal agents are becoming available: idarucizumab, a reversal agent for dabigatran, received European Medicines Agency/U.S. Food and Drug Administration approval in the fourth quarter of 2015, and reversal agents for factor Xa inhibitors are in development.
4. Some DOACs require twice-daily dosing, which may reduce adherence.

Characteristics of the DOACs are summarised in Table 22.3.

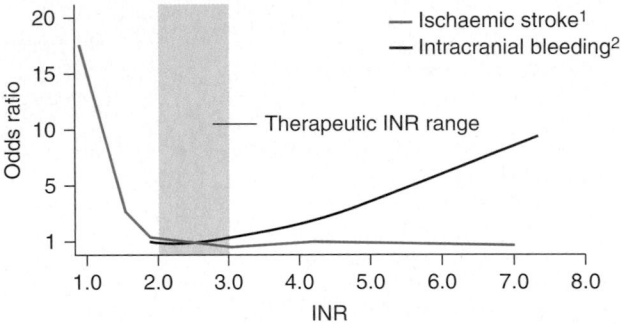

Fig. 22.12 The risk of stroke or intracranial bleeding according to the international normalised ratio (INR) in patients who are taking vitamin K antagonists. [1]Hylek et al. (1996); [2]Fang et al. (2004).

Each of the DOACs has been compared with warfarin in a prospective, randomised, multicentre clinical trial examining both efficacy for stroke risk reduction and safety in patients with AF and moderately increased stroke risk (Connolly et al., 2009; Giugliano et al., 2013; Granger et al., 2011; Patel et al., 2011). The results are summarised in Table 22.4.

Current European Society of Cardiology guidance (Kirchhof et al., 2016) is that where an oral anticoagulant is indicated for stroke risk reduction in AF:

- DOACs are recommended where there are difficulties in maintaining the INR within the therapeutic range with a VKA, where side effects are experienced with a VKA or where a patient is unable or unwilling to undertake INR monitoring.
- DOACs should be considered rather than VKAs for most patients with non-valvular AF based on their net clinical benefit.

Non-pharmacologic means of stroke risk reduction in atrial fibrillation. A majority of intracardiac thrombi occurring in the context of AF develop in the left atrial appendage. It is common practice to excise the left atrial appendage during surgical operations on the mitral valve, because patients with mitral valve disease requiring surgery are at high risk of development of AF. Left atrial appendage closure devices implanted percutaneously obviate the need for long-term treatment with an oral anticoagulant and have been shown to provide protection against stroke equivalent to that of warfarin in moderate-risk patients with AF. The medium- to long-term benefit of these devices is partially offset by a short-term risk of procedure-related complications.

Catheter ablation of AF may be curative. An important question is whether successful catheter ablation reduces stroke risk to the extent that it may no longer be necessary to take an oral anticoagulant. The results of several retrospective/observational studies suggest that this may indeed be the case (Bunch et al., 2013). The methodological limitations of this type of study are such that, pending the results of ongoing prospective trials addressing this question, current guidelines recommend

Table 22.3 Pharmacokinetic and pharmacodynamic properties of non-vitamin K antagonist oral anticoagulants

	Dabigatran[a]	Apixaban[a,b]	Rivaroxaban[a,c]	Edoxaban[d,e]
Mechanism of action	Oral direct thrombin inhibitor	Oral factor Xa Inhibitor	Oral factor Xa inhibitor	Oral factor Xa inhibitor
Bioavailability (%)	6	50	60–80	62
Plasma protein binding (%)	35	87	92–95	55
Time to peak levels (h)	0.5–2.0	3–4	2–4	1–2
Half-life (h)	12–14	12	5–13	10–14
Dosing				
Non-valvular atrial fibrillation	Twice daily	Twice daily	Once daily	Once daily

[a]Eriksson et al. (2009).
[b]Bristol Myers Squibb-Pfizer (2017).
[c]Bayer (2017).
[d]Bounameaux and Camm (2014).
[e]Daiichi Sankyo UK Limited (2017).

Table 22.4 Summary of the results of prospective randomised trials comparing non-vitamin K antagonist oral anticoagulant drugs with warfarin for stroke risk reduction in patients with non-valvular atrial fibrillation

Drug	Dosage	Trial outcome
Dabigatran[a]	150 mg twice a day 110 mg twice a day	**Efficacy:** both doses non-inferior to warfarin, higher dose superior to warfarin in preventing stroke and systemic embolism **Safety:** lower dose less major bleeding than warfarin, both doses less intracranial haemorrhage compared with warfarin
Rivaroxaban[b]	20 mg once a day 15 mg once a day	**Efficacy:** non-inferior to warfarin **Safety:** non-inferior to warfarin and less intracranial haemorrhage compared with warfarin
Apixaban[c]	5 mg twice a day 2.5 mg twice a day	**Efficacy:** superior to warfarin for stroke risk reduction and all-cause mortality **Safety:** less major bleeding or intracranial haemorrhage compared with warfarin
Edoxaban[d]	60 mg once a day 30 mg once a day	**Efficacy:** both doses non-inferior to warfarin **Safety:** less major bleeding or intracranial haemorrhage compared with warfarin

[a]Connolly et al. (2009).
[b]Patel et al. (2011).
[c]Granger et al. (2011).
[d]Giugliano et al. (2013).

the continuation of oral anticoagulants following catheter ablation of AF according to the CHA_2DS_2-VASc score (Camm et al., 2012).

Duration of treatment with oral anticoagulants. In trials comparing different drug-based treatment strategies for AF, a majority of strokes occurred in patients who had been considered to have good heart rhythm control and whose oral anticoagulants had therefore been stopped (Sherman et al., 2005). It is known that asymptomatic AF is commonplace, even in patients who also have symptomatic episodes of AF. Furthermore, the presence and prevalence of AF may be underestimated by many detection strategies. For these and other reasons it is rarely appropriate to discontinue oral anticoagulant treatment in those patients with a CHA_2DS_2-VASc score ≥ 1.

Emergency management of atrial fibrillation. AF associated with unstable angina, heart failure or hypotension requires emergency treatment. In most cases, the treatment of choice is DC cardioversion. Concerns about thromboembolism as the heart returns to sinus rhythm are valid but should not delay emergency treatment. Immediate DC cardioversion is appropriate when the onset of AF is clearly identified as within 48 hours of presentation or when the patient is already taking an oral anticoagulant with, in the case of warfarin, a therapeutic INR for at least 4 weeks. If facilities permit, a transoesophageal echocardiogram may be performed in patients not already receiving an oral anticoagulant to exclude intracardiac thrombus. Heparin should then be given immediately and continued until the patient is established on an oral anticoagulant. A DOAC would be an attractive choice in this situation because of the rapid onset of action of this class of drugs. Anticoagulant therapy should be continued for at least 3 months following cardioversion because the complete return of effective contraction of the atrial musculature may take several weeks following the restoration of sinus rhythm. The need for long-term stroke prophylaxis is guided thereafter by the CHA_2DS_2-VASc score.

If DC cardioversion is deemed inappropriate, rapid ventricular rate control may be achieved with intravenous β-blockers, verapamil or digoxin.

Long-term management of atrial fibrillation. There has been considerable debate about the pros and cons of a rate-control strategy focusing on achieving adequate control of the ventricular rate with drugs modifying the AV node versus a rhythm-control strategy, in which an attempt is made to restore and maintain sinus rhythm with antiarrhythmic drugs with or without DC cardioversion. These strategies have been compared in several large-scale prospective randomised trials, which have failed to demonstrate an advantage to a rhythm-control strategy. Sinus rhythm has been associated with a 47% reduction in all-cause mortality, although this benefit was offset by a 49% increase in mortality associated with the use of antiarrhythmic drugs (AFFIRM Investigators, 2004). In that study, a wide variety of antiarrhythmic drugs was used at the discretion of the investigator. These included several class I antiarrhythmic drugs, sotalol and amiodarone. A rhythm-control strategy may be more appropriate in (1) younger patients, (2) those with paroxysmal AF, (3) those with AF associated with heart failure, and (4) patients who remain symptomatic despite adequate ventricular rate control.

Ventricular rate control. The mainstay of a ventricular rate-control strategy is the use of drugs that prolong the AV nodal refractory period, thus reducing the ventricular rate. β-Blockers or CCBs (verapamil or diltiazem) are generally effective both at rest and on exertion, although a combination of these drugs is occasionally necessary. Digoxin may control the ventricular rate at rest but is less successful at controlling the rate during exertion, and therefore should only be considered in patients with non-paroxysmal AF who do no or little physical exercise. Where ventricular rate control cannot be achieved with drugs, catheter ablation of the AV node in combination with permanent pacemaker implantation can provide excellent symptom relief. The adverse effects of right ventricular apical pacing may offset some of the benefit of a slower ventricular rate and regular rhythm; therefore, biventricular pacing may be more appropriate in this situation.

Rhythm control. Rhythm control can be considered in terms of either restoration or maintenance of sinus rhythm. The most rapid and effective means of restoring sinus rhythm is DC cardioversion. Where AF is of short duration, well-tolerated and not associated with structural heart disease, class IC antiarrhythmic drugs such as flecainide and class III drugs such as amiodarone may be used intravenously to achieve chemical cardioversion. Stroke risk should be managed in the same way as described for the emergency management of AF.

Although sinus rhythm can be restored in most patients with DC cardioversion and/or antiarrhythmic drugs, most patients will revert to AF without further treatment. The SAFE-T trial examined 665 patients with AF of at least 72 hours' duration. Sinus rhythm was restored with antiarrhythmic drugs (sotalol or amiodarone) or placebo, supplemented where necessary by DC cardioversion (Singh et al., 2005). Patients were then maintained on placebo, sotalol or amiodarone. By 2 years, that probability of remaining in sinus rhythm was 10% (placebo), 30% (sotalol) and 50% (amiodarone). Another similar study (Roy et al., 2000) demonstrated equivalent efficacy of sotalol and the class Ic antiarrhythmic drug propafenone in the maintenance of sinus rhythm (40% at 2 years) and confirmed the superiority of amiodarone (60%). Most heart rhythm specialists consider that the toxicity of amiodarone precludes its long-term use for the management of AF. It was hoped that dronedarone would provide efficacy similar to amiodarone, but it has been shown to be less effective, although it has far fewer side effects and is not used widely. In practice, for long-term treatment, flecainide tends to be used in younger patients with structurally normal hearts and with no evidence of cardiac conduction system disease. Sotalol is preferred in patients with hypertensive or ischaemic heart disease, and amiodarone is generally reserved for elderly patients in whom there may be fewer concerns about the side effects of long-term amiodarone (Kirchhof et al., 2016).

Modern strategies for curative catheter ablation of AF followed the discovery in 1998 that paroxysmal AF is due, in most cases, to rapid firing by the musculature surrounding the pulmonary veins close to their junctions with the left atrium. The cornerstone of most current ablation strategies for paroxysmal AF is complete electrical isolation of all four pulmonary veins from the left atrium, using either radiofrequency ablation (cautery) or cryo-ablation to ablate in rings around the pairs of ipsilateral veins. Catheter ablation can cure a majority of paroxysmal AF but needs to be repeated in 20–25% of patients and carries risk, including stroke (2–3/1000) and pericardial effusion (1–2/100). Catheter ablation has been shown to be superior to antiarrhythmic drug therapy in maintaining sinus rhythm and improving symptoms and quality of life. Catheter ablation has also been shown in non-randomised studies to improve left ventricular ejection fraction and heart failure symptoms. The CASTLE-AF study (Marrouche et al., 2018) was the first to demonstrate that catheter ablation is associated with a reduction in mortality by comparison with standard medical therapy, in patients with severely impaired left ventricular systolic function and heart failure symptoms. No benefit has been convincingly demonstrated in terms of reduced stroke risk. The natural history of AF is for episodes of AF to increase in frequency and duration until persistent AF supervenes. This progression appears to occur as a result of atrial remodelling, a complex and incompletely understood process involving electrical and structural changes in the whole atrial myocardium predisposing to the development of AF independent of the pulmonary veins. Catheter ablation strategies for persistent AF are more complex than those for paroxysmal AF with a correspondingly higher rate of repeat procedures and a lower overall success rate. For all of these reasons, drug therapy remains the first-line treatment of AF, with catheter ablation reserved for patients with symptomatic AF that cannot be managed satisfactorily with drugs and whose symptoms trouble them enough to undergo ablation.

Ventricular tachyarrhythmias

Ventricular tachycardia

VT is a rapid, abnormal heart rhythm that originates in the ventricles. VT may present with palpitation, chest pain, breathlessness, presyncope, syncope or sudden cardiac death (death occurring suddenly and unexpectedly within 1 hour of the onset of symptoms from a presumed cardiac cause). It is clinically useful to subdivide VT in the following ways: VT complicating structural heart disease and 'normal heart' VT.

Ventricular tachycardia complicating structural heart disease. Most VT occurs in patients with significant structural heart disease. The predominant cause is healed myocardial infarction, but other important causes include hypertensive and valvular heart disease and a variety of cardiomyopathies including dilated cardiomyopathy, hypertrophic cardiomyopathy, or arrhythmogenic right ventricular cardiomyopathy. VT of this type is usually due to re-entry. Scarring of ventricular myocardium creates the central obstacle around which potential re-entry circuits develop forming the VT 'substrate'. In this setting, a single ventricular premature beat, the VT 'trigger', may induce VT. The importance of VT complicating structural heart disease is that there is a high chance of the VT recurring, and patients are at substantially increased risk of sudden cardiac death.

'Normal heart' ventricular tachycardia. These uncommon VTs occur in the context of a structurally normal heart and a normal ECG in sinus rhythm and are exemplified by right ventricular outflow tract (RVOT) tachycardia and fascicular tachycardia. The importance of recognising these VTs is that unlike VT associated with structural heart disease, they are associated with a normal prognosis, may be managed successfully with drugs (β-blockers, verapamil or flecainide for RVOT tachycardia, verapamil for fascicular tachycardia) and are curable by catheter ablation.

Ventricular fibrillation

Ventricular fibrillation (VF) comprises rapid and totally disorganised electrical activity in the ventricles such that effective contraction ceases and results in sudden death unless sinus rhythm is restored either spontaneously or by defibrillation. Acute myocardial ischaemia and infarction are probably responsible for most VF, although virtually any structural heart disease may also be complicated by VF. Other cases occur in the context of a group of conditions known as channelopathies.

Channelopathies. Channelopathies are a group of inherited conditions characterised by abnormal function of the protein channels present in the cardiac myocyte cell membrane that regulate the flow of ions responsible for generating the resting transmembrane potential and the action potential. These include the long QT syndromes, short QT syndrome, early repolarisation syndrome, Brugada syndrome and catecholaminergic polymorphic VT. A detailed description of these conditions is beyond the scope of this chapter, but there are certain key points:

- With the exception of catecholaminergic polymorphic VT, each is associated with characteristic abnormalities of the resting ECG in sinus rhythm.
- Each may be complicated by ventricular tachyarrhythmias and sudden cardiac death.
- β-Blockers reduce the likelihood of arrhythmia in long QT syndromes and catecholaminergic polymorphic VT.
- Many drugs lengthen the QT interval (Box 22.1) and are contraindicated in patients with long QT syndromes. A list of drugs known to prolong the QT interval can be found at http://www.crediblemeds.org.
- Class I antiarrhythmic drugs and a variety of other drugs are contraindicated in Brugada syndrome. A list of drugs to avoid in the Brugada syndrome can be found at http://www.brugadadrugs.org.
- Most patients with these conditions who experience syncope or cardiac arrest or who develop spontaneous ventricular arrhythmias will be considered for an implantable cardioverter-defibrillator (ICD).

Emergency management of ventricular arrhythmias

VF and pulseless VT should be managed according to Resuscitation Council (UK) guidelines for advanced life support, which are updated periodically and can be found at http://www.resus.org.uk.

VT associated with a pulse is also the subject of guidelines by the Resuscitation Council (UK) (http://www.resus.org.uk). If the patient is hypotensive in a low cardiac output state or has heart failure, the correct treatment is prompt DC cardioversion. If none of these features are present, chemical cardioversion may be attempted with intravenous amiodarone

---

Box 22.1 Drugs associated with prolonged QT intervals

Inhalational agents: halothane, isoflurane
Macrolide antibiotics: erythromycin, clarithromycin
Halofantrine
Lithium
Fosphenytoin
Mizolastine
Phenothiazines
Pentamidine
Sertindole
Antihistamines: terfenadine, astemizole, mizolastine
Antipsychotics: haloperidol, droperidol, pimozide
Tricyclic antidepressants: amitriptyline, imipramine
Class IA or III antiarrhythmics

Adapted from Crouch et al. (2003).

---

300 mg over 20–60 minutes followed by 900 mg over the next 24 hours. Amiodarone must be given via a central vein because it can cause thrombophlebitis when given peripherally and limb-threatening soft tissue damage if extravasation occurs.

Ongoing management of ventricular arrhythmias

Once stabilised, patients presenting with VT or VF should remain in hospital and their management should be discussed at an early stage with a specialist cardiac electrophysiology service. Investigations should be performed to establish the nature and extent of underlying heart disease, with emphasis on detecting structural heart disease, coronary artery disease, inducible myocardial ischaemia and consideration of channelopathies in those with structurally normal hearts.

Most patients with ischaemic heart disease should be treated with aspirin, statins, angiotensin-converting enzyme (ACE) inhibitors or angiotensin II receptor antagonists and β-blockers. β-Blockers and ACE inhibitors reduce somewhat the risk of sudden cardiac death. Although these patients remain at high risk of sudden cardiac death because of recurrent ventricular tachyarrhythmias, there is no role for the routine use of antiarrhythmic drugs. In patients with complex ventricular ectopy and impaired left ventricular systolic function following acute myocardial infarction, class Ic antiarrhythmic drugs including flecainide were shown in the Cardiac Arrhythmia Suppression Trial (CAST) (Echt et al., 1991) to increase mortality, whereas in other high-risk groups amiodarone has been shown to have no effect on all-cause mortality (Cairns et al., 1997; Julian et al., 1997). All patients should be considered for an ICD. These devices have been shown to improve prognosis following:

- cardiac arrest due to VT or VF in the absence of a reversible underlying cause,
- VT associated with syncope or significant haemodynamic compromise,
- VT with a left ventricular ejection fraction of less than 35%.

Although ICDs treat further episodes of VT and VF, they do not prevent these arrhythmias from recurring and resulting in device therapies including shocks that are psychologically traumatic and lead to premature battery depletion. In the case of frequently recurring ventricular arrhythmias, patients should be on the maximum tolerated dose of a β-blocker, and there is a role in this situation for antiarrhythmic drugs including amiodarone and mexiletine (mexiletine has a European license and is available by special order in the UK). Catheter ablation of VT is an important adjunctive treatment.

Bradycardia

Bradycardia is conventionally defined as a resting heart rate of less than 60 per minute when awake or 50 per minute when asleep. Bradycardia can be classified as sinus bradycardia, where the sinus node discharges too slowly, or AV block ('heart block'), where conduction between the atria and ventricles is impaired. AV block may be subdivided into three classes:

First degree. Every P wave conducts to the ventricles but takes longer than normal to do so. The PR interval on the ECG is prolonged to greater than 200 ms (one large square on a standard ECG recorded at 25 mm/s).

Second degree. Some, but not all, P waves conduct to the ventricles. Progressive PR interval prolongation followed by a non-conducted P wave is referred to as Mobitz type I or Wenckebach heart block and implies block occurring in the AV node. Mobitz type II heart block is the term used when a non-conducted P wave is not preceded by progressive PR interval prolongation and implies block occurring in the conducting system below the level of the AV node.

Third degree ('complete heart block'). No P waves conduct to the ventricles.

Bradycardia may be due to intrinsic cardiac disease or secondary to non-cardiac disease or drugs. In many cases, bradycardia due to intrinsic cardiac disease is idiopathic, that is, occurs without other identifiable heart disease. Bradycardia may also complicate acute myocardial infarction or virtually any form of structural heart disease and is also common following cardiac surgery. Non-cardiac causes of bradycardia include neurocardiogenic ('vasovagal') syncope (faints), hypothyroidism, hyperkalaemia, hypothermia and raised intracranial pressure. Complete heart block may occur as a complication of Lyme disease (tick-borne borreliosis). Drugs commonly associated with bradycardia include β-blockers, verapamil, diltiazem, digoxin and antiarrhythmic drugs of any class.

The management of bradycardia is as follows:
- Treat underlying medical conditions.
- Consider stopping or reducing the dose of causative drugs.
- Consider temporary or permanent pacemaker implantation. Permanent pacemaker implantation is indicated for symptomatic bradycardia as a result of sinus bradycardia or AV block, or on prognostic grounds for Mobitz type 2 second-degree or third-degree AV block.

In an emergency situation, drugs may be used in an attempt to support the heart rate until transvenous pacing can be established. The most useful drugs in this situation are atropine in 500-microgram boluses up to a total of 3 mg, adrenaline infused at a rate of 2–10 micrograms/min or isoprenaline 1–10 micrograms/min, titrated against heart rate. External pacing is another useful measure until transvenous pacing can be established. More detailed guidance on the emergency management of bradycardia may be viewed at http://www.resus.org.uk.

Drug therapy

Antiarrhythmic drug therapy is used to control the frequency and severity of arrhythmias, with the aim of maintaining sinus rhythm where possible. Although antiarrhythmic drug treatment has been the mainstay of arrhythmia treatment, many of these drugs have limited efficacy and important toxicity. Many arrhythmias are now curable by catheter ablation. Implantable devices such as permanent pacemakers and ICDs have assumed an increasingly important role in the treatment of arrhythmias, and in many cases, antiarrhythmic drugs have an adjunctive role. Antiarrhythmic drugs can be grouped according to their electrophysiological

effects at a cellular level, using the Vaughan–Williams classification (Vaughan-Williams, 1970). Alternatively, antiarrhythmic drugs may be classified according to their main sites of action within the heart.

Vaughan–Williams classification

All antiarrhythmic drugs act by altering the movement of electrolytes across the myocardial cell membrane. The Vaughan–Williams classification groups drugs according to their ability to block the movement of one or more of these ions across the myocardial cell membrane (Vaughan-Williams, 1970). Most drugs have several modes of action, and their effectiveness as antiarrhythmic agents depends upon the summation of these effects. The effect of the different drug classes on the various phases of the action potential are shown in Table 22.5. The choice of which drug to use is based upon the origin of the arrhythmia, regardless of its pattern. However, the preference of one class over another may vary, depending on a clinician's experience with particular drugs, on the presentation of the arrhythmia and on patient characteristics. Such factors also govern the choice of drug within a class. The drug chosen should have the dosing schedule and adverse effect profile that best suit the patient or inconvenience them least (see Tables 22.6 and 22.7). Thus, for example, a patient with glaucoma or prostatism should not be given disopyramide, which possesses marked anticholinergic properties, and a patient with obstructive airways disease should preferably not be prescribed a β-blocker (class II), although if considered essential they could have a cardio-selective agent.

The pharmacokinetic profiles of selected antiarrhythmic drugs are presented in Table 22.8.

Class I antiarrhythmic drugs

Class I antiarrhythmic drugs block sodium channels and therefore inhibit the inward sodium current I_{Na}, responsible for the upstroke of the action potential in cells other than those of the sinoatrial and AV nodes. The result of I_{Na} inhibition is to slow conduction velocity, which should promote re-entry, and thus be proarrhythmic. The antiarrhythmic effect of class I

Table 22.5 Effect of different drug classes on phases of action potential

Phase	Dominant ion movement	Drug class	Effect
0	Sodium inward	IA	Block ++
		IB	Block +
		IC	Block +++
2	Calcium inward	IV	Block
3	Potassium outward	III	Marked slowing
4	Sodium inward, potassium outward	I, II, IV	Slows

Table 22.6 Adverse effects of antiarrhythmic drugs (class I)

Drug	Cardiac	Non-cardiac	Caution or avoid in
Disopyramide	Torsade de pointes Myodepressant	Anticholinergic (urinary retention, constipation, dry mouth, blurred vision)	Glaucoma, prostatism, hypotension
Procainamide		Lupus, nausea, diarrhoea	Myasthenia gravis, slow acetylators (increased risk of lupus)
Quinidine	Torsade de pointes Vasodilation (i.v.)	Diarrhoea, nausea, tinnitus, headache, deafness, confusion, visual disturbances, blood dyscrasias	Myasthenia gravis
Lidocaine (lignocaine)		Convulsions in overdose, paraesthesiae	Liver failure (reduce dose)
Mexiletine		Nausea, paraesthesiae	Second- or third-degree heart block
Flecainide	Proarrhythmic	Paraesthesiae, tremor	Not recommended if any cardiac dysfunction
	Myodepressant		
Propafenone	Proarrhythmic Myodepressant	Gastro-intestinal disturbances	Not recommended if any cardiac dysfunction

Table 22.7 Adverse effects of antiarrhythmic drugs (classes II–IV)

Drug	Cardiac	Non-cardiac	Caution or avoid in
β-Blockers (general)	Myodepressant Heart block	Bronchoconstriction (β_2) Vasoconstriction Hallucinations/vivid dreams (greater with more lipophilic agents) Decreased renal blood flow Changes in serum lipid profile Drowsiness, fatigue	Asthma, COPD, Raynaud's disease, diabetes mellitus, depression
Dofetilide	Torsade de pointes		Combination with disopyramide or amiodarone or drugs in Table 22.5
Amiodarone	Torsade de pointes	Hyperthyroidism/hypothyroidism, pneumonitis, myopathy, neuropathy, hepatitis, corneal deposits, photosensitivity	Thyroid disease, liver dysfunction, lung disease (e.g. pneumonectomy)
Bretylium	Hypotension	Initial sympathomimetic response, nausea	
Verapamil	Heart block	Constipation, headaches, flushing, ankle oedema, light-headedness	Myasthenia gravis
Adenosine	Heart block	Bronchoconstriction, flushing, chest pain	Asthma, COPD, combination with dipyridamole Decompensated heart failure, patients with a history of convulsions/seizures or recent heart transplant (<1 year)

COPD, Chronic obstructive pulmonary disease.

Table 22.8 Pharmacokinetics of selected antiarrhythmics

	Oral absorption	Protein binding (%)	Elimination, metabolism, half-life (therapeutic range if recommended to be measured)
Amiodarone	Slow, variable	>95	Extensive metabolism, very variable rate, $t_{1/2}$ 2 days initially increasing to 40–60 days
Bretylium	Intravenous/intramuscular only	Unbound	Renal, $t_{1/2}$ 5–10 h
Digoxin	Variable, 70%	25	70% renal, variable, $t_{1/2}$ 36 h (0.8–2 ng/mL)
Diltiazem	40% absorbed	80	Hepatic, $t_{1/2}$ 3 h
Disopyramide	Rapid, >80%	30–90	50% renal, 15% bile, active metabolite, $t_{1/2}$ 4–10 h
Flecainide	Complete, slow	40	30% renal, $t_{1/2}$ 20 h
Lidocaine	Intravenous/intramuscular only	60–80	10% renal, rapid hepatic metabolism to central nervous system–toxic products, $t_{1/2}$ 8–100 min increases with duration of dosing
Mexiletine	>90%	60–70	10% renal, $t_{1/2}$ 10–12 h, hepatic metabolites mostly inactive
Procainamide	Rapid, >75%	15–20	50% renal, 25–40% converted to N-acetylprocainamide (active, $t_{1/2}$ 6 h), procainamide $t_{1/2}$ 2.5–4.5 h
Propafenone	Complete, rapid	>95	Extensive first-pass metabolism, capacity-limited, $t_{1/2}$ 2–12 h
Quinidine	Rapid, >80%	80–90	Mixed renal and hepatic, $t_{1/2}$ 6 h
Verapamil	Rapid, >90%	90	Hepatic, $t_{1/2}$ 4–12 h, marked first-pass effect

All values quoted are subject to marked interindividual variability. Most therapeutic ranges are poorly defined. Oral absorption does not account for drug lost by first-pass hepatic metabolism. Rapid absorption indicates a peak plasma concentration in less than 2 hours.
$t_{1/2}$, Elimination half-life at normal renal function.

drugs is attributed to critical depression of conduction in already slowly conducting areas such as the diastolic pathway of re-entry circuits associated with structural heart disease, resulting in conduction block and abolishing or preventing re-entry. The properties of class I antiarrhythmic drugs fall into three subgroups: class Ia, class Ib and class Ic antiarrhythmic drugs.

Class Ia antiarrhythmic drugs. Drugs in this class (quinidine, disopyramide and procainamide) have an intermediate inhibitory effect on the inward sodium current I_{Na}, generally causing significant slowing of conduction only at faster heart rates. Class Ia drugs also inhibit the rapid component of the delayed rectifier current I_{Kr}, resulting in prolongation of the cardiac action potential and hence effective refractory period. This property is responsible for a propensity to cause Torsade de pointes. Both quinidine and disopyramide additionally block muscarinic cholinoceptors, which may contribute to their efficacy for the treatment of arrhythmias in which the parasympathetic nervous system plays a role, such as AF.

Class Ia antiarrhythmic drugs have been used for the treatment of a variety of atrial and ventricular arrhythmias but are now rarely used because of their proarrhythmic and non-cardiac side effects and potential for drug interactions.

Class Ib antiarrhythmic drugs. Class Ib drugs (lidocaine, mexiletine) are the weakest sodium channel blockers, producing little change in the QRS duration in normal cardiac tissue, and also have no significant effect on repolarisation.

Lidocaine is occasionally used in the treatment of VT, particularly when VT occurs in patients already taking amiodarone and β-blockers. Lidocaine acts preferentially on ischaemic myocardium and is more effective in the presence of a high external potassium concentration. Therefore, hypokalaemia must be corrected for maximum efficacy. Lidocaine has no value in treating supraventricular tachyarrhythmias.

Mexiletine may be administered intravenously or orally to control VT. Frequent gastro-intestinal and central nervous system (CNS) side effects (dizziness, light-headedness, tremor, nervousness, difficulty with coordination) limit the dose and possible therapeutic benefit.

Class Ic antiarrhythmic drugs. Class Ic antiarrhythmic drugs (flecainide, propafenone) inhibit the inward sodium current I_{Na} with a slow time-constant for recovery, leading to marked slowing of conduction, which is most prominent in depolarised tissue. They also inhibit the ultra-rapid (I_{Kur}) and rapid (I_{Kr}) components of the delayed rectifier outward potassium current, prolonging the cardiac action potential and hence increasing the effective refractory period. This action is more prominent at higher heart rates ('use dependency'), which may help to explain the efficacy of these drugs for the treatment of AF. Propafenone is also a β-adrenoceptor antagonist.

Class Ic agents are potent antiarrhythmics used largely in the control of paroxysmal supraventricular and ventricular tachyarrhythmias resistant to other drugs, although they have acquired a particularly bad reputation as a result of the proarrhythmic effects seen in the CAST (Echt et al., 1991) and the Cardiac Arrest Study Hamburg (CASH) (Kuck et al., 2000) studies. Faster heart rates, increased sympathetic activity, and diseased or ischaemic myocardium all contribute to the proarrhythmic effects of these drugs. This has led to these drugs being contraindicated in patients with structural heart disease because poor systolic function exaggerates the proarrhythmic effects. However, flecainide is effective for the treatment of both supraventricular and ventricular arrhythmias in patients without structural heart disease and is moderately successful for maintenance of sinus rhythm after cardioversion of AF. Propafenone has mild β-blocking properties, especially in higher doses, so it should be avoided in patients with reversible obstructive airways disease.

Class II antiarrhythmic drugs: β-adrenoreceptor antagonists (β-blockers)

β-Adrenoceptors are widely distributed throughout the atrial and ventricular myocardium, with particularly high concentrations in the sinoatrial and AV nodes. β_1-Adrenoceptors account for 70–80% of the total, and β_2-adrenoceptors a majority of the remainder. Stimulation of β_1-adrenoceptors by binding of adrenaline or noradrenaline activates a G_s protein, which in turn activates adenylyl cyclase, which catalyses the formation of cAMP from adenosine triphosphate (ATP) (Fig. 22.13).

cAMP increases the inward current I_f, which increases the pacemaker rate, I_{Na}, which increases conduction velocity in tissue with an action potential upstroke carried by that current, and $I_{Ca,L}$, which is responsible for a positive inotropic effect, and increases the conduction velocity and reduces the refractory period in the AV node. cAMP also increases the repolarising current I_{Ks}, which shortens APD and hence effective refractory period. β-Blockers compete with adrenaline and noradrenaline for occupation of β-adrenoceptors and therefore reduce the sinus rate, slow conduction, and increase refractory period in the AV node; have a negative inotropic effect; and slightly prolong cardiac action potential and effective refractory period. The latter effect is probably clinically unimportant. Although some of the antiarrhythmic effects of β-blockers may be explained in terms of their acute effects on transmembrane currents, the effects of adrenergic stimulation, and hence those of β-blockers, are complex, differ between acute and chronic stimulation, and are modified by a variety of disease states. Furthermore, although many of the effects of β-blockers are as a direct result of changes in transmembrane currents, others result from changes in heart rate: for example, APD and effective refractory period are inversely proportional to heart rate.

β-Blockers licensed for the treatment of arrhythmias include propranolol, acebutolol, atenolol, esmolol, metoprolol and sotalol. The antiarrhythmic activity of the various β-blockers is reasonably uniform, the critical property being β_1-adrenoreceptor blockade. Atenolol, metoprolol, propranolol and esmolol are available for intravenous use. Esmolol, a selective β_1-adrenoreceptor antagonist, has a half-life of 9 minutes with full recovery from its β-blockade properties within 30 minutes. Esmolol is quickly metabolised in red blood cells, independent of renal and hepatic function, and due to its short half-life can be useful in situations where there are relative contraindications or concerns about the use of a β-blocker. Sotalol has some class III activity, as well as class II effects.

The use of β-blockers is somewhat constrained by their adverse effects. β_2-Adrenoreceptors on bronchial smooth muscle are tonically activated by circulating catecholamines to cause bronchodilation. β-Blockers can, therefore, cause bronchoconstriction and are contraindicated in patients with asthma, and should be used with caution in chronic obstructive pulmonary disease. β_2-Adrenoreceptors are also found on vascular smooth muscle and are tonically activated by circulating catecholamines to cause vasodilatation. β-Blockers may, therefore, cause vasoconstriction and exacerbate the symptoms of peripheral vascular disease.

Cardiac adverse effects of β-blockers include sinus bradycardia, exacerbation of AV conduction block, reduced exercise capacity, and exacerbation of acute heart failure. In patients with chronic, stable heart failure due to mild-to-moderate LV systolic dysfunction and already treated by ACE inhibitors and diuretics, however, β-blockers improve both symptoms and prognosis. Other adverse effects of β-blockers include nightmares and impotence.

β-Blockers vary in their lipid solubility. Agents such as propranolol and carvedilol are highly lipid-soluble, whereas others such as atenolol and nadolol are more hydrophilic. Lipid solubility determines the degree of drug penetration into the CNS and the utility of haemodialysis or haemofiltration. High lipid solubility is associated with a larger volume of distribution and better CNS penetration. Lipophilic β-blockers are primarily metabolised by the liver. Conversely, hydrophilic β-blockers have a small volume of distribution and are eliminated essentially unchanged by the kidneys; this property allows hydrophilic β-blockers to be removed by haemodialysis.

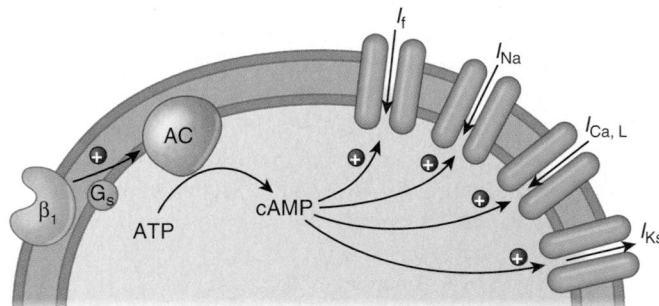

Fig. 22.13 Principal mechanisms of antiarrhythmic action of β-adrenoreceptor antagonists.
AC, adenylyl cyclase; ATP, adenosine triphosphate; cAMP, cyclic adenosine monophosphate.

Class III antiarrhythmic drugs

Class III antiarrhythmic drugs inhibit the delayed rectifier current I_K, which prolongs cardiac APD and hence effective refractory period. Most clinically important arrhythmias are as a result of re-entry. For re-entry to sustain, the activation wavefront must continuously meet electrically excitable tissue as it progresses around the re-entry circuit, the so-called excitable gap. Prolongation of the effective refractory period by a class III antiarrhythmic drug reduces or even abolishes the excitable gap, thus reducing the likelihood of sustained re-entry.

Class III drugs include sotalol, dofetilide, amiodarone and dronedarone. Sotalol and dofetilide selectively inhibit the rapid component of the delayed rectifier current I_{Kr}, whereas amiodarone and dronedarone are less specific, also inhibiting the slow component I_{Ks}. Selective I_{Kr} inhibitors are more effective at slower heart rates, a phenomenon termed reverse use dependence. It is this property that predisposes to the development of Torsade de pointes, a polymorphic VT that may be life-threatening. The development of Torsade de pointes is attributed to a combination of triggered activity as a result of EADs and increased transmural dispersion of repolarisation within the ventricles because action potential prolongation is not uniform across the ventricular wall. Hypokalaemia, hypomagnesaemia or bradycardia increase the likelihood of Torsade de pointes; therefore, sotalol, with marked class II activity, may be uniquely arrhythmogenic.

Amiodarone is a potent antiarrhythmic drug with additional class I, II and IV activity that is effective in treating a wide variety of atrial and ventricular arrhythmias, but its use is constrained by complex pharmacokinetics and concern about toxicity. Many heart rhythm specialists would consider that the side effect profile of amiodarone precludes its use for the long-term treatment of atrial arrhythmias. Amiodarone may be extremely effective in the emergency treatment of VT and VF, especially where recurrent. Amiodarone may also reduce the likelihood of recurrent ventricular arrhythmias when taken on a long-term basis but confers no prognostic benefit and should be considered as an adjunct to treatment with an ICD.

When rapid control of an arrhythmia is needed, the intravenous route is preferred, with 300 mg given over 30–60 minutes followed by 900 mg over 23–24 hours, administered through a central vein. Higher loading doses may cause hypotension. A concurrent oral loading regimen of up to 2400 mg daily in two to four divided doses is usually given for 7–14 days and then reduced to a maintenance dosage of 200 mg daily or less.

During the early stages of therapy with amiodarone (whether intravenous or oral), the kinetics of the drug are different from those after chronic administration. Amiodarone is highly lipid-soluble and thus has a very large volume of distribution. As the slowly equilibrating tissue stores are penetrated to a minimal extent during the early days of therapy, the effective elimination half-life ($t_{1/2}$) is initially dependent upon a more rapidly exchanging compartment, with a half-life of 10–17 hours, substantially shorter than the half-life seen during chronic administration. The short half-life becomes important during the acute phase and any intravenous to oral changeover period because the absorption of oral amiodarone is very slow, taking up to 15 hours. The combination of a relatively fast elimination and a poor rate of absorption could lead to a significant fall in serum amiodarone levels if intravenous therapy is stopped abruptly when oral therapy is initiated, with the period of maximum risk being the first 24 hours of oral therapy. It is therefore advisable to phase out intravenous therapy gradually and allow an intravenous/oral overlap period of at least 24 hours. Once amiodarone has reached saturation, amiodarone is eliminated very slowly, with a half-life of about 25–110 days. Because of the long terminal half-life of amiodarone, there is a potential for drug interactions to occur several weeks (or even months) after treatment with it has been stopped. Common interactions include antibacterials, other antiarrhythmics, lipid-regulating drugs and digoxin.

Amiodarone has been associated with toxicity involving the lungs, thyroid gland, liver, eyes, skin and peripheral nerves. The incidence of most adverse effects is related to total amiodarone exposure (i.e. dosage and duration of treatment). Therefore, practitioners must consider carefully the risk–benefit ratio of the use of amiodarone in each patient, use the lowest possible dose of amiodarone, monitor for adverse effects and, if possible, discontinue treatment if adverse effects occur.

Corneal microdeposits (reversible on withdrawal of treatment) develop in nearly all adult patients given prolonged amiodarone; these rarely interfere with vision, but drivers may be dazzled by headlights at night. However, if vision is impaired or if optic neuritis or optic neuropathy occur, amiodarone must be stopped to prevent blindness. Long-term administration of amiodarone is associated with a blue-grey discoloration of the skin. This is more commonly seen in individuals with lighter skin tones. The discoloration may revert upon cessation of the drug. However, the skin colour may not return completely to normal.

Individuals who are taking amiodarone may become more sensitive to the harmful effects of ultraviolet A (UV-A) light. Using sunblock that also blocks UV-A rays appears to prevent this side effect. Amiodarone contains iodine and can cause disorders of thyroid function. Both hypothyroidism and hyperthyroidism may occur. Clinical assessment alone is unreliable, and laboratory tests should be performed before treatment and every 6 months including tri-iodothyronine (T_3), T_4 and thyroid stimulating hormone (TSH). A raised T_3 and T_4 with a very low or undetectable TSH concentration suggests the development of thyrotoxicosis. Amiodarone-associated thyrotoxicosis may be refractory to treatment, and amiodarone should usually be withdrawn, at least temporarily, to help achieve control, although treatment with carbimazole is often required. Hypothyroidism can be treated safely with replacement therapy without the need to withdraw amiodarone if amiodarone is considered essential. Amiodarone is also associated with hepatotoxicity, and treatment should be discontinued if severe liver function abnormalities or clinical signs of liver disease develop.

The most serious adverse effect of amiodarone therapy is pulmonary toxicity, typically acute pneumonitis or more insidious pulmonary fibrosis. Although acute pneumonitis may respond to corticosteroids, pulmonary fibrosis is largely irreversible.

Class IV antiarrhythmic drugs (calcium channel blockers)

CCBs bind to and inhibit voltage-gated transmembrane calcium channels carrying an inward current $I_{Ca,L}$. This current is responsible for phase 0 depolarisation of the action potential in the sinoatrial and AV nodes. CCBs reduce the sinus rate and reduce conduction velocity and increase the effective refractory period of the AV node. By reducing calcium entry, CCBs have a negative inotropic effect. L-type calcium channels are also present in vascular smooth muscle, and CCBs therefore cause vasodilatation. In vivo, dihydropyridine CCBs such as nifedipine and amlodipine are relatively selective for vascular smooth muscle, with only minor cardiac effects, whereas phenylalkylamine (verapamil) and benzothiazepine (diltiazem) CCBs are considerably more cardioselective.

Verapamil possesses a chiral carbon and is marketed as a racemic mixture of R- and S-stereoisomers. In humans, both isomers share qualitatively similar negative chronotropic and dromotropic effects on the sinoatrial and AV nodes, respectively, but the S-stereoisomer is 10–20 times more potent than the R with respect to these effects. Hence the S-stereoisomer determines the negative chronotropic and dromotropic effects of verapamil, whereas the R-stereoisomer is of minor importance.

Verapamil also undergoes extensive stereoselective first-pass hepatic metabolism. S-verapamil is more rapidly metabolised than R-verapamil after oral administration, resulting in a lower bioavailability of the S-stereoisomer and a proportionally higher concentration of the R-stereoisomer in the systemic circulation (20% and 50%, respectively). However, because C_{max} is higher with the immediate-release formulation and S-verapamil is 10–20 times more potent than R-verapamil, it is unsurprising that this difference is also clinically significant. With the immediate-release formulation, a plot of PR-interval change versus time has the same shape as the concentration–time curve. The extended-release formulation does not have the same concentration–time effect relationship. This has been attributed to the difference in oral input rates, to the concentration-related saturable first-pass hepatic metabolism, or both.

Because the formulation of verapamil may play a role in the drug's complex pharmacokinetics and efficacy, one formulation of verapamil cannot be safely substituted for another. Immediate-release preparations are preferred to maximise bioavailability of the S-stereoisomer.

Class IV antiarrhythmic drugs should be avoided in sick sinus syndrome or second- or third-degree heart block unless the patient has a permanent pacemaker. Combined therapy with a CCB and β-blocker should be instituted with caution because of the risk of excessive AV block, and should be used where only where monotherapy is insufficient to control ventricular rate during atrial flutter or fibrillation. Verapamil causes greater arterial vasodilation than diltiazem and may be especially useful in patients with hypertension or angina. Both agents have a negative inotropic effect and are thus contraindicated in heart failure. Adverse effects are mostly predictable and include ankle oedema, flushing, dizziness, lightheadedness and headache. Constipation is common in patients receiving verapamil, whereas a rash is common with diltiazem.

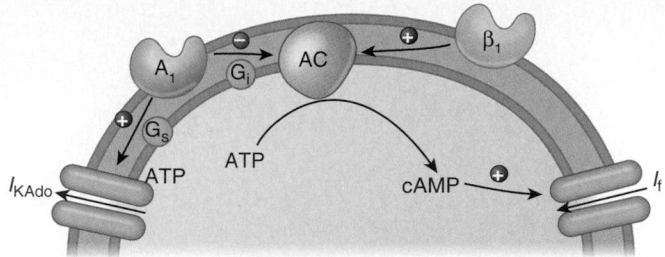

Fig. 22.14 Principal mechanisms of antiarrhythmic action of adenosine.
AC, adenylyl cyclase; ATP, adenosine triphosphate; cAMP, cyclic adenosine monophosphate.

Adenosine

The electrophysiological effects of adenosine are mediated by A_1 adenosine receptors in the cell membrane of atrial, sinoatrial and AV nodal, but not ventricular, myocytes. Binding of adenosine to the A_1 receptor activates a G protein that in turn activates an outward potassium current I_{KAdo}, resulting in hyperpolarisation, and inhibits the pacemaker current I_f and an inward calcium current I_{Ca}. Activation of A_1 receptors also has indirect electrophysiological effects mediated by an inhibitory G protein, which inhibits production of cAMP by adenylyl cyclase, thus opposing the action of catecholamines (Fig. 22.14). The effects of these actions are a reduction in the firing rate of cells with pacemaker activity (negative chronotropic effect), a reduction in conduction velocity in the AV node (negative dromotropic effect) manifest as varying degrees of AV block, and a shortening of atrial effective refractory period, occasionally manifest as the development of AF following the administration of adenosine.

The ultra-short duration of action (<10 seconds) of intravenous adenosine makes it very suitable as a diagnostic aid and for interrupting supraventricular arrhythmias in which the AV node is part of the re-entry pathway. Adenosine is, however, a bronchoconstrictor and causes dyspnoea, flushing, chest pain and further transient arrhythmias in a high proportion of patients, and its metabolism is inhibited by dipyridamole, a vasodilator drug that blocks adenosine uptake by cells, thereby reducing the metabolism of adenosine.

Ivabradine

Ivabradine is a selective inhibitor of the I_f current that plays an important role in pacemaker activity in cells of the cardiac conduction system. I_f is an inward depolarising current of sodium and potassium via specific membrane channels that are activated by hyperpolarisation. Predominantly as a result of I_f, the transmembrane potential in cells of the sinoatrial node becomes progressively less negative until the threshold potential for action potential generation is reached. The magnitude of I_f is increased by cAMP. The sinoatrial node is innervated by both sympathetic and parasympathetic (the vagus) nerves. Binding of catecholamines to β-adrenoceptors stimulates the production of cAMP and hence increases the rate of discharge of the sinoatrial node. Binding of acetylcholine to muscarinic cholinoceptors has the

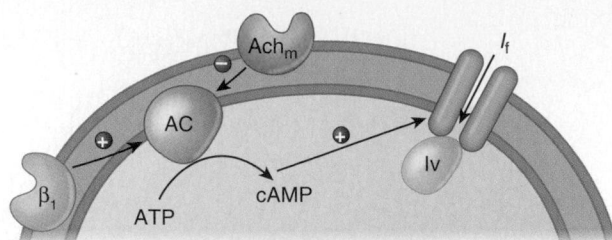

Fig. 22.15 Principal mechanisms of antiarrhythmic action of ivabradine. AC, Adenylyl cyclase; ATP, adenosine triphosphate; cAMP, cyclic adenosine monophosphate.

opposite effect (Fig. 22.15). Ivabradine selectively blocks I_f channels, resulting in a dose-dependent reduction in the slope of diastolic depolarisation in cells of the sinoatrial node, and hence a reduction in the sinus rate. Ivabradine exhibits use dependence, which means its effect is more pronounced at higher heart rates. Ivabradine was developed as an antianginal drug and is also used in patients with chronic heart failure associated with sinus tachycardia. It has been used for the treatment of inappropriate sinus tachycardia, although it is not currently licensed in the UK for that indication.

Digoxin

The therapeutic effect of digoxin results from central and peripheral augmentation of vagal tone, manifest as reduced conduction velocity and prolonged effective refractory period of the AV node. The latter property has the effect of reducing the ventricular rate during atrial tachyarrhythmias. The effect of digoxin is most pronounced under conditions of vagal predominance (i.e. rest and sleep), whereas the drug is relatively ineffective during conditions of sympathetic predominance, such as exercise or AF of acute onset.

Digoxin also directly inhibits the transmembrane Na^+-K^+-ATPase exchange pump. As a result there is a tendency for intracellular sodium concentration to increase, which in turn activates a Na^+-Ca^{2+} exchange pump, which extrudes sodium in exchange for calcium, increasing intracellular calcium concentration. The latter is responsible for the positive inotropic effect of digoxin but also, in overdose, for intracellular calcium overload, resulting in DADs, which may lead to triggered activity.

Digoxin is not indicated for the treatment of paroxysmal AF because it has no direct antiarrhythmic effect and neither terminates an episode of AF nor reduces the likelihood of further episodes of AF occurring. Furthermore, digoxin has limited efficacy for ventricular rate control at the start of an episode of AF, where sympathetic nervous system activity is often high.

The long half-life of digoxin (about 36 hours) warrants special consideration when treating arrhythmias as several days of constant dosing would be required to reach steady-state. Therefore, loading doses of up to 1.5 mg may be used rapidly to increase digoxin serum levels. Digoxin is given once daily thereafter, usually in 125- or 250-microgram doses, and has a narrow therapeutic window with the ideal blood concentration regarded as 1–2 micrograms/L. Because digoxin is excreted

predominantly by the kidney (70% renal elimination in normal renal function), renal function is the most important determinant of the daily digoxin dosage. Importantly, in severe renal insufficiency, there is also a decrease in the volume of distribution of digoxin; therefore, lower loading doses should be used.

Both the therapeutic and toxic effects of digoxin are potentiated by hypokalaemia and hypercalcaemia. There are also numerous drug interactions (Table 22.9), some of which are pharmacokinetic and some of which are pharmacological.

The occurrence of adverse drug reactions is common, because of the narrow therapeutic index of digoxin. Adverse effects are concentration dependent and are rare when serum digoxin concentration is less than 0.8 micrograms/L. Common adverse effects include loss of appetite, nausea, vomiting and diarrhoea as gastro-intestinal motility increases. Other common effects are blurred vision, visual disturbances (yellow-green halos and problems with colour perception), confusion and drowsiness. The often described adverse effect of digoxin, xanthopsia, the disturbance of colour vision (mostly yellow and green colour), is rarely seen.

Table 22.9 Interactions involving digoxin	
Effect	Offending agent or condition
Serum level increased by	Amiodarone, verapamil, diltiazem, quinidine, propafenone, clarithromycin, broad-spectrum antibiotics (erythromycin, tetracyclines), decreased renal blood flow (β-blockers, non-steroidal anti-inflammatory drugs), renal failure, heart failure
Serum level decreased by	Colestyramine, sulfasalazine, neomycin, rifampicin, antacids, improved renal blood flow (vasodilators), levothyroxine (thyroxine)
Therapeutic effect increased by	Hypokalaemia, hypercalcaemia, hypomagnesaemia, antiarrhythmic classes IA, II and IV, diuretics that cause hypokalaemia, corticosteroids, myxoedema, hypoxia (acute or chronic), acute myocardial ischaemia or myocarditis
Therapeutic effect decreased by	Hyperkalaemia, hypocalcaemia, thyrotoxicosis

Patient care

Patients with cardiac arrhythmia may experience considerable anxiety related to their condition. The symptoms typically occur unpredictably, may be extremely unpleasant and may result in the need for urgent medical attention. Many patients are worried that their condition may be life-threatening, whereas others presenting with arrhythmia are found to have prognostically important

Table 22.10 Common therapeutic problems in the management of arrhythmias

Problem	Comment
All antiarrhythmics are proarrhythmic	Prevention is better than cure. Minimise the requirement for drugs by careful attention to precipitating factors. Consider use of pacemakers or non-pharmacological therapies if appropriate.
Nausea and vomiting with blurred vision and visual discolouration on digoxin	These are symptoms and signs of digoxin toxicity noting digoxin has a narrow therapeutic range. Poor renal function may have also contributed.
β-Blockers are generally contraindicated in bronchial and peripheral vascular disease	Consider verapamil or diltiazem.
Calcium channel blockers–induced constipation	If it occurs, give regular osmotic laxatives.
Torsade de pointes may be precipitated by taking other medication with amiodarone or disopyramide	Patients should remind members of healthcare team that they are taking antiarrhythmic drugs; also consider electrolyte disturbance such as hypokalaemia.
Patients experiencing myopathy	Healthcare professionals involved in screening prescriptions for antiarrhythmics should be aware of the clinically relevant interactions and how to manage these. Patients who are taking statins will need regular monitoring for signs of myopathy, particularly those receiving high-intensity statin therapy.
Patient with severe asthma admitted with supraventricular tachycardia	Adenosine is contraindicated because of the risk of bronchospasm. Verapamil is a suitable alternative.
Amiodarone is commonly associated with an increased tendency to sunburn	Warn all patients to stay covered up when outdoors, use sun block or stay indoors.
Acutely treated patient with atrial fibrillation cardioverted initially with i.v. amiodarone, but on converting to oral therapy, reverted back to atrial fibrillation	Although amiodarone has a long terminal half-life once saturated, amiodarone has a very large volume of distribution, and because tissue stores are penetrated to a minimal extent during the early days of therapy, the effective elimination half-life ($t_{1/2}$) is initially dependent upon a more rapidly exchanging compartment, with a $t_{1/2}$ of 10–17 h, substantially shorter than the $t_{1/2}$ seen during chronic administration. The shorter $t_{1/2}$ becomes important during the acute phase and any intravenous to oral changeover period because the absorption of oral amiodarone is very slow, taking up to 15 h. The combination of a relatively fast elimination and a poor rate of absorption could lead to a significant fall in serum amiodarone levels if intravenous therapy is stopped abruptly when oral therapy is initiated, with the period of maximum risk being the first 24 h of oral therapy. It is, therefore, advisable to phase out intravenous therapy gradually and allow an intravenous/oral overlap period of at least 24 h.

underlying heart disease. The diagnosis of an inherited cardiac condition also raises concern for potentially affected relatives. An individual's anxiety may be exacerbated by the fact that most antiarrhythmic drugs work in only a proportion of patients, and several treatment options may be tried before the most appropriate one is identified.

Many patients therefore require considerable reassurance. The patient's family and friends may need to be advised on what to do in the event of an acute arrhythmia. Patients should give informed consent for all interventions, and prescribers must be prepared that a patient's views on the use of a medicine may differ from their own. Prescribers should seek and respect patients' views on treatment choices, rather than assume all patients are the same or that they will always agree with their own views.

Examples of some common therapeutic problems that may occur during the management of arrhythmias are set out in Table 22.10.

Case studies

Case 22.1

Ms AJ, a 25-year-old woman, presents to the hospital emergency department with a 2-hour history of palpitation and chest tightness. She has experienced several similar episodes in the past, all of which have started abruptly at rest and consisted of rapid, regular palpitations. Previous episodes have all stopped after a few minutes and between events she has been entirely well. Ms AJ has no history of heart disease or other ongoing medical problems and is on no regular drug treatment. She drinks alcohol within recommended weekly limits and takes no other recreational drugs. On examination Ms AJ is anxious, has a slightly cool periphery, her pulse is 190 beats/min and regular, and blood pressure is 130/90 mmHg. The remainder of the examination is unremarkable. A 12-lead ECG demonstrates a regular narrow-complex tachycardia with no discernible P waves.

Question

What is the most likely diagnosis, and how should Ms AJ be managed?

Answer

Ms AJ has the signs and symptoms of SVT. Non-pharmacological means of restoring sinus rhythm include carotid sinus massage, subjecting the patient to the Valsalva manoeuvre or eliciting the diving reflex by immersion of the face in ice-cold water. Either approach should result in a brief vagal discharge sufficient to block conduction in the AV node and terminate the tachycardia. If these manoeuvres are unsuccessful, intravenous adenosine can be given in doses of up to 12 mg as a rapid bolus injection followed quickly by a saline flush. Intravenous verapamil 5 mg may also be administered as a rapid bolus injection and is a good alternative where adenosine is contraindicated.

Case 22.2

Mr DS was admitted to hospital for an emergency laparotomy for a perforated gut. He has a history of paroxysmal AF for which he has recently been started on amiodarone 200 mg once daily.

Following the laparotomy Mr DS has new-onset AF that the medical team would like to treat pharmacologically. His only other current medication is thromboprophylaxis with enoxaparin 20 mg once daily.

Questions

1. What treatment plan would you initially suggest for Mr DS?
2. What longer-term monitoring would be appropriate for Mr DS if he was to remain taking amiodarone?

Answers

1. If Mr DS has any electrolyte abnormalities, these should be corrected. If he remains in AF he should be prescribed amiodarone by i.v. infusion, because acutely amiodarone can be effective in cardioversion. The reduced dose of enoxaparin is because Mr DS is a post-surgical patient and at high risk of bleeding.
Mr DS cardioverts back to sinus rhythm following a bolus dose of 300 mg amiodarone. The plan is to maintain him on amiodarone for a short period, for example, a week (600 mg daily) to try to keep him in sinus rhythm, with a view to stopping if he is maintained back in sinus rhythm during this period.

2. If Mr DS was to continue amiodarone therapy longer-term, then the following monitoring would be appropriate:

Chest X-ray: pulmonary	Baseline and if symptoms present
Thyroid function test	Baseline and every 3–6 months
Liver function tests	Baseline and every 3–6 months
Eye examination	Baseline and every 12 months
ECG	Baseline and as required
Clinical evaluation	Baseline and every 3 months

Case 22.3

Mr SB is 77 years of age. He attends the hospital emergency department with worsening shortness of breath. His medical history includes a myocardial infarction 10 years ago which left him with left ventricular dysfunction (ejection fraction <40%). He also has hypertension. Mr SB's current medication is:

- bisoprolol 2.5 mg daily,
- ramipril 5 mg daily,
- aspirin 75 mg daily,
- furosemide 80 mg each morning,
- atorvastatin 40mg daily.

His heart rate is 65 beats/min and irregular, and he has a blood pressure of 160/85 mmHg. Mr SB's ECG shows AF. It was decided to control his AF with an increased dose of bisoprolol.

Questions

1. What drug is most appropriate for stroke prevention in Mr SB?
2. Should anticoagulation be initiated along with aspirin or in place of it?

Answers

1. All patients presenting with AF (or atrial flutter) should undergo assessment of their risk of stroke. Although various risk-stratification schemes exist, the CHA_2DS_2-VASc score is widely used. For Mr SB the following is determined: Congestive cardiac failure 1; Hypertension 1; Age older than 75 years 2; Diabetes mellitus 0; Stroke 0; Vascular disease 1; Sex category 0. Given that Mr SB has a CHA_2DS_2-VASc score of 5, this suggests an annual stroke risk of 6.7% if no therapy is prescribed (Lip et al., 2010b). This risk will reduce to 5.4% if he is prescribed aspirin, or 2.2% if he is prescribed an anticoagulant. Assuming no contraindications or concerns, anticoagulation should be prescribed.

2. In patients with stable vascular disease, such as those with no acute ischaemic events or percutaneous coronary intervention/stent procedure in the preceding year, anticoagulation monotherapy should be used (Kirchhof et al., 2016). There is no need for concomitant aspirin, which could increase the risk of a major bleed. Therefore, concomitant antiplatelet therapy should not be prescribed for Mr SB. In patients with AF treated for acute coronary syndrome, and in those receiving a coronary stent, the doctor may consider a combination of an anticoagulant and aspirin (Kirchhof et al., 2016); however, it should be noted that such a combination will significantly increase the risk of a major bleed. Optimising the modifiable risk factors in HAS-BLED (e.g. blood pressure) will help minimise the risk of bleeding if a decision is taken to prescribe aspirin and an anticoagulant together.

References

ACTIVE Investigators, Connolly, S.J., Pogue, J., et al., 2009. Effect of clopidogrel added to aspirin in patients with atrial fibrillation. N. Engl. J. Med. 360, 2066–2078.

AFFIRM Investigators, 2004. Relationship between sinus rhythm, treatment, and survival in the atrial fibrillation follow-up investigation of rhythm management (AFFIRM) study. Circulation 109, 1509–1513.

Bayer, 2017. Xarelto: summary of product characteristics. Available at: http://www.medicines.org.uk/emc/medicine/21265.

Bounameaux, H., Camm, A.J., 2014. Edoxaban: an update on the new oral direct factor Xa inhibitor. Drugs 74, 1209–1231.

Bristol Myers Squibb-Pfizer, 2017. Eliquis: summary of product characteristics. Available at: http://www.medicines.org.uk/emc/medicine/24988.

Bunch, T.J., May, H.T., Blair, T.L., et al., 2013. Atrial fibrillation patients have long-term stroke rates similar to patients without atrial fibrillation regardless of CHADS2 score. Heart Rhythm 10, 1272–1277.

Cairns, J.A., Connolly, S.J., Roberts, R., et al., 1997. Randomised trial of outcome after myocardial infarction in patients with frequent or repetitive ventricular premature depolarisations: CAMIAT Canadian Amiodarone Myocardial Infarction Arrhythmia Trial Investigators. Lancet 349, 675–682.

Camm, A.J., Lip, G.Y.H., De Caterina, R., et al., 2012. Focused update of the ESC guidelines for the management of atrial fibrillation. Eur. Heart J. 33, 2719–2747.

Connolly, S.J., Ezekowitz, M.D., Yusuf, S., et al., 2009. Dabigatran versus warfarin in patients with atrial fibrillation. N. Engl. J. Med. 361, 1139–1151.

Crouch, M.A., Limon, L., Cassano, A.T., 2003. Drug-related QT interval prolongation: drugs associated with QT prolongation. Pharmacotherapy 23, 802–805.

Daiichi Sankyo UK Limited, 2017. Lixiana: summary of product characteristics. Available at: http://www.medicines.org.uk/emc/medicine/30513.

Echt, D.S., Liebson, P.R., Mitchell, L.B., et al., 1991. Mortality and morbidity in patients receiving encainide, flecainide, or placebo: the Cardiac Arrhythmia Suppression Trial. N. Engl. J. Med. 324, 781–788.

Eriksson, B.I., Quinlan, D.J., Weitz, J.I., 2009. Comparative pharmacodynamics and pharmacokinetics of oral direct thrombin and factor Xa inhibitors in development. Clin. Pharmacokinet. 48, 1–22.

Fang, M.C., Chang, Y., Hylek, E.M., et al., 2004. Advanced age, anticoagulation intensity, and risk of intracranial haemorrhage among patients taking warfarin for atrial fibrillation. Ann. Intern. Med. 141, 745–752.

Giugliano, R.P., Ruff, C.T., Braunwald, E., et al., 2013. Edoxaban versus warfarin in patients with atrial fibrillation. N. Engl. J. Med. 369, 2093–2104.

Granger, C.B., Alexander, J.H., McMurray, J.J.V., et al., 2011. Apixaban versus warfarin in patients with atrial fibrillation. N. Engl. J. Med. 365, 981–992.

Hart, R.G., Benavente, O., McBride, R., et al., 2007. Meta-analysis: antithrombotic therapy to prevent stroke in patients who have nonvalvular atrial fibrillation. Ann. Intern. Med. 146, 857–867.

Hylek, E.M., Skates, S.J., Sheehan, M.A., et al., 1996. An analysis of the lowest effective intensity of prophylactic anticoagulation for patients with nonrheumatic atrial fibrillation. N. Engl. J. Med. 335, 540–546.

Julian, D.G., Camm, A.J., Frangin, G., et al., 1997. Randomised trial of effect of amiodarone on mortality in patient with left ventricular dysfunction after recent myocardial infarction: EMIAT. European Myocardial Infarct Amiodarone Trial Investigators. Lancet 349, 667–674.

Kirchhof, P., Benussi, S., Kotecha, D., et al., 2016. 2016 ESC guidelines for the management of atrial fibrillation developed in collaboration with EACTS. Eur. Heart J. 37, 2893–2962.

Kuck, K., Cappato, R., Siebels, J., et al., 2000. Randomized comparison of antiarrhythmic drug therapy with implantable defibrillators in patients resuscitated from cardiac arrest. Circulation 102, 748–754.

Lip, G.Y., Nieuwlaat, R., Pisters, R., et al., 2010a. Refining clinical risk stratification for predicting stroke and thromboembolism in atrial fibrillation using a novel risk factor-based approach: the Euro Heart Survey on Atrial Fibrillation. Chest 137, 263–272.

Lip, G.Y.H., Frison, L., Halperin, J.L., et al., 2010b. Identifying patients at high risk of stroke despite anticoagulation. A comparison of contemporary stroke risk stratification schemes in an anticoagulated atrial fibrillation cohort. Stroke 41, 2731–2738.

Marrouche, N.F., Brachmann, J., Andresen, D., et al., 2018. Catheter ablation for atrial fibrillation with heart failure. N Engl. J. Med. 378, 417–427.

National Institute for Health and Care Excellence (NICE), 2014. Atrial fibrillation: management. Clinical Guideline (CG180), London, NICE. Available at: https://www.nice.org.uk/guidance/cg180.

Olesen, J.B., Lip, G.Y., Hansen, M.L., et al., 2011. Validation of risk stratification schemes for predicting stroke and thromboembolism in patients with atrial fibrillation: nationwide cohort study. Br. Med. J. 342, d1124.

Patel, M.R., Mahaffey, K.W., Garg, J., et al., 2011. Rivaroxaban versus warfarin in nonvalvular atrial fibrillation. N. Engl. J. Med. 365, 883–891.

Pisters, R., Lane, D.A., Nieuwlaat, R., et al., 2010. A novel user-friendly score (HAS-BLED) to assess 1-year risk of major bleeding in patients with atrial fibrillation: the Euro Heart Survey. Chest 138, 1093–1100.

Roy, D., Talajic, M., Doran, P., 2000. Amiodarone to prevent recurrence of atrial fibrillation. N. Engl. J. Med. 342, 913–920.

Sherman, D.G., Kim, S.G., Boop, B.S., et al., 2005. Occurrence and characteristics of stroke events in the atrial fibrillation follow-up investigation of sinus rhythm management (AFFIRM) study. Arch Intern Med. 165, 1185–1191.

Singh, B.N., Singh, S.N., Reda, D.J., 2005. Amiodarone versus sotalol for atrial fibrillation. N. Engl. J. Med. 352, 1861–1872.

Vaughan-Williams, E.M., 1970. The experimental basis for the choice of an anti-arrhythmic drug. Adv. Cardiol. 4, 275–289.

Further reading

Billman, G.E. (Ed.), 2010. Novel therapeutic targets for antiarrhythmic drugs. Wiley, Hoboken.

Fogoros, R.N., 2007. Antiarryhthmic Drugs: A Practical Guide, second ed. Wiley-Blackwell, Oxford.

Lip, G., Nieuwlaat, R., Pisters, R., et al., 2010. Refining clinical risk stratification for predicting stroke and thromboembolism in atrial fibrillation using a novel risk factor based approach: the Euro Heart Survey on Atrial Fibrillation. Chest 137, 263–272.

Useful websites

Current list of drugs known to cause QT interval prolongation: http://www.crediblemeds.org

Current list of drugs to avoid in patients with Brugada syndrome: http://www.brugadadrugs.org

UK Resuscitation Council website, with guidance on the management of peri-arrest tachy and bradyarrhythmias: http://www.resus.org.uk

European Society of Cardiology: https://www.escardio.org/

American Heart Association: http://www.heart.org

23 Thrombosis

Philip A. Routledge, Hamsaraj Shetty and Simon J. Wilkins

Key points

Venous thromboembolism

- Venous thromboembolism (VTE) is the development of a 'thrombus', principally containing fibrin and red blood cells, in the venous circulation. This most often occurs as a deep vein thrombosis (DVT) in the deep, as distinct from the superficial, veins of the legs.
- If part of a thrombus in the venous circulation breaks off and enters the right heart, it may become lodged in the pulmonary arterial circulation, causing pulmonary embolism (PE).
- Combinations of sluggish blood flow and hypercoagulability are the most common causes of VTE. Vascular injury is also a recognised causative factor.
- Treatment of VTE involves the use of anticoagulants and, in severe cases, thrombolytic drugs.
- Anticoagulant therapy often involves an immediate-acting agent, such as heparin, followed by maintenance treatment with an oral anticoagulant, such as warfarin.
- Another option is the use of a direct oral anticoagulant (DOAC), also sometimes known as a non–vitamin K antagonist oral anticoagulant/novel oral anticoagulant (NOAC), with a marketing authorisation for such use. The use of heparin in the early stages is not necessary with all of the DOACs, but requirements change, and thus product literature should be consulted.
- Unfractionated heparins increase the rate of interaction of thrombin with antithrombin III 1000-fold and prevent the production of fibrin from fibrinogen.
- Low-molecular-weight heparins inactivate factor Xa, have a longer half-life and produce a more predictable response than unfractionated heparins.
- Warfarin is the most widely used coumarin because of potency, reliable bioavailability and an intermediate half-life of elimination (36 hours).
- Warfarin consists of an equal mixture of two enantiomers, (R)- and (S)-warfarins, that have different anticoagulant potencies and routes of metabolism. The latter enantiomer is a much more potent anticoagulant.
- DOACs currently available include dabigatran etexilate, a direct thrombin (factor IIa) inhibitor, and apixaban, edoxaban and rivaroxaban, which are direct inhibitors of activated factor Xa.

Arterial thromboembolism

- Arterial thromboembolism is normally associated with vascular injury and hypercoagulability.

- Acute myocardial infarction is the commonest form of arterial thrombosis.
- Arterial thromboembolism affecting the cerebral circulation results in either transient ischaemic attacks (TIAs) or, in more severe cases, cerebral infarction (stroke).
- Arterial thrombosis is the development of a 'thrombus' consisting of platelets, fibrin, red blood cells and white blood cells in the systemic circulation.
- An embolus may result in peripheral arterial occlusion, either in the lower limbs or in the cerebral circulation (where it may cause thromboembolic stroke).

Venous thromboembolism

Epidemiology

Venous thromboembolism (VTE) is common, with an incidence of 2–5%. Deep vein thrombosis (DVT) may result in not only pulmonary embolism (PE) but also subsequent morbidity as a result of the post-phlebitic limb. Thrombosis and thromboembolism are the most common direct cause of maternal death in the UK (Knight et al., 2016). Thromboembolism appears to increase in prevalence past the age of 50 years, and the diagnosis is more often missed in this age group.

Aetiology

VTE occurs primarily due to a combination of stagnation of blood flow and hypercoagulability. Vascular injury is also a recognised causative factor but is not necessary for the development of venous thrombosis. In VTE, the structure of the thrombus is different from that in arterial thromboembolism. In the former, platelets seem to be uniformly distributed through a mesh of fibrin and other blood cell components, whereas in arterial thromboembolism the white platelet 'head' is more prominent, and it appears to play a much more important initiatory role in thrombus.

Sluggishness of blood flow may be related to bed rest, surgery or reduced cardiac output, for example, in heart failure. Factors increasing the risk of hypercoagulability include surgery, pregnancy, oestrogen administration, malignancy, myocardial infarction and several acquired or inherited disorders of coagulation (for further detail on genetic factors, see Rosendaal and Reitsma [2009]).

Protein C deficiency

Protein C deficiency is inherited through autosomal-dominant transmission and has a prevalence of 0.2–0.5% in the general population (Bauer et al., 2017). Such patients are at increased risk not only for VTE but also for warfarin-induced skin necrosis, which occurs because protein C (and its closely related cofactor, protein S) is a vitamin K–dependent antithrombotic factor that can be further suppressed by the administration of warfarin. Thrombosis in the small vessels of the skin may occur if large loading (induction) doses of warfarin are given to such patients when the suppression of the antithrombotic effects of these factors occurs before the antithrombotic effects of blockade of vitamin K–dependent clotting factor (II, VII, IX and X) production has occurred. The prevalence of protein C deficiency in individuals who have had a VTE is 2–5% (Bauer et al., 2017).

Protein S deficiency

Protein S deficiency is probably even rarer than protein C deficiency; the prevalence in the general population is unknown (Bauer et al., 2017). The familial form, inherited in an autosomal-dominant fashion, is a high-risk state, accounting for VTE in some individuals. The prevalence of protein S deficiency in individuals who have had a VTE is reported to be 1% (Bauer et al., 2017).

Factor V Leiden

The presence of factor V Leiden, a point mutation in the factor V gene, causes the activated factor V molecule to be resistant to deactivation by activated protein C (APC). This defect may have a prevalence of 4–5% in Caucasian populations (Bauer et al., 2017) and higher in patients with thromboembolic disease, and it may in itself be of little consequence until there is another risk factor, such as immobility or use of the contraceptive pill. In these circumstances, the combination of risks may be responsible for the increased predisposition to thromboembolism in a high proportion of affected individuals.

Antithrombin III deficiency

Antithrombin III deficiency is a rare autosomal-dominant inherited abnormality associated with a reduced plasma concentration of this protein. The defect may not result in clinical problems until pregnancy or until patients enter their fourth decade, when venous and, to a lesser extent, arterial thrombosis becomes more common. Nevertheless, its prevalence in individuals with VTE has been estimated to be between 1% and 7% (Bauer et al., 2017).

Lupus anticoagulant

Lupus anticoagulant, an antibody against phospholipid, is so named because it increases the clotting time in blood when measured by some standard coagulation tests. Patients affected are more prone to thromboembolism. It is also found in the primary antiphospholipid syndrome (PAPS), where it may signify an increased risk of venous and arterial thrombosis and for recurrent miscarriage (Derksen et al., 2001).

Prothrombin G20210A mutation

A mutation in part of the prothrombin gene (prothrombin G20210A) results in increased prothrombin concentrations and an increased risk of venous thrombosis by three- to fourfold over controls (Bauer et al., 2017).

Fibrinogen gamma 10034T

Approximately 6% of individuals carry this variant gene, which increases thrombotic risk approximately twofold (Rosendaal, 2009).

Oestrogens

Oestrogens increase the circulating concentrations of clotting factors I, II, VII, VIII, IX and X and reduce fibrinolytic activity. They also depress the concentrations of antithrombin III, which is protective against thrombosis. This effect is dose related, and venous thrombosis was more often seen with contraceptive pills containing high (50 micrograms) oestrogen than with the present lower-dose preparations (Rosendaal, 2009). Hormone replacement therapy, pregnancy and the puerperium (up to 6 weeks after delivery) are also recognised risk factors for VTE (National Institute for Health and Care Excellence [NICE], 2015a).

Malignancy

VTE is more common in malignancy, and the risk may be up to fivefold greater than in those without malignancy. Although first described in association with carcinoma of the pancreas, all solid tumours seem to be associated with this problem. The absolute risk seems to be related to the type of tumour and its stage and treatment with chemotherapy. The exact mechanisms responsible for the increased risk of VTE in malignancy are not known but may be related to the expression of tissue factor or factor X activators (Elyamany et al., 2014).

Surgery

The increased risk of VTE in surgery is related, in part, to stagnation of venous blood in the calves during the operation and recovery. Tissue trauma may also play a role because VTE appears to be more common in operations that involve marked tissue damage, such as orthopaedic surgery. This may in turn be related to release of tissue thromboplastin and to reduced fibrinolytic activity. The most important risk factors associated with VTE after surgery are duration of anaesthesia and procedure of more than 90 minutes (or 60 minutes if surgery involves lower limbs or pelvis), acute surgical admission with an inflammatory or intra-abdominal condition and expected significant reduction in mobility (NICE, 2015a). Other patient-related risk factors for VTE include age older than 60 years, dehydration, known thrombophilias, obesity (body mass index >30 kg/m^2), one or more significant comorbidities, personal history or first-degree relative with previous VTE, use of hormone replacement therapy or oestrogen-containing contraceptives and varicose veins with associated phlebitis. These will add to the risk, if present, but are also independent risk factors.

Clinical manifestations

DVT occurs commonly in the veins of the lower limbs and pelvis. In some patients, there may not be any local symptoms or signs, and the onset of PE may be the first evidence of the presence of VTE. In other cases, patients classically present with pain involving the calf or thigh, associated with swelling, redness of the overlying skin and increased warmth. In a large DVT that prevents venous return, the leg may become discoloured and oedematous. Massive venous thrombus can occasionally result in gangrene, although this occurs very rarely now that effective drug therapies are available.

PE may occur in the absence of clinical signs of venous thrombosis. It may be very difficult to diagnose because of the non-specificity of symptoms and signs. Clinical diagnosis is often made because of the presence of associated risk factors. Obstruction with a large embolus of a major pulmonary artery may result in acute massive PE, presenting with sudden shortness of breath and dull central chest pain, together with marked haemodynamic disturbance, for example, severe hypotension and right ventricular failure, sometimes resulting in death due to acute circulatory failure unless rapidly treated.

Acute submassive PE occurs when less than 50% of the pulmonary circulation is occluded by embolus, and the embolus normally lodges in a more distal branch of the pulmonary artery. It may result in some shortness of breath, but if the lung normally supplied by that branch of the pulmonary artery becomes necrotic, pulmonary infarction results, with pleuritic pain and haemoptysis (coughing up blood), and there may be a pleural 'rub' (a sound like Velcro being torn apart when the patient breathes in) as a result of inflammation of the lung. Patients may, rarely, develop recurrent thromboembolism. This may not result in immediate symptoms or signs, but the patient may present with increasing breathlessness and signs of pulmonary hypertension (right ventricular hypertrophy) and, if untreated, progressive respiratory failure.

Investigations

Deep vein thrombosis

A DVT is the most common cause of pain, swelling and tenderness within the leg, although other conditions, such as a Baker's cyst (which involves rupture of the posterior aspect of the synovial capsule of the knee), may mimic it. The two-level DVT Wells score is advocated as a helpful initial clinical screening test to ascertain whether DVT is likely or unlikely (NICE, 2015b). The clinical scoring tool for this approach is shown in Table 23.1.

A DVT Wells Score of 2 points or more means that a DVT is classified as *likely*. If this is the case, a proximal leg vein ultrasound scan should be carried out within 4 hours of being requested, and if the result is negative, a D-dimer test should be performed (D-dimer is a product formed in the body when blood is broken down). If a proximal leg vein ultrasound scan cannot be carried out within 4 hours, a D-dimer test should be performed and an interim 24-hour dose of a parenteral anticoagulant given while waiting for the proximal leg vein ultrasound scan to be carried out within 24 hours. The NICE (2015b) guidance also recommends that the proximal leg vein ultrasound scan should be repeated 6–8 days later for all patients with a positive D-dimer test and a negative proximal leg vein ultrasound scan.

Table 23.1 Two-level deep vein thrombosis Wells score

Clinical feature	Points
Active cancer (treatment ongoing, within 6 months, or palliative)	1
Paralysis, paresis or recent plaster immobilisation of the lower extremities	1
Recently bedridden for 3 days or more or major surgery within 12 weeks requiring general or regional anaesthesia	1
Localised tenderness along the distribution of the deep venous system	1
Entire leg swollen	1
Calf swelling at least 3 cm larger than asymptomatic side	1
Pitting oedema confined to the symptomatic leg	1
Collateral superficial veins (non-varicose)	1
Previously documented DVT	1
An alternative diagnosis is at least as likely as DVT	−2
Clinical probability simplified score	
DVT – likely	2 points or more
DVT – unlikely	1 point or less

DVT, Deep vein thrombosis.
Adapted from Wells et al. (2003) and NICE (2015b).

Ultrasound. Ultrasound is a non-invasive alternative to venography that does not involve exposure to ionising radiation or potentially allergenic contrast media. It is now the initial investigation of choice in clinically suspected DVT, although it is less sensitive for below-knee and isolated pelvic deep vein thrombosis.

Venography. Venography involves injection of radio-opaque contrast medium, normally into a vein on the top of the foot, and subsequent radiography of the venous system. Although specific, it is also invasive.

Magnetic resonance imaging. Magnetic resonance imaging (MRI) is also non-invasive and avoids radiation exposure. When used with direct thrombus imaging (DTI), which detects methaemoglobin in the clot, MRI DTI is sensitive and specific, even with below-knee and isolated pelvic deep vein thrombosis. However, it is not widely clinically available, and ultrasound remains the primary initial investigation.

Pulmonary embolism

If PE is suspected, and the two-level PE Wells Score indicates that PE is *likely* (more than 4 points using the two-level

Table 23.2 Two-level pulmonary embolism Wells Score

Clinical feature	Points
Clinical signs and symptoms of DVT (minimum of leg swelling and pain with palpation of the deep veins)	3
An alternative diagnosis is less likely than PE	3
Heart rate >100 beats/min	1.5
Immobilisation for more than 3 days or surgery in the previous 4 weeks	1.5
Previous DVT/PE	1.5
Haemoptysis	1
Malignancy (on treatment, treated in the last 6 months, or palliative)	1
Clinical probability simplified scores	
PE – likely	More than 4 points
PE – unlikely	4 points or less

DVT, Deep vein thrombosis; PE, pulmonary embolism.
Adapted from Wells et al. (2000).

PE Wells Score; Table 23.2), either an immediate computed tomography pulmonary angiogram (CTPA) should be performed or immediate interim parenteral anticoagulant therapy initiated, followed by a CTPA, if a CTPA cannot be carried out immediately. A proximal leg vein ultrasound scan should be considered if the CTPA is negative and DVT is suspected (NICE, 2015b).

Computed tomography pulmonary angiogram. CTPA is a minimally invasive test that has now largely superseded pulmonary angiography as the most specific test in the diagnosis of PE. It involves the intravenous administration of iodine-containing contrast media to allow sophisticated radiographic imaging to detect whether blood is flowing to all parts of the lungs or whether a PE is causing blockage in the pulmonary arterial vasculature.

Ventilation–perfusion scanning. Ventilation–perfusion scanning involves the injection of a radiolabelled substance into the vein and measurement of perfusion via the pulmonary circulation, using a scintillation counter. This is often combined with a ventilation scan in which radiolabelled gas, normally xenon, is inhaled by the patient. PE classically results in an area of under- or non-perfusion of a part of the lung that, nevertheless, because the airways are patent, ventilates normally. This pattern is called ventilation–perfusion mismatch and is a specific sign of PE. The preferred technique is a ventilation/perfusion single-photon emission computed tomography (V/Q SPECT) scan. If a V/Q SPECT scan is not available, a V/Q planar scan is an alternative, although it has lower sensitivity and specificity. NICE recommends that ventilation-perfusion scanning can be considered

as an alternative to CTPA in patients who are allergic to contrast media, or who have renal impairment or whose risk from irradiation is considered to be high, because total radiation exposure is lower than with CTPA (NICE, 2015b).

Other findings. Other findings occur in PE, such as changes in the chest radiograph, for example, a raised right hemidiaphragm as a result of the loss of lung volume (PE more commonly affects the right than the left lung). Hypoxia is also seen, and the larger the PE, the worse this is. The electrocardiogram may show signs of right ventricular strain. The echocardiogram may show right ventricular overload and dysfunction in massive PE. However, all these changes are relatively nonspecific and do not obviate the need for the specific tests mentioned previously.

Treatment

The aim of treatment of venous thrombosis is to allow normal circulation in the limbs and, wherever possible, to prevent damage to the valves of the veins, thus reducing the risk of the swollen post-phlebitic limb. Secondly, it is important to try to prevent associated PE and also the recurrence of either venous thrombosis or PE in the risk period after the initial episode.

In acute massive PE, the initial priority is to correct the circulatory defect that has caused the haemodynamic upset, and in these circumstances, rapid removal of the obstruction using thrombolytic drugs or surgical removal of the embolus may be necessary. In acute submassive PE, the goal of treatment is to prevent further episodes, particularly of the more serious acute massive PE. In both DVT and PE, a search must be made for underlying risk factors, such as carcinoma, and particularly in those with repeated episodes of VTE.

The treatment of VTE consists of the use of anticoagulants and, in severe cases, thrombolytic drugs. Anticoagulant therapy involves the use of immediate-acting agents (particularly heparin) and oral anticoagulants, the commonest of which is warfarin, but direct oral anticoagulant (DOACs) are also an option as alternatives. Anticoagulation may be necessary for some time after the initial event, depending on the persistence of risk factors for recurrent thromboembolism.

Prophylaxis

Prevention of initial episodes of VTE in those at risk is clearly of great importance. It has been estimated that around 25,000 people in the UK die from preventable hospital-acquired VTE annually, including patients admitted to hospital for medical care and surgery (House of Commons Health Committee, 2005). There is also widespread evidence of inconsistent use of prophylactic measures for VTE in hospital patients, including mechanical and pharmacological means of VTE prophylaxis. Some of the medicines described in the following sections contribute to those pharmacological measures. Guidelines on reducing the risk of VTE in patients admitted to hospital are available (NICE, 2015a).

Heparins

Conventional or unfractionated heparin (UFH) is a heterogeneous mixture of large mucopolysaccharide molecules ranging widely in molecular weight between 3000 and 30,000, with immediate anticoagulant properties. It acts by increasing the rate of the interaction of thrombin with antithrombin III by a factor of 1000. It, thus, prevents the production of fibrin (factor I) from fibrinogen. Heparin also inhibits the production of activated clotting factors IX, X, XI and XII, and these effects occur at concentrations lower than its effects on thrombin.

Unlike UFH, low-molecular-weight heparins (LMWHs) contain polysaccharide chains ranging in molecular weight between 4000 and 6000. Whereas UFH produces its anticoagulant effect by inhibiting both thrombin and factor Xa, LMWHs predominantly inactivate only factor Xa. In addition, unlike UFH, they inactivate platelet-bound factor Xa and resist inhibition by platelet factor 4 (PF4), which is released during coagulation. Dalteparin, enoxaparin and tinzaparin are LMWHs with similar efficacy and adverse effects.

Because UFH and LMWHs all consist of high-molecular-weight molecules that are highly ionised (heparin is the strongest organic acid found naturally in the body), they are not absorbed via the gastro-intestinal tract and must be given by intravenous infusion or deep subcutaneous (never intramuscular) injection. UFH is highly protein bound, and it appears to be restricted to the intravascular space, with a consequently low volume of distribution. It does not cross the placenta and does not appear in breast milk. Its pharmacokinetics are complex, but it appears to have a dose-dependent increase in half-life. The half-life is normally about 60 minutes but is shorter in patients with PE. It is removed from the body by metabolism, possibly in the reticuloendothelial cells of the liver, and by renal excretion. The latter seems to be more important after high doses of the compound.

LMWHs have a number of potentially desirable pharmacokinetic features compared with UFH. They are predominantly excreted renally and have longer and more predictable half-lives than UFH and so have a more predictable dose response than UFH. They can, therefore, be given once or, at the most, twice daily in a fixed dose, sometimes based on the patient's body weight, without the need for laboratory monitoring, except for patients given treatment doses and those at a high risk of bleeding.

The major adverse effect of all heparins is haemorrhage, which is more common in patients with severe heart or liver disease, renal disease, general debility and in women older than 60 years. The risk of haemorrhage is increased in those with prolonged clotting times and in those given UFH by intermittent intravenous bolus rather than by continuous intravenous administration. UFH is monitored by derivatives of the activated partial thromboplastin time (APTT), for example, the kaolin–cephalin clotting time (KCCT); in those patients with a KCCT three times greater than control, there is an eightfold increase in the risk of haemorrhage. The therapeutic range for the KCCT during UFH therapy, therefore, appears to be between 1.5 and 2.5 times the control values. Rapid reversal of the effect of UFH can be achieved using protamine sulphate, but this is rarely necessary because of its short duration of action. LMWHs may produce fewer haemorrhagic complications, and at the doses normally used for treatment, they do not significantly affect coagulation tests, so routine monitoring is not necessary (Baglin et al., 2006). Protamine sulfate can inhibit the prolongation in clotting time induced by LWMHs, but does not fully inhibit their anti-factor Xa activity.

Box 23.1 Guidelines to control unfractionated heparin treatment

Loading dose
5000 IU over 5 min

Infusion
Start at 1400 IU/h (e.g. 8400 IU in 100 mL of normal saline over 6 h). Check after 6 h.
Adjust dose according to ratio of the KCCT to the control value using the following values

KCCT ratio	Infusion rate change
>7.0	Discontinue for 30 min to 1 h and reduce by >500 IU/h
>5.0	Reduce by 500 IU/h
4.1–5.0	Reduce by 300 IU/h
3.1–4.0	Reduce by 100 IU/h
2.6–3.0	Reduce by 50 IU/h
1.5–2.5	No change
1.2–1.4	Increase by 200 IU/h
<1.2	Increase by 400 IU/h

After each dose change, wait 10 h before next KCCT estimation unless KCCT >5, when more frequent (e.g. 4-hourly) estimation is advisable. Developed using Diogen (Bell and Alton); local validation may be necessary.

KCCT, Kaolin–cephalin clotting time.
Modified from Fennerty et al. (1986).

Heparins, particularly UFH, may also cause thrombocytopenia (low platelet count). This may occur in two forms. The first occurs 3–5 days after treatment and does not normally result in complications. The second type of thrombocytopenia occurs after about 6 days of treatment and often results in much more profound decreases in platelet count and an increased risk of thromboembolism. LMWHs are thought to be less likely to cause thrombocytopenia, but this complication has been reported, including in individuals who had previously developed thrombocytopenia after UFH. For these reasons, patients should have a platelet count on the day of starting UFH, and alternate-day platelet counts should be performed from days 4–14 thereafter. For patients on LMWH, platelet counts should be performed at 2- to 4-day intervals from days 4–14 (Keeling et al., 2006). If the platelet count falls by 50% and/or the patient develops new thrombosis or skin allergy during this period, heparin-induced thrombocytopenia (HIT) should be considered; if HIT is strongly suspected or confirmed, heparin should be stopped and an alternative agent such as a heparinoid or hirudin commenced.

Heparin-induced osteoporosis is rare but may occur when the drug is used during pregnancy and may be dose related. The exact mechanism is unknown. Other adverse effects of heparin are alopecia, urticaria and anaphylaxis, but these are also rare.

It has been shown that there is a nonlinear relationship between the dose of UFH infused and the KCCT. This means that disproportionate adjustments in dose are required depending on the KCCT if under- or overdosing is to be avoided (Box 23.1). Because the half-life of UFH is 1 hour, it would take 5 hours (five half-lives of the drug) to reach a steady state. A loading dose is therefore administered to reduce the time to achieve adequate anticoagulation. UFH in full dose can also be given by repeated subcutaneous injection, and in these circumstances the calcium salt appears to be less painful than the sodium salt. Opinions differ as to whether the subcutaneous or intravenous route is preferable. The subcutaneous route may take longer to reach effective plasma heparin concentrations but avoids the need for infusion devices.

Use of a LMWH or fondaparinux is recommended in the immediate stages of proximal DVT and PE. UFH may be considered for use, with appropriate monitoring and care, in patients with severe renal impairment, at increased risk of bleeding or with haemodynamic instability. LMWH, UFH or fondaparinux should be administered with warfarin for at least 5 days or until the international normalised ratio (INR) has been in the therapeutic range for 2 successive days, whichever is the longer. Monitoring, as detailed previously, is essential to avoid the complications of HIT. Patients with previous exposure to heparin within the past 100 days should also have a platelet count performed before the second dose of heparin is administered (Winter et al., 2005). Requirements with DOACs differ, and not all require cover with a parenteral anticoagulant when used to treat a VTE.

Heparinoids

Danaparoid is a heparinoid that is licensed for prophylaxis of DVT in patients undergoing general or orthopaedic surgery. It is a mixture of the low-molecular-weight sulphated glycosami-noglycuronans: heparin sulphate, dermatan sulphate and a small amount of chondroitin sulphate. It acts by inhibiting factor Xa and, like LMWHs, is given by subcutaneous injection. It normally has a low cross-reactivity rate with heparin-associated antiplatelet antibodies, and if this is not present, it can be used in the treatment of individuals who develop HIT but still need ongoing anticoagulation. It is administered intravenously, with monitoring of anti-Xa activity only required in those at high risk of bleeding, for example, in renal insufficiency. It should be avoided in severe renal insufficiency and severe hepatic insufficiency.

Hirudins

Lepirudin, a recombinant hirudin, is licensed for anticoagulation in patients with type II (immune) HIT who require parenteral antithrombotic treatment. The dose of lepirudin is adjusted according to the APTT, and it is given intravenously by infusion. The risk of haemorrhage is greater in those with poor renal function. Severe anaphylaxis occurs rarely in association with lepirudin treatment and is more common in previously exposed patients (Keeling et al., 2006). Bivalirudin is an analogue of hirudin but acts as a direct thrombin inhibitor. It is licensed for anticoagulation in patients undergoing percutaneous coronary intervention (PCI). It has to be administered parenterally, and the activated clotting time (ACT) is used to assess its activity. Haemorrhage is also an important adverse effect of this agent.

Fondaparinux

Fondaparinux sodium is a synthetic pentasaccharide that binds to antithrombin III, thus inhibiting factor Xa but without effect on factor IIa. Therefore, at doses normally used for treatment, it does not significantly affect coagulation tests, and routine monitoring

of these is not necessary. It has to be given parenterally. It is used for prophylaxis of VTE in high-risk situations and for treatment of acute DVT and treatment of acute PE, except in haemodynamically unstable patients or patients who require thrombolysis or pulmonary embolectomy. It also has an indication for the treatment of unstable angina or non-ST-segment-elevation myocardial infarction (NSTEMI) and for the treatment of ST-segment-elevation myocardial infarction (STEMI). Haemorrhage is the most important adverse effect.

Oral anticoagulants

Warfarin. Although it is not the only coumarin anticoagulant available, warfarin is by far the most widely used drug in this group because of its potency, duration of action and more reliable bioavailability. When given by mouth, warfarin is completely and rapidly absorbed, although food decreases the rate (but not the extent) of absorption. It is extremely highly plasma-protein bound (99%) and, therefore, has a small volume of distribution (7–14 L). It consists of an equal mixture of two enantiomers, (R)- and (S)-warfarins. They have different anticoagulant potencies and routes of metabolism.

Both enantiomers of warfarin act by inducing a functional deficiency of vitamin K and thereby prevent the normal carboxylation of the glutamic acid residues of the amino-terminal ends of clotting factors II, VII, IX and X. This renders the clotting factors unable to cross-link with calcium and thereby bind to phospholipid-containing membranes. Warfarin prevents the reduction of vitamin K epoxide to vitamin K by epoxide reductase. (S)-warfarin appears to be at least five times more potent in this regard than (R)-warfarin. Because warfarin does not have any effect on already carboxylated clotting factors, the delay in onset of the anticoagulant effect of warfarin is dependent on the rate of clearance of the fully carboxylated factors already synthesised. The half-life of removal of factor VII is approximately 6 hours, that of factor IX is 24 hours, that of factor X is 36 hours and that of factor II is 50 hours. Some of the variability in response to warfarin may be related to genetic variations in the gene encoding the vitamin K epoxide reductase multiprotein complex (VKORC1 gene).

The effect of warfarin is monitored using the one-stage prothrombin time, for example, the INR. This test is sensitive chiefly to factors VII, II and X (and to a lesser extent factor V, which is not a vitamin K–dependent clotting factor). However, factor VII is the most important factor in the extrinsic pathway of clotting. The optimum therapeutic range for the INR differs depending on the clinical indication because the lowest INR consistent with therapeutic efficacy is the best in reducing the risk of haemorrhage. Examples of therapeutic ranges recommended for various indications are given in Table 23.3 (Keeling et al., 2011).

Warfarin is metabolised by the liver via the cytochrome P450 system. Only very small amounts of the drug appear unchanged in the urine. The average clearance is 4.5 L/day, and the half-life ranges from 20 to 60 hours (mean 40 hours). It thus takes approximately 1 week (around five half-lives) for the steady state to be achieved after warfarin has been initiated. The enantiomers of warfarin are metabolised stereo-specifically, (R)-warfarin being mainly reduced at the acetyl side chain into

Table 23.3 Recommended target INRs for different conditions

Indication	Target INR
Pulmonary embolus (first episode)	2.5
Proximal deep vein thrombosis (first episode)	2.5
Recurrence of venous thromboembolism while on warfarin therapy (and INR >2.0)	3.5
Antiphospholipid syndrome	2.5
Non-rheumatic atrial fibrillation	2.5
Atrial fibrillation associated with mitral stenosis or regurgitation	2.5
Cardioversion	2.5
Mechanical prosthetic heart valve (depends on prosthesis thrombogenicity; consult full guideline) Bioprosthetic valve (depends on valve affected and associated risk factors; consult full guideline)	

INR, International normalised ratio.
Adapted from Keeling et al. (2011); consult the full guideline for further information.

Table 23.4 Some clinically important drug interactions with warfarin

Interacting drug	Effect	Probable mechanism(s)
Carbamazepine Rifampicin St John's wort	Reduced anticoagulant effect	Induction of warfarin metabolism
Oral contraceptives, oestrogens and progestogens Vitamin K (e.g. in some enteral feeds)	Reduced anticoagulant effect	Pharmacodynamic antagonism of anticoagulant effect
Amiodarone Cimetidine Ciprofloxacin Clarithromycin Erythromycin Fibrates Fluconazole Fluvastatin Itraconazole Ketoconazole Leflunomide Metronidazole Miconazole Norfloxacin Ofloxacin Paracetamol Rosuvastatin Sulfinpyrazone Sulfamethoxazole Trimethoprim	Increased anticoagulant effect	Inhibition of warfarin metabolism
Danazol Tamoxifen	Increased anticoagulant effect	Pharmacodynamic potentiation of anticoagulant effect
Cranberry juice	Increased anticoagulant effect	Mechanism unknown
NSAIDs (including aspirin at all doses) Clopidogrel	Increased risk of bleeding	Additive effects on coagulation Haemostasis

NSAIDs, Non-steroidal anti-inflammatory drugs.

secondary warfarin alcohols, whereas (S)-warfarin is predominantly metabolised at the coumarin ring to hydroxywarfarin. The clearance of warfarin may be reduced in liver disease and during the administration of a variety of drugs known to inhibit either the (S) or (R), or both, enantiomers. The number of possible interactions and the potential severity of their outcome mean that it is essential not to prescribe any medicine concomitantly with warfarin until a thorough check on all possible interactions has been undertaken. The British National Formulary (BNF) contains comprehensive information on possible interactions between warfarin and other medicines. It is advised that the BNF is always consulted before the use of any other medication with warfarin. Some examples of significant interactions with warfarin are provided in Table 23.4.

Renal function is thought to have little effect on the pharmacokinetics of, or anticoagulant response to, warfarin. Some of the variability in warfarin dose requirement is related to genetic polymorphisms of the cytochrome (CYP2C9) mediating the rate of hepatic metabolism of (S)-warfarin. Individuals with the variant isoform (either heterozygotes or in particular homozygotes) metabolise this more active enantiomer more slowly and so require lower doses.

The major adverse effect of warfarin is haemorrhage, which often occurs at the site of a predisposing abnormality, such as an ulcer or a tumour. The risk of bleeding is increased by excessive anticoagulation, although this may not need to be present for severe haemorrhage to occur. Close monitoring of the degree of anticoagulation of warfarin is, therefore, important, and guidelines for reversal of excessive anticoagulation are shown in Box 23.2.

It is also important to reduce the duration of therapy of the drug to the minimum effective period to reduce the period of risk.

Skin reactions to warfarin may also occur but are rare. The most serious skin reaction is warfarin-induced skin necrosis, which may occur over areas of adipose tissue such as the breasts, buttocks or thighs, especially in women, and is related to relative deficiency of protein C or S. This is important because these deficiencies result in an increased risk of thrombosis, and therefore warfarin may more often be used in such subjects. Preventing excessive anticoagulation in the initial stages of induction of therapy may reduce the severity of the reaction. A dosing schedule which helps achieve this is shown in Table 23.5.

Warfarin may also be teratogenic, producing in some instances a condition called chondrodysplasia punctata. This is associated with 'punched-out' lesions at sites of ossification, particularly of

Box 23.2 Recommendations for management of bleeding and excessive anticoagulation in patients receiving warfarin

- Major bleeding – stop warfarin sodium; give phytomenadione (vitamin K_1) 5 mg by slow intravenous injection; give dried prothrombin complex (factors II, VII, IX and X) 25–50 units/kg; if dried prothrombin complex unavailable, fresh frozen plasma 15 mL/kg can be given but is less effective; recombinant factor VIIa is not recommended for emergency anticoagulation reversal.
- INR >8.0, minor bleeding – stop warfarin sodium; give phytomenadione (vitamin K_1) 1–3 mg by slow intravenous injection; repeat dose of phytomenadione if INR is still too high after 24 h; restart warfarin sodium when INR <5.0.
- INR >8.0, no bleeding – stop warfarin sodium; give phytomenadione (vitamin K_1) 1–5 mg by mouth using the intravenous preparation orally (unlicensed use); repeat dose of phytomenadione if INR is still too high after 24 h; restart warfarin when INR <5.0.
- INR 5.0–8.0, minor bleeding – stop warfarin sodium; give phytomenadione (vitamin K_1) 1–3 mg by slow intravenous injection; restart warfarin sodium when INR <5.0.
- INR 5.0–8.0, no bleeding – withhold 1 or 2 doses of warfarin sodium and reduce subsequent maintenance dose.
- Unexpected bleeding at therapeutic levels – always investigate the possibility of an underlying cause (e.g. unsuspected renal or gastro-intestinal tract pathology).

INR, International normalised ratio.
Based on Keeling et al. (2011), and adapted from information within the British National Formulary 2018.

Table 23.5 Suggested warfarin induction schedule

Day	INR	Warfarin dose (mg)
First	<1.4	10 (5 may be more appropriate for the elderly and those with low body weight, liver disease, cardiac failure or at high risk of bleeding)
Second	<1.8	10
	1.8	1
	>1.8	0.5
Third	<2.0	10
	2.0–2.1	5
	2.2–2.3	4.5
	2.4–2.5	4
	2.6–2.7	3.5
	2.8–2.9	3
	3.0–3.1	2.5
	3.2–3.3	2
	3.4	1.5
	3.5	1
	3.6–4.0	0.5
	>4.0	0 (predicted maintenance dose)
Fourth	<1.4	>8
	1.4	8
	1.5	7.5
	1.6–1.7	7
	1.8	6.5
	1.9	6
	2.0–2.1	5.5
	2.2–2.3	5
	2.4–2.6	4.5
	2.7–3.0	4
	3.1–3.5	3.5
	3.6–4.0	3
	4.1–4.5	Miss out next day's dose, then give 2 mg
	>4.5	Miss out 2 days' doses, then give 1 mg

INR, International normalised ratio.
Modified from Fennerty et al. (1984).

the long bones but also of the facial bones, and may be associated with the absence of the spleen. Although it has been associated predominantly with warfarin anticoagulation during the first trimester of pregnancy, other abnormalities, including cranial nerve palsies, hydrocephalus and microcephaly, have been reported at later stages of pregnancy if the child is exposed.

Other coumarin anticoagulants are available. Acenocoumarol (nicoumalone) has a much shorter duration of action than warfarin, and phenindione may be associated with a higher incidence of non-haemorrhagic adverse effects. In the vast majority of cases, these drugs have not been shown to have any clear benefits over warfarin, but they may be used occasionally where a patient does not tolerate warfarin. It is now the case that a patient who does not tolerate warfarin would be more likely to receive a DOAC rather than another vitamin-K antagonist instead.

The necessary duration of anticoagulation in venous thrombosis and pulmonary embolus is still uncertain. On the basis of the available evidence, therapy may be required for approximately 6 months after the first DVT or PE. It may be possible to reduce the duration of therapy in patients who have had a postoperative episode because it is likely that the risk factor has been reversed (unless immobility continues). In patients with a second episode, therapy may be required for even longer, and in patients with more than two episodes, lifelong treatment may be necessary to reduce the risk of recurrence (Keeling et al., 2011).

Direct acting oral anticoagulants. DOACs (e.g. apixaban, dabigatran, edoxaban and rivaroxaban) are highly effective agents, but like all anticoagulants, they can cause potentially life-threatening bleeding in some patients. The various DOACs have different marketing authorisations for use in different indications, and because these are relatively new agents, their authorisations are subject to regular change. Product literature and/or the BNF should be consulted before use to ensure that an appropriate agent is selected for the indication.

Although DOACs interact with fewer drugs than vitamin-K antagonists such as warfarin, some potentially significant interactions do occur. All of the available agents appear to be substrates for p-glycoprotein (p-GP), and so various inhibitors or inducers of this system will respectively increase or decrease the effect of the DOACs to different extents. A DOAC dose reduction is advised when certain other medicines are co-prescribed and some are contraindicated in combination. As with warfarin, the BNF should be consulted before the co-administration of any other medicine with a DOAC.

The relatively short half-lives of the DOACs means adherence to treatment is essential for them to be optimally effective. They are not, therefore, a panacea for a patient who is nonadherent to warfarin or other medicines.

There is sometimes a perception that there is no requirement for biochemical or physiological monitoring with DOACs. It is true that no routine anticoagulant monitoring is required; indeed, this is not currently possible. However, there is a requirement to assess renal function before initiation and periodically thereafter, particularly where a decline in renal function is suspected, and also to monitor for signs of suspected bleeding or anaemia.

The DOACs have been shown in clinical trials to be generally safe for use without routine anticoagulant monitoring; however, arguments for and against laboratory monitoring have been published (Kitchen et al., 2014). The absence of such monitoring may be a disadvantage in some cases, as it is not possible to identify signs of sub-therapeutic or supra-therapeutic plasma levels until a thromboembolism or haemorrhage occurs. Further information on the effects of DOACs on laboratory measures of anticoagulation can be found in the relevant British Society for Haematology guideline (Kitchen et al., 2014).

When considering the use of a DOAC, it is advised that the Cockroft–Gault formula is used to calculate an accurate creatinine clearance before initiation. Dose reductions are advised with DOACs at different levels of renal impairment, and they are also contraindicated at different levels of impairment. This is sometimes dependent on the indication for which they are prescribed. In patients with moderate to severe renal impairment, a drug which is not predominantly renally excreted, with a marketing authorisation for this use, should be used. Some further information is given in the following sections, but again, the product literature and/or the BNF should also be consulted.

Haemorrhage is the major adverse effect of the DOACs, and patients should be advised to seek urgent medical attention if they notice signs of bleeding. Idarucizumab, a monoclonal antibody fragment, is licenced in the UK for reversal of the anticoagulant effect of dabigatran (NICE, 2016). It binds to both free and thrombin-bound dabigatran, reversing the anticoagulant effect within minutes. Andexanet alfa, which is a recombinant modified human factor Xa decoy protein, has been shown to reverse the anticoagulant effects of apixaban and rivaroxaban (Connolly et al., 2016). It does not yet have a marketing authorisation in the UK.

Dabigatran. Dabigatran is an orally active inhibitor of both free and clot-bound thrombin (Wittkowsky, 2010). It has a rapid onset of action. Dabigatran etexilate is a prodrug which is hydrolysed to active dabigatran in the liver. Because 80% of activated dabigatran is excreted unchanged through the kidneys, it should be avoided in patients with severe renal impairment (creatinine clearance <30 mL/min), and the dose should be reduced in moderate renal impairment (creatinine clearance 30–50 mL/min). Dabigatran is a substrate for the transport protein p-GP, which facilitates renal elimination of certain drugs. Amiodarone, an inhibitor of p-GP, reduces the clearance of dabigatran, and so doses should be reduced in patients who are on concurrent treatment with amiodarone. In patients who are on strong p-GP inhibitors, such as verapamil and clarithromycin, dabigatran should be used with caution, and it should not be used together with quinidine. Drugs such as rifampicin and St John's wort, which are potent p-GP inducers, may potentially reduce its efficacy.

Rivaroxaban. Rivaroxaban is an orally active inhibitor of both the 'free' and prothrombinase complex-bound forms of activated factor X (Xa) (Wittkowsky, 2010). Two-thirds of the dose is metabolised, principally by CYP450 enzymes, and the remaining third is excreted unchanged in the urine. It should also be used with caution in patients with creatinine clearance less than 30 mL/min (severe renal impairment) and is contraindicated in those with creatinine clearance less than 15 mL/min.

Like dabigatran, rivaroxaban also appears to be a p-GP substrate, and it should be used with caution when prescribed concomitantly with p-GP inhibitors and potent p-GP inducers. Several CYP3A4 inhibitors and inducers have also been shown to affect its metabolism. Some CYP3A4 inhibitors significantly increase the area-under-the-curve (AUC) of rivaroxaban, particularly ketoconazole and other azole-antimycotics, such as itraconazole, voriconazole and posaconazole and also HIV protease inhibitors such as ritonavir. Therefore, the use of rivaroxaban is not recommended in patients receiving concomitant systemic treatment with these agents. The CYP3A4 inducer rifampicin (and possibly other inducers of this cytochrome) reduces the AUC for rivaroxaban.

Apixaban. Apixaban is an orally active direct inhibitor of activated factor X (factor Xa). Around 30% of the dose is excreted unchanged in urine. The normal elimination half-life is around 12 hours, but this is prolonged in renal dysfunction. It is not recommended if the creatinine clearance is less than 15 mL/min. The dose should be reduced if the eGFR is between 15 and 29 mL/min/1.73 m^2, or if serum-creatinine ≥133 mmol/L and the patient's age is ≥80 years or the patient's body weight is ≤60 kg.

Like dabigatran and rivaroxaban, apixaban also appears to be a p-GP substrate, and so it should be used with caution when prescribed concomitantly with p-GP inhibitors and potent p-GP inducers.

Edoxaban. Edoxaban is also an orally active direct inhibitor of activated factor X (factor Xa). Around 50% of the clearance of the drug is via the kidney as unchanged drug in the urine, the remainder being cleared by metabolism and biliary or intestinal excretion. The terminal elimination half-life of edoxaban following oral administration in health is around 10–14 hours. The manufacturer advises a reduction in edoxaban dose in moderate to severe renal impairment and to avoid using the medicine in end-stage renal disease or in dialysis.

Edoxaban is a substrate of p-GP, and co-administration of potent inhibitors like ciclosporin, dronedarone, erythromycin, ketoconazole, quinidine or verapamil increases edoxaban exposure, necessitating a recommended reduction in dose.

Fibrinolytic drugs

Thrombolytic therapy is used in life-threatening acute massive PE. It has been used in DVT, particularly in those patients where a large amount of clot exists and venous valvular damage is likely. However, fibrinolytic drugs are potentially more dangerous than anticoagulant drugs, and evidence is not available in situations other than acute massive embolism to show a sustained benefit from their use.

Streptokinase. Streptokinase was the first agent available in this class. It was produced from streptococci and is a large protein that binds to and activates plasminogen, thus encouraging the breakdown of formed fibrin to fibrinogen degradation products. It also acts on the circulating fibrinogen to produce a degree of systemic anticoagulation. Because it is a large protein molecule, it cannot be administered orally and has to be given by intravenous infusion. The half-life of removal from the body is 30 minutes. It is cleared chiefly by the reticuloendothelial system in the liver.

Its major adverse effect is to increase the risk of haemorrhage, but it may also be antigenic and produce an anaphylactic reaction. It may also cause hypotension during infusion, and in some patients, particularly those who have been administered the drug within the previous 12 months, a relative resistance to the drug may occur. Thrombolytic therapy is contraindicated in patients who have had major surgery or with active bleeding sites in the gastro-intestinal or genitourinary tract; those who have a history of stroke, renal or liver disease; and those with hypertension. It should also be avoided during pregnancy and the postpartum period.

Alteplase. Tissue plasminogen activator (rt-PA) or alteplase was developed using recombinant DNA technology. Although this agent is much more expensive than streptokinase, it can be used in those situations where streptokinase may be less effective because of development of antibodies, for example, within 1 year of previous streptokinase use or where allergy to streptokinase has previously occurred. Alteplase produces a lesser degree of systemic anticoagulation because it is more active against plasminogen associated with the clot; immediate use of heparin subsequently is necessary to prevent recurrence of thrombosis. Alteplase is also used for acute ischaemic stroke, where its prompt use may improve outcome in carefully selected individuals in whom cerebral haemorrhage has been excluded using appropriate imaging techniques (NICE, 2012). Currently, it is the only thrombolytic licensed for this indication (see discussion of arterial thromboembolism).

Reteplase and tenecteplase. Reteplase and tenecteplase are also fibrin-specific agents, and so heparin is required to prevent rebound thrombosis. They are indicated for the treatment of acute myocardial infarction. In this clinical situation, reteplase is administered as an intravenous bolus, followed by a second bolus 30 minutes later (double bolus), and tenecteplase is given as a single intravenous bolus. They, therefore, have the advantage of convenience of administration compared with alteplase, and they are the preferred option in pre-hospital settings, particularly when administered by paramedics (NICE, 2002).

Urokinase. Urokinase, like alteplase and streptokinase, can be used for the treatment of DVT and PE. It is also licensed to restore patency in intravenous catheters and cannulas blocked by fibrin thrombi.

Patient care

Patients taking oral anticoagulants should be given full information on what to do in case of problems and what circumstances and drugs to avoid. An anticoagulant card with previous INR values and doses should also be provided to those taking warfarin, and patients should be told of the colour codes for the different strengths of warfarin tablets and advised to carry their treatment card at all times. Similarly, patients taking a DOAC should be provided with an appropriate anticoagulant card for their treatment. The likely duration of any anticoagulant therapy should be made clear to the patient to avoid unnecessary and potentially dangerous prolongations of treatment. Patients who have received a fibrinolytic agent should also carry a card identifying the drug given and the date of administration.

Arterial thromboembolism

Acute myocardial infarction is the commonest clinical presentation of acute arterial thrombosis. Stroke is commonly caused by atherothromboembolism from the great vessels or embolism arising from the heart (approximately 80% of strokes). These two conditions are discussed elsewhere. Peripheral arterial thrombosis or thromboembolism may also occur, most often in the lower limb. Antiplatelet drugs are often used for prophylaxis, but surgical embolectomy and/or fibrinolytic therapy may be needed for treatment of acute thrombotic or thromboembolic events to avoid consequent ischaemic damage.

Aetiology

Arterial thromboembolism is normally associated with vascular injury and hypercoagulability. Vascular injury is most often due to atheroma, itself aggravated by smoking, hypertension, hyperlipidaemia or diabetes mellitus. Although the exact mechanism is not clear, it is thought that platelet aggregation may be induced by the shear stresses caused by the stenosis of an atherosclerotic vessel. This thrombotic material may embolise to cause occlusion further downstream. Hypercoagulability is also a risk factor. It may be associated with increased plasma fibrinogen levels and an increase in circulating cellular components, for example, polycythaemia or thrombocythaemia. As mentioned earlier, the thrombus formed in the artery contains a much larger proportion of platelets, possibly reflecting the fact that other blood components that are not as readily adherent may be dissipated by the higher flow rates in the arterial circulation. Oestrogens, by the mechanisms described earlier, are likely to increase the risk of arterial and venous thrombosis. Hyperlipidaemia may also increase the risk of hypercoagulability, as well as enhance thrombotic risk through its role in the progression of atheroma and vascular injury.

Treatment and prevention

Aspirin

Aspirin (acetylsalicylic acid) is a potent inhibitor of the enzyme cyclo-oxygenase, which catalyses the production of prostaglandins. It reduces the production of a pro-aggregatory prostaglandin, thromboxane A_2, in the platelet, an effect that lasts for the life of the platelet.

Aspirin is well absorbed after oral administration. It is rapidly metabolised by esterases in the blood and liver (so that its half-life is only 15–20 minutes) to salicylic acid and other metabolites that are excreted in the urine. In the doses used in prophylaxis against thromboembolism, aspirin is largely metabolised by the liver, but in overdose, urinary excretion of salicylate becomes a limiting factor in drug elimination.

The major adverse effect of aspirin is gastro-intestinal irritation and bleeding. This problem is much more common with higher doses of aspirin (300 mg or more) that were once used in the prevention of arterial thromboembolism but are less common with the doses (e.g. 75 mg) now used. Concomitant use of ulcer-healing drugs, particularly proton pump inhibitors, can reduce the risk of peptic ulceration induced by non-steroidal anti-inflammatory drug (NSAID) use in patients susceptible to the problem (NICE, 2015c). There is also little evidence that buffered or enteric-coated preparations of aspirin are safer in this respect. However, the vast majority of patients tolerate low-dose aspirin well, and it is normally given as a single oral dose of soluble aspirin. Aspirin may also, rarely, induce asthma, particularly in patients with co-existing reversible airway obstruction. Other patients have a form of aspirin hypersensitivity that may result in urticaria and/or angioedema. In this situation, there may be cross-reactivity with other NSAIDs.

Haemorrhagic stroke is a rare but very serious complication of therapy with aspirin (and with other antiplatelet agents). Aspirin must not be given to children or people younger than 16 years because of the risk of the rare but life-threatening possibility of Reye's syndrome, which may cause liver and renal failure.

Aspirin is an established treatment for the secondary prevention of cardiovascular events. However, a review of its use for primary prevention found that the risks and benefits are more finely balanced than previously thought, and low-dose aspirin is no longer routinely recommended for this indication, even in high-risk patients such as those with diabetes or hypertension (Anon., 2009). It should also be noted that it does not have a marketing authorisation for such use.

Clopidogrel

Clopidogrel is a prodrug that is metabolised in part to an active thiol derivative. The latter inhibits platelet aggregation by rapidly and irreversibly inhibiting the binding of adenosine diphosphate (ADP) to its platelet receptor, thus preventing the ADP-mediated activation of the glycoprotein IIb/IIIa receptor for the life of the platelet. It is an orally active prodrug and is given once daily for the reduction of atherosclerotic events in those with pre-existing atherosclerotic disease. In this respect, it may be a useful alternative to aspirin in aspirin-allergic subjects, but haemorrhage occurs with the same frequency as aspirin, and thrombocytopenia (sometimes severe) may be commoner than with aspirin therapy. Activation to its active metabolite may be subject to a genetic polymorphism of CYP450 2C19 and may also be reduced by the proton pump inhibitor omeprazole or esomeprazole, so the use of alternative gastroprotective agents may need to be considered if required.

Clopidogrel is licensed in the UK for the prevention of atherothrombotic events (myocardial infarction, ischaemic stroke, established peripheral arterial disease, and acute coronary syndrome in combination with aspirin) and the prevention of atherothrombotic and thromboembolic events in atrial fibrillation (Consilient Health, 2017).

Prasugrel

Prasugrel inhibits platelet activation and aggregation. It is a prodrug whose active metabolite irreversibly binds to P2Y12 class of ADP receptors on platelets. This prevents activation of the GPIIb/IIIa receptor complex and thus causes inhibition of ADP-mediated platelet activation and aggregation. In combination with aspirin, it is recommended by NICE as an option, within its marketing authorisation, for preventing atherothrombotic events in adults with acute coronary syndrome (unstable angina [UA], NSTEMI or STEMI) having primary or delayed percutaneous coronary intervention (NICE, 2014).

Ticagrelor

Like prasugrel and clopidogrel, ticagrelor blocks ADP receptors of subtype P2Y12. However, unlike the other antiplatelet drugs, it has a binding site different from ADP (it is an allosteric antagonist), and the blockade is therefore reversible. It is an active drug in its own right and does not require activation by metabolism. Ticagrelor in combination with low-dose aspirin is recommended for up to 12 months as a treatment option in adults with acute coronary syndromes (NICE, 2011).

Dipyridamole

Dipyridamole is prescribed as an adjunct to oral anticoagulation for prophylaxis of thromboembolism associated with prosthetic heart valves. Dipyridamole modified-release preparations 200 mg twice a day may be used in combination with aspirin 75 mg daily for long-term vascular prevention in people with ischaemic stroke or TIA without paroxysmal or permanent atrial fibrillation, but only if clopidogrel 75 mg daily cannot be used (Bowen et al., 2016). If clopidogrel and aspirin cannot be tolerated or are contraindicated, then modified-release dipyridamole 200 mg twice a day would be used by itself.

Dipyridamole is a phosphodiesterase inhibitor and, thus, elevates concentrations of cyclic AMP. It may also block the uptake of adenosine by erythrocytes and other cells. Adverse effects include headache (to which tolerance may gradually develop) gastro-intestinal problems, flushing and hypotension.

Glycoprotein IIb/IIIa inhibitors

Glycoprotein IIb/IIIa inhibitors prevent platelet aggregation by blocking the binding of fibrinogen to receptors on platelets.

Abciximab. Abciximab is a monoclonal antibody which binds to coronary glycoprotein IIb/IIIa receptors and to other related sites. It is recommended as an adjunct to heparin and aspirin for the prevention of ischaemic complications in high-risk patients undergoing percutaneous transluminal coronary intervention (NICE, 2010). Abciximab should be used once only to avoid further risk of thrombocytopenia.

Eptifibatide and tirofiban. Eptifibatide and tirofiban also inhibit glycoprotein IIb/IIIa receptors; they are licensed for use with heparin and aspirin to prevent early myocardial infarction in patients with unstable angina or NSTEMI.

Abciximab, eptifibatide and tirofiban all have to be administered parenterally and should be used by specialist clinicians only (NICE, 2010).

Patient care

Aspirin is normally well tolerated at the doses used for stroke prevention. However, it should not be given to patients with a history of gastro-intestinal ulceration. Because it may induce bronchospasm in susceptible individuals, it should be used cautiously in such circumstances. It is best tolerated if taken once daily as soluble aspirin after food.

Case studies

Case 23.1

Mr AJ, a 75-year-old patient receiving warfarin to prevent DVT, comes to the clinic with an INR of 12, despite taking the same dose of the drug. There is no evidence of bleeding. He was previously well controlled on warfarin.

Question

What should be done?

Answer

Because Mr AJ's INR is more than 8 (even if there is no bleeding), the national guidelines recommend that warfarin be stopped (Keeling et al., 2011). The patient should then be given phytomenadione (vitamin K$_1$) 1–5 mg by mouth using the intravenous preparation orally (unlicensed use). The dose of phytomenadione should be repeated if the INR is still too high after 24 hours. However, a single dose often helps the INR return to close to the target level at 24 hours without causing warfarin resistance subsequently. The warfarin can be restarted when the INR is less than 5.0. A search for clinical conditions or drugs which might cause warfarin sensitivity should also be made. Measurement of plasma warfarin concentration may help in difficult cases.

Case 23.2

A patient, Mr FG, receiving heparin for 7 days for extensive VTE develops arterial thrombosis.

Question

What would you suspect in this situation, and what should be done?

Answer

The rare but serious heparin-induced thrombocytopenia (HIT) may be responsible. The platelet count should be measured immediately, and if HIT is strongly suspected or confirmed, the heparin should be discontinued. An alternative anticoagulant should be started at full dose whilst specific confirmatory tests are being performed, unless there are significant contraindications. Danaparoid and lepirudin may be considered as alternative anticoagulants in these circumstances.

Case 23.3

Mr MT, admitted to an acute hospital with suspected myocardial infarction, says that he had a myocardial infarction 4 years ago and was treated with a drug to 'dissolve the clot in the coronary artery'. The chest pain started 4 hours earlier, and his electrocardiogram shows ST-segment elevation in the anterior leads.

Question

What relevance may Mr MT's previous treatment, present history and findings have to his management on this occasion?

Answer

Thrombolytic drugs are indicated for any patient with acute myocardial infarction, provided the likely benefits outweigh the possible risks. Trials have shown that the benefit is greatest in those with electrocardiogram (ECG) changes that include ST-segment elevation, especially in those with anterior infarction, and in patients with bundle branch block. The patient has received a thrombolytic, possibly streptokinase, in the past. Mr MT should be asked if he was given a card to carry with him with the identity of the therapy he was given. If the prior treatment was with streptokinase or anistreplase (no longer available), prolonged persistence of antibodies to streptokinase may reduce the effectiveness of subsequent treatment. Therefore, streptokinase should not be used again beyond 4 days of first administration of streptokinase (or anistreplase), and urgent consideration should be given to the use of an alternative thrombolytic agent such as alteplase, reteplase or tenecteplase.

Case 23.4

A 64-year-old male patient, Mr TS, is to be prescribed aspirin therapy following an acute myocardial infarction.

Question

What questions should you ask Mr TS before starting treatment with aspirin?

Answer

Mr TS should be asked if he has had aspirin before and, if so, whether he tolerated it. Caution is necessary in elderly patients, in those with uncontrolled hypertension and in patients taking other drugs that increase the risk of bleeding. Caution is also required in those with a previous history of peptic ulceration, and some manufacturers advise avoidance in such circumstances; active peptic ulceration is a definite contraindication. Other contraindications include severe hepatic impairment, severe renal failure, haemophilia and other bleeding disorders. Aspirin may induce bronchospasm or angioedema in susceptible individuals, for example, in asthmatics, and caution should be exercised in these circumstances.

Case 23.5

Mrs BC, a 56-year-old woman on warfarin therapy for atrial fibrillation with mitral stenosis, appears to become resistant to warfarin after previously good control on 5 mg daily. Her INR does not rise above 1.4 even when her warfarin dose is increased to 20 mg daily.

Question

What can be done to find the cause of the resistance?

Answer

Mrs BC should be asked about any new medications which might have been introduced recently, including over-the-counter and herbal preparations. Some proprietary medicines may contain vitamin K, which could cause resistance by pharmacodynamic mechanisms. Other medicines, including the herbal medicine St John's wort, might induce warfarin metabolism and result in resistance as a result of a pharmacokinetic interaction (see Table 23.4). One other cause of apparent resistance to warfarin is poor adherence, and this should, therefore, be considered. Supervised administration of the dose and/or measurement of plasma warfarin concentrations may be of value if this is suspected.

References

Anon, 2009. Aspirin for primary prevention of cardiovascular disease? Drugs Therapeut. Bull. 47, 122–125.

Baglin, T., Barrowcliffe, T.W., Cohen, A., et al., 2006. British Committee for Standards in Haematology, guidelines on the use and monitoring of heparin. Br. J. Haematol. 133 19–34.

Bauer, K.A., Leung, L.L.K., Tirnauer, J.S., 2017. Protein C deficiency. UpToDate. Available at: https://www.uptodate.com/contents/protein-c-deficiency.

Bowen, A., James, M., Young, G., 2016. Intercollegiate Stroke Working Party, national clinical guideline for stroke. Royal College of Physicians, London. Available at: https://www.strokeaudit.org/SupportFiles/Documents/Guidelines/2016-National-Clinical-Guideline-for-Stroke-5t-(1).aspx.

Connolly, S.J., Milling, T.J., Eikelboom, J.W., et al., 2016. Andexanet alfa for acute major bleeding associated with factor Xa inhibitors. New Engl. J. Med. 375, 1131–1141.

Consilient Health, 2017. Summary of product characteristics clopidogrel. Available at: https://www.medicines.org.uk/emc/medicine/24979.

Derksen, R.H.W.M., de Groot, P.G., Nieuwenhuis, H.K., et al., 2001. How to treat women with antiphospholipid antibodies in pregnancy? Ann. Rheum. Dis. 60, 1–3.

Elyamany, G., Alzahrani, A.M., Bukhary, E., 2014. Cancer-associated thrombosis: an overview. Clin. Med. Insights Oncol. 8, 129–137.

Fennerty, A., Dolben, J., Thomas, P., et al., 1984. Flexible induction dose regimen for warfarin and prediction of maintenance dose. Br. Med. J. 288, 1268–1270.

Fennerty, A.G., Renowden, S., Scolding, N., et al., 1986. Guidelines for the control of heparin treatment. Br. Med. J. 292, 579–580.

House of Commons Health Committee, 2005. The prevention of venous thromboembolism in hospitalised patients. The Stationery Office, London.

Keeling, D., Baglin, T., Tait, C., et al., 2011. For British Committee for Standards in Haematology, guidelines on oral anticoagulation with warfarin: fourth edition. Br. J. Haematol. 154, 311–324.

Keeling, D., Davidson, S., Watson, H., 2006. Haemostasis and Thrombosis Task Force of the British Committee for Standards in Haematology, the management of heparin induced thrombocytopenia. Br. J. Haematol. 133, 259–269.

Kitchen, S., Gray, E., Mackie, I., 2014. Measurement of non-coumarin anticoagulants and their effects on tests of haemostasis. Guidance from the British Committee for Standards in Haematology. Br. J. Haematol. 166, 830–841.

Knight, M., Nair, M., Tuffnell, D., et al. (Eds.), for MBRRACE-UK, 2016. Saving lives, improving mothers' care surveillance of maternal deaths in the UK 2012–14 and lessons learned to inform maternity care from the UK and Ireland Confidential Enquiries into Maternal Deaths and Morbidity 2009–14. National Perinatal Epidemiology Unit, Oxford. Available at: https://www.npeu.ox.ac.uk/downloads/files/mbrrace-uk/reports/MBRRACE-UK%20Maternal%20Report%202016%20-%20website.pdf

National Institute for Health and Care Excellence (NICE), 2002. Guidance on the use of drugs for early thrombolysis in the treatment of acute myocardial infarction. Technology Appraisal 52. NICE, London. Available at: http://www.nice.org.uk/guidance/ta52.

National Institute for Health and Care Excellence (NICE), 2010. Guidance on the use of glycoprotein IIb/IIIa inhibitors in the treatment of acute coronary syndromes. Technology Appraisal 47 NICE, London. Available at: http://www.nice.org.uk/guidance/ta47/.

National Institute for Health and Care Excellence (NICE), 2011. Ticagrelor for the treatment of acute coronary syndromes. Technology Appraisal Guidance TA236. NICE, London. Available at https://www.nice.org.uk/guidance/ta236/.

National Institute for Health and Care Excellence (NICE), 2012. Alteplase for treating acute ischaemic stroke. Technology Appraisal TA264. NICE, London. Available at: https://www.nice.org.uk/guidance/ta264/.

National Institute for Health and Care Excellence (NICE), 2014. Prasugrel with percutaneous coronary intervention for treating acute coronary syndromes. Technology Appraisal TA317. NICE, London. Available at: http://www.nice.org.uk/ta317.

National Institute for Health and Care Excellence (NICE), 2015a. Reducing the risk of venous thromboembolism (deep vein thrombosis and pulmonary embolism) in patients admitted to hospital. Clinical Guideline 92. NICE, London. Available at: http://www.nice.org.uk/guidance/cg92.

National Institute for Health and Care Excellence (NICE), 2015b. Venous thromboembolic diseases: diagnosis, management and thrombophilia testing. NICE, London. Available at: https://www.nice.org.uk/guidance/CG144.

National Institute for Health and Care Excellence (NICE), 2015c. Clinical knowledge summaries. Antiplatelet treatment. Available at: https://cks.nice.org.uk/antiplatelet-treatment#!scenario:1.

National Institute for Health and Care Excellence (NICE), 2016. Reversal of the anticoagulant effect of dabigatran: idarucizumab. Evidence summary [ESNM 73]. NICE, London. Available at: https://www.nice.org.uk/advice/esnm73/chapter/Key-points-from-the-evidence.

Rosendaal, F.R., 2009. In: Van Beek, E.J.R., Büller, H.R., Oudkerk, M. (Eds.), Deep Vein Thrombosis and Pulmonary Embolism. Wiley-Blackwell, Chichester.

Rosendaal, F.R., Reitsma, P.H., 2009. Genetics of venous thrombosis. J. Thromb. Haemostasis. 7 (Suppl. 1), 301–304.

Wells PS, Anderson DR, Rodger M, et al., 2000. Derivation of a Simple Clinical Model to Categorize Patients Probability of Pulmonary Embolism: Increasing the Models Utility with the SimpliRED D-dimer. Thromb. Haemost. 83, 416–420.

Wells, P.S., Anderson, D.R., Rodger, M., et al., 2003. Evaluation of D-dimer in the diagnosis of suspected deep-vein thrombosis. New Engl. J. Med. 349, 1227–1235.

Winter, M., Keeling, D., Sharpen, F., et al., 2005. Procedures for the outpatient management of patients with deep vein thrombosis. Clin. Lab. Haematol. 27, 61–66.

Wittkowsky, A.K., 2010. New oral anticoagulants: a practical guide for clinicians. J. Thromb. Thrombolysis. 29, 182–191.

Further reading

Kesieme, E., Kesieme, C., Jebbin, N., et al., 2011. Deep vein thrombosis: a clinical review. J. Blood Med. 2, 59–69.

Useful website

Thrombosis UK: http://www.thrombosisuk.org.

24 Dyslipidaemia

Helen Williams

Key points

- Elevated concentrations of total cholesterol (TC) and low-density lipoprotein cholesterol (LDL-C) increase the risk of cardiovascular disease (CVD), whereas high-density lipoprotein cholesterol (HDL-C) confers protection.

- Two-thirds of the UK adult population has a serum TC greater than 5 mmol/L. The average TC concentration is 5.6 mmol/L.

- Dyslipidaemia may develop secondary to disorders such as diabetes mellitus, hypothyroidism, chronic renal failure, nephrotic syndrome, obesity, high alcohol intake and some drugs.

- Understanding and managing dyslipidaemia is of particular importance to reduce cardiovascular (CV) events in patients with or at risk of CV disease, but dyslipidaemia can also predispose patients to other disorders; for example, severe hypertriglyceridaemia (>10 mmol/L) is responsible for up to 4% of cases of acute pancreatitis.

- Androgens, β-blockers, ciclosporin, oral contraceptives, diuretics, glucocorticoids and vitamin A derivatives are examples of drugs that can have an adverse effect on the lipid profile.

- There are five main classes of lipid-lowering agents: statins, fibrates, resins, nicotinic acid derivatives and absorption blockers. More recently, proprotein convertase subtilisin/kexin type 9 inhibitors have been introduced.

- Statins are the drugs of choice in the treatment of primary prevention and secondary prevention of CVD.

- The aim of treatment in primary prevention (≥10% risk of CVD over 10 years) is to reduce overall CV risk by treatment with a high-intensity statin, such as atorvastatin 20 mg. No specific target treatment levels are recommended in primary prevention, although a 40% or more drop in non-HDL-C should be used as a marker of adherence.

- In secondary prevention, treatment should be started with a high dose of a high-intensity statin, such as atorvastatin 80 mg daily. No specific target treatment levels are recommended in secondary prevention, although a 40% or more decline in non-HDL-C should be used as a marker of adherence.

Disorders of lipoprotein metabolism together with high-fat diets, obesity and physical inactivity have all contributed to the current epidemic of atherosclerotic disease seen in developed countries. Disorders of lipoprotein metabolism that result in elevated serum concentrations of total cholesterol (TC) and low-density lipoprotein cholesterol (LDL-C) increase the risk of development of cardiovascular disease (CVD). In contrast, high-density lipoprotein cholesterol (HDL-C) confers protection against CVD, with the risk reducing as HDL-C increases. It is, therefore, clear that the term hyperlipidaemia, which was formerly used to describe disorders of lipoprotein metabolism, is inappropriate. It is more appropriate to use the term dyslipidaemia, which encompasses both abnormally high levels of specific lipoproteins, for example, LDL-C, and abnormally low levels of other lipoproteins, for example, HDL-C, as well as disorders in the composition of the various lipoprotein particles. It is particularly appropriate when considering the individual at risk of CVD with a normal or high TC and low HDL-C (TC:HDL-C ratio).

Epidemiology

Lipid and lipoprotein concentrations vary among different populations, with countries consuming a Western type of diet generally having higher TC and LDL-C levels than those where regular consumption of saturated fat is low. The UK's cholesterol level is ninth highest in the world, slightly less than 5.5 mmol/L. However, UK men and women have both shown one of the largest drops in cholesterol in all high-income countries, from 6.2 to 5.4 mmol/L (Farzadfar et al., 2011). In contrast, in China and Japan, the average is reading is less than 5 mmol/L (Research Committee on Serum Lipid Level Survey 1990 in Japan, 1996; Yang et al., 2012).

The ideal serum lipid profile is unknown and varies between different populations, even across Europe, and also within a given population. Until recently, calculated LDL-C level was a key target for lipid lowering and monitoring, but in 2014 the National Institute for Health and Care Excellence (NICE) recommended the use of non-high-density lipoprotein cholesterol (non-HDL-C) rather than LDL-C. Non-HDL-C is TC minus HDL-C. LDL-C is not directly measured; it requires a calculation using a fasting sample and for the triglyceride levels to be less than 4.5 mmol/L (NICE, 2014). Measurement of non-HDL-C does not require either of these. Non-HDL-C represents the total of cholesterol circulating on apoprotein B (apoB) particles, that is, both LDL and triglyceride-rich lipoproteins, and represents the main atherogenic particles. A desirable value is less than 3 mmol/L.

The values presented in Table 24.1 represent what might be considered as an optimal lipid profile in the UK. Specific target levels for patients receiving treatment for primary or secondary

Table 24.1 Optimal serum lipid profile

Total cholesterol	<4.0 mmol/L
Low-density lipoprotein cholesterol	<2.0 mmol/L
Triglyceride	<1.7 mmol/L (fasting)
High-density lipoprotein cholesterol	>1.0 mmol/L in men >1.2 mmol/L in women

prevention of CVD are no longer recommended by NICE (2014); they state that a 40% reduction in non-HDL-C from pretreatment baseline is an indication of adherence to treatment.

Despite a 50% reduction in the death rate from CVD over the past 25 years, CVD remains the leading cause of death in the UK (NICE, 2014). The death rate from CVD is threefold higher in males than females, but because women live longer and are at increased risk of stroke after the age of 75 years, their lifetime risk of disease is greater (NICE, 2014). Death from CVD is responsible for one quarter of premature deaths in men and 17% of premature deaths in women (British Heart Foundation, 2015). The higher the levels of TC in an individual, the greater is the chance of development of CVD. For an individual, there appears to be no level below which a further reduction of TC or LDL-C is not associated with a lower risk of CVD.

Population-based approaches to vascular screening have the potential to provide significant health gain for society because most deaths from CVD occur in individuals who are not yet identified as at increased risk. Moreover, a small reduction in average population levels of TC and LDL-C/non-HDL-C can potentially prevent many deaths. In England, the NHS Health Checks scheme was introduced in 2009 for everyone between 40 and 74 years of age to receive a free health check every 5 years; this health check includes measurement of TC and the TC:HDL-C ratio and a calculation of cardiovascular (CV) risk. The intention is that individuals are given the necessary information about their health to make changes to lifestyle and avoid preventable disease.

Lipid transport and lipoprotein metabolism

The clinically important lipids in the blood (unesterified and esterified cholesterol and triglycerides) are not readily soluble in serum and are rendered miscible by incorporation into lipoproteins. There are six main classes of lipoproteins: chylomicrons, chylomicron remnants, very low-density lipoproteins (VLDL), intermediate-density lipoproteins (IDL), LDL and HDL.

The protein components of lipoproteins are known as apoproteins (apo), of which apoA-I, apoE, apoC and apoB are perhaps the most important. ApoB exists in two forms: B-48, which is present in chylomicrons and associated with the transport of ingested lipids; and B-100, which is found in endogenously secreted VLDL-C and associated with the transport of lipids from the liver (Fig. 24.1).

When dietary cholesterol and triglycerides are absorbed from the intestine they are transported in the intestinal lymphatics as chylomicrons. These are the largest of the lipoprotein particles of which triglycerides normally constitute approximately 80% of the lipid core. The chylomicrons pass through blood capillaries in adipose tissue and skeletal muscle, where the enzyme lipoprotein lipase is located, bound to the endothelium. Lipoprotein lipase is activated by apoC-II on the surface of the chylomicron. The lipase catalyses the breakdown of the triglyceride in the chylomicron to free fatty acid and glycerol, which then enter adipose tissue and muscle. The cholesterol-rich chylomicron remnant is taken up by receptors on hepatocyte membranes, and in this way dietary cholesterol is delivered to the liver and cleared from the circulation.

VLDL-C is formed in the liver and transports triglycerides, which again make up approximately 80% of its lipid core, to the periphery. The triglyceride content of VLDL-C is removed by lipoprotein lipase in a similar manner to that described earlier for chylomicrons, and forms IDL-C particles. The core of IDL-C particles is roughly 50% triglyceride and 50% cholesterol esters, acquired from HDL-C under the influence of the enzyme lecithin-cholesterol acyltransferase (LCAT). Approximately 50% of the body's IDL particles are cleared from serum by the liver. The other 50% of IDL-C are further hydrolysed and modified to lose triglyceride and apoE1, and become LDL-C particles. LDL-C is the major cholesterol-carrying particle in serum.

LDL-C provides cholesterol, an essential component of cell membranes, bile acid and a precursor of steroid hormones to those cells that require it. LDL-C is also the main lipoprotein involved in atherogenesis, although it appears to take on this role only after it has been modified by oxidation. For reasons that are not totally clear, the arterial endothelium becomes permeable to the lipoprotein. Monocytes migrate through the permeable endothelium and engulf the lipoprotein, resulting in the formation of lipid-laden macrophages that have a key role in the subsequent development of atherosclerosis. The aim of treatment in dyslipidaemia is normally to reduce concentrations of LDL-C (and consequently atherogenesis), and thus reduce TC at the same time.

Non-HDL cholesterol (TC minus HDL-C) is a measure of all the 'bad elements' of the lipid profile and is now used in preference to LDL-C, because it can be calculated without the need to take a fasting blood sample and is not affected by the presence of high triglyceride levels.

Whereas VLDL-C and LDL-C are considered the 'bad' lipoproteins, HDL-C is often considered to be the 'good' antiatherogenic lipoprotein. In general, about 65% of TC is carried in LDL-C and about 25% in HDL.

High-density lipoprotein

HDL-C is formed from the unesterified cholesterol and phospholipid removed from peripheral tissues and the surface of triglyceride-rich proteins. The major structural protein is apoA-I. HDL-C mediates the return of lipoprotein and cholesterol from peripheral tissues to the liver for excretion in a process known as reverse cholesterol transport.

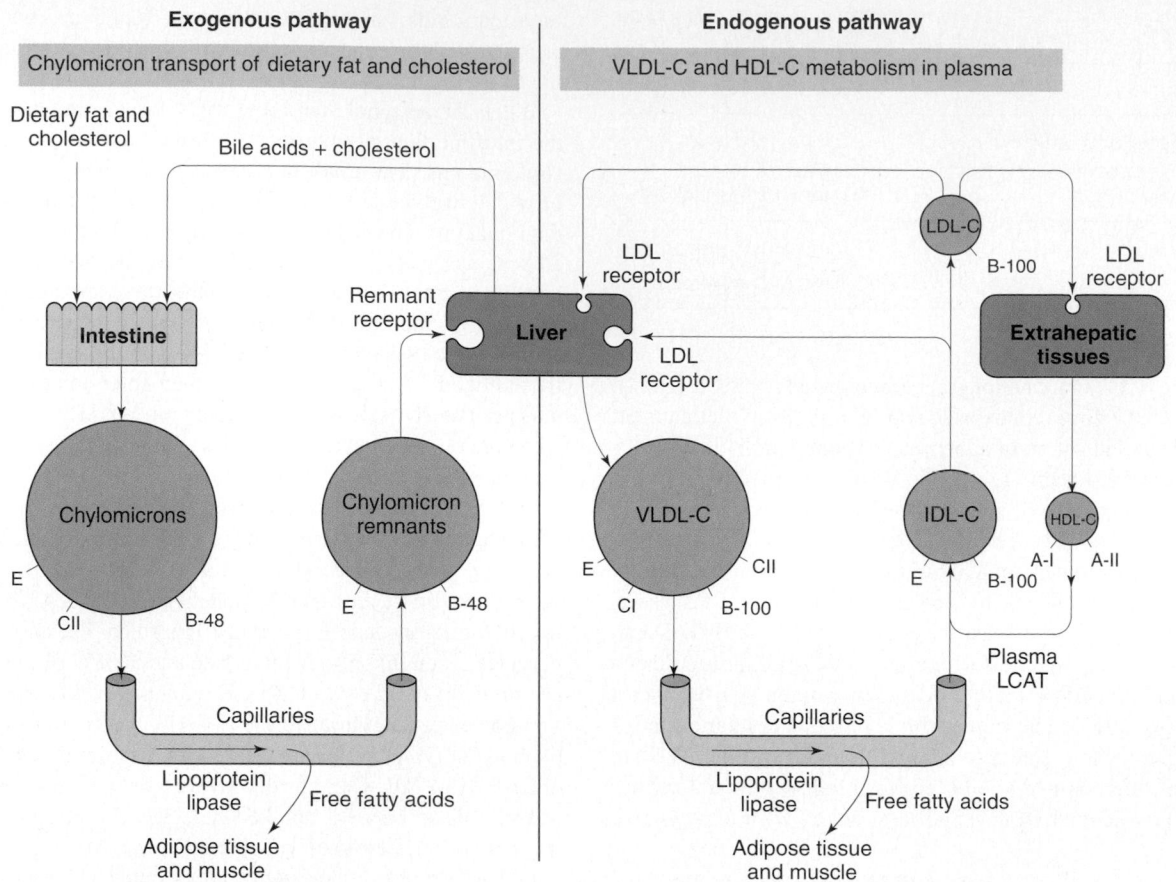

Fig. 24.1 Schematic representation of lipoprotein metabolism in plasma. Dietary cholesterol and fat are transported in the exogenous pathway. Cholesterol produced in the liver is transported in the endogenous pathway.
HDL-C, High-density lipoprotein cholesterol; IDL-C, intermediate-density lipoprotein cholesterol; LCAT, lecithin-cholesterol acyltransferase; LDL-C, low-density lipoprotein cholesterol; VLDL-C, very low-density lipoprotein cholesterol.

Reverse cholesterol transport pathway

The reverse cholesterol transport pathway (Fig. 24.2) controls the formation, conversion, transformation and degradation of HDL-C and is the target site for a number of drugs (Chapman et al., 2010).

The reverse cholesterol transport system involves lipoprotein-mediated transport of cholesterol from peripheral, extrahepatic tissues and arterial tissue (potentially including cholesterol-loaded foam cell macrophages of the atherosclerotic plaque) to the liver for excretion, either in the form of biliary cholesterol or bile acids. The ATP-binding cassette transporters, ABCA1 and ABCG1, and the scavenger receptor B1 are all implicated in cellular cholesterol efflux mechanisms to specific apoA-1/HDL acceptors. The progressive action of lecithin cholesterol acyltransferase (LCAT) on free cholesterol in lipid-poor, apolipoprotein A-I-containing nascent HDLs, including pre-β-HDL, gives rise to the formation of a spectrum of mature, spherical HDLs with a neutral lipid core of cholesteryl ester and triglyceride. Mature HDLs consist of two major subclasses, large cholesteryl ester-rich HDL_2 and small cholesteryl ester-poor, protein-rich HDL_3 particles; the latter represent the intravascular precursors of HDL_2. The reverse cholesterol transport system involves two key pathways: (1) the direct pathway (blue lines in Fig. 24.2), in which the cholesteryl

ester content (and potentially some free cholesterol) of mature HDL particles is taken up primarily by a selective uptake process involving the hepatic scavenger receptor B1; and (2) an indirect pathway (dotted blue lines in Fig. 24.2) in which cholesteryl ester originating in HDL is deviated to potentially atherogenic VLDL, IDL and LDL particles by cholesteryl ester transfer protein. Both the cholesteryl ester and free cholesterol content of these particles are taken up by the liver, predominantly via the LDL receptor, which binds their apoB100 component. This latter pathway may represent up to 70% of cholesteryl ester delivered to the liver per day. The hepatic LDL receptor is also responsible for the direct uptake of HDL particles containing apoE; apoE may be present as a component of both HDL_2 and HDL_3 particles, and may be derived either by transfer from triglyceride-rich lipoproteins or from tissue sources (principally liver and monocyte-macrophages). Whereas HDL uptake by the LDL receptor results primarily in lysosomal-mediated degradation of both lipids and apolipoproteins, interaction of HDL with scavenger receptor B1 regenerates lipid-poor apoA-I and cholesterol-depleted HDL, both of which may re-enter the HDL/apoA-I cycle.

From this description it is evident that HDL-C plays a major role in maintaining cholesterol homeostasis in the body. As a

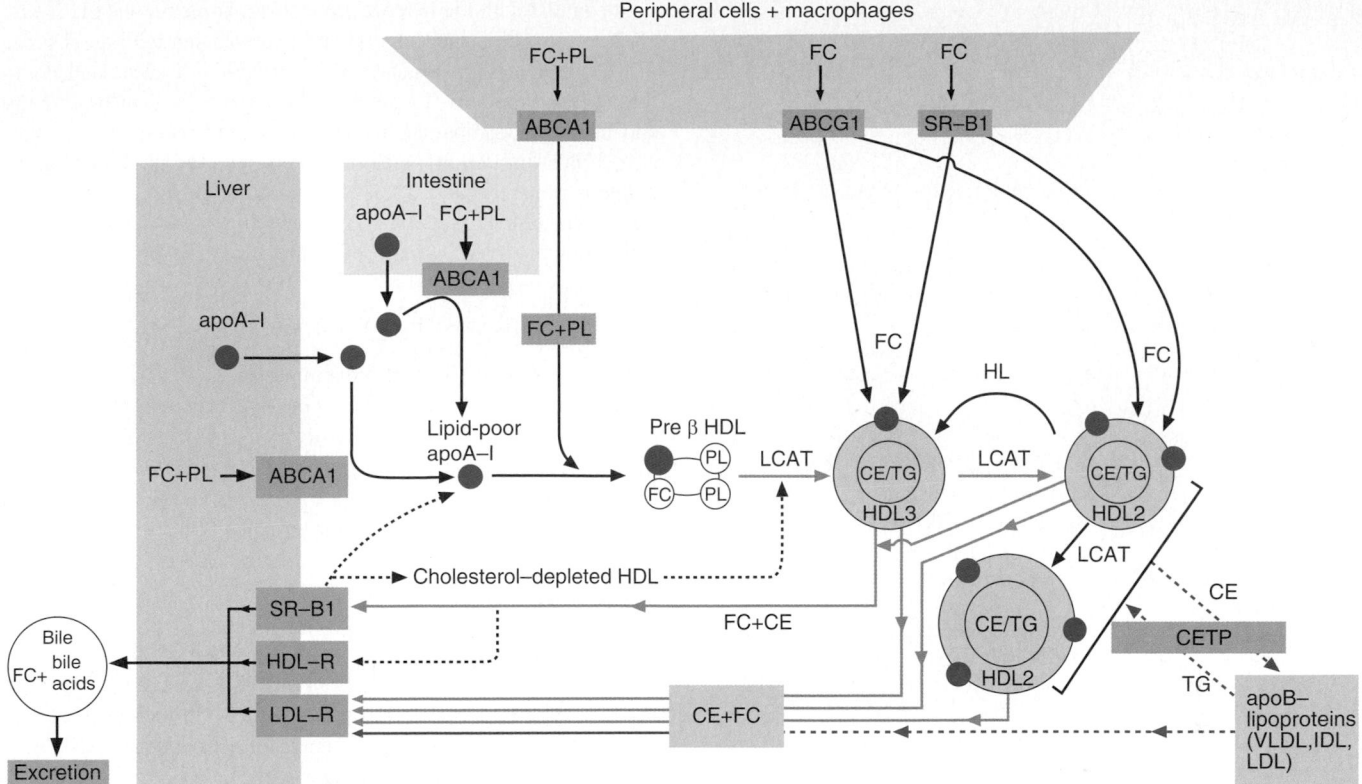

ABDA1 = ATP binding cassette transporter A1; ABDG1 = ATP binding casssette transporter G1; CE = cholesterol ester; CETP = cholesteryl ester transfer protein; FC = free cholesterol; HDL–R = holo HDL receptor; HL = hepatic lipase; LCAT = lecithin cholesterol acyltransferase; LPL = lipoprotein lipase; PL = phospholipids; SR–B1 = hepatic scavenger receptor B1; TG = triglycerides

Fig. 24.2 Pathways of reverse cholesterol transport in human. (Chapman et al., 2010, with kind permission from Oxford University Press, Oxford.)

consequence it is considered desirable to maintain both levels of the protective HDL-C and the integrity of the reverse cholesterol transport pathway. Low levels of HDL-C are found in 17% of men and 5% of women, and may be a risk factor for atherogenesis that is comparable in importance to elevated levels of LDL-C. Drugs that reduce HDL-C levels are considered to have an undesirable effect on lipid metabolism and increase the risk of development of CVD. Examples of drugs that can lower HDL-C include some progestins, anabolic steroids, danazol, β-blockers and first-generation antipsychotics (Herink and Ito, 2015).

Triglycerides

The role of hypertriglyceridaemia as an independent risk factor for atherosclerotic CVD is unclear because triglyceride levels are confounded by an association with low HDL-C, hypertension, diabetes and obesity, and a synergistic effect with LDL-C and/or low HDL-C. An isolated elevation of triglyceride may be the consequence of a primary disorder of lipid metabolism; it may be secondary to the use of medicines such as oestrogens, protease inhibitors, retinoids, corticosteroids, some immunosuppressants and some antipsychotics (Herink and Ito, 2015); or it may be a component of the metabolic syndrome or type 2 diabetes

mellitus. Many individuals have a mixed dyslipidaemia that includes elevated levels of triglycerides and LDL-C, but a reduction of LDL-C normally remains the primary focus of treatment. A recent analysis, in more than 73,000 individuals, of a genetic variant that regulates triglyceride concentrations has demonstrated a causal association between triglycerides and coronary heart disease (CHD) (Triglyceride Coronary Disease Genetics Consortium and Emerging Risk Factors Collaboration, 2010).

Aetiology
Primary dyslipidaemia

Up to 60% of the variability in cholesterol fasting lipids may be genetically determined, although expression is often influenced by interaction with environmental factors. The common familial (genetic) disorders can be classified as:
- the primary hypercholesterolaemias such as familial hypercholesterolaemias (FHs) in which LDL-C is raised;
- the primary mixed (combined) hyperlipidaemias in which both LDL-C and triglycerides are raised; or
- the primary hypertriglyceridaemias such as type III hyperlipoproteinaemia, familial lipoprotein lipase deficiency and familial apoC-II deficiency.

Box 24.1 Simon Broome criteria indicating familial hypercholesterolaemia (NICE, 2008a)

Definite FH is defined as:
1. TC >6.7 mmol/L or LDL cholesterol >4.0 mmol/L in a child <16 years old, or TC >7.5 mmol/L or LDL cholesterol >4.9 mmol/L in an adult (levels are either pretreatment or highest on treatment.)
   PLUS
2. Tendon xanthomas in patient, or in first-degree relative (parent, sibling, child), or in second-degree relative (grandparent, uncle, aunt)
   OR
3. DNA-based evidence of an LDL receptor mutation or familial defective apoB-100

Possible FH is defined as:
Above criteria PLUS one of the following:
- Family history of myocardial infarction: <50 years of age in second-degree relative or <60 years in first-degree relative
- Family history of raised cholesterol: >7.5 mmol/L in adult first- or second-degree relative or >6.7 mmol/L in child or sibling <16 years of age

DNA, Deoxyribonucleic acid; LDL-C, low-density lipoprotein cholesterol; TC, total cholesterol.

Familial hypercholesterolaemia

Heterozygous FH is an inherited metabolic disease, which NICE estimates to affect approximately 1 in 500 of the population (110,000 individuals in England and Wales) (NICE, 2008a). However, more recent data suggest a higher prevalence, with a Danish study of more than 69,000 people detecting a prevalence of 1 in 137 (Benn et al., 2012). FH is caused by a range of mutations, which vary from family to family, in genes for the pathway that clear LDL-C from the blood. The most common mutation affects the LDL receptor gene. Given the key role of LDL receptors in the catabolism of LDL-C, patients with FH may have serum levels of LDL-C two to three times higher than the general population. It is important to identify these individuals from birth and initiate treatment early in life; otherwise, they will be exposed to high concentrations of LDL-C and will suffer the consequences. FH is transmitted as a dominant gene, with siblings and children of a parent with FH having a 50% risk of inheriting it. It is important to suspect FH in people who present with TC greater than 7.5 mmol/L, particularly where there is evidence of premature CV disease within the family (NICE, 2014). The clinical criteria that indicate FH are listed in Box 24.1. Guidance on diagnosis, identifying affected relatives, and management are available, but it is important to seek specialist advice for this group of high-risk patients (NICE, 2008a).

In patients with heterozygous FH, CVD presents about 20 years earlier than in the general population, with some individuals, particularly men, dying of atherosclerotic heart disease often before the age of 40 years. The adult heterozygote typically exhibits the signs of cholesterol deposition such as corneal arcus (crescentic deposition of lipids in the cornea), tendon xanthoma (yellow papules or nodules of lipids deposited in tendons) and xanthelasma (yellow plaques or nodules of lipids deposited on eyelids) in their third decade.

In contrast with the heterozygous form, homozygous FH is rare (1–2 per 1 million individuals) and is associated with an absence of LDL receptors and almost absolute inability to clear LDL-C. In these individuals, involvement of the aorta is evident by puberty and usually accompanied by cutaneous and tendon xanthomas. Myocardial infarction (MI) has been reported in homozygous children younger than 5 years (Dumić et al., 2007; Gautschi et al., 2012; Widhalm et al., 2011). Up to the 1980s, sudden death from acute coronary insufficiency before the age of 20 years was normal.

Familial combined hyperlipidaemia

Familial combined hyperlipidaemia has a prevalence of 1 in 50–200 and is associated with excessive synthesis of VLDL-C (Gaddi et al., 2007). In addition to increases in triglyceride and LDL-C levels, patients also typically have raised levels of apoB and elevated levels of small, dense LDL particles. It is associated with an increased risk of atherosclerosis and occurs in approximately 10% of patients who present with CHD before the age of 60 years (Gaddi et al., 2007).

Familial type III hyperlipoproteinaemia

Familial type III hyperlipoproteinaemia has an incidence of 1 in 5000–10,000 (National Organization of Rare Disorder, 2005). It is characterised by the accumulation of chylomicron and VLDL remnants that fail to get cleared at a normal rate by hepatic receptors because of the presence of less active polymorphic forms of apoE. Triglycerides and TC are both elevated and accompanied by corneal arcus, xanthelasma, tuberoeruptive xanthomas (groups of flat or yellowish raised nodules on the skin over joints, especially the elbows and knees), and palmar striae (yellow raised streaks across the palms of the hand). The disorder predisposes to premature atherosclerosis.

Familial lipoprotein lipase deficiency

Familial lipoprotein lipase deficiency is characterised by marked hypertriglyceridaemia and chylomicronaemia, and usually presents in childhood. It has an incidence of 1 per 1 million individuals (Gotoda et al., 1991) and is due to a deficiency of the extrahepatic enzyme lipoprotein lipase, which results in a failure of lipolysis and the accumulation of chylomicrons in plasma. The affected patient presents with recurrent episodes of abdominal pain, eruptive xanthomas, lipaemia retinalis (retinal deposition of lipid) and enlarged spleen. This disorder is not associated with an increased susceptibility to atherosclerosis; the major complication is acute pancreatitis.

Familial apolipoprotein C-II deficiency

In the heterozygous state, familial apoC-II deficiency is associated with reduced levels of apoC-II, the activator of lipoprotein lipase. Typically, levels of apoC-II are 50–80% of normal. This level of activity can maintain normal lipid levels. In the rare homozygous state, there is an absence of apolipoprotein C-II and despite normal levels of lipoprotein lipase, it cannot be activated. Consequently, homozygotes have triglyceride levels from 15 to greater than 100 mmol/L (normal range <1.7 mmol/L) and may

Box 24.2 Examples of disorders known to adversely affect the lipid profile

- Anorexia nervosa
- Bulimia
- Type 1 diabetes
- Type 2 diabetes
- Hypothyroidism
- Pregnancy
- Inappropriate diet
- Alcohol abuse
- Chronic renal failure
- Nephrotic syndrome
- Renal transplantation
- Cardiac transplantation
- Hepatocellular disease
- Cholestasis
- Myeloma

Table 24.2 Typical effects of selected drugs on lipoprotein levels

Drug	VLDL-C	LDL-C	HDL-C
Alcohol	↑	0	↑
Androgens, testosterone	↑	↑	↓
Angiotensin-converting enzyme inhibitors	0	0	0
β-Blockers	↑	0	↓
Calcium channel blockers	0	0	0
Ciclosporin	↑	↑	↑
Oestrogens, oestradiol	↑	↓	↓
Glucocorticoids	↑	0	↑
Isotretinoin	↑	0	↓
Progestins	↓	↑	↓
Protease inhibitors	↑	0	0
Sertraline	↑	↑	0
Tacrolimus	↑	↑	↑
Thiazide diuretics	↑	↑	↓
Valproate	↑	0	↓

Effect seen may vary depending on dose, duration of exposure, and drugs within same class.
↓, Reduction; ↑, increase; 0, no change; HDL-C, high-density lipoproteins cholesterol; LDL-C, low-density lipoproteins cholesterol; VLDL-C, very low-density lipoproteins cholesterol.

experience development of acute pancreatitis. Premature atherosclerosis is unusual but has been described.

Lipoprotein(a)

There are many other familial disorders of lipid metabolism in addition to those mentioned earlier, but most are rare. However, a raised level of lipoprotein(a), otherwise known as Lp(a), appears to be a genetically inherited determinant of CVD. Lp(a) is an LDL-like particle synthesised by the liver and first described more than 40 years ago. It is found in the serum of virtually everyone in a wide concentration range (0.01–2 g/L), with up to 70% of the variation in concentration being genetically determined. The concentration of Lp(a) is not normally distributed, and the contribution of inheritance to circulating Lp(a) levels is more pronounced than for any other lipoprotein or apoprotein. A parental history of early-onset CVD is associated with raised concentrations of Lp(a), and these appear to play a role in both atherogenesis and thrombosis. An important component of Lp(a) is apo(a), which is structurally and functionally similar to plasminogen and may competitively bind to fibrin and impair fibrinolysis.

Concentrations of Lp(a) greater than 0.3 g/L occur in about 20% of Caucasians (von Depka et al., 2000) and increase the risk of coronary atherosclerosis and stroke. Under a wide range of circumstances, there are continuous, independent, and modest associations of Lp(a) concentration with the risk of CHD and stroke (Erqou et al., 2009).

Secondary dyslipidaemia

Dyslipidaemias that occur secondary to a number of disorders (Box 24.2), dietary indiscretion, or as a side effect of drug therapy (Table 24.2) account for up to 40% of all dyslipidaemias. Fortunately, the lipid abnormalities in secondary dyslipidaemia can often be corrected if the underlying disorder is treated, effective dietary advice implemented, or the offending drug withdrawn.

On occasion, a disorder may be associated with dyslipidaemia, but not the cause of it. For example, hyperuricaemia (gout) and hypertriglyceridaemia co-exist (Emmerson, 1998). In this particular example, neither is the cause of the other, and treatment of

one does not resolve the other. There are, however, two notable exceptions to the rule with this example: nicotinic acid and fenofibrate. Both drugs reduce triglyceride levels, but nicotinic acid increases urate levels, whereas fenofibrate reduces them by an independent uricosuric effect.

Some of the more common disorders that cause secondary dyslipidaemias include the following.

Diabetes mellitus

Premature atherosclerotic disease is the main cause of reduced life expectancy in patients with diabetes. The atherosclerotic disease is often widespread, and complications such as plaque rupture and thrombotic occlusion occur more often and at a younger age. The prevalence of CHD is up to four times higher among patients with diabetes, with more than 80% likely to die of a CV event (Haffner et al., 1998; Malmberg et al., 2000). LDL levels are a stronger predictor of CV risk in patients with diabetes than blood glucose control or blood pressure.

Type 1 diabetes. In patients with type 1 diabetes, HDL-C may appear high, but for reasons which are unclear it does not impart the same degree of protection against CVD as in those without diabetes. It is, therefore, not appropriate to use CV risk prediction charts that utilise the TC:HDL-C ratio in patients with type 1 diabetes. Patients with type 1 diabetes have a twofold to threefold increased risk of development of CVD. NICE (2014) recommends that people with type 1 diabetes should be considered for treatment with a statin if they are more than 40 years old or have had type 1 diabetes for more than 10 years, or have evidence of kidney disease or other CVD risk factors.

Type 2 diabetes. Patients with type 2 diabetes typically have increased triglycerides and decreased HDL-C. Levels of TC may be similar to those found in individuals without diabetes, but the patient with type 2 diabetes often has increased levels of highly atherogenic small, dense LDL particles.

Individuals with type 2 diabetes and older than 40 years, but without CVD, are often considered to have the same CV risk as patients without diabetes who have survived an MI. This assumption is generally appropriate but influenced by patient age, duration of diabetes and gender, and it holds better for women than men. This probably occurs because the impact of type 2 diabetes is more marked in women than men. In previous NICE (2008b) guidance, the criteria for at risk was age older than 40 years but with one other risk factor present, for example, hypertension, obesity, smoker, etc. NICE (2014) now recommends CV risk assessment using QRisk2 for individuals with type 2 diabetes to assess whether a statin should be considered.

Hypothyroidism

Abnormalities of serum lipid and lipoprotein levels are common in patients with untreated hypothyroidism. Hypothyroidism may elevate LDL-C because of reduced LDL receptor activity, and it frequently causes hypertriglyceridaemia and an associated reduction in HDL-C as a result of reduced lipoprotein lipase activity. Remnants of chylomicrons and VLDL-C may also accumulate. However, once adequate thyroid replacement has been initiated the dyslipidaemia should resolve.

Chronic renal failure

Dyslipidaemia is frequently seen in patients with renal failure in the predialysis phase, during haemodialysis, or when undergoing chronic ambulatory peritoneal dialysis. The hypertriglyceridaemia that most commonly occurs is associated with reduced lipoprotein lipase activity and often persists despite starting chronic maintenance renal dialysis. NICE (2014) recommends that people with chronic kidney disease and an estimate of glomerular filtration rate less than 60 mL/min/1.73 m^2 and/or albuminuria should be considered for a statin.

Nephrotic syndrome

In patients with the nephrotic syndrome, dyslipidaemia appears to be caused by an increased production of apoB-100 and associated VLDL-C along with increased hepatic synthesis of LDL-C and a reduction in HDL-C. The necessary use of glucocorticoids in patients with the nephrotic syndrome may exacerbate underlying lipoprotein abnormality.

Obesity

Chronic, excessive intake of calories leads to increased concentrations of triglycerides and reduced HDL-C. Obesity per se can exacerbate any underlying primary dyslipidaemia. Individuals with central obesity appear to be at particular risk of what has become known as the metabolic or DROP (dyslipidaemia, insulin resistance, obesity and high blood pressure) syndrome which represents a cluster of risk factors. Obesity and sedentary lifestyle coupled with inappropriate diet and genetic factors interact to produce the syndrome (Kolovou et al., 2005).

Alcohol

In the heavy drinker, the high-calorie content of beer and wine may be a cause of obesity with its associated adverse effect on the lipid profile. In addition, alcohol increases hepatic triglyceride synthesis, which in turn produces hypertriglyceridaemia.

Light-to-moderate drinkers (1–3 units/day) have a lower incidence of CVD and associated mortality than those who do not drink. This protective effect is probably due to an increase in HDL-C and appears independent of the type of alcohol. Men and women should be advised to limit their alcohol intake to 2–3 units/day with a maximum intake of 14 units/week. Everyone should be advised not to binge drink and aim to have two or more alcohol-free days a week (Department of Health, 2016).

Drugs

A number of drugs can adversely affect serum lipid and lipoprotein concentrations (see Table 24.2).

Antihypertensive agents. Hypertension is a major risk factor for atherosclerosis, and the beneficial effects of lowering blood pressure are well recognised. It is, however, a concern that, although treatment of patients with some antihypertensives has reduced the incidence of cerebrovascular accidents and renal failure, there has been no major impact in reducing the incidence of CHD. It has been suggested that some of these antihypertensive agents have an adverse effect on lipids and lipoproteins that override any beneficial reduction of blood pressure.

Diuretics. Thiazide and loop diuretics increase VLDL-C and LDL-C by mechanisms that are not completely understood. Whether these adverse effects are dose dependent is also unclear. Use of a thiazide for less than 1 year has been reported to increase TC by up to 7% with no change in HDL-C (Ames, 1988). However, short-term changes in lipids do not occur with the low doses in current use and in the longer-term there is little effect on TC levels.

β-Blockers. The effects of β-blockers on lipoprotein metabolism are reflected in an increase in serum triglyceride concentrations, a decrease in HDL-C, but with no discernible effect on LDL-C (Herink and Ito, 2015). β-Blockers with intrinsic sympathomimetic activity appear to have little or no effect on VLDL-C or HDL-C. Pindolol has intrinsic sympathomimetic activity but is rarely used as an antihypertensive agent because it may exacerbate angina. Alternatively, the combined α- and β-blocking effect of labetalol may be of use because it would appear to have a negligible effect on the lipid profile.

Overall, the need to use a diuretic or a β-blocker must be balanced against patient considerations. A patient in heart failure should receive a diuretic if indicated regardless of the lipid profile. Likewise, the patient with heart failure may also benefit from a β-blocker such as bisoprolol or carvedilol. Patients who have had an MI should be considered for the protective effect of a β-blocker, and again the benefits of use will normally override any adverse effects on the lipid profile.

If an antihypertensive agent without adverse effects on lipoproteins is required, angiotensin-converting enzyme (ACE) inhibitors, angiotensin II receptor antagonists, calcium channel blockers, or α-adrenoceptor blockers can be used.

Oral contraceptives. Oral contraceptives that contain an oestrogen and a progestogen provide the most effective contraceptive preparations for general use and have been well studied with respect to their harmful effects.

Oestrogens and progestogens both possess mineralocorticoid and glucocorticoid properties that predispose to hypertension and diabetes mellitus, respectively. However, the effects of the two hormones on lipoproteins are different. Oestrogens cause a slight increase in hepatic production of VLDL-C and HDL-C, and reduce serum LDL-C levels. In contrast, progestogens increase LDL-C and reduce serum HDL-C and VLDL-C (Herink and Ito, 2015).

The specific effect of the oestrogen or progestogen varies with the actual dose and chemical entity used. Ethinyloestradiol at a dose of 30–35 micrograms or fewer would appear to create few problems with lipid metabolism (Herink and Ito, 2015), while norethisterone is one of the more favourable progestogens even though it may cause a pronounced decrease in HDL-C.

Corticosteroids. The effect of glucocorticoid administration on lipid levels has been studied in patients treated with steroids for asthma, rheumatoid arthritis and connective tissue disorders. Administration of a glucocorticoid such as prednisolone has been shown to increase TC and triglycerides by elevating LDL-C and, less consistently, VLDL-C (Herink and Ito, 2015). The changes are generally more pronounced in women. Alternate-day therapy with glucocorticoids has been suggested to reduce the adverse effect on lipoprotein levels in some patients.

Ciclosporin. Ciclosporin is primarily used to prevent tissue rejection in recipients of renal, hepatic and cardiac transplants. Its use has been associated with increased LDL-C levels, hypertension and glucose intolerance (Herink and Ito, 2015). These adverse effects are often exacerbated by the concurrent administration of glucocorticoids. The combined use of ciclosporin and glucocorticoid contributes to the adverse lipid profile seen in transplant patients. Unfortunately, the administration of a statin to patients treated with ciclosporin increases the incidence of myositis, rhabdomyolysis (dissolution of muscle associated with excretion of myoglobin in the urine) and renal failure. Use of a statin is, therefore, contraindicated in patients who are receiving ciclosporin. Similar interactions between statins and other drugs used to prevent tissue rejection, including tacrolimus and sirolimus, have been reported, and hence concomitant use is not recommended (Wiggins et al., 2016).

Hepatic microsomal enzyme inducers. Drugs such as carbamazepine, phenytoin, phenobarbital, rifampicin and griseofulvin increase hepatic microsomal enzyme activity and can also increase serum HDL-C. The administration of these drugs may also give rise to a slight increase in LDL-C and VLDL-C. The overall effect is one of a favourable increase in the TC:HDL-C ratio.

Cardiovascular risk assessment

Primary prevention

It is recommended that CV risk assessment is carried out every 5 years for all adults from the age of 40 years, with no history of CVD or diabetes, and not receiving treatment for raised blood pressure or dyslipidaemia. A number of CVD risk calculators are available, including QRisk (UK and recommended by NICE; https://www.qrisk.org/), SCORE (Europe; https://www.escardio.org/Education/Practice-Tools/CVD-prevention-toolbox/SCORE-Risk-Charts#), Joint British Socities-3 (JBS-3; http://www.jbs3risk.com) and ASSIGN (Scotland; http://assign-score.com).

QRisk2

QRisk2 is based on a database, established in 2003, of anonymised UK primary care patients. It contains more than 20 million sets of encrypted patient records. A cohort of 1.28 million patients without evidence of diabetes mellitus or CVD was identified and followed up for more than 5 years looking for the first development of CVD as an endpoint (Hippisley-Cox et al., 2007).

The following parameters, with any missing values calculated by a complex averaging procedure, are used to calculate a patient's CV risk:

- patient age (35–84 years)
- patient sex
- smoking status
- family history of heart disease aged less than 60 years
- existing treatment with blood pressure agent
- postcode (postcode is linked to Townsend score measure of deprivation)
- body mass index (BMI) (height and weight)
- systolic blood pressure (use current, not pretreatment, value)
- TC and HDL-C
- self-assigned ethnicity (not nationality)
- rheumatoid arthritis
- chronic kidney disease
- atrial fibrillation

The QRisk2 risk assessment tool should be used to assess CVD risk of the primary prevention of CVD in people up to and including age 84 years. It calculates the risk of an individual having a heart attack or stroke in the next 10 years. Patients with a CV risk ≥10% over 10 years are considered to be at sufficient risk to warrant lipid-lowering therapy according to current NICE (2014) guidelines, although recommendations as to when to intervene with medication vary internationally. It should be noted that although NICE (2014) recommends using the tool for people with type 2 diabetes, it does not recommend using it for patients with type 1 diabetes.

Other risk assessment tools

Framingham. Up to 2008, risk charts and calculators based on Framingham data were the most widely used and researched approach for calculating CV risk and are the data on which the risk charts discussed earlier are based.

ASSIGN. ASSIGN is a risk calculator based on data from a Scottish population and includes many of the variables utilised in the Framingham-based model. It also takes into account social status, determined by postcode of residence in Scotland, and family history of CVD (Woodward et al., 2007).

SCORE. The European SCORE risk charts were developed from a large dataset tested thoroughly on European data. It operates with hard, reproducible endpoints (CVD death), and risk of CHD and stroke death can be derived separately. The SCORE risk function can be calibrated to each country's national mortality statistics. The SCORE database was developed through combining results from 12 European cohort studies with 250,000 patients' data equating to 3 million person-years of observation and 7000 fatal CV events recorded (European Society of Cardiology, 2017).

Secondary prevention

Patients with CVD and levels of TC greater than 4 mmol/L and LDL-C greater than 2 mmol/L are those most likely to benefit from treatment with lipid-lowering agents. Typical of individuals who fall into this category are patients with a history of angina, MI, acute coronary syndrome (ACS), coronary artery bypass grafting, coronary angioplasty, or cardiac transplantation, as well as patients with evidence of atherosclerotic disease in other vascular beds, such as patients post-stroke or transient ischaemic attack, and those with peripheral arterial disease.

As in the situation with primary prevention outlined earlier, if an individual is to receive a lipid-lowering agent as part of a secondary prevention strategy, the possibility of a familial dyslipidaemia and the need to assess other family members must not be overlooked (NICE, 2008b, 2014).

Treatment

Lipid profile

When a decision has been made to determine an individual's lipid profile, a random serum TC and HDL-C, from which non-HDL-C levels can be calculated, will often suffice. If a subsequent decision is made to commence treatment and monitor outcome, a more detailed profile may be obtained, although it may not be essential if non-HDL-C is used for monitoring. Treatment should not be initiated on the basis of a single random sample.

Serum concentrations of triglycerides increase after the ingestion of a meal and, therefore, if a full lipid profile is to be obtained, patients must fast for 12–15 hours before they can be measured. Patients must also be seated for at least 5 minutes before drawing a blood sample. TC level and HDL are little affected by food intake, and this is, therefore, not a consideration if only these are to be measured. However, it is important that whatever is being measured reflects a steady-state value. For example, during periods of weight loss, lipid concentrations decline as they do following

---

Box 24.3   Lifestyle targets

- Do not smoke.
- Maintain ideal body weight (BMI 20–25 kg/m^2).
- Avoid central obesity.
- Reduce total dietary intake of fat to ≤30% of total energy intake.
- Reduce intake of saturated fats to ≤7% of total fat intake.
- Reduce intake of dietary cholesterol to <300 mg/day.
- Replace saturated fats by an increased intake of monounsaturated fats.
- Increase intake of fresh fruit and vegetables to at least five portions per day.
- Regularly eat fish and other sources of omega-3 fatty acids (at least two portions of fish each week).
- Choose whole-grain varieties of starchy food.
- Reduce intake of sugar and food products that contain refined sugars including fructose.
- Eat at least four to five portions of unsalted nuts, seeds and legumes per week.
- Limit alcohol intake to <14 units/week (men and women).
- Restrict intake of salt to <100 mmol/day (<6 g of sodium chloride or <2.4 g sodium/day).
- Undertake regular aerobic exercise, aiming for 150 min of moderate-intensity aerobic activity or 75 min of vigorous-intensity aerobic activity per week.
- Avoid excess intake of coffee or other caffeine-rich products.

---

an MI. In the case of the latter, samples drawn within 24 hours of infarct onset will reflect the preinfarction state. In general, measurement should be deferred for 2 weeks after a minor illness and for 3 months after an MI, serious illness or pregnancy.

Once the TC and HDL-C are known, non-HDL-C can be calculated as follows:

$$\text{Non-HDL-C} = \text{TC} - \text{HDL-C}$$

If the TC, HDL-C and triglyceride values are known, then the value for LDL-C can be calculated using the Friedewald equation:

$$\text{LDL-C} = (\text{total cholesterol} - \text{HDL-C}) - (0.45 \times \text{triglyceride}) \text{ mmol/L}$$

The Friedewald equation should not be used in non-fasting individuals, it is less reliable in individuals with diabetes, and it is not valid if the serum triglyceride concentration is greater than 4.5 mmol/L.

Lifestyle

When a decision is made to start treatment with a lipid-lowering agent, other risk factors must also be tackled as appropriate, such as smoking, obesity, high alcohol intake and lack of exercise (Box 24.3). Underlying disorders such as diabetes mellitus and hypertension should be treated as appropriate. Issues around body weight, diet and exercise will be briefly covered in the following sections.

Body weight and waist measurement

The overweight patient is at increased risk of atherosclerotic disease and typically has elevated levels of serum triglycerides, raised LDL-C and a low HDL-C. This adverse lipid profile is often compounded by the presence of hypertension and raised blood glucose, that is, the metabolic syndrome. A reduction in body weight will generally improve the lipid profile and reduce overall CV risk.

It is useful to classify the extent to which an individual is overweight by calculating their BMI. The BMI (kg/m²) in all but the most muscular individual gives a clinical measure of adiposity.

- BMI 18.5: underweight
- BMI 18.6–24.9: ideal
- BMI 25–29.9: overweight
- BMI 30–40: obese
- BMI >40: morbidly obese

The distribution of body fat is also recognised as a factor that influences CVD risk. Measurement of waist circumference is perhaps the most accurate indicator of central obesity and correlates well with CVD risk. Target waist circumference should be less than 102 cm in white Caucasian men, less than 88 cm in white Caucasian women, less than 90 cm in Asian men and less than 80 cm in Asian women (World Health Organization, 2011).

Diet

Diet modification should always be encouraged in a patient with dyslipidaemia, but it is rarely successful alone in bringing about a significant improvement in the lipid profile. Reduction or modification of dietary fat intake has shown variable results on CV morbidity and mortality. Systematic review of dietary interventions to lower cholesterol in community settings indicates that mean reductions in TC of up to 6% can be achieved, although there is a wide variation in response to diet between individuals (Tang et al., 1998). The overall picture is that patients with dyslipidaemia should receive dietary advice, and a small number of those who adhere to the advice will experience a decline in TC.

There is a common misconception that a healthy diet is one that is low in cholesterol. However, generally it is the saturated fat content that is important, although many components of a healthy diet are not related to fat content. For example, the low incidence of CVD in those who consume a Mediterranean-type diet suggests an increased intake of fruit and vegetables is also important. The typical Mediterranean diet has an abundance of plant food (fruit, vegetables, breads, cereals, potatoes, beans, nuts and seeds), minimally processed, seasonally fresh and locally grown; fresh fruit as the typical daily dessert, with sweets containing concentrated sugars or honey consumed a few times per week; olive oil as the principal source of fat; dairy products (principally cheese and yoghurt) consumed daily in low-to-moderate amounts; 0–4 eggs consumed weekly; and red meat consumed in low-to-moderate amounts. This diet is low in saturated fat (<8% of energy) and varies in total fat content from less than 25% to greater than 35% of energy.

Fish. Regular consumption of the long-chain omega-3 fatty acids, principally eicosapentaenoic acid and docosahexaenoic acid, typically found in fatty fish and fish oils, has been linked to the low levels of CHD seen in Inuits (Eskimos). Hu et al. (2002) studied a group of 84,688 women enrolled in the Nurses' Health Study, all of whom were registered nurses aged 30–55 years and were free from CVD and cancer at baseline in 1980. During the 16-year follow-up, a significant inverse association between fish intake and incidence of CHD was observed. The Lyon Heart Study (de Lorgeril et al., 1999) was an intervention trial involving 605 survivors of first MI, of whom 303 were randomised to be control patients and 302 were advised to adopt a Mediterranean-style diet, including use of margarine with higher levels of linoleic acid and α-linoleic acid (ALA) than olive oil. In the experimental group the relative risk of MI-caused death was 0.44 and that of cardiac death and nonfatal MI was 0.28, whereas other clinical events such as unstable angina, heart failure and stroke were also less frequently observed.

Consumption of omega-3 fatty acids decreases triglyceride levels but has little effect on LDL-C or HDL-C. The proposed mechanisms are thought to involve the omega-3 fatty acids and their antiarrhythmic properties, ability to reduce blood pressure and heart rate, lower triglyceride levels, stimulate endothelial-derived nitric oxide, increase insulin sensitivity, decrease platelet aggregation and decrease proinflammatory eicosanoids. There would appear to be benefits in consuming at least two portions (portion = 140 g) of fish per week, including a portion of oily fish, particularly in those who have had an MI. Pregnant women are advised to limit their intake of oily fish to two portions per week because of the potential accumulation of low-level pollutants in the fish.

Trans fats. Trans fats are unsaturated fatty acids with at least one double bond in the trans configuration. They are formed when vegetable oils are hydrogenated to convert them into semi-solid fats that can be incorporated into margarines or used in commercial manufacturing processes. Trans fats are typically found in deep-fried fast foods, bakery products, packaged snack foods, margarines and crackers. When the calorific equivalent of saturated fats, cis unsaturated fats and trans fats are consumed, trans fats raise LDL-C, reduce HDL-C and increase the ratio of TC:HDL-C. In addition to these harmful effects, trans fats also increase the blood levels of triglycerides, increase levels of Lp(a) and reduce the particle size of LDL-C, all of which further increase the risk of CHD. It is, therefore, necessary to reduce the dietary intake of trans fatty acids to less than 0.5% of total energy intake, and this has led to calls for a complete ban on trans fats in foods.

Stanol esters and plant sterols. The availability of margarines and other foods enriched with plant sterols or stanol esters appears to increase the likelihood that LDL-C can be reduced by dietary change. Both stanol esters and plant sterols at a maximum effective dose of 2 g/day inhibit cholesterol absorption from the gastro-intestinal tract and reduce LDL-C by an average of 10%. They compete with cholesterol for incorporation into mixed micelles, thereby impairing its absorption from the intestine. However, as with other dietary changes, the reduction seen varies between individuals and is probably dependent on the initial cholesterol level and the total amount of stenol esters and/or plant sterols ingested. There is currently no evidence that ingestion lowers the risk of CV events, and as a result they are not recommended by NICE (2014).

Antioxidants. Antioxidants occur naturally in fruit and vegetables and are important components of a healthy diet. Their consumption is thought to be beneficial in reducing the formation of atherogenic, oxidised LDL-C. Primary and secondary prevention trials with antioxidant vitamin supplements, however, have not been encouraging. Neither vitamin E nor β-carotene supplements would appear to reduce the risk of CHD but likewise have not been shown to be harmful.

Salt. Dietary salt (sodium) has an adverse effect on blood pressure and, therefore, a potential impact on CHD and stroke. It is recommended that the average adult intake of sodium should be reduced from approximately 150 mmol (9 g) to 100 mmol (6 g) of salt or even lower. This intake can be reduced by consuming fewer processed foods, avoiding many ready meals and not adding salt to food during cooking and at the table.

Exercise

Moderate amounts of aerobic exercise (brisk walking, jogging, swimming, cycling) on a regular basis have a desirable effect on the lipid profile of an individual. These beneficial effects have been demonstrated within 2 months in middle-aged men exercising for 30 minutes, three times a week. Current advice from NICE (2014) is to advise people at high risk of or with CVD to do the following every week:

- at least 150 minutes of moderate-intensity aerobic activity, or
- 75 minutes of vigorous-intensity aerobic activity or a mix of moderate and vigorous aerobic activity.

People are also advised to do muscle strengthening activities on 2 or more days a week that work all major muscle groups (legs, hips, back, abdomen, chest, shoulders and arms). If people cannot perform moderate-intensity physical activity because of comorbidity, medical conditions or personal circumstances, then they need to exercise at their maximum safe capacity.

Exercise per se probably has little effect on TC levels in the absence of a reduction in body weight, body fat or dietary fat. Perhaps the most important effect of regular exercise is to raise levels of HDL-C in a dose-dependent manner according to energy expenditure.

Overall, comprehensive dietary and lifestyle changes (stopping smoking, stress management training and moderate exercise) can bring about regression of coronary atherosclerosis. Unfortunately, many find it difficult to attain or sustain the necessary changes. In others, dietary and lifestyle changes alone will never be adequate or will not bring about the necessary improvement in lipid profile quickly enough. As a consequence, the use of lipid-lowering drugs is widespread.

Drugs

If an individual is found to be at risk of CVD (primary prevention), including people with type 2 diabetes, then all other modifiable risk factors should be addressed, including dietary and lifestyle changes, before statin therapy is offered. CV risk assessment should then be repeated using QRisk2, and if the CV risk remains high, drug therapy in the form of a statin should be offered. In an individual who requires treatment for secondary prevention, a delay of several months in starting treatment is not appropriate and treatment will normally be commenced immediately with a lipid-lowering agent.

Primary prevention

In primary prevention, dyslipidaemia should not be treated in isolation, and management must be embarked upon with clear goals. In addition to lifestyle advice, this will not only address management of dyslipidaemia, but will also seek to optimise use of antihypertensive agents and other CV protective therapies, and achieve tight blood glucose control as appropriate. In patients without evidence of arterial disease, statin treatment must be considered if the risk of CVD is ≥10% over 10 years (NICE, 2014). Although some dispute the benefit of statins in primary prevention (Kausik et al., 2010), treatment will normally include:

- a lipid-lowering agent such as atorvastatin 20 mg/day (or alternative) with an aim of a 40% decline in non-HDL-C from baseline to indicate adherence to treatment (NICE, 2014);
- personalised information on modifiable risk factors including physical activity, diet, alcohol intake, weight and tight control of diabetes;
- advice to stop smoking; and
- advice (and treatment if appropriate) to achieve blood pressure below 140 mmHg systolic and 90 mmHg diastolic.

Some consider an isolated raised TC:HDL ratio greater than 6.5 warrants treatment regardless of the risk assessment outcome, but this approach has received little support in national treatment guidelines.

For primary prevention in patients with type 1 diabetes who are more than 40 years old or have had type 1 diabetes for more than 10 years or have established nephropathy or other CVD risk factors, atorvastatin 20 mg daily should be offered and lifestyle modifications made (NICE, 2014). Patients with type 2 diabetes who have a risk of CVD of ≥10% over 10 years should be offered atorvastatin 20 mg daily for primary prevention (NICE, 2014).

Secondary prevention

In individuals diagnosed with CVD or other occlusive arterial disease, treatment should include:

- a lipid-lowering agent such as atorvastatin 80 mg/day (or alternative) with an aim of a 40% decline in non-HDL-C from baseline to indicate adherence to treatment (NICE, 2014);
- advice to stop smoking;
- personalised information on modifiable risk factors including physical activity, diet, alcohol intake, weight and diabetes;
- advice and treatment to achieve blood pressure at least below 140 mmHg systolic and 90 mmHg diastolic;
- tight control of blood pressure and glucose in those with diabetes;
- low-dose aspirin (75 mg daily) or clopidogrel (75 mg daily);
- ACE inhibitors in selected groups, specifically those with left ventricular dysfunction, diabetes, chronic kidney disease or nephropathy;
- β-blocker for those who have had an MI and in those with heart failure; and
- anticoagulant therapy for those with atrial fibrillation and additional stroke risk factors.

In patients with chronic kidney disease, atorvastatin 20 mg daily should be offered for primary or secondary prevention of CVD (NICE, 2014).

Lipid-lowering therapy

Five well-established classes of lipid-lowering agents are available:

- statins
- cholesterol absorption inhibitors
- fibrates
- bile acid binding agents
- nicotinic acid and derivatives

Proprotein convertase subtilisin/kexin type 9 (PCSK9) inhibitors have recently been introduced for use in selected indications.

Agents such as soluble fibre and fish oils have also been used to reduce lipid levels. The choice of lipid-lowering agent depends on the underlying dyslipidaemia, the response required and patient acceptability. The various groups of drugs available have different mechanisms of action and variable efficacy depending on the lipid profile of an individual. Statins are currently the drugs of choice in the majority of patients with dyslipidaemia due to the overwhelming evidence that treatment with these agents reduces CV events.

Statins

The discovery of a class of drugs, the statins, which selectively inhibit 3-hydroxy-3-methylglutaryl-coenzyme A reductase (HMG-CoA reductase) was a significant advance in the treatment of dyslipidaemia. Their primary site of action is the inhibition of HMG-CoA reductase in the liver and the subsequent inhibition of the formation of mevalonic acid, the rate-limiting step in the biosynthesis of cholesterol. This results in a reduction in intracellular levels of cholesterol, an increase in expression of hepatic LDL receptor, and enhanced receptor-mediated catabolism and clearance of LDL-C from serum. Production of VLDL-C, the precursor of LDL-C, is also reduced. The overall effect is a reduction in TC, LDL-C, VLDL-C and triglycerides with an increase in HDL-C. The reduction in LDL-C occurs in a dose-dependent manner, with a lesser and dose-independent effect on VLDL-C and triglycerides.

Simvastatin was the first member of the group to be marketed in the UK, and it was followed by pravastatin, fluvastatin, atorvastatin, cerivastatin and rosuvastatin. Cerivastatin was withdrawn from the market in 2001 because of an observed increased risk of fatal rhabdomyolysis. Lovastatin is available in the USA and pitavastatin is available in Japan since 2003. The relative potencies of the statins available in the UK are shown in Table 24.3.

The efficacy of statins has been demonstrated in a number of landmark randomised placebo-controlled trials and evaluated by meta-analysis (Cholesterol Treatment Trialists, 2012). A greater absolute benefit was seen in those trials that involved established CVD, that is, secondary prevention studies, compared with those that involved individuals without established CVD, that is, primary prevention studies. Statins are currently the lipid-lowering agents of choice in both primary and secondary prevention of CVD. Over time there has been a shift towards more intensive lipid lowering, with the Cholesterol Treatment Trialist Collaboration (2010) undertaking a meta-analysis of 26 trials including more than 170,000 participants, concluding further

Table 24.3 Relative potency of statins

Dosage (mg/day)	% Reduction in low-density lipoprotein cholesterol				
	5	10	20	40	80
Fluvastatin	–	–	21	27	33
Pravastatin	–	20	24	29	–
Simvastatin	–	27	32	37	42[a]
Atorvastatin	–	37	43	49	55
Rosuvastatin	38	43	48	53	–

[a]The Medicines and Healthcare products Regulatory Agency advises that because there is an increased risk of myopathy associated with high-dosage 80 mg/day simvastatin, this dosage should be considered only in patients with severe hypercholesterolaemia and high risk of cardiovascular complications who have not achieved their treatment goals on lower doses, when the benefits are expected to outweigh the potential risks.
Adapted from NICE (2014).

reductions in LDL-C safely produce definite further reductions in the incidence of heart attack, of revascularisation and of ischaemic stroke, with each 1.0 mmol/L reduction reducing the annual rate of these major vascular events by just more than a fifth. There was no evidence of any threshold within the cholesterol range studied suggesting that reduction of LDL-C by 2–3 mmol/L would reduce risk by about 40–50%.

There is much debate around the statin of choice. Atorvastatin is currently the preferred agent because of its low cost, safety profile and evidence of efficacy. Of paramount importance is the need to identify patients who need treatment and ensure they receive an appropriate, effective dose of a statin and adhere to treatment. Despite overwhelming evidence of benefit, effectiveness is frequently compromised by poor adherence and persistence. For example, Helin-Salmivaara et al. (2008) studied persistence with therapy in more than 18,000 new statin users and reported 1-year persistence rate of 73% and 10-year persistence rate of 44%. Thirteen percent of patients stopped taking the statin after the first prescription. Patient factors that influence this include perception of risk, side effects of medication, expected treatment duration and socio-demographic factors.

Rosuvastatin is the most potent of the statins, with evidence of impact on morbidity and mortality (see Table 24.3) (Ridker et al., 2008). It is normally reserved for those individuals who have had an inadequate response to their first-line statin or failure to tolerate other statins. There remains concern about its safety profile, rhabdomyolysis in particular, when used at the higher dosage of 40 mg/day. It is recommended that this dosage should be used only under specialist supervision in individuals with severe FH and at high CV risk. In patients of Asian origin (Japanese, Chinese, Filipino, Vietnamese, Korean and Indian), the maximum dose should not exceed 20 mg/day because of their increased predisposition to myopathy and rhabdomyolysis.

All the statins require the presence of LDL receptors for their optimum clinical effect, and consequently they are less effective in patients with heterozygous FH because of the reduced number of LDL receptors. However, even in the homozygous patient where there are no LDL receptors, they can bring about some reduction of serum cholesterol, although the mechanism is unclear.

Adverse effects

Many side effects appear mild and transient. The commonest include gastro-intestinal symptoms, altered liver function tests and muscle aches. Less common are elevation of liver transaminase levels in excess of three times the upper limit of normal, hepatitis, rash, headache, insomnia, nightmares, vivid dreams and difficulty concentrating.

Myopathy (unexplained muscle soreness or weakness) leading to myoglobulinuria secondary to rhabdomyolysis is also a rare but serious potential adverse effect of all the statins that can occur at any dose. The risk of myopathy is increased:

- when there are underlying muscle disorders, a family history of muscle disorders, renal impairment, untreated hypothyroidism, alcohol abuse, or the recipient is aged over 65 years or female;
- where statins are co-prescribed with other lipid-lowering drugs, for example, fibrates or nicotinic acid;
- when there is a history of myopathy with another lipid-lowering drug or statin; or
- where there is co-prescription of simvastatin or atorvastatin with drugs that inhibit cytochrome P450 3A4 (CYP3A4).

The statins are a heterogeneous group metabolised by different cytochrome P450 (CYP450) isoenzymes. Simvastatin, atorvastatin and lovastatin are metabolised by CYP3A4, fluvastatin is metabolised by CYP2C9, and pravastatin and rosuvastatin are eliminated by other metabolic routes and less subject to interactions with CYP450 isoenzymes than other members of the family. Nevertheless, caution is still required because a 5- to 23-fold increase in pravastatin bioavailability has been reported with ciclosporin. Simvastatin and atorvastatin do not alter the activity of CYP3A4 themselves, but their serum levels are increased by known inhibitors of CYP3A4 (Table 24.4). Advice has been published on drug interactions with simvastatin (Medicines and Healthcare products Regulatory Agency, 2012) (Table 24.5).

Pleiotropic properties

Although the effect of statins on the lipid profile contributes to their beneficial outcome in reducing morbidity and mortality from CVD, other mechanisms, known as pleiotropic effects, may also play a part. These effects include plaque stabilisation, inhibition of thrombus formation, reduced serum viscosity, and anti-inflammatory and antioxidant activity. These pleiotropic properties, that is, cholesterol-independent effects, are far reaching and reveal a clinical impact beyond a process of reducing TC. For example, lowering TC produces only modest reductions of a fixed, atherosclerotic, luminal stenosis but results in a qualitative change of the plaque and helps stabilise it. This protects the plaque from rupturing and triggering further coronary events.

Inflammation is thought to play a prominent part in the development of atherosclerosis, and increased levels of C-reactive

Table 24.4 Examples of drug interactions involving statins and the cytochrome P450 enzyme pathway

CYP 450 isoenzyme	Inducers	Inhibitors
CYP3A4		
Atorvastatin	Phenytoin	Ketoconazole
Lovastatin	Barbiturate	Itraconazole
Simvastatin	Rifampicin	Fluconazole
	Dexamethasone	Erythromycin
	Cyclophosphamide	Clarithromycin
	Carbamazepine	Tricyclic antidepressants
	Omeprazole	Nefazodone
		Venlafaxine
		Fluoxetine
		Sertraline
		Ciclosporin
		Tacrolimus
		Diltiazem
		Verapamil
		Protease inhibitors
		Midazolam
		Corticosteroids
		Grapefruit juice
		Tamoxifen
		Amiodarone
CYP2C9		
Fluvastatin	Rifampicin	Ketoconazole
	Phenobarbitone	Fluconazole
	Phenytoin	Sulfaphenazole

protein have been used to identify individuals at risk of plaque rupture and consequent MI and stroke. Statins can reduce levels of C-reactive protein.

An important aspect of vascular endothelium dysfunction is the impaired synthesis, release and activity of endothelial-derived nitric oxide, an important and early marker of atherosclerosis. After the administration of a statin, one of the earliest effects observed (within 3 days) is an increased endothelial nitric oxide release, thereby mediating an improvement in vasodilation of the endothelium.

For some, although it has been thought that part of the beneficial effect of statins on CVD could be attributed to an effect on blood coagulation, it is now evident that statins, amongst their many actions, decrease platelet activation and activity, reduce prothrombin activation, factor Va generation, fibrinogen cleavage and factor XIII activation, and increase factor Va inactivation.

Over-the-counter sale

Low-dose (10 mg) simvastatin can be purchased from community pharmacies in the UK to treat individuals at moderate CV risk. Men aged 55–70 years with or without risk factors and men aged 45–54 years or women aged 55–70 years with at least one risk factor (smoker, obese, family history of premature CHD or of South Asian origin) are eligible for treatment. Simvastatin cannot be sold to individuals who have CVD, diabetes or familial dyslipidaemia, or are taking lipid-lowering agents or medication that may interact with simvastatin. The rationale for over-the-counter

Table 24.5 Advice on drug interactions with simvastatin

Avoid with simvastatin as contraindicated	HIV protease inhibitors Azole antifungals Erythromycin, clarithromycin, telithromycin Nefazodone Ciclosporin Danazol Gemfibrozil
Do not exceed a dose of simvastatin 10 mg daily	Other fibrates (except fenofibrate)
Do not exceed a dose of simvastatin 20 mg daily	Amiodarone Amlodipine Verapamil Diltiazem
Avoid when taking simvastatin	Grapefruit juice

Adapted from Medicines and Healthcare products Regulatory Agency (2012).

sale is to reduce the risk of a first major coronary event in adults at moderate risk, but sales have been low. Moreover, the evidence base to support the use of 10 mg simvastatin and achieve long-term CV benefit is limited.

Patient counselling

In patients who are receiving a statin, a once-daily regimen involving an evening dose is often preferred. Several of the statins (fluvastatin, pravastatin, simvastatin) are claimed to be more effective when given as a single dose in the evening compared with a similar dose administered in the morning. This has been attributed to the fact that cholesterol biosynthesis reaches peak activity at night. However, atorvastatin and rosuvastatin may be taken in the morning or evening with similar efficacy. A reduction in TC and LDL-C is usually seen with all statins within 2 weeks, with a maximum response occurring by week 4 and maintained thereafter during continued therapy.

Cholesterol absorption inhibitors

Ezetimibe is a 2-azetidinone derivative that interacts with a putative cholesterol transporter in the intestinal brush-border membrane and thereby blocks cholesterol re-absorption from the gastro-intestinal tract. It can reduce LDL-C by 15–20% when added to diet. Ezetimibe also brings about a small increase in HDL-C and a reduction in triglycerides. When added to a statin, ezetimibe lowers LDL-C by approximately 20% over and above that achieved by statin therapy alone (Kastelein et al., 2008).

Ezetimibe monotherapy is recommended by NICE (2016a) for the treatment of primary hypercholesterolaemia in patients where initial statin therapy is contraindicated or not tolerated. Ezetimibe plus statin therapy is recommended for the treatment of primary hypercholesterolaemia where the TC or LDL-C is not controlled, either after dose optimisation of statin therapy or where the dose

is limited by intolerance and a change to an alternative statin is being considered (NICE, 2016a).

Ezetimibe use has been limited because of a lack of CV outcomes data. The IMPROVE-IT study (Cannon et al., 2015) demonstrated that the addition of ezetimibe to simvastatin 40 mg in 18,144 patients following an ACS reduced the primary endpoint, a composite of CV death, MI, unstable angina requiring rehospitalisation, coronary revascularisation or stroke, by 6.4% (absolute risk reduction 2% over 7 years) when compared with patients who received simvastatin alone. As a result, ezetimibe is now licensed to reduce the risk of CV events in patients with CHD and a history of ACS when added to ongoing statin therapy or initiated concomitantly with a statin.

Ezetimibe should be prescribed at a dosage of 10 mg daily and can be taken at any time of the day, with or without food. Ezetimibe is contraindicated in patients who have a hypersensitivity to the active substance or excipients, are pregnant or lactating and, if co-administered with a statin, in patients with active liver disease or unexplained persistent elevations in serum transaminases.

Fibrates

The use of fibrates has waned over the last 10–15 years because of lack of efficacy data compared with the statins. However, some agents from this class, such as bezafibrate and fenofibrate, are still used in selected patients. Members of this group include bezafibrate, ciprofibrate, fenofibrate and gemfibrozil. They are thought to act by binding to peroxisome proliferator-activated receptor α on hepatocytes. This then leads to changes in the expression of genes involved in lipoprotein metabolism. Consequently, fibrates reduce triglyceride and, to a lesser extent, LDL-C levels, while increasing HDL-C. Fibrates take 2–5 days to have a measurable effect on VLDL-C, with their optimum effect present after 4 weeks. In addition to their effects on serum lipids and lipoproteins, the fibrates may also have a beneficial effect on the fibrinolytic and clotting mechanisms. The fibrates also produce an improvement in glucose tolerance, although bezafibrate probably has the most marked effect.

In the patient with elevated triglycerides and gout, only fenofibrate has been reported to have a sustained uricosuric effect on chronic administration. Overall, there appears little to differentiate members of the group with regard to their effect on the lipid profile, with fenofibrate and ciprofibrate being the most potent members of the group.

In patients with diabetes, the typical picture of dyslipidaemia is one of raised triglycerides, reduced HDL-C and near-normal LDL-C. Despite the effect of fibrates to reduce triglycerides and increase HDL-C, statins are first-line lipid-lowering agent in most guidelines because of a lack of clear evidence that fibrates prevent CVD in diabetes. Early data for fibrate monotherapy in primary and secondary prevention studies did show promise with a significant reduction in coronary events and stroke, and even a modest impact on CV mortality (Frick et al., 1987; Rubins et al., 1999). It was hoped that a 5-year study of fenofibrate in individuals with type 2 diabetes (Keech et al., 2005) would clarify the issue. However, in the final analysis the results provided little convincing evidence to change from recommending a statin, although they did confirm the safety of using a combination of a

Table 24.6 Typical drug interactions involving bile acid binding agents and fibrates[a]

Drug group	Interacting drug	Comment
Bile acid binding agents		
Colestyramine/colestipol		All medication should be taken 1 h before or at least 4 h after colestyramine/colestipol to reduce absorption caused by binding in the gut
	Acarbose	Hypoglycaemia enhanced by colestyramine
	Digoxin	Absorption reduced
	Diuretics	Absorption reduced
	Levothyroxine	Absorption reduced
	Mycophenolate mofetil	Absorption reduced
	Paracetamol	Absorption reduced
	Raloxifene	Absorption reduced
	Valproate	Absorption reduced
	Statins	Absorption reduced
	Vancomycin	Effect of oral vancomycin antagonised by colestyramine
	Warfarin	Increased anticoagulant effect due to depletion of vitamin K or reduced anticoagulant effect due to binding or warfarin in gut
Colesevelam		All medication should be taken at least 4 h before or 4 h after colesevelam to reduce absorption caused by binding in the gut
	Ciclosporin	Absorption reduced
	Digoxin	Absorption unchanged
	Glyburide	Absorption reduced
	Levothyroxine	Absorption reduced
	Oral contraceptive	Absorption reduced
	Statins	Absorption unchanged
	Valproate	Absorption unchanged
	Warfarin	Absorption unchanged Increased anticoagulant possible because of depletion of vitamin K
Fibrates	Antidiabetic agents	Improvement in glucose tolerance
	Ciclosporin	Increased risk of renal impairment
	Colestyramine/colestipol	Reduced bioavailability of fibrate if taken concomitantly
	Statin	Increased risk of myopathy
	Warfarin	Increased anticoagulant effect

[a]Absorption studies involve concomitant administration.

statin and fenofibrate. In contrast, gemfibrozil should not be used with a statin. Similarly, the ACCORD study (ACCORD Study Group, 2010) compared combination statin plus fibrate therapy with statin alone in patients with type 2 diabetes and concluded that the combination of fenofibrate and simvastatin did not reduce the rate of fatal CV events, nonfatal MI or nonfatal stroke, as compared with simvastatin alone.

Overall, fibrates should not be used first line to reduce lipid levels in either primary or secondary prevention of CVD (NICE, 2014). Fibrates may be considered first line in patients with isolated severe hypertriglyceridaemia, especially in individuals with triglyceride levels greater than 10 mmol/L where there is a risk of acute pancreatitis (Fortson et al., 1995). In those with mixed hyperlipidaemia, fibrates may be considered when a statin or other agent is contraindicated or not tolerated, or as an add-on therapy where monotherapy is ineffective.

Adverse effects

Overall, the side effects of fibrates are mild and vary between members of the group. Their apparent propensity to increase the cholesterol saturation index of bile renders them unsuitable for patients with gallbladder disease. Gastro-intestinal symptoms such as nausea and abdominal pain are common but transient, and often resolve after a few days of treatment. Myositis has been described and is associated with muscle pain, unusual tiredness or weakness. The mechanism is unclear, but it is thought that fibrates may have a direct toxic action on muscle cells in susceptible individuals.

Fibrates have been implicated in a number of drug interactions (Table 24.6), of which two in particular are potentially serious. Fibrates are known to significantly increase the effect of anticoagulants, while concurrent use with a statin is associated with an increased risk of myositis and, rarely, rhabdomyolysis.

Concurrent use of cerivastatin and gemfibrozil was noted to cause rhabdomyolysis, and this contributed to the withdrawal of cerivastatin from clinical use in 2001.

Bile acid binding agents

The three bile acid binding agents in current use are colestyramine, colestipol and colesevelam. Both colestyramine and colestipol were formerly considered first-line agents in the management of patients with FH but now have limited use. Colesevelam is the most recent of the bile acid binding agents to receive marketing authorisation (in 2004) and consequently has never had a first-line indication. Each of the bile acid binding agents reduce TC and increase triglyceride levels.

Following oral administration, neither colestyramine, colestipol nor colesevelam is absorbed from the gut. They bind bile acids in the intestine, prevent reabsorption and produce an insoluble complex that is excreted in the faeces. The depletion of bile acids results in an increase in hepatic synthesis of bile acids from cholesterol. The depletion of hepatic cholesterol upregulates the hepatic enzyme 7-α-hydroxylase which increases the conversion of cholesterol to bile acids. This increases LDL receptor activity in the liver and removes LDL-C from the blood. Hepatic VLDL-C synthesis also increases, and it is this which accounts for the raised serum triglycerides. There is little evidence that bile acid binders reduce the risk of CV events, and therefore they are not recommended for use for primary or secondary prevention of CVD (NICE, 2014). This class should only be considered for use by specialists as adjunctive therapy where first-line therapies for the management of dyslipidaemia are contraindicated or ineffective.

Colestyramine has a starting dosage of one 4-g sachet twice a day. Over a 3- to 4-week period the dosage should normally be built up to 12–24 g daily taken in water or a suitable liquid as a single dose, or up to four divided doses each day. Occasionally, 36 g/day may be required, although the benefits of increasing the dose above 16 g/day are offset by gastro-intestinal disturbances and poor patient adherence.

Colestipol is also available in a granular formulation and can be mixed with an appropriate liquid at a dose of 5 g once or twice daily. This dose can be increased every 1–2 months to a maximum of 30 g in a single- or twice-daily regimen.

Colesevelam is up to six times as potent as the other bile acid binding agents, probably because of a greater binding to glycocholic acid. Whether this translates into better clinical outcomes or more, or less, problems with drugs administered concurrently is unclear. Colesevelam is administered as a 625 mg tablet to a maximum dosage of 4.375 g/day (7 tablets). There is limited evidence to suggest it may achieve a higher adherence than colestyramine or colestipol. It can be taken as a single- or twice-daily regimen.

Adverse effects

With all three agents, side effects are more likely to occur with high doses and in patients older than 60 years. Bloating, flatulence, heartburn and constipation are common complaints. Constipation is the major subjective side effect, and although usually mild and transient, it may be severe.

Colestyramine, colestipol and colesevelam are known to interact with many drugs primarily by interfering with absorption (see Table 24.6). Whether these absorption-type interactions are qualitatively and quantitatively similar between the different agents is unclear, and the picture is confused when the absorption of a given drug is known to interact with one bile acid binding agent but has not been tested with other members of the group.

Long-term use of bile acid binding agents may also interfere with the absorption of fat-soluble vitamins, and supplementation with vitamins A, D and K is recommended.

Patient counselling

Palatability is often a major problem with the bile acid binding agents, and patients need to be well motivated and prepared for the problems they may encounter.

Both colestyramine and colestipol are available in an orange flavour and/or as a low-sugar (aspartame-containing) powder. Colestipol is without taste and is odourless. Each sachet of colestyramine or colestipol should be added to at least 150 or 100 mL of liquid, respectively, and stirred vigorously to avoid the powder clumping. The powder does not dissolve but disperses in the chosen liquid, which may be water, fruit juice, skimmed milk or non-carbonated beverage. Both may also be taken in soups, with cereals and with pulpy fruits with high moisture content, such as apple sauce.

All patients who are receiving a bile acid binding agent should be advised that reduced absorption with co-administered drugs should be anticipated. Medication that has to be taken should be administered 1 hour before (at least 4 hours for colesevelam) or at least 4 hours after the bile acid binding agent. As a consequence, for individuals receiving multiple-drug therapy, bile acid binding agents may not be appropriate for this reason alone.

Nicotinic acid and derivatives

Nicotinic acid in pharmacological doses (1.5–6 g) lowers serum LDL-C, TC, VLDL-C, apolipoprotein B, triglycerides and Lp(a), and increases levels of HDL-C (particularly the beneficial HDL$_3$ subfraction). While nicotinic acid and its derivatives may have beneficial effects on the lipid profile and did hold promise in terms of reducing CV events, these products have been withdrawn from the market in the UK due to safety concerns (European Medicines Agency, 2014), following a meta-analysis indicating increased risk of diabetes, myositis and infection. Only patients under the management of a lipid specialist should be prescribed nicotinic acid or nicotinic acid derivatives in line with NICE guidance for FH, with supplies imported on a named patient basis (NICE, 2008a).

The commonest side effect of nicotinic acid is flushing which is most prominent in the head, neck and upper torso and occurs in more than 90% of patients. It is cited as the major reason for discontinuation of treatment in 25–40% of patients. A number of strategies have been devised to overcome this, including co-administration of a cyclo-oxygenase inhibitor such as aspirin. Other strategies include regular consistent dosing, the use of extended-release formulations, patient education, dosing with meals or at bedtime, and the avoidance of alcohol, hot beverages, spicy foods, and hot baths or showers close to or after dosing. Less common side effects of nicotinic acid include postural hypotension, diarrhoea, exacerbation of peptic ulcers, hepatic dysfunction, gout and increased blood glucose levels.

Fish oils

Fish oil preparations rich in omega-3 fatty acids have been shown to markedly reduce serum triglyceride levels by decreasing VLDL-C synthesis, although little change has been observed in LDL-C or HDL-C levels. The effect is, however, inconsistent, and significant increases in LDL-C have also been reported to accompany the use of fish oils. Available commercial products contain omega-3-acid ethyl esters (Omacor) and omega-3-marine triglycerides (Maxepa). Either can be used as an alternative to a fibrate or in combination with a statin to manage hypertriglyceridaemia. However, they are not recommended by NICE (2014) for use in the primary or secondary prevention of CVD.

Soluble fibre

Preparations that contain soluble fibre, such as ispaghula husk, have been shown to reduce lipid levels. The fibre is thought to bind bile acids in the gut and increase the conversion of cholesterol to bile acids in the liver. However, their role in the management of dyslipidaemia is unclear, and they are much less effective than statins in reducing TC and LDL-C.

Proprotein convertase subtilisin/kexin type 9 inhibitors

Key to the removal of LDL cholesterol from the circulation is the LDL receptor PCSK9, a secreted protease that has a role in controlling the number of LDL receptors available by binding LDL-C receptors and preventing them from being expressed on the cell surface. High levels of PCSK9 suppress LDL-C receptor activity, reducing the number of available receptors, and result in raised circulating cholesterol. Inhibition of PCSK9 will facilitate increased LDL-C receptor activity through increased number of receptors, and hence lower circulating cholesterol levels.

Alirocumab and evolocumab, both monoclonal antibody PCSK9 inhibitors, have recently been licensed as options in the management of primary FH and non-FH. In the studies to date, evolocumab with or without background statin therapy has been shown to reduce LDL-L levels between 55% and 75% compared with placebo, and by up to 50% more than ezetimibe (Raal et al., 2015; Robinson et al., 2014; Stroes et al., 2014). Across five clinical trials involving 2476 patients with FH receiving optimal statin therapy, the average reduction in LDL-C with alirocumab ranged from 36% to 59%, compared with placebo (U.S. Food and Drug Administration, 2015). The first CV outcomes study investigated the impact of evolocumab in addition to statins in patients with atherosclerotic coronary disease (Sabatine et al., 2017). Over 2.2 years of follow-up, the addition of evolocumab to statin therapy demonstrated a significant reduction in CV events: 9.8% versus 11.3% for statins alone with an absolute risk reduction of 1.5%.

Currently, these drugs are recommended by NICE as an option for the treatment of primary hypercholesterolaemia or mixed dyslipidaemia provided a set of usage criteria are met, including minimum baseline LDL levels before initiation of treatment (NICE, 2016b, 2016c).

Both drugs are administered by subcutaneous injection and require storage in a refrigerator. Both are contraindicated in patients with known hypersensitivity to the active ingredient or excipients. In the trials to date, both drugs have been well tolerated with the most common side effects being symptoms of influenza, nasopharyngitis, upper respiratory tract infection, rash, nausea, backache, arthralgia and injection-site reactions.

Drugs in development

Cholesterol ester transfer protein inhibitors

Low levels of cholesterol ester transfer protein (CETP) are associated with increased levels of HDL-C and reduced CV risk. CETP transfers cholesterol from HDL-C to LDL-C and VLDL-C, thereby altering the HDL-C:LDL-C ratio in a potentially unfavourable manner. In epidemiological studies, higher circulating levels of HDL have been associated with reduced CV events, hence the CETP inhibitors were thought to be a promising therapeutic option. However, of the original four CETP inhibitors in development, three have been abandoned because of increased mortality (torcetrapib) or lack of impact on CV events despite adequate HDL increases (dalcetrapib and evacetrapib). Recently announced results of the REVEAL study of anacetrapib indicate a modest reduction in CV events when added to intensive statin therapy, with no major safety signals (Bowman et al., 2017). Whether this will result in a change to clinical practice in the future remains to be seen.

Other options

Low-density lipoprotein apheresis

Lipoprotein apheresis is a treatment option used in patients with severe treatment-resistant hypercholesterolaemia. Currently approximately 70 patients are receiving apheresis treatment in England and Wales. Lipoprotein apheresis removes LDL-C, Lp(a) and triglycerides from the plasma. Treatment can lower LDL-C by upwards of 75%, but the effect is transient, and hence treatment needs to be repeated at regular intervals (Thompson et al., 1995). The efficacy and superiority of lipoprotein apheresis in comparison with standard lipid-lowering therapies is well established; however, there is still uncertainty regarding the ability of lipoprotein apheresis to promote atherosclerotic plaque regression, because its effects are only transient. Furthermore, although LDL apheresis is a highly effective treatment, its uptake and application are somewhat restricted because of its limited availability at specialist centres only and the need for repeated treatments on a weekly or twice-weekly basis.

NICE (2008a) recommends that apheresis is considered for the management of people with clinical homozygous FH and also for those with heterozygous FH in exceptional circumstances, for example, progressive, symptomatic CHD despite maximal oral lipid-lowering therapy and optimal medical-surgical intervention.

Lomitapide

Lomitapide inhibits microsomal triglyceride transfer protein which plays a major role in the assembly and secretion of the lipoproteins in the intestine and liver. As a result, lomitapide inhibits the synthesis of triglyceride-rich chylomicrons in the intestine and VLDL (the precursor of LDL) in the liver. This results in an overall reduction in circulating cholesterol. Lomitapide has been studied extensively in patients with homozygous FH and at a dosage of 1 mg/kg/day lowered LDL-C by 50.9% from baseline (Cuchel et al., 2007). It is licensed for use only in patients with homozygous FH and may have a role in preventing progression to LDL apheresis or, in those already receiving apheresis, to reduce the frequency of sessions to minimise the impact on quality of life. It is an option for a very small cohort of patients across the country and at a cost of more than £200,000 per annum, usage will remain very low.

Lomitapide is initiated at a low 5 mg dose and increased gradually every 4 weeks to a maximum of 60 mg daily. It is contra-indicated where there is hypersensitivity to the active substance or any excipients, in patients with moderate or severe hepatic impairment and those with unexplained persistent abnormal liver function tests, in patients with a known significant or chronic bowel disease such as inflammatory bowel disease or malabsorption, where there is concomitant administration of greater than 40 mg simvastatin or strong or moderate CYP3A4 inhibitors and in pregnancy. Adverse events include gastro-intestinal (mainly diarrhoea), deranged liver function tests (increased levels of aspartate transaminase and/or alanine transaminase and alkaline phosphatase) and increased hepatic fat content and possible steatohepatitis.

Case studies

Case 24.1

Mr DF is a 43-year-old man who has been relatively fit and well for the past 20 years during which he has rarely visited his primary care doctor. Two weeks ago he was admitted to hospital having suffered an MI. On questioning it was revealed that his brother had died in a road traffic accident at the age of 19 and his father had died of CHD at age 54 years.

Examination of Mr DF revealed a corneal arcus and tendon xanthomas. Blood drawn within 2 hours of the onset of his MI revealed TC 7.8 mmol/L, HDL-C 0.9 mmol/L and triglycerides 2.3 mmol/L.

Questions

1. What is the likely diagnosis of Mr DF?
2. What are the treatment options?
3. Mr DF wants to know why he was not identified as being at high risk of CHD before he suffered his MI.

Answers

1. Mr DF has the signs and family history of classic heterozygous FH, most likely because of a genetic defect in the LDL receptor on hepatocytes. His presentation with an acute cardiac event at such an early age is indicative of the raised CV risk present for individuals with FH.
2. Mr DF has a high level of LDL-C, and action is required to reduce it. Appropriate lifestyle advice is necessary, but a high-dose high-intensity statin, such as atorvastatin 80 mg daily, will be required to achieve the desired outcome of at least a 50% reduction in LDL-C. In addition, this patient has recently suffered an MI, which in itself is an indication for a high-intensity statin first line. Mr DF should be managed by a lipid specialist in the first instance and relatives, including any children, should be screened for the presence of FH to allow early initiation of lipid-lowering therapy.

3. Unfortunately, Mr DF's father probably died of heart disease at a time when the practice of detecting affected families and screening first-degree relatives was not widespread. The early, unrelated death of his brother and Mr DF's previous good health would not have given an opportunity to identify any underlying familial disorder. From population data it is known that the prevalence of heterozygous FH is about 1 in 500. Consequently, 120,000 cases would be expected in the UK. However, far fewer cases are known, and cascade screening programmes to track cases in affected families are now recommended once an index case has been identified. A family history of elevated TC or death from CHD before the age of 55 years in a first-degree male relative, as in the case of Mr DF, is an important sign that should highlight the potential risk to other family members. The NHS Health Checks programme in England will assist in the identification of undetected FH.

Case 24.2

Mr PT is a 52-year-old active school teacher. Four years ago he was found to have a raised TC and elevated blood pressure for which he was started on 10 mg simvastatin and 2.5 mg ramipril. Over the years his dose of simvastatin has been gradually increased to 40 mg/day, but apart from this his medication has remained unchanged. He presents at the clinic complaining of aches and pains in his legs over the past 10 days. On questioning he reveals that over recent months he has been eating fresh grapefruit and consuming the occasional glass of grapefruit juice. A tentative diagnosis of myopathy is initially made.

Questions

1. What is the likelihood that grapefruit juice has contributed to Mr PT's problem?
2. Are any additional biochemical tests warranted?
3. Would atorvastatin, rosuvastatin or pravastatin be a more appropriate statin to prescribe if Mr PT wanted to continue with the occasional glass of grapefruit juice?

Answers

1. Grapefruit juice is known to interact with statins through its inhibition of the CYP3A4 enzyme. It has been suggested that it is the furanocoumarin in the grapefruit juice which binds to CYP3A4 and inactivates it in both the liver and the gastro-intestinal tract. As little as 200 mL of grapefruit juice may inhibit CYP3A4, thereby prolonging the half-life of the statin and increasing serum levels. When taken on a regular basis this can increase the risk of dose-related side effects such as rhabdomyolysis and increase the risk of myopathy. Current advice is that grapefruit juice should be avoided altogether when taking simvastatin, regardless of whether it is fresh grapefruit or grapefruit juice, grapefruit juice diluted from concentrate or frozen grapefruit juice.
2. A creatine kinase (CK) level should be checked in patients reporting significant muscle pain to exclude overt myopathy.
   - If CK is raised significantly (>5 times upper normal level), temporary withdrawal of the statin is warranted. Once the CK declines to normal levels, and in view of the suspicion that grapefruit intake was a precipitating factor, the statin could be reinitiated and the patient warned to avoid grapefruit and seek advice promptly should the muscle aches recur.
   - If the CK is normal, then this is a simple myalgia. Grapefruit should be avoided and hopefully the symptoms will resolve. If the pain does not resolve this may have an impact on adherence and an alternate statin should be considered. Of all the

agents currently on the UK market, simvastatin is most likely to cause myalgia and myopathy.

3. Atorvastatin is also metabolised by CYP3A4. Although the effect is less dramatic than with simvastatin, the concurrent intake of large quantities of grapefruit juice with atorvastatin is not recommended. Neither pravastatin nor rosuvastatin is substantially metabolised by CYP450 and may be better alternatives. However, when there is a history of myopathy, the need for caution remains because the risk of recurrence is enhanced whatever lipid-lowering agent is prescribed. There are separate concerns regarding the muscle toxicity of rosuvastatin, especially when used at the higher dose of 40 mg.

Because this patient is being treated with a statin for primary prevention, the NICE (2014) guidelines suggest that if a person is not able to tolerate a high-intensity statin, then one should aim to treat with the maximum tolerated dose. Patients should be reassured that any statin at any dose reduces CVD risk. Strategies for dealing with adverse effects include:

- stopping the statin and trying again when the symptoms have resolved to check whether the symptoms are related to the statin,
- reducing the dose within the same intensity group, or
- changing the statin to a lower intensity group.

Case 24.3

Mrs MC is a very active, 51-year-old Caucasian woman who for the past 6 months has been suffering from the classic symptoms of the menopause. Six months ago on a routine visit to her doctor she had her lipid profile measured and this revealed an HDL-C of 0.8 mmol/L and TC of 5 mmol/L. Her blood pressure was 140/80 mmHg. She is currently prescribed no medication but is receiving intensive lifestyle support to lower her cholesterol. She has no other medical history of note other than a record that her mother died at the age of 66 years from a heart attack.

Mrs MC would like to be prescribed hormone replacement therapy (HRT) to control her menopausal symptoms and reduce her risk of CVD.

Questions

1. Is it appropriate to prescribe HRT to reduce Mrs MC's CV risk?
2. What is the value of measuring HDL-C?
3. Does Mrs MC have a risk of CVD that requires treatment with a lipid-lowering agent?

Answers

1. The impact of HRT on CV risk has been a subject of much debate over many years. There are no compelling data to justify the use of HRT for the prevention or treatment of CVD in postmenopausal women. In fact, current evidence indicates that HRT may increase the risk of breast cancer, ovarian cancer, CVD and thromboembolic disease. NICE guideline NG23, "Menopause: Diagnosis and Management" (NICE, 2015), concluded that HRT does not increase CVD risk when started in women younger than 60 years and does not affect the risk of dying of CVD. In addition, NICE (2015) states that HRT with oestrogen alone is associated with no, or reduced, risk of CHD, whereas HRT with oestrogen and progestogen is associated with little or no increase in the risk of CHD. The presence of CV risk factors is not a contraindication to HRT as long as they are optimally managed. If Mrs MC is to be prescribed HRT, then this should be based on the need to control her menopausal symptoms and improve her quality of life.

2. HDL-C is a major fraction of cholesterol in serum and an important determinant of CV risk in men and women, even when the level of TC appears to be within the normal range. The incidence of MI is positively correlated with the cholesterol concentration and inversely related to the concentration of HDL-C. The TC:HDL-C ratio is another way to represent this risk and has been shown to have good predictive capabilities in women. Until the menopause, women generally have high levels of HDL-C as a result of the circulating oestrogen. However, following the menopause, HDL-C levels fall rapidly. Lifestyle advice may improve the TC:HDL ratio, especially via increased physical activity.

3. With reference to the Qrisk2 CV risk calculator, it can be determined that with a TC:HDL-C ratio of 6.25 (5/0.8) and a systolic blood pressure of 140 mmHg Mrs MC has a 8.2% risk of development of CVD over the next 10 years. This would not automatically make her a candidate for treatment with a lipid-lowering agent because her 10-year CV risk is not more than 10%. Knowledge of Mrs MC's BMI and blood glucose level would be useful additional information, as would a more detailed insight into her family history of CVD. It is only when all the relevant information has been gathered that a final decision on the use of a lipid-lowering agent can be made. It would also be of interest to determine whether the lifestyle support has brought about any improvement in Mrs MC's lipid profile or blood pressure. It is important to recognise that Mrs MC's CV risk will increase as she gets older; if nothing changes in 5 years' time her CV risk will be 11.9%, which is over the threshold for offering statin therapy. She should be offered advice and support to address all modifiable risk factors for CVD including optimising her diet, undertaking regular physical activity and taking steps to control her blood pressure.

Case 24.4

Mr EC is a 48-year-old Pakistani executive for a large, multinational company who works long hours and frequently has to travel abroad. He has a family history of CHD, and 9 months ago he attended a coronary screening clinic for a health check. At the clinic he was found to have a normal blood pressure (132/84 mmHg) but a blood screen revealed a TC of 5.7 mmol/L and triglycerides of 11.8 mmol/L. When he revisited the clinic 4 weeks later after trying to follow dietary advice, a fasting blood sample revealed a TC of 5 mmol/L and triglycerides of 2.7 mmol/L. Liver function tests were normal. He is a non-smoker and claims never to drink more than 10 units of alcohol per week. His BMI is 27 kg/m².

After repeated requests to revisit the clinic he eventually turned up stating he had been away from home for 6 months on a series of business trips. He was trying to keep to a low-fat diet and his blood profile revealed TC 5.7 mmol/L, triglycerides 4.3 mmol/L, HDL-C 0.7 mmol/L and LDL-C 3 mmol/L, non-HDL-C 5 mmol/L.

Questions

1. Is Mr EC at high risk of CHD?
2. Is Mr EC a candidate for lipid-lowering therapy?
3. Should Mr EC's children be screened for dyslipidaemia?

Answers

1. Mr EC has a TC:HDL-C ratio of 8.1 (5.7/0.7). Qrisk2 indicates a CVD risk score of 12.3%, which indicates he should be considered for statin therapy after other modifiable risk factors have been

addressed and if QRisk score remains ≥10. However, it should also be remembered that QRisk will underestimate the risk of CVD in those with familial hyperlipidaemia. Mr EC would appear to have a mixed lipidaemia, although it is difficult to interpret non-fasting triglycerides because of the influence of food intake. The low HDL-C and raised BMI indicate he is overweight and/or has a non-ideal lifestyle. Exclusion of diabetes, high alcohol intake, liver and renal impairment is necessary. The possibility of impaired glucose tolerance should not be overlooked and a haemoglobin A_{1c} level should be checked.

2. Given the elevated triglycerides and TC, Mr EC is certainly a candidate for lifestyle advice. The use of a statin should be considered if the lifestyle changes do not bring about the necessary improvements in the lipid profile. However, the dyslipidaemia may be secondary to obesity, alcoholism, diabetes or hypothyroidism. If any of these disorders are present, appropriate treatment may correct the underlying dyslipidaemia.

3. The family history of CHD is important but is only significant if the age of onset in a parent or sibling was younger than 60 years. In this case, the children should have CV risk assessment undertaken every 5 years from the age of 40 years. However, were a rare familial disorder, for example, familial dysbetalipoproteinaemia, be identified as the causative factor, his children should be screened after puberty because the offending gene may not express itself in the younger child.

Mr EC was subsequently found to have diabetes for which he initially received metformin together with a statin. In this scenario where a patient is diagnosed with type 2 diabetes, it is also important to consider advising children about lifestyle issues and the need to control weight throughout life.

Case 24.5

Mr JT is a 68-year-old man with stable angina. He is currently receiving simvastatin 40 mg daily with well-controlled lipid levels (TC 3.8 mmol/L, LDL-C 1.8 mmol/L, HDL-C 0.9 mmol/L, triglycerides 1.3 mmol/L, non-HDL-C 2.9 mmol/L). He has been receiving simvastatin for the past 7 years and has complained previously about muscle aches, but on this visit he states that his muscle pain has become more troublesome, to the extent that he wishes to stop taking the statin. He asks if there is anything else he can take to control his cholesterol.

Questions

1. What action would you take immediately?
2. What options are available for Mr JT?
3. What would you recommend to Mr JT?

Answers

1. A CK level should be checked to exclude myopathy in this patient, because this can occur at any time during statin treatment. Assuming the CK is normal and this is myalgia, then it is still essential to address Mr JT's concerns, because this muscle pain is likely to impact on his adherence over time. An important issue is to ensure that the patient understands why he is taking a statin. The emphasis should be on the expected reduction in the risk of death, heart attack or stroke, rather than on achieving specific cholesterol treatment targets. It may be worth temporarily stopping the statin to demonstrate the causal relationship. If the aches and pains remain despite cessation of simvastatin, then this is unlikely to be a statin-related issue. Many people report aches and pains, particularly as they get older, and it is easy to blame the statin for all of these complaints.

2. Options for Mr JT include:
   - Reducing the dose of simvastatin: Mr JT has been receiving simvastatin for many years and a simple reduction in dosage to 20 mg/day may improve tolerability without compromising the lipid control substantially. Although an increase in TC and LDL-C is expected with dose reduction, this is usually small (in the order of 6%) and should have little overall impact on risk.
   - Substituting an alternative statin: Simvastatin causes more myalgia and myopathy than other statins; therefore, an alternative agent may be better tolerated. Pravastatin is particularly well tolerated and may be a suitable alternative in this patient where potency is less of an issue. Where greater potency is required, atorvastatin (starting at a dosage of 10–20 mg daily and increasing as required to control lipids) or rosuvastatin is a possibility.
   - Switching to an alternative agent, such as ezetimibe: Non-statin agents could be used to lower cholesterol but should be reserved for patients who are unable to tolerate statins. Ezetimibe monotherapy may be a suitable alternative if Mr JT cannot tolerate statin therapy after dose reduction and a change in agent.
   - Using a low dose of statin plus an alternative agent, such as ezetimibe: This may be a suitable option if this patient can tolerate only small doses of statins and the ezetimibe is introduced to increase the degree of cholesterol lowering achieved. This is a useful combination in some patients, but every effort should be made to maximise the statin dose before adding ezetimibe to ensure maximal outcome benefits.

3. For Mr JT, a good starting point would be a reduction in the dosage of simvastatin to 20 mg daily, providing he is willing to continue to take this drug. Myalgia appears to be dose related, and the symptoms may resolve with the lower dose. An alternative is to try pravastatin, perhaps at a starting dosage of 20 mg daily, to see whether it is better tolerated. The dosage will probably need increasing to give adequate control of lipid levels. The use of ezetimibe should be reserved as an additional medicine if only low doses of statins can be tolerated or for monotherapy if that patient cannot be persuaded to take any statin at all. Mr JT should be reviewed regularly over the next few months, until his concerns regarding his lipid-lowering therapy have been addressed, to encourage ongoing adherence.

Case 24.6

Mrs RS is a 36-year-old care assistant from the Philippines with heterozygous FH. She has diffuse, symptomatic coronary artery disease and is currently taking rosuvastatin 20 mg daily and ezetimibe 10 mg daily. Her lipid levels are: TC 8.6 mmol/L (12.3 mmol/L before statin therapy), non-HDL-C 7.7 mmol/L, HDL-C 0.9 mmol/L and LDL-C 7.0 mmol/L.

Questions

1. What treatment options would you consider next for Mrs RS?
2. How would you monitor therapy?
3. What other issues should you consider?

Answers

1. Mrs RS needs a significantly greater reduction in her lipid levels than is currently being achieved with statin and ezetimibe. A higher statin dose is contraindicated in view of the ethnicity of Mrs RS. Whilst other classes of oral lipid-lowering therapies could be considered, they are unlikely to deliver a significant further

reduction in LDL. In this case, a lipid specialist may consider the use of a PCSK9 inhibitor, because it is the only drug class able to deliver the significant drop in cholesterol required here. Mrs RS meets the NICE criteria for use of a PCSK9 inhibitor (NICE, 2016b, 2016c); she has heterozygous FH and evidence of CVD, is at high risk of events and her LDL-C level remains greater than the 3.5 mmol/L threshold for use, despite statin and ezetimibe therapy.

2. Mrs RS will need to be willing to inject the PCSK9 inhibitor at two weekly intervals and will need adequate training to feel confident in doing this procedure. In the UK, supplies of these drugs are usually delivered by a homecare provider, and the companies offer nursing support to patients at home who require additional support with the injections. Mrs RS should also be followed up by the lipid specialist within 4–6 weeks of initiation to check she is managing the injections and is not experiencing significant side effects. Her lipid levels will fall rapidly on a PCSK9 inhibitor with a reduction in LDL-C of at least 30% expected within the first 3 months of therapy. If this is not achieved, injection technique and adherence should be checked initially, but if a poor response persists, ongoing treatment should be reviewed.

3. Lifestyle issues, particularly diet and physical activity, should be regularly reviewed with appropriate advice, support and/or signposting to enable Mrs RS to make any necessary changes. In view of the presence of heterozygous FH, her first-degree relatives should be screened for FH and offered appropriate advice and treatment.

References

ACCORD Study Group, 2010. Effects of combination lipid therapy in type 2 diabetes mellitus. N. Engl. J. Med. 362, 1563–1574.

Ames, R., 1988. Effects of diuretic drugs on the lipid profile. Drugs 36 (Suppl. 2), 33–40.

Benn, M., Watts, G.F., Tybjaerg-Hansen, A., et al., 2012. Familial hypercholesterolemia in the Danish general population: prevalence, coronary artery disease, and cholesterol-lowering medication. J. Clin. Endocrinol. Metab. 97, 3956–3964.

Bowman, L., Hopewell, J.C., Chen, F., et al.; The HPS3/TIMI55-REVEAL Collaborative Group, 2017. Effects of anacetrapib in patients with atherosclerotic vascular disease. N. Engl. J. Med. 377, 1217–1227.

British Heart Foundation, 2015. Cardiovascular disease statistics 2015. Available at: https://www.bhf.org.uk/publications/statistics/cvd-stats-2015.

Cannon, C.P., Blazing, M.A., Giugliano, R.P., et al.; for the IMPROVE-IT Investigators, 2015. Ezetimibe added to statin therapy after acute coronary syndromes. N. Engl. J. Med. 372, 2387–2397.

Chapman, M.J., Le Goff, W., Guerin, M., et al., 2010. Cholesterol ester transfer protein: at the heart of the action of lipid modulating therapy with statins, fibrates, niacin, and cholesteryl ester transfer protein inhibitors. Eur. Heart J. 31, 149–164.

Cholesterol Treatment Trialist Collaboration, 2010. Efficacy and safety of more intensive lowering of LDL cholesterol: a meta-analysis of data from 170 000 participants in 26 randomised trials. Lancet 376, 1670–1681.

Cholesterol Treatment Trialist Collaboration, 2012. The effects of lowering LDL cholesterol with statin therapy in people at low risk of vascular disease: meta-analysis of individual data from 27 randomised trials. Lancet 380, 581–590.

Cuchel, M., Bloedon, L.T., Szapary, P.O., et al., 2007. Inhibition of microsomal triglycerides transfer protein in familial hypercholesterolemia. N. Engl. J. Med. 356, 148–156.

de Lorgeril, M., Salen, P., Martin, J.L., et al., 1999. Mediterranean diet, traditional risk factors, and the rate of cardiovascular complications after myocardial infarction: final report of the Lyon Diet Heart Study. Circulation 99, 779–785.

Department of Health, 2016. UK Chief Medical Officers' low risk drinking guidelines. Available at: https://www.gov.uk/government/uploads/system/uploads/attachment_data/file/545937/UK_CMOs__report.pdf.

Dumić, M., Uroić, A.S., Francetić, I., et al., 2007. Three-year-old boy – a homozygote for familial hypercholesterolemia. Lijec Vjesn 129, 130–133.

Emmerson, B., 1998. Hyperlipidaemia in hyperuricaemia and gout. Ann. Rheum. Dis. 57, 509–510.

Erqou, S., Kaptoge, S., Perry, P.L., Emerging Risk Factors Collaboration, et al., 2009. Lipoprotein(a) concentration and the risk of coronary heart disease, stroke, and nonvascular mortality. J. Am. Med. Assoc. 302, 412–423.

European Medicines Agency, 2014. Acipimox only to be used as additional or alternative treatment to reduce high triglyceride levels. Available at: http://www.ema.europa.eu/ema/index.jsp?curl=pages/medicines/human/referrals/Nicotinic_acid/human_referral_prac_000020.jsp&mid=WC0b01ac05805c516f.

European Society of Cardiology, 2017. SCORE Risk Charts. The European cardiovascular disease risk assessment model. Available at: https://www.escardio.org/Education/Practice-Tools/CVD-prevention-toolbox/SCORE-Risk-Charts.

Farzadfar, F., Finucane, M.M., Danaei, G., et al., 2011. National, regional, and global trends in serum total cholesterol since 1980: systematic analysis of health examination surveys and epidemiological studies with 321 country-years and 3.0 million participants. Lancet 377, 578–586.

Fortson, M.R., Freedman, S.N., Webster 3rd, P.D., 1995. Clinical assessment of hyperlipidemic pancreatitis. Am. J. Gastroenterol. 90, 2134–2139.

Frick, M.H., Elo, O., Haapa, K., et al., 1987. Helsinki Heart Study: primary-prevention trial with gemfibrozil in middle-aged men with dyslipidemia. Safety of treatment, changes in risk factors, and incidence of coronary heart disease. N. Engl. J. Med. 317, 1237–1245.

Gaddi, A., Cicero, A.F.G., Odoo, F.O., et al.; on behalf of the Atherosclerosis and Metabolic Diseases Study Group, 2007. Practical guidelines for familial combined hyperlipidemia diagnosis: an up-date. Vasc. Health Risk Manag. 3, 877–886.

Gautschi, M., Pavlovic, M., Nuoffer, J.M., 2012. Fatal myocardial infarction at 4.5 years in a case of homozygous familial hypercholesterolaemia. JIMD Rep. 2, 45–50.

Gotoda, T., Yamada, N., Kawamura, M., et al., 1991. Heterogeneous mutations in the human lipoprotein lipase gene in patients with familial lipoprotein lipase deficiency. J. Clin. Invest. 88, 1856–1864.

Haffner, S.M., Lehto, S., Rönnemaa, T., et al., 1998. Mortality from coronary heart disease in subjects with type 2 diabetes and in nondiabetic subjects with and without prior myocardial infarction. N. Engl. J. Med. 339, 229–234.

Helin-Salmivaara, A., Lavikainen, P., Korhonen, M.J., et al., 2008. Long-term persistence with statin therapy: a nationwide register study in Finland. Clin. Ther. 30, 2228–2240.

Herink, M., Ito, M.K., 2015. Medication induced changes in lipid and lipoproteins. In: De Groot, L.J., Chrousos, G., Dungan, K., et al. (Eds.), Endotext. Available at: https://www.ncbi.nlm.nih.gov/books/NBK326739/.

Hippisley-Cox, J., Coupland, C., Vinogradova, Y., et al., 2007. Derivation and validation of QRISK, a new cardiovascular disease risk score for the United Kingdom: prospective open cohort study. BMJ 335, 136.

Hu, F.B., Bronner, L., Willett, W.C., et al., 2002. Fish and omega-3 fatty acid intake and risk of coronary heart disease in women. JAMA 287, 1815–1821.

Kastelein, J.J., Akdim, F., Stroes, E.S., et al., 2008. Simvastatin with or without ezetimibe in familial hypercholesterolemia. The ENHANCE study. N. Engl. J. Med. 358, 1431–1443.

Kausik, R.K., Sreenivasa, R.K.S., Erqou, S., et al., 2010. Statins and all-cause-mortality in high-risk primary prevention: a meta-analysis of 11 randomized controlled trials involving 65,229 participants. Arch. Intern. Med. 170, 1024–1031.

Keech, A., Simes, R.J., Barter, P., et al.; FIELD Study Investigators, 2005. Effects of long-term fenofibrate therapy on cardiovascular events in 9795 people with type 2 diabetes mellitus (the FIELD study): randomized controlled trial. Lancet 366, 1849–1861.

Kolovou, G.D., Anagnostopoulou, K.K., Cokkinos, D.V., 2005. Pathophysiology of dyslipidaemia in the metabolic syndrome. Postgrad. Med. J. 81, 358–366.

Malmberg, K., Yusuf, S., Gerstein, H.C., et al., 2000. Impact of diabetes on long-term prognosis in patients with unstable angina and non-Q-wave myocardial infarction: results of the OASIS (Organization to Assess Strategies for Ischemic Syndromes) Registry. Circulation 102, 1014–1019.

Medicines and Healthcare products Regulatory Agency, 2012. Simvastatin: updated advice on drug interactions. Drug Safety Update. Available at:

https://www.gov.uk/drug-safety-update/simvastatin-updated-advice-on-drug-interactions.

National Institute of Health and Care Excellence (NICE), 2008a. Identification and management of familial hypercholesterolaemia. Clinical guideline CG71 NICE, London. Available at: http://guidance.nice.org.uk/CG71/Guidance/pdf/English.

National Institute of Health and Care Excellence (NICE), 2008b. CG67: lipid modification: cardiovascular risk assessment and the modification of blood lipids for the primary and secondary prevention of cardiovascular disease. Clinical Guideline CG67 NICE, London. Available at: https://www.nice.org.uk/guidance/cg67.

National Institute for Health and Care Excellence (NICE), 2014. Cardiovascular disease: risk assessment and reduction, including lipid modification. Clinical guideline CG181 NICE, London. Available at: https://www.nice.org.uk/guidance/cg181.

National Institute for Health and Care Excellence (NICE), 2015. NG23: menopause: diagnosis and management. NICE, London. Available at: https://www.nice.org.uk/guidance/ng23/chapter/Recommendations#long-term-benefits-and-risks-of-hormone-replacement-therapy.

National Institute for Health and Care Excellence (NICE), 2016a. Ezetimibe for treating primary heterozygous-familial and non-familial hypercholesterolaemia. Technology appraisal guidance (TA385). NICE, London. Available at: https://www.nice.org.uk/guidance/ta385.

National Institute for Health and Care Excellence (NICE), 2016b. Evolocumab for treating primary hypercholesterolaemia and mixed dyslipidaemia. Technology appraisal guidance (TA394). NICE, London. Available at: https://www.nice.org.uk/guidance/ta394.

National Institute for Health and Care Excellence (NICE), 2016c. Alirocumab for treating primary hypercholesterolaemia and mixed dyslipidaemia. Technology appraisal guidance (TA393) NICE, London. Available at: https://www.nice.org.uk/guidance/ta393.

National Organization of Rare Disorder (NORD), 2005. Hyperlipoproteinemia type III. Available at: https://rarediseases.org/rare-diseases/hyperlipoproteinemia-type-iii/.

Raal, F.J., Honarpour, N., Blom, D.J., et al.; TESLA Investigators, 2015. Inhibition of PCSK9 with evolocumab in homozygous familial hypercholesterolaemia (TESLA Part B): a randomised, double-blind, placebo-controlled trial. Lancet 385, 331–340.

Research Committee on Serum Lipid Level Survey 1990 in Japan, 1996. Current state of and recent trends in serum lipid levels in the general Japanese population. J. Atheroscler. Thromb. 2, 122–132.

Ridker, P.M., Danielson, E., Fonseca, F.A.H., 2008. Rosuvastatin to prevent vascular events in men and women with elevated C-reactive protein. N. Engl. J. Med. 359, 2195–2207.

Robinson, J.G., Nedergaard, B.S., Rogers, W.J., et al.; LAPLACE-2 Investigators, 2014. Effect of evolocumab or ezetimibe added to moderate- or high-intensity statin therapy on LDL-C lowering in patients with hypercholesterolemia: the LAPLACE-2 randomized clinical trial. JAMA 311, 1870–1882.

Rubins, H.B., Robins, S.J., Collins, D., et al., 1999. Veterans Affairs High-Density Lipoprotein Cholesterol Intervention Trail. N. Engl. J. Med. 341, 410–418.

Sabatine, M.S., Guigliano, R.P., Keech, A.C., et al., 2017. Evolocumab and clinical outcomes in patients with cardiovascular disease. N. Engl. J. Med. 376, 1713–1722.

Stroes, E., Colquhoun, D., Sullivan, D., et al.; GAUSS-2 Investigators, 2014. Anti-PCSK9 antibody effectively lowers cholesterol in patients with statin intolerance: the GAUSS-2 randomized, placebo-controlled phase 3 clinical trial of evolocumab. J. Am. Coll. Cardiol. 63, 2541–2548.

Tang, J.L., Armitage, J.M., Lancaster, T., et al., 1998. Systematic review of dietary intervention trials to lower blood total cholesterol in free-living subjects. BMJ 316, 1213–1220.

Thompson, G.R., Maher, V.M.G., Kitano, Y., et al., 1995. Familial Hypercholesterolaemia Regression Study: a randomised trial of low-density-lipoprotein apheresis. Lancet 345, 811–816.

Triglyceride Coronary Disease Genetics Consortium and Emerging Risk Factors Collaboration, 2010. Triglyceride-mediated pathways and coronary disease: collaborative analysis of 101 studies. Lancet 375, 1634–1639.

U.S. Food and Drug Adminsitration, 2015. FDA approves Praluent to treat certain patients with high cholesterol. Available at: http://www.fda.gov/NewsEvents/Newsroom/PressAnnouncements/ucm455883.htm.

von Depka, M., Nowak-Göttl, U., Eisert, R., et al., 2000. Increased lipoprotein (a) levels as an independent risk factor for venous thromboembolism. Blood 96, 3364–3388.

Widhalm, K., Binder, C.B., Kreissl, A., et al., 2011. Sudden death in a 4-year-old boy: a near-complete occlusion of the coronary artery caused by an aggressive low-density lipoprotein receptor mutation (W556R) in homozygous familial hypercholesterolemia. J. Pediatr. 158, 167.

Wiggins, B.S., Saseen, J.J., Page, R.L., on behalf of the American Heart Association Clinical Pharmacology Committee of the Council on Clinical Cardiology; Council on Hypertension; Council on Quality of Care and Outcomes Research; Council on Functional Genomics and Translational Biology, et al., 2016. Recommendations for management of clinically significant drug-drug interactions with statins and select agents used in patients with cardiovascular disease: a scientific statement from the American Heart Association. Circulation 134, e468–e495. https://doi.org/10.1161/CIR.0000000000000456. Available at: http://circ.ahajournals.org/content/early/2016/10/17/CIR.0000000000000456.

Woodward, M., Brindle, P., Tunstall-Pedoe, H., for the SIGN group on risk estimation, 2007. Adding social deprivation and family history to cardiovascular risk assessment: the ASSIGN score from the Scottish Heart Health Extended Cohort (SHHEC). Heart 93, 172–176.

World Health Organization, 2011. Waist circumference and waist-hip ratio. Report of a WHO expert consultation 2008. WHO, Geneva. Available at: http://apps.who.int/iris/bitstream/10665/44583/1/9789241501491_eng.pdf.

Yang, W., Xiao, J., Yang, Z., et al., 2012. Serum lipids and lipoproteins in Chinese men and women. Circulation 125, 2212–2221.

Further reading

Aronis, K.N., Blumenthal, R.S., Martin, S.S., 2016. Expert analysis. Summarizing the current state and evidence on efficacy and safety of statin therapy. Available at: http://www.acc.org/latest-in-cardiology/articles/2016/11/17/09/03/summarizing-the-current-state-and-evidence-on-efficacy-and-safety-of-statin-therapy.

Gonzalez, L., Helkin, A., Gahtan, V., 2016. Dyslipidemia part 2: review of dyslipidemia treatment in patients with noncoronary vascular disease. Vasc. Endovascular Surg. 50, 119–135.

Helkin, A., Stein, J.J., Lin, S., et al., 2016. Dyslipidemia part 1: review of lipid metabolism and vascular cell physiology. Vasc. Endovascular Surg. 50, 107–118.

Henderson, R., O'Kane, M., McGilligan, V., et al., 2016. The genetics and screening of familial hypercholesterolaemia. J. Biomed. Sci. 23, 39.

Hendrani, A.D., Adesiyun, T., Quispe, R., et al., 2016. Dyslipidemia management in primary prevention of cardiovascular disease: current guidelines and strategies. World J. Cardiol. 8, 201–210.

Savarese, G., Gotto Jr., A.M., Paolillo, S., et al., 2013. Benefits of statins in elderly subjects without established cardiovascular disease: a meta-analysis. J. Am. Coll. Cardiol. 62, 2090–2099.

Useful websites

Cardiovascular risk calculators:
ASSIGN: http://assign-score.com
SCORE: https://www.escardio.org/Education/Practice-Tools/CVD-prevention-toolbox/SCORE-Risk-Charts#

QRISK: https://www.qrisk.org
JBS3: www.jbs3risk.com

25 Asthma

Kelly Atack and Ian Clifton

Key points

- Asthma is a common chronic inflammatory disorder of the airways.
- The common symptoms of asthma are breathlessness, wheeze and cough.
- Reversible airflow obstruction is the main physiological measure used in the diagnosis of asthma.
- Asthma triggers should be identified and avoided where possible.
- Poorly controlled asthma remains a significant health burden despite effective therapy.
- The keystone of pharmacological therapy in people with asthma is the delivery of effective anti-inflammatory drugs.
- Well-established national and international guidelines should be used to direct therapy.
- Asthma therapy should be titrated to the lowest effective dose to ensure control with minimal side effects.
- Inhaler technique is crucial to ensure that drug delivery is effective.
- People with asthma should be offered asthma education and self-management plans.

Introduction

Asthma is a chronic inflammatory condition of the airways. The airway inflammation is associated with hyper-responsiveness of the airways and variable airflow obstruction (Global Initiative for Asthma 2012). These physiological changes result in the classic symptoms of intermittent breathlessness, cough and wheeze.

Asthma was first formally described by Hippocrates approximately 2500 years ago. The term *asthma* is derived from the Greek word *aazein*, which describes panting or laboured breathing.

The modern treatment of asthma began with the use of epinephrine at the turn of the 20th century, followed by the introduction of xanthines, such as theophylline, in the 1920s. During the 1950s oral corticosteroids were introduced, with subsequent introduction of chromoglycate, inhaled corticosteroids and short-acting β-agonists in the 1960s. Subsequently, during the 1980s and 1990s long-acting β-agonists and leukotriene antagonists were introduced, respectively. Therapies, particularly for people with severe asthma, have advanced during the early 21st century with the introduction of targeted biological therapy such as omalizumab (anti-immunoglobulin E [IgE]) and mepolizumab (anti-interleukin-5 [IL-5]).

Epidemiology

Asthma is a common condition, with an estimated 300 million people affected worldwide. The prevalence of the condition varies widely in different populations, and it appears to lie in the range of 1–18% (Global Initiative for Asthma, 2012). One of the reasons for this variation in prevalence would appear to be the lack of a strict definition. There may also be overlap with other conditions, such as chronic obstructive pulmonary disease. During childhood, asthma tends to be commoner in boys; however, during adulthood, the condition tends to be more frequent in women (Global Initiative for Asthma, 2012).

Within the UK, the prevalence of asthma is thought to amongst the highest in the world, with an estimated 5.4 million people receiving asthma treatment. Asthma is estimated to affect 1 in 12 adults and 1 in 11 children in the UK. Approximately 900 individuals die from asthma each year in the UK. The National Review of Asthma Deaths identified that the majority of deaths occurred outside of the hospital environment, with only approximately a third (30%) occurring in hospital (Royal College of Physicians, 2014). A common theme in many studies examining asthma deaths is the underuse of personal asthma action plans (PAAPs), overuse of bronchodilators and underuse of corticosteroids.

Aetiology

The aetiology of asthma is complex and not fully elucidated. It is recognised that there is a complex interaction between multiple genetic and environmental factors. There is evidence for a hereditary component to asthma, and current data suggest that multiple genes are involved in the development of asthma. Numerous environmental factors have been identified as potential factors that influence the risk of developing asthma. These include exposure to allergens, infectious agents, occupational substances, air pollution and diet.

One hypothesis for the increasing prevalence of asthma is the 'hygiene hypothesis', which postulates that reduction in early childhood exposure to infectious agents increases the susceptibility to allergic diseases. There are other potential explanations for the increased incidence of asthma in the developing world, including air pollution.

Pathophysiology

Asthma is an inflammatory disorder of the airways, and various inflammatory cells and mediators have been identified as playing an important role in the pathophysiology of asthma.

Bronchial hyper-reactivity is recognised as a key feature of asthma pathophysiology. This results in the airways of people with asthma responding to exposure to particular triggers, which vary from person to person. Exposure to triggers causes constriction of the airway smooth muscle, resulting in bronchoconstriction.

Bronchoconstriction is a result of activation of the parasympathetic pathways of the autonomic nervous system. The release of acetylcholine by the postganglionic nerve fibres activates the M3 muscarinic receptors within the airway smooth muscle. Activation of these receptors results in contraction of the smooth muscle and, consequently, constriction of the diameter the airway.

The inflammatory process follows the bronchoconstriction, resulting in the production of excess mucus and oedema within the airway. The combination of bronchoconstriction and inflammatory process leads to narrowing of the airway calibre and the classic symptoms of breathlessness, wheeze and cough.

Some people with asthma have brittle asthma, which is classified into two types. Type I brittle asthma is defined by periods of prolonged peak flow variability, whereas type II is characterised by sudden deteriorations on a background of good control and relatively normal lung function.

Over the last few years there has been a paradigm shift in the understanding of asthma pathophysiology. This has led to asthma no longer describing a single disease but a collection of multiple subgroups referred to as phenotypes (Wenzel, 2012).

The majority of people with asthma have an inflammatory process driven by T_H2 processes that tend to be associated with atopy, allergy, type I hypersensitivity and eosinophilic inflammation. Asthma associated with an inflammatory process driven by eosinophilic inflammation has long been recognised to be responsive to treatment with corticosteroids (Brown, 1958). The understanding of non-T_H2-driven asthma is much less established than that of asthma driven by T_H2 pathways. This subgroup of people with asthma can be associated with a later age of onset, obesity and neutrophilic inflammation. Lack of response to treatment with corticosteroids tends to be a feature of non-T_H2-driven asthma.

Clinical signs and symptoms

Asthma can present with a number of different symptoms but classically presents with cough, wheeze and breathlessness, often induced by exposure to a wide variety of trigger factors. Individuals with asthma will commonly describe exposure to certain triggers resulting in an increase in symptoms (Table 25.1). The frequency and severity of these symptoms is highly variable between individuals and also within individuals. At times the person with asthma may be asymptomatic, whereas at other times the person may have a high level of symptoms potentially requiring hospital admission. Asthma tends to demonstrate diurnal variation, generally with increased symptoms at night and early in the morning.

Table 25.1 Potential triggers for asthma symptoms

Type of potential trigger	Trigger
Allergens	House dust mite Animal dander Moulds Pollens
Infectious agents	Influenza Rhinovirus
Drugs	Non-steroidal anti-inflammatory drugs Beta blockers Prostaglandins
Occupational	Isocyanates Wheat flour Soy caster bean Latex Formaldehydes Hair colourants
Other	Sulphites Nitrogen oxides Sulphur dioxide Exercise Cold air Stress

There are a number of signs of acute asthma, including tachypnoea (increased rate of respiration), wheeze on expiration and use of accessory muscles of respiration. In children there may also be indrawing of the intercostal muscles.

Investigations

The diagnosis of asthma is a clinical one; there is no standardised definition of the type, severity or frequency of symptoms, nor of the findings on investigation (British Thoracic Society [BTS] and Scottish Intercollegiate Guidelines Network [SIGN], 2016). A key part of the diagnostic process is to identify the characteristic symptoms of asthma from the patient. Due to the long-term nature of the condition, the history obtained from the patient is not sufficient to make the diagnosis, and it is important to use diagnostic tests to provide objective evidence of asthma.

Lung function testing

Lung function testing is a key part of the diagnosis and monitoring for people with asthma. Lung function testing in asthma aims to demonstrate the presence of reversible airflow obstruction. It can also provide a guide to response to treatment and detect deterioration in asthma control. There are a number of different methods for testing lung function, all of which have particular strengths and weaknesses.

Peak expiratory flow rate (PEFR) is the maximum airflow rate during forced expiration. A peak flow meter can measure

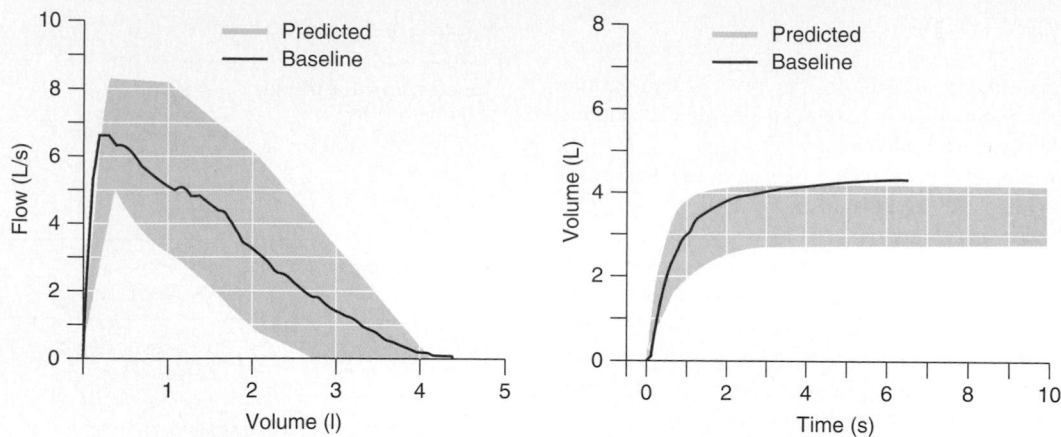

Fig. 25.1 Example flow–volume loop (A) and volume–time curve (B). FEV_1, Forced expiratory volume in 1 second; FVC, forced vital capacity.

Table 25.2 Spirometry parameters

Abbreviation	Term	Definition
FEV_1	Forced expiratory volume in 1 second	Volume of air forcibly expired in 1 second
FVC	Forced vital capacity	Total volume of air forcibly expired at maximum expiration
FEV_1%	Percent of predicted FEV_1	Calculated from normal values for gender, age, height and ethnic origin
FVC%	Percent of predicted FVC	
FEV_1/FVC	Ratio between FEV_1 and FVC	Normal ratio >0.7, if ratio <0.7, then spirometry in keeping with airflow obstruction

FEV_1, Forced expiratory volume in 1 second; FVC, forced vital capacity.

PEFR in a simple portable device that provides a simple and useful method for patients to monitor their asthma. When using a peak flow meter, the patient undertakes three forced expirations through the device and records the highest of the three values.

Measurements of spirometry provide a measure of lung function that is more reproducible than PEFR. Spirometry is preferable to PEFR because it provides a more accurate measure of airflow obstruction. When performing spirometry, an individual inhales to maximal inspiration, then exhales maximally to complete expiration. The spirometry provides a graphical representation of the manoeuvre as a volume–time curve and/or a flow–volume loop (Fig. 25.1). Examination of the spirometry trace as well as review of the spirometry values is important to ensure that the procedure has been performed appropriately. When performing spirometry, the forced expiratory volume in 1 second (FEV_1) and forced vital capacity (FVC) are recorded (see Table 25.2 for definitions of spirometry parameters). This then allows for calculation of the FEV_1/FVC ratio and also the percentage of predicted values.

Further investigations

Sometimes the combination of clinical assessment and measurement of lung function is not sufficient to confirm the diagnosis of asthma, and further investigations are required.

Reversibility testing

Reversibility testing measures the response to bronchodilators or corticosteroids to determine whether there is an improvement in lung function as demonstrated by a change in FEV_1 or PEFR. The use of reversibility testing in individuals with normal or near-normal lung function is limited because there is limited scope for improvement. Salbutamol reversibility is assessed by repeating spirometry after 20 minutes following the administration of 400 micrograms salbutamol. Corticosteroid reversibility can be undertaken by using oral prednisolone for 2 weeks or inhaled beclometasone for 6–8 weeks.

There are a number of definitions of a positive reversibility trial. The European Respiratory Society/American Thoracic Society (ERS/ATS) guidelines define a positive test as greater than 200 mL or 12% improvement in FEV_1 and/or FVC in response to treatment with bronchodilators or corticosteroids (Pellegrino et al., 2005). The National Institute for Health and Care Excellence (NICE) uses a higher threshold requiring greater than 400 mL improvement in FEV_1 (NICE, 2010).

Measurement of airway hyper-responsiveness

Testing of airway hyper-responsiveness has long been established as a research tool, and such testing is now starting to become more routine in clinical practice. These tests are generally more useful in patients with normal or near-normal spirometry. The tests aim to demonstrate bronchoconstriction in response to administration of an inhaled challenge. A number of substances can be used as challenges, including histamine, methacholine and mannitol.

Measures of airway inflammation

Eosinophilic airway inflammation can be determined using induced sputum differential counts or measurement of the fraction of exhaled nitric oxide (FeNO). Evidence of active eosinophilic airway inflammation is seen more commonly in people with asthma but also would seem to predict an increased response rate to corticosteroids (Green et al., 2002a).

Other tests

Other tests that can be useful in supporting the diagnosis include measurement of blood eosinophil count, measurement of serum IgE and testing for atopy through either skin-prick testing or IgE testing for specific allergens. For individuals with atypical features, consideration should be undertaken for a chest X-ray (BTS and SIGN, 2016).

Treatment

Chronic treatment

The aim of asthma management is to have complete control and have no exacerbations of the disease. The BTS defines complete asthma control as the following (BTS and SIGN, 2016):

- no daytime symptoms,
- no night-time wakening due to asthma symptoms,
- no requirement for rescue medication,
- no asthma attacks/exacerbations,
- no limitations on activity,
- normal lung function – FEV_1 and/or peak expiratory flow (PEF) greater than 80% predicted or best,
- minimal adverse effects from medication.

BTS guidelines recommend that treatment should begin at the most appropriate step to improve symptoms and lung function as quickly as possible (Fig. 25.2; BTS and SIGN, 2016).

Treatment must be balanced against the risk of adverse effects and should be titrated down where possible whilst keeping good control of asthma. Prior to moving treatment up a step, adherence and inhaler technique must be assessed and any triggers should be removed.

Inhaled corticosteroids

Corticosteroids bind to glucocorticoid receptors within the lung and decrease the formation of cytokines, which produce IgE and promote the expression of IgE receptors. They also inhibit the influx of eosinophils into the lung, therefore reducing overall inflammation. Inhaled corticosteroids (ICSs) are recommended as the second step as a regular preventative therapy in the BTS guidelines

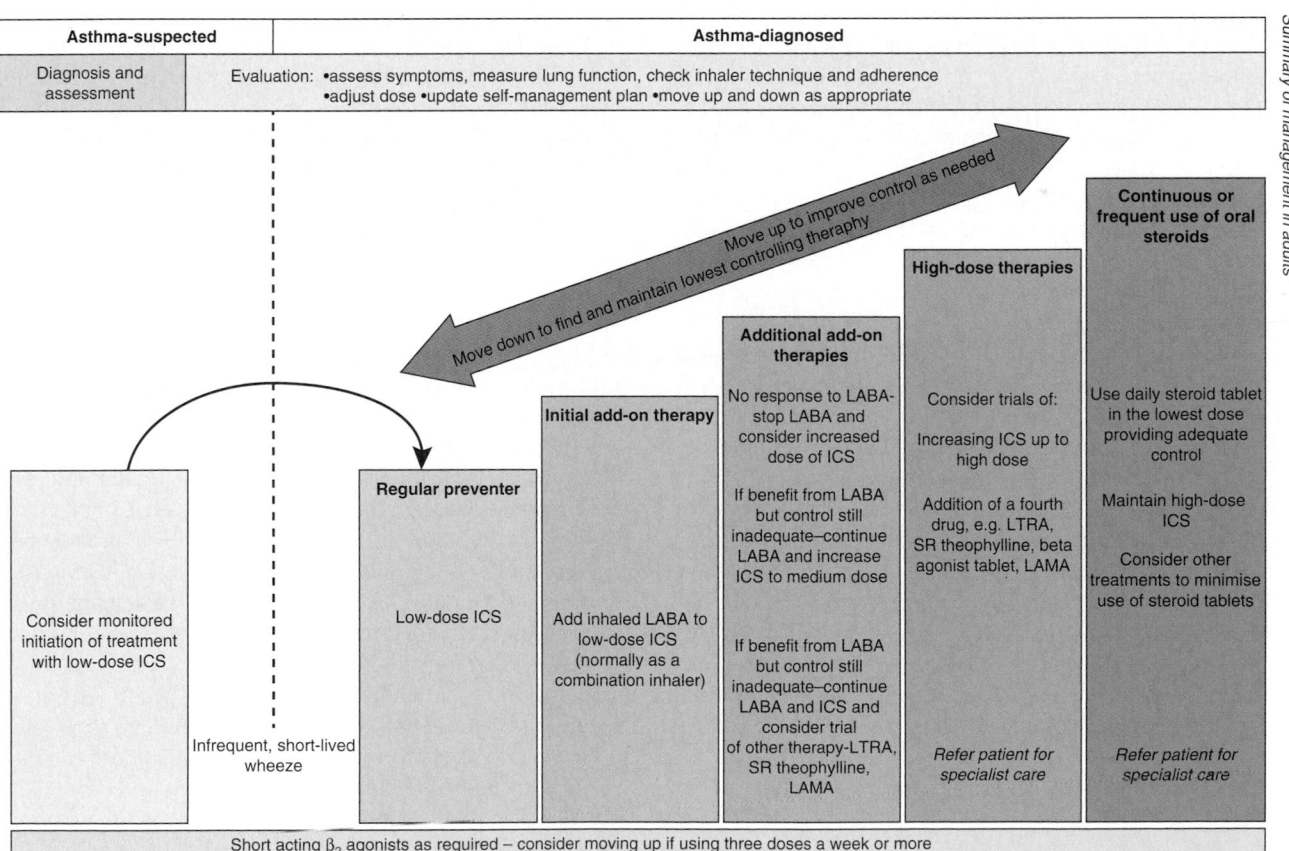

Fig. 25.2 Summary of stepwise management of asthma in adults (BTS and SIGN, 2016).
ICS, Inhaled corticosteroids; LABA, long-acting β-agonist; LAMA, long-acting antimuscarinics; LTRA, leukotriene antagonists; SR, sustained release.
Reproduced from BTS/SIGN British Guideline on the management of asthma by kind permission of the British Thoracic Society.

(BTS and SIGN, 2016), for all people with asthma, except those with very mild and occasional symptoms, where 'as-required' symptomatic treatment with short-acting β2-agonists alone may be sufficient. Standard doses of ICSs are suggested as 200–400 micrograms/day of beclometasone dipropionate (BDP) or equivalent in 24 hours. For adults, it is recommended that patients commence treatment at a dose of 200–800 micrograms/day of BDP or equivalent. This can be increased to up to 2000 micrograms/day of BDP or equivalent as a fourth step if patients have no response to the addition of a long-acting β-agonist (LABA) or a trial of alternative agents (BTS and SIGN, 2016). It should be noted, however, that at doses of 800 micrograms/day of BDP or equivalent, this will achieve 90% clinical benefit for the patient. At doses higher than this there is a significant increase in adverse effects (Holt et al., 2001). Budesonide, ciclesonide, fluticasone and mometasone are other ICSs that are available and widely used.

Administering drugs via the inhalation route allows the drug to be delivered directly into the lungs, allowing it to take action in the target organ and reducing systemic absorption and therefore the risk of adverse effects. It is imperative to note, however, that using corticosteroids in the inhaled form is not without risk. Patients on long-term, high-dose ICSs (i.e. at a dose of more than 1000 micrograms/day of beclometasone or equivalent) are encouraged to carry a steroid card with them and should be educated of the potential serious adverse effects (BTS and SIGN, 2016). ICSs can cause oral candidiasis and dysphonia; hence, encouraging patients to rinse the mouth after use is important. Long-term, high-dose ICS use will result in some of the steroid being absorbed systemically, potentially leading to adverse effects, including increased blood glucose and susceptibility to diabetes. ICSs can also lead to osteoporosis, increasing the risk of fractures, muscle wasting and impaired wound healing. They can also cause psychiatric reactions and mood disorders, as well as adrenal suppression, which may lead to the patient requiring steroid replacement therapy. Consequently, it is important to inform the patients of the risks associated with ICSs and consider the risk versus benefit of them, particularly in patients with medical conditions that may be exacerbated by the use of steroids.

ICSs are available in a variety of devices, in combination with a LABA or as individual agents. In some circumstances they are used in conjunction with a LABA as a reliever, such as in the 'Maintenance and Reliever Therapy' regimen. Traditionally, there were few devices containing ICSs available to patients. More recently there has been an influx of new devices into the UK market. This gives patients and healthcare professionals more choice with regard to selecting the most appropriate device. Care needs to be taken, however, when changing a patient's inhaled therapy due to the variety of different devices and doses currently available (Table 25.3).

Because there is some systemic absorption, ICSs also have interactions with other medicines. Itraconazole and ritonavir, in particular, interact significantly by inhibiting the metabolism of ICSs and can increase levels enough to induce adrenal suppression.

Short-acting β-agonists

Short-acting β-agonists (SABAs), such as salbutamol and terbutaline, are the first-line step and should be prescribed for all asthma patients and should be used on a when-required basis (BTS and SIGN, 2016). Patients with very infrequent signs and symptoms of asthma may require only a SABA. Excessive use of SABAs, defined as more than one canister per month, has been associated with an increased risk of asthma death.

Additionally, oral SABAs are not recommended due their higher risk of systemic side effects compared with administration via inhalation.

Long-acting β-agonists

LABAs act on the β2-receptors in the smooth muscle of the bronchi, aiding bronchodilation. Inhaled LABAs are a first-line addition to ICSs and can be administered as an individual ingredient or in a combination inhaler with an ICS. The addition of a LABA to a low-dose ICS has been shown to be as effective as increasing the ICS dose and may be associated with fewer side effects. LABAs, such as salmeterol, formoterol fumarate and vilanterol, are designed to be used regularly but have different characteristics in terms of onset and duration of action (Table 25.4). Indacaterol and olodaterol are LABAs designed for once-daily administration; however, they are not currently licensed for use in asthma.

LABAs can exert an effect on β-receptors elsewhere and are not completely selective to β2-receptors. Consequently, they also affect the β1-receptors in the cardiac muscle, increasing cardiac output and stimulation, leading to tachycardia and arrhythmias. Additionally, they can cause tremor and hypokalaemia. LABAs used alone have been associated with an increased risk of death and therefore should not be used without an ICS (Royal College of Physicians, 2014). The Medicines and Healthcare Products Regulatory Agency (MHRA) recommends that LABAs should ideally be administered in a combination inhaler to aid adherence (MHRA, 2008). There are not many interactions with LABAs, but care must be taken when using LABAs with other agents that cause hypokalaemia. Due to the cardiac risks associated with the use of LABAs, it is important to step down treatment where possible for safety.

The use of LABAs as monotherapy in asthma is associated with significantly worse asthma outcomes and increased asthma mortality compared with treatment with ICSs. This increased mortality is not seen when LABAs and ICSs are used concurrently. Consequently, national (BTS and SIGN, 2016) and international (Global Initiative for Asthma, 2012) guidelines are very clear that long-acting relievers should not be prescribed without an ICS and where possible should be prescribed as a combination ICS/LABA inhaler to prevent people inadvertently taking only the LABA. Table 25.5 demonstrates that there are a large number of ICS/LABA preparations and devices currently on the market and that it is important to be aware of the different strengths when swapping between devices. Some patients may require a regimen requiring the separate components in separate inhaler devices, for example, if ciclesonide is prescribed as an alternative to other ICSs due to oropharyngeal side effects. However, patients in this situation must be made aware of the importance of adhering to both the LABA and the ICS.

When added to an existing ICS, LABAs are used in preference to leukotriene receptor antagonists because they provide greater control and reduce exacerbation rates (Chauhan and Ducharme, 2014).

Table 25.3 Equivalent steroid doses for inhaled corticosteroids

Name	Device	Equivalence to 400 micrograms of beclometasone dipropionate
Beclometasone dipropionate		
Asmabec	Clickhaler	400 micrograms
Clenil	pMDI	400 micrograms
Easyhaler beclometasone	Easyhaler	200 micrograms
Fostair	pMDI and Nexthaler	200 micrograms
Qvar	Autohaler, Easi-Breathe and pMDI	200 micrograms
Budesonide		
Budelin	Novolizer	400 micrograms
DuoResp	Spiromax	200 micrograms
Easyhaler budesonide	Easyhaler	400 micrograms
Pulmicort	Turbohaler	400 micrograms
Symbicort	Turbohaler	400 micrograms
Ciclesonide		
Ciclesonide	pMDI	200–300 micrograms
Fluticasone furoate		
Relvar	Ellipta	200 micrograms
Fluticasone propionate		
Flixotide	Accuhaler and pMDI	200 micrograms
Flutiform	pMDI	200 micrograms
Seretide	Accuhaler and pMDI	200 micrograms
Sirdupla	pMDI	200 micrograms
Mometasone furoate		
Asmanex	Twisthaler	200 micrograms

pMDI, Pressurised metered dose inhaler.

Table 25.4 Pharmacokinetic characteristics of different long-acting β-agonists

Drug	Onset of action (min)	Duration of action (h)
Formoterol	2–3	12
Salmeterol	10–14	12
Vilanterol	5–15	24

Table 25.5 Approximate equivalent dose of combination inhaled corticosteroids/long-acting β-agonist inhalers

Name and device	Active ingredients	Low dose (micrograms per dose)	Medium dose (micrograms per dose)	High dose (micrograms per dose)
DuoResp Spiromax	Budesonide and formoterol	160/4.5 1 puff BD	160/4.5 2 puffs BD 320/9 1 puff BD	320/9 2 puffs BD
Flutiform pMDI	Fluticasone and formoterol	50/5 2 puffs BD	125/5 2 puffs BD	250/10 2 puffs BD
Fostair pMDI	Beclometasone and formoterol	100/6 1 puff BD	100/6 2 puffs BD 200/6 1 puff BD	200/6 2 puffs BD
Fostair NEXThaler	Beclometasone and formoterol	100/6 1 puff BD	100/6 2 puffs BD 200/6 1 puff BD	200/6 2 puffs BD
Relvar Ellipta	Fluticasone and vilanterol		92/22 1 puff OD	184/22 1 puffs OD
Seretide Accuhaler	Fluticasone and salmeterol	100/50 1 puff BD	250/50 1 puff BD	500/50 1 puff BD
Seretide pMDI	Fluticasone and salmeterol	50/25 2 puffs BD	125/25 2 puffs BD	250/25 2 puff BD
Sirdupla pMDI	Fluticasone and salmeterol		125/25 2 puffs BD	250/25 2 puffs BD
Symbicort Turbohaler	Budesonide and formoterol	100/6 1–2 puffs BD 200/6 1–2 puffs BD		400/12 1–2 puffs BD

BD, Twice daily; OD, once daily; pMDI, pressurised metered dose inhaler.

Leukotriene antagonists

Leukotriene antagonists work by reducing the inflammation in the bronchi, by inhibiting leukotriene receptors in the respiratory mucosa and reducing sputum eosinophilia. Leukotriene antagonists such as montelukast and zafirlukast are recommended for use in the UK when patients are not responding to a LABA or as an addition to an ICS/LABA combination inhaler in someone with persistent poor control.

There is some evidence for their use in addition to ICSs, and they have been shown to be particularly useful for people with exercise-induced asthma (Malmstrom et al., 1999) and potentially for patients with allergic rhinitis (Nathan, 2003). They can be taken orally, and there are a number of preparations available, including granules if patients have problems with swallowing solid oral dosage forms.

Leukotriene antagonists are commonly associated with relatively mild side effects of headaches and gastro-intestinal side effects. However, they are also rarely associated with the more serious eosinophilic granulomatosis with polyangiitis (previously known as Churg-Strauss syndrome). This is characterised by vasculitis and eosinophilia, and care should be taken to inform patients of this rare adverse effect. There are minimal drug interactions associated with the leukotriene antagonists.

Long-acting antimuscarinics

Long-acting antimuscarinics (LAMAs) work by binding to the muscarinic M3 receptors in the smooth muscle of the lung to aid bronchodilation. LAMAs may also be trialled in patients who have not responded to an ICS/LABA combination in the fourth step of the BTS guidelines (BTS and SIGN, 2016). Tiotropium

has been demonstrated to improve asthma control and quality of life as well as reduce exacerbation frequency in patients with severe asthma (Rodrigo and Castro-Rodriguez, 2015). The other currently marketed LAMAs – aclidinium, glycopyrronium and umeclidinium – are not currently licensed for use in asthma. It should be noted that they have antimuscarinic side effects throughout the body and can cause dry mouth, constipation, urinary retention and angle-closure glaucoma.

Theophylline preparations

Theophylline and aminophylline are methylxanthines and work as bronchodilators and stimulate respiration. The exact mechanism of action is unclear, and their effect is not specific to the lung. Oral theophylline and aminophylline can be used as an alternative in the same way as the leukotriene antagonists when patients are unresponsive to LABAs or as an addition to an ICS/LABA combination inhaler (BTS and SIGN, 2016).

Methylxanthines have a narrow therapeutic window and require close monitoring of serum theophylline levels to ensure a therapeutic dose and avoid toxicity. Levels should be taken 5 days after commencing treatment or changing doses and annually, with the aim of achieving a serum level of 10–20 mg/L. At toxic levels methylxanthines have effects on the central nervous system, causing tremor and action on cardiac muscle α-receptors that results in increased cardiac output and tachycardia, as well as constricting cerebral blood vessels. Because theophylline may also cause convulsions, care must be taken when prescribing for people with epilepsy. The use of theophylline should be reviewed regularly. The risk of cardiotoxicity and high plasma concentrations should be taken into consideration to ensure that the benefit outweighs the risk.

Table 25.6 Drug interactions with theophylline

Drug	Interaction
Azole antifungals (itraconazole, fluconazole)	May increase theophylline levels
Calcium-channel antagonists (diltiazem, verapamil)	May increase theophylline levels
Carbamazepine	May decrease theophylline levels
Cimetidine	May increase theophylline levels
Fluvoxamine	May increase theophylline levels
Isoniazid	May increase theophylline levels
Lithium carbonate	Increased lithium levels
Macrolide antibiotics (azithromycin, clarithromycin, erythromycin)	May increase theophylline levels
Phenytoin	May reduce theophylline and phenytoin levels
Primidone	Decreased theophylline levels
Quinolone antibiotics (ciprofloxacin, norfloxacin)	May increase theophylline levels
Rifampicin	Decreased theophylline levels
Ritonavir	May increase theophylline levels
St John's wort	May reduce theophylline levels

Theophylline is metabolised using the cytochrome P450 pathway; therefore, its plasma concentration can be decreased by enzyme inducers and increased by drugs that inhibit cytochrome P450 (Table 25.6). Unfortunately, antimicrobials that may be used for the treatment of respiratory tract infections, such as ciprofloxacin and clarithromycin, inhibit cytochrome P450. Therefore, patients should be informed to halve the dose of theophylline whilst taking these medicines, to ensure levels are not increased and cause toxicity. Care should be taken when prescribing medicines concurrently with theophylline, and interactions should be checked to assess the risk of toxicity.

Biological therapies

Biological therapies are slowly being introduced into the UK for treatment of allergic asthma. Omalizumab is a humanised monoclonal anti-IgE antibody. It works to reduce the amount of circulating IgE and reduce the inflammatory response. Omalizumab is being more widely used in particular and is licensed for use in patients with uncontrolled asthma where their asthma is mediated by the presence of IgE. In the UK, it is approved for people with allergic asthma who need continuous or frequent treatment with oral corticosteroids and had at least four courses in the last year (NICE, 2013). It has been shown to significantly reduce the number of exacerbations in patients with severe asthma who have not improved on standard treatments.

Omalizumab is administered as a subcutaneous injection two to four times weekly, and it can take up to 12–16 weeks before an effect is felt. The dose of omalizumab is calculated according to the individual's weight and serum IgE levels.

Mepolizumab is another humanised monoclonal antibody. It targets IL-5, which is responsible for activating eosinophils, and is used for patients with severe refractory eosinophilic asthma. It has recently been approved for use in the UK for people with severe eosinophilic asthma requiring frequent or daily oral corticosteroids (NICE, 2017).

Because biological therapies are not metabolised, there are minimal drug interactions, although there are concerns regarding the possibility of an anaphylactic reaction during therapy. Patients are therefore expected to have these injections administered in a specialist hospital setting (BTS and SIGN, 2016).

More biological therapies targeted at specific parts of the inflammatory response are being developed to reduce the need for oral steroids and their associated side effects. However, such therapies are likely to be expensive and therefore only used in specialist centres.

Oral corticosteroids

Oral corticosteroids, such as prednisolone, can be used for the treatment of both exacerbations and chronic asthma. A maintenance dose of oral corticosteroids is occasionally used for chronic asthma treatment for individuals requiring multiple courses of oral steroids who are on the fifth step of treatment (BTS and SIGN, 2016). Individuals who may require long-term oral corticosteroids should be referred to a specialist clinic for review of their asthma and treatment plan. These drugs should be used at the lowest dose possible and regularly reviewed, and patients should be monitored for risk of adverse effects. Corticosteroids will reduce lung inflammation; however, they also have systemic adverse effects. The risk of these serious adverse effects must be thoroughly considered to ensure that patients are gaining benefit from oral corticosteroid use. Patients should be fully informed of the risks of long-term oral steroids. Other treatments, such as calcium and vitamin D, bisphosphonates for bone protection and medicines for gastric protection, may also be required when the patient is prescribed oral corticosteroids.

Care must also be taken to consider interactions with oral corticosteroids because they can increase the risk of gastro-intestinal bleeding. Other medicines that increase the risk of this (e.g. non-steroidal anti-inflammatory drugs [NSAIDs] and selective serotonin re-uptake inhibitors [SSRIs]) should be used with caution.

Steroid-sparing agents

Steroid-sparing agents, such as methotrexate, ciclosporin and oral gold, have been used in some patients with difficult-to-treat asthma to reduce the risk of adverse effects from prolonged use of corticosteroids, despite a limited evidence base (Davies et al., 1998; Evans et al., 2000a,b). When used, they are prescribed on a 3-month trial after discussion with the patient about the potential

Table 25.7 Classification of acute asthma severity (BTS and SIGN, 2016)

Severity of exacerbation	Characteristics
Moderate asthma	Increased symptoms PEFR 50–75% of best or predicted No features of acute severe asthma
Acute severe asthma	Any one of the following features: • PEFR 33–50% of best or predicted • ≥25 breaths/min • Heart rate ≥110 beats/min • Inability to complete sentences in one breath
Life-threatening asthma	One of the following features in a patient with acute severe asthma: • PEFR <33% of best or predicted • PaO_2 ≤8 kPa • Normal $PaCO_2$ (4.6–6.0 kPa) • sO_2 <92% • Altered consciousness level • Exhaustion or poor respiratory effort • Haemodynamic instability as defined by cardiac arrhythmias or hypotension • Cyanosis • Silent chest
Near-fatal asthma	One of the following features: $PaCO_2$ >6.0 kPa Need for mechanical ventilation with raised inflation pressures

$PaCO_2$, Partial pressure of carbon dioxide in arterial blood; PaO_2, partial pressure of oxygen in arterial blood; PEFR, peak expiratory forced reserve.

Box 25.1 Factors lowering the threshold for admission to hospital

- People younger than 18 years
- Poor adherence to medication
- Person living alone
- Psychological problems, such as depression, and alcohol or drug misuse
- Physical or learning disability
- Previous near-fatal attack or brittle asthma
- Persistent exacerbation despite an adequate dose of oral corticosteroids before presentation
- Presentation at night or in the afternoon
- Pregnancy

risks. It is recommended they are only used under the supervision of a specialist severe asthma service (BTS and SIGN, 2016).

Cromones

Inhaled sodium cromoglicate and nedocromil have a limited role in the management of asthma, and they are significantly less effective than ICS therapy (BTS and SIGN, 2016). They are rarely used in current practice.

Acute treatment

When assessing a person with an acute exacerbation of asthma, it is important to ask about possible trigger factors, such as recent allergen exposure or upper respiratory tract viral infections (Green et al., 2002b). An acute exacerbation of asthma needs prompt assessment and appropriate treatment because it represents a potentially life-threatening condition.

Risk stratification and assessment

The severity of an acute exacerbation of asthma is determined by a number of different clinical factors and is categorised as moderate, acute severe, life-threatening or near-fatal (Table 25.7). This risk stratification provides guidance on the need for admission to

hospital. Patients with life-threatening or near-fatal asthma should be admitted to hospital for assessment and treatment. Patients with acute severe asthma who have responded to initial therapy and have no other concerning features do not need to be admitted to hospital. Patients should be assessed for a number of other factors because these may influence the threshold for referral for admission to hospital (see Box 25.1).

Treatment

Acute asthma can be life-threatening, and treatment aims to relieve immediate symptoms, improve bronchoconstriction and address airway inflammation. Acute asthma is stratified according to clinical observations and investigations (see Table 25.7). Acute severe asthma is defined as the patient's peak flow reduced to between 33–50% of the patient's best or predicted, increased respiratory rate of more than 25 breaths per minute, heart rate of more than 110 beats per minute and the patient is unable to complete a sentence in one breath. Life-threatening asthma is defined as the peak flow being less than 33% of the patient's best or predicted, oxygen saturation of less than 92%, silent chest, reduced respiratory effort, hypotension and an altered state of consciousness. Sufficient treatment with steroids and monitoring of the patient's condition are key factors in ensuring the patient's recovery. Overuse of β-agonist therapy has been associated with asthma death; therefore, care must be taken and monitoring undertaken.

Oxygen. Patients with severe or life-threatening acute asthma should have their oxygen saturation maintained at 94–98% to treat hypoxia. These patients should be administered oxygen via a face mask, Venturi mask or nasal cannulae as a matter of urgency. Pulse oximetry should be used to measure oxygen saturation where possible; however, this should not be a barrier to the use of oxygen in this situation if unavailable (BTS and SIGN, 2016; O'Driscoll et al., 2008).

Bronchodilators. Inhaled β-agonists should also be administered in emergency situations to treat bronchoconstriction. High doses should be given via the nebulised route where possible. However, if the patient is at home, they can administer 4–6 puffs at one time of a SABA into a large-volume spacer and take multiple breaths in and out of this device. Patients should have their potassium and heart rate monitored due to the potential adverse effects of hypokalaemia and tachycardia associated with nebulised β-agonist use (BTS and SIGN, 2016).

If their response to nebulised β-agonists is poor, or in cases of severe exacerbations, then there is evidence for the addition of nebulised ipratropium for increased bronchodilation (Lanes et al., 1998). Ipratropium is an antimuscarinic and works on the M3 receptors to relax the smooth muscle of the bronchi to induce bronchodilation.

Intravenous salbutamol and terbutaline have also been used; however, these are no longer recommended because nebulised salbutamol is a safer option. The only scenario where they could be considered would be where a patient was not responding to β-agonists via an inhaled route (BTS and SIGN, 2016; Travers et al., 2012).

Corticosteroids. Oral corticosteroids should be administered after an acute asthma attack at the earliest stage possible for the most benefit (Rowe et al., 2007). There is much evidence suggesting they will reduce the risk of another attack and aid recovery time, as well as decrease mortality (Rowe et al., 2007). Oral prednisolone should be administered at a dose of 40–50 mg daily, preferably in the morning to mimic the body's natural cortisol production and reduce adverse effects, including insomnia. If the oral route is unavailable, then intravenous hydrocortisone may be administered at a dose of 100 mg four times daily until the oral route is available again.

Corticosteroid therapy should be continued for at least 5 days but can be extended until the patient's condition has improved. Additionally, corticosteroids can be stopped without needing to wean down the dose unless they have been prescribed for longer than 2 weeks or if the patient is already taking maintenance corticosteroids because this poses a risk of adrenal suppression. The shortest course length possible should be used to protect patients from the adverse effects of corticosteroids (BTS and SIGN, 2016).

Intravenous magnesium. Patients who have not responded well to initial bronchodilator therapy can be administered a dose of intravenous magnesium at a dose of 1.2–2 g over 20 minutes. This can aid bronchodilation and reduce the requirement for admission to hospital (Rowe et al., 2000). It has minimal adverse effects unless repeated doses are administered and hypermagnesaemia develops. Blood pressure, respiratory rate and urine output should be monitored whilst intravenous magnesium is administered. Signs of toxicity, including weakness, nausea, drowsiness and slurred speech, should also be monitored.

Intravenous aminophylline. Intravenous aminophylline may be commenced in severe acute asthma to aid with bronchodilation, although evidence suggests it does not provide additional bronchodilation compared with SABAs (Travers et al., 2012). Care should be taken with regards to the dosing of intravenous aminophylline. A loading dose should be administered to patients who are not taking oral theophylline or aminophylline already. Smoking status also needs to be obtained because patients who smoke require a higher maintenance dose; conversely, patients with heart failure require lower loading doses as per Table 25.8. The risk of arrhythmias and toxicity due to high plasma concentrations should be taken into consideration before commencement. Patients require daily plasma concentration levels to ensure safety. Due

Table 25.8 Dosing of intravenous aminophylline

Patient characteristics	Loading dose
Adult already taking oral theophylline/aminophylline	No loading dose required
Adult not taking oral theophylline/aminophylline	5 mg/kg over 20 min
	Maintenance dose
Elderly adult/adult with heart failure	0.3 mg/kg/h
Nonsmoking adult	0.5 mg/kg/h
Smoking adult	0.7 mg/kg/h

to the risks involved with intravenous aminophylline and also the monitoring involved, this should not be commenced without specialist medical input.

Antibiotics. Acute asthma exacerbations are mostly caused by exposure to allergens or viruses. Consequently, antibiotics are not indicated and should not be commenced without clear evidence of a bacterial cause (Graham et al., 2001).

Patient care
Structure of an asthma review

There are a number of issues that should be addressed during an asthma review to ensure that it is as effective as possible. Firstly the degree of asthma control needs to be assessed. If the person's asthma symptoms are controlled, then potentially a step down in therapy may be indicated. Conversely, when the person's asthma is not at the appropriate level of control, a number of factors will need to be assessed prior to stepping up pharmacological therapy. These include assessment of trigger factors, concordance and inhaler technique (Fig. 25.3).

Assessment of asthma control

One key aspect of an asthma review is determining the level of control. The degree of asthma control can be assessed using a number of different methodologies.

There are several different definitions used to report symptoms in clinical practice. These include:
- Global Initiative for Asthma definition (Global Initiative for Asthma, 2012; Table 25.9),
- Royal College of Physicians 3 questions (Pearson and Bucknall, 1999),
- Asthma Control Questionnaire (Juniper et al., 1999),
- Asthma Control Test (Nathan et al., 2004).

Other physiological tests can be useful to help to monitor asthma control, including lung function (PEFR or FEV_1) or measures of eosinophilic airway inflammation (Green et al., 2002a).

Patient education

It is important to provide high-quality and accurate information to people with asthma. This information is crucial for achievement of adherence with therapy and improving patient outcomes. There are a number of organisations that can help provide information for patients (see Box 25.2).

Inhaler technique

Good inhaler technique is imperative in optimising asthma treatment. Many new devices are now available. This allows for more patient choice but also requires healthcare professionals to be trained in their use so that they can provide accurate patient training. Optimal inhaler technique is paramount in ensuring the drug is delivered into the lung for it to exert its action. Errors

in inhaler technique have been associated with reduced asthma control (Giraud and Roche, 2002). Inhaler technique should be reassessed during regular asthma reviews and should also be reassessed after an exacerbation. Inhaler devices should be chosen based on patient choice and the patient's ability to use them (BTS and SIGN, 2016). It should be appreciated that every inhaler has a different number of steps that need to be achieved to allow the drug to be accurately delivered. Simplifying information is a good approach to helping patients retain the correct technique.

The most common inhaler device prescribed in the UK is the pressurised metered dose inhaler (pMDI), which contains an aerosol, yet it has been shown that only 21% of patients are able to use pMDIs correctly even after expert training (Lenney et al., 2000). In stable patients, their inhaler technique should be checked at every asthma review. Patients should also be checked after an

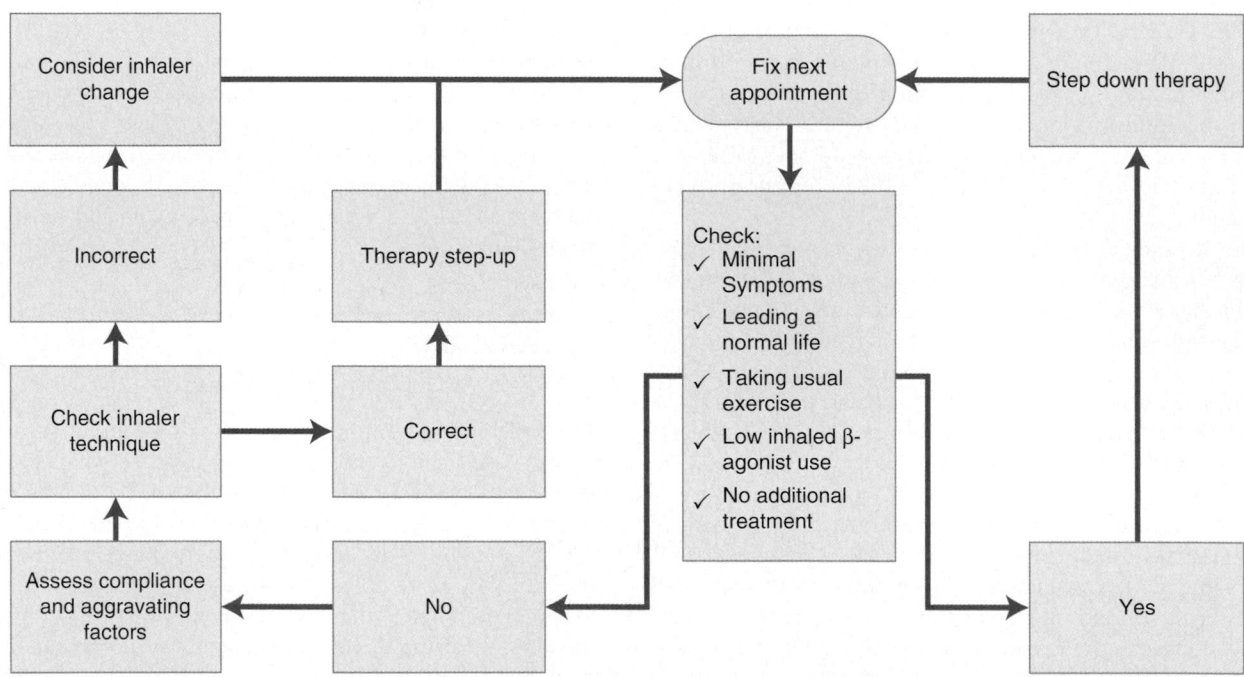

Fig. 25.3   Structure of an asthma review. (Adapted from Crompton et al., 2006.)

Table 25.9   Definition of asthma control

Characteristic	Controlled asthma	Partly controlled asthma	Uncontrolled
	All characteristics present	Any characteristic present	
Daytime symptoms	<2 per week	>2 per week	
Limitations of daily activity	None	Any	
Night-time symptoms or awakening from sleep	None	Any	3 or more characteristics of partly controlled asthma present in any week
Lung function as measured by PEFR or FEV$_1$	Normal	<80%	
Use of reliever inhaler	<2 per week	>2 per week	

FEV$_1$, Forced expiratory volume in 1 second; PEFR, peak expiratory flow rate.
Adapted from Global Initiative for Asthma (2012).

exacerbation and each time there is a decision made to switch inhalers. Inhalers should not be changed or the dose increased without ensuring that the patient can use the inhaler optimally. Additionally, using inhalers correctly will reduce waste, improve patient outcomes and reduce the risk of adverse effects such as oral candidiasis (Basheti et al., 2007; Capstick and Clifton, 2012).

Particle size, inspiratory flow and resistance all affect lung deposition of the inhaled drug. The particle size of the drug decides the location in which it will be deposited. Ideally, inhaled drugs should have a particle size of 1–5 micrometres for them to be deposited within the airways and have an effect on the receptors within the bronchi. There are some pMDIs that have been developed with extra-fine particles, allowing a reduced dose of corticosteroid to be used, and these have been shown to have improved lung deposition compared with standard pMDIs (Basheti et al., 2007; Capstick and Clifton, 2012).

Inspiratory flow also has an impact on lung deposition, and each device requires a different level. Dry powder inhalers (DPIs) require a quick inspiratory flow so that the dose is broken up into small enough particles to penetrate the airways, whereas pMDIs require a slower inspiratory flow. Failing to achieve the desired inspiratory flow for any device increases the likelihood that the drug will deposit into the mouth and oropharynx rather than the lungs, leading to a lack of efficacy and an increased risk of oral side effects. The inspiratory flow is determined by the effort of the patient during inspiration and the resistance to airflow within the device. pMDIs have a low resistance to airflow, meaning they require less effort on inhalation, whereas DPIs

have a high resistance to airflow, requiring more effort on inhalation (Capstick and Clifton, 2012).

Inhaler devices can be split into pMDIs, DPIs, breath-actuated metered-dose inhalers (BA-MDIs) and soft-mist inhalers (SMIs), with each device requiring a different technique (Table 25.10). Many patients using pMDIs find the coordination of pressing the canister down to deliver the dose whilst inhaling difficult. BA-MDIs or DPIs may be more appropriate for use in these patients, or the use of a spacer may be beneficial. These strategies remove the need for coordination. Additionally, spacer devices reduce the amount of resistance and decrease particle size, thus allowing improved drug deposition (Capstick and Clifton, 2012).

DPIs may involve the loading of a single capsule manually by the patient or be multiple-dose devices, which may require other manipulation by the patient to load the dose. The only SMI device available in the UK is the Respimat device. This device requires multiple steps to prepare the dose and administer the drug, but it removes the reliance on the patient's inspiratory flow to deliver the drug (Capstick and Clifton, 2012).

Prior to prescribing an inhaler, healthcare professionals must check the patient's inspiratory flow and inhaler technique. The In-Check Dial Inspiratory Flow Meter or inhaler device whistles can be used to test inspiratory flow. Placebo inhalers are also available to help train patients on how to use new devices (Capstick and Clifton, 2012).

Different inhaler devices

Pressurised metered dose inhaler

The pMDI (Fig. 25.4) is a cost-effective device used widely. It is a pressurised aerosol device and can be used with spacer devices if needed. It is available for several drugs, although a popular choice can be difficult to use due to the coordination required. Inhalation should be slow and deep for this device; if patients inhale too quickly using this device, the aerosol will hit the back of the pharynx rather than travel to the lungs and deposit in the desired area.

Box 25.2 Organisations that provide educational material for people with asthma

- Asthma UK: http://www.asthma.org.uk
- British Lung Foundation: http://www.lunguk.org
- Allergy UK: http://www.allergyuk.org
- Global Initiative for Asthma: http://www.ginasthma.org
- European Lung Foundation: http://www.europeanlung.org
- NHS Choices: http://www.nhs.uk/Conditions/Asthma

Table 25.10 Guide to suitability of inhaler devices according to the patient's inspiratory flow and ability to coordinate inhaler actuation and inhalation

Inspiratory flow	Good actuation–inhalation coordination		Poor actuation–inhalation coordination	
	>30 L/min	<30 L/min	>30 L/min	<30 L/min
pMDI	✓	✓	✓	✓
BA-MDI	✓		✓	
pMDI + spacer	✓	✓	✓	✓
Dry powder inhaler	✓		✓	
Soft-mist inhaler	✓		✓	✓
Nebuliser	✓	✓	✓	✓

BA-MDI, Breath-actuated metered dose inhaler; pMDI, pressurised metered dose inhaler.
Adapted from Voshaar et al. (2001).

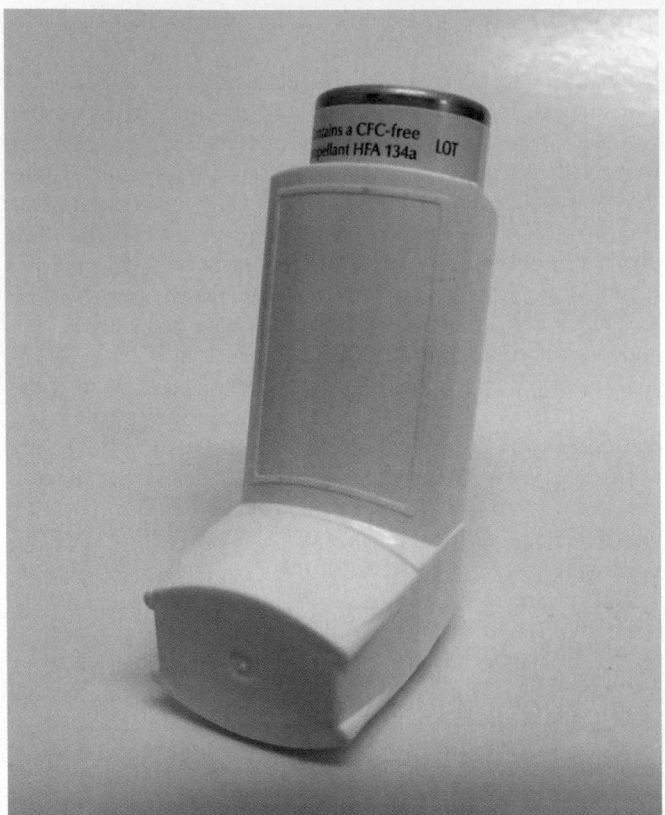

Fig.25.4 Pressurised metered dose inhaler. (Reproduced by kind permission of T. Capstick.)

Breath-actuated metered dose inhaler

Easi-Breathe. The Easi-Breathe device is a BA-MDI and is an aerosol inhaler. The Easi-Breathe device may be favourable for those patients who struggle with the coordination aspect of the pMDI. This device again requires slow and deep inhalation.

Autohaler. The Autohaler device is another type of breath-actuated inhaler that requires priming by pushing a lever into the vertical position prior to inhalation. Slow and steady inhalation is required for this device.

Dry powder inhalers

Ellipta. The Ellipta is a new, simple DPI that is primed by opening the cover completely until a click is heard. It has a dose counter; however, doses may be wasted if the cap is opened multiple times or if the device is not held upright. It requires deep and strong inhalation to achieve drug deposition into the lungs.

Nexthaler. The Nexthaler is a new DPI device (Fig. 25.5) that also requires priming by opening the cap completely. It requires strong and deep inhalation, and if this is achieved, a click should be heard. It has a dose counter and cannot be multi-dosed.

Novolizer. The Novolizer device is a DPI that requires priming by pressing the button down until it clicks. It has a coloured control window that patients may find useful; it changes from red to green as the inhaler is primed, then back to red once the dose is inhaled. It requires deep and strong inhalation, and patients cannot multi-dose using this device.

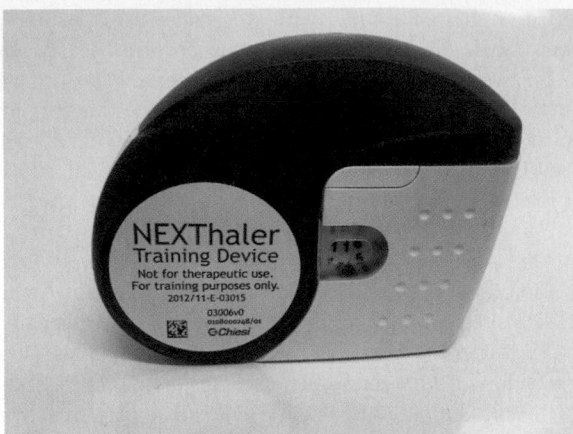

Fig. 25.5 Nexthaler device. (Reproduced by kind permission of T. Capstick.)

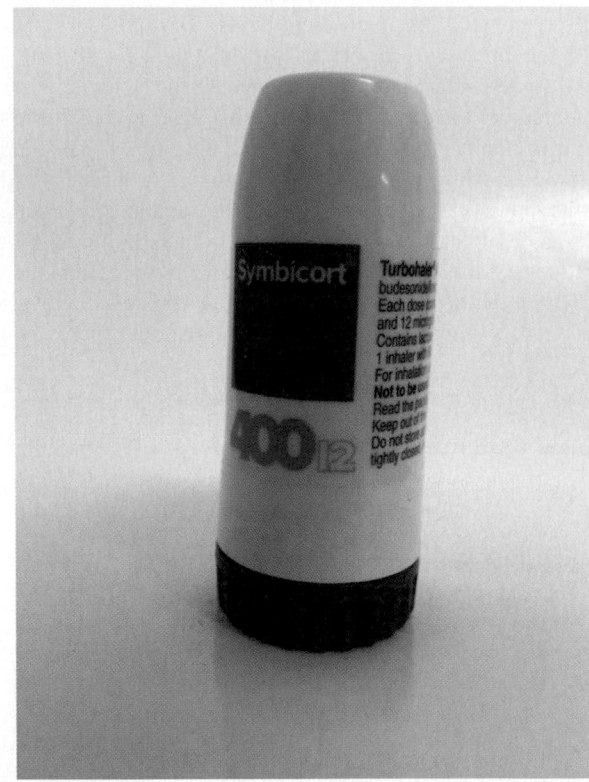

Fig. 25.6 Turbohaler device. (Reproduced by kind permission of T. Capstick.)

Spiromax. The Spiromax is a DPI and requires loading by opening the cap. It requires strong and deep inhalation, has a dose counter and patients cannot multi-dose when using this device.

Turbohaler. The Turbohaler device is another DPI (Fig. 25.6) that requires strong and deep inhalation to achieve deposition of the dose into the lungs. It has a dose counter and requires priming by twisting the bottom of the device to load it prior to inhalation. Fortunately, patients are unable to multi-dose because the counter will continue to count down but will not actually load multiple doses.

Twisthaler. The Twisthaler device is a DPI requiring strong and deep inhalation. It is primed by twisting the cap anticlockwise to remove it and ensuring the pointers on the device and the counter are aligned. It has a dose counter, which will count down with multiple actuations; however, the dose is not loaded multiple times.

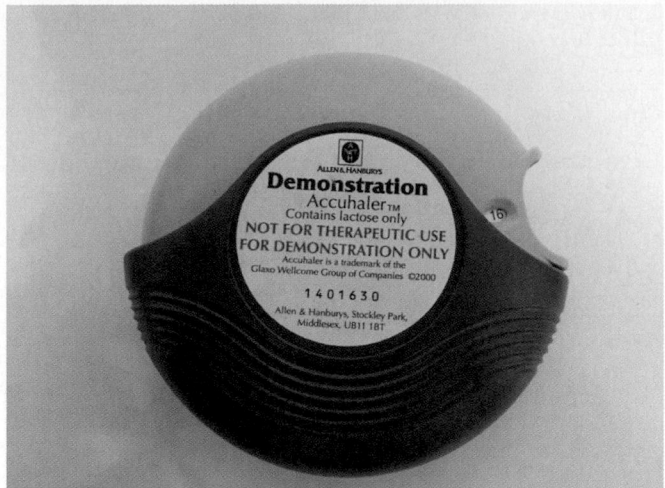

Fig. 25.7 Accuhaler device. (Reproduced by kind permission of T. Capstick.)

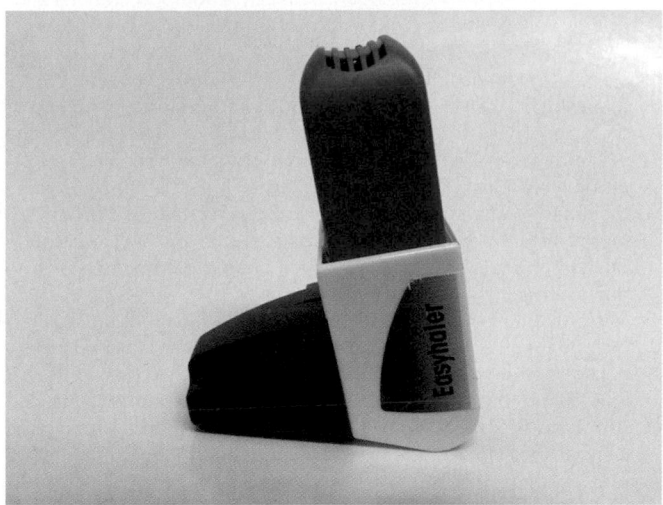

Fig. 25.8 Easyhaler device. (Reproduced by kind permission of T. Capstick.)

Accuhaler. The Accuhaler is a DPI (Fig. 25.7) that does not require coordination. It has a dose counter; therefore, it can aid patients in ensuring they do not run out of their inhaler. It has increased lung deposition compared with a pMDI and is useful for patients with poor dexterity. The Accuhaler does require loading by pushing down a lever; however, if this dose is loaded several times, there is potential to waste the dose if these doses are not inhaled. There is also potential to take too many doses if the lever has been pushed down multiple times. Inhalation should be strong and deep with this device.

Clickhaler. The Clickhaler device is a DPI and is primed by pushing the button down prior to inhaling; it does not require coordination. There is a risk of multi-dosing with this device if the button is pushed multiple times prior to inhalation.

Easyhaler. The Easyhaler is a DPI (Fig. 25.8) very similar to the Autohaler. It requires priming by pushing the button down in the upright position; however, patients are unable to load multiple doses, as with the Clickhaler. The dose may be lost if the device is not kept upright.

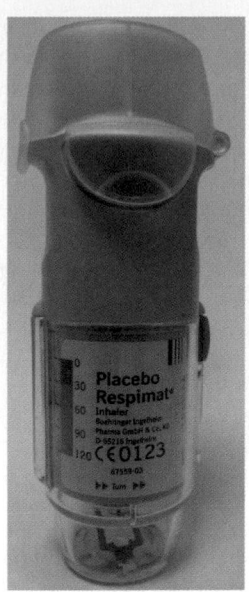

Fig. 25.9 Respimat device. (Reproduced by kind permission of T. Capstick.)

Soft-mist metered dose inhaler

Respimat. Respimat is a soft-mist metered dose inhaler (Fig. 25.9) that requires multiple steps to use efficiently. It requires slow and steady inhalation. Those with dexterity issues may find this device difficult to use due to the cartridge requiring insertion into the device and the requirement to then turn the base of the device and push the button during inhalation.

Adherence

Good adherence to asthma treatment is imperative in improving asthma outcomes and reducing exacerbations. A concordant decision must be made between the healthcare professional and the patient with regards to prescribing medicines. Adherence to treatment for any long-term condition has been shown to be poor, and there are a number of barriers to adherence. Consequently, patient adherence should be monitored regularly and interventions made if patients are having difficulty adhering to their medicines. Time should be taken to discuss barriers with patients, whether these are physical or psychological, intentional or unintentional, and concordant decisions made with regards to overcoming these. Treatment should not be stepped up with regard to treating asthma without assessing and improving adherence where possible.

Management plans

Self-management is a long-established practice in the care of people with asthma. When self-management is delivered to people (and/or their carers) with asthma, there is good evidence for reduced emergency healthcare utilisation, particularly emergency department attendance, hospital admission and unscheduled primary care consultations. From a patient perspective, self-management has been demonstrated to improve asthma control and quality of life, as well as reducing absenteeism from work and school (BTS and SIGN, 2016).

The key aspects of self-management are education that is strengthened by written PAAPs. The PAAPs include advice about recognising the loss of asthma control as defined by symptoms and peak flow. In response to recognition of deteriorating asthma control, there are then two or three action points. These action points can include increasing ICS dose, starting an oral corticosteroid and seeking immediate medical attention.

Case studies

Case 25.1

Mr DM is a 25-year-old man with a history of asthma since childhood. He has a background of poor asthma control; he uses his reliever most days and wakes at night approximately twice per week. He works full-time in a garage, smokes 10 cigarettes per day and has a pet dog at home. He has been admitted to hospital in January with an acute severe exacerbation of asthma. During his hospital stay his regular inhalers were changed from Symbicort 200/6 Turbohaler two puffs twice a day to Seretide 500/50 Accuhaler one puff twice a day.

Questions

1. What asthma reviews should Mr DM have following this exacerbation of his asthma?
2. What components are key to each asthma review?
3. What are the potential causes of Mr DM's poor asthma control?
4. What is the increase in Mr DM's inhaled steroid dose?

Answers

1. Mr DM should be reviewed by a respiratory specialist prior to discharge from hospital. He should also be seen by his primary care doctor or specialist primary care nurse two days following discharge. Subsequent to this he should be seen in a hospital asthma clinic 4 weeks following discharge.
2. At each review Mr DM's asthma control should be assessed, adherence with therapy should be reviewed, aggravating factors identified and inhaler technique checked.
3. Mr DM has a number of factors that may be worsening his asthma, including his smoking and exposure to pets. In view of the time of the year, the most likely cause of his exacerbation may be a viral infection. More information about his job should be elicited because exposure to isocyanates in car-paint fumes can be an asthma trigger.
4. Mr DM was initially taking Symbicort 200/6 Turbohaler two puffs twice daily. This is equivalent to 800 micrograms of beclometasone per day. His dose has been increased to Seretide 500/50 Accuhaler one puff twice daily, which is equivalent to 2000 micrograms beclometasone per day.

Case 25.2

Mrs ES is 36 years old. She weighs 76 kg, and her height is 170 cm. Her usual PEFR is 440 L/min. She does not smoke. Mrs ES is prescribed a Fostair 100/6 pMDI two puffs twice a day and salbutamol 100 micrograms/dose pMDI two puffs to be taken as required. She is admitted to hospital with an exacerbation of asthma. Mrs ES's initial observations demonstrate a PEFR of 100 L/min, respiratory rate of 30 breaths/min and sO$_2$ of 92% on room air.

She is started on nebulised bronchodilators and a steroid but fails to improve.

Questions

1. What severity of asthma exacerbation does Mrs ES have?
2. What bronchodilators and at what dose would be recommended?
3. What dose of steroid would be recommended?
4. Because she is failing to improve, what two other therapies could be considered, and at what dose?

Answers

1. Mrs ES has a life-threatening exacerbation as determined by her oxygen saturation and PEFR. Her oxygen saturation is ≤92%, and her PEFR is less than 33% of her normal value.
2. Mrs ES should be started on nebulised salbutamol 5 mg and ipratropium 500 micrograms as an immediate response. If she fails to respond clinically to the initial therapy, then repeated (or 'back-to-back') administration of salbutamol can be used until clinical improvement is seen in terms of routine observations and/or PEFR. Once she is more stable, the nebulised bronchodilators should be administered 6 hourly and stopped 24 hours prior to discharge from hospital.
3. She should receive 40–50 mg of oral prednisolone immediately, then once daily for a minimum of 5 days. Because her asthma exacerbation is life-threatening, she should be monitored in hospital until clinically stable for discharge. If she is unable to take the tablets orally, then an alternative would be hydrocortisone 100 micrograms intravenously. Once she is able to take medication orally, then the intravenous hydrocortisone should be swapped to oral prednisolone as previously described.
4. Mrs ES could be considered for intravenous magnesium 1.2–2 g over 20 minutes. Alternatively, she could receive intravenous aminophylline. Aminophylline would require a loading dose of 5 mg/kg (380 mg) over 20 minutes, followed by a maintenance infusion of 0.5 mg/kg/h (38 mg/h). If Mrs ES received intravenous aminophylline, then therapeutic drug monitoring would need to be undertaken daily.

Case 25.3

Mr CM is a 56-year-old man with a history of asthma over the preceding 5 years. His height is 177 cm and weight is 80 kg. He had one exacerbation of his asthma 3 years ago that required hospital admission, and he is currently prescribed Symbicort 200/6 Turbohaler two puffs twice daily. At his asthma review today, Mr CM reported minimal symptoms from his asthma and could not remember the last time he used his reliever inhaler. His peak flow was 580 L/min, which is at his best.

Questions

1. Is Mr CM's asthma controlled?
2. Should Mr CM's asthma treatment be altered?
3. What potential alterations could be used in Mr CM's treatment?

Answers

1. Mr CM's asthma is controlled because he is reporting minimal symptoms, has not had an exacerbation in the last 12 months and has a normal peak flow. He would fulfil the Global Initiative for Asthma (2012) definition of controlled asthma.

2. Mr CM's asthma treatment should be considered for a step down in treatment because he meets the current guideline definition for asthma control. He is currently on step 3 of the BTS guideline treatment.
3. Mr CM is currently taking Symbicort 200/6 two puffs twice daily. This is a medium-dose combination inhaled steroid and LABA inhaler. Potential changes to his therapy would be either to continue the LABA and reduce his ICS dose (i.e. change to Symbicort 100/6 Turbohaler two puffs twice a day) or, alternatively, to change his inhaler to an equivalent ICS dose as monotherapy.

Case 25.4

Miss CM is 45 years old. She presents with a 6-month history of intermittent breathlessness, wheeze and cough. Miss CM has found that she gets symptoms at least three or four times each week. She has also noticed that her symptoms are worse first thing in the morning, also significantly during the winter when she had a minor upper respiratory tract infection.

She is currently taking no regular medication. Apart from seasonal allergic rhinitis, Miss CM has no other health problems.

Questions

1. What is the likely diagnosis?
2. What investigations should be undertaken?
3. What treatment should be started?
4. What non-pharmacological measures should be considered?

Answers

1. Miss CM's history is suggestive of a diagnosis of asthma. The intermittent symptoms, diurnal variation and previous atopy (seasonal allergic rhinitis) would all be supportive of this diagnosis.
2. Miss CM should undertake a lung function test to confirm the presence of airflow obstruction. Ideally this should be spirometry measurements, although an alternative would be serial peak flow measurements. These measurements should be taken morning and evening for 2 weeks. If these investigations were not conclusive, then Miss CM may need to proceed to reversibility testing or be considered for referral to a hospital specialist for further investigation.
3. Initial therapy would be a regular ICS at a starting dose equivalent to beclometasone 400 micrograms per day.
4. The other key non-pharmacological interventions are to provide Miss CM with a PAAP. She should also receive education regarding her condition and training in the use of her inhaler device.

References

Basheti, I., Reddel, H.K., Armour, C.L., et al., 2007. Pharmacists' understanding of patient education on metered-dose inhaler technique. Ann. Pharmacother. 34, 1249–1256.

British Thoracic Society (BTS) and Scottish Intercollegiate Guidelines Network (SIGN), 2016. British Guideline on the Management of Asthma. SIGN, Edinburgh (QRG 153). Available at http://www.sign.ac.uk.

Brown, H.M., 1958. Treatment of chronic asthma with prednisolone; significance of eosinophils in the sputum. Lancet 2, 1245–1247.

Capstick, T.G., Clifton, I.J., 2012. Inhaler technique and training in people with chronic obstructive pulmonary disease and asthma. Expert Rev. Respir. Med. 6, 91–101.

Chauhan, B.F., Ducharme, F.M., 2014. Addition to inhaled corticosteroids of long-acting beta$_2$-agonists versus anti-leukotrienes for chronic asthma. Cochrane Database Syst. Rev. 2014 (1), Art. No. CD003137. https://doi.org/10.1002/14651858.CD003137.pub5.

Crompton, G.K., Barnes, P.J., Broeders, M., et al., 2006. The need to improve inhalation technique in Europe: a report from the Aerosol Drug Management Improvement Team. Resp. Med. 100, 1479–1494.

Davies, H., Olson, L., Gibson, P., 1998. Methotrexate as a steroid sparing agent for asthma in adults. Cochrane Database Syst. Rev. 1998 (3), Art. No. CD000391. https://doi.org/10.1002/14651858.CD000391.

Evans, D.J., Cullinan, P., Geddes, D.M., 2000a. Cyclosporin as an oral corticosteroid sparing agent in stable asthma. Cochrane Database Syst. Rev. 2000 (4), Art. No. CD002993. https://doi.org/10.1002/14651858.CD002993.

Evans, D.J., Cullinan, P., Geddes, D.M., 2000b. Gold as an oral corticosteroid sparing agent in stable asthma. Cochrane Database Syst. Rev. 2000 (4), Art. No. CD002985. https://doi.org/10.1002/14651858.CD002985.

Giraud, V., Roche, N., 2002. Misuse of corticosteroid metered-dose inhaler is associated with decreased asthma stability. Eur. Respir. J. 19, 246–251.

Global Initiative for Asthma, 2012. Global strategy for asthma management and prevention. Available at http://ginasthma.org.

Graham, V., Lasserson, T., Rowe, B.H., 2001. Antibiotics for acute asthma. Cochrane Database Syst. Rev. 2001 (2), Art. No. CD002741. https://doi.org/10.1002/14651858.CD002741.

Green, R.H., Brightling, C.E., McKenna, S., et al., 2002a. Asthma exacerbations and sputum eosinophil counts: a randomised controlled trial. Lancet 360, 1715–1721.

Green, R.M., Custovic, A., Sanderson, G., et al., 2002b. Synergism between allergens and viruses and risk of hospital admission with asthma: case-control study. Br. Med. J. 324, 763.

Holt, S., Suder, A., Weatherall, M., et al., 2001. Dose–response relation of inhaled fluticasone propionate in adolescents and adults with asthma: meta-analysis. Br. Med. J. 323, 253–256.

Juniper, E.F., O'Byrne, P.M., Guyatt, G.H., et al., 1999. Development and validation of a questionnaire to measure asthma control. Eur. Respir. J. 14, 902–907.

Lanes, S.F., Garrett, J.E., Wentworth, C.E., et al., 1998. The effect of adding ipratropium bromide to salbutamol in the treatment of acute asthma: a pooled analysis of three trials. Chest 114, 365–372.

Lenney, J., Innes, J.A., Crompton, G.K., 2000. Inappropriate inhaler use: assessment of use and patient preference of seven inhalation devices. EDICI Resp. Med. 94, 496–500.

Malmstrom, K., Rodriguez-Gomez, G., Guerra, J., et al., 1999. Oral montelukast, inhaled beclomethasone, and placebo for chronic asthma. A randomized, controlled trial. Montelukast/Beclomethasone Study Group. Ann. Intern. Med. 130, 487–495.

Medicines and Healthcare Products Regulatory Agency, 2008. Review on long-acting β$_2$ agonists for asthma. Available at https://www.gov.uk/drug-safety-update/review-on-long-acting-2-agonists-for-asthma.

Nathan, R.A., 2003. Pharmacotherapy for allergic rhinitis: a critical review of leukotriene receptor antagonists compared with other treatments. Ann. Allergy Asthma Immunol. 90, 182–190.

Nathan, R.A., Sorkness, C.A., Kosinski, M., et al., 2004. Development of the asthma control test: a survey for assessing asthma control. J. Allergy Clin. Immunol. 113, 59–65.

National Institute for Health and Care Excellence (NICE), 2010. Chronic obstructive pulmonary disease in over 16s: diagnosis and management (CG101). Available at https://www.nice.org.uk/guidance/cg101.

National Institute for Health and Care Excellence (NICE), 2013. Omalizumab for treating severe persistent allergic asthma (review of Technology Appraisal Guidance 133 and 201). Available at https://www.nice.org.uk/guidance/ta278.

National Institute for Health and Care Excellence (NICE), 2017. Mepolizumab for treating severe eosinophilic asthma. Available at https://www.nice.org.uk/guidance/ta431.

O'Driscoll, B.R., Howard, L.S., Davison, A.G., 2008. BTS guideline for emergency oxygen use in adult patients. Thorax 63 (Suppl. 6), 1–68.

Pearson, M., Bucknall, C., 1999. Measuring Clinical Outcomes in Asthma: A Patient Focused Approach. Royal College of Physicians, London.

Pellegrino, R., Viegi, G., Brusasco, V., et al., 2005. Interpretative strategies for lung function tests. Eur. Respir. J. 26, 948–968.

Rodrigo, G.J., Castro-Rodriguez, J.A., 2015. What is the role of tiotropium in asthma? A systematic review with meta-analysis. Chest 147, 388–396.

Rowe, B.H., Bretzlaff, J.A., Bourdon, C., et al., 2000. Magnesium sulfate for treating exacerbations of acute asthma in the emergency department. Cochrane Database Syst. Rev. 2000 (1), Art. No. CD001490. https://doi.org/10.1002/14651858.CD001490.

Rowe, B.H., Spooner, C., Ducharme, F.M., et al., 2007. Early emergency department treatment of acute asthma with systemic corticosteroids. Cochrane Database Syst. Rev. 2007 (3), Art. No. CD000195. https://doi.org/10.1002/14651858.CD000195.pub2.

Royal College of Physicians, 2014. Why Asthma Still Kills: The National Review of Asthma Deaths (NRAD) Confidential Enquiry Report. Royal College of Physicians, London.

Travers, A.H., Jones, A.P., Camargo, C.A., et al., 2012. Intravenous beta$_2$-agonists versus intravenous aminophylline for acute asthma. Cochrane Database Syst. Rev. 2012 (12), Art. No. CD010256. https://doi.org/10.1002/14651858.CD010256.

Voshaar, T., App, E.M., Berdel, D., et al., 2001. Recommendations for the choice of inhalatory systems for drug prescription. Pneumologie 55, 579–586.

Wenzel, S.E., 2012. Asthma phenotypes: the evolution from clinical to molecular approaches. Nat. Med. 18, 716–725.

Further reading

Barnes, P.J., Rodger, I.W., Thomson, N.C., 1998. Asthma: Basic Mechanisms and Clinical Management, third ed. Academic Press, London.

Mahmoudi, M., 2016. Allergy and Asthma: Practical Diagnosis and Management, second ed. Springer International Publishing, New York.

Wenzel, S.E., 2012. Asthma phenotypes: the evolution from clinical to molecular approaches. Nat. Med. 18, 716–725.

Useful websites

Asthma UK: http://www.asthma.org.uk
British Lung Foundation: http://www.blf.org.uk
Allergy UK: http://www.allergyuk.org

Global Initiative for Asthma: http://www.ginasthma.org
European Lung Foundation: http://www.europeanlung.org
NHS Choices: http://www.nhs.uk/conditions/asthma

26 Chronic Obstructive Pulmonary Disease

Trevor Rogers and Helen Meynell

Key points

- Chronic obstructive pulmonary disease (COPD) is a leading cause of morbidity and mortality worldwide.
- Reducing exposure to tobacco smoke as well as other recreational drugs, including cannabis, cocaine and heroin; occupational dusts; chemicals and pollutants is an important goal to prevent the onset and progression of COPD.
- Smoking cessation is the single most important intervention to reduce the risk of developing COPD and slow disease progression.
- Risk factors for COPD include host factors (α_1-antitrypsin deficiency and airway hyper-responsiveness) and exposure to tobacco smoke as well as socio-economic status.
- Pulmonary rehabilitation, incorporating exercise and education, is the intervention that has the greatest impact on quality of life.
- Drugs have an important role in maximising lung function and reducing exacerbations.

Definitions

Chronic obstructive pulmonary disease (COPD) is defined on the basis of airflow obstruction that is not fully reversible. Certainly, this clinical entity is highly prevalent and familiar, usually in older patients with a significant smoking history. It is associated with largely irreversible damage to the airways and lung parenchyma (emphysema). However, based as it is on physiology, this definition is likely also to include other pathologies. For example, there is a subset of patients who meet this definition who have varying degrees of eosinophilia and who share the important characteristic of corticosteroid responsiveness with the other highly prevalent condition in which airflow obstruction is a key feature: asthma. A diagnostic label is only of use if it is helpful in practice, and in this important aspect of corticosteroid responsiveness, the use of the unqualified terms of COPD, and indeed asthma, fail. Reflecting this, there has recently been a move away from these umbrella terms, instead identifying 'treatable traits', such as eosinophilic, steroid-responsive airway disease and those in which it is absent when the emphasis is on bronchodilatation. The term COPD is so firmly entrenched that its use will undoubtedly continue for the foreseeable future, but its limitations do need to be borne in mind.

Epidemiology

COPD is a leading cause of morbidity and mortality. In the UK an estimated 3 million people have the condition (a prevalence of about 5%), of whom only about 900,000 have been diagnosed; a substantial majority, an estimated 2 million people, have not. The diagnosis is usually not made before patients reach their 50s, with prevalence increasing with age. Worldwide prevalence is likely to vary between about 5% and 10%, with estimates varying according to the methods employed in identifying disease.

Aetiology

Whilst smoking is overwhelmingly the commonest cause, it is now well established that dust and fume exposure can also cause the condition. In the developed world this is most often seen in subjects exposed occupationally, as in mining, steel working and similar occupations. Globally, cooking using biomass in poorly ventilated houses is an important cause, especially in women. The rare homozygous α_1-antitrypsin deficiency predisposes to early-onset emphysema, mostly in smokers, revealing the importance of the balance between neutrophil-derived proteases and anti-proteases in the development of the condition. The major risk factors are summarised in Table 26.1.

Pathology and pathophysiology

The two pathological components of COPD are chronic bronchitis and emphysema, existing in the individual in greater or lesser proportions. Emphysema means dilatation of the airways distal to the terminal bronchiole, with loss of alveolar walls and consequent reduction in the surface area of the alveolar membrane. This impairs gas transfer and can be measured in the laboratory by a reduction in the carbon monoxide gas transfer coefficient (DL_{CO}). Another effect of this tissue damage is a reduction in the traction on airways, increasing lung compliance and making airways prone to collapse during expiration. The tendency is for emphysematous areas to coalesce, which can lead to the formation of large air cysts, called bullae. These are most commonly located in the upper

Table 26.1 Risk factors for the development of chronic obstructive pulmonary disease

Risk factor	Comment
Smoking (including tobacco, heroin, cannabis)	Risk increases with increasing consumption, but there is large inter-individual variation in susceptibility.
Age	Lung function impairment progresses with age.
Gender	Male gender was previously thought to be a risk factor, but this may be due to historical higher rates of smoking in men.
Occupation	Development of COPD is associated with occupational dust and fume exposure, including coal mining, farming, grain-handling and the cement and cotton industries.
Genetic factors	Alpha-1 antitrypsin deficiency is the strongest single genetic risk factor, accounting for 1–2% of COPD.
Air pollution	Death rates are higher in urban areas than in rural areas. Indoor air pollution from burning biomass fuel is also a risk factor, particularly in the developing world.
Socio-economic status	COPD has increased prevalence in individuals of low socio-economic status.

COPD, Chronic obstructive pulmonary disease.

zones, whereas in α_1-antitrypsin deficiency, emphysematous areas are more basally distributed. Occasionally giant bullae can develop and occupy over half of the volume of a lung.

The other pathological component is chronic bronchitis. This has been defined clinically, largely in epidemiologic studies, as a chronic cough with sputum production for at least 3 months per year for 2 consecutive years. Pathologically, chronic bronchitis refers to hypertrophy of the mucus-secreting goblet cells in airway walls. This in turn leads to worsening airflow obstruction by luminal obstruction of small airways, epithelial remodelling and alteration of airway surface tension, predisposing to collapse.

At a microscopic level the inflammation is predominantly neutrophilic, and as is usual, this is not responsive to corticosteroids. A relatively small proportion of COPD patients, however, have a significant eosinophilic component to their disease, which is steroid responsive (see later discussion).

Repeated bronchial infections can cause damage to bronchial walls, leading to loss of elasticity, and dilatation, a condition called bronchiectasis, which develops in a proportion of COPD patients. This tends to be associated with copious sputum production, with repeated infective exacerbations and frequently with the emergence of pathogens more resistant to first-line antibiotics.

Both emphysema and bronchitis combine to impair the ability to expel air from the lungs, leading to hyperinflation of the thorax. The consequent overstretching of intercostal muscles and diaphragm places them at a mechanical disadvantage, reducing their efficiency. Hyperinflation can be exacerbated by exercise, leading to further reduction in efficiency of the respiratory pump, a process known as dynamic hyperinflation.

The syndrome known as hypoxic cor pulmonale is widely misunderstood. It refers to peripheral oedema occurring in COPD with type 2 respiratory failure. It is not, as widely thought, due to simple right ventricular failure and pressure overload: pulmonary artery pressures are similar to those tolerated by many millions of people living at high altitude without difficulty over lifetimes, and right ventricular hypertrophy is rarely found at autopsy. In fact, cardiac output increases during acute episodes. It is likely that the systemic vasodilation caused by elevated carbon dioxide levels causes blood pressure to fall. Renal salt and fluid retention mediated by neurohumoral mechanisms are utilised by the body to maintain blood pressure, as in other forms of high-output cardiac failure. The onset of oedema is an important milestone in the natural history of COPD, suggesting a poor prognosis, albeit much improved by long-term oxygen therapy (LTOT). Whilst loop diuretics are necessary to control oedema, the improvement in gas exchange by optimal medical management is the real key to its treatment.

Clinical manifestations
Symptoms, signs and natural history

The earliest symptoms of COPD are cough and expectoration of sputum. These develop insidiously, often being disregarded as a 'smoker's cough'. Acute infections may lead to episodic breathlessness and increased expectoration, frequently with wheezing, which may be appreciated by the patient and by the clinician on auscultation of the chest. Lung function usually continues to decline at an accelerated rate, particularly whilst smoking continues, although it is likely that many COPD patients start from a lower baseline with reduced lung function from an early age. Due to the substantial reserve of respiratory function, which is only called on at times of stress, such as heavy exertion or respiratory tract infection, more persistent symptoms of breathlessness only occur when large amounts of lung have been destroyed. This is the explanation for the gross underdiagnosis of the condition, especially in its earlier stages. When pulmonary reserve is exhausted, patients often perceive that they have fairly suddenly developed a problem with persistent breathlessness. Thus, identification of early intermittent symptoms and performing spirometry to identify and quantify airflow obstruction can be helpful in concentrating efforts on smoking cessation, at a time when severe disability is completely avoidable.

If emphysema is prominent, the chest becomes visibly hyperinflated, which can also be appreciated by a hyper-resonant percussion note, as part of the clinical examination.

Other symptoms that may be experienced are sleep disturbance, dry mouth, lethargy and weight loss, the last of which is a poor prognostic sign, independent of lung function but more common in advanced disease. If respiratory failure develops, ankle oedema appears, comprising the clinical syndrome of hypoxic cor pulmonale. This may be associated with headache and drowsiness and is clinically associated with a bluish complexion ('cyanosis'), warm peripheries, a bounding pulse and flapping tremor.

Table 26.2	Assessment of severity of airflow obstruction
FEV$_1$	Severity
Greater than 80% predicted	GOLD stage 1: Mild
50–79% predicted	GOLD stage 2: Moderate
30–49% predicted	GOLD stage 3: Severe
<30% predicted	GOLD stage 4: Very severe

FEV$_1$, Forced expiratory volume in 1 second.
Adapted from GOLD (2017).

Table 26.3	Modified Medical Research Council dyspnoea scale
Grade	Degree of breathlessness related to activities
1	Not troubled by breathlessness except on strenuous exercise
2	Short of breath when hurrying or walking up a slight hill
3	Walks slower than contemporaries on level ground because of breathlessness, or has to stop for breath when walking at own pace
4	Stops for breath after walking about 100 m or after a few minutes on level ground
5	Too breathless to leave the house, or breathless when dressing or undressing

Adapted from Fletcher et al. (1959).

Two COPD stereotypes have been recognised, the so-called 'pink puffer' and 'blue bloater'. Pink puffers tend to have a more emphysematous phenotype, with marked hyperinflation. They maintain normal blood gases at the expense of a high work of breathing and severe breathlessness. These patients are typically thin. The blue bloater, in contrast, tends to have less obvious hyperinflation and slips into respiratory failure and hypoxic cor pulmonale. These patients are less breathless and tend to be obese. It should be emphasised that whilst these caricatures do exist, they are opposite ends of a spectrum, with many patients having elements of both. Interestingly, pathologically, the lungs of these two stereotypes are very similar, suggesting that the cause for the difference lies in the central respiratory control of breathing.

Investigations

Airflow obstruction is readily measured by spirometry, now conventionally performed, in the assessment of COPD, 10–20 minutes after bronchodilator treatment. Airflow obstruction is present when the ratio of the volume expired in the first second (FEV$_1$) to the total volume expired (FVC) falls below 70%. The severity of airflow obstruction is assessed by the post-bronchodilator FEV$_1$ expressed as the percentage of the predicted, according to age and height, and can be graded as shown in Table 26.2.

More detailed physiological evaluation is not usually required, but lung volume measurements and carbon monoxide gas transfer (DL$_{CO}$) can more precisely quantify the severity of air trapping and emphysema, respectively. When the diagnosis remains in doubt, including when lung function testing reveals features that may indicate interstitial lung disease (pulmonary fibrosis), computed tomography (CT) scanning can be helpful in identifying emphysema, and this is also useful when lung volume reduction treatment is being considered, including the surgical removal of giant bullae. CT scanning can also be useful in identifying the not infrequent co-existence of bronchiectasis. Plain chest radiography has both poor sensitivity and specificity for COPD but is recommended when the diagnosis is first being considered to exclude other pathologies. COPD is a strong risk factor for lung cancer, even after correction for smoking has been included. Therefore, when a smoker presents with persistent new respiratory symptoms, this is an important differential diagnosis in which the chest X-ray is useful. In COPD the chest X-ray can be normal but often shows hyperinflated lungs, increased lung markings due to bronchial wall thickening and regions of lucency corresponding to areas of emphysema/bullae.

Symptoms can be quantified with differing levels of precision. One of the simplest is the modified Medical Research Council (mMRC) dyspnoea score (Table 26.3), which is readily usable in clinical practice.

More complex and multidimensional instruments exist, generating indices of quality of life, the most widely used of which is the St George Respiratory Questionnaire (SGRQ), which was developed specifically for COPD and is mostly used in clinical trials (Jones et al., 1991). Functional assessments can also be used, including exercise tests, including the 6-minute walk and shuttle walks. Body mass index (BMI) is also prognostically important, with weight loss and cachexia being associated with a poor prognosis. Indeed, a combination of BMI, the severity of airflow obstruction, severity of breathlessness and walking distance can be used to assess prognosis having been incorporated into the Body-Mass Index, Airflow Obstruction, Dyspnoea, and Exercise (BODE) index (Celli et al., 2004).

Classification

COPD has historically been graded in severity according to the degree of airflow obstruction (see Table 26.2). Symptom severity correlates poorly with lung function. The Global Strategy for the Diagnosis, Management, and Prevention of Chronic Obstructive Pulmonary Disease guidelines (GOLD, 2017) have been updated to introduce the 'ABCD' algorithm. This is the first classification to combine risk assessment with symptoms to help determine the most effective treatments. This generates a 2 × 2 matrix (Fig. 26.1). It is important to note that there are two ways of qualifying as high risk: higher GOLD score (equating to poor lung function) or frequent exacerbations.

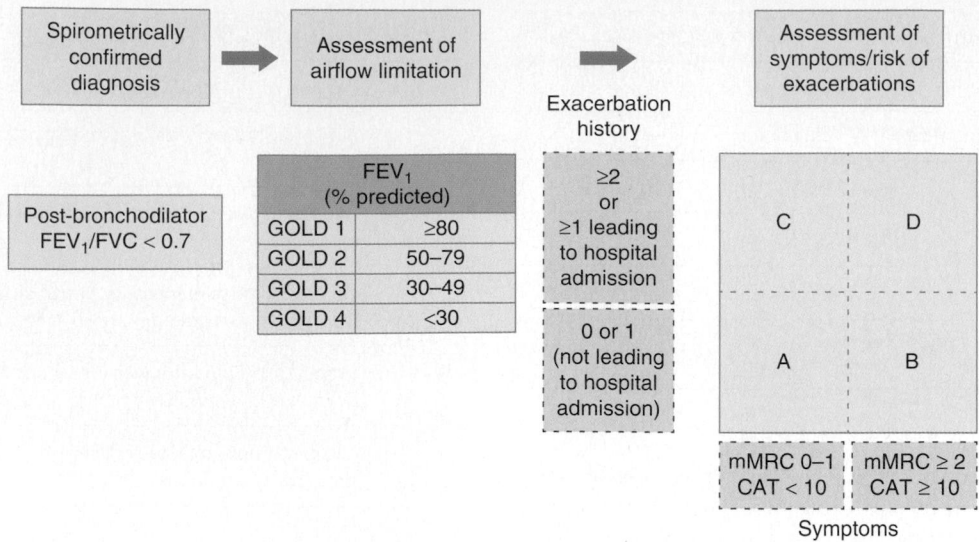

Fig. 26.1 GOLD refined ABC assessment tool. For mMRC definitions, see Table 26.3. The CAT score refers to the COPD Assessment Test (GlaxoSmithKline, 2009).
COPD, Chronic obstructive pulmonary disease; FEV$_1$, forced expiratory volume in 1 second; FVC, forced vital capacity; mMRC, Modified Medical Research Council.
(GOLD, 2017; with kind permission from GOLD.)

Treatment

Managing stable chronic obstructive pulmonary disease

The National Institute for Health and Care Excellence (NICE, 2010) guidance for the management of COPD has largely been superseded by the body of evidence that is outlined in the GOLD (2017) guidelines. As such, NICE is no longer favoured for the management of COPD, and GOLD (2017) is a comprehensive document that respiratory professionals should be referring to when managing these patients. The rate of progression of COPD does not change despite medication or rehabilitation, but the measures in the guidance can significantly improve a patient's quality of life and reduce the symptom burden. If the treatment plan is optimised, then this is likely to reduce symptoms, exacerbations and admissions to hospital. The aims of treatment with the pharmacological agents are shown in Box 26.1.

Fig. 26.1 outlines assessment of COPD dependent on symptom burden and exacerbation frequency.

A group A patient is one who is relatively symptom-free (mMRC 0–1 or CAT score <10) with no exacerbations in the previous year. For these patients, who are most likely to present in primary care, a bronchodilator should be prescribed. An as-required bronchodilator would only be recommended for those patients with very occasional breathlessness: it is preferable to use a long-acting bronchodilator in these circumstances. Once initiation with a bronchodilator has occurred, the patient should be re-assessed and an alternative bronchodilator prescribed if symptoms remain an issue.

Group B patients are those patients who are more symptomatic (mMRC >2 or CAT score >10) who also have not exacerbated in the previous year. For these patients, GOLD (2017) guidelines recommend the use of a long-acting β-agonist (LABA) or long-acting anti-muscarinic antagonists (LAMAs). This is very similar to the management of category A patients, with a step up in

> **Box 26.1** Treatment aims for patients with chronic obstructive pulmonary disease
>
> - Prevent disease progression
> - Relieve symptoms
> - Improve exercise tolerance
> - Improve quality of life and health status
> - Prevent and treat complications such as hypoxaemia
> - Prevent and treat exacerbations
> - Reduce mortality

therapy to a dual LABA-LAMA combination should symptoms continue. GOLD (2017) guidelines also give the flexibility to initiate treatment straight away with a LABA-LAMA combination.

Group C patients are those who are not particularly symptomatic but have experienced more than two exacerbations requiring antibiotics and/or steroids or more than one exacerbation requiring hospital admission in the previous year. For these patients, GOLD (2017) guidelines recommend a LAMA, escalating to a LABA-LAMA combination if further exacerbations occur. In this group, there is an option to add in a LABA/inhaled corticosteroid (ICS), but this is not the preferred choice of agent.

Group D patients are those with frequent exacerbations and severe symptoms. For these patients, the options are very flexible and would be based on individual patients. Ultimately, for these patients, so-called 'triple therapy' may be appropriate (i.e. LAMA plus LABA/ICS). Roflumilast has recently been approved by NICE (2017) as an add-on bronchodilator in this group of patients. It is generally thought that ICSs should be reserved for these patients with very debilitating symptoms and frequent exacerbations.

Pharmacological treatments do not change the underlying pathology. The common therapeutic problems associated with COPD are shown in Box 26.2.

Box 26.2 Common therapeutic problems associated with chronic obstructive pulmonary disease

- Failure of patient to stop smoking
- Inadequate inhaler technique, leading to subtherapeutic dosing and medicine wastage
- Poor adherence to the treatment regimen
- Inappropriate prescribing (or lack of prescribing) of antibiotics in an acute exacerbation of chronic obstructive pulmonary disease
- Failure to properly assess a patient for home nebulisation
- Failure to properly assess adherence to at least 15 h/day of oxygen therapy
- Failure to discontinue current inhalers when switching to new devices/regimens

Surgical treatments

Intervention to reduce lung volume can improve lung function and breathlessness in appropriately selected patients, with severe air trapping. This can be achieved by surgical removal of emphysematous regions, especially when these are located primarily in the upper zones, or more recently by the placement of endobronchial valves.

Lung transplantation is an option when lung function and quality of life become severely impaired, but the rigorous criteria applied in selection and the paucity of donor organ availability limit this to a very small proportion of patients.

Smoking cessation

Smoking is the most important and modifiable factor in the development of COPD. Smoking cessation interventions are effective in reducing ill health and prolonging life. All COPD patients who continue to smoke, regardless of age, should be given encouragement to stop smoking and be offered help to do so at every opportunity (GOLD, 2017). Even brief conversations between the patient and the healthcare professional can lead to quitting and, as a result, are one of the most cost-effective of all healthcare interventions. Once a quit date has been determined, it is the level of dependence rather than the motivation that influences the success rate, and this is where having professional support can help the individual to maintain his or her smoke-free status. For example, in the first few days after quitting, the cough and sputum production increase as the cilia start to recover from their paralysis due to the toxic effects of the smoke.

Fig. 26.2 summarises how lung function and symptoms are believed to be affected by continuing to smoke or stopping at any age. Estimates suggest that stopping smoking leads to a sustained 50% reduction in the rate of lung function decline; however, it should be remembered that the damage already sustained cannot be reversed.

Bronchodilators

Short-acting β-agonists and short-acting antimuscarinics. Bronchodilators in COPD are used to reverse airflow limitation. They are useful for easing symptoms such as wheeze and improve exercise tolerance. GOLD (2017) guidance recommends that the once the diagnosis of COPD is confirmed, the patient is assessed for symptom severity, either using the CAT score or mMRC dyspnoea score. In addition, the number of exacerbations in the past year should also be determined. Once these have been assessed, the patient can be initiated on appropriate treatment using the modified ABCD algorithm (see Fig. 26.1). Patients should be provided with a short-acting β_2-agonist (SABA) for use when required. Salbutamol and terbutaline are the principal SABAs available, although formoterol, which is long-acting, has an equally swift onset of action of approximately 5 minutes. Ipratropium, the only short-acting anti-muscarinic available (SAMA), is another option, provided the patient is not taking a LAMA, although its rate of onset is slower.

Long-acting bronchodilators. LAMAs and LABAs are the mainstay of treatment for patients with stable COPD. The evidence base is rapidly growing, and the role of bronchodilators and their position in therapy is also rapidly changing. The recent FLAME study (Jadwiga et al., 2016) has demonstrated that a combination product of indacaterol and glycopyrronium is superior to salmeterol plus fluticasone for all exacerbations, lung function and health-related quality of life in patients with a history of exacerbations. In addition, there was a lower incidence of pneumonia in the LABA/LAMA arm.

Long-acting muscarinic antagonists. Tiotropium has been a cornerstone of treatment and provides the most robust evidence of efficacy. The landmark trial UPLIFT showed that treatment with tiotropium in mild to severe disease can significantly sustain improvements in lung function over 4 years. It was also shown to delay time to first exacerbation, reduce the number of exacerbations per year and reduce the risk of exacerbations leading to hospital admission (Tashkin et al., 2008).

There was controversy over the cardiovascular safety of Tiotropium Respimat, which has been largely discounted following publication of TIOSPIR in 2013 (Wise et al., 2013), a randomised, double-blind, parallel group trial of around 17,000 patients. Patients were randomised to either tiotropium Respimat 2.5 micrograms, tiotropium Respimat 5 micrograms or tiotropium 18 micrograms in the HandiHaler device. End points were risk of death and time to first exacerbation, but cardiovascular safety was also assessed. The trial showed that 2.5-microgram and 5-microgram doses via the Respimat device had a similar safety profile and exacerbation rate to the HandiHaler mode of delivery. Other, newer LAMAs include aclidinium, umeclidinium and glycopyrronium, and new trial data are emerging regarding quality of life, exacerbations and improvement in lung function (Jones et al., 2012; Kerwin et al., 2012; Trivedi et al., 2014). Choice of LAMA is made by consideration of the patient's ability to use the device, adherence and tolerability.

Long-acting β2-adrenergic agonists. Salmeterol, indacaterol, olodaterol and formoterol are all available in the UK in a range of different inhaler devices and in combination with LAMAs or ICSs. There is emerging evidence that LABAs are also effective in reducing exacerbations and improving symptoms; however, asthma must be confidently excluded before initiating a LABA without an ICS. The TORCH study (Calverley et al., 2007) demonstrated that salmeterol significantly reduced exacerbation frequency.

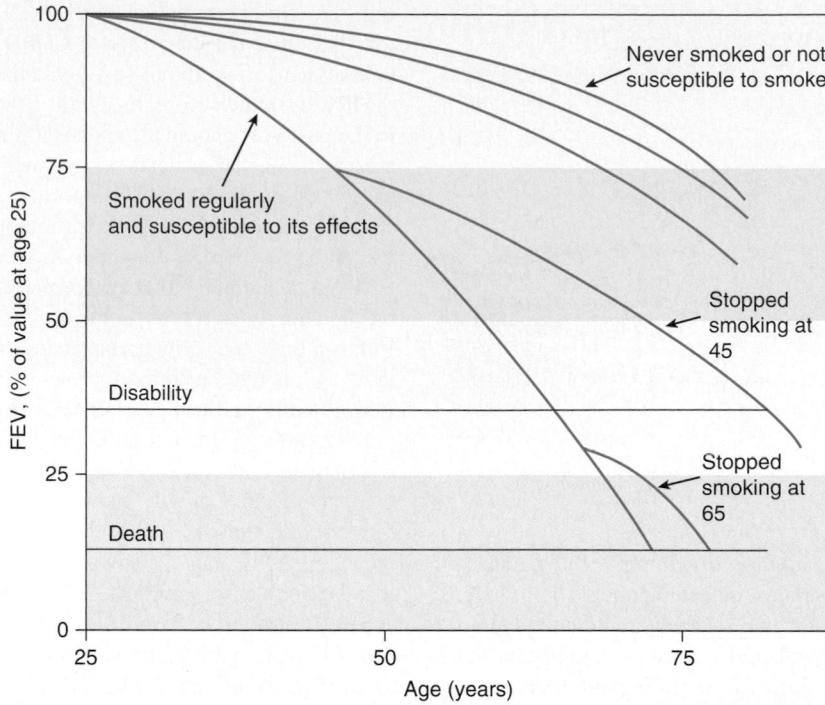

Fig. 26.2 Diagrammatic representation of the effects of smoking and smoking cessation in a man who is likely to develop COPD if he smokes. (Reproduced from Fletcher and Peto, 1977, with permission.)

Nebulised bronchodilator therapy. For those patients who suffer debilitating breathlessness, a home nebuliser has traditionally been offered for SABA and/or ipratropium bromide therapy. However, with the evidence of longer-term benefits conferred by the newer long-acting inhaler-delivered drugs, there has been a marked reduction in long-term nebuliser use. Very occasionally patients do seem to benefit from high-dose nebuliser treatment, and motivated patients are generally loaned a device to explore this aspect. Further consideration should be given to the very time-consuming nature of regular nebulisation on the patient's social well-being and fitness.

Combination long-acting β-agonist and long-acting muscarinic antagonist therapy. Numerous LABA-LAMA combinations have been introduced into the UK market. Available options are Anoro (umeclidinium/vilanterol), Spiolto (tiotropium/olodaterol), Duaklir (aclidinium/formoterol) and Ultibro Breezhaler (glycopyrronium/indacaterol). SPARK was a 64-week, double-blind, randomised, parallel group study comparing glycopyrronium/indacaterol versus tiotropium versus glycopyrronium (Wedzicha et al., 2013). SPARK showed that the dual combination decreased moderate to severe exacerbations compared with both tiotropium and glycopyrronium alone. The LABA-LAMA combinations offer value for money in comparison to the separate components and short-acting drugs, so it is reasonable to use a LABA-LAMA combination inhaler from the outset rather than to use monotherapy and add in a different inhaler at a later date. Thus, the availability of these LABA-LAMA combinations along with recognition that an identifiable (non-eosinophilic) majority do not benefit from inhaled steroids has effectively made the previous complex NICE (2010) guidance on escalation of therapy redundant. This also stratifies the treatment according to inhaler device rather than changing devices at each step of the guideline.

There is some concern around the use of these agents in patients who may have an asthmatic component to their disease. This is because the use of a LABA without an ICS increases the risk of death in asthma (Spitzer et al., 1992). It is, therefore, imperative that a firm diagnosis of COPD is made when considering these agents. The absence of eosinophilia may be helpful in identifying patients who are unlikely to require inhaled steroids, although the role of blood eosinophils has yet to be firmly established in clinical practice. Evidence for the so-called 'triple therapy' (LABA-LAMA-ICS) is limited, and cost per quality-adjusted life-year (QALY) is very high.

Long-acting β₂-adrenergic agonists and inhaled corticosteroid therapy

Several preparations are now available on the UK market and include Relvar Ellipta (vilanterol and fluticasone furoate), Seretide Accuhaler and AirFluSal Forspiro (salmeterol and fluticasone propionate), Symbicort Turbohaler and DuoResp Spiromax (formoterol and budesonide), and Fostair (formoterol and ultrafine beclometasone). One of the pivotal trials was the TORCH study (Calverley et al., 2007), which compared salmeterol to fluticasone to salmeterol/fluticasone and placebo. The primary end point of reduced mortality was not reached, despite a non-significant trend toward benefit. This was also important as being the first study to identify an increased risk of pneumonia in patients using ICSs, whether as monotherapy or in combination with a LABA. At this time, trials had not been designed to assess the risk of pneumonia, and where pneumonia was reported, there was variation in methods for diagnosis and how it was distinguished from COPD exacerbations. Patient demographics (e.g. smoking or vaccination status, concurrent or previous use of oral corticosteroids) were not recorded. It has now become clear that ICSs, alone or in combination with a LABA, can increase the number of serious pneumonias that require hospitalisation. Because patients receiving an ICS are no more likely to die overall compared with controls, the clinical implication of these findings is yet to be established (Kew and Seniukovich, 2014). There is also debate whether the increased risk of pneumonia is a class effect or if a particular ICS is implicated. An increased risk of pneumonia with Relvar Ellipta of approximately double compared with the LABA monotherapy arm (6% vs 3%) has been identified (Dransfield et al., 2013). The trial was designed to detect pneumonia as a primary end point and used radiographic techniques for diagnosis, which means that the diagnosis was robustly established. More information was also available with regard to participants' smoking status, pneumonia history and body mass index (which is a risk factor for pneumonia).

It is advised that the corticosteroid dose prescribed is the minimum to maintain symptom control and/or decrease exacerbations. A recent review by the European Medicines Agency (EMA) Pharmacovigilance Risk Assessment Committee (EMA, 2016) has concluded that ICSs in the treatment of COPD do significantly increase the risk of pneumonia, but the benefits of using ICSs continue to outweigh the risks overall. The committee also concludes that there is insufficient evidence to distinguish between different ICSs with regard to risk of pneumonia.

Triple therapy combination inhalers. Trimbow pMDI (ultra-fine beclometasone/formoterol/glycopyrronium) and Trelegy (fluticasone furoate/vilanterol/umeclidinium) have recently been licensed for the management of COPD in patients who continue to experience symptoms despite treatment with ICS/LABA.

Two efficacy studies using Trimbow have been completed. The TRILOGY study compared Trimbow to Fostair 100/6 over a 26 week period. This study identified that Trimbow improved pre- and post-dose FEV$_1$ compared to Fostair and also reduced the annual rate of exacerbations by 23% as a secondary end point (Singh et al., 2016). The TRINITY study compared Fostair plus tiotropium to Trimbow over a 52 week study period. As expected, Trimbow was superior to tiotropium alone for reduction in exacerbations and improvement in FEV$_1$. Trimbow was shown to be non-inferior (or equivalent) to the triple combination with regard to exacerbations and FEV$_1$ (Vestbo et al., 2017). In these studies pneumonia was seen in a small proportion of patients, similar to other ICS studies.

These combination inhalers may offer a simplified regimen for those patients that benefit from ICS, combined with a significant cost saving. It is important to recognise that existing patients on so-called triple therapy need a therapeutic review before switching to a combination inhaler device to assess inhaler technique and to review whether the ICS can be withdrawn safely from therapy for that individual.

Withdrawal of inhaled corticosteroids in patients with chronic obstructive pulmonary disease

From the emerging literature (Magnussen et al., 2014), there is increasing confidence that there is overuse of ICSs in the COPD patient population. It is far easier to change the therapy strategy in those patients newly diagnosed. How this is managed in the existing population is more challenging because of the evidence suggesting bronchodilation rather than suppression of inflammation is important in patients with a low eosinophil count. The recent WISDOM study by Magnussen et al. (2014) showed that in a severe to very severe COPD population without a tendency to exacerbate, gradual withdrawal of ICS did not increase exacerbation rates or result in loss of symptom control. Although the evidence is beginning to point toward ICS withdrawal in this phenotype, the practicalities of how this should be undertaken are yet to be determined, and there are many factors to be considered: for example, how this would be communicated across the primary/secondary care interface; how the patient would be counselled when being switched from one inhaler type to another; whether the patient should be switched to a LABA-LAMA device and a monotherapy (off-license) ICS to gradually reduce the steroid. The WISDOM study does provide a basis on which withdrawal regimens can be based (Magnussen et al., 2014), but it should be noted that the role of ICSs in these patients is currently very much debated within the respiratory community.

Roflumilast

Roflumilast is a PDE-4 inhibitor recommended by NICE (2017) for use in patients with severe or very severe COPD with a chronic bronchitic phenotype. These patients should have had two or more exacerbations in the last 12 months despite receiving treatment with triple inhaled therapy, that is, LABA/LAMA/ICS during that period. The evidence considered by NICE was based on two clinical trials REACT (Martinez et al., 2015) and RE(2) SPOND (Martinez et al., 2016). The primary endpoints, rates of moderate or severe exacerbations, did not reach statistical significance versus placebo in the intention to treat analysis. However, it did in a pre-defined sensitivity analysis using negative binomial regression and approval has been given by NICE (2017).

Roflumilast may have a role in those patients who are obese and of a chronic bronchitic phenotype. Currently roflumilast is considered to generally provide only a modest benefit in a small cohort of patients, rather than the whole population as recommended by NICE (2017). Moreover, not only is there small clinical benefit, roflumilast is associated with significant side effects: notably weight loss, diarrhoea and nausea. These would not be appropriate in an already cachectic patient meeting the treatment criteria. In addition, more patients taking roflumilast withdrew in both trials due to adverse effects (Martinez et al., 2015, 2016). There is also an increased risk of psychiatric disorders in patients with or without a history of depression, including suicidal ideation.

Controversy with the NICE (2017) guidance lies with the definition of triple therapy. To be eligible for roflumilast, a patient must demonstrate that triple therapy is entirely clinically appropriate.

There is a view that ICS is overused and that maximal bronchodilation is sufficient for symptom management and reduction in exacerbation rates for many patients. In addition, a patient has to have been adherent with the triple therapy for 12 months to be eligible. In the UK there are practical problems implementing the guidance because of challenges associated with assessing adherence to the triple therapy. This is coupled with difficulties in assessment of the number of exacerbations, particularly in those patients who have rescue packs at home. This, together with the equivocal evidence and side effect profile for roflumilast reduces the incentive for secondary care prescribers to adopt the NICE (2017) guidance. There is also debate about when to stop roflumilast, if the patient still exacerbates. Currently NICE has not provided practical advice on this management aspect.

Theophylline and aminophylline

Methylxanthines are weak bronchodilators with a narrow therapeutic index. It appears that the benefits of these compounds in COPD may involve other mechanisms, including increasing respiratory drive and exercise tolerance as well as some steroid-sparing and anti-inflammatory effects. These drugs are now being superseded due to their relative lack of effect and poor tolerability. If used, patients should be given a therapeutic trial of 6–8 weeks to see if there is any clinical benefit. Treatment should be discontinued if there is no improvement in breathlessness or lung function testing.

Care must be taken to ensure theophylline levels are measured, particularly if the patient is prescribed interacting medications such as ciprofloxacin or clarithromycin. Other comorbidities that can also affect the clearance of theophylline include heart failure and smoking.

Mucolytics

Carbocysteine, the most commonly prescribed mucolytic, provides some symptomatic benefit in those patients with a productive cough. Upon initiation, the carbocysteine should be trialled for 6–8 weeks and then assessed for clinical improvement (e.g. reduction in cough frequency and/or sputum production). If there is no perceived benefit, then the mucolytic should be stopped. A systematic review has shown that patients who take mucolytics are less likely to exacerbate (Poole et al., 2015). The benefit appears to be greatest in those patients who exacerbate frequently and/or who have prolonged exacerbations. There is little evidence to support the initiation of mucolytics in the acute phase.

Prophylactic antibiotics

Currently, prophylactic antibiotic therapy with azithromycin is not currently recommended in the GOLD (2017) guidance unless the patient is a former smoker with recurrent exacerbations despite optimal pharmacological therapy. Macrolide antibiotics appear to have immunomodulatory and anti-inflammatory effects. One study has shown that azithromycin in a dose of 250 mg daily (in addition to usual COPD medication) reduced exacerbation rates from 1.83 per patient-year in the placebo group to 1.48 per patient-year (Albert et al., 2011). However, azithromycin has been associated with prolonged QT intervals and ventricular arrhythmias. Probably more importantly, there is real concern regarding antibiotic resistance and the effect on the microbial flora in the community. Unfortunately, azithromycin appears to be particularly prone to causing transmissible antibiotic resistance, even when compared to other macrolides. Whilst the routine use of prophylactic azithromycin is not recommended, it may be considered in very severe patients who have a history of frequent exacerbations, whose medication regimens have been fully optimised, who are not at risk of ventricular arrhythmias and who have a normal QT interval on electrocardiography.

Pharmacological management of exacerbations of chronic obstructive pulmonary disease

Exacerbations of COPD are an acute deterioration beyond the day-to-day variation in symptoms, often precipitated by viral or bacterial infection. This can result in episodes of respiratory failure and may require admission to hospital, although patients can often be safely managed at home, with appropriate support and self-management plans.

Bronchodilators

These are used to treat the acute wheeze and breathlessness. After acute admission, hand-held inhalers plus spacer device is recommended where possible, but in practice, it is more pragmatic from a nursing workload perspective to administer bronchodilators via a nebuliser at least for the first day. Salbutamol 2.5 mg four times daily is usually adequate with the addition of ipratropium 500 micrograms four times daily as an adjunct. Doses above 1 mg of salbutamol confer small additional benefits and increase cost and side effects. It is usually preferable to use a mouthpiece for delivery of nebules where possible to decrease adverse effects and to improve lung deposition. This is particularly important with the use of ipratropium in patients with glaucoma. LAMAs and LABA-LAMAs should be suspended whilst on nebuliser therapy.

Antibiotics

Acute infective exacerbations may be bacterial or viral in origin. If the exacerbation is bacterial in origin, suggested by purulent sputum, then antibiotics should be prescribed. Common bacteria include *Streptococcus pneumoniae*, *Haemophilus influenzae* and *Moraxella catarrhalis*. First-line antibiotics include amoxicillin, doxycycline and clarithromycin, but local antibiotic policy should be followed. Antibiotic therapy is not indicated if sputum is non-purulent (or similar in colour to normal) unless there is other evidence or infection, such as infective consolidation, high fever or acute-phase response (i.e. a markedly raised C-reactive protein [CRP] or erythrocyte sedimentation rate [ESR]). Patients admitted to hospital should have sputum sent for culture and sensitivity to optimise therapy. Usually a 5- to 7-day course is

Table 26.4 Comparison of type 1 and type 2 respiratory failure

	Type 1 respiratory failure	Type 2 respiratory failure
PaO_2 level	Low	Low
$PaCO_2$ level	Low or normal	Raised
Pathophysiological cause	Impaired gas exchange (ventilation/perfusion mismatch)	Hypoventilation (may also be impaired gas exchange)
Common associated diseases	'Pink-puffer' variant of COPD Pneumonia Pulmonary embolism Asthma (unless moribund)	'Blue-bloater' variant of COPD Morbid obesity Neuromuscular diseases including respiratory muscle weakness, kyphoscoliosis
Treatment	Whatever concentration of oxygen needed (FiO_2) to achieve SaO_2 of 94–98% Treatment of the underlying cause	Controlled oxygen to achieve SaO_2 88–92% If $PaCO_2$ climbs, causing pH to fall below 7.35, consideration of non-invasive ventilation

COPD, Chronic obstructive pulmonary disease; FiO_2, fraction of inspired oxygen; $PaCO_2$, arterial carbon dioxide tension; PaO_2, arterial oxygen tension; SaO_2, percentage of oxygen saturation of arterial blood.

effective. It is prudent to monitor sputum volume and colour and temperature to ensure resolution of infection prior to discontinuing antibiotics. If the exacerbation follows influenza, then there is a risk of *Staphylococcal aureus* infection, when an agent with anti-staphylococcal properties should be used (e.g. flucloxacillin or co-amoxiclav).

Corticosteroids

GOLD (2017) recommends a course of prednisolone 30 mg for 5–7 days only. There is evidence to suggest that a shorter course of steroids does not increase the risk of relapse and minimises risk to the patient. Many clinicians favour the use of a 5-day course (Leuppi et al., 2013). ICSs are usually continued during this phase. Increasingly, an absence of eosinophilia is used to identify patients who may not benefit, but this is not presently supported by guidelines.

Aminophylline

On occasion, intravenous aminophylline may be used if there is an inadequate response to bronchodilators. If the patient is already on a theophylline compound, then the loading dose is not required. If the patient is unsure if he or she is on a theophylline and that information is not available, then it is best to omit the loading dose and give the maintenance dose only. Smoking status should be established because smoking increases the metabolism of theophylline. Once smoking stops, then continuing a patient on his or her usual theophylline dose will likely result in toxicity.

Thromboprophylaxis

All acutely unwell medical patients admitted to hospital should receive a prophylactic dose of low-molecular-weight heparin if there is no known contraindication.

Physiotherapy

When bronchiectasis complicates COPD, physiotherapy instruction on daily sputum clearance exercise is the mainstay of control, along with antibiotics for infective exacerbations. Otherwise, the input of the physiotherapist is generally limited to pulmonary rehabilitation, which is now widely available.

Management of acute respiratory failure in chronic obstructive pulmonary disease

The type of respiratory failure is important in the management of the acute exacerbation: patients with type 1 respiratory failure (that is, a low oxygen level without an increased carbon dioxide level) are not at risk of developing elevated carbon dioxide levels when receiving supplemental oxygen therapy and can safely be treated with whatever oxygen concentration is required to achieve normal oxygen saturation (94–98%). In contrast, patients with type 2 respiratory failure (when the carbon dioxide level is increased) can develop severe carbon dioxide retention with attendant narcosis, especially if treated with injudicious concentrations of oxygen; a target of 88–92% is sufficient. These two forms of respiratory failure are compared in Table 26.4.

Some patients live with undiagnosed type 2 respiratory failure, and its longstanding nature can be identified when the pH is normal. The respiratory acidosis is fully compensated by a metabolic alkalosis, reflected by a high standard bicarbonate level observed on arterial blood gas analysis.

When patients present acutely with a respiratory acidosis (i.e. the pH is less than 7.35 despite appropriate oxygen and bronchodilator therapy), the introduction of non-invasive ventilation (NIV) can be life-saving and may obviate invasive positive pressure ventilation (IPPV). It is important that a ceiling of escalation of treatment is established in the acute setting because severely disabled patients are unlikely to survive or benefit from IPPV and indeed would often decline this when its implications are explained.

Doxapram, a respiratory stimulant, has largely been superseded by NIV and is no longer recommended as a routine treatment. Doxapram must be infused at a rate of 1.5–4 mg/min in those patients where NIV is contraindicated and in patients with hypercapnic respiratory failure who are comatosed. It can sometimes enable the patient to become more rousable and more able to cooperate with therapy. Clinicians should be aware that doxapram can also be harmful in respiratory failure because it stimulates both respiratory and nonrespiratory muscles. As a consequence it must only be used under expert medical advice and in a suitably supervised clinical area to minimise risk. Overall, the recommendation is to avoid doxapram due to its very limited benefits.

Patient care

Pulmonary rehabilitation

The most effective treatment for improving quality of life and ameliorating breathlessness is pulmonary rehabilitation. It is composed of multiple interventions, not just exercise training. Thus, subjects receive education on self-management, nutrition, home exercise and medication use. Programmes typically run from 6–8 weeks, usually with two visits per week. Pharmacists are well placed to contribute to this programme of education regarding pharmacological management, including introducing the concept of medicines in the palliation of symptoms.

Vaccination

Whilst pneumococcal and influenza vaccinations are not 100% effective, all patients diagnosed with COPD should be offered them. Influenza vaccination is annual, and a single pneumococcal inoculation is advised unless there is another reason to be vaccinated more frequently (e.g. nephrotic syndrome). Patients should be reassured that the influenza vaccine is inactive and that they are not able to contract the illness from the vaccination itself.

Stopping smoking

The effects of smoking on health are well known and well publicised. As described previously, stopping smoking is the most important intervention patients can achieve no matter their age or how advanced their lung disease is. There are a number of therapeutic options to aid a quit attempt.

Nicotine replacement therapy

Nicotine replacement therapy (NRT) can be used to aid abrupt smoking cessation (e.g. whilst on a ward as an in-patient) or, alternatively, to reduce the number of cigarettes smoked in the lead-up to a specified quit date.

There are many different formulations available that can be prescribed. Many of these are now licensed to be used in combination with other NRT products with or without smoking and also in pregnancy. These are shown in Table 26.5.

The mode of action is directly on nicotine receptors in the brain, which release dopamine. This has the effect of reducing the nicotine withdrawal symptoms (e.g. agitation). Another significant influencing factor is the habit of putting a cigarette to the lips, and the use of some of the products that mimic this action can also be helpful, especially in social situations. NRT does not completely eliminate the effects of withdrawal because none of the available products can accurately reproduce the rapid and high levels of nicotine obtained from cigarettes.

There is no clear evidence that one formulation is more effective than another, and the effectiveness of any of these products will lie with the individual and his or her trigger points and habits. Choices are influenced by the number of cigarettes smoked, personal preference/previous/experience and tolerance of side effects. Another factor to consider, although unlikely with a diagnosis of COPD, is if the patient is pregnant. Patches should be avoided where possible due to the continuous level of nicotine in the plasma. As with any pharmacological therapy, the benefits should always outweigh the risks, and the use of nicotine patches is not contraindicated in pregnancy if the patient is able to maintain her smoke-free status as a result of using the product. For information on formulations available and their usage/side effects, please see Table 26.5.

Bupropion

Bupropion (amfebutamone hydrochloride) is licensed for smoking cessation and works by inhibiting uptake of noradrenaline and dopamine within the neuronal synapses. This reduces the withdrawal symptoms by increasing synaptic dopamine levels. Treatment is started 2 weeks prior to the quit date, and cigarettes should be stopped in the second week of treatment. If abstinence is not achieved or maintained by week 7 of treatment, it should be discontinued. Bupropion is contraindicated in epilepsy, acute alcohol or benzodiazepine withdrawal, bipolar disorder, central nervous system (CNS) tumour, eating disorders and hepatic cirrhosis. The main side effects include agitation, anxiety, dry mouth, allergic reactions and insomnia.

Varenicline

Varenicline is a selective nicotine receptor partial agonist at the a4b2 acetylcholine receptor. It alleviates the craving and withdrawal whilst reducing the rewarding and reinforcing effects of smoking by preventing binding of nicotine to a4b2 receptors if a cigarette is smoked. A recent trial, EAGLES, compared varenicline with bupropion, NRT patches and placebo. The trial showed that at weeks 12 and 24, varenicline provided superior abstinence rates in both psychiatric and nonpsychiatric patients (Anthenelli et al., 2016). Varenicline is usually started 1–2 weeks before quitting smoking and comprises a 12-week course. Medicines and Healthcare Products Regulatory Agency (MHRA)/Commission on Human Medicines (CHM) advice states that varenicline may be associated with increased risk of suicide, and patients should be counselled to discontinue treatment if they develop agitation, depression or suicidal thoughts. Any patient with a history of psychiatric illness should be monitored closely.

Electronic cigarettes

The use of electronic cigarettes has also received attention, with controversy over effectiveness and regulation. Initially, the

Table 26.5 Comparison of nicotine replacement products

Formulation	Use and comments	Specific side-effects
Patch 24 h: 7, 14, 21 mg 16 h: 5, 10, 15, 25 mg	Apply on waking to dry, clean and non-hairy skin on the hip, trunk or upper arm and held in position for 10–20 s. Remove the 16-h patch prior to bed. Place next patch on a different area and avoid using the same site for several days. Licensed for use over 12 years of age. Patch therapy can be useful in pregnancy if patient vomiting, otherwise intermittent therapy is preferable.	Local skin irritation and rash, insomnia. Do not use on broken skin or in patients with skin disorders.
Chewing gum: 2, 4 mg	Chew one piece of gum when urge to smoke occurs or to prevent cravings. No more than 15 pieces of 4 mg gum should be used in one day. The gum should be chewed until the taste becomes strong then should be rested between gum and cheek until taste has faded. The gum should then be chewed again. Repeat for 30 min or until taste dissipates. Avoid acidic drinks (e.g. coffee, fruit juice) for 15 min before and during treatment.	Gum may stick to dentures. Jaw ache, headache and mild burning in mouth and throat may occur.
Sublingual tablets: 2 mg	Place tablet under the tongue and allow to dissolve. Acidic drinks should be avoided for 15 min before and during treatment. Maximum 40 tablets per day.	Gastritis, oesophagitis and peptic ulcers can be aggravated by swallowing nicotine
Inhalator: 10, 15 mg cartridge	Inhale as required up to 5 min per session. Helps to satisfy the hand-to-mouth habit. The nicotine is absorbed through the oral mucosa rather than the lungs. No more than 12 cartridges of the 10 mg strength or 6 cartridges of the 15 mg strength per day. A 10 mg cartridge lasts approximately 20 min of intense use; a 15 mg cartridge lasts approximately 40 min of intense use.	Caution with asthmatics because can cause bronchospasm. Nasal irritation, rhinorrhea, sneezing, throat irritation and cough may occur.
Lozenges: 1, 1.5, 2, 4 mg	One lozenge every 1–2 h as required. Slowly allow the lozenge to dissolve in the mouth; periodically move the lozenge from one side of the mouth to the other. Lozenges last 10–30 min depending on their size. Maximum of 15 lozenges per day. Patients who smoke less than 20 cigarettes per day should use the lower-strength lozenges; patients who smoke more than 20 cigarettes per day or who have failed to quit on the low-strength should use the high-strength lozenge. Avoid acidic drinks for 15 min before and during treatment.	Gastritis, oesophagitis and peptic ulcers can be aggravated by swallowing nicotine. Nasal irritation, rhinorrhea, sneezing, throat irritation and cough may occur.
Oromucosal spray: 500 micrograms and 1 mg per actuation	One to two sprays when cravings occur, do not exceed 2 sprays per episode. Maximum 64 sprays per day. Avoid acidic drinks for 15 min before and during treatment. Spray should be released into the mouth by holding the spray as close to the mouth as possible and avoiding the lips. Do not inhale while spraying and avoid swallowing for a few seconds after use.	Gastritis, oesophagitis and peptic ulcers can be aggravated by swallowing nicotine.
Intranasal spray	One spray as required; can spray into each nostril when craving occurs. Maximum 64 sprays per day. More rapidly absorbed than other forms of nicotine replacement therapy.	Caution in asthma, nasal/sinus conditions or allergies.
Orodispersible film: 2.5 mg	Suitable for smokers who have their first cigarette of the day more than 30 min after waking up. Place one film on the tongue. Close the mouth and press the tongue gently to the roof of the mouth until the nicotine film dissolves (approximately 3 min). The film should not be chewed or swallowed whole. Users should not eat or drink while a nicotine film is in the mouth.	Gastritis, oesophagitis and peptic ulcers can be aggravated by swallowing nicotine.

Information taken from British National Formulary (2017).

stance from the professional bodies such as the MHRA was that electronic cigarettes could not be recommended due to the variation in product quality, although anecdotal reports do suggest that these are effective in helping to support a quit programme. Subsequently, there have been several papers published that appear to endorse the use of e-cigarettes (Public Health England, 2015a). Public Health England (2015b) issued a press release that concluded that e-cigarettes are 95% less harmful than tobacco with no evidence that they encourage children or nonsmokers to start smoking tobacco. However, there is no long-term information about the solvents used in the process of 'vaping' and the long-term clinical impact that this may have on the patient. There are also very real concerns around the risk of fire if the electronic cigarette is left charging, particularly with a noncompatible charger from a different brand. The use of an electronic cigarette is not considered safe in patients on long-term oxygen therapy (LTOT), and so electronic cigarettes are not permitted on hospital premises or in any area that may be oxygen enriched, for example, in the home of a patient with LTOT in place.

Effect of smoking on concomitant medications

When smoking is discontinued, this can have significant impact on how concomitant medications are metabolised. Areas of high risk include the previously common respiratory medication the-ophylline. Theophylline is a narrow-therapeutic-index medication that interacts with antibiotics such as clarithromycin and cipro-floxacin, causing the theophylline levels to significantly increase. It is imperative that an accurate smoking history is taken for patients prescribed theophylline because smoking increases its metabolism. Admission to hospital for an exacerbation of COPD means the patient is no longer able to smoke whilst an in-patient; therefore, theophylline metabolism is reduced, and the theophyl-line levels will become raised. Tachycardia and tremor are often attributed to salbutamol nebuliser therapy, but these should be recognised as a potential sign of likely theophylline toxicity. For patients who smoke, theophylline levels should be taken on admission to hospital and the doses reduced as appropriate.

Oxygen therapy

Large studies in the USA and Britain performed in the 1970s showed an important improvement in prognosis when LTOT is used for substantial proportions of the day in patients with stable hypoxaemia (Cooper et al., 1987; Medical Research Council Working Party, 1981; Nocturnal Oxygen Therapy Trial Group, 1980). The accepted criteria are as follows: patients with stable COPD and a resting PaO_2 ≤7.3 kPa or patients with stable COPD with a resting PaO_2 ≤8 kPa plus evidence of peripheral oedema, polycythaemia or pulmonary hypertension (British Thoracic Society [BTS], 2015). Oxygen is delivered via an oxygen con-centrator, which is usually piped to the living room and bedroom so that the patient can use oxygen for at least 15 hours/day at a flow rate sufficient to raise PaO_2 above 8 kPa.

Outside this setting, oxygen is usually unhelpful: there is no evidence that short-burst oxygen therapy improves breathless-ness, despite its powerful placebo effect. Occasionally patients are sufficiently motivated and benefit from portable oxygen to enable increased exercise capacity, but these are exceptions.

Patients with the typical 'pink-puffing' form of COPD tend to maintain normal blood gases until very late in the disease and so rarely meet the criteria for LTOT. Neither are they at risk of adverse effects from high concentrations of oxygen. In contrast, the 'blue-bloating' patients develop type 2 respiratory failure, meaning that that they develop elevated carbon dioxide levels and accommodate to surprisingly low oxygen levels. This group is the one that tends to benefit from LTOT. They are also, how-ever, susceptible to developing acute rises in carbon dioxide levels in response to acute exacerbations, especially when high concentrations of oxygen are administered. This life-threatening complication can cause initial headache and drowsiness, lead-ing on to coma and ultimately respiratory arrest. As a result, the BTS (2008) emergency oxygen guidelines recommend rela-tively low target oxygen saturation in the management of acute exacerbations, measured by pulse oximetry, of 88–92% in such patients, whereas those with normal or low carbon dioxide levels should have a normal target of 94–98%.

Acute episodes of type 2 respiratory failure may occur, with development of a respiratory acidosis as acute elevations of car-bon dioxide overtake the relatively slow process of compensation by renal metabolic alkalosis. Oxygen and drug therapy alone are often insufficient; indeed, even low flow rates of oxygen may make acidosis worse. It has been shown that non-invasive ven-tilation can be life-saving and can avoid the need for invasive ventilation in the relatively small proportion of patients who are otherwise fit enough to be eligible. It is recommended when the pH is less than 7.35. During the first 48 hours of therapy, the patient is encouraged to adhere to the therapy for as long as pos-sible to maximise the effectiveness of the intervention.

Some patients are prone to recurrent severe episodes of type 2 respiratory failure despite long-term oxygen therapy. They often have severe nocturnal hypoventilation and sleep poorly. Such patients may benefit from long-term domiciliary non-invasive ventilation as well as LTOT.

Antidepressants

It is widely recognised that depression is prevalent within the COPD population. It is also recognised that it is underdiagnosed, as it is in many chronic medical conditions. The selection of antidepres-sant should be made according to comorbidities, side-effect profile, interaction profile and patient choice. For example, for a cachectic patient, mirtazapine may be preferable because it can cause appe-tite stimulation. Likewise, if insomnia is a problem, then tricyclic antidepressants, trazodone or mirtazapine are good choices. For patients with a cardiac history, sertraline is the safest option.

Palliative care

Palliative care is defined by the World Health Organization (WHO, 2015) as follows:

an approach that improves the quality of life of patients and their families facing the problem associated with life-threatening illness, through the prevention and relief of suffering by means of early identification and impeccable assessment and treatment of pain and other problems, physical, psychosocial and spiritual.

Palliative care for COPD patients should start at the point of diagnosis: it is a progressive disease, and most patients con-tinue to deteriorate despite maximising pharmacological and non-pharmacological treatments. COPD contributes to the increasing population of patients diagnosed with life-limiting illnesses not related to malignancy. Any patient deemed to be in the last year of life is entitled to be managed symptomati-cally through the palliative route, but resources are currently limited for these patients. Often the most debilitating symptoms are breathlessness, depression and anxiety. It is seen as best practice to discuss preferred place of care, resuscitation status and the patient wishes as they approach the last year of life. For example, the patient's wish to have antibiotics and/or invasive and non-invasive ventilation in the event of a future severe exacerbation should be determined.

Management of breathlessness

Breathlessness is the primary symptom in the patient with COPD, reported in 90–95% of the COPD population. Breathlessness is not always related to exertion and correlates poorly with lung function. Other causes of breathlessness also frequently coexist. Heart failure, angina and dysfunctional breathing/panic should be diagnosed and treated appropriately. Unfortunately, the dyspnoea of COPD can be refractory to conventional treatment in up to 50% of patients.

Non-pharmacological methods are outlined as follows:

- addressing fear and anxiety through education and psychological support;
- use of a hand-held fan, or sitting near an open window, to stimulate the second and third trigeminal nerves, which reduces the sensation of breathlessness;
- activity-pacing advice;
- breathing exercises (e.g. pursed-lip breathing);
- complementary therapies (e.g. acupuncture, hypnosis, massage).

Opioids are the mainstay of treatment for breathlessness. The evidence base for the management of dyspnoea is not as established as for pain management, but patients do derive benefit. A Cochrane review has concluded that opioids can reduce dyspnoea irrespective of route of administration (Jennings et al., 2002). The mechanism is believed to be a central action on the respiratory control centre: it is well known that in higher doses opioids can reduce minute ventilation. They can reduce the perception of breathlessness in the same way as the perception of pain. It seems paradoxical to be giving a medication known to depress respiratory drive to a patient with an already-compromised respiratory function, but it is understood that the response to chronic hypoxia results in an abnormal perception of the symptom of breathlessness. This practice is also regarded as safe. No reports of respiratory depression were found in a study of the use of opioids for relief of dyspnoea in heart failure (Oxberry et al., 2011). To initiate opioids, the first-line choice is morphine sulfate. Often, very small doses are effective (e.g. 1.25–2.5 mg at night) initially, but it is also entirely appropriate to follow the NICE (2012) guidance for the management of pain (i.e. 2.5–5 mg every 4–6 hours or morphine sulfate MR 10 mg twice a day with 2.5 mg as required). There is no upper limit for dosing, provided relief is obtained and there are no signs of opiate toxicity, such as myoclonus, pinpoint pupils or respiratory depression. As with the initiation of any medication, it is very important that the patient understands the reason for prescribing opiates and that any misperceptions are explored. Patient should also be advised that drowsiness, especially when these drugs have recently been started, may affect fitness to drive; however, there is no restriction on driving in the UK (Department for Transport, 2013).

Benzodiazepines

There is a paucity of evidence to support the use of benzodiazepines for management of breathlessness, but it has been reported anecdotally that they are effective, and there is a trend towards benefit (Simon et al., 2010). Opioids would be first line, but benzodiazepines are used particularly in patients who suffer with panic/anxiety during an acute episode of breathlessness. Lorazepam is widely used, 0.5 mg when required up to a maximum of 4 mg daily in divided doses.

Case studies

Case 26.1

Mr B is a 67-year-old retired miner who presents to hospital as an emergency with acute shortness of breath and a cough productive of green sputum. Mr B has a past medical history of COPD and had a myocardial infarction 10 years ago. He smokes 35 cigarettes per day and has done so for the last 45 years. Spirometry has shown that his FEV_1 is 58% of predicted. He weighs 45 kg. When he is well his CAT score is 8. There are no known drug allergies.

Mr B's regular medication is:
- aspirin 75 mg daily,
- bisoprolol 10 mg daily,
- simvastatin 20 mg at night,
- salmeterol 25 microgram pressurised metered dose inhaler (pMDI) two puffs twice daily.

On examination:
- blood pressure (BP) 130/75 mmHg,
- temperature 38.6 °C,
- pulse 98 bpm,
- respiratory rate 28 breaths/min.

Investigations:
- white blood cell count 20.8×10^9 L,
- creatinine 140 mmol/L – his baseline was 93 mmol/L 3 months ago,
- Hb – normal,
- oxygen saturation 84% on 28% oxygen via Venturi mask,
- chest X-ray – no consolidation seen.

Arterial blood gases on 28% oxygen:

pH	7.30	(7.35–7.45)
pO_2	7.26 kPa	(10–13 kPa)
pCO_2	8.3 kPa	(4.7–6.0 kPa)
HCO_3	24 mmol/L	(22–26 mmol/L)

Questions

1. What is the diagnosis, and how was this determined?
2. What do the arterial blood gases show, and how would you suggest this is managed?
3. What would you expect to see on Mr B's prescription chart for acute management of his condition?

   Mr B shows no clinical improvement and appears to be tiring. He is transferred to the intensive care unit (ICU) in case ventilation (invasive or non-invasive) may be needed. In the ICU, the intensivists wish to increase his medical treatment.
4. What options are there?
5. How should aminophylline be administered?
6. What treatment options would you recommend for Mr B once he has recovered from his acute illness?
7. Are there any other medications that require optimisation?

Answers

1. Mr B has an infective exacerbation of COPD. The patient has a cough productive of green sputum and elevated temperature and white blood cell count. He is also tachypnoeic and has deranged arterial blood gases. Other potential diagnoses include anaemia, which has been excluded because his haemoglobin level is normal, community-acquired pneumonia and acute heart failure, which have also been excluded because the chest X-ray is currently clear. The patient has also developed an acute kidney injury, which should be considered when prescribing any new medications.

2. The low PaO_2 indicates significant hypoxia. The reduced pH and raised carbon dioxide constitute a respiratory acidosis and indicate hypoventilation. The normal bicarbonate indicates there has not yet been any metabolic compensation and that the condition has deteriorated in the last 1–2 days.

   The acidosis indicates a need for non-invasive ventilation. Administering higher concentrations of oxygen alone will exacerbate carbon dioxide retention and may precipitate narcosis. His arterial blood gases should be checked every 30–60 minutes after any change in oxygen therapy, and the carbon dioxide levels should be closely monitored. If there is any increase in the carbon dioxide concentration, then this may indicate a clinical deterioration.

3. In the acute phase, the aim of treatment is to optimise oxygen levels, bronchodilate to improve symptoms and treat any underlying infection. Other interventions include thromboprophylaxis at appropriate doses and frequencies according to local policy.

   The prescription should therefore include oxygen at a flow rate to maintain oxygen saturation between 88% and 92%. A salbutamol nebuliser 2.5 mg four times daily (or 10 puffs of salbutamol 100 micrograms/actuation via a spacer device four times daily) plus ipratropium 500 micrograms nebuliser four times daily will provide bronchodilation. An appropriate antibiotic such as amoxicillin or doxycycline should be prescribed for a total of 5–7 days (or as per local policy) given the green sputum and 30 mg oral prednisolone for a total of 5 days. There is no benefit in giving i.v. hydrocortisone if the patient is able to swallow; therefore, oral steroids will suffice.

4. The dose of nebulised salbutamol can be increased, but the main limitation is the side effects, including tremor, tachycardia and hypokalaemia. Ordinarily, if there has been an inadequate response to bronchodilators, then intravenous aminophylline may be considered.

5. Aminophylline is available in 250 mg/10 mL vials. The loading dose required is 5 mg/kg (i.e. 225 mg in his case). To make the dose practical for administration it should be rounded to the nearest millilitre. In this case, either 250 mg (10 mL) or 200 mg (9 mL) should be added to a 50 to 100 mL bag of either sodium chloride 0.9% or glucose 5% and given over 20 minutes. Immediately after giving the loading dose, the maintenance infusion must be started.

   - To calculate the maintenance dose = 500 microgram/kg/h. Convert to milligrams first so that everything is in the same units (i.e. 0.5 mg/kg/h). Dose to be given is therefore 22.5 mg/h.
   - Check if the is patient fluid restricted because this may dictate which fluid volume to use. In Mr B's case there is no evidence that fluid restriction is required. Add 500 mg of aminophylline to a 500 mL bag of compatible i.v. fluid. This gives a 1 mg/mL solution, which should be infused at 22.5 mL/h through an infusion pump.
   - To check aminophylline levels, the infusion should be stopped after 4–6 hours. After waiting 20 minutes a blood sample can be taken from a cannula different from the one the infusion

is running through. The infusion should then immediately be restarted. It is not necessary to wait for the result before restarting the infusion.

   - The rate should be adjusted according to level obtained.

6. Because Mr B has exacerbated, he would benefit from a full medication review. Mr B has continued to be symptomatic despite demonstrated adherence to his salmeterol therapy. GOLD (2017) guidelines suggest that a LAMA should be added to his current prescription. Mr B would fall in GOLD group C because he has had an exacerbation requiring hospital admission and his CAT score is less than 10 when he is feeling well. Alternatively, once inhaler technique has been assessed and recorded, a LABA-LAMA combination could be prescribed to maintain cost-effectiveness, for example, Anoro, Spiolto, Duaklir or Ultibro. Mr B's salmeterol should be discontinued, and this should be communicated to him and his primary care doctor.

   Whilst Mr B is an in-patient, it would be a good opportunity to offer him smoking cessation advice and pharmacological intervention to support his quit attempt. He should also be referred into the pulmonary rehabilitation service and be seen by a dietician, as he is underweight at 45 kg.

   Mr B should be offered a routine pneumococcal and annual flu vaccination and be given a self-management plan with reserve antibiotics and steroids with clear instruction on when to start these. Finally, at least 12 hours prior to discharge, he should be weaned from the oxygen and nebulisers and converted back to regular inhalers.

7. Mr B suffered a myocardial infarction 10 years ago. His medication could be reviewed. His simvastatin should be increased to a minimum of 40 mg at night. β-Blockers are not contra-indicated in COPD, and indeed, there is evidence to suggest that β-blockers may decrease mortality in patients with this condition, so this medicine should be continued. Addition of an angiotensin-converting enzyme (ACE) inhibitor should be considered once the acute kidney injury has resolved.

Case 26.2

Ms M is a 54-year-old woman who presents to hospital as an emergency, with shortness of breath and coughing up green sputum. She has a history of COPD and an FEV_1 of 44% of predicted. She smokes 50 cigarettes per day and has done so for the past 34 years. She normally finds it difficult to get herself dressed in the morning without becoming breathless. She is allergic to penicillin, which causes her tongue to swell. She has had antibiotics and steroids from her primary care doctor 5 times in the past 8 months.

Her usual medication is:

- Anoro Ellipta 55/22 micrograms one puff daily, started 6 months ago;
- salbutamol 100 micrograms pMDI two puffs when required (has been using this every 2 hours in the past 2 days);
- Uniphyllin 600 mg twice daily.

The doctor diagnoses Ms M with an infective exacerbation of COPD and prescribes:

- oxygen – target saturation 88–92%;
- dalteparin 5000 units daily;
- doxycycline 200 mg as a single stat dose followed by 100 mg daily, total course 5 days;
- salbutamol nebules 5 mg four times daily;
- ipratropium 500 micrograms four times daily;
- Anoro Ellipta 55 micrograms/22 micrograms one puff daily;
- Uniphyllin 600 mg twice daily;
- Prednisolone 30 mg daily for 5 days.

Questions

1. What is Ms M's MRC dyspnoea score?
2. What monitoring parameters would need to be measured, and why?

Ms M is admitted to a respiratory ward and appears to be doing well. On day 2, she starts to vomit, and the medical team prescribes i.v. cyclizine 50 mg three times daily to try to control this. Her BP has dropped to 90/52 mmHg, and her pulse is elevated at 135 bpm. She is tremulous, and her respiratory rate has increased to 40 breaths/min.

3. What is the cause of Ms M's vomiting, how can this be managed and why has this occurred?

Potassium levels come back as 3.0 mmol/L with no electrocardiogram (ECG) changes other than sinus tachycardia. After giving Ms M a bolus of 250 mL sodium chloride 0.9%, her BP improves to 110/60 mmHg. The medical team prescribes 40 mmol/L potassium in 1 litre sodium chloride 0.9% over 4 hours via an infusion pump with a plan to recheck potassium at the end of this period. All other electrolytes are within the normal range. The theophylline level comes back as 30 mg/L (range 10–20 mg/L). The plan is to continue to monitor Ms M on the cardiac monitor for 24 hours, repeat electrolytes and blood glucose every 6 hours and give i.v. potassium as and when required.

4. What pharmaceutical care planning should be made prior to Ms M's discharge?

Answers

1. 5, breathless whilst getting washed/dressed
2. Temperature, blood pressure, respiratory rate, pulse and arterial blood gases should be monitored to indicate if Ms M is clinically improving or deteriorating. WCC should be measured to monitor improvement in infection in conjunction with the basic observations outlined previously. The pulse rate and potassium level are important because the patient is receiving salbutamol, prednisolone and theophylline, all of which can lower potassium levels significantly. In addition, potassium is likely to drop further with her profuse and protracted vomiting. Platelets and creatinine need to be monitored because dalteparin can cause heparin-induced thrombocytopenia, and the dose is affected by renal function. Theophylline levels should be monitored on admission to hospital, particularly because Ms M is prescribed salbutamol nebules concurrently, which predisposes the patient to theophylline toxicity.
3. The most likely cause of Ms M's vomiting is theophylline toxicity. A theophylline level (even if one was taken on admission) should now be requested. Administration of theophylline should be stopped until the result is known. The most likely cause of theophylline toxicity is that Ms M has been unable to smoke whilst an in-patient. Stopping smoking reduces the metabolism of theophylline, so the patient requires a lower dose when smoking has stopped. This had not been identified as a risk factor when Ms M was admitted to hospital. Potassium, magnesium, calcium, blood glucose and phosphate levels need to be measured because profound and rapid hypokalaemia can develop with theophylline toxicity, particularly if salbutamol is being administered concurrently; i.v. replacement may be required. In the immediate situation, Ms M needs fluid resuscitation because her blood pressure is currently low; an arterial blood gas needs to be analysed to exclude metabolic acidosis or respiratory alkalosis. Salbutamol nebules need to be discontinued due to the tachycardia and likely hypokalaemia. Ms M needs to be placed on a cardiac monitor and a 12-lead ECG performed. Monitor for restlessness, agitation and convulsions. Ensure 4 mg i.v. lorazepam is prescribed as required in the event of convulsions. Beta blockers

can be considered if severe tachycardia persists. Monitor theophylline levels every 2 to 4 hours to ensure they are falling. Activated charcoal is not usually indicated if theophylline levels are less than 40 mg/L, but treatment of theophylline toxicity should be considered if symptoms do not resolve rapidly. Toxbase (www.toxbase.org) should be accessed for more detailed information.

Ondansetron is an alternative antiemetic should cyclizine be ineffective; therefore, 8 mg when required should be prescribed proactively.

4. Smoking cessation should be discussed with Ms M. She should be offered advice on support available and the pharmacological therapies that may aid her quit attempt. She should be referred to the smoking cessation team. If Ms M decides to quit, then the theophylline dose will need to be adjusted. Initially the theophylline dose should be halved to 300 mg twice daily and a level taken within a week, 4–6 hours post-dose. Ms M should also be offered pulmonary rehabilitation. She has also had five courses of oral prednisolone in the last 8 months, which increases the risk for osteoporosis. Osteoporosis prophylaxis should therefore be considered. For a patient of 54 years of age, a bone scan would usually need to be arranged. Ms M is already on Anoro, but due to her exacerbation history, she may benefit from ICS/LABA, particularly if her blood eosinophil levels are elevated. This would mean switching Anoro to a different inhaler. If her inhaler technique is good with the Ellipta device, then a suitable ICS/LABA would be Relvar 92 micrograms/22 micrograms one puff daily plus Incruse 55 micrograms one puff daily. Ms M would need to understand that the Anoro has been discontinued. Ms M should be provided with a self-management plan together with reserve steroids and antibiotics. Her vaccinations should also be checked to ensure they are up to date.

Case 26.3

Mrs K is a well-known COPD patient who has had very frequent admissions to hospital due to the symptoms related to end-stage COPD. She has no family support at home and is severely disabled by breathlessness. She is on LTOT and complies with the 15 h/day prescription. She is an ex-smoker. Mrs K is cachectic and extremely anxious, especially when she is acutely unwell and more breathless than usual. She finds it hard to sleep at night. She is adherent to her medications and knows precisely what each item is for and how often to take them. She is very reluctant for these medicines to be changed or altered. In the last few admissions, Mrs K has required non-invasive ventilation and prolonged courses of antibiotics. Mrs K has recognised herself that recently she has been more symptomatic and has been struggling to cope at home. She has decided that she does not want any more antibiotics or respiratory support should her condition acutely deteriorate once more. It has been recognised by the medical team that Ms K is entering into the last few weeks of her life, and a Do Not Attempt Cardiopulmonary Resuscitation form has been discussed with Mrs K and has been signed to be valid to the end of life.

Her regular medications are as follows:
- alendronic acid 70 mg weekly,
- betahistine 16 mg three times daily,
- carbocysteine 750 mg three times daily,
- domperidone 10 mg three times daily,
- furosemide 40 mg daily,
- gabapentin 800 mg three times daily,
- lansoprazole 30 mg daily,
- prochlorperazine 5 mg three times daily,
- quinine sulfate 300 mg at night,
- salbutamol 2.5 mg nebules four times daily,
- senna 15 mg at night,
- Seretide 500 Accuhaler one puff twice daily.

Questions

1. How would you rationalise Mrs K's current medication, and how would you persuade her to stop unnecessary medications?

   Upon talking to Mrs K, it becomes apparent that she is extremely low in mood. You suggest to her that an antidepressant may help her feel better, although it will not change her physical situation. She agrees that she feels 'down in the dumps', and she says she is willing to try a new tablet if it makes her feel better about herself.

2. Which antidepressants would you consider suitable?

3. Mrs K is breathless and anxious at rest. What suggestions could you make to help control these symptoms?

   Next time Mrs K is admitted, she is extremely unwell. Her opioid usage is equivalent to 60 mg morphine sulfate per day. She is confused and in type 2 respiratory failure. Her wish was not for further intervention, and reversible causes for the confusion are ruled out. There is no evidence of opioid toxicity (e.g. pinpoint pupils/myoclonic jerks). Mrs K is breathless, scared and agitated. She is now unable to take oral medication. Her doctor decides that she is progressing to the last few hours/days of life.

4. What would you suggest to manage her symptoms?

Answers

1. Alendronic acid, betahistine, prochlorperazine, domperidone and quinine should be stopped because these are now nonessential medications that will not significantly contribute to symptom management at this stage of her condition. A trusting relationship needs to be established with Mrs K and the risks and benefits of stopping all the medications discussed with her. Mrs K needs gentle support to understand that the medicines will not cause her symptoms to become worse and indeed may contribute to unnecessary side effects. It may be that one medicine at a time is stopped, with perhaps either the betahistine or the prochlorperazine being a suitable starting point. Betahistine and prochlorperazine are both used for vertigo, and therapeutic duplication is unnecessary, so a pragmatic starting point would be to stop one of these in the first instance. She should not take regular salbutamol in the nebuliser on top of Seretide, and instead this should be changed to as required.

2. Selective serotonin reuptake inhibitors such as citalopram would be suitable for Mrs K; mirtazapine or duloxetine would be other appropriate choices. Choosing which option is better will depend on side effects, interactions with her current medications and cost. Citalopram is licensed for panic disorder, whereas duloxetine is licensed for depression and generalised anxiety disorder. Mirtazapine is licensed for depression. Mrs K is cachectic and finds it hard to sleep at night because of her anxiety, so a suitable choice for Mrs K would be mirtazapine because this is an appetite stimulant and causes some drowsiness. It should be started at 15 mg at night and then titrated if tolerated.

3. A hand-held fan could be tried to relieve the breathlessness. Mrs K should be referred to physiotherapy to be taught coping techniques and to ensure there is no element of dysfunctional breathing. Opioids are an option to control breathlessness. Mrs K could be started on small doses of morphine sulfate solution (e.g. 2.5 mg every 4–6 hours). Often patients are initiated with morphine sulfate modified-release (MR) tablets/capsules 10 mg twice daily with 2.5 mg as a breakthrough dose to be taken if breathlessness occurs during the day. This is calculated by dividing the total daily dose of morphine by six. Laxatives and anti-emetics should also be prescribed as required. The 'as-required usage' of the breakthrough morphine should be monitored and the maintenance dose increased as appropriate dependent on clinical effect and side effects. This is calculated by adding up how much breakthrough morphine the patient has taken in the last 24 hours and adding this to the current maintenance dose. For example, if Mrs K had taken an additional 10 mg of morphine in the last 24 hours, then the total daily dose of morphine is added to the 10 mg twice-daily maintenance prescription. This makes the total daily dose of morphine 30 mg, which is then divided by 2 for the MR preparations (i.e. 15 mg twice daily). The use of benzodiazepines is also an alternative option to morphine, with lorazepam being the drug of choice. Mrs K could be started on 0.5 mg as required (max 4 mg/day). This can be used regularly if a good effect is seen. It is also appropriate to combine benzodiazepines with opioids for symptom control. Information should be provided on the hospital discharge letter to inform the primary care doctor of the newly started medications and their indications.

4. Ms K should be started on a continuous subcutaneous syringe driver containing both diamorphine (or morphine) and midazolam. Administration of midazolam and opioids via the subcutaneous route is off-license, and mixing of these products is also unlicensed. It is standard practice within palliative care to administer these medications in this manner. To calculate the equivalent dose of subcutaneous diamorphine, divide the total daily dose of oral morphine by 3. In Mrs K's case, she is taking a total daily dose of 60 mg oral morphine. To calculate the dose of diamorphine to add into the syringe driver, this total daily dose should be divided by 3. So, for Mrs K, the equivalent dose of diamorphine is 20 mg over 24 hours. If subcutaneous morphine is to be added to the syringe driver, then the total daily dose of oral morphine is divided by 2, so Mrs K would need 30 mg of subcutaneous morphine in the syringe driver over 24 hours. A small dose of midazolam should be added to the syringe driver (e.g. 5–10 mg over 24 hours). Appropriate breakthrough doses of both opioid and midazolam should be prescribed. In Mrs K's case, this would be 20 mg of diamorphine divided by 6, which is 3 mg or 30 mg of morphine divided by 6, which is 5 mg. Midazolam 2.5 mg should also be prescribed as required. Hyoscine butylbromide 20 mg subcutaneously every hour as required should be added to the prescription to reduce respiratory secretions. An anti-emetic (e.g. subcutaneous haloperidol 1.5–2.5 mg every 4 hours as required) should also be prescribed. During the dying phase, the usage of 'as-required medications' should be monitored daily as a minimum. Any medication that has been administered twice in the preceding 24 hours should be added to the syringe driver to maintain adequate symptom control. Compatibilities should be checked prior to mixing. At the end of life, it is not appropriate to continue with routine monitoring, such as blood pressure and temperature or blood glucose testing, because this does not add to the clinical management of the patient and can be distressing and uncomfortable.

References

Albert, R.K., Connett, J., Bailey, W.C., et al., 2011. Azithromycin for prevention of exacerbations of COPD. N. Engl. J. Med. 365 (8), 689–698.

Anthenelli, R.M., Benowitz, N.L., West, R., et al., 2016. Neuropsychiatric safety and efficacy of varenicline, bupropion, and nicotine patch in smokers with and without psychiatric disorders (EAGLES): a double-blind, randomised, placebo-controlled clinical trial. Lancet 387 (10037), 2507–2520.

British Thoracic Society, 2008. Guideline for emergency oxygen use in adult patients. Available at: https://www.brit-thoracic.org.uk/document-library/clinical-information/oxygen/emergency-oxygen-use-in-adult-patients-guideline/emergency-oxygen-use-in-adult-patients-guideline/.

British Thoracic Society, 2015. BTS guidelines for home oxygen use in adults. Available at: https://www.brit-thoracic.org.uk/document-library/clinical-information/oxygen/home-oxygen-guideline-(adults)/bts-guidelines-for-home-oxygen-use-in-adults/.

Calverley, P.M., Anderson, J.A., Celli, B., et al., 2007. Salmeterol and fluticasone propionate and survival in chronic obstructive pulmonary disease. N. Engl. J. Med. 356 (8), 775–789.

Celli, B.R., Cote, C.G., Marin, J.M., et al., 2004. The body-mass index, airflow obstruction, dyspnoea, and exercise capacity index in chronic obstructive pulmonary disease. N. Engl. J. Med. 350, 1005–1012.

Cooper, C.B., Waterhouse, J., Howard, P., 1987. Twelve year clinical study of patients with hypoxic cor pulmonale given long-term domiciliary oxygen therapy. Thorax 42, 105–110.

Department for Transport, 2013. Drugs and driving: the law. Available at: https://www.gov.uk/drug-driving-law.

Dransfield, M.T., Bourbeau, J., Jones, P.W., et al., 2013. Once-daily inhaled fluticasone furoate and vilanterol versus vilanterol only for prevention of exacerbations of COPD: two replicate double-blind, parallel-group, randomised controlled trials. Lancet Respir. Med. 1, 210–223. https://doi.org/10.1016/s2213-2600(13)70040-7.

European Medicines Agency, 2016. PRAC reviews known risk of pneumonia with inhaled corticosteroids for chronic obstructive pulmonary disease. Available at: http://www.ema.europa.eu/docs/en_GB/document_library/Press_release/2016/03/WC500203476.pdf.

Fletcher, C., Elmes, P., Fairbairn, M., et al., 1959. Significance of respiratory symptoms and the diagnosis of chronic bronchitis in a working population. Br. Med. J. 2, 257–266.

Fletcher, C., Peto, R., 1977. The natural history of chronic airflow obstruction. Br. Med. J. 1 (6077), 1645–1648.

GlaxoSmithKline, 2009. How is your COPD? Take the COPD assessment test. Available at: http://www.catestonline.org/images/pdfs/CATest.pdf.

GOLD (Global Initiative for Chronic Obstructive Lung Disease), 2017. Global strategy for diagnosis, management, and prevention of COPD. Available at: http://goldcopd.org.

Jadwiga, A., Wedzicha, M., Banerji, D., et al., 2016. Indacaterol–glycopyrronium versus salmeterol–fluticasone for COPD. N. Engl. J. Med. 374, 2222–2234.

Jennings, A.-L., Davies, A.N., Higgins, J.P.T., et al., 2002. A systematic review of the use of opioids in the management of dyspnoea. Thorax 57 (11), 939–944.

Jones, P.W., Quirk, F.H., Baveystock, C.M., 1991. The St. George's respiratory questionnaire. Respir. Med. 85 (Suppl. B), 2531.

Jones, P.W., Singh, D., Bateman, E.D., et al., 2012. Efficacy and safety of twice-daily aclidinium bromide in COPD patients: the ATTAIN study. Eur. Respir. J. 40, 830–836.

Kerwin, E., Hebert, J., Gallagher, N., et al., 2012. Efficacy and safety of NVA237 versus placebo and tiotropium in patients with COPD: the GLOW2 study. Eur. Respir. J. 40 (5), 1106–1114.

Kew, K.M., Seniukovich, A., 2014. Inhaled steroids and risk of pneumonia for chronic obstructive pulmonary disease. Cochrane Database Syst. Rev. 2014 (3), Art. No. CD010115. https://doi.org/10.1002/14651858.CD010115.pub2.

Leuppi, J.D., Schuetz, P., Bingisser, R., et al., 2013. Short-term vs conventional glucocorticoid therapy in acute exacerbations of chronic obstructive pulmonary disease: the REDUCE randomized clinical trial. JAMA 309 (21), 2223–2231.

Magnussen, H., Disse, B., Rodriguez-Roisin, R., et al., 2014. Withdrawal of inhaled glucocorticoids and exacerbations of COPD. N. Engl. J. Med. 371 (14), 1285–1294.

Martinez, F.J., Calverley, P.M.A., Goehring, U.-M., et al., 2015. Effect of roflumilast on exacerbations in patients with severe chronic obstructive pulmonary disease uncontrolled by combination therapy (REACT): a multicentre randomised controlled trial. Lancet 385 (9971), 857–866.

Martinez, F.J., Rabe, K.F., Sethi, S., et al., 2016. Effect of roflumilast and inhaled corticosteroid/long-acting β2-agonist on chronic obstructive pulmonary disease exacerbations (RE(2)SPOND). A randomized clinical trial. Am. J. Respir. Crit. Care Med 94 (5), 559–567.

Medical Research Council Working Party, 1981. Long-term domiciliary oxygen therapy in chronic hypoxic cor pulmonale complicating chronic bronchitis and emphysema. Report of the Medical Research Council Working Party. Lancet 317 (8222), 681–686.

National Institute for Health and Care Excellence (NICE), 2010. Chronic obstructive pulmonary disease in over 16s: diagnosis and management. Available at: https://www.nice.org.uk/guidance/CG101.

National Institute for Health and Care Excellence (NICE), 2012. Palliative care for adults: strong opioids for pain relief. Available at: https://www.nice.org.uk/guidance/cg140/resources/palliative-care-for-adults-strong-opioids-for-pain-relief-35109564116677.

National Institute for Health and Care Excellence (NICE), 2017. Roflumilast for treating chronic obstructive pulmonary disease. Technology appraisal guidance. Available at: https://www.nice.org.uk/guidance/ta461.

Nocturnal Oxygen Therapy Trial Group, 1980. Continuous or nocturnal oxygen therapy in hypoxemic chronic obstructive lung disease: a clinical trial. Ann. Int. Med. 93, 391–398.

Oxberry, S.G., Torgerson, D.J., Bland, J.M., et al., 2011. Short-term opioids for breathlessness in stable chronic heart failure: a randomized controlled trial. Eur. J. Heart Fail. 13 (9), 1006–1012.

Poole, P., Chong, J., Cates, C.J., 2015. Mucolytic agents versus placebo for chronic bronchitis or chronic obstructive pulmonary disease. Cochrane Database Syst. Rev. 2015 (7), Art. No. CD001287. https://doi.org/10.1002/14651858.CD001287.pub5.

Public Health England, 2015a. E-cigarettes: a new foundation for evidence-based policy and practice. Available at: https://www.gov.uk/government/uploads/system/uploads/attachement_data/file/454517/Ecigareetes_a_firm_foundation-for_evidence_based_policy_and_practice.pdf.

Public Health England, 2015b. E-cigarettes around 95% less harmful than tobacco estimates landmark review. Available at: https://www.gov.uk/government/news/e-cigarettes-around-95-less-harmful-than-tobacco-estimates-landmark-review.

Simon, S.T., Higginson, S.J., Booth, S., et al., 2010. Benzodiazepines for the relief of breathlessness in advanced malignant and non-malignant diseases in adults. Cochrane Database Syst. Rev. 2010 (1), Art. No. CD007354. https://doi.org/10.1002/14651858.CD007354.pub2.

Singh, D., Papi, A., Corradi, M., et al., 2016. Single inhaler triple therapy versus inhaled corticosteroid plus long-acting β2 agonist therapy for chronic obstructive pulmonary disease (TRILOGY): a double-blind, parallel group, randomised controlled trial. Lancet 10048 (388), 963–973.

Spitzer, W.O., Suissa, S., Ernst, P., et al., 1992. The use of beta-agonists and the risk of death and near death from asthma. N. Engl. J. Med. 326 (8), 501–506.

Tashkin, D.P., Celli, B., Senn, S., et al., 2008. A 4-year trial of tiotropium in chronic obstructive pulmonary disease. N. Engl. J. Med. 359 (15), 1543–1554.

Trivedi, R., Richard, N., Mehta, R., et al., 2014. Umeclidinium in patients with COPD: a randomised placebo-controlled study. Eur. Respir. J. 43, 72–81.

Vestbo, J., Papi, A., Corradi, M., et al., 2017. Single inhaler extrafine triple therapy versus long-acting muscarinic antagonist therapy for chronic obstructive pulmonary disease (TRINITY): a double blind, parallel group, randomised controlled trial. Lancet 389 (10082), 1919–1929.

Wedzicha, J.A., Decramer, M., Ficker, J.H., et al., 2013. Analysis of chronic obstructive pulmonary disease exacerbations with the dual bronchodilator QVA149 compared with glycopyrronium and tiotropium (SPARK): a randomised, double-blind, parallel-group study. Lancet Respir. Med. 1 (3), 199–209.

Wise, R.A., Anzueto, A., Cotton, D., et al., 2013. Tiotropium Respimat inhaler and the risk of death in COPD. N. Engl. J. Med. 369 (16), 1491–1501.

World Health Organization (WHO), 2015. WHO definition of palliative care. Available at: http://www.who.int/cancer/palliative/definition/en/.

Further reading

Bafadhel, M., McKenna, S., Terry, S., et al., 2012. Blood eosinophils to direct corticosteroid treatment of exacerbations of chronic obstructive pulmonary disease. Am. J. Respir. Crit. Care Med. 186 (1), 48–55.

Karner, C., Cates, C.J., 2011. The effect of adding inhaled corticosteroids to tiotropium and long-acting beta2-agonists for chronic obstructive pulmonary disease. Cochrane Database Syst. Rev. 2011 (9), Art. No. CD009039. https://doi.org/10.1002/14651858.CD009039.pub2.

McCarthy, B., Casey, D., Devane, D., et al., 2015. Pulmonary rehabilitation for chronic obstructive pulmonary disease. Cochrane Database Syst. Rev. 2015 (2), Art. No. CD003793. https://doi.org/10.1002/14651858.CD003793.pub3.

Suissa, S., Patenaude, V., Lapi, F., et al., 2013. Inhaled corticosteroids in COPD and the risk of serious pneumonia. Thorax 68, 1029–1036.

Vollenweider, D.J., Jarrett, H., Steurer-Stey, C.A., et al., 2012. Antibiotics for exacerbations of chronic obstructive pulmonary disease. Cochrane Database Syst. Rev. 2012 (12), Art. No. CD010257. https://doi.org/10.1002/14651858.CD010257.

Useful websites

COPD Assessment Test: http://www.catestonline.org/images/pdfs/CATest.pdf

British Lung Foundation: https://www.blf.org.uk/

British Thoracic Society: https://www.brit-thoracic.org.uk/

27 Insomnia

Deborah Baidoo and Michele Sie

Key points

- Hypnotic medicines do not cure insomnia but can provide useful short-term symptomatic treatment.
- Before starting medication, the primary cause of insomnia should be investigated and treated appropriately where possible.
- Non-pharmacological approaches should be considered first line.
- Hypnotic medicines should only be used short-term (2–4 weeks); long-term regular use leads to tolerance, dependence and other adverse effects.
- Sleep hygiene, relaxation techniques and psychological methods are more appropriate than hypnotics as long-term treatment for patients with insomnia.
- Nonbenzodiazepine hypnotics, such as zopiclone, zolpidem and zaleplon, have similar pharmacological and adverse effects to benzodiazepines.
- Promethazine, an antihistamine, can be used for the short-term management of insomnia in adults, but tolerance to its hypnotic effects can occur.
- A melatonin preparation is available for primary insomnia licensed in those older than 55 years. It is a naturally occurring hormone that stimulates sleep initiation but does not cause tolerance or dependence.

Definitions and epidemiology

Insomnia refers to difficulty in either falling asleep, remaining asleep or feeling refreshed from sleep. It is the most common sleep disorder and in the UK adult population; an annual prevalence of around 35% has been reported (Ellis et al., 2012). Insomnia has been significantly associated with increasing age, female gender, comorbid anxiety, depression and pain. By age 50, a quarter of the population is dissatisfied with their experience of sleep, rising to 30–40% (two-thirds of them women) among individuals older than 65 years (Sateia and Nowell, 2004).

Pathophysiology

The pathophysiology of insomnia is related to the overactivity of the arousal, emotional regulatory and cognitive sleep systems in the brain (Riemann et al., 2015). These systems are functionally interrelated, and their activity determines the degree and type of alertness during wakefulness and the depth and quality of sleep.

Sleep systems

The phenomenon of sleep is actively induced and maintained by neural mechanisms in several brain areas, including the lower brainstem, pons and parts of the limbic system. These mechanisms have reciprocal inhibitory connections with arousal systems so that the activation of sleep systems inhibits waking and vice versa. Normal sleep includes two distinct levels of consciousness, nonrapid eye movement (NREM) sleep and rapid eye movement (REM) sleep, which are promoted from separate neural centres.

NREM sleep normally takes up about 80% of sleeping time. It is divided into three stages (N1–N3), which merge into each other, forming a continuum of decreasing cortical and behavioural arousal (Fig. 27.1). Stage N3 represents the deepest phase of sleep and is also termed delta sleep (DS) due to the production of delta waves in the brain during this stage. Historically NREM sleep was defined as four stages (1–4) until 2007 when the American Academy of Sleep Medicine reclassified the sleep–wake cycle and changed the stages by amalgamating NREM stages 3 and 4 into stage N3 (Schulz, 2008).

REM sleep normally takes up about 20% of sleeping time and has characteristics quite different from NREM sleep. The electroencephalogram (EEG) shows desynchronised fast activity similar to that found in the alert conscious state, and the eyes show rapid, jerky movements. Peripheral autonomic activity is increased during REM sleep, which may result in changes in blood pressure, heart rate and respiration as well as sexual arousal. Atonia occurs, causing a temporary paralysis. Heightened cognition, resulting in vivid dreams and nightmares, most often occurs during REM sleep, although brief frightening dreams (hypnagogic hallucinations) can occur in NREM sleep, especially at the transition between sleeping and waking. Normally stage N3 sleep occurs primarily in the first few hours of the night, whereas REM sleep is most prominent towards the morning. Brief awakenings during the night are normal. Both DS and REM sleep are thought to be essential for brain function, and both show a rebound after a period of deprivation, usually at the expense of lighter (stage N1 and N2) sleep, which appears to be expendable. Many medicines can affect the different stages of sleep. Benzodiazepines suppress stage N3 of sleep but cause only a slight decrease in REM sleep.

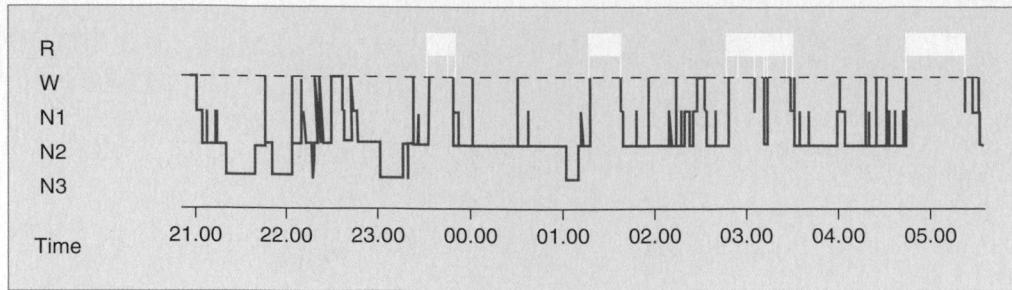

Fig. 27.1 The stages of sleep across a single night in adults.
N1, N2, N3, nonrapid eye movement sleep stages 1, 2 and 3; R, rapid eye movement sleep; W, wake.
(Keenan and Hirshkowitz, 2011, Principles and Practice of Sleep Medicine. Reprinted with permission from Elsevier.)

Z-hypnotics shorten stage N1 of sleep and prolong stage N2 of sleep but have little effect on stage N3 and REM sleep. Sedating antihistamines cause a reduction in the duration of REM sleep.

Aetiology and clinical manifestations

Insomnia may be caused by any factor that increases activity in arousal systems, which leads to decreased activity in sleep systems. Increased sensory stimulation (e.g. electronic media use) activates arousal systems, resulting in difficulty in falling asleep. Common physical health causes include chronic pain, gastric reflux, uncontrolled asthma and external stimuli such as noise, bright lights and extremes of temperature.

Mental health conditions often affect sleep. Anxiety may delay sleep onset as a result of increased emotional arousal. Difficulty in staying asleep is characteristic of depression. Patients typically complain of early waking, but sleep records show frequent awakenings, early onset of REM sleep and reduced NREM sleep. Alteration of sleep stages, increased dreaming and nightmares may also occur in schizophrenia, and recurring nightmares are a feature of posttraumatic stress disorder (PTSD). Interference with circadian rhythms, as in shift work or rapid travel across time zones, can cause difficulty in falling asleep or early waking.

Frequent arousals from sleep are associated with myoclonus, 'restless legs syndrome', muscle cramps, bruxism (tooth grinding), head banging and sleep apnoea syndromes. Reversal of the sleep pattern, with a tendency for poor nocturnal sleep but a need for daytime naps, is common in the elderly, in whom it may be associated with cerebrovascular disease or dementia. In general, decreased duration of sleep has been shown to increase the future risk of musculoskeletal pain conditions and myocardial infarction. Associations have also previously been identified with an increased risk of obesity and diabetes, but in larger studies, these have been shown not to be significant (Sivertsen et al., 2014). Sleep disturbances in the elderly are also associated with increased falls, cognitive decline and a higher rate of mortality (Cochen et al., 2009). There is growing concern that daytime sleepiness resulting from insomnia increases the risk of industrial, traffic and other accidents, medical errors and a general decrease in performance and functioning.

Difficulty in falling asleep may result directly from the action of stimulants, including caffeine, nicotine, theophylline, sympathomimetic amines, some antidepressants, levothyroxine and antimuscarinics. Some illicit substances, cocaine, amphetamines and anabolic steroids can also cause insomnia. Withdrawal after chronic use of central nervous system depressants, including hypnotics, anxiolytics and alcohol, commonly causes rebound insomnia with delayed or interrupted sleep, increased REM sleep and nightmares. With rapidly metabolised drugs, such as alcohol or short-acting benzodiazepines, duration of action is limited, which may result in early waking. Certain medicines, including antipsychotics, tricyclic antidepressants and propranolol, occasionally cause nightmares, which may result in insomnia.

Investigations and differential diagnosis

Many patients complaining of insomnia overestimate their sleep requirements. Although most people sleep for 7–8 hours daily, some healthy subjects require as little as 3 hours of sleep, and sleep requirements decline with age. Such 'physiological insomnia' does not usually cause daytime fatigue, although the elderly may take daytime naps. If insomnia is causing distress, primary causes such as pain, medicines that disturb sleep, psychiatric disturbance including anxiety and depression and organic causes such as sleep apnoea should be identified and treated before hypnotic therapy is prescribed.

Treatment
Non-pharmacological therapies

Explanation of sleep requirements, attention to sleep hygiene (Box 27.1), reduction in caffeine or alcohol intake and the use of analgesics where indicated may obviate the need for hypnotics. Medications that cause insomnia should also be avoided if possible. Sleep restriction, stimulus control and psychological techniques such as relaxation therapy and cognitive behavioural therapy (CBT) are also beneficial (Siebern et al., 2012). However, studies comparing psychological approaches to hypnotics are scarce (Riemann and Perlis, 2009).

Box 27.1 Principles of typical advice for good sleep hygiene

- Have a good bedtime routine; go to bed and get up at the same time every day, and avoid daytime naps.
- Avoid stimulants such as caffeine, nicotine, chocolate and alcohol 6 h before bedtime.
- Take regular exercise during the day, but avoid strenuous exercise within 4 h of bedtime.
- Avoid large meals close to bedtime.
- Associate bed with sleep. Do not watch TV or listen to music when retiring to bed.
- The bedroom should be a quiet, relaxing place to sleep; make sure the room is not too hot or too cold.
- If after 30 min you cannot get off to sleep, then get up. Leave the bedroom and try to do something else; return to bed when sleepy. This can be repeated as often as necessary until you are asleep.

Hypnotic medicines

Hypnotic medicines provide only symptomatic treatment for insomnia. Although often efficacious in the short-term they do little to alter the underlying cause, which should be sought and treated where possible. About 9 million prescriptions for hypnotics are issued each year in primary care in England, and there is a trend that prescribing of these medicines is reducing year on year. These medicines can improve the quality of life if used rationally.

The ideal hypnotic would:

- gently suppress brain arousal systems while activating systems that promote deep and satisfying sleep,
- have a rapid onset of action with no residual effects,
- have no ataxic or memory effects,
- not induce tolerance or dependence if used long-term
- not cause withdrawal effects when stopped,
- not depress respiration,
- be safe for use in the elderly patient.

Unfortunately, most available hypnotics are general central nervous system depressants which inhibit both arousal and sleep mechanisms. Thus, they do not induce normal sleep and often have adverse effects, including daytime sedation ('hangover') and rebound insomnia on withdrawal. They are unsuitable for long-term use because of the development of tolerance and dependence.

Benzodiazepines

By far the most commonly prescribed hypnotics are the benzodiazepines. Various benzodiazepines are available (Table 27.1). These medicines differ considerably in potency (equivalent dosage) and in rate of elimination but only slightly in clinical effects. All benzodiazepines have sedative/hypnotic, anxiolytic, amnesic, muscular relaxant and anticonvulsant actions, with minor differences in the relative potency of these effects.

Pharmacokinetics. Most benzodiazepines marketed as hypnotics are well absorbed and rapidly penetrate the brain, producing hypnotic effects within half an hour after oral administration. Rates of elimination vary, however, with elimination half-lives from 6 to 100 hours (see Table 27.1). These medicines undergo hepatic metabolism via oxidation or conjugation and some form pharmacologically active metabolites with even longer elimination half-lives.

Oxidation of benzodiazepines is decreased in the elderly, in patients with hepatic impairment and in the presence of some medication, for example, oral contraception, disulfram and propranolol.

Pharmacokinetic characteristics are important in selecting a hypnotic medicine. A rapid onset of action combined with a medium duration of action (elimination half-life about 6–8 hours) is usually desirable. Too short a duration of action may lead to, or fail to control, early morning waking, whereas a long duration of action (e.g. nitrazepam) may produce residual effects the next day and may lead to accumulation if the medication is used regularly. However, frequency of use and dosage are also important. For example, diazepam (5–10 mg) produces few residual effects when used occasionally, despite its slow elimination, although chronic use impairs daytime performance. Large doses of short-acting medicines may produce hangover effects, whereas small doses of longer-acting medicines may cause little or no hangover.

Mechanism of action. Most of the effects of benzodiazepines result from their interaction with specific binding sites associated with postsynaptic $GABA_A$ receptors in the brain. All benzodiazepines bind to these sites, although with varying degrees of affinity, and potentiate the inhibitory actions of GABA at these sites.

$GABA_A$ receptors are the major inhibitory transmitter receptor in the brain. They are multi-molecular complexes (Figs. 27.2 and 27.3) that control a chloride ion channel and contain specific binding sites for gamma aminobutyric acid (GABA), benzodiazepines and several other medicines, including many nonbenzodiazepine hypnotics and some anticonvulsant medicines (Richter et al., 2012). The various effects of benzodiazepines (hypnotic, anxiolytic, anticonvulsant, amnesic, muscle relaxant) result from GABA potentiation in specific brain sites and at different types of $GABA_A$ receptor. There are multiple subtypes of $GABA_A$ receptor, which may contain different combinations of at least 19 subunits (including α_{1-6}, β_{1-3}, γ_{1-3} and others), and the subtypes are differentially distributed in the brain.

Benzodiazepines predominantly bind to receptors containing α, β, and γ subunits, and it appears that their combination with α_1-containing subtypes mediates their sedative, amnesic and anticonvulsant effects whilst α_2-containing subtypes mediate their anxiolytic effects (Möhler, 2006).

Zopiclone

Zopiclone, a cyclopyrrolone, was the first nonbenzodiazepine to be approved for the treatment of insomnia in the European market. Although classed as a nonbenzodiazepine, it still binds to benzodiazepine receptors and is more selective for the α_1 subtype. It has been shown to be effective in promoting sleep initiation and sleep maintenance and is licensed in the UK for up to 4 weeks of use. It has an elimination half-life of approximately 5 hours. This medicine appears to have no particular advantages over benzodiazepines, although it may cause less alteration of sleep stages.

It has hypnotic effects similar to benzodiazepines and carries a similar potential for adverse effects including tolerance, dependence and abstinence effects on withdrawal. Psychiatric reactions, including hallucinations, behavioural disturbances and nightmares, have been reported to occur shortly after the first dose. Other common adverse reactions include a bitter taste, a dry mouth and difficulty arising in the morning (Zammit, 2009).

Table 27.1 Overview of the medication used for insomnia

Drug	Usual dose at night (adult) (mg)	Half-life in adults (h)	Licensed indication	Tolerance	Dependence
Benzodiazepines					
Diazepam	5–15	24–36	Insomnia (short-term use)	Yes	Yes
Loprazolam	1	11	Insomnia (short-term use)	Yes	Yes
Lorazepam	1–2	12–16	Insomnia (short-term use)	Yes	Yes
Lormetazepam	0.5–1.5	10	Insomnia (short-term use)	Yes	Yes
Nitrazepam	5–10	18–36	Insomnia (short-term use)	Yes	Yes
Temazepam	10–20	5–11	Insomnia (short-term use)	Yes	Yes
Z-Hypnotics					
Zaleplon	5–10	2	Insomnia (short-term use up to 2 weeks)	Yes	Yes
Zolpidem	5–10	2–3	Insomnia (short-term use up to 4 weeks)	Yes	Yes
Zopiclone	3.75–7.5	3.5–6	Insomnia (short-term use up to 4 weeks)	Yes	Yes
Orexin receptor antagonist					
Suvorexant	10	10–22	Insomnia up to 3 months	Yes	Yes
Chloral and derivatives (rarely used)					
Cloral betaine[a]	707–1414	Unclear	Insomnia (short-term use)	Yes	Yes
Clomethiazole					
Clomethiazole	192–384	4–5	Severe insomnia in elderly (short-term use)	Yes	Yes
Antihistamines					
Promethazine	25–50	10–19	Insomnia (short-term use)	Yes	No
Diphenhydramine	50	2.5–9	Relief of temporary sleep disturbance (short-term use up to 2 weeks)	Yes	No
Melatonin					
Melatonin (Circadin) Unlicensed products also available	2	3.5–4	Insomnia in adults older than 55 years (up to 13 weeks)	No	No

[a]Chloral betaine 707 mg is equivalent to 414 mg chloral hydrate tablets.

Eszopiclone

The S(+) enantiomer of zopiclone is available in the USA, but there are no current plans for it to be launched in the UK. The advantage that the isomer incurs over zopiclone is unclear. Eszopiclone has been shown to promote sleep onset and sleep maintenance. It has a mean elimination half-life of approximately 7 hours. There is no evidence of tolerance, rebound insomnia or serious withdrawal effects (Hair et al., 2008; Zammit, 2009).

Zolpidem

Zolpidem is an imidazopyridine that binds preferentially to the α_1 benzodiazepine receptor subunit thought to mediate hypnotic effects. It is an effective hypnotic with only weak anticonvulsant and muscle relaxant properties. It has a short elimination half-life (2–3.5 hours), reducing the risk of hangover effects, but rebound effects may occur in the later part of the night, causing early morning waking and daytime anxiety. Zolpidem can cause tolerance and a pharmacodependence, leading to a withdrawal

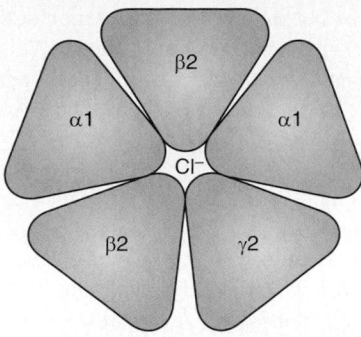

GABA_A receptor

6 different α subunits

4 different β subunits

3 different γ subunits

Most common mammalian
structure $(α1)_2(β2)_2(γ1)$

Fig. 27.2 The GABA_A receptor and subunits. The GABA_A receptor is a heteropentameric glycoprotein. A total of five distinct polypeptide subunits have been cloned to date—α, β, γ, d, and r—and multiple isoforms of these subunits are reported in the literature. Different conformations of the GABA_A receptor are found throughout the brain, and the most common mammalian arrangements of subunits is $(α_1)2(β_2)2(γ_1)$. The specific subunits in the GABA_A receptor confer functional diversity on the receptor. For example, the γ subunit needs to be co-expressed with the α and β subunits to observe the potentiation of the GABA_A receptor by benzodiazepines.

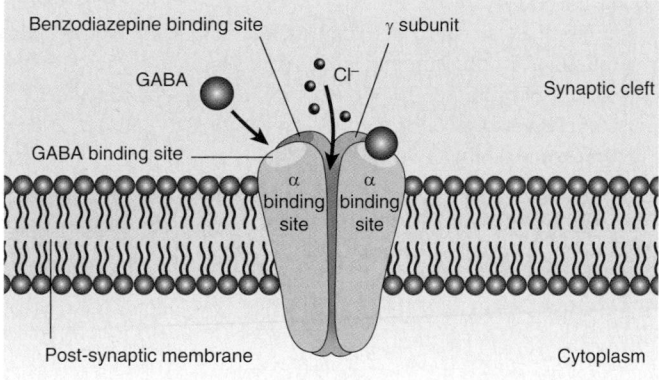

Fig. 27.3 Schematic representation of the GABA_A receptor. GABA is the major inhibitory neurotransmitter in the central nervous system. The GABA_A receptor is composed of five subunits—two α, two β and one γ subunit. Two molecules of GABA activate the receptor by binding to the α subunits. Once activated the receptor allows the passage of negatively charged ions (Cl⁻) into the cytoplasm, which results in hyperpolarisation and the inhibition of neurotransmission. (Source: www.CNSforum.com.)

syndrome and causing irritability, agitation, nervousness and, in severe cases, seizures. Anecdotal case reports have also associated zolpidem with complex sleep-related behaviours. These have included sleep-walking, 'sleep-driving', 'sleep self-intoxication', amnesia, making phone calls, preparing food and eating while asleep. Long-term use of zolpidem has been shown to increase the risk of major injury (head trauma or fracture). In the USA in 2013 zolpidem became the first medication to be prescribed

differently according to gender following evidence that women were more susceptible to next-day impaired alertness due to slower elimination (Farkas et al., 2013). A controlled-release version of zolpidem (zolpidem-CR) is available in some countries.

Zaleplon

Zaleplon is a pyrazolopyrimidine which, like zolpidem, binds selectively to the α₁ benzodiazepine receptor. It has been shown to effectively promote sleep initiation but is less effective in promoting sleep maintenance. It has a very short elimination half-life of 1 hour and appears to cause minimal residual effects on psychomotor or cognitive function after 5 hours.

There is little evidence of tolerance or withdrawal effects in short-term use, and the medicine appears suitable for use in the elderly.

Suvorexant

Suvorexant, a novel hypnotic, is a dual orexin-1 receptor and orexin-2 receptor antagonist. Suvorexant is structurally unrelated to benzodiazepines and other hypnotic agents. It has been shown to be effective in promoting sleep initiation and maintaining sleep and can be used for periods of up to 3 months. It has an elimination half-life of approximately 15 hours (range of 10–22 hours).

Clinical trial data showed no evidence of rebound insomnia on discontinuation, no evidence of physical dependence with prolonged use and no reports of withdrawal symptoms. However, further clinical trials may be required to determine tolerance and withdrawal effects in long-term use (Yang, 2014).

Other hypnotic medicines

The risk of adverse effects, including dependence and dangerous respiratory depression in overdose, generally outweighs the potential benefits of the older hypnotics – chloral derivatives, clomethiazole and barbiturates. Therefore, these treatments are best avoided. Antidepressants with sedative properties, such as mirtazapine or agomelatine, may be helpful if sleep disturbance is secondary to depression. Sedative antipsychotics are not recommended for the management of insomnia due to their adverse effects.

Antihistamines

Diphenhydramine and promethazine

Diphenhydramine and promethazine are H-1 receptor antagonists. Activating H-1 receptors promotes wakefulness, and therefore H-1 receptor antagonists promote sedation. The evidence for the efficacy in the management of acute or chronic insomnia is sparse. Diphenhydramine and promethazine have an elimination half-life of approximately 2–9 hours and 5–14 hours, respectively.

The long duration of action may lead to hangover effects, and antihistamines are associated with a potential for tolerance and abuse. Abrupt discontinuation can be associated with activation, insomnia and mild antimuscarinic withdrawal symptoms such as nausea, sweating and headache. Many antihistamines have potent anticholinergic activity, leading to adverse effects of sedation, dizziness, dry mouth, constipation, urinary retention, blurred vision and weight gain.

Melatonin

Melatonin is a naturally occurring hormone, produced by the pineal gland, which regulates the circadian rhythm of sleep. It begins to be released once it becomes dark and continues to be released until the first light of day. Melatonin release decreases with age, which may in part explain why older adults require less sleep. Melatonin supplementation promotes sleep initiation and helps reset the circadian clock, allowing uninterrupted sleep. It has also been shown to improve next-day functioning. Contrary to most other hypnotics, melatonin shows no abuse or tolerance potential and appears to have no next-day sedation problems (Riemann et al., 2015). Prolonged-release melatonin (Circadin) was launched in June 2008 and is available at a dose of 2 mg at night for up to 13 weeks. It is licensed as monotherapy in primary insomnia for adults older than 55 years old. Although the adverse-effect profile looks advantageous, there are currently no trials comparing melatonin against psychological or other hypnotic treatments. Circadin is also much more expensive than other currently prescribed hypnotics

Potential adverse effects of hypnotic use

Tolerance and dependence

Tolerance to the hypnotic effects of benzodiazepines, z-hypnotics and antihistamines develops rapidly and may lead to unprescribed dose escalation by users. Nevertheless, poor sleepers may report continued efficacy. Physical and psychological dependence are common with benzodiazepines and z-hypnotics, and despite safety recommendations for short-term use, these medicines are often used long-term because of difficulties on withdrawal. Prescribing hypnotics beyond limited short courses brings potential hazards, of dependence, adverse effects and adverse events, for example, falls. Targeted deprescribing of hypnotic medicines can lead to better health outcomes.

Rebound insomnia

Rebound insomnia, in which sleep is poorer than before pharmacological treatment, is common on withdrawal of benzodiazepines. Sleep latency (time to onset of sleep) is prolonged, intra-sleep wakenings become more frequent and REM sleep duration and intensity are increased, with vivid dreams or nightmares which may add to frequent awakenings. These symptoms are most marked when the medicines have been taken in high doses or for long periods but can occur after only a week of low dose administration. They are prominent with moderately rapidly eliminated benzodiazepines (temazepam, lorazepam) and may last for many weeks. With slowly eliminated benzodiazepines (diazepam), DS and REM sleep may remain depressed for some weeks and then slowly return to the baseline, sometimes without a rebound effect. Tolerance and rebound effects are reflections of a complex homeostatic response to regular use of medicines, involving desensitisation, uncoupling and internalisation

of certain GABA/benzodiazepine receptors and sensitisation of receptors for excitatory neurotransmitters (Allison and Pratt, 2003). These changes encourage continued hypnotic usage and contribute to the development of dependence.

Oversedation and hangover effects

Many benzodiazepines and z-hypnotics used to treat insomnia can give rise to a subjective 'hangover' effect, and after most of them, even those with short elimination half-lives, psychomotor performance, including driving ability and memory, may be impaired on the following day. Oversedation is most likely with slowly eliminated medicines, especially if used chronically, and is most marked in the elderly in whom drowsiness, incoordination and ataxia, leading to falls and fractures, and acute confusional states may result, even from small doses. Chronic use can cause considerable cognitive impairment, sometimes suggesting dementia. Paradoxical excitement may occasionally occur.

These medicines may also decrease alveolar ventilation and depress the respiratory response to hypercapnia, increasing the risk of cerebral hypoxia, especially in the elderly and in patients with chronic respiratory disease.

Drug interactions

Concomitant use of two or more medicines that cause central nervous system (CNS) depression result in additive effects that can increase drowsiness, cause marked sedation and reduce alertness, which may lead to accidents and severe respiratory depression. Medicines that can cause CNS depression include antidepressants, antiepileptics, antihistamines, antipsychotics, anxiolytics, benzodiazepines, barbiturates, hypnotics, opioid analgesics and skeletal muscle relaxants as well as alcohol (all amounts). (Zammit, 2009).

Suvorexant is metabolised via cytochrome P450 isoenzyme CYP3A, and therefore use with potent inhibitors of these enzymes (e.g. ketoconazole) is not recommended. Dose adjustment may be required when used with moderate inhibitors (e.g. fluconazole); conversely, concomitant use with potent CYP3A inducers (e.g. rifampicin) is likely to reduce efficacy of suvorexant (Yang, 2014).

Rational pharmacological treatment of insomnia

A hypnotic may be indicated for insomnia when it is severe, disabling, unresponsive to other measures or likely to be temporary. In choosing an appropriate agent, individual variables relating to the patient and to the medicine need to be considered (see Table 27.1).

Patient care

Type of insomnia

The duration of insomnia is important in deciding on a hypnotic regimen. Transient insomnia may be caused by changes of routine such as overnight travel, change in time zone, alteration of shift work or temporary admission to hospital. In these circumstances, a hypnotic with a rapid onset, medium duration of action and few residual effects could be used on one or two occasions.

Short-term insomnia may result from temporary environmental stress. In this case, a hypnotic may occasionally be indicated but should be prescribed in low dosage for 1 or 2 weeks only, preferably intermittently, on alternate nights or one night in three to prevent tolerance and dependence.

Chronic insomnia presents a much greater therapeutic problem. It is usually secondary to other conditions (organic or psychiatric) at which treatment should initially be aimed. In selected cases, a hypnotic may be helpful, but it is recommended that such medicines should be prescribed at the minimal effective dosage and administered intermittently (one night in three) or temporarily (not more than 2 or 3 weeks). Occasionally it is necessary to repeat short, intermittent courses at intervals of a few months.

The elderly

The elderly are especially vulnerable both to insomnia and to adverse effects from hypnotic medicines. They may have reduced metabolism of some medicines and may be at risk of cumulative effects. They are also more susceptible than younger people to CNS depression, including cognitive impairment and ataxia (which may lead to falls and fractures). They are sensitive to respiratory depression, prone to sleep apnoea and other sleep disorders and are more likely to have 'sociological', psychiatric and somatic illnesses which both disturb sleep and may be aggravated by hypnotics. For some of these elderly patients, hypnotics can improve the quality of life, but the dosage should be adjusted (usually half the recommended adult dose), and hypnotics with long elimination half-lives or active metabolites should be avoided.

A considerable number of elderly patients give a history of regular hypnotic use going back for 20 or 30 years. In many of these patients, gradual reduction of hypnotic dosage or even withdrawal may be indicated and can be carried out successfully, resulting in improved cognition and general health with no impairment of sleep or escalation of other symptoms.

The young

Traditional benzodiazepine-like hypnotics are generally contraindicated for children. Promethazine is the only licensed paediatric sedative for use in those aged 5 years or older. The use of promethazine in young children is usually unjustified, and there have been reports of a possible association between the use of phenothiazine antihistamines and sudden infant death syndrome (SIDS), although this has not been confirmed. The off-label use of melatonin is common particularly in those with attention-deficit/hyperactivity disorder (ADHD).

Disease states

Hypnotics are contraindicated in patients with acute pulmonary insufficiency, significant respiratory depression, marked neuromuscular respiratory weakness, sleep apnoea syndrome or severe hepatic impairment. In terminal conditions, the possibility of pharmacodependence becomes a less important issue, and regular use of hypnotics with a medium duration of action should not be denied if they provide symptomatic relief of insomnia.

Choice of pharmacological treatment

There is little difference in hypnotic efficacy between most of the available agents. The main factors to consider in the rational choice of a hypnotic regimen are duration of action and the risk of adverse effects, especially oversedation and the development of tolerance and dependence. There is no compelling evidence to distinguish z-hypnotics from the shorter-acting benzodiazepine hypnotics (National Institute for Health and Care Excellence, 2004). Patients who do not respond to either a benzodiazepine or z-hypnotic should not be prescribed the other. Cost may also be a factor when prescribing melatonin.

Rate of elimination

Slowly eliminated medicines should be avoided because of the risk of oversedation and hangover effects. Very short-acting drugs such as zaleplon carry the risk of late-night rebound insomnia and daytime anxiety. Medicines with a medium elimination half-life (6–8 hours) appear to have the most suitable profile for hypnotic use. These include temazepam and zopiclone, and as such, these are the medicines of first choice in most situations where hypnotics are indicated in adults. Sedative antihistamines are a reasonable second choice, followed by melatonin.

Duration and timing of administration

To prevent the development of tolerance and dependence, the maximum duration of treatment should be limited to between 2 and 4 weeks, and treatment should, where possible, be intermittent (one night in two or three). Dosage should be tapered slowly if hypnotics have been taken regularly for more than a few weeks to prevent potential withdrawal effects such as rebound insomnia, anxiety, loss of appetite, tremor, perspiration and seizures (Tapering advice is available in the British National Formulary.). Doses should be taken 20 minutes before retiring in order to allow dissolution in the stomach and absorption to commence before the patient lies down in bed.

Medicines and driving

In the UK the Department for Transport has introduced a new offence of driving with certain controlled drugs above specified limits in the blood. The new law came into force on 2 March 2015 and outlaws driving while under the influence of drugs. As well as illegal drugs, the new legislation also includes some prescription medicines. Medicines included in the new offence that might be used for insomnia include benzodiazepines (e.g. temazepam and diazepam). The legislation provides for a statutory 'medical defence', if patients are taking medicines in accordance with instructions and their driving is not impaired. Patients who are unsure about the effects of their medication or how the new legislation may affect them are advised to seek the advice of their doctor or pharmacist. Drivers who are taking prescribed medication at high doses are advised to carry evidence with them, such as prescriptions slips, when driving in order to minimise any inconvenience should they be asked to take a test by the police (Department for Transport, 2014).

Case studies

Case 27.1

Mr PH, aged 24, was hospitalised for 3 months after a serious motorcycle injury followed by painful complications. While in hospital he developed panic attacks and insomnia. He received no psychological support but was prescribed temazepam, initially in 20 mg doses but later increased to 60 mg because of continued insomnia. After discharge from hospital Mr PH continued to receive temazepam from his primary care doctor, and the dosage was increased over a period of years until he was taking 80 mg temazepam each night and 40–80 mg during the day. At the age of 30, Mr PH was removed from the practice list of his doctor after he altered a prescription. He later attended several different primary care doctors, obtaining multiple temazepam prescriptions. When he could no longer satisfy his need from prescriptions, he took to obtaining temazepam on the street, taking large and irregular doses by mouth. All this time, his anxiety levels increased. His behaviour became chaotic, and he was twice imprisoned for credit card fraud, but he was able to obtain temazepam and other drugs from his co-prisoners. When last heard of, Mr PH, aged 35, was again buying temazepam illicitly, as well as other addictive drugs, had started injecting intravenously and was involved in a court case for obtaining money under false pretences.

Question

How could the risk of creating dependence and subsequent personal tragedy have been avoided?

Answer

Mr PH's problematic situation could have been averted by judicial prescribing, supply and management of medicines likely to cause dependence or substance misuse.

- The risk of creating dependence could be reduced by not introducing medicines with an abuse potential unless absolutely necessary. Non-pharmacological approaches (e.g. sleep hygiene and/or cognitive behavioural therapy) should have been considered in the first instance.
- Rapid and large dose escalation of temazepam should be avoided, and the lowest effective therapeutic dose for hypnotics should be used. The appropriate dose of hypnotic should be reviewed at each opportunity because the signs of dependence, its effects, and withdrawal from medicines with abuse potential are not always obvious, so timely recognition and assessment may be difficult.
- The treatment and management of the underlying cause for insomnia should be investigated because Mr PH may have been experiencing PTSD or panic disorder. Along with psychological approaches, an antidepressant with sedative effects may have been a more appropriate prescription choice, instead of prolonged treatment with excessive doses of temazepam.
- A slow reducing-dose schedule for hypnotics should be implemented when the acute episode for insomnia has been managed. On discharge from hospital, Mr PH's primary care doctor should have been warned about his temazepam intake and a slow withdrawal schedule communicated.

- Signs of drug-seeking behaviour, such as visiting more than one doctor, fabricating stories and forging prescriptions, should be addressed. The series of primary care doctors who gave Mr PH prescriptions should have been aware that he was likely to attempt to obtain illicit supplies and should have referred him to a withdrawal clinic or substance misuse unit. Doses should be reduced steadily and/or weekly or even daily prescriptions issued for small amounts if dependence is suspected.
- Prescribers should closely monitor amounts prescribed for medicines with abuse potential to prevent patients or their carers from accumulating stocks. A minimal amount should be prescribed in the first instance, or when seeing a new patient for the first time. Patients seen by temporary care services should be given small amounts of medicines unless they present an unequivocal letter from their own primary care doctor.

Case 27.2

Mrs RS, a recently widowed woman aged 75, had difficulty sleeping after her bereavement. She was initially prescribed temazepam 10 mg at night, which was changed following reports of next-day hangover effect to zopiclone in a bedtime dose of 7.5 mg. This was very effective and was continued for over 4 weeks. Mrs RS lived alone but was visited occasionally by her daughter. On a visit 2 weeks after the zopiclone was started, Mrs RS seemed calm and said that she was sleeping well, but the daughter noticed her mother was unsteady on her feet. A few weeks later the daughter visited again and found her mother lying on the bedroom floor, in pain and unable to move. She said that she had lost her balance on getting out of bed. An ambulance was called, and it was found in hospital that Mrs RS had broken her hip.

Question

Should the doctor have prescribed temazepam or zopiclone for this patient, and what other treatment options are available?

Answer

- First-line treatment for insomnia should be non-pharmacological, such as sleep hygiene and relaxation techniques. The doctor should have completed a healthy sleep assessment to identify any contributory factors to Mrs RS's insomnia, such as using stimulant substances (e.g. caffeine) or taking other medicines that may have affected her sleep (e.g. diuretics in the evening).
- Benzodiazepines and z-hypnotics should be avoided in the elderly. If used, a medication with a short duration of action should be selected, and the dose of hypnotic should be reduced to ¼–½ of the adult dose. Zopiclone starting dose in the elderly is 3.75 mg at night.
- Hypnotics should be used on alternate nights or one night in three to prevent tolerance and dependence.
- The elderly are particularly prone to ataxia and light-headedness with benzodiazepines and z-hypnotics, and this can lead to falls and fractures.
- Benzodiazepines and z-hypnotics are not recommended, except acutely, for bereavement. Their amnesic effects may interfere with subsequent psychological adjustment.
- If a hypnotic was indicated, melatonin would have been a better option for Mrs RS because it has less adverse effects, has no tolerance or dependence risks, does not exhibit the increased risk of falls observed with other hypnotics and can be used for up to 13 weeks.

References

Allison, C., Pratt, J.A., 2003. Neuroadaptive processes in GABAergic and glutamatergic systems in benzodiazepine dependence. Pharmacol. Ther. 98, 171–195.

Cochen, V., Arbus, C., Soto, M.E., et al., 2009. Sleep disorders and their impact on healthy, dependent and frail older adults. J. Nutr. Health Aging 13, 322–330.

Department for Transport, 2014. Guidance for healthcare professionals on drug driving. Available at: https://www.gov.uk/government/publications/drug-driving-and-medicine-advice-for-healthcare-professionals

Ellis, J.G., Perlis, M.L., Neale, L.F., et al., 2012. The natural history of insomnia: focus on prevalence and incidence of acute insomnia. J. Psychiatr. Res. 46, 1278–1285.

Farkas, R.H., Unger, E.F., Temple, R., 2013. Zolpidem and driving impairment: identifying persons at risk. N. Engl. J. Med. 369, 689–691.

Hair, P.I., McCormack, P.L., Curran, M.P., 2008. Eszopiclone: a review of its use in the treatment of insomnia. Drugs 68, 1415–1434.

Keenan, S., Hirshkowitz, M., 2011. Monitoring and staging human sleep. In: Kryger, M.H., et al. (Ed.), Principles and Practice of Sleep Medicine, fifth ed. Elsevier Saunders, St. Louis, pp. 1602–1609.

Möhler, H., 2006. GABA$_A$ receptor diversity and pharmacology. Cell Tiss. Res. 326, 505–516.

National Institute for Health and Care Excellence, 2004. Guidance on the use of zaleplon, zolpidem and zopiclone for the short-term management of insomnia. Technology Appraisal 77. NICE, London. Available at: http://guidance.nice.org.uk/TA77/Guidance/pdf/English

Richter, L., De Graaf, C., Sieghart, W., et al., 2012. Diazepam-bound GABA$_A$ receptor models identify new benzodiazepine binding-site ligands. Nat. Chem. Biol. 8, 455–464.

Riemann, D., Nissen, C., Palagini, L., et al., 2015. The neurobiology, investigation, and treatment of chronic insomnia. Lancet Neurol. 14, 547–558.

Riemann, D., Perlis, M.L., 2009. The treatments of chronic insomnia: a review of benzodiazepine receptor agonists and psychological and behavioral therapies. Sleep Med. Rev. 13, 205–214.

Sateia, M.J., Nowell, P.D., 2004. Insomnia. Lancet 364, 1959–1973.

Schulz, H., 2008. Rethinking sleep analysis. J. Clin. Sleep Med. 4, 99–103.

Siebern, A.T., Suh, S., Nowakowski, S., 2012. Non-pharmacological treatment of insomnia. Neurotherapeutics 9, 717–727.

Sivertsen, B., Lallukka, T., Salo, P., et al., 2014. Insomnia as a risk factor for ill health: results from the large population based prospective HUNT study in Norway. J. Sleep Res. 24, 124–132.

Yang, L.P., 2014. Suvorexant: first global approval. Drugs 74, 1817–1822.

Zammit, G., 2009. Comparative tolerability of newer agents for insomnia. Drug Saf. 32, 735–738.

Further reading

Anon., 2009. Melatonin for primary insomnia. Drug Ther. Bull. 47, 74–77.

Bloom, H.G., Ahmed, I., Alessi, C.A., et al., 2009. Evidence-based recommendations for the assessment and management of sleep disorders in older persons: supplement. J. Am. Geriatr. Soc. 57, 761–789.

Schutte-Rodin, S., Broch, L., Buysse, D., et al., 2008. Clinical guideline for the evaluation and management of chronic insomnia in adults. J. Clin. Sleep. Med. 15 (4), 487–504.

Wilson, S.J., Nutt, D.J., Alford, C., et al., 2010. British Association for Psychopharmacology consensus statement on evidence-based treatment of insomnia, parasomnias and circadian rhythm disorders. J. Psychopharm. 24, 1577–1600. Available at: https://www.bap.org.uk/pdfs/BAP_Guidelines-Sleep.pdf

Winkelman, J.W., 2015. Insomnia disorder. N. Engl. J. Med. 373, 1437–1444.

Useful websites

The National Sleep Foundation was founded in 1990 by the leaders in sleep medicine. The website has a number of resources covering topics such as sleep science, healthy sleep habits, and sleep disorders for medical professionals, patients and the public: https://sleepfoundation.org

The Clinical Knowledge Summaries website from NICE is a concise summary of current evidence for primary care professionals: https://cks.nice.org.uk/insomnia

The Royal College of Psychiatrists' website provides information for professionals, patients and the public, including a number of health advice leaflets: http://www.rcpsych.ac.uk/

The NHS Choices website provides advice for patients and the public, including advice on the management on insomnia. https//www.nhs.uk

28 Anxiety Disorders

Stephen Bleakley and David S. Baldwin

Key points

- Benzodiazepines should typically only be used short-term (2–4 weeks) because long-term regular use can lead to tolerance, dependence and other adverse effects in some patients.
- If benzodiazepines are indicated, the smallest effective dose should be used along with intermittent dosing where possible. Start with small doses; increase if necessary. Use half the adult dose in elderly patients.
- Psychological therapies ('talking therapies') are generally considered first-line treatments in all anxiety disorders because they may provide lower relapse rates than pharmacotherapy.
- Some antidepressants are appropriate as long-term treatment for anxiety disorders.
- Selective serotonin reuptake inhibitors (SSRIs) are the recommended antidepressants in anxiety disorders but can worsen symptoms at the beginning of treatment, so patients should be monitored carefully in the first weeks.
- When antidepressants are used, they often require higher therapeutic doses in anxiety disorders than those used in patients with depression.

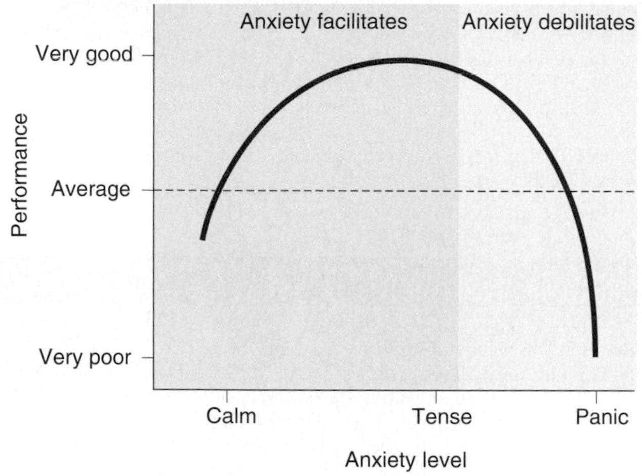

Fig. 28.1   The Yerkes–Dodson curve.

Definitions and epidemiology

Anxiety is a normal, protective, psychological response to an unpleasant or threatening situation. Mild to moderate anxiety can improve performance and ensure appropriate action is taken. However, excessive or prolonged anxiety can be disabling, lead to severe distress and cause much impairment in social functioning. Fig. 28.1 shows that as anxiety levels increase, performance and actions initially increase; however, as the anxiety level increases beyond acceptable or tolerated levels, performance declines.

The term *anxiety disorder* encompasses a variety of conditions that can either exist on their own or in conjunction with another psychiatric or physical illness. Symptoms of anxiety vary, but patients generally present with a combination of psychological, physical and behavioural symptoms (Fig. 28.2). Some of these symptoms are common to many anxiety disorders, whereas others are distinctive to a particular disorder. Anxiety disorders are broadly divided into generalised anxiety disorder (GAD), panic disorder, social anxiety disorder, specific phobias, separation anxiety disorder and illness anxiety disorder. Posttraumatic stress disorder (PTSD) and obsessive-compulsive disorder (OCD) were previously classified under the umbrella of anxiety disorders but

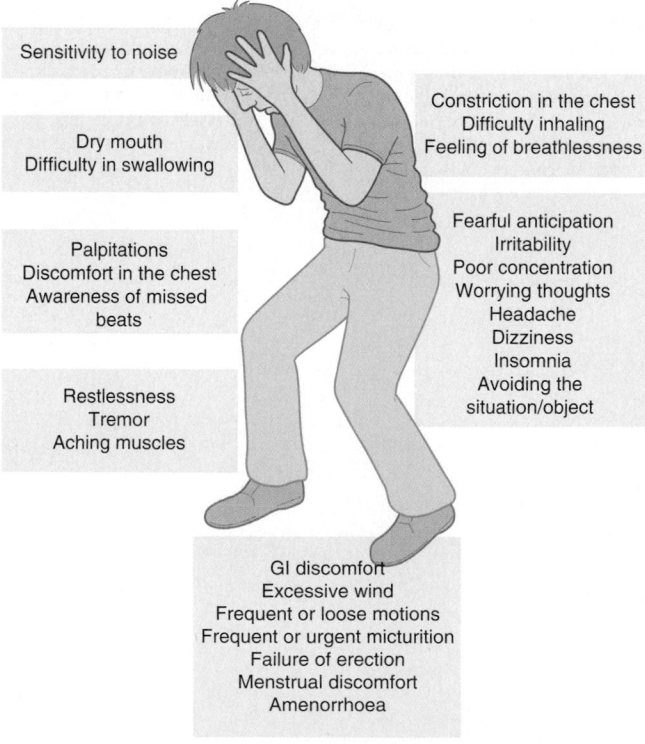

Fig. 28.2   The symptoms of anxiety.

Table 28.1 A brief description of anxiety and related disorders

Symptoms common to all anxiety disorders	Fear or worry, sleep disturbances, concentration problems, dry mouth, sweating, palpitations, GI discomfort, restlessness, shortness of breath, avoidance behaviour
Generalised anxiety disorder (GAD)	Persistent (free-floating), excessive and inappropriate anxiety on most days for at least 6 months. The anxiety is not restricted to a specific situation.
Panic disorder (with or without agoraphobia)	Recurrent, unexplained surges of severe anxiety (panic attack). Most patients develop a fear of repeat attacks or the implications of an attack. Often seen in agoraphobia (fear in places or situations from which escape might be difficult).
Social anxiety disorder (or social phobia)	A marked, persistent and unreasonable fear of being observed, embarrassed or humiliated in a social or performance situation (e.g. public speaking or eating in front of others)
Specific phobia	Marked and persistent fear that is excessive or unrealistic, precipitated by the presence (or anticipation) of a specific object or situation (e.g. flying, spiders). Sufferers avoid the feared object/subject or endure it with intense anxiety.
Posttraumatic stress disorder (PTSD)	Can occur after an exposure to a traumatic event which involved actual or threatened death or serious injury or threats to the physical integrity of self or others. The person responds with intense fear, helplessness or horror. Sufferers can re-experience symptoms (flashbacks) and avoid situations associated with the trauma. Usually occurs within 6 months of the traumatic event.
Obsessive-compulsive disorder (OCD)	Persistent thoughts, impulses or images (obsessions) that are intrusive and cause distress. The person attempts to get rid of these obsessions by completing repetitive, time-consuming purposeful behaviours or actions (compulsions). Common obsessions include contamination, and the compulsion may be repetitive washing or cleaning.

GI, Gastro-intestinal.

Box 28.1 Patient testimonies (NICE, 2005a, 2005b)

Symptoms described by a sufferer of posttraumatic stress disorder:
I would feel angry at the way the crash happened and that there was nothing I could do to stop it or help. I was physically exhausted, but was finding it hard to sleep. As soon as the bedroom light went out at night a light would come on in my head and all I could do was lie there and think. When I would eventually fall asleep, I would wake up with nightmares of the crash. I could not get away from it. It was all I could think about in the day and all I would dream about at night.

Thoughts from a sufferer of obsessive-compulsive disorder:
I've just arrived home from work. Tired and tense, I'm convinced my hands are contaminated with some hazardous substance and my primary concern now is to ensure that I don't spread that contamination to anything that I, or others, may subsequently touch. I will wash my hands, but first I will need to put a hand in my pocket to get my door keys, contaminating these, the pocket's other contents, and everything else I touch on my way to the sink. It will be late evening before I will have completed the whole decontamination ritual.

A slow recovery described by a posttraumatic stress disorder and panic attack sufferer:
Slowly I gained ground and as each new insight came I was able to see my symptoms diminish. The panic attacks tapered off, the intensity of the flashbacks dwindled, and my irritable bowel began to loosen some of its hold on me. I was able to breathe again.

are now considered to be separate illnesses. For completeness, though, these will also be discussed here. Table 28.1 presents a brief description of anxiety and related disorders. Patient testimonials are presented in Box 28.1. Approximately two-thirds of sufferers of an anxiety disorder will have another psychiatric illness. This is most commonly depression, and often successful treatment of an underlying depression will significantly improve the symptoms of anxiety. Many patients also present with symptoms of more than one anxiety disorder at the same time, which can further complicate treatment. Anxiety disorders are the most commonly reported mental disorders and as a whole have a lifetime prevalence of approximately 21% (Baldwin et al., 2014), with specific phobias the most commonly reported.

For all anxiety disorders together, the overall female-to-male ratio is 2:1. The age of onset of most anxiety disorders is in young adulthood (20s and 30s), although the maximum prevalence of generalised anxiety and agoraphobia in the general population is in the 50- to 64-year-old age group.

Pathophysiology

Anxiety occurs when there is a disturbance of the arousal systems in the brain. Arousal is maintained by at least three interconnected systems: a general arousal system, an 'emotional' arousal system and an endocrine/autonomic arousal system (Fig. 28.3). The general arousal system, mediated by the brainstem reticular formation, thalamic nuclei and basal forebrain bundle, serves to link the cerebral cortex with incoming sensory stimuli and provides a tonic influence on cortical reactivity or alertness. Excessive activity in this system, due to internal or external stresses, can lead to a state of hyperarousal as seen in anxiety. Emotional aspects of arousal, such as fear and anxiety, are contributed by the limbic system, which also serves to focus attention on selected aspects of the environment. There is evidence that increased activity in certain limbic pathways is associated with anxiety and panic attacks.

These arousal systems activate physical responses to arousal, such as increased muscle tone, increased sympathetic activity

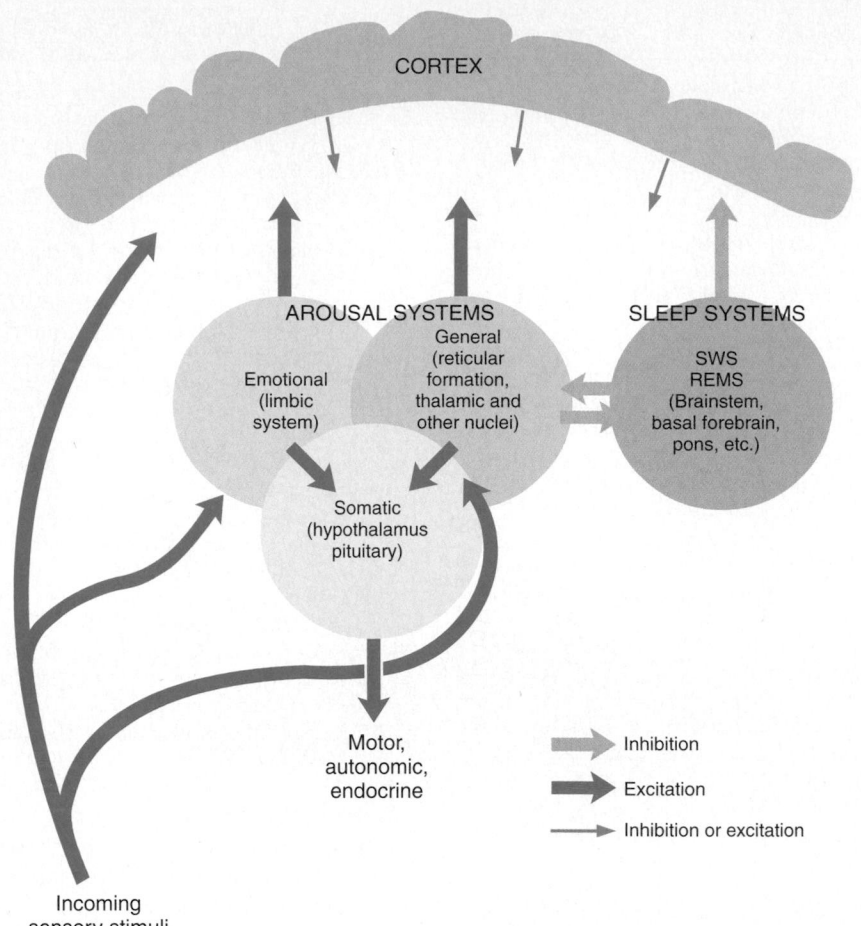

Fig. 28.3 Diagram of arousal and sleep systems. Arousal systems receive environmental and internal stimuli, cause cortical activation and mediate motor, autonomic and endocrine responses to arousal. Reciprocally connected sleep systems generate slow-wave sleep (SWS) and rapid eye movement sleep (REMS). Either system can be excited or inhibited by cognitive activity generated in the cortex.

and increased output of anterior and posterior pituitary hormones. Inappropriate increases in autonomic activity are often associated with anxiety states; the resulting symptoms (palpitations, sweating, tremor, etc.) may initiate a vicious circle that increases the anxiety.

Several neurotransmitters have been implicated in the arousal systems. Acetylcholine is the main transmitter maintaining general arousal, but there is evidence that heightened emotional arousal is particularly associated with noradrenergic and serotonergic activity. Drugs which antagonise such activity have anxiolytic effects. In addition, the inhibitory neurotransmitter γ-aminobutyric acid (GABA) exerts an inhibitory control on other transmitter pathways, and increased GABA activity may have a protective effect against excessive stress reactions. Many drugs which increase GABA activity, such as the benzodiazepines, are potent anxiolytics.

Aetiology and clinical manifestations

Anxiety is commonly precipitated by stress or adverse life events, but vulnerability to stress and trait anxiety also appear to be linked to genetic factors. Many patients presenting for the first time with anxiety symptoms have a long history of high anxiety levels going back to childhood. Anxiety may also be induced by central stimulant drugs (e.g. caffeine, amphetamines), withdrawal from chronic use of central nervous system depressant drugs (e.g. alcohol, hypnotics, anxiolytics) and metabolic or endocrine disturbances (e.g. hyperventilation, hypoglycaemia, thyrotoxicosis). Anxiety may form part of a depressive disorder or psychosis and may occur in temporal lobe lesions and in rare hormone-secreting tumours such as phaeochromocytoma or carcinoid syndrome.

Apart from the psychological symptoms of apprehension and fear, somatic symptoms may be prominent in anxiety and include palpitations, chest pain, shortness of breath, dizziness, dysphagia, gastro-intestinal disturbances, loss of libido, headaches and tremor. Panic attacks are experienced as storms of increased autonomic activity combined with a fear of imminent death or loss of control. If panic becomes associated with a particular environment, commonly a crowded place with no easy escape route, the patient may actively avoid similar situations and eventually become agoraphobic. When anxiety is precipitated by a specific cause, then behaviour can become altered to ensure the sufferer avoids the cause. This avoidance behaviour can maintain the often-irrational fear and strengthen the desire to avoid the threat.

Investigations and differential diagnosis

In patients presenting with symptoms and clinical signs of anxiety, it is important to exclude organic causes such as thyrotoxicosis, excessive use of stimulant drugs such as caffeine and the possibility of alcohol dependence or withdrawal effects from benzodiazepines. However, unnecessary investigations should generally be avoided if possible. Extensive gastroenterological, cardiological and neurological tests may increase anxiety by reinforcing the patient's fear of a serious underlying physical disease.

Treatment

Treatment for anxiety disorders often requires multiple approaches. The patient may need short-term treatment with an anxiolytic, such as a benzodiazepine, to help reduce the immediate symptoms combined with psychological therapies and an antidepressant for longer-term treatment and to prevent relapse of symptoms.

Psychological interventions

Psychological therapies ('talking therapies') are generally considered first-line treatments in all anxiety disorders because they may provide lower relapse rates than pharmacotherapy. Psychotherapy, however, is less readily available, is more emotionally demanding and takes longer to work than pharmacotherapy. If the patient is unable to tolerate the anxiety or associated distress, then medicines are often used before psychotherapy or while awaiting psychotherapy. The ideal treatment should be tailored to the individual and optimised treatment may involve the combination of psychotherapy and pharmacotherapy. The type of treatment should depend on symptoms, type of anxiety disorder, speed of response required, long-term goals and patient preference.

The specific psychotherapy with the most supporting evidence in anxiety disorders is cognitive behavioural therapy (CBT). CBT focuses on the 'here and now' and explores how individuals feel about themselves and others and how behaviour is related to these thoughts. Through individual therapy or group work, the patient and therapist identify and question maladaptive thoughts and help develop an alternative perspective. Individual goals and strategies are developed and evaluated with patients, who are encouraged to practise what they have learned between sessions. Therapy usually lasts for around 60–90 minutes every week for 8–16 weeks, or longer in more resistant cases. Cognitive behavioural therapists are usually health professionals such as mental health nurses, psychologists, primary care doctors, social workers, counsellors or occupational therapists who have undertaken specific training and supervision.

In PTSD, CBT is trauma focused, with the therapist helping patients confront their traumatic memories and people or objects associated with the trauma. At the same time, patients are taught skills to help them cope with the emotional or physical response to the trauma. One such skill includes relaxation training, which may involve systematically relaxing major muscle groups in a way that decreases anxiety. Another psychotherapy sometimes recommended in PTSD is eye movement desensitisation and reprocessing (EMDR). This involves briefly recounting the trauma or objects associated with the trauma to the therapist, who will then simultaneously initiate another stimulus, for example, moving a finger continuously in front of the patient's eyes or hand tapping. Over time, it enables the patient to focus on alternative thoughts when associations with the trauma occur. Routinely applied single- or multiple-session 'debriefing' following a traumatic event is not thought effective to prevent PTSD and, therefore, not recommended.

In OCD, CBT includes exposure and response prevention (ERP). This involves the therapist and the patient repeatedly facing the fears, beginning with the easiest situations and progressing until all the fears have been faced. At the same time the person must not perform any rituals or checks.

Specific phobias, illness anxiety disorder and separation anxiety disorder are also almost exclusively treated using psychological therapies. Only a few patients will require additional drug therapy, which is usually a selective serotonin reuptake inhibitor (SSRI).

Other psychotherapies (excluding those based on CBT techniques) are occasionally tried, but these have a poorer evidence base and are, therefore, not usually recommended. Self-help approaches are recommended (National Institute for Health and Care Excellence [NICE], 2011) for GAD and panic disorder. They usually involve using materials either alone or in part under professional guidance to learn skills to help cope with the anxiety. The materials, such as books, tapes or computer packages, can be accessed at home and at the patient's convenience. Some self-help material, however, is of poor quality, so it is probably best used in those who have mild symptoms and who do not need more intensive treatments.

Pharmacotherapy

Benzodiazepines

Benzodiazepines are often prescribed to provide an immediate reduction in the symptoms of severe anxiety. Various benzodiazepines are available (Table 28.2). These drugs differ considerably in potency (equivalent dosage) and in the rate of elimination but only slightly in clinical effects. All benzodiazepines have sedative/hypnotic, anxiolytic, amnesic, muscular relaxant and anticonvulsant actions, with minor differences in the relative potency of these effects.

Pharmacokinetics. Most benzodiazepines are well absorbed and rapidly penetrate the brain, producing an effect within half an hour after oral administration. Rates of elimination vary, however, with elimination half-lives from 8 to 35 hours (see Table 28.2). The drugs undergo hepatic metabolism via oxidation or conjugation and some form pharmacologically active metabolites with shorter or even longer elimination half-lives. An example of this effect is diazepam, which has active metabolites including temazepam and oxazepam. Oxidation of benzodiazepines is decreased in the elderly, in patients with hepatic impairment and in the presence of some drugs, including alcohol. Benzodiazepines are metabolised mostly through the cytochrome P450 3A4/3 enzyme system in the liver, so significant enzyme inducers (e.g. carbamazepine) may reduce levels, whereas enzyme inhibitors (e.g. erythromycin) may increase levels (Bazire, 2014).

Mechanism of action. Most of the effects of benzodiazepines result from their interaction with specific binding sites associated with postsynaptic $GABA_A$ receptors in the brain. All benzodiazepines bind to these sites, although with varying degrees of affinity, and potentiate the inhibitory actions of GABA at these sites. GABA is the most important inhibitory neurotransmitter in the central nervous system (CNS). Neuronal activity in the CNS is regulated by the balance between GABA inhibitory activity and excitatory neurotransmitters such as glutamate. If the balance swings towards more GABA activity, sedation, ataxia and amnesia occur. Conversely, when GABA is reduced arousal, anxiety and restlessness occur. $GABA_A$ receptors are multimolecular complexes that control a chloride ion channel and contain specific binding sites for GABA, benzodiazepines and several other drugs, including many nonbenzodiazepine hypnotics and some anticonvulsant drugs (Haefely, 1990) (Fig. 28.4). The various effects of benzodiazepines (hypnotic, anxiolytic, anticonvulsant, amnesic, muscle-relaxant) result from GABA potentiation in specific brain sites and at different $GABA_A$ receptor types. There are multiple subtypes of $GABA_A$ receptor which may contain different combinations of at least 17 subunits (including α_{1-6}, β_{1-3}, γ_{1-3}, and others), and the subtypes are differentially distributed in the brain (Christmas et al., 2008). Benzodiazepines bind to two or more subtypes, and it appears that combination with α_2-containing subtypes mediates their anxiolytic effects and α_1-containing subtypes their sedative and amnesic effects. There is some evidence that patients with anxiety disorders have reduced numbers of benzodiazepine receptors in key brain areas that regulate anxiety responses (Roy-Byrne, 2005). Secondary suppression of noradrenergic and/or serotonergic and other excitatory systems may also be of importance in relation to the anxiolytic effects of benzodiazepines.

Role in treating anxiety. Benzodiazepines have been used for more than 50 years in the treatment of anxiety and can provide rapid symptomatic relief from acute anxiety states.

Table 28.2 Profile of selected benzodiazepines (Bazire, 2014; Taylor et al., 2015)

Drug	Usual daily dose (mg)	Half-life hours (range)	Equivalent dose to diazepam 10 mg
Alprazolam	0.5–1.5	13 (12–15)	Unknown
Chlordiazepoxide	30	12 (6–30)	30 mg
Clonazepam	2–4	35 (20–60)	1–2 mg
Diazepam	5–30	32 (21–50)	—
Lorazepam	1–4	12 (8–25)	1 mg
Oxazepam	30	8 (5–15)	30 mg
Temazepam	10–20	8 (5–11)	20 mg

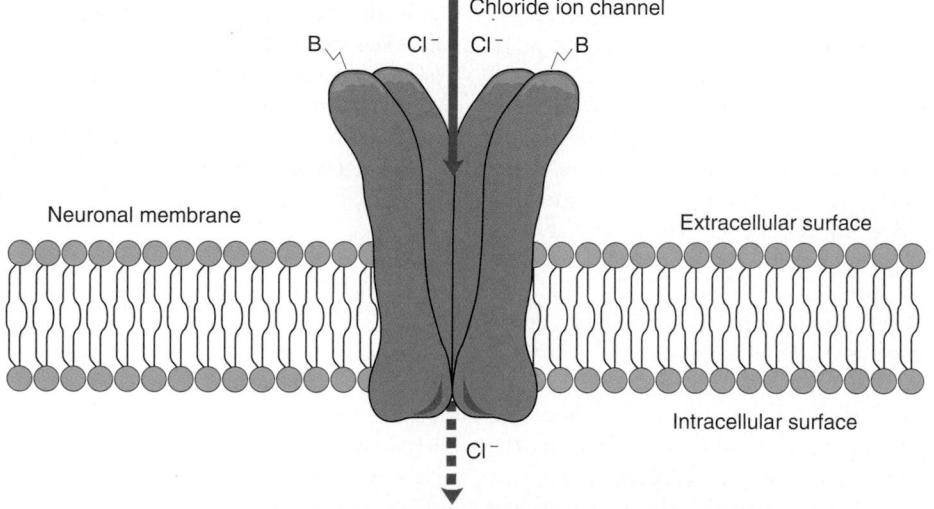

GABA activation of receptor opens channel gate, an effect enhanced by benzodiazepine binding to receptor subunits

Fig. 28.4 Schematic diagram of the $GABA_A$ receptor. This consists of five subunits arranged around a central chloride ion channel (one subunit has been removed in the diagram to reveal the ion channel, shown in the closed position). Some of the subunits have binding sites for benzodiazepines (B) and other hypnotics and anticonvulsants. Activation of the receptor by GABA opens the chloride channel, allowing chloride ions (Cl⁻) to enter the cell, resulting in hyperpolarisation (inhibition) of the neuron. Occupation of the benzodiazepine site, along with GABA, potentiates the inhibitory actions of GABA.

Concerns about dependence and tolerance largely restrict use to short-term treatment (Baldwin et al., 2013a). Many clinical trials have shown short-term efficacy in patients with anxiety disorders, although the efficacy shown is in part dependent on the year of publication of the study. Older randomised controlled trials appear to show a larger effect than more recent ones (Martin et al., 2007). Anxiolytic effects have also been reported in normal volunteers with high trait anxiety and in patients with anticipatory anxiety before surgery. However, in subjects with low trait anxiety and in nonstressful conditions, benzodiazepines may paradoxically increase anxiety and impair psychomotor performance.

Although useful for many anxiety disorders, benzodiazepines are not generally recommended for those with panic disorder (NICE, 2011). Some patients report worse panic attacks after the benzodiazepines are stopped. Benzodiazepines are also useful at the start of SSRI treatment in OCD and as hypnotics in PTSD (NICE, 2005a, 2005b). They should, however, be used at the lowest effective dose, prescribed intermittently where possible and used for no longer than 2–4 weeks.

Choice of benzodiazepine in anxiety. The choice of benzodiazepine depends largely on pharmacokinetic characteristics. Potent benzodiazepines such as lorazepam and alprazolam (Table 28.2) have been widely used for anxiety disorders but are probably inappropriate. Both are rapidly eliminated and need to be taken multiple times a day. Declining blood concentrations may lead to interdose anxiety as the anxiolytic effect of each tablet wears off. The high potency of lorazepam (~10 times that of diazepam), and the fact that it is available only in 1- and 2.5 mg tablet strengths, has often led to excessive dosage. Similarly, alprazolam (~20 times more potent than diazepam) has often been used in excessive dosage, particularly in the USA. Such doses lead to adverse effects, a high probability of dependence and difficulties in withdrawal.

A slowly eliminated benzodiazepine such as diazepam is more appropriate in most cases. Diazepam has a rapid onset of action, and its slow elimination ensures a steady blood concentration. Clonazepam, although long acting, is more potent than diazepam and in practice is often difficult to withdraw from. It is only indicated for epilepsy in the UK but is commonly used as an anxiolytic.

Parenteral administration of lorazepam or diazepam may occasionally be indicated for severely agitated patients.

Adverse effects. Adverse effects include drowsiness, lightheadedness, confusion, ataxia, amnesia, a paradoxical increase in aggression, an increased risk of falls and of road traffic accidents. They are also widely acknowledged as addictive and cause tolerance after more than 2–4 weeks of continuous use (Taylor et al., 2015). Respiratory depression is rare but possible following high oral doses or parenteral use. Flumazenil, a benzodiazepine receptor antagonist, can reverse the effects of severe reactions but requires repeated dosing and close monitoring because of its short half-life.

Psychomotor and cognitive impairment. Although oversedation is not usually a problem in anxious patients, there is evidence that long-term use of benzodiazepines can result in psychomotor and memory impairment in some patients. Some patients on long-term benzodiazepines complain of poor memory, and incidents of shoplifting have been attributed to memory lapses associated with benzodiazepine use. In elderly patients, the amnesic effects may falsely suggest the development of dementia. There is some evidence that benzodiazepines also inhibit the learning of alternative stress-coping strategies, such as behavioural treatments for agoraphobia. Additive effects with other CNS depressants, including alcohol, occur and may contribute to road traffic and other accidents.

Disinhibition, paradoxical effects. Rarely, benzodiazepines produce paradoxical stimulant effects. These effects are most marked in impulsive individuals and include excitement, increased anxiety, irritability and outbursts of rage. Violent behaviour has sometimes been attributed to disinhibition by benzodiazepines. This behaviour is normally suppressed by social restraints, fear or anxiety. Increased daytime anxiety can also occur with rapidly eliminated benzodiazepines and may be a withdrawal effect.

Affective reactions. Chronic use of benzodiazepines can worsen depression and may possibly provoke suicide attempts in impulsive patients. Aggravation of depression is a particular risk in anxious patients who often have mixed anxiety/depression. Benzodiazepines are taken alone or in combination with other drugs in 40% of self-poisoning incidents. Although relatively nontoxic in overdose, they can cause fatalities as a result of drug interactions and in those with respiratory disease.

Some patients on long-term benzodiazepines complain of 'emotional anaesthesia', the inability to experience either pleasure or distress. However, in some patients, benzodiazepines induce euphoria, and they are occasionally used as drugs of abuse.

Dependence. The greatest drawback of chronic benzodiazepine use is the risk of drug dependence. It is generally agreed that the regular use of therapeutic doses of benzodiazepines as hypnotics or anxiolytics for more than a few weeks (2–4 weeks) can give rise to dependence, with withdrawal symptoms on cessation of drug use in around 40% of patients. It is estimated that there are about 1 million long-term benzodiazepine users in the UK, and many of these are likely to be dependent. People with substance misuse histories or anxious or 'passive-dependent' personalities seem to be most vulnerable to dependence and withdrawal symptoms. Such individuals make up a large proportion of anxious patients in psychiatric practice, are often described as suffering from 'chronic anxiety' and are the type of patient for whom benzodiazepines are most likely to be prescribed. Such patients often continue to take benzodiazepines for many years because attempts at dosage reduction or drug withdrawal result in intolerable abstinence symptoms. Nevertheless, these patients continue to suffer from anxiety symptoms despite continued benzodiazepine use, possibly because they have become tolerant to the anxiolytic effects and may also suffer from other adverse effects of long-term benzodiazepine use such as depression or psychomotor impairment.

Abuse. Over the last 30 years, there has been much concern about benzodiazepine abuse. Some patients escalate their prescribed dosage and may obtain prescriptions from several doctors. These tend to be anxious patients with 'passive-dependent' personalities who may have a history of alcohol misuse; they may combine large doses of benzodiazepines with excessive alcohol consumption. In addition, a high proportion (30–90%) of illicit recreational drug abusers also use benzodiazepines, and some take them as euphoriants in their own right. Recreational use of most benzodiazepines has been reported in various countries; in the UK, temazepam is the most commonly abused anxiolytic drug. Exceedingly large doses (over 1g) may be taken and sometimes injected intravenously. Benzodiazepines became easily available due to widespread prescribing, which favoured their entrance into the illicit drug scene. Abusers can become dependent and suffer the same adverse effects and withdrawal symptoms as prescribed-dose users.

Benzodiazepine withdrawal. Many patients on long-term benzodiazepines seek help with drug withdrawal. Clinical experience shows that withdrawal is feasible in most patients if carried out with care. Abrupt withdrawal in dependent subjects is dangerous and can induce acute anxiety, psychosis or convulsions. However, gradual withdrawal, coupled where necessary with psychological treatments, can be successful in the majority of patients. The duration of withdrawal should be tailored to individual needs and may last many months. Dosage reductions may be of the order of 1–2 mg of diazepam per month. Even with slow dosage reduction, a variety of withdrawal symptoms may be experienced, including increased anxiety, insomnia, hypersensitivity to sensory stimuli, perceptual distortions, paraesthesia, muscle twitching, depression and many others (Box 28.2). These may last for many weeks, although diminishing in intensity, but occasionally, the withdrawal syndrome is protracted for a year or more. Transfer to diazepam, because of its slow elimination and availability as a liquid and in low-dosage forms, may be indicated for patients taking other benzodiazepines. Useful guidelines for benzodiazepine withdrawal are given in the British National Formulary, and detailed withdrawal schedules are also available (Lader et al., 2009).

The eventual outcome does not appear to be influenced by dosage, type of benzodiazepine, duration of use, psychiatric history, age, severity of withdrawal symptoms or rate of withdrawal. Hence, benzodiazepine withdrawal is worth attempting in patients who are motivated to stop, and most patients report that they feel better after withdrawal than when they were taking the benzodiazepine. Community pharmacists may be ideally suited to advise doctors and patients on the management of benzodiazepine withdrawal. Leading a benzodiazepine withdrawal clinic may also be a useful role for non-medical prescribers.

Drug interactions. In addition to the pharmacokinetic interactions listed earlier, benzodiazepines have additive effects with other CNS depressants. Combinations of benzodiazepines with alcohol, other hypnotics, tricyclic antidepressants (TCAs), sedative antipsychotics, antihistamines or opioids can cause marked sedation and may lead to accidents, collapse or severe respiratory depression.

Pregnancy and lactation. The regular use of benzodiazepines is not recommended in pregnancy because the drugs are concentrated in fetal tissue where hepatic metabolism is minimal. They have been associated with an increased risk of oral clefts following first-trimester exposure, a low birth weight, neonatal depression, feeding difficulties and withdrawal symptoms if given in late pregnancy. They also enter breast milk and may cause sedation, lethargy and weight loss in the infant. Long-acting benzodiazepines should particularly be avoided during lactation because of the potential for the infant to accumulate the drug. Short- to medium-acting benzodiazepines are occasionally used with enhanced monitoring of the infant.

Antidepressant drugs

Antidepressants can provide a long-term treatment option for those with an anxiety disorder. They are generally recommended for those who are unable to commit to or have not responded to psychological therapies. In addition, antidepressants are considered first-line treatment option either alone or in combination with CBT in patients suffering from OCD with moderate or severe impairment (NICE, 2005a). The number needed to treat (NNT) to see one benefit with antidepressants is around five in PTSD and GAD (NICE, 2005b, 2011).

The response rate to antidepressants in anxiety is often lower and takes longer than that seen in depression. Initial worsening of symptoms can occur, and high therapeutic doses are often required to improve response (Baldwin et al., 2014).

Selective serotonin reuptake inhibitors. The SSRIs have a broad anxiolytic effect and are considered the first drug option in GAD, panic disorder, social anxiety disorder, PTSD and OCD (Baldwin et al., 2014; NICE, 2005a, 2005b, 2011, 2013). Individual SSRIs have varying licensed indications across the anxiety disorders, but this does not necessarily mean others have no supporting evidence. Where more than one SSRI is licensed in a particular disorder, it is not possible to conclude which SSRI would be more effective because of the lack of direct head-to-head trials. The SSRIs differ in their interaction potential, side-effect profile and ease of discontinuation. Initial worsening of symptoms is common when starting an SSRI in anxiety,

---

Box 28.2	Benzodiazepine withdrawal symptoms
Symptoms common to anxiety states	Symptoms relatively specific to benzodiazepine withdrawal
Anxiety, panic	Perceptual distortions, sense of movement
Agoraphobia	
Insomnia, nightmares	Depersonalisation, derealisation
Depression, dysphoria	Hallucinations
Excitability, restlessness	Distortion of body image
Poor memory and concentration	Tingling, numbness, altered sensation
Dizziness, light-headedness	Skin prickling (formication)
Weakness, 'jelly legs'	Sensory hypersensitivity
Tremor	Muscle twitches, jerks
Muscle pain, stiffness	Tinnitus
Sweating, night sweats	Psychosis[a]
Palpitations	Confusion, delirium[a]
Blurred or double vision	Convulsions[a]
Gastro-intestinal and urinary symptoms	

[a]Usually only on rapid or abrupt withdrawal from high doses.

so beginning with half the dose than that used in depression is recommended, as is reassuring the patient that this is usually only experienced for the first few weeks of treatment. In view of these concerns, the NICE guidelines for GAD and panic disorder recommend that patients are reviewed every 2 weeks for the first 6 weeks of treatment to monitor for efficacy and tolerability (NICE, 2011). Although unlicensed, sertraline was recommended by NICE (2011) as the first-line SSRI in GAD because it was the most cost-effective drug. Sertraline and escitalopram are highlighted as appropriate first-choice SSRIs in social anxiety disorder (NICE, 2013).

Tricyclic antidepressants. Certain TCAs, such as clomipramine, imipramine and amitriptyline, are efficacious in some anxiety disorders. They are, however, associated with a greater burden of adverse reactions, such as antimuscarinic effects, hypotension and weight gain. Of particular concern is the TCAs' cardiac toxicity in overdose, which relegates their position to second line following the failure of an SSRI. They should be avoided in any patient at risk of suicide or those with an underlying cardiac disease. TCAs commonly cause sedation, which occasionally can prove useful in anxiety disorders. Clomipramine may also be slightly more effective in OCD compared with SSRIs.

Monoamine-oxidase inhibitors. The monoamine-oxidase inhibitors (MAOIs) are rarely used in practice because of their potentially severe interactions with other medicines and tyramine in the diet. Moclobemide is a reversible MAOI, so it causes fewer problematic interactions. Phenelzine and moclobemide are occasionally used by specialists in social anxiety disorder following the failure of an SSRI. Phenelzine is also recommended as a third-line treatment option in PTSD (NICE, 2005b).

Other antidepressants. The selective and noradrenaline reuptake inhibitor (SNRI) venlafaxine has some evidence to support its use in almost all the anxiety disorders but is only licensed for use in GAD, OCD and social anxiety disorder. Discontinuation symptoms are common following venlafaxine withdrawal and can be experienced after missing a single dose. Patients prescribed venlafaxine should be reminded of the importance of a slow withdrawal (over at least 4 weeks, sometimes longer) when discontinuation is necessary. Venlafaxine can increase blood pressure at higher doses in some patients and so is contraindicated in patients with a high risk of cardiac ventricular arrhythmia or uncontrolled hypertension. Duloxetine, another SNRI, is also licensed in GAD and can similarly increase blood pressure; withdrawal symptoms are also reported after abrupt discontinuation.

Mirtazapine, an α_2-adrenoreceptor antagonist, is recommended as an option for PTSD if patients do not wish to participate in trauma-focused CBT (NICE, 2005b). Mirtazapine has a lower incidence of nausea, vomiting and sexual dysfunction than the SSRIs but can commonly cause weight gain and sedation.

Agomelatine, a melatonin agonist and specific serotonin receptor antagonist, has proven efficacy in the acute treatment and prevention of relapse in GAD (Baldwin et al., 2014), although it is currently unlicensed for these conditions.

No other antidepressants are routinely recommended for anxiety disorders, although some, such as vortioxetine, have been evaluated in GAD to investigate potential future uses. To reduce the risk of symptoms returning, patients should be advised to continue the antidepressant for at least 6 months following improvement of symptoms in panic disorder and for 12 months in GAD, PTSD, OCD and social anxiety disorder (Baldwin et al., 2014; NICE, 2005a, 2011). Those with an enduring and recurrent illness, however, may continue for many years, depending on the risk of relapse and severity of symptoms.

For a complete review of the antidepressants, including adverse effects and interactions, see Chapter 29.

Other medications occasionally used in anxiety

Hydroxyzine, a sedating antihistamine, is licensed for the short-term treatment of anxiety in adults at a dose of 50–100 mg four times a day. The clinical evidence only supports its use in GAD (for up to 4 weeks) if sedation is required (Baldwin et al., 2014).

Antipsychotics have limited evidence and a high side effect burden when used in anxiety disorders. The first-generation (typical) antipsychotics are associated with movement disorders such as akathisia and tardive dyskinesia and so are rarely used in anxiety. The second-generation (atypical) antipsychotics are less likely to cause movement disorders but can have other physical health concerns. Antipsychotics (most commonly risperidone, olanzapine and quetiapine) are occasionally used by specialists for those with resistant symptoms in OCD, GAD, PTSD and social anxiety disorder (Baldwin et al., 2014).

Pregabalin has robust evidence and is licensed for GAD and has shown an anxiolytic effect over placebo after 1 week in adults or 2 weeks in the elderly (Montgomery et al., 2008). Two short-term studies in GAD (4 and 6 weeks) suggest that pregabalin 400–600 mg/day is as effective but better tolerated than venlafaxine 75 mg/day XL or lorazepam 6 mg/day. Pregabalin is most commonly used in GAD in combination with an SSRI or SNRI when initial treatments have failed (Baldwin et al., 2014). Emerging evidence also supports pregabalin in social anxiety disorders. Adverse effects of pregabalin include dizziness, somnolence and nausea, and there have been concerns raised over its abuse potential (Baldwin et al., 2013b; Schnerning et al., 2016).

Buspirone, a $5HT_{1A}$ partial agonist, is licensed for short-term use in anxiety. It is not a benzodiazepine and so does not treat or prevent benzodiazepine-withdrawal problems. In GAD, buspirone and other azapirones are superior to placebo in short-term studies (4–9 weeks) but less effective or acceptable than benzodiazepines (Chessick et al., 2006). Buspirone is occasionally used in GAD after nonresponse to the first-line treatments.

Propranolol and oxprenolol are both licensed for anxiety symptoms but are probably only useful for physical symptoms such as palpitations, tremor, sweating and shortness of breath. Beta blockers do not have sufficient evidence to support their inclusion in NICE guidelines, but intriguingly, small pilot studies indicate that giving an immediate course of propranolol following a traumatic event may prevent emerging PTSD (Pitman et al., 2002; Vaiva et al., 2003).

An overview of the recommended drug treatments in anxiety is provided in Table 28.3.

Table 28.3 Overview of the recommended drug treatments in anxiety

	Generalised anxiety disorder	Panic disorder	Social anxiety disorder (social phobia)	Obsessive-compulsive disorder	Posttraumatic stress disorder
Immediate management/ short-term treatment	Benzodiazepines (2–4 weeks only)	Benzodiazepines not recommended by NICE	Benzodiazepines (2–4 weeks only)	Benzodiazepines (only to counter initial worsening of symptoms with SSRIs)	Hypnotics may be considered for short-term use for insomnia
First-line pharmacotherapy[a]	SSRI Escitalopram Paroxetine	SSRI Citalopram Escitalopram– Paroxetine Sertraline	SSRI Citalopram– Escitalopram– Paroxetine	SSRI Escitalopram Fluoxetine Sertraline[b]	SSRI Escitalopram Fluoxetine– Fluvoxamine Paroxetine–Sertraline
Other drug treatments with supporting evidence	Agomelatine Buspirone Duloxetine Imipramine Pregabalin[c] Venlafaxine Quetiapine Vilazodone Vortioxetine	Clomipramine[b] Imipramine[b] Mirtazapine Moclobemide Venlafaxine	Moclobemide[c] Phenelzine[c] Venlafaxine Pregabalin[c]	Clomipramine Augmentation with aripiprazole, quetiapine or risperidone[c]	Amitriptyline[c] Augmentation with olanzapine or risperidone[c] Imipramine Mirtazapine[b] Phenelzine[c] Venlafaxine Prazosin[c]

[a]The licensed SSRI is indicated but other SSRIs may also be beneficial.
[b]Unlicensed but recommended by NICE (2005a, 2005b, 20011, 2013).
[c]Usually prescribed by mental health specialists only.
SSRI, Selective serotonin reuptake inhibitor.

Case studies

Case 28.1

Mrs DW is a 32-year-old with a 10-year history of 'emotional problems'. These have largely been dealt with by her primary care doctor, who has prescribed low-dose TCAs for the last 3 years. Mrs DW's life is severely restricted by a number of rituals which she obsessively carries out. They include washing of sinks, baths and toilets; disinfection of kitchen surfaces; and vacuuming. These activities occupy her up to 8 hours a day.

Current prescribed medication:
- diazepam 10 mg three times a day,
- amitriptyline 25 mg twice a day.

Both have been prescribed for 3 years.

Mrs DW is concerned about possible addiction to her medication, as previous attempts to stop it have been unsuccessful. In addition, both she and her family feel that more can be achieved and are willing to work at solving the problems faced by Mrs DW.

Questions

1. Is this appropriate therapy for OCD, and if not, what would be a better first choice?
2. Suggest possible drug therapies for Mrs DW and indicate for how long they should be continued.
3. Provided an alternative therapy is commenced, recommend an appropriate scheme for withdrawal of the diazepam.

Answers

1. Benzodiazepines are not recommended in OCD. The first choice is CBT or an SSRI.
2. Potential drug treatments include high-dose SSRIs or clomipramine. Augmentation strategies (e.g. antipsychotics) would also be a possibility. Treatment may need to be continued for a year before a dose reduction is tried.
3. Because Mrs DW is on a dose of 30 mg diazepam daily, it would be appropriate to consider reducing the diazepam by 2 mg/day every 1–2 weeks until a 20 mg/day dose is reached. Further reductions may need to be 1 mg every 1–2 weeks until stopped. Longer intervals between dose reduction may be necessary as the dose reduces towards zero. The patient may wish to adopt faster withdrawal and accept the consequences. All patients should be monitored for increased anxiety, restlessness, agitation and other effects, and may need slow withdrawal.

Case 28.2

Mrs AB, a previously well 30-year-old woman, had been treated with paroxetine 40 mg daily for anxiety/depression which had been precipitated by a traumatic marriage breakup. After taking paroxetine for 18 months, Mrs AB's problems had mainly resolved, and she was feeling well. She decided that she no longer needed the drug and stopped taking it. Within 3 days, her anxiety/depression returned, with insomnia and nightmares. Her mood lowered, and she became irritable and found herself weeping for no reason. A week later she returned to her doctor complaining of these symptoms, as well as depersonalisation and electric shock sensations. The doctor thought the original depression had returned and reinstated paroxetine, which cleared up her symptoms within a few days.

Questions

1. What alternative explanation could there be for Mrs AB's symptoms, and what other decision could the doctor have made?
2. What would be a suitable withdrawal schedule for her paroxetine?

Answers

1. All antidepressants can cause a discontinuation reaction. Mrs AB's symptoms are typical of SSRI withdrawal. This occurs most commonly with paroxetine, perhaps partly due to its rapid rate of elimination (half-life around 21 hours in chronic users).
2. In this previously well patient, who is no longer under marital stress, the doctor, after reinstating paroxetine, could have supplied a gradual tapering schedule of drug withdrawal – that is, reducing the dose by 10 mg/week, aiming to withdrawal in 4 weeks or longer depending on patient preference.

Case 28.3

Mr SB is a 22-year-old soldier. He has recently returned from his second active tour, where he was injured by a roadside bomb. Two of his squad were killed in the same blast, and although his physical injuries healed quickly, he has persistent and intense episodes of panic and flashbacks. He is especially aroused at night and has great difficulty getting to sleep. An initial prescription of an SSRI has proved ineffective, and he is currently on the waiting list for psychological therapies.

Question

1. What alternative drug treatment may be appropriate?

Answer

1. A sedating antidepressant such as mirtazapine or amitriptyline may be appropriate, ensuring adequate duration of therapy and effective dose. A short course of a benzodiazepine may prove useful but for no longer than 2–4 weeks. Alternatively, augmenting the antidepressant with a sedating antipsychotic such as olanzapine may be useful. For prolonged symptom treatment and relapse prevention, it is likely that the patient will need to fully engage with psychological therapies.

Case 28.4

Ms AC is a 32-year-old personal assistant to a director of a leading investment company. She has recently been promoted to this role and is now expected to entertain potential clients by dining out with the director at local restaurants. She has always preferred eating alone in the comfort of her own home, and the thought of eating in public while promoting the business fills her with dread, which brings on palpitations and shortness of breath.

Questions

1. What drug therapy is available which may provide some immediate relief of her anxiety symptoms?
2. What would be an appropriate choice of treatment for long-term control and prevention of symptoms?

Answers

1. β-Blockers such as propranolol may help with the shortness of breath and palpitations but will not treat the fear and dread. Benzodiazepines may be appropriate but may affect her performance and cause other adverse reactions.
2. For long-term control, a course of CBT including exposure techniques is appropriate or treatment with an SSRI such as escitalopram or sertraline.

References

Baldwin, D., Ajel, K., Masdraskis, V., et al., 2013a. Pregabalin for the treatment of generalized anxiety disorder: an update. Neuropsychiatr. Dis. Treat. 9, 883–892.

Baldwin, D., Anderson, I., Nutt, D., et al., 2014. Evidence-based guidelines for the pharmacological treatment of anxiety disorders, post-traumatic stress disorder and obsessive-compulsive disorder: a revision of the 2005 guidelines from the British Association for Psychopharmacology. J. Psychopharmacol. 28, 403–439.

Baldwin, D.S., Aitchison, K., Bateson, A., et al., 2013b. Benzodiazepines: risks and benefits. A reconsideration. J. Psychopharmacol 27 (11), 967–971.

Bazire, S., 2014. Psychotropic Drug Directory. Lloyd-Reinhold Publications, Shaftesbury.

Chessick, C.A., Allen, M.H., Thase, M.E., et al., 2006. Azapirones for generalized anxiety disorder. Cochrane Database Syst. Rev. 2006 (3), Art. No. CD006115. https://doi.org/10.1002/14651858.CD006115.

Christmas, D., Hood, S., Nutt, D., 2008. Potential novel anxiolytic drugs. Curr. Pharm. Des. 14, 3534–3546.

Haefely, W., 1990. Benzodiazepine receptor and ligands: structural and functional differences. In: Hindmarch, I., Beaumont, G., Brandon, S. (Eds.), Benzodiazepines: Current Concepts. John Wiley, Chichester, pp. 1–18.

Lader, M., Tylee, A., Donoghue, J., 2009. Withdrawing benzodiazepines in primary care. CNS Drugs 23, 19–34.

Martin, J., Sainz-Pardo, M., Furukawa, T., et al., 2007. Review: benzodiazepines in generalized anxiety disorder: heterogeneity based on systematic review and meta-analysis of clinical trials. J. Psychopharmacol. 21, 774–782.

Montgomery, S.A., Chatamra, K., Pauer, L., et al., 2008. Efficacy and safety of pregabalin in elderly people with generalised anxiety disorder. Br. J. Psychiatry 193, 389–394.

National Institute for Health and Care Excellence (NICE), 2005a. Obsessive compulsive disorder. Clinical Guideline 31. Available at: http://www.nice.org.uk/Guidance/CG31.

National Institute for Health and Care Excellence (NICE), 2005b. Post traumatic stress disorder (PTSD). Clinical Guideline 26. Available at: http://www.nice.org.uk/CG26.

National Institute for Health and Care Excellence (NICE), 2011. Generalised anxiety disorder and panic disorder in adults: management. Clinical Guideline 113. Available at: https://www.nice.org.uk/guidance/cg113/-resources/generalised-anxiety-disorder-and-panic-disorder-in-adults-management-35109387756997.

National Institute for Health and Care Excellence (NICE), 2013. Social anxiety disorder: recognition, assessment and treatment. Clinical Guideline 159. Available at: https://www.nice.org.uk/guidance/cg159.

Pitman, R., Sanders, K., Zusman, R., et al., 2002. Pilot study of secondary prevention of posttraumatic stress disorder with propranolol. Biol. Psychiatry 51, 189–192.

Roy-Byrne, P.P., 2005. The GABA-benzodiazepine receptor complex: structure, function and role in anxiety. J. Clin. Psychiatry 66 (Suppl. 2), 14–20.

Schjerning, O., Rosenzweig, M., Pottegård, A., et al., 2016. Abuse potential of pregabalin: a systematic review. CNS Drugs 30 (1), 9–25.

Taylor, D., Paton, C., Kapur, S., 2015. The Maudsley Prescribing Guidelines in Psychiatry, twelfth ed. Wiley-Blackwell, Chichester.

Vaiva, G., Ducrocq, F., Jezequel, K., et al., 2003. Immediate treatment with propranolol decreases posttraumatic stress disorder two months after trauma. Biol. Psychiatry 54, 947–949.

Further reading

Baldwin, D., 2008. Room for improvement in the pharmacological treatment of anxiety disorders. Curr. Pharm. Des. 14, 3482–3491.

Bleakley, S., 2013. Anxiety disorders: clinical features and diagnosis. Clin Pharmacist 5, 281–283.

Garner, M., Mohler, H., Stein, D., et al., 2009. Research in anxiety disorders: from the bench to the bedside. Eur. Neuropsychopharmacol. 19, 381–390.

Useful websites

British Association for Behavioural and Cognitive Psychotherapies has a list of therapists, training resources and general information for the public: http://www.babcp.com

Anxiety UK, a national charity for anyone affected by an anxiety disorder: http://www.anxietyuk.org.uk

No Panic, a national charity offering support for suffers of panic attacks, phobias, OCD and GAD: http://www.nopanic.org.uk

College of Mental Health Pharmacy, a national charity supporting the work and education of pharmacy staff in mental health: http://www.cmhp.org.uk

29 Affective Disorders

Alan Pollard

Key points

- Diagnosis of affective disorders should be made using standardised criteria, for example, *Diagnostic and Statistical Manual of Mental Disorders*, Fifth Edition, and *International Classification of Diseases*, 10th Revision.

- Target symptoms should be recorded and response to treatment monitored against these symptoms.

- In patients with mild depression, non-pharmacological strategies should be considered as first-line intervention.

- The evidence base for determining the choice of a particular antidepressant in an individual patient does not exist. For most patients, when an antidepressant is indicated, a generic selective serotonin reuptake inhibitor should be considered as a first-line treatment option.

- Currently, all antidepressants are considered equally effective but differ in their side effect profile, toxicity in overdose, need for dose titration, and monitoring.

- In the absence of a previous response or contraindication, antidepressant choice should be guided by evidence-based clinical guidelines and the clinician and patient's perception of the risks and benefits of available options. Resource implications should not be ignored.

- Emerging evidence and a greater understanding of the clinical application of pharmacogenomics may lead to the ability to individualise treatments in the future.

- Comprehensive assessment, accurate diagnosis, adequate duration of pharmacotherapy, and involvement of the patient in the treatment regimen are the cornerstones of effective medicines management of affective disorders.

- Valproate, antipsychotics, and benzodiazepines, sometimes in combination, are the treatments of choice in acute mania.

- Either lithium, valproate, or specific antipsychotics may be considered to be the first-line prophylactic agent of choice in bipolar I disorder.

The term *affect* relates to mood or emotional state, and this chapter therefore analyses mood disorders. These consist in clinical practice of depression and bipolar disorder. Within bipolar disorder, mood swings predominate so at times the person may present as 'high' or manic, which led to the historical description of manic depression for this condition. The issues addressed in this chapter relate to adults. Affective disorders in children and adolescents are more complex and are beyond the scope of this chapter.

Classification

Depression

The term *depression* is often used by people to describe a general feeling of being low in mood and negative, but in clinical practice, depression is more than just sadness or unhappiness in response to a life event. A diagnosis of depression is only made when key signs and symptoms are present. *International Classification of Diseases,* 10th Revision (ICD 10; World Health Organization [WHO]) and *Diagnostic and Statistical Manual of Mental Disorders,* Fifth Edition (DSM-5; American classification system) list their relevant diagnostic criteria. Much overlap exists, and both require a cluster of presenting features to be present for a defined period.

Depression is subclassified as mild, moderate or severe according to the intensity of presenting symptoms. This classification has implications for treatment options with milder forms of depression amenable to psychological-based interventions, whereas more severe forms of depression are likely to require more medically focused interventions, such as antidepressants or at the most severe end electroconvulsive therapy (ECT).

Mania and hypomania

When mood becomes abnormally elated, the terms *hypomania* or *mania* may be applied. Mania is the more extreme form and is often distinguished from hypomania by the presence of psychotic symptoms (see Chapter 30 for further information on psychosis) and the potential need for hospitalisation. In the early stages of hypomania, irritability may be more evident than overt symptoms of overactivity and elation.

Bipolar and unipolar disorders

Depression on its own is a unipolar disorder. Mania or hypomania on its own could also be defined as a unipolar disorder, but in the UK the term *bipolar disorder* is used from the outset because at some point it is expected that a depressive episode will ensue. Bipolar I identifies mania as the first episode that brought the patient in for treatment. Bipolar II is applied when depressive episodes dominate the presentation. Between episodes, patients may have a relatively level state of mood and can be clinically described as euthymic, although many will say that subjectively they may feel on the subdued side. Mood cycles are very

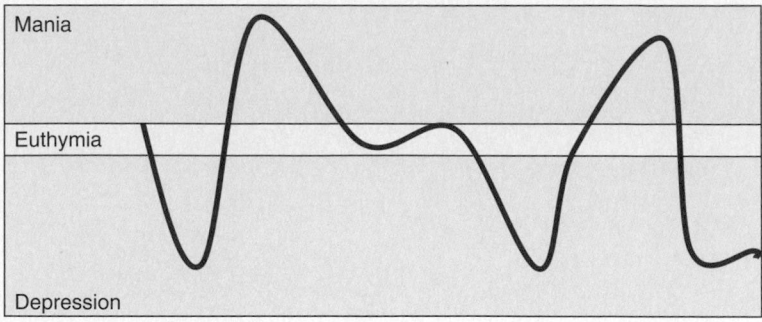

Fig. 29.1 Mood swings in bipolar disorder.

individual and often asymmetric, with the majority of patients having far more depressive episodes than manic episodes. Fig. 29.1 shows a diagrammatic representation of a pattern of mood swings in bipolar disorder. The time interval between mood episodes is also very variable, but to be identified as a rapid cycling as few as four episodes per year are needed.

Bipolar disorder is a cyclical mood disorder. Abnormally elevated mood or irritability alternates with depressed mood, but mood fluctuations are often asymmetric and for much of the time patients are never truly 'euthymic'.

Epidemiology

Nearly one-fifth of adults experience anxiety or depression, with the conditions affecting a higher proportion of women than men. Reported in 2012, the World Mental Health Survey, conducted in 17 countries, found that on average about 1 in 20 people reported having an episode of depression in the previous year. Depressive disorders may start at a young age; they reduce people's functioning and often are recurring. For these reasons, depression remains the leading cause of disability worldwide. In contrast, bipolar disorder is quite different. The aggregate lifetime prevalence rates have been identified as 0.6% for bipolar I disorder, 0.4% for bipolar II disorder, 1.4% for subthreshold bipolar and 2.4% for bipolar spectrum disorder. Twelve-month prevalence rates were 0.4% for bipolar I, 0.3% for bipolar II, 0.8% for subthreshold bipolar and 1.5% for bipolar spectrum disorder (Merikangas et al., 2011).

The incidence of bipolar I is generally reported to be the same for both men and women, whereas some studies suggest that bipolar II may be slightly more common in women. Although depression may occur at any age, including childhood, it is estimated that the average age of onset of depression is in the mid-20s. Some earlier studies found the incidence and prevalence of depression in women peaking at the age of 35–45 years. In bipolar disorder an earlier age of onset is suggested, perhaps in late adolescence, with most people experiencing their first episodes before 30 years of age.

Aetiology

Like most other psychiatric disorders, the causes of affective disorders remain unknown. In depression it is likely that genetic, environmental, biochemical, hormonal and social factors all have some role in determining an individual's susceptibility to development of the disorder, with major life events sometimes acting as a trigger for a particular episode. Although pharmacological treatments are clearly effective, there is no simple relationship between biochemical abnormalities and affective disorders.

Genetic causes

Evidence for a genetic component to mood disorders has been documented consistently using family, twin and adoption studies. The first genetic studies of mood disorders were conducted more than 70 years ago and included assessment of concordance rates for monozygotic and dizygotic twins with mood disorders. These early studies did not distinguish between bipolar depression and unipolar depression. A review in 2000 of twin studies in recurrent unipolar depression estimated heritability at 37%, with a substantial component of unique individual environmental risk but little shared environmental risk (Sullivan et al., 2000).

In depression one theory suggests that a variant of the gene responsible for encoding the serotonin transporter protein could account for early childhood experiences being translated into an increased risk of depression through stress sensitivity in adulthood. In bipolar disorder some genetic linkage has been proposed, but a precise marker remains elusive.

Following a large, comparative study of bipolar patients and healthy control subjects, five DNA regions were identified as risk regions associated with bipolar disorder. Of particular interest is the ADCY2 region because it codes an enzyme that has a role in sending signals to nerve cells.

The discovery of the ADCY2 risk region provides new insight into the biological mechanisms involved in the development of bipolar disorder (Muhleisen et al., 2014).

The incidence of affective disorder in first-degree relatives of someone with severe depression may be about 20%, which is almost three times the risk of relatives in control groups. Comparisons of the risk of affective disorder in the children of both parents with an affective disorder show a four times greater risk, and the risk is doubled in children with one parent with an affective disorder. Studies evaluating twins have found fairly strong evidence for a genetic factor. Evidence of a genetic link has also been found in studies of children from parents with affective disorder who were adopted by healthy parents. A higher incidence of affective disorder was found in the biological parents of adopted children with affective disorder than in the adoptive parents.

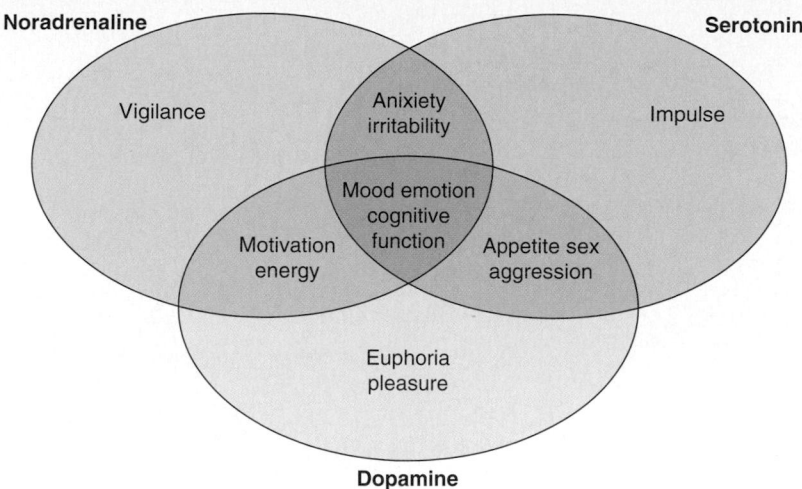

Fig. 29.2 Amine transmitters and association with behavioural response.

Environmental factors

Although environmental stresses can often be identified before an episode of mania or depression, a causal relationship between a major event in someone's life and the development of an affective disorder has not been firmly established. It may be that life events described as 'threatening' are more likely to be associated with depression. The lack of prospective studies makes it difficult to interpret data linking early life events, such as loss of a parent, to the development of an affective disorder. The fact that specific environmental stresses have not been identified should not lead to the conclusion that the environment or lifestyle is irrelevant to the course or development of affective disorders. Employment, higher socio-economic status and the existence of a close and confiding relationship have been consistently noted to offer some protection against the development of an episode.

Biochemical factors

In its simplistic form the biochemical theory of depression postulates a deficiency of neurotransmitter amines in certain areas of the brain. This theory has been developed to suggest that receptor sensitivity changes may be important. Alternative propositions suggest a central role of acetylcholine arising from dysregulation of the cholinergic and noradrenergic neurotransmitter systems. Although many neurotransmitters may be implicated, the theory focuses on an involvement of the neurotransmitters noradrenaline (norepinephrine), serotonin (5-hydroxytryptamine [5-HT]) and dopamine. This theory emerged from the findings that both monoamine oxidase inhibitors (MAOIs) and tricyclic antidepressants (TCAs) appeared to increase neurotransmitter amines, particularly noradrenaline (norepinephrine), at important sites in the brain. When it was found that reserpine, previously used as an antihypertensive, caused both a depletion of neurotransmitter and also induced depression, this was taken as further evidence of the monoamine theory. Newer antidepressants continue to pharmacologically promote serotonin and noradrenaline activity, albeit in more subtle ways. However, the amine transmitters do not work in isolation, and modifying the serotonin system will impact on noradrenergic (norepinephrinergic) and dopaminergic systems.

Fig. 29.2 shows the actions of each monoamine transmitter and their inter-relationship. Because the transmitters do not work in isolation, modification of one transmitter will impact across numerous behavioural domains. The overlap between transmitters linked to discrete behaviours helps account for why a single transmitter-focused antidepressant may produce a broad improvement in a range of depressive symptoms. Although less attention has been paid to dopaminergic activity, some studies have found reduced activity in patients with depression, and an overactivity has been postulated in mania. There remains no clear biochemical model to explain mania.

Endocrine factors

Stress triggers the hypothalamus to release corticotrophin-releasing factor. Corticotrophin-releasing factor interacts with the pituitary gland to release adrenocorticotrophic hormone. Adrenocorticotrophic hormone binds to adrenal glands on the kidney and releases stress hormones including cortisol. There is negative feedback under short-lived healthy conditions, but chronic stress may damage the switch off process (Fig. 29.3).

Patients with depression often have higher baseline cortisol levels and larger adrenal glands (the source of cortisol). Dexamethasone mimics cortisol, and it was postulated that this agent could provide a diagnostic marker for depression. Failure of a test dose of dexamethasone to suppress cortisol levels in the so-called dexamethasone suppression test was once thought to be a robust marker of depression. However, all severe and enduring mental health conditions chronically stress the hypothalamic–pituitary–adrenal axis, switch off the negative feedback and can result in failure of dexamethasone to suppress cortisol production.

Physical illness and side effects of medication

Disorders of mood, particularly depression, have been associated with several types of medication and a number of physical

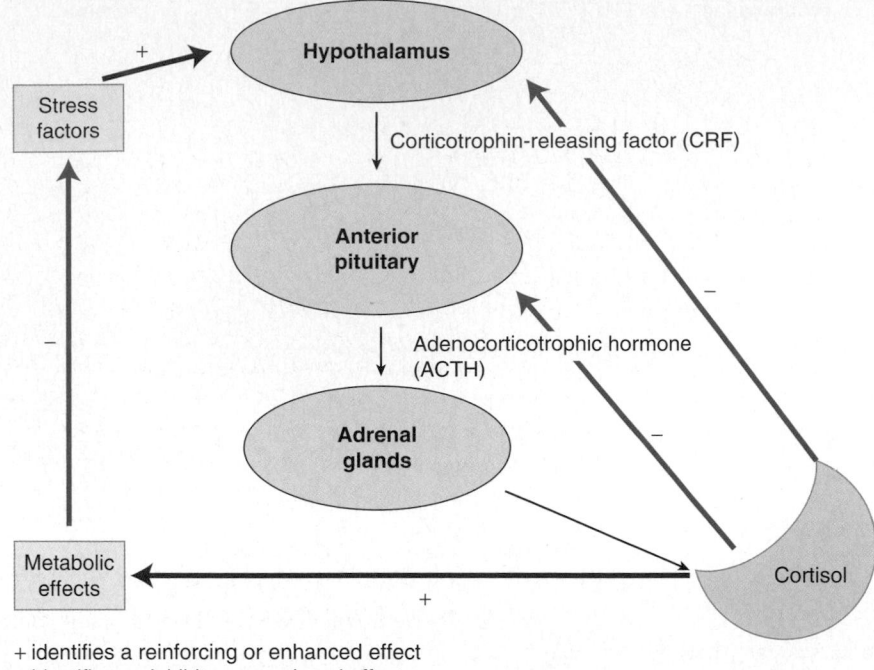

+ identifies a reinforcing or enhanced effect
− identifies an inhibitory or reduced effect

Fig. 29.3 The hypothalamic–pituitary–adrenal axis, key hormones and feedback mechanisms involved in regulating the body's response to stress.

illnesses (Box 29.1). Depression can affect the outcome in people with a range of physical problems. An increase in mortality rates has been found in those patients with comorbid depression. Many drugs can affect mood states and other risk factors such as underlying physical health condition that contribute to a syndromal episode. This is why in any patient assessment it is important to always look for any organic factors that may contribute to an altered mental state. For many long-term physical conditions (e.g. diabetes), the incidence of depression is higher than in controls. Altered or abnormal biochemistry may be another factor, particularly as presentation is more acute in onset. When medication is a main driver for mood-related changes, then a few drugs (e.g. interferon-alfa, corticosteroids and digoxin) can be identified as potentially more problematic with associated evidence to support this risk (Preda, 2012).

Clinical manifestations

Depression

A low mood is the central feature of depression. This is often accompanied by a loss of interest or pleasure in normally enjoyable activities. Thinking is pessimistic and in some cases suicidal. A depressed person may complain he or she has little or no energy. In severe cases psychotic symptoms such as mood-congruent hallucinations or delusions may be present. Anxiety or agitation frequently accompanies the disorder, and the so-called biological features of sleep disturbances, weight loss and loss of appetite are often present. Sexual drive is often reduced, and some people may lose interest in sex altogether. Depression in an older adult may present with more somatic symptoms, particularly gastric problems,

and non-specific aches and pains. In some cases, known as atypical depression, the biological symptoms are reversed and excessive eating and sleeping may occur. In contrast with anxiety and agitation, psychomotor retardation may be a presenting feature.

The following mnemonic may be useful in helping to identify the key signs and symptoms that present in depression. INSADCAGES describes the sense of being trapped in a prison of sadness (Box 29.2).

Bipolar disorder

Standardised diagnostic criteria vary. For an ICD 10 diagnosis of bipolar disorder, at least two mood episodes must occur, one of which must be manic or hypomanic (Box 29.3). According to DSM 5, at least one episode of mania must have occurred for a diagnosis of bipolar I disorder to be made; depression may also occur, but it is not essential.

Mania/Hypomania

In hypomanic states the mood is described as elated or irritable, and the accompanying overactivity is usually unproductive. Disinhibition may result in excessive spending sprees, inappropriate sexual activity and other high-risk behaviours. Driving may be particularly dangerous. Manic people may describe their thoughts as racing, with ideas rapidly changing from one topic to another. Speech may be very rapid or indeed stop as the rapid flow of thoughts is not able to be vocalised. Ideas may become grandiose, with patients embarking on expansive projects which lead nowhere and usually their projects are left incomplete and disjointed. Clothing may become flamboyant, and if makeup is

Box 29.1 Physical illnesses and drugs implicated in disorders of mood

Biochemical change	Effect on mental state	Mental health link
Hyperthyroid state	Overactivity, poor sleep	Hypomania
Hypothyroid state	Lethargy, reduced energy levels	Depression
Hypoglycaemia	Confusion, disorientation, tremor and unsteadiness	Alcohol intoxication

Drug group	Comment
Anticonvulsants	More prone to induce depressive episodes, but some agents can trigger a manic presentation and psychotic symptoms
Antidepressants	In bipolar patients unopposed antidepressants may trigger a manic episode
Antimalarials	Mefloquine carries a risk of depression, anxiety and psychosis
β-Blockers	Propranolol and some other β-blockers may contribute to depression
Corticosteroids	Long-term treatment reported to contribute to depression but also known in short-term and high doses to induce euphoria and manic presentations
HIV medicines	Non-nucleoside reverse transcriptase inhibitors may increase the risk of depression
Interferons	As many as 40% of people who are receiving interferon-alfa may experience depression
Isotretinoin	Has been associated with depression and proactive monitoring for signs of depression recommended
Methyldopa	An antihypertensive that may be used during pregnancy but has been associated with depression

Box 29.2 Mnemonic describing the key signs and symptoms present in depression

Insomnia – typically early morning wakening
Neurotic symptoms – anxiety/agitation with ruminations
Suicidality – thoughts/plans around self-harm
Appetite ↓ – leading to weight loss
Depressed mood – tearfulness, feeling low
Concentration ↓ – reading and staying focused, retaining information, concentrating on television more difficult
Anhedonia – loss of pleasure in usually rewarding pastimes
Guilt/worthlessness – pessimistic around the future; may not believe in being worthy of receiving help; exaggerated negativity around past misdemeanours
Energy ↓ – poor self-care, lack of motivation
Sex – loss of libido; amenorrhoea

Box 29.3 ICD 10 diagnostic criteria for bipolar affective disorder (WHO, 1992)

Bipolar affective disorder is characterised by repeated (at least two) episodes in which the patient's mood and activity levels are significantly disturbed. This disturbance consists on some occasions of an elevation in mood and increased energy and activity (mania or hypomania), and on others of a lowering of mood and decreased energy and activity (depression).

Manic episodes usually begin abruptly and last for between 2 weeks and 4–6 months (median 4 months). Depression tends to last longer (median about 6 months). Episodes of both kinds often follow stressful life events or other mental trauma, but the presence of such stress is not essential for the diagnosis.

worn it may become excessive and will often involve bright colours. Hypomania and mania are on a continuum, and in clinical practice mania is applied when the patient experiences psychotic symptoms and cannot be managed outside of a hospital environment or equivalent intervention.

Severity

The severity of depression may vary from mild through moderate to severe. In the UK more than 90% of depression cases are managed in primary care, and in most circumstances it is not necessary for people with milder forms of depression to be seen by specialist services. In the absence of a risk of serious self-harm, or other complex comorbidities, patients should be entirely managed by the primary healthcare team. Guidelines advise that a stepwise approach is taken on the management of depression; evidence supports antidepressant therapy as more effective in the moderate-to-severe cases (National Institute of Health and Care Excellence [NICE], 2009a, 2009b).

If left untreated, it is important to remember that affective disorders carry a risk of mortality. In addition to suicidal attempts by someone who is depressed, the lack of self-care and physical exhaustion resulting from mania may become life-threatening.

The social and financial consequences can have a devastating effect on both the patient with mania or hypomania and his or her family. Depression may also contribute to poorer outcomes of physical problems such as increased pain and worsening outcomes from cardiac disease and diabetes.

Investigations

No universally accepted biochemical or genetic tests exist that will confirm the presence of an affective disorder. Various rating scales have been developed that may help to demonstrate the severity of depressive disorder or distinguish a predominantly anxious patient from a depressed patient. In an older adult, distinguishing depression from early stages of dementia can also pose a challenge (see Chapter 33). Within the limits of our current understanding of the technology, biochemical or genetic tests are unlikely to be helpful in determining the treatment plan or management of affective disorders.

In the UK, mental and behavioural disorders are commonly classified using the ICD 10 (WHO, 1992). The American Psychiatric Association (2013) has developed a precise system of diagnosis based on the description of symptoms in the DSM 5.

A systematic approach to the diagnosis of affective disorders is important when considering the effectiveness of medication.

Box 29.4 ICD 10 diagnostic criteria for depressive disorder (WHO, 1992)

Usual symptoms
Depressed mood, loss of interest and enjoyment, and reduced
    energy leading to increased fatigability and diminished activity

Common symptoms
Reduced concentration and attention
Reduced self-esteem and self-confidence
Ideas of guilt and unworthiness (even in a mild type of episode)
Bleak and pessimistic views of the future
Ideas or acts of self-harm or suicide
Disturbed sleep
Diminished appetite

In a depressive episode the mood varies little from day to day and is often unresponsive to circumstances, yet may show characteristic diurnal variation as the day goes on. The clinical picture shows marked individual variations, and atypical presentations are particularly common in adolescence. In some cases anxiety, distress and motor agitation may be more prominent at times than the depression.

For depressive episodes of all grades of severity, a duration of 2 weeks is usually required for diagnosis, but shorter periods may be reasonable if symptoms are unusually severe and of rapid onset.

Mild depressive episode: For at least 2 weeks, at least two of the usual symptoms of a depressive episode plus at least two of the common symptoms listed earlier must be present. An individual with a mild depressive episode is usually distressed by the symptoms and has some difficulty in continuing with ordinary work and social activities, but will probably not cease to function completely.

Moderate depressive episode: For at least 2 weeks, at least two or three of the usual symptoms of a depressive episode plus at least three (preferably four) of the common symptoms listed earlier must be present. An individual with moderately severe depressive episode will have these symptoms to a marked degree, but this is not essential if a particularly wide variety of symptoms are present overall. These individuals will usually have considerable difficulties in continuing with social, work or domestic activities.

Severe depressive episode: For at least 2 weeks, all three of the usual symptoms of a depressive episode plus at least four of the common symptoms listed earlier, some of which should be of severe intensity, must be present. An individual with severe depressive episode may be unable or unwilling to describe many symptoms in detail, but an overall grading of severe may still be justified. These individuals will usually show considerable distress or agitation, unless retardation is a marked feature. Loss of self-esteem or feelings of uselessness or guilt are likely to be prominent. Suicide is a distinct danger, particularly in severe cases.

Most new clinical trials for antidepressants or antipsychotics require a DSM diagnosis as an entry criterion. In the UK the ICD 10 classification is commonly used, with the severity of depression determined by the presence of the number of symptoms (see Boxes 29.3 and 29.4). More recently, use of the symptom count as a single factor upon which to base treatment decisions has been cautioned against (NICE, 2009a, 2009b). Account should also be taken of the extent of impairment and disability associated with depression. Recognition of enduring subsyndromal symptoms of low mood and other depression-related symptoms is acknowledged by NICE as significant enough to warrant intervention.

National guidelines provide a sound framework for the management of depression (NICE, 2009a, 2009b) and bipolar disorder (NICE, 2014). It is important that people with depression are identified. A simple screening process for the presence of depression could involve asking the patient two questions about his or her mood and interest. For example, the patient could be asked: 'During the last month, have you often been bothered by feeling down, depressed or hopeless?' and 'During the last month, have you often been bothered by having little interest or pleasure in doing things?' If the answer to either question is no, it is unlikely the patient will be considered to have a depressive disorder. Patients who answer yes warrant further investigation. A follow-up question asking about any unusual periods of elation or overactivity is recommended to detect potential for bipolar disorder.

Identification of target symptoms may be useful in evaluating the response to treatment. In routine clinical practice, antidepressant medication should not generally be used to treat patients with mild depression. Non-pharmacological strategies are preferable in this group.

Rating scales

Various rating scales can be used to assist with the assessment of the severity of the disorder. Two of the more commonly used rating scales are the Beck Depression Inventory and the Hamilton Depression Rating Scale.

Beck depression inventory

This is a self-reporting scale that evaluates 21 depressive symptoms. Subjects are asked to read a series of statements and mark on a scale of 1–4 the severity of their symptoms. The higher the score, the more severely depressed a person may be.

Hamilton depression rating scale

This rating scale is used by a healthcare professional at the end of an interview to rate the severity of depression. It scores on 17 items, although 21 items are listed. The higher the score is, the more severe the depression. Moderate depression starts at 14, with severe depression scoring greater than 19.

Treatment

The aim of treatment is to promote recovery, and in unipolar depression a return to premorbid state is a realistic goal. In bipolar disorder the focus shifts to reducing intensity and duration of mood swings. In all cases quality of life is an important consideration. Pharmacological interventions alongside psychological interventions will be utilised in most patients.

Pharmacological management of unipolar depression, bipolar disorder (including bipolar depression) and manic states are quite distinct. In some cases medication used will be outside of its product licence but supported by a strong evidence base. Clinicians should be aware of the licensed indication of treatments, so that any off-label use is done knowingly and in line with current best practice.

Treatment of depression

In moderate and severe depression, pharmacological intervention is important, but this should never be considered in isolation from the social, cultural and environmental influences on the patient. Non-pharmacological therapies are effective, and in mild depression they are considered preferable to drug treatment. Non-drug treatments and antidepressant medication are not mutually exclusive, and in some cases it is preferable to use both in combination. Cognitive behavioural therapy (CBT) is frequently employed to support changes to unhelpful patterns of thinking that occur in depression.

The basis of CBT was developed more than 50 years ago and subsequently refined into a specific therapy in the 1970s. This type of treatment helps patients to address their unhelpful thoughts and actions associated with depression. Over a series of up to 20 sessions, the CBT therapist works with the patient either alone or in groups, to replace negative or self-critical thoughts and actions with more positive and helpful ones. CBT is not a 'quick fix' solution to depression; patients are often given 'homework' between sessions to try and put their positive actions into practice. Interpersonal psychotherapy is another form of psychotherapy which may help patients deal with more social aspects of their depression. This type of therapy explores relationships and their effect on mental health and well-being.

Drug treatment

In the treatment of depression all of the antidepressants currently available in the UK may be considered to be equally effective. Table 29.1 defines terminology often used when reporting outcomes of antidepressant treatment in the literature. A strong response to placebo is found in most of the studies of antidepressants. Tolerability is, therefore, an important factor in the choice of drug; patients who are unable to tolerate the side effects of antidepressants are likely to discontinue taking these drugs. Overall, the selective serotonin reuptake inhibitors (SSRIs) antidepressants appear to be better tolerated than tricyclics, and their improved safety profile in overdose may be an important consideration for use.

For most patients first-line treatment is a generic SSRI. For these agents the starting dose is often the treatment dose because these agents have a flat dose–response curve. This means increasing the dose serves only to increase adverse effects. Patients should notice some discernible improvement in symptoms by week 2, although full benefit is often not seen until 4–6 weeks into treatment. This delay is probably due to adaptive neurochemical changes that need to take place but are not fully understood. Some effects which are directly linked to primary transmitter effects will occur quickly. These are often side effects. Some such as increased sedation may be helpful, particularly if poor sleep is improved, whereas others such as dry mouth, blurred vision and constipation will not be welcome. In older adults and with MAOIs, this full benefit time frame may be extended to 12

Table 29.1	Different terms employed in reporting interventions in depression management
Term	Definition
Onset	A 20% improvement in depressive symptoms
Response	A 50% improvement in depressive symptoms
Remission	A return to premorbid baseline with minimal or no residual symptoms
Recovery	Usually declared when the patient has been in sustained remission for between 4 and 6 months

weeks. In monitoring a patient's progress, failure to see any onset of benefit at week 2 should prompt a review of treatment, and often this will be a change to an alternative agent. Patients may also switch antidepressants because of tolerability issues. When considering an antidepressant for a particular patient, many factors are likely to influence the choice of agent.

- Previous experience or response to treatment: If this is not the first occasion of taking an antidepressant, then it is useful to explore past outcomes with treatment, and if positive consider a previously successful antidepressant as first line.
- Dosing regimen: A big advantage of SSRIs is the once-daily dosing which often requires no further titration.
- Other medications or comorbidities: Patients with epilepsy and receiving anticonvulsant medication may be exposed to interactions with some antidepressants. All antidepressants lower seizure threshold, but this per se is not usually a problem in clinical practice for patients well stabilised on their anticonvulsant treatment. Those at risk of QTc prolongation may need to avoid antidepressants that carry a larger impact on QT prolongation. Any significant renal or hepatic impairment may also need to be taken into consideration.
- Formulary constraints: The local health economy may add its own additional formulary and prescribing restrictions.
- Cost: Resource implications are important because the volume of prescribing in depression means that small price differences can equate with significant savings.

For patients who obtain a partial response to a chosen antidepressant, augmentation options, as opposed to a switch to an alternative treatment, are available. The most common and universal antidepressant treatment used in augmentation is lithium. Evidenced-based antidepressant combinations have also been identified (NICE, 2009a, 2009b) and also included in the updated evidence based British Association for Psychopharmacology 2015 guidelines for treating depressive disorders with antidepressants (Cleare et al., 2015). Specialist texts such as Maudsley Prescribing Guidelines and Bazire's Psychotropic Drug Directory provide details of less commonly prescribed combinations.

Once a patient is in remission, then the question of when to stop treatment is likely to arise. For a first episode of depression, where the patient is well supported psychosocially, the evidence-based recommendation is to continue for a minimum of 6 months. Where patient support is less favourable or this is not the patient's first episode of depression, maintenance treatment should continue for 2 years. Any patient who has experienced three or more episodes within a 5-year period is likely to benefit from ongoing antidepressant treatment.

Given these time frames many patients express concerns about becoming addicted to antidepressants. It can be accurately stated that antidepressants are not addictive. Antidepressants do not cause the cravings associated with drugs of addiction. In addition the dose does not need to be increased to preserve ongoing benefit. Patients are also unlikely to become preoccupied with where the next dose is obtained, so addiction criteria are unmet. However, abrupt cessation of a course of antidepressant treatment can lead to unpleasant discontinuation effects. Patients may interpret such discontinuation effects as withdrawal. However, healthcare professionals can advise that a 4-week dose reduction strategy should minimise any adverse events resulting from discontinuation of treatment.

Monoamine oxidase inhibitors

Traditional monoamine oxidase inhibitors. The traditional MAOI group contains the earliest recognised antidepressants comprising isocarboxazid, phenelzine and tranylcypromine. Their antidepressant effect is understood to come about from promoting levels of biogenic amines serotonin, noradrenaline (norepinephrine) and dopamine, by blocking enzyme breakdown of these transmitters in key brain synapses. These agents are no longer early choices in depression for several reasons. Clinically they can be slow to provide noticeable benefit and do not provide any early symptom relief of associated anxiety or poor sleep. However, the main concern is the risk they introduce alongside tyramine-containing foods and medicines that may similarly release noradrenaline (norepinephrine) from peripheral nerve terminals, that is, indirectly acting sympathomimetics. These traditional MAOI agents block both MAO-A and MAO-B enzyme subtypes, rendering the patient vulnerable to the pressor effects of such compounds. MAO enzyme is present in many areas of the body including the gut, and normally tyramine found in cheese would be broken down by MAO in the gut. With no gut MAO available, the tyramine passes unhindered in to the circulation, where it displaces noradrenaline on to peripheral target sites. The cardiovascular system is most at risk, increasing heart rate with a vasoconstriction which leads to a dramatic rise in blood pressure. This hypertensive crisis, sometimes referred to as a 'cheese' reaction, is a medical emergency and is one of the few situations where hypertension produces key symptoms for the patient. Symptoms of a hypertensive crisis are likely to include pain and stiffness in the neck, an occipital headache and angina-like chest pain. In an emergency department, treatment is likely to involve the administration of a noradrenergic (norepinephergic) α receptor blocker such as phentolamine or phenoxybenzamine.

Therefore, patients should be aware of the dietary precautions and need to avoid purchasable medicines that carry similar risk. MAOI warning cards were produced, but these have now been discontinued. However, the patient leaflet contained with the medicines provides this written advice. Most patients receiving these treatments are likely to have been receiving them for some time and will be fully aware of food restrictions and the need to check the safety of any bought medicines with the pharmacist. As well as being used for depression, these agents may be in place as part of treatment for phobic disorders.

Of the three drugs in this category, tranylcypromine carries the highest risk of hypertensive crisis, whereas isocarboxazid is the weakest and safest. Although tranylcypromine is a reversible inhibitor of MAO and enzyme recovery may be seen in as little as 5 days following cessation of treatment, in clinical practice MAOI precautions should be maintained for a full 2 weeks after stopping treatment regardless of which MAOI has been taken.

Reversible inhibitors of monoamine oxidase. Monoamine oxidase exists in two forms, MAO-A and MAO-B. MAO-A is the major form found in monoamine neurones. MAO-A inhibition appears necessary for an antidepressant response. MAO-B inhibition helps preserve dopamine and has an anti-parkinsonian effect. MAO-A is also found in the gut and liver, where it acts to metabolise ingested tyramine. Moclobemide is a competitive reversible inhibitor of MAO-A and is displaced by large amounts of tyramine. There is therefore little risk of a potentially fatal hypertensive crisis, and the need for dietary caution or the avoidance of other medicines is reduced. MAO-B can also compensate physiologically for some loss of MAO-A activity. Moclobemide was introduced into clinical practice in the early 1990s as a safer option over traditional MAOIs. Patients can be reassured that dietary and medicinal restrictions associated with original MAOIs are not required. If an MAOI antidepressant is initiated, this is likely to be the agent of choice. In terms of clinical efficacy, timescales and unwanted effects, it shares many of the traditional MAOI characteristics.

Tricyclic antidepressants.
Pharmacologically, tricyclic agents act as serotonin, noradrenaline (norepinephrine) reuptake inhibitors, but with the additional property of blocking acetylcholine at muscarinic receptors. This additional antimuscarinic property is not believed to confer any therapeutic benefit but accounts for many predictable unwanted effects of this class of drugs.

Predictable antimuscarinic side effects are:
- Dry mouth: Caused by reduced saliva production. This is best countered by sips of cool water, chewing sugar-free gum or the application of saliva-enhancing sprays.
- Blurred vision: Accommodation is impaired early on in treatment, and patients should be reassured that this will settle and is not an indication of sight problems.
- Constipation: Reduced peristalsis may occur. Most patients are likely to require a laxative early on in treatment and this should be proactively managed. Depression itself caused by reduced mobility and poor diet may separately contribute.
- Difficulty passing urine: Reducing sphincter activity. Male patients with enlarged prostate may find this problematic, and in rare instances urinary retention may ensue.
- Confusion: Confusion is a central antimuscarinic effect. Older adults are more overtly vulnerable, but subtler effects in other patients may lead to reduced reaction times and pose increased driving risks. Depression itself will already have lowered reaction time. Doses of tricyclics should be titrated over several days to full treatment dose with these factors in mind.

A number of TCAs are in current clinical use. The basic chemical structures of these compounds are similar, but there are differences between them. All of the TCAs require dose titration to achieve optimum antidepressant dose. Most are significantly sedating and with central antimuscarinic effects; therefore, starting a patient on the full treatment dose would predictably induce a confusional state alongside unwanted sedation. Furthermore, the common property of postural hypotension and blurred vision further adds to an unpleasant experience and increases the risk of falls or other accidents.

Tricyclics can be taken as single daily doses because of their long half-lives and often at night so that peak levels occur during sleep. Tricyclics are toxic in overdose. The antimuscarinic effects on the vagus nerve can lead to the development of cardiac arrhythmias and these, in turn, may prove fatal. Children and older adults are especially vulnerable.

In low doses some tricyclics have other uses in clinical practice. For example, those with significant noradrenergic (norepinephrinergic) reuptake properties may be used to help with neuropathic pain. Low doses of particularly sedating agents are sometimes used for hypnotic purposes. This should not be supported because it represents unlicensed use and is employing an agent with many adverse properties to substitute for a single need.

Amitriptyline. Amitriptyline is one of the more sedating agents and in low doses is often employed to manage neuropathic pain. Its use in depression continues to decline because it is no longer a recommended first-line treatment option.

Imipramine. Imipramine is similar to amitriptyline, but less sedating. This agent may be employed in children to help manage nocturnal enuresis or again in children as part of attention-deficit/hyperactivity disorder treatment. Again use as an antidepressant is declining for the same reasons as amitriptyline.

Clomipramine. Pharmacologically clomipramine is a potent serotonin reuptake inhibitor with minimal noradrenergic (norepinephrinergic) reuptake inhibition, and this leads to some differences in clinical application outside of depression. For example, it has little or no value in neuropathic pain management, but as a serotonin-rich drug it has an established role in the management of obsessive-compulsive disorder (OCD).

Dosulepin. Formerly known as dothiepin (British Approved Name), dosulepin is the most cardiotoxic of the tricyclic agents and should now not be initiated in any new patients. Patients already established on this agent should not be automatically switched to another antidepressant. Instalment dispensing (i.e. dispensing only small quantities at a time) may be put in place if there are concerns about self-harming through overdosing.

Lofepramine. Within the tricyclic group, lofepramine carries a much-reduced toxicity profile. Antimuscarinic effects do occur with lofepramine, but these are less severe than with other tricyclics. Lofepramine does not have a significant sedative effect. For new patients who require a TCA to manage their depression, this is likely to be the drug of choice.

Selective serotonin reuptake inhibitors. In the mid-1980s these agents were developed in an attempt to reduce some of the problems associated with the TCAs. Overall, the SSRIs are better tolerated by most patients, and they are considerably less toxic in overdose; this means that they should be the first-line choice for the pharmacological management of moderate or severe depression (NICE, 2009a, 2009b). Compared with TCAs, they have less impairment on reaction time and there is less additional sedation if alcohol is consumed. Because generic versions of the drugs are available, the financial impact of using SSRIs first line is considerably reduced. The SSRIs have a broadly similar range of side

effects, but there are variations in the intensity or duration. The degree of specificity for serotonin reuptake differs between the SSRIs, but this does not correlate with clinical efficacy. When given in adequate doses for an adequate period of time, all of the drugs in this class appear to be equally effective. The two main clinical issues with SSRIs are nausea and their early alerting effects whereby patients are likely to feel more anxious or on edge during the first 2 weeks of treatment. Nausea is best addressed by advising patients to take their daily dose after breakfast. Nausea should decline within a few days, but for some patients it remains an intolerable adverse event and an alternative class of agent is required. Alerting effects may be addressed by exploring non-pharmacological strategies to promote relaxation (e.g. yoga or music). Alternatively, a short course (maximum 2 weeks) of a benzodiazepine such as diazepam could be prescribed. A hypnotic agent such as zopiclone or zolpidem could be prescribed if alerting effects occur at nighttime.

Some years ago the SSRI paroxetine was subject to media attention in the UK, and this led to the identification of three important medicines management issues with use of antidepressants: unpleasant events occurring on abrupt cessation of treatment, sexual dysfunction and increased risk of suicide.

It has now become standard practice to stop antidepressant treatment over a 4-week period by gradually reducing the dose. Patients who abruptly stop antidepressants may feel acutely quite unwell, and this should not be taken to indicate a recurrence of the depression. Left unchecked, symptoms will remit after some days, but a short-term reinstatement of dose and review of the discontinuation strategy is often all that is required.

Sexual dysfunction has now been identified as a feature of many other classes of antidepressant, linked to agonist effect on serotonin 5-HT$_2$ receptors. There are various pharmacological strategies identified in the literature to manage this, and some of the newer antidepressants carry less sexual dysfunction. It should also be remembered that depression itself reduces libido, but antidepressant impairment is more often associated with ejaculatory ability.

Self-harm and suicide are aspects of depression itself, and the suggestion that this class of antidepressants actually contributed to this mortality outcome was subject to much debate and review of evidence. The early alerting effects of SSRIs may allow a patient to carry out a suicidal intent. With the older TCAs, many patients receiving treatment experience significant sedation and are unable to act on these impulses. As the depression remits, the suicidal ideation reduces with effective treatment.

Since their launch as antidepressants, SSRIs have become treatment options for a range of anxiety-based disorders (e.g. panic disorder, OCD, general anxiety disorder, eating disorders, post-traumatic stress disorder), but generally the doses required are much higher than those employed in depression.

Fluvoxamine. The first SSRI launched in the mid-1980s, fluvoxamine was marketed at a high dose requiring a three times a day dosing. Many patients experienced severe nausea, and the drug has many interactions because it is a potent inhibitor of the cytochrome P450 drug metabolising system. It is unlikely to be seen very often in clinical practice today.

Fluoxetine. The main difference between fluoxetine and the other SSRIs is its long half-life. In the initial stages of treatment, some patients may experience a greater feeling of nervousness with fluoxetine than with the other SSRIs. The long half-life of fluoxetine, mediated through its major metabolite norfluoxetine, can be a problem if severe side effects develop. In other situations, the long half-life means that the risk of a patient experiencing discontinuation symptoms is minimal. This SSRI may be abruptly stopped because it will take about 5 weeks to clear from the body. Formulations of fluoxetine that can be taken on a weekly basis are available in some parts of the world.

Paroxetine. In contrast with fluoxetine, paroxetine has a relatively short half-life and no active metabolites. Therefore, this drug requires gradual dose reduction prior to stopping. It has some inhibitory activity at CYP4502D6, which may need to be considered in patients who are taking other medications.

Sertraline. The SSRI sertraline is preferred where a patient has comorbid cardiac disease because it does not increase the burden of the underlying condition and has very few drug interactions. It is also a popular choice within perinatal mental health because it does not independently add to any baseline risk of taking SSRIs. In pregnancy all SSRIs carry a slightly increased risk of neonatal septal heart defect. From week 20 there is an increased risk of the respiratory syndrome persistent pulmonary hypertension of the neonate. However, the absolute risk remains small at 0.3%, although subsyndromal respiratory states are more common. Exposure to SSRIs during the third trimester is likely to produce mild neonatal withdrawal reactions (e.g. irritability or tremor). These are minimal with sertraline but may be more problematic with paroxetine.

Citalopram and Escitalopram. Citalopram is a racemic mixture of *R*- and *S*-citalopram and predates escitalopram, the active *S* enantiomer of citalopram. Escitalopram was launched on the basis that the *R* enantiomer has no antidepressant effect, and it may even counteract some of the antidepressant effects of the *S* enantiomer of escitalopram. Citalopram carries a greater risk of clinically significant QT prolongation, prompting restrictions to be placed on doses especially in older adults. The QT prolongation effect is much less with escitalopram. In clinical practice several patients do find escitalopram much more tolerable, and now that escitalopram is available generically, the economic pressure to avoid using this SSRI as first-line treatment is much less.

Other Antidepressants

Trazodone. Trazodone is a little used antidepressant which requires adult dosages of 300 mg daily and above to treat depression. It is rapidly absorbed on an empty stomach, leading to profound dizziness, so it should always be taken with food. Its mechanism of action remains unclear. It does have some helpful anxiolytic properties and occasionally is used in older adults more for this property than to manage depression. Compared with the tricyclics it is much safer in overdose and lacks significant antimuscarinic properties. Priapism has also been noted as a rare but distressing side effect. This is almost certainly due to its potent α receptor–blocking properties.

In an attempt to improve on the benefits gained with SSRIs over TCAs, newer antidepressants were introduced from the late 1990s onward. These antidepressants include venlafaxine, duloxetine, reboxetine, mirtazapine, agomelatine and vortioxetine. Table 29.2 summarises the key practice points associated with these newer agents.

Venlafaxine. Venlafaxine possesses minimal antimuscarinic properties and greatly reduced toxicity compared with TCAs. At low doses the drug behaves more like an SSRI, but as the dose is increased venlafaxine adopts its serotonin noradrenaline reuptake inhibitor (SNRI) profile. Across all doses there is weak dopamine reuptake inhibition. Dose titration therefore is indicated. There is a low potential for postural hypotension, although the drug carries a risk of hypertension at higher doses. Discontinuation effects can be problematic, and careful gradual dosage reduction is required when stopping treatment.

Duloxetine. The SNRI profile of duloxetine remains constant and equal between the two transmitters, serotonin and noradrenaline (norepinephrine). This means that dose titration is not routinely indicated.

Medicine management issues including adverse events closely resemble SSRIs. In the UK duloxetine is also licensed separately for neuropathic pain and stress incontinence; this latter indication is under a different brand.

Reboxetine. Reboxetine is indicated for more reclusive and presentations where the patient is particularly lacking energy. The main side effects are dry mouth and insomnia. The drug is considered to have a low evidence base of independent effectiveness.

Mirtazapine. Compared with SSRIs, the antidepressant mirtazapine represents an agent with reduced alerting effects, minimal nausea and low incidence of sexual dysfunction. However, both sedation, which is more prominent at lower dose, and weight gain are significant. Use of mirtazapine has superseded mianserin to which it is chemically related.

Agomelatine. Advantages of agomelatine include restoration of sleep pattern without residual sedation and impaired reaction time, as well as minimal weight gain, gastro-intestinal upset and sexual dysfunction. Abnormal liver function tests are common and require regular liver function monitoring in accordance with the Summary of Product Characteristics. Variable efficacy has been seen in clinical trials.

Vortioxetine. The mechanism of action of vortioxetine is described descriptively, but the focus is on promoting serotonin activity. Nausea is the most common adverse effect. Sexual dysfunction is present but only at higher doses. Early alerting effects are likely to be less pronounced, and in remission patients appear to be less residually cognitively impaired with this agent. There is no evidence of QT prolongation. Patients show minimal weight gain and no evidence of significant discontinuation symptoms following abrupt cessation of treatment. NICE (2015) supports its use as a third-line option for the treatment of major depression.

Other treatments

Electroconvulsive therapy. When urgent intervention is indicated to manage severe depression, ECT may be considered. ECT involves inducing a seizure under controlled conditions. Unless a patient lacks capacity it requires their agreement and is prescribed by a psychiatrist. ECT involves the administration of an anaesthetic and muscle relaxant before the application of the treatment and thus is carried out under theatre-like conditions with full resuscitation facilities present. ECT is often delivered twice weekly as a course of six to eight treatments and for some patients provides a rapid resolution of the most severe symptoms,

Table 29.2 Newer antidepressants and key practice points

Name	Type	Practice points
Venlafaxine	SNRI	• Reduced toxicity compared with TCAs • At low doses, drug behaves like SSRI, adopting SNRI profile as dose increases; across all doses there is additional dopamine reuptake inhibition • Dose titration applicable • Low risk of postural hypotension, but risk of hypertension at high dose • Marked discontinuation effects
Duloxetine	SNRI	• A fixed ratio of serotonin to noradrenaline (norepinephrine) reuptake inhibition • Dose titration rarely indicated • Resembles SSRIs in clinical practice • Also licensed for neuropathic pain and for stress incontinence; in the UK duloxetine is marketed under a different brand name when prescribed for stress incontinence
Reboxetine	NARI	• Indicated for more reclusive and anergic presentations • Key side effects are dry mouth and insomnia • Low evidence base of independent effectiveness
Mirtazapine	NaSSA	• Reduced alerting effects • Minimal nausea • Low incidence of sexual dysfunction • Sedation is more prominent at lower dose • Weight gain is significant
Agomelatine	MT_1 MT_2 agonist $5-HT_{2c}$ antagonist	• Restoration of sleep pattern without residual sedation and impaired reaction time • Minimal weight gain, GI upset and sexual dysfunction • Abnormal LFTs are common and require regular monitoring • Variable efficacy in trials
Vortioxetine	Direct modulation of receptor activity and inhibition of the serotonin transporter	• Nausea is most common adverse effect • Sexual dysfunction present at higher doses only • Alerting effects less pronounced • Less residual cognitive impairment • No evidence of QT prolongation • Minimal weight gain • No significant discontinuation symptoms

GI, Gastro-intestinal; LFT, liver function test; NARI, noradrenaline reuptake inhibitor; NaSSA, noradrenaline-specific serotonin agonist; SNRI, serotonin noradrenaline reuptake inhibitor; SSRI, selective serotonin reuptake inhibitor; TCA, tricyclic antidepressant.

promoting enough improvement to provide ongoing treatment via pharmacological and non-pharmacological means. Although the treatment itself is very safe, patients must be risk assessed for safe receipt of an anaesthetic, and many patients experience short-term memory loss following treatment.

ECT remains controversial, but its speed of effect is not currently matched by any antidepressant medication. This situation may change because recently the immediate and beneficial effects of ketamine in treating depression have been identified.

St John's wort (Hypericum perforatum). In the UK herbal remedies such as St John's wort do not feature in prescribing guidelines, but this agent has become a popular option for self-medication. Extracts of hypericum have been shown to be as effective as standard antidepressants in the management of major depression (Linde et al., 2008). Herbal remedies can appear attractive because they sound and feel 'natural', and some patients assume that this exempts them from the serious side effects or interactions that characterise prescribed medicines. In reality St. John's wort has been identified as a cytochrome P450 enzyme inducer

responsible for oral contraceptive failure, breakthrough seizures and reducing the effectiveness of antirejection medication. Mental health stigma may lead some patients to self-medicate for anonymity of treatment. St John's wort is readily accessible, but information provided with the herbal medication will not provide specific information about use in depression. As a herbal product there is some variance in the quality and content of various active ingredients, which indicates inconsistency of dosing is likely. As with prescription antidepressants, treatment should continue for 6 months to minimise the risk of relapse. Once a patient is feeling better this may prove financially challenging if he or she is buying the product. Encouraging people to be aware of mental health issues together with the signs and symptoms of depression is beneficial. However, management of depression without professional support severely limits the options for other interventions (e.g. psychological support) and also objective monitoring.

Ketamine. Ketamine predominantly exerts its effect through an antagonist action on the glutamate N-methyl-D-aspartate receptor. Researchers are now looking for an alternative oral preparation with the same therapeutic effect but fewer of the adverse effects, less abuse potential and fewer problems of administration seen with ketamine. It also means that antidepressants of the future may depart from the traditional biogenic amines and focus on the glutamate pathway.

Treatment of mania

The treatment of acute mania often requires urgent intervention to reduce high arousal states and associated risks. Pharmacological agents employed include benzodiazepines, valproate, antipsychotics and lithium. Combinations of these agents may be used in the early management of such episodes. Lithium is now rarely used in the management of acute mania because it has a slow onset of effect and the dose required can result in high levels which are close to toxic. From a patient perspective, an early unpleasant experience with lithium is likely to deter a patient to agree to this agent being used as a longer-term strategy to help protect against further mood swings. At the same time any agents that could be exacerbating a manic episode should be reviewed. Depression associated with bipolar disorder should not be managed by using antidepressants in isolation because there is a risk of prompting a switch to a manic episode. Agents such as quetiapine or lamotrigine with or without lithium represent evidence-based preferred options. Therefore, antidepressants in bipolar patients should be urgently reviewed and strong consideration given to their withdrawal. Sometimes non-psychotropic drugs such as high-dose steroids (e.g. prednisolone) may precipitate an episode. Prescribing prednisolone in divided doses, as well as reducing the overall daily dose, may help mitigate the situation.

Benzodiazepines

Lorazepam, because of its high potency and availability in both tablet and injection form, is often the agent of choice for prompt sedation. As with other members of this group it works quickly to lower high arousal states and on its own may be enough to interrupt an emergent episode. Some patients have small quantities of benzodiazepine, or related agents, available to self-manage any early signs of such mood swings. In more urgent cases lorazepam may need to be given parenterally to a patient by a healthcare professional to effect treatment. In the UK this may be under the provision of the Mental Health Act legislation if the patient does not consent and there are clear risks of not treating the episode. An alternative parenteral agent to lorazepam is midazolam, which has the advantage of not requiring refrigeration or dilution 1:1 with water for injection prior to intramuscular injection. However, in the UK midazolam is a Schedule 3 Controlled Drug, and this requires additional processes relating to ordering, recording and auditing of stock levels.

Valproate semisodium

Valproate semisodium (divalproate) is licensed in the UK as a specific treatment for mania associated with bipolar disorder. This distinguishes it from the original sodium valproate which,

introduced into the UK in the 1970s, remains licensed only for the management of epilepsy.

Valproate semisodium is a 1:1 molar combination of sodium valproate and valproic acid. Following administration, valproate ion is released and subsequently absorbed. Any meaningful therapeutic differences between sodium valproate and valproate semisodium have not been established. The mechanism of action of valproate in mania is unclear but may be related to increased levels of γ-aminobutyric acid. The antimanic effects of valproate are seen within 3 days, but the full benefit of treatment may not be apparent for up to 3 weeks. Doses should be rapidly titrated to between 1000 and 2000 mg/day. Routine valproate serum levels are not necessary, but levels between 50 and 100 mg/L have been reported to be associated with optimal response in some patients. Although the risks for liver damage are greater in young children, liver function tests should be performed prior to initiation of therapy and periodically thereafter in all patients. In addition, the patient must be instructed to report any problems, such as unexplained bruising, that may indicate abnormalities in coagulation. Although valproate is well established as a prophylactic treatment to prevent relapse, this is an off-label use across all formulations. Valproate should not be used in women of childbearing potential because of its high risk of teratogenicity. These warnings have been strengthened in the UK through amended NICE guidance.

Antipsychotics

All antipsychotics are acknowledged as being intrinsically antimanic, although not all have this utility formally listed within their licensed indications. Most of the second-generation (atypical) antipsychotics, for example, olanzapine, risperidone, quetiapine, aripiprazole and asenapine, are licensed for use in the management of acute mania and in most cases prevention of new manic episodes.

Haloperidol is still commonly prescribed as part of the acute management of mania. It is less sedating than other antipsychotics, but because of its potent dopamine D_2 receptor blockade it carries a much higher risk of inducing acute extrapyramidal side effects. See Chapter 30 for more details around management of extrapyramidal side effects.

Longer-term management

Second-generation antipsychotics also have an established role in the longer-term management of bipolar disorder. Quetiapine in particular is now recognised as an evidence-based choice for management of bipolar depression. This paradox of an antipsychotic playing a key role in managing depression associated with bipolar disorder is linked to the limited understanding of the pharmacological mechanisms of newer antipsychotics in the management of affective disorders.

Continuation therapy with a prophylactic mood stabiliser should be considered in all bipolar patients who have had two or more acute episodes within 2–4 years. It may also be reasonable to consider prophylaxis in any patient following a severe manic episode. Because treatment is long-term the cooperation of the patient is essential; therefore, a thorough explanation of the risks and benefits of the treatment is vital.

Lithium. Lithium has two distinct roles within affective disorders:

- In unipolar depression it can augment the partial effect of an antidepressant. Adding lithium to the regimen can lead to remission within a few weeks.
- In bipolar disorder lithium remains for the UK the first-choice mood stabiliser.

It has a greater impact on manic episodes, but in bipolar depression its effectiveness can be improved when used alongside lamotrigine. Lithium has a significant impact on reducing suicide rates in bipolar disorder. The mechanism of action remains to be fully elucidated, but since its discovery lithium has been shown to act upon various neurotransmitter systems at multiple levels of signalling in the brain. It is suggested that lithium restores the balance among faulty signalling pathways in critical brain regions. Such effects are thought to trigger long-term changes in neuronal signalling patterns that account for the prophylactic properties of lithium in the treatment of bipolar disorder. Through its inhibitory effects on glycogen synthase kinase-3beta (GSK-3β) and β-arrestin-2, lithium may alter the level of phosphorylation of cytoskeletal proteins, which leads to neuroplastic changes associated with mood stabilisation (Malhi et al., 2013).

Lithium has a number of medicines management issues because it has a narrow therapeutic range, a low therapeutic index, a wide range of unpleasant side effects and may be involved in several clinically significant drug interactions. It is potentially very toxic, with a clear correlation between serum levels and efficacy, as well as toxicity. It was made the subject of a national patient safety alert in 2009 requiring all healthcare services to implement a five-point action plan. Before initiating treatment with lithium, certain tests should be performed:

- Check serum urea and electrolytes to identify fluid and salt balance.
- Measure serum creatinine to generate an estimate of glomerular filtration rate and assess renal function.
- Undertake thyroid function test and measure calcium levels to check on baseline activity of thyroid and parathyroid glands.
- Where clinically indicated, perform a full blood count. This would include patients with a history of blood disorders because lithium is likely to induce a benign increase in white cells.
- Conduct an electrocardiogram if cardiovascular risk factors are present or the patient has existing cardiovascular disease.

If no abnormalities are found in these parameters, lithium can then be initiated based on the premise that 1 g lithium carbonate produces a steady-state level of around 1.0 mmol/L.

Serum levels. At steady state, which is usually 7 days following initiation of treatment, blood samples are taken 12 hours after the last dose. The 12-hour standard lithium level range is routinely 0.4–1.0 mmol/L. For prophylaxis a plasma lithium level of 0.6–0.8 mmol/L is considered optimum whether lithium is being used in unipolar depression or within bipolar disorder management. The majority of a dose of lithium is excreted unchanged in the urine, making renal function the primary determinant of the treatment dose. The target range for prophylaxis should be routinely around 0.6 mmol/L, and so a dosage of around 600 mg daily for adult patients is appropriate. Older adults, who will invariably have some age-related reduced renal function, may be initiated at 200 mg daily, but target levels are the same, so under-dosing should be avoided.

When initiating lithium, or making a dose adjustment, it takes around 7 days for a revised steady state to develop. Therefore, unless assessment is required for toxicity, blood levels should not be measured any sooner because dosing adjustments would be based on inaccurate levels. Dose adjustments with lithium are straightforward because at steady-state lithium levels vary in direct proportion to dose; that is, a doubling of dose will double the blood level. However, should this empirical dosing lead to predictive doses above 1600 mg daily, adherence should be thoroughly assessed.

Doses are likely to need adjusting during the early stages of treatment according to patient response and measured serum levels. A number of predictable and unwanted effects can occur, such as polydipsia (increased thirst), polyuria (increased urine output of up to 3 L/day), mild stomach discomfort with some looseness of the bowels and fine tremor of the hands.

However, with the exception of polyuria, these early adverse effects usually resolve within 1–2 weeks. Patients usually adapt to the increased urine output. Monitoring should initially include routine lithium levels on a 3 monthly basis which may be reduced to 6 monthly after a year in patients who continue with stable levels and have no other comorbidities that could affect the body's handling of lithium. Assessment of renal function and thyroid status should be carried out 6 monthly or at least annually. A lithium treatment pack (National Patient Safety Agency [2009] lithium resource pack) should be made available to all patients who are prescribed lithium.

Some patients may notice a swelling in the neck (goitre). Lithium can reduce the output of thyroid hormone, but this is easily corrected with levothyroxine. Often any reduction in thyroid activity is identified in blood tests before the patient notices any discomfort. Weight gain is a significant side effect of lithium therapy.

Lithium toxicity. When lithium levels exceed 1.5 mmol/L signs of lithium toxicity begin to develop. Lithium toxicity is characterised by severe shaking of the hands, giddiness or loss of balance, slurred speech, unusual drowsiness or sleepiness, vomiting and/or diarrhoea. These symptoms should be seen as a medical emergency. Lithium levels may become high unintentionally and usually because of dehydration, diet and drugs. It is important to educate the patient on recognising and avoiding lithium toxicity.

Dehydration arising from extreme fluid loss because of feverish illness, sickness and diarrhoea should prompt a stopping of the lithium until the situation is improved. This will avoid high concentrations of lithium developing. In relation to diet, extreme changes to salt intake, particularly the exclusion of salt from the diet, may lead to the body retaining more lithium to compensate for the salt loss. Some medicines taken alongside lithium may interact. Patients should be advised to ask their pharmacist before purchasing any over-the-counter medicines. Some medications may push lithium levels into the toxic range. This applies not just to prescription drugs, where the diuretic bendroflumethiazide is a classic example, but also to some over-the-counter medications such as ibuprofen; this analgesic is best avoided unless there is good access to close monitoring of the lithium.

Formulation. As the absorption and bioavailability of lithium may vary from brand to brand, it is important that patients do not inadvertently change brands or dosage forms without levels being checked. Failing to correctly convert a tablet dose to the correct equivalent of the liquid formulations can also lead to dosing errors. The poor aqueous solubility of lithium carbonate (soluble 1 part in 100 parts water) compared with lithium citrate means that the citrate salt is used in all liquid formulations of lithium.

When converting from citrate formulations to carbonate, it should be noted that:

520 mg of lithium citrate = 200 mg of lithium carbonate.

Other anticonvulsants in bipolar disorder. Carbamazepine is a second-line prophylactic treatment which is likely to be prescribed when lithium is ineffective, contraindicated or not tolerated. The medicines management issues that apply when carbamazepine is employed as an anticonvulsant are the same as when it is used as an anticonvulsant. However, there is no robust evidence to confirm that such carbamazepine target serum levels are applicable for use in bipolar disorder.

There is a good evidence base to support the use of lamotrigine in bipolar depression. Specific drug-related monitoring is also not required. Lamotrigine should always be initiated slowly and at half the standard incremental regimen when valproate is also being taken. This is because valproate elevates lamotrigine levels and through this process increases the risk of development of serious skin reactions to lamotrigine. The use of lamotrigine in bipolar disorder remains unlicensed in the UK.

Patient care

Adherence to medication in patients with affective disorders may prove challenging. A patient with severe depression may feel that no treatment can help. At the height of a manic episode anything that will subdue great elation and well-being may be resisted. In these circumstances patients may be described as lacking insight, and in the UK their choice to refuse treatment overridden by the processes within the Mental Health Act. However, outside of an acute phase, good therapeutic discussions around treatment options can take place. Pharmacists are ideally placed to present balanced information on the medicines available to help patients identify treatments and regimens.

It is good practice to provide written information about the medicines. One source is the Choice and Medication website (http://www.choiceandmedication.org/cms/?lang=en) which provides access via subscription to independent medicines information on psychotropic agents. It is not restricted by licensed indications and is a resource for both healthcare professionals and patients.

In any patient consultation it should be remembered that concerns around stigma associated with a mental health condition and adherence to treatment may need to be addressed. During treatment selection shared decision making is likely to be much more successful than a unilateral decision made by a healthcare professional. The nature of bipolar disorder means that some patients value the option of advance decisions. This is encouraged as best practice with patients identifying and recording their preference(s) and dislikes for acute intervention which allow, unless circumstances dictate otherwise, their preferences to be honoured in a relapse situation. Exploring with patients their hopes and expectations around medication and actively listening to their concerns about treatment should help to ensure that rewarding conversations take place.

Many of the drugs used in the treatment of affective disorders have the potential to interact with other drugs that have been prescribed or purchased. Some of these are summarised in Table 29.3. Common therapeutic problems in the management of affective disorder are outlined in Table 29.4.

Table 29.3 Examples of important drug interactions with drugs used in the management of affective disorders

Drug group	Interacting drugs	Effects
Tricyclics	Adrenaline (epinephrine) and other directly acting sympathomimetics	Increased risk of hypertension and arrhythmias
	Alcohol	Enhanced sedation
	Antiarrhythmics	Risk of ventricular arrhythmias
	Anticonvulsants	Lowered seizure threshold and possible lowered tricyclic levels
	MAOIs	Severe hypertension, although some combinations are relatively safe and have been used in augmentation strategies
	Fluoxetine	Increased tricyclic serum levels
	Paroxetine	Increased tricyclic serum levels
SSRIs	Anticoagulants	Enhanced anticoagulant effects
	MAOIs	Central nervous system effects of SSRIs increased and risk of serotonin syndrome
	Lithium	Possible serotonin syndrome

Table 29.3 Examples of important drug interactions with drugs used in the management of affective disorders—cont'd

Drug group	Interacting drugs	Effects
MAOIs	Fermented beverages, tyramine-rich foods	Hypertensive crisis; nonfermented alcoholic beverages will not induce hypertensive event
	Antihypertensives	Increased hypotensive effect
	Anticonvulsants	Lowered seizure threshold
	Levodopa	Hypertensive crisis
	Sympathomimetics	Hypertensive crisis
Antipsychotics	Anaesthetic agents	Hypotension
	Anticonvulsants	Lowered seizure threshold
	Drugs that prolong QT interval	Risk of ventricular arrhythmias
Lithium	Non-steroidal anti-inflammatory drugs	Enhanced lithium serum levels
	SSRIs	Possible serotonin syndrome
	Diuretics	Enhanced lithium serum levels particularly with thiazides
	Angiotensin-converting enzyme inhibitors	Enhanced lithium serum levels
	Sumatriptan	Possible central nervous system toxicity; notably, some other triptans are cautioned alongside SSRIs and MAOIs for the same reason
St John's wort	Induces cytochrome P450 enzymes, particularly 1A2, 2C9 and 3A4	
	Indinavir	Reduced indinavir serum concentration (avoid)
	Warfarin	Reduced anticoagulant effect (avoid)
	SSRIs	Increased serotonergic effect (avoid)
	Carbamazepine (and other anticonvulsants)	Reduced serum concentrations (avoid)
	Digoxin	Reduced digoxin serum concentration (avoid)
	Oestrogens and progestogens	Reduced contraceptive effect (avoid)
	Theophylline	Reduced theophylline serum concentration (avoid)
	Ciclosporin	Reduced ciclosporin serum concentration (avoid)

Always check latest British National Formulary or other reference source for specific drug interaction information.
MAOI, Monoamine oxidase inhibitor; SSRI, selective serotonin reuptake inhibitor.

Table 29.4 Common therapeutic problems in the management of affective disorder

Problem	Possible solution
Antidepressants	
Treatment failure (30–40% of patients will not respond to first antidepressant)	Ensure adequate dose and duration of treatment Check adherence, engage the patient and develop therapeutic alliance Reassess response against target symptoms
Risk of self-harm	Reconfirm diagnosis and identify other risk factors, e.g. high levels of alcohol consumption in unsupervised situations
Discontinuation reactions	Re-introduce antidepressant and adopt slower tapering of dose
True relapse which develops much later than acute discontinuation events	Consider long-term treatment
Intolerance	Consider changing to a different class
Antimanic agents	
Treatment failure	Ensure adequate dose, check serum levels and adherence; consider drug combinations
Toxicity adverse effects	Determine dose by clinical response, guided by serum levels Ensure patient is well informed and able to recognise impending toxicity and adverse effects of treatment
Problematic weight gain	Dietary advice; structured exercise programmes; consider alternative pharmacotherapy, noting that most drugs used in affective disorders will cause some degree of weight gain
Lithium levels	Ensure serum levels are 12 h post-dose. This is facilitated by single night time dosing and a blood sample taken the following morning

Case studies

Case 29.1

Ms PS is a 21-year-old woman who presented to her primary care doctor with a 2-month history of difficulty in getting to sleep. She described herself as feeling generally unhappy. She was socialising much less but was able to perform most of her usual daily routines. She sometimes felt as though she had little energy and was spending more time just watching the television.

Question

What other questions would you want to ask of Ms PS before a diagnosis is made? What treatment options are indicated?

Answer

Firstly, it is important to explore with the patient if there are any other changes, especially with regard to signs and symptoms that present in depression. In a discussion with Ms PS it would be important to look for other symptoms of anxiety such as worrying thoughts, appetite changes and associated weight loss, suicidality, reduced concentration, loss of interest in hobbies and reduced libido (see mnemonic in main text).

On further questioning by her primary care doctor, Ms PS does not reveal any indicators of self-harm. She does not identify any significant weight loss, and her appetite has not reduced significantly. She does not demonstrate any signs of poor self-care, is in a supportive relationship, and although she has some financial concerns, these are not excessive.

It is likely that her depression is subthreshold or of mild severity. Referral to specialist services is not appropriate. Ms PS could be given advice on sleep hygiene. Sleep hygiene strategies include ensuring that the sleeping environment is comfortable and at an acceptable temperature and not too bright. Ms PS herself should be advised to avoid heavy meals, excessive exercise and stimulant (e.g. caffeine-based drinks) prior to bedtime. Associating bed with sleep and avoiding reading, watching TV or listening to the radio in bed is also recommended.

Active monitoring should be adopted and Ms PS asked to attend for a follow-up appointment in around 2 weeks.

At this stage antidepressants are not indicated. Non-pharmacological interventions to consider would be a structured group exercise programme, guided self-help based on the principles of CBT or computerised CBT. The specific intervention should be guided by Ms PS's preferences.

Case 29.2

Mr DD is a 50-year-old unemployed man with a long-standing history of bipolar disorder. He has been prescribed lithium for some time. His admission into hospital was prompted by a short period of increasingly disturbed behaviour. Mr DD's daughter had contacted the mental health services when she discovered that her father had just spent over £5000 on scientific instruments from an Internet auction site. Over the same period she had noticed that her father had lost interest in his self-care and become elated at the prospect of being on the verge of developing a special formula to solve the fuel crisis. On assessment Mr DD said he felt 'fine, fine all the time'. He told the visiting team that he did not need to be in hospital and it would keep him away from his top-secret mission. He also said that they could not admit him. Mr DD's speech was sometimes very rapid, and it was sometimes difficult to understand what he was saying. His

records showed that on his last admission he had been treated with haloperidol. He was not keen to take any medication offered and it was decided that admission to hospital was appropriate.

Question

What treatment is appropriate for Mr DD?

Answer

Although Mr DD has an established psychiatric diagnosis, it is still important to rule out any organic or physical causes or drivers for his presentation. Following a thorough physical and psychiatric examination, it was established that Mr DD had been relatively well since commencing treatment with lithium almost 4 years previously. However, it was identified that a few months ago he decided to stop taking lithium. It is important that symptoms of mania are promptly brought under control. Haloperidol would be a suitable choice, in view of his previous response. However, a review of Mr DD's medication history revealed that he had experienced several acute dystonic reactions to haloperidol during previous admissions. His daughter also reported that her father had commented on how awful it felt being given haloperidol during his last admission. Mr DD was, therefore, given the option to discuss alternative antipsychotic treatment. He agreed to take olanzapine which was prescribed at a dosage of 15 mg daily.

When Mr DD's manic symptoms are controlled, prophylactic treatment should be discussed with him. This should include a discussion about why he had discontinued lithium several months earlier. The opportunity should be taken to provide written information with the offer of a further discussion that should include his daughter.

Mr DD had stopped lithium because he felt he no longer needed it, but after discussion he was prepared to restart treatment. In line with results from renal and thyroid function tests, lithium carbonate may be re-introduced. A suitable starting dose is likely to be of the order 400 mg lithium carbonate at night.

One week later, a 12-hour standard serum lithium level should be performed and the dose of lithium adjusted to achieve the same lithium levels as before (0.6 mmol/L).

The side effects and signs of impending toxicity from lithium should be explained to Mr DD and, if possible, his daughter. They should be provided with the National Patient Safety Agency lithium resource booklet or any local hospital equivalent publication. In the UK this resource is used to provide important safety information around medicines management of lithium and includes the importance of regular lithium levels and other blood tests such as kidney and thyroid function, signs and symptoms of lithium toxicity, and actions that can be taken to avoid lithium toxicity. Once Mr DD is more settled, the olanzapine can be reduced with a view to discontinuation. This may take several weeks and can be done after he has been discharged from hospital. Further discussion with the patient and prescriber about having a supply of medication to help with any breakthrough symptoms that may occur in the future would be helpful and promote insight into the condition. This medication might be olanzapine or could be an agreed benzodiazepine or related sedative agent.

Case 29.3

Mr MA is a 49-year-old unemployed man. He was admitted to a psychiatric unit as an emergency admission. Mr MA had been prescribed fluoxetine 20 mg daily 2 months ago, and after no apparent response the prescriber had changed this to citalopram 20 mg daily 4 weeks earlier. On admission he was noted to be withdrawn, lacking motivation and just gave yes or no in response to questioning. He reported no interests in his life, and it was noted that he had attempted to harm himself in the past. Two weeks after admission there was no significant improvement in his symptoms. Mr MA is a non-smoker and takes no other medications. He has lost some weight but remains still mildly obese with a body mass index of 32 kg/m².

Question

What treatment options would you consider for Mr MA?

Answer

Mr MA demonstrates symptoms of severe depression with some risk factors, and ECT may be considered an early intervention pending review of antidepressant treatment. Mr MA must give his consent to this treatment because he is an informal patient and retains capacity to make treatment decisions.

Before considering a change in antidepressant treatment, previous adherence should be checked. Review of the medicine charts and discussion with nursing staff, relatives, key workers and the patient should enable a reasonable judgement to be reached. A dose increase is unlikely to be helpful unless the patient is a fast metaboliser or smoker because SSRIs have a flat dose–response curve. In this case, the patient had taken the majority of prescribed doses, is a non-smoker, and having received no apparent benefit, a change in treatment is warranted.

An in-depth review of his physical condition and previous medication should be undertaken. This should include discussion about any previous antidepressant treatment found to be particularly effective, or troublesome.

This review revealed that Mr MA had received several different antidepressants over the past 20 years. Three years ago he was treated with venlafaxine modified release 75 mg twice daily. The medical records confirmed Mr MA's view that this medication had helped him in the past, but on further questioning he stated that he had not taken medication for long after discharge from hospital because he did not want to get 'hooked' on it.

The importance of long-term treatment and the proposed treatment plan should be discussed with Mr MA. Particular issues to be addressed include an assessment of physical health including baseline blood pressure and the need for ongoing periodic monitoring. In view of Mr MA's concerns about dependence, particular attention should be given to discussion around 'antidepressant addiction'. Based on Mr MA's agreement to the treatment plan, his previous response, the lack of any physical contraindication and the ability to organise ongoing, periodic blood pressure monitoring, venlafaxine would be an appropriate treatment option.

Case 29.4

Ms YS is a 28-year-old student with a history of bipolar disorder. She recently moved to the area in the hope of continuing her studies. She was urgently assessed at the request of her key worker, who reported that Ms YS had recently become increasingly elated and her partner was very concerned about the increased credit card bills she was incurring. In the past Ms YS had been prescribed lithium but had refused to continue with it because of significant weight gain. She had been switched to valproate. Prescribed medication was valproate semisodium 1500 mg daily. However, Ms YS had become aware that this agent was very toxic in pregnancy. Being keen to start a family with her partner, Ms YS had stopped taking this treatment.

Question

Describe the treatment options available for Ms YS.

Answer

Cautions around the use of valproate in pregnancy have recently been strengthened in national guidance (NICE, 2016). However, in any perinatal mental health situation the wellness of the mother and the treatment(s) needed must be balanced against individualised risks of effective treatment. The fetal malformation risk of valproate use in pregnancy is dose dependent and non-linear (Eadie, 2016). Valproate semisodium at a dose of 1500 mg daily has a risk of around 18%. The risk is fetal malformation. At higher valproate doses of around 2000 mg/day the incidence of spina bifida is increased. The risk to Ms YS could be reduced by identifying a lower effective dose; for example, at 1000 mg daily the risk is around 10%.

Alternative agents for managing manic episodes include lithium, carbamazepine and antipsychotics. Carbamazepine is inherently less teratogenic, and at a dosage of 1000 mg daily fetal malformation risk is around 8%. However, because Ms YS has not previously been prescribed this drug its effectiveness for her bipolar management is unknown.

For both carbamazepine and valproate, supplementary high-dose folate (5 mg folic acid daily) might help mitigate some of the risk to the developing foetus including development of neural tube defect, but the protective effect of folate has recently been questioned if used pre-conception (Eadie, 2016).

Lithium, outside of first-trimester use, where there is a risk of around 1 in 1000 of causing a heart defect (Ebstein's anomaly), is now considered a suitable option with careful medicines management. Ms YS stopped treatment because of weight gain, not because of lack of efficacy, and her priorities may now be different. As part of pregnancy planning lithium is sometimes stopped during a low-risk period of relapse and this is timed to coincide with first trimester. For Ms YS and her hypomanic state, re-establishing lithium may take too long.

Second-generation antipsychotics with a license for use in and prevention of further manic episodes remain another option. There is no one particular agent to recommend and in line with the US Food and Drug Administration category C classification, benefits are considered to outweigh risks when used in pregnancy. If this option is selected, then choice of agent is best determined by consideration of other properties of each agent. Drugs that may be considered include aripiprazole, olanzapine and risperidone.

Benzodiazepines may also be considered as a short-term adjunct if additional sedation is required.

Case 29.5

Ms AB is a 55-year-old unemployed lady with a long-standing history of depression. She has been treated with several antidepressants over the years and is currently under the care of the community mental health team. The only treatment that appears to have had any effect on her depressive episodes has been dosulepin. She has taken several overdoses in the past, and her psychiatrist is reluctant to prescribe this drug.

Question

What measures could be taken to enable Ms AB to be treated effectively?

Answer

Ms AB does not have treatment-resistant depression. She has been successfully treated with dosulepin in the past, but seemingly impulsively takes an overdose from time to time. This case requires management of the overdose risk and exploring any triggers that prompt such action, or moving to an alternative untried regimen which carries a lower toxicity profile.

Although current guidelines (NICE, 2009a, 2009b) now advocate that no new patients should be commenced on dosulepin, this is not the same as switching patients for whom the drug is effective to an alternative agent.

If Ms AB is going to continue to take dosulepin, then practical measures for controlling the quantities of medication should be introduced. This could be ensuring she receives sufficient medication for only a few days' treatment at a time. An instalment dispensing arrangement requires good communication among all those involved in her care. When individualising the supply of medication in this way, all of those involved must be alert to the possibility that the system of supply may break down. In this case, an apparently routine prescription for 1 month's supply of medication may have fatal consequences.

References

American Psychiatric Association, 2013. Diagnostic and Statistical Manual of Mental Disorders, fifth ed. American Psychiatric Publishing Inc., Washington, DC.

Cleare, A., Pariante, C.M., Young, A.H., et al., 2015. Evidence-based guidelines for treating depressive disorders with antidepressants: a revision of the 2008 British Association for Psychopharmacology guidelines. J. Psychopharmacol. 29 (5), 459–525.

Eadie, M.J., 2016. Antiepileptic drug safety in pregnancy. Clin. Pharm. 8 (1), 24–31.

Linde, K., Berner, M.M., Kriston, L., 2008. St John's wort for major depression. Cochrane Database Syst. Rev. 2008 (4), CD000448. https://doi.org/10.1002/14651858.CD000448.pub3.

Malhi, G., Tanious, M., Das, P., et al., 2013. Potential mechanisms of action of lithium in bipolar disorder. Current understanding. CNS Drugs 27 (2), 135–153.

Merikangas, K.R., Jin, R., Jian-Ping, H., et al., 2011. Prevalence and correlates of bipolar spectrum disorder in the. World Mental Health Survey Initiative. Arch. Gen. Psychiatry 68 (3), 241–251.

Muhleisen, T.W., Leber, M., Schulze, T.G., et al., 2014. Genome wide association study reveals two new risk loci for bipolar disorder. Nat. Commun. 5, 3339. https://doi.org/10.1038/ncomms4339. Available at: http://www.nature.com/ncomms/2014/140311/ncomms4339/full/ncomms4339.html.

National Institute for Health and Care Excellence (NICE), 2009a. Depression. The treatment and management of depression in adults. Clinical Guidelines 90. NICE, London. Available at: http://www.nice.org.uk/guidance/CG90.

National Institute for Health and Care Excellence (NICE), 2009b. Depression. The treatment and management of depression in adults. Clinical Guidelines 91. NICE, London. Available at: http://www.nice.org.uk/guidance/CG91.

National Institute for Health and Care Excellence (NICE), 2014. Bipolar disorder. The management of bipolar disorder in adults, children and adolescents in primary and secondary care. Clinical Guideline 185. NICE, London. Available at: https://www.nice.org.uk/guidance/cg185.

National Institute for Health and Care Excellence (NICE), 2015. Vortioxetine for treating major depressive episodes. Technology appraisal guidance TA 367. NICE, London. Available at: https://www.nice.org.uk/guidance/ta367.

National Institute for Health and Care Excellence (NICE), 2016. Bipolar disorder: assessment and management: update to CG 185. Supporting toolkit on the risks of valproate medicines in female patients. Available at: http://www.medicines.org.uk/emc/RMM.421.pdf.

National Patient Safety Agency, 2009. Safer lithium therapy. Available at: http://www.nrls.npsa.nhs.uk/EasySiteWeb/getresorce.axd?AssetID=65428&.

Preda, A., 2012. Substance induced mood disorder. Available at: http://www.nrls.npsa.nhs.uk/EasySiteWeb/getresource.axd?AssetID=65428&....

Sullivan, P.F., Neale, M.C., Kendler, K.S., 2000. Genetic epidemiology of major depression: review and meta-analysis Am. J. Psychiatry 157 (10), 1552–1562.

World Health Organization (WHO), 1992. International Classification of Diseases and related health problems, 10th Revision (ICD 10). World Health Organization, Geneva.

Further reading

Bazire, S., 2016. Psychotropic Drug Directory 2016. Lloyd-Reinhold Communications, Cheltenham, UK.

Cipriani, A., Furukawa, T.A., Salanti, G., et al., 2009. Comparative efficacy and acceptability of 12 new-generation antidepressants: a multiple-treatments meta-analysis. Lancet 373, 746–758.

Cipriani, A., Pretty, H., Hawton, K., et al., 2005. Lithium in the prevention of suicidal behaviour and all-cause mortality in patients with mood disorders: a systematic review of randomised trials. Am. J. Psychiatry 162, 1805–1819.

Fournier, J., DeRubeis, R.J., Hollon, S., et al., 2010. Antidepressant drug effects and depression severity: a patient-level meta-analysis. J. Am. Med. Assoc. 303, 47–53.

Geddes, J.R., Burgess, S., Hawton, K., et al., 2004. Long-term lithium therapy for bipolar disorder: systematic review and meta-analysis of randomized controlled trials. Am. J. Psychiatry 161, 217–222.

Gelder, M., Andreasen, N., Lopez-Ibor, J., et al., 2012. New Oxford Textbook of Psychiatry, second ed. Oxford University Press, Oxford.

Goodwin, G., 2009. Evidence-based guidelines for treating bipolar disorder: revised second edition – recommendations from the British Association for Psychopharmacology. J. Psychopharmacol. 23, 346–388.

Halverson, J.L., 2016. Depression clinical presentation. Available at: http://emedicine.medscape.com/article/286759-clinical.

Kasper, S., Hamon, M., 2009. Beyond the monoaminergic hypothesis: agomelatine, a new antidepressant with an innovative mechanism of action. World J. Biol. Psychiatry 10, 117–126.

Shiloh, R., Stryjer, R., Weizman, A., et al., 2006. Atlas of Psychiatric Pharmacotherapy, second ed. Informa Healthcare, Abingdon, UK.

Taylor, D., Paton, C., Kapur, S., 2015. The Maudsley Prescribing Guidelines in Psychiatry, twelfth ed. Wiley-Blackwell, Oxford.

Walden, J., Heinz, G. (Eds.), 2014. Bipolar Affective Disorders: Etiology and Treatment. Thieme Publishing Group, Stuttgart.

Useful website

Choice and Medication: http://www.choiceandmedication.org/cms/subscribers/?lang=en

30 Schizophrenia

Caroline Parker

Key points

- Schizophrenia is a complex chronic illness which varies greatly in presentation (positive and negative symptoms).
- Positive symptoms such as hallucinations, delusions and thought disorder, which commonly occur in the acute phase of the illness, usually respond to treatment with antipsychotics.
- Negative symptoms such as apathy, social withdrawal and lack of drive, which occur commonly in the chronic phase of the illness, are more resistant to medication.
- The term 'atypical' or 'second generation' is used to describe the newer antipsychotics that generally do not cause the extra-pyramidal side effects (EPSE) or hyperprolactinaemia.
- However, the second generation antipsychotics are associated with a range of metabolic side effects including weight gain and diabetes, which in turn may have long-term effects on morbidity and mortality.
- The older 'typical' or 'first generation' antipsychotics are often associated with anticholinergic, sedative and cardiovascular side effects, in addition to EPSE.
- Long-term treatment with first generation antipsychotics is associated with the development of the movement disorder tardive dyskinesia.
- Most first generation and second generation antipsychotics have similar efficacy in the treatment of schizophrenia. The exception is clozapine, which has greater efficacy than all other antipsychotics and is therefore indicated for treatment-resistant schizophrenia. Its use is hampered by the mandatory requirement for regular full blood count checkups.
- Decisions about which antipsychotic to use should be a shared decision between patient and the prescriber, based on an informed discussion involving individual preference, previous efficacy of medication and potential side effects.

The concept of schizophrenia can be difficult to understand. People who do not suffer from schizophrenia can have little idea of what the experience of hallucinations and delusions is like. The presentation of schizophrenia can be extremely varied, with a great range of possible symptoms. It is a chronic disorder with a lifetime prevalence of 1 in 100 people. There are also many misconceptions about the condition of schizophrenia that have led to prejudice against sufferers of the illness. People with schizophrenia are commonly thought to have low intelligence and to be dangerous. In fact, only a minority shows violent behaviour, with social withdrawal being a more common picture. Up to 10% of people with schizophrenia commit suicide.

Classification

Since the late 19th century there have been frequent attempts to define the illness we now call schizophrenia. Kraepelin, in the late 1890s, coined the term 'dementia praecox' (early madness) to describe an illness where there was a deterioration of the personality at a young age. Kraepelin also coined the terms 'catatonic' (where motor symptoms are prevalent and changes in activity vary), 'hebephrenic' (silly, childish behaviour, affective symptoms and thought disorder prominence) and 'paranoid' (clinical picture dominated by paranoid delusions). A few years later Bleuler, a Swiss psychiatrist, introduced the term 'schizophrenia', derived from the Greek words *skhizo* ('to split') and *phren* ('mind'), meaning the split between the emotions and the intellect.

Two systems for the classification of schizophrenia are widely used: *Diagnostic and Statistical Manual of Mental Disorders*, Fifth Edition (DSM 5) (American Psychiatric Association, 2013) and the *International Classification of Diseases and Related Health Problems*, 10th Edition (ICD 10) (World Health Organization, 1992).

Symptoms and diagnosis

Schizophrenia is a chronic illness; the exact nature of the symptoms varies greatly in presentation between individuals. It comprises 'positive' and 'negative' symptoms. Positive symptoms include hallucinations (these may be auditory, visual or visceral), delusions, thought disorder (including thought insertion or deletion), paranoia, and grandiosity. Negative symptoms include apathy, social withdrawal and lack of drive and interest.

The intensity of an individual's positive and negative symptoms may vary over time. As with most chronic illness, a person with schizophrenia may always have some of these symptoms to some degree, but during an acute relapse they will be worse, and it is usually the positive symptoms that are more obvious to other people and may be problematic. During periods of remission between acute episodes, it is often the negative symptoms that are more problematic, and these are generally less responsive to treatment with antipsychotics.

Acute psychotic illness

An acute psychotic episode may occur in a number of disease states and for a range of reasons, and a single psychotic episode

Some mimic the impact of clozapine on a wide range of dopamine and serotonin receptors (e.g. olanzapine), some mimic the impact on particular receptors (e.g. $5\text{-HT}_2/\text{D}_2$ receptor antagonists such as risperidone), others focus on limited occupancy of D_2 receptors (e.g. quetiapine), and still others focus on alternative theories such as partial agonism (e.g. aripiprazole).

Selecting an antipsychotic and dose

Despite a wide selection of antipsychotics with different chemical structures, different suggested variation in mechanisms of action and different safety profiles, a number of studies and meta-analyses in recent years have demonstrated that all antipsychotics are of similar efficacy for the treatment of positive symptoms of schizophrenia, with the exception of clozapine which has superior efficacy, being effective for people with schizophrenia who did not successfully respond to treatment with other antipsychotics (Kane et al., 1988; Lieberman et al., 1994). There is no clear advantage of a second generation antipsychotic over a first generation antipsychotic (Hartling et al., 2012; Jones et al., 2006; Leucht et al., 2009, 2013; Lieberman et al., 2005; Stroup et al., 2007). They do, however, vary significantly in terms of potential side effects.

The choice of antipsychotic should always be informed by a patient's previous response to treatment, past experiences, including side effects, and preference, as well as any concurrent medical comorbidity and medication (National Institute for Health and Care Excellence [NICE], 2014).

Side effects

A large number of adverse effects are associated with antipsychotic medicines. In general the frequent or troublesome side effects of the older first generation antipsychotics include EPSE, tardive dyskinesia (TD), anticholinergic effects, cardiac effects and hypotension, hyperprolactinaemia and sexual dysfunction. In contrast, in general the frequent or troublesome side effects of the newer second generation antipsychotics, including metabolic changes such as diabetes, weight gain and sexual dysfunction, can affect adherence in many patients. Sedation remains a factor for many antipsychotics.

Beyond these generalisations there is great variation in side effects with each antipsychotic. Some effects, such as sedation and weight gain, may be beneficial for particular patients, but not for others. The susceptibility of individual patients to such adverse effects can vary significantly and is often a major factor in determining the choice of antipsychotic. When deciding on the most suitable antipsychotic for an individual patient, the relative potential of the individual antipsychotics to cause specific side effects such as EPSE, akathisia, metabolic side effects, weight gain and other unpleasant subjective experiences should be considered (NICE, 2014).

Extensive prescribing guidelines are available (Barnes et al., 2011; Bazire, 2016; Procyshyn et al., 2015; Taylor et al., 2015) providing detailed comparisons of the relative likelihood of side effects with the various antipsychotics. The major side effects are set out below.

Sedation. Of the commonly used antipsychotics, sedation is most prominent with olanzapine and clozapine, even when used at moderate doses. However, it is seen to a lesser extent with many other antipsychotics. Patients may become accustomed to the sedation after the initial period (i.e. the first few weeks of treatment), although for some individuals it may make that particular antipsychotic an unfeasible maintenance option.

Weight gain and diabetes. Weight gain was a common feature with the first generation phenothiazine antipsychotics, but is now seen to a greater extent with certain second generation antipsychotics, particularly olanzapine and clozapine. Weight gain is generally related to increased food intake driven by increased appetite and lack of satiation. In addition to weight gain, these two second generation antipsychotics have also been associated with increased incidence of diabetes and hyperlipidaemia. This is seen with some other second generation antipsychotics (e.g. quetiapine), but to a much lesser extent.

Schizophrenia itself is associated with increased incidence of diabetes and cardiovascular disease; therefore, any additional effect from an antipsychotic on increasing weight gain, lipids and adversely affecting glucose control is a significant concern. People with schizophrenia often suffer poorer physical health in addition to poor mental health and require regular and often proactive monitoring of physical health risk factors.

Cardiac side effects and QT prolongation. Postural hypotension may be relatively common with a number of antipsychotics. This is part of the rationale for slow-dose titrations when initiating treatment (e.g. olanzapine, risperidone, quetiapine, clozapine, chlorpromazine).

Some antipsychotics, particularly haloperidol, are associated with changes to the QTc interval measured on the electrocardiogram (ECG) and, if given in high doses, may increase the risk of sudden cardiac death. Although overall the risk is very low, monitoring the ECG has become part of normal practice. Maximum licensed doses should not be exceeded.

Extrapyramidal side effects and tardive dyskinesia. The EPSE such as akathisia, dystonia and parkinsonian symptoms are frequently associated with first generation antipsychotics, particularly trifluoperazine, fluphenazine and haloperidol (see Box 30.1). They are also seen with certain second generation antipsychotics, especially at higher doses (e.g. risperidone, amisulpride). These side effects can be managed by dosage reduction or by giving anticholinergics such as procyclidine or orphenadrine.

Attempts to treat TD have been many and varied. These strategies are rarely successful and the focus should be on avoiding development rather than treatment. Currently, the most successful strategies involve a gradual withdrawal of the causal first generation antipsychotic and replacement with a second generation antipsychotic.

Anticholinergics may be prescribed to counter the EPSE of antipsychotics. A number of studies have investigated the discontinuation of anticholinergic agents and reported re-emergence of the EPSE. The anticholinergics are not without problems, having their own range of side effects including dry mouth, constipation and blurred vision. They can cause euphoria and, therefore,

Box 30.1   Movement disorders associated with antipsychotics

Extrapyramidal symptoms consist of:

- *Parkinsonian symptoms* (usually present as tremor, rigidity, bradykinesia, stooping gait and poverty of facial expression): may appear gradually. These may remit if the antipsychotic is withdrawn and may be suppressed by the administration of anticholinergics; however, routine co-administration of anticholinergics is not justified because not all patients are affected. Anticholinergics are also associated with adverse effects and may unmask or worsen *tardive dyskinesia*.
- *Acute dystonic reactions* (abnormal face and body movements as a result of sustained muscle contraction) and *dyskinesia*: occurs more commonly in children or young adults and may appear after only a few doses. These are acute and painful and need immediate treatment with an anticholinergic, often in the parenteral form.
- *Akathisia* (inner restlessness): patients may pace up and down, constantly shifting their leg position or tapping their feet.
- *Tardive dyskinesia* (rhythmic, involuntary movements that usually affect the tongue, face, neck and jaw muscles, but can also affect extremities): usually develops after long-term use of antipsychotics or with high doses. It is of particular concern because it may be irreversible and there is no effective treatment. Withdrawal of the causal antipsychotic at the earliest signs may halt its full development.

have the potential for misuse. Withdrawal problems can include cholinergic rebound. One of the benefits of most second generation antipsychotics is the reduced need for co-prescription of anticholinergics.

Hormonal effects and sexual dysfunction. The side effects of hormonal effects and sexual dysfunction are primarily influenced by the effect of antipsychotics on inhibiting prolactin regulation leading to hyperprolactinaemia. This may become symptomatic; symptoms include amenorrhoea, galactorrhoea, gynaecomastia and loss of libido. Such effects are relatively common with the older first generation antipsychotics, as well as with certain second generation antipsychotics such as risperidone, paliperidone and amisulpride.

Neuroleptic malignant syndrome. The neuroleptic malignant syndrome is a rare but serious idiosyncratic adverse effect that can occur with any antipsychotic and with a few other related medicines (e.g. metoclopramide). The primary symptoms are related to loss of autonomic control (e.g. rigidity, fever, diaphoresis, confusion and fluctuating consciousness). There may also be a significant rise in creatinine kinase, although this is not a specific diagnostic indicator. Although unpredictable, the onset is particularly associated with the use of high-potency first generation antipsychotics such as haloperidol, recent and rapid-dose increases, and abrupt withdrawal of anticholinergics. Treatment usually requires urgent admission to a medical ward and immediate withdrawal of all antipsychotics.

Clozapine and refractory illness

Clozapine was developed as an antipsychotic during the 1960s. Unfortunately, it was associated with a 1–2% incidence rate of neutropenia, and this initially resulted in its withdrawal.

However, it was noted even at an early stage in trials that it was completely free from causing the debilitating extrapyramidal symptoms frequently seen with all the other existing antipsychotics. In the 1980s, clozapine was demonstrated to have a greater efficacy than other antipsychotics because it was effective for some patients for whom other antipsychotics had failed (Kane et al., 1988; Lieberman et al., 1994). It was subsequently reintroduced into clinical practice but with mandatory routine blood monitoring.

Clozapine is now established as the antipsychotic of choice in treatment-resistant schizophrenia (NICE, 2014), but it is not without problems (Bleakley and Taylor, 2013). Treatment-resistant schizophrenia is generally defined as a failure to respond to two antipsychotics used (in succession) at therapeutic doses for a reasonable period of time. The use of clozapine should not be delayed or viewed as a treatment option of 'last resort'. The earlier it is used the better is the patient's prognosis.

In addition to neutropenia, clozapine is associated with a greater risk of seizures, particularly at higher dosages (>600 mg daily); therefore, careful dose titration is required, as well as regular adherence to the daily doses. Other problematic side effects include initial hypotension and sedation. Later, significant weight gain, mediated through increased food intake driven by food craving, disturbed glucose control, and potentially the development of diabetes and excessive drooling can also present.

A regimen of gradual dose titration starting at 12.5 mg twice daily aiming to reach 300 mg in 2–3 weeks is normally recommended. If the titration is too rapid, tachycardia, sedation and seizures may be problems. Although tachycardia is a common and usually benign problem during the initiation, if it is associated with fever, chest pain or hypotension this may indicate a high risk of myocarditis, and clozapine should be stopped (Bleakley and Taylor, 2013).

When treatment with clozapine is perceived to be inadequate, or dose optimisation is limited due to side effects, the treatment plan can become complex. The theory behind the addition of a further medication is either to enhance the plasma concentration of clozapine, or for the second medication to enhance a particular receptor blockade which may be considered necessary in a specific patient (Barber et al., 2017; Paton et al., 2007). The augmentation strategy with the best evidence to support its use is the addition of sulpiride or amisulpride to clozapine. Other strategies include the addition of risperidone, lamotrigine or omega-3 fatty acids. However, many of the trials that support these augmentation strategies are small scale. A meta-analysis concluded that no single strategy was superior to another (Paton et al., 2007).

Using antipsychotics

As a general rule, a patient should be prescribed only one antipsychotic at a time. Exceptions would include the short periods of time when changing from one antipsychotic to another, because an antipsychotic should not be stopped abruptly, and the new one is likely to require titration to a therapeutic dose; therefore, there will often be a period of a few weeks of crossover. Another exception is augmentation of clozapine as described earlier.

If a person is being treated with an antipsychotic and it is not thought to be working sufficiently the following steps are recommended:

- consider the patient's adherence to the prescribed dose;
- optimise the dose;
- review the symptoms and diagnosis in case it has changed;
- consider changing to another antipsychotic;
- consider using clozapine if the patient has not responded successfully to two antipsychotics.

Prescribers should not keep increasing the dose of the existing antipsychotic beyond the BNF maximum or simply add a second antipsychotic for use alongside the first.

Maximum and equivalent doses

The consensus is that higher than licensed doses of antipsychotics do not improve the overall level of response which tends to plateau. Higher doses only increase the number and severity of side effects, because many are dose related; therefore, both acute and longer-term risks are increased (Royal College of Psychiatrists, 2014).

If more than one antipsychotic is used regularly, then prescribers should consider the total cumulative daily dose of antipsychotics and the BNF maximum should not be exceeded.

Antipsychotics vary in potency of D_2 receptor activity. However, this is known to be only part of the explanation for their efficacy. There is no definitive list of equivalent doses in terms of efficacy, but in terms of safety a standardised concept has been developed for calculating maximum doses. This widely accepted method is to calculate what proportion the current dose is of the maximum dose stated in the BNF. For example, a daily dose of 15 mg of olanzapine is 75% of the maximum dose of 20 mg a day. This method is not without its drawbacks because it generally reflects the maximum doses manufacturers used in trials, but not all manufacturers conducted dose ranging trials to establish the maximum beneficial dose.

Onset of effect

The full antipsychotic effect is not evident immediately. For the more sedating antipsychotics the sedating effects may be evident within hours and generally wears off after 2–3 weeks (Kapur et al., 2005). The actual antipsychotic effects on thought disorder, hallucinations and delusions may begin to be noticed within a week, but it may take several more weeks for full effects to be seen. If there has been no response at all within 2–3 weeks of adherence, then a change of antipsychotic or change of dose is probably indicated.

Long-acting formulations of antipsychotics

Oral antipsychotic medication should be offered to people with newly diagnosed schizophrenia. There may be circumstances where oral formulations of antipsychotics may not be suitable for an individual patient, for example, for those who struggle to remember to take medicines regularly and for those with swallowing problems. For such patients a 'depot' intramuscular formulation may be an alternative strategy for maintenance treatment (Fig. 30.2). Some patients also prefer to have a depot because this avoids the daily routine of taking oral medicines. Non-adherence with oral medicines is a major problem in patients with any long-term illness, and the administration of a depot formulation guarantees drug delivery.

Antipsychotics have been available in depot formulations since the 1960s; there are now a number available and they are widely used. Despite this increasing range of options in terms of treatment efficacy and overall adverse effects, there is minimal discernable difference between the depot formulations; however, there are notable practical differences (Shajahan et al., 2010).

Disadvantages of depots include reduced flexibility of dosage because it may be necessary to wait a few weeks until the next dose is due before any dose amendment can be made. Other disadvantages are the potentially painful nature of intramuscular injections and, for some antipsychotics, a high incidence of EPSE. In addition, risperidone long-acting injection has a considerable delay in onset, because there is no release of the active drug from the microsphere formulation until 3 weeks after injection. The olanzapine depot is associated with a post-injection syndrome consistent with olanzapine overdose; there is a requirement for patients to be observed for 3 hours after every injection.

Most long-acting (depot) formulations are esters which are lipophilic and soluble. These are dissolved in an oily vehicle such as sesame oil or a thin vegetable oil (Viscoleo). Once injected into muscle it is slowly released from the oil vehicle. Active drug becomes available following hydrolysis for distribution to the site of the action.

Although the ideal long-acting antipsychotic formulation should release the drug at a constant rate so that plasma level fluctuations are kept to a minimum, all of the available products produce significant variations. This can result in increased side effects at the time of peak plasma concentrations, usually after 5–7 days for oil-based depots after which plasma concentrations decline.

Four first generation and four second generation antipsychotics are currently licensed in the UK as long-acting depot formulations for intramuscular injection. The first generation depots are oily injections given every 1–5 weeks; the second generation depots (or long-acting injections) are aqueous suspensions, given every 2–4 weeks (Table 30.1).

Interactions and antipsychotics

There are claimed to be many interactions involving antipsychotics, but few appear to be clinically significant. Carbamazepine accelerates the metabolism of haloperidol, risperidone and olanzapine, and should not be used with clozapine because of the additional risk of neutropenia. Most antipsychotics increase the sedative effect of alcohol. The selective serotonin reuptake inhibitors fluoxetine, paroxetine and fluvoxamine interact with clozapine, resulting in increases in clozapine plasma concentration. Smoking tobacco increases the rate of metabolism of

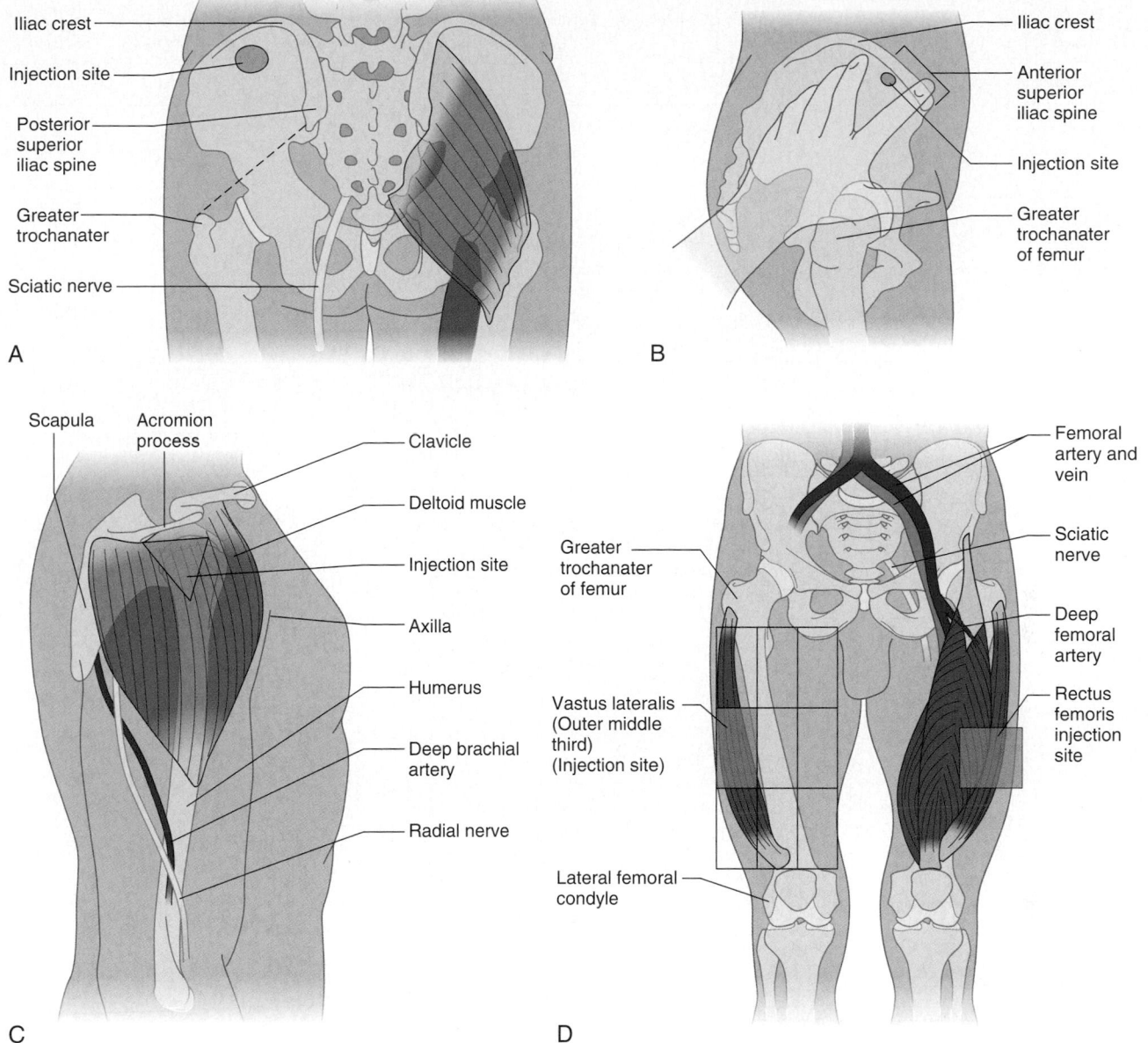

Fig. 30.2 Location of intramuscular injection site (deltoid and gluteal). A and B are both gluteal injection sites, viewed from different angles. C is a deltoid injection site. D is vastus lateralis and rectus femoris injection sites.

olanzapine and clozapine, and regular doses may need to be reduced if a person stops smoking. Clozapine levels should also be checked if a patient changes his or her smoking habits.

Therapeutic drug monitoring

Therapeutic drug monitoring is only of value if there is a reliable laboratory assay and a correlation exists between the concentration of the drug in any particular body compartment, usually blood/plasma, and its clinical effectiveness. Unfortunately, this is not the case for most antipsychotics, and the measurement of drug concentrations is not a part of routine clinical practice except with clozapine, although even with clozapine there is only a weak correlation between plasma levels and clinical effect. The general guidance is that individuals who have not adequately responded to clozapine and have a plasma level less than 350–500 micrograms/L may benefit from a dose increase. Those who suffer side effects and have a plasma level above this range may benefit from a dose reduction. Those with a plasma level greater than 1000 micrograms/L are more likely to suffer seizures, and antiepileptic cover using sodium valproate should be considered.

Table 30.1 Depot antipsychotics available in the UK

Trade name	Generic name	Formulation and vehicle	Administration (intramuscular) and comments	Time to peak (days)	Half-life (days)	Available since
First generation						
Clopixol	Zuclopenthixol decanoate	Thin vegetable oil	Upper outer buttock (gluteal) or upper lateral thigh, every 1–4 weeks	4–7	19	1978
Depixol	Flupentixol decanoate	Thin vegetable oil	Upper outer buttock (gluteal) or upper lateral thigh, every 1–4 weeks	7	17	1972
Haldol	Haloperidol decanoate	Sesame oil	Gluteal, every 4 weeks	3–9	21	1982
Modecate	Fluphenazine decanoate	Sesame oil	Gluteal, every 2–5 weeks	0.3–1.5	6–9	1968
Second generation						
Risperdal Consta	Risperidone	Powder for reconstitution with aqueous solution in a prefilled syringe, forms a suspension	Gluteal or deltoid, every 2 weeks Requires refrigeration	32	8–9	2002
Abilify Maintena	Aripiprazole	Prefilled syringe of aqueous prolonged-release suspension	Gluteal or deltoid, every month	7 after gluteal, and 4 after deltoid administration	47	2015
Xeplion	Paliperidone palmitate	Prefilled syringe of aqueous prolonged-release suspension	Gluteal or deltoid, every month (no refrigeration), active metabolite of risperidone	13	25–49	2011
ZypAdhera	Olanzapine pamoate	Powder for reconstitution with aqueous fluid, forms a suspension	Gluteal, every 2 or 4 weeks Observe patient carefully for symptoms of post-injection syndrome for 3 h after each dose	3	10	2010

Case studies

Case 30.1

Mr LT is a 20-year-old man. His childhood was disrupted by constant changes to family membership. From an early age his behaviour was difficult, but despite such changes at school he coped and performed academically well. At age 15 he started using cannabis and increasingly lost interest in his studies at school. His parents became concerned as he appeared to undergo a change of personality, communicating with them very little. He eventually dropped out of school and briefly took various short-term jobs. He was unable to sustain any long-term employment. When he was 17 he moved into a flat and seemed to live a twilight existence involving illicit drugs and all-night raves. Police were called to his flat after a violent disturbance. They found Mr LT living in squalor. He was surrounded by pieces of paper containing incomprehensible messages and was incoherent. He sat with a fixed stare, appearing quite inaccessible. He kept laughing and responding to imaginary people. He was very resistant to hospital admission, and had to be admitted under a section of the Mental Health Act 1983. On the ward he has remained quiet but appears to be in conversation with people who are not there.

....

Questions

1. Outline the medicine(s) of choice for Mr LT and the rationale for your selection.
2. What factors in his presentation are likely to influence his prognosis?

3. Outline the medicine(s) of choice if there is a short-term, immediate need to control aggressive behaviour.

Answers

1. The choice of medicine used (or not) will be influenced by the working diagnosis. So the first need is to ascertain whether Mr LT's behaviour results from abuse of cannabis and other illicit substances, or whether it is the onset of a psychotic illness such as schizophrenia. If the former, he would be expected to recover within a few days with little or no medication. If, however, this is the first presentation of a schizophrenic illness, the symptoms are likely to persist and it would be appropriate to prescribe an antipsychotic. For first episode psychosis an oral antipsychotic should be offered. The exact choice will partly depend on which is tolerable to the patient, the likelihood of certain side effects, the patient's age (there are additional considerations if the patient is aged <18 years) and the balance and risk of side effects. It would usually be a second generation antipsychotic such as aripiprazole or risperidone. Olanzapine may not be such a suitable choice because of the high likelihood of significant weight gain and metabolic symptoms. If there are concerns that he may not swallow the medications, then an orodispersible formulation may be useful. These formulations are available for aripiprazole and risperidone and some other medicines.

2. A number of factors in Mr LT's history indicate a poor prognosis:
   - there has been a deterioration in his overall functioning;
   - his age (quite young), which is typical for a first breakdown;
   - his poor work record;
   - his substance misuse history;
   - his grossly disorganised behaviour;
   - a number of positive symptoms such as hallucinations.

3. If whilst in hospital Mr LT becomes acutely aggressive because of the psychosis, other medicines may be needed in addition to the prescribed regular antipsychotic, to control his aggression to protect both him and other people. A decision would have to be made about whether to use antipsychotics or benzodiazepines in the short-term. This decision is separate from the longer-term treatment plan. Each hospital should have their own protocol for the management of such emergencies. The NICE guidelines on the management of violence (NICE, 2015) recommend that if a person will not take oral medicines, then use lorazepam injection or haloperidol plus promethazine injections (at the same time).

Case 30.2

Mr GL, aged 32 years, has relapsed for the third time this year. The pattern for the last two psychotic relapses is the same as this presentation, and both required brief admissions. On both previous occasions his positive symptoms responded rapidly to antipsychotics. The first antipsychotic, risperidone, was titrated up to 8 mg/day and he suffered distressing EPSE. This was subsequently changed to olanzapine, and he was stabilised and discharged on a dosage of 15 mg daily. However, he stopped taking this within a couple of weeks of discharge, claiming not to be ill and having gained notable weight. During his second relapse and admission he was successfully treated with amisulpride 400 mg twice daily but again stopped taking it soon after discharge.

Questions

1. Was Mr GL's medication treatment appropriate?
2. What strategies could be adopted to maintain Mr GL's treatment?

3. What would you recommend if Mr GL relapsed and was admitted again?

Answers

1. Mr GL has been treated with three oral second generation antipsychotics all with good effect. The initial treatment was with a fairly large dose of risperidone (8 mg). If this was his first episode and if he was antipsychotic naive, the dose was titrated straight up to this dose quite quickly, and it may well be considered excessive. The usual treatment dosage is 4–6 mg/day. EPSE are dose related and could be expected at a dosage of 8 mg/day. The second choice of olanzapine, another second generation antipsychotic was appropriate, because this rarely causes EPSE. The third choice of amisulpride was unlikely to cause weight gain (unlike olanzapine) but is quite likely to cause EPSE. Choosing a third oral antipsychotic was not addressing the potential issue of adherence.

2. Mr GL has no insight into his illness or the need for continuing treatment. Repeatedly stopping antipsychotics and having relapses leads to a worse prognosis. Therefore, it is really important to properly address Mr GL's repeated discontinuation of antipsychotic medication, which could be for a number of reasons including:
   - His lack of insight into the nature of his illness, and its need for treatment, is part of the illness itself, and his failure to gain insight is a sign of his incomplete recovery, which in turn drives poor adherence to medicines, and so a poorer response.
   - He needs a more supportive home environment with help to remind, encourage and prompt him to take his antipsychotic medication daily.
   - He is suffering from side effects that deter him from taking the antipsychotic regularly.

   Mr GL's opinion and preferences about medication should be sought, and the next antipsychotic should be selected accordingly. He should also be educated (again) about the need for ongoing treatment, as per any chronic illness.

3. If Mr GL were to relapse again it would be important to establish the reason. Repeated relapses will adversely affect his longer-term prognosis. Therefore, a depot formulation of antipsychotic should be considered. In most cases, the use of a depot antipsychotic injection would be the easiest way to ensure adherence in the short-term although if Mr GL is determined to avoid treatment, then this strategy is unlikely to be successful, because he simply would not attend the appointments for the depot injection. In his case, the response to each antipsychotic bodes well, and he is therefore fairly likely to respond to the next antipsychotic if given as a depot. However, because he has had EPSE with high doses of risperidone this may influence the choice of depot. He should be involved in the decision as to which depot. It could be worth trying a risperidone depot but at a moderate dose (not as high as the oral dosage of 8 mg daily). Alternatively, paliperidone, the active metabolite of risperidone, may be appropriate, although this too can induce EPSE in a dose-related manner. However, the patient may prefer this option because it is a monthly, rather than fortnightly, injection. Alternatively, it may be appropriate to try a first generation antipsychotic with a lower propensity to cause EPSE such as flupenthixol decanoate or zuclopenthixol decanoate. These also have great dose flexibility. Therefore, they could be started very gently at low doses to establish whether they are tolerated, before increasing the dose.

Case 30.3

Ms SW, aged 28 years, has a 5-year history of schizophrenia with many admissions to hospital. Throughout the period of her illness she has received a range of different oral antipsychotics including risperidone, olanzapine, quetiapine, amisulpride, as well as the depot formulations of flupenthixol and zuclopenthixol decanoate. For most of this time she has had fixed beliefs that she is being watched and spied on by gangs of men who want to sexually assault her when she is asleep and tarnish her name and reputation to everyone she knows. When she is ill these beliefs torment her and she rarely goes out of her flat, preferring to stay hidden at home. Until recently she has been treated with zuclopenthixol decanoate 500 mg by intramuscular injection every week at her home, plus olanzapine 10 mg at night, fluoxetine 20 mg daily, and procyclidine 5 mg three times daily. She was admitted to hospital 3 months ago. There is no sign of improvement in her mental state; however, she has greatly increased in weight, now approaching 127 kg.

Questions

1. Comment on Ms SW's current treatment plan.
2. What would you recommend next?
3. The team wishes to consider clozapine for Ms SW. What should be done before Ms SW can receive clozapine?

Answers

1. Although sometimes polypharmacy (the use of more than one antipsychotic) is used for patients when there has been poor or inadequate response, the practice is not evidence based and is potentially risky. Additional medicines are often added in a crisis or in the hope of achieving a greater degree of response. As in this case, the strategy is often unsuccessful. The particular issues of note with this patient's treatment regimen are:
   - The combination of two antipsychotics exceeds the BNF maximum dose. The maximum dose of zuclopenthixol decanoate depot is 600 mg/week; therefore, 500 mg weekly is 83% of the maximum dose. The maximum dose of olanzapine is 20 mg; therefore, 10 mg is 50% of the maximum dose. 83% + 50% = 133%. Doses greater than 100% confer greater risks for side effects, and the Royal College of Psychiatrists monitoring guidance should be followed. This includes a regular review of the dosage and regular blood tests and ECGs.
   - There is a combination of a first generation (zuclopenthixol decanoate) and a second generation (olanzapine) antipsychotic; this reduces the potential benefit of using a second generation antipsychotic with a very low incidence of EPSE because the patient is still suffering with EPSE to the extent that she requires the anticholinergic, procyclidine.
   - The use of a depot formulation suggests that there has been an issue with poor/incomplete/erratic adherence; however, the concurrent use of oral olanzapine means that she is expected to be adherent with this oral formulation. Therefore, the logic for this combination of formulations needs to be reviewed and her adherence assessed.
   - She is at risk of development of TD by being on an antipsychotic long term that is causing EPSE.
   - This regular dose of the anticholinergic procyclidine is likely to cause its own side effects.
   - The need for such frequent dosing of the intramuscular depot might not be necessary; administration at 2-weekly intervals would normally be appropriate.

- She is suffering severe weight gain. This is more likely to be caused by olanzapine by increasing her appetite, rather than by the zuclopenthixol decanoate.

2. Because Ms SW has not fully responded to (more than) two antipsychotics taken at proper therapeutic doses for reasonable periods of time, she meets the definition of treatment-resistant schizophrenia. Trying yet further alternative antipsychotics is not likely to be any more successful than the current treatment regimen, and clozapine is therefore indicated.

3. The preparation for starting treatment with clozapine involves a number of steps. These include:
   - First, discussing the potential treatment plan with Ms SW. This includes explaining that it is indicated for treatment-resistant schizophrenia and is more likely to be effective than any other antipsychotic. The need to have regular mandatory blood tests, initially weekly, to assess the full blood counts to monitor for any signs of neutropenia must be clearly explained.
   - We would need to consider that until now the use of a depot formulation has been considered necessary. Presumably she has had a history of problems with adherence to oral antipsychotics (this would be the indication for choosing a depot). Therefore, because clozapine is available only as an oral formulation, the team would need to review whether anything would now need to be put in place to support her long-term adherence with oral clozapine, as regular adherence is particularly important with this option; erratic compliance is particularly risky, increasing the likelihood of hypotension (potentially casing syncope), severe sedation and seizures. This may mean planning for additional services and support for Ms SW when she is discharged from hospital and reviewing her living accommodation arrangement (i.e. whether she has staff living with her or visiting who can support her adherence).
   - Ideally the team would want to get Ms SW's consent to having regular blood tests and starting an oral medicine. However, if she is very unwell she may not currently have capacity to agree to these things. If she does not agree and is detained in hospital under the Mental Health Act 1983, although it is legal to enforce blood tests this can be very traumatic and not favourable for the patient's therapeutic relationship with the care team. In addition it is not practically possible to force a patient to take oral tablets.
   - All patients prescribed clozapine and their consultant psychiatrist and the dispensing pharmacy service must be registered with a clozapine monitoring scheme (i.e. ZTAS [Zaponex Treatment Access System], CPMS [Clozaril Patient Monitoring Service] or DMS [Denzapine Monitoring System]). Only then may the clozapine be legally dispensed.
   - Once registered with a clozapine monitoring scheme and before starting clozapine a baseline full blood count and background checks are required to ensure that the patient is not already suffering from neutropenia or another blood disorder. Once these have been checked, clozapine can be prescribed.
   - The Summary of Product Characteristics for clozapine says that depot antipsychotics are contraindicated with it because of the small risk of neutropenia. This is compounded by the nature of the formulation, meaning that the depot antipsychotic remains present in the patient for some time (weeks). Therefore, further doses of this should be stopped before clozapine is started.
   - The prescriber should be aware of the interaction between fluoxetine and clozapine, noting that this causes an increase in clozapine's levels. It may be appropriate to continue the fluoxetine, but the patient may need lower doses of clozapine. Serum levels of clozapine can be checked to optimise the dose and avoid unnecessarily high levels, which are associated with toxicity.

- Once the depot is stopped, which was the cause of the EPSE, then the associated prescription for the anticholinergic procyclidine can also be gradually stopped. This should not be done immediately or abruptly, because the EPSE may continue for some time, and the depot antipsychotic may take weeks to no longer have effects. Furthermore stopping procyclidine abruptly can lead to symptoms of cholinergic rebound. However, the prescribing team should also be aware that clozapine has notable anticholinergic effects, which would be compounded by concurrent procyclidine.

- Ideally all other treatments would be stopped and clozapine prescribed alone. However, sometimes this is simply not practicable, because the patient would then be left untreated whilst the clozapine is titrated, which routinely takes 2–3 weeks. Therefore, the final steps of gradually withdrawing other medicines may occur alongside the gradual initial titration phase with clozapine.

References

American Psychiatric Association, 2013. Diagnostic and Statistical Manual of Mental Disorders, fifth ed. American Psychiatric Association, Washington, DC.

Barber, S., Olotu, U., Corsi, M., et al., 2017. Clozapine combined with different antipyschotic drugs for treatment-resistant schizophrenia. Cochrane Database Syst. Rev. 3, CD006324. https://doi.org/10.1002/14651858.CD006324.pub3.

Barnes, R.E., 2011. Schizophrenia Consensus Group of the British Association for Psychopharmacology, evidence-based guidelines for the pharmacological treatment of schizophrenia: recommendations from the British Association for Psychopharmacology. J. Psychopharmacol. 25 (5), 567–620.

Bazire, S., 2016. Psychotropic Drug Directory: The Professionals' Pocket Handbook and Aide Memoire. Lloyd-Reinhold Publications, Shaftesbury, UK.

Bleakley, S., Taylor, D., 2013. Clozapine handbook. Lloyd-Reinhold Publications, Shaftesbury, UK.

Hartling, L., Abou Setta, A.M., Dursun, S., et al., 2012. Antipsychotics in adults with schizophrenia: comparative effectiveness of first-generation versus second-generation medications. Ann. Intern. Med. 157 (7), 498–511.

Jones, P.B., Barnes, T.R., Davies, L., et al., 2006. Randomised controlled trial of the effect on quality of life of second- vs. first-generation antipsychotic drugs in schizophrenia. Cost utility of the latest antipsychotic drugs in schizophrenia study (CUtLASS-1). Arch. Gen. Psychiatry 63, 1079–1087.

Kane, J., Honigfield, G., Singer, J., Meltzer, H., 1988. Clozapine for the treatment-resistant schizophrenic. A double-blind comparison with chlorpromazine. Arch. Gen. Psychiatry 45, 789–796.

Kapur, S., Arenovich, T., Agid, O., et al., 2005. Evidence for onset of antipsychotic effects within the first 24 hours of treatment. Am. J. Psychiatry 162 (5), 939–946.

Leucht, S., Komossa, K., Rummel-Kluge, C., et al., 2009. A meta-analysis of head-to-head comparisons of second-generation antipsychotics in the treatment of schizophrenia. Am. J. Psychiatry 166, 152–163.

Leucht, S., Cipriani, A., Spineli, L., et al., 2013. Comparative efficacy and tolerability of 15 antipsychotic drugs in schizophrenia: a multiple-treatments metaanalysis. Lancet 382, 951–962.

Lieberman, J.A., Safferman, A.Z., Pollack, S., et al., 1994. Clinical effects of clozapine in chronic schizophrenia: response to treatment and predictors of outcome. Am. J. Psychiatry 15, 1744–1752.

Lieberman, J., Stroup, T.S., McEvoy, J., et al., 2005. Clinical Antipsychotics Trials of Intervention Effectiveness (CATIE) Investigators. Effectiveness of antipsychotic drugs in patients with chronic schizophrenia N. Engl. J. Med. 353 (12), 1209–1223.

National Institute for Health and Care Excellence (NICE), 2014. Clinical guideline: CG178 psychosis and schizophrenia in adults: treatment and management. Available at: https://www.nice.org.uk/guidance/cg178.

National Institute for Health and Care Excellence (NICE), 2015. NICE guidance: NG10. violence and aggression: short-term management in mental health, health and community settings. Available at: https://www.nice.org.uk/guidance/ng10.

Paton, C., Whittington, C., Barnes, T., 2007. Augmentation with a second antipsychotic in patients with schizophrenia who partially respond to clozapine: a meta-analysis. J. Clin. Psychopharmacol. 27, 198–204.

Procyshyn, R.M., Bezchlibnyk-Butler, K.Z., Jeffries, J.J. (Eds.), 2015. Clinical Handbook of Psychotropic Drugs, twenty first ed. Hogrefe Publishing, Gottingen.

Royal College of Psychiatrists (RCP), 2014. Consensus Statement on High-Dose Antipsychotic Medication. CR190. RCP, London.

Shajahan, P., Spence, E., Taylor, M., et al., 2010. Comparison of the effectiveness of depot antipsychotics in routine clinical practice. The Psychiatrist 34, 273–279.

Stroup, T.S., Lieberman, J.A., McEvoy, J., et al., 2007. Effectiveness of olanzapine, quetiapine, and risperidone in patients with chronic schizophrenia after discontinuing perphenazine: a CATIE study. Am. J. Psychiatry 164 (3), 415–427.

Taylor, D., Paton, C., Kapuar, S., 2015. The Maudsley Prescribing Guidelines, twelfth ed. Wiley-Blackwell, Chichester, UK.

World Health Organization, 1992. International Classification of Diseases and Related Health Problems, tenth ed. (ICD 10). World Health Organization, Geneva.

Further reading

National Institute for Health and Care Excellence (NICE), 2016. Clinical guideline CG185. Bipolar disorder: assessment and management. Available at: https://www.nice.org.uk/guidance/cg185.

National Institute for Health and Care Excellence (NICE), 2011. Clinical guideline CG120. Coexisting severe mental illness (psychosis) and substance misuse: assessment and management in healthcare settings. Available at: https://www.nice.org.uk/guidance/cg120.

National Institute for Health and Care Excellence (NICE), 2015. NICE guideline NG10. Violence and aggression: short-term management in mental health, health and community settings. Available at: https://www.nice.org.uk/guidance/ng10.

National Institute for Health and Care Excellence (NICE), 2016. Clinical guideline CG155. Psychosis and schizophrenia in children and young people: recognition and management. Available at: https://www.nice.org.uk/guidance/cg155.

Scottish Intercollegiate Guidelines Network (SIGN), 2013. Management of schizophrenia: SIGN publication number 131. Available at: http://www.sign.ac.uk/guidelines/fulltext/131/.

31 Epilepsy

Gonçalo Cação and Josemir W. Sander

Key points

- An epileptic seizure is a transient paroxysm of uncontrolled neuronal discharges causing an event which is discernible by the person experiencing the seizure and/or an observer.
- Epilepsy is a brain disorder characterised by an enduring predisposition to generate epileptic seizures.
- The annual incidence of epileptic seizures is around 50 cases per 100,000 of the population.
- About 60–70% of those who develop epilepsy will become seizure free on treatment, and about 50% will eventually withdraw their medication successfully.
- Generalised seizures present immediate involvement of both hemispheres and include different types of seizures: tonic-clonic, absence, myoclonic, clonic, tonic and atonic.
- Focal seizures arise from an area limited to one hemisphere and may evolve into a bilateral convulsive seizure.
- Treatment of epilepsy is usually for at least 3 years and, depending on circumstances, sometimes for life.
- Treatment aims to control seizures using one drug without causing side effects and minimising the use of polypharmacy.
- Management of epilepsy requires empowering the person to understand his or her condition and medication, and helping the person to develop effective partnerships with health professionals.

An epileptic seizure is a transient occurrence of signs and/or symptoms due to abnormal excessive or synchronous neuronal activity in the brain, causing an event that is discernible by the person experiencing the seizure and/or by an observer. Epilepsy is a disorder of the brain characterised by an enduring predisposition to generate epileptic seizures and by the associated neurobiologic, cognitive, psychological, and social consequences. According to the International League Against Epilepsy (ILAE) (Fisher et al., 2014), epilepsy is defined by any of the following conditions:

1. at least two unprovoked (or reflex) seizures occurring more than 24 hours apart;
2. one unprovoked seizure (or reflex) and a probability of further seizures similar to the general recurrence risk (at least 60%) after two unprovoked seizures, occurring over the next 10 years;
3. diagnosis of an epilepsy syndrome.

A person with epilepsy will show recurrent epileptic seizures that occur unexpectedly and stop spontaneously.

Epidemiology

There are problems in establishing precise epidemiological information for a heterogeneous condition such as epilepsy. Unlike most ailments, epilepsy is episodic; between seizures, individuals may be perfectly normal and have normal investigations. Thus, the diagnosis is essentially clinical, relying heavily on eyewitness descriptions of the events. There are also a number of other conditions in which consciousness may be transiently impaired and which may be confused with epilepsy. Another problem is that of case identification, because sometimes the person may be unaware of the nature of the attacks and so may not seek medical help. People with milder epilepsy may also not be receiving ongoing medical care and so may be missed in epidemiological surveys. Because there is some degree of stigma attached to epilepsy, people may sometimes be reluctant to admit their condition. In today's society, in high- and low-income countries, fear, misunderstanding, discrimination and social stigma still exist. These affect the quality of life for people with the disorder and their families.

Epilepsy does impact on an individual's human rights; for example, access to health and life insurance is often affected. A person who suffers from epilepsy may not be able to obtain a driving license, and it has an impact on the choice of career. A global campaign has been established to raise awareness about epilepsy, provide information and highlight the need to improve care and reduce the disorder's impact through public and private collaboration. This is supported through a partnership established between World Health Organization (WHO), ILAE and the International Bureau for Epilepsy.

Epilepsy is recognised as a priority in effective healthcare delivery, and there are still a number of issues that health professionals should consider (WHO, 2015):

- Epilepsy is a chronic neurological disorder that affects people of all ages.
- More than 50 million people worldwide have epilepsy.
- Nearly 80% of people with epilepsy are found in resource-poor settings.
- Epilepsy responds to treatment 70% of the time. Despite this, approximately more than two-thirds of people affected in poor countries are not treated.
- People with epilepsy and their families suffer from stigma and discrimination in many parts of the world.

Incidence and prevalence

Epileptic seizures are common. The incidence (number of new cases per given population per year) in high-income countries is estimated between 40 and 70 cases per 100,000 persons, and the cumulative incidence rate (the risk of having the condition at some point in life) is 2–5%. The incidence is higher in the first two decades of life but falls over the next few decades, only to increase again in late life, mainly because of cerebrovascular diseases. Currently, the elderly are the group in the population with the highest incidence of epilepsy. Most studies of the prevalence of active epilepsy (the number of cases in the population at any given time) in high-income countries provide figures in the range of 4–10 per 1000, with a rate of 5 per 1000 population most commonly quoted. In England, epilepsy has been estimated to affect between 362,000 and 415,000 people (National Institute for Health and Care Excellence [NICE], 2012).

In low-income countries, the prevalence is higher with rates of 10 per 1000 population cited and reported annual new cases twice those seen in high-income countries, presumably because of the higher risk of experiencing conditions that can lead to permanent brain damage. Overall, nearly 80% of epilepsy cases worldwide are found in resource-poor settings.

Prognosis

Up to 5% of all people will suffer at least one seizure in their lifetime. The prevalence of active epilepsy is, however, much lower, and most people who experience seizures have a very good prognosis as about 60–70% of all will eventually become seizure free. About half will successfully withdraw their medication. Once a substantial period of remission has been achieved, the risk of further seizures is greatly reduced. The probability of seizure freedom is particularly high in those with generalised epilepsy and a normal neurological examination. A minority of people (up to a third) will experience chronic epilepsy and in such cases, treatment is more difficult. People with symptomatic epilepsy, more than one seizure type, associated learning disabilities, or neurological or psychiatric disorders are more likely to have a poor outcome. For those who continue to have seizures, in appropriate candidates epilepsy surgery may render seizure freedom more than continued antiepileptic drugs (AEDs) alone. Of people with chronic epilepsy, fewer than 5% will be unable to live in the community or will depend on others for their day-to-day needs. Most people with epilepsy are entirely normal between seizures, but a small minority of people with severe epilepsy may suffer physical and intellectual deterioration.

Mortality

People with epilepsy, especially the young and those with severe epilepsy, are at an increased risk of premature death. Most studies have given overall standardised mortality ratios between two and three times that of the general population (Thurman et al., 2017). Common causes of death include accidents (drowning, head injury, road traffic accidents), status epilepticus, tumours, cerebrovascular disease, pneumonia, iatrogenic accidents and suicide. Sudden unexpected death in epilepsy (SUDEP) is defined as a sudden unexpected, witnessed or unwitnessed, non-traumatic and non-drowning death in people with epilepsy, with or without evidence for a seizure, and excluding documented status epilepticus, in which postmortem examination does not reveal a toxicological or anatomic cause for death. This entity remains unexplained, but identified risk factors are younger age at onset, frequent convulsions, long duration of epilepsy and refractory epilepsy. Its incidence is about 0.35 cases per 1000 person-years in a population-based incidence cohort of epilepsy (Tomson et al., 2005).

Aetiology

Epileptic seizures are produced by abnormal discharges of neurones that may be caused by any pathological process which affects the cortical layer of the brain. The idiopathic or genetic epilepsies are those in which there is a clear genetic component, and they probably account for a third of all new cases of epilepsy. In a significant proportion of cases, however, no cause can be determined, and these are termed as unknown or cryptogenic epilepsies. Possible explanations for unknown epilepsy include as yet unexplained metabolic or biochemical abnormalities and microscopic lesions in the brain resulting from brain malformation or trauma during birth or other injury. The term 'symptomatic' or structural/metabolic epilepsy indicates that a probable cause has been identified.

The likely aetiology depends upon age of onset and seizure type. The commonest causes in young infants are hypoxia or birth asphyxia, intracranial trauma during birth, metabolic disturbances, congenital malformations of the brain and infection. In young children and adolescents, genetic epilepsies account for the majority, although trauma and infection also play a role. In this age group, particularly in children aged between 6 months and 5 years, seizures may occur in association with febrile illness. These are usually short convulsions that occur during the early phase of a febrile disease. They must be distinguished from seizures that are triggered by central nervous system infections which produce fever, for example, meningitis or encephalitis. Unless febrile seizures are prolonged, focal and recurrent, or there is a background of neurological handicap, the prognosis is excellent and it is unlikely that the child will develop epilepsy.

The range of causes of adult-onset epilepsy is very wide. Both genetic epilepsies and those due to perinatal causes may also begin in early adulthood. Other important causes are trauma, developmental disorders (e.g. cortical dysplasias), brain tumours, cerebrovascular diseases, immunological disorders and degenerative conditions. Brain tumours are responsible for the development of epilepsy in up to a third of those between the ages of 30 and 50 years. Over the age of 50 years, cerebrovascular disease is the commonest risk factor for epilepsy and may be present in up to half of people developing the condition in this age group.

Pathophysiology

Epilepsy differs from other neurological conditions because it has no pathognomonic lesion. A variety of different electrical or chemical stimuli can easily give rise to a seizure in any normal brain. The hallmark of epilepsy is a rather rhythmic and repetitive hyper-synchronous discharge of neurones, either localised in an area of the cerebral cortex or generalised throughout the cortex, which can be observed on an electroencephalogram (EEG).

Neurones are interconnected in a complex network in which each individual neurone is linked through synapses with hundreds of others. A small electrical current is discharged by neurones to release neurotransmitters at synaptic levels to permit communication with each other. Neurotransmitters fall into two basic categories: inhibitory or excitatory. Therefore, a neurone discharging can either excite or inhibit neurones connected to it. An excited neurone will activate the next neurone, whereas an inhibited neurone will not. In this manner, information is conveyed, transmitted and processed throughout the central nervous system.

A normal neurone discharges repetitively at a low baseline frequency, and it is the integrated electrical activity generated by the neurones of the superficial layers of the cortex that is recorded in a normal EEG. If neurones are damaged, injured or suffer a chemical or metabolic insult, a change in the discharge pattern may develop. In the case of epilepsy, regular low-frequency discharges are replaced by bursts of high-frequency discharges usually followed by periods of inactivity. A single neurone discharging in an abnormal manner usually has no clinical significance. It is only when a whole population of neurones discharge synchronously in an abnormal way that an epileptic seizure may be triggered. This abnormal discharge may remain localised or it may spread to adjacent areas, recruiting more neurones as it expands. It may also generalise throughout the brain via cortical and subcortical routes, including callosal and thalamocortical pathways. The area from which the abnormal discharge originates is known as the epileptic focus. An EEG recording carried out during one of these abnormal discharges may show a variety of atypical signs, depending on which area of the brain is involved, its progression and how the discharging areas project to the superficial cortex.

Clinical manifestations

The clinical manifestation of a seizure will depend on the location of the focus and the pathways involved in its spread. ILAE has recently published a revised classification of seizure types (Fisher et al., 2017). It divides seizures into three main groups according to its onset (Box 31.1). If it involves initial activation of both hemispheres of the brain simultaneously, the seizures are termed 'generalised'. If a discharge starts in a localised area of the brain, the seizure is termed 'focal'. Lastly seizures are classified as 'unknown onset' if it is not possible to classify as focal or generalised.

Box 31.1 Classification of seizures (Fisher et al., 2017)

Focal onset
Aware/Impaired awareness
Motor onset: automatisms, atonic, clonic, epileptic spasms, hyperkinetic, myoclonic, tonic
Non-motor onset: autonomic, behaviour arrest, cognitive, emotional, sensory

Generalised onset
Motor: tonic-clonic, clonic, tonic, myoclonic, myoclonic-tonic-clonic, myoclonic-atonic, atonic, epileptic spasms
Non-motor (absence): typical, atypical, myoclonic, eyelid myoclonia

Unknown onset
Motor: tonic-clonic, epileptic spasms
Non-motor: behaviour arrest

Generalised seizures

Generalised seizures are subdivided in motor and non-motor (absence) types. The motor includes tonic-clonic, clonic, tonic, myoclonic, myoclonic-tonic-clonic, myoclonic-atonic, atonic and epileptic spasms. The non-motor includes typical absence, atypical absence and absence with special features (myoclonic, eyelid myoclonia).

Tonic-clonic seizures

Tonic-clonic seizures often begin with bilateral myoclonic jerks, followed by a tonic contraction of the extremities and trunk sustained by a short period. Then contractions become progressively longer and interrupted, resulting in clonic jerking. Cyanosis, incontinence and tongue biting may occur. The seizure ceases after a few minutes and may often be followed by a period of drowsiness, confusion, headache and sleep.

Typical absence seizures

Typical absence seizures happen almost exclusively in childhood and early adolescence, and are characterised by behavioural arrest for a few seconds. The child goes blank and stares; fluttering of the eyelids and flopping of the head may occur. The attacks last only a few seconds and afterwards normal activity is resumed as if nothing had happened. They are seen in developmentally normal people and are associated with a typical rhythmic 3-Hz spike and wave complexes on the EEG.

Atypical absence seizures

Atypical absence seizures differ from the previous types because they are mostly seen in people with developmental delay, the behavioural arrest may be longer, the EEG shows background abnormalities (diffuse slowing), and the spike and wave complexes are less than 3 Hz in frequency.

Absence seizures with special features

Absence seizures with special features are absence seizures associated with other characteristics such as eyes myoclonic (Jeavons syndrome) or myoclonic movements.

Myoclonic seizures

Myoclonic seizures are abrupt, very brief, involuntary, shocklike jerks, which may involve the extremities and/or axial trunk muscles. They usually happen in the morning, shortly after waking. They may sometimes cause the person to fall, but recovery is immediate. There are non-epileptic myoclonic jerks that occur in a variety of other neurological diseases and may also occur in healthy people, particularly when they are just going off to sleep (hypnic jerks).

Tonic seizures

Tonic seizures occur during sleep with a duration of approximately 20 seconds. They usually involve all or most of the brain, affecting both sides of the body. If the person is standing when the seizure starts, they may fall.

Clonic seizures

Clonic seizures are rare alone, but most often are part of a tonic-clonic seizure. They are characterised by a rapidly alternating contraction and relaxation of a muscle – clonus. Brief and infrequent clonic seizures in infants usually disappear on their own within a short time.

Atonic seizures

Atonic seizures comprise a sudden loss of muscle tone, causing the person to collapse to the ground. Recovery afterwards is quick. They are rare, accounting for less than 1% of the epileptic seizures seen in the general population, but more common in people with severe epilepsy starting in infancy.

Focal seizures

In focal seizures, discharges are localised, and manifestations often reflect activation of the underlying cortical areas. They are primarily divided according to awareness in focal aware and focal with impaired awareness. Then subdivided according to motor or non-motor onset. The motor onset includes automatism (e.g. chewing, lip smacking, fumbling), atonic, clonic, epileptic spasms, hyperkinetic, myoclonic and tonic seizures. The non-motor onset includes autonomic (e.g. pallor, tachycardia), behaviour arrest, cognitive, emotional and sensory seizures. Symptoms may vary widely from person to person but will normally be stereotyped in one person.

This seizure may progress into a bilateral tonic-clonic seizure, which is termed as focal to bilateral tonic-clonic.

Epileptic spasms

Previously considered a type of generalised epilepsy, it is now placed under both focal and generalised seizures because they are also seen in children with structural lesions confined to one hemisphere and where surgical treatment can often be curative. They occur in early infancy and are characterised by tonic flexion of the head, neck and trunk, with circumflexion of the upper extremities.

Diagnosis

Diagnosing epilepsy can be difficult because it is first necessary to demonstrate a tendency to recurrent epileptic seizures. The one feature that distinguishes epilepsy from other conditions is its unpredictability and transient nature. The diagnosis is clinical and depends on a reliable account of what happens during the events, if possible, from the individual and from an eyewitness. Investigations may help and the EEG is usually one of them. These investigations, however, cannot conclusively confirm or refute the diagnosis.

Other conditions may cause impairment or loss of consciousness which can be misdiagnosed as epilepsy; these include syncope, breath-holding attacks, transient ischaemic attacks and psychogenic attacks. People may also present with acute symptomatic seizures or provoked seizures as a result of other problems such as drugs, metabolic dysfunction, infection, head trauma or flashing lights (photosensitive seizures). These conditions have to be clearly ruled out before a diagnosis of epilepsy is made. Epilepsy must only be diagnosed when at least one of the three defining ILAE conditions given at the beginning of this chapter is present. The diagnosis must be accurate because the label 'suffering with epilepsy' carries a social stigma that has great implications.

An EEG recording is often the only examination required in typical generalised epilepsies, and it aims to record abnormal neuronal discharges. EEGs have, however, limitations that should be clearly understood. Up to 5% of people without epilepsy may have non-specific abnormalities in their EEG recording, while up to 40% of people with epilepsy may have a normal recording between seizures. The diagnosis of epilepsy needs to be strongly supported by a bona fide history of unprovoked seizures. The EEG is, however, invaluable in classifying epilepsy.

The chance of recording the discharges of an actual seizure during a routine EEG, which usually takes 20–30 minutes, is slight and because of this, ambulatory EEG monitoring and EEG video-telemetry are sometimes required. Ambulatory EEG allows recording in day-to-day circumstances using a small recorder. EEG video-telemetry is useful in the assessment of difficult cases, particularly if surgery is considered. The individual is usually admitted and remains under continuous monitoring. This is only helpful in a very few cases and best suited for people who have frequent seizures.

Neuroimaging with magnetic resonance imaging (MRI) is the most valuable investigation when structural abnormalities (e.g. stroke, tumour, developmental abnormalities, hydrocephalus) are suspected. MRI does not need to be done routinely in generalised epilepsy, but is particularly important in people who develop epilepsy before the age of 2 years or in adulthood, in those with any suggestion of focal onset and in those who continue with seizures despite first-line medication.

Other diagnostic investigations, such as functional MRI, magnetic resonance spectroscopy, single-photon emission computerised tomography and positron emission tomography studies, are normally performed only in specific cases, particularly when evaluating for surgical treatment.

Treatment

In 2004 the NICE issued guidance on the diagnosis and treatment of epilepsy in adults and children in primary and secondary care, which was updated in 2014 (NICE, 2014). This guidance covers issues such as when a person with epilepsy should be referred to a specialist centre, the special considerations concerning the care and treatment of women, and the management of people with learning disabilities. The key points of the guidance are summarised in Box 31.2.

Treatment during seizures

Convulsive seizures may look frightening, but the person is not in pain, will usually have no recollection of the event afterwards and is usually not seriously injured. Emergency treatment is seldom necessary, but the person should, however, be made as comfortable as possible, preferably lying down (ease to the floor if sitting), cushioning the head and loosening any tight clothing or neckwear. During seizures, the individual should not be moved unless he or she is in a dangerous place, for example, in a road, by a fire or hot radiator, at the top of stairs or by the edge of water. No attempt should be made to open the person's mouth or force anything between the teeth. This usually results in damage and broken teeth or other objects may be inhaled, causing secondary lung damage. When the seizure stops, the person should be turned over into the recovery position and the airway checked for any blockage.

Focal seizures are usually less dramatic. During automatisms, people may behave in a confused manner and should generally be left undisturbed. Gentle restraint may be necessary if the automatism leads to dangerous wandering. Attempts at firm restraint, however, may increase agitation and confusion. No drinks should be given after the seizure, nor should extra AEDs be given. It is commonly felt that seizures may be life-threatening, but this is seldom the case. After a seizure, it is important to stay with the person and offer reassurance until the confused period has completely subsided and the person has fully recovered.

Status epilepticus

Status epilepticus is traditionally defined as ongoing seizure activity for ≥ 30 minutes, but from a pragmatic point of view, a seizure that lasts longer than 5 minutes warrants pharmacological intervention. Initial management of status epilepticus is supportive and may include:

- secure airway and resuscitate,
- administer oxygen,
- assess cardiorespiratory function,
- establish intravenous access.

Buccal midazolam (10 mg) is first-line treatment in the community. Rectal diazepam is an alternative if preferred or if buccal midazolam is not available. If intravenous access is already established and resuscitation facilities are available, intravenous lorazepam is administered.

First-line AED for hospital management of status epilepticus is intravenous lorazepam. If unavailable, then intravenous diazepam should be administered or buccal midazolam if immediate intravenous access cannot be secured. If seizures continue, intravenous phenytoin or valproate or phenobarbital should be administered as second-line treatment. In the refractory status, general anaesthesia with propofol, midazolam or thiopentone may be necessary.

Febrile convulsions

Febrile convulsions may occur in the young without epilepsy. Brief events are managed conservatively with the primary aim of reducing the child's temperature. Tepid sponging and use of paracetamol is usual. Prolonged febrile convulsions lasting ≥ 10–15 minutes or in a child with risk factors, active management is required to avoid brain damage. The drug of choice is diazepam

---

Box 31.2 Key points on the diagnosis and management of epilepsy (NICE, 2012, 2014)

Diagnosis
- Diagnosis is to be made urgently by a specialist with an interest in epilepsy.

Management
- The individual with epilepsy, and their family and/or carers, should participate in all decisions, taking into account any specific need.
- All should have a comprehensive agreed-upon care plan.
- Treatment should be individualised according to seizure type, epilepsy syndrome, co-medication and comorbidity, the individual's lifestyle and personal preferences.

Prolonged or repeated seizures and convulsive status epilepticus
- Prescribe buccal midazolam or rectal diazepam for use in the community.
- Buccal midazolam is first-line treatment. Rectal diazepam is prescribed if the previous is not available or if it is preferred. Intravenous lorazepam is prescribed if intravenous access is established and resuscitation facilities are available.

Women and girls of childbearing potential
- They must be given accurate information and counselling about contraception, conception, pregnancy, caring for children, breastfeeding and menopause.

Review and referral
- Regular structured review should occur at least once a year.
- Individuals should be given all required information and referral if necessary.
- Individuals should be referred back to tertiary care if seizures are not controlled, uncertainty of diagnostic or treatment failure.

by intravenous or rectal administration. Prophylactic management of febrile convulsions may be required in some children, such as those with pre-existing risk factors or a history of previous prolonged seizures.

Long-term treatment

In most cases, epilepsy can only be treated by regular, long-term drug treatment aiming at suppressing seizures. Full seizure control can be obtained in most cases, and in others drugs may reduce seizure frequency or severity.

Initiating treatment with an AED is a major event in a person's life, and the diagnosis should be unequivocal. Treatment options must be considered with careful evaluation of all relevant factors, including the number and frequency of seizures, the presence of precipitants such as alcohol, drugs or flashing lights, and the presence of other medical conditions. Single seizures do not require treatment unless they are associated with a structural abnormality in the brain, a progressive brain disorder or there is a clearly abnormal EEG recording. If there are long intervals between seizures (>2 years), there is a case for not starting treatment. If there are more than two attacks that are clearly associated with a precipitating factor, fever or alcohol, for instance, then treatment may not be necessary.

Therapy is long-term, usually for at least 3 years and, depending on circumstances, sometimes for life. A full explanation of all of the implications must be given to the person, and the individual must be involved in all stages of the treatment plan. It is vital that the person fully understands the implications and agrees with the treatment goals. Empowerment of the person with epilepsy to be actively involved in the decision-making process will encourage adherence and is essential for effective clinical management. Support for people so that they understand the implications of the condition and why drug therapy is important is crucial to ensure effective clinical management.

Health professionals have a key role in supporting people with epilepsy to ensure they are able to manage their medicines appropriately. AED treatment will fail unless the person fully understands the importance of regular therapy. Poor adherence is still a major factor which results in hospital admissions and poor seizure control, and leads to the clinical use of multiple AEDs.

General principles of treatment

The primary aim of epilepsy treatment is to control seizures using one drug, with the lowest effective dose causing the fewest side effects possible. The established AEDs, those licensed before 2000, are still an important part of the antiepileptic armamentarium, and include carbamazepine, clobazam, clonazepam, ethosuximide, gabapentin, lamotrigine, phenobarbital, phenytoin, piracetam, primidone, sodium valproate, tiagabine, topiramate and vigabatrin. Since 2000, new AEDs such as eslicarbazepine acetate, brivaracetam, felbamate, lacosamide, levetiracetam, oxcarbazepine, perampanel, pregabalin, stiripentol, rufinamide and zonisamide have been introduced. The choice of drugs depends largely on the seizure type, and so correct diagnosis and

classification are essential. Table 31.1 lists the main indications for the more commonly used AEDs, and Table 31.2 summarises the clinical use of the newer AEDs.

Initiation of therapy in newly diagnosed epilepsy

A first-line AED suitable for the person's seizure type should be introduced slowly, starting with a small dose. A hasty introduction may induce side effects that may challenge the person's confidence. For most drugs, a gradual introduction will produce a therapeutic effect just as fast as a rapid introduction, and the person should be reassured about this.

Maintenance dosage

There is no single optimum dose of any AED that will suit all because the required dose varies from person to person

Table 31.1 Antiepileptic drugs for different seizure types

Seizure type	First-line treatment	Adjunctive anti-epileptic drugs
Focal seizures	Carbamazepine	Brivaracetam
	Lamotrigine	Clobazam
	Levetiracetam	Eslicarbazepine
	Oxcarbazepine	Gabapentin
	Sodium valproate	Lacosamide
		Perampanel
		Phenytoin
		Pregabalin
		Topiramate
		Zonisamide
Generalised seizures		
Tonic-clonic	Carbamazepine	Clobazam
	Lamotrigine	Levetiracetam
	Oxcarbazepine	Topiramate
	Sodium valproate	
Tonic or atonic	Sodium valproate	Lamotrigine
		Rufinamide
		Topiramate
Absence	Ethosuximide	Clobazam
	Lamotrigine	Clonazepam
	Sodium valproate	Levetiracetam
		Topiramate
		Zonisamide
Myoclonic	Levetiracetam	Clobazam
	Sodium valproate	Clonazepam
	Topiramate	Piracetam
	Zonisamide	

Table 31.2 Summary of newer antiepileptic agents

Antiepileptic drugs	Clinical use	Available formulation
Brivaracetam	Adjunctive for focal seizures	Tablets: 10, 25, 50, 75, 100 mg Oral solution: 10 mg/mL Injection solution: 10 mg/mL
Eslicarbazepine acetate	Adjunctive for focal seizures	Tablets: 800 mg
Lacosamide	Adjunctive for focal seizures	Tablets: 50, 100, 150, 200 mg Syrup: 10 mg/mL Infusion: 200 mg/20 mL
Levetiracetam	Monotherapy and adjunctive therapy for focal and generalised seizures	Tablets: 250, 500, 750, 1000 mg Syrup: 100 mg/mL Injection: 500 mg/5 mL Granules: 250 mg, 500 mg, 1 g
Oxcarbazepine	Monotherapy and adjunctive therapy for focal and generalised tonic-clonic seizures	Tablets: 150, 300, 600 mg Syrup: 60 mg/mL
Perampanel	Adjunctive for focal seizures	Tablets: 2, 4, 6, 8, 10, 12 mg
Pregabalin	Adjunctive for focal seizures	Tablets: 25, 50, 75, 100, 150, 200, 225, 300 mg Syrup: 20 mg/mL
Zonisamide	Monotherapy and adjunctive for focal seizures	Capsule: 25, 50, 100 mg

and from drug to drug. Drugs are introduced slowly and then increased incrementally to an initial target dose. Seizure control should then be assessed, and the dose of drug changed if necessary. For most AEDs, dosage increments are constant over a wide range. More care is, however, needed with phenytoin because the serum level–dose relationship is not linear and small dose changes may result in considerable serum level changes. Phenytoin is, however, currently rarely used. Generic prescribing for epilepsy remains controversial. Most specialists would prefer people to remain on the same brand because it provides consistency. This is also preferred by the majority of people with epilepsy and is recommended by NICE (2014). Different preparations of some AEDs may vary in bioavailability or pharmacokinetic profiles. This is obviously important in those people in whom the dosage has been carefully titrated to

achieve optimal control. The Medicines and Healthcare products Regulatory Agency (MHRA) has classified AEDs into three categories (MHRA, 2013):
- Category 1: phenytoin, carbamazepine, phenobarbital and primidone. People receiving these drugs should be maintained on a specific manufacturer's product.
- Category 2: valproate, lamotrigine, perampanel, rufinamide, clobazam, clonazepam, oxcarbazepine, eslicarbazepine, zonisamide and topiramate. The need for continued supply of a particular manufacturer's product is based on clinical judgement and consultation with the patient/carer, taking into account factors such as seizure frequency and treatment history.
- Category 3: levetiracetam, lacosamide, tiagabine, gabapentin, pregabalin, ethosuximide and vigabatrin. It is usually unnecessary to maintain the patient on a specific manufacturer's product.

Altering drug regimens

If the maximal tolerated dose of a drug does not control seizures or if it is not tolerated, the first drug should be replaced with another first-line AED. To do this, the second drug should be added gradually to the first. Once a good dose of the new drug is established, the first drug should then slowly be withdrawn.

Withdrawal of drugs

AEDs should not be withdrawn abruptly. Withdrawal of individual AEDs should be carried out in a slow, stepwise fashion to avoid the precipitation of rebound seizures (e.g. over 2–3 months). This risk is particularly great with barbiturates (phenobarbital and primidone) and benzodiazepines (clobazam and clonazepam). If a drug needs to be withdrawn rapidly, for example, if there are life-threatening side effects, a benzodiazepine can be used to cover the withdrawal phase.

Examples of withdrawal regimens are given below.
- Carbamazepine
  100–200 mg every 2 weeks (as part of a drug change)
  100–200 mg every 4 weeks (total withdrawal)
- Phenobarbital
  15–30 mg every 2 weeks (as part of a drug change)
  15–30 mg every 4 weeks (total withdrawal)
- Phenytoin
  50 mg every 2 weeks (as part of a drug change)
  50 mg every 4 weeks (total withdrawal)
- Sodium valproate
  200–400 mg every 2 weeks (as part of a drug change)
  200–400 mg every 4 weeks (total withdrawal)
- Ethosuximide
  125–250 mg every 2 weeks (as part of a drug change)
  125–250 mg every 4 weeks (total withdrawal)

Variations in the earlier regimens may be used in different settings. People must be monitored closely for any change in seizure frequency. The pace of withdrawal may be slower if the person is within the higher end of the quoted dose range and faster if the person is an in-patient.

When to make dose changes

Some AEDs have long half-lives and it may take time, normally five half-lives, before a change in dose results in a stable blood level. For example, phenobarbital has a half-life of up to 6 days and will take more than 4 weeks to produce a stable blood level. For this reason an assessment of the effectiveness of any dose change should be undertaken several weeks after the dose change has been made and be informed by knowledge of the half-life of the drug.

Newer antiepileptic drugs

The newer AEDs are generally used as second-line drugs when treatment with established first-line drugs has failed. Exceptions to this are levetiracetam and oxcarbazepine. Overall, newer AEDs are not more effective than the established drugs but seem to be better tolerated. Notwithstanding, the chronic side effect profile of the new AEDs has not yet been fully established.

Follow-up and monitoring of treatment

It is essential to follow up people in whom AED treatment has been started. The reason for this is essentially to monitor the efficacy and side effects of treatment, upon which drug dosage will depend, but also to encourage good adherence. This follow-up is particularly important in the early stages of treatment, when an effective maintenance dose may not have been fully established, when the importance of adherence may not have been recognised by the person and when the psychological adjustment to regular treatment may not be resolved.

Chronic epilepsy

The drug treatment of people with uncontrolled epilepsy despite initial attempts is much more difficult than that of those newly diagnosed. Prognosis is worse, drug resistance may have developed, and there may be additional neurological, psychological or social problems.

Assessment. The diagnosis of epilepsy should be reassessed before assuming seizures are intractable because misdiagnosis is common. Progressive neurological conditions should also be ruled out. A treatment history should be obtained and note made of previous drugs used which were helpful, unhelpful or of uncertain benefit. Serum level measurements should be obtained where appropriate, and drugs not previously tried should be identified.

Choice of drug and dosage. Treatment should always be started with one AED appropriate for seizure type and suitable for the individual. Only when attempts at monotherapy fail should a combination of two AEDs be tried. In the majority of people, there is no place for therapy with more than two drugs. The choice of drugs should be made according to seizure type and previous treatment history. Drugs that were helpful in the past or found to be of uncertain benefit, or which have not been used before, should be tried if appropriate to seizure type. The use of sedative AEDs should be minimised where possible.

Intractable epilepsy. It is important to realise that there are limits to AED treatment and that in some people, albeit a small group, seizure control is not possible with the drugs currently available. In such cases the goal of drug treatment changes, and the objectives are to reduce medication to minimise toxicity while providing partial control. The sedative drugs, for example, barbiturates or benzodiazepines, should be used only where absolutely necessary. In these persons, surgical treatment or the use of experimental antiepileptic agents may be considered. However, only a relatively small number of people with focal epilepsy are suitable for curative surgical treatment.

Stopping treatment

Withdrawing therapy should be considered in people who have been seizure free for a considerable period. In no individual case, however, can the safety of drug withdrawal be guaranteed, and the risk of relapse on withdrawal of medication in a person who has been seizure free for more than 2 years is about 40%. The longer the person has been free of seizures, the lower the risk of seizure recurrence when drugs are withdrawn. If a person has a learning disability, focal seizures or symptomatic epilepsy, neurological signs or other evidence of cerebral damage, this risk is much higher, and in such cases it may be best to continue drug treatment indefinitely. Drug withdrawal should be carried out only very slowly in staged decrements, and only one drug at a time should be withdrawn.

The risks of drug withdrawal should be clearly explained to the person, and the possible medical and social implications taken into account. There may be serious social or domestic consequences if seizures recur, and the attacks may be subsequently difficult to control, even if the original AED regimen is re-established. In the final analysis, the decision to withdraw therapy is an individual one, and the person should be made aware of the risks and benefits of withdrawal.

Monitoring antiepileptic therapy

Therapeutic drug monitoring (TDM) involves the measurement of serum drug levels and their pharmacokinetic interpretation. It is an integral component in the management of people who are taking phenytoin and carbamazepine but is less useful in people receiving other AEDs. Indeed, TDM has a very limited use for new AEDs, except in people who are acutely unwell, pregnant or in the elderly. It is also very useful to document AED side effects and in managing drug interactions. Adherence may also be a problem in these people, and hence TDM may be useful to establish treatment adherence.

TDM is indicated:

- at the onset of therapy,
- if seizure control is poor or sudden changes in seizure control occur,
- if toxicity is suspected,
- if poor or non-adherence is suspected,
- to monitor the timescale of drug interactions,
- when changing AED therapy or making changes to other aspects of a person's drug regimen that may interact with the AED.

The frequency of undertaking TDM varies. Those with stabilised epilepsy may require their serum levels to be checked only once a year. TDM may be used more often in some people, for one or more of the above indications. A number of the newer AEDs do not require routine TDM. However, because most are used as adjuvant therapy, it is useful to establish baseline levels of existing drugs before the new agent is introduced. Clinical effects should be monitored and TDM, where appropriate, carried out at 6- to 12-month intervals.

Drug development and action

Some of the established AEDs were developed in animal models in which the potential drugs were assessed in terms of their ability to raise seizure threshold or prevent spread of seizure discharge. The animals involved in these tests would not have epilepsy but would have seizures induced by, for instance, maximal electroshock or subcutaneous pentylenetetrazole. As a consequence the relevance of these models to epilepsy can be questioned.

Established AEDs such as phenytoin, phenobarbital, sodium valproate, carbamazepine, ethosuximide, clonazepam and diazepam are effective but have poor side-effect profiles, are involved in many interactions and have complex pharmacokinetics. Over the past 15 years, there has been renewed interest in the development of new AEDs, based on a better understanding of excitatory and inhibitory pathways in the brain. The main mechanisms of the available drugs are thought to involve:

- voltage-gated sodium channels: most common mechanism of action, shared by carbamazepine, eslicarbazepine, felbamate, lacosamide, lamotrigine, oxcarbazepine, phenytoin, rufinamide, topiramate, valproate and zonisamide;
- voltage-gated calcium channels: ethosuximide, lamotrigine, gabapentin, pregabalin, valproate and zonisamide;
- enhancement of the inhibitory γ-aminobutyric-acid (GABA)-ergic system (Fig. 31.1): benzodiazepines, barbiturates, stiripentol, tiagabine and vigabatrin;
- attenuation of glutamate-mediated excitatory neurotransmission: perampanel;
- synaptic vesicle protein 2A: levetiracetam and brivaracetam.

Unlike most of the older agents, levetiracetam, lacosamide, pregabalin and zonisamide are devoid of clinically significant enzyme-inhibiting or enzyme-inducing properties. Oral contraceptives may increase the metabolism of lamotrigine and topiramate, and oxcarbazepine may induce cytochrome P450 CYP3A4 which is responsible for the metabolism of oral contraceptives (Sabers and Gram, 2000).

Antiepileptic drug profiles

The maintenance doses for the used AEDs are given in Table 31.3, whereas pharmacokinetic profiles of some AEDs are presented in Table 31.4. Drug interactions are summarised in Table 31.5, and common side effects in Table 31.6.

Acetazolamide

Acetazolamide is occasionally used as an AED. It can be prescribed as a second-line drug for most types of seizures, but particularly for focal seizures, absence seizures and myoclonic seizures. Its intermittent use in catamenial seizures has also been suggested. Acetazolamide has only limited use as long-term therapy because of the development of tolerance in the majority of people. Side effects include skin rash, weight loss, paraesthesia, drowsiness and depression. Routine TDM is not available for this drug.

Brivaracetam

Brivaracetam is a new AED, recently approved by the European Medicines Agency and launched in the UK in 2016. It is indicated as adjunctive therapy in the treatment of focal epilepsy in adult and adolescents from 16 years of age. The initial dosage is 25–50 mg twice daily, with a usual maintenance dose of 25–100 mg twice daily. The most common side effects are somnolence, dizziness and fatigue. The clinical experience with this AED in the "real world" is still small, but initial experience suggests that it is effective for some people who had not benefitted from other AEDs.

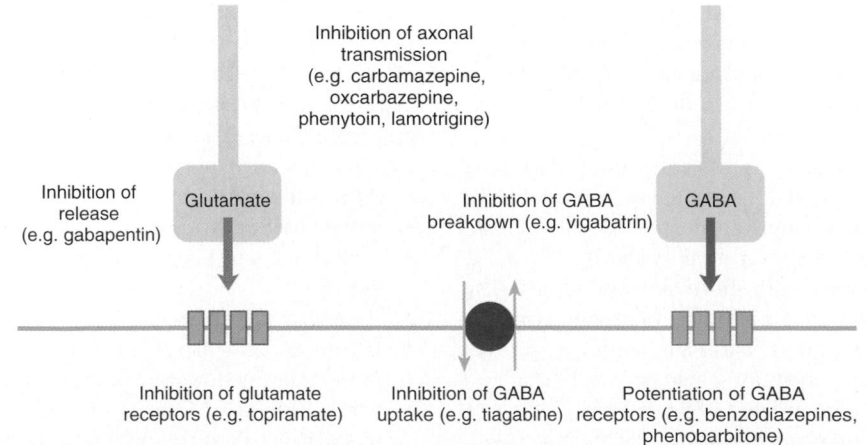

Fig. 31.1 Action of antiepileptic drugs. GABA, γ-Aminobutyric acid. (From Duncan et al., 2006.)

Carbamazepine

Carbamazepine is a first-line drug for generalised tonic-clonic seizures and focal seizures. It is not effective in absence seizures and myoclonic seizures, where it may even be deleterious. Carbamazepine acts through blockage of voltage-gated sodium channel. Tolerance to its beneficial effect does not usually develop. Adverse events may occur in up to a third of people treated with carbamazepine, but only about 5% of these events will require drug withdrawal, usually because of skin rash, gastro-intestinal disturbances or hyponatraemia. Dose-related adverse reactions including ataxia, dizziness, blurred vision and diplopia are common. Idiosyncratic reactions, such as skin rash, occur in up to 10%, but rarely cause severe skin eruptions as erythema multiform and Stevens–Johnson syndrome. Others serious adverse events including hepatic failure and bone marrow depression are extremely uncommon.

Carbamazepine exhibits auto-induction, that is, induces its own metabolism as well as inducing the metabolism of other drugs (see Table 31.7). It should, therefore, be introduced at low dosage, and this should be steadily increased over a period of a month. The target serum concentration therapeutic range is 4–12 micrograms/mL. In addition, a number of clinically important pharmacokinetic interactions may occur, and caution should be exercised when co-medication is instituted (see Table 31.5). The slow-release preparation of carbamazepine has distinct advantages, allowing twice-daily ingestion and avoiding high peak serum concentrations. A 'chewtab' formulation is also available, and pharmacokinetic studies have shown that it performs well even if inadvertently swallowed whole. Carbamazepine retard reduces fluctuations of serum levels and allows a twice-daily regimen, which can assist adherence.

Table 31.3 Commonly used starting and maintenance doses of antiepileptic drugs for adults

Antiepileptic drug	Starting dose (mg)	Average maintenance (total mg/day)	Doses/day
Acetazolamide	250	500–1500	2
Carbamazepine	200	800–2000	2–4 (retard 2)
Clobazam	10	10–40	1–2
Clonazepam	1	2–8	1–2
Eslicarbazepine	400	800–1200	1
Ethosuximide	250	500–2000	2
Gabapentin	300	1800–3600	3
Lacosamide	50	200–400	2
Lamotrigine	25	200–400[a]	1–2
Levetiracetam	250	1500–3000	2
Oxcarbazepine	300	600–2400	2–3
Perampanel	2	4–12	1–2
Phenobarbital	60	60–240	1–2
Phenytoin	200	200–500	1–2
Pregabalin	25	150–600	2–3
Primidone	250	250–1500	1–2
Rufinamide	200	400–1200	2
Sodium valproate	500	1000–2500	2–4
Tiagabine	5[b]	30–45	2–3
Topiramate	25	100–500	2
Vigabatrin	500	1000–3000	2
Zonisamide	50	200–500	2

[a]Reduce by 50% if receiving sodium valproate.
[b]If taking enzyme inducer.

Clobazam

Clobazam is a 1,5-benzodiazepine that is said to be less sedative than 1,4-benzodiazepine drugs such as clonazepam and diazepam. As with other benzodiazepines, it acts through activation of the ionotropic γ-aminobutyric acid ($GABA_A$) receptor. The development of tolerance is common, but clobazam is used as an adjunctive therapy for focal and generalised seizures that have proved unresponsive to other medication. Its intermittent use in catamenial epilepsy has also been suggested; it is also used in people with seizure clusters as a single dose of 20–30 mg because it can have a prophylactic action. Clobazam may produce less sedation than other benzodiazepines, but otherwise its adverse effects are similar, including dizziness, behavioural disturbances and dry mouth. Withdrawal may be difficult.

Clonazepam

Clonazepam, a 1,4-benzodiazepine, is a second-line drug for generalised tonic-clonic seizures, absences, myoclonic seizures and as adjunctive therapy for focal seizures, but as with clobazam, effectiveness often wears off with time as tolerance develops. It has limited use in epilepsy management and is almost restricted to refractory myoclonic seizures. It has an adverse effect profile similar to that of clobazam, but may be more sedating.

Diazepam

Diazepam is used mainly in the treatment of status epilepticus, intravenously or in the acute management of febrile convulsions as a rectal solution. Absorption from suppositories or following intramuscular injection is slow and erratic. The rectal solution may also be useful in status epilepticus if it is not possible to give the drug intravenously.

Table 31.4 Pharmacokinetic data of antiepileptic drugs

Drug	Absorption			Protein binding (% bound)	Elimination		
	F (%)	T_{peak} (h)	V_d (L/kg)		$T_{\frac{1}{2}}$ (h)	Renal excretion (%)	Active metabolite
Carbamazepine	75–85	1–5 (chronic dose)	0.8–1.6	70–78	24–45 (single), 8–24 (chronic)	<1	Yes
Diazepam	90	1–2	1–2	96	20–95	2	Yes
Clonazepam	80–90	1–2	2.1–4.3	80–90	19–40	2	–
Gabapentin	51–59	2–3	57.7	0	5–7	100	No
Lamotrigine	100	2–3	0.92–1.22	55	24–35 (induces its own metabolism)	<10	No
Ethosuximide	90–95	3–7	0.6–0.9	0	20–60	10–20	No
Phenobarbital	95–100	1–3	0.6	40–50	50–144	20–40	No
Phenytoin	85–95	4–7	0.5–0.7	90–95	9–40 (non-linear kinetics)	<5	No
Primidone	90–100	1–3	0.4–1.1	20–30	3–19	40	Yes
Sodium valproate	100	0.5–1.0	0.1–0.5	88–92	7–17	<5	No
Vigabatrin	60–80	2	0.6–1.0	0	5–7	100	No
Zonisamide	100	2–4	1.1–1.7	40	52–69	30	Yes

F, Bioavailability; T_{peak}, time to peak; V_d, volume of distribution.

Eslicarbazepine acetate

Eslicarbazepine acetate is a drug which is similar to oxcarbazepine and which is licensed as a second-line treatment for focal seizures. As with oxcarbazepine, its mode of action is thought to be by interacting with voltage-gated sodium channels. Currently, it is available only as a 800 mg tablet. It has a long half-life and can be used once per day. The recommended starting dosage is 400 mg once daily for 1–2 weeks, then increased to 800 mg once daily. The maximum dosage is 1200 mg daily. Its pharmacokinetic profile and side effects are also similar to those of oxcarbazepine.

Ethosuximide

Ethosuximide is a drug of first choice for generalised absence seizures, and it has no useful effect against any other seizure type. It mechanism of action is through blockage of low-voltage activated calcium channel. Tolerance does not seem to be a problem. The most commonly encountered adverse effects are gastrointestinal symptoms, which occur frequently at the beginning of therapy. Behaviour disorders, anorexia, fatigue, sleep disturbances and headaches may also occur. Idiosyncratic side effects include rash, Stevens–Johnson syndrome and aplastic anaemia.

The therapeutic range commonly quoted is 1–1.5 g daily in two divided doses, increased if necessary up to 2 g daily. The initial dosage is 500 mg daily in two divided doses and increased in steps of 250 mg every 5–7 days. The absorption of ethosuximide is complete, and the bioavailability of the syrup and capsule formulations is equivalent. An increase in daily dose may lead to disproportionately higher increases in average serum concentrations; therefore, careful monitoring is indicated at high doses.

Felbamate

Felbamate may be used as a drug of last resort in people with intractable epilepsy, particularly in those within the Lennox–Gastaut spectrum. It is licensed in the USA and most countries of the European Union, but not in the UK. Its mechanism of action is unknown. The usual dosage is between 2400 and 3600 mg/day. Felbamate exhibits significant pharmacokinetic interactions with phenytoin, carbamazepine and valproic acid. Side effects include diplopia, insomnia, dizziness, headache, ataxia, anorexia, nausea and vomiting. A major limiting problem is its potential to cause aplastic anaemia and liver failure. It, therefore, seems prudent to limit use to specialist centres and severe intractable cases.

Table 31.5 Examples of drug interactions involving antiepileptic drugs

Drug affected	Effect on serum level	Drug implicated	Possible mechanism
Carbamazepine	Increase	Valproate sodium Cimetidine Dextropropoxyphene Erythromycin Isoniazid Troleandomycin Danazol	Enzyme inhibition
	Decrease	Phenytoin, phenobarbital	Enzyme induction
Ethosuximide	Increase	Valproate sodium	Enzyme inhibition
	Decrease	Carbamazepine	Enzyme induction
Lamotrigine	Increase	Valproate sodium	Enzyme inhibition
	Decrease	Phenytoin, carbamazepine	Enzyme induction
Phenobarbital	Increase	Valproate sodium	Enzyme inhibition
	Decrease	Rifampicin	Enzyme induction
Phenytoin	Increase	Valproate sodium Chloramphenicol Isoniazid Disulfiram Fluconazole Flu vaccine Amiodarone Fluoxetine	Enzyme inhibition Mechanism unclear
	Decrease	Phenobarbital Rifampicin Carbamazepine Furosemide Acetazolamide	Enzyme induction Decreased responsiveness of renal tubules. Increased osteomalacia
Sodium valproate	Increase	Salicylates	Displacement from protein binding sites and possible enzyme inhibition
Topiramate	Decrease	Phenytoin, carbamazepine	Enzyme induction
	Decrease	Potential enzyme inducers	Enzyme induction
Zonisamide	Decrease	Carbamazepine, phenytoin, phenobarbital and primidone	Enzyme induction

Gabapentin

Gabapentin is occasionally used as a second-line treatment of focal seizures. Although initially developed as an AED, its main use currently is for the treatment of neuropathic pain. It exerts its effect through blockage of high-voltage activated calcium channels. In view of its pharmacokinetic profile, a three times daily dosage must be used; the usual dosage is 0.9–3.6 g daily. It should be started with 300 mg once daily on day 1, then 300 mg twice daily on day 2 and then 300 mg three times a day on day 3. To date, no clinically significant interactions with other AEDs, or other drugs, have been reported. The most frequently reported side effects are drowsiness, dizziness, diplopia, ataxia and headache. Idiosyncratic effects include increasing seizures.

Lacosamide

Lacosamide, a functionalised amino acid, is a second-line drug for focal epilepsy in people older than 16 years. Its putative mode of action is not shared with any other currently available AEDs. It is said to enhance the slow inactivation of sodium channels and to modulate collapsing response mediator protein-2. The maintenance dosage is 100 mg twice daily, and the maximum dosage is 200 mg twice daily. It should be started at 50 mg twice daily and increased by steps of 50 mg twice daily in weekly intervals. No drug interactions are known. Its commonest side effects are dizziness, headaches, nausea and diplopia. No idiosyncratic side effects have yet been associated with this drug. The drug should be used with caution in people with a history of cardiac conduction problems because it is known to increase PR intervals in some people.

Table 31.6 Side-effect profile of antiepileptic drugs

Drug	Dose related (predictable)	Non-dose related (idiosyncratic)
Brivaracetam	Drowsiness, dizziness, fatigue, nausea, ataxia, irritability	Not reported
Carbamazepine	Diplopia, drowsiness, headache, nausea, orofacial dyskinesia, arrhythmias	Photosensitivity, Stevens–Johnson syndrome, agranulocytosis, aplastic anaemia, hepatotoxicity, teratogenicity
Clobazam	Fatigue, drowsiness, dizziness, ataxia, irritability, hypersalivation, weight gain, psychosis	Rash
Clonazepam	Fatigue, sedation, drowsiness, ataxia	Rash, thrombocytopenia
Eslicarbazepine	Fatigue, drowsiness, diplopia, hyponatraemia, ataxia, nystagmus, tremor	Not reported
Ethosuximide	Nausea, vomiting, drowsiness, headache, lethargy	Rash, erythema multiform, Stevens–Johnson syndrome, aplastic anaemia
Gabapentin	Drowsiness, fatigue, diplopia, ataxia, headache	Increased seizures
Lacosamide	Nausea, vomiting, dizziness, headache, drowsiness, depression, diplopia, impaired memory, impaired coordination, tremor, fatigue, asthenia, pruritus	Not reported
Lamotrigine	Headaches, drowsiness, diplopia, ataxia, tremor, insomnia	Rash, liver failure, Stevens–Johnson syndrome, aplastic anaemia, toxic epidermal necrolysis, pancytopenia
Levetiracetam	Dizziness, drowsiness, irritability, behavioural problems, insomnia, ataxia headache, nausea	Not reported
Oxcarbazepine	Diplopia, ataxia, fatigue, hyponatraemia, headache, nausea, confusion, vomiting	Rash
Perampanel	Drowsiness, ataxia, lethargy, blurred vision, weight gain	Not reported
Phenobarbital	Fatigue, listlessness, depression, poor memory, impotence, irritability, hypocalcaemia, osteomalacia, folate deficiency	Maculopapular rash, exfoliation, hepatotoxicity, teratogenicity, Dupuytren's contracture, frozen shoulder
Phenytoin	Ataxia, nystagmus, drowsiness, diplopia, asterixis, orofacial dyskinesia, folate deficiency	Blood dyscrasias, rash, Dupuytren's contracture, hepatotoxicity, gingival hyperplasia, acne, coarse facies, hirsutism
Pregabalin	Dizziness, ataxia, weight gain, diplopia, tremor, abnormal thinking	Not reported
Piracetam	Diarrhoea, weight gain, insomnia, depression, hyperkinesia	Not reported
Primidone	Fatigue, depression, psychosis, impotence, hyperkinesia, nausea, nystagmus, ataxia, folate deficiency	Rash, agranulocytosis, thrombocytopenia, teratogenicity
Retigabine	Drowsiness, slurred speech, ataxia, tremor, diplopia	Urinary tract symptoms, skin and retinal discolouration
Sodium valproate	Tremor, weight gain, dyspepsia, nausea, vomiting, hair loss, drowsiness, peripheral oedema, hyperammonaemia	Acute pancreatitis, thrombocytopenia, hepatotoxicity, teratogenicity, polycystic ovarian syndrome
Tiagabine	Dizziness, nervousness, tremor, concentration difficulties	Increased seizures, non-convulsive status
Topiramate	Anorexia, weight loss, impaired concentration, impaired speech, paraesthesia, kidney stones	Not reported
Vigabatrin	Drowsiness, weight gain, nystagmus, diplopia, ataxia, irritability, depression, psychosis	Visual field defects, increased seizures
Zonisamide	Ataxia, dizziness, somnolence, anorexia, memory and concentration impairment, confusion	Rash, blood dyscrasias

Table 31.7 Practice points

Problem	Comment
Hepatic enzyme induction	Enzyme induction occurs with carbamazepine, phenytoin, phenobarbital, primidone and topiramate. Interactions occur with a large number of drugs including oral contraceptives.
Use of progesterone-only contraceptives with enzyme-inducing AED	Best avoided. If no acceptable alternative, women should take at least double usual dose of progesterone-only pill.
Use of combined oral contraceptive with enzyme-inducing AED	Preparations containing 50 micrograms of oestrogen should be used.
Continuation of AED during pregnancy	Should be reviewed before attempting pregnancy to determine whether reducing or discontinuing treatment is possible. Avoid use of sodium valproate in childbearing women.
Use of phenytoin as monotherapy	Less frequently considered first- or second-line monotherapy because of poor side-effect profile, narrow therapeutic index and saturation pharmacokinetics.
Changing between generic manufacturers	Because bioavailability or pharmacokinetic profiles may vary between different generic drugs, it is now recommended to prescribe a consistent brand of AED.

AED, Antiepileptic drugs.

Lamotrigine

Lamotrigine is a first-line drug for people with focal and generalised seizures. The main action is through blockage of voltage-gated sodium channel. Lamotrigine does not seem to interact with other concomitantly administered AEDs. However, hepatic enzyme inducers increase the metabolism of lamotrigine, reducing its half-life. Therefore, higher doses need to be administered if it is used in conjunction with enzyme inducers such as phenytoin and carbamazepine. Inhibitors of hepatic enzymes such as sodium valproate block the metabolism of lamotrigine, and reduced doses need to be used if both drugs are given in combination. The recommended starting dosage is 25 mg once daily when used as monotherapy and 25 mg on alternate days in people receiving concomitant sodium valproate, with a maximum recommended dosage of 500 mg daily, but no more than 200 mg daily if concomitant to valproate. It should be increased by 25 mg in 14-day intervals, as too rapid titration may be associated with an increased incidence of skin rash.

Headaches, drowsiness, ataxia and diplopia are the most commonly reported acute adverse effects, particularly during dose escalation. A skin rash is the commonest idiosyncratic side effect and affects up to 5% of individuals.

Levetiracetam

Levetiracetam is a broad-spectrum drug, indicated both as a first-line and as an add-on for the treatment of focal and generalised seizures. Mechanism of action is not fully understood, but it binds to the synaptic vesicle protein 2A. The usual dosage is between 1000 and 3000 mg/day, divided in two daily doses. It is usually started at 250 mg once daily for 1–2 weeks, then increased to 250 mg twice daily and then titrated upwards in incremental steps of 250 mg twice daily every 2 weeks. It is well tolerated, and the most frequent central nervous system adverse events are dizziness, irritability, asthenia, insomnia and ataxia. No idiosyncratic adverse events have yet been reported.

Oxcarbazepine

Oxcarbazepine is an analogue of carbamazepine. It is an inactive pro-drug that is converted in the liver to the active 10-hydroxy metabolite and bypasses the 10,11-epoxide, the primary metabolite of carbamazepine. The usual dosage is between 600 and 2400 mg daily in divided doses. The spectrum of efficacy and side effects is broadly comparable with carbamazepine, apart from hyponatraemia which is more pronounced with oxcarbazepine. The principal advantage over carbamazepine is the lack of induction of hepatic enzymes, with the consequence that there is no auto-induction of the metabolism of the drug and fewer pharmacokinetic interactions. In addition, more than two-thirds of people who are allergic to carbamazepine can tolerate oxcarbazepine.

Perampanel

Perampanel is licensed for the adjunctive treatment of focal-onset seizures with or without secondarily generalised seizures in people with epilepsy aged ≥12 years. It is a selective, non-competitive antagonist of the α-amino-3-hydroxy-5-methyl-4-isoxazolepropionic acid glutamate receptor. Effective dosage is between 4 and 12 mg/day, given in a once-a-day regimen. Commonest side effects are drowsiness, ataxia, lethargy, irritability, weight gain and blurred vision.

Phenobarbital

Phenobarbital, a barbiturate, may be used for the treatment of tonic-clonic and focal seizures. It may also be used in other seizure types. As with other barbiturates, it acts through activation of the ionotropic $GABA_A$ receptor. Its antiepileptic efficacy is similar to that of phenytoin or carbamazepine. Adverse effects on cognitive function, the propensity to produce tolerance and the risk of serious seizure exacerbation on withdrawal make it an unattractive option, and it should be used only as a last resort. In addition to cognitive effects, barbiturates may cause skin rashes, ataxia, folate deficiency, osteomalacia, behavioural disturbances (particularly in children) and an increased risk of connective tissue disorders such as Dupuytren's contracture and frozen shoulder. Phenobarbital is a potent enzyme inducer and is implicated in several clinically important drug interactions (see Table 31.5).

Phenytoin

In current practice, phenytoin is a second-line drug for focal seizures, tonic-clonic seizures, as well as atonic seizures and atypical absences. It is not effective in typical generalised absences and myoclonic seizures, where it may even be deleterious. It acts through blockage of voltage-gated sodium channel. Tolerance to its antiepileptic action does not usually occur. Phenytoin has non-linear kinetics and a low therapeutic index, and in some patients frequent drug serum level measurements may be necessary. Drug interactions (see Table 31.5) are common because phenytoin metabolism is very susceptible to inhibition by some drugs, whereas it may enhance the metabolism of others (see Table 31.7). Caution should be exercised when other medication is introduced or withdrawn. Effective dosages are between 200 and 500 mg/day.

Adverse events may occur in up to a half of those treated with phenytoin, but only about 10% will necessitate drug withdrawal, most commonly because of skin rash. Dose-related adverse reactions including nystagmus, ataxia and lethargy are common. Cosmetic effects such as gum hypertrophy, hirsutism and acne are well-recognised adverse effects and should be taken into account when prescribing for children and young women. Chronic adverse effects include folate deficiency, osteomalacia, Dupuytren's contractures and cerebellar atrophy. Serious idiosyncratic adverse events, including hepatic failure and bone marrow depression, are extremely uncommon.

Piracetam

Piracetam is indicated only for treatment of refractory myoclonus as an add-on drug. Effective dosages are between 12 and 24 mg/day. The most common side effects are diarrhoea, weight gain, insomnia and depression. There are no known idiosyncratic adverse effects or drug interactions.

Pregabalin

Pregabalin has been licensed for the adjunctive treatment of refractory focal epilepsy. It is closely related to gabapentin and a structural analogue of the neurotransmitter GABA but does not seem to affect transmitter response. It modulates calcium channels by binding to a subunit of Ca^{2+}, and this action is thought to be the basis of its antiepileptic mechanism. The recommended doses for pregabalin are between 150 and 600 mg divided into two doses, although some people may respond to doses outside this range. Pregabalin is normally started at 25 mg twice daily and increased in incremental steps of 50 mg daily every week up to 600 mg daily in two to three divided doses according to clinical need.

Overall, pregabalin is well tolerated, and so far no idiosyncratic side effects have been described. Dizziness, drowsiness, ataxia, tremor and diplopia are the most common side effects. Weight gain occurs particularly with higher doses. No pharmacokinetic interactions have yet been identified. In addition to its use in epilepsy, pregabalin has also been indicated for neuropathic pain and generalised anxiety disorders.

Primidone

Primidone is principally metabolised to phenobarbital and has similar effects but a more severe side-effect profile than phenobarbital. There is nothing to recommend primidone as an AED over phenobarbital.

Rufinamide

Rufinamide is licensed as an orphan drug for the adjunctive treatment of seizures in Lennox–Gastaut syndrome. It is a triazole derivative and is structurally unrelated to any other AED. Its mode of action is unknown. A serious hypersensitivity syndrome that may include rash, fever, lymphadenopathy, hepatic dysfunction, haematuria and multi-organ dysfunction has been reported upon initiation of therapy. Individuals should be warned to seek immediate medical assistance if signs or symptoms of hypersensitivity develop.

Sodium valproate

Sodium valproate is a broad-spectrum AED, effective over the complete range of seizures type, but with particular value in the idiopathic generalised epilepsies. This is mainly due to its broad mechanism of action, known to act on voltage-gated sodium and calcium channels, and also in the turnover of GABA. Tolerance to its antiepileptic action does not usually occur. Drug interactions with other AEDs may be problematic (see Table 31.5). Phenobarbital levels increase following co-medication with valproate, and a combination of these two drugs may result in severe sedation. Sodium valproate may also inhibit the metabolism of lamotrigine, phenytoin and carbamazepine. Enzyme-inducing drugs enhance the metabolism of sodium valproate, so caution should be exercised when other AEDs are introduced or withdrawn.

Up to a third of people may experience adverse effects, but fewer than 5% will require the drug to be stopped. Adverse effects include nausea, diarrhoea, weight gain, alopecia, skin rash and thrombocytopenia. Confusion, stupor, tremor and hyperammonaemia are usually dose related. Serious adverse events, including fatal pancreatic and hepatic failure, are extremely uncommon.

The usual therapeutic range quoted is 1–2 g daily with a maximum dosage of 2.5 g/day. Because of the lack of a good correlation between total valproate concentrations and effect, serum level monitoring of the drug has limited use. TDM should only be performed in cases of suspected toxicity, deterioration in seizure control, to check adherence or to monitor drug interactions. Sodium valproate is more teratogenic than other commonly used AEDs and should be avoided in women of childbearing age (see Table 31.7).

Stiripentol

Stiripentol is licensed as an orphan drug for severe myoclonic epilepsy of infancy (Dravet syndrome) when used in conjunction with sodium valproate and clobazam. It is an aromatic alcohol and is unrelated to any other AED. Its mode of action is unknown.

Tiagabine

Tiagabine is a drug with mild efficacy in seizure control. It is used as a second-line drug in focal seizures with or without secondary generalisation. It prevents the removal of GABA from the synaptic cleft by blockage of GABA transport. The usual dosage is between 30 and 45 mg daily in two to three divided doses, and it is normally started at 5–10 mg daily in one to two divided doses, with incremental steps of 5–10 mg every week. The most common adverse events are on the central nervous system and consist of sedation, tremor, headache, mental slowing, tiredness and dizziness. Confusion, irritability and depression may occur. Increases in seizure frequency and episodes of non-convulsive status have also been reported. Use in pregnancy is not recommended, although no teratogenicity has been reported in humans.

Topiramate

Topiramate is chemically unrelated to other AEDs and is a used as a first-line drug for people with focal seizures with or without secondary generalisation and for generalised seizure. It has multiple mechanism of action: voltage-gated sodium and calcium channels, GABA and glutamate receptors. Recommended dosages are between 75 and 300 mg/day. It has to be titrated slowly, starting with a dosage of 25 mg once daily, titrating upwards in 25- to 50 mg increments every 1–2 weeks up to a usual dosage of 100–200 mg daily in two divided doses. The maximum dosage is 500 mg/day in monotherapy or 400 mg/day as adjunctive therapy. It has no clinically significant interactions with other AEDs, although hepatic enzyme inducers accelerate its metabolism and doses need to be adjusted downwards if the patient is coming off carbamazepine or phenytoin.

Side effects include dizziness, drowsiness, irritability, impaired concentration, paraesthesias, nephrolithiasis and fatigue. People starting topiramate should increase their fluid intake to reduce the risk of kidney stones. Weight loss is seen in up to 40% of those who are taking topiramate.

Vigabatrin

Vigabatrin inhibits GABA degradation, but because of a poor safety profile it is a last resort drug for focal seizures. It is still a first-line treatment of infantile spasms, particularly if associated with tuberous sclerosis. Vigabatrin does not interact with other drugs apart from decreasing phenytoin levels, probably by blocking its absorption. The most common adverse events associated with vigabatrin are behavioural disturbances, ranging from agitation to frank psychosis and visual field defects, which had been associated with long-term treatment in up to 40–50% of patients. Other known adverse effects include drowsiness, headaches, ataxia, weight gain, depression and tremor. Careful monitoring for side effects, particularly ophthalmological, on initiation of therapy is essential.

Zonisamide

Zonisamide, a sulfonamide analogue which inhibits carbonic anhydrase, is a potent blocker of the spread of epileptic discharges. This effect is believed to be mediated through action also at voltage-sensitive sodium channels. It is used as a second-line drug for those with focal seizures with or without secondary generalisation. It can be effective in generalised seizures, particularly myoclonic seizures. Recommended dosages are between 200 and 500 mg/day, although some people may derive benefit from dosages outside this range. When used in monotherapy, the recommended starting dose is 100 mg once daily, titrating upwards every 2 weeks in 100 mg increments. The usual maintenance dosage is 300 mg once daily, and the maximum dosage is 500 mg/day. When used as adjunctive therapy, the recommended starting dosage is 50 mg daily in two divided doses for 7 days, then increased to 100 mg daily in two divided doses, and finally increased in steps of 100 mg every week. The usual maintenance dosage is 300–500 mg daily in one to two divided doses. Its long elimination half-life allows once-daily dosing.

It does not affect levels of carbamazepine, barbiturates or valproate, but may increase the serum concentration of phenytoin by about 10–15%. Zonisamide metabolism is, however, induced by carbamazepine, barbiturates and phenytoin, and higher zonisamide doses may be necessary during co-administration with these AEDs.

Side effects include dizziness, drowsiness, headaches, anorexia, weight loss, skin rashes, irritability, impaired concentration and fatigue. These are mostly transient and seem to be related to the dose and rate of titration. Nephrolithiasis has also been reported, particularly in Caucasians. It is not recommended for women of childbearing age because there are issues about its teratogenic potential.

Recent and future evidence for antiepileptic drugs

ILAE has published an updated review of AED efficacy and effectiveness as initial monotherapy for epileptic seizures and syndromes (Glauser et al., 2013). After a thorough review of published reports, they summarised the level of evidence for each seizure type and epilepsy syndrome. In adults with focal-onset seizures, carbamazepine, levetiracetam, phenytoin and zonisamide have level A evidence (highest supporting level of clinical trial evidence). Only oxcarbazepine has level A for children with focal-onset seizures, and gabapentin and lamotrigine have that level for the elderly with the same seizure type. There is no drug with level A evidence for generalised-onset tonic-clonic seizures in adults or in children. Ethosuximide and valproic acid have level A evidence in children with childhood absence epilepsy.

The new AEDs are still not capable of achieving the primary goal of epilepsy treatment – complete freedom of seizures – although some may have a more favourable profile, with lesser drug interactions and side effects. As such, this group of drugs will probably continue to expand, with new AEDs appearing in the quest of epilepsy cure.

Case studies

Case 31.1

Ms JB is a 31-year-old woman with a history of early-morning myoclonic jerks from age 14 years. When she was 18 years old she had her first convulsive seizure. A diagnosis of juvenile myoclonic epilepsy was made, and Ms JB was started on phenytoin with no results. She was then switched to topiramate, which also did not help her seizures. As a last resort, at age 18 years, she was switched to sodium valproate 1200 mg/day which fully controlled her seizures.

At the age of 21 years, she delivered a healthy baby and experienced no problems with epilepsy control. At age 22, she had her second pregnancy and delivered a healthy baby. Three weeks after delivery early-morning myoclonic seizures returned. The dose of sodium valproate was increased to 1500 mg/day to control jerks. However, 6 months later she experienced a recurrence of her convulsive attacks with no clear precipitating factor. Sodium valproate was increased to 2000 mg/day. Early-morning myoclonic seizures crept back and she had further convulsive seizures. Lamotrigine was started and she is now taking 100 mg daily. She has been completely seizure-free for the last 2 years and is now driving again.

Ms JB wants to discuss her medication with you and would like to stop treatment. She has no plans to increase her family.

Question

What advice would you give Ms JB?

Answer

Ms JB should be advised to continue on medication. She has juvenile myoclonic epilepsy, which tends to recur when medication is withdrawn. Because Ms JB has no intention of having further children, pregnancy need not be a consideration in the choice of her continued drug therapy with valproate. She is generally well, and hence it would be sensible to advise her to continue with the present regimen, because sodium valproate and lamotrigine have a synergistic effect in juvenile myoclonic epilepsy. If, however, Ms JB wants to reduce medication, then a slow decrease of sodium valproate with optimisation of treatment with lamotrigine should be considered.

Case 31.2

Mr OB is a 44-year-old man who suffers from focal epilepsy. An MRI scan shows a choroid cyst on the right temporal lobe, bilateral hippocampal sclerosis and cerebral atrophy. Seizures take the form of focal with impaired awareness and at night evolved to bilateral tonic-clonic. He has had trials of treatment with every single drug available and almost every combination.

Six months ago, he was taking 225 mg topiramate, 400 mg phenytoin and 10 mg clobazam each day. He could not tolerate a higher dose of topiramate. At this point levetiracetam was added and titrated up to 2000 mg/day. This led to a significant improvement in Mr OB's seizure control. Indeed, seizures have almost completely been abolished and he is only having occasional nocturnal events. He is, however, complaining of drowsiness and periods of unsteadiness.

Question

What treatment is appropriate for Mr OB?

Answer

Mr OB needs his drug regimen optimising. The decision should be made to reduce either the dose of topiramate or that of phenytoin. Usually phenytoin is reduced first, as it is an enzyme inducer. However, because Mr OB has had a bad experience in the past when an attempt was made to discontinue phenytoin, at which time he had a significant increase in seizure frequency, it would, therefore, be more appropriate to discontinue topiramate. This was done and his improvement has been maintained.

Case 31.3

Ms GD is a 28-year-old woman with a history of early-morning myoclonic jerks since age 14 years. At 16 years of age she presented with her first generalised tonic clonic convulsive seizure and was referred to a hospital specialist who diagnosed juvenile myoclonic epilepsy. At that time Ms GD was started on sodium valproate 1200 mg/day and within a few weeks her seizures were totally controlled. Ms GD has since remained on the same medication and has been well controlled. However, she now wishes to start a family and is concerned about the effects of the valproate on her baby.

Question

What advice would you give Ms GD?

Answer

Sodium valproate is teratogenic, with the most common malformation reported being neural tube defects. Ms GD has had no seizures for more than 5 years, and it must, therefore, be determined whether she still needs medication. The risk of recurrence is low because she has been seizure free for well over 5 years. An important consideration is whether she is a driver, because if she is taken off medication and has a seizure, she will be unable to hold a license. The other issue is the effect of pregnancy on her seizures because some women may experience an increase in seizures during pregnancy. The options that need to be considered include change of medication. The following drugs would be alternatives: lamotrigine, zonisamide and levetiracetam.

Case 31.4

Mr TD is a 41-year-old man who has cryptogenic focal epilepsy. Mr TD experienced his first seizure at age 14, and this was diagnosed as a secondary generalised attack, although discussing his history revealed he might have had focal with impaired awareness seizures. Two years ago Mr TD was referred for assessment, but it was determined that he was not a candidate for surgery. Mr TD was taking carbamazepine 1200 mg/day and could not tolerate higher doses. Previous trials of valproate, phenytoin, phenobarbital, vigabatrin, lamotrigine, oxcarbazepine and topiramate had demonstrated little benefit. Levetiracetam was started and increased to 2500 mg. Improvement in Mr TD's seizure control has been noted over the past 2 years, with only two nocturnal focal with impaired awareness seizures recorded. His current medication is levetiracetam 2500 mg/day and carbamazepine 1200 mg/day.

Question

Should TD's therapy be reduced to levetiracetam monotherapy?

Answer

If a person has been seizure free for 3 years, it is good practice to review therapy. There is a need to discuss with Mr TD whether he wishes to continue with his medication. Issues of relevance include a long history of epilepsy, the diagnosis and the range of drugs previously tried which may indicate an increased risk of seizure recurrence on coming off drugs. It also needs to be clear whether he wishes to drive, because a recurrence would lead to him having to surrender his driving license.

Case 31.5

Mr FD is a 23-year-old student who was involved in a road traffic accident and admitted to hospital with a head trauma. He was stabilised, but during his admission he had a seizure and was then discharged on no medication. Three months later Mr FD attended an outpatient hospital follow-up appointment and was identified to have had no further seizures.

Question

Was Mr FD's clinical management appropriate, and is there a role for prophylactic anticonvulsant medication?

Answer

Mr FD requires a full neurological review. The long-term use of antiepileptics following head injury is not indicated unless the person has a history of seizures, and Mr FD has had no seizures post-discharge.

Case 31.6

Mr RA is a 75-year-old retired teacher who lives alone. He has longstanding epilepsy, and his current medication includes phenytoin 300 mg daily. Mr RA suffered a recent fall and was rushed to hospital with a suspected fractured neck of femur. On admission he was stabilised and found not to have sustained a fracture. His other medication was furosemide 40 mg in the morning and enalapril 5 mg twice daily. Routine blood levels of the anticonvulsants revealed a toxic level of phenytoin of 40 mg/L (normal therapeutic range 10–20 mg/L).

Question

How long will it take for the toxic levels of phenytoin to fall within the therapeutic range?

Answer

Phenytoin exhibits non-linear pharmacokinetics. Usual management will involve withholding phenytoin and monitoring serum levels each day. One assumption that can be made is that if the hepatic enzymes are fully saturated with phenytoin, then at maximum metabolic capacity approximately 10 mg/L of the drug will be eliminated each day. Initially, however, the drug will redistribute into serum, so for the first few days phenytoin levels will fall slowly. It is usual for the levels to take 6–7 days to fall within the therapeutic range. Therapy will then need to be reviewed. On further investigation it was found that Mr RA had a severe chest infection and was prescribed ciprofloxacin. His antibiotic regimen was completed 5 days ago. Mr RA was suffering from phenytoin toxicity which may have resulted in ataxia and contributed to his fall.

References

Duncan, J.S., Sander, J.W., Sisodiya, S.M., Walker, M.C., 2006. Adult epilepsy. Lancet 367, 1087–1100.
Fisher, R.S., Acevedo, C., Arzimanoglou, A., et al., 2014. ILAE official report: a practical clinical definition of epilepsy. Epilepsia 55, 475–482.
Fisher, R.S., Cross, J.H., French, J.A., et al., 2017. Operational classification of seizure types by the International League Against Epilepsy: position paper of the ILAE Commission for Classification and Terminology. Epilepsia 58 (4), 522–530.
Glauser, T., Ben-Menachem, E., Bourgeois, B., et al., 2013. ILAE Subcommission on AED Guidelines. ILAE Subcommission on AED Guidelines. Updated ILAE evidence review of antiepileptic drug efficacy and effectiveness as initial monotherapy for epileptic seizures and syndromes. Epilepsia 54, 551–563.
Medicines and Healthcare products Regulatory Agency (MHRA), 2013. Formulation switching of antiepileptic drugs: a report on the recommendations of the Commission on Human Medicines from July 2013. Available at: http://webarchive.nationalarchives.gov.uk/20141205150130/http://www.mhra.gov.uk/home/groups/comms-ic/documents/websiteresources/con341226.pdf.

National Institute for Health and Care Excellence (NICE), 2012. Epilepsies: diagnosis and management. Clinical guideline [CG137]. Available at: https://www.nice.org.uk/guidance/cg137.
National Institute for Health and Care Excellence (NICE), 2014. Evidence update 53: the epilepsies. Available at: http://www.nice.org.uk/guidance/cg137/evidence/evidence-update-544389949.
Sabers, A., Gram, L., 2000. Newer anticonvulsants: comparative review of drug interactions and adverse effects. Drugs 60, 23–33.
Thurman, D.J., Logroscino, G., Beghi, E., et al., 2017. The burden of premature mortality of epilepsy in high-income countries: a systematic review from the Mortality Task Force of the International League Against Epilepsy. Epilepsia 58, 17–26.
Tomson, T., Walczak, T., Sillanpaa, M., et al., 2005. Sudden unexpected death in epilepsy: a review of incidence and risk factors. Epilepsia 46 (Suppl. 11), 54–61.
World Health Organization (WHO), 2015. Epilepsy, key facts. Fact Sheet Number 999. Available at: http://www.who.int/mediacentre/factsheets/fs999/en/.

Further reading

Nair, D.R., Nair, R., O'Dyer, R. (Eds.), 2010. Epilepsy. Clinical Publishing, Oxford.

National Institute for Health and Care Excellence (NICE), 2013. Epilepsy in adults. Available at: http://www.nice.org.uk/guidance/qs26.

National Institute for Health and Care Excellence (NICE), 2013. Epilepsy in children and young people. Available at: http://www.nice.org.uk/guidance/qs27.

Perucca, E., Tomson, T., 2011. The pharmacological treatment of epilepsy in adults. Lancet Neurol. 10 (5), 446–456.

Schmidt, D., Schachter, S.C., 2014. Drug treatment of epilepsy in adults. Br. Med. J. 348, g254.

Trinka, E., Cock, H., Hesdorffer, D., et al., 2015. A definition and classification of status epilepticus—report of the ILAE Task Force on Classification of Status Epilepticus. Epilepsia 56, 1515–1523.

Wyllie, E., 2015. Wyllie's Treatment of Epilepsy: Principles and Practice, sixth ed. Lippincott Williams and Wilkins, Philadelphia.

32 Parkinson's Disease

Emma Lane and Roger Barker

Key points

- Parkinson's disease is the second most common neurodegenerative disease, affecting 1% of the population older than 65 years.

- Parkinson's disease is characterised by bradykinesia, resting tremor, rigidity and, later in the disease course, postural instability.

- A range of non-motor features including psychiatric, cognitive and autonomic impairments contribute significantly to an impaired quality of life and are present from early in the disease course in many cases.

- Neuronal loss in the brainstem (substantia nigra) leads to a profound dopamine deficiency in the striatum. This provides the rationale for dopaminergic replacement therapies, although the pathology is not restricted to this site.

- Levodopa, coupled with an amino acid decarboxylase inhibitor, remains the most potent oral treatment for Parkinson's disease.

- End-of-dose wearing off and on–off fluctuations are motor complications synonymous with the ongoing use of levodopa. Despite advances in oral pharmacotherapy, the on–off phenomenon can be difficult to treat effectively.

- Other dopaminergic therapies are available for the management of Parkinson's disease. Dopamine agonists are used, sometimes as first-line therapy, in younger patients, although the increasing recognition of the neuropsychiatric problems that can arise with these agents has reduced their use. It is now therefore recommended that information regarding impulse control disorders is explicitly given to patients when such drugs are used.

- Dopamine agonists can also be given as adjunctive therapies to levodopa, when the primary aim is to smooth out motor fluctuations.

- Other interventions including surgical treatments of Parkinson's disease, such as deep brain stimulation of the subthalamic nucleus, are effective in certain patients with marked motor fluctuations.

- Advanced Parkinson's disease is difficult to manage, particularly the emerging dementia and neuropsychiatric problems. Reduction of dopaminergic therapy is the first approach, and rivastigmine and other cholinesterase inhibitors may be useful for the dementia associated with Parkinson's disease.

Parkinson's disease (PD) is the most common cause of Parkinsonism and is the second most common neurodegenerative disease, after Alzheimer's disease. Although descriptions of the condition appeared before the 19th century, it was James Parkinson's eloquent account in 1817 that fully documented the clinical features of the illness and Charcot in the late 19th century who named the condition after him. Identification of the dopamine deficiency and loss of pigmented neurons in the substantia nigra occurred in the middle part of the 20th century and was soon followed by the introduction of dopamine replacement therapy with levodopa. Although excellent at managing some of the motor features, levodopa is associated with the development of motor complications after some years in the form of on–off problems and dyskinesias. Such complications can now be treated using a range of other therapeutics including more invasive approaches such as deep brain stimulation.

In addition to these motor features, only some of which respond to dopaminergic agents, the identification of a host of non-motor symptoms from disease onset (and in some cases even ahead of them) is now known to contribute in a major way to the quality of life of patients with PD. This similarly presents a complex therapeutic challenge.

Background

PD affects 1% of the population that are more than 65 years of age, increasing to 2% over the age of 80 years. One in 20 patients is, however, diagnosed before their 40th year. It is estimated that PD affects around 127,000 people in the UK, with more than 6 million sufferers worldwide. Demographically the disease is believed to have a small male/female predominance (around 3:2). Prevalence is recorded as slightly higher in European and North and South American populations compared with Arabic, African and Asian countries. The biggest risk factor for the disease is age, which has major implications for public health as the lifespan of the world's population increases.

Parkinsonism describes the main motor features of the disease but can also be a feature of other, less common neurodegenerative conditions (multiple system atrophy [MSA], progressive supranuclear palsy and corticobasal degeneration), as well as a side effect of various medications.

Aetiology

Both genetic and environmental factors are likely to contribute to the risk of development of PD (Fig. 32.1), with environmental factors precipitating the onset of PD in a genetically susceptible individual.

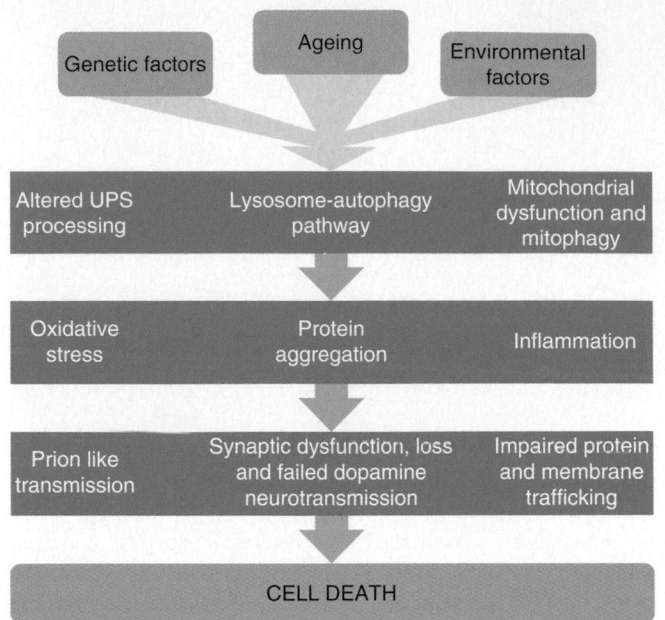

Fig. 32.1 Summary of pathophysiological processes considered to be central to Parkinson's disease.
UPS, Ubiquitin proteasome system.

Environment

The relevance of environmental factors came to the fore in the 1980s, when drug addicts attempting to manufacture pethidine accidently produced a toxin called MPTP (1-methyl-4-phenyl-1,2,3,6-tetrahydropyridine). The severe Parkinsonian state induced by inhalation or injection of the toxin produced a clinical syndrome that was indistinguishable from advanced PD. Similarities in the structure of MPTP to the commonly used herbicide paraquat opened up exploration of the role of chemicals used in the agricultural industry. Pesticide exposure, rural living, agricultural occupation and well water drinking alongside head injury are all associated with an increased risk of development of PD. Conversely, tobacco smoking, coffee drinking, non-steroidal anti-inflammatory drug use, calcium channel blocker use and alcohol consumption have all been linked to a reduced risk of the disease (Bellou et al., 2016).

Genetics

Single monogenic causes for PD account for a very small number of patients. The first gene of this nature to be discovered was that encoding a mutation in the synaptic protein α-synuclein (Polymeropoulos et al., 1997). Shortly after its identification as the causative gene in this familial form of PD, it was found to be the major component of the intracellular protein accumulations, Lewy bodies that characterise sporadic disease (Spillantini et al., 1997). This highlighted that this protein was central to what goes wrong in all cases of PD and was not just the preserve of a rare familial form of

the condition. Since this discovery, duplication and triplication in the α-synuclein gene, as well as further mutations in it along with mutations in many other genes, have been found to contribute to familial forms of the disease. However, the phenotypic nature of these forms of Parkinsonism is often different from idiopathic disease, causing atypical or early-onset forms of the disease, with the exception of the LRRK2 families.

Although these genes form very much the minority of cases, there is nevertheless clear genetic risk of the development of PD, as is evidenced by recent large genome-wide associated studies (Bras et al., 2015; Edwards et al., 2011). This has revealed a large number of genetic loci linked to an increased risk of development of the disorder.

More recently, through careful clinical observation in Gaucher's disease families, it was recognised that one of the strongest genetic risk factors is a heterozygous mutation in the *GBA* gene. This is found in between 5% and 10% of patients with so-called sporadic disease.

Pathophysiology

The two characteristic pathological features of PD are neuronal loss, especially in the pigmented brainstem nuclei, together with the presence of eosinophilic inclusion bodies, called Lewy bodies, in surviving cells. Dopaminergic neurones within the substantia nigra pars compacta, projecting to the striatum, are particularly affected by the disease, leading to a loss of dopamine in the terminal region. There is considerable reserve in this pathway, and a loss of more than 50% of nigral neurones occurs before overt motor features appear. The identification of Lewy bodies in other areas of the central nervous system (CNS) means that dopamine is not the only neurotransmitter system affected, and all of this correlates with the increasing recognition of the range of other clinical features seen in the course of the disease, some of which even precede the development of the motor phenotype.

Indeed, neuropathologically, the Braak hypothesis proposes that α-synuclein may first accumulate in the dorsal vagal nucleus of the lower brainstem and then gradually ascend rostrally to affect critical brain regions including the substantia nigra and ultimately the cerebral cortex (Braak et al., 2003). If true, this would suggest that prior to the loss of dopamine cells, other cell populations should be affected, resulting in changes in bowel control, mood, sleep and locomotion, all of which would fit with the prodromal features that many patients with PD report. In addition there is early pathology in the olfactory bulb which may also account for the loss of sense of smell that many patients experience ahead of them developing overt motor problems.

All of this not only accounts for the features of prodromal PD, but also the deficits that are reported as the disease evolves and which typically do not respond to dopaminergic replacement therapies.

Clinical features

Motor features

A prerequisite feature for a diagnosis of PD is the presence of bradykinesia. This is the slowness of initiation of voluntary movement, with progressive reduction in speed of repetitive actions. The other cardinal features of the disease are tremor when at rest (pill-rolling tremor), postural instability and cogwheel rigidity. Cogwheel rigidity describes the jerky resistance when limbs are moved. These are listed in most diagnostic guidelines for PD. The disease presents asymmetrically and patients continue to report a 'bad side' as the disease progresses, although pure unilateral disease is rare, and usually raises concerns that some other disease process is occurring if this is the case. It is important to note, however, that many patients (15–20%) never really develop a tremor, whereas up to 60% of people with PD may have a dominant postural tremor (tremor-dominant), worse with the arms held outstrctched, which can cause diagnostic confusion with essential tremor (ET). Postural instability is an important milestone in PD, and typically more than half of patients will reach this stage within 10 years of diagnosis. This problem comprises an impairment of righting reflexes, which leads to impaired gait and increased risk of falling.

Patients typically display a characteristic stooped posture and loss of arm swing when walking, which is often a very helpful early diagnostic sign when seeing patients for the first time. There is reduced blink frequency and facial expression (hypomimia), which, together with a low-volume (hypophonic), monotonous speech, may lead to significant difficulties in communication. All of this can easily be misdiagnosed as depression. Writing becomes small (micrographia) and barely legible, with the words falling off the line as the patient continues to write.

Non-motor features

A range of non-motor features encompassing autonomic, cognitive and psychiatric problems are seen in nearly all cases of PD and have a pronounced effect on quality of life. They can precede disease onset and tend to become more prominent as the condition evolves. Common autonomic problems include postural hypotension (falling blood pressure on standing) which may contribute to falls and blackouts later in the disease course and is a leading cause of hospitalisation for patients with PD. Constipation can be an ongoing problem that may precede the diagnosis of PD by up to 20 years and relates possibly to pathology in the enteric nervous system. In terms of psychiatric problems, depression affects approximately 40% of patients and is a major determinant of both carer stress and nursing home placement. Paranoia and hallucinations occur in many patients typically as a prelude of the dementia, but often are provoked and worsened by dopaminergic and related drugs used to treat PD. In addition some of the dopaminergic agonists can induce major behavioural problems in some patients, especially young male patients with PD.

Cognitive impairment at a very mild level is now thought to be present in many patients at diagnosis. However, the development of a frank dementia tends to occur later on in the disease course and is especially related to the age of the patient at disease onset. Younger onset patients may show cognitive impairment but evolve to a dementia at a slower rate compared with older patients. Longitudinal community-based studies indicate that dementia may ultimately develop in 80% of people with PD (Hely et al., 2008). The cognitive impairment that defines the dementia is often associated with the symptoms of hallucinations that are typically visual with delusional misinterpretation, including paranoid ideation, and rapid fluctuations in attention.

Finally many patients complain of sleep problems, with the major one being a REM sleep behavioural disorder that can occur ahead of the diagnosis of PD. This condition is characterised by patients acting out their dreams. In addition many patients complain of a restless leg syndrome and limb pain.

Differential diagnosis

Although PD is a common form of Parkinsonism, there are numerous other diseases that present with Parkinsonism. A detailed description of these different causes is beyond the scope of this chapter, but a few points should be highlighted. ET is a common condition but does not cause bradykinesia. Nevertheless, it may be very difficult to differentiate from tremor-dominant PD. In about 50% of cases of ET there is a positive family history and in a similar number a good response to a low dose of alcohol. If there are doubts, some form of nuclear medicine imaging looking at dopamine in the brain can help distinguish tremulous PD from ET.

Several clinical and clinicopathological series have highlighted the problems in making a correct diagnosis of PD. If clinical criteria, such as those produced by the UK Parkinson's Disease Brain Bank, are not applied, then the error rate (false-negative diagnosis) may be as high as 25–30%. These criteria are listed in Box 32.1. The common conditions misdiagnosed as PD, outside of ET or dystonic tremor, are other neurodegenerative disorders such as progressive supranuclear palsy, MSA and corticobasal degeneration, as well as small vessel disease affecting the brain.

Drug-induced Parkinsonism

An important differential diagnosis to consider when a patient presents with Parkinsonism is whether their symptoms and signs may be drug induced. This is because drug-induced Parkinsonism is potentially reversible upon cessation of the drug. Reports linking drug-induced Parkinsonism with the neuroleptic chlorpromazine were first published in the 1950s. Since then, numerous other agents have been associated with it. Many of these are widely recognised, although others are not (Table 32.1). Repeat prescription of vestibular sedatives and antiemetics such as prochlorperazine and cinnarizine are the most commonly encountered causes of drug-induced Parkinsonism. The pathogenesis of drug-induced Parkinsonism is likely due to dopamine receptor blockade, but only in part because there is no clear correlation in incidence and severity with the drug dosage and length of exposure. Sodium valproate is also now recognised to cause an encephalopathy dominated by Parkinsonism and cognitive impairment which is reversible upon drug cessation.

Box 32.1 Clinical criteria for diagnosis of Parkinson's disease

Step 1: Diagnosis of Parkinsonian syndrome
The patient has bradykinesia, *plus one or more* of the following:
a. classic rest tremor, 4–6 Hz
b. muscular rigidity
c. postural instability, without other explanation

Step 2: Exclusion criteria for PD suggesting an alternate diagnosis
a. history of repeated strokes
b. history of repeated head injury
c. history of definite encephalitis
d. oculogyric crises
e. dopamine receptor blocking agent exposure at onset of symptoms
f. more than one affected relative (often not applied)
g. sustained remission
h. strictly unilateral features after 3 years
i. supranuclear gaze palsy
j. cerebellar signs
k. early severe autonomic involvement
l. early severe dementia
m. extensor plantar
n. cerebral tumour or hydrocephalus on CT scan or MRI
o. negative response to large doses of levodopa
p. MPTP exposure

Step 3 Supportive prospective positive criteria for PD (three or more required for diagnosis of definite PD)
a. unilateral onset
b. rest tremor present
c. progressive disorder
d. progressive persistent asymmetry
e. an excellent (>70%) response to levodopa
f. a sustained (>5 years) response to levodopa
g. severe levodopa-induced dyskinesias
h. clinical course >10 years
For a diagnosis, step one should be fulfilled with no exclusion criteria and three supportive criteria should also be present.

CT, Computed tomography; MPTP, 1-methyl-4-phenyl-1,2,3,6-tetrahydropyridine; MRI, magnetic resonance imaging; PD, Parkinson's disease.

Table 32.1 Examples of non-neuroleptic drugs associated with drug-induced Parkinsonism

Medication	Comment
Cinnarizine, metoclopramide, prochlorperazine	Antiemetics
Antipsychotics	Dose-dependent effects; clozapine least associated with abnormal movements
Tetrabenazine	Used to treat chorea through a catecholamine-depleting action
Sodium valproate, Non-steriodal anti-inflammatory drugs, amiodarone, phenytoin, oral contraceptives	Unclear how they cause Parkinsonism
Lithium	Lithium causes postural tremor; reports of Parkinsonism occurring with lithium have usually been in the context of prior exposure to neuroleptics
Phenelzine 5-Fluorouracil Pethidine Vincristine-Adriamycin	Only single case reports of drug-induced Parkinsonism with these drugs
Amphotericin	One case report of drug-induced Parkinsonism in a child after bone marrow transplantation and a second in association with cytosine arabinoside therapy

Drug-induced Parkinsonism is more common in the elderly and in women. The clinical features can be indistinguishable from PD, although the signs in drug-induced Parkinsonism are more likely to be bilateral at onset. Withdrawal of the offending agent will lead to improvement and resolution of symptoms and signs in approximately 80% of patients within 8 weeks of discontinuation. Drug-induced Parkinsonism may, however, take up to 18 months to fully resolve in some cases. Further, in other patients, the Parkinsonism may improve after stopping the drug, only to then deteriorate. In this situation, the drug may have unmasked previously latent PD.

Investigations

The diagnosis of PD is a clinical one and should be based, preferably, upon validated criteria. In young-onset or clinically atypical PD, a number of investigations may be appropriate. These include copper studies and DNA testing to exclude Wilson's disease and Huntington's or mitochondrial disease, respectively. Brain imaging by computed tomography (CT) or magnetic resonance imaging (MRI) may be necessary to exclude hydrocephalus, cerebrovascular disease or basal ganglia abnormalities suggestive of an underlying metabolic cause. When there is difficulty in distinguishing PD from ET, a form of functional imaging called [123I]β-CIT (2ß-carbomethoxy-3β-(4-iodophenyl) tropane) single-photon emission computerised tomography (FP-CIT SPECT; also known as DaTSCAN) may be useful, because this technique can sensitively identify loss of nigrostriatal dopaminergic terminals in the striatum (Fig. 32.2). Thus, in ET, the SPECT scan is normal, whereas in PD, reduced tracer uptake is seen (Jennings et al., 2004).

Differentiating PD from MSA and progressive supranuclear palsy is not an uncommon clinical problem and may be very difficult, particularly in the early disease stages and especially in the case of MSA-Parkinsonism. FP-CIT SPECT cannot differentiate PD from these other forms of degenerative Parkinsonism. MRI brain scanning, anal sphincter electromyography, tilt table testing for orthostatic hypotension and eye movement recordings may all be of some help, although they are rarely diagnostic in their own right. Typically the diagnosis in these cases becomes apparent over time, and should always be considered when patients

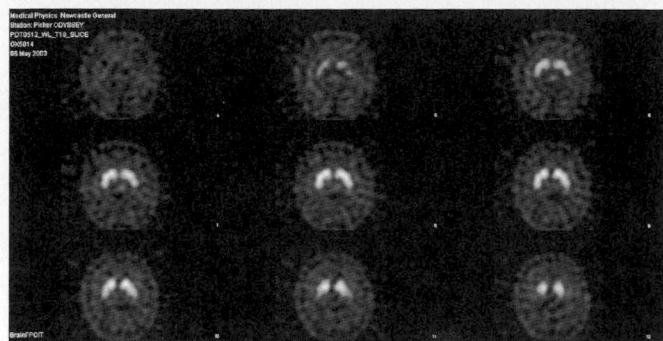

Fig. 32.2 A normal FP-CIT SPECT scan image, showing symmetric tracer uptake in both striata (mirror image commas). In Parkinson's disease, the tail of the comma is lost at an early stage, with the most severe loss being contralateral to the side most affected clinically.

respond poorly to dopaminergic therapies with early involvement of other systems outside the nigrostriatal system such as autonomic dysfunction.

Treatment

General approach

The treatment of PD at the current time is wholly symptomatic. No drug has proven to have significant disease-modifying or neuroprotective capabilities, although monoamine oxidase type B (MAO-B) inhibitors have been explored for such activity. At the present time there are several ongoing clinical trials looking at possible disease-modifying therapies which include the neurotrophic factor GDNF, as well as the GLP-1 agonists exenatide and liraglutide.

There is no accepted algorithm for the treatment of PD, although guidance has been produced by the National Institute for Health and Care Excellence (NICE, 2017). A number of factors may influence the first choice therapy for management of motor symptoms, including patient preference, quality of life, severity and type of disease (tremor-dominant vs akinetic rigid), comorbidities and potential benefits and harms of the medicines (Table 32.2).

The principles of treatment with levodopa have changed little in practice since its initial introduction in 1967, when the drug was started in low doses and gradually increased thereafter (Cotzias et al., 1967). The benefits that levodopa treatment confers make it the gold standard to this day, nearly 50 years on from its first introduction. Until quite recently it was not often the first-line approach in newly diagnosed patients, but this has changed of late with the recognition of the behavioural problems that dopamine agonists can induce. Thus, many clinicians will now start patients on low-dose levodopa in preference to dopamine agonists, even though this is likely to precipitate the well-recognised motor complications of long-term levodopa therapy earlier. These include a premature wearing off of the anti-Parkinsonian effects of levodopa and fluctuations in the response with the development of involuntary movements known as dyskinesias. These typically occur after a number of years of treatment and relate as much to the duration of disease as to the drug itself.

The first problem that patients typically describe with levodopa is a wearing-off effect, in which the patient finds that the effect of the medicine does not last until their next dose is due. This manifests itself as the patient starting to 'go off' as they approach their next dosing time. With time this evolves into more complex on–off problems, where patients can 'go off' for no obvious reason. This stage of the illness is also often accompanied by levodopa-induced dyskinesias. Dyskinesias are classed depending on their relationship to levodopa dosing occurring at the peak of levodopa response, so-called peak dose dyskinesia (the commonest type), 'diphasic dyskinesia' at the start and end of levodopa therapy, and the end of dose 'wearing off' dyskinesia. These problems emerge at a rate of approximately 10% per year, so that by 10 years into their illness all PD patients can expect to experience some motor fluctuations of this type. Notably, however, levodopa-induced dyskinesias and fluctuations develop earlier in younger patients with PD and relate to the dose of medication they are given (Rascol et al., 2000). On–off episodes may be extremely disabling and remain a major therapeutic challenge in the management of PD, although the development of deep brain stimulation and enteral delivery systems for dopaminergic agents have proven beneficial in managing this aspect of PD.

There are limited pharmacotherapeutic options for the management of dyskinesia, so management trends have shifted towards keeping the levodopa dose to a minimum or a 'levodopa-sparing approach'. This takes the form of either later administration of levodopa, provided alternative treatments can give adequate symptomatic control, or the use of combination therapies, in an effort to reduce the cumulative dose of levodopa given. However, the benefit of this approach beyond 5 years into the illness remains a matter of debate.

Drug treatment

Levodopa preparations

Immediate-release levodopa. Irrespective of the debate regarding when to start levodopa therapy, there is no doubt that levodopa remains the most effective oral symptomatic treatment for PD. It is administered with the peripheral dopa-decarboxylase inhibitors carbidopa or benserazide, where carbidopa plus levodopa is known as co-careldopa (Sinemet) and benserazide plus levodopa is co-beneldopa (Madopar). The decarboxylase inhibitor blocks the peripheral conversion of levodopa to dopamine and thereby allows a lower dose of levodopa to be administered. Levodopa readily crosses the blood–brain barrier and is converted by endogenous aromatic amino acid decarboxylase to dopamine and then stored in the surviving nigrostriatal nerve terminals.

Immediate-release co-beneldopa is usually commenced in a dosage of 50 mg, typically three times a day. The patient may be

Table 32.2 Potential benefits and harms of dopamine agonists, levodopa and monoamine oxidase type B inhibitors

	Levodopa	Dopamine agonists	Monoamine oxidase B inhibitors
Motor symptoms	More improvement in motor symptoms	Less improvement in motor symptoms	Less improvement in motor symptoms
Activities of daily living	More improvemet in activities of daily living	Less improvement in activities of daily living	Less improvement in activities of daily living
Motor complications	More motor complications	Fewer motor complications	Fewer motor complications
Adverse events	Fewer specified adverse events*	More specified adverse events*	Fewer specified adverse events*

*Excessive sleepiness, hallucinations and impulse control disorders (see the summary of product characteristics for full information on individual medicines).
With kind permission from NICE (2017).

instructed in the early stage of the illness to take the drug with food to minimise nausea. Paradoxically, in more advanced PD, it may be beneficial to take levodopa 30 minutes or so before food, as dietary protein can critically interfere with the absorption of the drug. If there is little or no response to 50 mg three times daily, the unit dose may be doubled to 100 mg. Should the patient's levodopa dose escalate to 600 mg/day with no significant response, the diagnosis of PD should be reviewed. Levodopa, commenced in the above way, is usually well tolerated. Nausea, vomiting and orthostatic hypotension are the most commonly encountered side effects. These adverse events may be circumvented by increasing the levodopa dose more slowly, or co-prescribing domperidone 10 or 20 mg three times daily; however, recently there have been some concerns with the cardiac safety of this agent. Later in the illness, and in common with all anti-Parkinsonian drugs, levodopa may cause vivid dreams, nightmares or even precipitate a confusional state, which tends to indicate that the patient is starting to develop a PD dementia.

Clinically relevant drug interactions with levodopa include hypertensive crises with MAO-A inhibitors. Levodopa should, therefore, be avoided for at least 2 weeks after stopping the inhibitor, although the non-selective forms of these drugs are rarely prescribed nowadays. Levodopa can also enhance the hypotensive effects of antihypertensive agents and may antagonise the action of antipsychotics. The absorption of levodopa may be reduced by concomitant administration of oral iron preparations.

Controlled-release levodopa. Both Sinemet and Madopar are available as controlled-release (CR) preparations. The nomenclature for Sinemet CR is confusing, as the drug is marketed as Sinemet CR (carbidopa/levodopa 50/200) and also as Half Sinemet CR (carbidopa/levodopa 25/100). Trying to prescribe Half Sinemet CR unambiguously can be difficult. If the instruction is misinterpreted and a tablet of Sinemet CR is halved, the slow-release mechanism is actually disrupted.

Levodopa in CR preparations has a bioavailability of 60–70%, which is less than the 90–100% obtained from immediate-release formulations. CR preparations have a response duration of 2–4 hours, compared with 1–3 hours for immediate release. Limited benefit has been shown for CR use over immediate-release levodopa in terms of dyskinesia development and response fluctuation frequency. However, CR preparations may be of help in simplifying drug regimens, in relieving nocturnal akinesia, and in co-prescribing with immediate-release levodopa during the day to relieve end-of-dose deterioration.

Two commonly encountered problems with CR preparations are, first, changing the patient from all immediate-release to all CR levodopa. This is poorly tolerated, because CR levodopa has a longer latency than immediate-release levodopa to turn the patient 'on' (typically 60–90 vs 30–50 minutes), and the patient's perception is that the quality of their 'on' period is poorer. Second, CR preparations should not be prescribed more than four times a day, because the levodopa may accumulate, causing unpredictable motor fluctuations and especially leading to dyskinesias later in the day.

Co-careldopa intestinal gel. An intestinal gel preparation of levodopa and carbidopa (Duodopa) is currently available that is administered directly into the small bowel (specifically, the jejunum) via a percutaneous route, using a portable electronic pump. Through continuous delivery in this way, motor fluctuations may be significantly reduced. Although effective, this treatment modality requires careful patient selection, and because of its cost, it is constantly being reviewed by central agencies authorising drug choice in PD. The endoscopic insertion of a percutaneous jejunostomy carries a definite morbidity and mortality. The treatment is also very expensive while mechanical problems with tube detachment and blockage have been reported. Thus, it is currently used only in advanced fluctuating patients who are deemed not to be suitable for deep brain stimulation or apomorphine infusions.

Other prolonged-release levodopa preparations that are in clinical trials include Rytary (IPX066) which is currently available in the USA. It utilises a mixed population of coated microspheres to vary the rate of release in a controlled fashion to provide the benefit of immediate relief as well as prolonging that benefit through slower release of the active agent. Two gastric retentive formulations are also in development, which slow down the passage of the drug through the pylorus aperture to improve levodopa uptake.

Dopamine agonists

In theory, dopamine agonists, which stimulate dopamine receptors both post- and pre-synaptically, would seem to be a very attractive therapeutic option in PD, because they may bypass the degenerating nigrostriatal dopaminergic neurones. Unfortunately, experience to date with the current oral agents reveals them to be less potent than levodopa and less well tolerated, with significant risks of side effects, for example, impulse control disorders, that have been more recognised since the beginning of this century.

Of the two main structural classes, the ergot- and non-ergot-derived dopamine agonists differ in their affinity for different members of the dopamine receptor families. Predominant activity is through the D2-like receptor class, whereas some express a preferential binding for D3 subtypes over D2. It is not known whether these differences are clinically significant, but experience to date would suggest not. Plasma half-lives vary considerably; cabergoline is an ergot dopamine agonist with a plasma half-life of 63–68 hours, meaning that once-daily dosing is possible, although it is now rarely used because of its fibrotic side effects. Ropinirole and pramipexole are non-ergot derivatives that originally had to be administered three times daily and have become the dopamine agonists of choice nowadays. Slow-release preparations of ropinirole (XL) and pramipexole (PR) are available for once-daily dosing. A transdermally administered non-ergot dopamine agonist, rotigotine, is also available as a 24-hour adhesive patch.

There have been very few comparative studies performed between the dopamine agonists, so it is not possible to be definitive as to which drug should be recommended. However, currently, ergot-derived dopamine agonists are avoided because of the side effects and the need, therefore, for annual screening of patients receiving these drugs. Thus, ropinirole, pramipexole and rotigotine are the most widely prescribed dopamine agonists, and if a patient does not get on with one of these, it may be worthwhile changing from one agonist to another, because there is variability in a given patient's tolerance to the different drugs.

Dopamine agonist side effects. The principal side effects of the dopamine agonists are nausea and vomiting, postural hypotension, hallucinations, confusion and, in some cases, major behavioural problems linked to impulse control disorders. These latter problems can be very significant and lead to major financial and social problems. Thus, there is a greater emphasis now on informing patients about these side effects when they are prescribed these drugs, with a recommendation that this advice is clearly documented in the hospital notes (NICE, 2017). Ergot derivatives run the risk of causing pleuropulmonary fibrosis and therefore are not routinely used anymore.

Ropinirole and pramipexole were previously implicated in causing 'sleep attacks', with sudden onset of drowsiness, leading to driving accidents in some cases. The term sleep attack is almost certainly a misnomer, however, as patients do have warning of impending sleepiness, although they may subsequently be amnesic for up to several minutes while in this state. Excessive sleepiness attributable to anti-Parkinsonian drugs is actually not a new phenomenon and is almost certainly a 'class effect' of all dopaminergic therapies. It is essential to advise patients who are taking all anti-Parkinsonian agents that they may be prone to excessive drowsiness. This may be compounded by the use of other sedative drugs and alcohol.

Dopamine agonists have also been associated with impulse control disorders. These disorders include pathological gambling, hypersexuality, punding and excessive shopping. The onset may relate to dopamine D2/3 receptor stimulation in predisposed individuals. Patients and their carers should be warned about these potential problems before the drug is prescribed, and patients should be regularly screened for abnormal behaviours while taking the agonist. However, in some cases, patients hide this information from their treating clinician, as well as family, and the problems are identified only when a major crisis emerges as a consequence of this behaviour, for example, house repossession, among others. This latter problem with impulse control disorders, although rare, has meant that these dopamine agonist therapies are now used less as first-line treatments, and this has been reflected in the NICE guidelines (NICE, 2017).

Apomorphine

Apomorphine is a specialised drug in the treatment of advanced PD, but almost certainly continues to be underused. It is the most potent non-selective dopamine agonist available but has a short half-life, a single bolus administration lasting for 45–60 minutes. It is therefore administered as either a bolus or subcutaneous infusion depending on the purpose. A bolus subcutaneous injection of apomorphine is suitable for patients who are optimised on their oral medications but who still suffer from troublesome, typically unpredictable 'off' periods or would benefit from rapid early-morning relief until their oral medication takes effect. Alternatively, continuous infusion is a useful therapeutic option in patients who are no longer well controlled by standard oral therapies and in whom apomorphine injections have proven effective. Frequent use of the injection (four to six times per day) is associated with increasing dyskinesia, so control is improved by the continuous infusional delivery of the drug (Trenkwalder et al., 2015).

Initiation of apomorphine therapy can be as an in-patient or as an outpatient by a nurse specialist, geriatrician or neurologist. Nausea and vomiting at the start of therapy can be treated with domperidone, usually 20 mg three times a day for 2–3 days before initiation. Other antiemetics such as prochlorperazine or metoclopramide cannot be used because they block dopamine receptors and make PD worse. Orthostatic hypotension can be managed with medication or with non-pharmacological interventions. Neuropsychiatric disturbance, probably at a lower frequency than with oral agonists, and skin reactions, including nodule formation, are other potential side effects. Apomorphine, in conjunction with levodopa, may, in rare cases, cause a Coomb's positive haemolytic anaemia, which is reversible. It is recommended that patients are screened before beginning treatment and at 6-monthly intervals thereafter.

Catechol-O-methyl transferase inhibitors

Inhibitors of the enzyme catechol-O-methyl transferase (COMT) represent a useful addition to the range of therapies available for

PD (Schrag, 2005). Use of the first agent in this class, tolcapone, was originally suspended in Europe because of fears over hepatotoxicity, although the drug became available again in 2005, accompanied by strict prescribing and liver function monitoring guidelines. Entacapone is also available, and studies have not shown derangement of liver function with this drug; thus, it is used much more.

COMT itself is a ubiquitous enzyme, found in the gut, liver, kidney and brain, among other sites. In theory COMT inhibition may occur both centrally, where the degradation of dopamine to homovanillic acid is inhibited, and peripherally, where conversion of levodopa to the inert 3-*O*-methyldopa is inhibited. In practice, both tolcapone and entacapone act primarily as peripheral COMT inhibitors and by so doing increase the amount of levodopa that enters the CNS.

Placebo-controlled studies in patients with fluctuating PD have confirmed the efficacy of entacapone in decreasing 'off' time and permitting a concomitant reduction in levodopa dose. A 20% reduction in 'off' time is reported, translating into nearly 1.5 hours less immobility per day. This reduction tends to occur towards the end of the day, a time when many patients with PD are at their worst in terms of motor function. A comparison of entacapone and tolcapone suggested that tolcapone may be the more potent COMT inhibitor, achieving up to an extra 1.5 hours of 'on' time per day (Entacapone to Tolcapone Switch Study Investigators, 2007).

When entacapone is prescribed, a 200 mg dose is usually given with each dose of levodopa administered, up to a frequency of 10 doses/day. The increased dyskinesias means an overall reduction of 10–30% in the daily dose of levodopa may be anticipated. Entacapone can be employed with any other anti-Parkinsonian drug, although caution may be needed with apomorphine. Entacapone is also marketed as a compound tablet containing levodopa and carbidopa (Stalevo). Although each tablet contains 200 mg of the COMT inhibitor, seven different doses of levodopa are available (50, 75, 100, 125, 150, 175 and 200 mg) to provide flexibility. The compound tablet may help adherence by significantly reducing the total daily number of tablets a patient needs to take.

Tolcapone is prescribed as a fixed 100 mg three times a day regimen, increasing if necessary to 200 mg three times a day. It may only be used after the patient has tried and not responded positively to entacapone and where provision for 2-weekly monitoring of liver function tests for the first 12 months, reducing in frequency thereafter, is available. Again, a concomitant reduction in levodopa may be necessary to offset an increase in dyskinesias.

The optimal way to use COMT inhibition is unknown. A patient experiencing end-of-dose deterioration, or generally underdosed, would seem to be the ideal candidate. However, few comparative studies of COMT inhibitors versus dopamine agonists are available to provide guidance as to which class of drug is best to use and when. The STRIDE-PD study (Stocchi et al., 2010) assessed the potential benefit of combined treatment with levodopa and entacapone in *de novo* PD patients to address whether this combined treatment was associated with a lower incidence of dyskinesias. Unfortunately, the opposite was actually found, with a higher incidence of dyskinesias in patients randomised to levodopa and entacapone compared with levodopa alone. Other than exacerbation of dyskinesias, COMT inhibitors may also cause diarrhoea, abdominal pain and dryness of the mouth. Urine discolouration is reported in approximately 8% of patients who are taking entacapone.

It is best to avoid non-selective MAO inhibitors or a daily dose of selegiline in excess of 10 mg (which in reality never happens in PD) when using entacapone. In addition, the co-prescribing of venlafaxine and other noradrenaline (norepinephrine) reuptake inhibitors is best avoided. Entacapone may potentiate the action of apomorphine. Patients who are taking iron preparations should be advised to separate this medication and entacapone by at least 2 hours.

Monoamine oxidase type B inhibitors

The propargylamines selegiline and rasagiline are inhibitors of MAO-B. Inhibition of this enzyme slows the breakdown of dopamine, effectively having a 'levodopa-sparing' effect in the striatum. The result of this is both a mild therapeutic effect and a possible delay in the onset of or reduction in existing motor complications. Both drugs may also have an antiapoptotic effect. Apoptosis is a form of programmed cell death thought to be important in several neurodegenerative conditions, including PD. Whether the drugs have a neuroprotective effect by this or some other means remains controversial, but the current consensus is that this is not the case. Different protocols and starting doses have made comparing outcomes from different trials impossible (Mínguez-Mínguez et al., 2013). However, their mild symptomatic effect, ease of use, relative absence of side effects and putative neuroprotection, in the absence of any other neuroprotective agents available, makes them still a common choice as first-line therapy for many doctors. A recent meta-analysis found a significant and comparable effect of the two drugs on Unified Parkinson's Disease Rating Scale scores in early PD (Jost et al., 2014).

A single daily dose of 5 or 10 mg of selegiline is prescribed. Higher doses are associated with only minimal additional inhibition of MAO. Selegiline may also be administered as a lyophilised freeze-dried buccal preparation. The dosage of rasagiline is 1 mg daily. Both selegiline and rasagiline may be used as *de novo* or adjunctive treatments in PD, although trial data for the latter indication is strongest for rasagiline and buccal selegiline.

Selegiline can rarely cause hallucinations and confusion, particularly in moderate-to-advanced disease, typically through enhancing the actions of levodopa centrally. The withdrawal of selegiline may then be associated with significant deterioration in motor function. Unlike selegiline, rasagiline is not metabolised to amphetamine-like products, so neuropsychiatric side effects are less frequent. A critical interaction occurs with opioid analgesics; selegiline in particular is associated with hyperpyrexia and CNS toxicity if administered concomitantly with pethidine. Selective serotonin reuptake inhibitors should be used with caution in combination with MAOB inhibitors because there remains a small theoretical risk of serotonin syndrome, although there has been only a single case report.

Amantadine

Amantadine was introduced as an anti-Parkinsonian treatment in the late 1960s. It has a number of possible modes of action, including facilitation of presynaptic dopamine release, blocking dopamine reuptake, an anticholinergic effect (nicotinic antagonist), and also may act as a weak *N*-methyl-ᴅ-aspartate (NMDA) receptor antagonist. Initially employed in the early stages of treatment, where its effects are mild and relatively short-lived, it is more commonly used as an antidyskinetic agent in advanced disease, the only drug licensed for such use.

Daily doses of 100–400 mg amantadine may be used. Some recommend even higher doses for improved antidyskinetic effect, although side effects become much more frequent at higher doses. These side effects include a toxic confusional state and peripheral and corneal oedema. Monitoring is not needed, but attention needs to be paid to patients reporting sudden visual changes. Livedo reticularis, a persistent patchy reddish-blue mottling of the legs, and occasionally the arms, is also a side effect.

Antimuscarinic drugs

The availability of antimuscarinic drugs such as trihexyphenidyl and orphenadrine predated the introduction of levodopa by nearly 90 years. Antimuscarinic drugs can have a moderate effect in reducing tremor but do not have any significant benefit upon bradykinesia. The use of antimuscarinic agents has declined because of troublesome side effects, including constipation, urinary retention, cognitive impairment and toxic confusional states. In selected younger patients, an antimuscarinic drug may still be helpful, but close monitoring is advised.

Surgical treatment

Surgical approaches for the management of PD include both lesioning (-otomies) and deep brain stimulation (a high-frequency signal that functionally turns off the nucleus being stimulated). The functional effects are similar, but deep brain stimulation is preferred clinically and has the advantage of being reversible and controllable to a degree. Various targets in the basal ganglia have been considered, but overwhelmingly deep brain stimulation of either the internal part of the globus pallidus or the subthalamic nucleus is the therapy of choice in most patients. The intervention is costly, but significant benefits can be gained, especially for patients who have previously had a good response to levodopa but are experiencing major motor fluctuations or dyskinesia. Careful case selection is essential for all forms of surgical intervention for PD: older and less biologically fit patients, those with active cognitive and/or neuropsychiatric problems, and patients with a suboptimal levodopa response are generally regarded as poor surgical candidates (Worth, 2013).

New potential surgical approaches also include the delivery of growth factors, dopamine cells and viral vectors (for the delivery of growth factors or enzymes required for dopamine synthesis). Clinical trials have demonstrated proof of principle for cell transplantation studies using fetal dopamine cells, and the future looks promising for stem cells as a more viable, quality-controlled source of transplantable cells (Barker et al., 2015). Hybridising these novel approaches with the more established deep brain stimulation is also being postulated in a multifaceted approach to managing this condition long-term.

Patient care

Common therapeutic solutions to problems encountered in the management of people with PD are presented in Table 32.3. After diagnosis, the provision of an explanation of the condition, education and support are essential. PD charities produce an excellent range of literature to help the newly diagnosed patient come to terms with the condition. Patients who drive are advised to inform their insurance company and also the UK Driver and Vehicle Licensing Agency.

A doctor will record impairments in the clinic, while the patient is more concerned with their disability and handicap. Thus, a patient can be noted to have seemingly marked impairment and yet may not complain about significant disability. The converse may also be true. Not all patients, therefore, require immediate treatment. Further, concomitant depression may distort the patient's perception of his or her disability, leading to inappropriate prescribing of anti-Parkinsonian therapy. In this situation, the use of an antidepressant may be more helpful. There is no good evidence base for which antidepressant should be used, and both the tricyclic agents and selective serotonin reuptake inhibitors have their advocates.

Accurate adherence with the timing of therapy may be particularly important in patients who are beginning to experience long-term treatment complications. It can be helpful for patients to keep diaries when they begin to experience problems with either bradykinesia or dyskinesia, so that these symptoms can be related to drug and food intake. Careful changes in timing of drug therapy or meals may initially be sufficient to reduce variation in performance. Some patients experience troublesome early-morning bradykinesia. It may then be beneficial to prescribe an initial dose of a rapidly acting agent, such as dispersible oral co-beneldopa, to take on first wakening so that the patient can then get up and dress. A combination of levodopa with dopamine agonists, which are more slow acting, may be useful in the patient with motor fluctuations. A combination of levodopa and a COMT inhibitor may be more appropriate in a patient with end-of-dose deterioration.

Other factors that need to be considered in patients with PD are the benefits of adequate sleep and rest at night, which may be made more difficult if they have urinary frequency or problems with nocturnal bradykinesia. Judicious use of hypnotic therapy may be appropriate, whereas a tricyclic antidepressant may offer the dual benefit of sedation with anti-muscarinic effects. Low friction sheets to assist turning in bed and encouragement of mobility through physiotherapy may also be helpful.

The treatment of the patient with severe disease remains one of the greatest challenges in the management of PD. On–off fluctuations may be refractory to oral dopaminergic therapies. Sudden freezing episodes compound failing postural stability, leading to

Table 32.3 Common therapeutic solutions in the management of Parkinson's disease

Problem	Cause	Possible solution
Early-onset dyskinesias in young patient with Parkinson's disease	Exposure to levodopa	Delay introduction of levodopa, use lowest possible dose, use alternative agent (e.g. dopamine agonist, MAOB inhibitor), or start amantadine
One dose of levodopa does not last until the next (wearing off)	Advanced disease (pre- and post-synaptic changes)	More frequent, smaller doses of levodopa, COMT inhibitor, dopamine agonist or MAOB-inhibitor Start slow-release levodopa in addition to immediate-release agents
Pain and immobility during the night	Evening dose of levodopa not lasting long enough	Use slow-release levodopa preparation or slow-release dopamine agonist last thing at night
Freezing episodes and/or unpredictable motor fluctuations	Advanced disease (pre- and post-synaptic changes)	Dopaminergic therapies, apomorphine, Duodopa or surgery Physiotherapy helpful for freezing; sensory cues can help (stripes on the floor, etc.). Some recent evidence to suggest rivastigmine may help some patients with freezing of gait
Mismatch between patient's symptoms and signs	Consider underlying depression	Consider antidepressant (e.g. citalopram)
Confusion and hallucinations with preserved cognition	Toxic (drug-related) psychosis	Exclude intercurrent infection or other medical problem Review and reduce anti-Parkinsonian therapy Consider atypical antipsychotic agent such as quetiapine
Fatigue and tiredness	Underlying brain pathology or dopamine agonists	Reduce or stop dopamine agonists; modafinil may help and should be tried
Poor sleep or RBD	Check no other cause for sleep problem such as going off at night, nocturia, sleep apnoea, etc.	For RBD, use clonazepam 0.25–0.5 mg at night or melatonin If insomnia is the major issue, try low-dose amitriptyline or a Z-drug
Confusion and hallucinations with impaired cognition	Underlying brain pathology and cholinergic deficit	Reduce anti-Parkinsonian therapy Cholinesterase inhibitor may be tried

COMT, Catechol-O-methyl transferase; MAOB, monoamine oxidase type B; RBD, REM sleep behavioural disorder.

increasing falls and injuries. In select patients, the use of apomorphine, either as bolus injection (via a penject device) or as a continuous subcutaneous infusion, may be helpful, as might the use of cholinesterase inhibitors (Worth, 2013).

The presence of reduced dexterity in virtually all people with PD means that thought needs to be given to the way in which medication is dispensed and stored. If the patient is taking a complex regimen of drugs or has early cognitive problems, the use of pre-packaged therapies may improve adherence.

Patients' relatives also need emotional and social support through what can be a very demanding period. It can be very difficult for relatives to cope with the patient's loss of physical mobility, together with a personality change. The involvement of occupational therapists, social workers and specialists in palliative care in this situation is important.

Psychosis and dementia

When cognitive impairment is problematic, the use of conventional antipsychotic medication is inappropriate because the pharmacological actions of such drugs, dopamine receptor antagonism, can precipitate a catastrophic worsening of Parkinsonism. Behavioural disturbances require discussion with carers and, if possible, with the patient themselves. A graded withdrawal of anti-Parkinsonian drugs is often indicated, aiming to simplify the regimen to levodopa monotherapy and especially removing drugs that are well known to cause neuropsychiatric problems such as amantadine and dopamine agonists. In rare cases, it may be necessary to reduce the dose or even completely withdraw levodopa therapy to control aggressive, sexually demanding or psychotic features. When reduction in dopaminergic therapy is ineffective or not tolerated because of unacceptable immobility, an atypical antipsychotic drug may be considered. In practice, the choice is restricted to quetiapine or clozapine, because risperidone and olanzapine are associated with worsening Parkinsonism, even in low doses (NICE, 2017). Further, both risperidone and olanzapine should not be used in cognitively impaired elderly people because of an increased risk of stroke. Clozapine is difficult to use for PD-associated psychosis because of the need to register the patient with a blood-monitoring programme. When quetiapine is used, it should be commenced at a low dose of 25 or 50 mg at night and increased slowly. The sedative effects may be helpful in promoting sleep.

Table 32.4 Management of autonomic/enteric problems in Parkinson's disease

	Symptom response to dopamine replacement therapy	Treatment options	Cautionary notes
Faecal incontinence	Unresponsive	None available	Check that this is not overflow diarrhoea from faecal impaction.
Urinary incontinence	Responsive	Antimuscarinic drugs; incontinence pads	Antimuscarinics agents could worsen cognitive impairments, constipation and produce a dry mouth.
Erectile dysfunction	Responsive	Consider sildenafil or similar agent	Consider if erectile dysfunction is part of a more general major autonomic problem.
Dysphagia (impaired swallowing) and speech	Responsive	Refer to speech and language therapists	Check no non-Parkinson's disease cause for problems with speech (e.g. dentures) or swallowing.
Nocturia		Consider antimuscarinic	Make sure there are no primary urological problems such as prostatism.
Sialorrhea (excessive drooling)	Responsive	Glycopyrronium bromide inhaler/oral medication; Botox injections into salivary glands If neither of the above work consider: • antimuscarinic such as a hyoscine patch • low-dose clonidine • sublingual atropine eye drops	
Excessive sweating	Unresponsive	β-Blockers can occasionally help	
Postural hypotension	May be induced by dopamine replacement therapy	Midodrine or fludrocortisone	May worsen with dopamine agonists and lead to falls; falls are a leading cause of hospitalisation in Parkinson's disease
Constipation	Responsive	Bulking agents, osmotic laxative, macrogol	May improve with a switch from oral therapy to rotigotine patch
Weight loss		Refer for nutritional advice	Make sure no other cause for this such as underlying malignancy

Many ongoing trials, see Schrag et al. (2015) for further information.

Cholinesterase inhibitors have shown promise in treating the neuropsychiatric features of PD and may also have modest cognitive-enhancing benefits. Visual hallucinations, delusions, apathy and depression seem to be particularly responsive to these agents. These effects have been demonstrated for rivastigmine, the only cholinesterase inhibitor licensed for use in PD dementia in a large, multicentre, double-blind, placebo-controlled study (Emre et al., 2004). Although not licensed, memantine has also been shown to be effective in smaller-scale clinical trials and can be used in combination with rivastigmine in some patients.

Autonomic problems

Treating the autonomic problems where possible is critical to improving a patient's quality of life. Understanding the root cause of the non-motor events is important because many are either unresponsive to dopamine replacement therapy or may actually be induced by them. Table 32.4 lists the main treatment options available for the major autonomic effects which commonly occur in patients. These include disorders of gut motility, constipation or difficulty with swallowing, disturbances of micturition, sometimes presenting as nocturia, and postural hypotension. Constipation can be managed in the usual way with osmotic laxatives and, if necessary, stimulant laxatives and stool-softening agents. The management of postural hypotension includes assessment of the patient's autonomic function to establish whether this is primarily drug-related or associated with an autonomic neuropathy. If the patient is dizzy on standing, simple measures such as advice on rising slowly may be adequate. The use of elastic stockings, to reduce pooling of the blood in the lower limbs, is sometimes helpful, although poorly tolerated. Pharmacological approaches include the use of midodrine (a selective α_1-adrenergic agonist) or fludrocortisone. It is also important to consider other therapies the patient is receiving that might contribute to such symptoms, for example, diuretics, and to stop these if possible.

Case studies

Case 32.1

Mr ST, a 35-year-old man, develops a worsening tremor of his right hand and has difficulty running on a treadmill at his local gym as his right leg will not keep up. His father developed PD in his early 70s.

On examination he has a bilateral tremor more on the right than the left and does not swing his right arm when walking. He has no other major deficits and no significant medical history.

Questions

1. What is the most likely diagnosis?
2. What other points do you need to consider?
3. What treatment, if any, would you recommend?

Answers

1. PD. The asymmetric onset of tremor, bradykinesia of the right leg and the loss of arm swing would all make one suspect this is the most likely diagnosis despite his young age.
2. In all patients with young-onset PD, it is important to exclude other causes. It is thus essential to take a medication history to ensure that this could not be drug induced, although the asymmetry of presentation would be against this. It is important to exclude a metabolic cause given his age, such as Wilson's disease, so relevant blood tests should be done, as well as an MRI scan of the brain to exclude signal change within the basal ganglia suggestive of a metabolic problem. Finally a genetic cause should be considered (e.g. Parkin mutation). However, even at this age most cases are sporadic and having a single family member with the condition who developed it late in life is not significant. Given the condition is quite common, one is allowed by chance to have another member of the family with PD.
3. Treatment options depend upon whether the motor symptoms impact on his quality of life. NICE (2017) suggests that if they do, levodopa should be offered, whereas if they do not impact on his quality of life, either a dopamine agonist, levodopa or an MAO-B inhibitor could be considered. He should also be told about the support networks that exist for PD and be encouraged to link up to

a research programme if possible, as he would be an ideal patient for emerging experimental therapies such as cell transplants or gene therapies.

Case 32.2

Mr HM, a 47-year-old man, with PD is well controlled with ropinirole XL 16 mg/day and rasagiline 1 mg once daily. He denies any problems when you review him in clinic, but his wife e-mails you to say that he spends a lot of time at night on eBay buying engine parts for a particular type of car that he has always been interested in.

Questions

1. What is being described here?
2. What is the cause of this behaviour?
3. How would you manage it?

Answers

1. Impulse control disorder.
2. This is likely to be driven by his premorbid personality and the use of the dopamine agonist.
3. Mr HM needs to be seen in the PD clinic, although this does not need to be done urgently (unless the level of expenditure on this activity is excessive). In clinic the patient should be given the opportunity to bring this issue up, and if not then it should be raised because often patients deny or do not recognise that this is an issue/problem. Once raised, it should be explained that this is a well-known side effect of the ropinirole, and that this drug should be stopped and replaced with levodopa. The rationale for this and the consequences of doing this need explaining, and the patient may require specialist input, such as cognitive behavioural therapy to help them wean off the dopamine agonist successfully.

Case 32.3

Mrs AB, a 63-year-old woman, has had PD for 5–6 years. She now finds her medication is not working as well as it used to, and that she takes a long time to get going in the morning and is rather fidgety last thing in the day. She is currently taking Madopar CR five times a day and selegiline 10 mg once daily, as well as 8 mg ropinirole XL once daily.

Questions

1. What is Mrs AB describing?
2. What is causing these symptoms?
3. How would you treat them?

Answers

1. Mrs AB has a combination of being 'off' in the morning and 'on' with dyskinesia in the evening.
2. She is on a regimen of drugs that is suboptimal for someone with PD for this length of time. Her dose of ropinirole is low; most patients experience an optimal response when receiving 16–20 mg daily of the drug. In addition, she has no immediate-release Madopar in the morning, so it takes her a while to get going and then during the day the use of only Madopar CR at this frequency means she is slightly overdosed in the evening.

3. She should reduce the Madopar CR to twice a day, increase the ropinirole to 16 mg/day and start an immediate release of Madopar (e.g. Madopar 62.5 or 125) three times a day.

Case 32.4

Mr CD, a 59-year-old man, has had PD for 12 years. He has responded well to levodopa in the past but now finds that he has unpredictable 'off' periods during the day and peak dose dyskinesias that are present for several hours every day. He has a medical history of hypertension and is known to have benign prostatic hypertrophy. His current regimen is Sinemet 110 six times a day; Half Sinemet CR twice a day, amantadine 100 mg three times a day and a rotigotine patch 12 mg once a day.

Question

What treatment would you recommend and why?

Answer

Mr CD has now entered the advanced stages of PD with marked motor fluctuations and as such is heading towards a more invasive therapeutic intervention.

In the first instance one could try fractionating his levodopa load, so, for example, one could put him on Sinemet CR twice a day and then Sinemet 62.5 eight times a day, while also increasing the amantadine up to the maximum dosage of 400 mg/day.

However, even if this is effective, the problems are likely to re-occur because his nigrostriatal pathway has now degenerated to the point that the uptake, release and post-synaptic effects of the levodopa are erratic. He will therefore need to be considered for:

- a subcutaneous apomorphine pump
- deep brain stimulation
- Duodopa infusion therapy (into the small bowel)

Given his age, response to therapy to date and the absence of major non-motor complications or comorbidities, he would be a good candidate for any one of these treatments. However, in the UK it is very difficult for him to have Duodopa treatment because of its expense, unless there are exceptionally good reasons for him not to have already been treated or offered treatment with apomorphine or deep brain stimulation treatment.

Case 32.5

Mrs EF, a 76-year-old woman, has had PD for about 10 years. She is well controlled on Madopar 125 four times a day, Madopar CR twice a day and amantadine 100 mg twice a day. However, over the last few months she has been seeing animals in her bedroom at night and on occasions thinks there is someone else in the house. She lives on her own, but her friend who comes with her to the clinic says she is becoming more withdrawn and suspicious of others.

Questions

1. What is being described here?
2. What investigations would you suggest?
3. What therapeutic management could be considered for Mrs EF?
4. What is likely to happen to Mrs EF in the next few years?

Answers

1. Mrs EF has developed neuropsychiatric problems with her PD that involves visual hallucinations with delusions and a degree of paranoia.
2. It is important to make sure that nothing else is causing this, such as a low-grade infection or some other comorbid condition or metabolic problem. Thus, an infective screen and a series of routine blood tests should be undertaken. It is unlikely to relate to a new intracranial problem such as encephalitis or a chronic subdural haematoma, but if there are focal neurological signs, then imaging of the brain is recommended with or without cerebrospinal fluid examination.

   However, the most likely cause is her underlying PD with cortical Lewy body pathology which with her medication is driving her current neuropsychiatric syndrome.
3. If no other cause is found, then the drugs should be reduced. The most likely agent is the amantadine, so this should be withdrawn over the next few weeks. If she does not improve with this change, then levodopa dose could be reduced, although this may make her unacceptably immobile and 'off'. If this occurs, the Madopar needs to be re-introduced and rivastigmine 1.5 mg twice a day needs to be started (after appropriate electrocardiogram screening) or alternatively quetiapine (25 mg at night).

   Mrs EF also needs to be closely followed up ideally by a specialist community nurse who can visit her at home.
4. Mrs EF is likely to progress to a PD dementia because these symptoms are typically an indication of this complication of PD.

References

Barker, R.A., Drouin-Ouellet, J., Marmar, M., 2015. Cell-based therapies for Parkinson's disease – past insights and future potential. Nat. Rev. Neurol. 11 (9), 492–503.

Bellou, V., Belbasis, L., Tzoulaki, I., et al., 2016. Environmental risk factors and Parkinson's disease: an umbrella review of meta-analyses. Parkinsonism Relat. Disord. 23, 1–9.

Braak, H., Del Tredici, K., Rüb, U., et al., 2003. Staging of brain pathology related to sporadic Parkinson's disease. Neurobiol. Aging 24, 197–211.

Bras, J., Guerreiro, R., Hardy, J., 2015. SnapShot: genetics of Parkinson's disease. Cell 160 (3), 570–572.

Cotzias, G.C., Van Woert, M.H., Schiffer, L.M., 1967. Aromatic amino acids and modification of parkinsonism. N. Engl. J. Med. 276, 374–379.

Edwards, Y.J.K., Beecham, G.W., Scott, W.K., et al., 2011. Identifying consensus disease pathways in Parkinson's disease using an integrative systems biology approach. PLoS One. 6 (2), e16917. https://doi.org/10.1371/journal.pone.0016917.

Emre, M., Aarsland, D., Albanese, A., et al., 2004. Rivastigmine for dementia associated with Parkinson's disease. N. Engl. J. Med. 351, 2509–2518.

Entacapone to Tolcapone Switch Study Investigators, 2007. Entacapone to Tolcapone switch: multicenter double-blind, randomized, active-controlled trial in advanced Parkinson's disease. Mov. Disord. 22 (1), 14–19.

Hely, M.A., Reid, W.G., Adena, M.A., et al., 2008. The Sydney multicenter study of Parkinson's disease: the inevitability of dementia at 20 years. Mov. Disord. 23, 837–844.

Jennings, D.L., Seibyl, J.P., Oakes, D., et al., 2004. (123I)beta-CIT and single-photon emission computed tomographic imaging vs. clinical evaluation in Parkinsonian syndrome: unmasking an early diagnosis. Arch. Neurol. 61, 1224–1229.

Jost, W.H., Friede, M., Schnitker, J., 2014. Comparative efficacy of selegiline versus rasagiline in the treatment of early Parkinson's disease. Eur. Rev. Med. Pharmacol. Sci. 18 (22), 3349.

Mínguez-Mínguez, S., Solís-García Del Pozo, J., Jordán, J., 2013. Rasagiline in Parkinson's disease: a review based on meta-analysis of clinical data. Pharmacol. Res. 74, 78–86.

National Institute for Health and Care Excellence (NICE), 2017. Parkinson's disease in adults. NICE guideline [NG71]. NICE, London. Available at https://www.nice.org.uk/guidance/ng71.

Polymeropoulos, M.H., Lavedan, C., Leroy, E., et al., 1997. Mutation in the alphasynculein gene identified in families with Parkinson's disease. Science 276, 2045–2047.

Rascol, O., Brooks, D.J., Korczyn, A.D., et al., 2000. A 5 year study of the incidence of dyskinesia in patients with early Parkinson's disease who were treated with ropinirole or levodopa. N. Engl. J. Med. 342 (20), 1484–1491.

Schrag, A., 2005. Entacapone in the treatment of Parkinson's disease. Lancet Neurol. 4, 366–370.

Schrag, A., Saubier, A., Chaudhuri, K.R., 2015. New clinical trials for nonmotor manifestations of Parkinson's disease. Mov. Disord. 30 (11), 1490–1503.

Spillantini, M.G., Schmidt, M.L., Lee, V.M., et al., 1997. Alpha-synuclein in Lewy bodies. Nature 388 (6645), 839–840.

Stocchi, F., Rascol, O., Kieburtz, K., et al., 2010. Initiating levodopa/carbidopa therapy with and without entacapone in early Parkinson disease: the STRIDE-PD study. Ann. Neurol. 68, 18–27.

Trenkwalder, C., Chaudhuri, K.R., García Ruiz, P.J., et al., 2015. Expert Consensus Group report on the use of apomorphine in the treatment of Parkinson's disease – clinical practice recommendations. Parkinsonism Relat. Disord. 21 (9), 1023–1030.

Worth, P.F., 2013. When the going gets tough: how to select patients with Parkinson's disease for advanced therapies. Pract. Neurol. 13 (3), 140–152.

Further reading

Ali, K., Morris, H.R., 2015. Parkinson's disease: chameleons and mimics. Pract. Neurol. 15, 14–15.

van der Brug, M.P., Singleton, A., Gasser, T., et al., 2015. Parkinson's disease: from human genetics to clinical trials. Sci. Trans. Med. 7, 305–320.

Walter, B.L., Vitek, J.L., 2004. Surgical treatment for Parkinson's disease. Lancet Neurol. 3, 719–728.

33 Dementia

Denise Taylor

Key points

- Globally, 47.5 million people live with dementia; 850,000 people in the UK have dementia, and this number is projected to rise to more than 1 million by 2025.
- In the UK, 62% of people with dementia are female, probably because life expectancy is higher in females and age is the biggest known risk factor for dementia.
- There is no cure for any form of dementia, except for the pseudo-dementias, which may respond to treatment.
- Risk reduction for dementia includes reducing modifiable cardio- and cerebrovascular risk factors.
- Early interventions include planning for the future in terms of advocacy and end-of-life care options.
- Pharmacological treatment is multifactorial and includes pharmacological support of cognitive function and non-pharmacological support of patients and their carer/family.
- Acetylcholinesterase inhibitors and memantine improve cognitive function, including improvements in social relationships, behaviour, engagement with the individual's environment, language and delay entry to nursing home care.
- Acetylcholinesterase inhibitors delay the neurodegenerative process.
- Future treatments include monoclonal antibodies and small molecule treatment.
- Maintaining physical and mental health by inclusion in socially and mentally stimulating activities is an important part of care.
- Healthcare professionals and carers need to adapt their communication style to best support the individual.

Definition

The word *dementia* is an umbrella term for a host of neurodegenerative diseases which cause progressive cognitive impairment, sufficient to interfere with work, social function and relationships. It is important to recognise that cognitive function is not just about memory but includes language, visuospatial and perceptual ability, thinking and problem solving, and personality. This progressive impairment is the root cause of distress for carers and family of people with dementia, as the person they love seems to change and disappear.

Epidemiology

Incidence and prevalence

Dementia is a global issue, with an estimated 47.5 million people living with dementia worldwide; this estimate is predicted to rise to more than 150 million by 2050 (Public Health England, 2016). In 2015, there were an estimated 856,700 people in the UK with dementia, with 720,251 living in England, 45,321 in Wales, 70,162 in Scotland and 20,966 in Northern Ireland (Alzheimer's Society, 2014). Established prevalence rates link the risk of dementia with increasing age, rising from 1 in 688 people younger than 65 years, to 1 in 14 people older than 65 years, to 1 in 6 older than 80 years and 1 in 3 of older than 90 years. However, in February 2016, the actual number of people in England with a recorded diagnosis in the record of their primary care doctor was 426,000, indicating a prevalence of 0.756% or 1 person in 132 (Health and Social Care Information Centre, 2016). Thus, about 41% of people with signs and symptoms of dementia in England are not yet diagnosed.

Furthermore, recent research suggests the proportion of people living with dementia has decreased by 20% over the last two decades, linked mainly to a reduction in male smoking, leading healthier lives and reduction of cardiovascular risks (Matthews et al., 2016). In the 1990s it was predicted there would be 250,000 new cases of dementia each year, whereas study findings put this at 210,000 per year (Winblad et al., 2016).

Prognosis

There is no cure for any of the dementias, with an average life expectancy post-diagnosis of 5–10 years; however, some people have survived for 20 years.

Annual UK societal costs of dementia are estimated at £26.3 billion: £4.5 billion on state social care, £11.6 billion on unpaid care, £4.3 billion on health care, £5.8 billion on individual social care and £100 million on other costs. These are higher than the cost of cancer, heart disease or stroke.

In the UK, up to one-third of Alzheimer's disease (AD) cases may be attributable to potentially modifiable risk factors, and 21.8% of AD cases could be attributed to physical inactivity. A 20% reduction in risk factors per decade could reduce UK prevalence rates by 16.2% (300,000 cases) by 2050 (Winblad et al., 2016). Table 33.1 describes the risk factors for dementia.

Table 33.1 Risk factors for dementia

Risk factors	Association
Age	Higher blood pressure in midlife Increased incidence of some diseases (encephalitis, delirium) Changes to nerve cells, DNA and cell structure Weakening of body's natural repair systems Changes in the immune system
Lifestyle factors	Smoking – doubles risk of dementia by increasing cardiovascular disease (stroke and diabetes), narrowing cerebro- and cardiovascular blood vessels, causing oxidative stress to the brain Lack of regular physical activity along with sedentary lifestyle Excessive alcohol consumption Diet high in saturated fat, sugar and salt and obesity in midlife
Concomitant disease	Parkinson's disease Stroke Type 2 diabetes High blood pressure
Genetic (small proportion of cases)	Early onset/younger people with dementia (40,000 people in UK with dementia <65 years) People with Down's syndrome are more likely to develop Alzheimer's disease in early 30s due to chromosome 21 missense Frontotemporal dementia (Pick's disease); Huntingdon's chorea

Table 33.2 Protective factors for dementia

Protective factor	Associated with...
Higher levels of education	Use it, don't lose it (brain function)
More mentally demanding occupations	Examples include teaching, research, mathematics, writers, accountants, lawyers, medicine
Cognitive stimulation	Doing puzzles, crosswords, learning a second language, dancing, singing
Social engagement	Being socially active improves mood, relieves stress, reduces risk of depression and reduces loneliness

Alzheimer's disease

AD is the most common form of dementia, accounting for 62% of people diagnosed with a dementia in the UK. AD was first described by Dr Lois Alzheimer in 1917 and includes early- and late-onset variants. It has been proposed that the prodromal period of AD is typically a 9-year decline in cognitive function, and part of that decline may possibly include a diagnosis of amnestic MCI. It is increasingly understood that taking active steps to reduce personal risk factors for dementia could affect this progression. There is no licensed treatment for MCI.

Causes of Alzheimer's disease

The majority of AD is of idiopathic or sporadic origin. Identified risk factors for developing AD are both modifiable and nonmodifiable and are described in Table 33.3.

Genetic research in families indicates that almost 50% of individuals with AD have at least one first-degree relative with a dementia. This statement has resulted in controversy, but researchers suggest that if the patient has late-onset AD, similarly affected relatives may have died of other causes before developing AD (Bateman et al., 2012). This has led other researchers to postulate that perhaps the formation of plaque and neurofibrillary tangles is not a process of normal aging at all but in fact the early stages of AD.

Pathophysiology of Alzheimer's disease

The pathophysiology of AD is associated with an excess of intracellular neurofibrillary tangles and extracellular amyloid-β. Amyloid precursor protein is a chain of 771 amino acids found widely throughout the body, including high concentrations in platelets, where it plays an as yet unknown function.

The cholinergic system is critical to normal memory and other cognitive functions. In AD there is a selective loss of cells in the basal forebrain, and the depletion of neurons in this area correlates with memory and cognitive decline in AD. When the first mild symptoms of AD occur, there is already a significant deficit in acetylcholine. Levels eventually reduce by 40–90% in

Subsequent public health strategies are aimed at people in their middle years reducing cardiovascular and cerebrovascular risks and maintaining brain function to decrease individual risks for dementia. Table 33.2 outlines these protective factors. A review of combined data for brain reserve and cognitive decline from 22 studies of more than 29,000 participants demonstrated a 46% lower risk of dementia in people with high levels of mental activity than in those with low levels (Valenzuela and Sachdev, 2006).

Clinical manifestations

It is now well established that a prodromal period exists in the development of dementia, whereas in people with a genetic missense mutation, the process may be established from birth. In those with sporadic disease, the process may be triggered some 20–30 years before the signs and symptoms are displayed. Symptoms, which may be termed mild cognitive impairment (MCI), may or may not progress to a dementia. However, findings suggest that individuals with predominantly memory problems (amnestic MCI) on presentation will progress to dementia.

Table 33.3 Nonmodifiable and modifiable risk factors for Alzheimer's disease

Non-modifiable	Modifiable
Gender – females have greater incidence than men, but this is related to the longevity of females as compared with men Increasing age Genetic risk • Early onset (40–55 years) linked to mutation of the amyloid precursor protein gene located on chromosome 21 (also referred to as AD1 genetic indicator) • Early onset (30–55 years) linked to mutation of the Presenilin 1 (PS1) gene located on chromosome 14; follows autosomal-dominant inheritance (also referred to as AD3 genetic indicator) • Onset (40–90 years) linked to mutation of the Presenilin 2 (PS2) gene located on chromosome 1; follows autosomal-dominant inheritance (also referred to as AD4 genetic indicator) • Familial Alzheimer's disease (onset 40–90 years or older) linked to the apolipoprotein E4 allele encoded on chromosome 19 (also referred to as AD2 genetic indicator)	Physical and cardiovascular health in middle years Head injury – amyloid is deposited in the brain within 24 h of injury Education – a high level of education is a protective factor in familial Alzheimer's disease High intraneuronal calcium levels lead to cell damage and ultimately cell death, which triggers amyloid deposition and formation of neurofibrillary tangles Ongoing intellectual activity – the 'use it or lose it' hypothesis suggests that continued learning is a protective factor in reducing the risk of developing Alzheimer's disease Environmental toxin as a neurotoxin rather than a causative factor (e.g. excessive alcohol intake, pesticides, aluminum levels in water or diet)

Adapted from Bateman et al., (2012).

moderate to severe AD. Other affected neurotransmitter systems are noradrenaline, dopamine, serotonin, glutamate and gamma-aminobutyric acid (GABA).

There are a number of hypotheses on the potential cause of the neuropathological processes that result in AD, and the most accepted are outlined in the following sections.

The neurofibrillary tangles hypothesis. It has been suggested that neurofibrillary tangles (NFTs) form due to the hyperphosphorylation of tau protein within the cell to form oligomers and then tangles. The tangles then impair the axonal flow of nutrients in and waste products out of the cell, resulting in cell death and dramatic loss in cholinergic neurons (Ballard et al., 2011). These cells produce acetylcholine and project diffusely into the hippocampus, basal nucleus of Meynert and entorhinal cortex.

NFTs have been found in brains of people with dementia pugilistica, in those with parkinsonism, in older people with Down's syndrome and in older people without dementia. It has been postulated that NFTs may be a pathological substrate for memory loss in AD, normal aging and MCI. Current research is focussed on the development and testing of a vaccine against NFTs which would, if successful, be aimed at preventing the AD process (Davtyan et al., 2016).

The amyloid hypothesis. The amyloid hypothesis suggests that the aberrant cleavage of amyloid precursor protein by β- and/or gamma-secretase enzymes results in amyloid-β, a peptide of 36–43 amino acids, toxic to nerve cells. AB40 is a soluble form of amyloid-β and associated with cerebrovascular plaques. A combination of the AB40 and the insoluble AB42, if not cleared, builds up to form early plaques via oligomerisation in the limbic and associated cortices. This blocks cell-to-cell transmission at synapses (Ballard et al., 2011). This affects synaptic efficacy, resulting in greater deposition of AB42, microglial and astrocyte activation and inflammatory response. This in turn leads to altered neuronal homeostasis, oxidative injury and tangle formation and ultimately in AD. Amyloid-β circulates in plasma, cerebrospinal fluid and brain interstitial fluid, mainly as soluble AB40. The extent of its presence is now used to improve the accuracy of AD diagnosis for clinical research studies (Albert et al., 2011).

The three dominantly inherited forms of early-onset AD (defined as occurring before 60 years of age) are associated with amyloid-β, presenilin 1 (PS1) and presenilin 2 (PS2) genetic missense mutations, which alter the role of gamma-secretase, leading to an increased production of AB42. In affected people this process remains unchecked throughout life, leading to early-onset dementia. For those with sporadic AD, there is a trigger which starts this process at a later stage in the individual's life, which ultimately leads to dementia (Bateman et al., 2012).

Genetic risk factors. The apolipoprotein E (APoE) gene enables the production of a protein, apolipoprotein E, which is responsible for linking lipids and proteins together to enable the removal of cholesterol and other fats from the bloodstream. If this process is blocked, then the risk of dementia increases. There are three well-known alleles of the APoE gene: e2, e3 and e4. Greater than 50% of the population carry e3, which has a neutral role in AD development. e2, however, is rare and thought to be protective, whereas e4 increases the risk of AD, and this risk increases with the number of alleles carried. These alleles are autosomal dominant and are inherited from both maternal and paternal parents, meaning people may carry any combination of e2 with e3 or e4 or both of each allele (Ballard et al., 2011; Bateman et al., 2012).

The presence of the e4 allele increases the risk of deposition of β-amyloid in the brain from birth and subsequent development of AD, although it must be stressed that this is not a 100% risk factor – environmental, dietary and physical properties may decrease this risk. In people without the e4 allele, there is a 10–15% risk of developing AD; this rises to greater than 75% if both alleles are e4. The genetic forms of AD are described in Table 33.3. Evidence suggests that AD is the sum of inherent host factors (a genetic predisposition) and external (environmental) factor(s) which act as a neurotoxin or catalyst for the neuropathological processes. Genetic testing is not recommended at this time, although it is often included as part of clinical trials.

Table 33.4 Progression and staging of Alzheimer's disease

Progression	Clinical presentation	Associated physical problems
Early stages (1–3 years)	Recent memory impairment, forgetting names, losing direction when out, depression, impaired activities of daily living, language difficulties	Visuospatial problems (e.g. walking into things)
Middle stages (2–10 years)	Amnesia, aphasia, inability to calculate solutions, inability to problem solve, personality change, behavioural changes (e.g. wandering); psychiatric changes such as delusions; inability to bathe, eat, toilet or dress without assistance	Falls, accidents involving cooking or other activities, impaired motor skills, may forget to eat and therefore have nutritional problems, may be unable to use the toilet correctly and develop chafing due to poor hygiene and soiling.
Late stages (8–12 years)	Short- and long-term memory loss, mutism or nonsensical speech, posture becomes rigid and in flexion, complete dependence on others, seizures	Inability to communicate needs (hunger, toileting); difficulty in swallowing or chewing food; decreased immune response, susceptibility to infections increased; double incontinence; bedridden patients are at risk of pressure sores and pneumonia

The progression and staging of AD are shown in Table 33.4. It is important to note that as cognitive impairment increases over time, there is matching physical deterioration, resulting in increasing frailty and vulnerability. Ultimately individuals move from relatively independent states of mobility to being bed-bound, mute and withdrawn.

Vascular dementia

Vascular dementia (VaD) is the result of ischaemic changes within the brain, associated with smoking, transient ischaemic attacks, strokes, long-term or poorly managed hypertension, atrial fibrillation and/or type II diabetes. Improved management of cardiovascular risks reduces the risk of vascular dementia.

Dementia with Lewy bodies

The cause of dementia with Lewy bodies (DLB) is not well understood, although there are proposed genetic links to the PARK11 gene, also associated with Parkinson's disease. Cases are sporadic, with no strong hereditary link, but the risk is heightened with the inheritance of the e4 allele of apolipoprotein E (APoE) as in AD.

Neuropathology

Neuropathology demonstrates the presence of abnormal collections of α-synuclein protein within the cytoplasm of Lewy bodies, which are similar in structure to those seen in Parkinson's disease. Lewy bodies are also found in Pick's disease and Huntington's chorea. Similarly, there are losses of dopamine-producing neurones in the substantia nigra and a loss of acetylcholine-producing neurones in the basal nucleus of Meynert as in AD.

There is increasing evidence to suggest that there may be a range of Lewy body disorders, with older patients more likely to develop cortical disease. Historically DLB had been viewed as a variant of AD, but it is a disorder in its own right and includes Lewy body dementia, Lewy body variant of AD, diffuse Lewy body disease, cortical Lewy body disease and senile dementia of Lewy body type.

People with DLB demonstrate an extreme sensitivity to the extra-pyramidal side effects of antipsychotic medication, with a two- to threefold increase in mortality even with atypical antipsychotics. This may be explained by deficits in nigrostriatal dopaminergic neurones and may be mediated via acute blockade of postsynaptic dopamine D_2 receptors in the striatum (McKeith et al., 2005).

The rarer dementias

There are more than 100 diseases that can cause dementia; however, many are rare, and the most common of these are presented in the following sections.

Parkinson's disease dementia

Long-term follow-up of people with Parkinson's disease (PD) suggests that up to 78% will eventually develop a dementia, with symptoms such as fluctuating cognition and visual hallucinations similar to DLB. Consensus guidelines suggest that DLB and Parkinson's disease dementia are overlapping clinical syndromes and lie on different points on the spectrum of Lewy body disease, sharing common underlying neuropathological processes (McKeith, 2006). Furthermore, distinguishing DLB and Parkinson's disease dementia as separate entities may be useful in clinical practice but is of limited value in terms of investigating and treating the underlying pathology.

Frontotemporal dementia

Frontotemporal dementia (FTD), previously known as Pick's disease, is the largest cause of dementia for younger people in the UK, usually affecting people between the ages of 45 and 64. However, 3 out of 10 people with FTD develop the condition at an older age. Autopsy studies show that neurodegeneration in the frontal and temporal lobes is linked to deposition of abnormal tau proteins inside neurons, which clump together in spherical arrangements known as 'Pick bodies'.

The frontal lobes regulate personality, emotions and behaviour, as well as reasoning, planning and decision-making. The temporal lobes are involved in the understanding and production of language.

Progression rates of FTD range from less than 2 years to greater than 10 years, with people living 8 years on average after symptom onset. About 10–15% of people with FTD have a strong family history, with several close relatives in different generations affected. Typically, in these cases, FTD is inherited from a parent as a genetic missense mutation in one of three genes: MAPT, GRN or C9ORF72. The children or siblings of a parent with genetic missense mutation have a 50% chance of inheriting it. These families should be offered referral to specialist genetics service for counselling with appropriate support. In comparison, inherited early-onset AD affects less than 1 in 1000 people with AD (Warren et al., 2013).

Corticobasal degeneration

Corticobasal degeneration is a rare disease, with neurodegeneration affecting the cortex and basal ganglia, and has some overlap with FTD. The cause is unknown, but neuropathology indicates high levels of tau protein. Onset is usually between the ages of 60 and 80, with a life expectancy of 8 years post-diagnosis.

Progressive supranuclear palsy

Progressive supranuclear palsy is a rare progressive movement disorder, also known as Steele–Richardson–Olszewski syndrome. It affects many brain areas, resulting in symptoms similar to those of Parkinson's disease. Onset is usually in the 60s, but it can affect younger people.

The cause of progressive supranuclear palsy is unknown but is associated with high levels of tau deposition in affected brain areas.

Creutzfeldt–Jakob disease

Creutzfeldt–Jakob disease (CJD) is a rare prion disease, with the most common sporadic variant normally affecting people older than 40 years. Estimates suggest the disease affects about 1 in every 1 million people each year. The trigger for sporadic CJD is unknown and could be inherited or transmitted from person to person.

More recently, the new variant CJD, typically affecting younger adults, was caused by eating meat from cattle infected with bovine spongiform encephalopathy. In new variant CJD, there may be many years between a person being infected and the development of symptoms.

HIV-associated neurocognitive disorder

HIV has adverse effects on the immune system. These include the development of neurocognitive disorders in up to half of people with HIV, called HIV-associated neurocognitive disorder (HAND). This may be a direct result of the virus's effects on a weakened immune system, enabling infections and cancers.

Huntington's disease

Huntington's disease is an inherited fatal genetic brain disease. Children of a parent with Huntington's disease have a 50% chance of inheriting it; however, in 1–3% of cases there is no history of the disease in family members. Genetic testing is available, but the family members need appropriate support. Huntington's disease is caused by mutations in the gene encoding the protein called huntingtin, resulting in misshaped huntingtin proteins which form aggregates with inclusion in neurons, resulting in cell death.

Multiple sclerosis

If multiple sclerosis occurs in the brain, those affected may experience varying degrees of cognitive impairment. However, the decline is not usually sufficiently severe or progressive to be termed 'dementia' but is referred to as 'cognitive difficulties'.

Niemann–Pick disease type C

Niemann–Pick disease type C is a rare inherited genetic disorder. Importantly, it is not related to FTD, which is also referred to as Pick's disease. It is caused by an inability to deal with cholesterol and other lipids. Lipid accumulates in all cells, including those in the brain.

Normal pressure hydrocephalus

Normal pressure hydrocephalus occurs when excess fluid accumulates in the brain. This does not cause pressure to build up within brain tissue.

Posterior cortical atrophy

Posterior cortical atrophy, also known as Benson's syndrome, is a rare neurodegenerative condition where damage occurs in the posterior brain region.

Alcohol-related brain damage

Binge drinking, or drinking excessive amounts of alcohol to become drunk, over a prolonged period of time can lead to a range of conditions known as alcohol-related brain damage (ARBD), the most common of which is alcoholic dementia, previously referred to as alcohol-related dementia. This includes Korsakoff's syndrome, also known as Korsakoff's psychosis (Zahr et al., 2011). Recent research suggests that APoE-e4 may be associated with a higher risk of Wernicke–Korsakoff in individuals who drink heavily (Harwood et al., 2010).

The exact number of people with ARBD is not known. It is likely to be under-diagnosed due to the stigma associated with alcohol misuse and people not seeking help, together with healthcare professionals' lack of awareness of the process of ARBD. UK postmortem studies suggest ARBD affects about 1 in 200 of the general adult population. Among those with alcoholic addiction, this figure rises to one in three. It is not clear why some people develop ARBD whereas others do not.

People with ARBD tend to be middle-aged, typically in their 40s or 50s, although they can be younger or older. ARBD is thought to cause more than 10% of dementia in younger people, defined as those aged under 65. ARBD is more prevalent in

Table 33.5 Differential diagnostic features of the main dementias

Feature	Onset and progression	Early symptoms	Late symptoms
Alzheimer's disease	Insidious onset with progressive decline of cognitive and physical function	Predominantly memory loss	Emergence of aphasia and agnosia
Vascular dementia	Sudden onset with stepwise progression Periods of stability followed by an episode of sharp decline	Person has insight Emotional lability and depression Focal neurological signs	Shuffling gait with a wide base, differentiated from Parkinson's disease as has preserved arm swing, presence of seizures and continued cerebral ischaemia
Dementia with Lewy bodies	Fluctuating periods of alertness and confusion Fluctuating cognitive function	Less severely impaired recent memory Early gait disturbance and parkinsonism with falls	Hallucinations, periods of confusion and psychotic symptoms
Fronto-temporal dementia	Gradual but progressive changes in behaviour, mood and personality	Apathy, poor judgement and insight, speech/language problems	Apathy, disinhibition – including sexual, depression, euphoria

people with poor socioeconomic backgrounds and affects men more frequently than women. However, affected women develop ARBD at a younger age than men and after fewer years of alcohol misuse.

Consequences of the dementia process

Behavioural changes in dementia

As the disease progresses, the resultant neuropathological damage is associated with changes in behaviour, mood, personality and the ability to communicate effectively. As a result of this, 95% of people with a dementia develop behavioural changes, and these can be found challenging to those that care for them (informal and formal carers). These challenging behaviours are also referred to as behavioural and psychological symptoms of dementia (BPSD). Symptoms include delusions, hallucinations, agitation or aggression, depression, anxiety, elation or euphoria, apathy or indifference, disinhibition, irritation or lability, a change in eating patterns and aberrant motor behaviour (wandering). As dementia progresses, people lose the sense of whether it is day or night and subsequently disrupt carers' sleep as they get up and dressed in the middle of the night. This is called sundowning. Formal and informal carers worry about people walking away from their chair/bed and 'wandering' around, going for walks on their own (because they can get lost). However, it is important to note that all people like to move around and enjoy a walk outside. Exercise should be built into the daily routine, and dementia care environments should include areas where people can walk safely on their own. A wide variety of behaviours can be displayed which in general are not harmful. However, they can be difficult to control and are a major reason for caregiver stress and admission to long-term care.

These symptoms may be caused by the disease affecting a particular area of the brain – for example, the sexual disinhibition observed in FTD, or the inability to convey a need for fluid, food, pain relief or other symptom. It is important to note that people

with dementia may express an emotion such as sadness or happiness but not be able to remember the reason. This is because factual memory for events and learning is stored in the hippocampus which is one of the first structures affected. However, emotional memory is stored in the amygdala which generally is only affected in the late stages.

Agitation. Agitation has been defined as behaviour which is seen as disruptive but nonaggressive (e.g. moaning, pacing, crying, arguing). It ranges to aggression in its severe forms, where the person may be aggressive or endanger others or him- or herself (e.g. kicking, screaming, throwing objects, self-injury, scratching). These behaviours can be very distressing to the caregiver and are the behaviours most likely to lead to institutionalisation. Therefore, support of the carer is key. Educational programmes for carers using behavioural techniques are more effective than most pharmacological treatments (Marriott et al., 2000).

Diagnosis of the dementias

There is considerable overlap of disease states, with dementias of mixed aetiology in combination of AD and VaD, or DLB and PDD being relatively common. Currently, computed tomography (CT) and/or magnetic resonance imaging (MRI) is used to exclude treatable forms of the symptoms (e.g. space-occupying lesions, hydrocephalus or ischaemic changes). These can also be used to give a 'probable' diagnosis of dementia with reference to consensus guidelines, clinical examination and test results. Information for differential clinical and disease features which may aid a probable diagnosis is described in Table 33.5.

At present, a definitive diagnosis can only be made at autopsy or if the individual takes part in a clinical trial where lumbar punctures (to check levels of *tau*), genetic testing and positron emission test (PET) scanning or high-volumetric MRI scanning is available.

Table 33.6 Possible signs of dementia

Sign	Change displayed
Day-to-day memory	Difficulty recalling events that happened recently Although long-term memory may remain relatively unaffected, short-term memory may become badly impaired and may be identified as repeating the same questions, forgetting names and routes, and losing/ misplacing items. People with dementia forget not only the specifics of an item or event but also the context.
Concentrating, planning or organising	Difficulties making decisions, solving problems or carrying out a sequence of tasks – e.g. cooking a meal, not knowing how to make a cup of tea or forgetting what order to put clothes on when getting dressed May begin to lose interest in people, objects and hobbies (e.g. sitting passively in front of the TV for hours, sleeping for long periods and neglect of personal care) Problems with tasks (e.g. working out change when paying in a shop, remembering appointments or paying bills)
Judgement	Inability to judge situations or people (e.g. putting on too many clothes on a hot day or too few on a cold day)
Language	Difficulties following a conversation or finding the right word for something. Conversations tend to be badly affected, with frequent pauses, forgetting very commonplace words, losing the thread of what is being said midsentence, and substituting unusual words (e.g. *hand clock* for *watch*).
Visuospatial skills	Problems judging distances (e.g. on stairs) and seeing objects in three dimensions. If distinct visual impairments such as inability to read or recognise signs, consider referral for occipital lobe scanning variant Alzheimer's disease.
Orientation	Losing track of the day or date, becoming confused about where they are or forgetting the way home from shopping or work
Changes in mood	Becoming frustrated or irritable, withdrawn, apathetic or anxious, easily upset or unusually sad, suspicious, depressed, or agitated. Dramatic mood swings which show noticeably more or less emotion than previously can indicate possible cause for concern. Patients may become angry if friends/family comment on such behaviour changes.
Visual hallucinations, delusions or paranoia[a]	Seeing things that are not really there and/or believing things that are not true and/or paranoid beliefs that people are stealing from them or trying to harm them in some way

[a]Hallucinations and paranoia are specific to certain forms of dementia, where it is the parts of the brain responsible for behaviour and emotional responses that are most affected.

General signs and symptoms of dementia

Dementia is neurodegenerative, so there is gradual onset, often noticed at times of stress or change (e.g. when admitted to hospital with an infection or when there is a change in environment such as going on holiday). The presentation of symptoms is influenced by pre-morbid personality, and those with good social skills can hide decline from relatives and carers.

Early symptoms include:
- memory loss, especially for recent events;
- difficulties with learning and/or retaining new information;
- being more repetitive;
- misplacing objects (e.g. car keys or spectacles);
- difficulty with complex tasks such as cooking, driving or dealing with finances;
- reduced ability to reason and problem-solve;
- impairment of spatial and visuospatial awareness (e.g. bumping into objects, driving accidents, getting lost in a familiar place);

- language problems, including inability to find the right word or difficulty following conversations;
- behavioural changes, including being more irritable, passive, withdrawn or suspicious.

All healthcare professionals are in a position to recognise early signs and symptoms of neurodegeneration and signpost or refer people appropriately (Table 33.6). It is also important to remember that at each stage of dementia, there is an associated decline in physical functioning, which may affect caring and require support from social services.

Classification of dementias

There is no definitive test for any dementia which is routinely available in primary care. It is a process of careful history taking; observation of the person's behaviour, cognition, mood, and

Table 33.7 Proportion of different forms of dementia in UK (Alzheimer's Society, 2014)

Different forms of dementia	%
Alzheimer's disease – includes posterior cortical atrophy	62
Vascular dementia	17
Mixed dementia – Alzheimer's disease and vascular dementia together	10
Dementia with Lewy bodies	4
Other rarer causes of dementia – includes corticobasal degeneration, Down's syndrome, HIV dementia, prion disease, Huntington's disease, alcohol-related brain disease	3
Parkinson's disease dementia	2
Frontotemporal dementia – common in people <65 years, associated with Pick's disease	2

Box 33.1 Differential diagnosis of dementia mnemonic

D	Drugs
E	Emotional problems, eyes, ears
M	Metabolic
E	Endocrine
N	Nutritional deficiency
T	Tumour
I	Infection
A	Anaemia or alcohol
S	Systemic disease

intellectual functioning; and then the systematic exclusion of all other possible causes (i.e. a diagnosis of exclusion). It is important to note that in each country there may be a different proportion of the dementias. AD is most prevalent in the UK, whereas in Japan it is vascular dementia. This is thought to be a product of cultural, genetic and environmental confounders. Table 33.7 provides details of the proportion of dementia types in the UK.

The screening process

Routine laboratory tests such as urea and electrolytes, full blood counts, thyroid function, folate, vitamin D, blood glucose or HbA1c are all undertaken to exclude possible treatable causes of cognitive decline (sometimes termed 'pseudo-dementias'), such as anaemia, thyroid disease, hyponatraemia, hypercalcaemia, hypo- or hyperglycaemia, renal impairment, serology (for venereal disease, including syphilis) and substance or alcohol misuse. Other exclusions include investigating confusion associated with the start or withdrawal of a medication or substance (legal or illegal). A midstream urine (MSU) test excludes delirium associated with urinary tract infections, and a chest and skull X-ray can exclude a chest infection or a space-occupying lesion (SOL). If available, head MRI for quantification of brain changes and the presence of space-occupying lesions, ischaemic lesions or other trauma should be undertaken. An MRI can also be used to identify the extent of neurodegeneration in a particular region of the brain, which can aid determination of the final diagnosis.

There is increasing sophistication in the use of positron emission tomography (PET) scanning, which allows greater accuracy of diagnosis by the distribution of neurodegeneration in brain regions and the deposition of β-amyloid and intracellular neurofibrillary tangles (NFTs) throughout the brain. Lumbar puncture samples are also often used to measure levels of various proteins, including tau and β-amyloid. However, these are not routinely used in practice due to cost, lack of expertise and possible adverse effects on the individual from invasive procedures. Consensus guidelines outline definitive ranges for such measurements and are used to establish diagnosis in people entered into clinical trials and define outcome measures of efficacy and appropriateness (Albert et al., 2011; Sperling et al., 2011).

The most important part of the diagnostic procedure is taking an accurate and detailed history, paying particular attention to intellectual functioning and neurological symptoms. Details of social and occupational history are important to discover. Athletes with a history of head injury or concussion (e.g. boxers) have a high risk of developing pugilistic dementia. Heavy alcohol drinkers may have ARBD. Interviewing carers or relatives is especially important because individuals may be unaware they have a memory or cognitive problem, and the process may also highlight a family history of dementia.

A useful mnemonic to remember the differential diagnosis of dementia is shown in Box 33.1.

Assessing cognitive function

Psychological tests, including a mini-mental state examination (MMSE), usually the Folstein (Folstein et al., 1975), assessment of perception (visuospatial deficits, mood, executive function, memory) and assessments for depression are also part of the differential diagnostic process. They are also used to monitor severity, progression of the disease and response to pharmacological and non-pharmacological treatments interventions. Examples are shown in Table 33.8 and also in the joint guidance on assessing cognition from the Alzheimer's Society and Royal College of General Practitioners (2015).

Diagnostic features of Alzheimer's disease

Key features include an insidious onset of symptoms, predominantly memory loss in the early stages. Progressive cognitive and physical decline is observed, with the emergence of aphasia and agnosia (failure of recognition) in later stages, where good principles of palliative care are needed. The 10 warning signs of AD are described in Table 33.9.

Ascertaining severity of Alzheimer's disease

The previously noted investigations can be supplemented by clinically based assessments such as biographical review, examples of which include the Clinician Interview Based Impression of

Table 33.8 Validated scales to test cognition

Scale	Overview of scale	Time to complete	Cutoff point for dementia
Abbreviated Mental Test Score (AMTS)	A 10-item scale, validated in hospital but used in UK primary care	<5 min	6–8/10
6-Item Cognitive Impairment Test (6CIT)	Three orientation items: count backwards from 20, months of the year in reverse, learn an address Validated in primary care	<5 min	8/24
Mini-Cog	Three-item word memory and clock drawing Validated in primary care Low sensitivity	2–4 min	5/8
General Practitioner Assessment of Cognition (GPCOG)	Developed for primary care and includes a carers' interview	5 min	Part 1: 5–8/9 complete part 2, 0–/9 cognitive impairment Part 2: 0–3/6 cognitive impairment
Montreal Cognitive Assessment Scale (MoCA)	Tasks are executive function and attention, with some language, memory and visuospatial skills Validated in many conditions, including mild cognitive impairment, Alzheimer's disease and Parkinson's disease dementia	10 min	26/30
Addenbrookes Cognitive Examination–III (ACE)	Validated in 5 domains: attention, memory, fluency, language, visuospatial	10–20 min	82–88/100
Folstein Mini-Mental State Examination (MMSE)	Eleven-item measure of cognitive functioning and its change that has been extensively studied and has good validity Less effective for dementia with Lewy bodies and frontotemporal dementia due to its focus on memory	10 min	≤24/30 Cut-point not valid in different cultures and in particularly highly educated or uneducated participants

Table 33.9 Ten warning signs for Alzheimer's disease

Warning sign	Signs of normal aging
Memory loss that disrupts daily life Forgetting recently learned or inability to learn new information; repeatedly asking for the same information	Sometimes forgetting names or appointments but remembering them later
Challenges in planning or problem solving Changes in managing finances or following a plan, taking longer to do things	Making occasional errors when balancing a chequebook or household accounts
Difficulty completing familiar tasks at home, work or leisure Getting lost driving to familiar places; difficulty with project management at work; difficulty remembering rules of a favourite game	Occasionally needing help with settings on microwave or television
Confusion with time or place Losing track of dates, seasons or passage of time; may forget where they are or how they got there	Getting confused about the day of the week but working it out later
Trouble understanding visual images and spatial relationships An early sign and includes trouble reading, judging distance and determining colour or contrast; may also present as hallucinations; distorted perceptions (e.g. passing a mirror and thinking someone else is in the room)	Vision changes related to cataracts
New problems with communication Difficulty following or maintaining conversation; problems finding or using the correct word	Sometimes having trouble finding the right word

Continued

Table 33.9 Ten warning signs for Alzheimer's disease—cont'd

Warning sign	Signs of normal aging
Misplacing items May put items in unusual places (spectacles in the fridge); may accuse people of stealing; cannot retrace steps to find the item	Misplacing things like spectacles or TV remote occasionally
Impaired or reduced judgement Make poor decisions, often involving money or large donations to telemarketers; less attention to personal grooming	Making a bad decision occasionally
Withdrawal from work or social activities May have trouble keeping up with favourite activities or remembering how to do them; may withdraw socially because of these changes	Sometimes feeling weary of work, family and social obligations
Changes in mood or personality May become confused, suspicious, depressed, fearful, anxious or even delusional; may be easily upset doing routine tasks when out of their comfort zone	Developing a specific way of doing things and being irritable when a routine is disrupted

Adapted from Alzheimer's Association (2009).

Severity (CIBIS) and the Clinician Interview Based Impression of Change (CIBC). The latter can be adapted to include input from the carer (CIBIC-plus).

Severity in AD has historically been defined by the Folstein Mini-Mental State Examination (MMSE) score:

- normal cognitive function: MMSE 27–30;
- mild AD: MMSE 21–26;
- moderate AD: MMSE 10–20;
- moderately severe AD: MMSE 10–14;
- severe AD: MMSE <10 (National Institute for Health and Care Excellence [NICE], 2016).

There is continued controversy about the use of the Folstein MMSE because it was originally designed to measure cognitive function in people with mental illness, including schizophrenia, but not dementia (Folstein et al., 1975). In March 2009 a judicial review highlighted the potential discriminatory effects of the MMSE as a rating scale for the start and withdrawal of treatment because of its limitations in people with previously poor intellect, non-white Caucasian ethnicity and low socioeconomic groups. This is due to the tendency for the MMSE to suggest false negatives in these groups. It has also been found to not be sensitive in people with previously high intellect because it gives false negatives. However, the Folstein MMSE is still used, but it is now copyrighted and incurs a charge for use (Folstein et al., 1975).

Diagnostic features of vascular dementia

VaD generally presents with sudden onset, and the dementia follows a stepwise progression. This means that there are periods of cognitive stability followed by periods of rapid decline. The neuropathology of VaD is distinctive, with either localised or generalised areas of brain atrophy and ventricular dilatation and associated areas of cerebral ischaemia and evidence of arteriosclerosis in major vessels. This cerebral damage results in focal neurological signs (absent in AD), and commonly associated clinical features include emotional lability, depression, early memory problems, apraxia, agnosia, dysarthria and dizziness.

The types of symptoms exhibited after damage to a particular area of the brain in VaD or any other dementia, which also influences behaviour, can be seen in Table 33.10.

Generally, insight is more preserved than in AD, but this often leads to increasing distress for patients because they are more aware of the prognosis of the disease. In late-stage VaD, there is a shuffling gait, which can be distinguished from Parkinson's disease by its broad base and preserved arm swing. Fitting and continued episodes of cerebral ischaemia are also late features of this disorder.

Diagnostic features of dementia with Lewy bodies

People with DLB exhibit typically delirium-like cognitive states with periods of fluctuating confusion, which vary in duration and severity from person to person and from time to time within an individual.

Visuospatial, visuo-perceptive and frontal deficits are common. Memory impairment is often less than in the other dementias in the early stages.

Compared with people with AD, people with DLB are more likely to have clouding of consciousness, significant Parkinsonism features, less severely impaired recent memory and a large number of different psychotic features. DLB is diagnosed on the presence of central features and core features; two of the latter are needed for a diagnosis of probable DLB and one for possible DLB (McKeith et al., 2005).

The central feature is progressive cognitive decline of sufficient magnitude to interfere with normal social and occupational function and including one or more of the following core features:

- fluctuating cognition,
- recurrent visual hallucinations (usually people or animals),
- spontaneous features of parkinsonism.

Other features which may support a diagnosis of DLB include repeated falls, syncope, transient loss of consciousness, systemised delusions, hallucinations in other modalities, rapid eye movement (REM) sleep behaviour disorder and depression. However, less likely to be present are a history of stroke or any

Table 33.10 Area of brain degeneration and associated behaviour change in the dementias

Site of brain degeneration/lesion	Change in behaviour exhibited
Frontal lobe Involving motor cortex Bilateral	Behaviour – disinhibited, over-familiar, tactless, over-talkative, jokes, pranks, errors of judgement, sexual indiscretions, disregard for the feelings of others Mood – fatuous and euphoric Concentration and attention – reduced Insight – impaired Contralateral spastic paresis or dysphasia, optic atrophy same side, anosmia, grasp reflex reduced Urinary incontinence
Parietal lobe Nondominant lobe affected Dominant lobe affected	Psychiatric changes less likely, neuropsychological disturbances often resembling hysteria Visuospatial difficulties Dysphasia, motor and dressing apraxias, right–left side disorientation, finger agnosia, agraphia, body image disorder
Temporal lobe Unilateral lesion/degeneration Bilateral If dominant lobe affected	Sometimes asymptomatic Personality change resembling frontal lobe symptoms but often accompanied by intellectual deficits and neurological signs Emotional instability and aggressive behaviour Associated with epilepsy and increasing schizophrenic-like disorder Specific learning impairment – in right-handed people, verbal skills affected; in left-handed people, nonverbal skills affected Amnesic syndrome and visual field defects Language and intellectual impairment
Occipital lobe	Disturbance in visual recognition, often misdiagnosed as hysteria Complex visual hallucinations, often mistaken for non-organic mental illness
Corpus callosum	Severe and rapid intellectual deterioration
Diencephalon and brainstem	Amnesic, hypersomnia, akinetic mutism Progressive intellectual deterioration, emotional lability with euphoria Abrupt outburst of temper, excessive eating, endocrine pituitary disorder

other physical illness or brain disorder sufficient enough to interfere with cognitive performance.

The fluctuation in cognition pattern is associated with:

- hallucinations, usually visual but also auditory;
- periods of confusion and attention deficit;
- other psychotic symptoms;
- early gait disturbances;
- extrapyramidal features, such as rigidity, bradykinesia, tremor and fixed posture (i.e. signs of parkinsonism and Parkinson's disease) (McKeith et al., 2005).

Diagnostic features of the rarer dementias

Diagnostic features of Parkinson's disease dementia

A differential diagnosis is made on the following criteria:

- Those people with Parkinson's disease who develop a dementia more than 12 months after the initial motor symptoms should be diagnosed with Parkinson's disease dementia.
- If the dementia precedes the motor symptoms or the duration of the motor symptoms is less than 12 months, then the diagnosis is DLB (McKeith, 2006).

Diagnostic features of frontotemporal dementia

Age is a diagnostic factor, with 7 out of 10 people with FTD aged between 45 and 64 years, as well as the presence of four main variants:

- behavioural variant;
- semantic dementia deficits in verbal and nonverbal understanding of memory;
- progressive non-fluent aphasia, a language disorder in which people have problems speaking;
- FTD associated with motor disorder, including motor neurone disease, corticobasal degeneration and progressive supranuclear palsy.

Diagnostic features of corticobasal degeneration

Early presenting symptoms affect movement and include stiffness, jerky movements and a unilateral inability to control hand movement. Eventually this affects other limbs, leading to loss of balance and coordination, and is also associated with cognitive deficits, including memory loss, perceptual difficulties and difficulties in swallowing and speaking.

Diagnostic features of progressive supranuclear palsy

The tau pathology results in paralysis of eye movements (causing double vision), affecting balance control and resulting in frequent falls. Other symptoms include stiff or slow movements, difficulties walking and speaking, swallowing problems and personality changes. A parkinsonian-like tremor may be present, but it is much less prominent than in Parkinson's disease.

A small proportion of people with progressive supranuclear palsy develop an overlapping condition with FTD, but the majority experience cognitive difficulties rather than a dementia syndrome. This cognitive impairment may affect the speed of thought processes and memory, but affected individuals will remain aware of what is going on around them.

Diagnostic features of Creutzfeldt–Jakob disease

In sporadic CJD, the disease progression is rapid over a few months, with early symptoms including minor lapses of memory, mood changes and loss of interest. Within weeks, the person may experience clumsiness, feel muddled, become unsteady when walking, and have slow or slurred speech. Symptoms progress to jerky movements, shakiness, stiffness of limbs, incontinence and loss of the ability to move or speak. By this stage, the person is unlikely to be aware of his or her surroundings or disabilities. The majority of people affected by CJD usually die within 6 months of their early symptom development.

Diagnostic features of HIV-associated neurocognitive disorder

Cognitive difficulties include mild deficits in short-term memory, learning, thinking, concentration and reasoning.

Diagnostic features of Huntington's disease

This neurodegeneration starts in the striatum, which is why first symptoms depict abnormal movements, including twitches and muscle spasms and problems with balance and coordination. Other symptoms include depression, mood swings, irritability and cognitive impairment, including difficulties with concentration, planning and organisational skills. The age of onset and disease course vary for each person, and dementia can occur at any stage of the illness. Some may experience short-term memory loss or develop obsessive behaviours. Unlike in AD, people with Huntington's disease dementia continue to recognise people and places until the very late stages of the disease.

Diagnostic features of multiple sclerosis cognitive difficulties

Symptoms include memory, concentration and problem solving. Emotional problems include mood swings and personality changes.

Diagnostic features of Niemann–Pick disease type C

Niemann–Pick disease type C mainly affects school-age children but can occur at any time, from early infancy to adulthood, and symptoms start with progressive loss of movement and difficulties with walking and swallowing.

Dementia occurs most commonly in those people who develop symptoms in late adolescence or early adulthood, with the main symptoms including confusion, memory problems and difficulties in concentrating and learning.

Diagnostic features of normal pressure hydrocephalus

Symptoms include difficulties with walking, dementia syndrome and urinary incontinence. Generally, there is no cause, but it may develop after recovery from a head injury, brain haemorrhage or severe meningitis.

Diagnostic features of posterior cortical atrophy

Initially, people with posterior cortical atrophy tend to have a relatively well-preserved memory but experience visual problems, such as difficulty recognising faces and objects in pictures, which then affect literacy and numeracy. Symptoms of posterior cortical atrophy occur in the mid-50s or early 60s, but diagnosis may take longer because of the subtle onset.

Diagnostic features of alcohol-related brain damage

ARBD is defined as long-term decline in memory or thinking caused by excessive alcohol use resulting in thiamine deficiency and neurodegeneration associated with the toxicity of alcohol itself on neurons. Associated alcohol misuse factors include repeated head injuries sustained from falls or fights and associated damage to the cardiovascular system, including raised blood pressure and cholesterol. However, these are all also risk factors for other dementias.

Treatment of dementia

Alzheimer's disease

Currently there are two pharmacological groups licensed for the treatment of the symptoms of AD: the acetylcholinesterase inhibitors (AChEIs) donepezil, rivastigmine and galantamine, and the N-methyl-D-aspartate (NMDA) receptor antagonist memantine. The NICE (2016) technology appraisal guidance for prescribing donepezil, galantamine, rivastigmine and memantine states that treatment aims are to promote independence, maintain function and treat symptoms, including cognitive, non-cognitive (hallucinations, delusions, anxiety, marked agitation and associated aggressive behaviour), behavioural and psychological symptoms. Donepezil, galantamine and rivastigmine are all recommended as treatment options for managing mild and moderate AD. Memantine is recommended as an option for managing moderate AD for people who cannot take AChEIs and as an option for managing severe AD. Information to guide the prescribing of medicines for dementia is shown in Table 33.11.

Acetylcholinesterase inhibitors

Acetylcholinesterase inhibitors exert their pharmacological activity by inhibiting the enzyme acetylcholinesterase to increase the concentration of acetylcholine at sites of neurotransmission.

Galantamine also enhances the action of acetylcholine on nicotinic receptors. Although these agents belong to the same group, they all produce their pharmacological effect in a slightly different way. Therefore, if a response to one agent is not seen, it is justifiable to try another. This also applies to the individual experience of adverse effects.

AD is progressive, which means that there will be less acetylcholine produced throughout the course of the disease. At the start of treatment with an AChEI, patients usually improve from

Table 33.11 Prescribing and monitoring medicines for dementia

	Donepezil	Rivastigmine	Galantamine	Memantine
Activity	Reversible acetylcholin-esterase inhibitor activity, dose-dependent activity Greater selectivity acetylcholinesterase	Pseudo-irreversible with greater selectivity acetylcholinesterase Dose-dependent activity	Reversible competitive AChEI with enhanced action of acetylcholine on muscarinic receptors Dose-dependent activity	Uncompetitive NMDA-receptor antagonist which modulates pathological levels of glutamate
Dosing	Start at 5 mg once daily and increase to 10 mg once daily after 4 weeks Evening dosing, just before retiring; if insomnia and vivid dreaming, change to morning.	Start 1.5 mg twice daily with morning and evening meals If well tolerated at 2 weeks, increase to 3 mg twice daily Subsequent increases to 4.5 mg and then 6 mg twice daily based on good tolerability and minimum 2 weeks of treatment before dose increase	Initially 4 mg twice daily for 4 weeks increasing to 8 mg twice daily for 4 weeks to maintenance dose of 12 mg twice daily	5 mg once daily, increasing by 5 mg/week to a maximum of 20 mg once daily If sedation occurs, change to an evening dose to aid sleep
Forms available (UK)	5 mg and 10 mg tablets Oral solution 1 mg/1 mL Orodispersible tablets 5 mg, 10 mg	Capsules 1.5 mg, 3 mg, 4.5 mg, 6 mg Oral solution 2 mg/1 mL Patches 4.6 mg/24 h, 9.5 mg/24 h, 13 .3 mg/24 h	Immediate-release tablets 8 mg or 12 mg twice-daily dosing Oral solution 4 mg/1 mL Modified release capsules; 8 mg, 16 mg, 24 mg once daily	Tablets 5 mg, 10 mg, 15 mg, 20 mg film Oral solution 10 mg/1 mL sugar-free
General	Low side-effect profile (nausea 14%, vomiting 8% and diarrhoea 12%)	Low side-effect profile but may cause severe anorexia in some and weight loss (nausea 47%, vomiting 31% and diarrhoea 19%) Licensed for use in Parkinson's disease dementia	Low side-effect profile (nausea 24%, vomiting 13% and diarrhoea 9%)	Low side-effect profile: constipation, dizziness, diarrhoea. Uncommon side effects include abnormal gait, confusion, fatigue, hallucinations
Pharmacokinetics	Peak concentration 3–4 h post-dose $t_{1/2}$ = 70 h (steady state in 3 weeks) Linear pharmacokinetics Metabolised in liver CYP450 system, modify dose in mild to severe hepatic impairment Renally excreted Food does not affect absorption 95% protein bound	$t_{1/2}$ approximately 2 h Inhibition lasts 10 h Renal excretion of rivastigmine and inactive metabolites involving cytochrome isoenzymes: CYP1A2, CYP2D6, CYP3A4/5, CYP2E1, CYP2C9, CYP2C8, CYP2C19 or CYP2B6 CYP450 minimally involved in metabolism Dose adjustment in moderate hepatic and renal impairment may be necessary Food delays absorption and affects AUC Protein binding 40%	Serum max 0.5 to 1 h $t_{1/2}$ 7–8 h Reduce dose in moderate hepatic impairment and avoid in severe impairment Avoid if eGFR <9 mL/min/1,73 m^2 Food affects absorption but does not affect extent of absorption Protein binding 18% Linear pharmacokinetics in dose range of 4–16 mg twice daily	t_{max} between 3 and 8 h Linear pharmacokinetics No CYP450 catalysed-metabolism 90% renally excreted If moderate renal impairment, titrate to 10 mg, and if tolerated, increase with monitoring to 20 mg In severe renal impairment, maximum dose 10 mg daily Food does not affect absorption 45% protein bound

Continued

Table 33.11 Prescribing and monitoring medicines for dementia—cont'd

	Donepezil	Rivastigmine	Galantamine	Memantine
Cautions	Asthma, COPD, sick sinus syndrome, supraventricular conduction disorders, susceptibility to peptic ulcers Common adverse effects mainly cholinergic, especially GI, also excessive mucous production and leg cramps	Asthma, COPD, sick sinus syndrome, supraventricular conduction disorders, susceptibility to peptic ulcers Common adverse effects mainly cholinergic, especially GI, also excessive mucous production and leg cramps If treatment is interrupted >3 days, re-initiate at 1.5 mg twice daily to reduce adverse effects (vomiting) Skin application-site reactions may occur with patch, mild or moderate in intensity Not an indication of sensitisation but may lead to allergic contact dermatitis	Asthma, COPD, sick sinus syndrome, supraventricular conduction disorders, susceptibility to peptic ulcers Common adverse effects mainly cholinergic, especially GI, also excessive mucous production and leg cramps Stevens–Johnson syndrome and acute generalised exanthematous pustulosis have been reported – informed patients to discontinue at the first sign of a rash	Avoid in severe hepatic impairment Avoid concomitant NMDA antagonists (e.g. amantadine, ketamine, dextromethorphan) Caution if history or diagnosis of epilepsy or seizures
Pharmaco-dynamic cautions	Cholinesterase inhibitors (cholinomimetics) should not be given concomitantly with other cholinomimetics, and they have the potential to antagonise the effect of anticholinergic medication. If anticholinergic medications such as atropine are abruptly stopped, there is a potential risk of exacerbation of cholinesterase inhibitors effects. Pharmacodynamic interactions with medicinal products that significantly reduce the heart rate, such as digoxin, β-blockers, certain calcium-channel blocking agents and amiodarone are possible, and caution should be taken with medicinal products that have potential to cause torsades de pointes. In such cases, an ECG should be considered. An exaggerated response to succinylcholine-type muscle relaxation during anaesthesia could occur.			

Always check in the latest Summary of Product Characteristics because this is more explicit than in the BNF for interactions with other medication.
AChEI, Acetylcholinesterase inhibitor; AUC, area under the curve; BNF, British National Formulary; COPD, chronic obstructive pulmonary disease; ECG, electrocardiogram; eGFR, estimate of glomerular filtration rate; GI, gastro-intestinal; NMDA, N-methyl-D-aspartate; t_{max}, time to maximal response; $t_{1/2}$, half-life of a drug.

pretreatment function and assessment scores. As the disease progresses, the amount of acetylcholine produced will be less than at pretreatment, so individual patient performance will decline, eventually to a stage where the agent will seem to have little clinical effect. One of the difficulties with measuring improvement or response to a treatment is that because the disease is progressing, signs and symptoms may seem to worsen rather than improve. However, AChEIs ensure that any acetylcholine that is produced (at any stage of the disease) will be available for neuronal transmission for longer. This means that the symptoms of AD, such as functions in activities of daily living, cognitive function and behaviour, will be alleviated to some extent for the time that the patient remains on treatment. Each of these agents has different formulations which may help people with swallowing difficulties or problems with dose titration.

Cautions for use. AChEIs should be prescribed with caution in patients with 'sick sinus syndrome' or other supraventricular cardiac conduction conditions, patients with concomitant asthma or obstructive pulmonary disease and those with, or at risk of, peptic ulcer disease. Rivastigmine should be prescribed with caution in patients with renal impairment or mild to moderate hepatic impairment.

All AChEIs cause gastro-intestinal effects such as diarrhoea, muscle cramps, fatigue, nausea, vomiting, insomnia and dizziness. These are generally mild and transient, and they often disappear within a few days of continued treatment. However, in some patients, these effects may be severe and result in significant weight loss. To reduce these effects, the medication can be taken after food, and/or an anti-emetic may be co-prescribed. Another approach is extending the time period required to reach the maximum therapeutic dose for such patients. If there is no history of Parkinson's disease or DLB, then long-acting metoclopramide may be given during the dose titration period. The alternative for those patients with Parkinson's disease or DLB is domperidone at 10–20 mg three or four times daily.

Selection of any concomitant medication for a person with dementia should include an analysis of its propensity to cause antimuscarinic effects because this interferes with memory and may exacerbate or cause confusion. Examples include hyoscine, oxybutynin, procyclidine, antipsychotics (including some atypicals), tricyclic antidepressants, furosemide, digoxin and cimetidine.

Controversies associated with treatment. Numbers needed to treat for AChEIs range from 3 to 7 at low dose and delay disease progression by at least 6 months, with increasing evidence from clinical practice that some patients benefit for periods of greater than 7 years (Livingston and Katona, 2000). There is robust evidence demonstrating that these agents delay the need for institutionalisation of the person with dementia by making it easier for the carer to provide care in the home environment (Geldmacher et al., 2003).

The heterogeneous nature of AD itself and the fact that many people have a mixed dementia syndrome imply that each patient may have a unique set of symptoms which one medication is not able to address.

Stopping and changing treatment. If a patient seems to have no improvement in objective scores but also no deterioration, it could be argued that the neurodegenerative process is being held at steady state. Therefore, the agent should be continued. If a patient has failed to tolerate the maximum effective dose of a particular agent over a 3-month assessment period, an alternative should be considered.

If withdrawing an AChEI, evidence suggests that patients should be carefully reviewed for the next 48–72 hours and for 2 weeks after discontinuation. This is because when an AChEI is withdrawn, the person with dementia can rapidly decline, and it then becomes apparent that the medication was producing effects in areas that had not been previously acknowledged. Dementia is a syndrome affecting many parts of a person's cognitive function, including personality, communication and behaviours, as well as memory. Just because a poor response in memory is seen, this does not mean the medicines are not being effective in other aspects. If the medicines are restarted within 2 weeks, patients often return to their level of function before withdrawal. If the period before restarting is longer than this, the deterioration appears to remain, although further progression may be halted for a further period of time if medication is restarted.

N-Methyl-D-aspartate receptor antagonist – memantine

Memantine is a voltage-dependent, moderate-affinity uncompetitive NMDA-receptor antagonist. It blocks excessive calcium ion influx into the neuron to prevent associated neuronal death but allows normal physiological functioning. It is licensed for the treatment of people with moderate through to severe AD. Studies demonstrate significant improvement in cognition and functioning (activities of daily living) global outcomes and also that fewer people taking memantine develop agitation (Hermann et al., 2011).

Memantine is licensed for use in patients with moderate and severe AD and may be co-prescribed with AChEIs dependent on specialist advice. It should also be considered at mild stages of AD if AChEIs cannot be tolerated or are contraindicated (NICE, 2016).

Emerging treatments for Alzheimer's disease

Since a Global Summit on Dementia in 2013, in response to the World Health Organization report (WHO, 2012), there has been wider international collaboration on potential treatments and sharing of information. Currently, there are several compounds in 3- to 4-year phase III clinical trials looking at the prevention of amyloid and tau deposition using monoclonal antibodies.

Monoclonal antibodies. Monoclonal antibodies clear toxic amyloid-β directly or by microglia and astrocyte activation. There are currently five fully human monoclonal antibodies in clinical trials (olanezumab, ducanumab, gentenerumab, crenezumab and Biogen/Eisai's BAN2401), all with slightly different modes of action. Some of the difficulties of treatment with monoclonal antibodies are that they possess limited brain bioavailability and can cause immunogenicity and serious adverse effects such as cerebral oedema.

Small molecules. Small molecules aid in prevention and treatment by reducing amyloid-β production, tau aggregation or neuroinflammation. Examples include gamma-secretase and β-secretase modulators to reduce aberrant cleavage of amyloid precursor protein (APP); inhibitors of tau aggregation; and tau vaccines and azeliragon, an antagonist of the receptor of advanced glycation end products (RAGE), which leads to inflammation and oxidative damage when occupied. RAGE also mediates transport of amyloid-β from the blood into the brain (Connelly, 2015).

Other targets. Other targets include the repositioning of agents currently used to treat hypertension (calcium channel blockers) and diabetes (pioglitazone), as well as exploring the effect of insulin resistance on brain function (Kim, 2015).

Treatment of rarer dementias

For all rarer dementias, there is currently no cure and generally no licensed treatment; consequently, management is symptomatic, combining medication, physiotherapy, occupational therapy and speech and language support. The exceptions are as follows:

- Rivastigmine is licensed for use in Parkinson's disease dementia.
- The current triad of antiretroviral medication regimen has resulted in a reduction in HIV-related dementia to approximately 2%, from 20% to 30% (Alzheimer's Society, 2015a).
- If normal pressure hydrocephalus is diagnosed and treated early with cranial surgery to drain excess fluid, symptoms generally improve after surgery, with some people making an almost complete recovery. In the majority of these cases, AD is the cause of posterior cortical atrophy; therefore, AChEIs and/or memantine may be of benefit.
- In ARBD, treatment is based on the person staying alcohol-free and rehabilitation from either dementia services, acquired brain injury services or the community mental health team. Any improvement in the person's abilities is usually greatest in the first 3 months of abstinence but can continue for 2–3 years. About 25% of people affected by ARBD make a very good recovery, with about 50% achieving partial recovery and needing support to manage their lives but possibly still being able to live in their own homes or in sheltered housing. The final 25% make no recovery and generally require long-term residential care (Alzheimer's Society, 2015b).

Treatment strategy for behavioural and psychological symptoms of dementia

First-line treatment for any challenging behaviour is either a psychological or alternative therapy intervention (NICE and Social Care Institute for Excellence [SCIE], 2011). These interventions should be given sufficient chance to exert an effect before trying

Box 33.2 Potential causes of behavioural change

- Depression
- Pain (remember that patients walk into objects)
- A superimposed acute confusional state (delirium) caused by infection (chest and urinary tract infections are most common)
- New medication being started or one stopped (including purchased and recreational, e.g. alcohol)
- Side effect or withdrawal effect of a medicine
- Communication problems (check glasses for correct prescription/clean; hearing aids [battery/turned on], denture use)
- Aggression might indicate the person wants to communicate but cannot and becomes frustrated
- Recent change in environment/staff/routine
- Review to determine if this is a common trigger (antecedent); linked to a behaviour
- Identify what changes this behaviour (e.g. distraction)

an alternative. If they are effective, then the person should just be monitored. It is important to remember that the disease is always progressing, and therefore challenging behaviours will stop or change. Box 33.2 details the possible causes of behavioural change.

Psychological and alternative therapies. Psychological and alternative therapies are first-line non-pharmacological treatment options and include adapting the environment (e.g. lighting, space to walk, colour schemes, access to outdoors). Behavioural interventions include distraction, reality orientation, occupational activities, reminiscence, cognitive stimulation and singing. Any possible underlying causes should be explored (e.g. pain, anxiety, depression, a recent change or upsetting event). Lavender oil (aromatherapy and massage) and melissa oil (aromatherapy) have both demonstrated significant improvement in agitation versus placebo (Fu et al., 2013).

Improving the staff knowledge of behavioural and psychological symptoms of dementia (BPSD) and how to manage them using non-pharmacological methods has been shown to result in a sustained 50% reduction in the use of antipsychotics over a year. In addition, improving social interaction also resulted in reduced rates of prescribing for patients with severe dementia (Fossey et al., 2006).

More importantly, treating unrecognised pain was found to reduce agitation significantly, as well as other neuropsychiatric symptoms (Husebo et al., 2011).

Behavioural treatment and carer support are priorities in managing sundowning. These are in addition to minimising napping during the day, regular exercise and establishing a day and night routine. Use of bright light (Lux) in the morning can reduce the incidence of agitation in the evening. Small studies have shown that people with dementia who receive light therapy in winter months display reduced behavioural problems such as agitation (NICE and SCIE, 2011).

Increasingly, forms of psychotherapy and modified cognitive-based therapy are being used with some success in people with dementia in the mild to moderate stages (Junaid and Hegde, 2006). Other psychosocial interventions include reminiscence and/or validation therapy; interactions with animals, music and children; and cognitive stimulation therapy (Toh et al., 2016).

Short-term pharmacological management of behavioural and psychological symptoms of dementia. If the behaviours are anxiety or mood related, then second-line treatment is low doses of selective serotonin reuptake inhibitors (SSRIs). These have reduced antimuscarinic effects compared with tricyclic antidepressants, and sertraline is the safest in terms of cardiovascular risks.

Occasionally an antipsychotic may be appropriate if all other avenues have been tried and the individual is a danger to him- or herself or others and/or is extremely distressed. Risperidone is the only licensed antipsychotic in the UK for the treatment of severe aggression in AD which has not responded to other treatments, but it can only be prescribed for a maximum period of 6 weeks. The Royal College of Psychiatrists (2016) recommend that the treatment decision is made by a specialist in dementia after discussion with the person's carer and/or family and the multidisciplinary team, and the reason recorded in the patient's medical record. The lowest dose producing the desired effect should be used, and the continued need should be reviewed regularly and the treatment discontinued when appropriate.

Longer-term prescribing of antipsychotics. If a challenging behaviour continues and requires longer-term management, then an alternative to an antipsychotic must be considered because rates of mortality are increased over those who do not take long-term antipsychotics. The long-term negative outcomes of being prescribed an antipsychotic in dementia were shown in the DAART-AD trial (Ballard et al., 2009). This study identified that at 24 months, the survival rate for those receiving an antipsychotic was 46% compared with 71% in the placebo arm; 36 months' survival was 30% compared with 50%; and at 42 months, it was 26% compared with 53%.

Potential alternatives include acetylcholinesterase inhibitors, memantine, citalopram, gabapentin and pregabalin. If highly antimuscarinic agents are initiated, monitoring is required because they reduce cognitive functioning by reducing cholinergic load and are linked with increased mortality and morbidity (Fox et al., 2011). People with dementia tend to be very sensitive to any centrally acting medication, and the prolonged action of sedatives increases the risk of falls. Therefore, if necessary, the smallest possible dose should be prescribed for the shortest time.

Patient care

Safer medicines use

Two-thirds of prescribing of antipsychotics in people with dementia is inappropriate and associated with increased morbidity and mortality for as long as it is prescribed. Both typical and atypical antipsychotics are associated with large side-effect profiles, with numbers needed to harm ranging from 4 to 13. Deaths related to antipsychotic prescribing are associated with cerebrovascular and cardiovascular events, as well as pneumonia (Wang et al., 2005).

If highly antimuscarinic agents are initiated, monitoring their effect is important because they reduce cognitive functioning by reducing cholinergic load and are linked with increased mortality and morbidity (Fox et al., 2011).

Medication should be reviewed regularly to reduce the presence of iatrogenic disease and to gain maximum benefit from medicines for dementia and cognitive functioning by lessening the use of highly antimuscarinic medication. It is important to ensure that the carer (with the permission of the person with dementia) is also involved in all aspects of medicines use because the carer is the person ensuring adherence with any medication regimen. For advice on medicines optimisation, please see Table 33.12. When the disease becomes end stage, then there should be a judicial review of all medication, and the principles of good palliative care should be put into place.

Preventing dementia

Reducing cardiovascular risk

If 1000 people with hypertension were treated with adequate treatment for 5 years, then 19 cases of dementia would be prevented (Kelly et al., 2009).

Aspirin does not improve cognitive functioning, but it will prevent further ischaemic events and should be prescribed if indicated.

Before and at all stages of dementia, people need advice on lifestyle changes to keep healthy and improve cerebrovascular and cardiovascular perfusion. There is robust evidence to

Table 33.12 Suggestions to enhance medicines optimisation and prescribing

Problem	Suggestions
Labelling issues	Carers appreciate complete directions such as 'at night' or 'after breakfast' so that they can plan dosing schedules according to mealtimes. If a medication is being taken for sleep, e.g. then directions such as 'take 1 h before bedtime' can help so that the medication is starting to take effect before the recipient actually goes to bed.
Disease progression	Disease progression effects physical functions as well and includes swallowing and chewing difficulties. Always ask if there is a problem because many carers just try to get the medication into the person any way they can, often mixing it with yoghurt, jam or mashed potato. Where possible, ensure liquid formulations are used if this is a problem. Carers value any support in this area because they have been told how important it is for the medicines to be taken but do not realise the potential effects of opening a long-acting capsule into yoghurt. Poor memory, a reduced sense of smell and the effects of medication may result in a reduced food and fluid intake, resulting in weight loss, dehydration and electrolyte disturbance. The provision of sip feeds may be useful in people at this stage of the disease. Control of bowels and bladder may reduce over time; in moderate to moderately severe stages, people may forget where the toilet is or not recognise the physical signs associated with bowel and bladder control. Regular toileting (on waking and after meals and before bed) may help, but also the provision of incontinence aids may be needed. Also think about the need for skin care to ensure that skin breakdown and possible pressure sores do not occur.
Simplifying medication regimens	Consider the use of long-acting preparations (e.g. galantamine XL) as an alternative to twice-daily dosing or patches if a long-acting form is needed. Long-acting preparations will take longer to reach steady state, but this often reduces the incidence of side effects and improves adherence to complex medication regimens.
Repeat dispensing issues	Concomitant medicines that run out at different times and may have different prescribers – try to rationalise prescribing and ordering to ensure a common quantity of medication is available. Prescriptions for the cognitive enhancer are often collected from a different place, increasing strain on the carer, especially if it means ringing a consultant's secretary to ensure a prescription is sent and sufficient quantities are ordered to last until the next appointment. You may be able to help ensure that the prescriber understands exactly what is needed and by when. Changing brands of concomitant medication can be confusing for any person, let alone someone with a memory problem who may just remember shape and/or colour. Great care is needed when making these changes to ensure that it is fully understood that it is the same medication and not another new one. Parallel imports may also be confusing.
Remembering medication	Memory and/or compliance aids may be a welcome addition to help make sense of the medication, as would a medication reminder card which also includes brief details of what to take and when. If you are helping individuals with a memory problem who live on their own, it is recommended to find out how they currently try to remember to take their tablets (many write notes for themselves and then tick things off the calendar or have a note on the fridge or a telephone call from a family member) and see if you can help improve the system. Try not to introduce anything too complex because they may not remember new information or routines. Suggestions that fit with their current daily activities may be most successful. It may also help to telephone them for a few days to see how they are getting on.

Continued

Table 33.12 Suggestions to enhance medicines optimisation and prescribing—cont'd

Problem	Suggestions
Medicines review	Discuss with the carer and person with dementia what they feel is most important; they will generally have one pressing issue which they would like to resolve. There is often at least one medication that people are not using either at all or as prescribed. Try to establish why. It may be that the behaviour has changed and the item is no longer needed or that an adverse event occurred which has put them off using the medication. If the latter, then a smaller dose or alternative medication may be more appropriate. Asking key questions can help identify what actually happened. Always communicate this with the prescriber (with the individual's permission) because this reduces waste and unnecessary prescribing and helps keep accurate records of medication regimens. Check that the time of day a dose is to be taken is appropriate if a side effect occurs (e.g. if insomania and/or nightmares occur in people on donepezil, ensure the dose is taken in the morning because this will improve sleep patterns).
Managing side effects	Diarrhoea, nausea, vomiting, anorexia and headache are common side effects on initiation and on dose titration of AChEIs. Carers need support to understand this is normal and that tolerance will generally develop. These may be transient (5–7 days), but if continuous, then a shared decision should be made on the balance of benefits and adverse reactions. Due to the different modes of action, another agent may be tried. **Antiemetics** For nausea/vomiting on initiation or dose titration of AChEIs, domperidone is preferred because it does not cross the blood–brain barrier or have anticholinergic side effects. Domperidone should be taken regularly three or four times daily for 3 or 4 days and then reduced to zero as symptoms subside. Long-acting metoclopramide is an option for those without movement disorders. **Diarrhoea** If diarrhoea is a problem, loperamide may be co-prescribed. The dose and frequency are generally titrated to the side effect and then taken regularly. Ensure that the dose is not so high or continued too long as to cause constipation. Donepezil is prescribed at night; however, it may cause vivid dreams interfering with sleep, in which case, this may be best administered in the morning. **Memantine** Side effects include dizziness, headache, confusion, hallucinations (which can also be part of the dementia process) and tiredness. Keeping a diary of tiredness is recommended because a short nap in the mid-afternoon may reduce the problem, as would administering the dose at night to aid sleep.
Referral of side effects	If side effects of AChEIs are severe and/or debilitating, then refer back to the prescriber. Referral should also be made if there are signs of urinary flow difficulties or worsening of asthma, COPD or cardiovascular symptoms, especially blackouts. With memantine, if hallucinations are distressing the individual, refer to specialist. NICE guidelines set out strict conditions to be met before the use of an antipsychotic.
Starting new medicines	If new medicines are started (including purchase of OTC products for coughs and colds), check whether they cause anticholinergic side effects because this will increase confusion, impair memory function and possibly antagonise the effect of the cholinesterase inhibitor. Dextromethorphan and memantine are contraindicated.
Concomitant prescribed medicines (for other medical conditions)	Ensure understanding of what each medication is for and common side effects associated with each, highlighting those that need to be reported immediately. It is often helpful to provide a medicine reminder chart which indicates what each is for, including common side effects and when to take them. Always check for interactions. Remember that any agent which has anticholinergic side effects will increase confusion and reduce cognitive functioning (as well as the other adverse effects, such as constipation, dry mouth, cardiovascular effects). Therefore, where possible, check for anticholinergic load (e.g. oxybutynin, antidepressants or antipsychotics) and recommend alternatives if possible. Remember that any medication with CNS effects (e.g. benzodiazepines, opiates or dopaminergic agents) may negatively affect cognitive functioning. Benzodiazepines are also amnestic. Any agent which has the potential to cause confusion, e.g. long-acting hypoglycaemic agents, non-steroidal anti-inflammatory agents and H_2 antagonists such as cimetidine, should be carefully monitored and/or withdrawn if possible. Side effects of aspirin are well known. Ask about gastro-intestinal problems, and check for excessive bruising after falls or knocks.
Stopping cognitive enhancers	Stopping cholinesterase inhibitors can produce a dramatic decline in cognitive and physical functioning which may require the agent to be restarted.

AChEIs, Acetylcholinesterase inhibitors; CNS, central nervous system; COPD, chronic obstructive pulmonary disease; NICE, National Institute of Health and Care Excellence; OTC, over-the-counter.

demonstrate that an active lifestyle and using the brain to learn a new language, dance or take part in gym activities alongside a healthy diet reduce the risk of dementia (Public Health England, 2016).

Herbal supplements, aromatherapy and social and behavioural interventions

People with dementia and family members may use various herbal supplements to try to prevent and/or delay the onset of dementia.

Claims of cognitive enhancement have been made for a number of supplements; the key ones are listed here. Cochrane Reviews on Dementia and Cognitive Improvement (http://dementia.cochrane.org/) hosts a number of systematic reviews on herbal supplements, aromatherapy and social and behavioural interventions for people with dementia. Another useful resource is the NICE-SCIE guideline on supporting people with dementia (NICE and SCIE, 2011).

Ginkgo biloba

The proposed mechanism of action of ginkgo biloba is to increase blood supply by dilating cerebral blood vessels and decreasing blood viscosity. There are some isolated reports of bleeding with ginkgo biloba with a theoretical interaction with aspirin or warfarin, possibly resulting in increased bleeding (Bent et al., 2005). The prescriber should be consulted before use in these circumstances. It is also proposed that the compound modifies neurotransmitter systems and decreases the density of oxygen free radicals. The evidence for improvement in cognitive functioning is inconsistent with three studies showing equivalence to placebo and one showing a substantial positive effect. However, it is known that ginkgo appears to be safe to use and is well tolerated; it is unknown whether long-term use has any effect on the onset of dementia (Birks and Grimley Evans, 2009).

Vitamin E

Vitamin E has an antioxidant effect, and it was thought this might reduce the onset of the neurodegenerative process. However, a review in 2012 stated there was no evidence of the efficacy of vitamin E in the prevention or treatment of people with AD or mild cognitive impairment and that the risks to individuals outweighed any benefits (Farina et al., 2012).

Folic acid, vitamin B_{12} and iron

The dietary supplement folic acid, vitamin B_{12} and iron are linked with cognitive dysfunction, confusion and/or memory problems, when there is a deficit. Older people may not eat sufficient fresh green vegetables or dietary protein to sustain normal levels. In addition, active transport mechanisms for vitamin B_{12} absorption are often impaired. However, if a deficiency has not been identified, supplementation with folic acid, vitamin B_{12} or iron will generally not have any clinical effect.

Supporting people with concerns about possible dementia

People often worry about the possibility of dementia if their memory seems to be less effective as they get older. With aging, our mental speed tends to decline, with thinking, problem solving and recall all becoming slower. Being very busy, depressed or anxious can impair the way in which short-term memories are laid down. If short-term memories are not laid down, then long-term memories will not be formed. For example, if you are not paying complete attention to a person when he or she is speaking, the information will not be retained completely, which results in reduced recall of the conversation, disruption of the short-term memory process and consequent inability to recall the conversation or interaction. Forgetting the occasional word or making a poor decision once in a while is nothing to be worried about. The time to seek help or refer to memory services is when changes in cognitive functioning impair an individual's ability to care for him- or herself or participate in work or social interactions. Healthcare professionals are often reluctant to discuss cognitive changes with people, but further information and signposting is welcomed so that they can address their own concerns.

Communicating with people with dementia and their carers

The most important thing to remember when talking to people with dementia is that they are still able to communicate and will probably enjoy the opportunity. The following points will aid effective communication, but supporting information may be necessary from relatives or caregiver(s) when accurate and reliable information is needed (e.g. an accurate medication history). People with dementia may make up answers if they think they should know but are unable to remember an answer.

Adapting communication skills

The fundamental principle of communication with people with dementia is to try to capitalise on the preserved memory systems. Therefore, the following strategies are advisable:
- Simplify sentences.
- Simplify vocabulary.
- Use yes-or-no, not multiple choice, questions.
- Talk about the here and now, not the abstract.
- Use direct language wherever possible.
- Avoid teasing and sarcasm.
- Check that what you say is understood.
- Summarise information.
- Provide written information.
- Use a slow speech rate.
- Speak clearly and audibly.
- Use a pleasant, accepting tone.
- Vary the pitch and tone of the voice.
- Limit the number of participants in the conversation.

Skilled communicators can establish a conversation with the person in a time and place that they remember and thus allow them to participate. It is also increasingly important to read the person's body language as the disease progresses. This is because often the person cannot communicate effectively with words, and physical exhibitions of agitation, depression, pain or frustration may be conveyed via pacing, withdrawal or shouting/hitting, for example.

Information provision for carers

The physical and psychological support of carers is very important; it is well evidenced that if they are not given the support they need, then the caring process breaks down, and early institutionalisation occurs (Eska et al., 2013). People need and want different advice at different stages of the illness, so always offer information even if it is not always accepted. Wide-ranging guidance for carers and healthcare professionals can be found in the NICE-SCIE (2011) guideline. As the disease progresses, carers may seek advice on how to manage behavioural changes and the reasons for their development. Useful information is provided by the Alzheimer's Society (2015c).

People with dementia and/or their carers may seek information on a number of issues to address before insight into care is lost. Awareness of any local dementia services and signposting people for information is therefore important. Topics may include:

* access to financial, social and healthcare advice and services;
* legal issues, such as continuing to drive or end-of-life care;
* occupational therapy for living aids, such as stair lift, stair gates, shower and bathing aids, walking and dressing aids;
* memory aids, including tools and prompts, as well as activities for improving cognitive and memory function;
* carer support and education on caring for a person with dementia.

Case studies

Case 33.1

Mrs LB is well known at your pharmacy because she organises the repeat prescriptions for her husband and collects these every 2 months. Mr TB, her husband, has hypertension and is prescribed losartan and simvastatin. Mr TB has recently retired; he was a banker, and you have only met him occasionally. Mrs LB has asked if she can speak with you. She seems quite upset and emotional. She says that over the last few months, her husband has been acting increasingly out of character. She has found him taking his tablets again because he was adamant he had not taken them earlier, although Mrs LB had watched him take them. In addition, he has been getting dressed as if he was going to work, in his suit with a packed briefcase. Mrs LB has had to remind him that he has retired and no longer needs to go to work. Of more concern is that Mr TB has started to have small accidents in the car – minor incidents such as hitting the garage door when reversing or the curb when driving. Mrs LB would like to know if these could be side effects of one his medicines. This is because on a few occasions recently he has taken double the dose of his medications.

Questions

1. What do you think could have potentially caused these behaviours?

    Three months later, Mr TB and Mrs LB arrive at the pharmacy looking shocked and a little upset. You take them to the counselling room. Mr TB gives you a prescription for donepezil 5 mg each evening and says that they have just been told that he probably has AD. Mr TB says he has had 'every test possible and that's what they've come up with'. It is a shock to both of them because no one in Mr TB's family has ever had a dementia. They both want to know more about this medicine.

2. What information should you provide Mr TB and Mrs LB about the benefits of treatment while also ensuring they understand this medicine is not a cure?

    The next weekend, Mr TB's daughter, their only child, visits the pharmacy and asks to speak to you. She is 32 years old, recently married and planning to start a family. She wants to know what her chances are of developing AD and whether she should consider not having a baby.

3. How do your respond to Mr TB's daughter?

Answers

1. Mr TB is neither delusional nor obsessive; these incidents are signs of short-term forgetfulness and changes in visuospatial co-ordination. Although simvastatin can cause depression and amnesia in some people, this is generally seen early in the treatment.

    Early recognition allows early diagnosis and the ability to rule out treatable pseudo-dementias. Depending on your local organisations and memory clinics available, you could suggest that Mrs LB makes an appointment for her husband to see his primary care doctor (with Mrs LB co-attending) to discuss possible referral for a memory clinic assessment. In some areas/countries, you may be able to refer Mr TB, or they could self-refer.

2. Mr TB and Mrs LB should be informed that acetylcholinesterase inhibitors (AChEIs), like donepezil, are not a cure for AD, or any dementia, but they can improve the symptoms associated with dementia. Importantly, these medicines work very well for one-third of people and somewhat well for another third; for the remaining third, they seem not to have an effect. AChEIs have linear kinetics; subsequently, effects are dose dependent, and it may take up to 3 weeks or longer to attain steady state. Therefore, if response appears to be negative, a dose increase should be tried and/or a change to another AChEI because they each have a slightly different mode of action. It should be explained to Mr TB and Mrs LB that the medicine needs to be taken at the same time of day. However, because donepezil can cause nightmares and affect sleeping, this would require a change to morning dosing. All AChEIs can cause nausea, vomiting and diarrhoea, so Mr TB and Mrs LB should be informed that because of this, doses are started low and titrated up over 2-week intervals to ensure that tolerance occurs. This titration will also affect the time taken for maximum efficacy to be reached. These effects can be managed with antispasmodics that do not act on the central nervous system, such as long-acting metoclopramide, domperidone or loperamide, as appropriate. It is always important to remember that any sedative medication, such as phenothiazines and sedative antihistamines, will impair cognitive functioning, especially if it is also highly antimuscarinic.

3. Because Mr TB's AD is not familial, you should explain to his daughter that there is unlikely to be a genetic risk (although this could be confirmed if needed). You could say that evidence shows that good public health interventions can reduce the risk of dementia. This includes reducing cardiovascular risks, appropriate treatment of ischaemic heart and vascular disease, keeping

fit and exercising three to four times weekly for 30–40 minutes to maintain an ideal body weight and engaging in social and mental activities to maintain good brain function. These can all reduce the risk of experiencing dementia. Environmental changes, such as avoiding centrally acting toxins and brain injury (sports such as boxing, rugby and football with repeated head trauma), can also reduce this risk. Although there are compounds being investigated in phase III studies for prevention of dementia, these are with populations with genetic risk factors. Currently, there are no pharmacological or herbal remedies which reduce the risk of idiosyncratic dementia.

Case 33.2

Mr SJ is a slim 65-year-old gentleman who has atrial fibrillation and is prescribed digoxin, enalapril, warfarin and simvastatin. He had been going to his primary care doctor for his warfarin tests – sometimes twice in the same day – and then forgetting about them a week later. His wife said he was also quite withdrawn and had lost interest in his garden and radio shows. It was the nurse in his local surgery who referred him to his primary care doctor for a dementia screen because she was concerned about his behaviour. Mr SJ was subsequently prescribed rivastigmine 1.5 mg capsules twice daily, and 2 weeks ago this was increased to 3 mg capsules twice daily. Today, he and his wife are at the pharmacy. They would like to know what Mr SJ can take for his nausea because it is putting him off his food, and he has already lost 2 kg in weight over the last 2 weeks.

Questions

1. What advice do you give Mr and Mrs SJ on managing the nausea and weight loss?

   Nine months later, Mr SJ is admitted to hospital for investigation into two recent falls at home, both of which resulted in extensive bruising because of the warfarin. Mr SJ did not fall or trip; Mrs SJ described the fall as though his legs just gave way. Mr SJ said he felt a little dizzy, and the next thing he could recall was that he was on the floor. The primary care doctor recently started atenolol 25 mg once daily because Mr SJ's blood pressure had increased to 150/95 mmHg. The rivastigmine he was prescribed has been successful because he is now socially engaged, able to complete activities of daily living and is very happy within himself. The consultant asks your opinion on whether the rivastigmine should be stopped because they consider it likely that Mr SJ's fall was due to bradycardia caused by rivastigmine.
2. What information could you provide to the consultant, and what treatment options would you recommend?

Answers

1. Nausea and vomiting are associated with dose increases of AChEIs and can be managed either by slowing down the rate of titration and/or co-prescription of an antiemetic such as metoclopramide. Because weight loss can impair physical strength, and resultant electrolyte imbalances may affect cognitive function in older people, it is important to address this issue. An alternative would be to consider rivastigmine patches to see if a more controlled dose release over 24 hours would have a reduced incidence of nausea. Mr SJ should be encouraged to eat small amounts more frequently until his body has time to develop tolerance to the dose increase, which usually takes about 2 weeks.
2. Rivastigmine is positively enhancing Mr SJ's life and therefore that of his wife and family. This is important because carer stress is

the key reason for people with dementia being admitted to care facilities.

Rivastigmine may cause bradycardia, which may contribute to the occurrence of torsade de pointes in patients with uncompensated heart failure, recent myocardial infarction, bradyarrhythmias, hypokalaemia or hypomagnesaemia or concomitant medicines which induce QT prolongation and/or torsade de pointes (e.g. antipsychotics, citalopram, antiarrhythmics). Rivastigmine therapy has been associated with hypertension. Atenolol is well known to cause bradycardia leading to syncope, which leads to falls.

Therefore, it would be appropriate to suggest withdrawing the atenolol used for blood pressure control, as it has led to bradycardia. An alternative would be to suggest increasing the dose of enalapril to control the rise in blood pressure, rather than adding a new medication. If the bradycardia still continued and the rivastigmine was still considered beneficial, then a pacemaker could be used to control heart rate and reduce falls.

Case 33.3

Mrs AS is a 76-year-old woman, and before her AD was diagnosed 5 years ago, she was fiercely independent and an active member of the community. Mrs AS now attends the local church service once a week and a coffee morning with her friends. However, she has resigned her previous secretarial position on a local women's group. She was started on galantamine XL 8 mg and subsequently increased to galantamine XL 24 mg once daily about 9 months ago. Her husband has been pleased with the effect because she is more sociable and plays with the grandchildren again. However, Mrs AS has started to get very agitated in the evening and refusing to sit down. She has been insisting that she wants to walk to post a letter and then gets very angry when her husband locks the door to prevent her from leaving the house. Last night, Mrs AS was so angry that she slapped her husband. He has asked your advice on what course of action he should take. He wants to know if he should encourage her to take an over-the-counter sleeping aid or if he should just persevere in trying to explain that she does not need to go out.

Questions

1. How do you respond to Mrs AS's husband's concerns?

   Eight months later, the primary care doctor for the local care home contacts you about Mrs AS. Mrs AS was admitted 2 months ago when her husband was unable to look after her following a small stroke. The staff have explained that Mrs AS has settled in well and enjoys her daily walk in the garden and her singing group sessions. She has always been friendly and polite and never gets angry. However, over the last 2 days, Mrs AS has lashed out at the same member of staff while he was helping her wash and dress. This morning, this staff member received a black eye, and the staff member wants Mrs AS's behaviour addressed. The primary care doctor asks if you think risperidone 500 micrograms at night would be an appropriate choice for Mrs AS.
2. How do you respond to the primary care doctor's question?

Answers

1. This behaviour sounds like 'sundowning', where people experience night–day reversal and associated agitation. This might be caused by too much napping during the day or inadequate exposure to bright light (dimmed lights, closed curtains or blinds or not being out of the house during the daytime) to suggest daytime,

leading to a loss of time orientation. As night approaches, there should be clear signals of closing curtains, turning down lights, calming the environment and establishing a routine which is suggestive of night time. Lavender and *Melissa officinalis* oils can be used as a massage (even only to the hands or feet) or used via a diffuser for inhalational effects to help decrease incidences of agitated behaviour. It is best if these are used before the expected behaviour, as part of a routine before bedtime and sleeping.

Short courses of small doses of z-hypnotics may also help if the oils are ineffective. However, tolerance quickly develops, and so does the potential for adverse effects such as postural hypotension, falls and decline in cognitive function, including memory impairment, as well as additional medication and possible interactions.

2. When behaviour changes occur, there should always be an ABC assessment. A = antecedent (what causes the behaviour), B = behaviour, and C = change (what changes the behaviour). This assessment needs to be undertaken to review Mrs AS's recent change in behaviour.

On further inquiry, the care home revealed that there has been a new male member of staff involved in helping Mrs AS to wash and dress. When Mrs AS's husband was contacted, he was very upset. He explained that his wife was a very private person with

respect to nudity, would not undress in front of him and had always insisted on washing and bathing herself. He said it was understandable that Mrs AS had become upset and angry when a male assistant was helping her, as this had never happened before, and she would have felt threatened. The recommendation is to ensure a female staff member helps Mrs AS when washing and dressing. Therefore, it is important to always question the reason behind a behavioural change and ensure that the family members are also informed. They may highlight possible reasons for the change. An antipsychotic should only be prescribed when the individual is a risk to him- or herself or others and after trialling non-pharmacological interventions. An antipsychotic should not be prescribed for sedation and in this situation would be unlikely to reduce Mrs AS's fear and distress. Good practice indicates that an antipsychotic should only be prescribed after a team discussion and further discussion with the patient and family outlining the associated increased risks for morbidity and mortality. The decision to prescribe should be documented in the patient's medical record and reviewed frequently to ensure it is still appropriate. The lowest possible dose to achieve the required effect should be prescribed. However, in this case, the cause of Mrs AS's changed behaviour was identified, and therefore no new medication was prescribed.

References

Albert, M.S., DeKosky, S.T., Dickson, D., et al., 2011. The diagnosis of mild cognitive impairment due to Alzheimer's disease: recommendations from the National Institute on Aging-Alzheimer's Association workgroups on diagnostic guidelines for Alzheimer's disease. Alzheimers Dement. 7270–7279. https://doi.org/10.1016/j.alz.2011.03.008.

Alzheimer's Association, 2009. 10 early signs and symptoms of Alzheimer's. Available at: http://www.alz.org/alzheimers_disease_10_signs_of_alzheimers.asp.

Alzheimer's Society, 2014. Dementia UK, Update 2014, second ed. Available at: https://www.alzheimers.org.uk/info/20025/policy_and_influencing/251/dementia_uk.

Alzheimer's Society, 2015a. Rarer causes of dementia. Available at: https://www.alzheimers.org.uk/download/downloads/id/1767/factsheet_rarer_causes_of_dementia.pdf.

Alzheimer's Society, 2015b. What is alcohol-related brain damage? Available at: https://www.alzheimers.org.uk/download/downloads/id/1765/factsheet_what_is_alchol-related_brain_damage.pdf.

Alzheimer's Society, 2015c. Changes in behaviour. Available at: https://www.alzheimers.org.uk/site/scripts/documents_info.php?documentID=159.

Alzheimer's Society and Royal College of General Practitioners, 2015. Helping you to assess cognition: a practical toolkit for clinicians. Available at: https://www.alzheimers.org.uk/downloads/download/1045/helping_you_to_assess_cognition_a_practical_toolkit_for_clinicians.

Ballard, C., Hanney, M.L., Theodoulou, M., et al., 2009. The dementia antipsychotic withdrawal trial (DART-AD): long-term follow up of a randomised placebo-controlled trial. Lancet Neurol. 8 (2), 151–157.

Ballard, C., Gauthier, S., Corbett, A., et al., 2011. Alzheimer's disease. Lancet 377 (9770), 1019–1031.

Bateman, R.J., Xiong, C., Benzinger, T.L.S., et al., 2012. Clinical and biomarker changes in dominantly inherited Alzheimer's disease. N. Engl. J. Med. 367 (9), 795–804.

Bent, S., Goldberg, H., Padula, A., et al., 2005. Spontaneous bleeding associated with ginkgo biloba: a case report and systematic review of the literature. J. Gen. Intern. Med. 20 (7), 657–666.

Birks, J., Grimley Evans, J., 2009. Ginkgo biloba for cognitive impairment and dementia. Cochrane Database Syst. Rev. 2009 (1), Art. No. CD003120. https://doi:10.1002/14651858.CD003120.pub3.

Connelly, D., 2015. Closing in on Alzheimer's disease. Pharm J. 295 (7876/7). https://doi.org/10.1211/PJ.2015.20069081.

Davtyan, H., Zagorski, K., Rajapaksha, H., et al., 2016. Alzheimer's disease Advax(CpG)-adjuvanted MultiTEP-based dual and single vaccines induce high-titer antibodies against various forms of tau and Aβ pathological molecules. Sci. Rep. 6 (28912). https://doi.org/10.1038/srep28912.

Eska, K., Graessel, E., Donath, C., et al., 2013. Predictors of institutionalization of dementia patients in mild and moderate stages: a 4-year prospective analysis. Dement Geriatr. Cogn. Dis. Extra. 3 (1), 426–445.

Farina, N., Isaac, M.G.E.K.N., Clark, A.R., et al., 2012. The use of vitamin E for Alzheimer's dementia and mild cognitive impairment. Cochrane Database Syst. Rev. 2012 (11) Art No., CD002854. https://doi:10.1002/14651858.CD002854.pub3.

Folstein, M.F., Folstein, S.E., McHugh, P.R., 1975. 'Mini-mental state'. A practical method for grading the cognitive state of patients for the clinician. J. Psychiatr. Res. 12 (3), 189–198.

Fossey, J., Ballard, C., Juszczak, E., et al., 2006. Effect of enhanced psychosocial care on people with severe dementia: cluster randomised trial antipsychotic use in nursing home residents. Br. Med. J. 332, 756–761.

Fox, C., Livingston, G., Maidment, I.D., et al., 2011. The impact of anticholinergic burden in Alzheimer's dementia – the Laser-AD study. Age Ageing. 40 (6), 730–735.

Fu, C.-Y., Moyle, W., Cooke, M., 2013. A randomised controlled trial of the use of aromatherapy and hand massage to reduce disruptive behaviour in people with dementia. BMC Complement Altern. Med. 13, 165. https://doi.org/10.1186/1472-6882-13-165.

Geldmacher, D.S., Provenzano, G., McRae, T., et al., 2003. Donepezil is associated with delayed nursing home placement in patients with Alzheimer's disease. J. Am. Geriatr. Soc. 51 (7), 937–944.

Harwood, D.G., Kalechstein, A., Barker, W.W., et al., 2010. The effect of alcohol and tobacco consumption, and apolipoprotein E genotype, on the age of onset in Alzheimer's disease. Int. J. Geriatr. Psych. 25 (5), 511–518.

Health and Social Care Information Centre, 2016. Patients in England with a record of dementia diagnosis on their clinical record: February 2016. Quality and Outcomes Framework dementia subset. Available at: http://content.digital.nhs.uk/media/20384/Dementia-Diagnosis-Summary-February-2016/pdf/qual-outc-fram-rec-dem-diag-feb-2016-sum.pdf.

Hermann, N., Li, A., Lanctôt, K., 2011. Memantine in dementia: a review of the current evidence. Expert Opin. Pharmacother. 12 (5), 787–800. https://doi.org/10.1517/14656566.2011.558006.

Husebo, B.S., Ballard, C., Sandvik, R., et al., 2011. Efficacy of treating pain to reduce behavioural disturbances in residents of nursing homes with dementia: cluster randomised clinical trial. Br. Med. J. 343, d4065.

Junaid, O., Hegde, S., 2006. Supportive psychotherapy in dementia. Adv. Psych. Treat. 13 (1), 17–23.

Kelly, S.P., Lawlor, B.A., Kenny, R.A., 2009. Blood pressure and dementia – a comprehensive review. Ther. Adv. Neurol. Disord. 2 (4), 241–260.

Kim, T.W., 2015. Drug repositioning approaches for the discovery of new therapeutics for Alzheimer's disease. Neurother. 12 (1), 132–142.

Livingston, G., Katona, C., 2000. How useful are cholinesterase inhibitors in the treatment of Alzheimer's disease? A number needed to treat analysis. Int. J. Geriatr. Psych. 15 (3), 203–207.

Marriott, A., Donaldson, C., Tarrier, N., Burns, A., 2000. Effectiveness of cognitive – behavioural family intervention in reducing the burden of care in carers of patients with Alzheimer's disease. B. J. Psych. 176 (6), 557–562.

Matthews, F.E., Stephan, B.C.M., Robinson, L., et al., 2016. A two decade dementia incidence comparison from the cognitive function and aging studies I and II. Nat. Commun. 7, 11398.

McKeith, I.G., 2006. Consensus guidelines for the clinical and pathologic diagnosis of dementia with Lewy bodies (DLB): report of the Consortium on DLB International Workshop. J. Alzheimers Dis. 9 (Suppl. 3), 417.

McKeith, I.G., Dickson, D.W., Lowe, J., et al., 2005. Diagnosis and management of dementia with Lewy bodies: third report of the DLB Consortium. Neurol. 65, 1863–1872.

National Institute for Health and Care Excellence (NICE), 2016. Donepezil, galantamine, rivastigmine and memantine for the treatment of Alzheimer's disease. Technology appraisal guidance [TA217]. Available at: https://www.nice.org.uk/guidance/ta217.

National Institute for Health and Care Excellence, Social Care Institute for Excellence (NICE-SCIE), 2011. The NICE-SCIE guideline on supporting people with dementia and their carers in health and social care. Available at: https://www.nice.org.uk/guidance/cg42/.

Public Health England, 2016. Health matters: midlife approaches to reduce dementia risk. Available at: https://www.gov.uk/government/publications/health-matters-midlife-approaches-to-reduce-dementia-risk/health-matters-midlife-approaches-to-reduce-dementia-riskhttps://publichealth matters.blog.gov.uk/2016/03/22/health-matters-midlife-approaches-to-reduce-dementia-risk/.

Royal College of Psychiatrists, 2016. FR/ID/09: psychotropic drug prescribing for people with intellectual disability, mental health problems and/or behaviours that challenge: practice guidelines. Available at: http://www.rcpsych.ac.uk/pdf/FR_ID_09_for_website.pdf.

Sperling, R.A., Aisen, P.S., Beckett, L.A., et al., 2011. Toward defining the preclinical stages of Alzheimer's disease: recommendations from the National Institute on Aging–Alzheimer's Association work groups on diagnostic guidelines for Alzheimer's disease. Alzheimers Dement. 7 (3), 280–292.

Toh, H.M., Ghazali, S.E., Subramaniam, P., 2016. The acceptability and usefulness of cognitive stimulation therapy for older adults with dementia: a narrative review. Int. J. Alzheimers Dis. Article ID 5131570.

Valenzuela, M.J., Sachdev, P., 2006. Brain reserve and dementia: a systematic review. Psychol. Med. 36, 441–454.

Wang, P.S., Schneeweiss, S., Avorn, J., et al., 2005. Risk of death in elderly users of conventional vs. atypical antipsychotic medications. N. Engl. J. Med. 353, 2335–2341.

Warren, J.D., Rohrer, J.D., Rossor, M.N., 2013. Frontotemporal dementia. Br. Med. J. 347, 4827.

Winblad, B., Amouyel, P., Andrieu, S., et al., 2016. Defeating Alzheimer's disease and other dementias: a priority for European science and society. Lancet Neurol. 15 (5), 455–532.

World Health Organization (WHO), 2012. Dementia a public health priority. Available at: http://www.who.int/mental_health/publications/dementia_report_2012/en/.

Zahr, N.M., Kaufman, K.L., Harper, C.G., 2011. Clinical and pathological features of alcohol-related brain damage. Nat. Rev. Neurol. 7, 284–294.

Further Reading

Taylor, D., 2013. Dementia. In: Dodds, L.J. (Ed.), Drugs in Use, fifth ed. Pharmaceutical Press, London.

National Institute for Health and Care Excellence, 2015. NICE advice: low-dose antipsychotics in people with dementia. Available at: https://www.nice.org.uk/advice/ktt7.

National Institute for Health and Care Excellence, 2015. NICE advice: management of aggression, agitation and behavioural disturbances in dementia: valproate preparations. Available at: https://www.nice.org.uk/advice/esuom41/chapter/Key-points-from-the-evidence.

National Institute for Health and Care Excellence, 2010. NICE advice: management of aggression, agitation and behavioural disturbances in dementia: carbamazepine. Available at: https://www.nice.org.uk/advice/esuom40/chapter/Key-points-from-the-evidence.

National Institute for Health and Care Excellence, 2013. NICE quality standard: dementia: independence and wellbeing. Available at: https://www.nice.org.uk/guidance/qs30.

National Institute for Health and Care Excellence, 2015. NICE pathways for dementia. Available at: https://pathways.nice.org.uk/pathways/dementia.

National Institute for Health and Care Excellence, 2015. NICE guideline: dementia, disability and frailty in later life – mid-life approaches to delay or prevent onset. Available at: https://www.nice.org.uk/guidance/ng16.

Seeley, W.W., Miller, B.L., 2013. Alzheimer's disease and other dementias. In: Hauser, S.L. (Ed.), Harrison's Neurology in Clinical Medicine, third ed. McGraw-Hill Medical, New York.

Taylor, D.A., Rajei-Dehkordi, Z., 2010. Practice guidance: pharmaceutical care in dementia. Available at: http://www.rpharms.com/public-health-resources/mental-health.asp.

Useful websites

Alzheimer's Association: http://www.alz.org/

Alzheimer's Society: http://alzheimers.org.uk/

Alzheimer's Society and Royal College of General Practitioners, Helping you to assess cognition: a practical toolkit for clinicians: https://www.alzheimers.org.uk/site/scripts/download_info.php?fileID=2532

Cochrane Reviews on Dementia – a number of systematic reviews of herbal supplements, aromatherapy and social and behavioural interventions for people with dementia: http://dementia.cochrane.org/our-reviews

CPPE Dementia Resources: https://www.cppe.ac.uk/programmes/l/dementia-e-01/

Alzheimer's Society Factsheet: driving and dementia: https://www.alzheimers.org.uk/site/scripts/download_info.php?downloadID=1118

World Health Organization (WHO) dementia resources: http://www.who.int/topics/dementia/en/

34 Pain

Roger David Knaggs and Gregory J. Hobbs

Key points

- Pain is multifactorial in its aetiology.
- Treatment often requires use of a combination of drugs with different mechanisms of action.
- Opioids are generally effective for acute pain and pain at the end of life. However, they are less effective for other types of pain, particularly low back pain and fibromyalgia. Adjuvant analgesics, such as tricyclic antidepressants or antiepileptic drugs, should be considered before opioids for persistent non-cancer pain.
- For cancer pain, the World Health Organization (WHO) analgesic ladder forms the basis for the use of analgesic drugs. Some clinicians prefer to omit weak opioids and start strong opioid therapy earlier.
- Breakthrough pain is treated with doses of immediate-release opioids, usually prescribed in addition to modified release formulations.
- Antiemetics and laxatives should be prescribed for patients taking opioids.
- Cancer pain may vary as the disease progresses. Drug therapy should be reviewed regularly to ensure that the most appropriate agent is being used for the type, site and intensity of pain.
- Most drugs are available in a range of different formulations, but whenever possible, the oral route should be used.
- When managing patients with chronic pain, analgesic drugs are used together with other non-pharmacological therapies as part of a biopsychosocial treatment framework.

Pain is defined as:

An unpleasant sensory and emotional experience associated with actual or potential tissue damage, or described in terms of such damage.
(International Association for the Study of Pain, 2012)

Acute pain may be thought of as a physiological process having a biological function, allowing the patient to avoid or minimise injury. Persistent or long-term pain, on the other hand, may be considered more as a disease in its own right than a symptom (Woolf, 2004).

Aetiology and neurophysiology

Neuroanatomy of pain transmission

The majority of tissues and organs are innervated by special sensory receptors (nociceptors) connected to primary afferent nerve fibres of differing diameters. Small myelinated Aδ fibres and unmyelinated C fibres are responsible for the transmission of painful stimuli to the spinal cord, where these afferent primary fibres terminate in the dorsal horn.

Pain transmission further within the central nervous system (CNS) is far more complex and understood less well. The most important parts of this process are the wide dynamic range cells in the spinothalamic tract that project to the thalamus and on to the somatosensory cortex. Modulation or inhibition of these neurones within the spinal cord result in less activity in the pain pathway. This modulatory action can be activated by stress or certain analgesic drugs, such as morphine, and is an important component of the gate theory of pain (Fig. 34.1).

The gate control theory recognises the pivotal role the spinal cord plays in the continual modulation of neuronal activity by the relative activity of large-diameter myelinated (Aβ) and smaller-diameter (myelinated Aδ and unmyelinated C) peripheral fibres and by descending inhibitory messages from the brain. Conversely, other influences can lead to an increased sensitivity to noxious stimuli. The most important of these is pain itself, and further painful stimuli can lead to increased pain sensitivity. This occurs through neurochemical and anatomical changes within the CNS. This enhancement of neuronal function is known as central sensitisation (Woolf, 2011) and manifests clinically as hyperalgesia (increased pain from a stimulus that usually provokes pain) and allodynia (pain from a stimulus that does not usually provoke pain).

Neurotransmitters and pain

Various neurotransmitters in the dorsal horn of the spinal cord are involved in pain modulation. These include amino acids such as glutamate and γ-aminobutyric acid (GABA), monoamines such as noradrenaline and 5-hydroxytryptamine (5-HT, serotonin) and peptide molecules, of which the opioid peptides are the most important. Opioid receptors are found in both the CNS and the periphery; in the CNS they are found in high concentrations in the limbic system, the brainstem and the spinal cord. The natural ligands (molecules that bind to the receptor) at opioid receptors are a group of neuropeptides including the endorphins.

Assessment of pain

Evaluation and diagnosis of pain requires a description of the pain and an assessment of its consequences. This should include a full

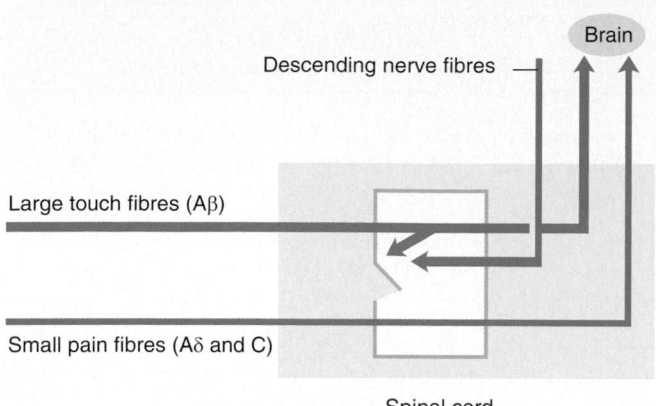

Fig. 34.1 Gate control theory of pain.

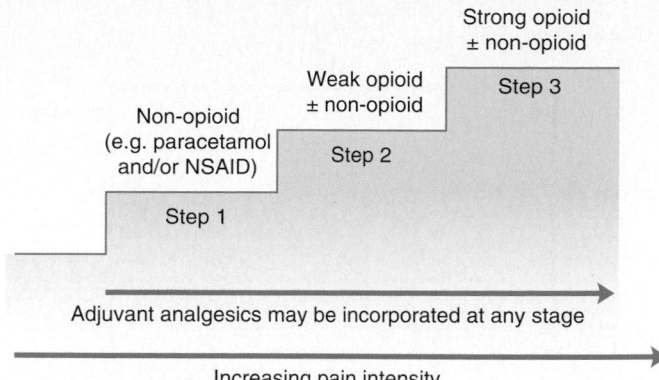

Fig. 34.2 World Health Organization three-step analgesic ladder. NSAID, Non-steroidal anti-inflammatory drug.

medical history, medication history and assessment of previous pain problems, paying attention to factors that influence the pain, for example, movement. An appropriate physical examination is usually performed. Additional diagnostic laboratory tests, imaging, including plain radiography, computed tomography (CT) and magnetic resonance imaging (MRI), and diagnostic nerve blocks may be used to confirm the diagnosis. Further, to develop an individualised management plan for people with chronic pain, a more detailed assessment of pain-related disability is usually required, including psychological and social assessment.

Pain is, however, a subjective phenomenon, and quantitative assessment is difficult (Breivik et al., 2008). The most commonly used instruments for acute pain are visual analogue and verbal rating scales. Visual analogue scales are 10-cm-long lines labelled with an extreme at each end, usually 'no pain at all' and 'worst pain imaginable'. The patient is required to mark the severity of the pain between the two extremes of the scale. Verbal rating scales use descriptors such as 'none', 'mild', 'moderate' and 'severe'. More elaborate questionnaires such as the Brief Pain Inventory (Cleeland and Ryan, 1994) and the McGill Pain Questionnaire (Melzack and Torgerson, 1971) help describe other aspects of the pain experience, and pain diaries may be used to record the influence of activity and medication on pain.

Management

Acute pain usually results from noxious stimulation as a result of tissue damage or injury. It can be managed effectively using analgesic drugs and is often self-limiting.

Long-term pain may be considered as pain which continues beyond the usual time required for tissue healing. Treatment may require involvement from specialist pain management services, hospices and a multidisciplinary approach that assesses and manages patients using a biopsychosocial approach. Initial treatment is usually directed at the underlying disease process where possible, for example, medicines, surgery or anti-tumour therapy. However, non-pharmacological treatments such as physical therapy and various psychological techniques including cognitive behavioural therapy may also form part of a multimodal treatment programme. In addition, pain can be modulated using techniques such as stimulation-based analgesia such as

transcutaneous electrical nerve stimulation (TENS), acupuncture and massage, or invasive procedures such as injections, neurolytic nerve blocks and spinal cord stimulation.

Research is progressing such that pain management is moving from symptom control towards mechanism-based pharmacological therapy (Baron et al., 2012; Woolf, 2004), although it can be difficult to apply in routine clinical practice.

Analgesic ladder

The World Health Organization (WHO) analgesic ladder (Fig. 34.2) forms the basis of many approaches to the use of analgesic drugs, particularly in pain at the end of life. There are essentially three steps: non-opioid analgesics, weak opioids and strong opioids. The analgesic efficacy of non-opioids, such as paracetamol and non-steroidal anti-inflammatory drugs (NSAIDs) (e.g. aspirin, ibuprofen and diclofenac), is limited by side effects and ceiling effects; that is, beyond a certain dose, no further pharmacological effect is seen. If pain remains uncontrolled, then a weak opioid, such as codeine or dihydrocodeine, may be helpful. There may be additional benefit in combining a weak opioid with a non-opioid drug, although many commercial preparations contain inadequate quantities of both components and are no more effective than a non-opioid alone. Strong opioids, of which morphine is considered the gold standard, have no ceiling effect, and therefore increased dosage continues to give increased analgesia, but side effects often limit the effectiveness. Adjuvant drugs, such as corticosteroids, antidepressants or antiepileptics, may be utilised at any step of the ladder.

Analgesic drugs
Paracetamol

Despite being used in clinical practice for more than 50 years and much investigation, the mechanism by which paracetamol exerts its analgesic effect remains uncertain. Inhibition of prostaglandin synthesis within the CNS has been proposed, although this is probably not the only mechanism. Interaction with the serotonin (Tjolsen et al., 1991) and endocannabinoid (Högestätt et al., 2005) neurotransmitter systems have been demonstrated in animal models.

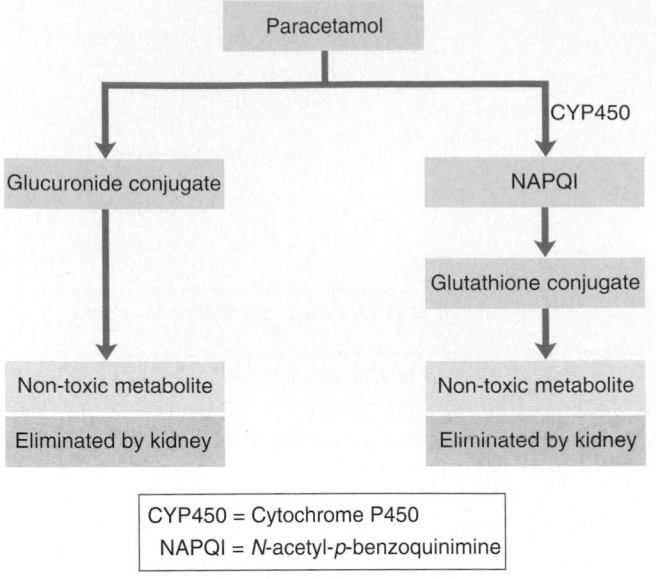

CYP450 = Cytochrome P450

NAPQI = *N*-acetyl-*p*-benzoquinimine

Fig. 34.3 Paracetamol metabolism in humans.

Box 34.1 'GRAB' mnemonic for serious, potentially fatal side effects of non-steroidal anti-inflammatory drugs

G – gastro-intestinal	Gastro-intestinal side effects are the most common unwanted effects of NSAIDs. These may be non-specific and less serious (e.g. dyspepsia, diarrhoea, nausea and vomiting) or more serious (e.g. ulceration, bleeding, intestinal obstruction).
R – renal	In susceptible individuals, especially the elderly, NSAIDs may cause acute renal failure. NSAIDs alter salt and water homeostasis, which may worsen heart failure and produce a small increase in blood pressure.
A – asthma	NSAIDs, particularly aspirin, may worsen asthma and cause bronchospasm in some patients.
B – blood disorders	All NSAIDs reduce platelet aggregation and increase the risk of bleeding, not just from the gastro-intestinal tract.

NSAID, Non-steroidal anti-inflammatory drug.

The bioavailability of paracetamol is around 60% after oral administration, but if given by the rectal route, it is much lower and much more variable. A formulation for intravenous infusion has been promoted more recently, and this has largely replaced the rectal route of administration. Therapeutic plasma levels are reached within 30 minutes of oral administration. The elimination half-life of paracetamol is relatively short ($t_{1/2}$ = 2–4 hours); hence, frequent dosing is required to maintain its analgesic effect.

With normal doses, the majority of a dose of paracetamol is metabolised and inactivated in the liver, undergoing a phase II conjugation reaction with glucuronic acid (Fig. 34.3). A small proportion of a dose is metabolised using a cytochrome P450 mediated reaction that forms a reactive intermediate, *N*-acetyl-*p*-benzoquinoneimine (NAPQI). Usually, NAPQI can be deactivated by conjugation with glutathione in the liver. However, after ingestion of a large amount of paracetamol, the hepatic stores of both glucuronic acid and glutathione become depleted, leaving free NAPQI, which causes liver damage.

The usual therapeutic dose for adults is paracetamol 1 g taken four times daily. It is very important that this dose is not exceeded; otherwise, hepatotoxicity is more common. This may be particularly problematic for malnourished adults with low body weight (Claridge et al., 2010). A reduced maximum daily dose (3 g/24 h) by intravenous infusion is recommended for patients with hepatocellular insufficiency, chronic alcoholism or dehydration. Paracetamol is also available as an over-the-counter (OTC) medicine and is a component of many cold and influenza remedies. Compared with other analgesics, paracetamol is not as potent; however, when taken in combination with an NSAID or opioid, there is an additive analgesic effect.

Non-steroidal anti-inflammatory drugs

Mechanism of action

NSAIDs exert their analgesic and anti-inflammatory effects through inhibition of the enzyme cyclo-oxygenase, responsible for the synthesis of prostaglandins. NSAIDs are used widely to relieve pain, with or without inflammation, in people with acute and persistent musculoskeletal disorders. In single doses, NSAIDs have superior analgesic activity compared with paracetamol (Hyllested et al., 2002). In regular higher doses, they have both analgesic and anti-inflammatory effects, which makes them particularly useful for the treatment of continuous or regular pain associated with inflammation. NSAIDs have been shown to be suitable for the relief of pain in dysmenorrhoea, toothache and some headaches and to treat pain caused by secondary bone tumours, which result from lysis of bone and prostaglandin release.

Side effects and tolerability

The side effects of NSAIDs are produced as a result of decreasing prostaglandin production required for normal body function, particularly in the gastro-intestinal and respiratory tracts, kidneys and platelets. Although effective in conditions in which there is an inflammatory contribution to pain, NSAIDs have serious, potentially fatal side effects that may be remembered by the acronym 'GRAB' (Box 34.1).

It has been estimated that there are 2000 deaths each year in the UK directly related to NSAID use, but the assumptions used in this estimate are hard to determine (Rainsford and Bjarnason, 2015). More widespread prescribing of proton pump inhibitors may have reduced this figure. Over recent years there have been increasing concerns regarding the cardiovascular side effects of nonselective NSAIDs, and there is increasing realisation that thromboembolic and ischaemic vascular events are not solely associated with COX-2 selective drugs (Coxib and Traditional NSAID Trialists' [CNT] Collaboration, 2013).

COX-2 selective drugs

Cyclo-oxygenase exists in two forms: cyclo-oxygenase-1 (COX-1) and cyclo-oxygenase-2 (COX-2). COX-1 is a constitutive enzyme that is expressed under normal conditions in a variety of tissues, including the gastro-intestinal tract and kidney, where it catalyses the production of prostaglandins required for homeo-static functions. It does not have a role in nociception or inflam-mation. COX-2 is an inducible enzyme that appears in damaged tissues shortly after injury and leads to the formation of inflam-matory prostaglandins within these tissues. COX-2 selective NSAIDs should, theoretically, inhibit the formation of inflamma-tory prostaglandins without affecting the activity of COX-1 in areas such as the gut. In practice, use of COX-2-specific drugs is associated with reduced risk of gastro-intestinal side effects when compared with non-selective drugs. However, their use has also been linked with adverse effects, particularly cardiovascular side effects, and this now limits their use.

Clinical considerations

The potential benefits of treatment with an NSAID or COX-2 selective drug must be weighed against the risks. Differences in anti-inflammatory activity between NSAIDs are small, but there is considerable variation in individual patient response as well as the incidence and type of side effects. In acute pain between 40% and 70% of patients will respond to any NSAID (Moore et al., 2013). Of the remaining patients, those who do not respond to one NSAID may well respond to another. An analgesic effect should normally be seen within a week, whereas an anti-inflammatory effect may not be achieved or assessable clinically for up to 3 weeks.

Guidance on NSAID use

The lowest effective dose of NSAID or COX-2 selective inhibi-tor should be prescribed for the shortest time necessary. The need for long-term treatment should be reviewed periodically. Prescribing should be based on the safety profiles of individual NSAIDs or COX-2 selective inhibitors, on individual patient risk profiles, for example, gastro-intestinal and cardiovascular. Prescribers should not switch between NSAIDs without careful consideration of the overall safety profile of the products and the patient's individual risk factors, as well as the patient's pref-erence (Medicines and Healthcare Products Regulatory Agency [MHRA], 2005).

Concomitant aspirin, and possibly other antiplatelet drugs, greatly increases the gastro-intestinal risks of using NSAIDs and severely reduces any gastro-intestinal safety advantages of COX-2 selective inhibitors. Aspirin should only be co-prescribed if absolutely necessary.

Other non-opioid analgesics

Nefopam is a drug which is chemically related to orphenadrine and diphenhydramine; however, it is not an opioid, anti-inflam-matory drug or antihistamine. The mechanism of analgesic action remains unclear. As a non-opioid, it is not associated with the problems of dependence and respiratory depression. The drug has a very high number of dose-related side effects in clini-cal use that may be linked to its antimuscarinic actions. Nefopam may be useful in asthmatic patients and in those who are intoler-ant of NSAIDs; however, it has become much more costly over recent years.

Opioid analgesics

Opioid analgesics mimic the actions of these natural ligands and exert their effect through the MOR (μ), DOR (δ) and, to a lesser extent, the KOR (κ) receptors.

Opioids for mild to moderate pain

Opioids for mild to moderate pain ('weak opioids') are prescribed frequently, either alone or in combination with other analgesics, for a wide variety of painful disorders. There are three major drugs in this group, codeine, dihydrocodeine and dextropropoxyphene, which are recommended as step 2 of the WHO analgesic ladder for pain that has not responded to non-opioid analgesics. Despite this recommendation, there is little data demonstrating that weak opioids are of any benefit in the relief of long-term pain, and it may be more beneficial to use a smaller dose of a more potent opioid.

Codeine. Codeine is the prototypical opioid for moderate pain. It is structurally similar to morphine, and about 10% of the dose is demethylated to form morphine, and the analgesic effects are likely to be due to this active metabolite. It is a powerful cough suppressant as well as being constipating. In combination with NSAIDs, the analgesic effects are usually additive, but the variability in response is considerable. A genetic polymorphism occurs within the population such that the hepatic microsomal enzyme CYP2D6 that is responsible for the conversion of codeine to morphine does not catalyse this conversion in approximately 8% of the Caucasian population. The duration of analgesic action is about 3 hours.

Dihydrocodeine. Dihydrocodeine is only available in a few countries and is chemically similar to codeine. It has similar properties to codeine when used at the same dosage and may be slightly more potent.

Dextropropoxyphene. Historically, dextropropoxyphene was prescribed in combination with other analgesics such as parace-tamol (co-proxamol). There are few data on its therapeutic value, and at least one review concluded that analgesic efficacy is less than aspirin and barely more than placebo. At best, dextropro-poxyphene failed to show any superiority over paracetamol (Li Wan Po and Zhang, 1997). At worst, it is a dangerous drug which has the potential for steadily developing toxicity. Patients with hepatic dysfunction and poor renal function are particularly at risk. It is associated with problems in overdose, notably a non-naloxone-reversible depression of the cardiac conducting sys-tem. Dextropropoxyphene interacts unpredictably with a number of drugs, including carbamazepine and warfarin. In 2005, the MHRA announced concerns about the safety and effectiveness of co-proxamol and directed that it should be withdrawn from clinical use in the UK; however, it still remains available as an unlicensed medicine for the small number of patients who do not obtain analgesia with other analgesic medicines.

Opioids for severe pain

Morphine. Morphine is the gold-standard opioid analgesic for severe pain ('strong opioid'). It is available for administra-tion by a range of administration routes, including oral, rectal and injectable formulations, and has a duration of action of about

4 hours after oral administration. Morphine is metabolised in the liver, and one metabolite, morphine 6-glucuronide, is pharmacologically active; this should be taken into consideration in patients who have renal failure.

A general protocol for morphine use to obtain rapid relief from acute pain is to use intravenous bolus doses of 2–5 mg titrated until pain relief is achieved. In the initial management of long-term pain, an oral regimen is more appropriate using an immediate-release formulation. A usual starting dose is 5–10 mg every 4 hours, and the patient should be advised to take the same dose as often as is necessary for breakthrough pain. It may be necessary to double the dose every 24 hours until pain relief is achieved, although a slower dose escalation will often suffice. After control is achieved, it is usual to change to an oral modified-release formulation, which allows less frequent dosing, either daily or twice daily.

Theoretically, there is no ceiling effect when the dose is increased. However, side effects usually prevent dose escalation; daily doses of up to oral morphine 1 or 2 g/day may be required for some cancer patients, but relatively few require more than about 200 mg daily.

Other strong opioids. Opioids such as pethidine and dextromoramide offer little advantage over morphine in that they are generally weaker in action with a relatively short duration of action (2 hours). Dipipanone is only available in a preparation which contains an antiemetic (cyclizine), and increasing doses lead to sedation and the risk of developing a tardive dyskinesia with long-term use. Methadone has a long elimination half-life of 15–25 hours, and accumulation occurs in the early stages of use. It has minimal side effects with long-term use, and some patients who experience serious adverse effects with morphine may tolerate methadone.

Oxycodone and hydromorphone are synthetic opioids that have been used for many years in North America and more recently in Europe. They are available in both immediate- and modified-release preparations. Some patients appear to tolerate these semi-synthetic opioids better than morphine, but there is no evidence to suggest which patients achieve better effect with either of these drugs.

Fentanyl is available as a transdermal formulation for long-term use. The patch is designed to release the drug continuously over 3 days. When starting the drug, alternative analgesic therapy should be continued for at least the first 12 hours until therapeutic levels are achieved, and an immediate-acting opioid should be available for breakthrough pain. Patches are replaced every 72 hours.

The relative potencies of the commonly used opioids are summarised in Table 34.1.

Clinical considerations. Use of opioids is almost universally accepted in cancer pain and acute pain after injury, trauma or surgery. There has been a marked and progressive rise in the prescribing of opioid drugs in the UK over the past decade. The trend of increased prescribing continues (Zin et al., 2014), with most prescriptions now for patients with non-cancer pain. However, most trials in this patient group have been for a limited duration, and for most patients, opioids only provide modest benefits for short periods. In other healthcare systems, there have been similar trends in increased opioid prescribing. The United States is considered currently to have a 'prescription opioid crisis'; in 2015, there were nearly as many deaths from unintentional overdose as deaths from road traffic accidents (Laderman and Martin, 2017).

Table 34.1 Relative potencies of opioid drugs

Drug	Potency (morphine = 1)
Codeine	0.1
Dihydrocodeine	0.1
Tramadol	0.2
Pethidine	0.1
Morphine	1
Diamorphine	2.5
Hydromorphone	7
Methadone	2–10 (with repeat dosing)
Fentanyl (transdermal)	150

The best outcomes are obtained in the long-term if the opioid dose can be kept low and particularly if use is intermittent. However, it is difficult to identify those people likely to experience good outcomes at the point of opioid initiation. As a general rule, strong opioid use is more likely to become problematic when patients have mental health problems (such as depression and anxiety) and/or a history of misuse of alcohol or other drugs, including opioids.

Agonist–antagonist and partial agonists

Most of the drugs in the agonist–antagonist category are either competitive antagonists at the μ opioid receptor, where they can bind to the site but exert no action, or they exert only limited actions; that is, they are partial agonists. Those that are antagonists at the μ opioid receptor can provoke a withdrawal syndrome in patients receiving concomitant opioid agonists such as morphine. These properties make it difficult to use these agents in the control of long-term pain, and the process of conversion from one group of drugs to another can be complex.

Buprenorphine

Buprenorphine is a semi-synthetic, highly lipophilic opioid that is a partial agonist at the μ opioid receptor and an antagonist at both the δ and κ receptors. It undergoes extensive metabolism when administered orally and to avoid this effect, it is given sublingually. It has high receptor affinity and, through this property, a duration of action of 6 hours.

A long duration of action and high bioavailability would suggest a role for buprenorphine in the management of long-term pain. Buprenorphine is also available as a transdermal formulation and may be an effective alternative to other strong opioids for long-term non-cancer pain. There is limited evidence of efficacy in osteoarthritis and low back pain. After sublingual or intravenous administration, the incidence of nausea and vomiting appears to be substantially higher than with morphine; however, respiratory depression and constipation are less frequent.

Pentazocine

Pentazocine, a benzomorphan derivative, is an agonist and at the same time a very weak antagonist at the μ opioid receptor. This drug became popular in the 1960s, when it was thought it would have little or no abuse potential. This is now known to be untrue, although its abuse potential is less than that of the conventional agonists such as morphine. It produces analgesia that is clearly different from morphine and is probably due to agonist actions at the κ receptor. There are no detailed studies of its use in long-term pain, but its short duration of action (about 3 hours) and the high incidence of psychomimetic side effects make it a totally unsuitable drug for such use.

Tramadol

Tramadol is a centrally acting analgesic that has opioid agonist activity and also has monoamine reuptake properties similar to many antidepressants. It is not as potent as morphine, and efficacy is limited by side effects, including an unfavourably high risk of drowsiness, nausea and vomiting. Its monoaminergic activity appears to be valuable in the management of neuropathic pain and hence may be an acceptable alternative to an opioid.

Tapentadol

Tapentadol is another centrally acting analgesic that combines opioid agonist activity and noradrenaline reuptake inhibition (NRI). In animal models, the NRI component is a key mechanism and may even predominate over opioid actions in chronic (and especially neuropathic) pain states. In humans there is a reduced incidence of some of the typical opioid-induced side effects compared with equianalgesic doses of classical opioids. This supports the hypothesis that tapentadol analgesia is only partially mediated by opioid agonist mechanisms.

Side effects of opioids

The adverse effects of opioids are nearly all dose related, and tolerance develops to the majority with long-term use.

Respiratory depression

Respiratory depression is potentially dangerous in patients with impaired respiratory function, but tolerance develops rapidly with regular dosing. It can be reversed by the MOR opioid antagonist, naloxone.

Sedation

Sedation is usually mild and self-limiting. Smaller doses, given more frequently, may counteract the problem. Rarely, dexamphetamine or methylphenidate has been used to counteract this effect.

Nausea and vomiting

Antiemetics should be co-prescribed routinely with opioids for the first 10 days. Choice of antiemetic will depend upon the cause, and a single drug will be sufficient in two-thirds of patients. Where nausea is persistent, additional causes should be sought and prescribing reviewed. If another antiemetic is used, it should have a different mechanism of action.

Constipation

Opioids reduce intestinal secretions and peristalsis, causing a dry stool and constipation. Unlike other adverse effects, constipation tends not to improve with long-term use, and when opioids are used on a long-term basis, most patients need a stool softener (e.g. docusate sodium) and a stimulant laxative (e.g. senna) regularly. Dosage should be titrated to give a comfortable stool. High-fibre diets and bulking agents do not work very well in preventing constipation in patients on opioids. Co-danthrusate (dantron + docusate sodium) and co-danthramer (dantron + poloxamer 188) are alternatives; however, because of the potential carcinogenicity and genotoxicity of dantron, they are only indicated for use in terminal care. More recent alternatives include methylnaltrexone, naloxegol, oral prolonged-release naloxone and peripherally restricted opioid antagonists. Each of these has greater affinity for MOR opioid receptors in the gastro-intestinal tract and prevents binding of the opioid agonist, allowing the agonist to reach the central nervous system.

Smooth muscle spasm

Opioids cause spasm of the sphincter of Oddi in the biliary tract and may cause biliary colic, as well as urinary sphincter spasm and urinary retention. Thus, in biliary or renal colic, it may be preferable to use another drug without these effects. Historically, pethidine was believed to be the most effective, but there is no evidence for this practice (Thompson, 2001).

Other side effects

There is increasing evidence that long-term opioid use may cause clinically significant adverse effects on the endocrine system. For example, opioid-induced pituitary dysfunction can lead to testosterone deficiency in men. Effects on the immune system are evident in animal studies and are also under scrutiny in humans.

Tolerance, dependence and addition

Treatment with opioids in the long-term may cause tolerance to the analgesic effect, although the mechanisms by which this happens remain unclear (Holden et al., 2005). When this occurs, the dosage may be increased or, alternatively, another opioid can be substituted. When switching to an alternative opioid, equivalence tables should be consulted but should only be considered a guide because there is significant variation for individuals. It is usual to reduce the equivalent dose by between 25% and 50% to ensure safety. Addiction is relatively uncommon when opioids are prescribed for pain relief.

Opioids and driving

In 2015 the law on driving whilst taking certain controlled drugs was strengthened. The new offence refers to driving with specified controlled drugs in the body, in excess of a specified limit. The new offence has a statutory 'medical defence' to protect patients who may test positive for certain specified drugs taken in accordance with the advice of a healthcare professional or the patient information leaflet that accompanies the medicine.

Special techniques for opioid administration

Patient-controlled analgesia

Patient-controlled analgesia (PCA) is a system which allows patients to titrate the dose of opioid to suit their individual analgesic requirements. The drug is delivered using a syringe attached to an electronic or elastomeric pump, which delivers a preset dose when activated by the patient depressing a button. A lockout period, during which the machine is programmed not to respond, ensures that a second dose is not delivered before the previous one has had an effect. Some devices allow an additional background infusion of drug to be delivered continuously. A maximum-dose facility ensures that the machine does not deliver more than a preset dose over a given time. PCA is a useful technique for the management of pain after surgery. The system is convenient and enjoys a high degree of patient acceptability.

The traditional intermittent intramuscular injection of opioids can be effective but is less versatile than titrated intravenous administration. The subcutaneous route is subject to most of the problems associated with intramuscular administration but tends to be less painful.

Opioid use via any route is associated with nausea, and antiemetics should be prescribed routinely. Administration of compound preparations containing both opioids and antiemetics is not recommended as few preparations contain drugs with similar pharmacokinetic profiles and accumulation, usually of the antiemetic, may occur.

Epidural analgesia

Epidural injections and infusions may be effective in relieving pain arising from both malignant causes and non-cancer diseases and are very effective in postoperative and labour pain. Various combinations of local anaesthetics, opioids or steroids can be administered into the epidural space near to the spinal level of the pain.

Epidural opioids

Effective analgesia can be obtained by administering small doses of opioids to the epidural space. Because there are opioid receptors in the spinal cord, smaller doses than administered by other parenteral routes are required and may be given with and without long-acting local anaesthetic drugs. However, severe respiratory depression, nausea and vomiting, urinary retention and pruritus can occur after their use. Life-threatening respiratory depression can occur when additional opioids are given by other routes to patients already receiving epidural opioids, and this practice should be actively discouraged. Respiratory depression which occurs soon after administration, due to intravascular absorption, is relatively common and simple to detect and treat. However, respiratory depression can also occur many hours after opioid administration. This is most common with morphine, probably because of its lower lipophilicity compared with fentanyl and diamorphine. Fentanyl has much greater stability than diamorphine, and it can be prepared with bupivacaine in a terminally sterilised formulation which minimises the risk of adding the incorrect dose to an infusion fluid in a clinical environment and maintains sterility.

Local anaesthetics

Local anaesthetic drugs, such as lidocaine and bupivacaine, produce reversible blockade of neural transmission in autonomic, sensory and motor nerve fibres by binding to sodium channels in the axon membrane from within, preventing sodium ion entry during depolarisation. The threshold potential is not reached, and consequently, the action potential is not propagated. The concentration of local anaesthetic and dose used determine the onset, density and duration of the block. There are marked differences in the recommended maximum safe doses of different local anaesthetic agents. If the maximum dose is exceeded, serious cardiovascular (arrhythmias) and CNS side effects (convulsions) may be observed.

Local anaesthetic drugs injected close to a sensory nerve or plexus will block the conduction of nerve impulses, including pain from sensory fibres, and provide excellent analgesia. Some local anaesthetics are given with adrenaline (epinephrine) to reduce systemic toxicity and increase the duration of action.

Local anaesthetics can be administered directly to wounds or by local infiltration to produce postoperative analgesia; however, these approaches will not normally block pain arising from deep internal organs. Local anaesthetic techniques are particularly useful in day-case surgery and children. Continuous infusions via a catheter will allow prolonged analgesia. More permanent neural blockade for the control of cancer pain may be achieved by using a neurolytic agent such as absolute alcohol or phenol.

A topical formulation of lidocaine has been marketed for the management of neuropathic pain caused by post-herpetic neuralgia. Up to three plasters may be worn for a 12-hour period each day.

Epidural local anaesthetics

Long-acting local anaesthetic drugs such as bupivacaine are most effective in relieving pain after major surgery. They work by blocking nerves in the spinal canal serving both superficial and deep tissues, and thus analgesia can be obtained in deep internal organs. Sensory and sympathetic nerves that maintain smooth muscle tone in blood vessels are blocked. As a result, vasodilation can occur, which may result in significant hypotension. Epidural catheters allow continuous infusions and long-term therapy by this route. Adverse effects may include muscle weakness in the area supplied by the nerve and, rarely, infection and haematomas.

Adjuvant medicines

To be an analgesic, a drug must relieve pain in animal models and give demonstrable and reliable pain relief in patients. Drugs such as the opioids and the NSAIDs clearly are analgesics. In some types of pain, such as cancer pain or neuropathic pain, the addition of non-analgesic drugs to analgesic therapy can enhance pain relief. A list of some adjuvant drugs is given in Table 34.2. It should be remembered that some drugs, such as tricyclic antidepressants (TCAs), have intrinsic analgesic activity, perhaps related to their ability to affect 5-HT and noradrenergic neurotransmission.

Antidepressants

Long-term pain is accompanied frequently by anxiety and depression. Thus, it is not surprising that the use of antidepressants and other psychoactive drugs is a routine component of pain management. There is evidence that some of these drugs have analgesic properties independent of their psychotropic effects.

The TCAs are frequently used for the treatment of long-term pain conditions with and without antiepileptic drugs, and there is a substantial body of literature about their analgesic action (McQuay et al., 1996).

The biochemical activity of the TCAs suggests that their main effect is on serotonergic and noradrenergic neurones. The TCAs inhibit the reuptake of the monoamines, 5-HT and/or noradrenaline in neurones found within in the brain and spinal cord. Through a rather complex mechanism, this causes an initial fall in the release of these transmitters followed by a sustained rise in the concentration of neurotransmitter at synapses in the pain neural pathways. This rise usually takes 2–3 weeks to develop. Tricyclic antidepressants are effective analgesics in headache, facial pain, low back pain, arthritis and, to a lesser degree, cancer pain.

Clinical use of antidepressants in long-term pain

When used in pain management, it is usual to start with a low TCA dose, for example, amitriptyline 10–25 mg at night and to titrate upwards according to response and adverse effects. Within clinical trials TCA doses have varied considerably, but most are lower than the doses used in psychiatry, in the order of amitriptyline 50–75 mg/day. Under specialist supervision, higher doses, for example, amitriptyline 150–200 mg/day, may be appropriate.

Tricyclic antidepressants have a wide range of adverse effects due to interaction with histamine and muscarinic acetylcholine receptors, and these may cause a marked reduction in patient adherence. Newer antidepressant drugs have generally been disappointing from the analgesic perspective. Outcomes with selective serotonin reuptake inhibitors (SSRIs) have been disappointing. Scientific (Sindrup and Jensen, 1999) and clinical evidence suggest that both noradrenergic and serotonergic transmission need to be enhanced for an analgesic effect to be seen (Sindrup et al., 2005). The serotonin/noradrenaline reuptake inhibitors (SNRIs) venlafaxine and duloxetine have effects on both monoamines and appear to possess analgesic activity in neuropathic pain conditions (e.g. diabetic neuropathy and

Table 34.2 Adjuvant drugs used in the treatment of pain

Drug class	Type of pain	Example
Antiepileptics	Neuropathic pain Migraine Cluster headache	Carbamazepine Sodium valproate Gabapentin Pregabalin Lamotrigine
Antidepressants	Neuropathic pain Musculoskeletal pain	Amitriptyline Imipramine Venlafaxine Duloxetine
Intravenous anaesthetic agents	Neuropathic pain Burn pain Cancer pain	Ketamine
Skeletal muscle relaxants	Muscle spasm Spasticity	Baclofen Dantrolene Botulinum toxin (type A)
Steroids	Raised intracranial pressure Nerve compression	Dexamethasone Prednisolone
Antibiotics	Infection	As indicated by culture and sensitivity
Antispasmodics	Colic Smooth muscle spasm	Hyoscine butylbromide Loperamide
Hormones/hormonal analogues	Malignant bone pain Spinal stenosis Intestinal obstruction	Calcitonin Octreotide
Bisphosphonates	Bone pain (caused by cancer or osteoporosis)	Pamidronate (for cancer pain) Alendronate

post-herpetic neuralgia). Some antidepressant compounds, including trazodone and mirtazapine, do not act via monoamine reuptake inhibition and do not appear to possess intrinsic analgesic activity. They are effective antidepressants and may have a place in the treatment of co-existing depression, but analgesia should be managed separately.

Antiepileptic drugs

The usefulness of this group of drugs is well established for the treatment of neuropathic pain (Wiffen et al., 2013). Conditions which may respond to antiepileptics include trigeminal neuralgia, postherpetic neuralgia and multiple sclerosis, glossopharyngeal neuralgia and similar pains that may follow amputation or surgery. Several classes of drugs show antiepileptic activity, and these can be broadly classed as sodium channel blockers (carbamazepine, phenytoin), glutamate inhibitors (lamotrigine), voltage-gated calcium channel ligands (gabapentin, pregabalin), gamma-aminobutyric acid (GABA) potentiators (sodium valproate, tiagabine) or drugs showing a mixture of these effects (topiramate). Failure to respond to one particular drug does not indicate that antiepileptics as a broad class will be ineffective. A drug with a different mechanism of action or combination therapy could be considered.

Antiepileptics are surprisingly effective in the prophylaxis of migraine and cluster headache. Their mode of action is unclear, but both of these conditions are associated with abnormal excitability of certain groups of neurones, and the neuronal depression caused by antiepileptics is probably important.

Ketamine

Ketamine is an intravenous anaesthetic agent with a variety of actions within the CNS. Many of its effects are related to its activity at central glutamate receptors, although it also has actions at certain voltage-gated ion channels and opioid receptors. Low doses of ketamine (0.1–0.3 mg/kg/h via the intravenous route) can produce profound analgesia, even in situations where opioids have been ineffective, such as neuropathic pain. Despite its variable oral availability, oral administration of ketamine can be surprisingly effective (Annetta et al., 2005; Mercadante, 1996). Its usefulness is limited by troublesome psychotropic side effects, although the simultaneous administration of benzodiazepines or antipsychotics can reduce these problems.

Anxiolytics

Benzodiazepines may be used for short-term pain relief in conditions associated with acute muscle spasm and are sometimes prescribed to reduce the anxiety and muscle tension associated with long-term pain conditions. Many authorities believe that they reduce pain tolerance and there is good evidence that they can reduce the effectiveness of opioid analgesics, although the mechanism by which this occurs is unclear. Clonazepam has been used in the management of neuropathic pain. Diazepam can be used to control painful spasticity, due to acute or spinal cord injury, but sedation may be troublesome, and tizanidine (see following discussion) is probably a more suitable choice.

Antihistamines

These agents were introduced into the management of long-term pain because of their sedative muscle relaxant properties. These actions are non-specific, and it is not clear whether the clinical effect is mediated centrally or peripherally. Most clinical studies have been carried out with hydroxyzine, which has shown benefit in acute pain, tension headache and cancer pain, but is not commonly used in current clinical practice.

Skeletal muscle relaxants

The drugs described in this section are used for the relief of muscle spasm or spasticity. It is essential that the underlying cause of the spasticity and any aggravating factors such as pressure sores or infections are treated. Skeletal muscle relaxants usually help spasticity, but this may be at the cost of decreased muscle tone elsewhere, which may lead to a decrease in patient mobility, which may make matters worse.

Baclofen, which has a peripheral site of action, working directly on skeletal muscle, is probably the most commonly prescribed skeletal muscle relaxant. It is a derivative of the inhibitory neurotransmitter GABA and appears to be an agonist at the $GABA_B$ receptor. Baclofen is used commonly in the treatment of spasticity caused by multiple sclerosis or other diseases of the spinal cord, especially traumatic lesions.

The α_2-adrenergic agonist tizanidine has potent muscle relaxant activity and is an alternative to baclofen. It may also have some direct analgesic effects.

Dantrolene is an alternative that is effective orally and which may have fewer, but potentially more serious, adverse effects. Its effect is due to a direct action on skeletal muscle and takes several weeks to develop.

Botulinum toxin

The bacterium *Clostridium botulinum* produces a potent toxin that interferes directly with neuromuscular transmission. Purified preparations of the type A toxin produce long-lasting relaxation of skeletal muscle. The effect often lasts in excess of three months and avoids the systemic side effects of agents such as baclofen. Great care must be taken in administering this drug because spread may occur to adjacent muscle groups, producing excessive weakness. Use of botulinum toxin has been approved by National Institute for Health and Care Excellence (NICE) for prophylaxis of migraine (NICE, 2014). Overdosage, with systemic absorption, may lead to generalised muscle weakness and even respiratory failure.

Clonidine

The α-adrenergic agonist clonidine has been shown to produce analgesia, and there is evidence that both morphine and clonidine produce a dose-dependent inhibition of spinal nociceptive transmission that is mediated through different receptors for each drug. This may explain why clonidine has been shown to work synergistically with morphine when given by the intrathecal or epidural routes. Clonidine also appears to be effective when given by other routes or even topically, but it may cause severe hypotension by any route.

Cannabinoids

Cannabis has been used as an analgesic for hundreds of years. Problems concerning the legal status of cannabis in most countries have hindered the scientific investigation of its analgesic properties. The active ingredient in preparations made from the hemp plant, *Cannabis sativa*, is δ-9 tetrahydrocannabinol. This compound has analgesic activity in animal models of experimental pain as well as in the clinical situation (Burns and Ineck, 2006). Overall, analgesic activity appears relatively weak, and it has not been possible to separate the analgesic activity from the potent psychotropic effects characteristic of these drugs, but a commercial preparation, Sativex, is now licensed for the management of spasticity in multiple sclerosis. There may be a clearer analgesic effect in neuropathic pain, but the evidence for this remains limited and must be considered along with the misuse potential when prescribing.

Stimulation-produced analgesia

Stimulation-produced analgesia can be used for trauma, postoperative pain, labour pain and various types of long-term pain.

Transcutaneous electrical nerve stimulation and acupuncture

Transcutaneous electrical nerve stimulation (TENS) machines are portable battery-powered devices that generate a small current to electrodes applied to the skin. The electrodes are placed at the painful site or close to the course of the peripheral nerve innervating the painful area, and the current is increased until paraesthesia is felt at the site of the pain. The current stimulates the large, rapidly conducting (Aβ) fibres which close the gating mechanism in the dorsal horn cells, and this inhibits the small, slowly conducting (Aδ and C) fibres. TENS, in particular, offers the patient a simple, noninvasive, self-controlled method of pain relief with relatively few adverse effects.

Acupuncture also works using a similar manner, although additional mechanisms, including stimulation of endogenous opioid release, may be involved. Acupuncture was recommended by NICE for several years for the treatment of low back pain but has been withdrawn in most recent guidance (NICE, 2016).

Treatment of selected pain syndromes

Postoperative pain

The majority of patients experience pain after surgery. The site and nature of surgery influences the severity of pain, although individual variation between patients does not allow prediction of the severity of pain by the type of operation.

Apart from the obvious humanitarian benefit of relieving suffering, pain relief is desirable for a number of physiological reasons after surgery or any form of major tissue injury. For example, poor-quality analgesia reduces respiratory function, increases heart rate and blood pressure, and amplifies the stress response to surgery. The use of intermittent and patient-controlled intermittent intravenous opioids injections has been described earlier in this chapter. However, opioids themselves may delay recovery and are associated with adverse events in the postoperative period (Kehlet et al., 1996). It is now common to treat postoperative pain using a 'multimodal approach', consisting of paracetamol, an NSAID, opioids and local anaesthetic blocks or wound infiltration. NSAIDs such as diclofenac and ketorolac must be used with caution in the postoperative period where there is a possibility of renal stress, such as blood loss, and the normal protective effect of prostaglandins on the kidney will be lost, culminating in acute renal failure. There is no evidence to support the pre-emptive use of either NSAIDs or local anaesthetic techniques, although there is some theoretical and clinical evidence suggesting that opioids given before surgery may be more effective than when given postoperatively.

Cancer pain

Cancer and pain are not synonymous. One-third of patients with cancer do not experience severe pain. Of the remaining two-thirds that do, about 88% can be controlled using basic principles of pain management (Scottish Intercollegiate Guidelines Network, 2008). Pain associated with cancer may arise from many different sources and may exhibit the characteristics of both acute and long-term pain. The mechanisms and sources of cancer pain may change with time, and regular assessment is required. Cancer occurs more frequently in the elderly, who may have a larger proportion of other painful conditions than the younger population. Pain may be arising from these sources too, and these require treatment at the same time.

Cancer pain can be treated both with drugs and other interventional techniques, such as radiotherapy and nerve blocks. Usually, drug treatment is based on the WHO analgesic ladder together with the use of adjuvant analgesics. Opioids are the mainstay for the treatment of cancer pain, although increasingly, some clinicians progress from non-opioid drugs to a strong opioid such as morphine, omitting the middle step of the analgesic ladder.

Although this chapter is concerned only with the management of pain, care of the patient with a terminal illness requires management of all aspects of the patient. The Liverpool Care Pathway (LCP) in England was promoted for many years as a resource to promote high-quality care in the last days of life (Ellershaw and Wilkinson, 2003). The LCP acknowledged that death was imminent and ensured the patient's comfort by omitting long-term non-essential medication and ensuring anticipatory prescribing in case the patient experienced pain, delirium, vomiting or breathlessness. However, in 2013, after much criticism in the media, it was phased out and replaced with an individual approach to end-of-life care for each patient (NICE, 2015).

Opioid use in cancer pain

Morphine remains the first-line opioid used for the management of cancer pain and may be given in immediate or modified release oral formulations. If not tolerated, alternatives such as oxycodone or hydromorphone, both having relatively long half-lives, may be considered. Optimal dosage is determined on an individual basis for each patient by titration against the pain. Patients requiring long-term modified-release opioids should have additional oral doses of rapidly acting opioid to act as an 'escape' medicine for incident or breakthrough pain. The British National Formulary recommends that the standard dose of a strong opioid for breakthrough pain is one-tenth to one-sixth of the regular 24-hour total daily dose. Methadone should not be used as first-line treatment of cancer pain but may be useful when alternatives have failed or the patient has experienced intolerable adverse effects.

When the oral route is unavailable, other routes of administration such as the buccal, rectal, transdermal or parenteral (subcutaneous, intravenous) or spinal (epidural or intrathecal) routes may be considered. Syringe drivers or implanted pumps may be used to provide analgesia in cases where conventional opioid delivery is ineffective. Morphine and oxycodone are available for parenteral administration, and in the UK, diamorphine is also suitable and readily available. Diamorphine hydrochloride has the advantage of being very water soluble, so a high dose may be given in a small volume, which reduces the frequency of changes of syringes and refills necessary to provide adequate pain relief. The proportion of patients who need an implanted pump for intrathecal drug delivery is extremely small and is confined largely to those who are persistently troubled with unacceptable adverse effects. Such patients may achieve pain relief with lower equivalent opioid doses and have few problems with side effects. Long-term maintenance of indwelling lines and catheters requires training for the patient and specialist expertise from physicians and nursing teams, but excellent long-term results are possible.

Use of adjuvant drugs and treatments for cancer pain

Neuropathic pain is common in cancer. As many as 40% of cancer patients may have a neuropathic component to their pain. Tricyclic antidepressants and antiepileptic drugs should be introduced early, but where these are ineffective, ketamine can have a beneficial effect.

Levomepromazine, a phenothiazine with analgesic activity, is a useful alternative when opioids cannot be tolerated. It causes neither constipation nor respiratory depression and has antiemetic and anxiolytic activity. It is sedative, which may be either a virtue or a problem in palliative care.

Corticosteroids are useful in managing certain aspects of acute and persistent cancer pain. They are particularly useful for raised intracranial pressure and for relieving pressure caused by tumours on the spinal cord or peripheral nerves. Dexamethasone is the most commonly used steroid to ameliorate raised intracranial pressure in patients with brain tumours. High steroid doses given for 1 or 2 weeks do not require a reducing-dosage regimen. Also, they may produce a feeling of well-being, increased appetite and weight gain, all beneficial for cancer patients, although these effects are usually transient.

It is essential that underlying causes of pain be treated; therefore, it is appropriate to use antibiotics to treat infections, radiotherapy to reduce tumour bulk or control bone pain, or surgery to achieve fracture fixation or to relieve bowel obstruction in conjunction with antispasmodics such as hyoscine N-butylbromide.

Specific cancer pain syndromes

Three types of malignant pain are briefly outlined to indicate various therapeutic approaches.

Cancer of the pancreas. Pain is caused by infiltration of the tumour into the pancreas as well as by obstruction of the bowel and biliary tracts and metastases in the liver. Patients may experience anorexia, nausea, vomiting and diarrhoea, and they also are often depressed. Surgery, radiotherapy and chemotherapy may relieve pain for long periods, as does neurolytic blockade of the coeliac plexus. Opioid analgesics are useful and may be administered by the intravenous or epidural routes by either bolus injection or continuous infusion.

Mesothelioma of the lung. Mesothelioma causes pain when the tumour penetrates surrounding tissues such as the pleura, chest wall and nerve plexuses. The WHO analgesic ladder should be used first, but it should be remembered that a NSAID may be beneficial because inflammation is often a component of the chest wall involvement. Adjuvants such as TCAs or steroids may be helpful. As the tumour progresses, nerve blocks or neurosurgery may be necessary, and invasion of the vertebrae can lead to nerve root or spinal cord compression. In the latter case, high-dose steroids such as dexamethasone may be given intravenously, but radiotherapy is also useful in reducing the size of the tumour.

Metastatic bone pain. Metastatic bone pain is usually treated with courses of chemotherapy and radiotherapy, but analgesics may also be beneficial. A prostaglandin-like substance has been isolated from bone metastases, and therefore an NSAID and, more recently, bisphosphonates are often used in bone pain. Steroids also interfere with prostaglandin formation, and dexamethasone, therefore, has a role, especially where there is nerve root or spinal cord compression.

Neuropathic pain

Neuropathic pain may be defined as 'pain arising as a direct consequence of a disease or lesion affecting the somatosensory system' and may occur as a result of pathological damage to nerve fibres in a peripheral nerve or in the CNS (Table 34.3). Neuropathic pain may be spontaneous in nature (continuous or paroxysmal) or evoked by sensory stimuli. Because the underlying aetiology

Table 34.3	Examples of causes of neuropathic pain
Cause of neuropathy	Examples
Trauma	Phantom limb Peripheral nerve injury Spinal cord injury Surgical
Infection/inflammation	Post-herpetic neuralgia HIV
Compression	Trigeminal neuralgia Sciatica
Cancer	Invasion/compression of nerve tissue by tumour
Ischaemia	Post-stroke pain Metabolic neuropathies (e.g. diabetic peripheral neuropathy)
Demyelination	Multiple sclerosis
Drugs	Vinca alkaloids Ethanol Taxols Antibacterials for TB and HIV

HIV, Human immunodeficiency virus; TB, tuberculosis.

is different from inflammatory types of pain, patients typically present with disturbances in sensory function often describing their pain as tingling, shooting or electric shocks. It is possible for patients to present with pain in the context of sensory loss. Unlike inflammatory pain, neuropathic pain serves no biological advantage and can be described as an illness in its own right.

Typically, neuropathic pain does not respond as well to conventional analgesics, such as paracetamol and NSAIDs. Guidelines for the pharmacological management of neuropathic pain in the non-specialist setting have been published (NICE, 2013).

Specific neuropathic pain syndromes

Postherpetic neuralgia. The pain associated with herpes zoster infection is severe, continuous and often described as burning and lancinating. Antiviral therapy, such as aciclovir, initiated at the first sign of the rash can reduce the duration of the pain, particularly post-herpetic pain, which follows the disappearance of the rash. Tricyclic antidepressants such as amitriptyline are the mainstay of treatment, commencing with low doses (e.g. amitriptyline 10–25 mg at night) and gradually increased according to pain relief (usual dose amitriptyline 50–75 mg at night). This may be combined with antiepileptic drugs if the response is poor or incomplete. Carbamazepine is historically important, but newer antiepileptic drugs, such as gabapentin and pregabalin, are considered first-line therapy and are often better tolerated. One study has demonstrated a significant difference in the incidence and, to a lesser extent, the intensity of pain in patients who received a single epidural methylprednisolone and bupivacaine injection compared with those who received antiviral therapy and analgesia as 'standard care' (van Wijck et al., 2006). However, given the modest clinical effects on acute pain and no effect on the incidence of postherpetic neuralgia, the routine use of epidural local anaesthetic and steroid injection is not widely supported.

Diabetic peripheral polyneuropathy. Nerve damage and neuropathy are among the long-term complications of diabetes mellitus (see Chapter 45) and are most prevalent in elderly patients with type II diabetes. Patients often describe numbness but also experience a burning sensation in their feet. The sensory loss can result in painless foot ulcers. Tricyclic antidepressants or SNRIs (duloxetine or venlafaxine) and antiepileptics, such as gabapentin and pregabalin, have been beneficial.

Trigeminal neuralgia. Trigeminal neuralgia presents as abrupt, intense bursts of severe, lancinating pain, provoked by touching sensitive trigger areas on one side of the face. The disorder may spontaneously remit for periods of several weeks or months. Antiepileptic drugs, particularly carbamazepine, have been used successfully. If drug therapy is ineffective, neurosurgical techniques such as decompression of the trigeminal nerve may be considered. If surgery is successful, antiepileptics should be withdrawn gradually afterwards.

Peripheral nerve injury and neuropathy. Damage to or entrapment of nerves can cause pain, unpleasant sensations and paraesthesiae. Tricyclic antidepressants and antiepileptic drugs,

such as gabapentin, have been used with some success to treat neuropathic pain (Moore et al., 2014). A neuroma occurs when damaged or severed nerve fibres sprout new small fibres in an attempt to regenerate. Pain develops several weeks after the nerve injury and is often due to the neuroma growing into scar tissue, causing pain as it is stretched or mobilised. Treatment of neuroma is very difficult, and few treatments are successful. Options include surgery and injections of steroid and local anaesthetic agents.

Complex regional pain syndromes. Complex regional pain syndromes are an important group of painful conditions that may follow trauma or damage to nerves and are characterised by neuropathic pain, trophic changes and motor dysfunction. The key elements of successful treatment are effective multimodal analgesia, including drugs with efficacy for neuropathic pain, and aggressive physiotherapy to facilitate a return to normal function. Sympathetic blockade using local anaesthetics may have a therapeutic role.

Back and neck pain

Back pain is one of the commonest reasons for seeing a medical practitioner. Despite this, the problem is poorly understood. The most practical classification is based on the duration of symptoms (BenDebba et al., 1997). Acute low pain is generally defined as pain that lasts for a few days or weeks. The majority of these problems tend to be self-limiting and resolve spontaneously. Typical treatments include rest, adequate analgesia with a NSAID and/or a weak opioid and maintaining physical activity.

Long-term back pain lasts for much longer and progressively leads to a chronic state associated with pain, depression, anxiety and disability. Early intervention is necessary to ensure good functional and vocational outcomes. If a patient is off work for as much as 6 months, then there is a less than 50% chance of the individual ever returning to work. The likelihood of returning to work falls to less than 25% after 1 year and is almost zero after 2 years. Although pharmacological therapies may aid rehabilitation, other treatment strategies have a greater role to play in the management of long-term back pain. Guidelines for the management of non-specific long-term low back pain and sciatica have been developed (NICE, 2016). It is essential for the patient to develop good self-management skills, and current recommendations emphasise the importance of using a biopsychosocial approach. Other treatment options include psychological therapies using a cognitive behavioural approach and manual therapy (spinal manipulation, mobilisation or soft tissue techniques such as massage) but only in combination with graded exercise programmes. Acupuncture is no longer recommended.

Osteoarthritis and rheumatoid arthritis

Pain often is a presenting symptom in osteoarthritis or the inflammatory arthritides, which include rheumatoid arthritis. The pathophysiology and management of osteoarthritis and rheumatoid arthritis is covered in Chapter 54.

Myofascial pain

Myofascial pain is pain arising from muscles and is associated with stiffness and neuropathic symptoms, such as tingling and paraesthesiae. It may occur spontaneously or after trauma, such as whiplash injury. Myofascial pain syndrome is sometimes also termed myositis, fibrositis, myalgia and myofascitis. Acute muscle injury can be treated using first aid techniques with the application of a cooling spray or ice to reduce inflammation and spasm, followed by passive stretching of the muscle to restore its full range of motion. Injection therapy with local anaesthetic or saline may be used to disrupt sensitive muscle trigger points. Local injections of botulinum toxin have also been shown to be effective where muscle spasm is prolonged and severe. TENS and acupuncture have an important role to play in reducing pain and muscle spasm. Treatment of long-term myofascial syndromes should always include a programme of physical therapy.

Postamputation and phantom limb pain

The majority of amputees suffer significant stump or phantom limb pain for at least a few weeks each year. Pain will be present in the immediate postoperative period in the stump, and this may be caused by muscle spasm, nerve injury and sensitivity of the wound and surrounding skin. As the wound heals, the pain generally subsides. If it does not, the reason may be vascular insufficiency or infection. Pain occurring a number of years after amputation may be caused by changes in the structure of the bones or skin in the stump. Reduction in the thickness of overlying tissue with age may expose nerve endings to increased stimuli or ischaemia. Usually, conventional analgesics are beneficial for stump pain, although sometimes relatively high doses may be required. Tricyclic antidepressants may also be helpful for stump pain, and surgery may be necessary to restore the vascular supply or reduce trauma to nerve endings.

Phantom pain is a referred pain which produces a burning or throbbing sensation, felt in the absent limb. Cramping sensations are caused by muscular spasm in the stump. The patient with phantom limb pain is often anxious, depressed and frightened, all of which exacerbate the pain. Conventional analgesic drugs alone are generally not adequate for phantom pain, but TCAs and antiepileptic drugs are useful adjuvants. Other therapy which can be effective includes TENS and sympathetic blockade. These patients frequently require management at specialist pain centres.

Headache

Everybody experiences the occasional tension headaches. They are caused by muscle contraction over the neck and scalp. Often they respond to simple analgesics available OTC, such as paracetamol and NSAIDs. They may also respond to TCA drugs given as a single dose at night as well as non-pharmacological treatments, such as TENS. NSAIDs may be indicated if the headache is associated with cervical spondylosis or neck injury.

Migraine

Most migraine attacks respond to simple analgesics such as aspirin or paracetamol. Soluble preparations are best because gut motility is reduced during a migraine attack, and absorption of oral medication may be delayed. Migraine treatment has improved markedly with the development of the triptan drugs, such as almotriptan, eletriptan, rizatriptan, sumatriptan, naratriptan and zolmitriptan (Goadsby, 2005). These are $5HT_{1B/1D}$-agonists that will often abort an attack, especially when given by the subcutaneous route. Their vasoconstrictor activity precludes their use in patients with angina or cerebrovascular disease, but the side effects are less serious than with the ergot derivatives they have replaced.

Prophylactic drug treatment of migraine includes α-adrenergic blockers, antiepileptics and TCAs. Long-term treatment is undesirable.

Cluster headache

Cluster headache is a disabling condition characterised by severe unilateral head pain occurring in clusters of attacks varying from minutes to hours. It shares some pathological features with migraine and treatment is similar, although high-resolution MRI studies have shown specific anatomical differences in the brains of people with cluster headache. Triptans are effective in acute attacks, as is inhalation of 100% oxygen. Prophylaxis is similar to that of migraine.

Dysmenorrhoea

Dysmenorrhoea is a common cause of pelvic pain in women. NSAIDs are effective as first-line therapy due to their effect on cyclo-oxygenase inhibition, but it can also be helped by the prescription of oral contraceptives because pain is absent in anovulatory cycles. Dysmenorrhoea due to endometriosis may require therapy with androgenic drugs such as danazol or regulators of the gonadotrophins such as norethisterone.

Burn pain

Patients with burns may require a series of painful procedures such as physiotherapy, debridement or skin grafting. Premedication with a strong opioid before the procedure and the use of Entonox (premixed 50% nitrous oxide and 50% oxygen) may be necessary to control the pain. Regular opioid administration may be useful to prevent the pain induced by movement or touch in the affected area. The anaesthetic drug ketamine has potent analgesic activity when used in subhypnotic doses. Its short duration of action may be beneficial to reduce the pain of dressing changes or other forms of incident pain. Even with low doses, a significant proportion of patients will experience side effects of dysphoria or hallucinations. These can be treated with benzodiazepines or antipsychotic compounds, such as haloperidol.

A summary of medicine indications and common therapeutic problems associated with analgesic use are presented in Table 34.4.

Table 34.4 Common therapeutic problems

Problem	Solution	Example
Neuropathic pain	Antiepileptics	Carbamazepine Sodium valproate Gabapentin Lamotrigine
	Antidepressants	Amitriptyline Imipramine
	Intravenous anaesthetic agents	Ketamine
Malignant bone pain	Bisphosphonates	Pamidronate Calcitonin
Muscle spasm/ spasticity	Skeletal muscle relaxants	Baclofen Dantrolene Botulinum toxin (type A)
Raised intracranial pressure	Corticosteroids	Dexamethasone Prednisolone
Nausea with morphine	Antiemetic	Cyclizine Droperidol Ondansetron
	Use an alternative route of administration	Topical or subcutaneous
Constipation	Determine if drug induced, e.g. opioids or tricyclic antidepressant	Co-prescribe laxatives (e.g. docusate sodium and senna)
Antidepressants in patients with ischaemic heart disease	Use a less cardiotoxic antidepressant	Duloxetine Venlafaxine
Drug interactions with carbamazepine	Use an antiepileptic which does not affect hepatic enzymes	Gabapentin
Renal failure	Morphine accumulates Use a drug which is not eliminated by kidney	Consider lower dose Fentanyl Buprenorphine
Sedation/impaired cognition	Identify any drug-related causes and adjust dose or stop drug	

Case studies

Case 34.1

Mrs NP is a 55-year-old care home assistant who has type 2 diabetes. Her current prescription is for metformin 500 mg three times a day and amitriptyline 50 mg at night. When collecting her repeat prescription, she mentions that she 'Can't get on with the new tablets' because they make her very drowsy in the mornings. You invite Mrs NP for a review of her medication. During the consultation, Mrs NP explains that for some time she has suffered from constant tingling and occasional shooting pain in her legs and feet, and 3 months ago amitriptyline 10 mg daily was prescribed. About one month ago, the dose of amitriptyline was increased to 50 mg daily. She takes the dose at night, as advised by her primary care doctor. When she works an early shift (about three times a week), she usually omits the dose of amitriptyline to be sure that she wakes up in time to get to work. Mrs NP says that she takes the metformin regularly and has no associated problems. She is keen to be fit enough to work because she is supporting her youngest son, who is studying to be a doctor.

Question

What advice should you give to this patient?

Answer

Mrs NP has developed diabetic peripheral neuropathy, a type of neuropathic pain. She is experiencing intolerable side effects from the increased dose of amitriptyline and therefore does not take it regularly. There are several options to improve tolerability. Firstly, Mrs NP should consider increasing the dose of amitriptyline more slowly. She may also benefit from taking her amitriptyline dose earlier in the evening, approximately 60–90 minutes before retiring to bed, so that it results in less hangover effect the following day. If neither of these strategies is beneficial, she should consult her primary care doctor about switching to an alternative drug to manage her neuropathic symptoms. Most recent guidance (NICE, 2013) recommends either gabapentin, pregabalin or duloxetine as alternatives to a tricyclic antidepressant as first-line therapy for neuropathic pain in the non-specialist setting.

Case 34.2

A 55-year-old lady, Mrs LT, with metastatic abdominal cancer from a probable primary in the pelvis, presents with an abdominal mass. Mrs LT's pain is uncontrolled despite regular prescription of oral opioids, and she has been sick for a week. Subacute bowel obstruction is present.

Question

How should Mrs LT be managed?

Answer

Management should begin with admission and rehydration. Mrs LT may be dehydrated and have marked electrolyte abnormalities which would need to be corrected. The oral route is unavailable for the delivery of adequate analgesia, and thus consideration should be given to the use of parenteral administration, either by the subcutaneous route or using patient-controlled analgesia. The sickness should be treated, and an underlying cause sought. This may be subacute obstruction which, in turn, may be due to constipation caused by the opioids or by the disease process. Abdominal masses that indent on palpation are faeces (not tumour). Abdominal radiographs would show fluid levels if there was obstruction rather than constipation. Other possible causes of vomiting are recent anticancer therapy, anxiety, dyspepsia from NSAIDs, raised intracranial pressure and vertigo. Surgery may be needed to relieve the obstruction, but the need may be avoided by use of hyoscine *N*-butylbromide, which may control colic with little additional sedation. If the problem is one of constipation, rectal measures may be necessary to re-establish function. These may include suppositories, enemas or digital disimpaction. Once control of pain has been achieved and bowel function has returned to normal, she must receive regular combination laxative therapy, ideally, a stimulant laxative, such as senna, and a faecal softener, such as docusate sodium. A high fluid intake and increased dietary fibre should be encouraged because this will help prevent stool from becoming hard. There has been interest in the use of peripheral opioid receptor antagonists to reduce opioid-induced constipation. Because they have higher affinity for the opioid receptor than the agonist, they bind preferentially to opioid receptors in the gastro-intestinal tract, allowing the agonist to continue to have its desired effect in the CNS. A combination of prolonged-release oxycodone and prolonged-release naloxone (Targinact) or naloxegol may be an alternative if maximal laxative therapy does not help this patient.

Attention should be paid to Mrs LT's emotional and spiritual needs at all times.

Case 34.3

A 28-year-old man, Mr FR, had a crush fracture of his ankle after falling from a roof. Fixation 9 months ago was described as satisfactory, but his leg is now very painful to even small stimuli, and he cannot use it or bear weight. Mr FR's lower leg has muscle wasting and is much colder than the opposite limb. The skin is very sensitive to touch, shiny and has a poor circulation.

Question

What is this condition, and how should this pain be treated?

Answer

Mr FR has presented with a complex regional pain syndrome. Management should be aggressive and directed towards functional restoration. Use of effective multimodal analgesia using pharmacological and non-pharmacological treatments is required. The aim is to facilitate aggressive physiotherapy and occupational therapy. There may be a burning component to the pain, which may respond to low doses of TCAs such as amitriptyline (10–25 mg at night initially, increased in small increments to 50–75 mg at night).

Aggressive treatment early in the course of the disease can reduce the length of time patients, such as Mr FR, have this problem, and early referral to seek specialised help is recommended. A small percentage of patients will continue to have problems whatever treatment is given.

Case 34.4

An 85-year-old man, Mr PL, is admitted to hospital after falling down a flight of stairs and landing heavily on his right side. On admission, Mr PL is in severe pain and finds breathing, and especially coughing, unbearably painful. A chest X-ray reveals that he has fractures of the 5th to 8th ribs on the right side.

Question

How should Mr PL's pain be managed, and what are the risks of under-treatment?

Answer

Multiple rib fractures are potentially very serious, and good analgesia can prevent potentially dangerous complications. Initial analgesia should include both potent opioids and NSAIDs (unless contraindicated). Opioids should be administered parenterally in the first instance, and subsequent use of patient-controlled analgesia would allow the patient to titrate his own analgesic requirements. The chest injury may well result in damage to the underlying lung, and it is essential to administer unrestricted high-flow oxygen to the patient because the combination of lung injury and ventilatory suppression secondary to either pain or the effects of opioids could lead to dangerous hypoxia. TENS may also prove helpful.

Arterial oxygen saturation (and preferably arterial blood gases) should be monitored. If pain remains poorly controlled or if Mr PL's oxygenation deteriorates, thoracic epidural analgesia using a mixture of local anaesthetic and opioid may be considered.

Failure to treat pain adequately in this situation may lead to a reduction in Mr PL's ability to cough and clear secretions from the chest. This can lead to respiratory failure and even death. Analgesia should be sufficient to allow regular physiotherapy to minimise the risk of such complications.

Case 34.5

A 45-year-old woman, Mrs SG, presents to her primary care doctor with a 2-day history of back pain after a lifting injury at work. The pain is constant and aching in character with radiation into the posterior aspect of both thighs as far as the knee. Physical examination shows Mrs SG to be maintaining a very rigid posture with some spasm of the large muscles of the back. Her range of movement is very poor, but there are no neurological signs in the legs.

Question

Which drugs may help Mrs SG's pain? What other advice should Mrs SG be given?

Answer

Acute back pain is very common and is rarely associated with serious spinal pathology. The absence of neurological signs is reassuring and indicates that early activity, possibly aided by a short course of analgesics, is the best way forward. A short course of regular NSAID (e.g. ibuprofen 400 mg three times a day) is recommended first-line treatment if not contraindicated. Paracetamol alone is not now recommended. If unable to take a NSAID, paracetamol in combination with a weak opioid is suggested. A muscle relaxant such as baclofen 20–40 mg/day in divided doses may be beneficial for short-term use only. The role of opioids is less clear. Short-term use (7–14 days) of a weak opioid such as codeine or tramadol is probably safe. Longer-term use is less satisfactory because there is no clear evidence of efficacy, and sedative side effects may reduce the patient's capacity and motivation to remain active.

Mrs SG should be advised to remain active and accept that some pain is likely during the recovery phase. Failure to remain active and, in particular, excessive bed rest are both associated with worse outcomes.

Case 34.6

A 50-year-old man, Mr TW, is admitted to hospital with an acute onset of severe mid-thoracic spinal pain. He is found to be anaemic, and investigations show that Mr TW has multiple myeloma with widespread bony lesions, including fresh spinal fractures.

Question

Which drugs may help Mr TW's pain? What particular hazards may occur in this condition?

Answer

Mr TW is extremely ill, and even with aggressive chemotherapy, he is unlikely to survive more than a few months. Most of his pain will be related to the destruction of bone, and the aim should be to provide pain relief via a 'central' mechanism through the use of opioids and to reduce the rate of bone destruction and associated inflammatory responses. A potent opioid will be required, and oral morphine would usually be the drug of first choice. In this situation, a combination of a modified-release preparation together with liberal 'as-required' dosing would be appropriate. The correct dose is the dose required to produce adequate pain relief without producing excessive sedation. Inflammatory pain may be improved by the use of NSAIDs and these should be given regularly, although they may be contraindicated in this condition (see following discussion). High-dose corticosteroids may achieve a similar effect and may also reduce the hypercalcaemia that is often seen in myeloma. Bone destruction and its associated pain may be reduced by the use of bisphosphonate compounds. In this case, intravenous pamidronate should be given.

Renal failure is common in myeloma. This may be due to obstruction of renal tubules by myeloma proteins or the effects of some chemotherapeutic agents. If renal impairment occurs, opioids should be used with caution so as to avoid problems with accumulation. Transdermal fentanyl may be a more appropriate drug. NSAIDs can precipitate acute renal failure in the presence of reduced renal blood flow. Finally, platelet function is often poor in patients with myeloma. This can be due to direct effects of myeloma proteins on platelets, bone marrow replacement by myeloma or the effects of chemotherapy. Use of NSAIDs may be associated with increased risk of gastrointestinal haemorrhage.

References

Annetta, M.G., Iemma, D., Garisto, C., et al., 2005. Ketamine: new indications for an old drug. Curr. Drug Targets. 6, 789–794.

Baron, R., Förster, M., Binder, A., 2012. Subgrouping of patients with neuropathic pain according to pain-related sensory abnormalities: a first step to a stratified treatment approach. Lancet Neurol. 11, 999–1005.

BenDebba, M., Torgerson, W.S., Long, D.M., 1997. Personality traits, pain duration, and severity, functional impairment, and psychological distress in patients with persistent low back pain. Pain. 72, 115–125.

Breivik, H., Borchgrevink, P.C., Allen, S.M., et al., 2008. Assessment of pain. Br. J. Anaesth. 101, 17–24.

Burns, T.L., Ineck, J.R., 2006. Cannabinoid analgesia as a potential new therapeutic option in the treatment of persistent pain. Ann. Pharmacother. 40, 251–260.

Claridge, L.C., Eksteen, B., Smith, A., et al., 2010. Acute liver failure after administration of paracetamol at the maximum recommended daily dose in adults. Br. Med. J. 341, c6764. https://doi.org/10.1136/bmj.c6764.

Cleeland, C.S., Ryan, K.M., 1994. Pain assessment: global use of the Brief Pain Inventory. Ann. Acad. Med. Singapore 23 (2), 129–138 .

Coxib and Traditional NSAID Trialists' (CNT) Collaboration, 2013. Vascular and upper gastrointestinal effects of non-steroidal anti-inflammatory drugs: meta-analyses of individual participant data from randomised trials. Lancet 382, 769–779.

Ellershaw, J., Wilkinson, S., 2003. Care of the Dying: A Pathway to Excellence. Oxford University Press, Oxford.

Goadsby, P.J., 2005. Advances in the understanding of headache. Br. Med. Bull. 73, 83–92.

Högestätt, E.D., Jonsson, B.A., Ermund, A., et al., 2005. Conversion on acetaminophen to the bioactive N-acylphenolamine AM404 via fatty acid hydrolase-dependent arachadonic acid conjugation in the nervous system. J. Biol. Chem. 280, 405–412.

Holden, J.E., Jeong, Y., Forrest, J.M., 2005. The endogenous opioid system and clinical pain management. AACN Clin. Issues. 16, 291–301.

Hyllested, M., Jones, S., Pedersen, J.L., et al., 2002. Comparative effect of paracetamol, NSAIDs or their combination in postoperative pain management: a qualitative review. Br. J. Anaesth. 88, 199–214.

International Association for the Study of Pain, 2012. IASAP taxonomy. Available at: https://www.iasp-pain.org/Taxonomy.

Kehlet, H., Rung, G.W., Callesen, T., 1996. Postoperative opioid analgesia: time for a reconsideration? J. Clin. Anesth. 8, 441–445.

Laderman, M., Martin, L., 2017. Health care providers must act now to address the prescription opioid crisis NEJM catalyst. Available at: http://catalyst.nejm.org/act-now-prescription-opioid-crisis/.

Li Wan Po, A., Zhang, W.Y., 1997. Systematic overview of co-proxamol to assess analgesic effects of addition of dextropropoxyphene to paracetamol. Br. Med. J. 315, 1565–1571.

McQuay, H.J., Tramer, M., Nye, B., et al., 1996. A systematic review of antidepressants in neuropathic pain. Pain 68, 217–227.

Medicines and Healthcare Products Regulatory Agency, 2005. Co-proxamol: Outcome of the review for risks and benefits. Available at: http://webarchive.nationalarchives.gov.uk/20141206131537/http://www.mhra.gov.uk/home/groups/pl-a/documents/websiteresources/con019462.pdf.

Melzack, R., Torgerson, W.S., 1971. On the language of pain. Anesthesiology 34, 50–59.

Mercadante, S., 1996. Ketamine in cancer pain: an update. Palliat. Med. 10, 225–230.

Moore, R.A., Wiffen, P.J., Derry, S., et al., 2014. Gabapentin for chronic neuropathic pain and fibromyalgia in adults. Cochrane DB Syst. Rev. 2014 (4), Art. No: CD007938. https://doi.org/10.1002/14651858.CD007938.pub3.

Moore, A., Derry, S., Eccleston, C., et al., 2013. Expect analgesic failure; pursue analgesic success. Br. Med. J. 346, f2690.

National Institute for Health and Care Excellence (NICE), 2013. Neuropathic pain in adults: pharmacological management in non-specialist settings. NICE Clinical Guideline 59. NICE, London. Available at: https://www.nice.org.uk/guidance/cg173.

National Institute for Health and Care Excellence (NICE), 2014. Botulinum toxin type A for the prevention of headaches in adults with chronic migraine. NICE Technology Appraisal Guidance TA260. NICE, London. Available at: https://www.nice.org.uk/guidance/ta260.

National Institute for Health and Care Excellence (NICE), 2015. Care of dying adults in the last days of life. NICE Guideline NG31. NICE, London. Available at: https://www.nice.org.uk/guidance/ng31.

National Institute for Health and Care Excellence (NICE), 2016. Low back pain and sciatica in over 16s: assessment and management. NICE Guideline 59. NICE, London. Available at: https://www.nice.org.uk/guidance/ng59.

Rainsford, K.D., Bjarnason, I., 2015. Gastrointestinal adverse reactions to ibuprofen. In: Rainsford, K.D. (Ed.), Ibuprofen: Discovery, Development and Therapeutics. Wiley, Chichester, pp. 363–429.

Scottish Intercollegiate Guidelines Network, 2008. Control of pain in adults with cancer. SIGN, Edinburgh. Available at: http://www.sign.ac.uk/pdf/SIGN106.pdf.

Sindrup, S.H., Jensen, T.S., 1999. Efficacy of pharmacological treatments of neuropathic pain: an update and effect related to mechanism of drug action. Pain 83, 389–400.

Sindrup, S.H., Otto, M., Finnerup, N.B., et al., 2005. Antidepressants in the treatment of neuropathic pain. Basic Clin. Pharmacol. Toxicol. 96, 399–409.

Thompson, D.R., 2001. Narcotic analgesic effects on the sphincter of Oddi: a review of the data and therapeutic implications in treating pancreatitis. Am. J. Gastroenterol. 96, 1266–1272.

Tjolsen, A., Lund, A., Hole, K., 1991. Antinociceptive effect of paracetamol in rats is partly dependent on spinal serotonergic systems. Eur. J. Pharmacol. 193, 193–201.

van Wijck, A.J., Opstelten, W., Moons, K.G., et al., 2006. The PINE study of epidural steroids and local anaesthetics to prevent postherpetic neuralgia: a randomised controlled trial. Lancet 367, 219–224.

Wiffen, P.J., Derry, S., Moore, R.A., et al., 2013. Antiepileptic drugs for neuropathic pain and fibromyalgia – and overview of Cochrane reviews. Cochrane Database Syst. Rev. (11), CD010567. doi:10.1002/14651858.CD010567.pub2.

Woolf, C.J., 2004. Pain: moving from symptom control toward mechanism-specific pharmacologic management. Ann. Intern. Med. 140, 441–451.

Woolf, C.J., 2011. Central sensitization: implications for the diagnosis and treatment of pain. Pain 152 (Suppl. 3), S2–S15.

Zin, C.S., Chen, L.-C., Knaggs, R.D., 2014. Changes in trends and pattern of strong opioid prescribing in primary care. Eur. J. Pain 18, 1343–1351.

Further reading

British Association for the Study of Headache, 2010. Guidelines for all healthcare professionals in the diagnosis and management of migraine, tension-type, cluster and medication-overuse headache. Available at: http://www.bash.org.uk/wp-content/uploads/2012/07/10102-BASH-Guidelines-update-2_v5-1-indd.pdf.

Brook, P., Connell, J., Pickering, T., 2011. Oxford Handbook of Pain. Oxford University Press, Oxford.

MacIntyre, P., Schug, S.A., 2015. Acute Pain Management: A Practical Guide, fourth ed. CRC Press, Boca Raton.

McMahon, S., Koltzenburg, M., Tracey, I., Turk, D.C. (Eds.), 2016. Melzack and Wall's Textbook of Pain, sixth ed. Elsevier Saunders, Philadelphia.

Melzack, R., Wall, P.D., 2003. Handbook of Pain Management: A Clinical Companion to Melzack and Wall's Textbook of Pain. Churchill Livingstone, Edinburgh.

Moore, R.A., McQuay, H.J., 2005. Prevalence of opioid adverse events in persistent non-malignant pain: systematic review of randomized trials of oral opioids. Arthritis Res. Ther. 7, R1046–R1051.

National Institute for Health and Care Excellence, 2004. Improving supportive and palliative care for adults with cancer. NICE Cancer Services Guideline 4. NICE, London. Available at: https://www.nice.org.uk/guidance/csg4.

National Institute for Health and Care Excellence, 2012. Palliative care for adults: strong opioids for pain relief. Clinical Guideline 140. NICE, London. Available at: https://www.nice.org.uk/guidance/cg140.

Schug, S.A., Palmer, G.M., Scott, D.A., et al., 2015. Acute Pain Management: Scientific Evidence, fourth ed. ANZCA & FPM, Melbourne.

Scottish Intercollegiate Guidelines Network, 2008. Management of chronic pain. SIGN 136. SIGN, Edinburgh. Available at: http://sign.ac.uk/guidelines/fulltext/136/index.html.

Useful websites

Oxford Pain: http://www.bandolier.org.uk/booth/painpag/index.html.

Change Pain: http://www.change-pain.co.uk/.

International Association for the Study of Pain: https://www.iasp-pain.org/.

PalliativeDrugs.com: http://www.palliativedrugs.com/.

Pain, Palliative and Supportive Care Group of Cochrane Library: http://papas.cochrane.org/.

Opioids Aware: https://www.fpm.ac.uk/faculty-of-pain-medicine/opioids-aware.

British Pain Society: https://www.britishpainsociety.org.

35 Nausea and Vomiting

Emma Mason and Philip A. Routledge

Key points

- Patients must be assessed carefully and, when necessary, reassessed frequently to identify the underlying cause of their nausea and/or vomiting.

- Antiemetics are symptomatic treatments only and do not treat the underlying cause.

- Choice of agent is based on an understanding of the likely pathophysiology, the receptors involved, the available route of administration and side effects.

- In certain situations, prophylactic regimens are beneficial, for example, motion sickness, postoperative nausea and vomiting, and chemotherapy-induced nausea and vomiting.

- Simple regimens are used when possible to prevent postoperative nausea and vomiting, such as parenteral cyclizine or prochlorperazine administered at induction. These and other antiemetics can be used for rescue therapy if vomiting occurs postoperatively.

- The choice of antiemetic to use in conjunction with cytotoxic chemotherapy depends on the 'emetogenicity' of the cytotoxic drugs used.

- Anticipatory emesis associated with chemotherapy can be treated with benzodiazepines, and dexamethasone may be useful in alleviating delayed emesis.

Nausea and vomiting are commonly (but not universally) associated symptoms. The word *nausea* is derived from the Greek *nautia*, meaning 'seasickness', and *vomiting* is derived from the Latin *vomere*, meaning 'to discharge'. Nausea is a subjective sensation, whereas vomiting is the reflex physical act of expulsion of gastric contents. Retching is defined as 'spasmodic respiratory movements' against a closed glottis with contractions of the abdominal musculature without expulsion of any gastric contents, that is, 'dry heaves' (American Gastroenterological Association, 2001). It is important to differentiate vomiting from regurgitation, rumination and bulimia. Regurgitation is the return of oesophageal or gastric contents into the hypopharynx with little effort. Rumination is the passive regurgitation of recently ingested food into the mouth followed by re-chewing, re-swallowing or spitting out. It is not preceded by nausea and does not include the various physical phenomena associated with vomiting. Bulimia involves overeating followed by self-induced vomiting.

Epidemiology

Nausea and vomiting from all causes have significant associated social and economic costs in terms of effects on quality of life and the need for extra medical care. In the community, nausea (with or without vomiting) is most likely to be associated with infection, particularly gastro-intestinal infection. Vestibular disorders may cause vomiting, as can motion sickness. Nausea and vomiting may be associated with pain, caused, for example, by migraine and severe cardiac pain. Many medicines cause nausea and occasionally also vomiting as a common dose-related (type A) adverse effect. This is particularly common with opioid use in palliative care. Nausea and vomiting also occur postoperatively or in association with cytotoxic chemotherapy or radiotherapy. These and other causes of nausea and vomiting are listed in Table 35.1.

Pathophysiology

Complex interactions between central and peripheral pathways occur in the production of the clinical features of nausea and vomiting. The most important areas involved peripherally are the gastric mucosa and smooth muscle (the enteric brain) and the afferent pathways of the vagus and sympathetic nerves. Centrally, the significant areas involved are the area postrema, the chemoreceptor trigger zone (CTZ), the nucleus tractus solitarus (NTS) and the vomiting centre.

From a pharmacotherapeutic point of view, the most important aspect of this complex pathophysiology is the variety of receptors involved, including histaminergic (H_1), cholinergic (muscarinic M_1), dopaminergic (D_2), serotonergic ($5HT_3$) and neurokinin-1 (NK_1) receptors. In the clinical situation, these become targets for various drugs directed at controlling the symptoms.

There are 10^8 neurons in the intestine, and a complex interaction occurs among these, the mucosa, the smooth muscle in the intestine, the parasympathetic (vagus nerve) and sympathetic nerves and the higher centres in the spinal cord and brain to result in normal gastro-intestinal peristaltic activity. The enteric brain and the vagus nerve monitor stimuli from mucosal irritation while smooth muscle monitors stretch, which may result in nausea and/or vomiting.

Table 35.1 Selected causes of nausea and vomiting

Central	
1. Intracranial	Migraine Raised intracranial pressure (tumour, infection, haemorrhage, hydrocephalus, etc.)
2. Labyrinthine	Iatrogenic Labyrinthitis, motion sickness, Ménière's disease, otitis media Cancer chemotherapy Many other medicines (e.g. opioids) Radiotherapy Postoperative
Endocrine/metabolic	Pregnancy, uraemia, diabetic ketoacidosis, hyperthyroidism, hyperparathyroidism, hypoparathyroidism, Addison's disease, acute intermittent porphyria
Infectious	Gastroenteritis (viral or bacterial) Other infections elsewhere
Gastro-intestinal disorders	Mechanical obstruction (gastric outlet or small bowel) Organic gastro-intestinal disorders (e.g. cholecystitis, pancreatitis, hepatitis) Functional gastro-intestinal disorders (e.g. non-ulcer dyspepsia, irritable bowel syndrome)
Psychogenic disorders	Psychogenic vomiting, anxiety, depression
Pain related	Myocardial infarction

Adapted from Quigley et al. (2001).

The area postrema in the floor of the fourth ventricle contains the CTZ and is a special sensory organ rich in dopaminergic, serotonergic, histaminergic and muscarinic receptors. It is located outside the blood–brain barrier, and it is likely that chemicals, toxins, peptides, drugs and neurotransmitters in the cerebrospinal fluid (CSF) and bloodstream interact with this area to cause nausea and vomiting. However, the precise mechanism is not known.

The vomiting centre is situated in the dorsolateral reticular formation close to the respiratory centre and receives impulses from higher centres, visceral efferents, the eighth (auditory) nerve (the latter two through the nucleus tractus solitarius) and from the CTZ (Fig. 35.1). It includes a number of brainstem nuclei required to integrate the responses of the gastro-intestinal tract, pharyngeal muscles, respiratory muscles and somatic muscles to result in a vomiting episode. The vomiting centre may be stimulated in association with, or in isolation from, the nausea process.

The vomiting reflex can be elicited either directly via afferent neuronal connections, especially from the gastro-intestinal tract, and is probably dependent on the integrity of the nucleus tractus solitarius, or from humoral factors dependent on the integrity of the area postrema. The sequence of muscle excitation and inhibition necessary for the act of vomiting is probably controlled by a central

pattern generator located in the nucleus tractus solitarius, and information from the CTZ and vagus nerve converges at this point.

The central causes of nausea and vomiting include increased intracranial pressure, dilation of cerebral arteries during migraine and stimulation of the labyrinthine mechanism or of the senses of sight, smell and taste.

The peripheral causes of nausea and vomiting include motion sickness, delayed gastric emptying and gastric mucosal irritation (e.g. ulceration, non-steroidal anti-inflammatory drugs [NSAIDs]). These mechanisms are all mediated through the vagal afferent neurons. The vomiting associated with distension or obstruction of the gastro-intestinal tract is mediated through both the sympathetic and vagal afferent neurons.

Patient management

Management of the patient with nausea and vomiting is approached in three steps:

1. Recognise and correct any complications. This includes correction of dehydration, hypokalaemia and metabolic alkalosis in the acute situation with symptoms of less than 4 weeks in duration. Weight loss and malnutrition are features of chronic nausea/vomiting, that is, when symptoms have been present for 4 weeks or longer.
2. Where possible, identify the underlying cause (see Table 35.1) and institute appropriate treatment. Here it is important to be aware that metabolic or endocrine conditions such as hypercalcaemia, hyponatraemia and hyperthyroidism can result in vomiting.
3. Implement therapeutic strategies to suppress or eliminate symptoms which are dependent on the severity and clinical context. Ideally, antiemetic drugs are prescribed only when the cause of the nausea and/or vomiting is known, because by suppressing symptoms, they may otherwise delay diagnosis. This is especially true in children. However, they may sometimes be necessary temporarily in situations when directly addressing the underlying cause will not bring symptom relief sufficiently rapidly.

Some scenarios illustrating common therapeutic problems in the management of nausea and vomiting are outlined in Table 35.2.

Antiemetic drugs

Several classes of antiemetic drugs are available that antagonise the neurotransmitter receptors involved in the pathophysiology of nausea and vomiting. These classes of drugs are generally distinguished from each other by the identity of their main target receptor, although some act at more than one receptor.

Antihistamines

Antihistamine medicines include cinnarizine, cyclizine, diphenhydramine and promethazine. They have some efficacy in nausea and vomiting caused by a wide range of conditions, including

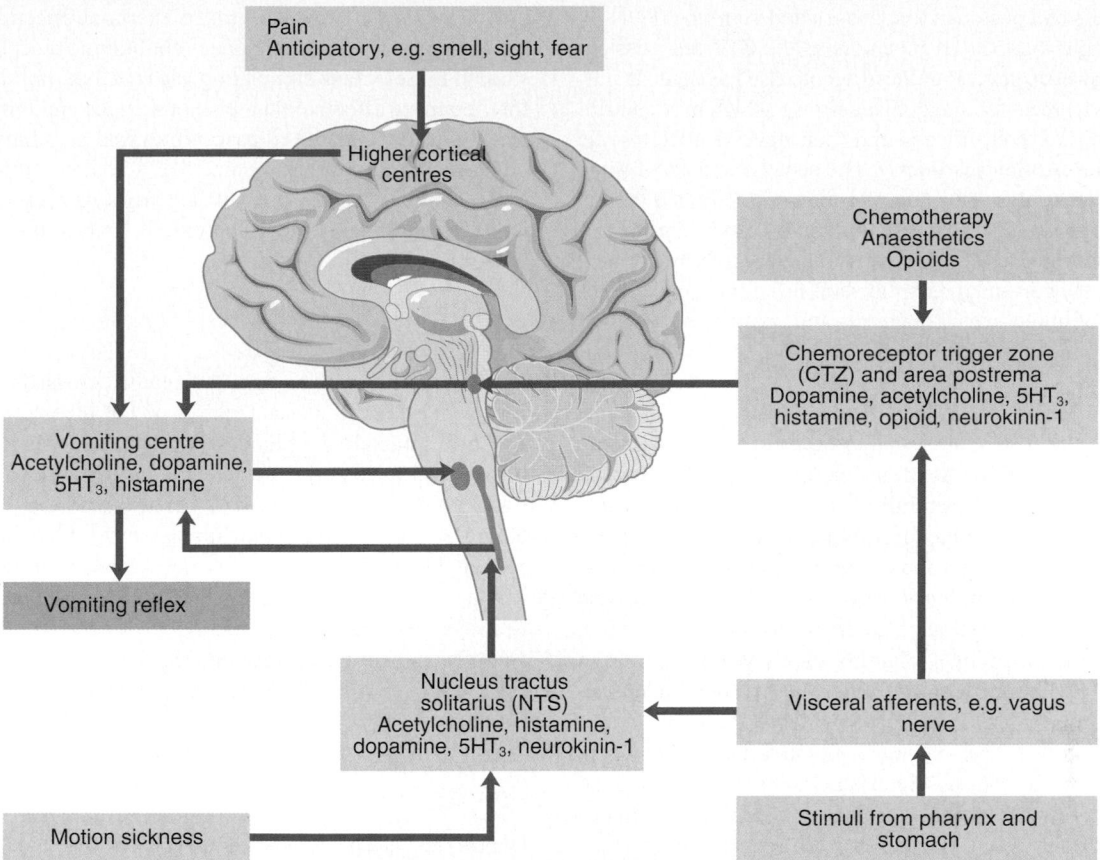

Fig. 35.1 Schematic representation of pathways involved in nausea and vomiting.

Table 35.2 Common therapeutic problems in managing patients with nausea and vomiting

Problem	Possible cause/solution
Persistent nausea and vomiting despite treatment	Is the cause correctly diagnosed? Review the antiemetic agent and the dose: if both correct, change to or add a second agent.
Patient with PONV is vomiting despite suitable antiemetic regimen	Check analgesia: pain may be causing nausea and vomiting, or patient-controlled analgesia may require adjustment downward to reduce analgesic dose.
Patient with bowel obstruction is passing flatus	Prokinetic drug is first-choice antiemetic. $5HT_3$ antagonists may also be effective.
Patient with bowel obstruction is not passing flatus	Spasmolytic drug is first choice. Prokinetic drugs are contraindicated. Similarly, bulk-forming, osmotic and stimulant laxatives are inappropriate; phosphate enemas and faecal softeners are better.
A terminally ill patient receiving diamorphine is vomiting, despite use of haloperidol	Levomepromazine given as a 24-h subcutaneous infusion can be very effective.
A patient with renal failure (uraemia) is vomiting	Consider a $5HT_3$ antagonist.
A patient develops an acute dystonic reaction to metoclopramide	Give an intramuscular injection of an antimuscarinic (e.g. procyclidine). Such extrapyramidal reactions to metoclopramide are more common in young adults (especially females), and this agent is best avoided in this group.

PONV, Postoperative nausea and vomiting.

motion sickness and postoperative nausea and vomiting (PONV). They are thought to block H_1 receptors in the CTZ and possibly elsewhere. However, several of these agents also have potent anticholinergic (M_1) receptor antagonist activity, which may contribute significantly to their efficacy and their adverse effect profile (see the section 'Antimuscarinics'). The sedative effects of some antihistamines may also contribute to antiemetic activity, although this property appears not to be essential, and it can be a particular problem when skilled tasks, such as driving, need to be performed. Nevertheless, the non-sedating antihistamines, for example, fexofenadine, are of limited value in nausea and vomiting.

Antimuscarinics

This is one of the oldest classes of antiemetics, of which many members are potent inhibitors of muscarinic receptor (M_1) activity, both peripherally and centrally. Antimuscarinic drugs such as atropine, hyoscine and glycopyrronium have been used preoperatively to inhibit salivation and excessive respiratory secretions during anaesthesia. Antimuscarinics act by inhibiting cholinergic transmission from the vestibular nuclei to higher centres within the cerebral cortex, thereby explaining their predominant use in the treatment of motion sickness. Hyoscine hydrobromide (scopolamine hydrobromide) is the most widely used agent, and it can be given orally, by subcutaneous or intramuscular injection, or transdermally for motion sickness. Inhibition of peripheral muscarinic receptors can cause drowsiness, dry mouth, dilated pupils and blurred vision, decreased sweating, gastro-intestinal motility and gastro-intestinal secretions and difficulty with micturition. Antimuscarinics agents may also precipitate closed-angle glaucoma in susceptible individuals.

Antidopaminergics

Phenothiazines and butyrophenones

Phenothiazines (e.g. prochlorperazine, perphenazine and trifluoperazine) and butyrophenones (e.g. haloperidol and droperidol) act as antagonists at dopamine (D2) receptors in the CTZ but may also have cholinergic receptor, muscarinic M_1 and histaminergic (H_1) receptor antagonist activity. As a consequence, they share several adverse effects with antihistamines and antimuscarinics, including drowsiness. In addition, the dopamine-blocking effects may be associated with acute dystonia (especially in children) and tardive dyskinesias or parkinsonism when used for prolonged periods. Prochlorperazine is less sedating and available as a buccal tablet and suppository for use when vomiting precludes oral administration. Phenothiazines are sometimes used for drug-associated emesis, including chemotherapy-induced nausea and vomiting (CINV), but like the butyrophenones, they have in many situations been superseded by more specific agents such as metoclopramide and the selective $5HT_3$ antagonists. Levomepromazine is sometimes used to relieve nausea and vomiting in terminal care.

Metoclopramide

At lower doses, metoclopramide acts as a selective D2 antagonist at the CTZ, and its effects mirror those of the phenothiazines and butyrophenones. However, it also exerts peripheral D2 antagonism at these doses and stimulates cholinergic receptors in gastric smooth muscle, thus stimulating gastric emptying. It may, therefore, be more effective than phenothiazines and butyrophenones when nausea is related to gastro-intestinal or biliary disease. At higher doses, it may exert some $5HT_3$-receptor antagonism, but at these doses, the incidence of acute dystonic reactions, particularly in young women and the elderly, may limit its usefulness in CINV.

Domperidone

Although domperidone does not readily cross the blood–brain barrier, it is a selective antagonist of D2 receptors at the CTZ, which lies outside the blood–brain barrier in the area postrema. It may also have peripheral effects that result in increased gastro-intestinal motility and faster gastric emptying. It is used in drug-associated vomiting, including CINV, and is relatively non-sedating. It can be given orally or by suppository. Acute dystonic reactions occur less frequently than with metoclopramide. It prevents nausea and vomiting during treatment with apomorphine and other dopamine agonists in Parkinson's disease and is also used to treat vomiting associated with emergency hormonal contraception.

Olanzapine

Olanzapine is an atypical antipsychotic that antagonises multiple neuroreceptors, including dopaminergic (D2), serotonergic ($5HT_3$), histaminergic (H_1), muscarinic and adrenergic receptors. Clinical studies suggest that olanzapine is effective in the prevention of CINV when used in combination with other antiemetics (Navari, 2014; Navari et al., 2011). The exact mechanism of olanzapine acting as an antiemetic is unclear, but its effects on the neuronal pathways involved in nausea and vomiting may partially explain its property. However, adverse effects such as akathisia and drowsiness may limit its use, and it is not licensed in Europe for this indication.

Selective $5HT_3$-receptor antagonists

Serotonin (5-hydroxytryptamine [5HT]) plays an important role in nausea and vomiting. The subtype $5HT_3$-receptors, which mediate the vomiting pathway, are located peripherally on vagal nerve endings in the gastro-intestinal tract and centrally in the brain, with high concentrations found in the area postrema and nucleus tractus solitarius. Highly emetogenic agents such as cisplatin are thought to disrupt gastric mucosa and initiate the release of 5HT from enterochromaffin cells, which stimulate the $5HT_3$-receptors on afferent vagal nerve endings and thus trigger the emetic reflex. Selective $5HT_3$-receptor antagonists that act centrally and peripherally are now commonly used to treat or prevent CINV (with drugs of moderate to high emetogenic potential) and PONV. They are also effective in radiotherapy-induced nausea and vomiting. Selective $5HT_3$ antagonists are generally well tolerated, with the most common adverse effects being constipation, headache, dizziness and sensation of warmth or flushing. Some available agents include granisetron, ondansetron and palonosetron. They are all more expensive than antihistamines, phenothiazines, antimuscarinics or dopamine antagonists.

Neurokinin-1 receptor antagonists

Substance P is a bioactive peptide that shares a common amino acid sequence with other bioactive peptides known as tachykinins. It appears to play an important role as a neurotransmitter in emesis, as well as in pain and a number of other inflammatory processes. Substance P binds to the subtype neurokinin-1 (NK_1) receptors, which are found in the area postrema and nucleus tractus solitarius. Selective NK_1 receptor antagonists, aprepitant and fosaprepitant (a prodrug of aprepitant), are now available for use as an adjunct to dexamethasone and a $5HT_3$ antagonist in preventing nausea and vomiting associated with moderately and highly emetogenic chemotherapy. A newer NK_1 receptor antagonist netupitant is now available as a fixed-dose combination with palonosetron (a $5HT_3$ antagonist) known as NEPA for the prevention of acute and delayed nausea and vomiting associated with moderately emetogenic chemotherapy and highly emetogenic cisplatin-based chemotherapy. They appear to be well tolerated, but NK_1 receptor antagonists are inhibitors, and sometimes inducers, of cytochrome P450 (CYP3A4) and inducers of CYP2C9 and glucuronidation. Therefore, potential drug interactions with chemotherapeutic agents and other concomitantly administered agents, for example, warfarin, may occur.

Cannabinoids

It is likely that the antiemetic activity of cannabinoids is related to stimulation of central and peripheral cannabinoid (CB1) receptors. Cannabinoids have modest antiemetic activity that is of similar magnitude to prochlorperazine in CINV, but they can cause a range of adverse CNS effects, including drowsiness and sometimes behavioural disturbances, which may at times be severe and which can persist for up to 72 hours after discontinuation. Thus, although the synthetic cannabinoid nabilone is indicated for nausea and vomiting caused by cytotoxic chemotherapy unresponsive to conventional antiemetics, it is recommended that patients are made aware of possible changes in their mood and other unwanted effects on their behaviour. In addition, nabilone should be used under close supervision, preferably in a hospital setting. A systematic review suggests that cannabinoids may have a role in refractory CINV (Smith et al., 2015).

Corticosteroids

Corticosteroids are known to have antiemetic effects. Their mechanism of action is unclear, but corticosteroid receptors are thought to exist in the area postrema. As single agents, they appear to be at least as effective as prochlorperazine in preventing nausea and vomiting associated with mild to moderately emetogenic cytotoxic chemotherapy. Dexamethasone, the most widely used corticosteroid in this context, improves the antiemetic activity of prochlorperazine and metoclopramide and may reduce some of the side effects associated with the latter. When combined with $5HT_3$ antagonists, corticosteroids are particularly effective in CINV associated with moderately emetogenic

chemotherapy or when used in delayed emesis. The same combination of dexamethasone and a $5HT_3$ antagonist, and sometimes with aprepitant, may also be effective in CINV associated with highly emetogenic chemotherapy regimens.

Complementary and alternative medicines

Systematic reviews support the use of stimulating wrist acupuncture point PC6 for preventing PONV as an alternative to conventional antiemetics (Lee et al., 2015), but the evidence for its use in combination with antiemetics for prevention of PONV is inconclusive. A systematic review of randomised trials has also demonstrated the efficacy of ginger (at least 1 g preoperatively) in PONV after certain types of surgery (Chaiyakunapruk et al., 2006). Ginger has also been claimed to be beneficial in motion sickness and pregnancy-associated nausea, but the evidence for each is limited (Ernst and Pittler, 2000).

Drug treatment in selected circumstances

Postoperative nausea and vomiting

PONV are common symptoms, with an incidence of 30% for vomiting and 50% for nausea. In high-risk groups the incidence can be as high as 80% (Gan et al., 2014). The aetiology is complex and multifactorial and includes patient-, medical-, surgical- and anaesthetic-related factors. Management is multimodal and involves strategies to reduce baseline risk, such as using less emetogenic induction agents, avoidance of volatile anaesthetic agents and use of opioids and consideration of the use of regional rather than general anaesthesia and adequate hydration.

Not all patients will experience PONV, but some are at higher risk. A simple scoring system is commonly used to risk stratify those who are likely to develop PONV so that prophylactic antiemetics can be given. The scoring system is based on the presence or absence of four factors:

- female gender,
- history of motion sickness or PONV,
- non-smoker,
- use of postoperative opioids.

The incidence of PONV with the presence of none, one, two, three or all four of these risk factors has been shown to be 10%, 20%, 40%, 60% and 80%, respectively (Apfel et al., 1999). Use of risk scores based on these criteria helps appropriately tailor antiemetic use and can significantly reduce the incidence of nausea and vomiting in clinical practice (Kovac, 2013).

Most antiemetic agents have some efficacy in PONV, but combination therapy with drugs from different classes may be needed in patients at medium to high risk of PONV (Gan et al., 2014). Prophylactic treatment with dexamethasone and/or $5HT_3$ antagonists (e.g. ondansetron, granisetron) are commonly used, as well as butyrophenones (e.g. haloperidol, droperidol) and antihistamines (e.g. cyclizine). NK_1 receptor antagonists (e.g. aprepitant) are also effective in the treatment and prophylaxis of PONV, but the cost may prohibit their routine use. The stimulation of acupuncture point PC6 appears to be safe but is rarely used, despite

Table 35.3 Classification of chemotherapy-induced nausea and vomiting

Classification	Definition
Acute	Occurring within the first 24 h after initiation of chemotherapy; generally peaks after 5–6 h
Delayed	Occurring from 24 h to several days (days 2–5) after chemotherapy
Breakthrough	Occurring despite appropriate prophylactic treatment
Anticipatory	Occurring before a treatment as a conditioned response to the occurrence of chemotherapy-induced nausea and vomiting in previous cycles
Refractory	Recurring in subsequent cycles of therapy, excluding anticipatory chemotherapy-induced nausea and vomiting

Reproduced by kind permission from Navari and Aapro (2016).

Table 35.4 Relative emetogenicity of chemotherapy drugs

Emetic risk (incidence of emesis without antiemetics)	Agent
High (>90%)	Cisplatin Mechlorethamine Streptozotocin Cyclophosphamide ≥1500 mg/m^2 Carmustine Dacarbazine Dactinomycin
Moderate (30–90%)	Oxaliplatin Cytarabine >1000 mg/m^2 Carboplatin Ifosfamide Cyclophosphamide <1500 mg/m^2 Doxorubicin Daunorubicin Epirubicin Idarubicin Irinotecan
Low (10–30%)	Paclitaxel Docetaxel Mitoxantrone Topotecan Etoposide Pemetrexed Methotrexate Mitomycin Gemcitabine Cytarabine ≤1000 mg/m^2 Fluorouracil Bortezomib Cetuximab Trastuzumab
Minimal (<10%)	Bevacizumab Bleomycin Busulfan 2-Chlorodeoxyadenosine Fludarabine Rituximab Vinblastine Vincristine Vinorelbine

From Kris et al. (2006).

some supporting evidence for its efficacy (Lee et al., 2015). Metoclopramide and cannabinoids appear to be of limited value in the management of PONV.

If PONV occurs despite prophylaxis therapy, then a further rescue antiemetic should be given, preferably from an alternative class to those given as prophylaxis.

Premedication with opioids increases the incidence of PONV, and this may be reduced by concurrent administration of either atropine or hyoscine, which are primarily used as anti-secretory drugs at premedication.

Chemotherapy-induced nausea and vomiting

There are different types of CINV identified depending on their onset and the possible underlying aetiology (see Table 35.3) Acute CINV is often associated with an increase in plasma serotonin concentrations for the most emetogenic agents, whereas delayed and anticipatory vomiting seem to be mediated by serotonin-independent pathways.

Management of CINV depends on the emetogenicity of the chemotherapy regimen and the use of combinations of antiemetic drugs based on their varying target receptors. Chemotherapy agents are divided into four emetogenic levels (Table 35.4) defined by the expected frequency of emesis (Kris et al., 2006).

5HT$_3$ and NK$_1$ receptor antagonists given as a combination with (or without) dexamethasone are the mainstay treatment for acute and delayed CINV in highly and moderate emetogenic chemotherapy regimens (Roila et al., 2016). Newer-generation 5HT$_3$ receptor antagonists, such as palonosetron, appear to be more effective than older 5HT$_3$ receptors, such as ondansetron and granisetron; this could be partly explained by their prolonged half-life and high affinity for 5HT$_3$ receptors (Rojas et al., 2008).

Evidence also points to synergism between 5HT$_3$ inhibition (e.g. by palonosetron) and NK$_1$ receptor inhibition (e.g. by netupitant) (Thomas et al., 2014), hence their therapeutic use in combination. A combined preparation such as netupitant and palonosetron (NEPA) is available for use.

Studies have also shown the use of olanzapine is effective in prevention of CINV when added to NK$_1$ receptor antagonists (Chiu et al., 2016).

In lower-level acute emesis, metoclopramide or prochlorperazine are commonly used and are often sufficiently effective. Dexamethasone can also be prescribed as a single agent for this indication, but its use in these circumstances appears to be uncommon in the UK.

Box 35.1 Factors that cause nausea and vomiting in their own right and may contribute to the failure of apparently appropriate prophylactic regimens for chemotherapy-induced nausea and vomiting

- Hypercalcaemia or other metabolic or endocrine disturbance
- Central nervous system metastases
- Antibiotics such as erythromycin/clarithromycin
- Gastro-intestinal obstruction
- Radiotherapy enteropathy

Dexamethasone is the most extensively evaluated steroid in the management of CINV. Used alone, it is not sufficiently effective for prevention of CINV in moderately or highly emetogenic chemotherapy. However, it enhances the effect of other agents such as $5HT_3$ and NK_1 antagonists in high-risk situations and, together with metoclopramide, it also appears to be useful in treating delayed emesis (Ioannidis et al., 2000).

The best management for anticipatory emesis is the avoidance of acute and delayed emesis during previous cycles. However, when anticipatory nausea and vomiting are a problem, a low dose of a benzodiazepine such as lorazepam is often effective.

When apparently appropriate antiemesis regimens fail, consideration should be given to the possibility of other underlying disease-related and medication-related issues (Box 35.1). Patients often derive benefit from antiemetics given as prophylaxis, and a further course at the same or a higher dose can be given. An alternative class of drug with a different pharmacological action (e.g. olanzapine or a cannabinoid) should also be considered if symptoms are not controlled.

Pregnancy-associated nausea and vomiting

Pregnancy-associated nausea and/or vomiting is defined as nausea and/or vomiting during early pregnancy where there are no other causes. It can affect up to 80% of pregnancies and typically starts around 4th to 7th week of gestation and peaks at around 9 weeks. Some women may continue to have nausea and or/vomiting into the second trimester, but in the majority of cases, symptoms are usually resolved by the 20th week of gestation (Shehmar et al., 2016). Risk factors for vomiting include a personal history of previous pregnancy-associated nausea/vomiting or motion sickness or migraine-associated nausea/vomiting and a family history of hyperemesis gravidarum or a large placental mass, for example, due to multiple pregnancy. First-trimester nausea and vomiting are not usually harmful to either the fetus or the mother and are not generally associated with a poor pregnancy outcome.

In contrast, hyperemesis gravidarum is a condition of intractable vomiting complicating between 0.3% and 3.6% of pregnancies (Shehmar et al., 2016). This is a serious condition characterised by dehydration, electrolyte imbalance and nutritional deficits with a body weight loss of more than 5% of pre-pregnancy weight. Patients will require hospital admission to correct the biochemical abnormalities.

In first-trimester nausea and vomiting, simple measures such as small, frequent, carbohydrate-rich meals and reassurance are sufficient to control symptoms. Ginger and PC6 acupressure have also been advocated, although the evidence base is equivocal in early pregnancy (Jewell and Young, 2003). Other studies on the use of acupuncture in pregnancy-associated nausea and vomiting remain unclear (King and Murphy, 2009). A recent Cochrane review was unable to recommend any intervention for nausea and vomiting in early pregnancy due to lack of robust evidence (Matthews et al., 2015). It is important to avoid antiemetic drugs when possible, and the measures outlined previously (carbohydrate-rich meal and reassurance) should be considered as first-line treatment.

Prescribing an antiemetic in the first trimester of pregnancy should only be done when the benefit outweighs the risks. Antihistamines (e.g. promethazine or cyclizine) or prochlorperazine should be given as first-line therapy and for a limited time period. If symptoms persist, then a limited course (no longer than 5 days) of metoclopramide or ondansetron could be considered.

In the serious condition of hyperemesis gravidarum, drug therapy may be used in addition to fluid and vitamin replacements (e.g. thiamine). In extreme cases, postpyloric feeding or enteral feeding is required. Corticosteroids have been found to be effective when all other treatment options have failed. There are few safety or efficacy data on which to select the most appropriate treatments, so the agents recommended for vomiting in pregnancy mentioned previously are generally those used in the UK.

Pyridoxine is no longer recommended for use in pregnancy-associated nausea and/or vomiting.

Migraine

Migraine is a paroxysmal disorder with attacks of headaches, nausea, vomiting, photophobia and malaise. Treatment is directed at:
- prophylaxis: trigger avoidance; β-blockers, pizotifen and, in severe cases, a 5HT1B/D-receptor agonist such as sumatriptan;
- analgesia, including aspirin, paracetamol, opioids and NSAIDs;
- antiemetics.

Nausea and vomiting in migraine are associated with headache intensity, and the concomitant gastric stasis aggravates the nausea and vomiting and may also delay absorption of oral analgesics. Metoclopramide and domperidone attenuate the autonomic dysfunction and promote gastric emptying, but the risk of acute dystonic crisis, especially with metoclopramide therapy, should be borne in mind, especially in young women and children but also in the elderly.

Labyrinthitis

Labyrinthine dysfunction results in vertigo, nausea and vomiting. Episodes may last a few hours or days. Causes include labyrinth viral infections, tumours and Ménière's disease. The onset of episodes is often unpredictable and disabling. Betahistine sometimes has some benefit. The antimuscarinics, antihistamines, phenothiazines or benzodiazepines can be used to suppress the vestibular system. Usually, hyoscine is sufficient, but if there is severe vomiting, prochlorperazine or metoclopramide may be of value.

Motion sickness

Motion sickness is a syndrome, a collection of symptoms without an identifiable cause. It is brought on by chronic repetitive movements which stimulate afferent pathways to the vestibular nuclei and lead to activation of the brainstem nuclei. Histaminergic and muscarinic pathways are involved. The symptoms include vague epigastric discomfort, headache, cold sweating and nausea which may culminate in vomiting. This is often followed by marked fatigue which can last hours or days. The onset of symptoms may be abrupt or gradual.

The antimuscarinics agent hyoscine is the prophylactic drug of choice, although there is no evidence of its benefit once motion sickness is established (Spinks and Wasiak, 2011). Antihistamine drugs may also be effective. The less sedating antihistamines cinnarizine or cyclizine are used. Promethazine, an antihistamine with sedative effects, is also effective, but phenothiazines, domperidone, metoclopramide and 5HT₃-receptor antagonists appear to be ineffective in this situation. Treatment should be started before travel; for long journeys, promethazine or transdermal hyoscine may be preferred for their longer duration (24 hours and 3 days, respectively). Otherwise, repeated doses will be needed.

The most important adverse effect of many drugs used is sedation, whilst for antimuscarinic drugs, it is blurred vision, urinary retention and constipation. In laboratory studies, the degree to which these effects impair performance, for example, driving a car, is highly variable, but subjects who take anti-motion sickness drugs should normally be deemed unfit for such tasks. These drugs also potentiate the effects of alcohol.

Many non-drug treatments have been advocated for the alleviation of motion sickness, including wristbands, which act on acupuncture points, variously positioned pieces of coloured paper or card, as well as plant extracts such as ginger. The evidence base for these interventions remains very limited.

Drug-associated nausea and vomiting

As well as chemotherapeutic agents, many commonly used medications for other disorders can cause nausea and vomiting (Quigley et al., 2001). Opioids are perhaps the most important group clinically, but dopamine agonists (used in Parkinson's disease), theophylline, digoxin and macrolide antibiotics such as erythromycin can all cause nausea and/or vomiting, often in a dose-related manner (type A toxicity). High-dose oestrogen, used in postcoital contraception, can produce these symptoms. Consideration should be given to altering the dose of the offending agent when possible and to administering the medication with food. With some agents, tolerance may develop. Thus, tolerance to the emetic effects of opioids often develops within 5–10 days, and therefore, antiemetic therapy is not generally needed for long-term opioid use.

Palliative care–associated nausea and vomiting

Nausea and vomiting are common and distressing symptoms in cancer patients. In most cases, the causes of nausea and vomiting are multifactorial, including concurrent infection, drugs and metabolic disturbances such as renal failure.

It is important to determine the predominant underlying cause for patients' symptoms by obtaining a careful history, conducting an examination and requesting appropriate investigations so that potentially reversible causes of nausea and vomiting can be treated (Box 35.2) and the most suitable antiemetic prescribed.

Oral antiemetic therapy is effective for treatment of nausea in patients with advanced cancer, but the subcutaneous route is preferred for those with severe persistent vomiting, either as a single-dose injection or a continuous infusion via a syringe driver. When patients' symptoms improve, switching from subcutaneous injection to the oral route may be preferable. Non-pharmacological interventions such as avoidance of certain food smells or unpleasant odours, relaxation techniques and use of acupuncture should be considered.

CINV is described in detail elsewhere in the chapter. Strong opioids such as morphine, diamorphine, oxycodone and fentanyl cause nausea and/or vomiting in up to one-third of patients after initiation of treatment, but the incidence is lower for weaker opioids such as codeine. Metoclopramide, cyclizine or haloperidol are often given for the relief of the nausea and vomiting induced by opioids.

Gastroduodenal or intestinal obstructions in advanced malignancy are usually caused by occlusion of the lumen (intrinsically and/or extrinsically) or by the absence of normal peristaltic propulsion. Surgery remains the definitive treatment for luminal occlusion due to cancer, but this is often inappropriate for patients who are frail or have advanced malignancy. The main aim of pharmacological interventions is symptom control. A prokinetic dopamine (D2) antagonist such as metoclopramide or domperidone should be used for patients with nausea and vomiting associated with functional gastric or intestinal stasis. Prokinetics are also used in patients with partial gastric outlet obstruction but can worsen patients' symptoms of abdominal pain in complete gastric outlet obstruction. Because prokinetics can exacerbate abdominal colicky pain associated with intestinal obstruction, their use should be avoided in that situation, and antiemetics such as cyclizine or haloperidol should be used for symptom control.

Dexamethasone has also been used for control of symptoms in malignant intestinal obstruction, not only for antiemetic effect but also to reduce inflammatory tumour oedema around the obstructive lesion. Antimuscarinics such as hyoscine butylbromide and somatostatin analogues such as octreotide have been used for symptom relief in intestinal obstruction by reducing gastro-intestinal secretion and motility and thus reducing the

---

Box 35.2 Potentially treatable causes of nausea and vomiting in palliative care

- Hypercalcaemia
- Constipation
- Renal failure
- Raised intracranial pressure
- Infection
- Bowel obstruction
- Peptic ulcer disease
- Drugs
- Anxiety

frequency and volume of vomitus. Olanzapine may also have a role in refractory nausea and vomiting caused by underlying malignancy, although this is an unlicensed (off-label) indication (Fonte et al., 2015).

Biochemical disturbances such as hypercalcaemia and renal failure can cause nausea and vomiting in patients with advanced malignancy, and correction of these may alleviate symptoms. However, aggressive treatment with bisphosphonates or insertion of nephrostomy tubes, respectively, would not often be appropriate for those who are in the terminal stages of their illness. Haloperidol and cyclizine appear to be effective for biochemical causes of nausea and vomiting. Levomepromazine has antidopaminergic, antihistaminergic, antimuscarinic and antiserotonergic activity. It is effective for most causes of nausea and vomiting and may help alleviate restlessness. It can also be given intramuscularly, intravenously or subcutaneously, including by continuous subcutaneous infusion. It may be considered if first-line antiemetics are insufficiently effective. Unfortunately, sedation and postural hypotension can be a problem in association with this agent.

Conclusion

Nausea and vomiting are symptoms caused by a variety of underlying causes. Thorough clinical assessment and appropriate investigations should be undertaken when prescribing a therapeutic trial of an antiemetic. The choice of agent(s) should be based on the likely cause and severity of the symptoms, the possible underlying pathophysiology, and the recommendations of evidence-based guidelines which take into account clinical effectiveness and cost-effectiveness.

Case studies

Case 35.1

Mr AN, a 30-year-old man, presents seeking a remedy for vomiting which had an acute onset, 12 hours previously.

Question

What questions should Mr AN be asked to determine the nature, cause and seriousness of these symptoms?

Answer

The cause of vomiting needs to be determined where possible to allow appropriate treatment to be initiated. The following questions should be asked:

- Are there symptoms or signs of infection, such as diarrhoea, sore throat, dysuria, photophobia, fever? Infection, often of the gastro-intestinal tract, is one of the commonest causes of vomiting.
- Is there headache? Raised intracranial pressure and meningitis can present with vomiting as an early symptom, usually without any nausea.

- Is there abdominal pain? Abdominal pain before vomiting usually means an organic gastro-intestinal cause. Pain after vomiting may be due to muscle tenderness.
- Has the patient started any new drugs (opioids, chemotherapeutic agents, digoxin, nicotine, NSAIDs, oral hypoglycaemics and some antibiotics are common causes) or drunk excess alcohol?
- Is there vertigo? If present, this is suggestive of a labyrinthine cause.

Case 35.2

Ms VW, a 19-year-old woman who is 12 weeks pregnant, presents to hospital with intractable nausea and vomiting which has not responded to home therapy and which has resulted in hypotension and dehydration.

Question

List, in order of importance, the therapeutic strategies for this problem.

Answer

Treatment would normally involve:
- intravenous rehydration and electrolyte replacement, vitamin replacement (e.g. thiamine),
- bed rest,
- antiemetics (e.g. cyclizine, promethazine or prochlorperazine) and review response after 24 hours,
- postpyloric feeding,
- corticosteroids,
- parenteral nutrition.

Case 35.3

Mrs MC, a 45-year-old woman, presents with ovarian carcinoma for which she is due to receive a course of cancer chemotherapy.

Question

What drugs might be appropriate, when should they be given, and what advice should be given to Mrs MC regarding monitoring of symptoms after treatment with the chemotherapy?

Answer

Mrs MC is likely to receive repeated cycles of emetogenic chemotherapy with carboplatin (moderate emetogenic risk) or cisplatin (high emetogenic risk) and, therefore, should be given prophylactic antiemetics before the start of chemotherapy. The choice of drugs includes 5HT3-receptor antagonists (ondansetron, granisetron or palonosetron) combined with dexamethasone for some moderate-emetic-risk situations and one of the 5HT3-receptor antagonists with an NK1-receptor antagonist (aprepitant or fosaprepitant) for high-risk situations, with or without dexamethasone to provide additional benefit. The monitoring of emesis and nausea both within and outside hospital for up to 5 days after treatment is useful in deciding which patients may need other therapies. It is also important to remember that patients should be given appropriate doses of antiemetics as rescue therapy to cover delayed-onset nausea.

Case 35.4

A hospital with a large number of surgical specialties, including major in-patient thoraco-abdominal and day-care procedures, wishes to update its PONV programme.

Question

What principles should be taken into account for a PONV programme?

Answer

The programme should contain a PONV risk score which can be used in preoperation assessment. A simplified score has been devised (Apfel et al., 1999), adding one point for each of the following: female gender, non-smoking status, history of PONV and opioid use. In low-risk individuals scoring 0 or 1 (less than 10% risk), prophylactic anti-emetic therapy is unnecessary. Moderate-risk subjects (score 1, risk 20%) may require single-agent antiemetic prophylaxis, whereas in high-risk subjects (score 3, risk 60%) two agents (one of them often dexamethasone) may be needed if intravenous anaesthesia is not possible. In very high-risk subjects (score 4, risk greater than 80%), intravenous anaesthesia should be considered when possible, and dexamethasone and another antiemetic agent should be administered. PONV rescue therapy should be chosen depending on the postoperative clinical situation.

References

American Gastroenterological Association, 2001. AGA medical position statement: nausea and vomiting. Gastroenterology 120, 261–262.

Apfel, C.C., Laara, E., Koivuranta, M., et al., 1999. A simplified risk score for predicting postoperative nausea and vomiting. Anesthesiology 91, 693–700.

Chaiyakunapruk, N., Kitikannakorn, N., Nathisuwan, S., et al., 2006. The efficacy of ginger for the prevention of postoperative nausea and vomiting: a meta-analysis. Available at: https://www.ncbi.nlm.nih.gov/pubmedhealth/PMH0023320/.

Chiu, L., Chow, R., Popovic, M., et al., 2016. Efficacy of olanzapine for the prophylaxis and rescue of chemotherapy induced nausea and vomiting (CINV). Support. Care Cancer 24, 2381–2392.

Ernst, E., Pittler, M.H., 2000. Efficacy of ginger for nausea and vomiting: a systematic review of randomized clinical trials. Br. J. Anaesth. 84, 367–371.

Fonte, C., Fatigoni, S., Roila, F., 2015. A review of olanzapine as an antiemetic in chemotherapy-induced nausea and vomiting and in palliative care patients. Crit. Rev. Oncol. Hematol. 95, 214–221.

Gan, T.J., Diemunsch, P., Ashraf, S.H., et al., 2014. Consensus guidelines for management of postoperative nausea and vomiting. Anesth. Analg. 118, 85–113.

Ioannidis, J.P., Hesketh, P.J., Lau, J., 2000. Contribution of dexamethasone to control of chemotherapy-induced nausea and vomiting: a meta-analysis of randomized evidence. J. Clin. Oncol. 18, 3409–3422.

Jewell, D., Young, G., 2003. Interventions for nausea and vomiting in early pregnancy. Cochrane Database Syst. Rev. 2010 (9), Art. No. CD000145. https://doi:10.1002/14651858.CD000145.pub2.

King, T.L., Murphy, P., 2009. Evidence-based approaches to managing nausea and vomiting in early pregnancy. J. Midwifery Womens Health 54, 430–444.

Kovac, A., 2013. Update on the management of postoperative nausea and vomiting. Drugs 73, 1525–1547.

Kris, M.G., Hesketh, P.J., Somerfield, M.R., et al., 2006. American Society of Clinical Oncology guideline for antiemetics in oncology: update. J. Clin. Oncol. 24, 2932–2947.

Lee, A., Chan, S.K., Fan, L.T., 2015. Stimulation of the wrist acupuncture point PC6 for preventing postoperative nausea and vomiting. Cochrane Database Syst. Rev. 2015 (11), Art. No. CD003281. https://doi:10.1002/14651858.CD003281.pub4.

Matthews, A., Haas, D.M., O'Mathúna, D.P., et al., 2015. Interventions for nausea and vomiting in early pregnancy. Cochrane Database Syst. Rev. 2015 (9), Art. No. CD007575. https://doi:10.1002/14651858.CD007575.pub4.

Navari, R.M., 2014. Olanzapine for the prevention and treatment of chronic nausea and chemotherapy-induced nausea and vomiting. Eur. J. Pharmacol. 722, 180–186.

Navari, R.M., Aapro, M., 2016. Antiemetic prophylaxis for chemotherapy-induced nausea and vomiting. N. Engl. J. Med. 374, 1356–1367.

Navari, R.M., Gray, S.E., Kerr, A.C., 2011. Olanzapine versus aprepitant for the prevention of chemotherapy-induced nausea and vomiting: a randomized phase III trial. J. Support. Oncol. 9, 188–195.

Quigley, E.M., Hasler, W.L., Parkman, H.P., 2001. A technical review on nausea and vomiting. Gastroenterology 120, 263–268.

Roila, F., Molassiotis, A., Herrstedt, J., et al., 2016. MASCC and ESMO guideline update for the prevention of chemotherapy- and radiotherapy-induced nausea and vomiting and of nausea and vomiting in advanced cancer patients. Ann. Oncol. 27 (Suppl. 5), v119–v133.

Rojas, C., Stathis, M., Thomas, A.G., et al., 2008. Palonosetron exhibits unique molecular interactions with the 5-HT3 receptor. Anesth. Analg. 107, 469–478.

Shehmar, M., MacLean, M.A., Nelson-Piercy, C., et al., 2016. The management of nausea and vomiting of pregnancy and hyperemesis gravidarum. Royal College of Obstetricians and Gynaecologists, London. Available at: https://www.rcog.org.uk/globalassets/documents/guidelines/green-top-guidelines/gtg69-hyperemesis.pdf.

Smith, L.A., Azariah, F., Lavender, V.T., et al., 2015. Cannabinoids for nausea and vomiting in adults with cancer receiving chemotherapy. Cochrane Database Syst. Rev. 2015 (11), Art. No. CD009464. https://doi:10.1002/14651858.CD009464.pub2.

Spinks, A.B., Wasiak, J., 2011. Scopolamine (hyoscine) for preventing and treating motion sickness. Cochrane Database Syst. Rev. 2011 (6), Art. No. CD002851. https://doi:10.1007/s00221-014-4017-7.

Thomas, A., Stathis, M., Rojas, C., et al., 2014. Netupitant and palonosetron trigger NK1 receptor internalization in NG108-15 cells. Exp. Brain Res. 232, 2637–2644.

Further reading

Carlisle, J., Stevenson, C.A., 2017. Drugs for preventing postoperative nausea and vomiting. Cochrane Database Syst. Rev. 2017 (7), Art. No. CD004125. https://doi:10.1002/14651858.CD004125.pub3.

Hatfield, A., 2014. Post-operative nausea and vomiting. In: Hatfield, A. (Ed.), The Complete Recovery Room, fifth ed. Oxford University Press, Oxford.

National Institute for Health and Excellence, 2016. Prevention of chemotherapy induced nausea and vomiting in adults: netupitant/palonosetron. Evidence Summary [ESNM69]. NICE, London. Available at: https://www.nice.org.uk/advice/esnm69/chapter/Key-points-from-the-evidence.

36 Respiratory Infections

Catherine Molyneux and Ali Robb

Key points

- Viral respiratory tract infections are usually mild and self-limiting, but influenza, severe acute respiratory syndrome (SARS) and Middle East respiratory syndrome (MERS) can have severe consequences for individuals, for public health and for economic activity.
- Exacerbations of chronic bronchitis are not always infective in origin; antibiotics are used when the sputum is purulent, but other therapeutic modalities are also valuable.
- *Streptococcus pneumoniae* remains the single most common cause of community-acquired pneumonia (CAP). Reduced susceptibility to penicillin can complicate the management of serious pneumococcal infections, but more significant degrees of resistance are currently not widespread among UK strains.
- CAP can be caused by a variety of pathogens, and this is reflected in the antimicrobial regimens recommended for initial treatment.
- There are many potential causes of hospital-acquired (nosocomial) pneumonia, and each unit with patients at risk will have its own resident bacterial flora. This will strongly influence the choice of antibiotics for empiric therapy.
- Patients with cystic fibrosis form a particularly high-risk population. Their respiratory tract flora becomes increasingly abnormal with age. Colonisation with *Staphylococcus aureus*, *Pseudomonas aeruginosa* and *Burkholderia cepacia* complex is associated with reductions in lung function.
- Antibiotic stewardship interventions, including close adherence to local guidelines, are important to maintain the effectiveness of antibiotic agents.

Respiratory tract infections are the most common group of infections seen in the UK and the commonest acute problem dealt with in primary care (National Institute for Health and Care Excellence [NICE], 2008a). Most are viral, for which (with some exceptions) only symptomatic therapy is available, and many are self-limiting. However, the term includes some serious bacterial infections for which prompt treatment is important.

The respiratory tract is divided into upper and lower parts: the upper respiratory tract consists of the sinuses, middle ear, pharynx, epiglottis and larynx, whereas the lower respiratory tract consists of the structures below the larynx, the bronchi, bronchioles and alveoli. Although there are anatomical and functional divisions both within and between these regions, infections do not always respect such boundaries. Nevertheless, it is clinically and bacteriologically convenient to retain a distinction between upper respiratory tract infections (URTIs) and lower respiratory tract infections (LRTIs).

Upper respiratory tract infections
Colds and flu

URTIs with coryzal symptoms, rhinitis, pharyngitis and laryngitis, associated with varying degrees of systemic upset, are extremely common; adults average 2–4 infections per year and children, 6–8, although up to 12 have been reported in some groups of children (NICE, 2015a).

These infections are usually caused by viruses. Rhinoviruses cause up to 50% of colds and up to 70% in the autumn. Various other viruses, including coronaviruses and the parainfluenza viruses, account for the rest.

Most viral URTIs are mild and self-limiting. However, new respiratory viruses continue to be identified, some of which produce more serious illness, for example, Middle East respiratory syndrome (MERS) coronavirus, first described in 2012, which can cause a spectrum of disease from asymptomatic infection to respiratory failure.

In general, the management of URTIs is symptomatic and consists of rest, adequate hydration, simple analgesics and antipyretics. Apart from one or two exceptional situations, antiviral drugs are not indicated and in most cases are not effective.

Antibacterial drugs have no activity against viral infections, although in the past they were widely prescribed, sometimes with spurious rationale, such as prophylaxis against bacterial superinfection, or simply because patients demanded them. In recent years, there has been heightened awareness of the adverse consequences of antibiotic overuse, the most serious of these being the promotion of antibiotic resistance.

Issuing antibiotic prescriptions for uncomplicated URTIs also reinforces the idea that these infections require medical intervention and is likely to lead to requests for an antibiotic in subsequent illnesses. This increased awareness of the harms of excessive antibiotic prescribing has led to national campaigns aimed at discouraging the public from seeking antibiotic treatment for viral infections, such as the National Health Service (NHS) antibiotic awareness campaign (Public Health England, 2015a).

Unfortunately, antibiotic prescription rates in the UK have plateaued after falling through the 1990s, and most people who request an antibiotic for an acute uncomplicated respiratory tract infection receive one (NICE, 2008a). Therefore, further work to educate and change the behaviour of both patients and prescribers is required.

Influenza

True influenza is caused by one of the influenza viruses (influenza A, B or, rarely, C). Influenza commonly causes a syndrome of fever (greater than 38 °C), myalgia, headache, sore throat and cough. It is usually self-limiting in healthy adults but can cause a severe pneumonitis and can be complicated by secondary bacterial infection. Serological studies in healthcare workers have suggested that 30–50% of infections in this group are asymptomatic, but this may vary with strain (Public Health England, 2015b).

Influenza tends to occur during the winter months, usually in an 8- to 10-week period; the timing, length and severity of this season can vary. The seasonality provides an opportunity to offer preventive vaccination in the autumn. In the UK the influenza vaccination strategy has changed in recent years. In 2012 the Joint Committee on Vaccination and Immunisation (JCVI) recommended extension of the programme to children aged between 2 and 17. A phased extension to the programme therefore began in 2013. The eligible cohorts are published each year. Children are vaccinated with a quadrivalent intranasal live attenuated vaccine; alternative authorised vaccines may be used for children in clinical risk groups for whom the intranasal vaccine is unsuitable (Public Health England, 2015b).

Vaccination with an inactivated quadrivalent vaccine is used in patients at higher risk of severe disease and healthcare workers. Patients at risk of severe influenza who are eligible for influenza vaccination in England are:

* people older than 65 years,
* people with chronic respiratory disease,
* people with chronic kidney disease,
* people with chronic liver disease,
* people who are immunosuppressed,
* people with chronic neurological disease,
* asplenic patients,
* pregnant women,
* people with a body mass index greater than 40.

Unfortunately, the virus mutates so rapidly that the circulating strains tend to change from season to season, necessitating annual revaccination against the prevailing virus (Public Health England, 2015b).

Influenza A and B infections are amenable to both prevention and treatment with neuraminidase inhibitors (NAIs) such as zanamivir and oseltamivir, although there is controversy about whether the benefits justify the cost. Zanamivir is administered by dry powder inhalation, whereas oseltamivir is given orally. There is an intravenous preparation of zanamivir which is unlicensed but available on a named patient basis. Oseltamivir is the first-line agent in most situations, but zanamivir is preferred where oseltamivir resistance is suspected or for severely immunocompromised patients when H1N1 is the predominant strain of influenza A in circulation (Public Health England, 2015c). H1N1 is a strain of influenza, where the *H* and *N* refer to antigens on the virus particle, the variants of which have been determined and identified by a number.

National guidelines for England recommend that NAIs can be used in secondary care for influenza at any time, but primary care doctors can only give NHS prescriptions for NAIs when the chief medical officer has confirmed that influenza is circulating and if the patient falls into a defined risk group (Public Health England, 2016a).

The group eligible for prophylaxis or treatment consists of those eligible for vaccination with inactivated vaccine as listed previously and women who are less than 2 weeks post-partum. The patient must be able to commence treatment within a defined time after the onset of symptoms or exposure to a patient with influenza.

Prophylaxis with NAIs is only offered to patients who are not protected by vaccination. This usually means those who have not been vaccinated, but in some years, the vaccine is poorly matched to the circulating strain and is therefore unlikely to be effective. In these years, vaccinated patients are eligible for prophylaxis (NICE, 2008b, 2009).

Whether oseltamivir treatment of people with symptoms of influenza can prevent the development of complications such as pneumonia is still a matter of vigorous debate, with two recent meta-analyses coming to different conclusions (Dobson et al., 2015; Jefferson et al., 2014).

The anti-Parkinsonian drug amantadine, which has activity against the influenza A virus, is not recommended for the treatment or prophylaxis of influenza because resistance emerges rapidly, and there is a high incidence of adverse effects.

Pandemics, or global epidemics, of influenza A occur around every 25 years and affect huge numbers of people. The 1918 'Spanish flu' pandemic is estimated to have killed 20 million people. Further pandemics took place in 1957–1958 (Asian flu), 1968–1970 (Hong Kong flu) and 1977 (Russian flu).

The World Health Organization (WHO) declared a worldwide influenza pandemic in June 2009 after the emergence of a novel H1N1 strain of swine lineage. In the UK, NICE guidance was superseded during the pandemic, and NAIs were given to all individuals with flu-like illness. A vaccine was also developed. Pandemic planning had been in operation for many years with plans for rapid vaccine development and stockpiling of antivirals. However, in retrospect, infections caused by the pandemic strain were generally associated with much milder disease than seen in previous pandemics, and some authorities have been accused of over-reaction.

There were also adverse outcomes of the widespread use of NAIs during the 2009 pandemic. Resistance to oseltamivir emerged in some units (Gulland, 2009). Some critics argued that the side effects of NAIs and uncertainty of benefit meant that the cure was worse than the disease (Strong et al., 2009). However, the relatively benign course of the 2009 pandemic should not provide false reassurance regarding the potential risks associated with future pandemics.

Avian influenza

An avian strain of influenza A, H5N1, emerged in South East Asia in 2003. It is now considered endemic in many parts of South East Asia and remains a concern for public health. A second avian strain, H7N9, was first detected in humans in 2013. To date, human cases have only been detected in China (WHO, 2014). Person-to-person spread of these strains remains limited, but they can cause severe disease, and there are concerns that they may mutate to become more easily transmissible between humans.

Sore throat (pharyngitis)

Causative organisms

Pharyngitis is a common condition. In most cases, it never comes to medical attention and is treated with simple therapy directed at symptom relief. Many cases are not due to infection at all but are caused by other factors, such as smoking. Where infection is the cause, most cases are viral and form part of the cold-and-flu spectrum. Epstein–Barr virus (EBV), which causes glandular fever (infectious mononucleosis), is a less common but important cause of sore throat because it may be confused with streptococcal infection.

The only common bacterial cause of sore throat is *Streptococcus pyogenes*, also known as the Lancefield group A β-haemolytic streptococcus. Other, less frequent bacterial causes include *Streptococcus dysgalactiae* (also known as Lancefield group C/G streptococci), *Arcanobacterium haemolyticum*, *Neisseria gonorrhoeae* and *Mycoplasma* sp.

In the past, prompt treatment of possible group A streptococcal infections was considered useful to prevent suppurative and non-suppurative complications. The suppurative complications include quinsy and mastoiditis, among many others. The most common non-suppurative (immune mediated) complications are rheumatic fever and glomerulonephritis, but there are others, including neurological complications such as Sydenham's chorea.

In the UK, complication rates are now low and the benefit of antibiotic treatment even in patients whose sore throat is caused by group A streptococci is therefore thought to be small (NICE, 2008a). A cohort study in UK general practice found more than 4000 people needed to be treated for URTI, otitis media or pharyngitis to prevent one serious complication (Petersen et al., 2007).

Although *C. diphtheriae* is rare in the UK, it should be considered when investigating travellers returning from parts of the world where diphtheria is common. *C. ulcerans* is as common a cause of clinical diphtheria in the UK as *C. diphtheriae* but usually runs a more benign course.

Clinical features

The presenting complaint is sore throat, often associated with fever and the usual symptoms of the common cold. The Centor score is a clinical scoring system used to identify those at higher risk of bacterial infection (Centor et al., 1981). The criteria are the presence of tonsillar exudate, history of fever, tender anterior surgical lymphadenopathy or adenitis and absence of cough. Each feature scores one point. Those with a Centor score of 3 or 4 have a 40–60% risk of group A streptococcal infection. Those with a Centor score of zero or one are unlikely to have group A streptococcal infection (Aalbers et al., 2011)

Scarlet fever, a toxin-mediated manifestation of streptococcal infection, is associated with a macular rash and sometimes considerable systemic illness. There has been an increased incidence of scarlet fever recently, with 14,387 cases in England between week 37 of 2014 and week 25 of 2015. Most of these cases were in children, with the peak incidence in those aged 1–4 (Public Health England, 2015d).

In the UK, there has been a recent increase in rates of group A streptococcal infection. This includes invasive group A streptococcal infection (iGAS), associated with infection in normally sterile sites such as blood or tissue. The UK experienced an upsurge in invasive group A streptococcal infection in 2008, and an enhanced surveillance protocol was put into place in 2009. These infections are extremely serious, and prompt antibiotic treatment is vital. The serotypes involved vary from year to year, with emm ST1, emm ST12 and emm ST89 most common in the 2015–16 season (Public Health England, 2016b).

Diagnosis

Microbiological diagnosis of the cause of pharyngitis is not usually required in a primary care setting. If a specific bacterial diagnosis is needed, a swab is sent for microbiological culture. Group A β-haemolytic streptococci are usually the organism sought, but if there is a history of treatment failure or recurrent infection, the plates are incubated for 48 hours to look for *Arcanobacterium haemolyticum* (Public Health England, 2015e). The main drawback to culture methods is that the results are not available for at least 24 hours. They also do not distinguish between infection and carriage.

Rapid antigen tests (RATs) for the detection of group A streptococcal antigens are available. Their performance depends on the skill of the user. The use of rapid antigen tests is one of the major points of disagreement in international guidelines. In the UK and the Netherlands, decisions on whether antibiotic treatment is appropriate depend on clinical severity, whereas in the USA, France and Finland, RATs are used (Pelucchi et al., 2012).

Treatment

Most people will recover from sore throat after 7 days. Analgesics such as paracetamol and ibuprofen are useful for reducing pain and fever. Under current guidance, most patients should not be prescribed an antibiotic. Delayed antibiotic prescriptions may be useful. In this scenario, the prescription is post-dated, or patients are advised only to use it if symptoms worsen or do not improve (NICE, 2008a).

NICE (2008a) guidelines suggest that patients with a Centor score of 3 or 4 are considered for an immediate or delayed antibiotic prescription. People who have marked systemic upset, those who are at increased risk of complications and those with valvular heart disease should be given an antibiotic. A low threshold for antibiotic prescribing is also recommended for those who are at risk of immunosuppression, those with previous rheumatic fever and those at risk of severe disease.

Penicillins such as penicillin V are recommended as first-line treatment for group A streptococcal pharyngitis. There is evidence that cephalosporins may be more effective clinically and in eradicating group A streptococci from the pharynx; however, given the higher cost and wider spectrum of activity, international guidelines (Pelucchi et al., 2012; Shulman et al., 2012) still favour penicillin V for 10 days. Aminopenicillins such as amoxicillin should be avoided if primary EBV infection is likely because, for reasons that are not understood, these drugs often cause skin rashes if used in this condition.

Five days of erythromycin or clarithromycin is recommended for patients with penicillin allergy. This is because a review of antibiotics for streptococcal pharyngitis in children found that this treatment was as effective as 10 days of penicillin V (Altamimi et al., 2012).

Acute epiglottitis

Causative organisms

Acute epiglottitis is a rapidly progressive cellulitis of the epiglottis and adjacent structures. Previously, almost all childhood cases and a high proportion of adult cases were caused by *Haemophilus influenzae* type b (Hib), with the rest being caused by other organisms such as pneumococci, streptococci and staphylococci. With the advent of routine vaccination against *H. influenzae* type b in October 1992, this disease has become uncommon.

Clinical features

The typical patient is a child between 2 and 4 years old with fever and difficulty speaking and breathing. The patient may drool because of impaired swallowing. Local swelling has the potential to cause rapid-onset airway obstruction, so the condition is a medical emergency.

Diagnosis

The diagnosis is made clinically, and initial management is concentrated on establishing or maintaining an airway. This takes priority over all other diagnostic and therapeutic manoeuvres. Thereafter, the diagnosis may be confirmed by visualisation of the epiglottis, typically described as 'cherry-red'. Microbiological confirmation may be obtained by culturing the epiglottis and the blood, but not until the airway is secure.

Treatment

In view of the high prevalence of amoxicillin resistance among encapsulated *H. influenzae*, the treatment of choice is a cephalosporin. It is customary to use a third-generation cephalosporin such as cefotaxime or ceftriaxone, but most infections should respond to a second-generation agent such as cefuroxime. If a sensitive organism is recovered, high-dose parenteral amoxicillin may be substituted.

Otitis media

Causative organisms

Inflammation of the middle ear (otitis media) is seen most frequently in children younger than 3 years. Most cases are due to bacteria, although viruses such as influenza virus and rhinoviruses have been implicated in a sizeable minority. *Streptococcus pneumoniae* and *H. influenzae* are the two most commonly encountered bacterial pathogens. *Moraxella catarrhalis* and *S. pyogenes* account for a smaller proportion of cases, perhaps 10%, and other bacteria are rarely seen.

Clinical features

Classically, otitis media presents with ear pain, which may be severe. If the drum perforates, the pain is relieved, and a purulent discharge may follow. There may be a degree of hearing impairment plus non-specific symptoms such as fever or vomiting. Complications include mastoiditis (which is now rare), meningitis and, particularly in the case of *H. influenzae* infection, septicaemia and disseminated infection. With the advent of routine vaccination against *H. influenzae* type b, these complications are uncommon.

Diagnosis

The diagnosis of otitis media is essentially made clinically, and laboratory investigations have little role to play. Unless the drum is perforated, sending a swab of the external auditory canal for microbiological culture is not required, and in fact, the results are likely to be unhelpful or misleading. For this reason, a causative organism is rarely isolated, and empirical treatment is provided.

Treatment

There has been much debate about whether or not antibiotics should be used for the initial treatment of acute otitis media (AOM). A Cochrane systematic review identified 12 trials covering 3854 episodes (Venekamp et al., 2015). Antibiotic treatment led to a statistically significant reduction in the number of children with pain in the first 7 days; however, symptoms spontaneously settled in 82% of children. Twenty children had to be treated for one to benefit; however, one child developed diarrhoea for every 14 treated, leaving the risk and benefit finely balanced. Antibiotics were most useful in patients under 2 with bilateral acute otitis media and patients with perforation and discharge. Therefore, antibiotics are currently only recommended for people who are systemically unwell, those who are at risk of serious complications and those whose symptoms have lasted more than 4 days and are not improving. They should also be considered for children under 2 with bilateral acute otitis media and for children with ear discharge (NICE, 2008a).

If antibiotic treatment is to be given, it should be effective against the three main bacterial pathogens: *S. pneumoniae*, *H. influenzae* and *S. pyogenes*. The streptococci are usually sensitive to penicillins, but these are much less active against *H. influenzae*, so the broader-spectrum agents amoxicillin and ampicillin are preferred. These drugs have identical antibacterial activity, but amoxicillin is recommended for oral treatment because it is better absorbed from the gastro-intestinal tract. About 20% of *H. influenzae* strains are resistant to amoxicillin due to production of β-lactamase, so if there is no response to amoxicillin, an alternative agent should be chosen.

Current national guidance suggests erythromycin or clarithromycin for patients with penicillin allergy; however, these drugs are much less active against *H. influenzae*, so alternatives to amoxicillin should only be used if the history of penicillin allergy is convincing (NICE, 2015b).

Pneumococcal conjugate vaccines, which are currently given routinely in the childhood vaccination schedule, may reduce the incidence of acute otitis media, although a review found only modest benefit when the 7-valent conjugate vaccine was used in healthy infants and no additional benefit in high-risk children (Fortanier et al., 2014). A small benefit was also found for influenza vaccination (Norhayati et al., 2015). Long-term antibiotic prophylaxis might have a role in some children, but any benefit has to be balanced against the risks, such as the development of antibiotic resistance and adverse effects of the antibiotics used (Leach and Morris, 2006).

Acute sinusitis

Causative organisms

Normally, the paranasal sinuses are sterile, but they can become infected after damage to the mucous membrane which lines them. This usually occurs after a viral URTI but is sometimes associated with the presence of dental disease. Sinusitis is caused by a virus in 98% of cases. Bacterial acute sinusitis is usually caused by the same organisms which cause otitis media (*S. pneumoniae* and *H. influenzae*), but occasionally other organisms such as *Staphylococcus aureus*, viridans streptococci (a term used to describe α-haemolytic streptococci other than *S. pneumoniae*) and anaerobes may be found.

Clinical features

The main feature of acute sinusitis is facial pain and tenderness, often accompanied by headache and a purulent nasal discharge. Complications include orbital involvement leading to periorbital cellulitis and intracranial involvement, including frontal bone osteomyelitis, meningitis and brain abscess. The average duration of the illness is 2.5 weeks, although most patients will be improving after 7–15 days (NICE, 2013a).

Bacterial infection should be suspected when three or more of the following criteria are present: discoloured or purulent discharge greater on one side, severe local pain greater on one side, a fever above 38 °C, deterioration after an initial milder illness and a raised erythrocyte sedimentation rate (ESR) or C-reactive protein (CRP) (NICE, 2013a). The condition may become chronic with persistent low-grade pain and nasal discharge, sometimes with acute exacerbations.

Diagnosis

This is usually clinical. However, in chronic cases, samples from sinus washouts may be sent for bacterial culture in an attempt to isolate the causative organism.

Treatment

Paracetamol or ibuprofen is used to alleviate pain. An intranasal decongestant may be useful if nasal congestion is problematic. Irrigating the nose with saline and applying warm face packs may also alleviate symptoms. If patients have severe or prolonged symptoms, intranasal corticosteroids may be considered.

If the patient is at high risk of complications or bacterial infection is thought likely, antibiotics should be prescribed. First-line agents are amoxicillin, phenoxymethyl penicillin and doxycycline. If there is no response after 48 hours or if the agent is poorly tolerated, second-line options include co-amoxiclav and azithromycin (NICE, 2008a).

Lower respiratory tract infections
Acute bronchitis

Acute bronchitis is acute inflammation of the bronchial tree leading to cough which lasts up to 3 weeks.

Causative organisms

Most cases are thought to be viral, but this is uncertain because no cause is identified in a large number of patients in clinical studies.

Clinical features

Patients may have sputum production, wheeze, dyspnoea and systemic upset. There are usually no focal signs on examination of the chest, although wheeze may be present.

Diagnosis

Diagnosis is usually clinical; microbiological investigation is not necessary in most cases. If symptoms persist for longer than 3 weeks, further investigation is indicated to rule out diagnoses such as chronic obstructive pulmonary disease (COPD) or tuberculosis. In smokers with persistent cough, malignancy must be considered.

Treatment

Treatment of acute bronchitis usually consists of analgesia, hydration and comfort measures. Antibiotics should be given if the patient has an impaired ability to fight infection or if the acute bronchitis is likely to worsen a pre-existing condition. If antibiotics are required, the first-line agent is amoxicillin, with doxycycline as an alternative (NICE, 2015c).

Pertussis

Pertussis is a highly infectious disease caused by *Bordetella pertussis*. *Bordetella parapertussis* causes a similar although usually milder infection. The illness classically begins with a coryza followed by a cough that becomes paroxysmal, usually within 1–2 weeks. The paroxysms of coughing may be followed by an inspiratory whoop or by vomiting. Infants may not develop the whoop. The disease usually lasts 2–3 months. Severe complications are most common in infants under 6 months of age and include bronchopneumonia, weight loss and cerebral hypoxia with resulting brain damage. Deaths are also most common in infants under 6 months.

Adults and older children who usually have received vaccination or have been infected previously often lack the classical picture of the disease. The inspiratory whoop and post-tussive vomiting are often absent, and they may simply present with prolonged cough. Cases in adults and older children are therefore often missed, increasing the risk of onward transmission.

In the 1950s there were more than 120,000 notifications of pertussis in England and Wales. Although there were periods of reduced vaccine uptake in the 1970s and 1980s, by 1992, 92% or more of children had been vaccinated by their second birthday, and notifications were down to fewer than 5000 a year. Although vaccine coverage remained above 95%, increased rates of pertussis were seen in 2011. This continued into 2012 when a national outbreak was declared. The reasons are unclear but may include the change to acellular vaccine, better case ascertainment and genetic changes in *B. pertussis* (Public Health England, 2016c).

During the 2012 outbreak, the highest rates of illness were in infants aged less than 3 months, and most became ill before they were old enough to receive their first vaccine. A maternal vaccination programme was therefore introduced. Pregnant women were immunised, ideally at between 28 and 32 weeks of gestation to allow time for maternal antibody to be produced and transferred to the baby (Public Health England, 2016c).

Diagnosis

There is a statutory duty in England to notify the local health protection team of suspected cases of pertussis to facilitate further public health action (Health Protection Agency, 2012).

Culture of a pernasal swab has traditionally been the method of diagnosis in the first 2 weeks of the illness; however, this is increasingly being replaced with polymerase chain reaction (PCR) techniques, which have increased sensitivity. Oral fluid testing for antitoxin immunoglobulin G (IgG) can be performed for patients between 5 and 16 years of age who have had a cough for more than 2 weeks and have not been vaccinated in the last year (Public Health England, 2013a). Serology testing for antitoxin IgG in serum samples is used to confirm the diagnosis in adults, if the date of symptom onset is more than 2 weeks before the date of the test and they have not been vaccinated recently. Serological testing is unable to distinguish between antibodies formed in response to disease and those formed in response to vaccination and so is unreliable in patients who have been recently vaccinated.

Treatment

Macrolides are the mainstay of treatment. A 3-day course of azithromycin or a 7-day course of erythromycin or clarithromycin is recommended. Erythromycin is not used in infants under 1 month old due to an association with pyloric stenosis. If the patient cannot take a macrolide, then co-trimoxazole is an alternative in patients older than 1 month. Cotrimoxazole cannot be used in pregnancy (Public Health England, 2013a).

Children are excluded from schools and nurseries until they have completed a course of treatment. If the diagnosis was made late and they have not been treated, they are excluded until 21 days have passed from the onset of symptoms (Public Health England, 2013a).

Because the paroxysmal cough is due to toxin-mediated damage, treatment does not eliminate the symptoms. The role of treatment is to reduce infectivity and onward transmission.

Bronchiolitis

Bronchiolitis is characterised by inflammatory changes in the small bronchi and bronchioles, but not by consolidation. It is particularly recognised as a disease of infants in the first year of life, in whom a small degree of airway narrowing can have a dramatic effect on airflow. However, the causal organisms are equally capable of infecting adults, who may then act as reservoirs of infection. Approximately one in three infants will develop bronchiolitis in their first year of life (NICE, 2015d).

Causative organisms

Most cases of bronchiolitis are caused by respiratory syncytial virus (RSV), which occurs in annual winter epidemics, but human metapneumovirus (hMPV), parainfluenza viruses, rhinoviruses, adenoviruses and occasionally *M. pneumoniae* have also been implicated.

Diagnosis

Bronchiolitis is characterised by a prodrome of fever and coryzal symptoms which progresses to wheezing, respiratory distress and hypoxia of varying degrees. Aetiological confirmation may be made by immunofluorescence and/or viral culture of respiratory secretions, although increasingly the diagnosis of respiratory syncytial virus is made using rapid antigen detection tests or by PCR.

Treatment

The treatment of bronchiolitis is mainly supportive and consists of oxygen, adequate hydration and ventilatory assistance if required. Nebulised ribavirin for the treatment of bronchiolitis is not mentioned in the NICE (2015d) guidelines.

Babies born earlier than 35 weeks of gestation or those less than 6 months of age at the onset of the RSV season are at high risk of the disease. Likewise, infants under 2 years old with congenital heart disease, chronic lung disease or with severe immunodeficiency are similarly at high risk. All such patients are candidates for prophylactic treatment with palivizumab. This is a humanised monoclonal antibody used for passive immunisation against respiratory syncytial virus (Public Health England, 2015f). There is currently no vaccine against RSV.

Exacerbations of chronic obstructive pulmonary disease

Chronic obstructive pulmonary disease (COPD) renders patients more vulnerable to respiratory infection, and infectious exacerbations cause significant morbidity and mortality. These acute exacerbations of COPD are a frequent cause of morbidity and admission to hospital. An exacerbation is defined as 'a sustained worsening of the patient's symptoms from his or her usual stable state that is beyond normal day-to-day variations, and is acute in onset' (NICE, 2010).

Diagnosis

Common symptoms include worsening breathlessness, cough, increased sputum production and change in sputum colour. It is important to remember that not all acute exacerbations of COPD have an infective aetiology and that many infective exacerbations will be triggered by viruses. Bacterial causes include *M. catarrhalis*, *H. influenzae* and *S. pneumoniae*.

Severe exacerbations can cause marked breathlessness, confusion, marked reduction in performance of activities of daily living and use of accessory muscles at rest. These patients require hospital admission. Milder exacerbations can be managed in the community. Sending sputum samples for culture as routine practice in primary care is not recommended.

Treatment

NICE recommends antibiotic therapy for exacerbations of COPD associated with purulent sputum or where there are clinical signs of pneumonia or consolidation on chest X-ray (NICE, 2010). Recommended treatment is with an aminopenicillin (e.g. amoxicillin), a macrolide or a tetracycline, according to local guidance with modification according to sputum culture results if sputum has been sent. However, routine sputum cultures are not recommended for patients managed in primary care.

Co-amoxiclav has the advantage of covering β-lactamase-producing strains of *H. influenzae* and *M. catarrhalis* that are therefore resistant to amoxicillin. However, this agent has a greater incidence of side effects, such as a higher risk of *Clostridium* (now named *Clostridioides*) *difficile* infection (CDI) and a much higher incidence of cholestatic jaundice.

Numerous other drugs are promoted for the treatment of COPD exacerbations. The activity of ciprofloxacin against *S. pneumoniae* is insufficient to justify its use as monotherapy against pneumococcal infections. However, it has useful activity against *H. influenzae* and *M. catarrhalis*. Levofloxacin, the active isomer of ofloxacin, does not seem to offer any great microbiological advantage. Moxifloxacin is a quinolone that retains activity against Gram-negative organisms such as *Haemophilus* and *Moraxella* but has greater activity against Gram-positives such as *S. pneumoniae*. It has been favourably compared with standard treatment in exacerbations of COPD (Wilson et al., 2004). However, its use has been limited by the high incidence of CDI

associated with quinolone use and, rarely, the development of life-threatening hepatic toxicity and prolonged QT syndrome.

Community acquired pneumonia

Pneumonia is infection of the lung parenchyma. The alveoli fill with bacteria, inflammatory cells and fluid in a process called consolidation. Mild pneumonia can be treated in the community, but patients with moderate to severe disease will require hospital admission. In hospitalised patients, the diagnosis is confirmed by the presence of consolidation on the chest X-ray. Diagnosing pneumonia in primary care is more complicated. Clinical studies have defined community-acquired pneumonia (CAP) differently, but fever greater than 38 °C, pleural pain, dyspnoea, tachypnoea and new signs on examination of the chest seem to be useful for separating CAP from bronchitis in the absence of a chest X-ray. The British Thoracic Society (BTS) guidelines (BTS Community Acquired Pneumonia in Adults Guideline Group, 2009) define CAP as symptoms of a lower respiratory tract infection (cough and at least one other), new focal signs on chest examination, at least one systemic feature and no other explanation for the illness. The NICE (2014) guidelines on community-acquired pneumonia suggested using a point-of-care CRP test to decide on antibiotic treatment in adult patients with LRTI if a clinical diagnosis of community-acquired pneumonia has not been made. Under these guidelines, antibiotics would not be given if CRP is less than 20, a delayed antibiotic prescription should be considered if CRP is greater than 20 but less than 100 and antibiotics should be offered if CRP is greater than 100 (NICE, 2014).

When community-acquired pneumonia is diagnosed clinically in an adult in the community, the 'CRB 65' mnemonic score is used to determine clinical risk. Table 36.1 describes the factors considered within the CRB score, where one point is scored for each of the following: confusion, respiratory rate, blood pressure and age. Patients with a CRB 65 score of 0 can be safely managed at home. Hospital assessment should be considered for patients with a score of 1 or more and especially if the score is 2 or more (NICE, 2014).

Severity scoring of community-acquired pneumonia in hospital patients uses the 'CURB 65' mnemonic score, which adds blood urea nitrogen of greater than 7 to the CRB 65 score. Patients with a CURB 65 of 0 or 1 are low risk and suitable for treatment at home. Patients with a CURB 65 score of 2 are at intermediate risk and should be considered for a short in-patient admission or outpatient treatment under hospital supervision. Patients with a CURB 65 score of 3 or more are at high risk and will require in-patient management (BTS Community Acquired Pneumonia in Adults Guideline Group, 2009; NICE, 2014).

In children, bacterial pneumonia should be considered where there is persistent or repetitive fever of greater than 38.5 °C with chest recession and a raised respiratory rate (BTS Community Acquired Pneumonia in Children Guideline Group, 2011).

Causative organisms

The most common cause of community-acquired pneumonia is *S. pneumoniae*. *H. influenzae* (usually noncapsulate strains) are another common cause. *S. aureus* can cause a severe necrotising pneumonia, classically occurring after an influenza infection.

Table 36.1 CRB score for assessing the severity of community-acquired pneumonia presenting in primary care

Marker	Explanation of marker
C	Confusion defined as AMTS <8 or new disorientation in person, place or time
R	Respiratory rate ≥30 breaths/min
B	Systolic blood pressure <90 mmHg or diastolic <60 mmHg
65	Age >65

Score	Each severity marker present scores 1 point
0	Low risk of mortality, <1%
1–2	Intermediate risk of mortality, 1–10%
3–4	High risk of mortality, >10%

AMTS, Abbreviated Mental Test Score developed and validated by Hodkinson (1972).

Table 36.2 Empirical treatment of community-acquired pneumonia in patients with no history of penicillin allergy

CAP severity	Antibiotic of choice
Mild	Amoxicillin oral
Moderate	Amoxicillin and clarithromycin i.v. or oral
Severe	Co-amoxiclav (i.v. until clinical improvement) and clarithromycin i.v. or oral

CAP, Community-acquired pneumonia; i.v., intravenous.

Organisms causing atypical pneumonia include *Legionella pneumophila*, *Mycoplasma pneumoniae*, *Chlamydophila pneumoniae*, *Chlamydophila psittaci*, *Coxiella burnetii* and viruses. It is not possible to determine the microbiological cause of pneumonia clinically or radiologically.

L. pneumophila is the cause of Legionnaire's disease, which occurs sporadically and in outbreaks often associated with contaminated air-conditioning or water systems. From 2002 to 2008, there were 300–600 new cases a year reported in England and Wales. Legionnaire's disease may be rapidly progressive, with very extensive consolidation and consequent respiratory failure.

Viral infections should not be forgotten as causes of pneumonia, although in practice it is unusual to make a definitive early diagnosis, so most cases are treated with antibacterials. Influenza can cause a primary viral pneumonia and can be complicated by secondary bacterial (particularly staphylococcal) pneumonia. Chickenpox can be complicated by primary varicella pneumonia, particularly in adults, and cytomegalovirus is capable of causing a variety of infections, including pneumonia, in patients with compromised cell-mediated immunity.

Diagnosis

Microbiological testing is not recommended as routine practice for adults or children with low-risk disease treated in the community. However, sputum culture may be useful in those who do not respond to first-line antibiotic treatment.

Adults with moderate- or high-severity CAP should have blood cultures and sputum cultures performed. The 2009 BTS guidelines also recommend pneumococcal antigen testing for all patients with moderate- or high-severity CAP (BTS Community Acquired Pneumonia in Adults Guideline Group, 2009). The success of sputum culture depends on the quality of the sample because samples from the upper respiratory tract will be contaminated with the normal regional flora. In patients who are severely ill and especially those requiring admission to an intensive care unit (ICU), more invasive sampling such as bronchoalveolar lavage may be required to tailor treatment.

The UK national guidelines for HIV testing in the UK recommend offering an HIV test to patients with bacterial pneumonia (British HIV Association et al., 2008). The BTS guidelines recommend that patients with high-severity CAP should have *Legionella* urinary antigen testing (BTS Community Acquired Pneumonia in Adults Guideline Group, 2009). The NICE (2014) guideline extends this to patients with moderate-severity pneumonia. However, because urine antigen testing only detects serogroup 1 *L. pneumophila*, a negative test does not exclude *Legionella* infection.

The other atypical pathogens may require serological diagnosis with complement fixation tests being performed in parallel on acute and convalescent serum. The convalescent sample should be taken 2 weeks after the onset of symptoms; however, these results are obviously too late to tailor treatment. Respiratory multiplex PCRs which detect agents such as *Mycoplasma*, *C. pneumoniae* and *C. psittaci* are increasingly commonly available and allow diagnosis of atypical infection during the acute illness.

Empirical treatment

Both the BTS and NICE have produced guidelines for the treatment of community-acquired pneumonia in adults. The BTS (BTS Community Acquired Pneumonia in Adults Guideline Group, 2009) and NICE (2014) guidelines make similar treatment recommendations (Table 36.2). Local guidelines may vary depending on local resistance rates and the demographics of the local population.

For mild disease, the recommended treatment is with amoxicillin, which provides activity against pneumococci and most strains of *H. influenzae*. Doxycycline or clarithromycin are the preferred alternatives in penicillin-allergic patients. However, for moderate or severe disease requiring admission to hospital, guidelines recommend that, until the aetiology is known, treatment should cover both 'typical' causes (e.g. *S. pneumoniae* and *H. influenzae*) and atypical causes (e.g. *M. pneumoniae*, *Chlamydophila* species and *Legionella*). For patients with moderate or severe CAP, the current national guidelines (BTS Community Acquired Pneumonia in Adults Guideline Group, 2009; NICE, 2014) therefore recommend a combination of a β-lactam drug plus a macrolide. For moderate disease, oral amoxicillin plus a macrolide is suggested, whereas for severe disease, a broad-spectrum β-lactamase stable penicillin (co-amoxiclav) and a macrolide should be given intravenously. In patients allergic to penicillin, a second-generation (e.g. cefuroxime) or third-generation (e.g. cefotaxime or ceftriaxone) cephalosporin can be used instead of co-amoxiclav, together with clarithromycin. For mild disease, the BTS guidelines (BTS Community Acquired Pneumonia in Adults Guideline Group, 2009) suggest a 7-day course, although the NICE (2014) guidance shortens this duration to 5 days. For more severe disease, a 7- to 10-day course is suggested, but this may need to be extended, for example, if the infection was caused by *S. aureus* or Gram-negative bacilli.

In children, a different approach is recommended. In the BTS guidance (BTS Community Acquired Pneumonia in Children Guideline Group, 2011), amoxicillin is recommended for all children, and oral administration is preferred unless the child cannot tolerate oral fluids, has problematic oral absorption or is showing signs of septicaemia. The agents recommended include amoxicillin, co-amoxiclav, cefuroxime, cefotaxime or ceftriaxone. Macrolides may then be added if the child does not respond to first-line treatment.

Targeted therapy

The treatment of choice for pneumococcal pneumonia is benzylpenicillin or amoxicillin. Erythromycin monotherapy may be used in penicillin-allergic patients, but resistance rates are rising. Macrolides are bacteriostatic rather than bactericidal, and the comparative efficacy of this approach is not known. There is retrospective evidence that combination therapy using both a β-lactam and a macrolide can reduce mortality in patients whose pneumonia is complicated by pneumococcal bacteraemia (Martinez et al., 2003). However, a Dutch study found that narrowing the spectrum of antibiotic cover in patients with a pneumococcal bacteraemia was associated with a lower mortality rate regardless of severity (Cremers et al., 2014).

Pneumococci with reduced susceptibility to penicillin are becoming increasingly common, particularly in continental Europe and the USA. In the UK, about 5–10% of strains express 'intermediate susceptibility' (minimum inhibitory concentration [MIC] 0.06–2 mg/L), but high-level resistance (MIC > 2 mg/L) remains uncommon. Intermediate susceptibility may result in treatment failure in conditions such as meningitis at sites where antibiotic penetration is reduced, but antibiotic penetration into the lungs is sufficiently good that penicillin and amoxicillin remain effective for pneumonia. Strains expressing high-level resistance are unlikely to respond to penicillins. However, such strains are often co-resistant to macrolides and other first-line agents and may require treatment with glycopeptides or linezolid. The European Respiratory Society and European Society

for Clinical Microbiology and Infectious Diseases (ESCMID) guidance on the treatment of LRTI reported no documented cases of treatment failure with adequate doses of penicillins in extrameningeal infection (Woodhead et al., 2011). A new formulation of amoxicillin/clavulanic acid (2 g/125 mg given 12 hourly) is reported to have successfully treated strains, with an amoxicillin MIC of 4–8 mg/L (Woodhead et al., 2011).

M. pneumoniae does not possess a cell wall and is therefore not susceptible to β-lactam agents. A tetracycline or a macrolide is a suitable alternative. Tetracyclines are also effective against *C. pneumoniae*, *C. psittaci* and *C. burnetii*, but erythromycin is probably less effective. Quinolones are highly active against these organisms.

Staphylococcal pneumonia is usually treated with flucloxacillin. Meticillin-resistant *S. aureus* (MRSA) pneumonia is being seen more commonly in the community and in hospital. Strains of *S. aureus* expressing Panton-Valentine Leukocidin, an exotoxin, are capable of causing a severe necrotising pneumonia and if clinically suspected should warrant urgent critical care and specialist microbiological input.

Treatment recommendations for Legionnaire's disease are based on a retrospective review of the famous Philadelphia outbreak of 1976 (Fraser et al., 1977), in which two deaths occurred among the 18 patients who were given erythromycin, compared with 16 deaths in 71 patients treated with penicillin or amoxicillin. This observation accords with the facts that *Legionella* is an intracellular pathogen and that macrolides penetrate more efficiently than β-lactams into cells. Azithromycin is probably the most effective of the macrolide/azalide derivatives, but clinical evidence to confirm this is lacking. Other agents with proven clinical efficacy and good intracellular activity against *Legionella* include rifampicin and quinolones. There have been no randomised controlled clinical trials comparing the new quinolones and the newer macrolides for the treatment of *L. pneumophila*. Guidance, based on observational studies, suggests non-severe cases should be treated with an oral fluoroquinolone (with a macrolide as an alternative). Severe cases are treated with a combination of a fluoroquinolone plus either a macrolide or rifampicin, de-escalating to a fluoroquinolone as the sole agent after the first few days (BTS Community Acquired Pneumonia in Adults Guideline Group, 2009). Treatment is not recommended for the non-pneumonic form of legionellosis (Pontiac fever), which presents as a self-limiting flu-like illness.

Prevention

Pneumococcal 23-valent polysaccharide vaccine and influenza vaccine should be offered to all those at risk of infection. For pneumococcal infection, this includes patients who fulfil the following criteria:
- asplenia or dysfunction of the spleen,
- chronic respiratory disease,
- chronic heart disease,
- chronic renal disease,
- chronic liver disease,
- diabetes,

- immunosuppressed,
- aged 65 years or older,
- cochlear implants,
- cerebrospinal fluid leaks.

In the UK, children are immunised with the 13-serotype conjugate vaccine as part of the normal childhood vaccination schedule. This should both protect them and reduce the circulation of these serotypes in the community; however, there is concern that vaccination may lead to serotype replacement, with serotypes not included in the vaccine filling the empty ecological niche (Public Health England, 2013b).

Hospital-acquired pneumonia

Hospital-acquired pneumonia (HAP) is defined as pneumonia developing more than 48 hours after admission and not incubating at the time of admission. It is a major cause of morbidity and mortality in hospital patients in the developed world. An important subset of HAP is ventilator-associated pneumonia (VAP), which is defined as pneumonia occurring more than 48 hours after endotracheal intubation.

The range of pathogens associated with HAP is wide. Traditionally, it has been divided into early infection, occurring after less than 5 days in hospital when more sensitive organisms are likely to be involved, and late infection, which carried a higher risk of multidrug-resistant organisms. However, these distinctions are not absolute.

Common pathogens include Gram-negative organisms such as *Pseudomonas aeruginosa*, *Escherichia coli*, *Klebsiella pneumoniae* and *Acinetobacter* spp. *S. aureus*, including MRSA is the main Gram-positive organism implicated. *S. pneumoniae* and *Haemophilus influenzae* are sometimes found in early-onset HAP, and the patient may have been incubating the infection at the time of admission; they are rare in late-onset HAP. HAP may be polymicrobial. It is rarely due to viruses or fungi unless the host is immunosuppressed. Hospital water supplies have been implicated in sporadic cases, and occasionally there have been outbreaks of *L. pneumophila*. Therefore, this possibility should be considered.

Clinical features

Nosocomial pneumonia accounts for 10–15% of all hospital-acquired infections, usually presenting with sepsis and/or respiratory failure. Up to 50% of cases are acquired on intensive care units. Predisposing features include stroke, mechanical ventilation, chronic lung disease, recent surgery and previous antibiotic exposure.

Diagnosis

Sputum is commonly sent for culture, but this is sometimes unhelpful because it may be contaminated by mouth flora. If the patient has received antibiotics, the normal mouth flora is often replaced by resistant organisms such as staphylococci or Gram-negative bacilli, making the interpretation of culture results difficult. Bronchoalveolar lavage is often more helpful. Blood cultures may be positive.

Treatment

The range of organisms causing nosocomial pneumonia is very large, so broad-spectrum empiric therapy is indicated. The choice of antibiotics will be influenced by preceding antibiotic therapy, the duration of hospital admission and, above all, by the individual unit's experience with hospital-acquired bacteria. It is important that units maintain surveillance systems and monitor their resistance rates so that guidelines can be modified over time. Both the British Society for Antimicrobial Chemotherapy (Masterton et al., 2008) guidelines and the NICE (2014) guidelines recommend following local policies based on local pathogen and susceptibility data.

Co-amoxiclav is sometimes used for early HAP but lacks pseudomonal cover. Agents such as piperacillin/tazobactam and meropenem have broad-spectrum activity including *Pseudomonas* sp. but do not cover MRSA, so an additional agent such as vancomycin or linezolid would be required in MRSA-colonised patients or in units with high rates of MRSA infection. With concerns about the spread of carbapenem-resistant *Enterobacteriaceae*, there has been a national attempt to control carbapenem use, with acute hospital trusts required to reduce their carbapenem prescribing below the 2014–15 baseline. The aim is to relieve the evolutionary selective pressure driving the development and spread of carbapenem resistance and therefore to reduce the spread of carbapenemase-producing organisms. There have also been attempts to use narrower-spectrum agents to reduce *C. difficile* risk. A study using amoxicillin and temocillin has been published; however, this combination lacks *P. aeruginosa* and *S. aureus* cover, and additional agents are therefore required in some circumstances (Habayeb et al., 2015).

Options in patients with type one hypersensitivity to penicillin include aztreonam or ciprofloxacin and an antibiotic with activity against Gram-positive bacteria (e.g. a glycopeptide or linezolid).

Prevention

General strategies for minimising the incidence of HAP include early postoperative mobilisation, analgesia, physiotherapy and promotion of rational antibiotic prescribing.

One of the Department of Health's (DH's) high-impact interventions (DH, 2011) is a care bundle for ventilated patients, aimed at reducing the prevalence of VAP. The high-impact interventions are a set of practice interventions introduced to provide NHS trusts with the tools to reduce serious healthcare-associated infections. Since 2008, the Health and Social Care Act controlling healthcare-associated infection has been a legal requirement for NHS trusts; it forms part of the code of practice all NHS trusts operate under. Implementation of care bundles such as this provides evidence that NHS trusts are complying with this obligation.

The recommendations in the ventilator care bundle include head-of-bed elevation, sedation holding to reduce the duration of mechanical ventilation, aspiration of secretions every 1–2 hours via a subglottic port in patients who have been intubated more than 72 hours, limiting stress ulcer prophylaxis to high-risk patients and good general hygiene of tubing management and suction.

Another strategy proposed for the prevention of VAP is selective decontamination of the digestive tract (SDD), based on the premise that the infecting organisms initially colonise the patient's oropharynx or intestinal tract. By administering non-absorbable antibiotics such as an aminoglycoside or colistin to the gut and applying a paste containing these agents to the oropharynx, it is proposed that the potential causative organisms will be eradicated and the incidence of pneumonia thereby reduced. In some centres, an antifungal agent such as amphotericin B is added; others also advocate addition of a systemic broad-spectrum agent such as cefotaxime.

The role of selective decontamination of the digestive tract remains controversial. A Cochrane review suggested that it did reduce respiratory tract infections, although mortality was only reduced if systemic antibiotics were also given (Di'Amico et al., 2009). However, questions remain about longer-term benefits and the potential effects on antibiotic resistance. The use of aerosolised antibiotics in this context has been considered; agents which would be suitable for administration by this route and with the appropriate antimicrobial spectrum include aminoglycosides (particularly tobramycin) and the polymyxin drug colistin. There are no published data available at present, and therefore this approach cannot be universally recommended.

Aspiration pneumonia

One further condition which may be seen either in hospital or in the community is aspiration pneumonia, initiated by inhalation of stomach contents contaminated by bacteria from the mouth. Risk factors include alcohol, hypnotic drugs and general anaesthesia; all of these may induce a patient to vomit while unconscious. Gastric acid is very destructive to lung tissue and leads to severe tissue necrosis. Damaged tissue is then prone to secondary infection, often with abscess formation. Anaerobic bacteria are particularly implicated, but these are often accompanied by aerobic organisms such as viridans streptococci.

Treatment

Treatment with amoxicillin and metronidazole is usually adequate. However, broader-spectrum drugs may be used if there are reasons to suspect Gram-negative involvement, for example, if the patient has been in hospital or has previously been exposed to antibiotics. Options for treatment in such patients include co-amoxiclav, piperacillin/tazobactam and carbapenems.

Novel coronaviruses

Most coronaviruses cause mild URTIs, but two have emerged in recent years which are more serious.

Severe acute respiratory syndrome

Clinically, the severe acute respiratory syndrome (SARS) coronavirus causes pneumonitis, presenting with a flu-like prodrome and progressing to dyspnoea, dry cough and often adult respiratory distress syndrome, requiring ventilatory support. Treatment of SARS is largely supportive. It was first described in 2003 after a large outbreak originating in China spread throughout the

Box 36.1 Middle East respiratory syndrome coronavirus epidemiological and clinical criteria

Epidemiological criteria
- Patient has lived in or travelled to an area where it could have been acquired in the last 14 days (as of February 2016, Bahrain, Jordan, Iraq, Iran, Kingdom of Saudi Arabia, Kuwait, Oman, Qatar, United Arab Emirates, and Yemen).
OR
- The patient has had close contact with a patient with MERS in the 14 days before the patient became ill and that patient had symptoms at the time of contact.
OR
- The patient is a healthcare worker on ICU caring for patients with respiratory distress.
OR
- The patient is part of a cluster of epidemiologically linked cases requiring ICU admission.
AND

Clinical case description
- The patient has a fever >38 °C or history of fever and cough and has evidence of disease of the lung parenchyma (e.g. chest X-ray changes) with no alternative explanation.

ICU, Intensive care unit; MERS, Middle East respiratory syndrome.
From Public Health England, 2018

Americas, Europe and Asia. The outbreak terminated that year, with only small numbers of cases occurring since. Many experts predict that SARS will re-emerge.

Middle East respiratory syndrome coronavirus

This novel coronavirus was first identified in 2012 and causes Middle East respiratory syndrome (MERS). The clinical picture ranges from asymptomatic infection to severe respiratory distress and death. Common symptoms include fever, cough and shortness of breath (Box 36.1). Some patients have gastro-intestinal symptoms such as diarrhoea; pneumonia is common but not universal. In 36% of identified cases, the patients have died (WHO, 2017). Camels appear to be a common host. Human-to-human transmission requires close contact, but there has been transmission to healthcare workers, and there have been nosocomial outbreaks (WHO, 2017). The risk in these patients is low, but they should be tested to exclude the possibility (Public Health England, 2018). Treatment is still under investigation and is currently supportive and includes supplemental oxygen and ventilation if required. No antiviral drugs are recommended at present.

Cystic fibrosis

Cystic fibrosis (CF) is an inherited, autosomal-recessive disease which, at the cellular level, is caused by a defect in the transport of ions in and out of cells. This leads to changes in the consistency and chemical composition of exocrine secretions. In the lungs, this is manifest by the production of very sticky, tenacious mucus which is difficult to clear by mucociliary action. The production of such mucus leads to airway obstruction and infection. These repeated infections lead to lung damage and bronchiectasis, which in turn predisposes to further infection. The pattern in CF is of a progressive decline in lung function with episodes of acute worsening known as pulmonary exacerbations. The features of these exacerbations include increased cough, increased sputum production, shortness of breath, chest pain, loss of appetite and decline in respiratory function.

Infective organisms

It had been thought that the microbiology of respiratory infections in cystic fibrosis involved a few key pathogens, but this is now acknowledged over recent years to be increasingly complex.

H. influenzae is frequently encountered in early childhood and has been reported to be the most common organism at 1 year of age. LRTI is sometimes difficult to distinguish from upper respiratory tract colonisation. As in healthy children, most of the infections in children with cystic fibrosis are with non-capsulate strains. *S. aureus* is a common pathogen and may be isolated from early infancy. In the UK, continuous anti-staphylococcal prophylaxis is recommended up to the age of 3, although some centres continue beyond this time. Prophylaxis has been with flucloxacillin, but MRSA rates vary between units and this may affect the choice of agent.

P. aeruginosa is the most common pathogen isolated from people with cystic fibrosis, and its prevalence increases with age. It is possible to clear 80% of early infections with aggressive antibiotic therapy (e.g. ciprofloxacin and an inhaled aminoglycoside) and so delay the onset of chronic colonisation. Once chronic colonisation with *P. aeruginosa* is established, it is associated with faster decline in lung function, increased hospitalisation and reduced survival. Long-term suppressive therapy with inhaled antibiotics is used in these patients to slow the decline in lung function.

An important feature of those *P. aeruginosa* strains which infect patients with cystic fibrosis is their production of large amounts of alginate, a polymer of mannuronic and glucuronic acid. This seems to be a virulence factor for the organism because it inhibits opsonisation and phagocytosis and enables the bacteria to adhere to the bronchial epithelium, thus inhibiting clearance. It does not confer additional antibiotic resistance. Strains which produce large amounts of alginate have a wet, slimy appearance on laboratory culture media and are termed 'mucoid' strains.

P. aeruginosa acquisition by CF patients had been thought to involve sporadic acquisition of environmental strains. However, some strains of *P. aeruginosa* are transmissible between CF patients. Guidelines recommend molecular fingerprinting to identify these epidemic strains (Cystic Fibrosis Trust Microbiology Laboratory Standards Working Group, 2010).

Other Gram-negative bacteria can also infect the lungs of patients with CF, with the *Burkholderia cepacia* complex being the most important. Outbreaks of these organisms occurred in CF centres in the 1980s and 1990s, leading to many deaths. Therefore, interaction between non-related CF patients, either socially or in healthcare settings, is strongly discouraged. Colonisation with genomovar IIIA of the *B. cepacia* complex (*cenocepacia*) precludes lung transplantation because of high postoperative mortality rates. Correct identification of the organism is therefore

vital, and because biochemical methods are unreliable, PCR methods are recommended (Cystic Fibrosis Trust Microbiology Laboratory Standards Working Group, 2010). The impact of other Gram-negative bacteria and also of organisms such as anaerobes which had traditionally not been thought to be pathogenic is still unresolved.

In recent years there has been an increase in the number of patients in Europe and the USA found to be colonised with non-tuberculous mycobacteria. Transmission of *Mycobacterium abscessus* complex has been recorded (Cystic Fibrosis Trust *Mycobacterium abscessus* Infection Control Working Group, 2013). Poorer outcomes after lung transplantation have been described in patients colonised with *M. abscessus* (Floto et al., 2015). The *Mycobacterium avium* complex is most frequently isolated, but the number of *M. abscessus* complex isolated is increasing rapidly. There are concerns that this may be related to widespread use of azithromycin prophylaxis. Consensus guidelines from the European Cystic Fibrosis Society and the US Cystic Fibrosis Foundation recommend annual screening for carriage of non-tuberculous mycobacteria and strict infection control precautions (Floto et al., 2015).

Fungi have also been increasingly recognised as important pathogens in cystic fibrosis. Aspergillus colonisation leading to allergic bronchopulmonary aspergillosis (ABPA) has been recognised for many years, but it has now also been suggested that it can cause exacerbations by producing a fungal bronchitis. *Scedosporium apiospermum* and *Wangiella (Exophiala) dermatitidis* are being isolated more commonly (Cystic Fibrosis Trust Antibiotic Working Group, 2009).

Treatment

Although this section concentrates on antibiotic therapy, it should be noted that other treatments such as physiotherapy play a vital part. In addition, lung transplantation can be lifesaving.

Acute respiratory exacerbations of CF caused by *P. aeruginosa* are usually treated with dual antibiotic therapy with two agents that act by different mechanisms (Table 36.3). The length of treatment course is usually 2 weeks. Sensitivity testing of *Pseudomonas* spp. and other non-fermenting Gram-negative bacilli should not be used in isolation to guide treatment because it is frequently unreliable in this setting. The choice of antibiotics will therefore be guided by the patient's response.

B. cepacia complex is often very difficult to treat, and strains may be resistant to all available antibiotics. Under these circumstances, combination therapy is often required.

The use of inhaled (usually nebulised) antibiotics as an adjunct to parenteral therapy has attracted attention, both for treatment of acute exacerbations and for longer-term use in an attempt to reduce the pseudomonal load. Agents which have been administered in this way include colistin, aminoglycosides and aztreonam. The best evidence that long-term administration can be beneficial comes from a large multi-centre trial of nebulised tobramycin (Moss, 2001). Patients were randomised to receive once-daily nebulised tobramycin or placebo in on–off cycles for 24 weeks, followed by open-label tobramycin to complete 2 years of study. Nebulised tobramycin was safe and well tolerated and was associated with a reduction in hospitalisation and

Table 36.3 Antibiotics with activity against *Pseudomonas*

Antibiotic	Comment
β-Lactams and related drugs	
Ureidopenicillins	Piperacillin, formulated in combination with the β-lactamase inhibitor tazobactam, is the only one of these agents currently available in the UK.
Cephalosporins	Ceftazidime is the third-generation cephalosporin active against *Pseudomonas*; it is very active against other Gram-negative bacilli but has rather lower activity against Gram-positive bacteria. Ceftobiprole is a new cephalosporin with activity against *Pseudomonas* and MRSA.
Carbapenems	Broad-spectrum agents with good Gram-negative activity. Imipenem was the first of these drugs, but CNS toxicity and its requirement for combination with the renal dipeptidase inhibitor cilastatin have largely led to its replacement by meropenem. Doripenem is a newer carbapenem with similar activity to meropenem. Ertapenem has poor activity against *Pseudomonas aeruginosa*.
Monobactams	Aztreonam is the only monobactam available and offers good activity against Gram-negative organisms but no activity against Gram-positive organisms.
Other antibiotic classes	
Aminoglycosides	Gentamicin and tobramycin have very similar activity against *Pseudomonas*; tobramycin is perhaps slightly more active. Netilmicin is less active, whereas amikacin may be active against some gentamicin-resistant strains.
Quinolones	Ciprofloxacin can be given orally and parenterally, but as with ceftazidime, resistance can develop while the patient is on treatment. Other quinolones, such as ofloxacin, its L-isomer levofloxacin, and moxifloxacin, have better Gram-positive spectrum but concomitantly less activity against *Pseudomonas*.
Polymyxins	Colistin (polymyxin E) can be given by inhalation and intravenously; it is usually reserved for more resistant cases due to its toxicity.

CNS, Central nervous system; MRSA, meticillin-resistant *Staphylococcus aureus*.

improvements in lung function. This was at the expense of a degree of tobramycin resistance, although this did not appear to be clinically significant. In patients who are intolerant of nebulised treatment, tobramycin and colistin dry powder inhalers can be used (NICE, 2013b).

Case studies

Case 36.1

A 40-year-old woman, Mrs LH, presents to her primary care doctor with a 1-week history of sore throat. She is normally fit and well and has had no other symptoms other than some lethargy.

Questions

1. What are the likely causes of Mrs LH's sore throat?
2. Should Mrs LH be prescribed antibiotics?
   The primary care doctor decides to prescribe a 10-day course of penicillin V to cover a possible streptococcal infection. Two weeks later, the patient returns. Mrs LH is feeling worse and is now experiencing difficulty in swallowing. Examination of her throat reveals widespread white plaques.
3. What is the likely diagnosis?
4. What other investigations might be indicated?

Answers

1. A viral aetiology is the most likely cause. These are usually the same viruses that cause colds. Bacterial infection with group A streptococci usually presents with a more severe infection. The Centor score can be used to help determine whether bacterial infection is likely; because there is no tonsillar exudate, history of fever, tender anterior surgical lymphadenopathy or adenitis and no cough, the score would be 0, indicating that bacterial infection is unlikely.
2. Antibiotics are not recommended for routine use. Treatment is directed at symptomatic relief, and most people recover within 7 days.
3. The likely cause is of Mrs LH's symptoms is oral candidiasis. The presence of dysphagia is concerning and raises the question of oesophageal involvement. If the dysphagia is significant, hospital admission may be indicated, and endoscopy may be required to elucidate the extent of the infection.
4. Mrs LH maybe immunocompromised, and this must be considered. Therefore, all patients with oral candidiasis should be offered HIV testing (British HIV Association et al., 2008).

Case 36.2

A 65-year-old man, Mr. NP, is found collapsed at home. He is brought into hospital. His family said that he complained of flu-like symptoms a few days before. Mr. NP is pyrexial, tachypnoeic, tachycardic and hypoxic. On examination, he is found to have reduced air entry at the right base.

Questions

1. What is the likely diagnosis?
2. What are the possible infecting organisms?
3. What empirical antibiotics would you choose?

Answers

1. Mr NP is likely to have community-acquired pneumonia.
2. The most likely causative organisms are *S. pneumoniae* and *H. influenzae*. However, *S. aureus* should also be considered in post–influenza pneumonia.
3. The choice of treatment for Mr NP should be guided by the 'CURB' 65 score. Given the history, the CURB 65 score is likely to be at least 3, indicating severe disease. A broad-spectrum β-lactam, such as co-amoxiclav, and a macrolide antibiotic are usually used. The β-lactam should be given intravenously initially.

Case 36.3

A 4-year-old girl, Miss GR, attends an appointment with her primary care doctor. Her mother explains that Miss GR is complaining of ear pain over the past 2 days. She is systemically well and playing in the consultation room. On examination she is afebrile, but the tympanic membrane is inflamed.

Questions

1. What is the likely diagnosis?
2. Should Miss GR be prescribed antibiotics?

Answers

1. It is likely that Miss GR has otitis media.
2. Immediate antibiotic treatment should not be necessary given that the infection is unilateral and the patient is over 2 years old. However, a delayed prescription could be considered, dated for 2 days after the consultation if the girl has not improved. Amoxicillin for 7 days would be a reasonable choice. The dose would depend on the patient's weight.

Case 36.4

A 30-year-old man, Mr SH, is found collapsed at home. He had complained of a sore throat over the past few days. On arrival at hospital, Mr SH is pyrexial (38.5 °C), hypotensive with a blood pressure of 80/50 mmHg and tachycardic with a heart rate of 130 beats/min.

Questions

1. What is the likely diagnosis?
2. What antibiotics should be prescribed for Mr SH?
3. What other treatments could be considered?

Answers

1. Invasive group A streptococcal infection seems the most likely diagnosis based on the clinical presentation.
2. A β-lactam antibiotic, for example, amoxicillin 1 g three times a day i.v. and clindamycin up to 1200 mg four times a day depending on weight, would be the usual therapy for a severe group A streptococcal infection. Because the patient has presented in septic shock, a broader-spectrum combination such as piperacillin and tazobactam and clindamycin would be used until the causative organism had been identified. The clindamycin could be stopped once the patient has stabilised, usually after 48–72 hours.
   If a group A streptococcus is isolated from clinical samples, the therapy can be rationalised to amoxicillin. Amoxicillin would usually be given for 10 days, but this could be switched to oral therapy once the patient has been afebrile for 24 hours, his haemodynamic parameters have returned to normal, and his inflammatory markers are falling.
3. Intravenous immunoglobulin has been used in group A streptococcal infection causing toxic shock. A single dose of 2 g/kg should be prescribed.

Case 36.5

A 72-year-old man, Mr AD, with a known history of COPD presents at the hospital emergency department with increasing breathlessness. Mr AD has a productive cough of cream-coloured sputum, which is normal for him. He has not noticed an increase in purulence or volume. Chest X-ray showed hyperinflated lungs but no focal consolidation, and a diagnosis of acute exacerbation of COPD was made.

Questions

1. Does Mr AD require antibiotics?
2. What investigations would inform the diagnosis?

Answers

1. Many exacerbations of COPD are non-infective. Therefore, antibiotics should be reserved for when sputum has become more purulent.
2. The diagnosis of an exacerbation of COPD is clinical. Sputum cultures should only be performed if antibiotics are required and if the patient is unwell enough to require referral to secondary care or if an initial empirical course of treatment has been ineffective.

Case 36.6

A 7-year-old girl, Miss TL, is seen in the hospital paediatric outpatient clinic for a routine appointment. She is known to have cystic fibrosis and has had several exacerbations in the past which have been treated with flucloxacillin. On this visit, Miss TL is stable, but the report of sputum culture received 2 days after the clinic shows a growth of *P. aeruginosa*.

Questions

1. What treatment should be started?
2. What other options are available?
3. One week later, you receive a telephone call from Miss TL's parents that she has become unwell. They suspect Miss TL has another chest infection. What agents might be appropriate for treating this infection?

Answers

1. Pseudomonas colonisation is associated with more rapid decline in lung function, and therefore decolonisation should be attempted, for example, using ciprofloxacin 20 mg/kg twice a day for 14 days and an inhaled aminoglycoside.
2. Non-pharmacological measures such as physiotherapy should also be included.
3. Combination treatment is usually favoured, depending on individual susceptibility results. This might include a β-lactam antibiotic such as ceftazidime or piperacillin/tazobactam in combination with an aminoglycoside such as tobramycin. In this case, Miss TL became unwell while on the original decolonisation regime; therefore, an alternative regime would be indicated.

Case 36.7

A 4-year-old boy, Master SW, presents with bouts of paroxysmal coughing which often end in vomiting. The previous week, Master SW had been unwell, with coryzal symptoms. Master SW has missed several of his standard vaccinations because his parents were concerned about 'overloading' his immune system.

Questions

1. What is the likely diagnosis?
2. What treatment should Master SW be offered?
3. What public health measures are necessary?

Answers

1. Pertussis should be considered as a possible diagnosis. This could be confirmed by culture or PCR if Master SW has been unwell for less than 2 weeks or by oral fluid IgG testing if he has been unwell for more than 2 weeks.
2. A 3-day course of azithromycin or a 7-day course of erythromycin or clarithromycin is the usual treatment for pertussis.
3. Pertussis is a notifiable disease, and in England, the local health protection team should be informed when the diagnosis is suspected. Because pertussis is highly infectious, Master SW should be excluded from nursery until 5 days after he starts treatment or 21 days after the cough started in line with Public Health England (2016c) guidance.

References

Aalbers, J., O'Brien, K.K., Chan, W.S., et al., 2011. Streptococcal pharyngitis in adults in primary care: a systematic review of the diagnostic accuracy of symptoms and signs and validation of the Centor score. BMC Med. 9 (67). Available at: https://bmcmedicine.biomedcentral.com/articles/10.1186/1741-7015-9-67.

Altamimi, S., Khalil, A., Khalalaiwi, K.A., et al., 2012. Short-term late generation antibiotics versus longer term penicillin for acute streptococcal pharyngitis in children. Cochrane Database Syst. Rev. 2012 (8). https://doi.org/10.1002/14651858.CD004872.pub3. Art. No. CD004872.

British HIV Association, British Association of Sexual Health and HIV, British Infection Society, 2008. UK national guideline for HIV testing, 2008. Available at: http://www.bhiva.org/documents/guidelines/testing/glineshivtest08.pdf.

British Thoracic Society (BTS) Community Acquired Pneumonia in Adults Guideline Group, 2009. Guideline for the management of community acquired pneumonia in adults. Thorax 64 (Suppl. 3). Available at: https://www.brit-thoracic.org.uk/document-library/clinical-information/pneumonia/adult-pneumonia/bts-guidelines-for-the-management-of-community-acquired-pneumonia-in-adults-2009-update/.

British Thoracic Society (BTS) Community Acquired Pneumonia in Children Guideline Group, 2011. Guidelines for the management of community acquired pneumonia in children. Thorax 66 (Suppl. 2). Available at: https://www.brit-thoracic.org.uk/document-library/clinical-information/pneumonia/paediatric-pneumonia/bts-guidelines-for-the-management-of-community-acquired-pneumonia-in-children-update-2011/.

Centor, R.M., Witherspoon, J.M., Dalton, H.P., et al., 1981. The diagnosis of strep throat in adults in the emergency room. Med. Decis. Making 1 (3), 239–246.

Cremers, A., Sprong, T., Schouten, J.A., et al., 2014. Effect of antibiotic streamlining on patient outcome in pneumococcal bacteraemia. J. Antimicrob. Chemother. 69, 2258–2264.

Cystic Fibrosis Trust Antibiotic Working Group, 2009. Antibiotic treatment for cystic fibrosis. Available at: https://www.cysticfibrosis.org.uk/the-work-we-do/clinical-care/consensus-documents.

Cystic Fibrosis Trust Microbiology Laboratory Standards Working Group, 2010. Laboratory standards for processing samples from people with cystic fibrosis. Available at: https://www.cysticfibrosis.org.uk/the-work-we-do/clinical-care/consensus-documents.

Cystic Fibrosis Trust *Mycobacterium abscessus* Infection Control Working Group, 2013. *Mycobacterium abscessus* suggestions for infection prevention and control. Available at: https://www.cysticfibrosis.org.uk/the-work-we-do/clinical-care/consensus-documents.

Department of Health (DH), 2011. High impact interventions: ventilator associated pneumonia. Available at: http://webarchive.nationalarchives.gov.uk/20120118164404/http://hcai.dh.gov.uk/files/2011/03/2011-03-14-HII-Ventilator-Associated-Pneumonia-FINAL.pdf.

Di'Amico, R., Pifferi, S., Torri, V., et al., 2009. Antibiotic prophylaxis to reduce respiratory tract infections and mortality in adults receiving intensive care. Cochrane Database Syst. Rev. 2009 (4). https://doi.org/10.1002/14651858.CD000022.pub3. Art. No. CD000022.

Dobson, J., Whitely, R.J., Pocock, S., et al., 2015. Oseltamivir treatment for influenza in adults: a meta-analysis of randomised controlled trials. Lancet 385, 1729–1737.

Floto, R.A., Olivier, K.N., Saiman, L., et al., 2015. US Cystic Fibrosis Foundation and European Cystic Fibrosis Society consensus recommendations for the management of nontuberculous mycobacteria in individuals with cystic fibrosis. Thorax 71, i1–i22.

Fortanier, A.C., Venekamp, R.P., Boonacker, C.W.B., et al., 2014. Pneumococcal conjugate vaccines for preventing otitis media. Cochrane Database Syst. Rev. 2014 (4). https://doi.org/10.1002/14651858.CD001480.pub4. Art. No. CD001480.

Fraser, D.W., Tsai, T.R., Orenstein, W., et al., 1977. Legionnaires' disease: description of an epidemic of pneumonia. N. Engl. J. Med. 297 (22), 1189–1197.

Gulland, A., 2009. First cases of spread of oseltamivir resistant swine flu between patients are reported in Wales. Br. Med. J. 339, b4975.

Habayeb, H., Sajin, B., Patel, K., et al., 2015. Amoxicillin plus temocillin as an alternative empiric therapy for severe hospital acquired pneumonia: results from a retrospective audit. Eur. J. Clin. Microbiol. Infect. Dis. 34, 1693–1699.

Health Protection Agency, 2012. Guidelines for the public health management of pertussis. Available at: https://www.gov.uk/government/uploads/system/uploads/attachment_data/file/323098/HPA_Guidelines_for_the_Public_Health_Management_of_Pertussis_2012_PB65.01-_Oct_2012.pdf.

Hodkinson, H.M., 1972. Evaluation of a mental test score for assessment of mental impairment in the elderly. Age Aging 1 (4), 233–238.

Jefferson, T., Jones, M., Doshi, P., et al., 2014. Oseltamivir for influenza in adults and children: systematic review of clinical study reports and summary of regulatory comments. Br. Med. J. 348, 2545. Available at: http://www.bmj.com/content/348/bmj.g2545.

Leach, A.J., Morris, P.S., 2006. Antibiotics for the prevention of acute and chronic suppurative otitis media in children. Cochrane Database Syst. Rev. 2006 (4). https://doi.org/10.1002/14651858.CD004401.pub2. Art. No. CD004401.

Martinez, J.A., Horcajada, J.P., Almela, M., et al., 2003. Addition of a macrolide to a β-lactam based empirical antibiotic regimen is associated with lower in-hospital mortality for patients with bacteremic pneumococcal pneumonia. Clin. Infect. Dis. 36 (4), 389–395.

Masterton, R.G., Galloway, A., French, G., et al., 2008. Guidelines for the management of hospital-acquired pneumonia in the UK: Report of the Working Party on Hospital-Acquired Pneumonia of the British Society for Antimicrobial Chemotherapy. J. Antimicrob. Chemother. 62 (1), 5–34.

Moss, R.B., 2001. Administration of aerosolized antibiotics in cystic fibrosis patients. Chest 120 (Suppl. 3), 107S–113S.

National Institute for Health and Care Excellence (NICE), 2008a. Respiratory tract infections (self-limiting): prescribing antibiotics [CG69]. Available at: https://www.nice.org.uk/guidance/cg69.

National Institute for Health and Care Excellence (NICE), 2008b. Oseltamivir, amantadine (review) and zanamivir for the prophylaxis of influenza [TA158]. Available at: https://www.nice.org.uk/guidance/ta158.

National Institute for Health and Care Excellence (NICE), 2009. Oseltamivir, amantadine (review) and zanamivir for the treatment of influenza [TA168]. Available at: https://www.nice.org.uk/guidance/ta168.

National Institute for Health and Care Excellence (NICE), 2010. Chronic obstructive pulmonary disease in over 16s diagnosis and management section 1.3.1 [CG101]. Available at: https://www.nice.org.uk/guidance/cg101.

National Institute for Health and Care Excellence (NICE), 2013a. Clinical knowledge summary: sinusitis. Available at: http://cks.nice.org.uk/sinusitis.

National Institute for Health and Care Excellence (NICE), 2013b. Colistimethate sodium and tobramycin dry powders for inhalation for treating pseudomonas lung infection in cystic fibrosis [TA276]. Available at: https://www.nice.org.uk/guidance/ta276.

National Institute for Health and Care Excellence (NICE), 2014. Pneumonia in adults – diagnosis and management [CG191]. Available at: https://www.nice.org.uk/guidance/cg191.

National Institute for Health and Care Excellence (NICE), 2015a. Common cold. Available at: http://cks.nice.org.uk/common-cold.

National Institute for Health and Care Excellence (NICE), 2015b. Otitis media – acute. Available at: http://cks.nice.org.uk/otitis-media-acute.

National Institute for Health and Care Excellence (NICE), 2015c. Chest infection – adults. Available at: http://cks.nice.org.uk/chest-infections-adult.

National Institute for Health and Care Excellence (NICE), 2015d. Bronchiolitis in children diagnosis and management [NG 9]. Available at: https://www.nice.org.uk/guidance/ng9.

Norhayati, M., Ho, J., Azman, M., 2015. Influenza vaccines for preventing acute otitis media in infants and children. Cochrane Database Syst. Rev. 2015 (3). https://doi.org/10.1002/14651858.CD010089.pub2. Art. No. CD010089.

Pelucchi, C., Grigoryan, L., Galeone, C., ESCMID Sore Throat Guideline Group, et al., 2012. Guideline for the management of acute sore throat. Clin. Microbiol. Infect. 18 (Suppl.), 1–27. Available at: https://www.ncbi.nlm.nih.gov/pubmed/22432746.

Petersen, I., Johnson, A.M., Islam, A., et al., 2007. Protective effects of antibiotics against serious complications of common respiratory tract infections: retrospective cohort study with the UK general practice research database. Br. Med. J. 335, 982. Available at: http://www.bmj.com/content/335/7627/982.

Public Health England, 2013a. Pertussis factsheet for health professionals. Available at: https://www.gov.uk/government/uploads/system/uploads/attachment_data/file/562472/HCW_Factsheet_Pertussis.pdf.

Public Health England, 2013b. Pneumococcal in immunisation against infectious diseases. The Green Book, chapter 25. Available at: https://www.gov.uk/government/uploads/system/uploads/attachment_data/file/596441/green_book_chapter__25.pdf.

Public Health England, 2015a. Antibiotic guardian and antibiotic awareness key messages. Available at: https://www.gov.uk/government/uploads/system/uploads/attachment_data/file/564516/antibiotics_awareness_key_messages.pdf.

Public Health England, 2015b. Influenza in immunisation against infectious diseases. The Green Book, chapter 19. Available at: https://www.gov.uk/government/uploads/system/uploads/attachment_data/file/456568/2904394_Green_Book_Chapter_19_v10_0.pdf.

Public Health England, 2015c. Guidance on the use of antiviral agents for the prophylaxis and treatment of seasonal influenza (2015–2016). Available at: https://www.gov.uk/government/uploads/system/uploads/attachment_data/file/457735/PHE_guidance_antivirals_influenza_2015_to_2016.pdf.

Public Health England, 2015d. Health Protection Report group A streptococcal infections sixth update on seasonal activity 2014/2015. Available at: https://www.gov.uk/government/uploads/system/uploads/attachment_data/file/377520/hpr4414_SF.pdf.

Public Health England, 2015e. Standards for microbiology investigations investigation of throat related specimens. Standards Unit, Microbiology Services. Available at: https://www.gov.uk/government/uploads/system/uploads/attachment_data/file/423204/B_9i9.pdf.

Public Health England, 2015f. Respiratory syncytial virus in immunisation against infectious diseases. The Green Book, chapter 27a. Available at: https://www.gov.uk/government/uploads/system/uploads/attachment_data/file/458469/Green_Book_Chapter_27a_v2_0W.PDF.

Public Health England, 2016a. PHE guidance on use of antiviral agents for the treatment and prophylaxis of seasonal influenza. Available at: https://www.gov.uk/government/uploads/system/uploads/attachment_data/file/580509/PHE_guidance_antivirals_influenza_2016_2017.pdf.

Public Health England, 2016b. Health Protection Report group A streptococcal infections second update on seasonal activity 2015/2016. Available at: https://www.gov.uk/government/uploads/system/uploads/attachment_data/file/508127/hpr1016.pdf.

Public Health England, 2016c. Pertussis in immunisation against infectious diseases. The Green Book, chapter 24. Available at: https://www.gov.uk/government/uploads/system/uploads/attachment_data/file/514363/Pertussis_Green_Book_Chapter_24_Ap2016.pdf.

Public Health England, 2018. Investigation and public health management of people with possible Middle East Respiratory Syndrome Coronavirus (MERS-CoV) infection. Available at: https://www.gov.uk/government/uploads/system/uploads/attachment_data/file/678219/Algorithm_case_Jan2018.pdf.

Shulman, S.T., Bisno, A.L., Clegg, H.W., et al., 2012. Clinical practice guideline for the diagnosis and management of group A streptococcal pharyngitis: 2012 update by the Infectious Diseases Society of America. Available at: https://www.idsociety.org/uploadedFiles/IDSA/Guidelines-Patient_Care/PDF_Library/2012%20Strep%20Guideline.pdf.

Strong, M., Burrows, J., Redgrave, P., 2009. Letters A/H1N1 pandemic. Oseltamivir's adverse events. Br. Med. J. 339, b3249. https://doi.org/10.1136/bmj.b3249.

Venekamp, R.P., Sanders, S.L., Glaziou, P.P., et al., 2015. Antibiotics for acute otitis media in children (Cochrane review). Cochrane Database Syst. Rev. 2015 (6). https://doi.org/10.1002/14651858.CD000219.pub4. Art. No. CD000219.

Wilson, R., Allegra, L., Huchon, G., et al., 2004. Short-term and long-term outcomes of moxifloxacin compared to standard antibiotic treatment in acute exacerbations of chronic bronchitis. Chest 125, 953–964.

Woodhead, M., Blasi, F., Ewig, S., et al., 2011. Joint Taskforce of the European Respiratory Society and European Society for Clinical Microbiology and Infectious Diseases. Guidelines for the management of adult lower respiratory tract infections – full version. Clin. Microbiol. Infect. 17 (Suppl. 6), 1–59. Available at: https://www.ncbi.nlm.nih.gov/pubmed/21951385.

World Health Organization (WHO), 2014. Avian and other zoonotic influenza factsheet. Available at: http://www.who.int/mediacentre/factsheets/avian_influenza/en/.

World Health Organization (WHO), 2017. Middle East respiratory syndrome coronavirus (MERS-CoV) factsheet. Available at: http://www.who.int/mediacentre/factsheets/mers-cov/en/.

Further reading

Bennett, J.E., Dolin, R., Blaser, M.J. (Eds.), 2015. Mandell, Douglas and Bennett's Principles and Practice of Infectious Disease, eighth ed. Elsevier, New York, pp. 748–885.

Kalil, A.C., Meterski, M.L., Klompas, M., et al., 2016. Management of adults with hospital-acquired and ventilator-associated pneumonia: 2016 Clinical Practice Guidelines by the Infectious Diseases Society of America and the American Thoracic Society. Clin. Infect. Dis. 63 (5), e61–e111.

37 Urinary Tract Infections

Neil J. B. Carbarns

Key points

- Urinary tract infection (UTI) is one of the most common complaints seen in general practice, is one of the most common reasons for prescribing antibiotics and accounts for about one-third of hospital-acquired infections.
- *Escherichia coli* is the most frequent pathogen, accounting for more than three-quarters of community-acquired UTIs.
- Antimicrobial sensitivity patterns are changing. *E. coli* and other bacteria are becoming increasingly resistant to amoxicillin, cephalosporins, trimethoprim and the quinolones, both in healthcare-related and community-acquired infection.
- Symptoms are variable; many UTIs are asymptomatic and some present atypically, particularly in children and the elderly.
- The concept of significant bacteriuria (at least 100,000 organisms/mL of urine) is generally used to distinguish between contamination and infection, but fewer organisms than this can still cause symptoms and disease. One-third of young women with cystitis have lower counts.
- Asymptomatic UTI should be treated in children and pregnant women, but first it should be confirmed by having two urine cultures with significant numbers of the same pathogen. Treatment options are reduced because some antibiotics are contraindicated in these patient groups.
- Catheter-related UTI should be treated only when the patient has systemic evidence of infection.
- A 3-day treatment course is usually sufficient in uncomplicated lower UTI in women. Longer, 7- to 14-day courses are recommended for men, children and pregnant women.
- Although it is not always necessary to send urine samples for laboratory analysis unless empirical treatment fails, they provide local epidemiology and antibiotic resistance data. Urine dipsticks for pyuria and bacteriuria are useful screening tests.
- Antibiotic prophylaxis may be beneficial in women with recurrent UTIs and in children with structural or functional abnormalities. Non-antimicrobial prevention measures include probiotics and cranberry products.

The term urinary tract infection (UTI) usually refers to the presence of organisms in the urinary tract together with symptoms, and sometimes signs, of inflammation. However, it is more precise to use one of the following terms.

- *Significant bacteriuria:* defined as the presence of at least 100,000 bacteria/mL urine. A quantitative definition such as this is needed because small numbers of bacteria are normally found in the anterior urethra and may be washed out into urine samples. Counts of fewer than 100 bacteria/mL are normally considered to be urethral contaminants unless there are exceptional clinical circumstances, such as a sick immunosuppressed patient.
- *Asymptomatic bacteriuria:* significant bacteriuria in the absence of symptoms in the patient.
- *Cystitis:* a syndrome of frequency, dysuria and urgency, sometimes with suprapubic tenderness, which usually suggests infection restricted to the lower urinary tract, that is, the bladder and urethra.
- *Urethral syndrome:* a syndrome of frequency and dysuria in the absence of significant bacteriuria with a conventional pathogen.
- *Acute pyelonephritis:* an acute infection of one or both kidneys with flank pain, tenderness and fever. Usually, the lower urinary tract is also involved.
- *Chronic pyelonephritis:* a potentially confusing term used in different ways. It can refer to continuous excretion of bacteria from the kidney, to frequent, recurring infection of the renal tissue or to a particular type of pathology of the kidney seen microscopically or by radiographic imaging, which may or may not be caused by infection. Although chronic infections of renal tissue are relatively rare, they do occur in the presence of kidney stones and in tuberculosis.
- *Relapse and reinfection:* relapse is recurrence of a UTI caused by the same organism that caused the original infection. Reinfection is recurrence caused by a different organism and is, therefore, a new infection.
- *Urosepsis:* includes clinical evidence of UTI with two or more criteria of a systemic inflammatory response, for example, abnormal temperature, white blood cell count, heart rate or respiratory rate.

Epidemiology

UTIs are among the most common infectious diseases occurring in either the community or healthcare setting. Uncomplicated UTIs typically occur in healthy adult non-pregnant women, whereas complicated UTIs are found in either sex and at any age, frequently associated with structural or functional urinary tract abnormalities.

Infants

UTI is a problem in all age groups, although its prevalence varies markedly. In infants up to 6 months of age, symptomatic UTI has a prevalence of about 2 cases per 1000 and is much more common in boys than in girls. In addition to these cases, asymptomatic UTI is much more common than this, occurring in around 2% of boys in their first few months of life.

Children

In preschool children, UTIs become more common and the sex ratio reverses, such that the prevalence rate is 5% in girls and 0.5% in boys. In older children, the prevalence of bacteriuria falls to 1.2% among girls and 0.03% among boys. Overall, about 3–5% of girls and 1–2% of boys will experience a symptomatic UTI during childhood. However, in girls, about two-thirds of UTIs are asymptomatic. The occurrence of bacteriuria during childhood appears to correlate with a higher incidence of bacteriuria in adulthood.

Adults

When women reach adulthood, the prevalence of bacteriuria rises to between 3% and 5%. Each year, about a quarter of these women with bacteriuria clear their infections spontaneously and are replaced by an equal number of newly infected women, who are often those with a history of previous infections. On average, about 10% of adult women have a symptomatic UTI each year, and more than half of adult women report that they have had a symptomatic UTI at some time. Two to five percent of women have recurrent UTIs, with the peak age of incidence in their early 20s and with a genetic predisposition. UTI is uncommon in young healthy men, with 0.5% of adult men having bacteriuria. Structural or functional abnormality is associated with UTI in men. The rate of symptomatic UTI in men rises progressively with age, from 1% annually at age 18 to 4% at age 60 years.

Elderly

In the elderly of both sexes, the prevalence of bacteriuria increases dramatically, reaching at least 20% among women and 10% among men. Asymptomatic bacteriuria in older persons does not seem to have any harmful effects, and there is no evidence that treating it is beneficial, including no decrease in urinary incontinence. Therefore, routine treatment of asymptomatic bacteriuria in older persons is not indicated (Nicolle, 2009).

Aetiology and risk factors

More than 95% of uncomplicated UTIs are caused by a single bacterial species. In acute uncomplicated UTI acquired in the community, *Escherichia coli* is by far the most common causative bacterium, being responsible for about 80% of infections. The remaining 20% are caused by other Gram-negative enteric bacteria such as *Klebsiella* and *Proteus* species, and by Gram-positive cocci, particularly enterococci and *Staphylococcus saprophyticus*. The latter organism is almost entirely restricted to infections in young, sexually active women.

Recurrent and complicated UTIs associated with underlying structural abnormalities, such as congenital anomalies, neurogenic bladder and obstructive uropathy, are often caused by more resistant organisms such as *Pseudomonas aeruginosa*, *Enterobacter* and *Serratia* species. In complicated UTI there is an increased rate of isolation of multiple organisms. Organisms such as these are also more commonly implicated in hospital-acquired urinary infections, including those in patients with poor urinary catheter care, which are an important source of cross-infection.

Rare causes of urinary infection, nearly always in association with structural abnormalities or catheterisation, include anaerobic bacteria and fungi. Urinary tract tuberculosis is an infrequent but important diagnosis that may be missed through lack of clinical suspicion. A number of viruses are excreted in urine and may be detected by culture or nucleic acid amplification methods, but symptomatic infection is confined to immunocompromised patients, particularly children following peripheral blood stem cell transplant, in whom adenoviruses and polyomaviruses such as BK virus are associated with haemorrhagic cystitis.

In hospitals, a major predisposing cause of UTI is urinary catheterisation. With time, even with closed drainage systems and scrupulous hygiene, bacteria can be found in almost all catheters, and this is a risk of the development of symptomatic infection.

Pathogenesis

There are three possible routes by which organisms might reach the urinary tract: the ascending, blood-borne and lymphatic routes. There is little evidence for the last route in humans. Blood-borne spread to the kidney can occur in bacteraemic illnesses, most notably *Staphylococcus aureus* septicaemia, but by far the most frequent route is the ascending route.

In women, UTI is preceded by colonisation of the vagina, perineum and periurethral area by the pathogen, which then ascends into the bladder via the urethra. Uropathogens colonise the urethral opening of men and women. That the urethra in women is shorter than in men and the urethral meatus is closer to the anus are probably important factors in explaining the preponderance of UTI in females. Further, sexual intercourse appears to be important in forcing bacteria into the female bladder, and this risk is increased by the use of diaphragms and spermicides, which have both been shown to increase *E. coli* growth in the vagina. Whether circumcision reduces the risk of infection in adult men is not known, but it markedly reduces the risk of UTI in male infants.

Organism

E. coli causes most UTIs, and although there are many serotypes of this organism, only a few of these are responsible for a disproportionate number of infections. Although there are as yet no molecular markers that uniquely identify uropathogenic *E. coli*, some strains possess certain virulence factors that enhance their ability to cause infection, particularly infections of the upper urinary tract. Recognised factors include bacterial surface structures called P-fimbriae, which mediate adherence to glycolipid receptors on renal epithelial cells, possession of the iron-scavenging aerobactin system, and increased amounts of capsular K antigen, which mediates resistance to phagocytosis.

Host

Although many bacteria can readily grow in urine, and Louis Pasteur used urine as a bacterial culture medium in his early experiments, the high urea concentration and extremes of osmolality and pH inhibit growth. Other defence mechanisms include the flushing mechanism of bladder emptying, because small numbers of bacteria finding their way into the bladder are likely to be eliminated when the bladder is emptied. Moreover, the bladder mucosa, by virtue of a surface glycosaminoglycan, is intrinsically resistant to bacterial adherence. Presumably, in sufficient numbers, bacteria with strong adhesive properties can overcome this defence. Finally, when the bladder is infected, white blood cells are mobilised to the bladder surface to ingest and destroy invading bacteria. The role of humoral antibody-mediated immunity in defence against infection of the urinary tract remains unclear. Genetic susceptibility of individual patients to UTI has been reviewed (Lichtenberger and Hooton, 2008).

Abnormalities of the urinary tract

Any structural abnormality leading to the obstruction of urinary flow increases the likelihood of infection. Such abnormalities include congenital anomalies of the ureter or urethra, renal stones and, in men, enlargement of the prostate. Renal stones can become infected with bacteria, particularly *Proteus* and *Klebsiella* species, and thereby become a source of 'relapsing' infection. Vesicoureteric reflux is a condition caused by failure of physiological valves at the junction of the ureters and the bladder which allows urine to reflux towards the kidneys when the bladder contracts. It is probable that vesicoureteric reflux plays an important role in childhood UTIs that lead to chronic renal damage (scarring) and persistence of infection. If there is a diminished ability to empty the bladder such as that due to spinal cord injury, there is an increased risk of bacteriuria.

Clinical manifestations

Most UTIs are asymptomatic. Symptoms, when they do occur, are principally the result of irritation of the bladder and urethral mucosa. However, the clinical features of UTI are extremely variable and to some extent depend on the age of the patient.

Infants

Infections in newborns and infants are often overlooked or misdiagnosed because the signs may not be referable to the urinary tract. Common but non-specific presenting symptoms include failure to thrive, vomiting, fever, diarrhoea and apathy. Further, confirmation may be difficult because of problems in obtaining adequate specimens. UTI in infancy and childhood is a major risk factor for the development of renal scarring, which in turn is associated with future complications such as chronic pyelonephritis in adulthood, hypertension and renal failure. It is therefore vital to make the diagnosis early, and any child with a suspected UTI should receive urgent expert assessment.

Children

Children older than 2 years with UTI are more likely to present with some of the classic symptoms such as frequency, dysuria and haematuria. However, some children present with acute abdominal pain and vomiting, and this may be so marked as to raise suspicions of appendicitis or other intra-abdominal pathology. Again, however, it is extremely important that the diagnosis of UTI is made promptly to pre-empt the potential long-term consequences. National guidance has been published in the UK on paediatric UTIs to promote a more consistent clinical practice by ensuring prompt, accurate diagnosis and appropriate management (National Institute for Health and Care Excellence [NICE], 2007). A key feature of the guidance is that children with unexplained fever should have their urine tested within 24 hours and attention is given to avoiding over- or under-diagnosis, appropriate investigation and the prompt start of antibiotic treatment.

Adults

In adults, the typical symptoms of lower UTI include frequency, dysuria, urgency and haematuria. Acute pyelonephritis (upper UTI) usually causes fever, rigors and loin pain in addition to lower tract symptoms. Systemic symptoms may vary from insignificant to extreme malaise. Importantly, untreated cystitis in adults rarely progresses to pyelonephritis, and bacteriuria does not seem to carry the adverse long-term consequences that it does in children.

In about 40% of women with dysuria, urgency and frequency, the urine sample contains fewer than 100,000 bacteria/mL. These patients are said to have the urethral syndrome. Some have a true bacterial infection but with relatively low counts (100–1000 bacteria/mL). Some have urethral infection with *Chlamydia trachomatis*, *Neisseria gonorrhoeae*, mycoplasmas or other 'fastidious' organisms, any of which might give rise to symptoms indistinguishable from those of cystitis. In others, no known cause can be found by conventional laboratory techniques. It is important to consider the possibility of urinary tract tuberculosis, because special methods are necessary for its detection. Sometimes the symptoms are of non-infectious origin, such as menopausal oestrogen deficiency or allergy. However, most cases of urethral syndrome will respond to standard antibiotic regimens as used for treating confirmed UTI.

Elderly

Although UTI is frequent in the elderly, most cases are asymptomatic, and even when present, symptoms are not diagnostic because frequency, dysuria, hesitancy and incontinence are fairly common in elderly people without infection. Further, there may be non-specific systemic manifestations such as confusion and falls, or alternatively the infection may be the cause of deterioration in pre-existing conditions such as diabetes mellitus or

be appreciated that the MSU is not an infallible guide to the presence or absence of urinary infection. True infections may be associated with low counts, particularly when the urine is very dilute because of excessive fluid intake or where the pathogen is slow growing. Although the quantitative criterion for 'significant' bacteriuria is generally taken as greater than 100,000/mL, in some specific groups, it is less: for men, it is greater than 1000/mL, and for women with symptoms of UTI, it is greater than 100/mL (Scottish Intercollegiate Guidelines Network [SIGN], 2012).

Most genuine infections are caused by one single bacterial species; mixed cultures usually suggest contamination. If a patient is taking an antibiotic when a urine specimen is obtained for culture, growth of bacteria may be inhibited. The laboratory may perform a test to detect antimicrobial substances in the urine, and this may be useful information to clarify circumstances in which the culture is negative but a significant pyuria is present.

Treatment

Although many, and perhaps most, cases clear spontaneously given time, symptomatic UTI usually merits antibiotic treatment to eradicate both symptoms and pathogen. Asymptomatic bacteriuria may or may not need treatment depending upon the circumstances of the individual case. Bacteriuria in children and in pregnant women requires treatment, as does bacteriuria present when surgical manipulation of the urinary tract is to be undertaken, because of the potential complications. On the other hand, in non-pregnant, asymptomatic bacteriuric adults without any obstructive lesion, screening and treatment are probably unwarranted in most circumstances. Unnecessary treatment will lead to selection of resistant organisms and puts patients at risk of adverse drug effects including bowel infection with *Clostridium difficile*, which has been particularly associated with the use of quinolones, cephalosporins and co-amoxiclav. A number of common management problems are summarised in Table 37.1.

Non-specific treatments

Advising patients with UTI to drink a lot of fluids is common practice on the theoretical basis that more infected urine is removed by frequent bladder emptying. This is plausible, although not evidence based. Some clinicians recommend urinary analgesics such as potassium or sodium citrate, which alkalinise the urine, but these should be used as an adjunct to antibiotics. They should not be used in conjunction with nitrofurantoin, which is active only at acidic pH.

Antimicrobial chemotherapy

The principles of antimicrobial treatment of UTI are the same as those of the treatment of any other infection: From a group of suitable drugs chosen on the basis of efficacy, safety and cost, select the agent with the narrowest possible spectrum and administer it for the shortest possible time. In general, there is no evidence that bactericidal antibiotics are superior

Table 37.1 Common management problems with urinary tract infections

Problem	Comments
Asymptomatic infection	Asymptomatic bacteriuria should be treated where there is a risk of serious consequences (e.g. in childhood), where there is renal scarring, and in pregnancy. Otherwise, treatment is not usually required.
Catheter in situ, patient unwell	Systemic symptoms may result from catheter-associated UTI and should respond to antibiotics, although the catheter is likely to remain colonised. Local symptoms such as urgency are more likely to reflect urethral irritation than infection.
Catheter in situ, urine cloudy or smelly	Unless the patient is systemically unwell, antibiotics are unlikely to achieve much and may give rise to resistance. Interventions of uncertain benefit include bladder washouts or a change of catheter.
Penicillin allergy	Clarify 'allergy': vomiting or diarrhoea are not allergic phenomena and do not contraindicate penicillins. Penicillin-induced rash is a contraindication to amoxicillin, but cephalosporins are likely to be tolerated. Penicillin-induced anaphylaxis suggests that all β-lactams should be avoided.
Symptoms of UTI, but no bacteriuria	Exclude urethritis, candidosis, etc. Otherwise, likely to be urethral syndrome, which usually responds to conventional antibiotics.
Bacteriuria, but no pyuria	May suggest contamination. However, pyuria is not invariable in UTI and may be absent particularly in pyelonephritis, pregnancy, neonates, the elderly, and *Proteus* infections.
Pyuria but no bacteriuria	Usually, the patient has started antibiotics before taking the specimen. Rarely, a feature of unusual infections (e.g. anaerobes, tuberculosis).
Urine grows *Candida*	Usually reflects perineal candidosis and contamination. True candiduria is rare and may reflect renal candidosis or systemic infection with candidaemia.
Urine grows two or more organisms	Mixed UTI is unusual; mixed cultures are likely to reflect perineal contamination. A repeat should be sent unless this is impractical (e.g. frail elderly patients), in which case best guess treatment should be instituted if clinically indicated.
Symptoms recur	May represent relapse or reinfection. A repeat urine culture should be performed shortly after treatment.

UTI, Urinary tract infection.

to bacteriostatic agents in treating UTI, except perhaps in relapsing infections. Blood levels of antibiotics appear to be unimportant in the treatment of lower UTI; what matters is the concentration in the urine. However, blood levels probably are important in treating pyelonephritis, which may progress to bacteraemia. Drugs suitable for the oral treatment of cystitis include trimethoprim; the β-lactams, particularly amoxicillin, co-amoxiclav and cefalexin; fluoroquinolones such as ciprofloxacin, norfloxacin and ofloxacin; and nitrofurantoin. Where intravenous administration is required, suitable agents include β-lactams such as amoxicillin and cefuroxime, quinolones, and aminoglycosides such as gentamicin.

In renal failure, it may be difficult to achieve adequate therapeutic concentrations of some drugs in the urine, particularly nitrofurantoin and quinolones. Further, accumulation and toxicity may complicate the use of aminoglycosides. Penicillins and cephalosporins attain satisfactory concentrations and are relatively non-toxic, and are therefore the agents of choice for treating UTI in the presence of renal failure.

Antibiotic resistance

Antimicrobial resistance is a major concern worldwide. The susceptibility profile of commonly isolated uropathogens has been constantly changing. Highly antibiotic-resistant organisms such as *Acinetobacter* and coliform bacteria of many species that produce extended-spectrum β-lactamase (ESBL) enzymes have emerged in recent years. They are particularly of concern as a cause of UTI in community-based patients because oral treatment options are limited. Previously, most ESBL-producing bacteria were hospital-acquired and occurred in specialist units.

ESBL-producing bacteria are clinically important because they produce enzymes that destroy almost all commonly used β-lactams except the carbapenem class, rendering most penicillins and cephalosporins largely useless in clinical practice. Some ESBL enzymes can be inhibited by clavulanic acid, and combinations of an agent containing it, for example, co-amoxiclav, with other oral broad-spectrum β-lactams, for example, cefixime or cefpodoxime, have been used to treat UTIs caused by ESBL-producing *E. coli*. These combinations are unlicensed and their effectiveness is variable.

In addition, many ESBL-producing bacteria are multiresistant to non-β-lactam antibiotics as well, such as quinolones, aminoglycosides and trimethoprim, narrowing treatment options. ESBL *E. coli* is often pathogenic, and a high proportion of infections result in bacteraemia with resultant mortality. Some strains cause outbreaks both in hospitals and in the community. Empirical treatment strategies may need to be reviewed in settings where ESBL-producing strains are prevalent, and it may be considered appropriate to use a carbapenem in seriously ill patients until an infection has been proved not to involve an ESBL producer.

Recently, even more resistant strains have emerged in India and Pakistan, with subsequent transfer to the UK, that carry a gene for a novel New Delhi metallo-β-lactamase-1 that also confers resistance to carbapenems. This *bla*NDM-1 gene was mostly found among *E. coli* and *Klebsiella*, which were highly resistant to all antibiotics except to colistin and tigecycline, which is not effective for UTI because it is chemically unstable in the urinary tract (Kumarasamy et al., 2010).

Uncomplicated lower urinary tract infections

The problem with empirical treatment is that more than 10% of the healthy adult female population would receive an antibiotic each year. The use of antibiotics to this extent in the population has implications for antibiotic resistance, a major focus of public health policy worldwide. This highlights the tension between maximising the benefit for individuals and minimising antibiotic resistance at a population level. Strategies have included diagnostic algorithms to predict more precisely who has a UTI, as well as issuing delayed prescriptions (Mangin, 2010).

Therapeutic decisions should be based on accurate, up-to-date antimicrobial susceptibility patterns. Among almost 2500 *E. coli* isolates in a European multicentre survey, the resistance rates were 30% for amoxicillin, 15% for trimethoprim, 3.4% for co-amoxiclav, 2.3% for ciprofloxacin, 2.1% for cefadroxil and 1.2% for nitrofurantoin (Kahlmeter, 2003). These figures are lower than most routine laboratory data would suggest, but it should be remembered that the experience of diagnostic laboratories is likely to be biased by the overrepresentation of specimens from patients in whom empirical treatment has already failed. It is important to be aware of local variations in sensitivity pattern and to balance the risk of therapeutic failure against the cost of therapy.

Adults

The preference for best guess therapy would seem to be a choice between trimethoprim, an oral cephalosporin such as cefalexin, co-amoxiclav or nitrofurantoin, with the proviso that therapy can be refined once sensitivities are available. The quinolones are best reserved for treatment failures and more difficult infections, because overuse of these important agents is likely to lead to an increase in resistance, as has been seen in countries such as Spain and Portugal. These recommendations are summarised in Table 37.2.

Other drugs that have been used for the treatment of UTI include co-trimoxazole, pivmecillinam, fosfomycin and earlier quinolones such as nalidixic acid. Co-trimoxazole was recognised as a cause of bone marrow suppression and other haematological side effects, and in the UK, its use is greatly restricted. Further, despite superior activity in vitro, there is no convincing evidence that it is clinically superior to trimethoprim alone in the treatment of UTI caused by strains susceptible to both. Pivmecillinam is an oral prodrug that is metabolised to mecillinam, a β-lactam agent with a particularly high affinity for Gram-negative penicillin-binding protein 2 and a low affinity for commonly encountered β-lactamases, and which therefore has theoretical advantages in the treatment of UTI. Pivmecillinam has been extensively used for cystitis in Scandinavian countries, where it does not seem to have led to the development of resistance, and for this reason, there have been calls for wider recognition of its usefulness, particularly for UTI caused by ESBL-producing strains. Fosfomycin is a broad-spectrum antibiotic with pharmacokinetic and pharmacodynamic properties that favour its use for treatment of cystitis

Table 37.2 Oral antibiotics used for lower urinary tract infections

Antibiotic	Dose (adult)	Side effects	Contraindications	Comments
Amoxicillin	250–500 mg three times a day	Nausea, diarrhoea, allergy	Penicillin hypersensitivity	High levels of resistance (>50%) in *Escherichia coli* not used empirically
Co-amoxiclav	375–625 mg three times a day	See amoxicillin	See amoxicillin	Amoxicillin in combination with clavulanic acid
Cefalexin	250–500 mg four times a day	Nausea, diarrhoea, allergy	Cephalosporin hypersensitivity, porphyria	
Trimethoprim	200 mg twice a day	Nausea, pruritus, allergy	Pregnancy, neonates, folate deficiency, porphyria	
Nitrofurantoin	50 mg four times a day	Nausea, allergy, rarely pneumonitis, pulmonary fibrosis, neuropathy	Renal failure, neonates, porphyria, glucose-6-phosphate dehydrogenase deficiency	Modified-release form may be given as 100 mg twice daily; inactive against *Proteus*
Ciprofloxacin	100–500 mg twice a day	Rash, pruritus, tendinitis	Pregnancy, children	Reserve for difficult cases

with a single oral dose (Falagas et al., 2010). Finally, older quinolones such as nalidixic acid and cinoxacin were once widely used, but generally these agents have given ground to the more active fluorinated quinolones.

Duration of treatment

The question of duration of treatment has received much attention. Traditionally, a course of 7–10 days has been advocated, and this is still the recommendation for treating men, in whom the possibility of occult prostatitis should be borne in mind. For women, though, there has been particular emphasis on the suitability of short-course regimens such as 3-day or even single-dose therapy. The consensus of an international expert working group was that 3-day regimens are as effective as longer regimens in the cases of trimethoprim and quinolones. β-Lactams have been inadequately investigated on this point, but short courses are generally less effective than trimethoprim and quinolones, and nitrofurantoin requires further study before definite conclusions can be drawn. Single-dose therapy, with its advantages of cost, adherence and the minimisation of side effects, has been used successfully in many studies but in general is less effective than when the same agent is used for a longer period.

In the urethral syndrome, it is worth trying a 3-day course of one of the agents mentioned earlier. If this fails, a 7-day course of tetracycline could be tried to deal with possible chlamydia or mycoplasma infection.

Children

In children, the risk of renal scarring is such that UTI should be diagnosed and treated promptly, even if asymptomatic. The drugs of choice include β-lactams, trimethoprim and nitrofurantoin. Quinolones are relatively contraindicated in children because of the theoretical risk of causing cartilage and joint problems. Children should be treated for 7–10 days.

Renal scarring occurs in 5–15% of children with UTI, who should be identified so that appropriate treatment can be instituted. Unfortunately, the subgroup at high risk cannot be predicted, and for this reason, many clinicians choose to investigate all children with UTI, for example, using ultrasound and radio-isotope scanning.

Acute pyelonephritis

Patients with pyelonephritis may be severely ill and, if so, will require admission to hospital and initial treatment with a parenteral antibiotic. Suitable agents with good activity against *E. coli* and other Gram-negative bacilli include cephalosporins such as cefuroxime and ceftazidime, some penicillins such as co-amoxiclav, quinolones, and aminoglycosides such as gentamicin (Table 37.3). A first-choice agent would be parenteral cefuroxime, gentamicin or ciprofloxacin. When the patient is improving, the route of administration may be switched to oral therapy, typically using a quinolone. Conventionally, treatment is continued for 10–14 days, although shorter courses of 7 days have been proven effective in patients who are less severely ill at the outset.

In hospital-acquired pyelonephritis, there is a risk that the infecting organism may be resistant to the usual first-line drugs. In such cases it may be advisable to start a broad-spectrum agent such as ceftazidime, ciprofloxacin or meropenem.

Relapsing urinary tract infection

The main causes of persistent relapsing UTI are renal infection, structural abnormalities of the urinary tract and, in men, chronic prostatitis. Patients who do not respond positively on a 7- to 10-day course should be given a 2-week course, and if that fails, a 6-week course can be considered. Structural abnormalities may need surgical correction before a cure can be maintained. It is essential that prolonged courses (i.e. >4 weeks) are managed

Table 37.3 Parenteral antibiotics used for pyelonephritis

Antibiotic	Dose (adult)	Side effects	Contraindications	Comments
Cefuroxime	750 mg three times a day	Nausea, diarrhoea, allergy	Cephalosporin hypersensitivity, porphyria	Implicated in *Clostridium difficile* diarrhoea
Ceftazidime	1 g three times a day	See cefuroxime	See cefuroxime	See cefuroxime
Co-amoxiclav	1.2 g three times a day	Nausea, diarrhoea, allergy	Penicillin hypersensitivity	
Gentamicin	80–120 mg three times a day or 5 mg/kg once daily	Nephrotoxicity, ototoxicity	Pregnancy, myasthenia gravis	Monitor levels
Ciprofloxacin	200–400 mg twice a day	Rash, pruritus, tendinitis	Pregnancy, children	Implicated in *Clostridium difficile* diarrhoea
Piperacillin with tazobactam	4.5 g three times a day	Nausea, allergy	Penicillin hypersensitivity	
Meropenem	500 mg three times a day	Nausea, rash, convulsions		Reserve for multiresistant cases

under bacteriological control, for example, with monthly cultures. In men with prostate gland infection, it is appropriate to select antibiotics with good tissue penetration such as trimethoprim and the fluoroquinolones.

Catheter-associated infections

In most large hospitals, 10–15% of patients have an indwelling urinary catheter. Even with the very best catheter care, most will have infected urine after 10–14 days of catheterisation, although most of these infections will be asymptomatic. Antibiotic treatment will often appear to eradicate the infecting organism, but as long as the catheter remains in place, the organism, or another more resistant one, will quickly return. The principles of antibiotic therapy for catheter-associated UTI are therefore as follows:
• Do not treat asymptomatic infection.
• If possible, remove the catheter before treating symptomatic infection.

Although it often prompts investigation, cloudy or strong-smelling urine is not *per se* an indication for antimicrobial therapy. In these situations, saline or antiseptic bladder washouts are often performed, but there is little evidence that they make a difference. Similarly, encrusted catheters are often changed on aesthetic grounds, but it is not known whether this reduces the likelihood of future symptoms.

Following catheter removal, bacteriuria may resolve spontaneously, but more often it persists (typically for longer than 2 weeks in more than half of patients) and may become symptomatic, although usually it will respond well to short-course treatment.

Antimicrobial catheters

Several different types of novel catheters with anti-infective properties have been developed with the aim of reducing the ability of bacteria to adhere to the material, which should lead to a decreased incidence of bacteriuria and symptomatic infection. Several studies of the effect of incorporating antibiotics such as rifampicin and minocycline or silver-based alloys into the catheter have shown benefit. Although clearly more costly than standard catheters, economic evaluation shows silver alloy catheters to be cost efficient when used in patients who need catheterisation for several days. The effect of these catheters on clinical outcomes such as bacteraemia remains to be determined.

Bacteriuria of pregnancy

The prevalence rate of asymptomatic bacteriuria of pregnancy is about 5%, and about a third of these women proceed to development of acute pyelonephritis, with its attendant consequences for the health of both mother and pregnancy. Further, there is evidence that asymptomatic bacteriuria is associated with low birth weight, prematurity, hypertension and pre-eclampsia. For these reasons, it is recommended that screening be carried out, preferably by culture of a properly taken MSU, which should be repeated if positive for confirmation (NICE, 2008).

Rigorous meta-analysis of published trials has shown that antibiotic treatment of bacteriuria in pregnancy is effective at clearing bacteriuria, reducing the incidence of pyelonephritis and reducing the risk of preterm delivery. The drugs of choice are amoxicillin or cefalexin or nitrofurantoin, depending on the sensitivity profile of the infecting organism. Co-amoxiclav is cautioned in pregnancy because of relative lack of clinical experience in pregnant women. Trimethoprim is contraindicated without folate supplementation (particularly in the first trimester) because of its theoretical risk of causing neural tube defects through folate antagonism. Nitrofurantoin should be avoided close to the time of expected delivery because of a risk of haemolysis in the baby. Ciprofloxacin is contraindicated because it may affect the growing joints. There are insufficient data concerning short-course therapy in pregnancy, and 7 days of treatment remains the standard. Patients should be followed up for the duration of the pregnancy to confirm cure and to ensure that any reinfection is promptly addressed.

Prevention and prophylaxis

There are a number of folklore and naturopathic recommendations for the prevention of UTI. Most of these have not been put to statistical study, but at least they are unlikely to cause harm.

Cranberry juice

Cranberry juice (*Vaccinium macrocarpon*) has long been thought to be beneficial in preventing UTI, and this has been studied in a number of clinical trials. Cranberry is thought to inhibit adhesion of bacteria to urinary tract cells on the surface of the bladder. In sexually active women, a daily intake of 750 mL of cranberry juice was associated with a 40% reduction in the risk of symptomatic UTI in a double-blinded 12-month trial. Many studies have been criticised for methodological flaws, and currently there is only limited evidence that cranberry juice is effective at preventing recurrent UTI. There have been no randomised controlled trials of the use of cranberry products (juice, tablets or capsules) in the treatment of established infection, or comparing it with established therapies such as antibiotics for preventing infection. In spite of the suggestive in vitro data and early reviews that suggested a benefit of cranberry for UTI, recent meta-analyses are conflicting in their support of its efficacy. A Cochrane review of 24 studies concluded that there was only a slight but nonsignificant reduction in the occurrence of symptomatic UTI overall (Jepson et al., 2012). However, another review of 13 studies concluded that cranberry-containing products are associated with a protective effect against UTIs (Wang et al., 2012).

A hypothetical benefit in using cranberry instead of antibiotics for this purpose is a reduced risk of the development of antibiotic-resistant bacteria. A significant hazard is an interaction of cranberry with warfarin, with a risk of bleeding episodes, and available products are not available in standardised formulations. Further, cranberry juice is unpalatable unless sweetened with sugar and therefore carries a risk of tooth decay, although ironically it is reported to prevent dental caries by blocking adherence of plaque bacteria to teeth.

Antibiotic prophylaxis

In some patients, mainly women, reinfections are so frequent that long-term antimicrobial prophylaxis with specific antibiotics is indicated. If the reinfections are clearly related to sexual intercourse, then a single dose of an antibiotic after intercourse is appropriate. In other cases, long-term, low-dose prophylaxis may be beneficial. One dose of trimethoprim (100 mg) or nitrofurantoin (50 mg) at night will suffice. These drugs are unlikely to lead to the emergence of resistant bacteria, although breakthrough infection with strains intrinsically resistant to the chosen prophylactic antibiotic is possible.

Children

In children, recurrence of UTI is common and the complications potentially hazardous, so many clinicians recommend antimicrobial prophylaxis following documented infection. The evidence in favour of this practice is not strong, and although it has been shown to reduce the incidence of bacteriuria, there is no good-quality evidence that prophylactic antibiotics are effective in preventing further symptomatic UTIs, and they have not been shown to reduce the incidence of renal scarring complications, which are the most important outcomes for the patient (Mori et al., 2009). Further, important variables remain to be clarified, such as when to begin prophylaxis, which agent to use and when to stop. Guidelines have abandoned the time-honoured recommendation for routine antibiotic prophylaxis following a first infection, although it may be considered when there is recurrent UTI (NICE, 2007).

Although evidence is limited for some recommendations, there are many common-sense general measures aimed at reducing the risk of recurrence of infection, particularly in girls. They include advice on regular bladder emptying, cleaning the perineal/anal area from front to back after urinating, treating constipation adequately and avoiding both bubble baths and washing the hair in the bath.

Case studies

Case 37.1

Mr FG, a 70-year-old man, has consulted his primary care doctor three times in the past 3 months and seems to have the same *E. coli* infection on each occasion. A short course of antibiotics clears up the symptoms, but a clinical relapse is soon apparent. Mr FG is admitted to hospital for transurethral resection of the prostate and 2 days after the operation he becomes unwell with rigors, fever and loin pain. Microscopy of his urine shows more than 200 white cells/mm³. Blood cultures are taken and rapidly become positive, with Gram-negative bacilli seen on microscopy.

Questions

1. Is there any way of predicting which UTIs are likely to go on to cause further problems such as pyelonephritis or prostatitis?
2. What antibiotic therapy is indicated now?

Answers

1. Progression of a simple UTI is much more common in patients other than young women. Foreign bodies such as catheters and stents, or physiological problems such as neurogenic bladder increase the risk of a complicated UTI. In men, persistent or recurrent infection with the same organism is highly suggestive of prostatitis and should prompt an extended course of treatment. Pyelonephritis is more difficult to predict. Frequency, dysuria and haematuria indicate lower tract infection. Fever, vomiting, rigors and flank pain are more suggestive of upper renal tract involvement.

2. Mr FG should be started on intravenous antibiotic therapy for presumed prostatitis or pyelonephritis and consequent bacteraemia. The antibiotic should cover Gram-negative organisms found in the hospital environment such as *Klebsiella*, *Enterobacter* and *Pseudomonas*. Appropriate agents would be piperacillin-tazobactam, ceftazidime, ciprofloxacin or meropenem. An alternative would be an aminoglycoside such as gentamicin, provided the patient has satisfactory renal function.

Case 37.2

A pregnant woman, Ms SL, aged 26 years is found to have bacteriuria at her first antenatal visit. No white or red cells are seen in her urine. Urine culture demonstrates *E. coli* at a count of more than 100,000 bacteria/mL, sensitive to trimethoprim, nitrofurantoin and cefalexin, but resistant to amoxicillin. Other than a degree of urinary frequency, which Ms SL ascribes to the pregnancy itself, the patient does not complain of any urinary symptoms.

Question

Does Ms SL need antibiotic treatment, and if so, which medicines could be safely prescribed?

Answer

Ms SL may be correct that her urinary frequency is a consequence of pregnancy. However, because of the consequences of untreated infection during pregnancy, even asymptomatic bacteriuria should be treated. A repeat urine specimen should be obtained to confirm the persistent finding of more than 100,000 bacteria/mL, and treatment started with either cefalexin or co-amoxiclav for 7 days. Trimethoprim should be avoided during early pregnancy because of its theoretical risk of teratogenicity, and nitrofurantoin should be avoided in late pregnancy because it may cause neonatal haemolysis. Following treatment, Ms SL should be reviewed throughout the pregnancy to ensure eradication of the bacteriuria and to permit early treatment of any relapse or reinfection.

Case 37.3

A 2-year-old boy is admitted to hospital with vomiting and abdominal pain. His mother reports that he was treated for a UTI 6 months previously but was not investigated further at the time. A clean-catch urine sample shows more than 50 white cells/mm³, and bacteria are seen on microscopy.

Question

What action should be taken?

Answer

It seems that this child is suffering from a recurrent UTI. An intravenous antibiotic such as cefuroxime should be started, because the child will not tolerate oral antibiotics at present. If the organism proves to be sensitive to amoxicillin, the treatment could be changed accordingly. Further investigations, for example, ultrasonography and radioisotope scan, may be carried out to determine any underlying cause of the infection and to look for already established renal scarring. The child may require long-term prophylaxis to prevent a further recurrence.

Case 37.4

Mrs EH, a 62-year-old woman, has been troubled by recurrent symptoms of UTI. She has been taking an oral oestrogen preparation for menopausal symptoms for some years. She is currently on an orthopaedic ward and catheterised because of incontinence. Mrs EH is afebrile but has been confused since her hip replacement 5 days earlier; she remains on cefuroxime, which was started as prophylaxis at the time of the operation. The urine in her catheter bag is cloudy, has a high white cell count and grows *Enterococcus faecalis* sensitive to amoxicillin but resistant to cephalosporins.

Questions

1. How should Mrs EH be managed?
2. In older women, is there any association with the use of different types of oestrogen delivery systems and UTIs?

Answers

1. Mrs EH's confusion may have a number of causes, including her recent surgery, sleep disturbance, drug toxicity, deep venous thrombosis or infection. If, following clinical examination and investigation, which should include blood cultures, her catheter-associated infection is thought to be contributing to her systemic problems, it should be treated with amoxicillin. If possible, the catheter should be removed, even if this is inconvenient for the nursing staff. Unless it has been prescribed for another indication, the cefuroxime is achieving nothing and may be stopped.
2. In post-menopausal women, there have been trials assessing the merits of topical oestrogen creams. Topical intravaginal oestriol cream has significant benefits in reducing the number of UTIs in those suffering recurrent infections. In a placebo-controlled trial, the rate of UTI was 12-fold less in the group receiving active oestrogen cream. This effect is not seen with oral oestrogens (Perrotta et al., 2008).

Case 37.5

Ms MD, a 45-year-old woman, suffers from recurrent episodes of cystitis. Examination is unremarkable. On the occasions when a specimen has been sent, the urine has contained few white cells and no significant growth of organisms.

Question

How should the patient be managed?

Answer

Ms MD is suffering from the urethral syndrome, in which symptoms of infection are not associated with objective evidence of UTI. It may be felt necessary to investigate her to exclude less common causes of UTI such as herpes simplex virus, *Chlamydia trachomatis*, *Neisseria gonorrhoeae*, *Gardnerella vaginalis*, *Mycoplasma hominis* and *Lactobacilli*. Otherwise, her symptoms are likely to respond to conventional courses of antibiotics. Consider non-infective causes, for example, psychological factors or trauma from intercourse.

Case 37.6

Ms LT, a 23-year-old woman, has recurrent symptoms of UTI temporally related to sexual intercourse, despite following advice to empty her bladder as soon as possible after sex.

Question

What do you think of the use of antibiotics such as trimethoprim for women who get recurrent problems after sexual intercourse?

Answer

Post-coital voiding does not have any prospective data to support it, but it is a simple, harmless intervention. Long-term continuous antimicrobial prophylaxis is unquestionably an effective treatment but may be overtreating those in whom UTIs follow intercourse. Post-coital prophylaxis, a single dose within 2 hours of intercourse, has the advantage of using less antibiotic overall. One small, placebo-controlled, double-blind trial assessed the efficacy of post-coital co-trimoxazole in preventing recurrent UTI and found that 12% of the active treatment patients developed a UTI in 6 months, compared with 82% of the control group. Other studies have shown nitrofurantoin, cefalexin and ciprofloxacin also to be effective.

Case 37.7

A 45-year-old woman, Mrs DG, was hospitalised in India a few weeks ago while undergoing cosmetic surgery. She now has severe symptoms of UTI and is admitted to hospital with a diagnosis of 'urosepsis'.

Question

What particular consideration is there in relation to the potential for Mrs DG's UTI to be an antibiotic-resistant strain?

Answer

Hospitalised patients in a number of countries are at risk of becoming colonised with coliform bacteria that are extremely resistant to commonly used antibiotics, as well as to those that are often used empirically for patients with sepsis. In the Indian subcontinent there have been particular problems with strains that are resistant to the carbapenem class of antibiotics such as meropenem, because the bacteria produce a transmissible hydrolyzing carbapenemase enzyme. Such strains are usually resistant to virtually all classes of antibiotics and it may be necessary to administer intravenous combination therapy including colistin or fosfomycin. Patients who have been hospitalised in areas where such resistant strains are prevalent should be screened for potential carriage of the organism if readmitted to hospital so that assiduous infection control precautions can be implemented.

References

Falagas, M.E., Vouloumanou, E.K., Togias, A.G., et al., 2010. Fosfomycin versus other antibiotics for the treatment of cystitis: a meta-analysis of randomized controlled trials. J. Antimicrob. Chemother. 65, 1862–1877.

Gopal Rao, G., Patel, M., 2009. Urinary tract infection in hospitalized elderly patients in the United Kingdom: the importance of making an accurate diagnosis in the post broad-spectrum antibiotic era. J. Antimicrob. Chemother. 63, 5–6.

Jepson, R.G., Williams, G., Craig, J.C., 2012. Cranberries for preventing urinary tract infections. Cochrane Database Syst. Rev. 2012 (10), CD001321. https://doi.org/10.1002/14651858.CD001321.pub5.

Kahlmeter, G., 2003. An international survey of the antimicrobial susceptibility of pathogens from uncomplicated urinary tract infections: the ECO SENS Project. J. Antimicrob. Chemother. 51, 59–76.

Kumarasamy, K.K., Toleman, M.A., Walsh, T.R., et al., 2010. Emergence of a new antibiotic resistance mechanism in India, Pakistan, and the UK: a molecular, biological, and epidemiological study. Lancet Infect. Dis. 10, 597–602.

Lichtenberger, P., Hooton, T.M., 2008. Complicated urinary tract infections. Curr. Infect. Dis. Rep. 10, 499–504.

Mangin, D., 2010. Urinary tract infection in primary care. Br. Med. J. 340, 373–374.

Mori, R., Fitzgerald, A., Williams, C., et al., 2009. Antibiotic prophylaxis for children at risk of developing a urinary tract infection: a systematic review. Acta Paediatrica. 98, 1781–1786.

National Institute for Health and Care Excellence (NICE), 2007. Urinary tract infection in children: diagnosis, treatment and long-term management. NICE, London. Available at: http://www.nice.org.uk/nicemedia/pdf/CG54fullguideline.pdf.

National Institute for Health and Care Excellence (NICE), 2008. Antenatal care for uncomplicated pregnancies. NICE, London. Available at: http://www.nice.org.uk/guidance/cg62.

Nicolle, L.E., 2009. Urinary tract infections in the elderly. Clin. Geriatr. Med. 25, 423–436.

Perrotta, C., Aznar, M., Mejia, R., et al., 2008. Oestrogens for preventing recurrent urinary tract infection in postmenopausal women. Cochrane Database Syst. Rev. 2008 (2), CD005131. https://doi.org/10.1002/14651858.CD005131.pub2.

Scottish Intercollegiate Guidelines Network (SIGN), 2012. Management of suspected bacterial urinary tract infection in adults. SIGN, Edinburgh. Available at: http://www.sign.ac.uk/guidelines/fulltext/88/index.html.

Wang, C.H., Fang, C.C., Chen, N.C., et al., 2012. Cranberry-containing products for prevention of urinary tract infections in susceptible populations: a systematic review and meta-analysis of randomized controlled trials. Arch. Intern. Med. 172, 988–996.

Further reading

Hooton, T.M., 2015. Nosocomial urinary tract infections. In: Mandell, G.L., Bennett, J.E., Dolin, R. (Eds.), Principles and Practice of Infectious Diseases, eighth ed. Elsevier, London, pp. 3334–3346.

Sobel, J.D., Kaye, D., 2015. Urinary tract infections. In: Mandell, G.L., Bennett, J.E., Dolin, R. (Eds.), Principles and Practice of Infectious Diseases, eighth ed. Elsevier, London, pp. 886–913.

Scottish Medicines Consortium and Scottish Prescribing Advisory Group, 2016. Guidance on management of recurrent urinary tract infection in non-pregnant women. NHS Scotland, Glasgow. Available at: https://www.scottishmedicines.org.uk/files/sapg1/Management_of_recurrent_lower_UTI_in_non-pregnant_women.pdf.

National Institute for Health and Care Excellence, 2015. Urinary tract infections in adults: quality standard QS90. NICE, London. Available at: https://www.nice.org.uk/guidance/qs90.

38 Gastro-Intestinal Infections

Jim Gray

Key points

- There are many different microbial causes of gastro-intestinal infections.
- Gastroenteritis is the most common syndrome of gastro-intestinal infection, but some gastro-intestinal pathogens can cause systemic infections.
- Fluid and electrolyte replacement is the mainstay of management of gastroenteritis.
- Antibiotic resistance in gastro-intestinal pathogens is an escalating problem.
- Most cases of gastroenteritis that occur in developed countries are mild and self-limiting and do not require antibiotic therapy. Unnecessary use of antibiotics simply promotes antibiotic resistance.
- Antibiotic therapy should be considered for patients with underlying conditions that predispose to serious or complicated gastroenteritis, or where termination of faecal excretion of pathogens is desirable to prevent further spread of the infection.
- *Clostridium difficile* is a very important cause of diarrhoea in hospitals. Strict control measures are required; cases are usually initially treated with oral metronidazole or oral vancomycin.
- Fidaxomicin is a new treatment for *C. difficile* that may be associated with a lower recurrence rate. Faecal microbiota transplantation is another treatment option that is becoming mainstream.
- Antibiotic therapy is also essential for life-threatening systemic infections, such as enteric fever.
- Where possible, antibiotic therapy should be delayed until a microbiological diagnosis has been established.

Gastro-intestinal infections represent a major public health and clinical problem worldwide. Many species of bacteria, viruses and protozoa cause gastro-intestinal infection, resulting in two main clinical syndromes. Gastroenteritis is a non-invasive infection of the small or large bowel that manifests clinically as diarrhoea and vomiting. Other infections are invasive, causing systemic illness, often with few gastro-intestinal symptoms. *Helicobacter pylori* and its association with gastritis, peptic ulceration and gastric carcinoma are discussed in Chapter 12.

Epidemiology and aetiology

In Western countries, the average person probably experiences one or two episodes of gastro-intestinal infection each year. Infections are rarely severe, and the vast majority of cases never reach medical attention. Nevertheless, they are of considerable economic importance. In the UK, viruses, especially noroviruses, are the most common cause of gastroenteritis. *Campylobacter*, followed by non-typhoidal serovars of *Salmonella enterica*, are the most common reported causes of bacterial gastroenteritis. Cryptosporidiosis is the most commonly reported parasitic infection. In developing countries, the incidence of gastro-intestinal infection is at least twice as high and the range of common pathogens is much wider. Infections are more often severe and represent a major cause of mortality, especially in children.

Gastro-intestinal infections can be transmitted by consumption of contaminated food or water or by direct faecal–oral spread. Airborne spread of viruses that cause gastroenteritis also occurs. The most important causes of gastro-intestinal infection, and their usual modes of spread, are listed in Table 38.1. In developed countries, the majority of gastro-intestinal infections are food-borne. Farm animals are often colonised by gastro-intestinal pathogens, especially *Salmonella* and *Campylobacter*. Therefore, raw foods such as poultry, meat, eggs and unpasteurised dairy products are commonly contaminated and must be thoroughly cooked to kill such organisms. Raw foods also represent a potential source of cross-contamination of other foods, through hands, surfaces or utensils that have been inadequately cleaned. Food handlers who are excreting pathogens in their faeces can also contaminate food. This is most likely when diarrhoea is present, but continued excretion of pathogens during convalescence also represents a risk. Food handlers are the usual source of *Staphylococcus aureus* food poisoning, where toxin-producing strains of *S. aureus* carried in the nose or on skin are transferred to foods. Bacterial food poisoning is often associated with inadequate cooking and/or prolonged storage of food at ambient temperature before consumption. Water-borne gastro-intestinal infection is primarily a problem in countries without a sanitary water supply or sewerage system, although outbreaks of water-borne cryptosporidiosis occur from time to time in the UK. The spread of pathogens such as *Shigella* or enteropathogenic *Escherichia coli (E.coli)* by the faecal–oral route is favoured by over-crowding and poor standards of personal hygiene. Such infections in developed countries are most common in children and can cause troublesome outbreaks in paediatric wards, nurseries and residential children's homes.

Treatment with broad-spectrum antibiotics alters the bowel flora, creating conditions that favour superinfection with microorganisms (principally *Clostridium difficile*) that can cause diarrhoea. *C. difficile* infection (CDI) may be associated with any

Table 38.1 Important causes of gastro-intestinal infection, their modes of spread and pathogenic mechanisms

Causative agent	Chief mode(s) of spread	Pathogenic mechanisms
Bacteria		
Campylobacter	Food, especially poultry, milk	Mucosal invasion, enterotoxin
Salmonella enterica, non-typhoidal serovars	Food, especially poultry, eggs, meat	Mucosal invasion, enterotoxin
Salmonella enterica serovars Typhi and Paratyphi	Food, water	Systemic invasion
Shigella	Faecal–oral	Mucosal invasion, enterotoxin
Escherichia coli		
Enteropathogenic	Faecal–oral	Mucosal adhesion
Enteroaggregative	Faecal–oral, food	Mucosal toxicity
Enterotoxigenic	Faecal–oral, food, water	Enterotoxin
Enteroinvasive	Faecal–oral, food	Mucosal invasion
Verotoxin-producing	Food, especially meat	Verotoxin
Staphylococcus aureus	Food, especially meats, dairy produce	Emetic toxin
Clostridium perfringens	Food, especially meat	Enterotoxin
Bacillus cereus		
Short incubation period	Food, especially rice	Emetic toxin
Long incubation period	Food, especially meat and vegetable dishes	Enterotoxin
Vibrio cholerae O1, O139	Water	Enterotoxin
Vibrio parahaemolyticus	Seafoods	Mucosal invasion, enterotoxin
Clostridium difficile	Faecal–oral (nosocomial)	Cytotoxin, enterotoxin
Clostridium botulinum	Inadequately heat-treated canned/preserved foods	Neurotoxin
Protozoa		
Giardia lamblia	Water	Mucosal invasion
Cryptosporidium	Water, animal contact	Mucosal invasion
Entamoeba histolytica	Food, water	Mucosal invasion
Viruses		
Rotavirus, norovirus, astrovirus, sapovirus, adenovirus	Food, faecal–oral, respiratory secretions	Small-intestinal mucosal damage

antibiotic, but clindamycin, the cephalosporins and the fluoro-quinolones are most commonly implicated. CDI is most common in patients with serious underlying disease and in the elderly. Although some sporadic cases are probably due to overgrowth of endogenous organisms, person-to-person transmission also occurs in hospitals and care homes, sometimes resulting in large outbreaks.

Pathophysiology

Development of symptoms after ingestion of gastro-intestinal pathogens depends on two factors. First, sufficient organisms must be ingested and then survive host defence mechanisms; and second, the pathogens must possess one or more virulence mechanisms to cause disease.

Host factors

Healthy individuals possess a number of defence mechanisms that protect against infection by enteropathogens. Therefore, large numbers of many pathogens must be ingested for infection to ensue; for example, the infective dose for *Salmonella* is typically around 10^5 organisms. Other species, however, are better able to survive host defence mechanisms; for example, infection with *Shigella* or verotoxin-producing *E. coli* (VTEC) can result from ingestion of fewer than 100 organisms. VTEC (principally *E. coli* O157) are especially important because of the risk of the life-threatening complication haemolytic uraemic syndrome (HUS).

Gastric acidity

Most microorganisms are rapidly killed at normal gastric pH. Patients whose gastric pH is less acidic, as, for example, following treatment with antacids or ulcer-healing drugs, are more susceptible to gastro-intestinal infections. There is a particularly strong association between proton pump inhibitor use and CDI.

Intestinal motility

It is widely held that intestinal motility helps to rid the host of enteric pathogens, and that anti-motility agents are therefore potentially hazardous in patients with infective gastroenteritis. Despite this, self-medication with antidiarrhoeals is commonly practised, and in otherwise healthy individuals is probably safe.

Resident microflora

The resident microflora of the lower gastro-intestinal tract, largely composed of anaerobic bacteria, help to resist colonisation by enteropathogens.

Immune system

Phagocytic, humoral and cell-mediated elements are important in resistance to different pathogens. Individuals with inherited or acquired immunodeficiencies are therefore susceptible to specific gastro-intestinal infections, depending on which components of their immune system are affected.

Organism factors

The first requirement of gastro-intestinal pathogens is that they are able to adhere to the gut wall and colonise the intestine. The symptoms of gastro-intestinal infection can then be mediated by various mechanisms (see Table 38.1).

Toxins

Toxins produced by gastro-intestinal pathogens can be classified as enterotoxins, neurotoxins and cytotoxins. Enterotoxins act on intestinal mucosal cells to cause net loss of fluid and electrolytes. The classic enterotoxin-mediated disease is cholera, the result of infection with toxigenic serotypes of *Vibrio cholerae*. Many other bacteria produce enterotoxins, including enterotoxigenic *E. coli* and *Clostridium perfringens*. The emetic toxins of *S. aureus* and *Bacillus cereus* are neurotoxins that induce vomiting by an action on the central nervous system. The symptoms of botulism are mediated by a neurotoxin that blocks release of acetylcholine at nerve endings. Cytotoxins cause mucosal destruction and inflammation (see later). The pathogenicity of *C. difficile* is mediated by two exotoxins, TcdA and TcdB, both of which are potent cytotoxic enzymes that damage the human colonic mucosa. Verotoxins are potent cytotoxins that cause direct damage to small-vessel endothelial cells, which is exacerbated by stimulation of production of inflammatory mediators by non-endothelial cells. This causes multiorgan microvascular injury, expressed most commonly as haemorrhagic colitis and HUS.

Mucosal damage

Cytotoxins are important in mediating mucosal invasion, but other mechanisms are also involved. Enteropathogenic *E. coli* causes diarrhoea by damaging microvilli when it adheres to the intestinal mucosa. Organisms such as *Shigella* and enteroinvasive *E. coli* express surface proteins that facilitate mucosal invasion. Diarrhoea due to mucosal damage may be caused by reduction in the absorptive surface area or the presence of increased numbers of immature enterocytes which are secretory rather than absorptive.

Systemic invasion

The lipopolysaccharide outer membrane and possession of an antiphagocytic outer capsule are important virulence factors in invasive *Salmonella* infections.

Clinical manifestations

Many cases of gastro-intestinal infection are asymptomatic or cause subclinical illness. Gastroenteritis is the most common syndrome of gastro-intestinal infection, presenting with symptoms such as vomiting, diarrhoea and abdominal pain. The term 'dysentery' is sometimes applied to infections with *Shigella* (bacillary dysentery) and *Entamoeba histolytica* (amoebic dysentery), where severe colonic mucosal inflammation causes frequent diarrhoea with blood and pus. Table 38.2 lists the most important causative agents of gastroenteritis together with a brief description of the typical illness that each causes. However, the symptoms experienced by individuals infected with the same organism can differ considerably. This is important because it means that it is rarely possible to diagnose the cause of gastroenteritis on clinical grounds alone.

Gastro-intestinal manifestations of infection with VTEC range from non-bloody diarrhoea to haemorrhagic colitis. In addition, VTEC are the most important cause of HUS, a serious complication which is most common in young children and the elderly. HUS is defined by the triad of microangiopathic haemolytic anaemia, thrombocytopenia and acute renal dysfunction. The mortality rate is about 5%, and up to half of the survivors suffer long-term renal damage.

Table 38.2 Characteristic clinical features of various causes of gastroenteritis

Causative agent	Incubation period	Symptoms (syndrome)
Campylobacter	2–5 days	Bloody diarrhoea Abdominal pain Systemic upset
Salmonella	6–72 h	Diarrhoea and vomiting Fever; may be associated bacteraemia
Shigella	1–4 days	Diarrhoea, fever (bacillary dysentery)
Escherichia coli		
Enteropathogenic	12–72 h	Infantile diarrhoea
Enteroaggregative	1–3 days	Childhood diarrhoea, traveller's diarrhoea
Enterotoxigenic	1–3 days	Traveller's diarrhoea
Enteroinvasive	1–3 days	Similar to *Shigella*
Verotoxin-producing	1–3 days	Bloody diarrhoea (haemorrhagic colitis) Haemolytic uraemic syndrome
Staphylococcus aureus	4–8 h	Severe nausea and vomiting
Clostridium perfringens	6–24 h	Diarrhoea
Bacillus cereus		
Short incubation period	1–6 h	Vomiting
Long incubation period	6–18 h	Diarrhoea
Vibrio cholerae O1, O139	1–5 days	Profuse diarrhoea (cholera)
Vibrio parahaemolyticus	12–48 h	Diarrhoea, abdominal pain
Clostridium difficile	Usually occurs during/just after antibiotic therapy	Diarrhoea, abdominal pain, pseudomembranous enterocolitis
Giardia lamblia	1–2 weeks	Watery diarrhoea
Cryptosporidium	2 days to 2 weeks	Watery diarrhoea
Entamoeba histolytica	2–4 weeks	Diarrhoea with blood and mucus (amoebic dysentery), liver abscess
Viruses	1–2 days	Vomiting, diarrhoea Systemic upset

The clinical spectrum of CDI ranges from asymptomatic carriage to life-threatening pseudomembranous colitis (so called because yellow-white plaques or membranes consisting of fibrin, mucus, leucocytes and necrotic epithelial cells are found adherent to the inflamed colonic mucosa).

Enteric fever, resulting from infection with *S. enterica* serovars Typhi and Paratyphi, presents with symptoms such as headache, malaise and abdominal distension after an incubation period of 3–21 days. During the first week of the illness, the temperature gradually increases, but the pulse characteristically remains slow. Without treatment, during the second and third weeks, the symptoms become more pronounced. Diarrhoea develops in about half of cases. Examination usually reveals splenomegaly, and a few erythematous macules (rose spots) may be found, usually on the trunk. Serious gastro-intestinal complications such as haemorrhage and perforation are most common during the third week. Symptoms begin to subside slowly during the fourth week. In general, paratyphoid fever is less severe than typhoid fever.

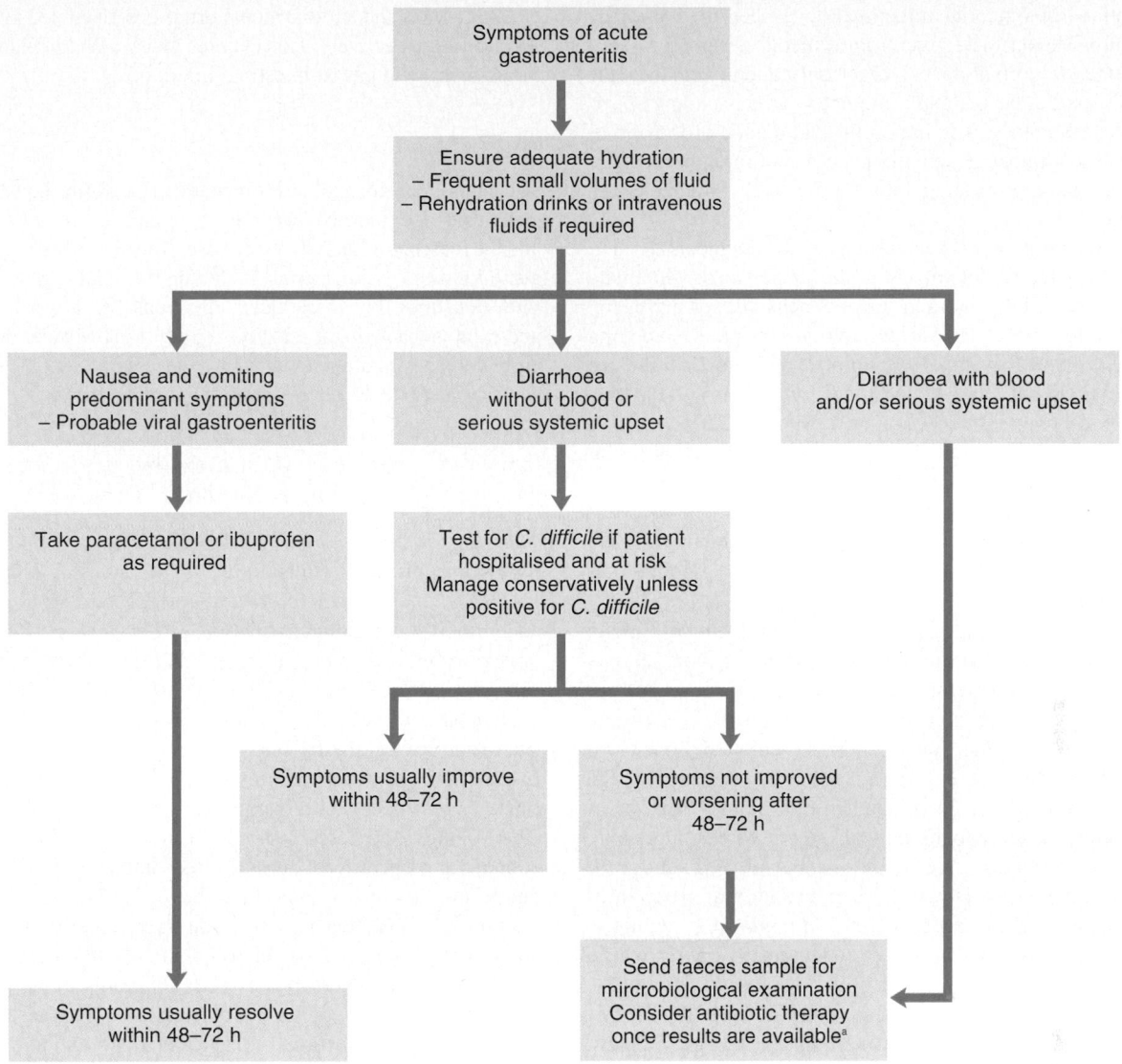

Fig. 38.1 Pathway for the investigation and management of patients with symptoms of acute gastroenteritis.

[a]Antibiotic therapy may have to be commenced empirically if patient has serious systemic upset

Botulism typically presents with autonomic nervous system effects, including diplopia and dysphagia, followed by symmetrical descending motor paralysis. There is no sensory involvement.

Gastro-intestinal infections are often followed by a period of convalescent carriage of the pathogen. This usually lasts for no more than 4–6 weeks but can be for considerably longer, especially for *Salmonella*.

Investigations

Many cases of gastroenteritis outside hospital are mild and short-lived, and microbiological investigation may not be necessary. However, investigations are always recommended where antibiotic therapy is being considered (Fig. 38.1), where

there are public health concerns (e.g. if the sufferer works in the food industry) and for gastro-intestinal infections in hospitalised patients.

The mainstay of investigation of diarrhoeal illness is examination of faeces. Conventional faecal microbiology is one of the most complex aspects of diagnostic microbiology. A range of different, often labour-intensive techniques have been required to test for different bacteria, viruses and protozoa. However, laboratory diagnostic strategies are changing; increasingly laboratories are using molecular methods (e.g. multiplex polymerase chain reaction [PCR]) to detect the full range of enteric pathogens (bacteria, viruses and parasites) more quickly and more accurately than by conventional methods. Results can be available in as little as an hour, compared with 2 or more days with conventional methods, which can assist with antibiotic stewardship and infection prevention and control.

Conventionally, bacterial infections have been diagnosed by stool culture. Various selective culture media designed to suppress growth of normal faecal organisms and/or enhance the growth of a particular pathogen are used. When sending specimens to the laboratory, it is important that details of the age of the patient, the clinical presentation and recent foreign travel are provided so that appropriate media for the likely pathogens can be selected.

A two-stage approach is recommended for diagnosis of CDI. Diarrhoeal stools are screened for the presence of glutamate dehydrogenase (GDH) antigen, an inexpensive, sensitive, but non-specific test; PCR is also suitable as an initial screening test, but it is more expensive. Samples that are positive for GDH, or by PCR, are then tested for *C. difficile* toxin. Patients who are toxin-positive have CDI; those who are GDH- or PCR-positive are *C. difficile* excretors. *C. difficile* excretors are at risk of development of CDI, especially if they are exposed to antibiotics; they also present an infection-control risk because they may spread toxigenic *C. difficile* to other patients who may develop CDI. Sigmoidoscopy is used to diagnose pseudomembranous colitis.

Various other procedures are sometimes useful in investigating patients with suspected bacterial gastroenteritis. Blood cultures should be taken from patients with severe systemic upset and are especially important when enteric fever is suspected. In enteric fever, the causative organism may also be cultured from urine or bone marrow. In *S. aureus* and *B. cereus* food poisoning, the pathogen can sometimes be isolated from vomitus. In cases of food poisoning, suspect foods may also be cultured. In general, serological investigations are of little value in the diagnosis of bacterial gastroenteritis. However, demonstration of serum antibodies to *E. coli* O157 can be helpful in confirming the cause of the HUS. Botulism is diagnosed by demonstration of toxin in serum.

Parasitic infestations are conventionally detected by microscopic examination of faeces, but PCR appears to be more sensitive. Molecular methods have to a large extent superseded electron microscopy and immunological tests for detection of enteric viruses.

Treatment

Many gastro-intestinal infections are mild and self-limiting and never reach medical attention. Where treatment is required, there are three main therapeutic considerations. Fluid and electrolyte replacement is the cornerstone of treatment of diarrhoeal disease. Most patients can be managed with oral rehydration regimens, but severely dehydrated patients require rapid volume expansion with intravenous fluids. Symptomatic treatment with antiemetics and anti-motility (antidiarrhoeal) agents is sometimes used, especially as self-medication. Antimicrobial agents may be useful both in effecting symptomatic improvement and in eliminating faecal carriage of pathogens, and therefore reducing the risk of transmitting infection to others.

Antiemetics and antidiarrhoeal drugs are discussed in Chapters 35 and 14, respectively. This chapter focuses on the place of antibiotic therapy in gastro-intestinal infections.

Antibiotic therapy

The requirement for antibiotic treatment in gastro-intestinal infection depends on the causative agent, the type and severity of symptoms, and the presence of underlying disease. Antibiotics are ineffective in some forms of gastroenteritis, including bacterial intoxications and viral infections. For many other infections, such as salmonellosis and campylobacteriosis, effective agents are available, but antimicrobial therapy is often not clinically necessary. Serious infections, such as enteric fever, always require antibiotic therapy.

Conditions for which antibiotic therapy is not available or not usually required

The symptoms of *S. aureus* and short incubation period *B. cereus* food poisoning and botulism are usually caused by ingestion of preformed toxin, and therefore antibiotic therapy would not influence the illness. Pathogens such as *C. perfringens*, *Vibrio parahaemolyticus*, and enteropathogenic *E. coli* usually cause a brief, self-limiting illness that does not require specific treatment.

None of the presently available antiviral agents are useful in gastroenteritis caused by viruses such as rotaviruses or noroviruses. Although most viral infections are self-limiting, chronic infections can occur in immunocompromised patients. Where possible, immunosuppression should be reduced. Immunoglobulin-containing preparations, administered orally or directly into the duodenum via a nasogastric tube, have also been reported to be effective in managing chronic viral gastroenteritis in immunocompromised patients. As well as human serum immunoglobulin, antibodies from other species (e.g. immunised bovine colostrum) have been used. Immunotherapy of viral gastroenteritis for severely immunocompromised patients remains experimental. Where these preparations are used, dosages and frequency of administration of immunoglobulin preparations must be determined locally, based on expert opinion (Pammi and Haque, 2011). Occasionally, where viruses such as cytomegalovirus or adenoviruses cause enteritis in immunocompromised patients, antiviral treatment, under specialist supervision, may be indicated.

At least one study has found that the risk of HUS in children with diarrhoea caused by VTEC was much higher in those who received antibiotics (Wong et al., 2000). On that basis, it is advised in the UK that antibiotics are contraindicated in children with VTEC infection (National Collaborating Centre for Women's and Children's Health, 2009). However, it has been suggested that some antibiotics, especially fosfomycin and quinolones, may prevent the development of HUS, and these treatments are used in some other countries (Corogeanu et al., 2012).

Conditions for which antimicrobial therapy may be considered

The place for antibiotics in the management of uncomplicated gastroenteritis due to bacteria such as *Salmonella* and

Campylobacter is not clear-cut. Certain antibiotics are reasonably effective in reducing the duration and severity of clinical illness and in eradicating the organisms from faeces. However, many microbiologists are cautious about the widespread use of antibiotics in diarrhoeal illness because of the risk of promoting antibiotic resistance (Pollack et al., 2013). Another difficulty with respect to antibiotic prescribing is that it is not usually possible to determine the aetiological agent of diarrhoea on clinical grounds, and stool culture takes at least 48 hours. Although an aetiological diagnosis can be established much faster using PCR, antibiotic susceptibility results are not provided. Patients with severe illness, especially systemic symptoms, may require antibiotic therapy before the aetiological agent, or its antibiotic susceptibilities, are established. In such circumstances, a fluoroquinolone antibiotic such as ciprofloxacin would usually be the most appropriate empiric agent, at least in patients in whom CDI is considered unlikely or has been excluded. Otherwise, it is reasonable to limit antibiotic use to microbiologically proven cases where there is serious underlying disease and/or continuing severe symptoms. Antibiotics may also be used to try to eliminate faecal carriage, for example, in controlling outbreaks in institutions, or in food handlers who may be prevented from returning to work until they are no longer excreting gastro-intestinal pathogens.

Campylobacteriosis. Erythromycin is effective in terminating faecal excretion of *Campylobacter*. Some studies have shown that treatment commenced within the first 72–96 hours of illness can also shorten the duration of clinical illness, especially in patients with severe dysenteric symptoms. The recommended dosage for adults is 250–500 mg four times a day orally for 5–7 days, and for children 30–50 mg/kg/day in four divided doses. Clarithromycin 250–500 mg (children <1 year of age, 7.5 mg/kg; 1–2 years, 62.5 mg; 3–6 years, 125 mg; 7–9 years, 5–7 days) twice a day orally or azithromycin 500 mg (children 10 mg/kg) once daily for 3 days is also effective. Ciprofloxacin, at a dosage of 500 mg twice daily orally for adults, may also be effective in *Campylobacter* enteritis. However, resistance rates to erythromycin have generally remained less than 5%, whereas resistance to ciprofloxacin has emerged, exceeding 10% in the UK and 50% in some other countries (Dingle et al., 2005).

Salmonellosis. Most cases of *Salmonella* gastroenteritis are self-limiting, and antibiotic therapy is unnecessary. However, antimicrobial therapy of salmonellosis is routinely recommended for infants younger than 6 months and immunocompromised patients, who are susceptible to complicated infections. Most antibiotics, even those with good in vitro activity, do not alter the course of uncomplicated *Salmonella* gastroenteritis. However, the fluoroquinolones, such as ciprofloxacin, can often shorten both the symptomatic period and the duration of faecal carriage. Ciprofloxacin resistance is now seen in up to 10% of non-typhoidal serovars of *S. enterica* in some countries but is still uncommon in the UK (Al-Mashhadani et al., 2011). The recommended dosage of ciprofloxacin for adults is 500 mg twice daily orally for 1 week. Fluoroquinolones are not licensed for this indication in children, although there is increasing evidence that they can safely be given to children. The recommended dosage of ciprofloxacin in childhood is 7.5 mg/kg twice daily orally. Trimethoprim at a dosage of 25–100 mg twice daily orally may be used in children if it is preferred not to use a fluoroquinolone.

Ciprofloxacin given orally at a dosage of 500–750 mg twice daily in adults (7.5–12.5 mg/kg twice daily in children) or 200 mg intravenously twice daily in adults (5–7.5 mg/kg twice daily in children) is recommended for invasive salmonellosis. Alternative agents include ampicillin or amoxicillin, trimethoprim or chloramphenicol (see later section Enteric Fever). However, resistance to these agents is more common than resistance to ciprofloxacin, and they are not recommended as empiric therapy.

E. coli **infections.** Most cases of enteropathogenic *E. coli*–associated diarrhoea are self-limiting and are managed conservatively; indeed, until recently few microbiology laboratories in Western countries have tested for these bacteria. However, increasingly laboratories are using PCR tests to investigate samples from patients with diarrhoea, and some of the commercially available PCR panels test for enteropathogenic *E. coli*. Consequently, some patients with chronic diarrhoea are now being reported to have enteropathogenic *E. coli*, the significance of which is uncertain (Duda-Madej et al., 2013). Specialist advice should be obtained before considering treatment of such patients. On the basis that enteroinvasive *E. coli* are closely related to *Shigella* and cause a similar clinical syndrome, similar therapy may be appropriate. Antibiotic therapy for traveller's diarrhoea caused by enterotoxigenic or enteroaggregative *E. coli* infections is often unnecessary, but troublesome symptoms will often respond to a single dose of ciprofloxacin or azithromycin; the need for further doses depends on clinical response. Alternatively, a 3- to 5-day course of trimethoprim may be given, although resistance is becoming increasingly common in some areas. Rifaximin is a new non-absorbable antibiotic that is available in a number of countries. It appears to be as effective as ciprofloxacin in treating *E. coli*–predominant traveller's diarrhoea but is ineffective in patients with inflammatory or invasive enteropathogens (Hopkins et al., 2014). The dosage for adults is 200 mg three times per day for 3 days.

Conditions for which antimicrobial therapy is usually indicated

Shigellosis. *Shigella sonnei*, which accounts for most cases of shigellosis in the UK and most other industrialised countries, usually causes a mild, self-limiting illness. Even if not required on clinical grounds, antibiotic therapy for shigellosis is usually recommended to eliminate faecal carriage, and therefore prevent person-to-person transmission. In contrast with salmonellosis, a number of antibiotics may be effective in shortening the duration of illness and terminating faecal carriage. This is especially true of strains of *S. sonnei* that are endemic in industrialised countries, whereas in developing countries, *Shigella* species that are multiple antibiotic resistant are an increasing problem. The fluoroquinolones are highly effective in shigellosis, and resistance is rare; therefore, they are often considered to be the treatment of choice, especially in adults and/or for treating imported infections. The dosage of ciprofloxacin is 500 mg twice daily orally in adults (7.5 mg/kg twice daily in children). Amoxicillin is an alternative first-line drug for *S. sonnei* infections acquired in the UK, where around 90% of isolates are susceptible. The dosage of amoxicillin is 250–500 mg three times daily in adults and 62.5–125 mg three times daily in children. Azithromycin (doses as for campylobacteriosis) is increasingly recommended as an alternative agent for shigellosis, especially in children (Jain et al., 2005). Third-generation cephalosporins such as ceftriaxone are another option for severe shigellosis. Trimethoprim resistance is now common, so this agent can no longer be recommended as empiric therapy. Antibiotic therapy is usually given for a maximum of 5 days.

Enteric fever. Treatment should be commenced as soon as a clinical diagnosis of enteric fever is made. Fluoroquinolones have been widely used as the first-choice treatment for typhoid and paratyphoid fevers. When treating isolates that are fully sensitive, the clinical response is at least as rapid as with the older treatments, there is a lower relapse rate and convalescent faecal carriage is shortened. However, the proportion of isolates with reduced susceptibility to fluoroquinolones has increased to around 75%. Although most of these isolates have minimum inhibitory concentration values below those regarded as fully resistant, treatment failures have been reported. For this reason, fluoroquinolones are no longer recommended as first-line treatment unless it is known that the isolate is fully sensitive. Resistance to other antibiotics that have been commonly used to treat enteric fever, such as co-trimoxazole, chloramphenicol and ampicillin, is now frequent. These agents therefore cannot be recommended as alternatives to fluoroquinolones for empiric treatment of enteric fever, but may be useful in patients with bacterial isolates that are confirmed as sensitive. Doses of ciprofloxacin are as outlined for non-typhoidal salmonellosis. The usual dosage of chloramphenicol is 50 mg/kg/day in four divided doses, and for ampicillin 100 mg/kg/day in four divided doses. Two weeks of antibiotic therapy is usually recommended, although shorter courses of ciprofloxacin (7–10 days) may be as effective.

The majority of cases of enteric fever diagnosed in the UK are related to travel to the Indian subcontinent, where multidrug resistance is common (Wain et al., 2015). Third-generation cephalosporins are the recommended first-choice agents to treat such infections, for example, cefotaxime (100–150 mg/kg daily in two to four divided doses in children; 6–8 g daily in three to four divided doses in adults) or ceftriaxone (50–80 mg/kg/day in children; 1–2 g/day in adults). Alternative agents for multidrug-resistant strains are intravenous carbapenems or oral azithromycin at a dosage of 20 mg/kg/day (maximum 1000 mg) for at least 5 days. Time taken for clearance of bacteraemia may be longer with azithromycin, but the relapse rate appears to be lower than with β-lactam antibiotics.

Chronic carriers of Salmonella. Patients may become chronic carriers after *Salmonella* infection, especially in the presence of underlying biliary tract disease. Oral ciprofloxacin 500–750 mg twice daily continued for 2–6 weeks is usually effective in eradicating carriage and has largely superseded the use of oral amoxicillin at a dosage of 3 g twice daily.

Cholera. Fluid and electrolyte replacement is the key aspect of the management of cholera. However, antibiotics do shorten the duration of diarrhoea, and therefore reduce the overall fluid loss, and rapidly terminate faecal excretion of the organism. Effective agents include tetracyclines, erythromycin, trimethoprim, ampicillin or amoxicillin, chloramphenicol, ciprofloxacin and furazolidone. However, antibiotic resistance is being increasingly seen; in particular, *V. cholerae* O139 is intrinsically resistant to furazolidone and trimethoprim. The choice of antibiotics is therefore governed by knowledge of local resistance patterns, which may vary between outbreaks. Tetracycline 250 mg four times daily or doxycycline 100 mg once daily by mouth is probably the most widely used therapy in adults. Ampicillin, amoxicillin or erythromycin is generally the preferred agent for children. Although clinical cure can be achieved after a single dose of antibiotics, treatment is usually given for 3–5 days to ensure eradication of *V. cholerae* from faeces.

C. difficile infection. The first objective is to diagnose CDI as soon as possible so that appropriate treatment and infection control measures can be put in place. Clinicians must consider the diagnosis in any patient in whom there is no clear alternative diagnosis for his or her diarrhoea. Stool samples must be sent to the laboratory immediately, and the laboratory must make testing available 7 days per week. Once the diagnosis is confirmed, attention must be paid to the patient's hydration and nutrition, non-essential antibiotic therapy or gastro-intestinal active drugs must be stopped and the patient's condition closely monitored. Although mild cases may resolve without specific therapy, treatment of all hospitalised patients with diarrhoea due to *C. difficile* is recommended, to shorten the duration of illness and to reduce environmental contamination and, therefore, the risk of nosocomial transmission.

Oral metronidazole 400 mg three times daily for 10 days is widely used as the first-line treatment for mild-to-moderate CDI. For severe CDI, oral vancomycin is recommended at a dosage of 125 mg four times daily for 10 days. In patients who are unable to take oral medication, either drug can be administered via a nasogastric tube. However, there is growing evidence that vancomycin is superior to metronidazole in CDI of all grades of severity (Nelson et al., 2017). Where there is no response to initial treatment, the dosage of vancomycin can be increased up to 500 mg four times daily, together with intravenous metronidazole 500 mg three times daily. Oral fidaxomicin 200 mg twice a day for 10 days was approved for CDI treatment in Europe in 2012. This drug is considerably more expensive than vancomycin, which is itself more expensive than metronidazole. Fidaxomicin has been shown in clinical trials to be at least non-inferior to vancomycin for the initial cure of CDI, but is clearly associated with a lower rate of recurrence. It is therefore recommended for treatment of patients deemed to be at high risk of recurrence; individual hospitals must make their own assessment of the cost-effective use of fidaxomicin (Wilcox, 2013).

Recurrence of symptoms occurs in about 20% of patients treated for CDI. Although some recurrences are due to germination of spores that have persisted in the colon since the original infection, it is recognised that some of these cases are due to reinfection, rather than relapse caused by the original strain (Loo et al., 2004). Most recurrences do respond to a further 10- to 14-day course of metronidazole or vancomycin, but increasingly fidaxomicin is seen as first-line treatment for this indication. A few patients experience repeated recurrences. Faecal microbiota transplantation is being increasing used in managing these patients. However, questions remain concerning regulatory matters, donor selection, the optimal mixture of the transplant and the preferred route of administration.

Pharmaceutical approaches to managing patients with multiple recurrences where fidaxomicin has failed include:

- a supervised trial of anti-motility agents alone (if there are no abdominal symptoms or signs of severe CDI),
- tapering or pulse therapy with oral vancomycin given for 4–6 weeks,
- a 2-week course of oral vancomycin 125 mg four times daily and oral rifampicin 300 mg twice daily,
- intravenous immunoglobulin, especially if the patient's albumin status worsens.

Trial data do not currently support the use of probiotics for the treatment or prevention of CDI (Department of Health and Health Protection Agency, 2009).

Cryptosporidiosis. Cryptosporidiosis in immunocompetent individuals is generally self-limiting. However, in immunosuppressed patients, severe diarrhoea can persist indefinitely and can even contribute to death. HIV-infected patients who are receiving highly active antiretroviral therapy now have a much lower incidence of cryptosporidiosis due to immune reconstitution and possibly a direct anti-cryptosporidium effect of protease inhibitors. There is no reliable antimicrobial therapy. Azithromycin, which is readily prescribable, is partially effective at a dosage of 500 mg once daily (10 mg/kg once daily in children). Treatment should be continued until *Cryptosporidium* oocysts are no longer detectable in faeces (typically 2 weeks), to minimise the risk of relapse post-treatment. Occasionally, therapy has to be continued indefinitely to prevent relapse. Most other agents that have been recommended for treatment of cryptosporidiosis, for example, nitazoxanide, spiramycin, paromomycin and letrazuril, are not licensed in the UK. These can usually be sourced from special-order manufacturing or importing companies (Smith and Corcoran, 2004). Of these agents, nitazoxanide has US Food and Drug Administration approval in the USA and has been shown to be effective in clinical trials at a dosage of 500 mg twice daily (adults and children aged ≥12 years) for 3 days (children 1–3 years: 100 mg twice daily; 4–11 years: 200 mg twice daily). Clinical cure rates of 72–88% have been reported in immunocompetent patients (Fox and Saravolatz, 2005), but are probably lower in immunosuppressed patients.

Giardiasis. Metronidazole is the treatment of choice for giardiasis. Various oral regimens are effective, for example, 400 mg three times daily (7.5 mg/kg in children) for 5 days, or 2 g/day (children: 500 mg to 1 g) for 3 days. Alternative treatments are tinidazole 2 g as a single dose, or mepacrine hydrochloride 100 mg (2 mg/kg in children) three times daily for 5–7 days. Nitazoxanide is a new thiazolide antiparasitic drug (discussed in the earlier Cryptosporidiosis section) that has also been licensed for treatment of giardiasis in some countries, but is not currently available in the UK. A single course of treatment for giardiasis has a failure rate of up to 10%. A further course of the same or another agent is often successful. Sometimes repeated relapses are due to reinfection from an asymptomatic family member. In such cases, all affected family members should be treated simultaneously.

Amoebiasis. The aim of treatment in amoebiasis is to kill all vegetative amoebae and also to eradicate cysts from the bowel lumen. Metronidazole is highly active against vegetative amoebae and is commonly the treatment of choice for acute amoebic dysentery and amoebic liver abscess. The dosage for adults is 800 mg (children 100–400 mg) three times daily for 5–10 days. To eradicate cysts, metronidazole therapy is followed by a 5-day course of diloxanide furoate 500 mg three times daily (20 mg/kg daily in three divided doses for children). Tinidazole has been shown to reduce clinical failure and be better tolerated than metronidazole (Gonzales et al., 2009). The dosage of tinidazole for adults is 2 g daily for 2–3 days, and for children is 50–60 mg/kg daily for 3 days.

Asymptomatic excretors of cysts living in areas with a high prevalence of *E. histolytica* infection do not merit treatment because most individuals quickly become reinfected. However, asymptomatic excretors of cysts in Europe or North America are usually treated with diloxanide furoate for 5–10 days; metronidazole and tinidazole are relatively ineffective in this situation.

Patient care

Individuals who are excreting gastro-intestinal pathogens are potentially infectious to others. Liquid stools are particularly likely to contaminate the hands and the environment. All cases of gastro-intestinal infection should be excluded from work or school at least until the patients are symptom free; hospitalised patients should be isolated in a single room. Patients should be advised on general hygiene, and in particular, on thorough handwashing and drying after visiting the toilet and before handling food.

In most countries, many gastro-intestinal infections are statutorily notifiable. Following notification, the authorities will judge whether the implications for public health merit investigation of the source of infection, contact screening or follow-up clearance stool samples from the original case.

Common therapeutic problems in the management of gastro-intestinal infection are summarised in Table 38.3. Problems associated with specific gastro-intestinal infections are summarised in Table 38.4.

Case studies

Case 38.1

A 12-year-old boy, Master RH, is admitted to hospital with a history of fever, weight loss and malaise 1 week after returning from visiting relatives in Pakistan. Whilst there he was diagnosed as having typhoid fever, and although details are sketchy, it seems that Master RH received treatment with ciprofloxacin. The only other medical history of note is that he experienced an anaphylactic reaction after taking penicillin 4 years ago. Twenty-four hours after admission, *S. enterica* serovar Typhi is isolated from a blood culture.

....

Questions

1. Why might Master RH not have fully responded to the treatment given in Pakistan?
2. Which antibiotic would now be most appropriate as empiric therapy?

Table 38.3   Practice points: general problems with treatment of gastro-intestinal infections

Problems	Resolution
Difficult or impossible to make a rapid aetiological diagnosis	New rapid and more sensitive diagnostic techniques (polymerase chain reaction) are being introduced Hospital laboratories are expected to offer rapid testing for *Clostridium difficile* 7 days per week
Antibiotic resistance in bacterial causes of gastroenteritis is increasing in prevalence	With no or few antibiotic agents on the horizon, good antibiotic stewardship is essential to preserve the effectiveness of existing treatments
Clinical effectiveness and cost-effectiveness of antibiotic therapy for many bacterial gastro-intestinal infections are not clearly established	Without reliable data showing benefit, antimicrobial therapy is not used in the majority of infections
No specific therapies for viral gastroenteritis	Infections in otherwise healthy individuals are generally self-limiting
Up to 20% of patients with *C. difficile* infection experience at least one recurrence	Fidaxomicin is a new treatment for *C. difficile* infection that may be associated with a lower rate of recurrence
Few other recent improvements in the diagnosis of bacterial or parasitic infections	Various non-evidence-based experimental treatments have been used to manage immunocompromised patients with protracted diarrhoea; faecal microbiota transplantation is being increasingly used to manage *C. difficile* infection
Acute illness may be followed by a period of non-infective diarrhoea	Cautious use of antidiarrhoeal medication may be indicated at this stage

Table 38.4   Practice points: problems with treatment of specific gastro-intestinal infections

Infection	Antibiotic	Problems	Resolution
Campylobacteriosis	Macrolides (e.g. erythromycin)	Not always effective, especially if commenced >72 h after onset of symptoms	Reserve therapy for cases where symptoms are severe or worsening at time of diagnosis
	Ciprofloxacin[a]	Up to 50% of strains are resistant	Use only as a second-line agent for isolates that have been shown to be sensitive
Salmonellosis	Ciprofloxacin[a]	Not always effective Resistance is increasing	Reserve therapy for cases where symptoms are severe or worsening at time of diagnosis
Enteric fever	Ciprofloxacin[a]	Resistance is increasing	None of these agents is now considered to be a suitable first-line therapy for enteric fever in the UK
	Ampicillin or amoxicillin	Resistance to these agents is now common	
	Chloramphenicol	Higher incidence of chronic carriage and relapse than with ciprofloxacin Resistance is now common	
Shigellosis	Trimethoprim	Resistance is increasing	Therapy should be guided by antibiotic sensitivities of the isolate; most trimethoprim-resistant strains are ciprofloxacin sensitive
Clostridium difficile	Metronidazole	Relapse rate up to 20%	Repeat course of treatment, or treatment with another agent, e.g. fidaxomicin, or consider faecal microbiota transplantation
	Vancomycin (oral)	More expensive than metronidazole Risk of promoting vancomycin-resistant enterococci Relapse rate up to 20%	Reserve for more serious cases; in the case of relapse, repeat course of treatment, or treatment with another agent, e.g. fidaxomicin, or consider faecal microbiota transplantation
Cryptosporidiosis	Azithromycin or nitazoxanide	Not always effective	Long-term therapy may be required to control symptoms

[a]Ciprofloxacin is not licensed for general paediatric use; it is widely used to treat gastro-intestinal infections in children.

Answers

1. Strains of *S. enterica* serovar Typhi that have reduced susceptibility to fluoroquinolones are common in the Indian subcontinent. Although these strains are not usually fully fluoroquinolone resistant, treatment failures have been reported, even when an appropriate dose regimen has been used. In this case, there is not even any assurance that the treatment regimen in Pakistan was adequate.
2. Given the lack of assurance of the adequacy of the ciprofloxacin treatment in Pakistan, one option would be to re-treat with ciprofloxacin. However, given the high likelihood that the strain will have reduced susceptibility to ciprofloxacin, it would be more logical to use an alternative agent. Of those, carbapenems and cephalosporins are β-lactam antibiotics that would be best avoided, given the history of anaphylaxis following penicillin exposure. Azithromycin would appear therefore to be the empiric treatment of choice in this case. If the patient was seriously unwell and/or unable to take oral medication, then a carbapenem antibiotic might have to be used under specialist supervision.

Case 38.2

A mother brings her 6-year-old daughter, Miss MF, to her primary care doctor because she has a 2-day history of bloody diarrhoea and abdominal pain. The family had been on a farm visit the previous weekend and had eaten food when there. The mother is anxious for her child to be treated with antibiotics because they will be going on their summer holiday in 1 week.

Questions

1. Give three possible infective causes of Miss MF's symptoms.
2. How should the primary care doctor respond to the mother's request for antibiotics?

Answers

1. The two commonest bacterial gastro-intestinal infections, campylobacteriosis and salmonellosis, can both present in this way. Many other bacterial and protozoan causes of gastroenteritis can also cause similar symptoms. One bacterium that is especially important to consider in this case, where there is a history of a farm visit, is *E. coli* O157. Every effort should be made to obtain a stool sample from the patient for microbiological examination.
2. It would not be appropriate to treat Miss MF's symptoms empirically with antibiotics for a number of reasons. Firstly, antibiotic therapy may make no difference to the speed of clinical resolution. Secondly, where antibiotics are justified, the choice of drug will depend on the aetiological agent. Thirdly, antibiotics are contraindicated in infection with *E. coli* O157, which must feature in the differential diagnosis in this case.

Case 38.3

An adult liver transplant patient, Mr EJ, presented with diarrhoea (up to 15 times per day), which has been ongoing for 10 days since he returned from a camping holiday. The microbiology laboratory has just called to say that Cryptosporidium oocysts were seen in his faeces sample.

Question

What treatment management can be offered to Mr EJ?

Answer

There is no reliable antimicrobial therapy for cryptosporidiosis. Azithromycin is readily prescribable, and as such may be used at a dosage of 500 mg once daily as a first-choice agent. If symptoms do abate, treatment should be continued until *Cryptosporidium* oocysts are no longer detectable in faeces (typically 2 weeks), to minimise the risk of relapse post-treatment. Occasionally, therapy has to be continued indefinitely to prevent relapse. Of the alternative agents for treatment of cryptosporidiosis, nitazoxanide appears to be the most effective. Although not licensed in the UK, it can usually be sourced from special-order manufacturing or importing companies. However, nitazoxanide treatment is also not always effective in patients who are unable to mount an appropriate immune response.

Case 38.4

A businessman, Mr JM, is planning a short trip to Egypt. During previous visits to the area, he has experienced troublesome diarrhoea despite being careful about hygiene. Although the diarrhoea has not made him seriously unwell, it has caused him considerable inconvenience during business discussions.

Question

Are there any antimicrobials that Mr JM could take to prevent this problem?

Answer

Although traveller's diarrhoea is not usually serious, it can cause considerable inconvenience whether the sufferer is travelling for leisure or business reasons. Simple measures that can help prevent traveller's diarrhoea include taking care with food and drinks (only bottled water from reputable sources should be used). There are two approaches to antibiotic use in traveller's diarrhoea. Either the drug can be taken prophylactically to try to prevent development of diarrhoea, or treatment can be commenced with the onset of diarrhoea. The latter approach is generally preferred because it limits unnecessary exposure to antibiotics, and the response to treatment is usually rapid. However, there are instances such as in this case where the inconvenience of even short-lived diarrhoea may be great enough to justify use of prophylaxis.

The choice of antibiotics for traveller's diarrhoea has been made more complicated by the increasing prevalence of antibiotic resistance in many developing countries. Drugs such as amoxicillin or trimethoprim no longer have a role. A fluoroquinolone, such as ciprofloxacin, still represents a reasonable first choice, with azithromycin as a possible alternative in areas where fluoroquinolone resistance is known to be common. For travellers from countries where it can be prescribed, rifaximin may be the agent of choice. For travellers to areas where infections such as amoebic dysentery or giardiasis are common, it may be appropriate to take a supply of metronidazole that can be started if there is no response to the first-line antibacterial prophylaxis.

Case 38.5

A 75-year-old woman, Mrs CS, on an elderly care ward experiences watery diarrhoea and abdominal pain 4 days after commencing therapy with ciprofloxacin for a urinary tract infection. C. difficile toxin is detected in a stool sample. She has had two previous episodes of CDI in the past year.

Question

How should Mrs CS be managed?

Answer

Firstly, treatment with ciprofloxacin should be discontinued. Four-day antibiotic therapy for a urinary tract infection will often suffice, but if further treatment is required, an antibiotic that is less likely to disturb the bowel flora should be prescribed. Secondly, Mrs CS requires treatment for her CDI. Metronidazole is often regarded as the preferred first-line treatment for mild-to-moderate CDI, whereas oral vancomycin would be a more expensive, but possibly more effective, alternative; either treatment would be on option here. However, because Mrs CS has recurrent CDI, many prescribers would now choose to treat with fidaxomicin. Although fidaxomicin is much more expensive, it is associated with a lower risk of CDI recurrence. Another treatment option that would be considered in some centres is faecal microbiota transplantation. Mrs CS should be closely monitored for the frequency and severity of the diarrhoea to ensure that she does not experience life-threatening complications of CDI. Finally, the patient should be isolated to reduce the risk of spread of the infection.

References

Al-Mashhadani, M., Hewson, R., Vivancos, R., et al., 2011. Foreign travel and decreased ciprofloxacin susceptibility in *Salmonella enterica* infections. Emerg. Infect. Dis. 17, 123–125.

Corogeanu, D., Willmes, R., Wolke, M., et al., 2012. Therapeutic concentrations of antibiotics inhibit Shiga toxin release from enterohemorrhagic *E. coli* O104:H4 from the 2011 German outbreak. BMC Microbiol. 12, 160.

Department of Health and Health Protection Agency, 2009. *Clostridium difficile* infection: how to deal with the problem. Department of Health, London.

Dingle, K.E., Clarke, L., Bowler, I.C., 2005. Ciprofloxacin resistance among human *Campylobacter* isolates 1991–2004: an update. J. Antimicrob. Chemother. 55, 395–396.

Duda-Madej, A., Gościniak, G., Andrzejewska, A., et al., 2013. Association of untypeable enteropathogenic *Escherichia coli* (EPEC) strains with persistent diarrhea in children from the region of lower Silesia in Poland. Pol. J. Microbiol. 62, 461–464.

Fox, L.M., Saravolatz, L.D., 2005. Nitazoxanide: a new thazolide antiparasitic agent. Clin. Infect. Dis. 40 (8), 1173–1180.

Gonzales, M.L.M., Dans, L.F., Martinez, E.G., 2009. Antiamoebic drugs for treating amoebic colitis. Cochrane Database Syst. Rev. 2009 (2), CD006085. https://doi.org/10.1002/14651858.CD006085.pub2.

Hopkins, K.L., Mushtaq, S., Richardson, J.F., et al., 2014. In vitro activity of rifaximin against clinical isolates of *Escherichia coli* and other enteropathogenic bacteria isolated from travellers returning to the UK. Int. J. Antimicrob. Agents 43, 431–437.

Jain, S.K., Gupta, A., Glanz, B., et al., 2005. Antimicrobial-resistant *Shigella sonnei*: limited antimicrobial treatment options for children and challenges of interpreting in vitro azithromycin susceptibility. Pediatr. Infect. Dis. J. 24, 494–497.

Loo, V.G., Libman, M.D., Miller, M.A., et al., 2004. Clostridium difficile: a formidable foe. Can. Med. Assoc. J. 171, 47–48.

National Collaborating Centre for Women's and Children's Health, 2009. Diarrhoea and vomiting caused by gastroenteritis: diagnosis, assessment and management in children younger than 5 years. RCOG Press, London.

Nelson, R.L., Suda, K.J., Evans, C.T., 2017. Antibiotic treatment for *Clostridium difficile*-associated diarrhoea in adults. Cochrane Database Syst. Rev. 2017 (3), CD004610. https://doi.org/10.1002/14651858. CD004610.pub5.

Pammi, M., Haque, K.N., 2011. Oral immunoglobulin for the prevention of rotavirus infection in low birth weight infants. Cochrane Database Syst. Rev. 2011 (11), CD003740. https://doi.org/10.1002/14651858.CD003740. pub2.

Pollack, L.A., Gould, C.V., Srinivasan, A., 2013. If not now, when? Seizing the moment for antibiotic stewardship. Infect. Control. Hosp. Epidemiol. 34, 117–118.

Smith, H.V., Corcoran, G.D., 2004. New drugs and treatment for cryptosporidiosis. Curr. Opin. Infect. Dis. 17, 557–564.

Wain, J., Hendriksen, R.S., Mikoleit, M.L., et al., 2015. Typhoid fever. Lancet 385, 1136–1145.

Wilcox, M., 2013. Updated guidance on the management and treatment of *Clostridium difficile* infection. Public Health England, London.

Wong, C.S., Jelacic, S., Habeeb, R.L., et al., 2000. The risk of the hemolytic uremic syndrome in children during a large outbreak of *Escherichia coli* O175:H7 infections. N. Engl. J. Med. 342, 1930–1936.

Further reading

DuPont, H.L., 2005. What's new in enteric infectious diseases at home and abroad. Curr. Opin. Infect. Dis. 18, 407–412.

Florez, I.D., Al-Khalifah, R., Sierra, J.M., et al., 2016. The effectiveness and safety of treatments used for acute diarrhea and acute gastroenteritis in children: protocol for a systematic review and network meta-analysis. Syst. Rev. 5, 14.

Goldenber, S.D., 2016. Faecal microbiota transplantation for recurrent *Clostridium difficile* infection and beyond: risks and regulation. J. Hosp. Infect. 92, 115–116.

Lübbert, C., 2016. Antimicrobial therapy of acute diarrhoea: a clinical review. Expert. Rev. Anti Infect. Ther. 14, 193–206.

Mohan, P., Haque, K., 2002. Oral immunoglobulin for the prevention of rotavirus infection in low birth weight infants. Cochrane Database Syst. Rev. 2002 (3), CD003740. https://doi.org/10.1002/14651858.CD003740.

Munnink, B.B., Hoek, L.V., 2016. Viruses causing gastroenteritis: the known, the new and those beyond. Viruses 8 (2), 42.

Toaimah, F.H., Mohammad, H.M., 2016. Rapid intravenous rehydration therapy in children with acute gastroenteritis: a systematic review. Pediatr. Emerg. Care 32, 131–135.

Useful websites

National Institute for Health and Care Excellence. Clinical Knowledge Summaries: Gastroenteritis: https://cks.nice.org.uk/gastroenteritis

Public Health England. Gastrointestinal infections: guidance, data and analysis: https://www.gov.uk/government/collections/gastrointestinal-infections-guidance-data-and-analysis

39 Infective Meningitis

Jim Gray

Key points

- The causative agents of meningitis are related to the age of the patient and the presence of underlying disease.
- The most common cause of early-onset neonatal meningitis is the group B streptococcus. Other important causes of neonatal meningitis include *Escherichia coli* and *Listeria monocytogenes*.
- Outside the neonatal period, *Neisseria meningitidis* and *Streptococcus pneumoniae* are the major causes of infective meningitis, accounting for around 75% of confirmed cases.
- Antibiotic treatment of meningitis requires attainment of adequate concentrations of bactericidal antibiotics in the cerebrospinal fluid.
- Suitable empiric therapies for neonatal meningitis are ampicillin or amoxicillin, combined with a third-generation cephalosporin such as cefotaxime.
- Increasing multidrug resistance in Gram-negative bacteria means that carbapenem antibiotics, especially meropenem, have an increasing role in the empiric treatment of neonatal meningitis.
- Increasing resistance to penicillins and concerns about the toxicity of chloramphenicol have led to the widespread use of cefotaxime or ceftriaxone as empiric therapy for meningitis outside the neonatal period.
- Because of the potentially rapid progression of the disease, patients with suspected meningococcal infection should receive emergency therapy with penicillin before admission to hospital.
- Close contacts of patients with meningococcal, and in some circumstances *Haemophilus influenzae* type b disease, should receive chemoprophylaxis and be considered for immunisation.
- There is increasing evidence of the benefit of steroids as adjunctive therapy in the management of some forms of bacterial meningitis.
- Introduction into the routine immunisation schedule of vaccines against *H. influenzae* type b, *N. meningitidis* group C and common *S. pneumoniae* serotypes has markedly reduced the incidence of meningitis caused by these bacteria. Immunisation against *N. meningitides* group B was introduced in the UK in 2015.

The brain and spinal cord are surrounded by three membranes, which from the outside inwards are the dura mater, the arachnoid mater and the pia mater. Between the arachnoid mater and the pia mater, in the subarachnoid space, is found the cerebrospinal fluid (CSF) (Fig. 39.1). This fluid, of which there is around 150 mL in a normal individual, is secreted by the choroid plexuses and vascular structures, which are in the third, fourth and lateral ventricles. CSF passes from the ventricles via communicating apertures to the subarachnoid space, after which it flows over the surface of the brain and the spinal cord (see Fig. 39.1). The amount of CSF is controlled by resorption into the bloodstream by vascular structures in the subarachnoid space, called the arachnoid villi. Infective meningitis is an inflammation of the arachnoid and pia mater associated with the presence of bacteria, viruses, fungi or protozoa in the CSF. Meningitis is one of the most emotive of infectious diseases, and for good reason: even today, infective meningitis is associated with significant mortality and risk of serious sequelae in survivors.

Aetiology and epidemiology

The annual incidence of acute bacterial meningitis in developed countries is 2–5 per 100,000 of the population. Viruses are the most common cause of meningitis, but because laboratory confirmation of the aetiological agent is often not achieved there are no reliable data on the incidence of viral meningitis.

Bacterial meningitis

Although bacterial meningitis occurs in all age groups, it is predominantly a disease of young children, with 40–50% of all cases occurring in the first 4 years of life. The pattern of micro-organisms causing meningitis is related to the age of the patient and the presence of underlying disease. Development of vaccines against the major causes of bacterial meningitis has dramatically changed the epidemiology of the condition outside the neonatal period. Following the introduction of vaccination against *Haemophilus influenzae* type b (Hib) into national childhood immunisation programmes in the early 1990s, invasive disease meningitis caused by that pathogen has almost been eliminated. Routine vaccination against *Streptococcus pneumoniae* and *Neisseria meningitidis* serogroup C (MenC) was subsequently adopted, and in 2015 the UK became the first country in the world to introduce the *N. meningitidis* serogroup B (MenB) vaccine into a national childhood immunisation programme (Salisbury and Ramsay, 2013).

N. meningitidis is the most common cause of bacterial meningitis from infancy through to middle age, with peaks of incidence in the less than 5-year age group and in adolescents. There are several serogroups of *N. meningitidis*, including A, B, C, W135

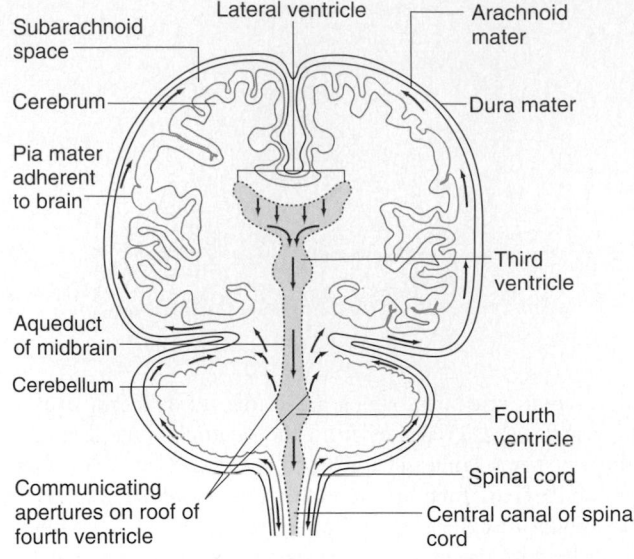

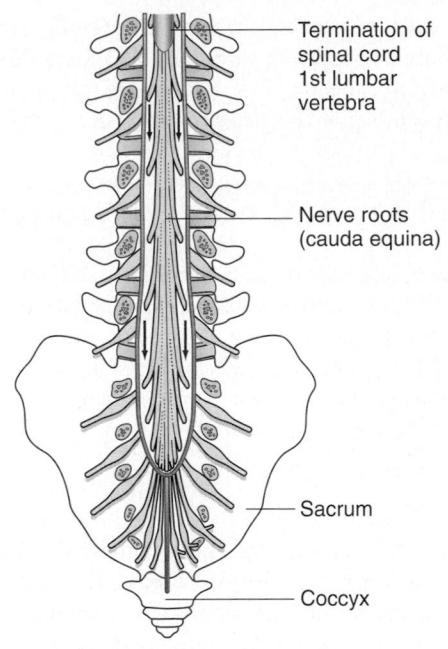

Fig. 39.1 The meninges covering the brain and spinal cord and the flow of cerebrospinal fluid (arrowed). (Modified from Ross and Wilson [1981], and reproduced with permission of Elsevier Ltd.)

and Y. In the late 20th century, serogroups B and C accounted for 60–65% and 35–40% of infections in the UK, respectively. However, with the introduction of vaccination against MenC into the routine immunisation programme in 1999, serogroup B now accounts for well more than 80% of all meningococcal disease. Moreover, in recent years an increase in other serogroups, especially W135, has been observed; based on this rise the former adolescent MenC dose has been replaced with a quadrivalent ACWY conjugate vaccine. The same vaccine is available to protect travellers to countries where other serogroups predominate, for example, in Africa and the Middle East where serogroups A and W135 prevail.

S. pneumoniae is the most common cause of meningitis in adults older than 45 years, but almost half of all cases of pneumococcal meningitis occur in children younger than 5 years. It has a poorer outcome than meningococcal meningitis. Vaccination against the most common serotypes of S. pneumoniae using a conjugate vaccine was added to the routine childhood immunisation programme in the UK in 2006; the original 7-valent vaccine was then replaced by a 13-valent vaccine in the spring of 2010. A different 23-valent polysaccharide vaccine is available for certain patient groups at risk of pneumococcal infection.

Hib was once the major cause of bacterial meningitis in children aged 3 months to 5 years but, as noted earlier, has been almost eliminated in the UK and other developed countries since the introduction of the vaccine.

Although patients with meningococcal or Hib meningitis are potentially infectious, most cases of meningitis due to these bacteria are acquired from individuals who are asymptomatic nasopharyngeal carriers (Health Protection Agency, 2012; Public Health England, 2013). People who live in the same household as a patient with meningococcal disease have a 500- to 1200-fold increased risk of development of infection if they do not receive chemoprophylaxis. Susceptible young children who are household contacts of an individual with Hib disease have a similarly increased risk of becoming infected. Epidemics of meningococcal disease sometimes occur. In developed countries, these take the form of clusters of cases among people living in close proximity (e.g. in schools or army camps) or in a particular geographical area. In Africa, large epidemics with many thousands of cases occur, usually during the dry season.

In the neonatal period, group B streptococci are the most common cause of bacterial meningitis. Other causes of neonatal meningitis include Escherichia coli and other Enterobacteriaceae, and rarely, Listeria monocytogenes. Most cases of early-onset infection (within the first 7 days of life) are acquired from the maternal genital tract around the time of delivery; late-onset infections may still be maternal in origin, but they can also be acquired from a variety of other sources.

L. monocytogenes is also an occasional cause of meningitis in immunocompromised patients. Meningitis can also occur as a complication of neurosurgery, especially in patients who have ventriculoatrial or ventriculoperitoneal shunts. Coagulase-negative staphylococci are the major cause of shunt-associated meningitis, but other bacteria are important, including Enterobacteriaceae and Staphylococcus aureus. Meningitis caused by S. aureus may also be secondary to trauma, or local or haematogenous spread from another infective focus. Meningitis may also be a feature of multisystem bacterial diseases such as syphilis, leptospirosis and Lyme disease.

The decline in the incidence of tuberculous meningitis in developed countries has mirrored the fall in the incidence of tuberculosis in these countries. Tuberculous meningitis may occur as part of the primary infection or as a result of recrudescence of a previous infection.

Viral meningitis

Human enteroviruses, such as echoviruses and Coxsackie viruses, account for about 70% of cases of viral meningitis in the UK. Parechoviruses are another important cause of meningitis in infants, especially neonates. Herpes simplex and varicella zoster viruses account for most other cases. Occasional causes of viral meningitis include mumps virus and human immunodeficiency viruses (HIVs).

Fungal meningitis

In Europe, fungal meningitis is rare in individuals without underlying disease. *Candida* species are an occasional cause of shunt-associated meningitis. *Cryptococcus neoformans* emerged as an important cause of meningitis in patients with late-stage HIV infection and other severe defects of T-cell function. With greater use of fluconazole for oral candidiasis, and especially the advent of highly active antiretroviral therapy, cryptococcosis has become much less common in developed countries. However, in sub-Saharan African countries with the highest HIV prevalence, cryptococcus is the leading cause of infective meningitis. In certain other areas of the world, infections with fungi such as *Coccidioides immitis* and *Histoplasma capsulatum* are endemic.

Pathophysiology

Most cases of bacterial meningitis are preceded by nasopharyngeal colonisation by the causative organism. In most colonised individuals, infection will progress no further, but in susceptible individuals, the organism invades the submucosa by circumventing host defences (e.g. physical barriers, local immunity, phagocytes) and gains access to the central nervous system (CNS) by invasion of the bloodstream and subsequent haematogenous seeding of the CNS. Other less common routes by which microorganisms can reach the meninges include:
- direct spread from the nasopharynx;
- blood-borne spread from other foci of colonisation or infection;
- abnormal communications with the skin or mucous membranes, for example, skull fractures, anatomical defects or a meningocoele;
- spread from an infected adjacent focus, for example, brain abscess, tuberculoma, infected paranasal air sinus or infection of the middle ear.

Once in the subarachnoid space, the infection spreads widely and incites a cascade of meningeal inflammation. The cerebral tissue is not usually directly involved, although cerebral abscess may complicate some types of meningitis.

The micro-organisms that most frequently cause meningitis are capable of doing so because they have a variety of virulence factors, including mechanisms for:
- attachment to host mucosal surfaces,
- evasion of phagocytosis and other host defences,
- meningeal invasion,
- disruption of the blood–brain barrier,
- induction of pathophysiological changes in the CSF space,
- secondary brain damage.

Overall, the net result of infection is vascular endothelial injury and increased blood–brain barrier permeability leading to the entry of many blood components into the subarachnoid space. This contributes to cerebral oedema and elevated CSF protein levels. In response to the cytokine response, neutrophils migrate from the bloodstream into the CSF. Cerebral oedema contributes to intracranial hypertension and a consequent decrease in cerebral blood flow. Anaerobic metabolism ensues, which contributes to increased lactate and decreases glucose concentrations. If this uncontrolled process is not modulated by effective treatment, transient neuronal dysfunction or permanent neuronal injury results.

Clinical manifestations

Acute bacterial meningitis usually presents with sudden-onset headache, neck stiffness, photophobia, fever and vomiting. On examination, Kernig's sign may be positive. This is resistance to extension of the leg when the hip is flexed, due to meningeal irritation in the lumbar area. Where meningitis is complicated by septicaemia, there may be septic shock. The presence of a haemorrhagic skin rash is highly suggestive, but not pathognomonic, of meningococcal infection. Untreated patients with bacterial meningitis deteriorate rapidly, with development of seizures, focal cerebral signs and cranial nerve palsies. Finally, obtundation and loss of consciousness herald death.

In infants with meningitis, the early physical signs are usually non-specific and include fever, diarrhoea, lethargy, feeding difficulties and respiratory distress. Focal signs such as seizures or a bulging fontanelle usually only occur at a late stage.

Viral meningitis usually presents with acute onset of low-grade fever, headache, photophobia and neck stiffness. Unless encephalitis develops, patients usually remain alert and oriented.

Although tuberculous and fungal meningitis sometimes present acutely, these infections typically have a more indolent course. The early stages of the diseases are dominated by general symptoms such as malaise, apathy and anorexia. As they progress, symptoms and signs more typical of meningitis usually appear.

Diagnosis

The definitive diagnosis of meningitis is established by detection of the causative organism and/or demonstration of biochemical changes and a cellular response in CSF. CSF is obtained by lumbar puncture, where a needle is inserted between the posterior space of the third and fourth lumbar vertebrae into the subarachnoid space. Before performing lumbar puncture, the possibility of precipitating or aggravating existing brain herniation in patients with intracranial hypertension must be considered. A computed tomography (CT) scan should be performed before undertaking lumbar puncture if any neurological abnormalities are present.

In health, the CSF is a clear colourless fluid which, in the lumbar region of the spinal cord, is at a pressure of 50–150 mm H_2O. There may be up to 5 cells/microlitre, the protein concentration is up to 0.4 g/L and the glucose concentration is at least 60% of the blood glucose (usually 2.2–4.4 mmol/L). Table 39.1 shows how the cell count and biochemical measurements can be helpful in determining the type of organism causing meningitis.

In bacterial and fungal meningitis, organisms may be visible in Gram-stained smears of the CSF. The common causes of bacterial meningitis are easily distinguished from each other by their

Table 39.1 Cellular and biochemical responses in different forms of infective meningitis

Type of meningitis	Cell count	Protein (g/L)	Glucose
Bacterial	Predominantly polymorphs, 500–2000 per microlitres (lymphocytes may predominate in early or partially treated cases)	1–3	<50% blood glucose
Tuberculous	Predominantly lymphocytes, 100–600 per microlitres	1–6	<50% blood glucose
Viral	Predominantly lymphocytes, 50–500 per microlitres	0.5–1	Usually normal
Cryptococcal	Predominantly lymphocytes, 50–1000 per microlitres	1–3	<50% blood glucose

Gram stain appearance. Special stains, such as the Ziehl–Neelsen method, are necessary to visualise mycobacteria. However, only small numbers of mycobacteria are present in the CSF in tuberculous meningitis, and direct microscopy is often unrevealing. Although cryptococci can be visualised by Gram staining, they are often more easily seen with India ink staining, which highlights their prominent capsules.

Regardless of the microscopic findings, CSF should be cultured to try to confirm the identity of the causative organism and to facilitate further investigations such as antibiotic sensitivity testing and typing. Special cultural techniques are required for mycobacteria, fungi and viruses. Cultures of other sites are sometimes helpful. In suspected bacterial meningitis, blood for culture should always be obtained. Bacteraemia occurs in only 10% of patients with meningococcal meningitis but is more common in most other forms of meningitis. In suspected meningococcal disease, culture of a nasopharyngeal swab may be helpful because antibiotic penetration at this site is less. It increases the chances of isolating meningococci when antibiotics were administered to the patient before presentation to hospital.

Non-culture-based methods are increasingly used to investigate the aetiology of meningitis. Molecular amplification techniques, such as polymerase chain reaction (PCR), have been widely used for some years now to detect specific pathogens, especially meningococci, pneumococci, *Mycobacterium tuberculosis* and various viruses, including herpes simplex viruses and enteroviruses. An important recent development has been the introduction of multiplex PCR tests that can detect 10 or more different bacterial, viral or fungal CNS pathogens in the same assay, giving results in about 1 hour.

Serum antibodies to *N. meningitidis* and various viruses may be detected, but these investigations usually depend on demonstration of seroconversion between two samples collected a week or more apart and are, therefore, undertaken more for public health than clinical reasons. Patients with tuberculous meningitis may have a positive Mantoux test or an interferon-γ release assay.

Drug treatment

Acute bacterial meningitis is a medical emergency that requires urgent administration of antibiotics. Other considerations in some forms of meningitis include the use of adjunctive therapy such as steroids and the administration of antibiotics to prevent secondary cases.

Antimicrobial therapy

Pharmacokinetic considerations

The antimicrobial therapy of meningitis requires attainment of adequate levels of bactericidal agents within the CSF. The principal route of entry of antibiotics into CSF is by the choroid plexus; an alternative route is via the capillaries of the central nervous system into the extracellular fluid and hence into the ventricles and subarachnoid space (see Fig. 39.1). The passage of antibiotics into CSF is dependent on the degree of meningeal inflammation and integrity of the blood–brain barrier created by capillary endothelial cells, as well as the following properties of the antibiotic:

- lipid solubility (the choroidal epithelium is highly impermeable to lipid-insoluble molecules),
- ionic dissociation at blood pH,
- protein binding,
- molecular size,
- concentration of the drug in the serum.

Antimicrobials fall into three categories according to their ability to penetrate the CSF:

- those that penetrate even when the meninges are not inflamed, for example, chloramphenicol, metronidazole, isoniazid and pyrazinamide;
- those that generally penetrate only when the meninges are inflamed, and are used in high doses, for example, most β-lactam antibiotics, the quinolones and rifampicin;
- those that penetrate poorly under all circumstances, including the aminoglycosides, vancomycin and erythromycin.

Recommended regimens

Clinical urgency determines that empirical antimicrobial therapy will usually have to be prescribed before the identity of the causative organism or its antibiotic sensitivities are known. Consideration of the epidemiological features of the case, together with microscopic examination of the CSF, is often helpful in identifying the likely pathogen. However, empiric therapy is usually with broad-spectrum antimicrobial therapy to cover all likely pathogens, at least until definitive microbiological information is available. For the purpose of selecting empiric antimicrobial therapy, patients with acute bacterial meningitis can be categorised into four broad groups: neonates and infants younger than 3 months; immunocompetent older infants, children and adults; immunocompromised patients; and those with ventricular shunts.

Table 39.2 Suitable antibiotic regimens for treatment of acute bacterial meningitis in different age groups

Age group	First-choice antibiotic therapy	Alternative therapies
Neonates, aged <8 days	Ampicillin 50 mg/kg twice daily or amoxicillin 25 mg/kg twice daily and cefotaxime 50 mg/kg twice daily or ceftazidime 50 mg/kg twice daily	Benzylpenicillin 50 mg twice daily and ampicillin 50 mg/kg twice daily or amoxicillin 25 mg/kg twice daily and gentamicin 2.5 mg/kg twice daily[a]
Neonates, aged 8–28 days	Ampicillin 50 mg/kg four times daily or amoxicillin 25 mg/kg three times daily and cefotaxime 50 mg/kg three times daily or ceftazidime 50 mg/kg three times daily	Meropenem 40 mg/kg two or three times daily[b]
Infants, aged 1–3 months	Ampicillin 50 mg/kg four times daily or amoxicillin 25 mg/kg three times daily and cefotaxime 50 mg/kg three times daily or ceftriaxone 75–100 mg/kg once daily	
Infants and children, aged >3 months[c]	Cefotaxime 50 mg/kg three times daily or ceftriaxone[d] 75–100 mg/kg once daily	Ampicillin 50 mg/kg four times daily or amoxicillin 25 mg/kg three times daily or benzylpenicillin[e] 30 mg/kg 4-hourly and chloramphenicol[f] 12.5–25 mg/kg four times daily
Adults	Cefotaxime[g] 2 g three times daily or ceftriaxone[d,g] 2–4 g once daily	Benzylpenicillin 2.4 g 4-hourly or ampicillin 2–3 g four times daily or amoxicillin 2 g three or four times daily and chloramphenicol[f] 12.5–25 mg/kg four times daily

[a]Benzylpenicillin is suitable for treating group B streptococcus meningitis, but this regimen is not recommended for Gram-negative bacterial meningitis.
[b]Use meropenem where multidrug-resistant Gram-negative bacterial meningitis is suspected or confirmed.
[c]Calculated doses for children should not exceed maximum recommended doses for adults.
[d]Ceftriaxone should not be administered to neonates within 48 h of completion of infusions of calcium-containing solutions; caution should be exercised in older age groups.
[e]Benzylpenicillin is inactive against *Haemophilus influenzae* and should therefore not be used in children aged <5 years.
[f]Monitoring of serum chloramphenicol levels is recommended, especially in children aged <4 years.
[g]Add ampicillin or amoxicillin to cover *Listeria monocytogenes* in elderly patients or where Gram-positive bacilli seen in cerebrospinal fluid.

Antibiotics for meningitis in neonates and infants younger than 3 months. The most important pathogens in neonates include group B streptococci, *E. coli* and other *Enterobacteriaceae* and *L. monocytogenes*. Where meningitis in a neonate is suspected, the recommended empiric treatment is with a third-generation cephalosporin, usually cefotaxime, along with amoxicillin or ampicillin (Galiza and Heath, 2009). Cephalosporins penetrate into CSF better than aminoglycosides, and their use in Gram-negative bacillary meningitis has contributed to a reduction in mortality rate to less than 10%. Where neonates present with sepsis without evidence of meningitis it is common practice to prescribe an aminoglycoside, such as gentamicin, together with benzylpenicillin, ampicillin or amoxicillin (in early-onset sepsis), or flucloxacillin (in late-onset sepsis) as empiric therapy. This cephalosporin-sparing approach is preferred because cephalosporins are potent selectors of antibiotic-resistant bacteria such as meticillin-resistance *S. aureus* (MRSA), vancomycin-resistant enterococci and multidrug-resistant Gram-negative bacteria (MDRGNB), and also predispose to secondary candidiasis. If a baby treated with a penicillin and aminoglycoside combination is subsequently suspected or confirmed to have meningitis, then their antibiotic therapy should be altered to ensure good CSF penetration of antibiotics (National Institute for Health and Care Excellence, 2012). Likewise, empiric antibiotic therapy must be reviewed in all cases of neonatal meningitis once a pathogen has been identified. MDRGNB are becoming more prevalent, especially as a cause of hospital-acquired infection.

These bacteria include AmpC and extended-spectrum β-lactamase producers that are resistant to cephalosporins; a carbapenem, such as meropenem, is the usual treatment of choice for such infections. Suitable dosages are listed in Table 39.2.

In infants outside the immediate neonatal period, the classic neonatal pathogens account for a decreasing number of cases of meningitis, and the common bacteria of meningitis in childhood become increasingly important. Amoxicillin or ampicillin plus cefotaxime or ceftriaxone is the recommended treatment. Therapy with amoxicillin or ampicillin and gentamicin is unsuitable for this age group because it provides inadequate cover against *H. influenzae*.

Antibiotics for meningitis in older infants, children and adults. Antimicrobial therapy has to cover *S. pneumoniae*, *N. meningitidis* and, in children younger than 5 years, *H. influenzae* (Brouwer et al., 2010). Achievable antibiotic CSF concentrations are compared with the susceptibilities of the common agents of meningitis in Table 39.3. Third-generation cephalosporins, such as cefotaxime or ceftriaxone, are now widely used in place of the traditional agents of choice, chloramphenicol, ampicillin, amoxicillin and penicillin (see Table 39.2). This change has stemmed from concern over the rare but potentially serious adverse effects of chloramphenicol and the emergence of resistance to penicillin, ampicillin and chloramphenicol among *S. pneumoniae* and *H. influenzae* in particular. Chloramphenicol resistance and reduced susceptibility to penicillin have also been reported in

Table 39.3 Achievable cerebrospinal fluid concentrations of antibiotics in meningitis and minimum inhibitory concentration values for common central nervous system pathogens

Antibiotic	CSF/serum ratio	Peak CSF level (mg/L)	MIC$_{90}$ (mg/L)		
			N. meningitidis	H. influenzae	S. pneumoniae
Ampicillin	1:10	10	0.02	0.25	0.05
Benzylpenicillin	1:20	1.5	0.02	1.0	0.02
Cefotaxime	1:20	10	0.01	0.06	0.25
Ceftriaxone	1:15	15	0.01	0.06	0.12
Chloramphenicol	1:2	15	1.0	1.0	2.5
Ciprofloxacin	1:5	0.6	0.004	0.015	1.0
Daptomycin	1:20	3.0	>4.0	>4.0	0.25
Gentamicin	1:40	<0.5	2.0	0.5	16
Imipenem	1:15	2.0	0.1	1.0	0.05
Linezolid	1:1.25	5.0	>8.0	>8.0	2.0
Meropenem	1:15	4.0	0.03	0.1	0.1
Rifampicin	1:20	1.0	0.5	1.0	2.0
Vancomycin	1:40	1.0	>4.0	>4.0	0.2

CSF, Cerebrospinal fluid; MIC$_{90}$, minimum concentration of antibiotic that is inhibitory for 90% of isolates.

N. meningitidis. The third-generation cephalosporins, cefotaxime or ceftriaxone, have a broad spectrum of activity that encompasses not only the three classic causes of bacterial meningitis, but also many other bacteria that are infrequent causes of meningitis. Because of the potential for calcium chelation in vivo, ceftriaxone must not be administered within 48 hours of the completion of infusions of calcium-containing solutions in neonates. The risk of precipitation is much lower in patients more than 28 days of age. Nevertheless, caution should still be exercised when treating older age groups, especially in the early treatment of meningococcal infections (where calcium-containing products are commonly used for resuscitation).

Cephalosporins are inactive against *L. monocytogenes*, and amoxicillin or ampicillin should be added where it is possible that the patient may have listeriosis, for example, in elderly patients, or where Gram-positive bacilli are seen on Gram stain; it is not necessary to routinely prescribe ampicillin or amoxicillin in all cases of suspected bacterial meningitis. Although earlier-generation cephalosporins such as cefuroxime achieve reasonable CSF penetration and are active against the agents of meningitis in vitro, they do not effectively sterilise the CSF and should not be used to treat meningitis. Addition of vancomycin should be considered for patients who have received recent prolonged or frequent antibiotic therapy, or who have travelled to an area with a high prevalence of penicillin-resistant pneumococci in the preceding 3 months.

In meningitis due to *N. meningitidis* and *H. influenzae*, prompt administration of chemoprophylaxis to close contacts of the case should be prescribed to eliminate nasopharyngeal carriage and hence reduce the risk of secondary cases.

N. meningitidis. In view of the potentially rapid clinical progression of meningococcal disease with a non-blanching rash, it is recommended that treatment should begin with the emergency administration of benzylpenicillin. Primary care clinicians should give penicillin while arranging transfer of the patient to hospital. The dose is 1200 mg for adults and children aged 10 years and older, 600 mg for children aged 1–9 years and 300 mg for children younger than 1 year. Ideally this should be given intravenously. The intramuscular route is less likely to be effective in shocked patients but can be used if venous access cannot be obtained. The only contraindication is in people who have a clear history of anaphylaxis after a previous dose; a history of a rash following penicillin is not a contraindication.

Strains of *N. meningitidis* with reduced sensitivity to penicillin are well known and presently account for 5–10% of isolates in Europe and the USA. In general, these cases respond to treatment with adequate doses of benzylpenicillin, and failure of penicillin treatment has rarely been reported. Nevertheless, cefotaxime and ceftriaxone are now widely used in preference to benzylpenicillin or chloramphenicol. Meningococcal meningitis should be treated for 7 days.

S. pneumoniae. Benzylpenicillin was once widely regarded as the treatment of choice for pneumococcal meningitis. However, pneumococci resistant to penicillin have emerged across the world, presenting a major therapeutic challenge in view of the severity of pneumococcal meningitis.

Although currently only about 5% of pneumococci in the UK are penicillin resistant, the frequency of resistance is increasing, and resistance rates of more than 50% have been reported in other countries, including Spain, Hungary and South Africa. Penicillin resistance in pneumococci is defined in terms of the minimum inhibitory concentration (MIC) of penicillin. Most strains have an MIC value of 0.1–2.0 mg/L and are defined as having moderate resistance; strains with an MIC value of more than 2 mg/L are considered highly resistant. This distinction is relevant for less serious infections with moderately resistant strains, which may still respond to adequate doses of some β-lactam antibiotics, such as cefotaxime, ceftriaxone or a carbapenem. However, the clinical outcome of meningitis with penicillin-resistant pneumococci treated with a β-lactam antibiotic as monotherapy is less good. For this reason many guidelines, including those produced by the Infectious Diseases Society of America, have for some years recommended therapy with a combination of a third-generation cephalosporin and vancomycin (McIntosh, 2005). This approach has not been adopted universally in the UK but should certainly be considered for patients who might have acquired their infection in a location where the incidence of penicillin resistance is high. Where vancomycin is given intravenously to treat meningitis, it is important to aim for trough serum levels of 15–20 mg/L because of the limited CSF penetration of vancomycin. Another problem is the emergence of pneumococci that are tolerant to vancomycin; that is, they are able to survive, but not proliferate, in the presence of vancomycin. Although such strains are uncommon, the outcome of meningitis treated with vancomycin is poor (Cottagnoud and Tauber, 2004).

Other antibiotics may be useful in treating pneumococcal meningitis. Use of rifampicin in combination with a cephalosporin and/or vancomycin is sometimes recommended, but there are few data confirming this improves the response rate in either penicillin-sensitive or -resistant pneumococcal meningitis. The dosage of rifampicin is 600 mg twice daily in adults or 10 mg/kg (maximum 600 mg) twice daily in children. Chloramphenicol is a suitable alternative to penicillin for treatment of meningitis due to penicillin-sensitive strains, for example, in patients who are penicillin allergic. However, chloramphenicol is not recommended for treating penicillin-resistant pneumococcal meningitis: although isolates may appear to be sensitive to chloramphenicol on routine laboratory testing, bactericidal activity is often absent, and the clinical response is usually poor.

Consideration of alternative antibiotics for treatment of penicillin-resistant pneumococcal meningitis is largely based on case reports rather than clinical trials. Success has been reported with meropenem as monotherapy and in conjunction with rifampicin. Moxifloxacin is a new-generation quinolone antibiotic with enhanced activity against Gram-positive bacteria, including *S. pneumoniae*, that is a suitable second-line agent for treating penicillin-resistant pneumococcal meningitis. Linezolid has excellent CSF penetration but does not have bactericidal activity, and clinical experience in treating meningitis has been variable (Rupprecht and Pfister, 2005).

The unpredictable nature of the response to therapy of penicillin-resistant pneumococcal meningitis means that patients require close observation during treatment, for example, monitoring of C-reactive protein. Repeat examination of CSF during therapy should also be considered.

Box 39.1 Indications for chemoprophylaxis in contacts of cases of infection with *Neisseria meningitidis* or *Haemophilus influenzae* type b

N. meningitidis
- Household and other close contacts (boyfriends/girlfriends) during the 7 days before onset of illness, irrespective of vaccination status (Prophylaxis is usually initiated as soon as possible by clinicians caring for the patient.)
- The index case when able to take oral medication and before discharge from hospital, unless the disease has already been treated with ceftriaxone (Those treated with cefotaxime should still receive prophylaxis because it is not known that cefotaxime eradicates carriage.)
- Healthcare workers whose mouth or nose was directly exposed to large-particle droplets/secretions from the respiratory tract of a probable or confirmed case of meningococcal disease during acute illness until completed 24 h of systemic antibiotics (Prophylaxis should only be initiated after consultation with hospital infection control team or public health doctor.)
- Other contacts (Prophylaxis should be initiated by a public health doctor.)
  - School pupils in the same dormitory or university students sharing a kitchen in a hall of residence
  - Schools, nurseries, universities and other closed communities where two or more linked cases have occurred
Vaccination is also recommended for close contacts (other than healthcare workers) of cases of serogroups A, C, W135 and Y.

Invasive Hib infection
- Household and other close contacts where there is a vulnerable person in the household (any child aged <10 years or an immunosuppressed or asplenic person of any age) (Prophylaxis usually initiated as soon as possible by clinicians caring for the patient.)
- The index case (if age <10 years) when able to take oral medication and before discharge from hospital
- Other contacts: prophylaxis is rarely necessary and should only be initiated by a public health physician
Vaccination is also recommended for the index patient and vulnerable household contacts.

H. influenzae. A third-generation cephalosporin, such as cefotaxime or ceftriaxone, is generally the treatment of choice for *H. influenzae* meningitis. These agents have superseded the traditional therapies of chloramphenicol and/or ampicillin or amoxicillin.

Other bacteria. Meningitis in immunocompetent individuals is rarely due to other bacteria. The definitive treatment for these individuals should be determined on an individual basis in light of careful clinical and microbiological assessment.

Chemoprophylaxis against meningococcal and *H. influenzae* type b infection. In meningococcal meningitis, spread between family members and other close contacts is well recognised; these individuals should receive chemoprophylaxis as soon as possible, preferably within 24 hours. Sometimes, chemoprophylaxis may be indicated for other contacts, but the decision to offer prophylaxis beyond household contacts should be made only after obtaining expert advice (Box 39.1). Of the antibiotics conventionally used to treat meningococcal infections, only ceftriaxone reliably eliminates nasopharyngeal carriage; where another antibiotic has been used for treatment, the index case also requires chemoprophylaxis. A number of antibiotics are suitable as prophylaxis (Box 39.2).

| **Box 39.2** | Recommended prophylactic regimens for contacts of cases of infection with *Neisseria meningitidis* or *Haemophilus influenzae* type b |

Meningococcal infection

Ciprofloxacin[a] (oral)

Children aged 1 month to 4 years	125 mg as a single dose
Children aged 5–12 years	250 mg as a single dose
Adults	500 mg as a single dose

Rifampicin (oral)

Children aged <1 year	5 mg/kg twice daily on 2 consecutive days
Children aged 1–12 years	10 mg/kg (maximum 600 mg) twice daily on 2 consecutive days
Adults	600 mg twice daily on 2 consecutive days

Azithromycin[a] (oral)

Pregnant women	500 mg as a single dose

Ceftriaxone[a] (intramuscular)

Children aged <12 years	125 mg as a single dose
Adults	250 mg as a single dose

Invasive Hib infection

Rifampicin (oral)

Children aged 1–3 months	10 mg/kg once daily for 4 days
Children aged >3 months	20 mg/kg once daily (maximum 600 mg) for 4 days
Adults	600 mg once daily for 4 days

Ceftriaxone[a] (intravenous or intramuscular)

Children aged <12 years	50 mg/kg once daily for 2 days
Adults	1 g once daily for 2 days

[a]Not licensed for this indication.

Ciprofloxacin is recommended for contacts of all ages (including pregnant and breastfeeding women) because of the convenience of single-dose administration, and unlike rifampicin, it does not interact with oral contraceptives and is readily available in community pharmacies. Although anaphylactoid reactions have been reported to occur in individuals receiving ciprofloxacin as chemoprophylaxis, none of these reactions have been fatal. If the strain is confirmed as group C (or A, W135 or Y), vaccination is normally offered to contacts who were given prophylaxis. Currently group B vaccination is not recommended for contacts. Appropriate immunisation should be given to any eligible unimmunised or partially immunised index case according to the recommended national schedule.

Chemoprophylaxis against Hib infection is usually indicated only for contacts where there is a vulnerable individual in the household (see Box 39.1). Only rifampicin has been proved to be effective in eliminating nasopharyngeal carriage (see Box 39.2). Ceftriaxone is recommended as an alternative agent if an individual is unable to tolerate or experiences an adverse reaction to rifampicin. Vulnerable individuals who are household contacts should also receive vaccination against Hib. The index case (if aged <10 years) should always receive rifampicin to eliminate nasopharyngeal carriage before discharge from hospital and should be considered for immunisation as follows.

Unimmunised or partially immunised index cases younger than 10 years (or of any age with asplenia or splenic dysfunction) should complete their primary course of Hib immunisation.

Fully vaccinated index cases are managed as follows (Public Health England, 2013):

- Age 5–10 months: Give one dose of Hib vaccine before discharge from hospital to cover them until they receive their routine 12-month booster dose.
- Older infants and children aged less than 10 years: Measure anti-Hib antibodies 4 weeks post-infection and give an additional dose of Hib vaccine if antibody levels are less than 1 mg/mL. If this is not feasible, give a dose of Hib vaccine before discharge from hospital.
- Aged ≥10 years with asplenia or splenic dysfunction: Give an extra dose of Hib vaccine if they completed their scheduled Hib immunisation more than 1 year previously.

Antibiotics for meningitis in special groups

Immunocompromised host. In the immunocompromised patient with neutropenia, the meninges can become infected. Possible causes of meningitis include *Enterobacteriaceae* and *Pseudomonas aeruginosa*, as well as the classic bacterial causes of meningitis. The choice of therapy is governed by the need to attain broad-spectrum coverage, using agents with good CSF penetration. Meropenem may now be the drug of choice for meningitis in this setting, although many other regimens are also appropriate.

Patients with cellular immune dysfunction are vulnerable to meningitis caused by *L. monocytogenes* and *C. neoformans*. Ampicillin or amoxicillin, along with cefotaxime or ceftriaxone, is recommended as empirical antibacterial therapy for meningitis in these patients. Definitive treatment of listeria meningitis is normally with high-dose ampicillin (3 g four times daily) or amoxicillin (2 g four times daily), with the addition of gentamicin to obtain a synergistic effect. The most appropriate treatment for patients who are penicillin allergic – or in the rare circumstance of infection with a strain that is ampicillin resistant – is uncertain and specialist microbiological advice should be sought. Specific therapies for cryptococcal meningitis are described in detail later in this chapter.

Patients who have had a splenectomy are susceptible to invasive infections with encapsulated bacteria, including *S. pneumoniae* and Hib. Standard therapy with either cefotaxime or ceftriaxone is appropriate.

Post-neurosurgery meningitis. The majority of cases are aseptic meningitis secondary to a local inflammatory reaction to blood breakdown products or to tumor antigens, but it is not usually possible to distinguish between aseptic meningitis and infective meningitis until culture results are available after 48–72 hours. Post-operative infective meningitis is usually due to micro-organisms introduced into the meninges at the time of surgery. The range of potential pathogens is wide, with staphylococci, enteric bacteria (e.g. *E. coli*) and respiratory bacteria (e.g. *Haemophilus* species) each accounting for around one-third of cases. Broad-spectrum empiric therapy, usually with a carbapenem antibiotic, is indicated; vancomycin should be added if the patient is at risk of infection with MRSA

Table 39.4 Antimicrobial regimens for treatment of shunt meningitis

Type of infection	First-choice antibiotic regimen	Other antibiotic regimens	Duration of therapy before reshunting
Internal shunt infection caused by Gram-positive bacteria	Intraventricular vancomycin + intravenous or oral rifampicin	Substitute flucloxacillin or intravenous vancomycin for rifampicin in cases of rifampicin resistance, except in the case of enterococci, where an aminoglycoside (e.g. gentamicin) should be used	7–10 days intravenous
External shunt infection caused by *Staphylococcus aureus*	As mentioned in the section, 'Shunt-associated meningitis', with the addition of intravenous flucloxacillin	Substitute intravenous vancomycin for flucloxacillin in the case of meticillin resistance (meticillin-resistant *S. aureus*)	12–14 days
Enterobacteriaceae	Intravenous cefotaxime ± an aminoglycoside + intraventricular aminoglycoside	Substitute ceftazidime or meropenem for cefotaxime in the case of cefotaxime resistance	14 days
Polymicrobial ventriculoperitoneal shunt infections	Intravenous amoxicillin, metronidazole, cefotaxime ± intravenous and/or intraventricular aminoglycoside	Seek specialist advice	14 days
Candida	Intravenous amphotericin B + flucytosine	Intravenous fluconazole or voriconazole ± flucytosine	10–14 days (antifungal fungal therapy should continue for 1 week after reshunting)

(Alnimr, 2012). Antibiotic therapy should be reviewed once culture results are available, to determine whether treatment can be discontinued (if a diagnosis of aseptic meningitis is established) or de-escalated.

Shunt-associated meningitis. Patients who have a ventricular shunt are at increased risk of meningitis. Shunt-associated infections are classified according to the site of initial infection. Internal infections, where the lumen of the shunt is colonised, constitute the majority of cases. External shunt infections involve the tissues surrounding the shunt. Most internal shunt infections are caused by coagulase-negative staphylococci. *S. aureus* and *Enterobacteriaceae* account for most external infections. It is generally held that management of shunt infections should include shunt removal, as well as systemic therapy with or without intraventricular antibiotics (Wells and Allen, 2013). Although the need for shunt removal has been questioned (Arnell et al., 2007), there is also evidence that shunts that are not removed are associated with subsequent shunt revisions because of complications from the infection. Appropriate antimicrobial regimens are listed in Table 39.4.

Tuberculous meningitis. The outcome in tuberculous meningitis relates directly to the severity of the patient's clinical condition on commencement of therapy. A satisfactory response demands a high degree of clinical suspicion such that appropriate chemotherapy is initiated early, even if tubercle bacilli are not demonstrated on initial microscopy. Most currently used antituberculous agents achieve effective concentrations in the CSF in tuberculous meningitis. Detailed discussion of antituberculous therapy is given in Chapter 41. Adjunctive steroid therapy is of value in patients with more severe disease, for example, in the presence of increased intracranial pressure,

altered consciousness, focal neurological findings, spinal block and tuberculous encephalopathy. However, routine use of steroids is not recommended. They may suppress informative changes in the CSF and interfere with antibiotic penetration by restoring the blood–brain barrier. Early neurosurgical management of hydrocephalus by means of a ventriculoperitoneal or ventriculoatrial shunt is also important in improving the prospects for neurological recovery.

Cryptococcal meningitis. The standard treatment of cryptococcal meningitis is amphotericin B. Traditionally, amphotericin B deoxycholate has been the preferred formulation given intravenously at a dose of 0.7–1.0 mg/kg per day. However, there is growing evidence that lipid formulations of amphotericin B are as effective, with less nephrotoxicity; AmBisome at a dosage of 4 mg/kg per day or Abelcet at a dosage of 5 mg/kg per day are suitable alternatives to amphotericin B deoxycholate (Nelson et al., 2011). Amphotericin B formulations should be combined with flucytosine 100 mg/kg per day in four divided doses. Addition of flucytosine results in quicker clearance of yeasts from the CSF and may be associated with an improved clinical outcome. Therapy with amphotericin B and flucytosine is normally continued for 6–10 weeks. As an alternative to prolonged therapy with two potentially toxic drugs, 2 weeks of therapy with amphotericin B and flucytosine may be given, followed by consolidation therapy with fluconazole 400 mg/day for at least 10 weeks. Initial treatment with fluconazole 400–800 mg/day plus flucytosine is clinically inferior to amphotericin B–based regimens, and in any case is no better tolerated than amphotericin B–based regimens. Regular haematological and biochemical monitoring is recommended during treatment, along with measurement of serum concentrations of flucytosine (which should not exceed 80 mg/L).

The clinical response to treatment of cryptococcal meningitis is slow, and it often takes 2 or 3 weeks to sterilise the CSF. Monitoring of intracranial pressure is essential, with large-volume CSF drainage indicated if the opening pressure reaches 250 mmHg. Serial CSF cultures are occasionally helpful in following the response to treatment, but monitoring of cryptococcal antigen titres in serum or CSF is of little value.

Patients with HIV infection who are treated for cryptococcal meningitis should then receive fluconazole indefinitely, or at least until immune reconstitution occurs. The dosage of fluconazole may be reduced to 200 mg/day, depending on the patient's clinical condition (Bicanic and Harrison, 2004). Itraconazole offers less good CSF penetration than fluconazole and is clinically inferior. However, it is sometimes used as maintenance therapy at a dosage of 200–400 mg/day for patients who are unable to tolerate fluconazole. Clinical data with newer triazoles, such as voriconazole and posaconazole, remain limited, but these agents may be useful, especially in the rare situation of fluconazole-resistant cryptococcal meningitis. The echinocandin class of antifungals does not possess useful activity against *Cryptococcus*.

Viral meningitis. None of the currently available antiviral agents has useful activity against human enteroviruses, the commonest causes of viral meningitis (Big et al., 2009). Fortunately, however, the condition is usually self-limiting. The viruses that commonly cause this condition, herpes simplex and varicella zoster meningoencephalitis, are treated with high-dose aciclovir 10 mg/kg three times daily for at least 10 days (adults and children aged ≥12 years). For younger children, the recommended dosages are 20 mg/kg three times daily for infants up to age 3 months and 500 mg/m^2 three times daily for those aged 3 months to 12 years.

Steroids as adjunctive therapy in bacterial meningitis. In pharmacological doses, corticosteroids, and in particular dexamethasone, regulate many components of the inflammatory response and also lower CSF hydrostatic pressure. However, by reducing inflammation and restoring the blood–brain barrier, they may reduce CSF penetration of antibiotics. The benefits of steroids in the initial management of meningitis caused by *M. tuberculosis* and Hib are well established, although in other forms of bacterial meningitis the evidence has been less compelling. However, a 2015 Cochrane review of corticosteroid use for acute bacterial meningitis concluded that corticosteroids significantly reduced hearing loss and neurological sequelae without serious adverse effects, although they did not reduce overall mortality (Brouwer et al., 2015). The use of adjunctive intravenous dexamethasone is now recommended for children and adults with community-acquired bacterial meningitis, regardless of bacterial aetiology. Adjunctive therapy should ideally be initiated within 4 hours of the first dose of antibiotic; do not start dexamethasone more than 12 hours after starting antibiotics (National Institute for Health and Care Excellence, 2015). The recommended dosage for adults is 10 mg intravenously four times daily for 4 days (for children 0.15 mg/kg four times daily for 4 days).

Intrathecal and intraventricular administration of antibiotics. Intrathecal administration, that is, administration into the lumbar subarachnoid space, of antibiotics was once widely used to supplement levels attained by concomitant systemic therapy. However, there is little evidence for the efficacy of this route of delivery, and it is now rarely used. In particular, it produces only

Table 39.5 Daily[a] doses (mg) of gentamicin and vancomycin for intraventricular administration

Antibiotic	Adult	Child ≥2 years old	Child <2 years old
Gentamicin	1.0[b]	1.0	1.0
Vancomycin	15–20	10[c]	10[c]

[a]If cerebrospinal fluid is not draining freely, reduce dose frequency to once every 2–3 days.
[b]Dose can be increased to up to 5 mg in the most severe cases.
[c]Reduce dose to 5 mg if ventricular size is reduced, or increase to 15–20 mg/day if ventricular size is increased.

low concentrations of antibiotic in the ventricles and, therefore, does little to prevent ventriculitis, one of the most serious complications of meningitis. Direct intraventricular administration of antibiotics in meningitis is important in certain types of meningitis, especially where it is necessary to use an agent (e.g. vancomycin or an aminoglycoside) that penetrates CSF poorly (Shah et al., 2004). The most common situation is in shunt-associated meningitis, where multiple antibiotic-resistant coagulase-negative staphylococci are the major pathogens, and where conveniently the patient will often have an external ventricular drain through which antibiotics can be administered.

There are considerable differences in recommended doses of antibiotics for intrathecal or intraventricular administration. A dose of 15–20 mg vancomycin per day is recommended for treatment of shunt-associated meningitis in adults with an extraventricular drain and 10 mg/day for neonates and children. The paediatric dose may need to be reduced to 5 mg/day if ventricular size is reduced, or increased to 15–20 mg/day if the ventricular size is increased. In all patients, the dose frequency should be decreased to once every 2–3 days if CSF is not draining freely. The CSF vancomycin concentration should be measured after 3–4 days, aiming for a trough concentration less than 10 mg/L. Recommended doses of antibiotics are otherwise largely based on anecdotal experience (Table 39.5).

Patient care

Common problems in the treatment of meningitis are set out in Table 39.6.

Prevention of person-to-person transmission

Patients with meningitis may be infectious to others. Neonates with meningitis usually have generalised infections, and the causative organisms can often be isolated from body fluids and faeces. Babies with meningitis should therefore be isolated to prevent infection spreading to other patients. Patients with meningococcal or Hib meningitis should be isolated until after at least 48 hours of antibiotic therapy. Contacts of these patients may be asymptomatic carriers and potentially infectious to others and/or at risk of development of invasive infection themselves. Chemoprophylaxis and vaccination can reduce these risks. Patients with most other types of meningitis do not represent a

Table 39.6 Practice points in infective meningitis

Infection	Antibiotic	Common problems	Resolution
Bacterial meningitis	Chloramphenicol	Risk of serious toxicity, especially in neonates	Avoid use if possible Close monitoring of serum levels where use essential
Neonatal meningitis	Aminoglycosides (e.g. gentamicin)	Poor CSF penetration provides unreliable activity for Gram-negative bacterial meningitis Unpredictable neonatal pharmacokinetics (especially preterm neonates)	Substitute with, or add, an antibiotic with better CSF penetration (e.g. a cephalosporin) Close monitoring of serum levels
Streptococcus pneumoniae meningitis	Penicillin Cefotaxime or ceftriaxone Vancomycin (intravenous)	Resistance is increasing Treatment failure in meningitis due to penicillin-resistant strains Unreliable CSF penetration	Use cefotaxime or ceftriaxone ± vancomycin as empiric therapy Add rifampicin or vancomycin Consider one of the newer antibiotics with good activity against multidrug-resistant Gram-positive bacteria
Listeria monocytogenes meningitis	Any	Relapse rate up to 10% after short courses of therapy	Give prolonged therapy (usually 3–4 weeks)
Cryptococcal meningitis	Amphotericin B Flucytosine Fluconazole	High incidence of side effects, e.g. fever, nausea, vomiting, anaemia, hypokalaemia, impaired renal function Risk of side effects, e.g. deranged liver function, bone marrow depression Low cure rate when used as monotherapy (except as consolidation therapy)	Change to lipid-based preparation of amphotericin B, or replace with fluconazole Close monitoring of serum levels Combine with flucytosine

CSF, Cerebrospinal fluid.

significant infectious hazard, and enhanced infection control precautions are not usually necessary.

Case studies

Case 39.1

A 3-week-old preterm infant was born at 25 weeks gestation and is being cared for on the hospital neonatal intensive care unit. He becomes unwell, with poor feeding, fever and increasing drowsiness. Sepsis, with possible meningitis, is diagnosed, and the baby is commenced empirically on amoxicillin and cefotaxime. A lumbar puncture reveals 1200 white blood cells/microlitre (80% of which are polymorphs) and low glucose and elevated protein levels, but no organisms are seen on a Gram-stained smear of the CSF.

On the following day the microbiology laboratory telephones the unit to tell them that Gram-negative bacilli have been grown from blood cultures and the CSF culture; the baby has not improved clinically.

Questions

1. What are the most likely aetiological agents in a 3-week-old baby with acute purulent meningitis?
2. Why might the baby's condition not have improved 24 hours after commencing antibiotic therapy?
3. Would you change the baby's antibiotic therapy once it was known that the baby had Gram-negative sepsis and meningitis?

Answers

1. At 3 weeks of age, the possible causes of meningitis include neonatal pathogens (group B streptococci, *E. coli* and *L. monocytogenes*), nosocomial pathogens such as *S. aureus* and Gram-negative bacilli, and even occasionally the usual causes of meningitis in older infants (especially *N. meningitidis* and *S. pneumoniae*). Most group B streptococcal disease presents in the first few days of life, whilst listeria meningitis is very uncommon, meaning that of the neonatal pathogens there is a greater likelihood of Gram-negative bacillary meningitis. Indeed on the second day it was confirmed that the baby did have Gram-negative bacillary meningitis.
2. Gram-negative sepsis is a serious condition, and it may take longer than 24 hours for a baby to begin to recover. However, it is important to consider the possibility of infection with multidrug-resistant Gram-negative bacteria (MDRGNB). Bacteria such as *E. coli*, *Klebsiella*, *Enterobacter* or *Serratia* may produce β-lactamases that destroy cephalosporins. *P. aeruginosa* is another Gram-negative bacterium that is always resistant to cefotaxime.
3. If the baby's condition is stable, it might be reasonable to observe him closely and defer any review of antibiotic treatment until more microbiology results are available. However, many prescribers would change antibiotic therapy to a carbapenem at this stage; this would be mandatory if either the baby's condition had deteriorated, or if the baby was known to be colonised with an MDRGNB.

Case 39.2

Mr HP, a 70-year-old man, is being treated for meningitis caused by *S. pneumoniae* that is moderately resistant to penicillin (MIC value 1.0 mg/L). Despite 7 days of treatment with intravenous vancomycin and cefotaxime, there has been little improvement in his clinical condition. A CT scan has shown meningeal inflammation consistent with meningitis, but no evidence of intracranial complications that might explain his poor clinical response. The most recent trough (pre-dose) serum vancomycin concentration was 5.3 mg/L.

Questions

1. Why might there have been an inadequate response to treatment with cefotaxime and vancomycin?
2. What options are there to modify Mr HP's antimicrobial therapy?

Answers

1. Cefotaxime alone may not adequately treat meningitis caused by penicillin-resistant pneumococci. CSF penetration of vancomycin is poor; the serum vancomycin concentration in this case is low, meaning that there is little prospect of drug concentration in the CSF being effective. Even if the vancomycin concentration in CSF were adequate, the infection may be due to a vancomycin-tolerant strain of *S. pneumoniae*. Tolerant strains appear fully sensitive to vancomycin by routine laboratory antimicrobial susceptibility sensitivity testing.
2. It is important to optimise Mr HP's treatment as quickly as possible. He might respond to increasing the dose of vancomycin with or without addition of rifampicin. However, these strategies give little assurance of success. It would probably be preferable to switch to an alternative agent. Meropenem would not be a good choice, and certainly not as monotherapy, because there has already been an inadequate response to another β-lactam antibiotic. Linezolid or a quinolone with good activity against Gram-positive bacteria (e.g. moxifloxacin) would be the most appropriate drugs.

Case 39.3

Mr KT, an 18-year-old man, is referred as an emergency with suspected meningitis. He was given intravenous penicillin by the primary care doctor before admission to hospital. On examination he is fully conscious, and neck stiffness is elicited. He is haemodynamically stable, and no rash is present.

Questions

1. What investigations would you undertake to establish the diagnosis?
2. What treatment would you give Mr KT?
3. What further action will be required if a diagnosis of meningococcal meningitis is either confirmed or considered likely?

Answers

1. Blood cultures and a nasopharyngeal swab for culture should be collected. There are no clinical contraindications to lumbar puncture, and in most centres this would be undertaken without a prior CT scan. The white cell count and glucose and protein concentrations in the CSF should be measured. A Gram stain should be undertaken, which may give immediate information on the likely identity of the pathogen, as well as culture. Blood and CSF should be tested for *N. meningitidis* and *S. pneumoniae* by PCR. In the

UK these tests are provided by national reference laboratories. In addition, some laboratories may undertake multiplex PCR testing or antigen testing locally to try to establish an early aetiological diagnosis.
2. Antibiotic treatment should be with a third-generation cephalosporin (cefotaxime or ceftriaxone). The latter should be entirely safe to use in this situation given that it sounds unlikely that the patient will have required resuscitation with calcium-containing fluids. There is no clinical indication to add amoxicillin. In addition, adjunctive therapy with dexamethasone (IV 10 mg four times a day for 4 days), for which there appear to be no contraindications, should be considered.
3. Meningitis is a notifiable disease. If a diagnosis of meningococcal meningitis is considered likely, then chemoprophylaxis should be offered to the patient and to close contacts as soon as possible (preferably within 24 hours) to eliminate nasopharyngeal carriage and prevent secondary cases. If a diagnosis of meningococcal disease is confirmed, immunisation may also be indicated for the contacts, depending on the strain's serogroup.

Case 39.4

Mrs GT, an 88-year-old woman who lives on her own, presents with a 3-day history of fever, headache and vomiting, and a 1-day history of altered consciousness. She was taking seven different dugs, including furosemide for heart failure. On examination she was ill-looking and had altered consciousness (Glasgow Coma Scale score 9/15). She was febrile (39.2 °C) and had marked neck stiffness. The remainder of the physical examination was unremarkable.

A brain CT scan demonstrated no parenchymal abnormality. For further assessment, a lumbar puncture was then performed. CSF analysis showed leucocytosis (90% polymorphs), high protein concentration and low glucose level with a decreased CSF/serum glucose ratio. No organisms were seen on Gram or acid-fast stains.

Questions

1. What are the likely causes of Mrs GT's meningitis?
2. What antimicrobial treatment would you prescribe?
3. If after 24 hours Gram-positive bacteria were isolated from the CSF, how would this change your management?

Answers

1. The CSF findings (polymorph leucocytosis, low glucose) are strongly suggestive of bacterial meningitis. Increasing life expectancy means we are likely to see more cases like this. As well as possibly being due to one of the usual causes of bacterial meningitis, the elderly are at greater risk of listeria meningitis. Tuberculous meningitis is unlikely because the history of illness is relatively brief.
2. Empiric treatment with amoxicillin or ampicillin together with a third-generation cephalosporin (e.g. cefotaxime) would be appropriate.
3. Isolation of Gram-positive bacilli is consistent with listeria meningitis. The treatment of listeria meningitis is with high-dose amoxicillin or ampicillin, combined with an aminoglycoside (e.g. gentamicin). In this patient the dose of amoxicillin or ampicillin will need to be based on an assessment of her renal function. The decision to add an aminoglycoside will need to consider the risks for toxicity in an elderly patient who is receiving furosemide, as well as the clinical condition of the patient. Because cephalosporins are high-risk antibiotics for *Clostridium difficile*, this treatment should be discontinued.

References

Alnimr, A., 2012. A protocol for diagnosis and management of cerebrospinal shunt infections and other infectious conditions in neurosurgical practice. Basic Clin. Neurosci. 3, 61–70.

Arnell, K., Enblad, P., Wester, T., et al., 2007. Treatment of cerebrospinal fluid shunt infections in children using systemic and intraventricular antibiotic therapy in combination with externalization of the ventricular catheter: efficacy in 34 consecutively treated infections. J. Neurosurg. 107, 213–219.

Bicanic, T., Harrison, T.S., 2004. Cryptococcal meningitis. Br. Med. Bull. 72, 99–118.

Big, C., Reineck, L.A., Aronoff, D.M., 2009. Viral infections of the central nervous system: a case-based review. Clin. Med. Res. 7, 142–146.

Brouwer, M.C., McIntyre, P., Prasad, K., et al., 2015. Corticosteroids for acute bacterial meningitis. Cochrane Database Syst. Rev. 9, CD004405. https://doi.org/10.1002/14651858.CD004405.pub5.

Brouwer, M.C., Tunkel, A.R., van de Beek, D., 2010. Epidemiology, diagnosis, and antimicrobial treatment of acute bacterial meningitis. Clin. Microbiol. Rev. 23, 467–492.

Cottagnoud, P.H., Tauber, M.G., 2004. New therapies for pneumococcal meningitis. Exp. Opin. Invest. Drugs 13, 393–401.

Galiza, E.P., Heath, P.T., 2009. Improving the outcome of neonatal meningitis. Curr. Opin. Infect. Dis. 22, 229–234.

Health Protection Agency Meningococcus and Haemophilus Forum, 2012. Guidance for public health management of meningococcal disease in the UK, updated March. Health Protection Agency, London. https://www.gov.uk/government/uploads/system/uploads/attachment_data/file/322008/Guidance_for_management_of_meningococcal_disease_pdf.pdf.

McIntosh, E.D., 2005. Treatment and prevention strategies to combat pediatric pneumococcal meningitis. Exp. Rev. Anti Infect. Ther. 3, 739–750.

National Institute for Health and Care Excellence, 2012. Neonatal infection: antibiotics for prevention and treatment. Clinical Guideline 149. Available at: http://www.nice.org.uk/guidance/cg449.

National Institute for Health and Care Excellence, 2015. Meningitis (bacterial) and meningococcal septicaemia in under 16s: recognition, diagnosis and management. Clinical guideline 102. Available at: https://www.nice.org.uk/guidance/cg102.

Nelson, M., Manji, H., Wilkins, E., 2011. Central nervous system opportunistic infections. In: British HIV Association and British Infection Association Guidelines for the Treatment of Opportunistic Infection in HIV-Seropositive Individuals 2011. HIV Med. 12 (Suppl. 2), 8–24.

Public Health England, 2013. Revised recommendations for the prevention of secondary *Haemophilus influenzae* type b (Hib) disease, updated July. Public Health England, London. https://www.gov.uk/government/uploads/system/uploads/attachment_data/file/231009/Revised_recommendations_for_the_preventions_of_secondary_Haemophilus_influenzae_type_b_disease.pdf.

Ross, J.S., Wilson, K.J.W., 1981. Foundations of Anatomy and Physiology, fifth ed. Churchill Livingstone, Edinburgh, pp. 172–173.

Rupprecht, T.A., Pfister, H.W., 2005. Clinical experience with linezolid for the treatment of central nervous system infections. Eur. J. Neurol. 12, 536–542.

Salisbury, D., Ramsay, M., 2013. Immunisation against infectious disease. Department of Health, London. Available at: https://www.gov.uk/government/collections/immunisation-against-infectious-disease-the-green-book.

Shah, S.S., Ohlsson, A., Shah, V.S., 2004. Intraventricular antibiotics for bacterial meningitis in neonates. Cochrane Database Syst. Rev. 4, CD004496. https://doi.org/10.1002/14651858.CD004496.pub2.

Wells, D.M., Allen, J.M., 2013. Ventriculoperitoneal shunt infections in adult patients. AACN Adv. Crit. Care. 24, 6–12.

Further reading

Chang, L., Phipps, W., Kennedy, G., et al., 2005. Antifungal interventions for the primary prevention of cryptococcal disease in adults with HIV. Cochrane Database Syst. Rev. 3, CD004773, pub2. https://doi.org/10.1002/14651858.CD004773.pub2.

Chaudhuri, A., Martinez-Martin, P., Kennedy, P.G., et al., 2008. EFNS guideline on the management of community-acquired bacterial meningitis: report of an EFNS Task Force on acute bacterial meningitis in older children and adults. Eur. J. Neurol. 15, 649–659.

Chavez-Bueno, S., McCracken, G.H., 2005. Bacterial meningitis in children. Pediatr. Clin. N. Am. 52, 795–810.

Correia, J.B., Hart, C.A., 2004. Meningococcal disease. Clin. Evid. 12, 1164–1181.

Ihekwaba, U.K., Kudesia, G., McKendrick, M.W., 2008. Clinical features of viral meningitis in adults: significant differences in cerebrospinal fluid findings among herpes simplex virus, varicella zoster virus, and enterovirus infections. Clin. Infect. Dis. 47, 783–789.

Perfect, J.R., Dismukes, W.E., Dromer, F., et al., Clinical practice guidelines for the management of cryptococcal disease: 2010 update by the Infectious Diseases Society of America. Clin. Infect. Dis. 50, 291–322.

Riordan, A., 2010. The implications of vaccines for prevention of bacterial meningitis. Curr. Opin. Neurol. 23, 319–324.

Tunkel, A.R., Hartman, B.J., Kaplan, S.L., et al., 2004. Practice guidelines for the management of bacterial meningitis. Clin. Infect. Dis. 39, 1267–1284.

Zunt, J.R., 2010. Infections of the central nervous system in the neurosurgical patient. Handb. Clin. Neurol. 96, 125–141.

40 Surgical Site Infection and Antimicrobial Prophylaxis

Philip Howard and Jonathan Sandoe

Key points

- Surgical site infection is a major cause of mortality and morbidity.
- Development of surgical site infection is a complex process influenced by host, operative and microbial factors.
- The microbial cause of surgical site infection varies with type of procedure, but Enterobacteriaceae (coliforms) have replaced *Staphylococcus aureus* as the predominant organism grown from surgical site infections for many procedures.
- Surveillance of surgical site infection is necessary to benchmark and improve prevention strategies.
- Antimicrobial prophylaxis is just one of many approaches to reduce surgical site infection.
- Not all operations require antimicrobial prophylaxis.
- Antimicrobial prophylaxis should be used only where there is evidence of efficacy or expert consensus that benefits outweigh risks.
- The choice of antimicrobial prophylaxis depends on the operation, pharmacokinetics, pharmacodynamics and patient factors.
- The timing of antimicrobial administration is key to reducing surgical site infection.
- Pharmacists are unlikely to see many patients before surgery; they must therefore develop systems to ensure that appropriate antimicrobial prophylaxis is given at the right time.

Surgery is the branch of medical science that treats injury or disease, or improves bodily function through operative procedures. Surgery has been used for thousands of years but has always been complicated to some extent by infection. Currently, surgery is an integral part of the management of many medical conditions and remains the definitive treatment for many cancers. Infections developing at the site of invasive surgical procedures are frequently referred to as surgical site infections. Surgical site infections occur when pathogenic microorganisms contaminate a surgical wound, multiply and cause tissue damage. The term 'surgical site infection' encompasses not only infection at the site of incision, but also infections of implants, prosthetic devices and adjacent tissues involved in the operation.

Epidemiology

In England, more than 11 million operations and interventions are undertaken each year. More than 50% of these are performed as day cases, and many patients are admitted on the day of surgery (Health and Social Care Information Centre, 2016).

Healthcare-associated infections (HCAIs), including surgical site infections, complicate around 6% of all hospital admissions (Health Protection Agency, 2012). Surgical site infections are of major clinical importance because they account for 14–16% of all HCAIs (Health Protection Agency, 2012; Health Protection Scotland, 2015; Public Accounts Committee, 2009) and are associated with considerable morbidity and mortality. One-third of peri-operative deaths are related to surgical site infections (Astagneau et al., 2001). It has been estimated that surgical site infections double the length of hospital stay (Coello et al., 2005). Although surgical site infections can be common in some procedures, the incidence can be minimised by the care provided before and after the operation, together with the skill of the surgeon (Health Protection Scotland, 2015).

Surveillance

Monitoring the incidence of surgical site infections is hampered by the lack of agreed measuring systems. In particular, to monitor the rates of surgical site infection within an organisation, or to benchmark between organisations, there needs to be a standard approach to diagnosis. Criteria for such a definition have been developed by the Centers for Disease Control and Prevention (Mangram et al., 1999), and these are presented in Table 40.1. More detailed surgical site infection scoring systems have been developed, but these are time consuming to use.

Mandatory surveillance for surgical site infections in orthopaedic surgery in the UK was introduced in 2004. In addition, Scotland and Wales monitor caesarian section surgical site infections (http://www.hps.scot.nhs.uk and http://www.wales.nhs.uk). England has a voluntary reporting system for a broader range of operations (https://www.gov.uk/guidance/surgical-site-infection-surveillance-service-ssiss). All report their findings annually. Many surgical site infections, especially those involving prosthetic joints, often develop late (>28 days post-operation), so post-discharge surveillance schemes are essential. Patients need to be aware how a surgical site infection may present after discharge from hospital. Surveillance of surgical site infections and feedback to the surgical team has been shown to reduce rates of infection (Gastmeier et al., 2005).

Table 40.1 Criteria for defining surgical site infection (Mangram et al., 1999)

Type	Level	Signs and symptoms
Superficial incisional	Skin and subcutaneous tissue	Localised (Celsian) signs such as redness, pain, heat or swelling at the site of the incision or by the presence of pus within 30 days
Deep incisional	Fascial and muscle layers	Presence of pus or an abscess, fever with tenderness of the wound, or a separation of the edges of the incision exposing the deeper tissues within 30 days (or 1 year if an implant is used)
Organ or space infection	Any part of the anatomy other than the incision that is opened or manipulated during the surgical procedure, e.g. joint or peritoneum	Loss of function of a joint, abscess in an organ, localised peritonitis or collection; ultrasound or computed tomography scans confirm infection; within 30 days of surgery if no implant is used or within 1 year of surgery if an implant is used.

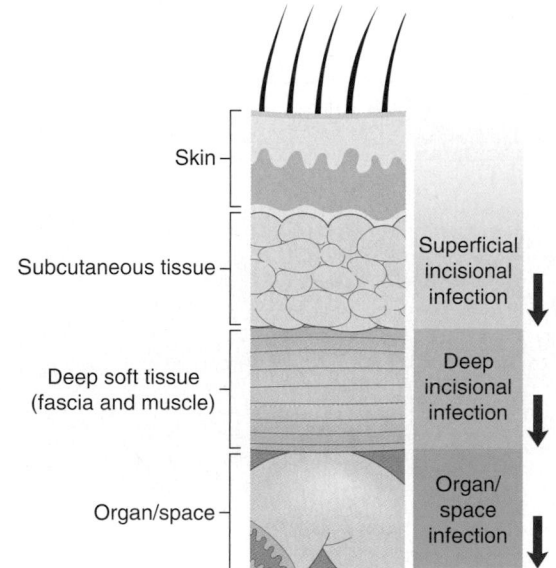

Fig. 40.1 Schematic representation of the anatomical classification of surgical site infection (Horan et al., 1993). (Reproduced with permission from the University of Chicago Press.)

Risk factors

Surgical site infections can be categorised into three groups: superficial incisional, deep incisional and organ or space (Fig. 40.1). Whether a wound infection occurs after surgery depends on a complex interaction among the following:

- procedure-related factors, for example, implantation of foreign bodies, degree of trauma to host tissues and experience of surgeon;
- patient-related factors, for example, host immunity, nutritional status and the presence or absence of diabetes;
- microbial factors (tissue adherence and invasion);
- peri-operative antimicrobial prophylaxis.

A system to stratify operative wounds by the expected level of bacterial contamination (Table 40.2) was developed to help predict likely infection rates (Mangram et al., 1999). A number of other factors have also been found to affect the incidence of surgical site infection and are discussed later.

Prosthetic implants

Medical implants have a detrimental effect on host defences such that a lower bacterial count is needed to initiate infection. Hence there is a greater risk of infection during implant surgery. Bacteria growing on an abiotic surface, such as a prosthetic hip implant or heart valve, together with a protective layer of microbial polymers are known as a biofilm (Donlan and Costerton, 2002). Antimicrobials are frequently ineffective against microorganisms growing in biofilms, making treatment of implant infections problematic and their prevention even more important.

Duration of surgery

The longer the operation, the greater the risk of wound infection. This, in turn, may be influenced by the experience (Fig. 40.2), speed and skill of the surgeon, and is additional to the classification of the operation by risk of infection, for example, clean, contaminated, dirty or infected.

Patient-related factors

A number of patient-related factors are known to influence the likelihood of developing a surgical site infection and include the following:

- wound potential for infection, for example, clean, contaminated, dirty or infected site,
- physical status of patient (Table 40.3),
- duration of procedure.

For each surgical procedure, a score of 0–3 is allocated to represent the number of risk factors present. Patients with a score of 0 are at the lowest risk of development of a surgical site infection, whereas those with a score of 3 have the greatest risk (Table 40.4). Use of this risk index allows comparison of similar patient groups in terms of surgical site infection risk over time. The risk index is a significantly better predictor of surgical wound risk than the traditional wound classification system and performs well across a broad range of operative procedures.

Table 40.2 Classification of surgical procedures by risk of infection (Mangram et al., 1999)

Type of procedure	Definition	Wound infection rate (%)	Example	Need for prophylaxis
Clean	Atraumatic; no inflammation encountered, no break in technique; gastro-intestinal, genitourinary and respiratory tracts not entered	1.5–4.2	Inguinal hernia repair	Not usually required
Contaminated	Gastro-intestinal or respiratory tract entered but without spillage; oropharynx, appendectomy, sterile genitourinary or biliary tract entered; minor break in technique	<10	Cholecystectomy (no spillage)	Usually required
Clean-contaminated	Acute inflammation; infected bile or urine; gross spillage from gastro-intestinal tract; major lapse in technique; fresh traumatic wound (12–24 h)	10–20	Appendicectomy	Required
Dirty and infected	Established infection; transection of clean tissues to enable collection of pus; traumatic wound with retained devitalised tissue; faecal contamination; delayed treatment	20–40	Sigmoid colectomy (Hartmann's procedure) for faecal peritonitis	Treatment required (not prophylaxis)

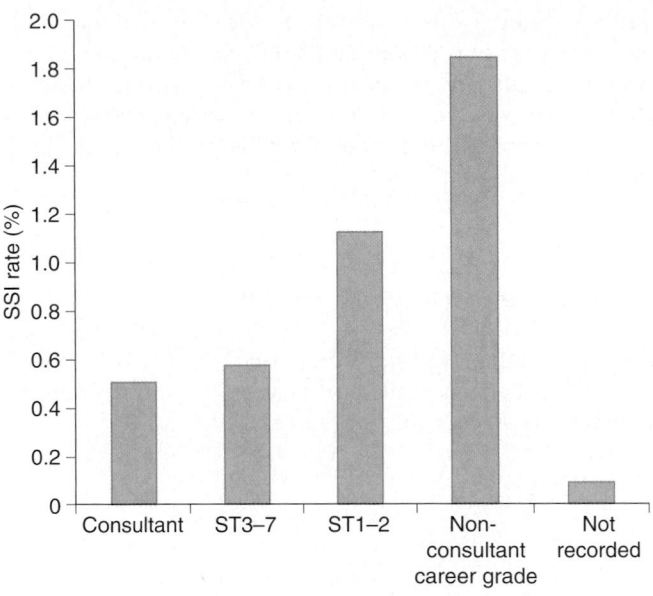

ST = Speciality registrar grade, number represents years of training

Fig. 40.2 Surgical site infection (SSI) rate by grade of operator for orthopaedic surgery in 2008 (Health Protection Scotland, 2009). (Reproduced with kind permission from Health Protection Scotland.)

Table 40.3 American Society of Anesthesiology classification of physical status (Mangram et al., 1999)

American Society of Anesthesiology score	Physical status
1	A normal, healthy patient
2	A patient with mild systemic disease
3	A patient with a severe systemic disease that limits activity but is not incapacitating
4	A patient with an incapacitating systemic disease that is a constant threat to life
5	A moribund patient who is not expected to survive 24 h with or without operation

Table 40.4 Risk index based on presence of co-morbidity and duration of operation (Culver et al., 1991)

Risk index	Infection rate (%)
0	1.5
1	2.9
2	6.8
3	13.0

Other factors

There are a number of other risk factors that may increase the risk of a surgical site infection (Table 40.5) for an individual patient, but the impact has not been quantified to the same extent as the risk factors discussed earlier. Some are modifiable; others such as age are not.

Table 40.5 Patient and operative risk factors for surgical site infection

Patient risk factors	Operative risk factors
Advanced age	Tissue ischaemia
Malnutrition	Lack of haemostasis
Obesity	Tissue damage, e.g. crushing by surgical instruments
Concurrent infection	Presence of necrotic tissue
Diabetes mellitus	Presence of foreign bodies including surgical materials
Liver impairment	
Renal impairment	
Immune deficiency states	
Prolonged preoperative stay	
Blood transfusion	
Smoking	

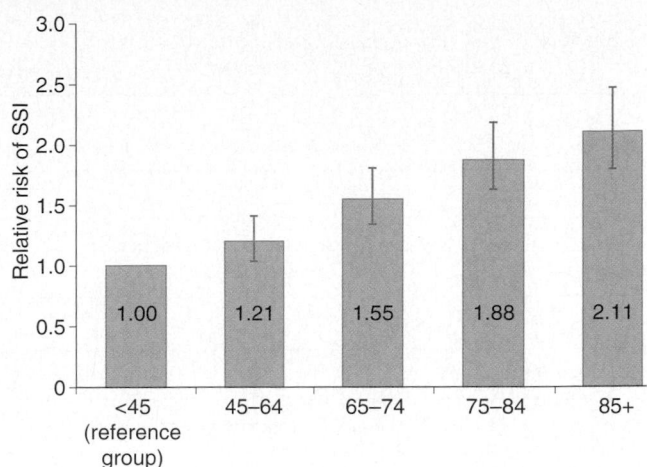

Fig. 40.3 Relative risk of surgical site infection (SSI) by age group, 2003–2007, adjusted for surgical category (reference age group is <45 years) (Health Protection Agency, 2008). (Reproduced with kind permission from Health Protection Agency.)

Smoking

Smoking increases the risk of development of a wound infection (Myles et al., 2002). The mechanism is not known, but tobacco use may delay wound healing via the vasoconstricting effects of nicotine, and thus increase the risk of infection (Myles et al., 2002). Smoking cessation for 30 days prior to surgery is recommended because it decreases post-operative morbidity and mortality (Sharma et al., 2013).

Diabetes mellitus

Long-term diabetes does not appear to have any impact on the risk of development of a surgical site infection. However, perioperative fluctuations in blood glucose for up to 48 hours have been shown to double the infection risk in cardiac patients (Latham et al., 2001).

Age

Increasing age is associated with an increased risk of surgical site infection. However, there is debate whether age serves simply as a marker for underlying disease or whether the decline in immune function with age is the significant factor. A study of 72,000 patients in the USA, which adjusted for hospital type, procedure, duration, wound class and physical status of the patient, showed a 1.1% increase in surgical site infection per year of age from the age of 18–65 years, but a 1.2% decrease in individuals older than 65 years (Kaye et al., 2005). In contrast, the findings of the English surgical site infection surveillance scheme (Fig. 40.3) indicated that the chance of acquiring a surgical site infection was 37% higher for a 65-year-old person compared with a 45-year-old person (Health Protection Agency, 2008).

Pathogenesis

Most surgery involves an incision through one of the body's protective barriers, typically the skin or other epithelial surface

such as the conjunctiva or tympanic membrane. When intact, these provide an excellent barrier to entry of both exogenous and endogenous bacteria. Other epithelial surfaces including the mucosal surfaces of the gastro-intestinal and genitourinary tracts, when intact, prevent entry of the luminal contents into the surrounding tissues and organs.

Any surgical operation will breach at least one of the surfaces mentioned and allow entry of bacteria. Whether an infection follows, depends on the ability of other defences to kill the invading bacteria. Important host mechanisms include antibodies, complement and phagocytes.

Development of a surgical site infection depends on survival of the contaminating microorganism in a wound site at the end of a surgical procedure, the pathogenicity and number of these microorganisms, and the host's immune response. Most microorganisms are from the host (endogenous), but they are occasionally introduced via surgical instruments, the environment or contaminated implants (exogenous). The likely invading microorganism varies according to the type of surgery (Table 40.6). Data for England from 2004 to 2016 show that Enterobacteriaceae (coliforms) have replaced *Staphylococcus aureus* as the predominant organism grown from surgical site infections for many procedure types (Public Health England, 2016). They accounted for 28% of all surgical site infections and were the prominent cause of surgical site infections in two categories: large-bowel surgery (53%) and coronary artery bypass graft (26%). *S. aureus* has steadily decreased to 13% from 39% in 2006/2007 (Fig. 40.4), primarily because of a reduction in meticillin-resistant *S. aureus* (MRSA) strains. The proportion of MRSA reduced from 25% to 4% of all *S. aureus* cases. Infection control measures including the introduction of mandatory MRSA screening for elective patients in 2009 may have contributed to this because known or previous MRSA carriers can be 'decolonised'.

The proportion of surgical site infections caused by *S. aureus* was highest in open reduction of long-bone fracture (44%), followed by knee prosthesis (42%), then hip hemiarthroplasty (34%) (Public Health England, 2016).

Table 40.6 Likely pathogens in post-operative wound infections

Category of surgery	Most likely pathogen(s)
Clean	
Cardiac/vascular/ orthopaedic	Coagulase-negative staphylococci, *Staphylococcus aureus*, Gram-negative bacilli
Breast	*S. aureus*
Clean-contaminated	
Burns	*S. aureus*, *Pseudomonas aeruginosa*
Head and neck	*S. aureus*, *Streptococcus* spp., anaerobes (from oral cavity)
Gastro-intestinal tract	Coliforms, anaerobes (*Bacteroides fragilis*)
Urogenital tract	Coliforms, *Enterococcus* spp.
Dirty	
Ruptured viscera	Coliforms, anaerobes (*B. fragilis*)
Traumatic wound	*S. aureus*, *Streptococcus pyogenes*, *Clostridium* spp.

Prevention of surgical site infection

The evidence that supports interventions to minimise surgical site infection has been highlighted in national guidelines (National Institute for Health and Care Excellence [NICE], 2017) and categorised into four areas: information to patients, preoperative phase, peri-operative phase and post-operative phase (Table 40.7). When selecting antimicrobial prophylaxis regimens or evaluating potential prophylaxis failures, it is important to ensure that all four aspects of prevention have been addressed.

Antimicrobial prophylaxis

In the early 1960s, it was demonstrated, using a guinea-pig model, that surgical-wound infection could be reduced by administration of an antimicrobial just before an incision was made, but the beneficial effect disappeared if antimicrobial administration was delayed by 3–4 hours after the incision (Burke, 1961). Since then, many clinical trials have indicated the benefit of maintaining adequate antimicrobial tissue levels from the time of initial surgical incision until closure.

There are potential adverse consequences to the administration of antimicrobials for both the individual and the population. For the individual, side effects range from antimicrobial-associated diarrhoea or thrush to life-threatening allergic reactions. From the population perspective, the development of antimicrobial

resistant bacteria is a concern. Antimicrobial prophylaxis should, therefore, only be offered to patients when there is evidence or, in the absence of evidence, expert consensus that the potential benefits of prophylaxis outweigh the risks.

The numbers of patients who need to be treated with antimicrobial agents to prevent one infection in the different types of surgery are presented in Table 40.8.

The infection risk associated with a particular surgical procedure and evidence of efficacy should be used to determine whether antimicrobial prophylaxis is to be administered. Not all surgical procedures warrant antimicrobial prophylaxis.

Choice of antimicrobial

Once it has been determined that antimicrobial prophylaxis is required, the next step is to select an appropriate agent(s). The choice of antimicrobial should take into account the following:
- likely infecting organisms (procedure specific);
- local susceptibility of potential pathogens to antimicrobials;
- pharmacokinetics, for example, penetration of antimicrobial to the site(s) in question;
- patient allergy to penicillins or other antimicrobials;
- administration time (bolus better than infusion);
- drug cost;
- carriage of resistant organisms, for example, MRSA;
- prevalence of *Clostridium difficile* infection in hospital.

The majority of clinical trials that have demonstrated the benefit of antimicrobial prophylaxis are outdated and probably do not reflect current surgical practice. First- and second-generation cephalosporins (cefazolin and cefuroxime) have been the mainstay of agents studied (Bratzler et al., 2013). There are advantages and disadvantages with using cephalosporins. The advantages include a low anaphylaxis risk, but they have the disadvantage of excessive or inadequate spectrum of cover depending on the operation (Morgan, 2006) and a strong association with *C. difficile* infection. Many antimicrobials used in prophylaxis have not been extensively studied in clinical trials but are selected on a theoretical basis of their antimicrobial spectrum (Tables 40.9–40.11).

Timing and duration

The timing of antimicrobial administration is one of the most important aspects of prophylaxis delivery. Animal studies, and latterly clinical observational studies, have shown that prophylaxis is most effective when given immediately before an operation (within 30 minutes of induction of anaesthesia), so that antimicrobial activity is present for the duration of the operation and for about 4 hours afterwards. Antimicrobials given too early prior to surgery are associated with prophylaxis failure, presumably because serum and tissue levels are not sustained during the surgical procedure. Similarly, for each hour antimicrobial administration was delayed after the start of the operation there was an increased rate of wound infection (Classen et al., 1992). This suggests bacterial replication, once commenced, cannot be eliminated by antimicrobial regimens designed for prophylaxis. The microbiological basis for these observations is likely to be that bacterial reproduction at a logarithmic rate follows a lag phase of relatively little increase in bacterial population. The

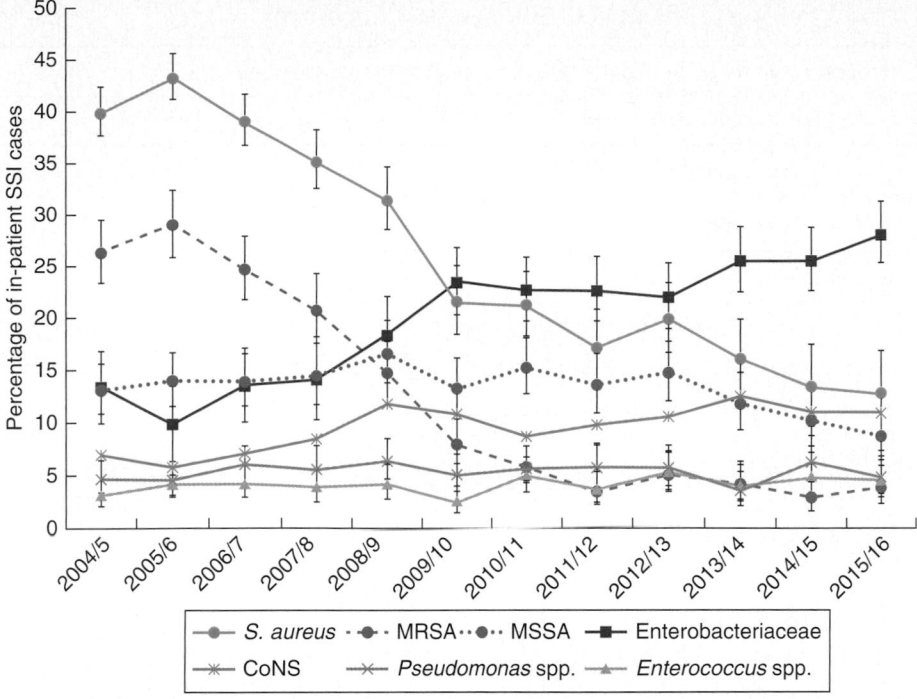

Fig. 40.4 Surgical site infection (SSI) isolated organisms 2004–16 (Public Health England, 2016). CoNS, Coagulase negative *Staphylococcus*; MRSA, meticillin-resistant *Staphylococcus aureus*; MSSA, meticillin sensitive *S. aureus*. (Reproduced with permission from Public Health England.)

Table 40.7 Recommendations for the prevention and treatment of surgical site infections (NICE, 2017)

Category	Recommendation
Information for patients and carers	How to recognise a surgical site infection and what to do
Preoperative phase	Patient preparation: preoperative washing, hair removal, nasal meticillin-resistant *S. aureus* decontamination and bowel preparation Antimicrobial prophylaxis guidance Staff preparation and theatre movement
Intra-operative phase	Operating team preparation Patient skin preparation Maintaining patient homeostasis Wound dressings
Postoperative phase	Dressing and cleansing the wound Antimicrobial treatment for surgical site infection Debridement of surgical site infections

lag phase for wound infection bacteria lasts typically 3–4 hours. If bacteria inoculated into a wound can be killed or inhibited by antimicrobials given early, the immune system can kill the remaining organisms. However, if antimicrobials are given only when the growth curve has entered the logarithmic phase, the chances of successful prophylaxis are reduced.

Formerly, protocols for prophylaxis extended for several post-operative days. Now, single-dose schedules are increasingly common with greater emphasis on ensuring immediate preoperative administration. Because surgery may be delayed at short notice, sometimes between the time the patient leaves the ward and arrives at the theatre, it is sensible for the responsibility for administration of antimicrobials to be transferred from ward staff to the operating team, allowing prophylaxis to be given around the time of induction of anaesthesia.

National guidelines recommend administration of prophylactic antimicrobials on starting anaesthesia, or earlier if a tourniquet is being used (NICE, 2017). Fig. 40.5 represents the two major studies undertaken to identify the optimum time for administration of prophylaxis. Both studies determined that post-incision administration of antimicrobials significantly increased the risk of surgical site infection (Classen et al., 1992; Steinberg et al., 2009). A large randomised controlled trial of pre-operative prophylaxis in more than 5000 general, vascular and orthopaedic surgical patients has recently found there was no difference in surgical site infection rates between patients given their preoperative antibiotics in the operating theatre (median time before administration 16 minutes) or in the anaesthetic room (median time to administration 42 minutes) (Weber et al., 2017). Historically, the only occasion where antimicrobial administration has been delayed to after the incision is caesarian section, where antimicrobials are given after cross-clamping the umbilical cord to prevent drug delivery to the neonate. However, it is recognised that this does not provide the mother with adequate tissue levels at the time of incision, and several studies have shown that antimicrobials can be given safely before incision without adversely affecting the neonate (Mackeen et al., 2014; Sullivan et al., 2007; Thigpen et al., 2005).

Table 40.8 Example of number needed to treat for antimicrobial prophylaxis (SIGN, 2014)

Type of surgery	Operation	NNT	Outcome
Upper GI surgery	Stomach and duodenal surgery	5	Wound infection
Lower GI surgery	Colorectal surgery	4	Wound infection and intra-abdominal abscesses
Obstetric	Caesarian section	19	Wound infection
Orthopaedic	Arthroplasty (hip replacement)	42	Hip infection

Number needed to treat is the number of patients who need to be treated to prevent one infection compared with receiving no antimicrobials.
GI, Gastro-intestinal.

Table 40.9 Antimicrobial susceptibility of common pathogens

Surgical site infection for a skin wound at any site	
Staphylococcus aureus	Highly variable (30–60% susceptible) to flucloxacillin; therefore, meticillin-resistant *S. aureus* screening essential
β-Haemolytic streptococci	90% susceptible to penicillins, macrolides or clindamycin
Additional pathogens by site of infection	
Head and neck surgery	
Oral anaerobes	95% susceptible to metronidazole or co-amoxiclav
Operations below the diaphragm	
Anaerobes	95% susceptible to metronidazole or co-amoxiclav
Escherichia coli and other Enterobacteriaceae	80–90% of *E. coli* sensitive to cefuroxime, co-amoxiclav (or other β-lactam with inhibitor combination) or gentamicin
Insertion of a prosthesis, graft or shunt	
Coagulase-negative *Staphylococcus* (CNS) *S. aureus*, diphtheroids	Two-thirds of CNS are meticillin resistant, but β-lactams may still be used but preferably with a second agent with staphylococcal cover, e.g. gentamicin, or a glycopeptide used instead see above for *S. aureus*.

Adapted from SIGN (2014).

Table 40.10 Microorganisms commonly isolated from surgical site infections and prophylactic antimicrobials used in common surgical procedures (Prtak and Ridgway, 2009)

Surgical procedure	Most common microorganisms	Examples of prophylactic intravenous antimicrobials
Gastro-intestinal	**Bowel flora**	
• Upper gastro-intestinal tract	*Staphylococcus aureus*, Gram-negative bacilli	Co-amoxiclav or cefuroxime or gentamicin
• Biliary	*S. aureus*, Gram-negative bacilli (enterococci, anaerobes)	Co-amoxiclav or cefuroxime and metronidazole or gentamicin and metronidazole
• Colorectal/appendicectomy	*S. aureus*, Gram-negative bacilli, anaerobes	Co-amoxiclav or cefuroxime and metronidazole or gentamicin and metronidazole

Continued

Table 40.10 Microorganisms commonly isolated from surgical site infections and prophylactic antimicrobials used in common surgical procedures (Prtak and Ridgway, 2009)—cont'd

Surgical procedure	Most common microorganisms	Examples of prophylactic intravenous antimicrobials
Urogenital		
• Transrectal biopsy	S. aureus, Gram-negative bacilli, anaerobes	Co-amoxiclav or cefuroxime and metronidazole or gentamicin and metronidazole
• Transurethral resection of prostate	S. aureus, Gram-negative bacilli, enterococci	Co-amoxiclav or cefuroxime or gentamicin
Obstetric/gynaecological		
• Caesarean section	S. aureus, Gram-negative bacilli, streptococci (anaerobes)	Co-amoxiclav or cefuroxime and metronidazole
• Hysterectomy	S. aureus, Gram-negative bacilli, anaerobes	Co-amoxiclav or cefuroxime and metronidazole
Vascular		
• Reconstructive arterial surgery	Skin flora: primarily staphylococci	Co-amoxiclav or cefuroxime
• Amputation	S. aureus, anaerobes if gangrenous	Co-amoxiclav or cefuroxime and metronidazole or vancomycin and metronidazole
Orthopaedic		
• Joint replacement surgery	Skin flora: primarily staphylococci	Co-amoxiclav or cefuroxime or flucloxacillin and gentamicin

If patient has previously had meticillin-resistant S. aureus or is at high risk (e.g. nursing home resident), use teicoplanin or other glycopeptide. For β-lactam allergy, replace co-amoxiclav or cefuroxime with teicoplanin with or without ciprofloxacin.

Table 40.11 Suggested cephalosporin-free antimicrobial prophylaxis for surgical site infection

Type of surgery	Suggested antimicrobials	Alternatives for penicillin allergy
Cardiothoracic	Flucloxacillin +/− gentamicin	Teicoplanin or co-trimoxazole
ENT, maxillofacial and oral	Amoxicillin + metronidazole or co-amoxiclav	Clarithromycin +/− metronidazole or clindamycin
Gynaecology	Gentamicin + metronidazole	
Lower GI	Gentamicin + metronidazole	
Obstetrics	Co-amoxiclav	Clarithromycin +/− metronidazole or clindamycin
Orthopaedic	Flucloxacillin +/− gentamicin	Teicoplanin or co-trimoxazole
Thoracic	Flucloxacillin or co-amoxiclav	
Upper GI	Gentamicin	
Urology	Gentamicin	
Vascular	Flucloxacillin +/− gentamicin (+metronidazole for amputations)	Co-trimoxazole or teicoplanin

ENT, Ears, nose and throat; GI, gastro-intestinal.
Adapted from SIGN (2014).

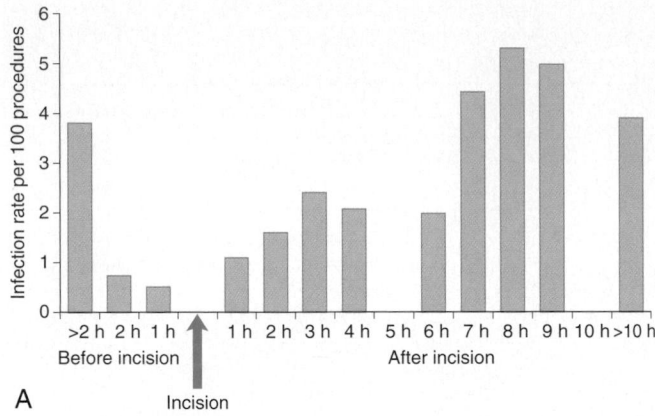

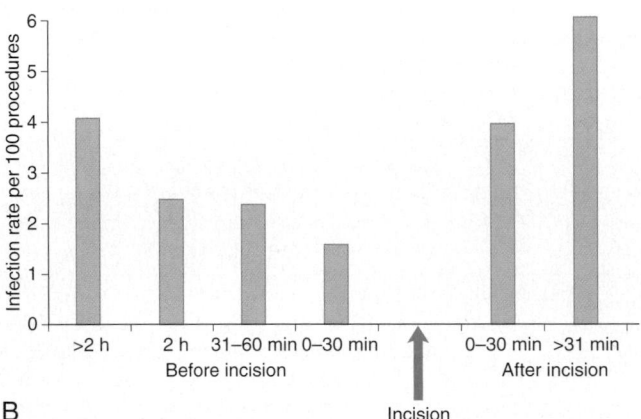

Fig. 40.5 Timing of antimicrobial prophylaxis administration and infection rate. Study A: The timing of prophylactic administration of antibiotics and the risk of surgical wound infection (Classen et al., 1992). Study B: Trial to reduce antimicrobial prophylaxis errors (Steinberg et al., 2009). (Taken from Mandell et al. [2010]. Reproduced with kind permission of Elsevier.)

When a tourniquet is used during orthopaedic procedures to minimise bleeding, the antimicrobial should be infused before inflating the tourniquet. This ensures adequate tissue levels are achieved at the site of surgery (Bratzler et al., 2013).

Certain practical issues should be considered when selecting an antimicrobial, for example, the requirement for intravenous infusion or safe intravenous bolus administration. An antimicrobial, which requires to be administered over a long period, for example, vancomycin 1 g over nearly 2 hours, is much less likely to be given completely compared with teicoplanin, which is administered as a bolus.

To improve the timing of antimicrobial prophylaxis administration, the World Health Organization (WHO) has introduced a question in their surgical safety checklist. The question 'Has antimicrobial prophylaxis been given within the last 60 minutes?' is to be asked aloud before incision (WHO, 2009).

Repeat doses

Although single-dose prophylaxis regimens are widely advocated (Department of Health and Health Protection Agency, 2008; NICE, 2017; Scottish Intercollegiate Guideline Network [SIGN], 2014),

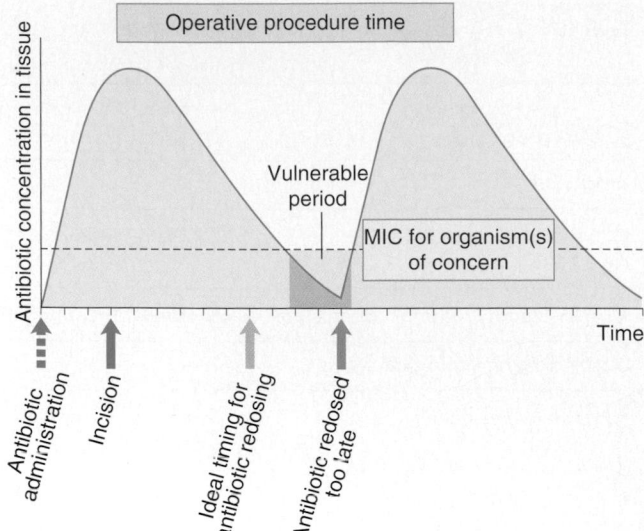

Fig. 40.6 Schematic presentation of tissue antibiotic concentration over time (Mandell et al., 2010). MIC, Minimum inhibitory concentration. (Reproduced with kind permission of Elsevier.)

many surgeons continue to use prolonged courses of 'prophylaxis' often for several days, without a clear evidence base. For some procedures, the optimum duration of prophylaxis is not known and 24- to 48-hour prophylaxis is considered acceptable, for example, for open heart surgery (SIGN, 2014).

Where single-dose prophylactic regimens have been adopted, the need for dosage adjustment in patients with reduced ability to excrete the drug (usually because of renal impairment) becomes unnecessary. This is because it is unlikely that single doses will have significant dose-related adverse effects. Although the half-life of many drugs used is relatively short (1–2 hours in normal volunteers), surgical patients often have slower clearance of antimicrobials from the blood. This concept will probably also hold true for prophylactic regimens lasting up to 48 hours.

There are some situations in which it is necessary to prescribe additional doses of antibiotics to achieve the aim of adequate tissue levels at the time of wound closure. The additional doses may be needed when there is significant blood loss (>1500 mL) because plasma is effectively diluted by intra-operative transfusions and fluid replacement. Long operations may also need extra antimicrobial doses during the operation, but additional doses post-operatively do not provide an additional prophylactic benefit.

Antimicrobial administration by hospital theatre staff has practical implications for the route of administration. Ward-based administration of prophylaxis can be given orally if appropriate preparations exist, but this is impractical in sedated or unconscious patients. The oral route tends to suffer from variable absorption, especially in the presence of anaesthetic premedication, and this also makes it unsatisfactory. The intravenous route is the most reliable way of ensuring effective serum levels and is the only route supported by a substantial body of evidence.

A schematic model for the tissue concentration time profile of an antimicrobial agent used to prevent surgical site infection is presented in Fig. 40.6. After an initial dose of the antimicrobial agent, tissue concentrations reach their peak rapidly, with a

Table 40.12 Time for peri-operative re-dosing of antimicrobials

Antimicrobials	Peak serum level (mg/L)	Half-life (h)	Time to redose (h)
Cefuroxime 1.5 g i.v.	100	1–2	4
Ciprofloxacin 400 mg i.v.	4.6	3–7	8
Co-amoxiclav 1.2 g	Unknown	1.4 AM/1.1 CL	2
Co-trimoxazole 960 mg i.v.	9 TMP/105 SMX	11 TMP/9 SMX	12
Flucloxacillin 1 g i.v.	120–350	0.75–1.5	3
Gentamicin	N/A as many doses used	2–3	6 unless >2 mg/kg; then do not redose
Metronidazole 500 mg i.v.	20–25	6–8	8
Vancomycin 1 g i.v.	20–50	4–8	12
Teicoplanin 400 mg i.v.	20	90–157	12

AM, Amoxicillin; CL, clavulanic acid; i.v., intravenous; N/A, not applicable; SMX, sulfamethoxazole; TMP, trimethoprim.
Adapted from Bratzler et al. (2013).

subsequent decline over time. The goal of prophylaxis is for the antimicrobial tissue concentration to remain above the minimum inhibitory concentration for the specific pathogens at the time of incision and throughout the procedure. The antimicrobial should be re-administered during prolonged procedures to prevent a period where tissue concentrations are less than the minimum inhibitory concentration (grey area). Failure to re-administer antimicrobials appropriately may result in a period during which the wound is vulnerable. Recommendations for peri-operative re-dosing schedules are presented in Table 40.12. General guidance is to repeat doses of antimicrobials at intervals of one to two half-lives; however, not all guidance recommends repeat dosing outside of cardiac surgery (SIGN, 2014).

β-Lactam allergy

Penicillin and cephalosporin antibiotics have been the cornerstone of antimicrobial prophylaxis to prevent surgical site infections. Patients reported to be allergic to β-lactam antibiotics or other antimicrobials need to be carefully assessed, because alternatives may not be optimal. Alternatives are often glycopeptides, for example, teicoplanin or vancomycin, which are more expensive, often need to be given by infusion (vancomycin) and can increase selection for resistant bacteria. The prevalence of true penicillin allergy in the general population is unknown. The incidence rate of self-reported penicillin allergy is approximately 10%, with the frequency of life-threatening anaphylaxis estimated at 0.01–0.05% (or 1–5 in 10,000) (NICE, 2014). More than 80% of patients with a self-reported allergy to penicillin have no evidence of allergy on skin testing. Important details of an allergic reaction include signs, symptoms, severity, history of prior reaction, time course of allergic event, temporal proximity to administered drug, route of administration, other medication being taken and adverse events to other medication (Park and Li, 2005). Reactions to penicillins and other β-lactams can occur because of allergy

to the parent compound or its metabolites. The cross-sensitivity between penicillins and cephalosporins is unknown but has been variably reported to be up to 10%. Early cephalosporin preparations were contaminated with penicillins probably leading to an overestimate of cross-sensitivity (Saxon et al., 1987). As the generation of the cephalosporin increases, the likelihood of cross-sensitivity decreases (Pichichero and Casey, 2007). Those with a penicillin allergy showed an increased risk of allergic reaction to a first-generation cephalosporin. First-generation cephalosporins share a similar side chain to penicillin and amoxicillin. However, cross-sensitivity to second- and third-generation cephalosporins was lower. The different side chains appear to play a more dominant role than the β-lactam ring in allergy.

Prospective studies have shown that the cross-reactivity to carbapenems and monobactams is very small. It is around 1% for imipenem and meropenem, and no cross-reaction has been reported for penicillins and aztreonam (Frumin and Gallagher, 2009).

The increased use of penicillins rather than first- or second-generation cephalosporins for surgical site infection prophylaxis is increasing the potential for adverse reactions. In addition, the current nomenclature for penicillin combinations, for example, co-amoxiclav, can often make it more difficult for staff to recognise penicillin-containing antimicrobials. Current guidance on the use of β-lactams in patients with penicillin allergy is detailed in Table 40.13.

Topical or local antimicrobial prophylaxis

Many surgical procedures involving the use of implants or prostheses now use topical antimicrobials to prevent late surgical site infection. Examples include antimicrobial-loaded cement for fixing hip and knee joint replacements into bone. Gentamicin and clindamycin are the only antimicrobials in commercially available products in the UK. Surgeons do add other antimicrobial agents, especially if replacing an infected prosthesis with choice based on prior knowledge of the pathogen and its sensitivity profile.

Table 40.13 Guidance on the use of β-lactam antibiotics in patients with penicillin allergy recommended by British National Formulary (Joint Formulary Committee, 2017)

Allergic reaction	Action
Immediate hypersensitivity reaction to a penicillin	Avoid penicillins and cephalosporins
Minor rash, localised or widespread but delayed (>72 h)	Avoid penicillins, but cephalosporins are safe to use

In vascular surgery, synthetic grafts bonded with or soaked in rifampicin are frequently used, despite evidence showing that there was no decrease in infection rates at 1 month and 2 years (Stewart et al., 2006). There is some evidence to support the local delivery of gentamicin into wounds via collagen fleece impregnated with gentamicin, and further research into this was recommended; however, two recent randomised controlled trials have shown it not to be efficacious (Bennett-Guerrero et al., 2010a, 2010b). The use of topical cefotaxime in contaminated surgery has been shown not to decrease peritonitis and should not be used.

Case studies

Case 40.1

A patient is due to have an elective total hip replacement. As part of the routine, pre-admission screening is done, during which swab samples are taken. The patient is identified as being MRSA-positive. The patient receives a 5-day course of nasal mupirocin and topical chlorhexidine washes as 'decolonisation therapy' prior to the admission. The unit normally uses single-dose co-amoxiclav as prophylaxis.

Question

Should there be a change to the routine antimicrobial prophylaxis for this patient?

Answer

A change to the routine antimicrobial prophylaxis should be recommended because co-amoxiclav is not active against MRSA. The commonly used terms 'decolonisation therapy' and 'MRSA eradication' falsely give the impression that this regimen eradicates MRSA carriage. In reality, it should be called 'suppression therapy' because these agents reduce the numbers of bacteria present but often fail to eradicate MRSA carriage. S. aureus is still a common cause of surgical site infection, and this patient remains at risk of an MRSA surgical site infection. As a consequence, an agent that is active against MRSA should be used. Glycopeptides are the recommended antimicrobial class in this situation, and there are two options: teicoplanin and vancomycin. Vancomycin needs to be given as an infusion at a maximum rate of 10 mg/min, which means that administering a 1 g dose will take nearly 2 hours and may be impractical before skin incision. Teicoplanin can be given as a bolus and so is the best choice. Where bone cement is required to secure the prosthesis, a commercially prepared bone

cement containing gentamicin should also be used. Ideally, all antimicrobial prophylaxis guidelines or protocols should contain an option for MRSA-positive patients. Administration of appropriate regimens is facilitated by MRSA screening of all elective patients.

Case 40.2

A patient with a severe allergy to penicillin is admitted for a hemicolectomy for cancer of the colon. The unit uses a single-dose co-amoxiclav regimen as antimicrobial prophylaxis for large-bowel surgery.

Question

The junior hospital doctor asks your advice as to the antimicrobials to use instead of co-amoxiclav? What advice would you give?

Answer

Colorectal surgery still carries one of the highest surgical site infection rates of up to 10% for elective procedures. The usual bacteria found in these surgical site infections are S. aureus, Gram-negative bacilli (e.g. Escherichia coli) and anaerobes. Options for treatment include gentamicin and metronidazole, or ciprofloxacin and metronidazole; centres that have a problem with C. difficile infection may prefer to use the former regimen.

Case 40.3

Mrs AJ, a 73-year-old woman, is seen in pre-admission clinic for assessment prior to a knee replacement. She has recently had C. difficile infection in the community after being treated with a 1-week course of co-amoxiclav. She is asymptomatic now. The surgical team is reluctant to use its usual antimicrobial prophylaxis regimen of co-amoxiclav, or cefuroxime or ciprofloxacin.

Question

The anaesthetist assessing Mrs AJ in the pre-assessment clinic asks your advice about what to prescribe. Mrs AJ is currently being screened for MRSA. What advice would you give?

Answer

The most common pathogens in knee replacement surgical site infections are S. aureus and coagulase-negative staphylococci, although infection rates are low. Depending on the result of the MRSA screening test, there will be different answers. If Mrs AJ is colonised with MRSA, she could receive a single dose of teicoplanin. Options for prophylaxis include flucloxacillin with gentamicin or teicoplanin, although the latter does not cover Gram-negative bacteria. The use of gentamicin-containing cement would be recommended.

Case 40.4

Mr LP, a 72-year-old man, is due for elective transurethral resection of the prostate (TURP) and is currently well with no signs of a urinary tract infection. Routine prophylaxis for surgical site infections on the unit is co-amoxiclav. The patient is known to have had a mitral valve replacement 2 years ago.

Question

You are asked whether the antimicrobial prophylaxis should be amended because of his valve replacement? What advice would you give?

Answer

NICE guidelines no longer recommend routine prophylaxis for patients at risk of endocarditis who are undergoing investigations involving the oral, gastro-intestinal or urogenital tract, in the absence of local infection (NICE, 2015). The usual prophylaxis for TURP should be recommended. If the patient had a urinary tract infection, this should ideally be treated before surgery.

References

Astagneau, P., Rioux, C., Golliot, F., et al., 2001. Morbidity and mortality associated with surgical site infections: results from the 1997–1999 INCISO surveillance. J. Hosp. Infect. 48, 267–274.

Bennett-Guerrero, E., Ferguson, T.B., Lin, M., et al., 2010a. Effect of an implantable gentamicin-collagen sponge on sternal wound infections following cardiac surgery: a randomized trial. J. Am. Med. Assoc. 304, 755–762.

Bennett-Guerrero, F., Pappas, T.N., Koltun, W.A., et al., 2010b. Gentamicin-collagen sponge for infection prophylaxis in colorectal surgery. N. Engl. J. Med. 363, 1038–1049.

Bratzler, D.W., Dellinger, E.P., Olsen, K.M., et al., 2013. Clinical practice guidelines for antimicrobial prophylaxis in surgery. Am. J. Health Syst. Pharm. 70, 195–283.

Burke, J., 1961. The effective period of preventative antibiotic action in experimental incisions and dermal lesions. Surgery 50, 161–168.

Classen, D., Evans, R.S., Pestotnik, S.L., et al., 1992. The timing of prophylactic administration of antibiotics and the risk of surgical-wound infection. N. Engl. J. Med. 326, 281–286.

Coello, R.C.A., Wilson, J., Ward, V., et al., 2005. Adverse impact of surgical site infections in English hospitals. J. Hosp. Infect. 60, 93–103.

Culver, D.H., Horan, T.C., Gaynes, R.P., et al., 1991. Surgical wound infection rates by wound class, operative procedure, and patient risk index. Am. J. Med. 91, S152–S157.

Department of Health and Health Protection Agency, 2008. *Clostridium difficile* infection: how to deal with the problem. DH/HPA, London. Available at: http://webarchive.nationalarchives.gov.uk/20140714084352/http://www.hpa.nhs.uk/web/HPAwebFile/HPAweb_C/1232006607827.

Donlan, R.M., Costerton, J.W., 2002. Biofilms: survival mechanisms of clinically relevant microorganisms. Clin. Microbiol. Rev. 15, 167–193.

Frumin, J., Gallagher, J.C., 2009. Allergic cross-sensitivity between penicillin, carbapenem, and monobactam antibiotics: what are the chances? Ann. Pharmacother. 43, 304–315.

Gastmeier, P.S.D., Brandt, C., et al., 2005. Reduction of orthopaedic wound infections in 21 hospitals. Arch. Orthop. Trauma Surg. 125, 526–530.

Health and Social Care Information Centre, 2016. Hospital episodes statistics (England): main procedures and interventions: summary, 2015–16. Department of Health, London. Available at: http://www.hesonline.nhs.uk.

Health Protection Agency, 2008. Surveillance of healthcare associated infections report 2008. HPA, London. Available at: http://webarchive.nationalarchives.gov.uk/20140714084352/http://www.hpa.nhs.uk/web/HPAwebFile/HPAweb_C/1216193833496.

Health Protection Agency, 2012. English National Point Prevalence Survey on Healthcare-Associated Infections and Antimicrobial Use, 2011. Available at: http://webarchive.nationalarchives.gov.uk/20140714084352/http://www.hpa.org.uk/Publications/InfectiousDiseases/AntimicrobialAndHealthcareAssociatedInfections/1205HCAIEnglishPPSforhcaiandamu2011prelim/.

Health Protection Scotland, 2009. Surveillance of surgical site infection. 2009 Annual Report. Health Protection Scotland, Glasgow. Available at: http://www.hps.scot.nhs.uk/resourcedocument.aspx?id=708.

Health Protection Scotland, 2015. Surveillance of surgical site infection. 2015 Annual Report. Health Protection Scotland, Glasgow. Available at: http://www.hps.scot.nhs.uk/resourcedocument.aspx?id=5763.

Horan, T.C., Culver, D.H., Gaynes, R.P., 1993. Surgical Site Infection (SSI) risk stratum rates: what they are and how to compare them using aggregated data from the National Nosocomial Infections Surveillance (NNIS) System. Am. J. Infect. Control. 21 (2), 99.

Joint Formulary Committee, 2017. British National Formulary, seventy third ed. British Medical Association and Royal Pharmaceutical Society, London.

Kaye, K.S., Schmit, K., Pieper, C., et al., 2005. The effect of increasing age on the risk of surgical site infection. J. Infect. Dis 191, 1056–1062.

Latham, R., Lancaster, A.D., Covington, J.F., et al., 2001. The association of diabetes and glucose control with surgical site infections among cardiothoracic surgery patients. Infect. Control Hosp. Epidemiol. 22, 607–612.

Mackeen, A., Packard, R.E., Ota, E., et al., 2014. Timing of intravenous prophylactic antibiotics for preventing postpartum infectious morbidity in women undergoing cesarean delivery. Cochrane Database Syst. Rev. 2014 (12), CD009516. https://doi.org/10.1002/14651858.CD009516.pub2.

Mandell, G.L., Bennett, J.E., Dolin, R., 2010. Principles and Practice of Infectious Diseases, seventh ed. Elsevier, Philadelphia.

Mangram, A.J., Horan, T., Pearson, M.L., et al., 1999. Guideline for prevention of surgical site prevention, 1999. Hospital Infection Control Practices Advisory Committee. Infect. Control Hosp. Epidemiol. 20, 250–255.

Morgan, M., 2006. Surgery and cephalosporins: a marriage made in heaven or time for divorce? Intern. J. Surg. 8. Available at: http://ispub.com/IJS/8/1/3613.

Myles, P.S., Iacono, G.A., Hunt, J.O., et al., 2002. Risk of respiratory complications and wound infection in patients undergoing ambulatory surgery: smokers versus nonsmokers. Anesthesiology 97, 842–847.

National Institute for Health and Care Excellence, 2014. Drug allergy: diagnosis and management of drug allergy in adults, children and young people. 183. NICE clinical guideline. Available at: https://www.nice.org.uk/Guidance/CG183.

National Institute for Health and Care Excellence, 2015. Prophylaxis against infective endocarditis: antimicrobial prophylaxis against infective endocarditis in adults and children undergoing interventional procedures. NICE, London. Available at: http://www.nice.org.uk/guidance/CG64.

National Institute for Health and Care Excellence, 2017. Surgical site infection: prevention and treatment of surgical site infection. Clinical Guideline 74. NICE, London. Available at: https://www.nice.org.uk/guidance/CG74.

Park, M.A., Li, J.T., 2005. Diagnosis and management of penicillin allergy. Mayo Clin. Proc. 80, 405–410.

Pichichero, M.E., Casey, J.R., 2007. Safe use of selected cephalosporins in penicillin-allergic patients: a meta-analysis. Otolaryngol. Head Neck Surg. 136, 340–347.

Prtak, L.E., Ridgway, E.J., 2009. Prophylactic antibiotics in surgery. Surgery (Oxford) 27, 431–434.

Publics Account Committee, 2009. Reducing healthcare associated infections in hospitals in England. In: Commons House. Hansard, London.

Public Health England, 2016. Surveillance of surgical site infections in NHS hospitals in England 2015/16. Public Health England, London. Available at: https://www.gov.uk/government/uploads/system/uploads/attachment_data/file/577418/Surgical_site_infections_NHS_hospitals_2015_to_2016.pdf.

Saxon, A., Beall, G.N., Rohr, A.S., et al., 1987. Immediate hypersensitivity reactions to beta-lactam antibiotics. Ann. Intern. Med. 107, 204–215.

Scottish Intercollegiate Guideline Network, 2014. Antibiotic prophylaxis in surgery. SIGN, Edinburgh. Available at: http://www.sign.ac.uk/assets/sign104.pdf.

Sharma, A., Deeb, A.P., Iannuzzi, J.C., et al., 2013. Tobacco smoking and postoperative outcomes after colorectal surgery. Ann. Surg. 258 (2), 296–300.

Steinberg, J.P., Braun, B.I., Hellinger, W.W., et al., 2009. Timing of antimicrobial prophylaxis and the risk of surgical site infections: results from the trial to reduce antimicrobial prophylaxis errors. Ann. Surg. 250 (1), 10–16.

Stewart, A., Eyers, P.S., Earnshaw, J.J., 2006. Prevention of infection in arterial reconstruction. Cochrane Database Syst. Rev. 2006 (3), CD003073. https://doi.org/10.1002/14651858.CD003073.pub2.

Sullivan, S.A., Smith, T., Chang, E., et al., 2007. Administration of cefazolin prior to skin incision is superior to cefazolin at cord clamping in preventing postcesarean infectious morbidity: a randomized, controlled trial. Am. J. Obstet. Gynecol. 196, 455e1–455e5.

Thigpen, B.D., Hood, W.A., Chauhan, S., et al., 2005. Timing of prophylactic antibiotic administration in the uninfected laboring gravida: a randomized clinical trial. Am. J. Obstet. Gynecol. 192, 1864–1871.

Weber, W.P., Mujagic, E., Zwahlen, M., et al., 2017. Timing of surgical antimicrobial prophylaxis: a phase 3 randomised controlled trial. Lancet 17, 605–614.

World Health Organization (WHO), 2009. WHO surgical safety checklist. Available at: http://www.who.int/patientsafety/safesurgery/checklist/en/.

Further references

Anderson, D.J., Kaye, K.S., Classen, D., et al., 2008. Strategies to prevent surgical site infections in acute care hospitals. Infect. Control Hosp. Epidemiol. 29 (Suppl. 1), S51–S56.

Elgohari, S., Wilson, J., Saei, A., et al., 2017. Impact of national policies on the microbial aetiology of surgical site infections in acute NHS hospitals in England: analysis of trends between 2000 and 2013 using multi-centre prospective cohort data. Epidemiol. Infect. 145, 957–969.

Nelson, R.L., Gladman, E., Barbateskovic, M., 2014. Antimicrobial prophylaxis for colorectal surgery. Cochrane Database Syst. Rev. 2014 (5), CD001181. https://doi.org/10.1002/14651858.CD001181.pub4.

Useful websites

Health Protection Scotland – surgical site infections: http://www.hps.scot.nhs.uk
Health in Wales – surgical site infections: http://www.wales.nhs.uk

Surgical site infection surveillance service: https://www.gov.uk/guidance/surgical-site-infection-surveillance-service-ssiss

41 Tuberculosis

Toby Capstick and Paul Whitaker

Key points

- Clinical manifestations of active tuberculosis (TB) disease are varied because *Mycobacterium tuberculosis* can infect any organ in the body, but common non-specific symptoms include malaise, weight loss, fever and night sweats.

- Diagnosis of TB is based on the context of clinical signs and symptoms and investigations such as radiography and microbiological results.

- Risk factors for TB include close contact with an infectious person, living in a country with a high incidence of TB, immunocompromise because of drugs or disease and previous under-treatment of TB.

- Treatment of active TB with single anti-TB drugs must never be attempted, and a single drug must never be added to a failing regimen, because of the risks for development of further drug resistance.

- Adherence to the full treatment course is essential to achieve cure, prevent relapse, prevent the development of drug resistance and prevent transmission to other people.

- Fixed-dose combination drugs are preferred to using separate drugs because they reduce pill burden and prevent selective non-adherence.

- Adverse effects of anti-TB drugs are common. Patients should be advised on common and serious adverse drug reactions, how to manage them and when to refer to their named healthcare professional.

- All patients should have a risk assessment for their likely adherence, and Directly Observed Therapy should be considered for patients thought likely to be non-adherent.

- The management of drug-resistant TB is highly complex and should only be managed by a multidisciplinary team with experience in managing such cases.

Introduction

Tuberculosis (TB) is a bacterial infection caused by *Mycobacterium tuberculosis* complex. It is a global problem and still accounts for millions of deaths every year. Unfortunately, the burden of TB disproportionately affects developing countries, and this effect is also compounded by co-infection with HIV. Advances in diagnostics and treatment have led to a reduction in TB mortality by 47% since 1990, with an estimated 53 million lives saved between 2000 and 2016. However, many new challenges are facing healthcare systems. The biggest concern has been the increase in multidrug-resistant tuberculosis (MDR-TB).

In 2006, the emergence of extensively drug-resistant tuberculosis (XDR-TB) was also reported. The treatment of drug-resistant TB is complex, costlier and of a longer duration than drug-susceptible cases.

Adequate and effective treatment is essential, both clinically for patients and also to control TB, because the Bacille Calmette-Guérin (BCG) vaccine does not prevent infection. Successful control depends on a close working collaboration between clinical, microbiological, pharmacy, infection control and public health teams in managing patients and their contacts.

Epidemiology

The global incidence of TB has declined steadily with rates now around 18% lower than in 2000. Reporting of patients with TB to national surveillance systems is variable between countries, but it is estimated that 10.4 million people experienced symptoms of TB worldwide in 2016 (World Health Organization [WHO], 2017); this number includes more than 1 million children. Ten percent of all patients were also positive for HIV. In 2016, despite the fact that all patients can potentially be cured, 1.3 million people died. In addition, a further 374,000 had TB-HIV co-infection (deaths among HIV-positive TB cases are classified as HIV deaths according to *International Classification of Diseases*, 10th Revision). Alongside HIV, TB remains a leading cause of death worldwide.

The highest annual incidence of TB (>100 cases per 100,000 population) is seen in sub-Saharan Africa, India and Southeast Asia. Intermediate rates of TB (26–100 cases/100,000) occur in China, South America, Eastern Europe and northern Africa. Lower rates (<25 cases per 100,000 inhabitants) occur in the USA, Western Europe, Canada, Japan and Australia.

In 2016, it was estimated that 490,000 cases of MDR-TB occurred; however, only about a quarter of these were detected and reported. Almost half of all of these cases occurred in India, China and the Russian Federation. In some areas of the world more than one in four people have drug-resistant TB; this is a problem especially in Eastern European countries such as Belarus and Lithuania.

A total of 5664 TB cases were reported in England during 2016 (Public Health England, 2017). The overall incidence across all population groups was 10.2 per 100,000 population. This rate has declined over the past 5 years because of a reduction in migrants from high-incidence countries, as well as improved pre-entry TB screening. The majority of TB cases in the UK were in the population born outside of the UK. The incidence amongst UK-born individuals remains stable at around 3.2 per 100,000 population.

Aetiology

M. tuberculosis complex contains five different species; however, it is *M. tuberculosis*, *M. bovis* and *M. africanum* that are associated with human disease. *M. tuberculosis* is the most notable cause of TB and accounts for the majority of cases worldwide. *M. africanum* is responsible for up to half of the cases of TB in West Africa but is not a major pathogen outside of this geographical area. *M. bovis* is the causative organism in bovine TB and accounts for between 5% and 10% of human TB. Its impact has fallen since the introduction of pasteurised milk. Both *M. bovis* and *M. africanum* can give rise to clinical features of disease that are indistinguishable from *M. tuberculosis*.

TB is an airborne disease, and the source of infection is from another individual with active pulmonary disease. Patients should be considered infectious if they have sputum smear-positive pulmonary disease (i.e. they produce sputum containing sufficient tubercle bacilli to be seen on microscopic examination of a sputum smear) or laryngeal TB. Patients with smear-negative pulmonary disease, on three sputum samples, are less infectious than those who are smear positive. When coughing, droplets containing the tubercle bacilli are aerosolised and subsequently inhaled by other people. The greatest risk is to prolonged, mainly household contacts.

Inhalation of *M. tuberculosis* and deposition in the lungs leads to one of three possible outcomes: immediate clearance of the organism, primary active disease, or latent infection (with or without subsequent reactivation of disease). Active TB develops in around 10% of patients who do not clear the organism, and latent TB develops in around 90%. In latent TB the infectious bacilli trigger an immune response and T lymphocytes become sensitised to the mycobacterium. The immune system forms granulomas around the infection to limit spread, and these latent bacilli can remain in this state for a long period. If there is a change in the inflammatory response, then the latent bacilli can be released, triggering reactivation of disease. It is estimated that there are 2 billion people worldwide who have latent TB and are at risk of reactivation. There is a 10% lifetime risk that latent TB will reactivate; however, factors that further increase the risk include HIV, immunosuppressant drugs, diabetes mellitus, chronic kidney disease and poor nutrition. The estimated annual risk of TB in those with HIV infection and TB co-infection is around 10%, as opposed to a 10% lifetime chance in someone infected with TB, but not HIV.

Clinical features

The classic symptoms related to TB are those of prolonged (>2 weeks) respiratory symptoms. These usually include chronic cough, weight loss, fevers and night sweats. Patients can be productive of purulent sputum as well as haemoptysis (Lawn and Zumla, 2011). Although this accounts for the majority of cases, between 10% and 40% of individuals can have extrapulmonary disease. In these patients they will often have the systemic symptoms of TB, such as weight loss and sweats, but will have focal signs and symptoms elsewhere. Common sites for extrapulmonary TB include the lymph nodes, pleura, skeletal sites, abdominal sites and the central nervous system (CNS). In the UK the commonest sites for extrapulmonary TB are the lymph nodes in the neck and the chest. Miliary TB is the widespread dissemination throughout the body due to spread through the bloodstream and is seen in around 3% of TB cases. It is more common in infants and the elderly, as well as immunocompromised individuals. In miliary TB the CNS is affected in around 20% of cases.

In patients with HIV the manifestations of TB can be atypical. Extrapulmonary disease is more common, and patients with advanced HIV can have very few signs and symptoms despite extensive and disseminated TB.

Diagnosis

Latent infection

Screening for latent *M. tuberculosis* infection is indicated for groups in which the prevalence of latent infection is high or in those who are at higher risk of reactivation. High-risk groups include foreign-born persons from endemic areas and contact screening during an investigation of an active TB case. The diagnosis and treatment of latent TB is important because this will result in a reduction in the numbers of active infectious cases in the future.

There are two ways of identifying latent TB: the first is a tuberculin skin test and the second an interferon-γ release assay (IGRA). Both methods are a test of the person's immunological memory against TB.

The only tuberculin skin test now used is the Mantoux test. The standard Mantoux test consists of an intradermal injection of 2 TU of Statens Serum Institute tuberculin RT23 in 0.1 mL of solution for injection. The results are read 48–72 hours later, although a valid reading can be obtained up to 96 hours later. The transverse diameter of the area of induration is measured with a ruler and the result recorded in millimetres. A diameter of induration ≥5 mm is considered positive and represents an immune response against the tuberculin (National Institute for Health and Care Excellence [NICE], 2016). A false-positive result can be caused by previous BCG vaccination or nontuberculous environmental mycobacterium. A false-negative result can occur if the patient has a lowered immune system and cannot mount an inflammatory response.

The IGRA measures the immune response following the exposure of the patient's blood cells to proteins from *M. tuberculosis*. After incubation for 16–24 hours the levels of interferon-γ are quantified. The advantages include that it is not affected by prior BCG vaccination and no second visit is required to read the test.

If either the tuberculin skin test or the IGRA is positive, an assessment of the patient has to be made to ensure he or she has no features of active TB. Only when it is confirmed that the patient is symptom free and has a normal chest radiograph can he or she be confirmed as having latent disease.

Active tuberculosis

Awareness of TB amongst healthcare professionals is essential for its control. Early diagnosis, especially of pulmonary TB, followed by prompt commencement of treatment can reduce the period of infectivity to other people, especially susceptible contacts, who might be at risk of the more serious forms of TB disease. TB should be considered part of the differential diagnosis in a range of clinical presentations. These include cough, pleural effusions, lymphadenopathy, skeletal pain, abdominal pain and fever of unknown origin.

Basic investigations include sputum microbiology, as well as chest radiograph; however, with the complexity of presentations many patients will require more extensive diagnostics to confirm TB. Confirmation is important to avoid unnecessary treatment, as well as to obtain appropriate specimens for testing drug susceptibilities. At present there is only a limited role for IGRAs and tuberculin skin testing in the diagnosis of active disease.

Microbiological testing

Sputum microscopy and mycobacterial culture are considered to be the gold standard tests for the diagnosis of pulmonary disease. The staining and microscopy of the sputum smear is a reliable and cost-effective way of identifying a patient with active TB. If positive, there is usually a high burden of disease, and these patients are more infectious. A negative smear cannot be relied upon and, in many cases, because *M. tuberculosis* is a slow-growing organism, culture positivity can take several weeks. A minimum of three sputum samples, one of which needs to be from early morning, should be collected from patients with suspected pulmonary TB. In many patients, treatment will be commenced on clinical suspicion before cultures become positive.

If conventional culture methods are used, such as the Lowenstein–Jensen medium, growth may take between 3 and 8 weeks. Modern liquid cultures can produce results more quickly, often in 1–3 weeks. Once the culture does become positive it allows for drug-susceptibility patterns to be identified, allowing appropriate treatment.

More recently, polymerase chain reaction–based tests can also detect *M. tuberculosis* complex in clinical specimens. These assays use nucleic acid probes to amplify specific target RNA or DNA. Using these probes, it is possible, with high sensitivity, to identify both *M. tuberculosis* and rifampicin resistance mutations (*rpoB* gene). These tests do not replace routine culture, but they may shorten the time interval before effective treatment is commenced.

In patients who do not have pulmonary TB, samples can be collected and processed in a similar way. These may include fluid from pleural effusions or tissue biopsies, for example, from lymph nodes. In tissue biopsies it is also possible to send them for histological diagnosis, and the typical features seen in TB are those of caseating granulomatous inflammation.

Radiology

Chest radiography is an essential part of the diagnostic workup in TB. It is important both for the initial diagnosis as well as to risk stratify, to determine how infectious the patient may be. Classic features on chest radiograph include focal infiltration of the upper

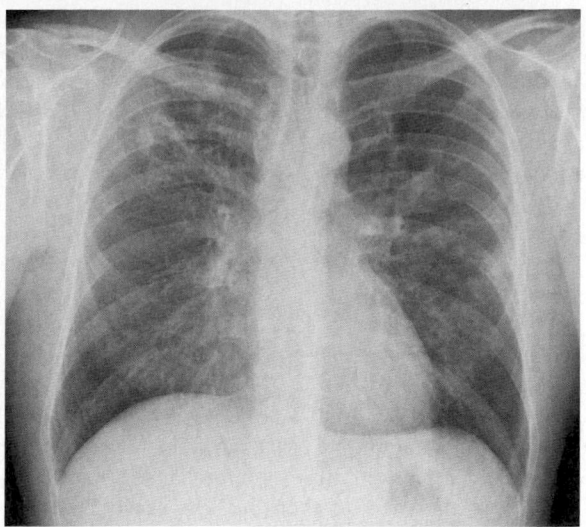

Fig. 41.1 Chest radiograph of a 45-year-old male patient with sputum heavily smeared positive for *Mycobacterium tuberculosis*. Chest radiograph shows increased airspace shadowing in both upper lobes with a cavity in the right upper lobe.

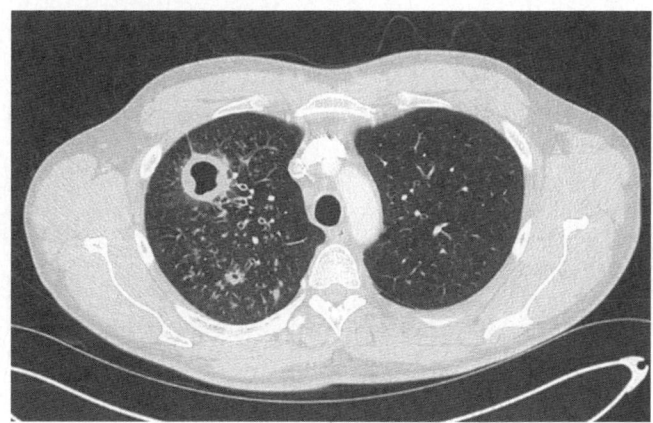

Fig. 41.2 Computed tomography (CT) of a 45-year-old male patient with sputum heavily smeared positive for *Mycobacterium tuberculosis*. CT scan shows thick-walled 4-cm cavity and nodular inflammation in the right upper lobe.

lobes, often with cavitation and lymph node enlargement (Fig. 41.1). However, in many cases, the features are not typical and may present with masses, nodules and pleural effusions. In patients with HIV atypical chest radiograph appearances are common.

Chest computed tomography (CT) is more sensitive than plain chest radiography and has a role in the atypical or the subtler cases (Fig. 41.2). In these cases the CT scan may indicate further investigations, such as bronchoscopy, to obtain microbiological samples.

Further imaging may also be required depending upon the presentation or symptoms, for example, a CT or magnetic resonance imaging scan of the brain in someone with neurological symptoms.

Public health action

TB is a statutorily notifiable communicable disease in the UK. Cases should be notified on clinical suspicion by the attending doctor to the local authority or a local Public Health England centre for communicable disease control. Notification enables public health action to be initiated and involves investigation of prolonged, close contacts who might be at risk of infection, mainly those living in the same household as the patient, to assess them for latent or active TB disease. It may also enable the source of the infection to be found and treated.

Latent TB infection is not infectious and does not require notification.

Bacille Calmette-Guérin Vaccination

The BCG vaccine contains a live attenuated strain of *M. bovis* and is 70–80% effective against the most severe forms of TB, such as TB meningitis in children, but is less effective in adults. The current (Public Health England, 2013) UK vaccination strategy targets the at-risk population rather than the entire UK population. In brief, BCG immunisation is offered to infants at high risk of TB exposure (e.g. those living in local areas of high incidence or with close relatives from high-incidence countries), children (where active TB is excluded) who are contacts of people diagnosed with pulmonary TB and people younger than 35 years who are at occupational risk of TB (e.g. healthcare workers, veterinary staff, prison staff and staff of hostels for homeless people).

Treatment

The aims of TB treatment are the following:
- cure the patient of TB disease,
- prevent death from active TB,
- prevent relapse of disease,
- prevent development of drug resistance,
- prevent the transmission of the disease to other patients or contacts.

M. tuberculosis is a slow-growing obligate pathogen that exists in different populations, making it difficult to target with antibacterials. It exists mostly as extracellular actively growing organisms, slowly growing organisms within macrophages under microaerobic and acidic conditions, and as dormant organisms in anaerobic conditions. The presence of organisms in pulmonary cavities, caseous necrotic foci or pus may reduce antibiotic penetration. Antibacterial activity may be reduced by the persistence of organisms within low pH environments, their long generation time, dormancy and low metabolic activity. Consequently, treatment of TB requires combinations of several anti-TB drugs, because monotherapy is liable to generate resistance, as demonstrated in the original trials of streptomycin. If untreated there is a 5-year mortality rate of 65%.

Drug-sensitive tuberculosis

Most patients with drug-sensitive TB can be treated in outpatient settings and do not require admission to hospital. The treatment of fully sensitive TB requires the use of four first-line anti-TB drugs: isoniazid, rifampicin, pyrazinamide and ethambutol (NICE, 2016). Streptomycin was previously used as an alternative to ethambutol but is no longer recommended for uncomplicated cases.

Isoniazid and rifampicin are the most effective bactericidal drugs, and they are most effective at preventing the emergence of drug resistance. Rifampicin and pyrazinamide have sterilising activity and kill semi-dormant persistent bacteria, and pyrazinamide is particularly effective in acid environments. Ethambutol is bacteriostatic and may prevent or delay the emergence of resistant strains.

Most patients with a fully sensitive strain of TB (including adults and children regardless of whether they are HIV positive) require a 6-month course of isoniazid and rifampicin, supplemented with pyrazinamide and ethambutol for the first 2 months (NICE, 2016). This is often referred to as the 'standard recommended regimen', and the use of fixed-dose combination (FDC) regimens (e.g. Voractiv, Rifater and Rifinah) is recommended to reduce pill burden and improve adherence. The recommended doses of first-line drugs are listed in Table 41.1.

Active tuberculosis without central nervous system involvement

The 'standard recommended regimen' is recommended for all people with active TB without CNS involvement. This includes pulmonary TB, which is defined as TB affecting the lungs, pleural cavity, mediastinal lymph nodes or larynx, and those with all forms of extrapulmonary TB, for example, peripheral lymph node, bone and joint, pericardial and disseminated (including miliary) TB.

Glucocorticoids are also recommended in the treatment of pericardial TB (at an initial dosage of prednisolone 60 mg daily (1 mg/kg/day in children) and then gradually tapered after 2–3 weeks (NICE, 2016).

Active tuberculosis with central nervous system involvement

Active TB affecting the CNS is associated with high rates of morbidity and mortality, and thus treatment is extended to 12 months, that is, 12 months of isoniazid and rifampicin, supplemented with pyrazinamide and ethambutol for the first 2 months. Rifampicin, isoniazid and ethambutol penetrate the cerebrospinal fluid (CSF) poorly; rifampicin achieves CSF concentrations that are only 10–20% of that in the blood. Isoniazid has good CSF penetration in patients with inflamed meninges, but achieves CSF concentrations that are only 20% of that in the blood when the meninges are not inflamed. Ethambutol has poor CSF penetration and may only be useful when the meninges are inflamed.

Glucocorticoids are also recommended for the treatment of TB of the CNS because they have been demonstrated to reduce mortality and disabling residual neurological deficit (Prasad and Singh, 2008). High doses of prednisolone or dexamethasone are recommended, with NICE recommending an initial dosage in adults of intravenous dexamethasone

Table 41.1 First-line antituberculosis drugs

Drug	Preparations	Daily unsupervised dose		Daily supervised dose	
		Adults	Children	Adults	Children
Individual drugs					
Isoniazid	**Oral:** 50 mg, 100 mg tablets Liquid (as a manufactured special) **Parenteral:** 50 mg/2 mL ampoules	300 mg once a day Consider 5 mg/kg once a day if low body weight	10 mg/kg (max. 300 mg) once a day	15 mg/kg (max. 900 mg) three times a week	15 mg/kg (max. 900 mg) three times a week
Rifampicin	**Oral:** 150 mg, 300 mg capsules 100 mg/5 mL syrup **Parenteral:** 600 mg powder for reconstitution	**<50 kg:** 450 mg once a day **≥50 kg:** 600 mg once a day	15 mg/kg (max. 450 mg if <50 kg; 600 mg if ≥50 kg) once a day	600–900 mg three times a week	15 mg/kg (max. 900 mg) three times a week
Pyrazinamide[a]	**Oral:** 500 mg tablets Liquid (as a manufactured special)	**<50 kg:** 1.5 g once a day **≥50 kg:** 2 g once a day	35 mg/kg (max. 1.5 g if <50 kg; 2 g if ≥50 kg) once a day	**<50 kg:** 2 g three times a week **≥50 kg:** 2.5 g three times a week	50 mg/kg (max. 2 g if <50 kg; 2.5 g if ≥50 kg) three times a week
Ethambutol[a,b]	**Oral:** 100 mg, 400 mg tablets	15 mg/kg once daily	20 mg/kg once daily	30 mg/kg three times per week	30 mg/kg three times per week
Fixed-dose combination drugs					
Voractiv	**Oral:** rifampicin 150 mg, isoniazid 75 mg, pyrazinamide 400 mg, ethambutol hydrochloride 275 mg	**30–39 kg:** 2 tablets daily **40–54 kg:** 3 tablets daily **55–69 kg:** 4 tablets daily **≥70 kg:** 5 tablets daily	Not recommended	Not recommended	Not recommended
Rifater	**Oral:** rifampicin 120 mg, isoniazid 50 mg, pyrazinamide 300 mg	**<40 kg:** 3 tablets daily **40–49 kg:** 4 tablets daily **50–64 kg:** 5 tablets daily **≥65 kg:** 6 tablets daily	Not recommended	Not recommended[c]	Not recommended
Rifinah	**Oral:** Rifinah 300/150 mg (rifampicin 300 mg, isoniazid 150 mg) Rifinah 150/100 mg (rifampicin 150 mg, isoniazid 100 mg)	**<50 kg:** Rifinah 150/100 mg 3 tablets daily **≥50 kg:** Rifinah 300/150 mg 2 tablets daily	Not recommended[d]	Not recommended[c]	Not recommended

[a]Dose adjustment may be required in renal impairment.
[b]Use IBW plus 40% of the excess weight in markedly obese patients.
- Male IBW (kg) = 50 + (2.3 × height in cm above 152.4)/2.54 (i.e. IBW = 50 kg + 2.3 kg for each inch over 5 feet).
- Female IBW (kg) = 45.5 + (2.3 × height in cm above 152.4)/2.54 (i.e. IBW = 45.5 kg + 2.3 kg for each inch over 5 feet)
[c]The BNF for Children advises that the use of Rifinah or Rifater in older children may be considered outside of license, provided that the respective dose of each drug is appropriate for the weight of the child.
[d]Rifinah is often used in supervised regimens to reduce tablet burden, but may require additional isoniazid to make up the full dose.
max., Maximum; IBW, ideal body weight.

Table 41.2   Treatment regimens for mono-resistant tuberculosis (NICE, 2016)

Drug resistance	Initial phase (2 months' duration)	Continuation phase
Rifampicin	Treat using multidrug-resistant tuberculosis regimen	
Isoniazid	Rifampicin, pyrazinamide, ethambutol	Rifampicin and ethambutol for 7 months (up to 10 months in extensive disease)
Pyrazinamide	Rifampicin, isoniazid, ethambutol	Rifampicin and isoniazid for 7 months
Ethambutol	Rifampicin, isoniazid, pyrazinamide	Rifampicin and isoniazid for 4 months

0.3–0.4 mg/kg once daily, then gradually tapered over 4–8 weeks (NICE, 2016).

Drug-resistant tuberculosis

Drug-resistant TB is most commonly caused by non-adherence to the full treatment regimen, prescribing of inappropriate treatment regimens or lack of availability of high-quality drugs. In one meta-analysis, the risk of development of MDR-TB in patients in whom treatment was unsuccessful after being prescribed an inappropriate treatment regimen was increased 27-fold (van der Werf et al., 2012). Although the number of drug-resistant cases of TB in the UK is relatively low, resistance to anti-TB drugs is becoming an increasing problem in many countries including the UK.

There are varying degrees of drug resistance that are encountered:

- mono-resistance: resistance to one anti-TB drug;
- MDR-TB: resistance to at least isoniazid and rifampicin;
- XDR-TB: resistance to any fluoroquinolone, and at least one injectable second-line drug (capreomycin, kanamycin or amikacin), in addition to multidrug resistance.

The treatment of drug-resistant TB is complex, with a paucity of randomised controlled trials to guide treatment regimen selection, and second-line anti-TB drugs are generally less effective than first-line drugs and often have poor adverse effect profiles.

Mono-resistant tuberculosis

In 2016 in England, 7.5% of cases had resistance to at least one first-line antibiotic, comprising 7.0% resistant to isoniazid, 1.7% to rifampicin, 1.2% to ethambutol and 0.6% to pyrazinamide (Public Health England, 2017). Treatment of mono-resistant TB requires the remaining first-line anti-TB drugs to be used for longer durations, as outlined in Table 41.2.

Multidrug-resistant tuberculosis

The treatment of MDR-TB is complex and requires prolonged courses of treatment. Only specialist doctors with experience in treating drug-resistant TB should manage these cases. Newly diagnosed patients require admission to hospital into a negative pressure isolation room until they become non-infectious, to prevent transmission to other people. Because the precise pattern of drug resistance can be highly variable in MDR-TB, there are limited clinical trials to guide treatment decisions and drug regimens need to be individualised. The treatment of MDR-TB is significantly more expensive than treating drug-sensitive TB, with drug costs of approximately £18,000 for a 20-month course of treatment compared with £260 for standard treatment. However, the costs of prolonged admissions, outpatient clinic appointments, staffing and testing will drive overall costs much higher.

MDR-TB is relatively uncommon in the UK, with just 1.5% cases reported in England in 2016 (Public Health England, 2017). Because there are relatively few doctors in the UK with experience in managing MDR-TB, it is recommended that cases are registered with the British Thoracic Society MDR-TB Clinical Advice Service to allow other registered healthcare professionals to provide advice. Guidelines for managing MDR-TB have been produced by the WHO (2016), and drug information is available from the UK TB Drug Monographs (http://www.tbdrugmonographs.co.uk).

Treatment regimens for MDR-TB are based on known drug sensitivity data, and it is of critical importance that just one drug is not added to failing treatment regimens, because this could result in further resistance developing to the new drug. The principles of treating MDR-TB with second-line drugs (Table 41.3) are complex, but treatment regimens usually comprise at least five effective drugs during the intensive phase (WHO, 2016):

- one group A drug: a fluoroquinolone (moxifloxacin most effective);
- one group B drug: a parenteral agent (amikacin or capreomycin);
- two group C drugs: prothionamide, cycloserine linezolid or clofazimine;
- usually pyrazinamide (unless resistant);
- if five drugs cannot be selected, one drug from group D2 (bedaquiline or delamanid) and others from group D3 (e.g. p-aminosalicylic acid, meropenem-clavulanate) are used;
- ethambutol and/or high-dose isoniazid may be used in addition.

The intensive phase of treatment should last 8 months, at which time the parenteral agent is stopped and the remaining drugs continued for a total of 20 months. If the regimen appears to be failing (often an indicator of poor adherence or increased resistance), at least two new drugs should be commenced. This is because adding a single drug is liable to result in further resistance developing.

Table 41.3 Second-line antituberculosis drugs (WHO, 2016)

WHO grouping	Drug	Route	Adults[a]	Children[a]
Group A: fluoroquino-lones	Levofloxacin (not licensed to treat TB in the UK)	Oral	10–15 mg/kg once daily (usually 750–1000 mg once daily)	**Age >5 years:** 10–15 mg/kg once daily **Age ≤5 years:** 7.5–10 mg/kg twice a day (limited experience)
	Moxifloxacin (not licensed to treat TB in the UK)	Oral, intrave-nous	Usual dose 400 mg once daily WHO recommendations for MDR-TB short course regimen (safety of the higher doses not verified): Weight <30 kg: 400 mg once a day Weight 30–50 kg: 600 mg once a day Weight >50 kg: 800 mg once a day	7.5–10 mg/kg once a day
Group B: second-line injectable agents	Streptomycin (unlicensed in the UK)	Intravenous	**Age ≤59 years** 15 mg/kg daily (usual max. 1 g daily, but can be increased if necessary in large, muscular adults) **Age >59 years:** 10 mg/kg daily (max. 750 mg daily) **All ages:** after initial period: 15 mg/kg three times per week	20–40 mg/kg daily (max. 1 g daily) After initial period: 20–40 mg/kg three times per week
	Amikacin (not licensed to treat TB in the UK)	Intravenous or intramuscular injection	**Age ≤59 years:** 15 mg/kg daily (usual max. 1 g daily, but can be increased if necessary in large, muscular adults) **Age >59 years:** 10 mg/kg daily (max. 750 mg daily) **All ages:** after initial period: 15 mg/kg three times per week	15–22.5 mg/kg daily (usual max. 1 g daily) After initial period: 15–30 mg/kg three times per week
	Capreomycin	Intramuscular injection There is expe-rience using as an intravenous infusion	**Age ≤59 years:** 15 mg/kg daily (usual max. 1 g daily, but can be increased if necessary in large, muscular adults) **Age >59 years:** 10 mg/kg daily (max. 750 mg daily) **All ages:** after initial period: 15 mg/kg three times per week	15–30 mg/kg daily (usual max. 1 g daily) After initial period: 15–30 mg/kg three times per week
Group C: other core second-line agents	Prothionamide (unlicensed in the UK)	Oral	15–20 mg/kg (max. 1 g) once daily Once-daily dosing is preferred to maximise peak levels, particularly for daily doses ≤750 mg; consider twice-daily dosing if patients are unable to tolerate once-daily regimens	15–20 mg/kg (max. 1 g) once daily Once-daily dosing is preferred to maximise peak levels, particularly for daily doses ≤750 mg; consider twice-daily dosing if patients are unable to tolerate once-daily regimens
	Cycloserine	Oral	Initially 250 mg twice a day, increased to 500 mg twice a day depending on serum con-centrations. The usual target dose is 10–20 mg/kg/day once or twice per day; max. 1 g/day	The usual target dose is 10–20 mg/kg/day once or twice per day; max. 1 g/day
	Linezolid (not licensed to treat TB in the UK)	Oral, intrave-nous	600 mg once a day Consider reducing to 300 mg once daily if serious adverse effects develop	**Age ≤11 years:** 10 mg/kg three times daily **Age >11 years:** 10 mg/kg twice daily (max. 600 mg in 24 h)
	Clofazimine (unlicensed in the UK)	Oral	100–200 mg once daily Doses of 200 mg daily for 2 months, then 100 mg daily have been used	Limited data, recommendation is based on experience and expert opinion and suggests 1 mg/kg/day

Continued

Table 41.3 Second-line antituberculosis drugs (WHO, 2016)—cont'd

WHO grouping	Drug	Route	Adults[a]	Children[a]
Group D: add-on agents	Bedaquiline	Oral	400 mg daily for the first 2 weeks, followed by 200 mg three times per week for the remaining 22 weeks	Not recommended; limited experience
	Delamanid	Oral	100 mg twice a day for 24 weeks	Not recommended; limited experience
	p-Aminosalicylic acid	Oral	150 mg/kg/day in two to four divided doses; usual dose is 8–12 g/day	200–300 mg/kg/day p-Aminosalicylic acid is only available in 4 g sachets; the GranuPAS brand comes with a dosage scoop graduated in milligrams to aid dosing in children
	Co-amoxiclav (not licensed to treat TB in the UK)	Oral, intravenous	Oral: 625 mg three times daily Intravenous: 1.2 g three times daily	Limited data, consult the UK TB Drug monographs
	Imipenem/cilastatin (not licensed to treat TB in the UK)	Intravenous	**Body weight >50 kg:** 1 g twice a day **Body weight (≤50 kg):** 15 mg/kg twice a day (dose is based on the imipenem component)	20–40 mg/kg (max. 2 g) three times a day
	Meropenem (not licensed to treat TB in the UK)	Intravenous	1 g three times a day Should be used in combination with clavulanate (as co-amoxiclav) 625 mg three times a day	1 month to 12 years: 20–40 mg/kg every 8 h (max. 6000 mg in 24 h)
	Thiacetazone (unlicensed in the UK)	Oral	150 mg once daily	No information

[a]Consult product literature or the UK TB Drug monographs (http://www.tbdrugmonographs.co.uk) for dose adjustment recommendations in marked obesity, renal impairment, or in response to serum levels.
max., Maximum; TB, tuberculosis; WHO, World Health Organization.

An alternative, shorter 9- to 12-month regimen has been proposed by WHO (2016) for patients with MDR-TB who have not previously been treated with second-line drugs and in whom resistance to fluoroquinolones and second-line injectable agents has either been excluded or is considered highly unlikely. In Western Europe, this regimen is likely to be suitable only for a minority of patients based on current drug-resistance patterns.

The short regimen comprises two phases of treatment:
- 4-month intensive phase (extended up to a maximum of 6 months in case of lack of sputum smear conversion): gatifloxacin (or moxifloxacin), kanamycin, prothionamide, clofazimine, high-dose isoniazid, pyrazinamide and ethambutol;
- 5-month continuation phase: gatifloxacin (or moxifloxacin), clofazimine, pyrazinamide and ethambutol.

Extensively drug-resistant tuberculosis

There is a lack of evidence for suitable treatment regimens for people with XDR-TB, and very limited experience in the UK. Cases should be managed only at specialist TB centres, advice should be sought from multidisciplinary teams, and cases must be registered with the British Thoracic Society MDR-TB Clinical Advice Service.

Treatment regimens are likely to comprise any or all remaining anti-TB drugs to which the isolate is likely to be sensitive, and drug costs may exceed £70,000. Bedaquiline and delamanid are two drugs with novel modes of action that have recently been licensed in the UK for the treatment of drug-resistant TB and may have a role when treating XDR-TB. Currently, however, there are very limited data on the safety of combining bedaquiline and delamanid in treatment regimens.

HIV/tuberculosis co-infection

Patients with TB/HIV co-infection should be managed by a multidisciplinary team that includes physicians with expertise in the treatment of both TB and HIV infection (Pozniak et al., 2011). First-line anti-TB drugs are recommended, and non-interacting antiretrovirals (ARVs) should be used where possible. TB treatment should only be modified where intolerance, severe toxicity or genotypic resistance limits ARV choice.

ARVs should ideally be commenced early during TB treatment, because delayed treatment may prolong or worsen immunosuppression. However, the treatment of HIV/TB co-infection is complicated because of overlapping toxicities, drug interactions, immune reconstitution disease and high pill burdens. Potential interactions between ARVs and anti-TB drugs must be checked before administration, using either manufacturer's summaries of product characteristics, the British HIV Association 2011 guidelines (Pozniak et al., 2011) on the treatment of TB/HIV co-infection or the University of Liverpool HIV drug interactions website (http://www.hiv-druginteractions.org).

The British HIV Association provides recommendations for commencing ARVs in patients with TB:
- CD4 less than 100 cells/microlitre: Start as soon as practical within 2 weeks after starting TB therapy, because there is an increased risk of further AIDS-defining events and increased mortality.
- CD4 100–350 cells/microlitre: Commence as soon as practical, but can wait until after completion of 2 months of TB treatment, especially when there are difficulties with drug interactions, adherence and toxicities.
- CD4 consistently greater than 350 cells/microlitre: Begin at physician discretion, because there is a low risk of HIV disease progression.

Latent tuberculosis infection

Latent TB infection can be successfully eradicated with appropriate courses of anti-TB drugs; however, these are not without risks due to their side effect profile. Treatment is recommended for children and adults aged up to 65 years, including those with HIV infection, confirmed to have latent TB infection after active TB disease is excluded (NICE, 2016). UK treatment regimens include either 3 months of isoniazid and rifampicin or 6 months of isoniazid alone.

The choice of treatment depends on each individual's circumstances, such that 3 months of isoniazid and rifampicin is recommended for people younger than 35 years, if hepatotoxicity is a concern after assessment of both liver function and risk factors, whereas 6 months of isoniazid alone may be preferred where drug interactions with rifamycins are a concern (e.g. with ARVs, contraceptives, immunosuppressants). Because the risk of hepatotoxicity increases with age, adults aged between 35 and 65 years should receive treatment only if there are no concerns of hepatotoxicity.

Treatment of latent TB infection in people who are contacts of patients with infectious MDR-TB is currently not recommended because of the lack of data demonstrating efficacy of any potential regimen.

Adverse effects

Paradoxical reactions

Occasionally patients treated for active TB may experience an exacerbation of signs or symptoms of disease (e.g. worsening lymph node swelling), or radiological manifestations of TB despite otherwise responding to anti-TB treatment. This is known as a paradoxical reaction or immune reconstitution inflammatory syndrome, and is thought to be due to an exaggerated immune response to dead bacilli. Patients may respond to treatment with high-dose prednisolone, such as 30 mg once daily (increased if on rifampicin), which is gradually reduced after 1–2 weeks. Non-pharmacological treatment options include recurrent needle aspiration of lymph nodes or abscesses.

Adverse drug reactions

Side effects from anti-TB drugs are common and patients should be advised of the common and serious effects, and how to manage them. This may be supplemented with patient information leaflets (PILs) such as those produced by TB Alert (http://www.thetruthabouttb.org/professionals/patient-support/). Common and serious adverse drug reactions of first- and second-line anti-TB drugs are listed in Table 41.4.

In drug-sensitive TB, rifampicin will cause an orange-red discolouration of urine and other body secretions throughout treatment, but is harmless. Gastro-intestinal side effects, such as nausea and vomiting, are common, particularly with pyrazinamide, but also with rifampicin and isoniazid. Whilst this is often mild and transient, some patients may experience severe symptoms that require antiemetics. Skin reactions including itching and rashes may occur with any first-line anti-TB drug; mild cases may require antihistamines, but if severe may require treatment interruption or systemic corticosteroid treatment.

Rifampicin, isoniazid and pyrazinamide are all potentially hepatotoxic, and liver function tests (LFTs) should be checked before commencing treatment. Many centres will also recheck LFTs periodically throughout treatment. If transaminases rise greater than five times the upper limit of normal, or greater than three times normal with symptomatic liver disease, all potentially hepatotoxic drugs (i.e. rifampicin, isoniazid and pyrazinamide) should be stopped immediately. LFTs should be closely monitored and the advice of a liver specialist sought if necessary. If the patient is well and sputum smear negative (i.e. non-infectious), no treatment is required until after LFTs return to normal. However, if the patient is unwell or sputum smear positive, TB treatment must continue using two anti-TB drugs with low risk of hepatotoxicity, such as streptomycin and ethambutol, with or without a fluoroquinolone (levofloxacin or moxifloxacin). Once liver function has returned to normal, the first-line anti-TB drugs can be reintroduced sequentially at full dose over a period of no more than 10 days, usually in the order of ethambutol, isoniazid, rifampicin, then pyrazinamide. Some guidelines advise against reintroducing pyrazinamide if the hepatotoxic reaction was particularly severe and prolonged, but continuing with ethambutol, rifampicin and isoniazid initially and extending the course duration to 9 months.

Peripheral neuropathy is a rare side effect of isoniazid and is more common in patients who are malnourished, immunocompromised, diabetic, elderly, alcoholic or have renal impairment. At-risk groups should be prescribed prophylactic doses of pyridoxine 10–50 mg once a day, although some guidelines recommend prescribing pyridoxine routinely for all patients. If symptomatic neuropathy occurs, larger pyridoxine doses may be required.

Ethambutol can rarely cause optic neuritis, resulting in blurred vision or red/green colour blindness, and patients should be advised to report any changes in vision. The risk is increased with large dosages greater than 15 mg/kg/day and with prolonged courses. Visual acuity and colour vision should be checked using a Snellen chart and Ishihara plates at the start of treatment and during treatment.

Monitoring of treatment

Adherence is possibly the most important aspect of monitoring of anti-TB drug treatment. It can be assessed in community settings simply by patient interview, tablet counts, reviewing prescription collection data or even by taking urine samples to assess for a red-orange colouration due to taking rifampicin, or with isoniazid urine test strips.

Anti-TB drugs are associated with a range of adverse effects that require routine monitoring. Routine tests for monitoring adverse effects of treatment include:

- urea and electrolytes, LFTs: repeated every 2–4 weeks for 2 months;
- baseline uric acid;
- baseline vitamin D level;
- baseline full blood count, clotting;
- HIV and hepatitis screen;
- baseline visual acuity and colour vision testing;
- nutritional assessment.

Table 41.4 Adverse drug reactions

WHO grouping	Drug	Common side effects	Serious side effects
First-line agents	Isoniazid	**Neurological:** peripheral neuropathy **Hepatic:** transient increases in LFTs	**Dermatological:** skin reactions, e.g. urticaria (uncommon) **Haematological:** agranulocytosis, megaloblastic anaemia, thrombocytopaenia **Hepatic:** hepatotoxicity (rare) **Immunological:** drug-induced lupus (rare) **Musculoskeletal:** arthralgia, rhabdomyolysis **Neurological:** seizure, psychosis (rare)
	Rifampicin	Reddish discolouration of urine, sweat, sputum, tears **Gastro-intestinal:** anorexia, nausea, vomiting, heartburn **Hepatic:** transient increases in LFTs Flu-like syndrome	**Haematological:** agranulocytosis (rare), haemolytic anaemia (rare, usually intermittent therapy), thrombocytopaenia (rare, usually high-dose/intermittent therapy) **Hepatic:** hepatotoxicity (rare) **Renal:** nephrotoxicity (rare)
	Pyrazinamide	**Hyperuricaemia** **Arthralgia** **Gastro-intestinal:** anorexia, nausea, vomiting **Hepatic:** transient increases in LFTs **Dermatological:** rash	**Haematological:** sideroblastic anaemia (rare), thrombocytopaenia (rare) **Hepatotoxicity**
	Ethambutol	**Endocrine:** hyperuricaemia **Gastro-intestinal:** nausea, vomiting	**Ophthalmic:** Optic neuritis (1–6%; greatest risk at doses >25 mg/kg/day, or >2 months of treatment) Red/green colour blindness
Group A: fluoroquinolones	Fluoroquinolones (e.g. levofloxacin, moxifloxacin)	**Cardiovascular:** QTc prolongation (risk: hypokalaemia, proarrhythmic conditions, in combination QT-prolonging drugs) **Gastro-intestinal:** nausea, vomiting, diarrhoea **Hepatic:** transient increases in LFTs **Other:** dizziness, headache	**Cardiovascular:** QTc prolongation **Dermatological:** SJS or TEN (rare) **Haematological:** (uncommon) agranulocytosis, aplastic anaemia, haemolytic anaemia, thrombocytopaenia **Hepatic:** acute hepatitis (rare) **Immunological:** anaphylaxis, immune hypersensitivity (uncommon) **Metabolic:** hypoglycaemia (in patients receiving hypoglycaemic drugs, uncommon) **Musculoskeletal:** tendon inflammation and rupture **Neurological:** seizures **Renal:** renal impairment (rare) **Respiratory:** extrinsic allergic alveolitis (rare) **Other:** serum sickness (rare)

Table 41.4 Adverse drug reactions—cont'd

WHO grouping	Drug	Common side effects	Serious side effects
Group B: second-line injectable agents	Injectable agents (e.g. amikacin, capreomycin, streptomycin)	**Nephrotoxicity:** accumulation if renal impairment **Ototoxicity:** irreversible vestibulo-cochlear nerve damage **Drug-induced eosinophilia** (capreomycin): usually subsides with intermittent dosing	**Dermatological:** induration and local pain with intramuscular injection **Endocrine:** hypocalcaemia, hypomagnesaemia and hypokalaemia **Neurological:** neuromuscular blockade and respiratory paralysis (more common in neuromuscular disease; usually dose-related and self-limiting) **Audiological:** ototoxicity: auditory > vestibular (higher with amikacin, prolonged use and older age) **Renal:** nephrotoxicity (higher with prolonged use)
Group C: other core second-line agents	Prothionamide	**Hepatic:** transient increases in LFTs **Gastro-intestinal:** nausea, vomiting, diarrhoea, anorexia, excessive salivation, metallic taste, stomatitis, and abdominal pain	**Hepatic:** acute hepatitis (rare) **Neurological** (maybe increased with cycloserine): dizziness, encephalopathy, peripheral neuropathy **Ophthalmic:** optic neuritis (rare) **Psychiatric:** psychotic disturbances, depression **Metabolic:** gynaecomastia, hypoglycaemia, hypothyroidism
	Cycloserine	**Neurological:** confusion, disorientation, dizziness, somnolence (increased risk if peak serum level >35 mg/L)	**Cardiovascular:** sudden development of congestive heart failure (doses >1–1.5 g daily [rare]) **Dermatological:** rash and photosensitivity, SJS (rare) **Haematological:** vitamin B_{12} and/or folic acid deficiency, megaloblastic anaemia or sideroblastic anaemia (rare) **Psychiatric:** depression, seizure, psychotic disturbances (increased risk if peak serum level >35 mg/L)
	Linezolid	**Gastro-intestinal:** diarrhoea (4%), nausea (3%), vomiting **Neurological:** headache (2%) **Infections:** candidiasis, particularly oral and vaginal (1%) **Hepatic:** transient increases in LFTs	**Metabolic:** lactic acidosis **Dermatological:** urticaria, rash; (rare) bullous disorders, e.g. SJS and TEN **Haematological:** myelosuppression **Neurological:** peripheral neuropathy, seizure, serotonin syndrome **Ophthalmic:** optic neuropathy: risk with prolonged treatment
	Clofazimine	**Dermatological:** pink to brownish-black skin discolouration within 1–4 weeks in 75–100% of patients; gradually disappears within 6–12 months after stopping treatment. Ichthyosis and dry skin (8–38%), pruritus (5%), rash (1–5%), photosensitivity reactions (wear protective clothing and sunscreens) **Gastro-intestinal** (up to 50% of patients): abdominal pain, nausea, vomiting, diarrhoea, weight loss	**Gastro-intestinal** (<1%): bowel obstruction, gastrointestinal haemorrhage **Ophthalmic:** conjunctival pigmentation (38–57%), subjective dimness of vision (12.3%), and dry eyes, burning and other ocular irritation (24.6%) **Psychiatric:** reactive depression due to skin discolouration **Other:** splenic infarction, discolouration of body fluids
	p-Aminosalicylic acid	**Gastro-intestinal:** nausea, vomiting, diarrhoea, abdominal pain **Immunological:** hypersensitivity reactions (5–10%) including rash and fever	**Metabolic:** hypothyroidism **Haematological:** haemolytic anaemia (patients with G6PD deficiency), agranulocytosis, eosinophilia, leucopaenia and thrombocytopaenia **Hepatic:** acute hepatitis (rare)

Table 41.4 Adverse drug reactions—cont'd

WHO grouping	Drug	Common side effects	Serious side effects
Group D: add-on agents	Bedaquiline	**Arthralgia** **Chest pain** **Gastro-intestinal:** nausea **Neurological:** headache **Respiratory:** haemoptysis	**Cardiovascular:** QTc prolongation (more common in hypokalaemia, proarrhythmic conditions, in combination with other drugs that prolong the QT interval such as clofazimine, fluoroquinolones or macrolides) **Hepatic:** increases in LFTs
	Delamanid	**Dermatological:** dermatitis and urticaria **Gastro-intestinal:** nausea, vomiting, diarrhoea **Neurological:** dizziness, insomnia, paraesthesia, tremor **Respiratory:** haemoptysis	**Cardiovascular:** QTc prolongation; increased risk if: hypoalbuminaemia (especially <28 g/L), known congenital prolongation of the QTc interval, any condition or concomitant drug that may prolong the QTc interval **Haematological:** anaemia, eosinophilia, thrombocytopaenia, leucopaenia **Hepatic:** increases in LFTs **Metabolic:** hypertriglyceridaemia, hypercholesterolaemia **Psychiatric:** psychotic disorder, agitation, anxiety, depression, restlessness
	p-Aminosalicylic acid	**Gastro-intestinal:** nausea, vomiting, diarrhoea, abdominal pain **Immunological:** hypersensitivity reactions (5–10%) including rash and fever	**Metabolic:** hypothyroidism **Haematological:** haemolytic anaemia (patients with G6PD deficiency), agranulocytosis, eosinophilia, leucopaenia and thrombocytopaenia **Hepatic:** acute hepatitis (rare)

G6PD, Glucose-6-phosphate dehydrogenase; LFT, liver function test; SJS, Stevens–Johnson syndrome; TB, tuberculosis; TEN, toxic epidermal necrolysis.
Adapted from the UK TB Drug Monographs.

Drug interactions

Rifampicin is a potent inducer of cytochrome P450 enzymes, and drug interactions are common, resulting in accelerated drug metabolism and reduced plasma concentrations. An accurate medication history must be taken, including herbal and over-the-counter remedies. Common significant drug interactions frequently encountered in clinical practice, resulting in reduced efficacy, include opiate analgesics, anticoagulants, antiepileptics, antifungals, antivirals, corticosteroids, immunosuppressants and hormonal contraceptives.

The absorption of isoniazid and rifampicin is reduced in the presence of food, and both should both be taken on an empty stomach, 30–60 minutes before food or 2 hours after food.

Isoniazid is also associated with a possible increased risk of headache, sweating, palpitations, flushing and hypotension when eating certain foods rich in histamine or tyramine such as cheese, skipjack tuna or other tropical fish, or red wine. In practice, no dietary restrictions are usually required unless symptoms are experienced. This reaction is thought to be due to an exaggerated histamine poisoning reaction following inhibition of histamine metabolism, or to the sympathomimetic action of tyramine resulting from inhibition of monoamine oxidase.

Adherence

Ensuring full adherence to treatment is critical to achieving treatment success, because non-adherence risks not only treatment failure, but also disease relapse, development of drug resistance and transmission to other people. Factors that affect adherence to treatment include communication barriers, size and number of tablets, adverse events of treatment and cost of prescriptions.

Approximately three-quarters of new cases of TB in England are born outside the UK (Public Health England, 2017), and language barriers may exist. Communication and adherence can be supported by the provision of PILs, such as those produced by TB Alert, which contain photographs of the tablets that the patient takes, and are available in a range of foreign languages.

To reduce tablet burden to support adherence, FDC tablets are recommended in TB treatment regimens, to prevent patients from being selective about which drugs to take and prevent drug resistance from developing, which may occur with separate drugs. Although there is a lack of evidence on adherence with different treatment regimens in TB, studies have demonstrated that FDC tablets are easier to swallow and more convenient to take than taking the four drugs given separately (Bartacek et al., 2009).

Supervised versus unsupervised treatment

Most patients diagnosed with active TB in the UK do not need to have their treatment supervised, but all should have a risk assessment for their likely adherence, and Directly Observed Therapy (DOT) should be considered for patients thought likely to be non-adherent. DOT should be considered for people who:

- have a history of non-adherence;
- have been treated previously;

- have a history of homelessness, drug or alcohol misuse;
- are currently in prison or have been in the past 5 years;
- have a major psychiatric, memory or cognitive disorder;
- are in denial of the diagnosis;
- have MDR-TB.

DOT is performed by directly observed swallowing of medication, and for drug-sensitive TB this is usually given three times weekly (often on Mondays, Wednesdays and Fridays) rather than daily (see doses in Table 41.1). Healthcare workers are usually responsible for observing medication being swallowed, although relatives or friends may be suitable observers in some situations. Although in the UK TB nurses frequently provide the DOT service, this can also be performed by community pharmacies as an enhanced service subject to local funding arrangements. The use of DOT (either given daily or intermittently) has been demonstrated to have similar outcomes in terms of cure and cure plus treatment completion in a systematic review (Karumbi and Garner, 2015).

Patient education

When commencing treatment, all patients should receive verbal and written information on their diagnosis, whether active or latent TB infection, and their treatment. Although all patients must be issued with a PIL provided by the manufacturer, these may be hard for some patients to read because of the complexity of language and size of the text. Consequently, many patients find the TB Alert PILs easier to read and understand, particularly because these are available in many languages.

Patients should be advised of the benefits of treatment, emphasising that complete adherence to treatment will ensure that they will be cured, but whilst they may begin to feel better within a few weeks, the full treatment course will take months to prevent relapse of disease. All patients should be advised that they may experience side effects, and whilst some may be harmless or temporary, others may be more serious and require the patient to contact a named healthcare professional.

Special circumstances

Renal disease

Several anti-TB drugs are eliminated by the renal route and consequently may require dose adjustment in moderate to severe kidney disease (Milburn et al., 2010). Of the first-line drugs, pyrazinamide and ethambutol should have their dose interval extended to three times weekly dosing in stage 4 and 5 chronic kidney disease, whereas isoniazid and rifampicin may be continued at the full daily dose. The dose and/or frequency of a number of second-line anti-TB drugs should also be adjusted, including all injectable agents, prothionamide, cycloserine and *p*-aminosalicylic acid. Patients with chronic kidney disease should be closely monitored for adverse effects, and therapeutic drug monitoring may be utilised to ensure that a safe and effective dose is used, particularly for ethambutol, aminoglycosides and cycloserine.

Liver disease

The incidence of active TB is increased in people with chronic liver disease, but is complicated by the fact that many anti-TB drugs are potentially hepatotoxic. The frequency of hepatotoxicity is also increased in the presence of liver cirrhosis, chronic hepatitis B and chronic hepatitis C. Such patients should be closely monitored with regular and frequent checks of LFTs, and treatment suspended if there is a rise in plasma aspartate aminotransferase or alanine aminotransferase greater than five times the upper limit of normal, or three to five times the upper limit if also symptomatic.

Pregnancy and breastfeeding

Active TB during pregnancy poses risks to both the mother and fetus, as well as to any close contacts. Complications of TB in pregnancy include spontaneous abortion, preterm labour, low birth weight and increased neonatal mortality. The first-line anti-TB drugs isoniazid, rifampicin, pyrazinamide and ethambutol are all considered compatible with use in pregnancy, and any risks of harm from these drugs are outweighed by the risks of untreated active TB. Many second-line drugs are not compatible with use in pregnancy, in particular the aminoglycosides, which are associated with hearing and/or balance problems.

Pregnant women who are diagnosed with latent TB infection may choose to delay commencing chemoprophylaxis until after delivery, provided that active TB is definitively excluded.

Breastfeeding is considered safe whilst taking anti-TB drugs, and all mothers should take supplemental pyridoxine 10–50 mg daily whilst taking isoniazid given the small risk of neurotoxicity to the feeding infant.

Elderly

The use of anti-TB drugs may be complicated in elderly patients because of the presence of comorbidities, drug interactions and increased incidence of adverse effects of treatment compared with younger people. In particular, healthcare professionals should be alert for the presence or worsening of renal or liver disease, and adverse effects of anti-TB drugs. Where necessary, doses may need to be adjusted and potential drug interactions managed by altering existing treatment plans.

Children

The treatment of TB in children is similar to that of adults, requiring a 2-month intensive phase of four drugs followed by a 4-month continuation phase of two drugs (extended to 12 months for TB affecting the CNS). See Table 41.1 for recommended doses. Adverse effects of treatment tend to be less frequent in children than in adults, and consequently LFTs do not need to be routinely monitored unless there is clinical suspicion of hepatotoxicity. Furthermore, because isoniazid may cause pyridoxine deficiency, supplementation is recommended in children at higher risk of experiencing symptoms, particularly malnourished children, HIV-infected children, breastfeeding infants and pregnant adolescents.

Treatment in children is also complicated by the lack of availability of drug preparations suitable for use in children. Of the FDCs, Rifater (rifampicin, isoniazid, pyrazinamide) may not be appropriate as the dose of each drug is not suitable for recommended doses in children; Voractiv (rifampicin, isoniazid, pyrazinamide, ethambutol) is not licensed for children younger than 8 years or less than 30 kg body weight; and Rifinah (rifampicin, isoniazid) is licensed only for use in adults. Consequently children diagnosed with TB frequently receive treatment with the four anti-TB drugs given separately. However, some UK specialist paediatric TB centres do use FDCs, but only after careful consideration of individual doses, which may require dose supplementation with individual drugs.

There is a lack of suitable preparations to use if children are unable to swallow large tablets. Rifampicin syrup is the only licensed liquid preparation available for treating TB, whilst isoniazid, pyrazinamide and ethambutol must all be ordered as an unlicensed special.

Case studies

Case 41.1

Mr SD is a 25-year-old man with a history of drug use, for which he is prescribed daily supervised methadone. He was released from prison 2 years ago. He has been referred to a chest physician with a cough productive of sputum and a fever (2 months in duration). A sputum sample, obtained by his primary care doctor, is positive for acid, alcohol-fast bacilli, and a chest radiograph shows right upper lobe cavities. A diagnosis of TB is made.

Questions

1. What risk factors does Mr SD have for TB?
2. What effects might TB treatment have on methadone, and how should this be managed?
3. How should Mr SD's TB treatment be managed?

Answers

1. Mr SD may be at risk of TB because of his lifestyle. He has the potential for chronic poor health and nutrition due to drug and alcohol abuse, which could result in a weakened immune system. The risk of TB in prisoners and people who have recently been discharged from prison in the UK is not currently clear, although prisoners are more likely to have other risk factors for TB (such as social exclusion and drug abuse). Recently, TB in UK prisoners has increased.
2. Rifampicin is a potent inhibitor of cytochrome P450 enzymes and will accelerate the metabolism of methadone, which can result in withdrawal symptoms. It is likely that most patients will require significant increases in methadone dose (as much as twofold to threefold dose increases) whilst being prescribed rifampicin. Consequently, the drug addiction service that prescribes Mr SD's methadone should be advised of the TB diagnosis and asked to monitor withdrawal symptoms and adjust the methadone dose accordingly. An appointment with the drug addiction service should ideally be arranged within 24 hours of commencing TB treatment.

An alternative option would be to use rifabutin instead of rifampicin, because it appears to interact to a lesser extent.
3. Due to his history, Mr SD would be considered high risk of non-adherence to TB treatment, and a DOT regimen should be strongly considered. This could be provided by local TB nurses, or alternatively the community pharmacist who supervises Mr SD's methadone treatment could be asked to provide this role. Community pharmacists may provide DOT as an enhanced service, with an agreement between the TB service and pharmacist about each other's responsibilities, including when the pharmacist should refer back to the TB service, for example, because of side effects or non-adherence.

Case 41.2

Ms RW is a 28-year-old Lithuanian woman who has lived in England for 3 years. She has been referred to the TB clinic with a 2-month history of weight loss, fever, night sweats and productive cough. Chest X-ray shows upper lobe infiltrates and cavities on both sides. A diagnosis of pulmonary TB is made.

Questions

1. Is Ms RW at low or high risk of drug-resistant TB?
2. Should she be in isolation?
3. What microbiological investigations are required?
4. What treatment should she receive?

Answers

1. Data collated by the WHO show that 12% of new TB cases in Lithuania are MDR-TB (WHO, 2017). Consequently Ms RW would be assumed to be at high risk of having MDR-TB.
2. Because there is a high risk of MDR-TB, Ms RW should be admitted to a negative pressure isolation room until she is demonstrated to be either not drug-resistant or non-infectious.
3. Sputum samples should be taken and undergo smear to test for the presence of acid, alcohol-fast bacilli. If positive, they should then undergo rapid diagnostic nucleic acid amplification tests for rifampicin resistance. Tests should also be done to assess susceptibility to other drugs.
4. Treatment should incorporate at least four second-line anti-TB drugs that are likely to be effective, in addition to pyrazinamide. In the absence of any history of contact with other cases of drug-resistant TB, a suitable regimen is likely to initially comprise pyrazinamide, a fluoroquinolone (e.g. moxifloxacin), an injectable agent (e.g. capreomycin), prothionamide and cycloserine. This should be supplemented with pyridoxine, to reduce neurological side effects from cycloserine, and an antiemetic.

Case 41.3

Mr KP is a 40-year-old man who was born in India. Six weeks ago, he was referred to the TB clinic with a productive cough and fever. Chest X-ray film showed patchy upper lobe consolidation, and sputum smear was positive for acid, alcohol-fast bacilli. He was commenced on Voractiv treatment as an outpatient.

Mr KP subsequently failed to turn up for his weeks 2 and 4 outpatient appointments, and so the local TB nurses had scheduled a home visit, but Mr KP was not at home at the appointed time.

His wife was at home, and she telephoned Mr KP on his mobile phone so that the TB nurses could speak to him. He admitted that he had taken only a few days of treatment and did not intend to take any more. The TB nurses advised him that if he did not take his treatment, he would need to be admitted to hospital.

Questions

1. What form of TB does Mr KP have?
2. How can Mr KP be forced into hospital admission?
3. Which groups of healthcare staff should be involved in arrangements for his admission to hospital?

Answers

1. Mr KP has sputum-smear-positive pulmonary TB, and thus would be considered to be and potentially pose an infection risk to others.
2. In the UK legal measures are allowed for compulsory admission of people with infectious pulmonary TB under section 37 of the Public Health (Control of Disease) Act 1984. Two separate applications to the magistrates court are required for compulsory hospital admission: the first for the admission, and the second for detention under section 38 of the Public Health (Control of Disease) Act 1984. This allows an infectious person to be isolated and prevent transmission; however, compulsory treatment of TB is not allowed.
3. Because Mr KP is infectious, admission to a hospital side room is required. A multidisciplinary approach should be taken to prepare and plan for the compulsory admission, including the ward nursing staff, doctors and public health representatives. This should be discussed with the patient, including the reasons why he will need to be kept in isolation.

Case 41.4

Mr FR, a 50-year-old man being treated for pulmonary TB, is reviewed in the outpatient clinic at week 4 of his standard anti-tuberculous treatment (isoniazid, rifampicin, pyrazinamide and ethambutol). He reports feeling generally run-down with some increased nausea. Routine blood tests are performed and his alanine transaminase (ALT) has risen from 37 to 230 U/L.

Questions

1. Should Mr FR's treatment be stopped?
2. What is the likely causative medicine?
3. How should the medicines be re-introduced?

Answers

1. Once the ALT has risen to five times the upper limit of normal (>200 U/L), then the medicines should be discontinued.
2. Unfortunately, all of the drugs used can cause liver toxicity. The least likely cause is ethambutol.
3. Mr FR's liver function should be monitored off treatment to ensure it is returning to baseline. At the same time it is important to assess for factors that may have increased risk of liver toxicity, such as viral hepatitis. When the ALT is less than two times the upper limit of normal (<80 U/L) reintroduction can take place in a sequential fashion starting with ethambutol plus either isoniazid or rifampicin. Pyrazinamide is reintroduced last, because it may be the most likely culprit. Latest NICE guidelines (NICE, 2016) recommend that the reintroduction regimen should take place quickly over no more than 10 days.

References

Bartacek, A., Schütt, D., Panosch, B., et al., 2009. Comparison of a four-drug fixed-dose combination regimen with a single tablet regimen in smear-positive pulmonary tuberculosis. Int. J. Tuberc. Lung Dis. 13, 760–766.

Karumbi, J., Garner, P., 2015. Directly observed therapy for treating tuberculosis. Cochrane Database Syst. Rev. 2015 (5), CD003343. Available at: http://onlinelibrary.wiley.com/doi/10.1002/14651858.CD003343.pub4/otherversions.

Lawn, S.D., Zumla, A.I., 2011. Tuberculosis. Lancet 363, 1050–1058.

Milburn, H., Ashman, N., Davies, P., 2010. Guidelines for the prevention and management of Mycobacterium tuberculosis infection and disease in adult patients with chronic kidney disease. Thorax 65, 559–570.

National Institute for Health and Care Excellence (NICE), 2016. NICE Guideline 33. Tuberculosis. NICE, London. Available at: https://www.nice.org.uk/guidance/ng33/.

Pozniak, A.L., Coyne, K.M., Miller, R.F., et al., 2011. British HIV Association guidelines for the treatment of TB/HIV coinfection 2011. HIV Med. 12, 517–524.

Prasad, K., Singh, M.B., 2008. Corticosteroids for managing tuberculous meningitis. Cochrane Database Syst. Rev. 2008 (1), CD002244. Available at: http://onlinelibrary.wiley.com/doi/10.1002/14651858.CD002244.pub3/abstract.

Public Health England, 2013. The 'Green Book' Immunisation against infectious disease. Available at: https://www.gov.uk/government/collections/immunisation-against-infectious-disease-the-green-book.

Public Health England, 2017. Tuberculosis in England 2017 report (presenting data to end of 2016). Available at: https://www.gov.uk/government/uploads/system/uploads/attachment_data/file/654152/TB_Annual_Report_2017.pdf.

van der Werf, M.J., Langendam, M.W., Huitric, E., et al., 2012. Multidrug resistance after inappropriate tuberculosis treatment: a meta-analysis. Eur. Respir. J. 39, 1511–1519.

World Health Organization. 2016. WHO treatment guidelines for drug-resistant tuberculosis. 2016 update. October 2016 revision. WHO/HTM/TB/2016.04. WHO, Geneva. Available at: http://www.who.int/tb/areas-of-work/drug-resistant-tb/treatment/resources/en/.

World Health Organization, 2017. Global Tuberculosis Report 2017. WHO/HTM/TB/2017.23. WHO, Geneva. Available at: http://apps.who.int/iris/bitstream/10665/259366/1/9789241565516-eng.pdf?ua=1.

Useful websites

TB Drug Monographs: http://www.tbdrugmonographs.co.uk/
Liverpool HIV Pharmacology Group. HIV Drug interactions: http://www.hiv-druginteractions.org

TB Alert: http://www.tbalert.org/
The Truth About TB: http://www.thetruthabouttb.org/

42 HIV Infection

Sheena Castelino, Alison Grant and Katie Conway

Key points

- As a result of effective combination antiretroviral therapy (cART), infection with the human immunodeficiency virus (HIV) has changed from being a terminal illness to a long-term manageable chronic infection, and many people living with HIV can enjoy a good quality of life, with essentially normal life expectancy.

- Untreated infection with HIV leads to a progressive deterioration in the cellular immune response. After primary HIV infection (PHI), or 'seroconversion', the infected individual may appear asymptomatic for a number of years before experiencing development of symptomatic disease and/or acquired immune deficiency syndrome.

- Complications arising from untreated HIV infection can manifest in a variety of ways, usually as opportunistic infections or malignancies that are uncommon in the immunocompetent population.

- The aim of the treatment of HIV infection is to suppress viral replication to prevent further deterioration of the immune system and allow immune reconstitution, thereby reducing morbidity and mortality associated with chronic HIV.

- Currently available antiretroviral agents are classified by their mechanism of actions as nucleoside or nucleotide analogue reverse transcriptase inhibitors, non-nucleoside reverse transcriptase inhibitors, protease inhibitors, integrase inhibitors and entry inhibitors.

- Antiretroviral agents are given in combination, usually of at least three agents, to improve efficacy and reduce the development of viral resistance. A high level of adherence to therapy is vital to ensure efficacy and prevent the emergence of resistant virus.

- Treatment regimens have improved both in terms of efficacy and tolerability over time, with the majority of people living with HIV experiencing virological suppression and good treatment outcomes. There are some important toxicities related to ART, and drug–drug interactions remain a challenge, particularly when faced with an aging HIV population and increasing poly-pharmacy.

- Effective treatment and virological suppression also significantly reduce the onward transmission of HIV.

Epidemiology

In June 1981 five cases of *Pneumocystis jiroveci* (formerly known as *carinii*) pneumonia (PCP) were described in homosexual men in the USA. Reports of other unusual conditions, such as Kaposi's sarcoma (KS), followed shortly. In each of these patients, there was found to be a marked impairment of cellular immune response, and so the term acquired immune deficiency syndrome, or AIDS, was coined. In 1984 a new human retrovirus, subsequently named human immunodeficiency virus (HIV), was isolated and identified as the cause of AIDS.

Although initially described in homosexual men, it soon became apparent that other population groups were affected, including intravenous drug users and individuals with haemophilia. During the first decade, the epidemic grew and the importance of transmission via heterosexual intercourse and from mother to child (vertical transmission) was increasingly recognised. There are two types of HIV: HIV-1, which is the predominant type worldwide; and HIV-2, which is less pathogenic and mainly found in West Africa.

Globally there are more than 36.9 million people living with HIV (UNAIDS, 2015), with the main burden of disease affecting sub-Saharan Africa. Heterosexual transmission of infection is most commonly seen worldwide. In the UK there are more than 100,000 people living with HIV and this number continues to rise, mainly because of effective HIV treatment, an aging HIV population and increased levels of testing. The number of those living with undiagnosed HIV has declined since 2010 (25% to 17% in 2014). There remain high and increasing levels of new infections amongst men who have sex with men (MSM), and prevention strategies are more important than ever. Amongst heterosexuals in 2014, the overall prevalence of HIV is 1 in 1000, but amongst black African men and women rates are 1 in 56 and 1 in 22, respectively. There are declining levels of new infections, in particular from those acquiring HIV abroad particularly from sub-Saharan Africa. However, there is a stable number of heterosexuals acquiring HIV within the UK. Within the heterosexual population, late diagnosis is still a significant problem. In 2014, 55% of cases were diagnosed late (i.e. CD4 cell count <350 cells/mm^3), and therefore at a 10-fold increased risk of death over the next year compared with those diagnosed early. The increasing proportion of individuals with HIV who are living into older age leads to an increase in comorbidities, such as cardiovascular disease, osteoporosis and osteopaenia, cancer, cognitive impairment, and hepatic and renal dysfunction. It is postulated that HIV directly and some antiretroviral therapies may contribute to the development of these comorbidities.

The impact of treatment advances on reducing the incidence of AIDS-related illnesses and mortality has been dramatic. However, the absolute numbers of new AIDS diagnoses and HIV-related deaths in the UK have plateaued and are largely due to late presentation, failure to diagnose HIV infection amongst the asymptomatic population and those disengaged from care.

Although the number living with HIV globally continues to rise, there are encouraging trends which include many low- and middle-income countries having declining incidence (35% decrease since 2000) and fewer AIDS-related deaths (42% decrease since 2004). There has also been an increase in access to available antiretroviral agents (ARVs; 84% increase since 2010). However, challenges remain, with 17.1 million people unaware of their infection and 22 million who still need access to treatment. In resource-poor settings, choice of agents and facilities for monitoring may be limited, and locally produced generic formulations are often used.

The virus has been isolated from a number of body fluids, including blood, semen, vaginal secretions, saliva, breast milk, tears, urine, peritoneal fluid and cerebrospinal fluid (CSF). However, not all of these are important in the spread of infection, and the predominant routes of transmission remain: sexual intercourse (anal or vaginal); sharing of unsterilised needles or syringes; blood or blood products in areas where supplies are not screened or treated; and vertical transmission in utero, during labour or through breastfeeding.

Pathogenesis

HIV, in common with other retroviruses, possesses the enzyme reverse transcriptase and consists of a lipid bilayer membrane surrounding the capsid (Fig. 42.1). Its surface glycoprotein molecule (gp120) has a strong affinity for the CD4 receptor protein found predominantly on the T helper/inducer lymphocytes. Monocytes and macrophages may also possess CD4 receptors in low densities and can therefore also be infected. The process of HIV entry is more complex than originally thought, and in addition to CD4 attachment, subsequent binding to co-receptors such as C-C chemokine receptor type 5 (CCR-5) or C-X-X chemokine receptor type 4 (CXCR-4) and membrane fusion also occur (Fig. 42.2).

After penetrating the host cell, the virus sheds its outer coat and releases its genetic material. Using the reverse transcriptase enzyme, the viral RNA is converted to DNA using nucleosides. The viral DNA is then integrated into the host genome in the cell nucleus, where it undergoes transcription and translation, enabling the production of new viral proteins. New virus particles are then assembled and bud out of the host cell, finally

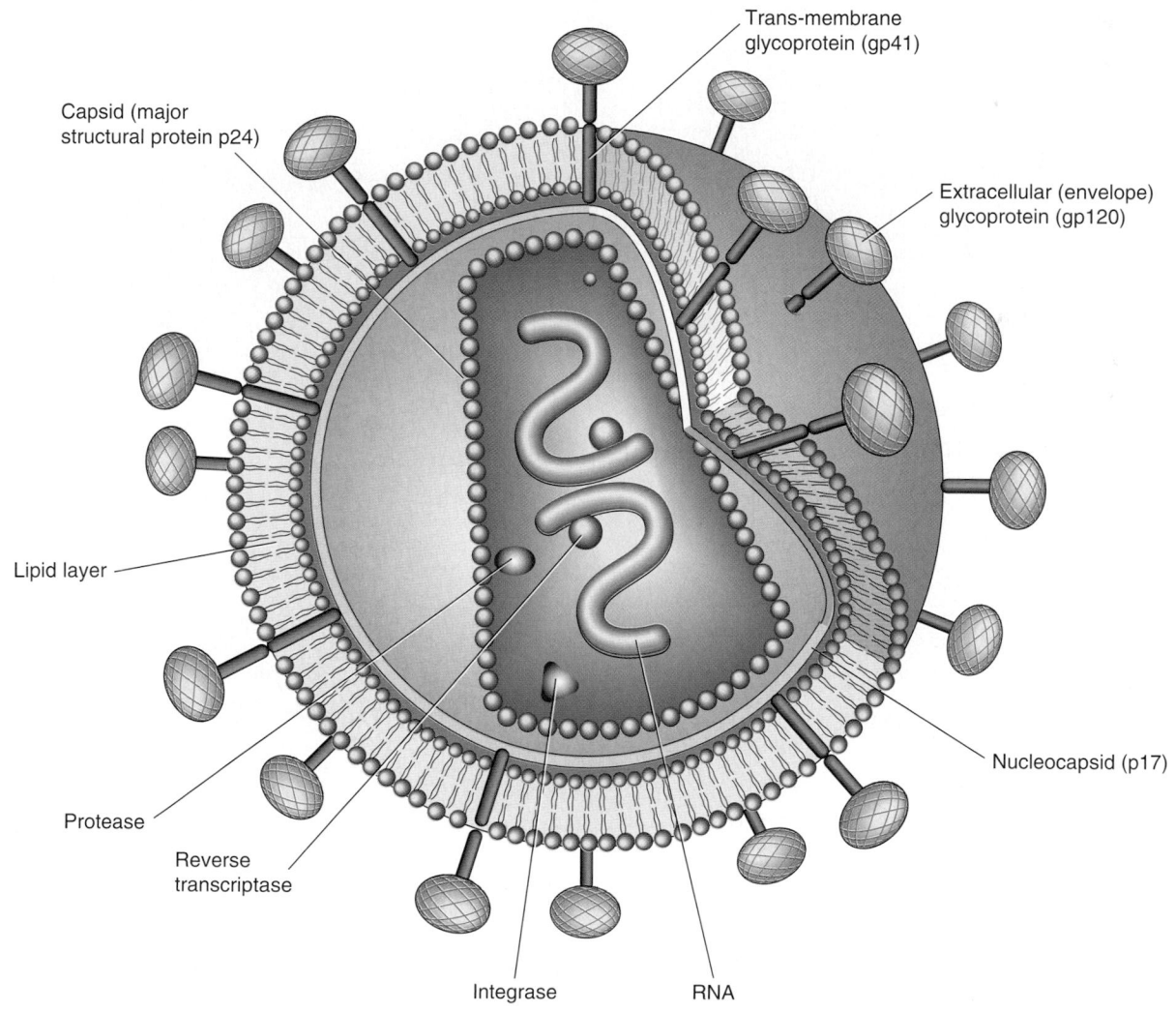

Trans-membrane glycoprotein (gp41)

Capsid (major structural protein p24)

Extracellular (envelope) glycoprotein (gp120)

Lipid layer

Nucleocapsid (p17)

Protease

Reverse transcriptase

Integrase

RNA

Fig. 42.1 Structure of the human immunodeficiency virus.

maturing into infectious virions under the influence of the protease enzyme.

During primary HIV infection (PHI), there is a very high rate of viral turnover and a subsequent drop in CD4 count as these cells are depleted. As the host immune system responds to this new infection, an equilibrium is then reached, which brings the level of the virus down to a 'set point', which is a relatively stable level of virus in the body and will vary between individuals. The CD4 count stabilises and may improve, but to a lower level than before infection occurred. At this stage the infection may appear

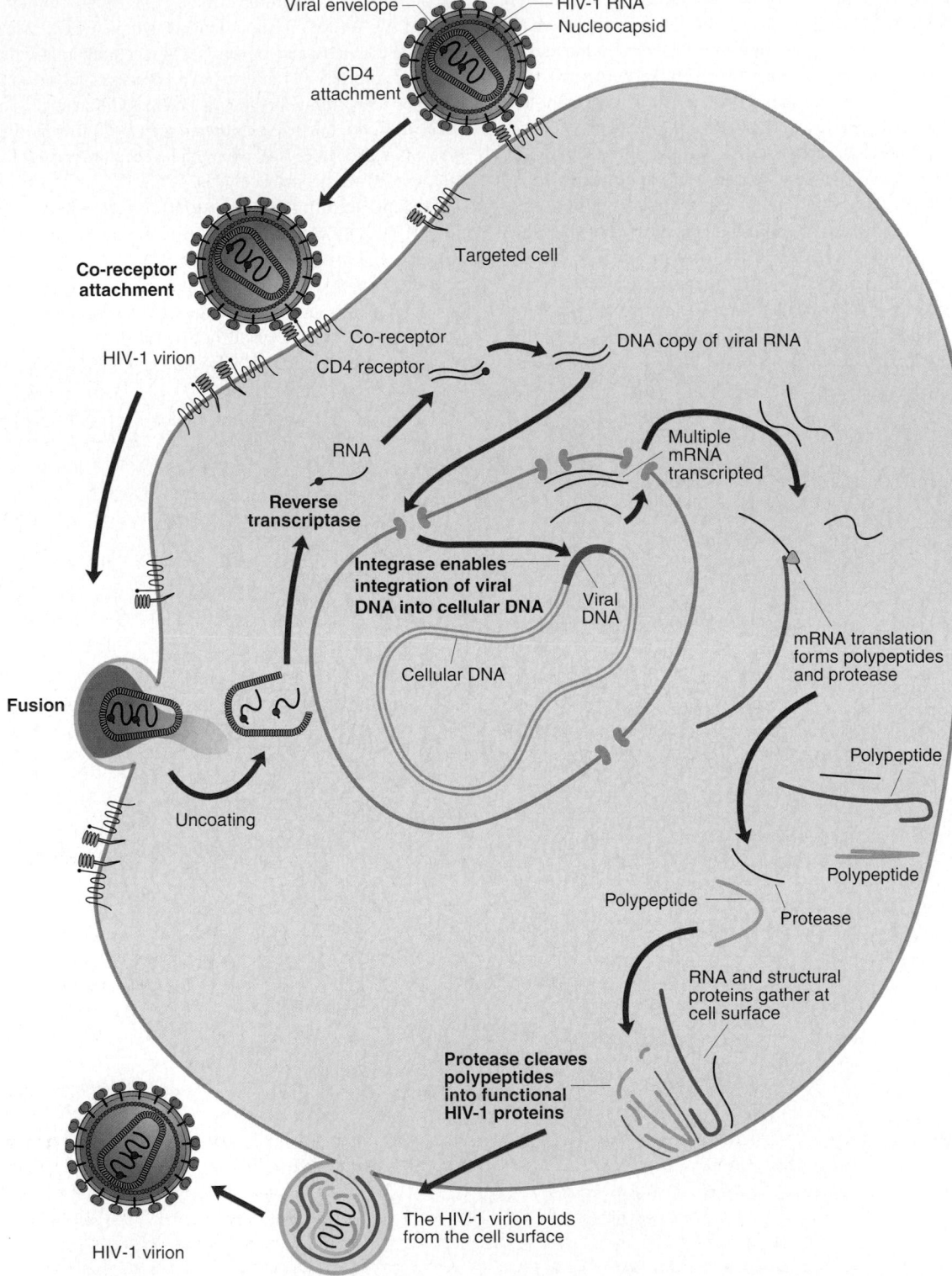

Fig. 42.2 Life cycle of human immunodeficiency virus (HIV) and the sites of action of currently available antiretroviral agents (in bold).

to be clinically latent, but in fact, as many as 10,000 million new virions are produced each day.

Over time, as chronic infection ensues, cells possessing CD4 receptors, particularly the T helper lymphocytes, are depleted from the body. The T helper cell is often considered to be the conductor of the 'immune orchestra', and thus as this cell is depleted, the individual becomes susceptible to a myriad of infections and tumours. The rate at which this immunosuppression progresses is variable, and the precise interaction of factors affecting it is still not fully understood. It is well recognised that some individuals rapidly develop severe immunosuppression, whereas others may have been infected with HIV for many years whilst maintaining a relatively intact immune system. It is likely that a combination of viral, host (genetic) and environmental factors contributes to this variation.

Clinical manifestations

Approximately 80% of individuals develop a flu-like illness during PHI, and this is characterised most commonly by a combination of some or all of the symptoms, such as fever, pharyngitis, rash, myalgia and headache/aseptic meningitis. Rarely, the degree of associated CD4 count depletion may be sufficient to result in development of an opportunistic illness such as oropharyngeal/ oesophageal candidiasis or *P. jiroveci* pneumonia. During this stage testing is of great importance for the individual's health both to avoid late diagnosis and to reduce onward transmission of the virus because PHI is the most infectious phase.

Although the clinical course of HIV disease varies with each individual, there is a fairly consistent and predictable pattern that enables appropriate interventions and preventive measures to be adopted. Patients can be classified into one of three groups according to their clinical status: asymptomatic, symptomatic or AIDS. This clinical progression generally relates to a decline in CD4 count and advancing immunosuppression.

Asymptomatic disease usually follows PHI and can last for a number of years. Symptomatic disease is characterised by non-specific symptomatology such as fevers, night sweats, lethargy and weight loss, or by complications including oral candidiasis, oral hairy leucoplakia, and recurrent herpes simplex or herpes zoster infections. AIDS is defined by the diagnosis of one or more specific conditions including *P. jiroveci* pneumonia, *Mycobacterium tuberculosis* infection and cytomegalovirus (CMV) disease. The World Health Organization (WHO, 2007) has produced a comprehensive guide to the clinical staging of HIV/AIDS and a full list of HIV-related and AIDS-defining conditions.

The sequelae of untreated HIV infection can be broadly considered in five categories:
- infections that can occur in immunocompetent patients but tend to occur more frequently, more severely and often atypically in the context of underlying HIV infection, for example, *Salmonella*, herpes simplex and *M. tuberculosis*;
- opportunistic infections, that is, infections that would not normally cause disease in an immunocompetent host, for example, *P. jiroveci* pneumonia and CMV;
- malignancies, particularly those that occur rarely in the immunocompetent population, for example, KS and non-Hodgkin's lymphoma;

- direct manifestations of HIV infection, for example, HIV encephalopathy, HIV myelopathy and HIV enteropathy;
- consequences of chronic immune activation, including premature cardiovascular disease, neurocognitive dysfunction and bone mineral density loss.

Investigations and monitoring
Current and previous infections

The initial diagnosis of HIV infection is made using a fourth-generation serological test, which tests for HIV antibodies and antigen simultaneously, and will detect the vast majority of individuals who have been infected with HIV at 4 weeks after specific exposure. A further test at 8 weeks post-exposure need only be considered following an event assessed as carrying a high risk of infection. Many of the rapid 'point-of-care tests' which test in real time, using finger prick or saliva, test only for HIV antibodies and may miss early infection hence have a 'window period' and need to be repeated 3 months after exposure. After confirmation of HIV infection, the patient is usually tested for prior exposure to a number of potential pathogens, including syphilis; hepatitis A, B and C; CMV; varicella zoster virus (VZV) and *Toxoplasma gondii*. This can enable subsequent treatment (in the case of undiagnosed syphilis), vaccination (if no prior exposure to hepatitis A, hepatitis B or VZV), prevention (if no prior exposure to *Toxoplasma* and CMV) and prophylaxis (if previous exposure to *Toxoplasma*), and can aid subsequent diagnosis (according to CMV or *Toxoplasma* status).

CD4 count

The level of immunosuppression is most easily estimated by monitoring a patient's CD4 count. This measures the number of CD4$^+$ T lymphocytes in a sample of peripheral blood. The normal range can vary between 500 and 1500 cells/mm^3. As HIV disease progresses, the number of cells declines. Particular complications of HIV infection usually begin to occur at similar CD4 counts (Fig. 42.3), which can assist in differential diagnoses and enable the use of prophylactic therapies. For example, patients with a CD4 count less than 200 cells/mm^3 should always be offered prophylaxis against *P. jiroveci* pneumonia. The CD4 count is also used to monitor response to antiretroviral treatment.

Viral load

The measurement of plasma HIV RNA (viral load) estimates the amount of circulating virus in the blood. This has been proven to correlate with prognosis, with a high viral load predicting faster disease progression (Mellors et al., 1997). Conversely, a reduction in viral load after commencement of antiviral therapy is associated with clinical benefit. This measure, in combination with the CD4 count, allows patients and clinicians to make informed decisions regarding which antiretrovirals to start, because some perform better at higher viral loads, to ensure that the medications are working (maintaining a fully supressed viral load) and when to change antiretroviral therapies (i.e. virological failure), enabling the most effective use of such agents.

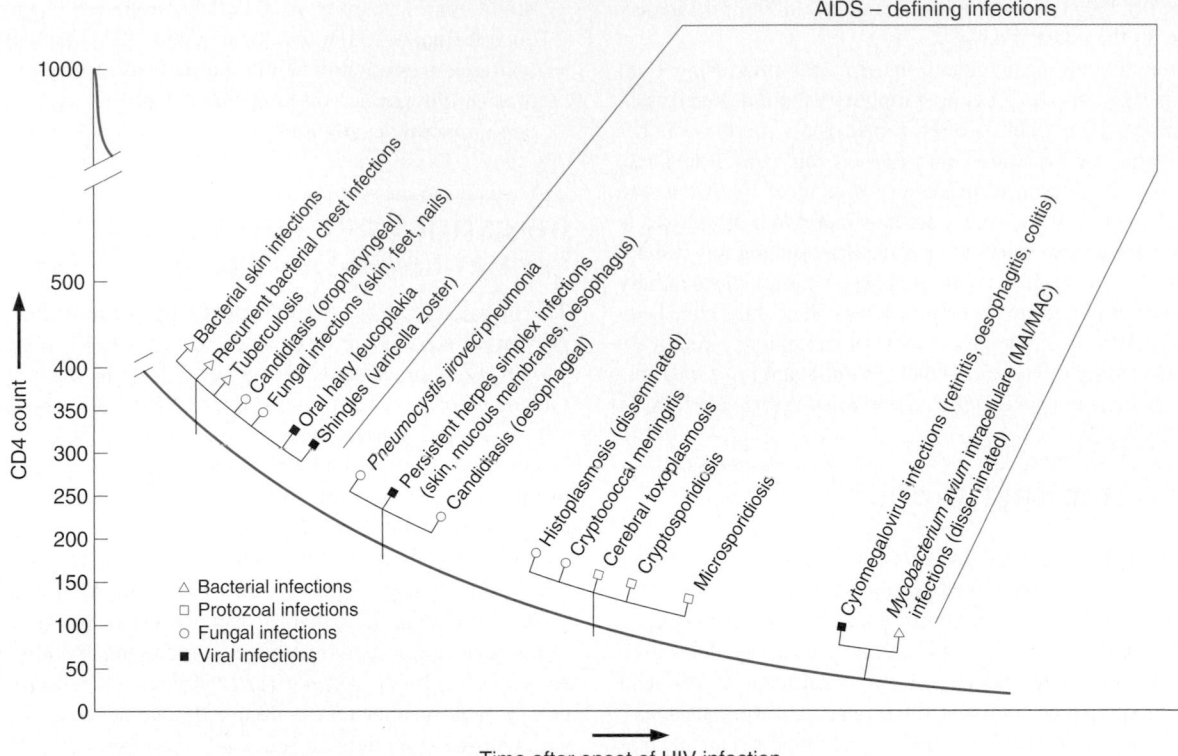

Fig. 42.3 Opportunistic complications of human immunodeficiency virus (HIV) infection and the CD4 count ranges at which they commonly occur.

Resistance testing

Certain mutations in the HIV virus confer resistance to certain antiretrovirals. Due to the implications of transmitted (primary) resistance, it is recommended that all patients have a genotypic HIV resistance test performed soon after diagnosis; this will ensure that appropriate initial therapy is selected. Further resistance tests should be performed at any subsequent virological failure to direct therapy choice.

Tropism testing

Viruses may enter the CD4 cell using the CCR5 co-receptor, the CXCR4 co-receptor or both co-receptors. Those that just use one co-receptor are known as CCR5-tropic or CXCR4-tropic viruses; those that can use both receptor types are called dual-tropic. Where a mixture of virus populations is present, the term mixed-tropic is used. Different methods of determining tropism are currently under evaluation. The tests must be performed in real time because viral tropism changes as the disease progresses. If CCR5 inhibitors are to be used, it is essential to determine that the virus is CCR5 tropic; that is, that there is no significant use of the CXCR4 receptor.

Drug treatment

The drug treatment of HIV disease can be classified as antiretroviral therapy, the management of opportunistic infections or malignancies, the management of 'non-HIV-related' comorbidities and

symptom control. For the first decade of the epidemic, most of the available drugs and therapeutic strategies were aimed at treating or preventing opportunistic complications and alleviating HIV-related symptoms. Since the advent of effective combination antiretroviral therapy (cART) the main aim is to suppress the HIV viral load, restore immune function and reduce the potential consequences of comorbidities. Unfortunately some opportunistic infections are still seen, as well as malignancies, often because of late diagnosis and because patients are from populations which are disengaged from care. Management of comorbidities is becoming much more important because the majority of people with HIV are living to an older age.

The speed at which new antiretroviral agents are developed means that there is often a lack of comprehensive data on drug interactions, side effects, etc. Thus, the ability to apply general pharmacological and pharmacokinetic principles, together with common sense, is required.

The treatment of many of the opportunistic complications of HIV comprises an induction phase of high-dose therapy, followed by maintenance and/or secondary prophylaxis using lower doses. This is due to the high rate of relapse or progression after a first episode of diseases such as *P. jiroveci* pneumonia, cerebral toxoplasmosis, systemic cryptococcosis and CMV retinitis. Where a cost-effective agent with an acceptable risk/benefit ratio exists, primary prophylaxis may be offered to individuals who are deemed to be at high risk of development of a particular opportunistic infection, for example, PCP prophylaxis. Discontinuation of prophylaxis, both primary and secondary, is possible in individuals who demonstrate immunological restoration on cART.

Paradoxically, this immunological restoration may result in apparent clinical deterioration with opportunistic infections during the first few weeks after initiation of highly active antiretroviral therapy. This is known as immune reconstitution inflammatory syndrome and usually occurs in those with a low baseline CD4 count.

The goals of therapy in people living with HIV are to:
- improve the quality and duration of life,
- prevent deterioration of immune function and/or restore immune status,
- treat and/or prevent opportunistic infections,
- relieve symptoms.

Antiretroviral therapy

Antiretroviral therapy is one of the fastest evolving areas of medicine. The specific details of treatment will therefore continue to change as new drugs emerge, although it is likely that the following general principles will remain:
- A combination of three antiretroviral agents, selected on the basis of treatment history and resistance tests, should usually be prescribed to increase efficacy and reduce the development of drug-resistant virus.
- Treatment strategies should be adopted that sequence drug combinations, being mindful of potential cross-resistance and future therapy options.
- Given the crucial importance of a high level of adherence to these therapies, the regimen adopted for a particular individual should, wherever possible, be tailored to suit his or her daily lifestyle.

Many organisations, such as the British HIV Association (BHIVA), the European AIDS Clinical Society, the International AIDS Society and the WHO, produce regularly updated guidelines on the use of antiretroviral therapy. These guidelines include the most up-to-date considerations of:
- when to start therapy;
- what to start with;
- how to monitor, including use of therapeutic drug monitoring (TDM) and resistance testing;
- when to switch therapy;
- what therapy to switch to;
- treating individuals who have been highly exposed to multiple agents;
- managing individuals with significant comorbidities, for example, tuberculosis (TB) or hepatitis B/C.

Most studies that evaluate triple combinations of antiretrovirals have been designed with so-called surrogate marker endpoints, measuring the effect on laboratory parameters such as CD4 count and HIV viral load. These trials are generally smaller and shorter in duration than clinical endpoint studies that are powered to measure the impact on survival and disease progression. Hammer et al. (1997) undertook the first large clinical endpoint trial that demonstrated the superiority of a triple combination over dual therapy. Following the results of this trial, the standard approach, where treatment is indicated, has been to use a combination of at least three agents. The reduction

in morbidity and mortality associated with triple therapy has been confirmed in routine clinical practice, as well as in other trials (e.g. Palella et al., 1998; Smit et al., 2006). Subsequent clinical trials have largely been for licensing purposes and/or have served to refine therapeutic choices rather than to change the paradigm of treatment. The concept of intermittent rather than continuous therapy was evaluated in the SMART study but shown to be linked with an increased risk of comorbidities not previously thought to be associated with HIV (such as cardiovascular disease, hepatic failure and renal failure), as well as HIV disease progression (El-Sadr et al., 2006).

There are studies which have evaluated novel strategies, such as monotherapy/dual-therapy approaches to reduce drug exposure and cost. The current BHIVA guidelines (BHIVA, 2015) advise triple therapy in those initiating cART and advise against boosted protease inhibitor (PI) monotherapy because of lower rates of virological efficacy (Delfraissy et al., 2008). Specific dual therapy can be used (darunavir [boosted with ritonavir] plus raltegravir) if there is a need to avoid certain nucleoside/nucleotide reverse transcriptase inhibitors (NRTIs), but with specific CD4 and viral load boundaries. Switching those patients who have achieved virological suppression because of toxicity, interactions or personal preference usually ensures patient adherence and subsequent maintenance on triple therapy. However, there are dual-therapy strategies should drug toxicities become problematic with a boosted PI plus lamivudine as the recommended alternative to triple therapy.

When to start therapy

Current UK guidelines (BHIVA, 2015) recommend starting antiretrovirals in all patients living with HIV regardless of their CD4 count. This is a change from previous guidelines, which recommended starting therapy when the CD4 count declined to ≤350 cells/mm³. This change was based on a large global study (INSIGHT START Study Group, 2015) which showed the risk of development of AIDS, serious non-AIDS events or death (combined as the primary endpoint) after 3 years was reduced by 57% in those who started at a higher CD4 count compared with patients who waited until their CD4 declined to ≤350 cells/mm³. In the UK, current funding is lagging behind guideline advice; therefore, patients are offered treatment with a CD4 ≤350 cells/mm³, hepatitis B/C co-infection and specific conditions (e.g. HIV-associated nephropathy, malignancy, pregnancy) and treatment as prevention. Treatment as prevention is the use of ARVs to suppress viral load to undetectable levels, to reduce the likelihood of onward transmission. This has been demonstrated to be highly effective in a number of large randomised control trials (Cohen et al., 2011; Rodger et al., 2014).

Choosing and monitoring therapy

The majority of individuals are currently commenced on a combination of two NRTIs and a third agent: either a boosted PI, an integrase inhibitor (INI) or a non-nucleoside reverse transcriptase inhibitor (NNRTI). The term 'boosted PI' refers to a combination of one PI combined with a low dosage (usually 100–200 mg once or twice daily) of ritonavir, another PI. The ritonavir does not directly add to the antiretroviral activity of the regimen; it is used purely as a pharmacokinetic enhancer of the other PI, by increasing the maximum plasma concentration, C_{max}, due to inhibition of cytochrome P450 enzymes and P-glycoprotein in the gut wall and/or extending the half-life ($t_{\frac{1}{2}}$) by inhibition of hepatic cytochrome P450 enzymes. Triple NRTI therapy is no longer recommended because it is associated with unacceptable rates of virological failure.

The aim of initial therapy is to achieve viral load suppression in the plasma to levels less than the detection limits of available assays (50 copies/mL). Such virological suppression is almost invariably accompanied by an elevation in CD4 count and clinical evidence of immune reconstitution. Whilst sustained suppression over many years is usually possible, viral rebound may occur and is often accompanied by the development of resistance to one or more agents in the combination. Upon confirmed virological failure, a resistance test is performed which will help to identify to which agents the virus may have adapted and the extent to which any such resistance mutations may confer cross-resistance to other available drugs. A second-line regimen is then constructed, wherever possible, utilising a new class of drug to which the individual has not previously been exposed. Upon virological failure of subsequent regimens, the available therapeutic options become increasingly complex, but with the availability of more agents targeting different parts of the virus life cycle, virological suppression is still usually possible and should remain the goal of treatment.

General prescribing guidelines for antiretrovirals are presented in Box 42.1, whereas details of common side effects and interactions of the currently available agents are summarised in Table 42.1.

The routine use of TDM is not recommended, but blood levels of PIs and NNRTIs should be measured in selected patients, for example, where there is liver impairment, suspected non-adherence, in pregnancy and children, or where there are concerns regarding potentially interacting drugs.

HIV mutates readily, and resistance to some antiretrovirals develops rapidly in the face of suboptimal treatment, for example, monotherapy or subtherapeutic blood levels. A high level of adherence to treatment is crucial to the sustained, successful outcome of antiretroviral regimens. In view of this, patients should be advised to take cART as close as possible to the same time every day and ideally within 2 hours of the agreed time each day. If they forget a dose, it should be taken as soon as they remember and then return to the original schedule. There are variations in the genetic barrier to resistance of different antiretrovirals. Many are fragile in terms of development of drug resistance in that a single point mutation will confer drug resistance, which can cross the drug class (NRTIs, NNRTIs and some INIs). cART with boosted PIs (particularly darunavir) and dolutegravir (INI) allow more latitude because it takes a number of mutations to reduce their efficacy and as such will be more appropriate for patients who struggle with adherence or who have historical drug resistance.

There has been significant progress over the years in reducing some of the physical burden of therapy, through the development of combination tablets and the use of strategies such as ritonavir boosting to reduce dietary restrictions and dosing frequency.

> **Box 42.1** General prescribing and monitoring information for antiretroviral agents
>
> - The Liverpool University HIV Drug interaction website is an invaluable tool and should be consulted, and other clinicians managing people living with HIV should be informed of this resource (http://www.hiv-druginteractions.org).
> - The Summary of Product Characteristics, current British National Formulary and national guidelines should be consulted when managing the treatment of an HIV-positive patient.
> - Adverse events should be reported. With greater exposure and long-term use, it is likely that more adverse events will be recognised. Some of these may be class effects associated with particular groups of antiretrovirals and should therefore be monitored even in new agents within a class. Examples include dyslipidaemia and diabetes mellitus with PIs, mitochondrial myopathy and lipoatrophy with NRTIs, and rash with NNRTIs.
> - There are limited data on the safety of many antiretroviral drugs when taken during pregnancy and their long-term effects on babies/children. Updated safety information from the Antiretroviral Pregnancy Register is published twice yearly. Caution should therefore be exercised with all agents. Treatment of women who are planning conception or who are pregnant must be discussed with the relevant experts and guidelines consulted (BHIVA, 2014). All pregnant women who are treated with antiretrovirals should be reported prospectively to the Antiretroviral Pregnancy Register.

Adherence aids such as pillboxes, medication record cards and alarms (e.g. on mobile phone) can also help to support adherence. However, practical issues are not the only barriers to adherence, and the individual's health beliefs and motivation, particularly around HIV and antiretroviral therapy, should also be addressed before treatment is commenced, because these are likely to have a significant impact on outcome (Horne et al., 2004). Although there is little evidence to demonstrate what the optimal interventions to improve adherence are, multidisciplinary and multiagency approaches appear to be most useful (Poppa et al., 2004).

Treatment interruptions

For many reasons, including toxicity, cost and adherence, patients and clinicians have been interested in considering 'drug holidays' or treatment interruptions. However, this strategy is no longer recommended in routine practice (El-Sadr et al., 2006). It is now recognised that there are dangers associated with this approach because of CD4 decline, disease progression, mortality related to comorbidities, for example, cardiovascular disease, and viral load rebound associated with increased transmission risk and a seroconversion-like syndrome. Further, because different anti-HIV medications have different half-lives, there may be a risk of functional monotherapy, particularly with NNRTIs, and the development of resistance if combinations are stopped abruptly in an unplanned fashion.

Post-exposure prophylaxis

Post-exposure prophylaxis (PEP) involves the use of antiretroviral drugs to prevent infection with HIV after possible

Table 42.1 Commonly used antiretroviral drugs: adult dosing information and general prescribing points

Drug and formulation	Dosage	Side effects	Main interactions/caution
NRTIs			
abacavir (ABC) 300 mg tablets 300 mg/15 mL oral solution Ziagen	300 mg twice a day/600 mg once a day	Nausea, vomiting, diarrhoea Rash (without systemic symptoms) Fatigue, fever, headache HSR: in clinical studies and post-marketing surveillance ~6–8% of patients developed this usually within the first 6 weeks (but may occur anytime) with symptoms indicating multi-organ system involvement – fever with or without a rash (maculopapular or urticarial), respiratory symptoms, gastro-intestinal symptoms, malaise, fever, myalgia, elevated LFTs; symptoms worsen with continued therapy and resolve on stopping; once suspected, the patient must not be rechallenged – a second reaction can be life threatening. **The risk of HSR is high in patients who test positive for the HLAB*5701 allele; therefore, it should not be used in these patients** **Take with or without food**	Caution with drugs inhibiting or metabolised by alcohol dehydrogenase or UDP transferase (i.e. disulfiram, chlorpromazine, isoniazid, chloral hydrate, alcohol, retinoids) Caution with potent enzyme inducers of UDP transferase (e.g. rifampcin, phenobarbitone, phenytoin) – may reduce levels of abacavir Monitor for evidence of withdrawal if given with methadone Abacavir and ribavirin share the same phosphorylation pathway and may compete for phosphorylation which could lead to a reduction in intracellular phosphorylated metabolite of ribavirin and reduced sustained virological response to hepatitis C treatment
emtricitabine (FTC) 200 mg capsule 10 mg/mL oral solution 200 mg capsule = 240 mg solution Emtriva	200 mg once a day Adjust dose in renal impairment CrCl < 50 mL/min	Headache, nausea and vomiting, diarrhoea, ↑ creatine kinase Insomnia, dizziness, neutropenia and anaemia, ↑ amylase, rash, ↑ LFTs Skin hyperpigmentation has been reported **Take with or without food**	Do not give concurrently with other cytidine analogues like lamivudine In patients co-infected with hepatitis B, discontinuation of emtricitabine may result in a rebound hepatitis – monitor LFTs and markers of HBV replication
lamivudine (3TC) 150 mg tablets 300 mg tablets 150 mg/15 mL oral solution Epivir	150 mg twice a day/300 mg once a day Adjust dose in renal impairment CrCl < 50 mL/min	Headache, insomnia, nausea and vomiting, gastro-intestinal disorders, cough and nasal symptoms, neutropenia and anaemia (in combination with zidovudine), ↑ amylase, rash, alopecia, arthralgia **Take with or without food**	Avoid high-dose co-trimoxazole (trimethoprim increases lamivudine levels by 40%, dosage adjustment needed in renal impairment) In patients co-infected with hepatitis B, discontinuation of lamivudine may result in a rebound hepatitis – monitor LFTs and markers of HBV replication
zidovudine (AZT) 100 mg and 250 mg capsules Syrup 50 mg/5 mL Retrovir	250 mg twice a day/200 mg three times a day (up to 250 mg four times a day) Adjust dose in renal impairment CrCl ≤ 10 mL/min	Anaemia, neutropenia, leucopenia, myalgia, nausea and vomiting, anorexia, rash, headache, insomnia, nail and skin pigmentation **Take with or without food**	↑ Risk of myelotoxicity with ganciclovir, high-dose co-trimoxazole, pyrimethamine, dapsone, flucytosine, vinblastine, doxorubicin, interferon-α Caution with potentially nephrotoxic drugs – pentamidine, amphotericin, aminoglycosides, ribavirin Monitor if receiving phenytoin (reports of changes in phenytoin levels) Do not use with ribavirin (increased risk of anaemia) Clarithromycin reduces the absorption of zidovudine (give 2 h apart) Reports of lactic acidosis and mitochondrial toxicity

Continued

Table 42.1 Commonly used antiretroviral drugs: adult dosing information and general prescribing points—cont'd

Drug and formulation	Dosage	Side effects	Main interactions/caution
NTRTIs			
tenofovir disoproxil (TDF) 245 mg (tenofovir disoproxil fumarate 300 mg) Viread	245 mg once a day Adjust dose in renal impairment CrCl <50 mL/min **Take with or after food**	Gastro-intestinal upset (diarrhoea, flatulence, nausea and vomiting), renal impairment, hypophosphatemia, proximal tubulopathy (including Fanconi syndrome) have been reported, decrease in bone mineral density	Monitoring renal function recommended before starting and 2–4 weeks of treatment, at 3 months, and thereafter every 3–6 months; more frequent monitoring required in patients with renal impairment Avoid giving with potentially nephrotoxic drugs (e.g. pentamidine, amphotericin, aminoglycosides) Avoid concomitant use of cidofovir which is secreted by the same renal pathway as tenofovir In patients co-infected with hepatitis B, discontinuation of tenofovir disoproxil may result in a rebound hepatitis – monitor LFTs and markers of HBV replication
tenofovir alafenamide (TAF) **Available only in combination products** F/TAF 200 mg/10 mg emtricitabine 200 mg/tenofovir alafenamide 10 mg Descovy 200 mg/10 mg F/TAF 200 mg/25 mg emtricitabine 200 mg/tenofovir alafenamide 25 mg Descovy 200 mg/25 mg R/F/TAF 25 mg/200 mg/25 mg rilpivirine/emtricitabine/tenofovir alafenamide Odefsey emtricitabine 200 mg, elvitegravir 150 mg/cobicistat 150 mg/tenofovir alafenamide 10 mg Genvoya	F/TAF 200 mg/10 mg recommended with boosted PIs (e.g. atazanavir/ritonavir or darunavir/ritonavir or Kaletra) F/TAF 200 mg/25 mg recommended with unboosted third agents (e.g. dolutegravir, raltegravir, rilpivirine, efavirenz, nevirapine) **F/TAF can be taken with or without food** **E/C/F/TAF should be taken with or after food** **R/F/TAF must be taken with a meal (390 kcal)** TAF is not recommended if eGFR < 30 mL/min	Better safety profile on bone and kidneys relative to tenofovir disoproxil fumarate	In patients co-infected with hepatitis B, discontinuation of TAF may result in a rebound hepatitis – monitor LFT and markers of HBV replication
NNRTIs[a]			
etravirine (ETR) 100 mg 200 mg Tablets Intelence	200 mg twice a day or 400 mg once a day Take with or after food The 100 mg tablets may be dispersed in water	Skin rash, diarrhoea, nausea, headache	Significantly reduces plasma concentrations of dolutegravir Can only be used with dolutegravir when co-administered with atazanavir/ritonavir, darunavir/ritonavir or lopinavir/ritonavir Clarithromycin levels reduced, but concentration of its active metabolite increased (which has reduced activity against Mycobacterium avium complex, so alternatives e.g. azithromycin, are recommended)

Drug	Dose/administration	Side effects	Interactions
efavirenz (EFV) 200 mg capsules 600 mg tablets efavirenz oral solution 30 mg/mL 600 mg tablet or capsule = 720 mg in 24 mL oral solution Sustiva	600 mg once a day Take at bedtime to minimise CNS side effects **Take on an empty stomach to minimise the risk of CNS side effects**	Skin rash, CNS effects (e.g. dizziness, light-headedness, insomnia, abnormal dreaming) – generally resolves after the first 2–4 weeks Depression Psychiatric adverse reactions	Reduces levels of anticonvulsants carbamazepine, phenobarbital, phenytoin Rifampicin decreases levels of etravirine Rifabutin decreases levels of etravirine and increases levels of rifabutin Reduces levels of antiarrhythmics Increases levels of warfarin Reduces levels of tacrolimus and ciclosporin Reduces the effect of hormonal contraceptives Do not give with terfenadine, astemizole, cisapride, triazolam, midazolam Efavirenz is an inducer of CYP3A4 and an inhibitor of other cytochrome P450 isoenzymes With clarithromycin ↑ risk of rash and 39% ↓ in clarithromycin concentration, whereas 34% ↑ in concentration of active metabolite of clarithromycin; therefore, use alternatives (e.g. azithromycin) Potential for increase or decrease in levels of phenytoin, phenobarbitone, carbamazepine, methadone – monitor for signs of withdrawal With rifampicin, 26% ↓ in efavirenz concentration; therefore, increase dosage of efavirenz to 800 mg once a day With rifabutin, decrease in rifabutin concentration – increase rifabutin dose by 50% Reduces levels of tacrolimus and ciclosporin Reduces the effect of hormonal contraceptives
rilpivirine (RPV) 25 mg tablets Edurant	25 mg once a day **Must be taken with a meal (390 kcal)**	Skin rash, headache, dizziness, insomnia, depression, abdominal pain Causes mild decrease in creatinine clearance	Antacids (aluminium, magnesium, calcium) should be taken 2 h before or 4 h after rilpivirine Do not use with proton pump inhibitors (loss of therapeutic effect of rilpivirine); can use with H₂ antagonists if dosed once a day and given 12 h before or 4 h after rilpivirine
nevirapine (NVP) 200 mg tablets 400 mg prolonged-release tablets Suspension 10 mg/mL Viramune	200 mg once a day for 2 weeks (lead-in period to lessen the frequency of rash), then 200 mg twice a day or 400 mg prolonged release once a day Note: Dose escalation should not occur if rash observed during the lead-in period, until rash resolves Adjust dose in renal impairment CrCl < 20 mL/min **With or without food**	Skin rash (skin reactions including Stevens–Johnson syndrome and toxic epidermal necrolysis have been reported – discontinue immediately if severe or accompanied by constitutional symptoms [fever, blistering, oral lesions]), nausea, headache and abnormal LFTs **Patients should be intensively monitored during the first 18 weeks to disclose the potential appearance of severe skin or hepatic reactions** Do not initiate nevirapine in female adults if CD4 > 250 cells/mm³ and in male adults if CD4 count > 400 cells/mm³ and detectable HIV viral load because of the risk of serious and life-threatening hepatotoxicity	Not recommended with rifampicin; with rifabutin, monitor for toxicity – some patients may experience large increases in rifabutin levels because of high interpatient variability Nevirapine is a hepatic enzyme inducer; careful monitoring of the effectiveness of other drugs that are metabolised by the cytochrome P450 enzyme system is recommended when taken in combination Methadone levels may be reduced With warfarin has the potential to ↑ or ↓ coagulation time Reduces the effect of hormonal contraceptives

Continued

Table 42.1 Commonly used antiretroviral drugs: adult dosing information and general prescribing points—cont'd

Drug and formulation	Dosage	Side effects	Main interactions/caution
PIs[b]			
atazanavir (ATV) 150 mg capsules 200 mg capsules Reyataz	300 mg once a day + ritonavir 100 mg once a day **Take with or after food**	Nausea, vomiting, headache, diarrhoea, rash, scleral icterus and jaundice, fatigue Asymptomatic QTc prolongation Nephrolithiasis	Do not give with rifampicin; with rifabutin, reduce dosage by 75% (if rifabutin dosage is 300 mg once a day, then reduce it to 150 mg three times a week) Do not give with terfenadine, astemizole, pimozide, ergot derivatives, cisapride, quinidine, bepridil, quetiapine, alfuzosin Caution with amiodarone, lidocaine (↑ levels of these drugs) Caution with drugs known to induce PR prolongation on ECG Not recommended with simvastatin or lovastatin (↑ risk of myopathy including rhabdomyolysis); caution with atorvastatin Caution with sildenafil (↑ in sildenafil levels) With warfarin, monitor anticoagulation parameters Not recommended with apixaban, dabigatran and rivaroxaban (increase in concentration of anticoagulant) With diltiazem, ↓ initial dose of diltiazem by 50% and titrate; caution with verapamil (↑ verapamil levels) Levels of ketoconazole and itraconazole, ciclosporin, tacrolimus may be ↑ With tenofovir ↓ in atazanavir levels; must be used boosted (i.e. atazanavir 300 mg once a day with ritonavir 100 mg once a day) With efavirenz ↓ in atazanavir levels; use 400 mg atazanavir boosted with ritonavir 100 mg once a day Not recommended with nevirapine (↓ atazanavir levels) With antacids or products containing buffers, administer atazanavir + ritonavir 2 h before or 1 h after the buffered product (atazanavir levels reduced because of ↑ gastric pH) Do not give with proton pump inhibitors (e.g. with omeprazole 76% decrease in atazanavir levels due to increase in gastric pH); caution with H₂ receptor antagonists; give atazanavir 2 h before or 10 h after ranitidine (which should be dosed as 300 mg once a day)
fosamprenavir (FPV) 700 mg tablets 50 mg/mL suspension Telzir	fosamprenavir 700 mg twice a day + ritonavir 100 mg twice a day **Take with or after food**	Nausea, vomiting, diarrhoea, headache, dizziness, rash Contains sulfonamide moiety – caution in sulfonamide allergy	Do not give with rifampicin; with rifabutin, reduce dosage by 75% (if rifabutin dosage is 300 mg once a day, then reduce it to 150 mg three times a week) Do not give with terfenadine, astemizole, pimozide, ergot derivatives, cisapride, quinidine, bepridil, quetiapine, alfuzosin, lidocaine Caution with amiodarone and other antiarrhythmics (darunavir ↑ levels of these) Not recommended with simvastatin or lovastatin (↑ risk of myopathy including rhabdomyolysis); caution with atorvastatin Caution with sildenafil (↑ in sildenafil levels) With warfarin, monitor anticoagulation parameters Not recommended with apixaban, dabigatran and rivaroxaban (increase in concentration of anticoagulant) Levels of ketoconazole and itraconazole, ciclosporin closporin, tacrolimus may be ↑

Drug	Dose	Side effects	Interactions
darunavir (DRV) 800 mg 600 mg Tablet 100 mg/mL suspension Prezista	darunavir 800 mg once a day + ritonavir 100 mg once a day darunavir 600 mg twice a day + ritonavir 100 mg twice a day (in patients with drug resistance) **Take with or after food**	Rash, nausea, vomiting, headache, dizziness, insomnia Contains sulfonamide moiety – caution in sulfonamide allergy	Do not give with rifampicin; with rifabutin, reduce dosage by 75% (if rifabutin dosage is 300 mg once a day, then reduce it to 150 mg three times a week) Do not give with terfenadine, astemizole, pimozide, ergot derivatives, cisapride, quinidine, bepridil, quetiapine, alfuzosin Caution with amiodarone, lidocaine (↑ levels of these drugs) Not recommended with simvastatin or lovastatin (↑ risk of myopathy including rhabdomyolysis); use lowest dose of atorvastatin Caution with sildenafil, dose of sildenafil should not exceed 25 mg in 48 h Levels of ketoconazole and itraconazole, ciclosporin, tacrolimus may be ↑ With warfarin, monitor anticoagulation parameters Not recommended with apixaban, dabigatran and rivaroxaban (increase in concentration of anticoagulant) Do not give with ticagrelor (increased levels of ticagrelor)
lopinavir/ritonavir (LPV/RTV) 200 mg/50 mg Tablets Liquid lopinavir 400 mg/ritonavir 100 mg in 5 mL Kaletra	2 tablets twice a day/4 tablets once a day/5 mL twice a day **Take with or after food**	Nausea, vomiting, diarrhoea; increase in LFTs, triglycerides and cholesterol	Do not give with rifampicin; with rifabutin, reduce dosage by 75% (if rifabutin dosage is 300 mg once a day, then reduce it to 150 mg three times a week) Do not give with terfenadine, astemizole, midazolam, triazolam, pimozide, ergot derivatives, flecainide, propafenone, cisapride Not recommended with simvastatin or lovastatin (↑ risk of myopathy including rhabdomyolysis); caution with atorvastatin Caution with sildenafil, dose of sildenafil should not exceed 25 mg in 48 h With warfarin, monitor anticoagulation parameters Not recommended with apixaban, dabigatran and rivaroxaban (increase in concentration of anticoagulant) Levels of calcium channel blocking agents may be ↑ Levels of ketoconazole and itraconazole, ciclosporin, tacrolimus may be ↑ Dexamethasone, phenobarbitone, phenytoin, carbamazepine may ↓ lopinavir levels With methadone, methadone levels may be ↓ With clarithromycin, consider ↓ dose of clarithromycin if renal or hepatic impairment Because it contains ritonavir there is the risk of Cushing's syndrome with potent corticosteroids metabolised by cytochrome P450 pathways (e.g. triamcinolone, fluticasone, budesonide) and subsequent risk of iatrogenic adrenal suppression when corticosteroid is discontinued

Continued

Table 42.1 Commonly used antiretroviral drugs: adult dosing information and general prescribing points—cont'd

Drug and formulation	Dosage	Side effects	Main interactions/caution
ritonavir (RTV) 100 mg tablets Solution 400 mg/5 mL Norvir	**Used as a pharmacokinetic enhancer** at a dosage of 100 mg once a day when taken in combination with atazanavir 300 mg once a day or darunavir 800 mg once a day 100 mg twice a day when taken with darunavir 600 mg twice a day **Take with or after food**	Nausea and vomiting, diarrhoea, asthenia, taste perversion, circumoral (around the mouth) and peripheral paraesthesia, fatigue and vasodilatation	Do not give with rifampicin and rifabutin Do not give with terfenadine, astemizole, cisapride, some sedatives (alprazolam, clorazepate, diazepam, flurazepam, triazolam, midazolam, zolpidem), some analgesics (piroxicam, dextropropoxyphene [contained in co-proxamol], pethidine), some antiarrhythmics (flecainide, amiodarone, quinidine, propafenone), clozapine, pimozide, bupropion, meperidine, ergot derivatives Caution with sildenafil, dose of sildenafil should not exceed 25 mg in 48 h Levels of ketoconazole and itraconazole, ciclosporin, tacrolimus may be ↑ With methadone or morphine, ↑ in methadone or morphine dose may be needed Do not give the oral solution with metronidazole (oral solution contains 40% alcohol), avoid with the capsules (12% alcohol) With theophylline, ↑ dose of theophylline may be required With warfarin, monitor anticoagulation parameters With clarithromycin, adjust dose of clarithromycin if renal impairment Not recommended with apixaban, dabigatran and rivaroxaban (increase in concentration of anticoagulant) Not recommended with salmeterol Risk of Cushing's syndrome with potent corticosteroids metabolised by cytochrome P450 pathways (e.g. triamcinolone, fluticasone, budesonide) and subsequent risk of iatrogenic adrenal suppression when corticosteroid is discontinued
Other pharmacokinetic enhancers			
cobicistat (COBI) 150 mg Tablet Tybost	150 mg once a day In combination with atazanavir 300 mg once a day or darunavir 800 mg once a day **Take with or after food**	Nausea, diarrhoea, fatigue	Do not give with rifampicin; with rifabutin, reduce dosage by 75% (if rifabutin dosage is 300 mg once a day, then reduce it to 150 mg three times a week) Do not give with amiodarone, quinidine, carbamazepine, phenobarbitone, phenytoin, ergot derivatives, cisapride, pimozide, midazolam, triazolam, lovastatin, simvastatin, alfuzosin, St. John's wort Not recommended with salmeterol, rivaroxaban With warfarin and dabigatran, monitor anticoagulation parameters Caution with sildenafil, dose of sildenafil should not exceed 25 mg in 48 h

			Reduces eGFR due to inhibition of tubular secretion of creatinine Contains azo colouring agent sunset yellow which may cause allergic reactions Risk of adrenal suppression and Cushing's syndrome with corticosteroids metabolised by cytochrome P450 pathways (e.g. fluticasone, budesonide) Reduces the effect of hormonal contraceptives Concentration of immunosuppressants (e.g. ciclosporin and tacrolimus) may be increased Do not use with the herbal remedy St. John's wort Risk of Cushing's syndrome with potent corticosteroids metabolised by P450 pathways (e.g. triamcinolone, fluticasone, budesonide) and subsequent risk of iatrogenic adrenal suppression when corticosteroid is discontinued
Entry inhibitor			
enfuvirtide injection (T-20) 90 mg/mL Fuzeon	90 mg twice a day by subcutaneous injection (upper arm, anterior thigh or abdomen) Alternate sites Use immediately after reconstitution; if not used immediately, store in the fridge (2–8 °C) for a maximum of 24 h and protect from light	Injection-site reactions (discomfort/pain at the injection site, induration, erythema, nodules and cysts, pruritus), diarrhoea, nausea, peripheral neuropathy	No clinically significant interactions expected with products metabolised by cytochrome P450 enzymes
maraviroc (MVC) 150 mg tablets 300 mg tablets Celcentri	Confirm that virus is CCR5 tropic before starting maraviroc 300 mg twice a day Reduce dosage to 150 mg once a day if CrCl < 80 mL/min and on a potent CYP3A4 inhibitor With efavirenz and rifampicin, increase dosage to 600 mg twice a day **Take with or without food**	Rash, abdominal pain, flatulence, nausea, depression, insomnia Delayed HSRs Cases of syncope caused by postural hypotension; caution in patients with severe renal impairment and in patients who have risk factors for or history of postural hypotension	With potent CYP3A inhibitors (e.g. cobicistat, rifabutin + PI, clarithromycin, itraconazole, ketoconazole), other PIs reduce dosage to 150 mg twice a day Not recommended with fosamprenavir/ritonavir Not recommended with St. John's wort
Integrase inhibitors			
raltegravir (RAL) 400 mg tablets Isentress	400 mg twice a day **Take with or without food**	Dizziness, headache, nausea and vomiting, insomnia, abnormal dreams, depression	Rifampicin reduces levels of raltegravir; if co-administration is unavoidable, double the dose of raltegravir Aluminium and magnesium hydroxide antacids reduce raltegravir levels – give 6 h apart

Continued

Table 42.1 Commonly used antiretroviral drugs: adult dosing information and general prescribing points—cont'd

Drug and formulation	Dosage	Side effects	Main interactions/caution
dolutegravir (DTG) 50 mg tablets Tivicay	50 mg once a day **Take with or without food**	Headache, nausea and diarrhoea, rash, ↑ creatinine kinase, insomnia, abnormal dreams, depression 10–14% decrease in creatinine clearance	Efavirenz, etravirine, nevirapine and rifampicin decrease dolutegravir levels – increase dolutegravir dosage to 50 mg twice a day Magnesium, aluminium, calcium, iron and multivitamins should be taken 2 h after or 6 h before dolutegravir Metformin levels increase (area under the curve increased by 79% with dolutegravir 50 mg once a day) – adjust metformin dose when starting and stopping dolutegravir
elvitegravir (EVG) 85 mg tablets 150 mg tablets Vitekta	85 mg once a day (in combination with atazanavir 300 mg once a day/ritonavir 100 mg once a day or lopinavir 400 mg/ritonavir 100 mg twice a day) 150 mg once a day (in combination with darunavir 600 mg twice a day + ritonavir 100 mg twice a day or fosamprenavir 700 mg twice a day + ritonavir 100 mg twice a day) **Take with or without food**	Diarrhoea, nausea, headache, rash, fatigue	Do not give with rifampicin; with rifabutin, reduce dosage by 75% (if rifabutin dosage is 300 mg once a day, then reduce it to 150 mg three times a week) Do not give with carbamazepine, phenobarbitone, phenytoin, St. John's wort Magnesium- and aluminium-containing antacids and multivitamins should be separated 4 h apart from elvitegravir With warfarin, monitor anticoagulation parameters

This information is not exhaustive – refer to the Summary of Product characteristics for further information. For combination products, see the individual drugs.
aNon-nucleoside reverse transcriptase inhibitors (NNRTIs) have a long half-life. Patients should be warned that if they discontinue them for whatever reason they should do so in consultation with their clinic which may recommend continuing the other drugs, e.g. the nucleotide analogue reverse transcriptase inhibitor (NRTI), for 2 weeks, or switching the NNRTI to a p'otease inhibitor (PI) for 2 weeks to prevent drug resistance. Do not use the herbal remedy St. John's wort.
bProtease inhibitors (PIs) reports of new or exacerbated diabetes mellitus and hyperglycaemia. There are reports of lipodystrophy with PIs. There are reports of increased bleeding in patients with haemophilia with PIs. Do not use the herbal remedy St. John's wort with PIs. PIs reduce the effect of hormonal contraceptives.
CNS, Central nervous system; CrCL, creatinine clearance; ECG, electrocardiogram; eGFR, estimate of glomerular filtration rate; HBV, hepatitis B virus; HSR, hypersensitivity reaction; LFT, liver function test; PI, protease inhibitor; UDP, uridine diphosphate.

exposure, which may be recommended after occupational injuries (Department of Health, 2008) or sexual exposure (Cresswell et al., 2016). Whilst PEP is a largely unproven and unlicensed indication for the drugs used, it is supported by animal model data and case–control studies. Where recommended in guidelines, PEP is usually commenced as a 3- to 5-day starter regimen of two NRTIs and an INI (tenofovir disoproxil fumarate, emtricitabine and raltegravir), followed by an ongoing course for a total of 4 weeks post-exposure. It is believed this will reduce the likelihood of infection by at least 80%. The decision to prescribe or take PEP must reflect a careful risk–benefit evaluation.

Pre-exposure prophylaxis

Pre-exposure prophylaxis (PrEP) uses one or two antiretroviral drugs (tenofovir disoproxil fumarate +/− emtricitabine) to prevent acquisition of HIV in high-risk populations. Many studies (Grant et al., 2010; McCormack et al., 2015) have shown a reduction in those at risk of acquiring HIV; those with less efficacious results are generally attributable to lower levels of adherence. The PROUD study (Dolling et al., 2016) found that PrEP conferred higher protection than in placebo-controlled trials, reducing HIV incidence by 86% in a population with sevenfold higher HIV incidence than expected. Although available in many countries, PrEP is not currently funded by the National Health Service.

Women with HIV

In addition to the general points covered elsewhere in this chapter, there are specific issues for women with HIV. These include:
- Cervical screening should be carried out at least annually, to check for gynaecological manifestations of HIV because cervical intraepithelial neoplasia/cervical cancer has a higher incidence in women living with HIV.
- Drug interactions between antiretrovirals and some oral contraceptives and contraceptive implants are important and should be discussed with women.
- Guidelines are available from the Faculty of Sexual and Reproductive Healthcare Clinical Guidance (http://www.fsrh.org) on drugs that reduce contraceptive efficacy and from the University of Liverpool HIV drug interactions website (http://www.hiv-druginteractions.org).
- All ritonavir boosted PIs and the NNRTIs nevirapine and efavirenz may reduce the efficacy of hormonal contraception by enzyme induction.
- There is a potential reduction in efficacy of the progesterone-only subdermal implant etonogestrel (Nexplanon). The long-acting injectable progesterones, depot medroxyprogesterone acetate (DMPA; Depo-Provera) and depot norethisterone enanthate (NET-EN; Noristerat), are not affected and can be used.
- There are no interactions with the intrauterine device (IUD) (copper coil) or the levonorgestrel-releasing intrauterine system (Mirena).
- The NRTIs etravirine, rilpivirine, raltegravir, dolutegravir and maraviroc do not have clinically significant interactions with hormonal contraceptives.

- A barrier method of contraception should also be recommended in addition to hormonal contraception, to prevent transmission of HIV and other sexually transmitted infections.
- Because women living with HIV are living longer, menopause and hormone replacement therapy (HRT) will become more of a prominent issue. There is currently a lack of data; therefore, potential drug interactions between HRT and ARVs need to be considered.

Mother-to-child transmission. The introduction of routine antenatal testing in the UK for HIV has made mother-to-child transmission a rare occurrence. Guidelines set out the management of HIV infection in pregnant women and the prevention of mother-to-child transmission (de Ruiter et al., 2014). In general, intervention reflects a risk–benefit evaluation between the efficacy of reducing transmission and the potential harmful effects to both mother and fetus.

The BHIVA pregnancy guidelines (2014) identify that women who require ART for their own health should commence treatment as soon as possible. Women who need ART solely to reduce transmission should start two NRTIs and a boosted PI by week 24 of pregnancy. Consideration should be given to starting ART at the beginning of the second trimester (viral load >30,000 copies/mL) or even earlier (viral load >100,000 copies/mL). Zidovudine monotherapy can be used in women planning a caesarean section who have a baseline viral load less than 10,000 copies/mL and a CD4 count greater than 350 cells/mm^3. However, because the BHIVA (2015) guidelines for the treatment of HIV-1$^+$ adults with antiretroviral therapy recommend starting ART at any CD4 count once they are ready to commit to taking therapy, this is likely to change.

Decisions regarding type of birth should be made after review of plasma viral loads at 36 weeks. Vaginal delivery is recommended if the plasma viral load is less than 50 copies/mL. A pre-labour caesarian section is recommended if plasma viral load is greater than 400 copies/mL. This should also be considered if plasma viral load is between 50 and 399, taking into account the decline of the HIV viral load trajectory time of ART, adherence issues, obstetric factors and the woman's views.

Infant post-exposure prophylaxis. Four weeks of zidovudine monotherapy is recommended if the maternal viral load is less than 50 copies/mL at 36 weeks' gestation and thereafter before delivery. Triple-drug therapy is recommended for all other circumstances. All infants should be exclusively formula fed from birth. Where a mother who is receiving effective ART and has repeated undetectable viral load chooses to breastfeed, this should be exclusive (except during the weaning period) and should be completed by the end of 6 months. This is because foods and fluids introduced to the gut of mixed-fed babies damage the bowel and may facilitate the entry into the body tissues of the HIV present in these mothers' breast milk. Maternal ART should be closely monitored up to 1 week after breastfeeding has ended.

Ethnicity

It is now recognised that ethnicity, as well as gender, can affect drug handling and response to treatment. This is due, in part, to epidemiological differences in gene expression. For example, reduced activity of cytochrome P450 2B6, one of the key enzymes involved in the metabolism of the NNRTI efavirenz, appears to be more common amongst African than Caucasian individuals. These drugs, therefore, have a significantly longer plasma half-life in those affected, which may impact on efficacy, toxicity and treatment interruptions. The prevalence of the HLA*B5701 gene, associated with abacavir hypersensitivity, also varies in different ethnic groups, although the clinical implications of this have yet to be fully researched.

As pharmacogenomics becomes more widely incorporated into clinical trials and routine patient care, it is hoped that a greater understanding will be gained of differences in response to treatment, enabling treatment strategies to be individualised and optimised.

Nucleoside and nucleotide analogue reverse transcriptase inhibitors

NRTIs must be phosphorylated within host cells to be activated. The active form resembles the host nucleotides and is used in reverse transcriptase chain elongation. This false substrate terminates the chain and viral replication ceases.

The NRTIs commonly used are:
- abacavir (ABC; Ziagen),
- emtricitabine (FTC; Emtriva),
- lamivudine (3TC; Epivir),
- tenofovir disoproxil fumarate (TDF; Viread).

Combination formulations of NRTIs are also available:
- abacavir + lamivudine (Kivexa),
- tenofovir disoproxil fumarate + emtricitabine (Truvada).

Older NRTIs are rarely used, but patients may have been exposed to these in the past. These include:
- didanosine (ddI; Videx),
- stavudine (d4T; Zerit),
- zalcitabine (ddC; Hivid),
- zidovudine (AZT; Retrovir),
- zidovudine + lamivudine (Combivir),
- zidovudine + lamivudine + abacavir (Trizivir).

There are two mechanisms by which resistance to NRTIs can occur. The first involves mutations (e.g. M184V, K65R, Q151M) which occur at or near the drug-binding site of the reverse transcriptase gene conferring drug resistance. The second, known as pyrophosphorolysis, is when the chain-terminating residue is removed, enabling viral replication to resume.

Non-nucleoside reverse transcriptase inhibitors

NNRTIs inhibit the reverse transcriptase enzyme by binding to its active site. They do not require prior phosphorylation and can act on cell-free virions, as well as infected cells. The NNRTIs available include:
- efavirenz (EFV; Sustiva),
- etravirine (ETR; Intelence),
- nevirapine (NVP; Viramune),
- rilpivirine (RPV; Edurant),
- Delavirdine (DLV; Rescriptor) is no longer available, but patients may have been exposed to this in the past.

Resistance to NNRTIs occurs rapidly in incompletely suppressive regimens, and it is therefore essential that they are prescribed with at least two NRTIs or a combination of NRTIs and PIs. Cross-resistance between nevirapine and efavirenz is high. Second-generation NNRTIs, like etravirine and rilpivirine, are active against some viruses resistant to nevirapine and efavirenz.

The NNRTIs have much longer plasma half-lives than PIs and NRTIs, so when stopping an NNRTI-containing combination, consideration should be given to either continuing the other agents for a period (e.g. 2 weeks after cessation of the NNRTI) or switching to a boosted PI before discontinuation.

Protease inhibitors

PIs bind to the active site of the HIV-1 protease enzyme, preventing the maturation of the newly produced virions so that they remain non-infectious. Commonly used PIs include:
- atazanavir (ATV; Reyataz),
- darunavir (DRV; Prezista),
- low-dose ritonavir (RTV; Norvir) as a booster (1100 mg) together with other PIs.

Less commonly used PIs include:
- fosamprenavir (FPV; Telzir),
- lopinavir co-formulated with ritonavir (LPV/RTV; Kaletra),
- saquinavir (SQV; Invirase).

Other PIs are no longer available, but patients may have been exposed to them in the past. These include:
- indinavir (IDV; Crixivan),
- nelfinavir (NFV; Viracept),
- tipranavir (TPV; Aptivus).

Second-generation PIs, like darunavir, are effective against many viruses resistant to the earlier PIs. Darunavir is used in first-line PI therapy as a once-daily boosted regimen (800 mg with 100 mg ritonavir); for patients with significant PI resistance, a higher dosage of 600 mg twice daily, boosted with ritonavir 100 mg twice a day is used. An alternative booster to ritonavir is cobicistat, which has no activity against HIV but is used as a booster at a dose of 150 mg once a day. Cobicistat is co-formulated with some PIs (e.g. darunavir [Rezolsta] and atazanavir [Evotaz]) and with an INI (e.g. elvitegravir [Genvoya and Stribild]).

Integrase inhibitors

INIs bind to the integrase enzyme, thus blocking the integration of viral DNA into host DNA. Raltegravir and elvitegravir have a lower genetic barrier to resistance than dolutegravir. In general, INIs must be used within a fully suppressive regimen to minimise the risk of drug resistance. INIs include:
- dolutegravir (DTG; Tivicay),
- raltegravir (RAL; Isentress),
- dolutegravir co-formulated with abacavir + lamivudine (Triumeq),
- elvitegravir (EVG) co-formulated with cobicistat + tenofovir disoproxil fumarate + emtricitabine (Stribild).

Entry inhibitors

There are currently two types of entry inhibitors: fusion inhibitors and CCR5 inhibitors. Fusion inhibitors block the structural rearrangement of HIV-1 gp41, and thus stop the fusion of the viral cell membrane with the target cell membrane, preventing viral

RNA from entering the cell. CCR5 inhibitors selectively bind to the human chemokine receptor CCR5, preventing CCR5-tropic HIV-1 from entering cells.

Enfuvirtide (T-20; Fuzeon), a fusion inhibitor, is administered subcutaneously and is primarily used in heavily treatment-experienced patients. The main side effect is injection-site reactions. The need to administer enfuvirtide by injection and the availability of other groups of drugs means it is rarely used.

Maraviroc (MVC; Celsentri), a CCR5 inhibitor, is indicated for use in patients with only CCR5-tropic virus, which is determined by a tropism test just before commencing treatment. It is usually used in patients with resistance to one or more other antiretroviral classes.

The different groups of drugs are co-formulated as fixed-dose combinations, and this helps reduce pill burden and may make them more acceptable to patients and also support adherence. Fixed-dose combinations are not suitable for patients with renal dysfunction who require dose modification. Currently available combinations include:

- Atripla (emtricitabine/tenofovir disoproxil fumarate/efavirenz),
- Eviplera (emtricitabine/tenofovir disoproxil fumarate/rilpivirine),
- Triumeq (abacavir/lamivudine/dolutegravir),
- Stribild (emtricitabine/tenofovir disoproxil fumarate/elvitegravir/cobicistat),
- Descovy (F/TAF; emtricitabine/tenofovir alafenamide),
- Odefsey (R/F/TAF; rilpivirine/emtricitabine/tenofovir alafenamide),
- Genvoya (E/C/F/TAF; elvitegravir/cobicistat/emtricitabine/tenofovir alafenamide),
- Rezolsta (darunavir/cobicistat),
- Evotaz (atazanavir/cobicistat),
- Dutrebis (raltegravir/lamivudine).

A combination not currently licensed in the UK is:

D/C/F/TAF: darunavir/cobicistat/emtricitabine/tenofovir alafenamide

As HIV drug patents expire many of these drugs are now available as cheaper generics with potential savings for drug budgets.

Toxicity of antiretroviral therapies

The availability and use of the different groups of antiretroviral drugs have led to decreased morbidity and mortality from HIV infection due to immune reconstitution and HIV viral suppression. However, there is also recognition of side effects and toxicities associated with ART. Patients who experience significant side effects may become non-adherent or refuse to take ART. A proactive approach to discussion with patients on how to recognise and manage side effects will support successful treatment (Max and Sherer, 2000). With all people living longer, managing ageing people living with HIV who have comorbidities requires healthcare staff to be mindful of the toxicities of ART and the impact of this on an ageing patient. Bone mineral density loss, kidney dysfunction, cardiovascular disease and neurocognitive disorders are more frequent in older patients, and these must be considered when choosing an HIV drug regimen.

Whilst there are many individual drug toxicities, there are also a number of class-specific or drug-related toxicities (Carr and Cooper, 2000).

Non-nucleoside reverse transcriptase inhibitors. Abacavir can cause a hypersensitivity reaction in 6–8% of individuals. The use of pharmacogenomics testing for HLA B*5701 status and only using abacavir in patients who are B*5701-negative has dramatically reduced the incidence of this hypersensitivity reaction (Mallal et al., 2008).

Tenofovir disoproxil fumarate can rarely cause proximal renal tubular dysfunction (Fanconi syndrome). This is characterised by glycosuria, hypophosphatemia and renal tubular acidosis from reduced bicarbonate reabsorption. Tenofovir disoproxil fumarate has also been shown to potentially reduce the estimate of glomerular filtration rate in certain patients. Caution should be observed when using tenofovir disoproxil fumarate in patients with pre-existing renal dysfunction or when patients are also taking other nephrotoxic drugs. Regular monitoring of renal function and checking for proteinuria is recommended for all patients receiving tenofovir disoproxil fumarate. Clinical observations have revealed a correlation between tenofovir disoproxil fumarate use and a reduction in bone mineral density, especially in young children and adolescents. This risk should be considered with patients who have risk factors for osteoporosis.

Tenofovir alafenamide is a novel targeted prodrug of tenofovir. It enters the cells, including HIV-infected cells, more efficiently and produces higher intracellular levels with lower doses. There are lower concentrations in the bloodstream and less exposure for the kidneys, bone and other organs and tissues. While the long-term clinical effects will be known by post-marketing surveillance, there is currently a strong suggestion that it is safer for the kidneys and bone than is tenofovir disoproxil fumarate.

The older NRTIs like didanosine, stavudine and zidovudine caused mitochondrial toxicity which may manifest as peripheral neuropathy, myopathy, lipoatrophy (fat loss particularly from the face, upper limbs and buttocks), hepatic steatosis, pancreatitis and lactic acidosis (McComsey and Lonergan, 2004). This is less common with the NRTIs which are now routinely prescribed (e.g. lamivudine, emtricitabine and tenofovir disoproxil fumarate).

Non-nucleoside reverse transcriptase inhibitors. NNRTIs cause rash, which frequently resolves early in therapy. In rare cases, Stevens–Johnson syndrome and toxic epidermal necrolysis have occurred. For patients who are taking nevirapine, the risk of rash is highest with a higher CD4 count; therefore, it should not be initiated if the CD4 count is greater than 250 cells/mm^3 for women and greater than 400 cells/mm^3 for men. There is also the small risk of serious hepatic toxicity. These factors make nevirapine a less favourable choice as first-line therapy.

Efavirenz is associated with central nervous system (CNS) toxicity including insomnia and mood problems. Caution is advised when considering initiating efavirenz in patients who have pre-existing depression or other mood problems. Patients with the homozygous G516T genotype of the enzyme CYP2B6 may metabolise it more slowly and have greater efavirenz exposure leading to higher rates of neuropsychiatric adverse reactions. The G516T genotype is more common in African individuals. Exposure to efavirenz is also significantly higher in women than in men and in non-Caucasian patients (Burger et al., 2006). This increased exposure is independent of body composition, use of hormonal contraceptives that may inhibit the metabolism of efavirenz and genetic polymorphism, and further research is needed to identify other factors.

Protease inhibitors. All PIs are associated with metabolic abnormalities including dyslipidaemias, insulin resistance, diabetes, lipodystrophy (abnormal fat distribution particularly affecting the abdomen and neck) and are well reported in HIV studies (Smith et al., 2010). These abnormalities may result in risk of coronary and/or cerebral vascular morbidity and mortality which is increased because people living with HIV have chronic inflammation as a result of long-term exposure to the virus.

Cardiovascular risk associations of antiretroviral agents

Observational studies have reported an increased risk of myocardial infarct with abacavir (Worm et al., 2010). A US Food and Drug Administration (FDA) meta-analysis of 26 randomised controlled trials, however, showed no association between abacavir and myocardial infarct (Ding et al., 2012). In spite of this conflicting evidence and uncertainty, in clinical practice abacavir tends to be avoided in patients with high cardiovascular risk (≥20% risk over 10 years).

Cumulative exposure to the older PIs, Kaletra and indinavir, has also been associated with increasing risk of myocardial infarct. A similar association exists for fosamprenavir (Worm et al., 2010). No association has been reported between the use of atazanavir/ritonavir and the risk of myocardial infarct, and there was insufficient evidence to include darunavir/ritonavir in the analysis (Monforte et al., 2013).

Maraviroc can cause postural hypotension. Therefore, care should be taken in patients with a history of postural hypotension, renal impairment or those taking antihypertensives. In view of limited data, maraviroc should be used with caution in patients with high cardiovascular risk.

Identifying and managing cardiovascular risk is an essential part of HIV care. National Institute for Health and Care Excellence (NICE) recommends the QRISK2 calculator for the English population (NICE, 2014). There is no HIV-specific cardiovascular risk calculator for those of non-white ethnicity.

One approach suggested is to use the QRISK2 equation with a correction for HIV status of 1.6 (Islam et al., 2012). As in the general population, encouraging patients to adopt modifiable lifestyles including smoking cessation, healthy diets and exercise will reduce the risk. Baseline cardiovascular risk assessment is recommended by BHIVA, and an annual cardiovascular risk assessment is recommended if the patient is a smoker, is diabetic and or has a body mass index greater than 30 and age greater than 40 years.

People who are living with HIV are at higher risk of non-alcoholic fatty liver disease. Factors associated with this include older age, overweight and waist circumference, lipodystrophy, insulin resistance, previous use of the older NRTIs (e.g. ddI, d4T, AZT) or PI use (e.g. indinavir and ritonavir) (Capeau et al., 2012).

Specific HIV drug choice

HIV treatment usually involves a three-drug regimen that contains either an NNRTI or a PI plus a 'backbone' consisting of two NRTIs. When selecting an NRTI backbone, factors such as efficacy, potential side effects and toxicities, patient preference and cost should be considered. Choosing the appropriate drug combination, monitoring patient parameters and switching to drugs that have a more favourable profile based on patient factors will ensure safety and success of treatment. Therefore, based on current evidence:

- Abacavir or abacavir-containing combinations (e.g. Kivexa) should be used with caution in patients whose baseline HIV viral load is greater than 100,000 copies/mL (except when used in combination with dolutegravir) because of the risk of virological failure. Abacavir-containing regimens should not be used in patients with high risk of CVD (≥20%) and if they are HLA*B5701-positive.
- Rilpivirine should not be used in patients whose baseline HIV viral load is greater than 100,000 copies/mL because of the risk of virological failure.
- Tenofovir disoproxil fumarate should not be used in patients with stage 3–5 chronic kidney disease (CKD) or they have a high risk of progression to CKD. It should also be avoided in individuals older than 40 years with osteoporosis, a history of fragility fracture or a FRAX score greater than 20% (major osteoporotic fracture).
- There is a theoretical advantage of using emtricitabine rather than lamivudine because of its longer half-life and in vitro potency. It is also incorporated more efficiently into proviral DNA.
- Zidovudine/lamivudine is considered for use only in specific circumstances (e.g. short-term use in pregnancy) because of its association with mitochondrial toxicity.

Third agent choice. As similar critical treatment outcomes are obtained, atazanavir/ritonavir, darunavir/ritonavir, raltegravir, dolutegravir, rilpivirine and elvitegravir/cobicistat are all recommended in current guidelines. Rilpivirine is recommended only in patients whose baseline HIV viral load is less than 100,000 copies/mL. In patients who tend to be non-adherent to their HIV medicines and have treatment interruptions, a PI/ritonavir-based regimen is recommended because it may be associated with less frequent selection for drug resistance (BHIVA, 2015).

The availability and use of effective ARV combinations has resulted in a decline in the incidence of severe HIV-associated cerebral disease. However, subtle forms of brain disorders, known as HIV-associated neurocognitive disorders, remain prevalent. Attempts have been made to correlate the pharmacokinetics of ARVs with respect to CNS penetration (clinical effectiveness penetration scores) and CSF HIV-RNA with change in neurocognitive function. However, results have been conflicting. Table 42.2 shows the clinical effectiveness scores that have been assigned to the various HIV drugs. Based on limited evidence, switching to ARV combinations that have higher clinical effectiveness penetration scores may be considered in clinical practice in patients who have neurocognitive disorders (Letendre et al., 2010).

Local guidance may recommend the rationale for choosing third agents which would include patient acceptability to a particular regimen. Interventions to address adherence and potential barriers should be embedded in the roles of all members of the HIV multidisciplinary team. This should include being mindful of patient's beliefs that may affect adherence, patient preferences with regard to practical barriers (e.g. pill burden and tablet size) and

Table 42.2 Central nervous system penetration effectiveness of human immunodeficiency virus drugs

HIV drug group	CNS penetration effectiveness scores[a]			
	4	3	2	1
NRTIs	Zidovudine	Abacavir, emtricitabine	Lamivudine	Tenofovir
NNRTIs	Nevirapine	Efavirenz	Etravirine	
PIs		Darunavir/ritonavir Fosamprenavir/ritonavir Lopinavir/ritonavir	Atazanavir/ritonavir	Saquinavir/ritonavir
Entry inhibitors		Maraviroc		Enfuvirtide
Integrase inhibitors		Raltegravir		

[a]A score of 4 is the highest and 1 is the lowest.
CNS, Central nervous system; HIV, human immunodeficiency virus; NNRTI, non-nucleoside reverse transcriptase inhibitor; NRTI, nucleotide analogue reverse transcriptase inhibitors; PI, protease inhibitor.
Adapted from Letendre et al., (2010).

the requirement to take some medicines with food which can be restrictive to those with busy lifestyles. Accommodating medicine taking into account a patient's individual lifestyle and use of appropriate adherence aids should be considered. This would include the use of multi-compartment compliance aids (e.g. Dossette boxes). Peer support, use of buddies and outreach services into the community can also augment strategies to support adherence.

HIV drug–drug interactions

Absorption

The absorption of some HIV drugs may be altered by the presence or absence of food. For example, rilpivirine needs 390 kcal for optimal absorption. Increase in pH by antacids (aluminium, magnesium hydroxide, calcium carbonate), H_2 antagonists or proton pump inhibitors can reduce some HIV drug levels (e.g. atazanavir and rilpivirine). Chelation caused by polyvalent ions like calcium, magnesium or iron can reduce levels of some HIV drugs (e.g. dolutegravir and elvitegravir). It is therefore important that patients who are prescribed these medicines understand how to manage these drug–drug interactions, for example, timing separation when taking multivitamins containing iron and magnesium (4 hours apart from dolutegravir) or completely avoiding proton pump inhibitors like omeprazole with rilpivirine.

Metabolism

Some HIV drugs, especially NNRTIs and PIs, are metabolised by the cytochrome P450 enzyme system. The enzyme responsible for the majority of drug metabolism is CYP3A4, although CYP2C19 and CYP2D6 are also common. Table 42.3 shows the HIV drugs that are major CYP450 enzyme inducers, inhibitor and substrates. Drugs may interact with the CYP450 enzymes through induction, inhibition or acting as a substrate. Some drugs act as inducers and inhibitors of different CYP450 enzymes. CYP450 enzymes are in the liver and in the small intestine. Ritonavir inhibits CYP3A4 in the liver and the intestine. This is one of the mechanisms that allows

Table 42.3 HIV drugs that are major CYP450 enzyme inducers, inhibitors and substrates

Type of action	CYP enzyme			
	1A2	2C19	2D6	3A4
Inducers	Ritonavir	Ritonavir Efavirenz		Nevirapine Efavirenz Etravirine Ritonavir
Inhibitors	Atazanavir	Etravirine	Ritonavir Cobicistat	Protease inhibitors Cobicistat
Substrates		Etravirine		Nevirapine Efavirenz Elvitegravir Etravirine Rilpivirine Maraviroc Protease inhibitors Cobicistat

it to act as a pharmacokinetic booster. Drugs that inhibit CYP450 enzymes decrease the metabolism of other drugs metabolised by the same enzyme. This can result in higher drug levels and an increase in the potential for drug toxicities. Inhibition usually occurs quickly.

Induction of CYP450 enzymes causes increased clearance of drugs metabolised by the same enzyme, with the maximum effect taking 1–2 weeks. Some drugs, like nevirapine, induce their own metabolism, and the starting dose (200 mg once a day for 2 weeks) is increased after this period (400 mg once a day). The herbal remedy St. John's wort is a strong inducer of CYP3A and will reduce levels of NNRTIs, PIs and cobicistat. Therefore, co-administration is not recommended.

The most important antiretroviral drugs to consider when evaluating drug–drug interactions are the pharmacoenhancers ritonavir and cobicistat. These agents can increase levels of many commonly used medicines including some statins, antidepressants, anticonvulsants, corticosteroids and cardiac drugs. One significant drug–drug interaction is between PIs and steroids metabolised by CYP3A enzymes (e.g. budesonide, fluticasone, methylprednisolone and triamcinolone). This interaction can result in adrenal insufficiency and iatrogenic Cushing's syndrome (Saberi et al., 2013). Despite well-documented case reports, patients continue to inadvertently receive these combinations. Therefore, HIV healthcare staff should obtain a complete medication history for any patient exhibiting signs and symptoms of Cushing's syndrome. Inhaled corticosteroids are used extensively in asthma and allergic rhinitis, and injectable corticosteroids in rheumatology and surgical patients.

Conducting a thorough medication history at each visit, including asking direct questions about prescribed medicines in other healthcare settings (e.g. by primary care doctors, other specialist hospital departments) and use of over-the-counter, herbal and recreational drugs is an important strategy in preventing significant drug–drug interactions which may result in virological failure or drug toxicity. Patients need to be counselled to explain that they are taking HIV medicines when in other healthcare settings to minimise this risk. Patient should also be advised to check drug–drug interactions before commencing new medicines.

Mycobacterium treatment results in complex drug–drug interactions. Rifampicin is a potent CYP3A4 inducer, although rifabutin has less effect. Therefore, rifabutin is the drug of choice in patients who require treatment for *M. tuberculosis* or *Mycobacterium avium* complex, to avoid significant reduction in HIV drug levels of, for example, nevirapine and the PIs. Rifampicin is also a strong inducer of the metabolising enzyme of the glucuronidation pathway UGT-1A1. Raltegravir is metabolised by UGT-1A1-mediated glucuronidation. Rifampicin will therefore reduce raltegravir levels, and co-administration is not recommended.

Tenofovir alafenamide (TAF) is a substrate for intestinal P-glycoprotein. Ritonavir and cobicistat both inhibit intestinal P-glycoprotein, thereby increasing tenofovir alafenamide exposure. For this reason a lower dose of tenofovir alafenamide (10 mg) is recommended when used with ritonavir- or cobicistat-boosted PIs. The standard dose of tenofovir alafenamide (25 mg) is recommended when administered with efavirenz, nevirapine, raltegravir, dolutegravir and maraviroc.

Excretion

Rilpivirine, dolutegravir and cobicistat inhibit renal transporters of creatinine, causing mild-to-moderate increase in serum creatinine and reduction in estimated creatinine clearance. Healthcare staff must correctly interpret these changes on initiating these drugs and differentiate this from clinically significant renal toxicities.

Tenofovir disoproxil fumarate undergoes active renal tubular secretion via organic anionic transporters in the renal proximal tubule cells, and this plays a role in the aetiology of nephrotoxicity. Tenofovir alafenamide is not a substrate for organic anionic transporters and is likely to be associated with reduced tenofovir levels in the proximal renal tubule cells.

The NRTIs in general tend to be renally cleared and require dose modification in renal impairment.

Hepatitis B co-infection

Hepatitis B virus (HBV) co-infection is less likely to be cleared spontaneously and more likely to become chronic in the HIV-positive population. It is likely to be associated with higher hepatitis B DNA levels and faster fibrosis progression rate, end-stage liver disease and hepatocellular carcinoma (Wilkins et al., 2013). People who are co-infected with HBV should be treated with tenofovir-, disoproxil-, fumarate-, and emtricitabine- or lamivudine-based cART, because these are effective against both HBV and HIV.

Response to hepatitis B vaccination is less with the standard dose; therefore, a higher dose (HBVAXPRO and Engerix B dose 40 micrograms, Fendrix 20 micrograms) is recommended (Geretti et al., 2015).

Hepatitis C co-infection

Hepatitis C virus (HCV) co-infection is cleared spontaneously in an estimated 10–25% of people, and chronic infection of HCV will develop in the majority. Patients with HCV/HIV co-infection have higher hepatitis C RNA levels and an accelerated liver fibrosis progression rate. It increases the risk of hepatocellular carcinoma, which tends to occur at a younger age and within a shorter period since infection. A global epidemic of acute hepatitis in HIV-infected MSM has been observed in the past decade. Transmission appears to be associated with high-risk traumatic sexual practices, presence of sexually transmitted infections and recreational drug use.

Early ART initiation is recommended to slow the fibrosis progression rate. The ART regimen should be selected to suit the planned hepatitis C treatment. Efficacy, side-effect profile and the duration of treatment have significantly improved since the introduction of HCV direct-acting antiviral agents, with sustained virological response rates of more than 90%. The choice of regimen and duration of HCV treatment are based on HCV genotype, HCV RNA, liver fibrosis stage, prior treatment history and drug–drug interaction (NICE, 2015).

Opportunistic infections

Treatment guidelines are produced by many different countries and may differ slightly; one example of UK guidelines are those produced by the BHIVA. Examples of guidelines available from BHIVA are for the management of opportunistic infections (Nelson et al., 2011), HIV-associated malignancies (Bower et al., 2014), hepatitis viruses (Wilkins et al., 2013) and TB (Pozniak et al., 2011). Such guidance should be consulted for further detailed information on the management of people living with HIV.

Fungal infections

Pneumocystis jirovecii pneumonia

P. jirovecii is an atypical fungus causing pneumonia in immuno-compromised individuals. It remains a major pathogen in those unaware of their HIV status, in people not seeking medical care for HIV and in those non-adherent to antiretroviral medication and/or prevention therapy (Miller and Huang, 2004; Morris and Gingo, 2015). It is thought to mainly cause clinical disease by exposure to an exogenous source, with likely transmission being via inhalation of airborne spores. In people living with HIV, PCP most commonly occurs in those with a CD4 T-cell count less than 200 cells/microlitre (or CD4 T-cell percentage <14%) (Nelson et al., 2011). Presentation is typically a gradual progression over several weeks, with principal symptoms being fatigue, fever, chills, sweats, non-productive cough and dyspnoea. Physical examination findings are non-specific and include fever, tachypnoea and tachycardia. Signs of pulmonary consolidation or changes in pulmonary signs are uncommon (Morris and Gingo, 2015; Nelson et al., 2011).

Presence of oxygen desaturation supports the diagnosis of PCP along with a typical chest radiographic appearance of bilateral interstitial shadowing; however, radiological imaging is not specific for PCP and can, in some cases, appear normal. Therefore, for a definitive diagnosis of PCP, this requires either an induced sputum for visualisation of the fungi (if routinely available) or bronchoscopic examination with bronchoalveolar lavage (BAL) (Morris and Gingo, 2015).

Treatment is instigated in patients with a proven diagnosis, or empirically where there is suspicion before confirmation (Table 42.4). Oxygen is essential for patients with compromised respiratory function. First-line therapy is high-dose trimethoprim-sulfamethoxazole (co-trimoxazole) for 21 days. In cases of co-trimoxazole intolerance, several alternative treatment choices are available.

Adjunctive corticosteroids should be given where PaO$_2$ <9.3 kPa or SpO$_2$ <92% to prevent further deterioration. Oral prednisolone is given at high doses for 21 days. Alternatively, intravenous methylprednisolone can be substituted if the patient is unable to take oral medication.

PCP can be prevented in people living with HIV by initiating ART, with the aim of restoring and preserving immunological function (Morris and Gingo, 2015). In patients with a CD4 T-cell count less than 200 cells/microlitre, CD4 T-cell percentage less than 14%, oral candidiasis or previous AIDS-defining illness, PCP prophylaxis should be started. First-line therapy is co-trimoxazole, which also provides prevention against toxoplasmosis; however, other regimens are available if this is contraindicated or not tolerated (see Table 42.4). Prophylaxis can be discontinued when CD4 T-cell count is sustained at greater than 200 cells/microlitre and suppression of HIV replication for more than 3 months on ART.

Oropharyngeal/oesophageal candidiasis

Candida species are common commensals in the general population, and candidiasis is a frequent manifestation of HIV infection, which may occur in early disease. It is usually characterised by white plaques on the oral mucosa, but may present as erythematous patches or as angular cheilitis. If swallowing is difficult (dysphagia) or painful (odynophagia), oesophageal involvement may be suspected. Oesophageal candidiasis without oral plaques is not common; therefore, any patient presenting with oesophageal symptoms without oral candidiasis should be considered for alternative diagnoses (Nelson et al., 2011). Diagnoses of oral and oesophageal candidiasis are made clinically because microbiological confirmation is likely to give a positive result in the absence of clinical disease. Cultures should be requested only in patients who are not responding to standard treatment (Nelson et al., 2011).

Treatment regimens are described in Table 42.5. Systemic azole antifungals are first-line therapy for oral and oesophageal candidiasis with higher doses and longer treatment courses generally used in oesophageal candidiasis. Topical treatment with nystatin is effective for oropharyngeal candidiasis; however, it is associated with a slower clearance of yeast from the mouth and a higher relapse rate. First-line azole therapy is fluconazole with other azoles or antifungal classes being reserved in cases of drug resistance. Routine prophylaxis is not recommended and is associated with the emergence of resistance (Nelson et al., 2011).

Cryptococcus neoformans

Cryptococcus is an encapsulated yeast present in the environment. People become exposed to the yeast after inhalation of fungal spores, although this rarely causes infection in immunocompetent individuals (Centers for Disease Control and Prevention, 2015). In patients with a compromised immune system, the yeast can localise to the lungs and cause infection. This can rapidly disseminate to the blood and develop into cryptococcal meningitis (Nelson et al., 2011).

Symptoms are dependent on site of infection. Meningitis is the most common presentation in people who are living with HIV. Symptoms include fever and headache, often without the characteristic symptoms of meningism such as photophobia and neck stiffness. Raised intracranial pressure may be associated with nausea, vomiting, confusion and coma. Other symptoms may be respiratory secondary to pulmonary disease or dermatological lesions resembling molluscum in skin disease.

The principal test is serum cryptococcal antigen which, if negative, generally excludes disseminated disease. In the presence of a positive result, all patients should have a lumbar puncture for CSF culture after cerebral imaging with computed tomography (CT) or magnetic resonance imaging (MRI). Manometry via lumbar puncture should be performed to exclude raised intracranial pressure. Blood cultures should also be performed and if positive for *Cryptococcus*, sensitivity testing may be performed if available (Nelson et al., 2011).

Treatment consists of an induction phase and a maintenance phase (Table 42.6). First-line treatment in the induction phase is intravenous liposomal formulation of amphotericin 4 mg/kg/day (once daily dosing) plus intravenous flucytosine 100 mg/kg/day (four times daily dosing). This is continued for at least 2 weeks or until CSF culture is negative for *Cryptococcus*. Liposomal amphotericin is the preferred formulation to reduce drug toxicity (Nelson et al., 2011).

Table 42.4 Treatment and prophylaxis of *Pneumocystis jirovecii* pneumonia

Drug	Dosage: route, frequency, duration	Common or significant side effects	Significant interactions	Monitoring	Comments
Atovaquone	**Treatment (mild to moderate):** 750 mg PO twice daily (with food) for 21 days Prophylaxis (unlicensed indication): 750 mg PO twice daily (with food)	Anaemia, neutropenia, hyponatraemia, insomnia, headache, nausea, diarrhoea, vomiting, elevated liver enzyme levels, hypersensitivity reactions including angioedema, bronchospasm and throat tightness, rash, pruritus, urticaria, fever	Drugs known to reduce atovaquone: rifampicin, rifabutin, metoclopramide, efavirenz, boosted protease inhibitors, tetracycline Drugs known to be increased by atovaquone: zidovudine	LFTs, renal function, FBC	Absorption improved by taking with food (especially high-fat food); reduced by diarrhoea
Clindamycin	**Treatment (severe):** 600 mg IV/PO four times daily or 900 mg IV/PO three times daily for 21 days (given with primaquine 15–30 mg PO once daily)	Clindamycin: abdominal pain, diarrhoea, pseudomembranous colitis, abnormal LFTs, nausea, vomiting, rash, urticaria, blood dyscrasias, dysgeusia (IV), thrombophlebitis (IV) Primaquine: nausea, vomiting, methaemoglobinaemia, haemolytic anaemia (especially in G6PD deficiency), bone marrow suppression	Neuromuscular blocking agents, erythromycin, neostigmine, pyridostigmine, oestrogens (risk of interaction is small)	LFTs, renal function, FBC, diarrhoea	Change in bowel habit should be investigated for *Clostridium difficile* Check G6PD status before use of primaquine
Co-trimoxazole (trimethoprim–sulfamethoxazole)	**Treatment: Moderate to severe:** 120 mg/kg/day IV/PO for 3 days, then reduced to 90 mg/kg/day for 18 days in three or four divided doses **Mild to moderate:** 1920 mg three times a day or 90 mg/kg/day in 3 divided doses for 21 days **Prophylaxis:** 480 mg (preferred) or 960 mg once daily or 960 mg three times a week	Hyperkalaemia, headache, nausea, diarrhoea, skin rash (rare: blood dyscrasias, drug fever, serious skin reactions, e.g. Stevens–Johnson syndrome and toxic epidermal necrolysis)	Ciclosporin (deterioration in renal function); rifampicin (can reduce plasma half-life of trimethoprim, although not thought to be significant); diuretics, in particular thiazide (increased risk of thrombocytopenia); pyrimethamine (risk of megaloblastic anaemia); warfarin (potentiates anticoagulant activity); phenytoin (prolongs phenytoin half-life); methotrexate (increases plasma levels of methotrexate); lamivudine (increases plasma levels of lamivudine in doses >960 mg); sulphonylureas (could potentiate hypoglycaemic effect)	LFTs, renal function, FBC, monitoring for rash	Caution in G6PD deficiency

Dapsone	**Treatment (mild to moderate):** 100 mg PO once daily (given with trimethoprim 20 mg/kg/day PO for 21 days **Prophylaxis:** 50–200 mg PO once daily (100 mg preferred)	Rash, photosensitivity, pruritus, haemolysis and methaemoglobinaemia are rare in dosages >100 mg daily or in individuals not G6PD deficient, 'dapsone syndrome' may occur 3–6 weeks after therapy, anorexia, headache, hepatitis, jaundice, abnormal LFTs, insomnia, nausea, psychosis, tachycardia and vomiting are infrequent	Probenecid, rifampicin	LFTs, FBC	Check G6PD status before use
Pentamidine	**Treatment:** 4 mg/kg IV once daily for 21 days **Prophylaxis:** 300 mg nebulised every 4 weeks	IV: leucopenia, thrombocytopenia, anaemia, azotaemia, hypoglycaemia, hyperglycaemia, hypocalcaemia, hypomagnesaemia, dizziness, hypotension, flushing, nausea, vomiting, taste disturbance, abnormal LFTs, rash, renal impairment, macroscopic haematuria; rare: pancreatitis, QT interval prolongation Nebulised: local respiratory reactions (including bronchospasm), taste disturbance, nausea	Foscarnet, drugs that prolong QT interval	Renal function, blood glucose, blood pressure, LFTs, FBC, blood urea nitrogen, calcium and magnesium, ECG for QT interval prolongation	Nebulised: pretreat with a bronchodilator and use an appropriate nebuliser

ECG, Electrocardiogram; FBC, full blood count; G6PD, glucose-6-phosphate dehydrogenase; IV, intravenous; LFT, liver function test; PO, oral.

Table 42.5 Treatment of oropharyngeal/oesophageal candidiasis

Drug	Dosage: route, frequency, duration	Common or significant side effects	Significant interactions	Monitoring	Comments
Azole antifungals					
Fluconazole	50–100 mg PO once daily for 7–14 days	Headache, abdominal pain, vomiting, diarrhoea, nausea, elevated LFTs, rash	Inducers and inhibitors of CYP3A4	LFTs	Duration of treatment will be less for oropharyngeal candidiasis Use with caution with medicines known to prolong QTc interval because some azole antifungals have been associated with prolongation of the QTc interval
Itraconazole	200 mg PO once daily for 7–14 days (or twice daily in fluconazole refractory candidiasis)	Headache, dyspnoea, abdominal pain, vomiting, nausea, diarrhoea, dysgeusia, elevated LFTs, rash, pyrexia	Inducers and inhibitors of CYP3A4	LFTs, FBC, renal function	Oral solution has higher bioavailability than capsule formulation
Voriconazole	Loading dose: IV: 6 mg/kg twice daily PO: 400 mg twice daily (if >40 kg) for 1 day Maintenance dosage: IV: 4 mg/kg twice daily PO: 200 mg twice daily (if >40 kg) for 7–14 days in total	Sinusitis, deranged FBC, peripheral oedema, hypoglycaemia, hypokalaemia, hyponatraemia, psychiatric disorders, headache, convulsion, syncope, tremor, hypertonia, paraesthesia, somnolence, dizziness, visual impairment, retinal haemorrhage, cardiac arrhythmias, hypotension, respiratory distress, diarrhoea, vomiting, abdominal pain, nausea, deranged LFTs, rash, alopecia, back pain, renal dysfunction, pyrexia	Inducers, inhibitors and substrates of CYP3A4, CYP2C19, CYP2C9	LFTS, FBC, renal function	Only for use in fluconazole resistance, where fluconazole has been shown to be ineffective or the patient is intolerant to fluconazole Use with caution with medicines known to prolong QTc interval because some azole antifungals have been associated with prolongation of the QTc interval
Posaconazole	Loading dose: 300 mg twice daily PO for 1 day Maintenance dosage: 300 mg once daily for 7–14 days in total	Neutropenia, anorexia, decreased appetite, hypokalaemia, hypomagnesaemia, paraesthesia, dizziness, somnolence, headache, dysgeusia, hypertension, nausea, vomiting, abdominal pain, diarrhoea, dyspepsia, dry mouth, flatulence, constipation, anorectal discomfort, deranged LFTs, rash, pruritus, pyrexia	Substrates of CYP3A4, rifabutin, efavirenz, fosamprenavir, phenytoin, digoxin, sulfonylureas	LFTs, FBC, renal function	Only for use in fluconazole resistance, where fluconazole has been shown to be ineffective or the patient is intolerant to fluconazole Use with caution with medicines known to prolong QTc interval because some azole antifungals have been associated with prolongation of the QTc interval
Echinocandins					
Anidulafungin	Loading dose: 200 mg once daily IV for 1 day Maintenance dose: 100 mg once daily IV for 7–14 days in total	Hypokalaemia, hyperglycaemia, convulsions, headache, hypo/hypertension, bronchospasm, dyspnoea, diarrhoea, nausea, vomiting, abnormal liver function, rash, pruritus, increased creatinine	Nil	LFTs, renal function, blood sugar	Only for use in fluconazole resistance, where fluconazole has been shown to be ineffective or the patient is intolerant to fluconazole

	Dosage	Side effects	Interactions	Monitoring	Notes
Caspofungin	Loading dose: 70 mg once daily IV for 1 day. Maintenance dosage: >80 kg: 70 mg once daily IV; <80 kg: 50 mg once daily IV for 7–14 days in total	Local injection-site reactions including phlebitis, reduced haemoglobin, reduced white cell count, hypokalaemia, headache, dyspnoea, nausea, diarrhoea, vomiting, elevated LFTs, rash, pruritus, erythema, hyperhidrosis, arthralgia, pyrexia, chills	Ciclosporin, tacrolimus, rifampicin	LFTs, renal function, FBC	Only for use in fluconazole resistance, where fluconazole has been shown to be ineffective or the patient is intolerant to fluconazole
Micafungin	150 mg once daily IV (if >40 kg) for 7–14 days	Leukopenia, neutropenia, anaemia, hypokalaemia, hypomagnesaemia, hypocalcaemia, headache, phlebitis, nausea, vomiting, diarrhoea, abdominal pain, elevated LFTs, rash, pyrexia, rigors	Itraconazole, sirolimus, nifedipine, amphotericin	FBC, renal function, magnesium, calcium, LFTs	Only for use in fluconazole resistance, where fluconazole has been shown to be ineffective or the patient is intolerant to fluconazole
Others					
Liposomal amphotericin	1–3 mg/kg once daily IV for 7–14 days	Hypokalaemia, hyponatraemia, hypocalcaemia, hypomagnesaemia, hyperglycaemia, headache, tachycardia, hypotension, vasodilation, flushing, dyspnoea, nausea, vomiting, abnormal LFTs, rash, back pain, renal impairment, rigors, pyrexia, chest pain	Nephrotoxic medication, drugs that may potentiate hypokalaemia, antineoplastic agents	Renal function, magnesium, LFTs, FBC	Only for use in fluconazole resistance, where fluconazole has been shown to be ineffective or the patient is intolerant to fluconazole

FBC, Full blood count; IV, intravenous; LFT, liver function test; PO, oral.

Table 42.7 Treatment and maintenance of toxoplasmosis

Drug	Dosage: route, frequency, duration	Common or significant side effects	Significant interactions	Monitoring	Comments
Treatment					
Sulfadiazine + pyrimethamine (+ calcium folinate)	Sulfadiazine: 1.5 g PO four times daily (≤60 kg) or 2 g PO four times daily (>60 kg) Pyrimethamine: 200 mg PO loading dose followed by 50 mg PO once daily (≤60 kg) or 75 mg PO once daily (>60 kg) Calcium folinate: 15 mg PO once daily for 6 weeks	Sulfadiazine: blood disorders, hypersensitivity reactions, hypoglycaemia, hypothyroidism, depression, psychosis, hallucinations, neurological reactions, tinnitus, cough, dyspnoea, GI symptoms, hepatitis, jaundice, purpura, rash, crystalluria Pyrimethamine: anaemia, leucopenia, thrombocytopenia, headache, giddiness, vomiting, nausea, diarrhoea, rash, abnormal skin pigmentation, fever	Sulfadiazine: thiopentone anaesthetics, warfarin, sulfphonylureas, clozapine, aspirin, ciclosporin, diuretics, methotrexate, oestrogen-containing oral contraceptives, probenecid Pyrimethamine: agents that depress folate metabolism, agents that cause myelosuppression, antacids, highly protein-bound drugs, methotrexate	LFTs, renal function, FBC	Ensure fluid intake of 2 L/day to reduce the risk of crystalluria Caution in G6PD deficiency Calcium folinate to counteract myelosuppressive effects of pyrimethamine
Clindamycin + pyrimethamine (+ calcium folinate)	Clindamycin: 600 mg PO/IV four times daily Pyrimethamine: 200 mg PO loading dose followed by 50 mg PO once daily (≤60 kg) or 75 mg PO once daily (>60 kg) Calcium folinate: 15 mg PO once daily for 6 weeks	Clindamycin: abdominal pain, diarrhoea, Pseudomembranous colitis, abnormal LFTs, nausea, vomiting, rash, urticaria, blood dyscrasias, dysgeusia (IV), thrombophlebitis (IV) Pyrimethamine: anaemia, leucopenia, thrombocytopenia, headache, giddiness, vomiting, nausea, diarrhoea, rash, abnormal skin pigmentation, fever	Clindamycin: neuromuscular blocking agents, erythromycin, neostigmine, pyridostigmine, oestrogens (risk of interaction is small) Pyrimethamine: agents that depress folate metabolism, agents that cause myelosuppression, antacids, highly protein-bound drugs, methotrexate	LFTs, renal function, FBC, diarrhoea	Change in bowel habit should be investigated for Clostridium difficile Caution in G6PD deficiency Calcium folinate to counteract myelosuppressive effects of pyrimethamine
Maintenance					
Sulfadiazine + pyrimethamine (+ calcium folinate)	Sulfadiazine: 500 mg PO four times daily (preferred) or 1 g twice daily (if reduced adherence is suspected) Pyrimethamine: 25 mg PO once daily Calcium folinate: 15 mg PO once daily continued until CD4 T-cell count >200 cells/microlitre for 6 months and suppression of HIV replication	Sulfadiazine: blood disorders, hypersensitivity reactions, hypoglycaemia, hypothyroidism, depression, psychosis, hallucinations, neurological reactions, tinnitus, cough, dyspnoea, GI symptoms, hepatitis, jaundice, purpura, rash, crystalluria Pyrimethamine: anaemia, leucopenia, thrombocytopenia, headache, giddiness, vomiting, nausea, diarrhoea, rash, abnormal skin pigmentation, fever	Sulfadiazine: thiopentone anaesthetics, warfarin, sulphonylureas, clozapine, aspirin, ciclosporin, diuretics, methotrexate, oestrogen-containing oral contraceptives, probenecid Pyrimethamine: agents that depress folate metabolism, agents that cause myelosuppression, antacids, highly protein-bound drugs, methotrexate	LFTs, renal function, FBC	Ensure fluid intake of 2 L/day to reduce the risk of crystalluria Caution in G6PD deficiency Calcium folinate to counteract myelosuppressive effects of pyrimethamine
Clindamycin + pyrimethamine (+ calcium folinate)	Clindamycin: 300 mg PO four times daily (preferred) or 600 mg three times daily (if reduced adherence is suspected) Pyrimethamine: 25 mg PO once daily Calcium folinate: 15 mg PO once daily continued until CD4 T-cell count >200 cells/microlitre for 6 months and suppression of HIV replication	Clindamycin: abdominal pain, diarrhoea, Pseudomembranous colitis, abnormal LFTs, nausea, vomiting, rash, urticaria, blood dyscrasias, dysgeusia (IV), thrombophlebitis (IV) Pyrimethamine: anaemia, leucopenia, thrombocytopenia, headache, giddiness, vomiting, nausea, diarrhoea, rash, abnormal skin pigmentation, fever	Clindamycin: neuromuscular blocking agents, erythromycin, neostigmine, pyridostigmine, oestrogens (risk of interaction is small) Pyrimethamine: agents that depress folate metabolism, agents that cause myelosuppression, antacids, highly protein-bound drugs, methotrexate	LFTs, renal function, FBC, diarrhoea	Change in bowel habit should be investigated for Clostridium difficile Caution in G6PD deficiency Calcium folinate to counteract myelosuppressive effects of pyrimethamine

FBC, Full blood count; G6PD, glucose-6-phosphate dehydrogenase; GI, gastro-intestinal; IV, intravenous; LFT, liver function test; PO, oral.

be considered in patients where there is evidence of raised intra-cranial pressure. Adjunctive anticonvulsants may be indicated if a patient presents with or develops seizures; however, there is no evidence to support routine prescribing (Nelson et al., 2011).

Cryptosporidiosis

Cryptosporidium is a protozoan parasite, which is ubiquitous in the environment. Transmission is via ingestion of cryptospo-ridium oocysts from contaminated water supplies, which leads to transmission of the parasite. Transmission may also occur during sexual intercourse, particularly via the faecal-oral route. Symptoms are profuse, non-bloody watery diarrhoea. This may be accompanied by nausea, abdominal cramps and pyrexia.

Diagnosis is via detection of cryptosporidium oocysts in a stool sample. Several samples may need to be checked because oocyst excretion can be intermittent, especially in less severe infections (Nelson et al., 2011).

Treatment options are described in Table 42.8. No specific treatments are available that target cryptosporidium. Optimal management is to restore immune function via initiation of ART. Several therapeutic options have been investigated for treatment; however, low study numbers and lack of promising results in immunocompromised individuals make ART the first choice of management. If treatment is considered worth using, nitazoxanide is the preferred agent; however, it should be rec-ognised that efficacy is limited in patients with compromised immune function. Patients should also be offered symptomatic and supportive therapy with fluid replacement, adequate hydra-tion and anti-motility agents.

Bacterial infections

Mycobacterium tuberculosis

In individuals who are living with HIV, *M. tuberculosis* (TB) is characterised by increased likelihood of reactivation of latent dis-ease, more rapid progression to clinical disease following acqui-sition, more frequent extrapulmonary manifestations of TB and more rapid progression of HIV disease if the individual is not receiving ART. The management of co-infection with TB and HIV requires specialist knowledge, and it is therefore mandatory to involve specialists in both HIV and respiratory and/or infec-tious diseases (Nelson et al., 2011).

Both clinical and radiographic presentation of TB may be atypical. Patients may have a normal chest radiograph and a

sputum-smear-negative result with positive culture. Definitive diagnosis is reliant on culture of the organism from biological specimens but may be complicated by atypical clinical features and reduced response to tuberculin testing. It is often necessary to initiate treatment empirically. Molecular diagnostics can rap-idly confirm if acid-fast bacilli from a body fluid smear test are not TB, which may avoid unnecessary treatment and infection-control measures. The increased incidence of multidrug-resistant TB and the emergence of extremely drug-resistant disease are a cause for concern and raise many infection-control issues. They also highlight the need for antibiotic therapy driven by bacterio-logical sensitivities (Nelson et al., 2011).

Recommendations for the treatment of *M. tuberculosis* are simi-lar to those in HIV-negative adults, and the appropriate guidelines should be consulted, for example, NICE (2016). The potential for drug–drug interactions and overlapping toxicities are greater in those receiving ART, and this should be considered when initiat-ing *M. tuberculosis* treatment (Table 42.9). Further information can be obtained from the University of Liverpool HIV drug inter-action website (http://www.hiv-druginteractions.org).

M. avium intracellulare/M. avium complex

M. avium intracellulare (MAI) or *M. avium* complex (MAC) are commonly found in the environment and are thought to enter individuals via the respiratory route and gastro-intestinal tract. With the increasing use of ART, the incidence of MAI/MAC has decreased significantly in people who are living with HIV because it typically occurs in severe immunosuppression with CD4 T-cell count less than 50 cells/microlitre. Infection usually presents as a systemic febrile illness with sweating, fatigue, abdominal pain, weight loss and diarrhoea. Lymphadenopathy, hepatosplenomeg-aly and/or splenomegaly may be present. Clinical presentation may vary with site of infection, for example, pulmonary MAI/MAC may present with respiratory symptoms (Temesgen, 2015). Diagnosis should be made based on culture of the organism from blood and sputum samples. In specific cases, it may be neces-sary for further investigations such as lung or lymph node tissue biopsy or bone marrow aspirate.

First-line treatment should be with a macrolide antibiotic (azithromycin is preferred secondary to less drug–drug interaction potential than other macrolide antibiotics), ethambutol and, ide-ally, rifabutin as a third agent. Treatment should be continued for at least 12 months and until individuals remain culture-negative, asymptomatic and have a sustained CD4 T-cell count greater than 100 cells/microlitre for at least 3 months (Nelson et al., 2011).

Table 42.8 Treatment of cryptosporidium

Drug	Dosage: route, frequency, duration	Common or significant side effects	Significant interactions	Monitoring	Comments
Nitazoxanide	500 mg orally twice daily for 3 days; course duration may be required for up to 12 weeks	Abdominal pain, diar-rhoea, nausea, vomit-ing, headache	Nil known	Full blood count, liver function tests, renal function	Take with food

Table 42.9 Drug–drug interactions between antiretroviral therapy and rifampicin/rifabutin

Antiretroviral	Rifampicin	Rifabutin
NRTIs/NTRTIs		
There are no interaction with any NRTIs/NTRTIs and rifamycins	Use standard doses	Use standard doses
NNRTIs		
Efavirenz	Efavirenz levels decreased: **Consider increasing efavirenz dosage to 800 mg once daily in patients >50 kg (may also consider TDM)**	Rifabutin levels decreased: **Increase daily dose of rifabutin by 50%**
Nevirapine	Nevirapine levels decreased: **Do not co-administer**	Rifabutin levels increased: **Use standard doses** **Caution: High intersubject variability means some patients may experience larger increases and may be at risk of rifabutin toxicity**
Etravirine	No data available: **Do not co-administer**	Limited data: **Use standard doses** **Caution: Etravirine and rifabutin levels both decreased**
Rilpivirine	Rilpivirine levels decreased: **Do not co-administer**	Rilpivirine levels decreased: **Increase rilpivirine dose by 100%**
Protease inhibitors		
Atazanavir/ritonavir	Atazanavir levels decreased: **Do not co-administer**	Rifabutin levels increased: **Reduce rifabutin dosage to 150 mg three times weekly (TDM advised because this dosage may be too low in some patients)**
Darunavir/ritonavir	Darunavir levels decreased: **Do not co-administer**	Rifabutin levels increased: **Reduce rifabutin dosage to 150 mg three times weekly (TDM advised because this dose may be too low in some patients)**
Fosamprenavir/ritonavir	Fosamprenavir levels decreased: **Do not co-administer**	Rifabutin levels increased: **Reduce rifabutin dosage to 150 mg three times weekly (TDM advised because this dose may be too low in some patients)**
Lopinavir/ritonavir	Lopinavir levels decreased: **Do not co-administer**	Rifabutin levels increased: **Reduce rifabutin dosage to 150 mg three times weekly (TDM advised because this dose may be too low in some patients)**
Saquinavir/ritonavir	Saquinavir levels decreased: **Do not co-administer**	Rifabutin levels increased: **Reduce rifabutin dosage to 150 mg three times weekly (TDM advised because this dose may be too low in some patients)**
Integrase inhibitors and entry inhibitors		
Dolutegravir	Dolutegravir levels decreased: **Increase dolutegravir dosage to 50 mg twice daily**	Use standard doses
Elvitegravir/cobicistat	Elvitegravir and cobicistat levels decreased: **Do not co-administer**	Elvitegravir and cobicistat levels decreased and rifabutin levels increased: **Use not recommended; however, no alternative; reduce rifabutin to 150 mg three times weekly**
Raltegravir	Raltegravir levels decreased: **Increase raltegravir dosage to 800 mg twice daily** **Caution: C_{min} still reduced at increased dosage**	Use standard doses

Table 42.9 Drug–drug interactions between antiretroviral therapy and rifampicin/rifabutin—cont'd

Antiretroviral	Rifampicin	Rifabutin
Maraviroc	Maraviroc levels decreased: **Increase maraviroc dosage to 600 mg twice daily**	Use standard doses
Enfuvirtide	Use standard doses	Use standard doses

TDM, Therapeutic drug monitoring.

In patients with a CD4 T-cell count less than 50 cells/microlitre, prophylaxis azithromycin 1250 mg once weekly should be considered. The addition of ART is considered essential to the management to restore a weakened immune function.

Viral infections

Herpes simplex and varicella zoster

The herpes viruses are a large family with three phases of infection: primary infection, latency and reactivation. Herpes simplex viruses 1 and 2 (HSV) and VZV are classified as α herpes viruses. VZV is usually transmitted via the respiratory route and causes both varicella (chickenpox) and zoster (shingles). HSV is transmitted via contact with infectious secretions and causes genital or orolabial ulcers. VZV cutaneous presents as localised, erythematous, maculopapular eruptions usually along a single dermatome, but may be multi-dermatomal. They then crust over a few days and typically last for 2–3 weeks. VZV eye disease causes visual loss, keratitis, anterior uveitis, severe post-herpetic neuralgia and necrotising retinopathy. Herpes zoster can disseminate and cause CNS disease and present with neurological disease.

Orolabial HSV is most commonly caused by HSV-1 and presents with sensory prodromal symptoms (usually a tingling), which typically precede development of vesicles that ulcerate and crust. Left untreated, they will usually resolve within 7–10 days. Genital HSV is caused by both HSV-1 and -2. Anogenital lesions develop and usually resolve untreated within 5–10 days; however, they may not resolve spontaneously and require treatment. Systemic HSV infection can result in pneumonia, hepatitis, oesophagitis and CNS disease.

VZV is usually diagnosed based on appearance of lesions, especially cutaneous disease. Swabs of infected lesions can also be checked for detection of expression viral antigens. CSF analysis can be performed; a positive result for VZV DNA supports the diagnosis of CNS disease. Swabs of infected lesions can be tested for identification of HSV-1 or -2, and in systemic disease appropriate samples should be obtained for analysis to identify HSV.

First-line treatment should be with aciclovir. Alternative treatment options which may be considered are valaciclovir and famciclovir. Oral aciclovir can be used for the treatment of local VZV (zoster), orolabial HSV and genital HSV if severe or recurrent disease. Systemic aciclovir is required for VZV (varicella), systemic VZV (zoster) and systemic HSV. Regular suppressive use of oral aciclovir at lower doses can be used in cases of recurrent disease (Nelson et al., 2011).

Cytomegalovirus

CMV is a member of the β-herpes viruses which infects greater than 50% of the human population. After infection the virus has the ability to establish lifelong, latent infection (Bronke et al., 2005). In individuals with advanced immunodeficiency, typically with a CD4 T-cell count less than 50 cells/microlitre, this can result in reactivation of the virus (viraemia) and clinical end-organ disease in a proportion of patients. Major sites of CMV disease are the retina (75%), gastro-intestinal tract, lung, liver and biliary tract, heart, adrenal glands and the nervous system (<1%) (Nelson et al., 2011).

Symptoms are dependent on the site of infection. Viral infection of the retina may be asymptomatic or present with floaters, scotomata, peripheral or central visual field defects and decreased visual acuity. In the gastro-intestinal tract symptoms are likely to be colitis, weight loss, anorexia, abdominal pain, diarrhoea, malaise and perforation. Oesophagitis presents with odynophagia, nausea and epigastric/retrosternal discomfort. Presentation in lung infection is similar to many other respiratory conditions: non-productive cough, exertional dyspnoea, fever and marked hypoxaemia. However, pneumonitis is uncommon. When the CNS is involved symptoms are dementia, ventriculoencephalitis, polyradiculomyelitis, lethargy, confusion and fever (Centers for Disease Control and Prevention, 2015).

CMV viraemia, as detected by polymerase chain reaction, may be positive in the absence of end-organ disease and, therefore, may be of negligible diagnostic use. If a positive result is obtained, evidence of end-organ disease should be considered depending on the patient's clinical symptoms.

For retina infections, diagnosis is usually based on clinical symptoms and visualisation of the retina. Endoscopy can reveal ulceration of the gut mucosa, and a biopsy can identify characteristic inclusions to aid diagnosis. Pneumonitis is hard to differentiate from CMV shedding in respiratory secretions. Therefore, BAL may reasonably exclude CMV pneumonia with a negative result; however, a positive result should be interpreted alongside clinical symptoms. Radiological imaging of the brain performed by MRI is a more sensitive test and, therefore, the preferred method over CT scanning. A lumbar puncture, if not contraindicated, can be performed for CSF examination to assess CNS infection.

Treatment of CMV is outlined in Table 42.10. For gastro-intestinal infection, treatment should be given with IV therapy because oral drugs may not be fully absorbed. Maintenance treatment is not recommended. However, for retinitis both induction and maintenance treatment should be given with either oral or IV therapy. A ganciclovir implant may be considered if systemic

Table 42.10 Treatment and maintenance of cytomegalovirus

Drug	Dosage: route, frequency, duration	Common or significant side effects	Significant interactions	Monitoring	Comments
Treatment					
Ganciclovir	5 mg/kg IV twice daily GI: 2–4 weeks Retinitis: 2–4 weeks Lung: 3 weeks	Sepsis, cellulitis, urinary tract infection, oral candidiasis, neutropenia, anaemia, thrombocytopenia, leucopenia, pancytopenia, appetite decreased, anorexia, depression, anxiety, confusion, abnormal thinking, headache, insomnia, dysgeusia, hypoaesthesia, paraesthesia, peripheral neuropathy, convulsions, dizziness, macular oedema, retinal detachment, vitreous floaters, eye pain, ear pain, dyspnoea, cough, diarrhoea, nausea, vomiting, abdominal pain, constipation, flatulence, dysphagia, dyspepsia, elevated LFTs, dermatitis, night sweats, pruritus, back pain, myalgia, arthralgia, muscle cramps, renal impairment, fatigue, pyrexia, rigors, pain, chest pain, malaise, asthenia, injection-site reactions, decreased weight	Imipenem-cilastin, probenecid, zidovudine, didanosine, mycophenolate, nephrotoxic drugs, bone marrow–suppressive agents	FBC, LFTs, renal function	Caution when handling; women of childbearing potential must be advised to use effective contraception during treatment; male patients should be advised to practise barrier contraception during and for at least 90 days following treatment
Valganciclovir	900 mg PO twice daily Retinitis: 2–4 weeks Lung: 3 weeks	See ganciclovir, similar potential side effects (except those associated with IV administration)	Imipenem-cilastin, probenecid, zidovudine, didanosine, mycophenolate, nephrotoxic drugs, bone marrow–suppressive agents	FBC, LFTs, renal function	Caution when handling; women of childbearing potential must be advised to use effective contraception during treatment; male patients should be advised to practise barrier contraception during and for at least 90 days following treatment
Foscarnet	90mg/kg IV twice daily GI: 2–4 weeks Lung: 3 weeks	Granulocytopenia, anaemia, leucopenia, thrombocytopenia, neutropenia, sepsis, decreased appetite, hypokalaemia, hypomagnesaemia, hypocalcaemia, hyperphosphataemia, hyponatraemia, hypophosphataemia, increased ALP, increased LDH, aggression, agitation, anxiety, confusional state, depression, nervousness, dizziness, headache, paraesthesia, abnormal coordination, convulsion, hypoaesthesia, involuntary muscle contractions, peripheral neuropathy, tremor, hypertension, hypotension, thrombophlebitis, diarrhoea, nausea, vomiting, abdominal pain, constipation, dyspepsia, pancreatitis, elevated LFTs, rash, pruritus, myalgia, renal impairment, genital discomfort and ulceration, asthenia, chills, fatigue, pyrexia, malaise, oedema	Nephrotoxic drugs, drugs that inhibit renal tubular secretion, IV pentamidine, ritonavir	Renal function, magnesium, bone profile, FBC, blood pressure, LFTs	Good hydration, prompt correction of electrolyte abnormalities and dose adjustment for renal function are vital Wash genital area after micturition to reduce risk of ulceration Reduce infusion rate if infusion-related side effects
Cidofovir	5 mg/kg IV once weekly Retinitis: 2 weeks Lung: 3 weeks	Renal impairment, neutropenia, ocular hypotony, iritis/uveitis, nausea, vomiting, alopecia, rash, asthenia, fever, chills, headache	Nephrotoxic drugs, drugs contraindicated with probenecid, tenofovir	Renal function (including urine protein), FBC	Must be co-administered with probenecid and IV fluids to minimise nephrotoxicity; caution with handling (potential carcinogen)

Maintenance

Ganciclovir	5 mg/kg IV once daily for 5 days of the week GI: no maintenance recommended Retinitis: continue until CD4 T-cell count >100 cells/microlitre and suppressed HIV viral load	Sepsis, cellulitis, urinary tract infection, oral candidiasis, neutropenia, anaemia, thrombocytopenia, leucopenia, pancytopenia, appetite decreased, anorexia, depression, anxiety, confusion, abnormal thinking, headache, insomnia, dysgeusia, hypoaesthesia, paraesthesia, peripheral neuropathy, convulsions, dizziness, macular oedema, retinal detachment, vitreous floaters, eye pain, ear pain, dyspnoea, cough, diarrhoea, nausea, vomiting, abdominal pain, constipation, flatulence, dysphagia, dyspepsia, elevated LFTs, dermatitis, night sweats, pruritus, back pain, myalgia, arthralgia, muscle cramps, renal impairment, fatigue, pyrexia, rigors, pain, chest pain, malaise, asthenia, injection-site reactions, decreased weight	Imipenem–cilastin, probenecid, zidovudine, didanosine, mycophenolate, nephrotoxic drugs, bone marrow–suppressive agents	FBC, LFTs, renal function	Caution when handling; women of childbearing potential must be advised to use effective contraception during treatment; male patients should be advised to practise barrier contraception during and for at least 90 days following treatment
Valganciclovir	900 mg PO once daily GI: no maintenance recommended Retinitis: continue until CD4 T-cell count >100 cells/microlitre and suppressed HIV viral load	See ganciclovir, similar potential side effects (except those associated with IV administration)	Imipenem–cilastin, probenecid, zidovudine, didanosine, mycophenolate, nephrotoxic drugs, bone marrow–suppressive agents	FBC, LFTs, renal function	Caution when handling; women of childbearing potential must be advised to use effective contraception during treatment; male patients should be advised to practise barrier contraception during and for at least 90 days following treatment
Foscarnet	90 or 120 mg/kg IV once daily for 5 days of the week GI: no maintenance recommended Retinitis: continue until CD4 T-cell count >100 cells/microlitre and suppressed HIV viral load	Granulocytopenia, anaemia, leucopenia, thrombocytopenia, neutropenia, sepsis, decreased appetite, hypokalaemia, hypomagnesaemia, hypocalcaemia, hyperphosphataemia, hyponatraemia, hypophosphataemia, increased ALP, increased LDH, aggression, agitation, anxiety, confusional state, depression, nervousness, dizziness, headache, paraesthesia, abnormal coordination, convulsion, hypoaesthesia, involuntary muscle contractions, peripheral neuropathy, tremor, hypertension, hypotension, thrombophlebitis, diarrhoea, nausea, vomiting, abdominal pain, constipation, dyspepsia, pancreatitis, elevated LFTs, rash, pruritus, myalgia, renal impairment, genital discomfort and ulceration, asthenia, chills, fatigue, pyrexia, malaise, oedema	Nephrotoxic drugs, drugs that inhibit renal tubular secretion, IV pentamidine, ritonavir	Renal function, magnesium, bone profile, FBC, blood pressure, LFTs	Good hydration, prompt correction of electrolyte abnormalities and dose adjustment for renal function are vital Wash genital area after micturition to reduce risk of ulceration Reduce infusion rate if infusion-related side effects
Cidofovir	5 mg/kg IV every 2 weeks GI: no maintenance recommended Retinitis: continue until CD4 T-cell count >100 cells/microlitre and suppressed HIV viral load	Renal impairment, neutropenia, ocular hypotony, iritis/uveitis, nausea, vomiting, alopecia, rash, asthenia, fever, chills, headache	Nephrotoxic drugs, drugs contraindicated with probenecid, tenofovir	Renal function (including urine protein), FBC	Must be co-administered with probenecid and IV fluids to minimise nephrotoxicity Caution with handling (potential carcinogen)

ALP, Alkaline phosphatase; FBC, full blood count; GI, gastro-intestinal; IV, intravenous; LDH, lactate dehydrogenase; LFT, liver function test; PO, oral.

treatment is contraindicated. Evidence for treatment for CNS infection is limited; however, ganciclovir with or without addition of foscarnet may be considered. In the cases of CNS infection, correcting immunodeficiency with ART is critical.

Most individuals with a lung infection will not require treatment, and the decision to treat should be based on positive BAL results, as well as clinical symptoms with no alternative cause.

Impact of antiretroviral therapy and clinical infections

The widespread use of ART has had a dramatic effect on the incidence, prognosis and clinical aspects of opportunistic infections, with a major reduction in the vast majority of opportunistic infections. As a consequence, there has been a reduction in mortality rates and hospital admissions. ART, although vital in the overall management of opportunistic infections, can be associated with some complications, for example, overlapping toxicities, drug–drug interactions and occasionally a severe immune reconstitution inflammatory syndrome.

Cancers

HIV increases the risk of many malignancies but is associated with three AIDS-defining malignancies: KS, high-grade B-cell non-Hodgkin's lymphoma and invasive cervical cancer.

Kaposi's sarcoma

KS is the most common malignancy in people who are living with HIV and is caused by the KS herpes virus. Individuals present with cutaneous or mucosal lesions, and visceral disease is uncommon. Lesions appear as raised purple papules and may be single or multiple, and in severe cases may result in oedema, ulceration and infection. These lesions are often characteristic in appearance, but diagnosis should be confirmed by histology. Plasma level of KS herpes virus DNA can also be used as a surrogate marker of tumour burden. Local therapy can be used for troublesome or local disease; however, this is limited to treating only small areas. Radiotherapy, intralesional vinblastine and topical retinoids have all demonstrated some treatment success. In more widespread disease, systemic treatment is required.

Initiation of ART can result in an improvement and in some cases resolution of KS. However, in patients with advanced, symptomatic or rapidly progressive disease, administration of systemic cytotoxic chemotherapy is required, and liposomal anthracyclines and taxanes are the established standard treatment.

High-grade B-cell non-Hodgkin's lymphoma

High-grade B-cell non-Hodgkin's lymphoma is the second most common malignancy in people who are living with HIV, although incidence has declined since the introduction of ART. Diagnosis should be based on histological confirmation from a tissue biopsy. Treatment should be according to conventional chemotherapy regimens; however, potential drug–drug interactions with ART should be considered because this can increase the toxicity of some chemotherapy combinations (e.g. PIs), increase the levels of some chemotherapy agents and increase the risk of neutropenia.

Invasive cervical cancer

Worldwide, cervical cancer is the second most common cancer in women overall and is associated with infection with human papillomavirus (HPV). Women who are living with HIV are more likely to have HPV infection, and therefore a higher prevalence of cervical cancer is seen in women living with HIV. Diagnosis is based on histopathological examination of cervical biopsies, and women with HIV should have an annual cervical cytology. Management should be the same as HIV-negative women according to national guidelines.

Neurological manifestations

Neurological symptoms may be caused by opportunistic infections, tumours or the primary neurological effects of the disease. HIV encephalopathy or HIV-associated cerebral disease is believed to result from direct infection of the CNS by HIV. This has dramatically declined with the effective use of ART; however, more subtle forms of brain disease, known as HIV-associated neurocognitive disorders, are reported. Initiation of ART should be immediate in individuals demonstrating any signs of neurocognitive disorders. Patients with any level of neurocognitive deficit should start standard ART; the level of CNS drug penetration should not influence therapeutic choice of ART because data of improvement in neurocognitive function are not conclusive (Churchill et al., 2015).

Progressive multifocal leucoencephalopathy

Progressive multifocal leucoencephalopathy is associated with the presence of JC virus. Transmission of the virus is not well understood, but it is thought to spread via respiratory secretions and tonsillar tissue, probably in childhood (Nelson et al., 2011). The virus disseminates after primary transmission and becomes latent. Following immune suppression, the virus replicates and is transported to the brain via B lymphocytes, where it infects permissive oligodendrocytes via the serotonin receptor (Nelson et al., 2011). Patients present with severe immunodeficiency over a period of weeks to months. Focal neurology, motor deficit, altered mood or mental status, ataxia and cortical visual symptoms may be present. Seizures occur rarely. The presence of focal features helps to distinguish progressive multifocal leucoencephalopathy from HIV encephalopathy. Radiological brain imaging using MRI combined with JC virus detection in a CSF sample are sufficient to confirm a diagnosis, rather than having to consider a brain biopsy. In many cases, introduction of ART prevents progression of disease, but it is unlikely to reverse the functional deficit. Adjunctive cidofovir or cytarabine, although active in vitro against JC virus, has not been shown to provide any additional benefit over ART alone (Nelson et al., 2011).

Case studies

Case 42.1

Miss F is a 32-year-old legal secretary, originally from Zimbabwe, and has lived in the UK for 10 years. She was diagnosed with HIV-1 2 years ago during a routine sexual health screen. Her baseline CD4 count was 320 cells/mm^3 and her viral load was 37,000 copies/mL. She had no baseline resistance and was hepatitis B immune and hepatitis C-negative. She was otherwise fit and well, taking only the combined oral contraceptive pill and had no allergies. She had a male partner who tested HIV-negative and they used condoms. She declines primary care doctor disclosure around her HIV status, as she is worried about confidentiality.

In view of her CD4 count less than 350 cells/mm^3 she was offered treatment. She was keen on a single-tablet regimen and Eviplera (tenofovir disoproxil fumarate, emtricitabine and rilpivirine) was started as a 1-pill once-a-day combination. This was chosen because there are no significant interactions with the combined oral contraceptive pill and it suited her lifestyle. In addition her viral load was less than 100,000 copies/mL, above which rilpivirine is not recommended in people starting cART because of higher rates of virological failure. She tolerated this well and achieved an undetectable viral load after 3 months, her CD4 count increased to greater than 600 cell/mm^3 and she remained stable.

She is recalled to clinic due to her viral load rising to 5697 copies/mL. A repeat sample confirms virological failure (viral load 7812 copies/mL), and a resistance test confirms an E138K mutation which confers resistance to rilpivirine.

Questions

1. What are the possible reasons for the rise in her viral load?
2. What ARV therapy change would you recommend?
3. What would you advise her to do regarding the combined oral contraceptive pill?

Answers

1. There are three main reasons for virological failure. Firstly, the patient has shown poor adherence to therapy, which should be explored in detail at this patient's appointment and support given around adherence if this has been the main issue. Secondly, rilpivirine has a significant food requirement of 390 calories to aid absorption and ensure adequate drug levels, so if she has been taking her Eviplera without food, this could put her at risk of virological failure. Thirdly, a full drug history needs to be taken. On discussion she reports that her primary care doctor prescribed her omeprazole 20 mg daily for the last 3 months due to new onset of dyspepsia. Omeprazole significantly decreases the rilpivirine plasma concentrations caused by an increase in gastric pH; therefore, co-administration in not recommended. This is the likely cause of virological failure in this patient. It is important that patients are supported to disclose to their primary care doctors/other clinicians and if they do not, that they seek advice from the specialist HIV pharmacy team if they are prescribed a new drug or buy over-the-counter medication.
2. She needs to switch her antiretroviral therapy because she is no longer receiving an effective combination. If she remains taking Eviplera, she is at risk of acquiring further drug resistance. The E138K mutation compromises rilpivirine and also has cross-class resistance, so the other NNRTIs are no longer an option. Tenofovir disoproxil fumarate and emtricitabine are still active; therefore, only the third agent needs

to be altered. The best option would be switching to a boosted PI. As a class, the PIs are much more robust and require multiple mutations to confer resistance; this strategy is recommended in the BHIVA (2015) guidelines. Atazanavir should be avoided because it also interacts with proton pump inhibitors. Therefore, ritonavir-boosted darunavir would be the third agent of choice, particularly if there were any adherence concerns. Other third agent choices would include an INI (raltegravir, elvitegravir or dolutegravir) or maraviroc if the patient was CCR5 tropic. These agents would not be recommended if there was any evidence of concurrent NRTI resistance.
3. Her contraception needs are important to consider because she is taking the combined oral contraceptive pill. Rilpivirine did not interact; however, darunavir/ritonavir will reduce its efficacy. Therefore, if she switches to this as a third agent, then she would have to be counselled and offered alternative contraception options. Medroxyprogesterone intramuscularly and the IUD/IUS are viable options, but the combined oestrogen/progesterone and other progesterone-based methods are less efficacious. If she switched to either raltegravir, dolutegravir or maraviroc, she could continue with the combined oral contraceptive pill because there are no significant drug–drug interactions.

Case 42.2

In 1997, Mr B, a 27-year-old man, presented with PCP. He had a CD4 count of 123 cells/mm^3, and plasma HIV RNA was unknown because viral load testing was not routinely available in clinics at the time. He had a good response to treatment with high-dose co-trimoxazole and was subsequently commenced on triple-combination therapy with stavudine, didanosine and indinavir. He continued receiving this regimen for 2 years, until HIV RNA testing became available and he was found to have a suppressed viral load and CD4 count of 412 cells/mm^3. His full antiretroviral therapy history, with reasons for switching, is detailed as follows (Table 42.11).

In April 2017 (now aged 47 years) his viral load remained <40 copies/mL, with CD4 count 670 cells/mm^3. However, his creatinine clearance (calculated using Cockcroft–Gault equation) was 41 mL/min and urine protein/creatinine ratio (UPCR) was significantly raised, at 86 mg/mmol (normal <30 mg/mmol). Both were normal when last monitored 4 months previously. On questioning, he revealed that he had been taking regular ibuprofen (400 mg three times a day) for the past month, following a wrist fracture. His QRISK2 score was calculated at 3.5%, and he is HLA-B*5701-negative.

Two weeks after stopping the ibuprofen, Mr B's creatinine clearance is now 52 mL/min and he is restarted on Atripla 1 tablet daily. His repeat UPCR, 1 week after stopping ibuprofen was 42 mg/mmol (improving), with normal urine albumin/creatinine ratio. His serum phosphate was low and fractional excretion of phosphate was 35% (normal <25%). Although his renal function was improving, it was decided to recommend changing his antiretroviral therapy to Kivexa 1 tablet daily and efavirenz 600 mg daily.

Questions

1. What are the possible drug-related causes of Mr B's renal dysfunction and what alterations, if any, to his drug therapy would you recommend?
2. What information should Mr B be given about the proposed change of his regimen to Kivexa plus efavirenz?

Answers

1. Tenofovir disoproxil fumarate use has been associated with renal dysfunction; the first sign of which may be a raised UPCR, although there are other causes. Mr B has a raised UPCR and

Table 42.11 Mr B's antiretroviral therapy treatment history (Case 42.2)

Start date	Drug name, dose and frequency	Stop date	Viral load and CD4 at switch	Reason for changing
May 1997	Stavudine 40 mg twice a day Didanosine 200 mg twice a day Indinavir 800 mg three times a day	Apr 1999	Viral load <200 copies/mL (lower limit of detection at that time) CD4 count 412 cells/mm^3	Renal stones (indinavir)
Apr 1999	Stavudine 40 mg twice a day Didanosine 200 mg twice a day Efavirenz 600 mg once a day	Jan 2002	Viral load <50 copies/mL (lower limit of detection at that time) CD4 count 503 cells/mm^3	Lactic acidosis (stavudine and didanosine)
Jan 2002	Tenofovir disoproxil fumarate 300 mg once a day Lamivudine 300 mg once a day Efavirenz 600 mg once a day	Mar 2008	Viral load <40 copies/mL CD4 count 633 cells/mm^3	Simplification (reducing pill burden)
Mar 2008	Atripla 1 tablet once a day			

reduced creatinine clearance, suggesting moderate renal dysfunction, which may be tenofovir disoproxil fumarate related. However, regular concomitant non-steroidal anti-inflammatory drugs may increase the risk of renal dysfunction. It is possible that the addition of regular ibuprofen has precipitated the renal dysfunction. Therefore, he would be advised to change to an alternative analgesic, if one is still required, starting with regular paracetamol.

Tenofovir disoproxil fumarate has also been associated with hypophosphataemia, a decrease in bone mineral density and other bone abnormalities (infrequently contributing to fractures). With Mr B's recent fracture, this should be investigated via annual DEXA scanning. Atripla is not recommended for patients with creatinine clearance less than 50 mL/min, because the doses of emtricitabine and tenofovir disoproxil fumarate need to be adjusted. For creatinine clearance 30–49 mL/min, a dosage of 200 mg emtricitabine and 300 mg tenofovir disoproxil fumarate (245 mg tenofovir disoproxil) every 48 hours is required. The efavirenz dosage remains 600 mg daily. However, Mr B's renal function must be closely monitored, for example, twice a week, to ensure that the dosages are adjusted promptly to reflect any change. This is to avoid over-dosing or under-dosing, and the associated risks of toxicity and antiretroviral therapy failure. If the renal dysfunction continued or worsened, despite stopping the ibuprofen and dose-adjusting his antiretroviral therapy, then a change of antiretroviral therapy might be warranted.

2. Mr B is being switched from Atripla 1 tablet daily to Kivexa 1 tablet daily and efavirenz 600 mg daily. The efavirenz component of his new regimen is also contained in Atripla, and therefore is not new in terms of drug exposure, merely as form of drug delivery. However, Kivexa is new for this patient. Points to include when counselling Mr B on this new drug regimen are:

   a. Why this change is being made: Mr B is demonstrating some toxicities of tenofovir disoproxil fumarate, and it has been decided to stop treatment with this drug to prevent any further renal deterioration. He also has a low phosphate level with a recent bone fracture which may have been contributed to by tenofovir disoproxil fumarate.

   b. How to take this combination: It is best to take efavirenz at night to avoid any disturbance in daily activities if Mr B has any CNS effects after taking his dose. He is used to taking Atripla; therefore, both new drugs should be taken at the same time as he has been used to taking his medication.

   c. Adverse effects: Mr B is HLA-B*5701-negative and is therefore very unlikely to develop a hypersensitivity reaction to abacavir (a component of Kivexa); however, he should still be aware of this reaction. Hypersensitivity reaction is characterised by fever and/or rash. Other symptoms associated may include

gastro-intestinal discomfort, respiratory symptoms, lethargy, malaise, headache, elevated liver function tests and myalgia. Symptoms usually appear within the first 6 weeks of initiation with abacavir, although they can occur anytime. General side effects such as nausea, vomiting, diarrhoea, fever, lethargy and rash are also present. Therefore, if Mr B has any of these symptoms he should be carefully evaluated for the presence of a hypersensitivity reaction. If Mr B experiences any worrying adverse effects, he should present for review.

   d. Monitoring and follow-up: Because Mr B is switching medication, he will need to return within 2 weeks to be monitored for tolerance to the new medication. This is in the form of a consultation, ideally with a pharmacist, to check whether he is experiencing any side effects. He will also have a safety blood test (usually liver function tests) at this stage to check for further potential adverse effects to new medication and subsequently (usually at 4 weeks) more safety bloods tests (usually liver and renal function tests) for viral suppression. At every review, patients should be made aware of the ongoing plan for their care and ensure they have enough medication to avoid any breaks in treatment.

Case 42.3

Mr C is a 58-year-old MSM who was recently diagnosed HIV through routine sexual health testing at his local genitourinary clinic. He is a smoker of 12 cigarettes a day and has hypertension which is under control (blood pressure 120/95 mmHg) on ramipril and bendroflumethiazide and is also taking pravastatin 40 mg once a day for high lipids. His fasting lipids were total cholesterol 5.9 mmol/L, low-density lipoprotein cholesterol 4.5 mmol/L, high-density lipoprotein 1.0 mmol/L, triglycerides 3.3 mmol/L. His height is 175 cm and his weight is 82 kg.

His CD4 count is 320 cells/mm^3 and his viral load is 70,000 copies/mL. He has agreed to start ART, and baseline blood samples for renal function and liver function tests, HIV drug resistance and HLAB5701 status have been done. His calculated creatinine clearance (Cockcroft–Gault equation) was 73 mL/min. He has no drug resistance.

Questions

1. What assessments would you do to decide which NRTI backbone (Kivexa or Truvada) Mr C should be prescribed?
2. What are the limitations of using the QRISK2 calculator? Is the calculated risk likely to be an overestimate or underestimate?

3. Mr C is concerned about the implications of his cardiovascular risk review. What information and advice should he be given?
4. Having considered all the issues, which backbone would you recommend?
5. What aspects need to be considered when determining the most suitable third agent to prescribe for Mr C?

....

Answers

1. To determine the most appropriate medicine, Mr C's HIV viral load should first be reviewed. Because it is less than 100,000 copies/mL, both backbones would be appropriate. If it was more than 100,000 copies/mL, Kivexa would be excluded. This would be followed by a cardiovascular risk assessment using the QRISK2-2016 calculator (http://qrisk.org) to determine whether he would be suitable for Kivexa (abacavir, one of the drugs in Kivexa, may be associated with an increased risk of cardiovascular disease and would be best avoided if the cardiovascular risk is >20%). His HLAB*5701 status would be reviewed and Kivexa would only be considered if it was HLA-negative. Mr C would be assessed for any renal or osteoporosis risks to establish whether Truvada would be suitable. His renal function would be determined using the Cockcroft–Gault equation to ascertain whether the combination Truvada was appropriate. His drug resistance results would be reviewed to ascertain that whatever combination was prescribed would result in viral suppression.

2. The main limitation of using the QRISK2 is that the population data underpinning the calculator come from individuals whose HIV status was not recorded. HIV infection itself is thought likely to increase the risk of cardiovascular disease, and therefore the cardiovascular risk may need to be increased by a factor of, for example, 1.6. Mr C's calculated 10-year risk rate is 25.3%, and this is likely to be an underestimate. Because abacavir may be associated with an increased risk of cardiovascular disease and is best avoided if the cardiovascular risk is greater than 20%, Kivexa may not be an appropriate choice.

3. Mr C should be given general lifestyle advice, especially to give up smoking, follow a healthy, balanced diet and regular exercise. Specific lipid-lowering dietary advice could be given. It would be useful to establish whether Mr C has changed his lifestyle in the last 4–6 months, for example, change in adherence to lipid-lowering therapy and/or change in diet. He should be encouraged to see his primary care doctor for review of his lipid-lowering agent to optimise his lipids.

4. Given Mr C's high cardiovascular risk, Kivexa would not be ideal, but Truvada could be considered as a backbone.

5. Aspects to consider with respect to a third agent are Mr C's concerns about pill burden, how medicine taking would fit into his lifestyle, whether he would be able to take raltegravir because this needs to be taken twice a day. If efavirenz is being considered, then its potential to cause CNS side effects would need to be reviewed with respect to Mr C's work and whether this could compromise safety in the workplace. In addition, if Mr C has had any mood problems they should be explored because they can be exacerbated by efavirenz. Resistance to drugs like efavirenz occurs if doses are missed. Therefore, if there was any likelihood that Mr C is going to miss doses, which would result in drug resistance, it would be better if Mr C was changed to a more robust regimen, for example, a PI-containing regimen – darunavir/ritonavir or atazanavir/ritonavir. If Mr C was taking any other concomitant medicines (e.g. stomach ulcer medicines like proton pump inhibitors) then atazanavir/ritonavir would not be an appropriate choice because of the drug–drug interactions. Therefore, the patient's wishes, concerns, lifestyle, as well as additional information (e.g. drug interactions), would be considered when determining a suitable third agent in line with local policy for the most cost-effective ARV therapy.

Case 42.4

Ms D is a 50-year-old social worker who was referred to the hospital accident and emergency department by her primary care doctor following a 4-week history of worsening respiratory symptoms, despite empirical treatment with amoxicillin, followed by clarithromycin. She has lost 3 kg in the last 2 months, has had a non-productive cough for 6 weeks and gets breathless climbing the stairs at home. Pulse oximetry showed desaturation to 91% on exercise, and her arterial blood gas sample had a PaO_2 of 8.1 kPa. Chest radiograph showed bilateral interstitial infiltrates. Her medical history includes irritable bowel syndrome (diagnosed 5 years ago), recurrent vaginal candidiasis for the past 7 years and allergic rhinitis, for which she uses fluticasone nasal spray. She works in an inner-city area and has no history of foreign travel outside mainland Europe. The hospital has recently introduced routine (opt out) HIV testing for all acute medical admissions, as a result of which Ms D was found to be HIV-positive, with a CD4 count of 47 cells/mm³.

....

Questions

1. What are the most likely HIV-related differential diagnoses for her respiratory symptoms?
2. How should her respiratory symptoms be managed?
3. When should she start antiretroviral therapy?
4. What drug interactions would you need to consider when managing Ms D both in the first few weeks and also in the longer-term?

....

Answers

1. The history, signs and symptoms (gradual onset, failure to respond to treatment for community-acquired pneumonia, weight loss, non-productive cough, breathlessness on exertion, oxygen desaturation, low PaO_2 and chest radiograph appearance) are all suggestive of PCP. However, some of these could also be consistent with TB which she may have been exposed to as a result of the nature of her job. TB would need to be excluded. Because Ms D has a significant degree of immunosuppression, the possibility of more than one pathogen/diagnosis must always be considered.

2. Until TB has been excluded, Ms D should be nursed in a negative pressure room. A bronchoscopy should ideally be performed to assist diagnosis. She should be started on treatment for PCP immediately with high-dose co-trimoxazole and systemic corticosteroid (see text and Table 42.4 for doses and administration details). Following induction treatment (usually 3 weeks in duration), she should receive secondary prophylaxis until her CD4 count on fully suppressive antiretroviral therapy is maintained above 200 cells/mm³ for 3–6 months.

   If she responds well to PCP treatment and bronchial washings are negative for acid-fast bacilli, then it would be reasonable for her to be managed expectantly with regard to the possibility of TB, that is, not kept in isolation and not started on TB treatment unless relevant symptoms persist or worsen, or new ones develop. If TB treatment were required, the standard four-drug (rifampicin, isoniazid, pyrazinamide, ethambutol) 2-month induction regimen, followed by 4 months of rifampicin and isoniazid plus pyridoxine would be recommended.

3. With a CD4 count of 47 cells/mm³, treatment with antiretroviral therapy would be recommended as soon as possible. Depending on how well she tolerated and responded to the PCP treatment, and whether TB treatment was also needed, antiretroviral therapy would usually be started within 2–4 weeks of diagnosis. For more information, refer to BHIVA guidelines for management of opportunistic infections (Nelson et al., 2011) and TB/HIV co-infection (Pozniak et al., 2011).

4. If Ms D did require TB treatment, the hepatic enzyme induction effect of rifampicin would need to be considered and a thorough review of drug–drug interactions would be advised.

The choice and dose of antiretroviral therapy would also be affected if treatment was started after the HIV genotypic resistance test result was known; if no resistance had been found, then efavirenz-containing antiretroviral therapy would be possible. If co-administered with rifampicin, the efavirenz dose should be increased to 800 mg once daily if her weight was greater than 60 kg; if less than 60 kg, standard dosage of 600 mg should be used. If she is experiencing side effects from efavirenz, TDM of efavirenz is recommended.

If PI-based antiretroviral therapy were initiated, either because of the presence of resistance mutations or whilst awaiting the HIV resistance test result, then TB therapy (if required) would need to be altered. Rifabutin (150 mg three times a week e.g. Monday, Wednesday and Friday) would be used instead of rifampicin. PIs also interact with intranasal and inhaled fluticasone and budesonide, resulting in increased levels of these steroids, due to inhibition of cytochrome 4503A4 in the gut wall and the liver and risk of increased steroid side effects and Cushing's syndrome. Beclometasone nasal spray would be a suitable alternative preparation for Ms D's allergic rhinitis and should be substituted.

Acknowledgements

The authors acknowledge the contribution of H. Leake-Date and M. Fisher to versions of this chapter which appeared in previous editions.

References

Bower, M., Palfreeman, A., Alfa-Wali, M., et al., 2014. British HIV Association guidelines for HIV-associated malignancies. HIV Med. 15 (Suppl. 2), 1–92. Available at: http://bhiva.org/documents/Guidelines/Malignancy/2014/MalignancyGuidelines2014.pdf.

British HIV Association (BHIVA), 2014. British HIV Association guidelines for the management of HIV infection in pregnant women 2012 (2014 Interim review). Available at: http://www.bhiva.org/documents/Guidelines/Pregnancy/2012/BHIVA-Pregnancy-guidelines-update-2014.pdf.

British HIV Association (BHIVA), 2015. BHIVA guidelines for the treatment of HIV-1-positive adults with antiretroviral therapy 2015. Available at: http://www.bhiva.org/documents/Guidelines/Treatment/2016/treatment-guidelines-2016-interim-update.pdf.

Bronke, C., Palmer, N.M., Jansen, C.A., et al., 2005. Dynamics of cytomegalovirus (CMV)-specific T cells in HIV-1–infected individuals progressing to AIDS with CMV end-organ disease. J. Infect. Dis. 191, 873–880.

Burger, D., van der Heiden, I., la Porte, C., et al., 2006. Interpatient variability in the pharmacokinetics of the HIV non-nucleoside reverse transcriptase inhibitor efavirenz: the effect of gender, race and CYP2B6 polymorphism. Br. J. Clin. Pharmacol. 61, 148–154.

Capeau, J., Bouteloup, V., Katlama, C., et al., 2012. Ten-year diabetes incidence in 1046 HIV-infected patients started on a combination antiretroviral treatment. AIDS 26 (3), 303–314.

Carr, A.M., Cooper, D.A., 2000. Adverse effects of antiretroviral therapy. Lancet 356 (9239), 1423–1430.

Centers for Disease Control and Prevention, 2015. C. neoformans infection. Available at: http://www.cdc.gov/fungal/diseases/cryptococcosis-neoformans/health-professionals.html.

Churchill, D., Waters, L., Ahmed, N., et al., 2015. BHIVA guidelines for the treatment of HIV-1-positive adults with antiretroviral therapy. Available at: http://bhiva.org/documents/Guidelines/Treatment/2015/2015-treatment-guidelines.pdf.

Cohen, M.S., Chen, Y.Q., McCauley, M., et al., 2011. Prevention of HIV-1 infection with early antiretroviral therapy. N. Engl. J. Med. 365, 493–505.

Cresswell, F., Waters, F., Briggs, E., et al., 2016. UK National Guideline for the use of HIV post-exposure prophylaxis following sexual exposure (PEPSE). Int. J. STD AIDS 27 (9), 713–738.

Delfraissy, J.F., Flandre, P., Delaugerre, C., et al., 2008. Lopinavir/ritonavir monotherapy or plus zidovudine and lamivudine in antiretroviral-naive HIV-infected patients. AIDS 22 (3), 385–393.

Department of Health, 2008. HIV post-exposure prophylaxis guidance from the UK Chief Medical Officers' Expert Advisory Group on AIDS. Department of Health, London.

de Ruiter, A., Taylor, G., Clayden, P., et al., 2014. British HIV Association guidelines for the management of HIV infection in pregnant women 2012 (2014 interim review). HIV Med. 15 (Suppl. 4), 1–77. Available at: http://www.bhiva.org/documents/Guidelines/Pregnancy/2012/BHIVA-Pregnancy-guidelines-update-2014.pdf.

Ding, X., Andraca-Carrera, E., Cooper, C., et al., 2012. No association of myocardial infarction with abacavir use: an FDA meta-analysis. J. Acquir. Immune Defic. Syndr. 61 (4), 441–447.

Dolling, D.I., Desai, M., McCowan, A., et al., 2016. An analysis of baseline data from the PROUD study: an open-label randomised trial of pre-exposure prophylaxis. Trials 17, 163.

El-Sadr, W.M., Lundgren, J.D., Neaton, J.D., et al., 2006. CD4+ count-guided interruption of antiretroviral treatment. N. Engl. J. Med. 355, 2283–2296.

Grant, R., Lama, J., Anderson, P., et al., 2010. Pre-exposure chemoprophylaxis for HIV prevention in men who have sex with men. N. Engl. J. Med. 363, 2587–2599.

Geretti, A., Brook, G., Cameron, C., et al., 2015. British HIV Association guidelines on the use of vaccines in HIV-positive adults 2015. Available at: http://www.bhiva.org/documents/Guidelies/Immunisation/consultation/BHIVA-Immunisation-Guidelines-2015-Consultation.pdf.

Hammer, S.M., Squires, K.E., Hughes, M.D., et al., 1997. A controlled trial of two nucleoside analogues plus indinavir in persons with human immunodeficiency virus infection and CD4 cell counts of 200 per cubic millimeter or less. N. Engl. J. Med. 337, 725–733.

Horne, R., Buick, D., Fisher, M., et al., 2004. Doubts about necessity and concerns about adverse effects: identifying the types of beliefs that are associated with non-adherence to HAART. Int. J. STD AIDS 15, 38–44.

INSIGHT START Study Group, 2015. Initiation of antiretroviral therapy in early asymptomatic HIV infection. N. Engl. J. Med. 373, 795–807.

Islam, F.M., Wu, J., Jansson, J., Wilson, D.P., 2012. Relative risk of cardiovascular disease among people living with HIV: a systematic review and meta-analysis. HIV Med. 13, 446–453.

Letendre, S., Ellis, R., Deutsch, R., et al., 2010. Correlates of time-to-loss-of-viral-response in CSF and plasma in the CHARTER cohort. 17th Conference on Retroviruses and Opportunistic Infections 2010, poster 430, February 16–19, 2010, San Francisco.

Mallal, S., Phillips, E., Carosi, G., et al., 2008. HLA-B*5701 screening for hypersensitivity to abacavir. N. Engl. J. Med. 358, 568–579.

Max, B., Sherer, R., 2000. Management of the adverse effects of antiretroviral therapy and medication adherence. Clin. Infect. Dis. 30 (Suppl. 2), S96–S116.

McComsey, G., Lonergan, J.T., 2004. Mitochondrial dysfunction: patient monitoring and toxicity management. J. Acquir. Immune Defic. Syndr. 37, S30–S35.

McCormack, S., Dunn, D.T., Desai, M., et al., 2015. Pre-exposure prophylaxis to prevent the acquisition of HIV-1 infection (PROUD): effectiveness results from the pilot phase of a pragmatic open-label randomised trial. Lancet 387, 53–60.

Mellors, J.W., Munoz, A., Giorgi, J.V., et al., 1997. Plasma viral load and CD4 lymphocytes as prognostic markers of HIV-1 infection. Ann. Intern. Med. 126, 946–954.

Miller, R., Huang, L., 2004. Pneumocystis jirovecii infection. Thorax 59, 731–733. Available at: http://thorax.bmj.com/content/59/9/731.full.

Monforte, A., Reiss, P., Ryom, L., et al., 2013. Atazanavir is not associated with an increased risk of cardio- or cerebrovascular disease events. AIDS 27, 407–415.

Morris, A., Gingo, M.D., 2015. BMJ Best Practice: *Pneumocystis jirovecii* pneumonia. Br. Med. J., 9. Available at: http://bestpractice.bmj.com/best-practice/monograph/19.html.

National Institute for Health and Care Excellence (NICE), 2014. Cardiovascular disease: risk assessment and reduction, including lipid modification. Available at: https://www.nice.org.uk/guidance/cg181.

National Institute for Health and Care Excellence (NICE), 2015. Sofosbuvir for treating chronic hepatitis C: technology appraisal guidance [TA330]. Available at: https://www.nice.org.uk/guidance/ta330.

National Institute for Health and Care Excellence (NICE), 2016. Tuberculosis. Available at: https://www.nice.org.uk/guidance/ng33/resources/tuberculosis-1837390683589.

Nelson, M., Dockrell, D.H., Edwards, S., on behalf of the BHIVA Guidelines Subcommittee, 2011. British HIV Association and British Infection Association guidelines for the treatment of opportunistic infection in HIV-seropositive individuals. HIV Med. 12 (Suppl. 2), 1–5. Available at: http://bhiva.org/documents/Guidelines/OI/hiv_v12_is2_Iss2Press_Text.pdf.

Palella Jr., F.J., Delaney, K.M., Moorman, A.C., 1998. Declining morbidity and mortality among patients with advanced human immunodeficiency virus infection. N. Engl. J. Med. 338, 853–860.

Poppa, A., Davidson, O., Deutsch, J., et al., 2004. British HIV Association (BHIVA) and British Association for Sexual Health and HIV (BASHH) guidelines on provision of adherence support to individuals receiving antiretroviral therapy (2003). HIV Med. 5 (Suppl. 2), 46–60.

Pozniak, A.L., Coyne, K.M., Miller, R.F., on behalf of the BHIVA Guidelines Subcommittee, et al., 2011. British HIV Association guidelines for the treatment of TB/HIV coinfection. HIV Med. 12, 517–524. Available at: http://bhiva.org/documents/Guidelines/TB/hiv_954_online_final.pdf.

Rodger, A., Bruun, T., Cambiano, V., et al., 2014. HIV transmission risk through condomless sex if HIV+ partner on suppressive ART: PARTNER study. 21st Conference on Retroviruses and Opportunistic Infections, abstract 153LB, 2014, Boston.

Saberi, P., Phengrasam, T., Nguyen, D.P., 2013. Inhaled corticosteroid use in HIV-positive individuals taking protease inhibitors: a review of pharmacokinetics, case reports and clinical management. HIV Med. 14, 519–529.

Smit, C., Geskus, R., Walker, S., et al., 2006. Effective therapy has altered the spectrum of cause-specific mortality following HIV seroconversion. AIDS 20, 741–749.

Smith, C., Sabin, C.A., Lundgren, J.D., et al., 2010. Data collection on Adverse Events of Anti-HIV drugs (D:A:D) Study. AIDS 24, 1537–1548.

Temesgen, Z., 2015. BMJ Best Practice: *Mycobacterium avium*-intracellulare. Br. Med. J., 7. Available at: http://bestpractice.bmj.com/best-practice/monograph/559.html.

UNAIDS, 2015. AIDS by the numbers 2015. Available at: http://www.unaids.org/sites/default/files/media_asset/AIDS_by_the_numbers_2015_en.pdf.

Wilkins, E., Nelson, M., Agarwal, K., et al., 2013. British HIV Association guidelines for the management of hepatitis viruses in adults infected with HIV 2013. HIV Med. 14 (Suppl. 4), 1–71. Available at: http://www.bhiva.org/documents/Guidelines/Hepatitis/2013/HepatitisGuidelines2013.pdf.

World Health Organization, 2007. WHO case definitions of HIV for surveillance and revised clinical staging and immunological classification of HIV-related disease in adults and children. Available at: http://www.who.int/hiv/pub/guidelines/HIVstaging150307.pdf.

Worm, S.W., Sabin, C., Weber, R., et al., 2010. Risk of myocardial infarction in patients with HIV infection exposed to specific individual antiretroviral drugs from the 3 major drug classes: the data collection on adverse events of anti-HIV drugs (D:A:D) study. J. Infect. Dis. 201, 318–330.

Further reading

Adler, M.W., Edwards, S.G., Miller, R.F., et al., 2012. ABC of HIV and AIDS. Wiley-Blackwell, Hoboken, NJ.

Crum-Cianflone, N., Huppler Hullsiek, K., Marconi, V., et al., 2009. Trends in the incidence of cancers among HIV-infected persons and the impact of antiretroviral therapy: a 20-year cohort study. AIDS 23, 41–50.

Marcus, J.L., Leyden, W.A., Chao, C.R., et al., 2014. HIV infection and incidence of ischemic stroke. AIDS 28, 1911–1919.

Rasmussen, L.D., Engsig, F.N., Christensen, H., et al., 2011. Risk of cerebrovascular events in persons with and without HIV: a Danish nationwide population-based cohort study. AIDS 25, 1637–1646.

Saag, M.S., Chambers, H.F., Eliopoulos, G.M., et al., 2016. The Sanford Guide to HIV/AIDS Therapy 2016–17 Pocket Edition, twenty fourth ed. Antimicrobial Therapy Inc., Sperryville, VA.

Taiwo, B., Zheng, L., Gallien, S., ACTG A5262 Team, et al., 2011. Efficacy of a nucleoside-sparing regimen of darunavir/ritonavir plus raltegravir in treatment-naive HIV-1-infected patients (ACTG A5262). AIDS 25, 2113–2122.

Useful websites

University of Liverpool HIV drug interaction website: http://www.hiv-druginteractions.org

University of Liverpool HEP drug interactions website: http://www.hep-druginteractions.org

QRISK2 Prediction algorithm for cardiovascular disease: https://www.qrisk.org

Clinical Care Option: https://www.clinicaloptions.com

British HIV Association (BHIVA): http://www.bhiva.org

HIV Pharmacy Association: http://www.hivpa.org

NAM aidsmap: http://www.aidsmap.com

Centers for Disease Control and Prevention: https://www.cdc.gov/hiv

British Association for Sexual Health and HIV: https://www.bashh.org

43 Fungal Infections

Manjusha Narayanan

Key points

- Fluconazole, a triazole, is considered to be standard therapy for oropharyngeal, oesophageal and vaginal candidiasis.
- Itraconazole and terbinafine are efficacious, non-toxic alternatives to griseofulvin when systemic treatment of dermatophytosis is required.
- Fungi can cause overwhelming deep-seated or systemic infections in immunocompromised hosts that are refractory to antifungal treatment alone.
- Incidence of non-Aspergillus mould infections has increased in transplant recipients over the past decade, and these can be lethal.
- Most therapy for deep-seated fungal infection in the immunocompromised host is empirical due to the difficulties in reaching a rapid, accurate diagnosis of systemic fungal infection.
- Lipid-complexed formulations of amphotericin offer a less toxic alternative to conventional amphotericin in the treatment of systemic fungal infection.
- Voriconazole, a triazole, appears to be an effective alternative to amphotericin in the treatment of invasive aspergillosis.
- Caspofungin is an alternative agent to amphotericin for invasive aspergillosis and may have a role to play in the empirical treatment of febrile neutropenic patients.
- Anidulafungin is an alternative to fluconazole in treatment of invasive candidiasis in adult non-neutropenic patients.

Introduction

Fungi are ubiquitous micro-organisms that differ from bacteria in their cellular structure, and this makes them naturally resistant to antibacterial agents (Table 43.1). Fungi are broadly divided into yeasts and moulds. Yeasts are typically round or oval-shaped microscopically; grow flat, round colonies on culture plates; and reproduce by forming buds from their cells. Moulds (e.g. *Aspergillus*, *Mucor*) appear as a collection or mass (mycelium) of individual tubular structures called hyphae that grow by branching and longitudinal extension. They appear as a fuzzy growth on appropriate conducive medium (e.g. *Penicillium* colonies on stale bread or Sabouraud's agar). The most commonly seen yeast, *Candida*, occasionally produces pseudohyphae.

Hundreds of species of fungi are in the environment, but only the important human fungal pathogens and their treatment will be discussed in this chapter. The fungi of medical importance can be divided into four groups (Table 43.2).

Some fungi like *Histoplasma capsulatum*, *Coccidioides immitis* and *Blastomyces dermatitidis* are known as dimorphic fungi (see Table 43.2) because they are found in the infected host in yeast form at 35–37 °C temperature but grow as moulds, in vitro, at room temperatures (22 °C incubation).

Fungi mainly reproduce by forming spores through mitosis giving rise to two daughter cells. They are known by names given to this imperfect state (asexual reproduction), but the same fungus, for example, *Scedosporium apiospermum* (asexual form), is also known as *Pseudoallescheria boydii* (sexual form). However, for all practical purposes, only the oldest and best-established name for the fungi is used in diagnostic laboratories.

Fungal spore are spread by air, water and direct contact with infected source. Humans usually become infected by inhalation of airborne spores or by inoculation into traumatised skin and mucous membrane.

Laboratory diagnosis

Microscopical examination and culture of fungi is the mainstay of laboratory diagnosis. Appropriate staining of histological sections of affected tissue is helpful in making a diagnosis when culture growth may or may not be positive. Yeast colonies and moulds are characteristic in their appearance on culture plates and can be preliminarily identified by their shape, colour and temperatures at which they grow. For the genus and species identification of yeasts, microscopic examination and biochemical tests are necessary. Moulds are identified by their morphology and the nature of sporulation on agar medium.

Antifungal sensitivity testing for yeast is done by determining the minimum inhibitory concentration (MIC) of the antifungal agent in the E-test strip method, which has now replaced the measurement of 'inhibition zone' by disc testing. E-test strips are also available for determining sensitivity of antifungal agents against moulds. Molecular diagnosis utilising polymerase chain reaction is not available for use in routine practice, but it can be available as a send-away test to specialised laboratories. Serological diagnosis to look for antibodies in patient's blood is of use only in *Coccidioides* infection. Enzyme-linked immunosorbent assay methods to look for galactomannan antigen in deep *Aspergillus* infection are available but not fully evaluated. A positive test needs to be interpreted in conjunction with other findings. Antigen detection is useful in disseminated *Histoplasmosis* and *Cryptococcosis*.

Table 43.1 Important characteristics of a fungal cell

Fungi	Bacteria
Eukaryotes	Prokaryotes, eubacteria
Cell and cytoplasm	Cell and cytoplasm
Nucleus with multiple chromosomes enclosed in a nuclear membrane	No nucleus or nuclear membrane has single chromosome
Contains endoplasmic reticulum, Golgi apparatus, mitochondria and ribosomes	Other structures absent except ribosomes
Cytoplasmic membrane	Cytoplasmic membrane
Contains phospholipids and sterols	Contains phospholipids and no sterols
Cell wall	Cell wall
Contains chitins, mannans,+/− cellulose	Contains peptidoglycan, lipids and proteins

Fungal infection

It is important to distinguish harmless colonisation with fungi and significant clinical infection, because only the latter would benefit from antifungal treatment.

More often, fungi are a cause of superficial infections of the skin and mucous membranes.

In some susceptible hosts whose immune system is heavily compromised, deep-seated infections involving organs like lungs and brain can manifest as 'difficult to cure' infections, for example, pulmonary aspergillosis or cryptococcal meningitis.

Antifungal agents

Topical and systemic antifungal agents are available to treat mucocutaneous candidiasis, various forms of tinea (ringworm) and other dermatophytosis, onychomycosis and deep-seated systemic infections (e.g. candidaemia, mucor mycoses, fungal endocarditis, osteomyelitis). Some infective conditions and their treatment are dealt with in the sections that follow. The side effects of a range of antifungal agents are set out in Table 43.3.

Table 43.2 Classification of fungi of medical importance

Group	Examples	Infections caused
Yeast	*Candida* spp.	Oral and vaginal thrush Deep seated: candidaemia, empyema
	Cryptococcus neoformans *Saccharomyces cerevisiae* *Malassezia furfur*	Meningitis Rare systemic infection in immunocompromised host
Yeastlike	*Geotrichum candidum* *Trichosporon beigelii*	
Dimorphic fungi	*Blastomyces dermatitidis*	For first three: deep systemic organ involvement, more commonly in the immunocompromised host
	Coccidioides immitis *Histoplasma capsulatum* *Paracoccidioides brasiliensis* *Sporothrix schenckii*	Deep subcutaneous infection following trauma
Moulds		
1. Hyaline a. Zygomycoses	*Rhizopus* *Mucor* *Absidia*	Infections in patients with neutropenia and those with diabetic ketoacidosis
b. Hyalohyphomycosis	*Aspergillus fumigatus* and other *Aspergillus* spp. *Fusarium* *Scedosporium apiospermum*	Systemic infection: invasive pulmonary or central nervous system involvement Fusarium keratitis Deep infection in immunocompromised host, e.g. transplant patients
2. Dermatophytes	*Trichophyton* spp. *Microsporum* spp. *Epidermophyton*	For all three: various skin (ringworm), hair and nail infections
3. Dematiaceous	*Alternaria* spp. *Cladophialophora* spp.	Deep tissue infection with granulomas Chromomycosis, mycetomas

Table 43.3 Side effects of systemic antifungal agents

Drug	Side effects
Griseofulvin	Mild: headache, gastro-intestinal side effects; hypersensitivity reactions such as skin rashes, including photosensitivity Moderate: exacerbation of acute intermittent porphyria; rarely, precipitation of systemic lupus erythematosus Contraindicated in acute porphyria, systemic lupus erythematosus, pregnancy and severe liver disease
Terbinafine	Usually mild: nausea, abdominal pain; allergic skin reactions; loss and disturbance of sense of taste Not recommended in patients with liver disease
Amphotericin	Immediate reactions (during infusion) include headache, pyrexia, rigors, nausea, vomiting, hypotension; occasionally, there can be severe thrombophlebitis after the infusion Nephrotoxicity and hypokalaemia Anaemia due to reduced erythropoiesis Cardiac failure (exacerbated by peripheral neuropathy [rare] hypokalaemia due to nephrotoxicity) Immunomodulation (the drug can both enhance and inhibit some immunological functions)
Flucytosine	Mild: gastro-intestinal side effects (nausea, vomiting); occasional skin rashes Moderate: myelosuppression (dose related), hepatotoxicity
Fluconazole	Mild: nausea, vomiting and occasional skin rashes; occasionally, elevated liver enzymes (reversible) Moderate or severe: rarely, hepatotoxicity and severe cutaneous reactions, especially in patients with AIDS
Itraconazole	Mild: nausea and abdominal pain; occasional skin rashes Moderate or severe: rarely, hepatotoxicity
Voriconazole	Similar to fluconazole and itraconazole Mild: reversible visual disturbances occur in about 30% of patients
Caspofungin, anidulafungin	Mild: gastro-intestinal side effects; occasional skin rashes

AIDS, Acquired immune deficiency syndrome.

Superficial infection

Candida infections
Epidemiology

Candida is a normal commensal of the human gastro-intestinal tract and skin. Loss of skin and mucosal integrity or use of broad-spectrum antibiotics which alter normal bacterial flora allow overgrowth of endogenous *Candida*. There are more than 100 species of *Candida*, but only a few are important as common human pathogens.

Thrush is candidal infection of the mucous membrane. It can manifest as oral infection, for example, oral thrush in various patient groups, vulvovaginal thrush in females, balanitis in the uncircumcised man or intertrigo infection in moist skin surfaces in close proximity, for example, groin area. Patients with diabetes and corticosteroid users, whether inhaled or oral, are also prone to infections. Dysphagia due to candidal oesophagitis presents in patients with acquired immune deficiency syndrome (AIDS) and cancer.

Clinical presentation

Oral thrush typically presents as a sore mouth with white curd-like patches on the tongue or oral mucosa which can bleed on scraping. Females with vaginal thrush present with itching and a creamy vaginal discharge. Skin infection in babies can present as pustular body rash or nappy rash in the moist perianal area.

Candida folliculitis may present in unkempt, bearded men. Nail infection with *Candida* (onychomycosis) or subcutaneous tissue involvement under the nail (paronychia) is seen in people whose occupation involves prolonged hand immersion in water.

In severe oesophageal candidiasis, ulceration or formation of pseudomembranes and, rarely, perforation of the lower third of the oesophagus may occur.

Candida can be a cause of hospital-acquired infection in patients, because it is found in the hospital environment on inanimate objects or on skin of healthcare workers.

Treatment

Oral and vaginal candidiasis may be treated by either topical or systemic antifungal agents. The drugs currently available for topical use fall into two groups: the polyenes, of which only amphotericin and nystatin are used clinically; and the imidazoles, such as econazole, clotrimazole, miconazole and fenticonazole. These agents are essentially identical in their antifungal activity, and the only reasons to choose between them are price and differing preparations. The two first-line systemic agents are both triazoles (fluconazole and itraconazole) and can be given by mouth. Voriconazole, a triazole, should be considered as second-line treatment if the *Candida* is resistant to first-line triazoles. Skin infections may also be treated topically, but nail infections are unlikely to respond to a topical antifungal agent alone and require systemic treatment. Oesophagitis will invariably require systemic treatment.

Topical treatment. The polyenes are broad-spectrum antifungal agents that are virtually insoluble in water and which are not absorbed from the gastro-intestinal tract or from skin or mucous membranes. Both nystatin and amphotericin (but particularly nystatin) are available in a wide range of formulations including pessaries, creams, gels, tablets, pastilles, etc. The choice of formulation clearly depends on the site of infection and patient preference.

Systemic treatment. Three triazole agents – fluconazole, itraconazole and voriconazole – are available for systemic treatment of oral and vulvovaginal candidiasis. A good source of advice on treatment is that from the Infectious Diseases Society of America (Pappas et al., 2009)

Vulvovaginal candidiasis.

- Several topical antifungal agents provide effective therapy; no agent is clearly superior.
- A single 150 mg dose of fluconazole is recommended for the treatment of uncomplicated cases.
- Complicated vulvovaginal candidiasis requires topical therapy for 7 days or multiple doses of fluconazole (150 mg every 72 hours for 3 doses). Recurrent infections with non-albicans *Candida*, for example, *C. glabrata*, may be more difficult to treat.

Candida balanitis.

- *Candida* balanitis can be treated with topical polyenes or imidazoles, or with systemic fluconazole at the same dose as for vaginal infection (e.g. fluconazole 150 mg for 1 dose).

It is sometimes stated that when treating a woman with vaginal candidiasis, the male partner should be treated simultaneously to prevent reinfection. Although there is no evidence to support this approach, it may be considered in women who suffer from repeated vaginal candidiasis.

Guidance on the treatment of topical and systemic therapy (Pappas et al., 2009) is also available for treatment of mild, moderate and severe oropharyngeal and oesophageal candidiasis and suppressive therapy for patients with human immunodeficiency virus (HIV) infection.

Dermatophytosis

Epidemiology

Dermatophytosis, or tinea, is a condition caused by three genera of dermatophyte fungi: *Trichophyton*, *Epidermophyton* and *Microsporum*. Unlike *Candida*, these are moulds which have a predilection for keratinised tissue such as skin, nail and hair. These fungi are very widely distributed throughout the world and may be acquired from the soil (anthrophilic, e.g. *Trichophyton rubrum*), from animals (zoophilic) or from humans (geophilic) infected with the fungus.

Some species are prevalent throughout the world, for example, *Microsporum canis*, whereas some are area specific, for example, *Trichophyton mentagrophytes* in Europe and New Zealand.

Clinical presentation

The classical clinical presentation of dermatophyte infection of the skin is ringworm (tinea), a circular, inflamed lesion with a raised edge and associated skin scaling. However, presentation is influenced by the site of infection, for example, tinea pedis (athlete's foot) between the toes or tinea cruris on the body, and by the actual species of fungus causing the infection. In general, less severe lesions are produced by human fungal strains, whereas those acquired from animals can produce quite intense inflammatory reactions.

Dermatophytosis of the nail results in thickened, discoloured nails, whereas in the scalp, infection presents with itching, skin scaling and inflammation, and patchy hair loss (alopecia).

Rarely, deep dermatophytosis may be seen in immunocompromised patients with involvement of subcutaneous tissue (granuloma).

Diagnosis

The diagnosis of dermatophyte infection is confirmed by collecting appropriate specimens such as material from infected nails and skin. The fungi can be seen microscopically and specimens may also be cultured, but antifungal susceptibility testing is not required.

Treatment

Small or medium areas of skin infection can be treated with topical therapy, but nail, hair and widespread skin infection should be systemically treated with oral antifungal agents.

The most commonly used topical agents are the imidazoles, of which a wide variety is available, including clotrimazole, econazole, miconazole and tioconazole. There is little to choose between these agents, all of which are usually applied two or three times daily, continuing for up to 2 weeks after the lesions have healed. Side effects are uncommon and usually consist of mild skin irritation. Other topical agents include amorolfine, terbinafine and tolnaftate.

The main oral antifungals used for dermatophytosis are terbinafine, itraconazole and fluconazole. Griseofulvin is an alternative treatment for tinea capitis.

Terbinafine. Terbinafine was the first member of a new class of antifungal agents, the allylamines, which became available for systemic use. These agents act by inhibition of the fungal enzyme squalene epoxidase, an enzyme involved in the synthesis of ergosterol, an essential component of the fungal cytoplasmic membrane. Although terbinafine has a very broad antifungal spectrum in the laboratory, its in vivo efficacy does not correspond to its in vitro activity, and it is used only for the treatment of dermatophyte infection.

About 70% of an oral dose of terbinafine is absorbed, and the drug appears in high concentrations in the skin. The half-life is about 16–17 hours; therefore, the drug can be given once per day. Terbinafine is metabolised in the liver and the metabolites are excreted in the urine so that hepatic or renal dysfunction will prolong the elimination half-life.

Terbinafine is the treatment of choice for tinea infections at 250 mg/day for 2–6 weeks, depending upon the infection. However, for nail infections a longer course of terbinafine is required (e.g. fingernails infections may be for ≥6 weeks at 250 mg/day and for toenail infections it may need to be continued for 12 weeks).

Itraconazole is the second preferred agent at 200 mg twice a day for 1 week and longer with repeated courses for finger and toenail involvement.

Griseofulvin. The first orally administered treatment for dermatophytosis was griseofulvin, which has been available since the late 1950s. Griseofulvin is active only against dermatophyte fungi, and it is inactive against all other fungi and bacteria. To exert its antifungal effect, it must be incorporated into keratinous tissue, where levels are much greater than serum levels; therefore, it has no effect if used topically.

Griseofulvin is well absorbed and absorption is enhanced if taken with a high-fat meal. In children, it may be given with milk. A 1000 mg dose produces a peak serum level of about 1–2 mg/L after 4 hours, with a half-life of at least 9 hours. An ultra-fine preparation of griseofulvin exists which is almost totally absorbed and permits the use of lower dosages (typically 330–660 mg daily). This preparation is not available in the UK. Elimination is mainly through the liver, and inactive metabolites are excreted in the urine. Less than 1% of a dose is excreted in urine in the active form, but some active drug is excreted in the faeces.

The usual adult dosage is 500 mg daily or 1 g for severe infections. The duration of treatment will depend upon the infection; it may require 6 weeks for treatment of larger lesions in tinea corporis.

The duration of treatment with griseofulvin is dependent entirely on clinical response. Skin or hair infection usually requires 4–12 weeks of therapy, but nail infections respond much more slowly; 6 months of treatment is often required for fingernails and a year or longer for toenail infections. Unfortunately, the rate of treatment failure or relapse in nail infection is high and may reach up to 60%; hence terbinafine and itraconazole may be preferred agents.

Pityriasis versicolor

Pityriasis versicolor is a common superficial skin infection caused by a yeastlike fungus, *Malassezia furfur*. The organism is a member of the normal skin flora and lives only on the skin because it has a growth requirement for medium-chain fatty acids present in sebum.

Clinical presentation

Pityriasis versicolor usually appears as patches scattered over the trunk, neck and shoulders. These patches produce scales and may be pigmented in light-skinned individuals, appearing light brown in colour. In dark-skinned patients, the lesions may lose pigment and appear lighter than normal skin.

In some patients, Malassezia yeast is also associated with dandruff and seborrhoeic dermatitis, although the exact role of the yeast in causing this condition remains uncertain. In patients with AIDS, seborrhoeic dermatitis may be quite extensive and sudden in onset. Malassezia folliculitis can appear as greasy papules or pustules on the trunk or face of an HIV-infected individual.

Diagnosis

The diagnosis of pityriasis versicolor is made by microscopy of scrapings from the lesion. The specimen is examined for the presence of yeast cells and short hyphae. Culture is not usually required for diagnosis and, because it requires special culture media, is not routinely attempted.

Treatment

Pityriasis versicolor is treated with topical terbinafine cream or a topical imidazole cream such as clotrimazole, econazole or miconazole. Cheaper topical alternatives are 2% selenium sulphide lotion or 20% sodium thiosulphate applied daily for 10–14 days. Relapses are common, and treatment may need to be repeated. In severe cases, oral itraconazole (200 mg once daily for 7 days) may be given. Treatment of seborrhoeic dermatitis and folliculitis is undertaken with topical azole creams and 1% hydrocortisone. This condition can also often relapse.

Ear infection

Fungi sometimes infect the external auditory canal, causing otitis externa, with the most common causative organisms being various species of *Aspergillus* (such as *A. niger* and *A. fumigatus*) and *C. albicans* and other *Candida* species. A variety of other fungi found in the environment can also cause this condition. The use of topical antibacterial agents in the ear may predispose to local fungal infection.

Clinical presentation

Fungal infection of the ear usually presents as pain and itching in the auditory canal, sometimes with a reduction in hearing caused by blockage of the canal. There may be an associated discharge from the ear. Clinical examination shows a swollen red canal, and the fungal mycelium is sometimes visible as an amorphous white or grey mass.

Diagnosis

The diagnosis of a fungal infection of the external canal can be made by microscopy and culture of material obtained from the ear.

Treatment

Aural toilet with removal of obstructing debris is very important in the management of fungal infections of the external auditory canal. A topical antifungal agent such as nystatin or amphotericin, or an imidazole can also be applied.

Infections with saprophytic fungi

Most mouldy fungi are saprophytes; they obtain their nutrition from dead organic matter. Some saprophytic fungi can cause significant human infections. An example of such an infection in a host with a normal immune system is fusarium keratitis in contact lens wearers. *Penicillium marneffei* can cause skin infection and disseminated fatal infection in HIV-infected patients in South East Asia. *Scedosporium* pulmonary infections are seen in lung transplant recipients. A large trial of retrospective data from the USA revealed that the three most common non-*Aspergillus* saprophytic moulds that cause invasive fungal infection among patients receiving haemopoietic stem cell transplants (HSCT) were *Fusarium*, *Scedosporium* and *Zygomycetes* (Marr et al., 2002).

Table 43.4 Conditions predisposing to systemic or deep-seated fungal infection

Infection	Predisposing conditions
Systemic candidiasis	Neutropenia from any cause (disease or treatment) Use of broad-spectrum antibiotics which eliminate the normal body flora Indwelling intravenous cannulae, especially when used for total parenteral nutrition Haematological malignancy and hematopoietic stem cell transplantation Solid organ transplantation AIDS (particularly associated with severe mucocutaneous infection) Intravenous drug abuse Cardiac surgery and heart valve replacement, leading to *Candida* endocarditis Gastro-intestinal tract surgery Oesophagectomy leak leading to pleural space infection (empyema)
Aspergillosis	Neutropenia from any cause, especially if severe and prolonged Acute leukaemia Solid organ transplantation (mainly lungs) Chronic granulomatous disease of childhood (defect in neutrophil function) Pre-existing lung disease (usually leads to aspergillomas; fungus balls form in the lung rather than invasive or disseminated infection)
Cryptococcosis	AIDS Systemic therapy with corticosteroids Renal transplantation Hodgkin's disease and other lymphomas Sarcoidosis Collagen vascular diseases
Zygomycosis	Diabetic hyperglycaemic ketoacidosis (leading to rhinocerebral infection) Severe, prolonged neutropenia Burns (leading to cutaneous infection)

AIDS, Acquired immune deficiency syndrome.

Deep-seated fungal infections

Most deep-seated or systemic fungal infections seen in the UK are the result of some breakdown in the normal body defences, which may be due to disease or medical treatment. Fungi that cause superficial infections can also cause deep-seated infection in immunocompromised patients with leukaemia and lymphoma, and those in the post-transplant period of immunosuppression. There are, however, a group of fungi, often referred to rather misleadingly as the pathogenic fungi, which are able to cause systemic infection in a previously healthy person. These infections, which are usually due to dimorphic fungi, include diseases such as histoplasmosis, blastomycosis and coccidioidomycosis. They are rare in the UK but rather more common in the USA and other parts of the world.

Fungal infections in the compromised host

Common mycoses
Epidemiology and predisposing factors

A large number of conditions may predispose the individual to systemic or deep-seated fungal infection. These are summarised in Table 43.4. A breach in the body's mechanical barriers may predispose to fungal infection. For example, fungal infection of the urinary tract occurs most commonly in catheterised patients who have received broad-spectrum antibiotics, whereas total parenteral nutrition (TPN) is strongly associated with fungaemia, sometimes with unusual fungi such as *Malassezia furfur*. This is due to the use of TPN infusions containing lipids, which are a growth requirement of this organism. Most cases of systemic fungal infection, however, are associated with a defect in the patient's immune system, and the nature of the organisms encountered is often related to the nature of the immunosuppression. Neutropenia, for example, is usually associated with *Candida* species, *Aspergillus* and mucormycosis, whereas defects of cell-mediated immunity, for example, HIV infection, are strongly associated with infection by *Cryptococcus neoformans*. Prolonged diabetic ketoacidosis is a risk factor for development of rhinocerebral zygomycosis, where mortality rates can be as high as 100% if there is significant underlying disease.

Many different fungi have been described as causing systemic fungal infection, but the most common organisms encountered and the conditions they cause are listed in Table 43.5. Of these, *Candida* and *Aspergillus* are by far the most common in the UK.

Table 43.5 Common causes of systemic and deep-seated fungal infection in the UK

Condition/organism	Common clinical presentations
Candidiasis (*Candida albicans, C. glabrata, C. krusei, C. tropicalis* other *Candida* species)	Fungaemia Colonisation of intravenous cannulae Pneumonia Meningitis Bone and joint infections Endocarditis Endophthalmitis Peritonitis in chronic ambulatory peritoneal dialysis
Aspergillosis (*Aspergillus fumigatus, A. flavus,* other *Aspergillus* species)	Invasive pulmonary aspergillosis Disseminated aspergillosis Aspergilloma Endocarditis
Cryptococcosis (*Cryptococcus neoformans*)	Meningitis Pneumonia Cutaneous infection
Zygomycosis (various species of the genera *Rhizopus, Mucor, Absidia*)	Rhinocerebral infection Pulmonary mucormycosis Surgical wound and burns infection
Malassezia furfur	Cutaneous infection (especially in burn patients) Fungaemia associated with total parenteral nutrition

Clinical presentation

Symptoms can be non-specific, such as low-grade fever, night sweats, weight loss, cough, chest pain and septic shock in extreme cases (Table 43.6).

Diagnosis

Organ-specific radiological findings backed by laboratory tests, as discussed earlier in this chapter, are the mainstay of diagnosis.

Treatment

Compared with the vast array of antibacterial agents available to treat bacterial infections, very few systemic antifungal agents are available and these comprise four major categories: the polyenes (conventional and lipid formulations of amphotericin B), the triazoles (fluconazole, itraconazole, voriconazole and posaconazole), the echinocandins (caspofungin, anidulafungin and micafungin) and flucytosine. To provide optimal therapy to the patient, it is necessary to understand the profile, properties and toxicity of these agents. Table 43.7 details the antifungal spectrum of activity against common fungi.

Antifungal prophylaxis is commonly used to prevent invasive fungal infections in the 'at-risk' group of patients.

Polyenes

Amphotericin B. Amphotericin, a member of the polyene group, is obtained from various species of *Streptomyces*. Chemically, it is a large carbon ring of 37 carbon atoms closed by a lactone bond. One side of the molecule contains seven

Table 43.6 Clinical presentation of systemic fungal infection

Condition	Clinical presentation
Fungaemia (the presence of fungi in the bloodstream), usually due to *Candida* species	Fever, low blood pressure and sometimes other features of septic shock, especially in patients with neutropenia Relatively low-grade fungaemias such as those associated with colonised intravenous cannulae often present only with fever Disseminated infection to multiple organ systems is quite common with *Candida* species, leading to central nervous system disease, endocarditis, endophthalmitis, skin infections, renal disease, and bone and joint infection
Pneumonia, most frequently due to *Aspergillus* species	Fever, chest pain and cough which may be non-productive; may progress rapidly, especially with *Aspergillus* infection, to severe respiratory distress, necrosis of the lung and pulmonary haemorrhage Formation of fungal balls in pre-existing lung cavities with or without invasion
Meningitis and other central nervous system infection	*Candida* infection may present as a typical meningitis, although it is often more insidious Aspergillosis is associated with headache, confusion and focal neurological signs due to the presence of brain infarcts Cryptococcosis most frequently presents as a chronic, insidious meningitis with headache and alteration in mental state
Mucormycosis	Angioinvasive; the most common presentation of mucormycosis is rhinocerebral infection Initially an infection of the sinuses, it then spreads locally to the palate, orbit and eventually into the brain, leading to encephalitis Pulmonary disease can present as fungal balls radiologically with symptoms of haemoptysis

Table 43.7 Antifungal spectrum of activity against common fungi

Organism	AmB[a]	Flu	Itr	Vor	Pos	Anidulafungin	Caspofungin	Micafungin	Flucytosine
Aspergillus species	+	−	+	+	+	+	+	+	−
A. flavus	±	−	+	+	+	+	+	+	−
A. fumigatus	+	−	+	+	+	+	+	+	−
A. niger	+	−	±	+	+	+	+	+	−
A. terreus	−	−	+	+	+	+	+	+	−
Candida species	+	+	+	+	+	+	+	+	+
C. albicans	+	+	+	+	+	+	+	+	+
C. glabrata	+	±	±	+	+	+	+	+	+
C. krusei	+	−	±	+	+	+	+	+	±
C. lusitaniae	−	+	+	+	+	+	+	+	±
C. parapsilosis	+	+	+	+	+	±	±	±	+
C. tropicalis	+	+	+	+	+	+	+	+	+
Cryptococcus neoformans	+	+	+	+	+	−	−	−	+
Coccidioides species	+	+	+	+	+	±[b]	±[b]	±[b]	−
Blastomyces	+	+	+	+	+	±[b]	±[b]	±[b]	−
Histoplasma species	+	+	+	+	+	±[b]	±[b]	±[b]	−
Fusarium species	±	−	−	+	+	−	−	−	−
Scedosporium apiospermum	±	−	±	+	+	−	−	−	−
Scedosporium prolificans	−	−	−	±	±	−	−	−	−
Zygomycetes	±	−	−	−	+	−	−	−	−

Plus signs (+) indicate that the antifungal agent has activity against the organism specified. Minus signs (−) indicate that the antifungal agent does not have activity against the organism specified. Plus/minus signs (±) indicate the agent has variable activity against the organism specified.
[a]Includes lipid formulations.
[b]In vitro data show that the echinocandins (specifically, micafungin) may have variable activity against the dimorphic fungi, depending on whether they are in the mycelial or yeastlike form.
AmB, Amphotericin B; Flu, fluconazole; Itr, itraconazole; Pos, posaconazole; Vor, voriconazole.
Adapted from Dodds Ashley et al. (2006).

carbon-to-carbon double bonds (polyene), and the other side contains seven hydroxyl groups. It dissolves in organic polar solvents but forms a colloidal suspension of micelles in water which is rendered stable by the addition of the surfactant sodium deoxycholate.

Amphotericin B binds to the ergosterol in fungal cytoplasmic membrane affecting its integrity by forming pores and, therefore, cell death. Nystatin, the other polyene, is only used topically because of toxicity associated with its systemic use.

Amphotericin is active against a vast majority of fungi, and this is the same for all formulations. Development of resistance is uncommon, although primary resistance has been identified for *Aspergillus terreus*, *Scedosporium* spp., *Trichosporon* spp. and *Candida lusitaniae*.

Pharmacodynamically, the ratio of the peak serum concentration to the MIC is important for its efficacy.

Amphotericin B deoxycholate. Released in 1950, colloidal in nature, amphotericin B deoxycholate is highly protein bound (99%) and insoluble in water. It penetrates poorly into cerebrospinal fluid (CSF). Initial elimination of the drug occurs with a half-life of 24–48 hours, but this is followed by very slow elimination (half-life about 14 days). As a consequence, it may take 10 weeks for the drug to disappear from the circulation.

Amphotericin B deoxycholate is given by slow intravenous (IV) infusion (manufacturer recommends between 2 and 6 hours) in 5% dextrose with a dose range of 0.25–1 mg/kg increased to 1.5 mg/kg for serious invasive infections. The duration of treatment can vary from 1 to 2 weeks to longer, depending on the severity of the infection and the organ system involved.

The most serious side effect of amphotericin is nephrotoxicity. Renal failure should be monitored regularly at least every other day, and if the serum creatinine exceeds 250 mmol/L, the drug should be discontinued until the creatinine level is below this limit. Hypokalaemia is also a problem and may be severe, necessitating replacement therapy.

Azotaemia may be seen in patients after the first few infusions of amphotericin B deoxycholate. Chills, fever and tachypnoea may occur but can be avoided by prescribing hydrocortisone 25–50 mg.

The manufacturer recommends that before commencing treatment, a 1 mg test dose should be given in 50 mL of 5% dextrose over a 20- to 30-minute period and the patient monitored for fever, rigors and hypotension. True allergic reactions are rare.

Amphotericin B lipid formulations. The advantage of delivering amphotericin encapsulated in liposomes or as a complex with lipid molecules is that a higher unit dose can be given and there is reduction in toxic effects. Three such preparations are currently available: liposomal amphotericin B (AmBisome), amphotericin B lipid complex (Abelcet) and amphotericin B colloidal dispersion (Amphocil).

Liposomal amphotericin B. In liposomal amphotericin B (AmBisome), the drug is contained in small vesicles, each consisting of a phospholipid bilayer enclosing an aqueous environment. This permits the delivery of higher doses (3 mg/kg once daily is recommended, but doses up to 10 mg/kg have been used in some centres) compared with conventional amphotericin, with very little of the immediate toxicity which is such a problem with the conventional formulation. Higher peak serum concentrations are obtained with the liposomal formulation compared with equivalent doses of the conventional drug, although it is not certain whether this is clinically relevant. Liposomal amphotericin is concentrated mainly in the liver and spleen, where it is taken up by cells of the reticuloendothelial system. Concentrations in the lung and kidneys are much lower, which may or may not be clinically important.

There is reduced nephrotoxicity with this formulation, and some of the renal dysfunction which has been described in clinical trials of liposomal amphotericin may have been due to concomitant drugs. Comparative clinical trials of liposomal amphotericin versus conventional amphotericin B have shown reduced toxicity because of the liposomal preparation (Cagnoni, 2002; Hamill, 2013; Walsh et al., 1999). It is this comparative lack of toxicity which accounts for much of the popularity of this agent, despite its expense. This agent performs as well as the conventional preparation in patients with febrile neutropenia (Cagnoni, 2002).

Amphotericin B lipid complex and amphotericin B colloidal dispersion. Amphotericin B lipid complex (Abelcet) is not a liposomal formulation, but consists of large sheets of amphotericin combined with phospholipids. This formulation gives lower peak serum levels compared with the conventional drug because it is rapidly taken up by tissue macrophages, whereas concentrations in the lungs and the liver are much higher. Patients seem to experience more immediate side effects than with liposomal amphotericin. There is less clinical trial evidence for the use of this agent compared with the liposomal preparation. Amphotericin B colloidal dispersion (Amphocil) is a formulation consisting of tiny discs of amphotericin and cholesterylsulphate. Like the lipid complex, it too produces low peak serum levels but high liver concentrations compared with the conventional drug. There is less clinical experience with this preparation than with the liposomal preparation, and it appears to have a higher incidence of certain adverse reactions than conventional amphotericin.

Choosing a lipid preparation. At present, the greatest clinical experience is with liposomal amphotericin B, and by reason of this and the reduced incidence of side effects it is the preferred agent of the three in many UK centres. Ideally all patients who require amphotericin would receive the conventional preparation initially, being changed to a lipid formulation only if they do not respond to or cannot tolerate the side effects of the conventional form. However, the incidence of side effects and the difficulty in administration of conventional amphotericin have in practice led to its replacement in most centres with a lipid formulation.

Other Antifungal Agent

Flucytosine. Amphotericin B and griseofulvin were the only systemic antifungal agents available until the early 1970s, when flucytosine became available for patient use.

Flucytosine (5-fluorocytosine) is a synthetic fluorinated nucleotide analogue. The mode of action is twofold. Following uptake by the cell, which is dependent on the presence of cytosine permease, flucytosine is deaminated to 5-fluorouracil by cytosine deaminase. This in turn is incorporated into fungal RNA in place of uracil, leading to impairment of protein synthesis. Further metabolism of 5-fluorouracil leads to a metabolite that inhibits the enzyme thymidylate synthetase, leading to inhibition of DNA synthesis. Mammalian cells have absent or weak cytosine deaminase activity which accounts for the selective toxicity of flucytosine.

For all practical purposes, flucytosine is only active against yeasts and yeastlike fungi. Inherent resistance occurs in approximately 10% of clinical isolates of *Candida* species, and acquired resistance develops rapidly if the drug is used alone. There are several resistance mechanisms, some of which result from a single-step mutation giving a high frequency of acquired resistance in organisms exposed to the drug. For this reason, flucytosine should always be given in combination with another agent such as amphotericin, with which it is synergistic.

Flucytosine is highly soluble in water, and more than 90% of an oral dose is absorbed from the gastro-intestinal tract. Virtually all of the absorbed dose is excreted unchanged in the urine by glomerular filtration. The elimination half-life is about 4 hours, but this is greatly prolonged in renal failure, and dosage modification is required in patients with renal dysfunction. The degree of protein binding is very low and flucytosine penetrates well into all tissues, including the aqueous humour of the eye, where about 10% of the serum level is achieved, and the cerebral spinal fluid, where about 80% of the serum level is achieved.

Flucytosine is given orally or by short IV infusion. The dosage administered by either route in patients with normal renal function is 100–200 mg/kg per day in four divided doses. This must be reduced in renal failure, but the degree of reduction depends on the degree of renal impairment, and it is obligatory to monitor the serum levels of flucytosine. Unfortunately, because the flucytosine assay is now rarely carried out routinely in UK laboratories, the sample is sent to a specialist laboratory. Monitoring is usually only carried out if there is a concern about the patient's renal function. Flucytosine is usually given in conjunction with amphotericin, which will probably cause some degree of renal dysfunction, therefore requiring modification of the flucytosine dose. Blood levels should be taken as per local guidelines to avoid dose-related marrow toxicity.

Some of the side effects of flucytosine are given in Table 43.3. The most important toxic effect is a dose-related myelosuppression with neutropenia and thrombocytopenia. This is usually reversible and can be avoided by monitoring serum levels of flucytosine and adjusting the dose accordingly. Hepatotoxicity is also probably a result of high serum levels, and liver function tests should be performed regularly. The drug is teratogenic in some animals and is not recommended in pregnant women for relatively trivial infections such as a fungal urinary tract infection. In cases of a life-threatening fungal infection, which is rare in pregnancy, the potential benefits of flucytosine must be weighed against the possible risks.

Azoles

Systemic azoles: Triazoles. Four triazoles are licensed in the UK: fluconazole, itraconazole, voriconazole and posaconazole. They differ substantially from one another in their pharmacokinetic and antifungal activity (Table 43.8). Their main side effects are listed in Table 43.3.

The basic chemical structure of the triazoles is the azole ring, a five-membered ring containing three nitrogen atoms. Their principal mode of action involves one of the nitrogen atoms of the azole ring binding to fungal cytochrome P450 enzymes. This inhibits the demethylation of lanosterol and leads to a reduced concentration of ergosterol necessary for a normal fungal cytoplasmic membrane.

Table 43.8 Comparative pharmacokinetics of antifungal agents

Pharmacokinetic parameter	Antifungal agent											
	AmB	ABCD	ABLC	LAB	Flu	Itra	Vor	Pos	Anidu-lafungin	Caspo-fungin	Mica-fungin	Flucyto-sine
Oral bioavailability (%)	<5	<5	<5	<5	95	50	96	ND	<5	<5	<5	80
Food effect	NA	NA	NA	NA	NE	ES	ES	Food	NA	NA	NA	NE
Distribution												
Total C_{max} (micrograms/mL)	0.5–2	4	131	0.1	0.7	11	4.6	7.8	0.83	0.27	0.24	80
AUC (mg × h/L)	17	43	14	555	400	29.2	20.3	8.9	99[b]	119	158[b]	62
Protein binding (%)	>95	>95	>95	>95	10	99.8	58	99	84	97	99	4
CSF penetration (%)	0–4	<5	<5	<5	>60	<10	60	NR	<5	<5	<5	75
Vitreal penetration (%)	0–38[c,d]	0–38[c,d]	0–38[c,d]	0–38[c,d]	28–75[c,d]	10[c]	38[c]	26[c,d]	0[d]	0[c]	<1[d]	49[d]
Urine penetration (%)[e]	3–20	<5	<5	4.5	90	1–10	<2	<2	<2	<2	<2	90
Metabolism	Minor Hep	Unknown	Unknown	Unknown	Minor Hep	Hep	Hep	Hep	None	Hep	Hep	Minor intestinal
Elimination	Faeces	Unknown	Unknown	Unknown	Urine	Hep	Renal	Faeces	Faeces	Urine	Faeces	Renal
Half-life (h)	50	30	173	100–153	31	24	6	25	26	30	15	3–6

[a]Data are for oral solution.
[b]For dosages of 100 mg/day.
[c]Human.
[d]Animal.
[e]Percentage of active drug or metabolites.
ABCD, Amphotericin B colloidal dispersion; ABLC, amphotericin B lipid complex; AmB, amphotericin B; AUC, area under the concentration curve; C_{max}, peak drug concentration; CSF, cerebrospinal fluid; ES, empty stomach; Flu, fluconazole, Hep, hepatic; Itra, itraconazole; LAB, liposomal amphotericin B; NA, not applicable; ND, no data; NE, no effect; NR, not reported; Pos, posaconazole; Vor, voriconazole.
Adapted from Dodds Ashley et al. (2006).

The propensity, in humans, to also inhibit the metabolism of drugs by cytochrome P450 results in a considerable number of drug interactions.

Fluconazole. Fluconazole is available both orally and parenterally and is used only in the treatment and prophylaxis of infections due to yeasts and yeastlike fungi. It is not used for the treatment of infections caused by moulds. It is highly effective in the treatment of *Cryptococcus* infection, but the first-line treatment of cryptococcosis of the central nervous system (CNS) is the combination of amphotericin B plus flucytosine for CNS infection caused by this organism. This may be followed by fluconazole, which in HIV-infected patients will be required lifelong as suppressive treatment to prevent relapse. In immunocompetent hosts, fluconazole may be used as the primary treatment for disease not involving the CNS, such as pulmonary infection.

In patients with candidaemia due to colonised IV cannulae, the most important treatment is removal of the infected cannula, but it is common practice to give a short course of fluconazole (until *Candida* speciation and susceptibility results are available) to prevent disseminated infection elsewhere. Although not proven in randomised clinical trials, changing potentially infected central-line catheters in patients with candidaemia is probably the most important part of therapy.

In non-neutropenic patients, studies have shown fluconazole and caspofungin to be as efficacious as and less toxic than conventional amphotericin B. In such patients, where the infecting organism and its susceptibility to fluconazole are known, it would be reasonable to commence treatment with fluconazole; caspofungin is a potential alternative. In patients with neutropenia and in patients infected with fluconazole-resistant organisms, amphotericin continues to be the treatment of choice. Fluconazole has also been successfully used as prophylaxis against *Candida* infections in patients with neutropenia and patients with AIDS, but this in turn has been associated with an increasing incidence of systemic infections with fluconazole-resistant strains.

Some units that use fluconazole extensively have noted an increase in the isolation of yeasts resistant to the drug, with the prevalence of resistance related to the extent of use of fluconazole. Resistance in *Candida* species is mainly seen in patients who are given long-term prophylactic fluconazole. This selects out those *Candida* species such as *C. krusei* and *C. glabrata* that are inherently less susceptible to fluconazole. Resistance in *C. albicans*, the most common species infecting humans, is seen mainly in patients with AIDS, partly because of the extensive use of fluconazole in treating severe oral and pharyngeal candidiasis in such patients and partly because of the very large numbers of yeasts in the oropharynx of patients with AIDS with candidiasis, which increases the chance of resistance due to spontaneous mutation.

Depending on the type of deep infection and the organ involved, fluconazole is used between the range of 200 and 800 mg/day. It is available for oral and IV use. Oral fluconazole has very good bioavailability (nearly 90%) and with a long half-life of about 34 hours, it is given once a day. It has good penetration in most tissues and all body fluids including the CSF. Because there is good correlation between clinical outcome and fluconazole's pharmacokinetic/pharmacodynamics parameters, therapeutic drug monitoring is not required. Fluconazole is a substrate for inhibition of CYP450 isoenzymes, including CYP3A4, CYP2C9, and CYP2C19; therefore, medications should be reviewed for potential drug interactions. Amongst antibiotics, rifampicin is the single CYP450 inducer that has been shown to markedly reduce fluconazole serum concentrations.

Itraconazole. Itraconazole is available for both oral and IV use (IV formulation may not always be available). The drug is available as capsules and as a liquid; however, the liquid formulation gives better absorption and pharmacokinetic profile than the capsule preparation, leading to significantly greater bioavailability and higher serum levels. Systemic bioavailability of itraconazole oral solution is around 55% optimised under fasting conditions. Itraconazole is extensively metabolised by the liver, predominantly by the CYP 3A4 isoenzyme system, and is known to undergo enterohepatic circulation. This is a broad-spectrum antifungal which is effective against yeasts, dermatophytes, the 'pathogenic' fungi and some filamentous fungi, such as *Aspergillus*.

In deep-seated infection, itraconazole is used to treat infections caused by the 'pathogenic' fungi, but there is less published evidence of its use in the treatment of systemic candidiasis, and it cannot be recommended for this purpose (Maertens and Boogaerts, 2005). However, although not a first-line agent for systemic candidiasis, it may be useful in patients who are infected with strains resistant to fluconazole, some of which may remain sensitive to itraconazole, and in patients who are for some reason unable to tolerate fluconazole. It has also been used to treat cryptococcosis, despite its poor penetration of CSF, and in that condition it is an alternative to fluconazole for patients who cannot take the latter drug.

There is now considerable evidence to support the use of itraconazole as a prophylactic agent in immunocompromised patients. It has been shown to be effective in reducing the incidence of systemic fungal infection compared with placebo and to be more effective than fluconazole, although this is due to a greater reduction in infections caused by filamentous fungi, including *Aspergillus*.

A loading dose of itraconazole 200 mg three times a day for 3 days is administered to achieve steady-state serum concentration, followed by 200 mg daily or twice a day. Therapeutic drug monitoring is essential to optimise clinical efficacy for prophylaxis or for treatment of invasive fungal infection.

Voriconazole. Voriconazole is available for both oral and IV administration. It has advantages over itraconazole in that its absorption from the gastro-intestinal tract is significantly better and is not affected by reductions in gastric acidity due to disease or concomitant medication. Its spectrum of activity is similar to that of itraconazole, but it is more active against *Fusarium* species, a mould which causes superficial infection of the nails and cornea, and occasionally systemic infection in immunocompromised patients.

Voriconazole given orally is rapidly and almost fully absorbed (oral bioavailability >90%), with a maximum serum concentration being achieved in about 2 hours after administration under fasting conditions. It is extensively distributed into tissue and penetrates well into the CSF and into vitreous and aqueous humour.

It is cleared by hepatic cytochrome P450 metabolism and is involved in many clinically relevant drug–drug interactions. Therapeutic drug monitoring may be indicated in some clinical settings.

The main clinical indication for the use of voriconazole is aspergillosis (Karthaus, 2011). Studies have shown improved efficacy compared with conventional amphotericin B in systemic *Aspergillus* infection. The largest randomised control trial demonstrates that voriconazole is superior to amphotericin B deoxycholate as primary therapy of aspergillosis (Walsh et al., 2008). One particular indication is cerebral aspergillosis. Although rare, this carries a high mortality rate (≥90%), and one study has shown this to be reduced by voriconazole, presumably because of its better penetration into the CNS (Schwartz et al., 2005). In addition to aspergillosis, voriconazole is also licensed for the treatment of *Fusarium* infection and for the management of patients infected with strains of *Candida* resistant to fluconazole. It has been shown to be as efficacious as amphotericin B followed by fluconazole in the treatment of candidaemia in patients who were not neutropenic, but it is not licensed for this indication.

For invasive pulmonary aspergillosis, a loading dose of 6 mg/kg IV every 12 hours for 2 doses was given followed by 4 mg/kg every 12 hours and converted to oral therapy 200 mg every 12 hours depending on clinical review to decide duration of treatment.

Voriconazole has a side-effect profile similar to that of other triazoles. Two adverse effects associated with voriconazole are visual disturbance (appearance of bright lights, colour changes or wavy lines) in 45% of patients and cutaneous phototoxicity (rash) in 8% patients. Both side effects are reversible after discontinuation of therapy.

Posaconazole. Posaconazole is the latest triazole to be made available for clinical use. It has activity against a wide range of yeasts (including *Cryptococcus* and many species of *Candida*) and a variety of moulds. Like itraconazole, it is absorbed slowly, is highly protein bound (>98%) and reaches a steady state after a period of 7–10 days. In contrast with voriconazole, optimal absorption is achieved when taken with a high-fat meal. It is available for oral use only in the form of tablets and oral suspension. Posaconazole penetrates very well in most tissues and fluid including CSF and the eye.

In adults it is indicated for treatment of invasive aspergillosis and fusariosis refractory to amphotericin, chromoblastomycosis and mycetoma refractory to itraconazole, and for prophylaxis of invasive fungal infections in patients with HSCT with graft-versus-host disease and haematological malignancies with prolonged neutropenia.

Posaconazole oral suspension is used 200 mg four times daily or 400 mg twice daily, and tablets are used 300 mg twice daily on first day followed by 300 mg daily.

Echinocandins. The echinocandin group of antifungal agents acts by inhibiting synthesis of fungal cell wall glucan.

Caspofungin. Caspofungin was the first of the echinocandins to become available for routine use; others, such as micafungin and anidulafungin, are now available. These agents interfere with the production of the fungal cell wall by inhibiting the synthesis of an important component, 1,3-β-D-glucan. This is a target which does not exist in mammalian cells, providing selective toxicity against fungi. Caspofungin has a significant advantage over the triazoles in that it does not inhibit the cytochrome P450 system and, therefore, is not associated with such a wide range of drug interactions.

The drug has a rather unusual spectrum of activity. It is active against most species of *Candida*, although some are less susceptible than others, but *Cryptococcus* is resistant. The commonly encountered species of *Aspergillus* are susceptible, but the drug is inactive against the dermatophytes, and activity against other fungi is variable.

Caspofungin is available only for administration via the IV route and does not penetrate into the CSF. Due to its spectrum of activity, caspofungin is indicated only for empirical treatment (in patients with neutropenia) and targeted treatment of candidiasis and aspergillosis. A comparative study showed caspofungin to be as efficacious as conventional amphotericin B in invasive candidiasis (Mora-Duarte et al., 2002). It has been shown to be effective in patients with aspergillosis who did not respond to or could not tolerate other antifungal agents. Finally, caspofungin was also shown to be as effective as liposomal amphotericin B in the empirical treatment of fungal infection in patients with neutropenia, and it had a lower incidence of unwanted effects (Walsh et al., 2004). The dosage for adults is 70 mg on the first day, then 50 mg once daily (70 mg once daily if body weight is more than 80 kg).

Anidulafungin. Anidulafungin is only available for administration via the IV route and is used in the treatment of invasive candidiasis in adult non-neutropenic patients (Reboli et al., 2007). Like caspofungin, it does not penetrate into the CSF. It is given as a single 200 mg loading dose by IV infusion on day 1, followed by 100 mg daily thereafter. No dose adjustment is required for renal or hepatic impairment.

Micafungin. Micafungin is very similar to caspofungin and anidulafungin. It is used for treatment of candidaemia, invasive candidiasis in adults and children if other antifungals are not appropriate. It is also used for treatment of oesophageal candidiasis if IV therapy is required and for prophylaxis of *Candida* infections in immunocompromised patients following HSCT. It is used between 1 and 3 mg/kg per day in patients ≤40 kg body weight and between 50 and 100 mg/day in greater than 40 kg body weight. No dose adjustment is necessary for renal or mild-to-moderate hepatic failure.

Choice of treatment

A recent development has been the use of combinations of antifungal agents to improve on the results of single agents. Currently, there is little firm evidence to support the use of such combinations. Amphotericin B plus flucytosine in the treatment of cryptococcosis is the only combination where evidence exists of increased efficacy over either agent alone. However, faced with a seriously ill patient who is not responding to single agents, it is not surprising that many clinicians attempt the use of a combination of antifungals, even though the evidence is that the results are no better than monotherapy.

Practice points regarding the drug toxicity in systemic antifungal agents are detailed in Table 43.9.

Table 43.9 Practice points

Drug toxicity in systemic antifungal agents	
Infusion-related side effects	• Particularly with conventional amphotericin B • Lipid-based preparations also show these, but to a lesser extent
Nephrotoxicity	• Particularly with conventional amphotericin B • Results in renal dysfunction • Cessation of treatment may be required • Drug-level monitoring is not helpful in prevention • Potassium loss and hypokalaemia are a serious complication • Renal toxicity may be potentiated by concomitant nephrotoxic agents
Hepatotoxicity	• Associated with the azole antifungals • Was particularly severe with ketoconazole • The newer triazoles may also cause serious liver damage
Bone marrow suppression	• Associated with flucytosine • Dose-related problem, so drug-level monitoring may help prevent it • Tends to preclude the use of flucytosine in patients whose marrow is already damaged (e.g. in haematological malignancy or following bone marrow transplant)
Drug interactions	• Associated particularly with the azoles • Due to their mode of action in inhibiting the cytochrome P450 system • A wide range of drugs may be affected, some with serious interactions

Difficulties in drug administration	
Drug precipitation	• Amphotericin B will precipitate out if given in electrolyte-containing infusions • This may also happen in 5% dextrose due to acidity resulting from the manufacturing process
Need for a test dose	• Required for all amphotericin B preparations
Long infusion times and/or large infusion volumes	• A particular problem with conventional amphotericin • Long infusion times mean reduced access to intravenous cannulae for other purposes • Large infusion volumes may be undesirable in patients with renal or cardiac dysfunction
Variable absorption when taken by mouth	• A known problem with itraconazole • Absorption is reduced in the presence of raised gastric pH (e.g. following the use of antacids or drugs such as omeprazole) • Absorption is increased in the presence of food or if taken with a cola drink • Subtherapeutic levels may occur because of poor absorption • Therapeutic drug monitoring is recommended to avoid low levels

Resistance to antifungal agents	
Amphotericin B	• Usually seen as a very broad-spectrum antifungal, but inherent resistance is seen in several clinically significant species: *Aspergillus terreus* *Candida lusitaniae* *Scedosporium apiospermum* • Acquired resistance developing during treatment is very uncommon • Lipid preparations have identical in vitro antifungal activity to the conventional form

Table 43.9 Practice points—cont'd

Flucytosine	• Acquired resistance during treatment is very common in *Candida* species
	• Monotherapy promotes the rapid development of resistance
	• Combination therapy with amphotericin will reduce the possibility of acquired resistance developing during treatment
Fluconazole	• Some species of *Candida* are inherently resistant or less susceptible to fluconazole: *C. krusei* *C. glabrata*
	• Long-term use of fluconazole may result in increased infections with these more resistant strains
	• Long-term use may also result in reduced susceptibility in strains of *C. albicans*

Case studies

Case 43.1

Ms TH, a 66-year-old woman with carcinoma of the oesophagus, undergoes sub-total oesophagectomy. She spends the early postoperative period on surgical intensive therapy unit (ITU) and is sent to the surgical ward for further management. On day 6 post-operation, she begins to show signs of sepsis, for which antibiotics are commenced. However, 48 hours later she has difficulty in breathing, takes a turn for the worse and is transferred to ITU. Chest imaging revealed a leak from the oesophagectomy site and fluid collection in the pleural space. Gram stain of aspirated pleural fluid reveals budding yeast cells, and mucopurulent sputum culture grows *Candida albicans*.

Question

How should Ms TH's infection be managed?

Answer

The immediate management of this patient would involve drainage of pleural fluid through an intercostal drain and commencement of systemic antifungal therapy. The source is very likely to be oral thrush. Fluconazole at 800 mg once a day, normally for 14–21 days, should be commenced awaiting antifungal sensitivity result. Urgent patient review is indicated to discuss surgical intervention to close the leak. Re-collection of yeasts in inadequately treated spaces can be a problem. It may be useful to consider the addition of a second antifungal agent to fluconazole.

Case 43.2

Mrs DM, a 38-year-old woman with diabetes, sustained severe trauma to the right leg requiring total knee replacement and insertion of metal rod into the right femur. She had an uneventful postoperative course. Four months later, she had to undergo washout and debridement of her prosthetic joint, thigh tissues and removal of the metal rod. Ten deep specimens grew *Candida tropicalis*.

Question

How should Mrs DM's infection be managed?

Answer

Fungal infections of prosthesis and deep subcutaneous tissues are difficult to treat. Mrs DM will need a two- or three-stage procedure. The prosthetic joint will need removal, and antifungal treatment (depending on sensitivity results) will be required for an 8- to 12-week period. Complete debridement of infected tissues, temporary stabilisation of the femur and thorough washout of the joint will be required. In some instances, the antifungal agent in orthopaedic cement can be used to pack the joint space along with systemic antifungal treatment. A new total knee replacement can be planned for a minimum of 3 months (or longer if antifungal treatment is prolonged beyond 3 months for satisfactory clearance of the infection).

Case 43.3

Ms KR, a 27-year-old woman, visits her primary care doctor reporting that her toenails have become distorted and discoloured. It looks unattractive, so she would like it corrected before her summer beach holiday. The primary care doctor makes the clinical diagnosis of tinea unguium (dermatophytosis of the nail), which is confirmed by laboratory culture of nail scrapings. The doctor knows that this condition is unlikely to respond to topical treatment and therefore consults the British National Formulary for a systemic agent. He finds that griseofulvin, terbinafine and itraconazole are all available for this condition. However, the situation is complicated by the fact that his patient tells him that she is trying to become pregnant and does not want to take anything which might harm a baby. At this point, the doctor seeks specialist advice.

Question

What is the most appropriate and safe treatment for Ms KR?

Answer

This is a complex decision. Griseofulvin is contraindicated in pregnancy because of its known teratogenicity in animals; therefore, it is not an appropriate choice for Ms KR. Itraconazole should only be used in life-threatening situations where the potential benefits to the mother outweigh the potential harm to the foetus (Actavis, 2016a). Therefore, it would be difficult to recommend itraconazole to Ms KR.

Terbinafine could be used if the potential benefit outweighs the risk (Actavis, 2016b); foetal toxicity and fertility studies in animals suggest no adverse effects. However, because this is not a serious condition, treating Ms KR with terbinafine would be difficult to justify.

After some discussion, Ms KR decided that she wanted the condition treated more than she wanted to become pregnant and returned to using her oral contraception. Griseofulvin decreases the effectiveness of oral contraceptives, and there are reports of contraceptive failure with imidazoles and oestrogens. Therefore, following this discussion Ms KR decided to take a course of terbinafine.

Case 43.4

Mr DF, an 18-year-old boy with acute myeloblastic leukaemia, sustained 20% accidental burns injury on face, upper body and right arm at a family barbecue. (He had only just recently left hospital after successful antibiotic treatment for a febrile neutropenic episode post-chemotherapy.)

Two weeks after admission to ITU for management of burns, Mr DF underwent a septic episode with septic shock. A blood culture was taken through a central line which showed Gram-negative bacilli. He was commenced on broad-spectrum antibiotics. His peripheral blood count was 3×10^9/L, and he had a markedly raised C-reactive protein level. Mr DF suffered a moderate degree of renal failure. Two days later another blood culture was taken through an arterial line and showed yeast cells on Gram stain. IV fluconazole was added to his treatment. Culture growth from the central line blood culture revealed *Pseudomonas aeruginosa* and *C. albicans*. The arterial blood culture grew *Candida krusei*. Antifungal sensitivities have been requested.

Question

How should Mr DF be managed?

Answer

Treatment of infections in burn patients can be challenging because the loss in skin integrity increases the risk of being colonised with various endogenous and hospital-acquired bacteria and fungi. Patients with haematological malignancies and chemotherapy treatment are more vulnerable to opportunistic infections.

Ideally antibiotics should be avoided in a patient who has an invasive fungal infection because it is believed that killing the bacterial flora helps fungi thrive in the absence of commensal competition. In this case, Mr DF has concomitant Gram-negative sepsis and lacks a strong bodily defence system because of his underlying disease condition.

Candida krusei is known to be resistant to fluconazole. It is difficult to treat IV catheter and other line infections with systemic antibiotics and antifungals alone. It is imperative that these lines are removed and treatment given through temporary peripheral lines for at least 48 hours before a new central line is inserted. New lines are very likely to become colonised with the same micro-organisms if inserted too early. Both *C. albicans* and *C. krusei* can be treated with a lipid formulation of amphotericin. The use of non-lipid conventional formulations of amphotericin should be avoided because Mr DF has a moderate degree of renal failure. The duration of treatment should be decided by reviewing the patient daily; this would include imaging and echocardiograms for up to 2 weeks to look for seeding of *Candida* in other organs. Choice of antifungals can be reviewed after antifungal sensitivity is available, and amphotericin can be switched to caspofungin if necessary.

Case 43.5

Mr TH, a 78-year-old male gardener, sustained an eye injury while cleaning out old dried plants from his client's garden. He sustained a laceration to the cornea and presented to eye casualty 48 hours after the incident. He was started on topical and systemic antibiotics. A corneal scrape revealed no organisms on Gram stain but grew *Fusarium* species on culture plates 4 days later.

Question

How will Mr TH be managed, and what are the further associated risks to his eye?

Answer

If there is no bacterial growth, the antibiotics can be stopped. Topical antifungal agents in the form of eye drops like natamycin or amphotericin B (if available) should be commenced and administered frequently.

The associated risk is from the spread of infection to the back of the eye with development of endophthalmitis. Urgent surgical vitrectomy and washout, with instillation of intravitreal antifungal agent (amphotericin B 5 micrograms) would be indicated, along with systemic antifungal therapy with amphotericin B 1.5 mg/kg or voriconazole 4 mg/kg every 12 hours and converted to oral therapy 200 mg every 12 hours.

References

Actavis, 2016a. Itraconazole 100 mg capsules. Available at: https://www.med icines.org.uk/emc/medicine/24176#CLINICAL_PARTS.

Actavis, 2016b. Terbinafine 250 mg tablets. Available at: https://www.medic ines.org.uk/emc/medicine/18150.

Cagnoni, P.J., 2002. Liposomal amphotericin B versus conventional amphotericin B in the empirical treatment of persistently febrile neutropenic patients. J. Antimicrob. Chemother. 49 (Suppl. 1), 81–86.

Dodds Ashley, E.S., Lewis, R., Lewis, S.J., et al., 2006. Pharmacology of systemic antifungal agents. Clin. Infect. Dis. 43, S28–S39.

Hamill, R.J., 2013. Amphotericin B formulations: a comparative review of efficacy and toxicity. Drugs 73, 919–934.

Karthaus, M., 2011. Prophylaxis and treatment of invasive aspergillosis with voriconazole, posaconazole and caspofungin – review of the literature. Eur. J. Med. Res. 16, 145–152.

Maertens, J., Boogaerts, M., 2005. The place for itraconazole in treatment. J. Antimicrob. Chemother. 56, i33–i38.

Marr, K.A., Carter, R.A., Crippa, F., et al., 2002. Epidemiology and outcome of mould infections in hematopoietic stem cell transplant recipients. Clin. Infect. Dis. 34, 909–917.

Mora-Duarte, J., Betts, R., Rotstein, C., et al., 2002. Comparison of caspofungin and amphotericin B for invasive candidiasis. N. Engl. J. Med. 347, 2020–2029.

Pappas, P.G., Kauffman, C.A., Andes, D., et al., 2009. Clinical practice guidelines for the management of candidiasis: 2009 update by the Infectious Diseases Society of America. Clin. Infect. Dis. 48, 503–553.

Reboli, A.C., Rotstein, C., Pappas, P.G., et al., 2007. Anidulafungin versus fluconazole for invasive candidiasis. N. Engl. J. Med. 356, 2472–2482.

Schwartz, S., Ruhnke, M., Ribaud, P., et al., 2005. Improved outcome in central nervous system aspergillosis, using voriconazole treatment. Blood 106, 2641–2645.

Walsh, T.J., Finberg, R.W., Arndt, C., et al., 1999. Liposomal amphotericin B for empirical therapy in patients with persistent fever and neutropenia. N. Engl. J. Med. 340, 764–771.

Walsh, T.J., Tepple, R.H., Donowitz, G.R., et al., 2004. Caspofungin versus liposomal amphotericin B for empirical antifungal therapy in patients with persistent fever and neutropenia. N. Engl. J. Med. 351, 1391–1402.

Walsh, T.J., Anaissie, E.J., Denning, D.W., et al., 2008. Treatment of aspergillosis: clinical practice guidelines of the Infectious Diseases Society of America. Clin. Infect. Dis. 46, 327–360.

Further reading

Bennett, J.E., 2010. Introduction to mycoses. In: Mandell, G.L., Bennett, J.E., Dolin, R. (Eds.), Principles and Practice of Infectious Diseases, seventh ed. Elsevier, Philadelphia, pp. 3221–3240.

Hay, R.J., 2010. Dermatophytosis and other superficial mycoses. In: Mandell, G.L., Bennett, J.E., Dolin, R. (Eds.), Principles and Practice of Infectious Diseases, seventh ed. Elsevier, Philadelphia, pp. 3345–3355.

Pfaller, M.A., Pappas, P.G., Wingard, J.R., 2006. Invasive fungal pathogens: current epidemiological trends. Clin. Infect. Dis. 43, S3–S14.

Mandell, G.L., Bennett, J.E., Dolin, R. (Eds.), 2014. Principles and Practice of Infectious Diseases, eighth ed. Elsevier, Philadelphia.

Winn, W., Allen, S., Janda, W., et al., 2006. Mycology. Koneman's Colour Atlas and Textbook of Diagnostic Microbiology, sixth ed. Lippincott Williams and Wilkins, Philadelphia, pp. 1153–1232.

Useful websites

British Society for Medical Mycology – for fungal updates access: http://www.bsmm.org

Centers for Disease Control and Prevention – for fungal updates access: http://www.cdc.gov/fungal

44 Thyroid and Parathyroid Disorders

Atul Kalhan and Mike D. Page

Key points

- Thyroid dysfunction is extremely common in clinical practice, with estimated prevalence rate of primary hypothyroidism and hyperthyroidism stated to be 1–2% and 0.4–2% of the population, respectively, based on epidemiological studies.

- Iodine deficiency remains the commonest cause of thyroid dysfunction worldwide, leading to enlarged and underactive thyroid gland while autoimmune thyroid disorders are more common in iodine-replete areas.

- The treatment of hypothyroidism requires lifelong levothyroxine therapy and monitoring. Commonly used medications such as antacids, iron, calcium tablets, and proton pump inhibitors may interfere with absorption of levothyroxine therapy.

- Thyroxine replacement therapy should be introduced with caution in the elderly, particularly those with cardiac disease.

- Thyroxine replacement therapy can be given weekly in patients who forget their daily doses or who are unable to self-medicate.

- Thyrotoxicosis can be treated with thionamide therapy, radioiodine, or surgery. The choice will largely be determined by the age of the patient, the cause of the thyrotoxicosis, the severity of the condition, comorbidity and patient preference.

- Patients treated with thionamide therapy require careful counselling about the symptoms and management of agranulocytosis and should be given written guidance.

- Elective parathyroidectomy is indicated in a select group of patients with primary hyperparathyroidism based on the age of the patient and/or evidence of end organ damage (osteoporosis, renal stones, renal impairment, etc.).

- Hypoparathyroidism can occur after thyroid surgery. It is managed with vitamin D analogues and requires lifelong monitoring.

Thyroid physiology

The thyroid gland consists of two lobes and is situated in the lower neck. The gland synthesises, stores and releases two major metabolically active hormones: tetra-iodothyronine (thyroxine $[T_4]$) and tri-iodothyronine (T_3). Regulation of hormone synthesis is by variable secretion of the glycoprotein hormone thyroid-stimulating hormone (TSH) from the anterior pituitary. In turn TSH is regulated by hypothalamic secretion of the tripeptide

thyrotrophin-releasing hormone (TRH) (Fig. 44.1). Low circulating levels of thyroid hormones initiate the release of TSH and probably also TRH. Rising levels of TSH promote increased iodide trapping by the gland and a subsequent increase in thyroid hormone synthesis. The increase in circulating hormone levels feeds back on the pituitary and hypothalamus, shutting off TRH, TSH and further hormone synthesis.

Both T_4 and T_3 are produced within the follicular cells in the thyroid. The stages in synthesis are shown in Fig. 44.2. In summary:

- Thyroglobulin and thyroid peroxidase are synthesised by follicular cells.
- Hydrogen peroxide (H_2O_2) is synthesised at the luminal membrane.
- Dietary inorganic iodide is trapped from the circulation and transported to the follicular lumen, where it is oxidised by H_2O_2.

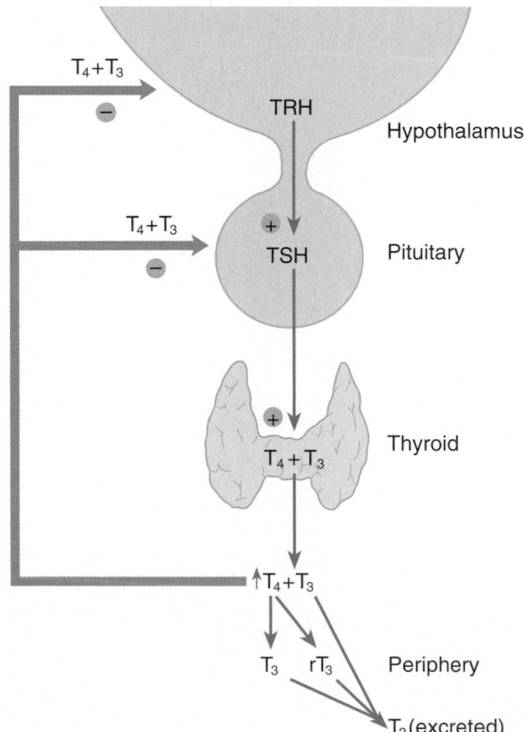

Fig. 44.1 Control of thyroid hormone secretion.
TRH, thyrotrophin-releasing hormone; TSH, thyroid-stimulating hormone.

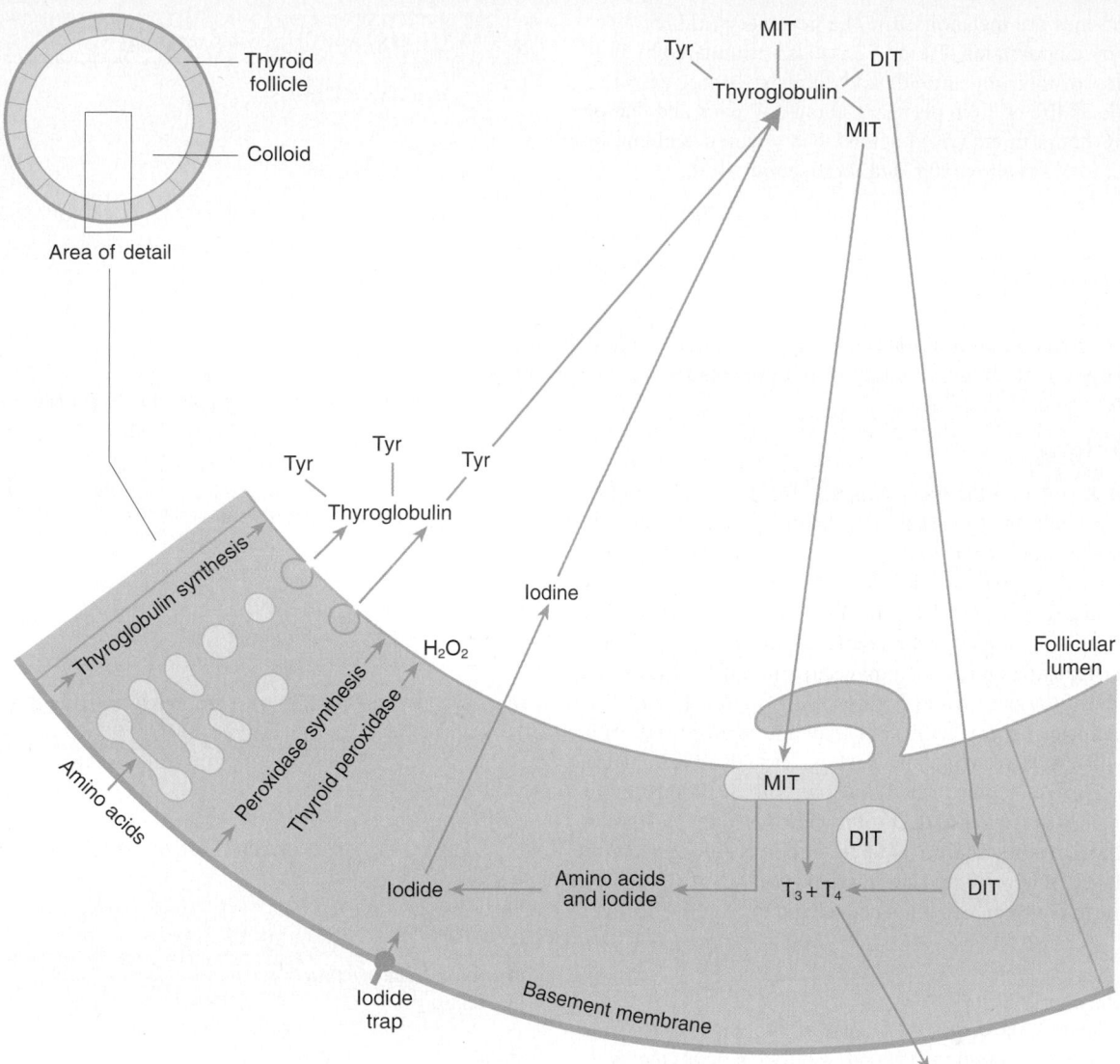

Fig. 44.2 Synthesis of thyroid hormones.
DIT, Diiodotyrosine; MIT, monoiodotyrosine; TRH, thyrotrophin-releasing hormone; TSH, thyroid-stimulating hormone; Tyr, tyrosine.

- Iodine is then transferred onto the tyrosine residues in thyroglobulin by iodinase enzymes forming mono-iodotyrosine (MIT) and di-iodotyrosine (DIT).
- Subsequently the formation of T_4 occurs as a result of the coupling of two DIT residues and of T_3 by coupling a DIT and an MIT residue. The hormones are then stored within the gland until their release into the circulation.
- Finally, thyroglobulin is resorbed into the follicular cell, hydrolysed, and its amino acids and remaining iodine re-used.

The T_4:T_3 ratio secreted by the thyroid gland is approximately 10:1. Consequently the gland secretes approximately 80–100 micrograms of T_4 and 10 micrograms of T_3 per day. However, only 10% of circulating T_3 is derived from direct thyroidal secretion, the remaining 90% being produced by peripheral conversion from T_4. T_4 can therefore be considered a prohormone that is converted in the peripheral tissues (liver, kidney and brain) either to the active hormone T_3 or to the biologically

Table 44.1 Plasma protein binding of thyroid hormones

Carrier protein	Plasma concentration	Proportion of T_4 and T_3 bound (%)
Thyroid-binding globulin	15 mg/L	75
Transthyretin (formerly thyroid-binding prealbumin)	250 mg/L	10
Albumin	40 g/L	15

inactive reverse T_3 (rT_3). In the circulation the hormones exist in both the active free and inactive protein-bound forms. T_4 is 99.98% bound, with only 0.02% circulating free. T_3 is slightly less protein bound (99.8%), resulting in a considerably higher circulating free fraction (0.2%). Details of protein binding are listed in Table 44.1.

The hormones are metabolised in the periphery (kidney, liver and heart) by deiodination. T_4 and T_3 are also eliminated by biliary secretion of their glucuronide and sulphate conjugates (15–20%). The half-life of T_4 in plasma is about 6–7 days and that of T_3 is 24–36 hours in euthyroid adults. The apparent volume of distribution for T_4 is about 10 L and for T_3 about 40 L.

Hypothyroidism

Hypothyroidism is the clinical state resulting from decreased production of thyroid hormones or rarely from tissue resistance.

Epidemiology

Accurate assessment of the prevalence and incidence of hypothyroidism is difficult due to variation in definitions and population samples. The prevalence rate of spontaneous primary hypothyroidism is estimated to be around 1–2% of the total population, with a female preponderance (10:1 female/male ratio). The prevalence of hypothyroidism is higher in the elderly population. A significant proportion of the adult population may show raised TSH levels in the presence of normal thyroid hormone levels (free T_4 and T_3). This biochemical abnormality may or may not be associated with hypothyroidism-related symptoms and is termed as subclinical hypothyroidism. According to the Whickham survey (Vanderpump et al., 1995), 8% of women and 3% of men in the study population had subclinical hypothyroidism. Despite a relatively high incidence and prevalence of hypothyroidism, mass population screening for autoimmune hypothyroidism is not considered to be cost-effective.

Aetiology

Iodine deficiency is the commonest cause of hypothyroidism globally and is especially common in Himalayan mountainous region in South East Asia, Central Africa and Latin America. In iodine-replete regions autoimmune disease is the common cause of primary hypothyroidism (Vanderpump, 2011) and accounts for more than 95% of adult cases. It is usually due to a failure of the thyroid gland itself as a result of autoimmune destruction, or the effects of treatment of thyrotoxicosis. Hypothyroidism may be drug induced. Amiodarone and lithium cause hypothyroidism in around 10% of patients treated (see later). Secondary disease is due to hypopituitarism, and tertiary disease is due to failure of the hypothalamus. Peripheral hypothyroidism is due to tissue insensitivity to the action of thyroid hormones. A more extensive classification is shown in Box 44.1.

Iodides may produce hypothyroidism in patients who are particularly sensitive to their ability to block the active transport pump of the thyroid gland. Iodine absorption from topical iodine-containing antiseptics has been shown to cause hypothyroidism in neonates. This is potentially very dangerous at a critical time of neurological development in the newborn infant. Transient hypothyroidism may be seen in 25% of iodine-exposed infants.

Clinical manifestations

Hypothyroidism can affect multiple body systems, but symptoms are mainly non-specific and gradual in onset (Box 44.2). Symptoms

---

Box 44.1 Classification of hypothyroidism

Primary hypothyroidism
Congenital hypothyroidism
    Agenesis
    Inherited enzyme defects
Immune
    Hashimoto's thyroiditis
    Spontaneous hypothyroidism in Graves' disease
    Postpartum hypothyroidism
Iatrogenic
    Postoperative hypothyroidism
    Hypothyroidism after radioactive iodine
    External neck irradiation
    Drugs: antithyroid thionamides, amiodarone, lithium, elemental iodide
Iodine deficiency
Subacute (viral)

Secondary/tertiary hypothyroidism
Hypopituitarism: any cause
Hypothalamic disease

Peripheral hypothyroidism
Insensitivity to thyroid hormones

Box 44.2 Signs and symptoms of hypothyroidism

Skin and appendages
Dry, cool, flaking, thickened skin
Reduced sweating
Yellowish complexion
Puffy facies and eyes
Sparse, coarse, dry hair
Brittle nails

Neuromuscular system
Slow speech
Poor memory and reduced cognitive function
Somnolence
Carpal tunnel syndrome
Psychiatric disturbance
Hearing loss
Depression
Muscle pain and weakness
Delayed deep tendon reflexes

Metabolic abnormalities
Raised total and low-density lipoprotein cholesterol
Macrocytic anaemia

Gastro-intestinal
Weight gain with decreased appetite
Abdominal distension and ascites
Constipation

Cardiovascular
Reduced cardiac output
Bradycardia
Cardiac enlargement

---

are frequently vague, especially in the early stages. It is common for symptoms to be incorrectly attributed by patients and their relatives to increasing age. The reverse is also common in that patients who have read about or have friends/family with hypothyroidism will assume that it is responsible for symptoms of fatigue and weight gain. Thus, hypothyroidism is often confused with simple obesity and depression. Mercifully, simple thyroid function tests (TFTs) give accurate diagnosis in all cases (see later).

The most useful clinical signs are myotonic (slow relaxing) tendon reflexes, bradycardia, hair loss and cool, dry skin. Effusions may occur into pericardial, pleural, peritoneal or joint spaces. Mild anaemia of a macrocytic type is quite common and responds to thyroxine replacement. Pernicious anaemia is a frequent concomitant finding in hypothyroidism. Other, organ-specific autoimmune diseases such as Addison's disease may be associated.

Myxoedema coma

Myxoedema coma is a rare but potentially fatal complication of severe, untreated hypothyroidism. Coma can be precipitated by hypothermia, stress, infection, trauma and certain drugs, notably β-blockers and respiratory depressants, including anaesthetic agents, narcotics, phenothiazines and hypnotics. The condition is a medical emergency and should be treated rapidly and aggressively.

The term 'myxoedema' used to be synonymous with hypothyroidism. It is now reserved for advanced disease in which there is swelling of the skin and subcutaneous tissues.

Investigations

The laboratory investigation of hypothyroidism is extremely simple. Usually clinical assessment, combined with a single estimation of thyroid hormones and TSH, is sufficient to make the diagnosis. In primary disease, the levels of free T_4 and T_3 are low, and the TSH level rises markedly. Some laboratories offer only TSH as a first-line test of thyroid function, although this can result in delayed diagnosis of secondary or tertiary hypothyroidism, which should be suspected on the basis of a low free T_4 along with low TSH levels.

Elevation of the TSH level occurs early in the course of thyroid failure and may be present before overt clinical manifestations appear. It is important to appreciate that hypothyroidism is not one disease but a spectrum. Early hypothyroidism may be asymptomatic or the symptoms less obvious and non-specific, but a normal TSH with normal free T_4 effectively excludes the diagnosis.

A chest radiograph may detect the presence of effusions, and an electrocardiogram is useful, especially in patients with angina or coronary heart disease, in whom replacement therapy needs to be introduced gradually.

Testing thyroid function: Pitfalls for the unwary

As indicated earlier (and in the section, Hyperthyroidism/thyrotoxicosis), a clinical assessment and measurement of free T_4 and TSH are usually all that is necessary to arrive at an accurate diagnosis of thyroid state. All modern TSH assays now use double antibody immunometric techniques, which are robust and highly reliable. Moreover, these assays are now so sensitive that they are able to identify thyrotoxic patients with TSH levels below the normal euthyroid range. Commercial free T_4 and free T_3 assays, however, are all indirect methods and are subject to interference from drugs and other disease states. As such, both T_3 and T_4 can be decreased as a non-specific consequence of systemic illness (the euthyroid

Table 44.2 Drug effects on thyroid function

	Clinical/Biochemical effects
Decrease TSH secretion	
Dopamine	Hypothyroidism (rarely clinically important)
Glucocorticoids	
Octreotide	
Alter thyroid hormone secretion	
Iodide (amiodarone, contrast agents)	Both hyperthyroidism and hypothyroidism
Lithium	Hypothyroidism
Decrease T_4 absorption	
Cholestyramine/colestipol	Increased levothyroxine dose requirement
Aluminium hydroxide	
Ferrous sulphate	
Calcium carbonate	
Multivitamins	
Sevelamer	
Proton pump inhibitors	
Sucralfate	
Alter T_4 and T_3 metabolism	
Increased hepatic metabolism	Low T_4 and T_3 levels
Phenobarbital	Normal or increased TSH
Phenytoin	
Rifampicin	
Carbamazepine	
Reduce conversion of T_4 to T_3	
β-Blockers	Lower T_3 levels
Propylthiouracil	Normal or increased TSH
Amiodarone	
Glucocorticoids	
Reduce T_4 and T_3 binding	
Furosemide	Increased measured free T_4 in some assays
Salicylates and non-steroidal anti-inflammatory drugs	
Heparin	
Increase thyroglobulin levels	
Oestrogen and tamoxifen	Increased total T_4
Opiates and methadone	
Others	
Cytokines: interferon and interleukin-2	Thyroiditis; can produce hypothyroidism and thyrotoxicosis

T_3, tri-iodothyronine; T_4, thyroxine; TSH, thyroid-stimulating hormone.

sick syndrome) and depression, along with a host of drugs (Surks and Sievert, 1995) that can interfere with thyroid hormone metabolism and free hormone assays (Table 44.2). Such patients require specialist assessment and collaboration with the local laboratory to rule out confounding disease and pituitary failure.

Treatment

The aims of treatment with levothyroxine are to ensure that patients receive a dose that will restore well-being and which usually returns the TSH level to the normal range. All patients with symptomatic hypothyroidism require replacement therapy.

T_4 is usually the treatment of choice except in myxoedema coma, where T_3 may be used in the first instance. Before commencing T_4 replacement the diagnosis of glucocorticoid deficiency must be excluded to prevent precipitation of a hypoadrenal crisis. If in doubt, hydrocortisone replacement should be given concomitantly until cortisol deficiency is excluded.

The initial dose of T_4 will depend on the patient's age, severity and duration of disease, and the coexistence of cardiac disease. In young, healthy patients with disease of short duration, T_4 may be commenced in a dosage of 50–100 micrograms of levothyroxine daily. Because the drug has a long half-life it should be given once daily. The most convenient time is usually in the morning. After 6–8 weeks on the same dose (not a shorter interval because TSH takes this time to stabilise after a dose change) TFTs should be checked. The TSH concentration is the best indicator of the thyroid state, and this should be used for further dosage adjustment. A raised TSH concentration indicates either inadequate treatment, poor adherence or both. Commonly used medications such as antacids, iron, calcium tablets and proton pump inhibitors (PPIs) may also interfere with absorption of levothyroxine therapy, and it is useful to advise the patients to take levothyroxine tablets separately from these medications (Zamfirescu and Carlson, 2011). The majority of patients will be controlled with dosages of 100–200 micrograms of levothyroxine daily, with few patients requiring more than 200 micrograms daily. In adults the median dose required to suppress TSH to normal is 125 micrograms daily. In the majority of patients once the appropriate dosage has been established it remains constant. During pregnancy, an increase in the dose of levothyroxine by 25–50% is needed to maintain TSH levels in a trimester-specific reference range.

Exacerbation of myocardial ischaemia, infarction and sudden death are all well-recognised complications of T_4 replacement therapy. Patients with coronary heart disease may be unable to tolerate full replacement doses because of palpitations, angina or heart failure. Elderly patients may have undiagnosed ischaemic heart disease (IHD). In these two groups of patients, treatment should therefore be started with 25 micrograms of levothyroxine daily and increased slowly by 25 micrograms every 4–6 weeks. During this time the patient's clinical progress should be carefully monitored. There is insufficient evidence supporting use of combination of T_4 and T_3 therapy over T_4 monotherapy in patients with primary hypothyroidism (Okosieme et al., 2016).

It is important to avoid both under-treatment and over-treatment. Hypothyroidism is rarely life-threatening, but adverse effects may result from prolonged over-treatment. This is indicated by a TSH level suppressed below the normal range. Although T_4 exerts an effect on many organs and tissues, it is the effect on bone and the heart that give the greatest cause for concern. There is evidence that bone density is reduced in patients who are taking excessive T_4 replacement therapy (Faber and Galloe, 1994; Uzzan et al., 1996), and that atrial fibrillation is more common if TSH is suppressed (Sawin et al., 1994). To minimise the risk of development of these complications, the dose should be carefully tailored to the needs of each individual patient. A proportion of patients may remain persistently symptomatic in spite of receiving an optimum dose of thyroxine replacement therapy despite the TSH levels being in the normal range. In these patients alternate aetiologies such as anaemia, renal and liver impairment, vitamin D/B_{12}/folate deficiency, adrenal insufficiency and depression, among others, should be considered. There is no convincing evidence supporting further increasing levothyroxine dose or use of thyroid extracts, T_3 (monotherapy or in combination with T_4) or over-the-counter dietary supplements in this subgroup of patients.

Patient care

The treatment of hypothyroidism requires lifelong treatment with T_4. Patients receiving long-term drug therapy are recognised to have a low adherence with their medication regimen. Treatment with T_4 is often terminated because patients feel well and think that treatment is no longer required. Patients should be educated to understand the effects of drug holidays on their health and TFTs, and should know that a normal TSH indicates adequate dosage. Written advice should be provided and monitoring of dosage should continue annually. A series of excellent patient information leaflets is available on the British Thyroid Association website (http://www.british-thyroid-association.org).

An official website of the Society of Endocrinology (http://www.yourhormones.info) also provides useful and relevant information for patients and caregivers.

Despite adequate counselling, some patients persistently forget to reliably take their tablets, leading to variable thyroid state and wildly fluctuating test results. Other patients lack the capacity to reliably self-medicate. There is evidence to show that weekly dosing with T_4 is a safe and acceptable way to manage this type of patient, for whom family members or community staff can supervise treatment (Grebe et al., 1997; Rangan et al., 2007). No guidelines have yet been published, although a weekly dose of levothyroxine which is sevenfold higher than the usual daily dose is considered a safe and efficacious way of bringing clinical and biochemical improvement in this sub-group of patients. Dosage changes are made in exactly the same way by assessing TSH levels after 6–8 weeks of stable dosing.

Rarely, patients are seen in whom TSH levels fluctuate or remain elevated despite high doses of levothyroxine and in whom adherence seems to be very good. There are a number of possible causes for this including malabsorption of levothyroxine, which can be due to coeliac or inflammatory bowel disease, or a number of commonly prescribed drugs (see Table 44.2). Such patients will need a careful sequential assessment by an endocrine service (Morris, 2009).

Prevention

Currently, nothing can be done to prevent autoimmune thyroid failure from developing; however, much can be done to ensure early detection and treatment. Careful follow-up of patients who have undergone radioiodine treatment, subtotal thyroidectomy, or completed a course of treatment for thyrotoxicosis is essential, along with monitoring of those prescribed amiodarone and lithium. An increase in TSH with normal concentrations of T_3 and T_4 will indicate the onset of hypothyroidism before the patient becomes symptomatic. Box 44.3 shows the prevalence of hypothyroidism after treatment for thyrotoxicosis.

Hyperthyroidism/thyrotoxicosis

Hyperthyroidism is defined as the production by the thyroid gland of excessive amounts of thyroid hormones. Thyrotoxicosis refers to the clinical syndrome associated with prolonged exposure to elevated levels of thyroid hormone. This distinction is important when evaluating TFTs (Table 44.3).

Box 44.3 Prevalence of thyroid disturbance after treatment for thyrotoxicosis

Thyroidectomy
6–75% hypothyroidism over their lifetime, dependent on the amount of remnant tissue.
Risk highest during first year after surgery

Antithyroid drugs (>6-month course)
43% relapse with thyrotoxicosis in the first year
13–21% relapse with thyrotoxicosis in the next 4 years

^{131}I therapy
24–90% develop hypothyroidism over their lifetime, depending on dose given

---

Epidemiology

Hyperthyroidism is a common condition. The Wickham survey identified 4.7/1000 women with active disease (Tunbridge et al., 1977). When previously treated cases were included, the population prevalence rose to 20/1000 women. As for hypothyroidism, it is much less common in men, who have a lifetime prevalence of around 2/1000.

Aetiology

Hyperthyroidism is a disorder of various aetiologies. In clinical terms, thyrotoxicosis is the result of persistently elevated levels of thyroid hormones.

Graves' disease

Graves' disease is the commonest cause of thyrotoxicosis. It is an autoimmune condition and results from production of an abnormal immunoglobulin G (IgG) that is able to occupy the TSH receptor on the thyroid follicular cell. Here it mimics the effect of TSH, causing cell division and stimulating thyroid hormone secretion. These stimulatory immunoglobulins

Table 44.3 Aetiology of hyperthyroidism

Condition	Frequency	Clinical features	I^{131} uptake
Thyrotoxicosis (increased hormone synthesis)			
Graves' disease	70%	Antibody mediated (TRABs) 90% are young women Diffuse goitre Ophthalmopathy (30%) Pretibial myxoedema Acropachy Transmissible to neonate	Increased
Multinodular goitre	20%	Benign autonomous nodules Often secrete T_3 Older women Always relapse after withdrawal of thionamides	Increased
Toxic single adenoma	5%		Increased
Iodine induced	<1%	Increased urine iodine	Variable
HCG induced	Rare	Molar pregnancy or choriocarcinoma	Increased
TSH dependent	Rare	Pituitary tumour	Increased
Thyroiditis (thyroid destruction and leakage of stored thyroid hormones)			
Acute	2%	Probably viral Neck pain: often severe	Absent
Silent	2%	Viral Autoimmune	Absent
Amiodarone induced	<1%	Increased urine iodine	Absent

HCG, human chorionic gonadotropin; T_3, triiodothyronine; TRAB, thyroid receptor antibody; TSH, thyroid-stimulating hormone.

are known as thyroid receptor antibodies (TRABs). Rarely are the TRABs inhibitory to the TSH receptor, resulting in hypothyroidism.

Ninety percent of patients with Graves' disease are young women often with a family history of the condition. In addition to the effects of thyrotoxicosis, around 30% of patients experience additional features including a congestive ophthalmopathy which is thought to result from antibody-mediated inflammation of orbital contents. Pretibial myxoedema, gynaecomastia and thyroid acropachy are rare manifestations.

In pregnancy the maternal TRABs can pass across the placenta to the foetus, resulting in transient neonatal thyrotoxicosis.

Nodular disease

Toxic multinodular goitre is also common but more often affects older women in whom an euthyroid nodular goitre may have been present for many years. Individual nodules become autonomous, producing T_3 and/or T_4. Clinically the thyrotoxicosis is generally less severe and more gradual in onset. Often only T_3 levels are elevated, although the TSH will be suppressed in all cases. Thyrotoxicosis may also be caused by single autonomous thyroid adenomas. These are benign, well-differentiated tumours that secrete excessive amounts of thyroid hormones.

Thyroiditis

If the thyroid is inflamed by viral or rapid autoimmune attack, the resulting follicular cell death will result in the release of pre-formed thyroid hormones. This usually presents as a painful mildly enlarged and tender thyroid. There is a brief period of hyperthyroidism before thyroid hormone levels fall to subnormal. Most often this period of hyperthyroidism does not lead to clinically apparent thyrotoxicosis and in any event is brief, but it is common for these patients to be prescribed thionamides which compound the ensuing hypothyroidism. It is therefore necessary to be aware of these conditions. Neck pain with disturbed TFTs should prompt referral for specialist assessment which will usually include a request for an iodine uptake scan. Iodine uptake is absent in hyperthyroidism associated with thyroiditis.

Clinical manifestations

Thyrotoxicosis is characterised by increases in metabolic rate and activity of many systems due to excessive circulating quantities of thyroid hormones. There is a wide spectrum of clinical disturbance. The signs and symptoms reflect increased adrenergic activity, especially in the cardiovascular and neurological systems (Box 44.4). Not all manifestations will be seen in every patient. Additional clinical features will depend on the underlying cause of the thyrotoxicosis (see Table 44.3).

The clinical features of thyrotoxicosis in the elderly may not be so obvious. Signs and symptoms of cardiovascular disturbance tend to predominate, atrial fibrillation is frequent and the patient may experience congestive heart failure. Unexplained heart failure after middle age should always arouse suspicion of thyrotoxicosis.

The extrathyroidal manifestations of Graves' disease deserve separate mention. Most frequent is ophthalmopathy due to inflammation and expansion of the contents of the orbit. The eye is pushed forward (proptosis) such that white sclera appears between the iris and the lower lid. Congestive changes develop including peri-orbital oedema, conjunctival swelling and redness. The extraocular muscles are swollen and become tethered, leading to failure of movement of the globe of the eye and thus diplopia. Severe disease causes pressure in the orbit, which can compress the optic nerve leading to blindness. The cutaneous features of Graves' disease include thickening of the pretibial skin (myxoedema), onycholysis (separation of the nail from the nail bed) and acropachy (similar to finger clubbing).

Investigations

In those with suspected thyrotoxicosis it is good practice to document the diagnosis with two sets of TFTs. If the diagnosis is in doubt, treatment should be withheld because unless severe, thyrotoxicosis can usually be safely observed whilst awaiting the results of investigations. Plasma free T_4 (and/or T_3) levels are elevated. The TSH level is suppressed to subnormal levels in all causes of thyrotoxicosis, except the exceptionally rare cases of TSH-secreting pituitary adenomas.

In the overwhelming majority of patients, the combination of the clinical findings and simple investigations is sufficient to make a firm diagnosis. Radioactive iodine uptake scans will differentiate those patients with thyroiditis. Measurement of TRABs

Box 44.4 Signs and symptoms of thyrotoxicosis
Skin and appendages
Warm, moist skin
Thinning or loss of hair
Increased sweating
Heat intolerance
Nervous system
Insomnia
Irritability, nervousness
Lid retraction – staring eyes
Symptoms of an anxiety state
Psychosis
Musculoskeletal
Fine motor tremor
Proximal muscle weakness
Rapid deep tendon reflexes
Osteoporosis
Gastro-intestinal
Weight loss despite increased appetite
Thirst
Diarrhoea
Cardiovascular
Palpitations, tachycardia
Shortness of breath on exertion
Atrial fibrillation
Congestive heart failure
Worsening angina

will identify patients with Graves' disease. If the diagnosis is still equivocal, the clinical findings should be reassessed and particular attention paid to the patient's drug history. A number of drugs, such as amiodarone, lithium, corticosteroids, interferons and levodopa, may modify the clinical features or interfere with the tests.

Treatment

A number of factors need to be considered when choosing the most appropriate form of therapy for an individual patient (Table 44.4). Usually a number of therapeutic options are available, and the patient should be involved in the decision on what treatment to have. The decision may also be influenced by physician preference, which in turn can depend on the facilities available. Three forms of therapy are available, including antithyroid drugs, surgery and radioactive iodine. There is no general agreement as to the specific indications for each form of therapy, and none of them is ideal, because all are associated with both short- and long-term sequelae. Neither surgery nor radioactive iodine should be given until the patient has been rendered euthyroid because of the risk of inducing a thyroid crisis (see later).

In children, surgery may be difficult and the complication rate is higher. Also radioiodine has been avoided because of concern about the potential development of thyroid malignancy, although there are no data which suggest this to be a problem. In pregnancy, radioiodine is not used because of the likelihood of the neonate having hypothyroidism. Thyroid surgery during pregnancy should be deferred until the second trimester if possible, and most patients' symptoms can be controlled with drugs. Thionamide doses should be kept as low as possible, especially in the last 2 months of pregnancy, because excessive treatment may produce goitre in the foetus. Aplasia cutis is said to occur after carbimazole therapy, so propylthiouracil is usually preferred over the former during the first trimester of pregnancy. Pregnant patients with thyrotoxicosis should be under the care of a specialist endocrine unit.

Immediate treatment of thyrotoxicosis

Patients need to have their symptoms addressed and their thyrotoxicosis controlled. Non-selective β-blockers in standard antihypertensive doses are effective within a matter of hours and should be offered to all non-asthmatics with severe thyrotoxicosis. These agents help to alleviate symptoms such as tremors, palpitations and anxiety which are generally associated with sympathetic over-activity. Carbimazole (40 mg once a day) or propylthiouracil (150 mg twice a day) will render most patients euthyroid within 6 weeks. Adjunctive treatment of cardiac disease and anxiety/sleeplessness may be required.

Graves' disease

A proportion (40–50%) of patients with Graves' disease will achieve a long-lasting remission after a period of euthyroidism while receiving thionamides. The optimal duration of antithyroid treatment is unknown and remains a controversial issue (Maugendre et al., 1999), but in most units the length of the treatment course has fallen to between 6 and 12 months. It is not appropriate to discuss complex treatment decisions with a thyrotoxic patient, so most are well into this period when discussions of their options occur. Remission of Graves' disease is much less likely in those with very large goiters, those who require high-dose thionamide treatment to maintain euthyroidism, those with high TRAB titres and patients who have relapsed once after a course of drug treatment. Such patients should therefore be rendered euthyroid and then have a discussion about either surgical or radioiodine thyroid ablation.

Nodular thyroid disease

As the nodules function autonomously and thyrotoxicosis will always recur when thionamides are stopped, there is no value in attempting to achieve a remission of nodular thyroid disease using prolonged medical treatment. Patients should be rendered euthyroid with drugs and then have a discussion about radioiodine ablative (RIA) therapy.

Antithyroid drugs

The thionamides, propylthiouracil, thiamazole (methimazole) and its precursor carbimazole, are equally effective

Table 44.4	Treatments available for thyrotoxicosis		
	Adverse effects (%)	Contraindications	Cautions

Thionamides
  Carbimazole
  Propylthiouracil
	Rash/arthropathy (5%)
	Agranulocytosis (0.3%)
	Hepatitis (rare)
		Previous severe allergy
		Cross-reactivity in 10%
			Pregnancy: propylthiouracil is preferred
			Do not use block/replace regimens

Radioiodine	Hypothyroidism requiring lifelong T_4	Pregnancy	Ensure euthyroid first Ophthalmopathy may deteriorate
Surgery	Hospital stay Neck scar Surgical/anaesthetic risk 10–75% requires T_4		Ensure euthyroid first Ophthalmopathy may deteriorate

T_4, thyroxine.

Table 44.5 Adverse effects of thionamides

	Adverse effect	Comments
Skin	Pruritic, maculopapular rash	Most common in first 6 weeks May disappear spontaneously with continued treatment Can be treated with an antihistamine Change to alternative agent Occurs in 5% of patients
	Urticarial rash with systemic symptoms, i.e. fever, arthralgia	Discontinue drug Alternative treatment required
Haematological	Agranulocytosis	Most common in first 6 weeks Incidence increases with age Discontinue drug Reversible Consider alternative treatment Occurs in 0.3% of patients
	Leucopenia	Transient Continue treatment Does not predispose to agranulocytosis
Other	Hepatitis	Rare
	Vasculitis Hypoprothrombinaemia Aplastic anaemia Thrombocytopenia	Discontinue drug

pharmacological therapies for thyrotoxicosis. In the UK carbimazole is usually used. These drugs prevent thyroid hormone synthesis by inhibiting the oxidative binding of iodide and its coupling to tyrosine residues. Propylthiouracil, but not carbimazole, inhibits the peripheral deiodination of T_4 to T_3. Thionamides may also have an immunosuppressive action.

Adverse effects. The most common adverse effect of antithyroid treatment is rash and arthropathy (5%) and less commonly agranulocytosis, hepatitis, aplastic anaemia and lupus-like syndromes (Table 44.5). Overall, serious effects such as these occur in approximately 0.3% of patients treated. These side effects usually occur during the first 6 weeks of treatment, but this is not invariable. Cross-sensitivity between carbimazole and propylthiouracil is around 10%, and the patient can often be safely changed to the alternative agent if an adverse event occurs.

Regular monitoring of white cell counts has been advocated, but is not warranted. Agranulocytosis is a rare event and even if it does occur, it happens rapidly such that routine monitoring of white cell counts may miss it. At the time of prescription, all patients should be counselled about the possible implication of sore throat, mouth ulcers and pyrexia, and instructed to seek an urgent (within hours) full blood count. This verbal information should be backed up by written advice which should specify where the patient should go for the blood test. An abnormal white cell count should prompt urgent admission under a specialist endocrine team.

The regimen

Carbimazole is usually given initially at a dosage up to 40–60 mg daily, depending on the severity of the condition. It can be given as a single daily dose in multiples of 20 mg tablets to aid adherence. Although the plasma half-life is short (4–6 hours), the biological effect lasts longer (up to 40 hours). T_4 concentrations are checked at 6-week intervals until the patient is clinically euthyroid and the T_4 and T_3 levels are normalised. (TSH remains suppressed for at least 4 weeks after resolution of significant thyrotoxicosis, so TSH levels are unhelpful in the early stages of treatment.)

At this point a decision is made about ongoing treatment. It is simplest to continue a high dose of carbimazole to suppress endogenous thyroid hormone production and to give a standard replacement dose of levothyroxine to maintain euthyroidism, the "block and replacement" regimen. This combination results in a steadier thyroid state, reduces the need for blood monitoring and requires fewer hospital attendances. Because adverse drug effects are allergic and not dose related, it is no riskier than tailored dose regimens.

Pregnancy is a specific situation, however, in which tailored-dose propylthiouracil is preferred over carbimazole during the first trimester. Both the immunoglobulins, which cause Graves' disease, and thionamide drugs cross the placenta and will affect the fetal thyroid, but maternal levothyroxine is not able to reach the foetus. Thus, the lowest possible dose of propylthiouracil or carbimazole in pregnancy should be used and the foetus closely monitored for heart rate and growth. Breastfeeding is considered to be safe when mothers are taking thionamides.

Patient counselling

Box 44.5 outlines counselling points for patients receiving antithyroid drugs. Patients should be advised of the importance of regular clinic attendance. This is necessary to monitor both therapeutic outcome and the development of adverse effects. As indicated earlier, the development of skin rashes, mouth ulcers or a sore throat should be immediately investigated and a full blood count performed. It may be dangerous to treat these symptoms with over-the-counter medication before carrying out further investigations.

It is important for the patient to understand the difference between specific antithyroid therapy and symptomatic treatment. The patient should also be advised about the timing of doses to aid adherence. Following completion of a course of treatment, the patient should understand that relapse may occur, and medical help should be sought if the initial symptoms recur.

Box 44.5 Counselling points for patients who are receiving
antithyroid drugs

1. Carbimazole can be given as a single daily dose.
2. Identify anticipated duration of treatment.
3. Explain block and replacement regimens.
4. Explain use of adjuvant therapy, e.g. β-blockers.
5. Encourage reporting of skin rashes, sore throat or mouth ulcers. Provide written guidance.
6. Ensure the patient understands the need for regular review.
7. Outline management of relapse.

Thyroid ablative therapy

Thyroid ablation is required for all patients with toxic multinodular goiters, those who have relapsed or are likely to relapse after drug therapy for Graves' disease, and those who are allergic to thionamides. Thyroid ablation can be achieved by radioiodine or surgery.

Radioactive iodine. Radioiodine therapy is extremely easy to administer by mouth and is very effective for a large majority of patients. It is contraindicated in pregnancy and breastfeeding, and is usually avoided in children. It is known to make ophthalmopathy worse in some patients with Graves' disease, but giving prednisolone 0.5 mg/kg for 3 weeks and commencing thyroxine replacement early (3 weeks after radioiodine) can mitigate this. Despite public concern in relation to radioactivity, accumulated experience over more than 60 years has not demonstrated any discernible risk of genetic, leukaemic or lymphoma risk (Vanderpump et al., 1996).

The commonest complication is the development of hypothyroidism. Doses sufficient to cause thyrotoxicosis to remit will result in virtually 100% of patients given radioiodine for Graves' disease becoming hypothyroid and around 50% of those treated for multinodular disease. Patients should be counselled to expect to require lifelong levothyroxine treatment after radioiodine therapy.

Antithyroid drugs must be withdrawn 1 week prior to radioiodine is given and should not be restarted for at least 3 days afterwards (otherwise the isotope will not be trapped by the thyroid). Because the ablative effect of radioiodine usually commences within 2–3 months, many patients with mild or moderate disease will not need to restart their drug treatments, although close patient monitoring is required. Patients with severe thyrotoxicosis should restart their antithyroid drugs on day 3. Treatment is then withdrawn periodically to assess the effects of the radioiodine.

The patient who is receiving radioiodine treatment is effectively radioactive for 6 weeks without ill effect. Because the patients are not at risk from this radioactivity, it seems inherently unlikely that the public faces any risk at all to health. Nevertheless, there are regulations governing exposure to radiation, which must be followed. After a standard 555 MBq dose a patient must for 14 days avoid close continuous contact (2 m) with other persons for periods of more than 1 hour, undertake to be careful in disposing of urine and must not work. For 24 days they must avoid close contact with children and pregnant women. In practice it is these regulations and the concerns they engender in the patient that result in a proportion of patients preferring a surgical approach.

Surgery. Surgery is required for those patients with very large goiters, patients who cannot be persuaded of the safety of radioiodine and those who have reacted adversely to both thionamides in pregnancy. The patient with hyperthyroidism to be treated surgically should first be rendered biochemically euthyroid whenever possible, but occasionally surgery needs to be performed as a semi-urgent procedure. This may require urgent patient preparation with a combination of antithyroid drugs and β-blockers, and iodide given as Lugol's solution. Iodide exerts a (usually) transient inhibitory effect on the ability of the gland to trap iodide, and it may also reduce the vascularity of the gland. In doses of 800–1200 mg/day, lithium is an effective antithyroid drug for patients who have reacted to thionamides. Lithium levels should be monitored to minimise toxicity. β-Blockers should be introduced and the dose titrated to reduce the pulse rate to less than 80 beats/min. They are usually continued for 1 week postoperatively. It is imperative that treatment is given right up to the time of operation, and the operation deferred if the pulse rate is not adequately controlled. Inadequate pretreatment can result in the occurrence of a thyroid crisis.

Complications of surgery include the generic ones of anaesthetic risk, bleeding, thromboembolic disease and infection. Specific risks of thyroid surgery include damage to recurrent laryngeal nerves (which may be particularly important to actors, singers and teachers) and hypoparathyroidism as a result of interference of the blood supply to the parathyroids or their inadvertent removal during surgery. If this occurs, tetany will begin within 48 hours of the operation, and treatment should be initiated with intravenous calcium gluconate. All patients who have undergone partial thyroidectomy should have serum calcium estimation 3 months after the operation because the development of hypoparathyroidism can be delayed. Later complications of thyroidectomy include hypothyroidism and recurrent thyrotoxicosis.

Treatment of complications

Ophthalmopathy

In most patients with Graves' disease, no specific treatment is required for the eyes. The commonest complaint is of 'grittiness', which can be treated with hypromellose eye drops or gel. If lid retraction is severe, inadequate lid closure can result in early-morning soreness. This can be alleviated by the short-term use of 5% guanethidine eye drops instilled each night and morning. The eyes should be monitored for any signs of infection and treated appropriately.

Fortunately, severe eye involvement occurs in less than 2% of patients with Graves' disease. Progressive ophthalmopathy-producing severe complications from proptosis, diplopia or visual failure should be treated with high-dose corticosteroid therapy (prednisolone 60 mg daily) until symptoms resolve. Failure to respond is an indication for orbital irradiation or surgical decompression, but such patients should be under the care of a highly specialised ophthalmic surgeon.

Treatment of localised myxoedema

Myxoedema is usually localised to small areas and is asymptomatic. More extensive disease causes difficulty in walking and considerable discomfort. Probably the most effective therapy is the nightly topical application of corticosteroid creams, such as betamethasone, under occlusive polythene dressings.

Thyroid Crisis

Thyroid crisis can develop in any patient with significant untreated thyrotoxicosis, but it is most common in those with severe Graves' disease. It is precipitated in such patients by infection, injury, trauma, anaesthetics, surgery and radioiodine. There is rapidly progressive tachycardia, muscle weakness (including cardiomyopathy), hyperthermia, sweating and vomiting compounding hypotension with ensuing circulatory collapse. In addition, patients are extremely anxious and often psychotic. It should be managed as a medical emergency in a high care area. In addition to supportive measures, specific antithyroid therapy is required along with drugs, which inhibit deiodination of T_4 to T_3. Propylthiouracil (inhibits deiodinase) is given orally (or via nasogastric tube) in high dose along with Lugol's iodine. Glucocorticoids should be given intravenously because they also inhibit deiodinase. Effective β-blockade is required by an intravenous infusion (propranolol is preferred because it also inhibits deiodinase).

Drugs and the thyroid

From the previous pages it will be evident that many commonly used drugs can affect the thyroid. This section draws together the most frequently encountered problems. In clinical practice drug effects and interactions produce thyrotoxicosis or hypothyroidism or disturb TFTs. It is worth specifically noting amiodarone, which contains large quantities of iodide which is released into the circulation during drug metabolism. Amiodarone's effects on the thyroid are extensive and complex.

Drugs and thyrotoxicosis

Table 44.2 indicates drug treatments associated with thyrotoxicosis. Amiodarone-induced thyrotoxicosis (AIT) is caused by two entirely different mechanisms. Type 1 AIT is similar to iodide-induced thyrotoxicosis and results from activation of nodular disease or of latent Graves' disease in patients with thyroid autoimmunity. In this condition the thyroid is actively synthesising hormone and treatment is with thionamides. Type 2 AIT has features similar to thyroiditis with leakage of pre-formed thyroid hormone, low uptake of radiolabel on scanning and is treated with glucocorticoids. AIT is an extremely challenging condition to manage for multiple reasons. These include difficulty in discrimination between type 1 and 2 diseases, each of which have different treatments, and the fact that most patients are taking amiodarone for serious cardiac dysrhythmias and amiodarone

has a very long tissue half-life. These patients should be under the care of a specialist endocrinology team.

A recent observation has been increased frequency of Graves' disease in patients who are undergoing bone marrow transplantation, after administration of alemtuzumab (a monoclonal antibody to CD52 cells) or α-interferon for multiple sclerosis and during highly active anti-retroviral treatment of HIV infection. It is thought that these cases all have immunological reconstitution as an underlying factor in aetiology (Weetman, 2009).

Drugs and hypothyroidism

Amiodarone is frequently associated with the development of hypothyroidism, particularly in those patients with positive thyroperoxidase (TPO) antibodies, indicative of latent Hashimoto's disease. Such patients seem particularly sensitive to the high levels of iodine liberated by drug metabolism, and it is thought that hypothyroidism occurs because of a failure of the patient's thyroid to escape from the suppressive effect of iodine on thyroxine synthesis (the Wolff–Chaikoff effect). If amiodarone can be withdrawn, hypothyroidism will resolve over a period of months. More often, however, amiodarone is continued and levothyroxine treatment is required.

Lithium inhibits T_4 and T_3 release from the thyroid (making it a useful adjunctive treatment for thyrotoxicosis in patients who react to thionamides) and causes a goitre in 40% of patients and hypothyroidism in 20%; again, this is more common in those with positive TPO antibodies. Like amiodarone, lithium is usually continued and these patients are treated with levothyroxine.

Drug-related interference with absorption of levothyroxine is one of the causes of hypothyroidism in patients treated with levothyroxine. Table 44.2 indicates the agents which may be implicated.

Calcium and parathyroid hormone
Physiology

Calcium ion plays a key role in multiple physiological functions in the human body including skeletal and cardiac muscle contraction, synaptic transmission, coagulation apart from acting as a second messenger intracellularly to regulate cell division, motility and signal transduction essential for homeostasis. Around 99% of total body calcium is stored in the bones, with only 1% of the rest of extracellular calcium being available for essential metabolic functions. Half of the calcium in extracellular fluid is bound to albumin, and it is the remaining ionised calcium that is biologically active.

The calcium levels in the body are dependent upon its absorption from the gastro-intestinal tract, turnover from the bones and excretion from the kidneys. Parathyroid hormone (PTH), vitamin D and magnesium levels play a role in controlling the calcium levels in the body. PTH is an 84-amino acid polypeptide which acts on hormone-specific receptors on target tissue cells and is secreted from parathyroid glands. Most individuals possess four parathyroid glands situated posterior to the upper and lower lobes of the thyroid with an extra fifth gland being present in around

10% of the population. PTH acts on the renal tubular transport of calcium and phosphate, and also stimulates the renal synthesis of 1,25-dihydroxycolecalciferol. Low levels of ionised (unbound) calcium stimulate PTH secretion, whereas high levels suppress its secretion.

PTH increases distal tubular reabsorption of calcium and decreases proximal and distal tubular reabsorption of phosphate. The effects of PTH on bone are complex. The two major cell types in bone are osteoblasts and osteoclasts. Osteoblasts are responsible for the synthesis of extracellular bone matrix and priming of its subsequent mineralisation. Osteoclasts decalcify and digest the protein matrix of bone, liberating calcium. PTH stimulates osteoclast-mediated bone resorption, but in addition has an anabolic effect on bone, with an increase in osteoblast number and function.

Vitamin D (calciferol) can either be derived from plant sources (vitamin D_2 or ergocacliferol) or animal sources (vitamin D_3 or cholecalciferol), or produced in epidermis of skin from cholesterol precursors. Vitamin D_3 needs hydroxylation in liver and kidney to get converted into the biologically active form 1,25-dihydroxycholecalciferol. Vitamin D increases calcium as well as phosphate absorption from the gastro-intestinal tract and influences PTH-mediated reabsorption of calcium from renal tubules.

Hypoparathyroidism/hypocalcaemia

Hypoparathyroidism is the clinical state which may arise either from failure of the parathyroid glands to secrete PTH, or from failure of its action at the tissue level.

Aetiology

Hypoparathyroidism most commonly occurs as a result of surgery for thyroid disease or after neck exploration and resection of adenoma-causing hyperparathyroidism. In experienced hands, the incidence of permanent hypoparathyroidism is less than 1% for all thyroid and parathyroid surgery. Other causes include autoimmune parathyroid destruction either as an isolated idiopathic disorder or as part of a multiple endocrine deficiency characterised by hyposecretion of several endocrine glands. Transient hypoparathyroidism with symptomatic hypocalcaemia can occur in neonates. The condition pseudo-hypoparathyroidism occurs in patients with defects of the PTH receptor such that although PTH levels are normal (or raised), calcium is low. Increasingly reports are identifying acute symptomatic hypocalcaemia and hypomagnesaemia complicating the use of omeprazole and other PPIs. These patients are severely magnesium depleted and have an acquired hypoparathyroidism which is reversible on stopping the offending drug (Cundy and Dissanayake, 2008).

Clinical manifestations

Most of the clinical features of hypoparathyroidism are due to hypocalcaemia. The decrease in ionised plasma calcium levels leads to increased neuromuscular excitability. The major signs and symptoms are shown in Box 44.6.

Box 44.6 Signs and symptoms of hypocalcaemia

Numbness and tingling in the extremities and around the mouth
Muscle spasm (tetany)
Epilepsy
Irritability
Cataracts (prolonged hypocalcaemia)
Chvostek's sign (facial spasm on tapping the seventh cranial nerve)
Trousseau's sign (spasm of hand when blood pressure cuff inflated above systolic pressure)

Box 44.7 Causes of hypocalcaemia

- Hypoparathyroidism
- Pseudohypoparathyroidism
- Vitamin D deficiency/malabsorption/insensitivity
- Acute and chronic renal failure
- Chronic alcoholism
- Hypomagnesaemia
- Drug induced (proton pump inhibitors)
- Acute pancreatitis

Investigations

Hypocalcaemia associated with undetectable or low plasma PTH levels is consistent with hypoparathyroidism. Total plasma calcium levels should always be corrected for any abnormality in the plasma albumin concentration using the following equation:

$$\text{corrected calcium} = \text{measured calcium} + (0.02 \times [40 - \text{plasma albumin}])$$

Hyperphosphataemia is often present. It should be noted that there are many other causes of hypocalcaemia (Box 44.7). Pseudohypoparathyroidism is easily distinguished because it is associated with excessive PTH secretion and reduced target organ responsiveness. Drugs that may produce hypocalcaemia include calcitonin, phosphate, bisphosphonates, phenytoin, phenobarbital, cholestyramine, cisplatin, 5-fluorouracil and high-dose intravenous citrate or lactate.

Treatment

Severe, acute hypocalcaemia with tetany should be treated with intravenous calcium gluconate. Initially, 10 mL of 10% calcium gluconate is given by slow intravenous injection, preferably with electrocardiographic monitoring. If the patient can swallow, oral therapy should then be commenced. If further parenteral therapy is required, 20 mL of 10% injection should be added to each 500 mL of intravenous fluid and given over 6 hours. The plasma magnesium level should always be measured in patients with hypocalcaemia and if low, magnesium therapy instituted.

For chronic treatment, PTH therapy is not currently a practical option because the hormone (recombinant human PTH) has to be administered parenterally, and the current high cost is prohibitive. Maintenance treatment for hypoparathyroidism is easily achieved with a vitamin D preparation to increase intestinal calcium absorption, often in conjunction with calcium supplementation. Many preparations, in a variety of formulations, are available including tablets, capsules, oral drops and injections. Ergocalciferol (vitamin D_2) is difficult to use and is not recommended. It has a long pharmacological and biological half-life, takes 4–8 weeks to restore normocalcaemia and its effects can persist for up to 4 months following withdrawal. In contrast, calcitriol and its synthetic analogue alfacalcidol are much easier to use. Alfacalcidol restores normocalcaemia within 1 week and its effects persist for only 1 week following withdrawal, permitting greater flexibility in dosage manipulation. The usual daily dose is 0.5–1 micrograms. Patients need close monitoring initially until stable normocalcaemia is achieved and thereafter at a minimum of 6-monthly intervals indefinitely.

Hyperparathyroidism

Hyperparathyroidism occurs when there is increased production of PTH by the parathyroid gland. Primary hyperparathyroidism causes hypercalcaemia. Secondary hyperparathyroidism reflects a physiological response to hypocalcaemia or hyperphosphataemia.

Epidemiology

Recent studies in the USA and Europe indicate an incidence rate for primary hyperparathyroidism of 25 cases per 100,000 of the population per year. The incidence is two to three times higher in women than in men, and the disease most commonly presents between the third and fifth decades of life.

Aetiology

Primary hyperparathyroidism is due to the development of either single parathyroid adenomas or rarely (<5%) hyperplasia of all four glands. It may occur as part the dominantly inherited multiple endocrine neoplasia syndromes.

Several conditions are associated with secondary hyperparathyroidism, including chronic renal failure and vitamin D deficiency. Chronic renal failure is the commonest cause. In the early stages of the disease a rise in the plasma phosphate concentration causes stimulation of PTH release, and in more advanced renal impairment reduced 1α-hydroxylation of vitamin D results in reduced intestinal calcium absorption, hypocalcaemia and further stimulation of the parathyroid glands. Tertiary hyperparathyroidism occurs in a minority of patients with end-stage renal disease, when hyperplastic parathyroid glands become autonomous and secrete PTH in levels that raise calcium levels above normal.

Clinical manifestations

The clinical features of primary hyperparathyroidism are shown in Box 44.8. These are related to the effects of hypercalcaemia itself, plus the effects of mobilisation of calcium from the skeleton and excretion in the urine. With increasingly early recognition of the biochemical abnormalities of primary hyperparathyroidism largely due to automated measurement of plasma calcium, most patients are identified at an early stage with mild or asymptomatic disease. The classical presenting features of bone disease and renal stones are now relatively uncommon. Although radiological evidence of

---

Box 44.8 Signs and symptoms in hyperparathyroidism

Anorexia, weight loss
Polydipsia, polyuria
Mental changes: poor concentration and memory
Fatigue
Nausea, dyspepsia and vomiting
Constipation
Hypertension
Renal stones
Conjunctival and corneal deposits
Bone pain and deformity
Pathological fractures

---

bone disease is now rare in these patients, measurement of bone mineral content by densitometry (dual-energy X-ray absorptiometry) scanning usually indicates that bone loss is accelerated, and the risk of osteoporotic fractures later in life is increased.

Investigations

Hypercalcaemia is the primary biochemical abnormality in primary hyperparathyroidism. Phosphate levels are often decreased and PTH levels are either inappropriately normal in the face of hypercalcaemia or elevated. In a patient with borderline elevation of calcium and a normal or only marginally elevated PTH, the benign condition familial hypocalciuric hypercalcaemia must be excluded. Urine calcium excretion is increased in primary hyperparathyroidism and low in familial hypocalciuric hypercalcaemia.

There are many other causes of hypercalcaemia, including malignancy (including myeloma), drugs (thiazides, excess vitamin D), thyrotoxicosis, immobilisation and sarcoidosis. In all these situations PTH levels are undetectable because the normal parathyroid glands appropriately switch off production of PTH in the face of hypercalcaemia. The most common cause of symptomatic hypercalcaemia in clinical practice is that associated with malignancy, and this diagnosis must always be excluded.

Localisation of parathyroid tumours is required only in those listed for neck exploration. Most parathyroid surgeons request a neck ultrasound prior to performing a neck exploration. Isotope scanning (technicium-99m sestamibi scan), computed tomography, magnetic resonance imaging and selective venous sampling are reserved for those patients (around 1% in experienced hands) in whom the adenoma cannot be located at the first operation.

Treatment

Surgical removal of the adenoma or removal of all hyperplastic tissue is the only curative treatment for primary hyperparathyroidism; however, the natural history of hyperparathyroidism is not fully documented. Some studies have indicated that more than 50% of untreated patients with primary hyperparathyroidism show no deterioration over 5 years, but the longer-term effects on renal function and bone mass remain unknown. In practice many patients are observed and their specific problems separately addressed. Tables 44.6 and 44.7 list current recommendations for initial evaluation and monitoring of patients with primary asymptomatic hyperparathyroidism, respectively. 25-Hydroxyvitamin

Table 44.6 Initial evaluation of patients with primary hyperparathyroidism

Investigation	Parameter
Blood test	Corrected calcium Phosphate Alkaline phosphatase Creatinine and urea 25 hydroxyvitamin D PTH
Urine test	urinary calcium/creatinine excretion or 24 h urinary calcium
Bone mineral density	DXA scan
Radiology	Abdominal X-ray or ultrasound renal tract

PTH, parathyroid hormone; DXA, dual energy X-ray absorptiometry.

Table 44.7 Monitoring of patients with primary hyperparathyroidism managed medically

Measurement	Recommendation
Bone mineral density	DXA scan every 1-2 years
Serum calcium	Annually
Renal function	eGFR and serum creatinine annually

DXA, dual energy X-ray absorptiometry; eGFR, estimated glomerular filtration rate.

Table 44.8 Guidelines for surgery in patients with primary hyperparathyroidism

Measurement	Recommended cutoff for surgery
Age	<65 years
Bone mineral density	1. T score <−2.5 at lumber spine, total hip, femoral neck and distal one-third radius 2. Radiological evidence of vertebral fracture
Renal function	1. Creatinine clearance <60 mL/min 2. 24 h urinary Ca >400 mg 3. Radiological evidence of nephrocalcinosis or nephrolithiasis
Serum calcium	>2.85 mmol/L
Dialysis	

Table 44.9 Treatment of hypercalcaemia

Mechanism	Treatment
Increase urinary calcium excretion	Normal saline plus loop diuretic
Reduce bone resorption	Bisphosphonates Calcitonin Gallium, mithramycin
Reduce gastro-intestinal absorption	Glucocorticoids if calcitriol dependent (vitamin D excess, sarcoid and some lymphoma patients)
Chelation Dialysis	Intravenous ethylenediaminetet-raacetic acid or phosphate

D replacement therapy is recommended in patients with primary hyperparathyroidism having co-existent vitamin D deficiency to maintain levels greater than 50 nmol/L. Bisphosphonate therapy (weekly alendronic acid or monthly zoledronic acid) should be prescribed in patients with primary hyperparathyroidism deemed unsuitable for elective parathyroidectomy who have evidence of osteoporosis on dual-energy X-ray absorptiometry scan (Bilezikian et al., 2014).

The main indications for surgical treatment are persistent hypercalcaemia greater than 2.85 mmol/L, symptomatic hypercalcaemia, renal impairment, renal stones and progression of osteoporosis (Table 44.8). Postoperatively temporary hypocalcaemia ("hungry bones") is common. In patients with bone disease, treatment with alfacalcidol and calcium supplements should be started on the day before the operation. Approximately 10% of surgically treated patients experience permanent hyperparathyroidism.

Treatment of hypercalcaemia

Severe hypercalcaemia is a common medical emergency. It must be corrected whilst investigation continues to identify the cause. Table 44.9 lists the available treatments. In practice rehydration and parenteral bisphosphonates (e.g. pamidronate 60–90 mg in 250 mL of normal saline over 60–90 minutes) will normalise calcium over 72 hours in most patients.

Case studies

Case 44.1

Mrs AD, a 38-year-old woman with known primary hypothyroidism, was reviewed in the endocrine clinic because of persistently elevated TSH levels of 24.5 mIU/L (0.4–4.5 mIU/L) despite being prescribed a high dosage of levothyroxine (350 micrograms/day) therapy. She was diagnosed to have primary autoimmune hypothyroidism around 3 years ago, although TSH levels were never well controlled despite gradual increase in her levothyroxine dose. She had not noticed any alteration in bowel habits and reported having normal appetite. Mrs AD denied poor adherence with levothyroxine tablets and was not taking any other medications.

On examination, she had a pulse rate of 58 beats/min, dry skin and non-pitting oedema at ankles. Her routine blood tests including full blood count, renal and liver function, and bone profile were within normal range.

Questions

1. What is the most likely cause of Mrs AD's persistently elevated TSH levels?
2. How would you investigate and manage her further?

Answers

1. Poor adherence with prescribed levothyroxine therapy remains the most common cause of persistently elevated TSH levels in a patient with primary hypothyroidism in clinical practice. The mean dosage of oral levothyroxine therapy most patients require is 1.6–1.8 micrograms/kg/day. Most patients respond well to this dose. Apart from poor adherence, one needs to consider malabsorption and drug-related interference with levothyroxine absorption if TSH levels remain persistently elevated despite optimum levothyroxine dose.

2. A careful history should focus on intake of over-the-counter medications such as antacids, calcium supplements, iron tablets and herbal remedies which can potentially interfere with absorption of levothyroxine therapy. Patient should be evaluated for malabsorption-related syndromes such as coeliac disease, and anti–tissue transglutaminase antibodies should be measured if indicated. Because poor adherence remains one of the most common causes of persistently elevated TSH levels in patients with hypothyroidism, once-weekly supervised levothyroxine therapy remains a useful strategy to treat such patients. Levothyroxine has an elimination half-life of around 7 days with a single dose up to 3 mg being well tolerated. The weekly supervised levothyroxine therapy is an efficacious, as well as safe, way to treat patients with non-adherence with therapy in primary care.

Stepwise approach to manage patients with hypothyroidism with persistently elevated TSH

Step 1: Confirm the diagnosis.
Repeat the blood test; exclude assay interference due to presence of heterophile antibodies. If free T_4 and free T_3 levels are normal in the presence of elevated TSH, consider TSH-secreting tumour or thyroid hormone resistance, although these are quite rare.

Step 2: Take medication history.
Check the patient's prescription and enquire about over-the-counter medication intake.

Step 3: Perform clinical evaluation.
Assess clinically for malabsorption syndromes such as coeliac disease and short bowel syndromes, and investigate accordingly.

Step 4: Assess adherence.
Evaluate adherence with the prescribed levothyroxine tablets because this remains the most common reason for persistently elevated TSH levels in clinical practice. Box 44.9 shows the possible causes of persistently elevated TSH levels in patients with hypothyroidism despite thyroxine therapy.

Case 44.2

Mrs NR, a 43-year-old school teacher, presented to her primary care doctor with ongoing symptoms of lethargy and gradual weight gain. On examination she had a body mass index of 30 kg/m². Her pulse rate was 68 beats/min; general physical, as well

---

Box 44.9 Causes of persistently elevated thyroidstimulating hormone (TSH) levels in patients with hypothyroidism

Impaired absorption
- Malabsorption syndromes
- Proton pump inhibitors
- Iron and/or calcium tablets
- Antacids
- Herbal remedies

Increased metabolism
- Barbiturates
- Carbamazepine
- Phenytoin
- Rifampicin
- Tyrosine kinase inhibitors, e.g. sunitinib

Increased demand
- Weight gain
- Pregnancy

Other causes
- Poor adherence (commonest cause)
- Nephrotic syndrome (rare)

---

as systemic, examination was unremarkable. Her investigations showed an free T_4 of 11.8 pmol/L (10–25 pmol/L) and TSH of 5.9 mIU/L (0.4–4.5mIU/L).

Questions

1. What is the likely diagnosis?
2. How would you like to investigate and manage Mrs NR further?

Answers

1. Mrs NR has primary subclinical hypothyroidism which is estimated to have a prevalence rate of 3–8% in the general population. The hypothalamic-pituitary-thyroid axis is extremely sensitive to even minor changes in thyroid hormone with a twofold change in free T_4 levels associated with 100-fold change in TSH levels. Gender, ethnic origin and body mass index also influence TSH values. The TSH levels also show an increase with age with values of 6–7 mIU/L considered normal at age of 70 years.

2. The first step is to confirm the diagnosis and exclude possibility of assay interference, silent thyroiditis and recovery from non-thyroidal illness by repeating the TFTs in 6–12 weeks. Measurement of anti-TPO antibodies can help predict development of overt hypothyroidism in the near future (estimated 4.3% risk of development of overt hypothyroidism if TPO antibodies are positive).
   Subclinical hypothyroidism is further subdivided into two categories based on TSH levels: (1) TSH >10 mIU/L and (2) TSH of 4.5–10 mIU/L. A therapeutic trial of levothyroxine can be considered in patients with TSH > 10 mIU/L (Pearce et al., 2013), although if the TSH levels are 4.5–10 mIU/L, levothyroxine therapy should be considered in the following cases:
   - history of infertility or miscarriages,
   - younger patients with increased risk of development of cardiovascular disease,
   - presence of goitre,
   - history of bipolar disease,
   - patient preference as a therapeutic trial.

Case 44.3

Mr RK, a 71-year-old man, was incidentally detected to have TSH <0.01 mIU/L (0.4–4.5 mIU/L) and FT$_4$ of 14.4 pmol/L (10–25 pmol/L) on routine blood tests done on an annual follow-up. He had a background history of type 2 diabetes mellitus and hypertension. He had no family history of thyroid dysfunction. On examination his pulse rate was 76 beats/min with regular rhythm. His general physical and systemic examination was unremarkable with no visible or palpable goitre.

Questions

1. What is the most likely diagnosis?
2. How would you like to investigate and manage Mr RK further?

Answers

1. Mr RK has subclinical hyperthyroidism (SHyper) which is estimated to have a prevalence rate of 0.6–16% of population based on age, TSH assay used and iodine intake. Solitary toxic adenoma, multinodular goitre and Graves' disease remain the commonest aetiologies leading to SHyper, with the first two being relatively more common in the elderly population as compared with Graves' disease which predominantly is seen in younger patients (more common in women as compared with men).
2. The management approach for a patient with suspected SHyper should include the following steps:
   Step 1: Confirm the diagnosis.
   Repeat the TFTs after 1–3 months in asymptomatic patients with no risk factors for ischaemic heart disease (IHD) or atrial fibrillation. In patients with symptoms (palpitations, weight loss, tremors, increased sweating, etc.) and/or presence of risk factors for IHD, the TFTs should be repeated within 2 weeks.
   Step 2: Evaluate the severity.
   Biochemically: SHyper can be subdivided into two categories, grade 1 (TSH 0.1–0.4 mIU/L) and grade 2 (TSH <0.1 mIU/L).
   Clinically: Patients with SHyper are considered to be high risk if:
   - aged >65 years;
   - presence of hyperthyroidism related symptoms;
   - presence of comorbidities such as arrhythmias, heart disease and osteoporosis.

   Step 3: Establish the aetiology.
   Toxic solitary thyroid adenoma, multinodular goitre, viral thyroiditis and Graves' disease are the commonest aetiologies leading to SHyper. Iatrogenic hyperthyroidism can be seen in patients receiving levothyroxine, amiodarone, lithium, corticosteroids, alemtuzumab (used in the treatment of multiple sclerosis) and interferon therapy.
   Step 4: Assess for complications.
   Atrial tachycardia, atrial fibrillation, heart failure and osteoporosis are associated with untreated severe SHyper.
   Step 5: Initiate appropriate treatment.
   Treatment is indicated in high-risk patients with SHyper who have persistent grade 2 disease (TSH <0.1 mIU/L), with RIA therapy being the modality of choice (Biondi et al., 2015). Patients who are deemed unsuitable or refuse RIA therapy can be managed with low-dose thionamide therapy (preferably carbimazole because of better tolerability and fewer side effects as compared with propylthiouracil).
   In contrast, the treatment of subclinical hypothyroidism in patients with TSH 4.5–10 mIU/L has limited benefits.

Case 44.4

Mrs. GE, a 78-year-old woman, was incidentally detected to have elevated calcium levels of 2.82 mmol/L (2.2–2.6 mmol/L) on routine blood tests. She has a background history of hypertension, osteoarthritis and chronic obstructive pulmonary disease. She was receiving amlodipine, ramipril and long-acting β-agonist inhaler therapy. Her mobility is limited because of breathing difficulties, and she mostly is confined indoors. Her subsequent investigations showed:

PTH	7.8 pmol/L (1.5–6.5 pmol/L)
Estimated glomerular filtration rate	65 mL/min per 1,73 m²
25-Hydroxyvitamin D	14 nmol/L (>50 nmol/L)
Bone mineral density scan	Severe osteoporosis

Questions

1. What is Mrs GE's likely diagnosis?
2. What is the definitive treatment for Mrs GE's underlying condition, and when should it be considered?
3. What other treatment options are available?

Answers

1. Mrs GE has elevated calcium and PTH levels suggestive of underlying primary hyperparathyroidism. It is a relatively common condition with prevalence of around 4/1000 women older than 60 years. The majority of patients with primary hyperparathyroidism may be asymptomatic, although it can lead to increased bone resorption leading to osteoporosis. Increased calcium may predispose to renal stone formation (mostly calcium oxalate stones) and contribute to gradual decline in renal function.
2. The definitive therapy for primary hyperparathyroidism includes an elective removal of the parathyroid gland after localising the gland using radiological investigations such as sestimibi scan. The 2014 consensus guidelines for elective parathyroidectomy include the presence of one or more of the following (Marcocci et al., 2014):
   - calcium >2.85 mg/dL,
   - decline in estimated glomerular filtration rate <60 mL/min,
   - age <50 years,
   - osteoporosis,
   - calcium excretion over 24 hours >400 mg.

   Elective parathyroidectomy is also recommended in patients with primary hyperparathyroidism who are deemed unsuitable for medical surveillance or who wish to opt for surgical treatment (in the absence of any medical contraindication for surgery).
3. Mrs GE is frail and elderly with multiple comorbidities; as a result, elective parathyroidectomy may not be a feasible option in her case. She can be managed conservatively by giving her bisphosphonates for osteoporosis and vitamin D supplements for her co-existent vitamin D deficiency. Her calcium levels can be lowered by using calcimimetic agents such as cinacalcet. Cinacalcet is a calcimimetic agent which acts as an allosteric modulator of calcium-sensing receptors which reduces the PTH secretion resulting in lowering of serum calcium levels. The calcium-sensing receptors are trans-membrane G-protein–coupled receptors present in parathyroid gland, bone, intestine, kidneys and vascular endothelium. These play a key role in regulation of serum calcium concentration. Cinacalcet use was approved by the European Medicine Agency in June 2008 for treatment of patients with primary hypercalcaemia who are deemed unsuitable for surgery. Cinacalcet tablet is usually initiated orally at a

dosage of 30 mg twice a day with the titration of the dose (every 2–4 weeks) based on serum calcium levels (maximum dose 90 mg four times a day). It is contraindicated in patients younger than 18 years, during pregnancy and in patients with hypocalcaemia; cautious use is suggested in epilepsy, heart and liver failure. Cinacalcet has been shown to be an efficacious agent in reducing serum calcium concentration, although it has modest impact on lowering PTH levels (Khan et al., 2015). It has also been shown to have no significant effect on bone density.

Cinacalcet along with low-dose vitamin D has been shown to attenuate vascular and cardiac valve calcification in patients with secondary hyperparathyroidism with chronic kidney disease stage 5 who were undergoing haemodialysis (Raggi et al., 2011). Cinacalcet use in patients with secondary hyperparathyroidism due to renal failure who were undergoing haemodialysis was not associated with reduced risk of cardiovascular death or non-fatal myocardial infarction. Although after adjustment to baseline characteristics were made in intention-to-treat analysis, a 12% reduction in risk of cardiovascular death or non-fatal myocardial infarction in patients receiving cinacalcet therapy was noticed. There was also a 50% reduction in need for elective parathyroidectomy in the group of patients receiving cinacalcet therapy (Chertow et al., 2012).

Case 44.5

Mr ML, a 38-year-old man, was admitted to a medical assessment unit at the hospital with weakness and cramps in the hands. He had a background history of gastro-oesophageal reflux disease and had been taking omeprazole (40 mg once a day) intermittently for the last 3 years.

On examination he had evidence of carpopedal spasm and paraesthesia on face.

Investigations showed serum calcium level of 1.92 mmol/L (2.2–2.6 mmol/L) and serum magnesium level of 0.35 mmol/L (0.7–12 mmol/L).

Questions

1. What is the likely diagnosis?
2. How should Mr ML be managed?

Answers

1. The most likely diagnosis in this patient is PPI-induced hypomagnesaemia and hypocalcaemia. This was first reported by Epstein et al. (2006), who described two patients receiving PPI therapy presenting with symptomatic hypocalcaemia and hypomagnesaemia that resolved on stopping PPI therapy. Since then multiple case reports and observational studies have been published suggestive of chronic PPI use predisposing to low magnesium and associated symptoms which may include arrhythmias, tetany and seizures. The exact mechanism leading to PPI-induced hypomagnesaemia is yet to be established, although it is believed to be linked to reduced absorption of magnesium from the gastrointestinal tract.

2. The PPI therapy needs to be stopped and substituted with a H$_2$ receptor antagonist such as ranitidine. The patient needs to be given a magnesium replacement (oral or intravenous depending upon symptoms and severity of hypomagnesaemia). Hypomagnesaemia needs to be corrected before hypocalcaemia because low magnesium levels render hypocalcaemia refractory to calcium replacement. Because there is widespread use of PPIs, apart from non-specific signs and symptoms associated with hypomagnesaemia, as well as hypocalcaemia, a high index of suspicion is required to diagnose these potentially life-threatening electrolyte abnormalities in patients receiving long-term PPI therapy.

Case 44.6

Mr. GD, a 55-year-old man of South East Asian origin, presented to his primary care doctor with generalised aches and pains. He had background history of dyslipidaemia and was receiving atorvastatin therapy. His subsequent blood tests showed:

25-Hydroxyvitamin D	15 nmol/L (<50 nmol/L)
Calcium	2.25 mmol/L (2.2–2.6 mmol/L)
Renal function	Normal
PTH	10.3 pmol/L (1.5–6.5 pmol/L)

Questions

1. What is the likely diagnosis?
2. What further treatment should Mr GD receive?

Answers

1. Mr GD has secondary hyperparathyroidism caused by vitamin D deficiency. Vitamin D deficiency is believed to have a prevalence rate varying from 15% to 25% of the population and is more common in elderly people living in nursing or residential homes, pregnant or breastfeeding women and individuals with low or no exposure to the sun. Vitamin D deficiency is also common in individuals of Afro-Caribbean and South East Asian ethnic origin because pigmented skin hampers sunlight-mediated conversion of cholesterol precursors to vitamin D in deeper layers of the epidermis. Vitamin D deficiency has been associated with increased risk of falls and osteoporosis in the elderly population. It has been linked with conditions such as multiple sclerosis, tuberculosis, bronchial asthma and diabetes, although the evidence linking it with these disorders is inconclusive.

2. According to National Osteoporosis Society guidelines (Francis et al., 2013), patients with serum 25-hydroxy vitamin D levels less than 30 nmol/L are considered to be vitamin D deficient, whereas levels of 30–50 nmol/L may be inadequate in some individuals. Oral vitamin D3 remains the treatment of choice in vitamin D deficiency. In patients with symptomatic disease, a loading regimen comprising 300,000 IU vitamin D (given as parenteral weekly or oral daily doses) is recommended. Subsequently, patients can be switched to maintenance dose comprising 800–2000 IU/day vitamin D. The maintenance doses are often continued lifelong. Serum calcium levels should be assessed 1 month after initiation of loading regimen or after initiation of maintenance therapy. Once a patient is receiving vitamin D replacement therapy, repeat routine monitoring of PTH levels is not indicated. Vitamin D toxicity is seen only occasionally in patients who are erroneously taking much higher than the recommended dose (>50,000 IU/day taken for several weeks to months), and doses less than 10,000 IU/day are generally considered to be safe.

References

Bilezikian, J.P., Brandi, L.M., Eastell, R., et al., 2014. Guidelines for the management of asymptomatic primary hyperparathyroidism: summary statement from the fourth international workshop. J. Clin. Endocrinol. Metab. 99 (10), 3561–3569.

Biondi, B., Bartalena, L., Cooper, D., et al., 2015. The 2015 European thyroid association guidelines on diagnosis and treatment of endogenous subclinical hyperthyroidism. Eur. Thyroid. J. 4 (3), 149–163.

Chertow, G.M., Block, G.A., Correa-Rotter, R., et al., 2012. Effect of cinacalcet on cardiovascular disease in patients undergoing dialysis. N. Engl. J. Med. 367, 2482–2494.

Cundy, T., Dissanayake, A., 2008. Severe hypomagnesaemia in long-term users of proton-pump inhibitors. Clin. Endocrinol. 69, 338–341.

Epstein, M., McGrath, S., Law, F., 2006. Proton-pump inhibitors and hypomagnesemic hypoparathyroidism. N. Engl. J. Med. 355, 1834–1836.

Faber, J., Galloe, M., 1994. Changes in bone mass during prolonged treatment subclinical hyperthyroidism due to l-thyroxine treatment: a meta analysis. Eur. J. Endocrinol. 130, 350–356.

Francis, R., Aspray, T., Fraser, W., et al., 2013. Vitamin D and Bone Health: A Practical Clinical Guideline for Patient Management. National Osteoporosis Society, Bath, UK.

Grebe, S.K., Cooke, R.R., Ford, H.C., et al., 1997. Treatment of hypothyroidism with once weekly thyroxine. J. Clin. Endocrinol. Metab. 82, 870–875.

Khan, A., Bilezikian, J., Bone, H., et al., 2015. Cinacalcet normalizes serum calcium in a double-blind randomized, placebo-controlled study in patients with primary hyperparathyroidism with contraindications to surgery. Eur. J. Endocrinol. 172 (5), 527–535.

Marcocci, C., Bollerslev, J., Khan, A.A., et al., 2014. Medical management of primary hyperparathyroidism: proceedings of the fourth international workshop on the management of asymptomatic primary hyperparathyroidism. J. Clin. Endocrinol. Metab. 99 (10), 3607–3618.

Maugendre, D., Gatel, A., Campion, L., et al., 1999. Antithyroid drugs and Graves' disease: prospective randomised assessment of long-term treatment. Clin. Endocrinol. 50, 127–132.

Morris, J.C., 2009. How do you approach the problem of TSH elevation in a patient on high-dose thyroid hormone replacement? Clin. Endocrinol. 70, 671–673.

Okosieme, O., Gilbert, J., Abraham, P., et al., 2016. Management of primary hypothyroidism: statement by the British Thyroid Association Executive Committee. Clin. Endocrinol. (Oxf) 84 (6), 799–808.

Pearce, S.H.S., Brabant, G., Duntas, L.H., et al., 2013. ETA guideline: management of subclinical hypothyroidism. Eur. Thyroid J. 2 (4), 215–228.

Raggi, P., Chertow, G.M., Torres, P.U., et al., 2011. The ADVANCE study: a randomized study to evaluate the effects of cinacalcet plus low-dose vitamin D on vascular calcification in patients on hemodialysis. Nephrol. Dial. Transplant. 26, 1327–1339.

Rangan, S., Tahrani, A., Macleod, A., et al., 2007. Once weekly thyroxine treatment as a strategy to treat non-compliance. Postgrad. Med. J. 83, e3.

Sawin, C.T., Geller, A., Wolf, P.A., et al., 1994. Low serum thyrotropin concentrations as a risk factor for atrial fibrillation in older persons. N. Engl. J. Med. 331, 1249–1252.

Surks, M.I., Sievert, R., 1995. Drugs and thyroid function. N. Engl. J. Med. 333, 1688–1694.

Tunbridge, W.M., Evered, D.C., Hall, R., et al., 1977. The spectrum of thyroid disease in a community: the Wickham survey. Clin. Endocrinol. 7, 481–493.

Uzzan, B., Campos, J., Cicherat, M., et al., 1996. Effects on bone mass of long-term treatment with thyroid hormones: a meta-analysis. J. Clin. Endocrinol. Metab. 81, 4278–4289.

Vanderpump, M.P., 2011. The epidemiology of thyroid disease. Br. Med. Bull. 99, 39–51.

Vanderpump, M.P., Alquist, J.A.O., Franklyn, J.A., et al., 1996. Consensus statement for good practice and audit measures in the management of hypo and hyperthyroidism. Br. Med. J. 313, 539–544.

Vanderpump, M.P., Tunbridge, W.M., French, J.M., et al., 1995. The incidence of thyroid disorders in the community: a twenty-year follow-up of the Whickham Survey. Clin. Endocrinol. (Oxf.) 43 (1), 55–68.

Weetman, A., 2009. Immune reconstitution syndrome and the thyroid. Clin. Endocrinol. Metab. 23, 693–702.

Zamfirescu, I., Carlson, H.E., 2011. Absorption of levothyroxine when coadministered with various calcium formulations. Thyroid 21 (5), 483–486.

Further reading

Beckerman, P., Silver, J., 1999. Vitamin D and the parathyroid. Am. J. Med. Sci. 317, 363–369.

Brown, A.J., 1998. Vitamin D analogues. Am. J. Kidney Dis. 32 (2 Suppl. 2), S25–S39.

Eskes, S.A., Wiersinga, W.M., 2009. Best Practice and Research: Clinical Endocrinology and Metabolism 23(6), 735–751.

Hanna, F.W.F., Lazarus, J.H., Scanlon, M.F., 1999. Controversial aspects of thyroid disease. Br. Med. J. 319, 894–899.

Lazarus, J.H., 2009. Best Practice and Research: Clinical Endocrinology and Metabolism 23(6), 723–733.

Lourwood, D.L., 1998. The pharmacology and therapeutic utility of bisphosphonates. Pharmacotherapy 18, 779–789.

Newman, C.M., Price, A., Davies, D.W., et al., 1998. Amiodarone and thyroid: a practical guide to the management of thyroid dysfunction induced by amiodarone therapy. Heart 79, 121–127.

Woeber, K., 2000. Update on the management of hyperthyroidism and hypothyroidism. Arch. Intern. Med. 160, 1067–1071.

Useful websites

British Thyroid Association: www.british-thyroid-association.org

Society of Endocrinology: www.yourhormones.info

45 Diabetes Mellitus

Sallianne Kavanagh and Jackie Elliott

Key points

- Diabetes is one of the most common chronic diseases in the UK, with an estimated 3.2 million individuals diagnosed in the UK, equivalent to more than 4% of the population.

- Up to 15–20% of hospital in-patients will have diabetes.

- The number of people with diabetes increased by 53% between 2006 and 2013.

- The life expectancy of a person with diabetes is shortened by approximately 15 years.

- Macrovascular complications are the cause of 75% of diabetes-related deaths.

- The cost of treating diabetes and its related complications is around £9 billion, equating to 10% of the total National Health Service (NHS) budget.

- Effective control of diabetes (glycaemic levels, blood pressure, dyslipidaemia) reduces the risk of developing long-term complications and saves both lives and money.

- Extreme hyperglycaemia and hypoglycaemia may lead to diabetic emergencies, both of which carry risks for morbidity and mortality.

- Dietary modifications and oral medicines may maintain adequate glycaemic control in type 2 diabetes, but in time, many patients will eventually require insulin.

- There is a wide variety of insulins and other medication classes, allowing regimens to be tailored to individual need.

Diabetes is one of the largest global health emergencies of the 21st century. Each year, more and more people are living with the condition, which leads to significant morbidity and mortality. Worldwide estimates are that 415 million adults have diabetes, with a further 318 million with impaired glucose tolerance and thus at high risk of developing the disease in the future (International Diabetes Federation, 2015).

Introduction

Diabetes mellitus is the most common of the endocrine disorders. It is a chronic metabolic condition, characterised by hyperglycaemia due to impaired insulin production and secretion with or without insulin resistance. Diabetes mellitus may be classified according to aetiology, by far the most common types being type 1 and type 2 diabetes (Box 45.1). In 2013, more than 3.2 million adults in the UK had a diagnosis of diabetes, with a prevalence of 6% and 6.7% in England and Wales, respectively. In 2014 the global prevalence of diabetes in adults was estimated to be 9%, and it is estimated that by 2030, diabetes will be the seventh leading cause of death (Mathers and Loncar, 2006).

Type 1 diabetes is a disease characterised by the destruction of the insulin-producing pancreatic β-cells. In more than 90% of cases, β-cell destruction is associated with autoimmune disease. Type 1 diabetes usually develops in children or young adults, although it can develop at any age and is associated with a faster onset of symptoms, leading to dependency on extrinsic insulin for survival.

Type 2 diabetes is more common and traditionally occurs in adults older than 40 years, with a peak onset between 60 and 70 years of age in developed countries. Regrettably, it is being increasingly seen in younger people, including adolescents and children. The prevalence of type 2 diabetes varies widely in different populations, being six times more common in those of South Asian origin compared with those of Northern European origin. It is caused by a relative insulin deficiency and the body's inability to effectively use insulin. The pancreas is able to produce some insulin; however, as insulin resistance increases, the effectiveness of circulating insulin decreases, and the amount produced is not sufficient to meet the body's requirements. Symptoms are generally slower in onset and less marked than those of type 1. Type 2 diabetes may be undiagnosed for many years, and during this period, the excessive glucose levels may lead to complications such as cardiovascular disease. Type 2 disease often progresses to the extent that extrinsic insulin is required to maintain blood glucose levels. The differences between type 1 and type 2 diabetes are highlighted in Table 45.1. Sometimes the type of diabetes is not clear, and additional tests are required to try to establish the correct diagnosis. However, there may be uncertainty even after further testing, so it is predominantly the degree of metabolic abnormality that is the key determinant of the form of treatment.

In high-income countries, one in seven births is affected by gestational diabetes. Gestational diabetes is hyperglycaemia that is first detected during pregnancy. Overt symptoms of hyperglycaemia are difficult to distinguish from normal symptoms of pregnancy; consequently, screening is performed in high-risk individuals. The risk of gestational diabetes should be assessed during early pregnancy for women with a body mass index (BMI) greater than 30 kg/m^2, a previous macrocosmic baby weighing 4.5 kg or greater, previous gestational diabetes, family

---

Box 45.1 Aetiological classification of diabetes mellitus

Type 1
- β-Cell destruction, usually leading to absolute insulin deficiency
- Autoimmune
- Idiopathic

Type 2
- Ranges from mild to significant secretion of insulin deficiency, with or without insulin resistance

Other specific types
- Gestational diabetes
- Maturity onset diabetes of the young
- Genetic defects in β-cell function or insulin action
- Diseases of the exocrine pancreas (e.g. neoplasia, hereditary haemochromatosis, cystic fibrosis)
- Endocrinopathies (e.g. acromegaly, Cushing's)
- Drug or chemical induced (e.g. alcohol, glucocorticoid steroids, high-dose thiazides)

Table 45.1 Differences between type 1 and type 2 diabetes

Type 1 diabetes	Type 2 diabetes
Autoimmune-mediated β-cell destruction	No autoimmune-mediated β-cell destruction
Islet cell antibodies present	No islet cell antibodies present
Genetic link	Very strong genetic link
Age of onset usually younger than 30 years	Age of onset usually older than 40 years
Faster onset of symptoms	Slower onset of symptoms
Insulin must be administered	Diet control and oral hypoglycaemic agents often sufficient control
Patients usually not overweight	Patients usually overweight
Extreme hyperglycaemia causes diabetic ketoacidosis	Extreme hyperglycaemia causes hyperosmolar hyperglycaemic state

history of diabetes or minority ethnic family origin with a high prevalence of diabetes. Testing for gestational diabetes should be offered to women with any of these risk factors (National Institute for Health and Care Excellence [NICE], 2015a). Hyperglycaemia in pregnancy is associated with adverse outcomes, including hypertension and foetal macrosomia. Women with gestational diabetes may respond to changes in diet and exercise; however, the majority of women will need oral blood glucose lowering agents or insulin therapy. Usually, gestational diabetes resolves after birth, but these women are at greater risk of developing gestational diabetes in subsequent pregnancies and type 2 diabetes in later years. Babies born to mothers with gestational diabetes have a higher risk of developing type 2

diabetes in adolescence and early adulthood. To minimise the potential adverse outcomes for the woman and baby, the targets for blood glucose control during pregnancy are tighter than for non-pregnant women.

Two other varieties of nontypical diabetes that may be seen are latent autoimmune diabetes in adults (LADA) and maturity-onset diabetes of the young (MODY). LADA occurs in younger, leaner individuals who appear to have type 2 diabetes because they do not become ketotic, and they may manage without insulin for a time. Antiglutamic acid decarboxylase (GAD) antibodies may be present, and the individual usually progresses to insulin more rapidly than those with other varieties of type 2 diabetes. MODY was noted more than 30 years ago and described a subset of type 2 diabetes of young onset, often with a positive family history. Genetic studies have now identified this to be a monogenic autosomal-dominant form of diabetes. MODY related to a mutation in the glucokinase gene typically causes a resetting of the glucose level with a 'mild' nonprogressive hyperglycaemia in which diet treatment is usually sufficient. Other types of MODY are related to mutations in the hepatocyte nuclear factor genes and usually develop during adolescence or the third decade of life. Pharmacological treatment is required, but sulfonylureas are often extremely effective, and the need for insulin can usually be avoided.

Secondary diabetes arises due to complications of other diseases, such as diseases of the pancreas or hormone disturbances such as in Cushing's disease and acromegaly.

Epidemiology

The incidence of type 1 diabetes, whilst less common, is increasing by around 3% every year worldwide. The causality is unknown, although it is speculated that environmental changes may be causing modification to the diabetes-associated alleles. Also, since the introduction of insulin in the 1920s, an increasing number of people with type 1 diabetes have had children.

More than half a million children are estimated to be living with type 1 diabetes worldwide; however, there are major ethnic and geographical differences in the incidence. In Northern Europe, the prevalence is approximately 0.3% in those younger than 30 years; the UK is ranked fifth in rates of prevalence. Figures are highest in Caucasians, especially Scandinavians, whereas the disorder is rare in Japan and the Pacific area (International Diabetes Federation, 2015).

Type 1 diabetes may present at any age, but there is a sharp increase around the time of puberty and a decline thereafter. Approximately 50–60% of patients with type 1 will present before 20 years of age. Type 2 diabetes is much more common than type 1, accounting for approximately 90% of people with diabetes. Currently it is estimated that worldwide, 1 in 11 adults has diabetes, with an anticipated increase to 1 in 10 by 2040 (International Diabetes Federation, 2015). Estimates in the UK suggest that type 2 diabetes currently affects approximately 3.2 million adults with a confirmed diagnosis, and a further 500,000 are thought to be undiagnosed (Diabetes UK, 2016). The incidence of type 2 rises with age, increasing obesity and physical inactivity, and it is associated with hypertension and disturbed lipid profiles. As with type 1, there are major ethnic and geographical variations. Type 2 diabetes is more common in people of African, African-Caribbean and South Asian family origin. The highest prevalence (1 in 8 adults) per capita is found in the North American and Caribbean region (International Diabetes Federation, 2015), increasing to values as high as 50% in the Pima Indians of Arizona (Bogardus, 1993). Diabetes is five times more common among Asian immigrants in the UK than in the indigenous population (Montesi et al., 2016). World studies indicate that type 2 diabetes is increasing in response to increased urbanisation and social changes; this is evident when considering the rapid economic growth and Westernisation observed in Asia, which is now emerging as an epicentre for diabetes prevalence (Chan et al., 2009; Gavin et al., 2002).

Aetiology

Both genetic and environmental factors are relevant in the development of type 1 diabetes, but the exact relationship between the two is still unknown. There is a strong immunological component to type 1 and a clear association with many organ-specific autoimmune diseases. Circulating islet cell antibodies (ICAs) are present in 70–90% of those with type 1 at the time of diagnosis. Family studies have shown that the appearance of ICAs often precedes the onset of clinical diabetes by several years. However, most patients diagnosed with type 1 diabetes do not have a positive family history. Type 1 diabetes is a disease of clinically rapid onset, but the physiological development is related to slowly progressive immunological damage. However, it is not currently possible to use screening methods to reliably identify patients who will develop diabetes in the future. The final event that precipitates clinical diabetes may be caused by sudden stress, such as an infection when the mass of β-cells in the pancreas falls to less than 5–10%, but more usually is unknown.

Studies have been carried out in which patients with newly diagnosed type 1 were treated with immunosuppressive therapies such as ciclosporin, azathioprine, prednisolone and anti-thymocyte globulin. When started soon after diagnosis, these therapies showed transient improvements in clinical measures and increased the rate of remissions in which insulin was not required. However, their use is limited in an otherwise healthy and young population due to potential toxicity and the risks associated with immune suppression. Studies of potentially less toxic immunosuppressives are ongoing (Chatenoud et al., 2012).

Studies have investigated the use of anti-CD3 monoclonal antibodies. When newly diagnosed type 1 patients are treated with short courses of anti-CD3 monoclonal antibodies, smaller insulin doses are required. This relates to better preservation of β-cell function (Herold and Taylor, 2003).

Type 2 diabetes has a stronger genetic predisposition. Identical twins have a concordance rate approaching 100%, suggesting the relative importance of inheritance over environment. If a parent has type 2, the risk of a child eventually developing type 2 is 15%, increasing to 50% if both parents, compared with 2–6% for type 1 (American Diabetes Association, 2013). Type 2 diabetes occurs because of the progressive development of insulin resistance and β-cell dysfunction, the latter leading to an inability of the pancreas to produce enough insulin to overcome the insulin

resistance. About 80% of people with type 2 diabetes are obese. This highlights the clear association between type 2 and obesity, with obesity causing insulin resistance. In particular, central obesity, where adipose tissue is deposited intra-abdominally rather than subcutaneously, is associated with the highest risk. Body mass index (BMI) has been used as an indicator for predicting type 2 risk; however, it does not take fat distribution into account, so waist circumference measurements are more reliable and are now being increasingly used.

Pathophysiology

The islets of Langerhans form the endocrine component of the pancreas, constituting 1–2% of the total pancreatic mass. Insulin is synthesised in the pancreatic β-cells, initially as a polypeptide precursor, preproinsulin. The latter is rapidly converted in the pancreas to proinsulin. This forms equal amounts of insulin and C-peptide through the removal of four amino acid residues. Insulin consists of 51 amino acids in two chains (the A chain contains 21 amino acids; the B chain contains 30), connected by two disulphide bridges. In the islets, insulin and C-peptide (and some proinsulin) are packaged into granules. Insulin associates spontaneously into a hexamer containing two zinc ions and one calcium ion.

Glucose is the major stimulant to insulin release. The response is triggered both by the intake of nutrients and the release of gastro-intestinal peptide hormones. After an intravenous injection of glucose, there is a biphasic insulin response. There is an initial rapid response in the first 2 minutes, followed after 5–10 minutes by a second response which is smaller but sustained over 1 hour. The initial response represents the release of stored insulin, and the second phase reflects discharge of newly synthesised insulin. Glucose is unique; other agents, including sulfonylureas, do not result in insulin biosynthesis, only release. Once released from the pancreas, insulin enters the portal circulation. The liver rapidly degrades it, and only 50% reaches the peripheral circulation. In the basal state, insulin secretion is at a rate of approximately 1 unit/h. The intake of food results in a prompt 5- to 10-fold increase in insulin release. Total daily secretion of insulin into the circulation in healthy individuals ranges from 30 to 50 units.

Insulin circulates free as a monomer, has a half-life of 3–5 minutes and is primarily metabolised by the liver and kidneys. In the kidneys, insulin is filtered by the glomeruli and reabsorbed by the tubules and degraded. In both renal and hepatic disease, there is a decrease in the rate of insulin clearance, which may necessitate dosage reduction for those using exogenous insulin. Peripheral tissues such as muscle and fat also degrade insulin, but this is of minor quantitative significance.

The interaction of insulin with the receptor on the cell surface sets off a chain of messengers within the cell. This opens up transport processes for glucose, amino acids and electrolytes.

In type 1 diabetes, there is an acute deficiency of insulin that leads to unrestrained hepatic glycogenolysis and gluconeogenesis with a consequent increase in hepatic glucose output. Also, glucose uptake is decreased in insulin-sensitive tissues such as adipose tissue and muscle; hence, hyperglycaemia ensues. Either as a result of the metabolic disturbance itself or secondary to

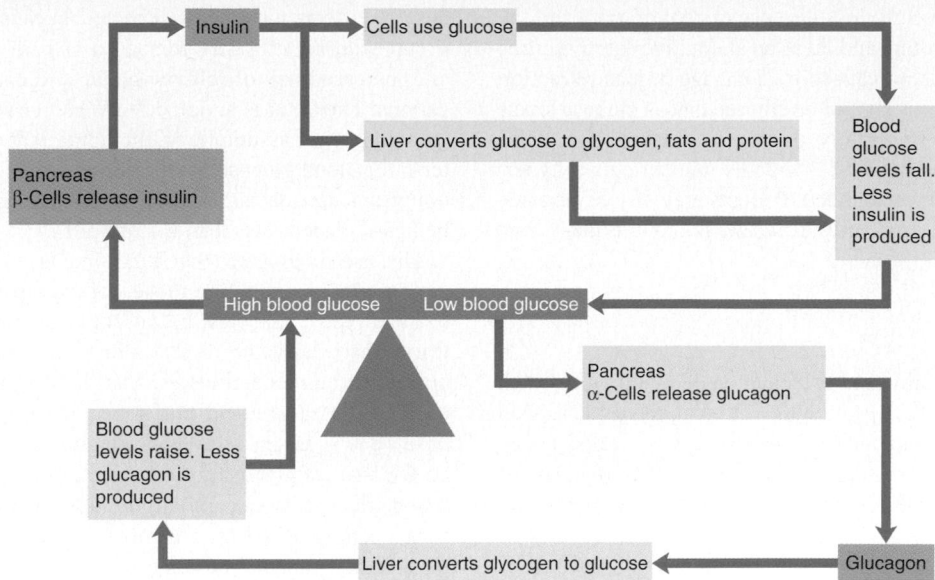

Fig. 45.1 Insulin–glucose relationship detailing the actions of insulin.

infection or other acute illness, there is increased secretion of the counter-regulatory hormones glucagon, cortisol, catecholamines and growth hormone. All of these will further increase hepatic glucose production (Fig. 45.1)

In type 2 diabetes, the process is usually less acute because relative insulin deficiency decreases over a sustained period of time. The initial response to hyperglycaemia is increased insulin production enabling euglycaemia. This hyperinsulinemia is able to maintain glucose levels for a period of time, but as insulin resistance increases, eventually not enough insulin can be produced, and β-cell function deteriorates, leading to a relative deficiency in insulin, and hyperglycaemia ensues. If this cycle is not interrupted, type 2 diabetes develops. Impaired glucose tolerance (IGT), impaired fasting glucose or hyperinsulinemia may be detected before overt diabetes develops, and if so, a strict diet and exercise regimen leading to weight loss and improved insulin sensitivity may delay or even prevent the onset of diabetes. At the time of diagnosis, those with type 2 diabetes may have already lost about 50% of their β-cell function. Irrespective of treatment, β-cell function continues to decline with time, often leading to the need for exogenous insulin therapy.

Type 2 diabetes is also associated with metabolic syndrome, although the relevance of this 'syndrome' continues to be debated in the literature (Khan et al., 2005). Metabolic syndrome is a group of risk factors commonly found in those with type 2 diabetes, including insulin resistance, glucose intolerance (type 2 diabetes or IGT), hyperinsulinemia, hypertension, dyslipidaemia, central obesity, atherosclerosis and increased levels of procoagulant factors, for example, plasminogen activator inhibitor-1 and fibrinogen.

Pathophysiology of insulin resistance

Abdominal fat is metabolically different from subcutaneous fat due to excess lipids in non-adipose tissue, which leads to cell dysfunction and death and subsequently lipotoxicity. Abdominal fat is resistant to the antilipolytic effects of insulin, resulting in the release of excessive amounts of free fatty acids, which in turn leads to insulin resistance in the liver and muscle. The effect is an increase in gluconeogenesis in the liver and an inhibition of insulin-mediated glucose uptake in the muscle. Both of these result in increased levels of circulating glucose. Further, excess fat itself may contribute to insulin resistance because when adipocytes become too large, they are unable to store additional fat, resulting in fat storage in the muscles, liver and pancreas, causing insulin resistance in these organs.

Additionally, the excess intra-cavity adipose tissue causes the oversecretion of some cytokines (adipokines or adipocytokines) associated with inflammation, endothelial dysfunction and thrombosis. Examples of such adipokines include plasminogen activator inhibitor-1 (prothrombotic), tumour necrosis factor-α and interleukin-6 (proinflammatory) and resistin (causes insulin resistance). The atherosclerosis associated with insulin resistance is considered to be due to hypercoagulability, impaired fibrinolysis and the toxic combination of endothelial damage, caused by chronic, subclinical inflammation, oxidative stress and hyperglycaemia. Excess adipose tissue is also thought to cause undersecretion of a beneficial adipokine called adiponectin. Adiponectin suppresses the attachment of monocytes to endothelial cells, thereby protecting against vascular damage. People with type 2 diabetes have lower levels of adiponectin than those without diabetes, and weight reduction increases adiponectin levels.

Clinical manifestations

The symptoms of both type 1 and type 2 diabetes are similar, but they usually vary in intensity. Those associated with type 1 diabetes are more severe and faster in onset. The symptoms are related to the osmotic effects of glucose and the abnormalities of energy partitioning. Common symptoms include polyuria and polydipsia, accompanied by fatigue due to an inability to utilise glucose and marked weight loss because of dehydration, and the breakdown of body protein and fat as an alternative energy source to glucose. Blurred vision caused by a change in lens refraction often occurs, and patients should be advised that as glucose levels are normalised, vision normally improves, and new spectacles should be avoided for the first 3 months until effective hyperglycaemia treatment is established. Patients may also experience higher infection rates, especially *Candida*, skin and urinary tract infections.

Type 1 diabetes

The metabolic abnormalities at presentation of an individual with type 1 diabetes are often profound. The symptoms mentioned earlier are usually extreme and of recent (days or weeks) onset. In a significant proportion, the presenting symptoms are those of diabetic ketoacidosis (DKA): nausea, vomiting, abdominal pain, dehydration, and shortness of breath (secondary to an attempt by the respiratory system to compensate for the metabolic acidosis caused by ketones) and, in extreme cases, coma. Without prompt treatment, DKA can be fatal.

Type 2 diabetes

Many patients with type 2 diabetes have an insidious onset of hyperglycaemia, with few or no classic symptoms. This is particularly true in obese individuals, whose diabetes may be detected only after glycosuria or hyperglycaemia is found during routine investigations or when they seek medical help for a problem they were unaware is a recognised complication of diabetes. Some patients are unaware of the disease even with marked classic symptoms because they begin so gradually and over such a long period of time. Recurring infections (e.g. urinary tract, chest, soft tissue) are common because sustained hyperglycaemia can result in severe impairment of phagocyte function, and raised glucose levels provide a growth medium for bacteria.

Generalised pruritus and symptoms of vaginitis, which may be due to candidal infection, are frequently the initial complaints of women with type 2 diabetes. Patients often present when the complications of sustained hyperglycaemia have already developed, for example, cardiovascular disease or renal disease. Retinopathy may be detected on routine ophthalmological examination. Alternatively, a combination of neuropathy, peripheral vascular disease (PVD) and infection may manifest as foot ulceration or gangrene. In some cases, patients present with hyperosmolar hyperglycaemic state (HHS), where glucose levels in excess of 35 mmol/L are found and excessive dehydration has occurred. Occasionally, patients with type 2 diabetes present with diabetic ketoacidosis, especially in severe infection or in those of African/Caribbean descent.

Diagnosis

In 2006 the World Health Organization (WHO, 2006) recommended that a glycated haemoglobin (HbA$_{1c}$) threshold of 48 mmol/mL (6.5%) may be used to diagnose diabetes. The current criteria have been accepted because they distinguish a group with significantly increased risk of premature mortality and increased risk of microvascular and cardiovascular complications. The UK has adopted the WHO criteria, which are based on a number of assumptions, including that normoglycaemia is a term for blood glucose levels associated with low risk of developing diabetes or cardiovascular disease, generally accepted to be blood glucose less than 6.1 mmol/L.

The use of glycated haemoglobin is not appropriate for all patient groups, including those, for example, who are suspected to have type 1 diabetes, gestational diabetes, haemoglobinopathies, anaemia, acute illnesses or with renal disease. As such, current recommendations are that the diagnosis is confirmed by a glucose measurement performed in an accredited laboratory on a venous serum sample. A diagnosis should never be made on the basis of glycosuria or a capillary reading of a finger-prick blood glucose alone, although such tests are commonly used for screening purposes. Diagnosis of type 1 diabetes is usually on clinical grounds, presence of hyperglycaemia, ketosis, rapid weight loss, younger age of onset, BMI less than 25 kg/m^2 and personal and/or family history of autoimmune disease. Do not discount the possible diagnosis of type 1 diabetes in patients who are older or have a raised BMI; it can occur at any age, with any BMI. A person is normally thought to have type 2 diabetes if he or she does not have type 1 diabetes, but as mentioned earlier, there are several other causes which ought to be considered (Table 45.2).

Diabetic emergencies

Hypoglycaemia and extreme hyperglycaemia, causing diabetic ketoacidosis or hyperosmolar hyperglycaemic state, constitute the three acute emergencies associated with diabetes.

Hypoglycaemia

Hypoglycaemia is the commonest side effect in the treatment of diabetes, resulting from the imbalance between glucose supply and insulin levels. It can occur both with insulin treatment and some oral agents, especially the longer-acting sulfonylureas (Table 45.3). Definitions of hypoglycaemia vary, but it is generally defined as being mild when blood glucose levels decrease and the person self-treats and as severe if intervention from a third party is required. Biochemical hypoglycaemia for hospital in-patients is specifically defined as a blood glucose less than 4.0 mmol/L. Physiologically, the defence to hypoglycaemia is the release of counter-regulatory hormones adrenaline (epinephrine), noradrenaline (norepinephrine) and glucagon. This tends to occur when the venous serum glucose drops to less than 3.5 mmol/L in healthy individuals. The symptoms people experience are non-specific and categorised as autonomic (adrenergic) symptoms and are the result of activation of the sympatho-adrenal system, whereas the neuroglycopenic symptoms are due to cerebral glucose deprivation (Table 45.4). These are a normal physiological response to hypoglycaemia and should alert the person to consume carbohydrates.

Table 45.2 Diagnostic criteria for the type 1, type 2 and gestational diabetes

Type 2 diabetes		Gestational	Type 1
Symptomatic	Asymptomatic		
A single fasting plasma glucose ≥7 mmol/L OR A single random plasma glucose ≥11.1 mmol/L	Positive results for two of the following on 2 different days: • A fasting glucose ≥7 mmol/L • A random plasma glucose ≥11.1 mmol/L • HbA$_{1c}$ ≥48 mmol/mol OR A single random plasma glucose ≥11.1 mmol/L OR A fasting glucose ≥7 mmol/L + HbA$_{1c}$ ≥48 mmol/mol	Fasting plasma glucose level of 5.6 mmol/L or greater OR A 2-h plasma glucose level of 7.8 mmol/L or greater	Based on clinical grounds Hyperglycaemia plus two out of three of: • Short history of symptoms • Ketones • Rapid weight loss

Table 45.3 Pharmacokinetic properties of non-insulin hypoglycaemic agents

Drug	Main elimination route	Elimination half-life (h)	Duration of action	Daily dose range	Doses per day
Sulfonylureas					
Tolbutamide	Hepatic	4–24	6–10	0.5–2 g	1–3
Chlorpropamide	Hepatic (80%) Renal (20%)	24–48	24–72	100–500 mg	1
Glibenclamide	Hepatic (40%) Biliary (60%)	2–4	16–24	2.5–15 mg	1–2
Glipizide	Hepatic	2–4	6–24	2.5–40 mg	1–3
Gliclazide	Hepatic	10–12	10–24	40–320 mg	1–2
Gliclazide MR	Hepatic	12–20	24	30–120 mg	1
Glimepiride	Renal (60%) Hepatic (40%)	5–8	12–24	1–6 mg	1
Biguanides					
Metformin	Renal	1–5	5–8	1–3 g	2–3
Metformin MR	Renal	6.5	10–16	0.5–2 g	1
Meglitinides					
Repaglinide	Hepatic	1	4–6	1–16 mg	3
Nateglinide	Hepatic	1	3–4	180–540 mg	3
Thiazolidinediones					
Pioglitazone	Hepatic	5–6	16–24	15–45 mg	1
Dipeptidyl peptidase 4 inhibitors					
Sitagliptin	Renal	10–12	12–24	100 mg (reduce in renal impairment)	1
Vildagliptin	Renal	3	10–12	50 mg	1–2
Saxagliptin	Renal/hepatic	2–3	24	5 mg	1

Continued

Table 45.3 Pharmacokinetic properties of non-insulin hypoglycaemic agents—cont'd

Drug	Main elimination route	Elimination half-life (h)	Duration of action	Daily dose range	Doses per day
Linagliptin	Hepatic	12	24+	5 mg	1
Alogliptin	Renal	21	24+	6.25–25 mg (reduce in renal impairment)	1
Sodium glucose co-transporter 2 inhibitors					
Dapagliflozin	Renal/hepatic	12–13	12–18	10 mg 5 mg (hepatic impairment)	1
Canagliflozin	Hepatic	8–18	24+	100–300 mg	1
Empagliflozin	Renal/hepatic	12	24+	10–25 mg	1
GLP1 agonist					
Exenatide twice daily	Renal	2–3	Data not available	5–10 microgram	2
Exenatide weekly	Renal	Depot	Depot	2 mg	Once weekly
Liraglutide	No main organ identified	13	Data not available	0.6–1.8 mg	1
Lixisenatide	Renal	3	Data not available	10–20 micrograms	1
Dulaglutide	No main organ	Depot	Depot	0.75–1.5 mg	Once weekly

GLP-1, Glucagon-like peptide 1 receptor agonist.

Table 45.4 Symptoms of hypoglycaemia

Adrenergic effects/autonomic (early symptoms)[a]	Neuroglycopenic effects (late symptoms)
Sweating	Confusion
Tachycardia	Slurred speech
Palpitations	Drowsiness
Pallor	Numbness of nose, lips or fingers
Hunger	Abnormal behaviour (anxiety, agitation, aggression)
Restlessness	Visual disturbances
Trembling	Loss of consciousness, seizures, coma and death

[a]These effects may be suppressed in people taking non-cardioselective β-blockers.

Hypoglycaemia unawareness is the term for when individuals do not counter-regulate to hypoglycaemia as effectively as normal. The reasons for the development of unawareness are multifactorial but are predominately due to a smaller counter-regulatory response with longer duration of diabetes and to previous recurrent episodes of hypoglycaemia suppressing the counter-regulatory response. These are exacerbated by a poor understanding of hypoglycaemia and the importance of effective treatment and, indeed, the rationale for preventing hypoglycaemia. If the serum glucose falls to approximately 2.8–3.2 mmol/L, there are acute changes in cerebral function which lead initially to cognitive dysfunction and which may present as confusion. As glucose levels fall further, the person is at risk of seizures, coma and even death. In patients who can detect hypoglycaemia, the autonomic symptoms of sweating, shaking and so forth occur above the level of cerebral dysfunction, and so they are able to self-treat. However, in patients with impaired awareness of hypoglycaemia, the autonomic symptoms occur below the level of neuroglycopaenic symptoms, and so patients may be very confused before any adrenergic symptoms occur, and therefore they are less likely to be able to self-treat. Thus, hypoglycaemia unawareness is associated with a much higher rate of severe hypoglycaemic episodes.

The ability to respond to the symptoms of hypoglycaemia are masked by alcohol intoxication, autonomic neuropathy and medications that supress the autonomic nervous system. There is evidence that the symptoms can be regained if, for a period of a few weeks/months, the serum glucose level can be maintained out of the hypoglycaemic range; this can be achieved without worsening glycaemic control (De Zoysa et al., 2014).

It is imperative, therefore, that people with diabetes who are prescribed medication which is known to cause hypoglycaemia

Table 45.5 Causes of hypoglycaemia

	Lifestyle factors		Medical factors
Diet	Reduced carbohydrate intake not matched with medication adjustment, e.g. due to missed or delayed meals and snacks	Insulin-/glucose-lowering drugs	Inappropriate use of one-off and when-required insulin doses Incorrect insulin or oral secretagogue pre-scribed Intravenous insulin infusion prescribed without concomitant glucose Incorrect timing of medication
Age	More likely in older people and those with longer duration of disease (decreased counter-regulatory response) Signs and symptoms may be misinterpreted because of age of patient (e.g. confusion)	Problems with blood glucose monitoring	Lack of education about how to interpret and use the results Monitoring not offered
Exercise/physiotherapy	Increase levels of exercise not matched with medication or dietary adjustment Mobilisation after illness Symptoms of hypoglycaemia may be misinter-preted as symptoms of exercise (e.g. sweating, tachycardia)	Changes in health status	Recovery from acute illness or stress, often re-lated to changes in eating habits and reduced carbohydrate intake Bariatric surgery, leading to reduced carbohy-drate consumption
History of severe hypoglycaemia	Inadequate treatment of previous event	Medication inter-actions	Discontinuation of long-term steroids Medication may need altering/stopping, dis-cuss with the multidisciplinary healthcare team responsible for the patient
Hypoglycaemia unawareness	Recurrent hypoglycaemia not adequately ad-dressed in patients on insulin or a sulfonylurea	Renal impairment/hepatic impair-ment	Dialysis Acute kidney injury (AKI) Medication may need stopping or the dose reducing – this will depend on the level of impairment and the product licence
Periods of fasting (e.g. Ramadan)	Reduced dietary intake and changes of meal-time need to be considered in conjunction with medication timing and doses		

should be educated about the autonomic symptoms so that they may take action to avoid further decline of serum glucose and are taught how to prevent future episodes.

Causes of hypoglycaemia

Hypoglycaemia occurs when insulin levels are higher than physi-ologically required to maintain a normal glucose (euglycaemia). Aside from changes in medication, the most common causes of hypoglycaemia are either a decrease in carbohydrate consump-tion or excess glucose utilisation from unexpected physical activ-ity (Table 45.5.).

If individuals have good control of their diabetes (as measured by HbA_{1c}), it would not be surprising that they may have one or two daytime mild episodes of hypoglycaemia each week. If hypoglycaemia is occurring more often than that, then possible contributory factors need to be reviewed: inappropriate insu-lin regimen; too high a dose of a sulfonylurea; meal and activ-ity patterns, including alcohol; injection techniques and skills (including insulin resuspension); injection site problems; organic causes such as gastroparesis; changes to insulin sensitivity (drugs affecting the renin–angiotensin system, weight loss, renal impair-ment); and psychological problems.

Nocturnal hypoglycaemia

Sometimes, hypoglycaemia occurs during the night, which may or may not wake the person with diabetes. Not unsurprisingly, blood glucose levels are often lower than detected during day-time hypoglycaemia, as the counter-regulatory response is less marked, and a more pronounced counter-regulatory response is required to wake the individual from sleep. Symptoms may include restlessness, although this may not be identified unless observed by another person. When nocturnal hypoglycaemia occurs, the person often wakes feeling unrested, unwell or with a headache. If nocturnal hypoglycaemia is suspected, then blood glucose should be measured at night, for example, 2.00–3.00 a.m. If confirmed, the patient should either have a snack before bedtime, reduce the evening/night-time dose of insulin or alter the timing of administration of the evening dose of intermedi-ate or long-acting insulin to delay the peak of bioavailability or change the intermediate-acting insulin to a peakless analogue as

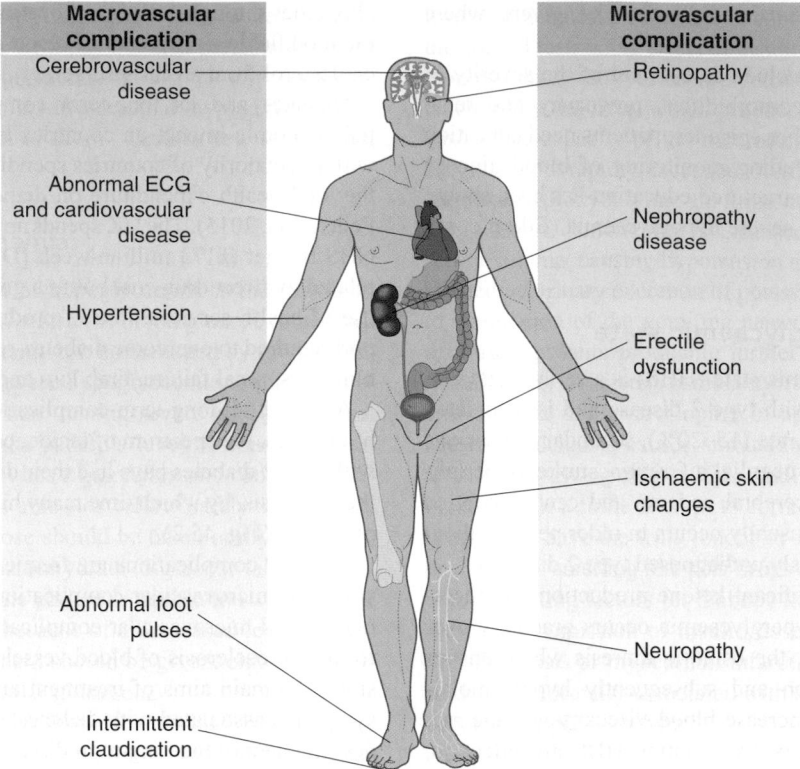

Fig. 45.2 Complications of diabetes. ECG, Electrocardiogram.

Hypertension

Hypertension is twice as common amongst the diabetic population compared with the general population, occurring in more than 80% of those with type 2 diabetes. Hypertension is associated with the development of macro- and microvascular complications; hence, the treatment target ranges for people with diabetes are generally lower than those for people without diabetes. For people with type 2 diabetes, hypertension is a feature of metabolic syndrome and is associated with insulin resistance. For those with type 1 disease, it is closely associated with renal disease. First-line antihypertensive drug treatment should be once-daily angiotensin-converting enzyme (ACE) inhibitors; exceptions to this are patients of African or Caribbean family origin and women who may become pregnant. Patients of African and Caribbean family origin should be offered an ACE plus diuretic or calcium channel blocker; women seeking to become pregnant should be offered a calcium channel blocker (NICE, 2015d).

Peripheral vascular disease

PVD affects more than 30% of people with diabetes who are older than 50 years. PVD particularly affects the arteries of the legs and may give rise to intermittent claudication, a cramping pain experienced on walking that is due to reversible muscle ischaemia secondary to atherosclerosis. The iliac vessels can be affected, causing buttock pain and erectile dysfunction. If PVD is present, the risk of cardiovascular disease increases, with approximately 20% of people suffering from a fatal myocardial infarction within 2 years of symptom onset. PVD is also responsible for much of the morbidity associated with diabetic foot problems.

Microvascular disease

Microvascular complications include retinopathy, nephropathy and neuropathy.

Retinopathy

Diabetic retinopathy is one of the leading causes of blindness in the UK and is the most common cause of blindness among people of working age in industrialised countries. Persistently high levels of blood glucose damage the network of blood vessels that supply the retina. The resulting retinopathy is initially symptomless in the early stages and may be advanced before it affects vision; therefore, screening is essential for early detection and subsequent treatment. Twenty years from the onset of diabetes, more than 90% of people with type 1 and more than 60% of people with type 2 will have diabetic retinopathy. Tight glycaemic control has been shown to prevent and delay the progression of retinopathy in patients with type 1 disease (Diabetes Control and Complications Trial Research Group [DCCT], 1993). Likewise, for patients with type 2 diabetes, both tight glycaemic control and tight blood pressure control reduce the risk of developing retinopathy (Kohner et al., 1998). When retinopathy is detected early, sight may be saved by laser photocoagulation. In advanced cases, surgery may be required.

Pregnancy may worsen moderate to severe retinopathy, particularly if there is poor or sudden improvement in glycaemic control. However, tight glycaemic control during pregnancy reduces the risk of foetal abnormalities.

Nephropathy

In diabetic renal disease, the kidneys become enlarged, and the glomerular filtration rate (GFR) initially increases. However, as nephropathy progresses, the GFR starts to decline. The GFR can be estimated (eGFR), but serum creatinine used alone to estimate renal function has limitations. The most popular method is the modified Modification of Diet in Renal Disease (MDRD) formula, which requires serum creatinine, age, sex and ethnicity. Creatinine clearance is often used for medication review and dose optimisation and may be calculated using the Cockcroft and Gault formula:

$$\text{C}_{\text{r}}\text{Cl (mL/min)} = \frac{(140 - \text{age}) \times \text{weight (kg)}}{\text{serum creatinine (mmol/L)}} \quad \begin{array}{l} (\times 1.23 \text{ if male,} \\ 1.04 \text{ if female}) \end{array}$$

The presence of nephropathy is indicated by the detection of microalbuminuria (small amounts of albumin present in urine). If higher amounts of albumin are detected, this is termed proteinuria or macroalbuminuria and signifies more severe renal damage. Microalbuminuria is defined as an albumin/creatinine ratio (ACR) greater than or equal to 3 mg/mmol. Proteinuria may be defined as an ACR greater than 30 mg/mmol or albumin concentration greater than 200 mg/L. Proteinuria may progress to end-stage renal disease and require dialysis. Albumin in the urine increases the risk of cardiovascular disease, with microalbuminuria associated with two to four times the risk, proteinuria with nine times the risk and end-stage renal disease increasing risk by 50 times.

Tight control of both glycaemic levels and blood pressure reduces the risk of developing nephropathy. ACE inhibitors or angiotensin receptor blockers (ARBs) are the treatments of choice because both have been proven to delay the progression to proteinuria in patients with macroalbuminuria, a renal protective outcome additional to their antihypertensive effects. Although not proven for all individual drugs in these classes, it is considered to be a class effect. These drugs should be used with care if there is a risk of renovascular disease.

Peripheral neuropathy

Peripheral neuropathy is the progressive loss of functional peripheral nerve fibres. Diabetic neuropathies can lead to a wide variety of sensory, motor and autonomic symptoms. The most common is the symmetrical distal sensory type, which is particularly evident in the feet and may slowly progress to a complete loss of feeling. Distal motor neuropathy can lead to symptoms of impaired fine coordination of the hands and/or foot slapping. Painful diabetic neuropathy is another manifestation of sensory neuropathy; it can be extremely disabling and may cause considerable morbidity. Guidance on the treatment of painful neuropathy is available (NICE, 2013). Diabetic proximal motor neuropathy is a relatively rare condition which is rapid in onset and involves weakness and wasting, principally of the thigh muscles. Muscle pain is common and may require multiple analgesic agents.

Autonomic neuropathy may affect any part of the sympathetic or parasympathetic nervous systems. The most common manifestation is erectile dysfunction. Bladder dysfunction usually manifests as loss of bladder tone with a large increase in volume. Diabetic diarrhoea is uncommon, but can be troublesome as it tends to occur at night. Gastroparesis may cause vomiting and delayed gastro-intestinal transit and variable food absorption, causing difficulty in the insulin-treated patient. There is no strong evidence that available antiemetic therapy is effective, although some people may benefit from domperidone, erythromycin or metoclopramide. Domperidone has the strongest evidence; however, the safety profile and cardiac risks must be considered. Postural hypotension due to autonomic neuropathy is uncommon but can be severe and disabling. Disorders of the efferent and afferent nerves controlling cardiac and respiratory function are more common but are rarely symptomatic. Autonomic neuropathy may also cause dry skin and lack of sweating, both of which may contribute to diabetic foot problems.

Macro- and microvascular disease combined

Diabetic foot problems

It is estimated that 10% of people with diabetes will develop a foot ulcer during their lifetime. Infected diabetic foot ulcers account for the largest number of diabetes-related hospital bed-days and are the most common non-trauma cause of amputations. Diabetic foot ulcers precede more than 80% of amputations in people with diabetes and are associated with poor morbidity and mortality, with approximately 50% of patients dying within 5 years. The rate of lower-limb amputation in people with diabetes is nearly 25 times higher than in the general population (NICE, 2015e). Diabetic foot ulcers impose immense medical and financial burdens on health care, as well as tremendous impact on the patient well-being and quality of life. Foot problems often develop as a result of a combination of sensory and autonomic neuropathy, PVD, poor foot care and hyperglycaemia. Development of foot ulcers may be partly preventable by patient education. People with diabetes need to learn that their feet are particularly vulnerable, and if problems arise, they must seek immediate professional advice.

There are three main types of foot ulcers: neuropathic, ischaemic and neuroischaemic. Neuropathic ulcers occur when peripheral neuropathy causes loss of pain sensation. The ulcers can be deep but are usually painless and are caused by trauma to the foot which is not noticed until after significant damage has occurred. Ischaemic ulcers result from PVD and poor blood supply causing a reduction in available nutrients and oxygen required for healing. Ischaemic ulcers may be painful and usually occur on the distal ends of the toes or the sides of the feet. Most ulcers have elements of both neuropathy and ischaemia and are termed neuroischaemic.

Diabetic foot ulcers are prone to infection, with the most common pathogens being staphylococci and streptococci. Wounds with an ischaemic component are commonly infected with anaerobic organisms. Resistant organisms are becoming common, and

Table 45.6 Glycaemic targets for patients with diabetes

	Fasting	Pre-meal	1 h post-meal	2 h post-meal	HbA$_{1c}$
Type 1 (NICE, 2015c)	5–7 mmol/L on waking	4–7 mmol/L		5–9 mmol/L (at least 90 min after eating)	48 mmol/mol
Type 2 (NICE, 2015d)		4–7 mmol/L		<8.5 mmol/L	48 mmol/mol (monotherapy) OR 58 mmol/mol (dual + therapy)
Gestational diabetes (NICE, 2015a)	<5.3 mmol/L		<7.8 mmol/L	<6.6 mmol/L	<48 mmol/mol

as such, antibiotic stewardship in the management of diabetic foot care is becoming increasingly important.

Charcot arthropathy. Charcot arthropathy is an uncommon foot complication caused by severe neuropathy, usually in a person with palpable foot pulses. It results in chronic, progressive destruction of joints with marked inflammation. Disorganised bone remodelling leads to fractures, altered foot shape and gross deformity. Because of the deformity which occurs, excess pressure over malpositioned bone frequently leads to ulceration unless footwear is extensively modified.

Treatment of diabetes

Treatment for people with diabetes includes advice on nutrition, physical activity, weight loss and smoking cessation. Drug therapy is prescribed where necessary, and a patient-centred approach should be undertaken, based on consideration of the individual needs, treatment aims and comorbidities.

The aim of treatment for most people is to achieve blood glucose as close to normal as possible. The current treatment target for people with type 2 diabetes is to achieve an HbA$_{1c}$ of 48 mmol/mol (6.5%), unless on multiple treatments or prescribed a drug associated with hypoglycaemia, in which case the aim is 53 mmol/mol (7.0%) (Table 45.6). Treatment targets may be further moderated for patients unlikely to achieve long-term risk reduction due to reduced life expectancy or significant comorbidities, where tight control poses a risk of significant hypoglycaemia, impaired hypoglycaemia awareness, or the person drives or operates machinery.

Structured education programmes

Diabetes is a chronic condition that is predominately managed by the person with diabetes. Accordingly, understanding of diabetes and successful self-management are imperative in achieving optimal outcomes. Evidence-based structured education that empowers patients to manage their own diabetes is now considered standard care. Group education is often utilised because it offers economic advantages over one-to-one education, as well as peer support. Examples of such programmes include Dose Adjustment for Normal Eating (DAFNE) in type 1 diabetes and Diabetes Education for Self-Management in the Ongoing and Newly Diagnosed (DESMOND) in type 2 diabetes (Box 45.2).

Diet

Dietary control is the mainstay of treatment for type 2 diabetes, and carbohydrate counting plays an integral part in the management of type 1. Dietary recommendations have undergone extensive review in recent years, and considerable changes have been made. Healthy eating advice for people with diabetes is the same as for the general population, and dietary interventions should be part of a personalised plan that addresses the individual's nutritional needs, personal choice, cultural preferences and willingness to change (Box 45.3).

Carbohydrates and sweeteners

The blood glucose level is closely affected by carbohydrate intake. Current guidance for carbohydrate consumption emphasises the importance of total carbohydrate intake, with a focus on selecting carbohydrates with a lower glycaemic index. Low-glycaemic-index carbohydrates give sustained release of glucose over time; examples include beans, pulses and starchy foods like whole-meal pasta and whole-grain bread. High-glycaemic-index carbohydrates that give high peaks in blood glucose concentration are best avoided or eaten in small quantities. Total carbohydrate consumption should not exceed 45–60% of energy intake, with monounsaturated fat and carbohydrate combined making up 60–70% of energy intake.

Sucrose or 'sugar' may be included in the diet but should account for no more than 10% of total energy and should be spaced throughout the day, rather than being consumed all in one go. Sugar alcohols, for example, sorbitol, maltitol and xylitol, are often used as sugar substitutes in diabetic foods and may cause diarrhoea. They are therefore considered to confer little advantage over sucrose. Non-nutritive or intense sweeteners such as aspartame, saccharin, acesulphame K, cyclamate and sucralose may be useful, especially for those who are overweight.

Alcohol

Alcohol contains carbohydrates and, if consumed in excess, may cause hyperglycaemia. However, more dangerously, it is also associated with later-onset (up to 16 hours post-alcohol) hypoglycaemia and hypoglycaemia unawareness. Alcohol should be restricted to the same maximum weekly quantities as for the general population (14 units/week).

Box 45.2 Essential topics to be included in patient diabetes education programmes

The disease
Signs and symptoms

Hyperglycaemia
Signs and symptoms
- Frequent urination
- Extreme thirst
- Fatigue

Hypoglycaemia
Signs and symptoms
- Hungry
- Palpitations/fast heartbeat
- Sweating/clammy skin
Treatment choices
- Small carton of full sugar juice
- 5 Jellybeans or similar sweets
- Glucose tablets or gel

Exercise
- Benefits and effect on blood glucose control

Diet
- Carbohydrate awareness
- Benefits of a well-balanced diet

Insulin therapy
- Injection technique
- Types of insulin
- Onset and peak actions
- Storage
- Stability

Urine testing
- Glucose
- Ketones

Home blood glucose and ketone testing
- Technique
- Interpretation

Oral hypoglycaemic agents
- Mode of action
- Dosing
- Need for multiple therapies

Foot care
- Checking feet daily for cuts, sores, redness or infection
- Daily washing of feet
- Keeping the skin smooth and soft

Management during illness
- Sick-day rules
- Importance of maintaining hydration

Cardiovascular risk factors
- Smoking
- Hypertension
- Obesity
- Hyperlipidaemia

Eye care
- Regular medical and ophthalmological examinations

Box 45.3 General dietary advice for people with diabetes

- Eat regular meals based on starchy foods such as bread, pasta, potatoes, rice and cereals. Whenever possible, choose high-fibre varieties of these foods, e.g. whole-meal bread and whole-meal cereals, which have a lower glycaemic index.
- Try to cut down on fat, particularly saturated (animal) fats. Monounsaturated fats such as olive oil are preferred. Use less butter, margarine and cheese and eat fewer fatty meals. Choose low-fat dairy foods, e.g. skimmed milk and low-fat yoghurt. Grill, steam or oven bake instead of frying or cooking with oil or other fats.
- Try to eat at least five portions of fruit and vegetables every day. This provides vitamins and fibre and helps balance the overall diet.
- Cut down on sugar and sugary foods. Sugar can still be used as an ingredient in foods and baking as part of a healthy diet. Use sugar-free, low-sugar or diet squashes and fizzy drinks because sugary drinks cause blood glucose levels to rise quickly.
- Use less salt because high intake can raise blood pressure. Food can be flavoured with herbs and spices instead of salt.
- Drink alcohol in moderation. Two units/day for women and men. A small glass of wine or half a pint of normal-strength beer is one unit. Never drink on an empty stomach. Excess alcohol can cause hypoglycaemia.

Fats

Because obesity is a major factor in type 2 diabetes and fats contain more than twice the energy content per unit mass than either carbohydrate or protein, consumption of fats should be limited. Intake of fat should be less than 35% of total energy consumption, with saturated and trans-unsaturated fats accounting for less than 10% of energy intake. Saturated fats are chiefly of animal origin; however, some are found in plants, such as cocoa butter, coconut oil and palm oil. Trans-unsaturated fats are found in hydrogenated vegetable oils and hard margarines.

Protein

For adults without nephropathy, protein intake is recommended as less than 1 g/kg of body weight, equivalent to about 10–20% of total energy intake. For those with nephropathy, protein intake may need to be further restricted, but this requires expert dietetic advice and supervision.

Fibre

Dietary fibre has useful properties in that it is physically bulky, and it delays the digestion and absorption of complex carbohydrates, thereby minimising hyperglycaemia. For the average person with type 2 diabetes, 15 g of soluble fibre from fruit, vegetables or pulses is likely to produce a 10% improvement in fasting blood glucose, glycated haemoglobin and low-density lipoprotein cholesterol (LDL-C). Insoluble fibre from cereals, whole-meal bread, rice and pasta has no direct effect on glycaemia or dyslipidaemia, but it has an overall benefit on gastro-intestinal health and may help in weight loss by promoting satiety.

Salt

Evidence shows that a modest reduction in salt consumption can significantly reduce both systolic and diastolic blood pressure in both hypertensive and normotensive individuals. Reducing salt intake from 9–12 to 5–6 g/day has a major effect on blood pressure, with the evidence supporting that a larger reduction in salt has the greatest impact on blood pressure reduction (He et al., 2013).

Obesity management in type 2 diabetes

Obesity management is an important issue in type 2 diabetes because of the insulin resistance which occurs as a consequence of excess adipose tissue. Weight loss in those who are overweight or obese is associated with an improvement in dyslipidaemia, hypertension and glycaemic control. Bariatric surgery can lead to profound improvements, with studies showing that laparoscopic banding can induce remission of type 2 diabetes in 48% of individuals and that Roux-en-y bypass procedures can induce remission in 84% (Vetter et al., 2009). More importantly, bariatric surgery is associated with a 92% relative risk reduction in diabetes-specific mortality and consequently should be offered to those with diabetes who have a BMI of 35 kg/m^2 or higher (NICE, 2014). For those with a BMI of 28 kg/m^2 or greater, it is recommended that the pancreatic and gastric lipase inhibitor orlistat be considered because the modest weight reduction which can be achieved with this agent yields benefits in diabetes control.

Insulin therapy in type 1 diabetes

Insulin replacement is the mainstay of treatment for all patients with type 1 diabetes. Exogenous insulin is used to mimic the normal physiological pattern of insulin secretion as closely as possible for each individual patient. However, a balance is required between tight glycaemic control and hypoglycaemia risk. If the risk of hypoglycaemia is high, then it may be necessary to aim for less tight glycaemic control. There is a wide variety of insulin preparations available which differ in species of origin, onset of action, time to peak effect and duration of action (Table 45.7).

Adults with type 1 diabetes should be supported to achieve a target HbA$_{1c}$ of 48 mmol/mol (6.5%) to minimise the risk of long-term vascular complications. Ideally this should be achieved through a flexible insulin regimen of self-injecting multiple daily doses of insulin, adjusted based on physical activity, food intake and current blood glucose. Blood glucose may be tested up to 10 times a day, with target blood glucose levels of 5–7 mmol/L on waking and 4–7 mmol/L before meals at other times of the day. Bedtime targets should be individually set. Adults who wish to test post-meals should aim for a plasma glucose 5–9 mmol/L at least 90 minutes after eating (see Table 45.6). Adults with type 1 diabetes who are unable to obtain good control of their diabetes or who have significant problems with hypoglycaemia may benefit from insulin pump therapy (NICE, 2008a). If, despite insulin pump therapy, adults with type 1 diabetes have recurrent severe hypoglycaemic episodes unresponsive to treatment, islet cell or pancreas transplantation may be considered. This option

Table 45.7 Common insulin nomenclature

Type of insulin	Description	Additional Information
Endogenous insulin	The natural insulin produced by the pancreas	
Human insulin	Laboratory synthesised insulin – equivalent to endogenous insulin	Available as two forms: • Short-acting soluble • Intermediate acting
Short-acting soluble insulin	A human insulin with a moderately fast onset and short duration of action	Often given with meals (prandial)
Intermediate-acting neutral protamine Hagedorn (NPH) Isophane	A suspension of human insulin with a more sustained duration of action	Given as background (basal) insulin
Premixed insulin	A mixture of the short- or rapid-acting insulin with the intermediate-acting insulin in predetermined concentrations	Human biphasic Analogue biphasic
Analogue insulin	Laboratory synthesised and modified insulin to alter how quickly or slowly it acts	Available as two forms: • Rapid acting • Long acting
Rapid-acting analogue	Modified synthetic insulin with rapid onset and short duration of action	Given with meals (prandial)
Long-acting analogue	Modified synthetic insulin with slow onset of action and sustained duration of action	Given as background (basal) insulin

is more widely offered if the patient has already received a renal transplant and is therefore currently taking immunosuppressive therapy.

Insulin species of origin

Until the 1980s, insulin was obtained and purified from the pancreas of pigs and cows. Many of the animal-derived products have been withdrawn, but some continue to be available. Porcine insulin only differs from human insulin in one amino acid at the end of the B chain (position B30). Human sequence insulins have subsequently been developed using recombinant DNA technology and are now the most common insulins in use. Human insulin may be produced semi-synthetically by enzymatic modification of porcine insulin (emp) or using genetic engineering and recombinant DNA technology. This is done by inserting either synthetic genes for the insulin A chain and B chain, or the proinsulin gene, or a proinsulin-like precursor into *Escherichia coli* (crb, prb) or yeast cells (pyr). The cells are fermented, resulting in large amounts of the recombinant protein, which is then converted into insulin and purified. More recently, human insulin analogues have been developed through genetic and protein engineering, producing insulin molecules with differing pharmacokinetic properties. In recent years, biosimilar insulin products have also been introduced; this is a biological copy of an existing insulin, but it cannot be said to be identical.

It is now standard practice to commence all patients requiring insulin on human insulin. Historically, in those who have been changed from animal to human insulin, there was a concern regarding an increased risk of hypoglycaemia and hypoglycaemic unawareness, although this was much less likely if the dose was reduced appropriately. Human insulin may be more potent dose for dose than animal insulin due to the formation of antibodies; hence, doses need to be reduced by 25% or more when changing from animal to either human or analogue insulin.

Insulin preparations

The onset of action, peak effect and duration of action are determined by the insulin type and by the physical and chemical form of the insulin, as detailed in Table 45.8.

Fast-acting insulins. Conventional fast-acting insulins are soluble insulins (also known as neutral insulins). After subcutaneous injection, soluble insulin starts to appear in the circulation within 10 minutes. The concentration rises to a peak after about 2 hours and then declines over a further 4–8 hours. This absorption curve can be contrasted with the physiological insulin concentration curve, where peak concentrations are reached 30–40 minutes after a meal and decline rapidly to 10–20% of peak levels after about 2 hours.

The fast-acting recombinant insulin analogues (insulin lispro, insulin aspart and insulin glulisine) offer greater convenience and flexibility, due to a more rapid absorption and shorter duration of action. They can be given immediately before a meal rather than the 30 minutes before recommended for human soluble insulin. The pharmacokinetic differences arise because the short-acting analogues remain as monomers (single units), unlike regular soluble human insulins, which self-associate into a hexameric (6-unit) form. Hexamers need to dissociate into dimers and monomers to be readily absorbed from subcutaneous tissue, which causes delayed absorption. However, in those people aiming for very tight glycaemic control (e.g. during pregnancy), there is benefit in injecting these short-acting insulin analogues 15–30 minutes pre-meals.

Intermediate-acting insulins. Conventional intermediate-acting insulins are insoluble, cloudy suspensions of insulin complexed with either protamine (also known as isophane or NPH insulin) or zinc (lente insulin). Over time, insulin dissociates from the complex, which gives the preparation its extended activity. The onset of action is usually 1–2 hours, with the peak effect being seen at 4–8 hours. There is considerable inter-patient variation in the duration of action, but it usually requires twice-daily administration to adequately cover a 24-hour period. Protamine

insulin and soluble insulin do not interact when mixed together. Therefore, ready-mixed (biphasic) preparations are available that contain both isophane and soluble insulin.

Long-acting insulins. More recently, long-acting insulin analogues, such as insulin glargine (Lantus), detemir (Levemir) and degludec (Tresiba), have been developed using recombinant DNA technology. They have a sustained duration of action, with more predictable, flat profiles of action with no pronounced peaks and less inter- and intra-subject dosing variability.

Insulin glargine differs from human insulin because two arginine molecules have been added to the B chain at the C-terminal end. This alters the isoelectric point from pH 5.4 to 6.7. Also, the neutral amino acid glycine replaces the asparagine residue at position A21. The changes mean that insulin glargine remains soluble at a slightly acidic pH. The product is buffered at a pH of 4. Once it is injected into subcutaneous tissue, it forms a microprecipitate in the more neutral surrounding pH. This allows slow absorption from the injection site. The recent introduction of glargine 300 units/mL (Toujeo), which forms a more compact microprecipitate, has a longer duration of action and less variable release profile.

Insulin detemir is formulated at neutral pH. It differs from human insulin by omission of the amino acid threonine at position B30 and the attachment of a fatty acid chain (myristic acid) to lysine at position B29. The modification allows the insulin molecule to reversibly bind to albumin, via the fatty acid chain, after absorption from subcutaneous injection. This reduces the amount of free, active insulin detemir because bound insulin is inactive. The long duration of action is produced by dissociation of the insulin molecule from albumin.

Insulin degludec forms soluble multihexamers upon subcutaneous injection, resulting in a depot that is continuously, slowly and evenly absorbed, with a duration of action beyond 42 hours. The sustained duration of action offers flexibility in dosing time, which may, for example, be particularly helpful for shift workers. In addition, due to its long half-life, it has been shown to reduce episodes of ketosis (Thalange et al., 2015).

Historically, insulin has been available in the UK as standard 100 units/mL. In recent years there have been increasing numbers of high-strength insulins developed. It is important to understand the insulin strength and how to use insulin correctly to minimise medication errors.

Combination products. Combined formulations of basal insulin and glucagon- (GLP-1–like peptide 1) receptor agonist are now commercially available. These offer the advantage of a single injection.

Insulin delivery

All the currently licensed insulin products are available only by injection. The subcutaneous route is routinely used for patients to self-administer their maintenance therapy and can be injected into the outer aspect of the thigh, abdominal wall, buttocks or upper arm. However, injecting into the arm safely over a long period of time is difficult and is therefore not usually a site of choice. Subcutaneous administration cannot be regarded as physiological because it delivers insulin to the systemic rather than portal circulation.

Table 45.8 Insulin preparations

Preparation	Origin	Onset (h)	Peak (h)	Duration (h)	Comments
Soluble insulin					
Actrapid (pyr)	H	0.5	2–5	8	Given at meal times (three times a day), usually with once-daily or twice-daily Humulin I Insulatard Levemir Lantus Tresiba Toujeo
Humulin S	H	0.5	1–3	5–7	
Insuman Rapid (crb)	H	0.5	1–3	7–9	
Hypurin Bovine Neutral	B	0.5–1	2–5	6–8	
Hypurin Porcine Neutral	P	0.5–1	2–5	6–8	
Apidra (glulisine)	H A	0.25	1	3–4	
Humalog (lispro)	H A	0.25	1–1.5	2–5	
NovoRapid (aspart)	H A	0.25	1–3	3–5	
Isophane insulin					
Hypurin Porcine Isophane	P	2	6–12	24	Once daily or twice daily Usually at bedtime and/or breakfast Occasionally pre-tea Used as monotherapy or with pre-meal quick-acting insulin
Insuman basal (crb)	H	1	3–4	12–20	
Insulatard (pyr)	H	2	4–12	24	
Humulin I	H	0.5	2–8	18–20	
Hypurin Bovine Isophane	B	2	6–12	24	
Long-acting analogues					
Levemir (detemir)	H A	2–4	6–14	16–20	Once daily or twice daily Usually at bedtime and/or breakfast Occasionally pre-tea Used as monotherapy or with pre-meal quick-acting insulin
Lantus (glargine 100 units/mL)	H A	2–4	6–12	20–24	
Toujeo (glargine 300 units/mL)	H A	2–4	No peak	24–26	
Tresiba (degludec)	H A	1	No peak	24–42	
Premixed insulin					
Humulin M3 (prb)	H	0.5	1–8.5	14–15	Usually twice daily Usually pre-breakfast and tea Rarely once a day NEVER at bedtime
Novomix 30	H A	0.25	1–4	Up to 24 h	
Humalog Mix 25	H A	0.25	1–2	22	
Humalog Mix 50	H A	0.25	1–2	22	
Hypurin Porcine 30/70	P	0.5	4–12	24	
Insuman Comb 15 (prb)	H	0.5	2–4	12–20	
Insuman Comb 25 (prb)	H	0.5	2–4	12–19	
Insuman Comb 50 (prb)	H	0.5	1–4	12–16	

Insulin preparation are classified as being human (H), beef (B), or pork (P) in origin. Analogue (A) denotes modified to alter onset and duration of action. crb, chain recombinant bacteria; prb, proinsulin recombinant bacteria; pyr, precursor yeast recombinant.

Insulin is available in a number of administration devices, including vials with syringes, cartridges for reusable pens and disposable pens.

Intravenous insulin delivery should be used in the management of ketoacidosis and hyperosmolar states. The intravenous route is also preferable for people with diabetes due to have major surgery and who may be 'nil by mouth' after surgery. The short half-life of insulin (3–5 minutes) means that changes in infusion rate have a rapid effect on insulin action and glycaemic control. Intravenous insulin is commonly delivered as a variable-rate insulin infusion (VRII), referred to as a 'sliding-scale' insulin regimen, in which the rate of infusion is adjusted according to frequent blood glucose readings, usually hourly. It is administered with a co-infusion of glucose (with potassium, unless patient is hyperkalaemic). Intravenous insulin regimens are not routinely recommended for patients who are eating and drinking.

Insulin regimens

Standard insulin regimens for managing type 1 disease vary between two and five injections daily. They must be tailored to the individual patient and will depend on lifestyle, willingness to achieve the best control and ability to cope with both injecting insulin and monitoring of blood glucose. The chosen insulin regimen is negotiated between patient and healthcare professional and may change throughout life according to priorities and patient preference. Starting doses of insulin and the ratio of short- to intermediate-acting insulin are very variable. In patients who are very active, such as manual workers and those who exercise regularly, lower doses are usually required.

Mealtime plus basal regimens. The best control for type 1 diabetes may be attained using a mealtime bolus plus basal regimen, also referred to as a basal-bolus regimen. This mimics normal physiological insulin release more closely than other regimens. A mealtime bolus plus basal regimen requires mealtime injections of insulin with a fast-acting preparation, preferably with an analogue, plus one or two injections of a basal (intermediate- or long-acting) insulin. This may require up to five injections a day. As a general rule, with this regimen, the soluble insulin injections given before each meal usually comprise 40–60% of the total daily dosage.

Current UK guidance is that newly diagnosed adults with type 1 diabetes should be offered multiple daily injections (basal bolus), including a rapid-acting analogue at mealtimes and twice-daily detemir, unless well managed on an alternative product, or twice-daily basal injections is not acceptable to the person (NICE, 2015c). Some individuals may benefit from delivery of fast-acting analogue insulin via a continuous subcutaneous insulin infusion administered via a pump worn on their person. The pump can be programmed to give a different basal rate of infusion at different times of day, and boluses are then provided by the pump at mealtimes. There are specific indications for pump therapy (NICE, 2008b).

These regimens offer the most flexibility of dosing and eating habits, and they often result in better blood glucose control. Individuals are taught to count mealtime carbohydrates and calculate their own insulin dose on the basis of the preprandial blood glucose concentration, which allows greater scope for 'normal eating'. An example is the DAFNE programme (DAFNE Study Group, 2002), in which patients are required to attend structured group education for 5 days.

The disadvantage of mealtime plus basal regimens is that they require multiple injections, unless a pump is in situ, and require regular blood glucose monitoring and the ability of the patient to match insulin doses according to carbohydrate intake, exercise levels and prevailing glucose levels. For some people, this is either too difficult or unsuitable.

Twice-daily regimens. The basal-bolus regimen may be too demanding for some to manage; as such, a twice-daily regimen may be more suitable. The simplest and most effective twice-daily regimens use premixed insulin, comprising a short- or rapid-acting plus an intermediate-acting insulin. Regular human insulin mixes and analogue mixes are available. The regular human insulin mixes should be given 30 minutes before breakfast and 30 minutes before the evening meal, whereas analogue mixes may be given immediately before these meals. The longer-acting component of the insulin mix given at breakfast time spans the lunchtime meal, and the evening dose bridges the night time. Twice-daily regimens using intermediate- or long-acting insulins alone are not usually sufficient for optimal control of type 1 diabetes.

Insulin dose adjustment. The information on which insulin dosage adjustment is based should be derived from blood glucose self-monitoring and the incidence and timing of hypoglycaemia. The frequency of monitoring usually mirrors the frequency of insulin injections, so the glucose concentration can be taken as a measure of the appropriateness of the previous insulin dose.

Adjustments to a dose of insulin should depend on the degree of insulin resistance present. To determine a suitable adjustment dose, the effect of other dosage adjustments in the same patient should be taken into consideration, as should the total insulin dose. For example, a 2-unit dose increase in someone taking 6 units of insulin would be a 33% dosage increase; however, a 2-unit dose increase in someone taking 60 units of insulin would be proportionately much less and make less impact. If monitoring shows persistent hyperglycaemia, then dose increases of 10–20% are usually required.

Storage of insulin

Insulin formulations are stable if kept out of light and not subject to freezing or extremes of heat. Loss of potency of 5–10% occurs in vials kept at high ambient room temperatures for 2–3 months. Insulin should therefore be stored in a domestic refrigerator except for the vial, cartridge or pen in current use, which, depending on the individual preparation, may be stable for 4–6 weeks (see manufacturers' recommendations). When pen injector devices are in use, they should never be stored in a refrigerator because there have been reports of devices 'seizing up' when stored in the cold. Also, the injecting of cold or refrigerated insulin is undesirable because it is more painful and the insulin absorption profile is altered.

Adverse effects of insulin

Hypoglycaemia is a common physiological complication of insulin therapy and is often a source of great anxiety to patients and carers. The symptoms may occur at different blood glucose levels in different individuals.

Thickening of subcutaneous tissues can occur at injection sites because of recurrent injection in the same area, known as lipohypertrophy. As well as looking unsightly, it can result in impaired and erratic insulin absorption, leading to poor glycaemic control. Good injection-site rotation reduces the incidence and impact. Bruising is usually a sign of superficial injections. Localised skin reactions occasionally occur but resolve even with continued use of the same insulin preparation.

Systemic allergic reactions rarely occur with the current highly purified insulins. Although reactions are not usually species specific, it is worthwhile to try insulin of a different species if allergy occurs. Also, some patients may experience allergy to the excipients within the insulin product or to the needle used for administration. If this is suspected, it is helpful to seek the advice of an immunologist and try an insulin product with different excipients.

Management of type 2 diabetes

About 85% of patients with type 2 diabetes are overweight at diagnosis, and this is known to cause insulin resistance; obese individuals also require higher doses of medication to control blood glucose levels. Education about healthy eating and weight loss through increased physical exercise and calorie restriction is required. Targets for weight should be to maintain a normal BMI of between 20 and 25 kg/m^2 or a waist circumference of less than 88 cm in women and 102 cm in men, which lowers the risk of developing insulin resistance. In those who are already overweight or obese, however, an achievable target of 10–15% body weight loss should be discussed because, if achieved, this will have significant benefits in overall diabetes control.

Some people are able to normalise their glycaemic control by weight loss and attention to diet (diet controlled). Nevertheless, such individuals still invariably have diabetes and are at risk of developing diabetic complications. Hyperglycaemia may still occur, especially in times of stress or if dietary control is lost, and consequently, they should be monitored regularly.

For more than 75% of people with type 2 diabetes, dietary measures and exercise alone do not produce adequate glycaemic control, and oral hypoglycaemic therapy is required. In the UK, there are seven classes of oral agents currently available: a biguanide (metformin), sulfonylureas (glibenclamide, gliclazide, glimepiride, glipizide, tolbutamide), meglitinides (repaglinide and nateglinide), a thiazolidinedione (pioglitazone), an α-glucosidase inhibitor (acarbose), the dipeptidyl peptidase-4 inhibitors (saxagliptin, sitagliptin, linagliptin, alogliptin and vildagliptin) and most recently the sodium-glucose co-tansporter-2 inhibitors (canagliflozin, dapagliflozin and empagliflozin).

When choosing and optimising the medication, it is important to adopt an individualised approach, not only considering the evidence base for the medication but also the individual circumstances. Factors to consider include degree of hyperglycaemia, weight, renal function, personal preference, comorbidities, risks from polypharmacy, ability to benefit from long-term interventions because of reduced life expectancy and also consideration of any disabilities such as visual impairment.

Metformin remains the foundation of oral treatment for type 2 diabetes (NICE, 2015d). The sulfonylureas and meglitinides are known as insulin secretagogues because they both enhance secretion of insulin from the pancreatic β-cells. The relatively recent introduction of the dipeptidyl peptidase inhibitors (DPP-4 inhibitors) and sodium-glucose co-tansporter-2 inhibitors (SGLT-2s) has been welcomed; these are useful classes of drugs, particularly for those in whom weight is a problem because they do not cause weight gain. Likewise, the injectable incretin mimetics (exenatide, liraglutide, lixisenatide and dulaglutide) are often helpful for the obese population because they are associated with weight reduction (Table 45.9)

In type 2 diabetes, the progressive decline in β-cell function with time and increasing insulin resistance means people with this disease show a progressive loss of glycaemic control and usually require two or three drugs with different modes of action to maintain control before ultimately requiring insulin (Fig. 45.3).

Biguanides

Mode of action. Metformin is the only biguanide available in the UK. The full mechanism of action of biguanides is still not completely understood. However, the principal mode of action is via potentiation of insulin action at an unknown intracellular locus, resulting in decreased hepatic glucose production by both gluconeogenesis and glycogenolysis. Metformin also stimulates tissue uptake of glucose, particularly in muscle, and is thought to reduce gastro-intestinal absorption of carbohydrate. The action of metformin does not involve stimulation of pancreatic insulin secretion, and therefore it is still a beneficial agent when β-cell function has declined. Metformin also offers the advantage that it does not cause hypoglycaemia and is not associated with weight gain. Metformin has a short duration of action, with a half-life of between 1.3 and 4.5 hours, and does not bind to serum proteins. It is not metabolised and is totally renally eliminated.

It has been shown that diabetes-related death was reduced by 42% in overweight subjects who took metformin for 10 years compared with those who took conventional therapies such as a sulfonylurea or insulin. Myocardial infarction was also reduced by 39% over the 10-year follow-up period. Consequently, metformin has become the first-line therapy for glycaemic control when oral agents are indicated, especially in overweight and obese patients (UK Prospective Diabetes Study Group [UKPDS], 1998a).

Adverse effects. The most common adverse effects of metformin, affecting about a third of patients, result from gastro-intestinal disturbances including anorexia, nausea, abdominal discomfort and diarrhoea. In some patients, diarrhoea can be extreme and can preclude metformin use. However, the gastro-intestinal side effects are usually transient and can be minimised by starting with a low dose, increasing the dose slowly and administering the drug with or after food. A suggested regimen is to start with 500 mg daily for 1 week, then 500 mg twice daily for 1 week, increasing the dosage at weekly intervals until the desired glycaemic response is achieved or intolerance occurs. The

Table 45.9 Factors to consider for dual therapy with metformin + additional agent (NICE, 2015d)

	Sulfonylurea	Thiazolidinedione	DPP-4 inhibitor	SGLT-2 inhibitor	GLP-1 agonist[a]	Insulin (basal)
Efficacy	High	High	Intermediate	Intermediate	High	High
Hypoglycaemia risk	Moderate	Low	Low	Low	Low	Moderate to high
Weight	Gain	Gain	Neutral	Loss	Loss	Gain
Side effects	Hypoglycaemia Rash Urticaria Liver enzyme disturbances	Oedema Heart failure, Fractures Bladder cancer, Respiratory tract infections Hypoesthesia	Hypoglycaemia Pancreatitis Headaches	Urinary tract Infections Dehydration Hypotension DKA	Gastrointestinal disturbances Pancreatitis Nausea and vomiting	Hypoglycaemia Injection site reactions Lipohypertrophy, rarely lipoatrophy
Relative cost	Low	Low	High	High	High	Variable

[a]NICE does not specifically recommend this combination at first intensification. Specialised and European practice does recognise this place in therapy
DKA, Diabetic ketoacidosis; DPP-4, dipeptidyl peptidase-4; GLP-1, glucagon-like peptide 1; SGLT-2, sodium-glucose co-tansporter-2.

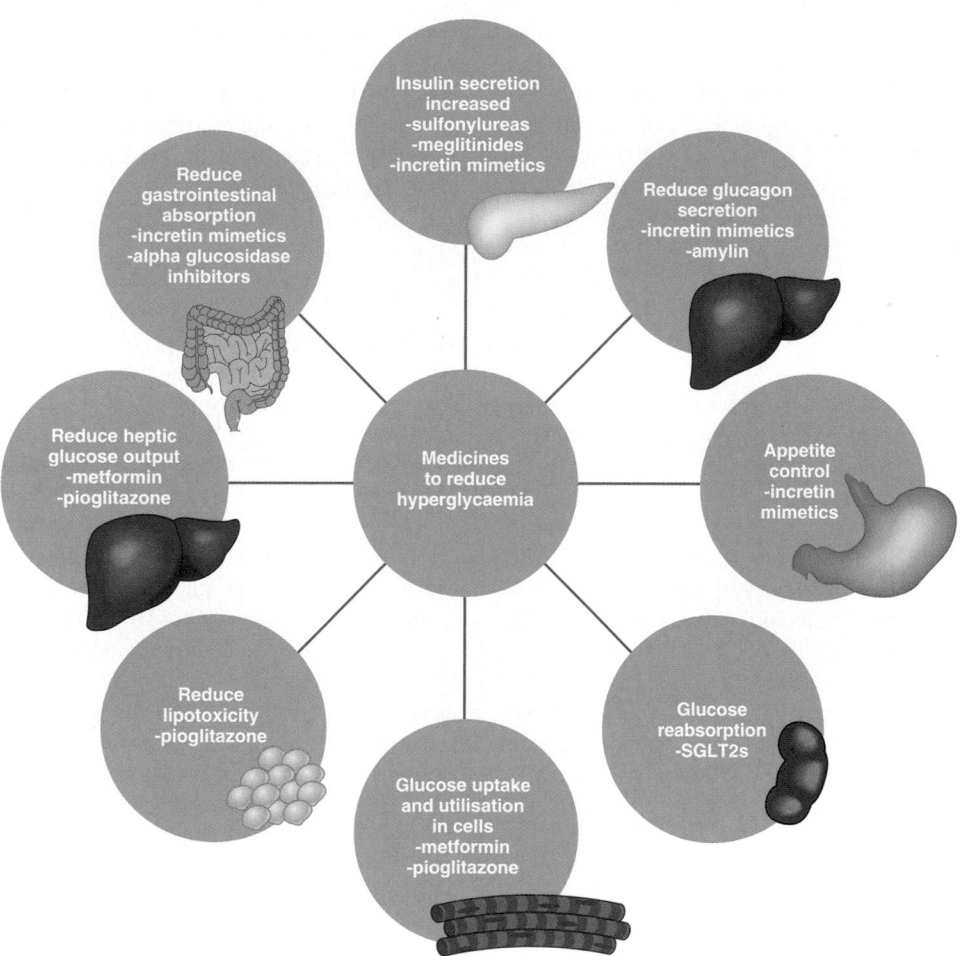

Fig. 45.3 Mode and place of action of the oral hypoglycaemic agents.

maximum licensed dose is 3 g/day, but doses of more than 2 g/day often cause intolerance and are not generally recommended.

Modified-release metformin preparations are now available and permit once-daily dosing. Clinical evidence suggests that these formulations cause fewer problems with gastro-intestinal side effects. The maximum licensed dose of the modified-release preparations (2 g daily) differs from the standard preparation.

The two previously available biguanides, phenformin and buformin, were withdrawn due to deaths associated with lactic acidosis. Lactic acidosis is a rare but potentially life-threatening complication with metformin, with an estimated incidence of five cases per 100,000 patient-years. Patients at most risk are those with renal insufficiency in whom the drug accumulates, individuals with co-existing conditions where lactate accumulates, and those who are unable to metabolise lactate. In practice, metformin should be used with caution for patients who have renal impairment (eGFR <45 mL/min/1.73 m^2) and should be stopped in anyone with an eGFR less than 30 mL/min/1.73 m^2. Metformin should also be stopped in severe liver disease, uncontrolled cardiac failure or severe pulmonary insufficiency. It should be withdrawn in patients with severe intercurrent illness, for example, acute myocardial infarction or septicaemia, or those undergoing major surgery or requiring investigation using radiographic contrast media and should only be restarted once renal function has been evaluated and determined as within acceptable limits.

Role of metformin. Metformin is recommended as the first-line drug for people with type 2 diabetes and is particularly useful in obese patients because it is weight neutral. Because it has a different mode of action than the other oral agents, it can be valuable when prescribed in combination.

Current NICE (2015c) guidance for type 1 diabetes states to consider metformin as an adjunct to insulin therapy if an adult has a BMI greater than or equal to 25 kg/m^2 (23 kg/m^2 in South Asian or related ethnic group).

Sulfonylureas

Mode of action. The major action of this class of drug relies on the ability of the pancreas to secrete insulin and hence requires functioning β-cells to exert a beneficial effect. Sulfonylureas lower blood sugar by increasing pancreatic β-cell sensitivity to glucose, allowing more insulin to be released from storage granules for a given glucose load. Sulfonylurea therapy is also associated with increased tissue sensitivity to insulin, resulting in improved insulin action. Studies also suggest that sulfonylureas may promote an increased systemic bioavailability of insulin due to reduced hepatic extraction of insulin secreted from the pancreas.

Pharmacokinetics. The pharmacokinetic parameters of oral hypoglycaemic agents are shown in Table 45.3. Chlorpropamide is the slowest and longest-acting agent, but it is now very rarely used. Although glibenclamide has been shown to have a short elimination half-life, it has a prolonged biological effect. All sulfonylureas are metabolised by the liver to some degree, and some may have active metabolites.

Choice of drug. There are few well-controlled long-term clinical comparisons between sulfonylureas; it would appear that when dosage is individualised and governed by the effect on fasting blood glucose, there is little or no difference in clinical efficacy between different agents. Therefore, choice is governed by the drug profile, the patient and the prescriber's clinical experience. In general, if a patient is not well controlled on the maximum dosage of one sulfonylurea, it is not worthwhile to change to another one.

Adverse effects. The frequency of adverse effects from sulfonylureas is low. They are usually mild and reversible on drug withdrawal. The most common adverse effects are weight gain and hypoglycaemia. Hypoglycaemia may be profound and long lasting and is often misdiagnosed, particularly in the elderly. The major risk factors for the development of hypoglycaemia include the use of a long-acting agent, increasing age, renal or hepatic dysfunction and inadequate carbohydrate intake.

Sulfonylurea dosage. The dosage should be individualised for each patient. The lowest possible dose required to attain the desired levels of blood glucose, without producing hypoglycaemia, should be used. Treatment should start with a low dose and be increased if necessary approximately every 2 weeks. For many agents, the maximum effect is seen if the dose is taken half an hour before a meal, rather than with or after food. The number of daily doses required will depend on the agent used and the total daily dose.

A modified-release preparation of gliclazide is available. A dose of 30 mg of the modified-release product is equivalent to 80 mg of the standard-release preparation.

Drug interactions. Several drugs can interfere with the efficacy of sulfonylureas by influencing either their pharmacokinetics or pharmacodynamics, or both. Despite much literature about displacement interactions with sulfonylureas, the clinical significance is doubtful. Many reported cases involve first-generation agents, which have a different protein-binding site from the second-generation agents, which bind in a non-ionic fashion and are not readily displaced. Ingestion of alcohol can cause hypoglycaemia in itself and can also prolong the hypoglycaemic effect of sulfonylureas.

Meglitinides

The meglitinides are insulin-releasing agents (insulin secretagogues), also called 'post-prandial glucose regulators'. They are characterised by a more rapid onset and shorter duration of action than sulfonylureas. Their site of action is pharmacologically distinct from that of the sulfonylureas. Repaglinide, a benzoic acid derivative, is licensed for use as a single agent when diet control, weight reduction and exercise have failed to regulate glucose levels, or in combination with metformin. Nateglinide is a derivative of the amino acid D-phenylalanine, licensed for combination therapy with metformin when metformin alone is inadequate.

Mode of action. Like the sulfonylureas, the meglitinides stimulate first-phase insulin secretion by inhibiting adenosine triphosphate (ATP)–sensitive potassium channels in the membrane of the pancreatic β-cells. This causes depolarisation and gating of the calcium channels (which are voltage sensitive), increasing the intracellular concentration of calcium and stimulating insulin release. The release of insulin only occurs in the presence of glucose. As glucose levels drop, less insulin is secreted. Conversely, if carbohydrates are consumed and glucose levels rise, insulin secretion is enhanced.

Pharmacokinetics. The pharmacokinetic properties of meglitinides confer a rapid onset and a short duration of action (see Table 45.3). Meglitinides are extensively metabolised in the liver, repaglinide by oxidative biotransformation and direct conjugation with glucuronic acid. The cytochrome P450 enzymes CYP2C8 and CYP3A4 have been shown in vitro to be involved its metabolism. Nateglinide is metabolised predominantly by cytochrome P450 enzyme CYP2C9 and to a lesser extent by CYP3A4. Repaglinide has no active metabolites, but nateglinide has partially active metabolites, one-third to one-sixth the potency of the parent compound. Meglitinides should be taken immediately before main meals, although the time can vary up to 30 minutes before a meal. The pharmacokinetic profile of meglitinides offers some advantages in patients with poor renal function or irregular eating habits.

Adverse effects. Meglitinides may cause a range of side effects, most commonly hypoglycaemia, weight gain, visual disturbances, abdominal pain, diarrhoea, constipation, nausea and vomiting. More rarely, hypersensitivity reactions and elevation of liver enzymes can occur.

Dosage. The recommended starting dose for repaglinide is 500 micrograms before or with each meal, increasing as necessary (depending on blood glucose measurements) every 1–2 weeks to a maximum single dose of 4 mg and a maximum daily dose of 16 mg. When patients are transferred from other therapies, the recommended starting dose is 1 mg preprandially. The recommended starting dose of nateglinide is 60 mg three times a day before meals, which may be subsequently increased to 120 mg three times a day. The maximum single dose is 180 mg, which may be given with the three main meals of the day.

Drug interactions. Drugs which induce or inhibit the cytochrome P450 enzymes CYP2C8 and CYP3A4 interact with repaglinide. Examples of drugs which enhance or prolong the hypoglycaemic effect include gemfibrozil, clarithromycin, ketoconazole, itraconazole, trimethoprim, other hypoglycaemic drugs, monoamine oxidase inhibitors, non-selective β-blockers, ACE inhibitors, salicylates, NSAIDs, octreotide, alcohol and anabolic steroids. Drugs which induce cytochrome P450 enzymes may also interact, for example, rifampicin and phenytoin, and may decrease repaglinide serum levels. Drugs that inhibit CYP2C9 may interact with nateglinide. Drugs that may enhance or prolong the hypoglycaemic effect include ACE inhibitors, gemfibrozil and fluconazole. The hypoglycaemic effects of nateglinide may be reduced by diuretics, corticosteroids and β-blockers.

Role of meglitinides. Meglitinides are an effective hypoglycaemic therapy in type 2 diabetes. They may be most beneficial in patients who experience problems with post-prandial glucose elevation and as single therapy in patients who eat at unpredictable times or have a tendency to miss meals.

Thiazolidinediones

Research into the action of the thiazolidinediones, also known as glitazones, has led to greater understanding of the development of type 2 diabetes. Pioglitazone has been shown to have a significant benefit on macrovascular morbidity and mortality, demonstrating the benefit of a glucose-lowering agent on macrovascular disease (Dormandy et al., 2005).

Mode of action. Glitazones act as agonists of the nuclear peroxisome proliferator-activated receptor-γ (PPAR-γ). PPAR-γ is mostly expressed in adipose tissue but is also found in pancreatic β-cells, vascular endothelium and macrophages. It is also expressed weakly in those tissues that express predominantly PPAR-α, for example, skeletal muscle, liver and heart. Thiazolidinediones lower fasting and post-prandial glucose levels in addition to lowering free fatty acid and insulin concentrations. They enhance insulin sensitivity and promote glucose uptake and utilisation in peripheral tissues. They also suppress gluconeogenesis in the liver and, by increasing insulin sensitivity in adipose tissue, suppress free fatty acid concentrations. The indirect effects of glitazones on adipose tissue are due to alterations in the regulation of gene expression. Various adipokines (adiponectin, tumour necrosis factor-α, resistin and 11β-hydroxysteroid dehydrogenase 1) are regulated by PPAR-γ agonists in animal studies.

Pharmacokinetics. Pioglitazone is metabolised extensively in the liver to both active and inactive metabolites.

Adverse effects. Congestive cardiac failure is an adverse effect. Therefore, because of the potential worsening of heart failure, pioglitazone should not be used in patients with a history of or pre-existing heart failure. Combination therapy with insulin and thiazolidinediones has been found to result in a higher incidence of oedema. There is also an increased risk of bone fracture with pioglitazone, and it should be used with caution in post-menopausal women. Approximately 1% of patients show a small decrease in the haemoglobin concentration during the first 4–12 weeks of therapy, possibly due to dilutional effects caused by an increase in serum volume. Pioglitazone caused weight gain of around 3.6 kg during clinical trials (Cheng and Kashyap, 2011). Some patients also experience headache, abdominal pain, myalgia and upper respiratory infection. Pioglitazone may also elevate liver transaminases. Studies have identified that there is a potential increase in the risk of bladder cancer. Pioglitazone should not be used in individuals with a history of bladder cancer, and the risk factors for bladder cancer should be assessed before initiating pioglitazone treatment (risks include age, smoking history, exposure to some occupational or chemotherapy agents, e.g. cyclophosphamide or prior radiation treatment in the pelvic region). Any macroscopic haematuria should be investigated before starting pioglitazone therapy, and patients should be advised to seek the attention of their doctor if haematuria or symptoms such as dysuria or urinary urgency develop during treatment.

Dosage. Pioglitazone is started at a dose of 15 or 30 mg and may be increased to 45 mg once daily. In combination with metformin or a sulfonylurea, the current dose can be continued. Dosage adjustment is not necessary in patients with mild or moderate renal impairment or in the elderly. Discontinue treatment in patients with severe renal impairment or in those with hepatic impairment.

Drug interactions. Pioglitazone is metabolised by cytochrome P450 CYP3A4. Therefore, ketoconazole, itraconazole, erythromycin and fluconazole increase serum concentrations, whereas rifampicin and phenytoin decrease serum levels of pioglitazone.

Role of thiazolidinediones. Thiazolidinediones improve glycaemic control in patients, especially in those with insulin resistance, by reducing HbA$_{1c}$ levels up to 1.5% compared with a sulfonylurea or metformin alone.

Glitazones may be used after lifestyle modification and the use of metformin monotherapy. Treatment should only be continued if, after 6 months of treatment, the HbA$_{1c}$ has reduced by 0.5% of its starting value.

Monotherapy with a thiazolidinedione may be a valuable treatment option for patients who are known to be insulin resistant. Triple therapy can be an alternative to transferring a patient to insulin, but the modest reduction in HbA$_{1c}$ usually means that many patients will eventually require insulin. It is important to be aware that because of their mode of action, which involves changes in gene transcription, thiazolidinediones take up to 3 months to have their maximum effect on glycaemic control.

Sodium-glucose co-tansporter-2 inhibitors

The SGLT-2s are a new class of oral medications for the treatment of type 2 diabetes. They are commonly referred to as the 'gliflozins'. They work by lowering the renal threshold to glucose, which leads to its urinary excretion. There are currently three licenced products: canagliflozin, dapagliflozin and empagliflozin.

Mode of action. Orally active, they selectively and reversibly inhibit the sodium-glucose co-transporter 2 (SGLT-2), which is selectively expressed in the proximal renal tubules of the kidney. SGLT-2 is the predominant transporter responsible for reabsorption of glucose from the glomerular filtrate back into the circulation. By inhibiting SGLT-2 the reabsorption of glucose is reduced. The amount of glucose excreted is dependent on blood glucose concentration and GFR. The reduction of renal reabsorption leading to urinary increased excretion of glucose improves both fasting and post-prandial glucose levels. Urinary glucose excretion is associated with calorific loss and reduction in weight, max 280 kcal/day and max 70 g/day, respectively.

Pharmacokinetics. The efficacy of SGLT-2s is dependent on renal function, and efficacy is reduced in renal impairment; dapagliflozin is not recommended if eGFR is less than 60 mL/min/m^2. Canagliflozin and empagliflozin require dose reduction in impaired renal function (eGFR less than 60 mL/min/m^2) and should be discontinued if eGFR is less than 45 mL/min/m^2. No dose adjustment is required in mild to moderate hepatic impairment; severe impairment requires discontinuation. They are not licensed in adults older than 75 years or children younger than 18 years of age.

Dapagliflozin and canagliflozin are metabolised via glucuronide conjugation mediated by UDP glucuronosyltransferase 1A9 (UGT1A9). Canagliflozin is also metabolised by UGT2BA and transported by P-glycoprotein and breast cancer resistance protein (BCRP).

In studies dapagliflozin neither inhibited cytochrome P450 (CYP) 1A2, CYP2A6, CYP2BB, CYP2C8, CYP2C9, CYP2C19, CYP2D6 CYP3A4 nor induced CYP1A2, CYP2BB or CYP3A4. Therefore, it is not expected to alter the metabolic clearance of co-administered medicinal products.

Empagliflozin is primarily metabolised by glucuronidation by uridine 5 diphosphoglucuronosyltransferases UGT1A3, UGT1A8, UGT1A9 and UGT2B7. It is a substrate of P-glycoprotein and breast cancer resistance protein (BRP), but medicinal interactions are not considered significant.

Adverse effects. Serious and life-threatening cases of DKA have been reported in people taking SGLT-2 inhibitors; the exact mechanism remains unclear. This atypical presentation in people with type 2 diabetes and near-normal blood glucose may delay diagnosis and treatment. As such, blood ketone tests should be undertaken in patients with acidosis symptoms, even if plasma glucose levels are near normal.

The most commonly reported side effects are infections and infestations, especially urinary tract infections, vulvovaginitis, balanitis and related genital infections. There may be a decrease in creatinine clearance, especially if taking other medication known to increase the risk of renal impairment, and it can lead to osmotic diuresis and volume-depletion reactions in elderly patients and those on diuretics. Caution should be applied if used with pioglitazone due to potential increases in the incidence of bladder cancer.

Drug interactions. Co-administration with diuretics may lead to dehydration and hypotension. Canagliflozin clearance is increased by enzyme inducers such as St John's wort, rifampicin, barbiturates, phenytoin, carbamazepine, ritonavir and efavirenz. If it is to be co-administered, the dose of canagliflozin may need to be increased, and glycaemic control monitored. Canagliflozin has been noted to inhibit P-glycoprotein (P-gp); therefore, patients taking digoxin and other cardiac glycosides should be monitored closely. The impact of the inhibition of the breast cancer resistance protein (BCRP) cannot be excluded, and therefore caution should be exerted when administering other medicinal products transported by BCRP such as rosuvastatin and anti-cancer medicinal products.

Role. The SGLT-2s are licensed for use in monotherapy or in combination with other glucose-lowering medicinal products, including insulin. Because they offer an alternative mechanism of action that is not insulin related, they are useful for patients with significant β-cell decline. They are also of particular benefit in patients where calorific reduction and weight loss would be valuable. It has also been identified that patients at high risk of cardiovascular events taking empagliflozin have a lower rate of cardiovascular outcomes and death compared with those receiving standard care (Zinman et al., 2015).

Dipeptidyl peptidase-4 inhibitors

The dipeptidyl peptidase-4 (DPP-4) inhibitors are a class of drugs that work on the incretin system. They are also commonly referred to as the 'gliptins' – sitagliptin, vildagliptin, saxagliptin, alogliptin and linagliptin.

Mode of action. DPP-4 inhibitors block the normal enzymatic inactivation of incretins, glucagon-like peptide-1 (GLP-1) and glucose-dependent insulinotropic peptide (GIP). Incretins play a role in increasing endogenous insulin in response to a high glucose load post-prandially. They also reduce the amount of glucose produced by the liver when glucose levels are sufficiently high. By blocking DPP-4, these drugs prolong incretin activity and inhibit glucagon release. This in turn causes a decrease in blood glucose and an increase in insulin secretion.

Pharmacokinetics. DPP-4 inhibitors are predominantly renally excreted. However, there is also a degree of hepatic metabolism involved in the elimination process, which varies with each drug. Sitagliptin is mainly excreted as unchanged drug in the urine, with a small metabolic contribution from the liver via the cytochrome P450 system. The kidney is thought to be mainly responsible for metabolic hydrolysis of vildagliptin to an inactive compound. Although saxagliptin is mainly eliminated renally, some hepatic biotransformation does occur via the cytochrome P450 system (CYP3A4/5), which results in a metabolite with half the potency of the parent compound. The dose guidance and pharmacokinetic parameters of the DPP-4 inhibitors are detailed in Table 45.3. In people with renal impairment, the significance of renal clearance for each of the DPP-4 inhibitors should be considered. The choice of agent and dose must be adjusted in accordance with the manufacturers' guidance.

Adverse effects. All DPP-4 inhibitors have been linked to gastro-intestinal side effects and upper respiratory tract infection. DPP-4 inhibitors do not cause hypoglycaemia, but they have the potential to cause hypoglycaemia when prescribed with other agents that can produce this effect. Vildagliptin has been associated with rare reports of liver dysfunction. Therefore, it is recommended that liver function tests are performed before starting treatment, at 3-month intervals for the first year and then periodically thereafter.

Drug interactions. DPP-4 inhibitors have a low potential for interaction with other medicines. However, because both sitagliptin and saxagliptin are metabolised by cytochrome P450 3A4/5 (and CYP2C8 for sitagliptin), they have the potential to interact with potent inducers or inhibitors of these enzyme. In practice, few drugs have been formally assessed. Therefore, general advice is to monitor blood glucose levels carefully if one of these drugs is co-prescribed with sitagliptin or saxagliptin.

Role of dipeptidyl peptidase-4 inhibitors. DPP-4 inhibitors are useful for those who still do not have adequate control or cannot tolerate treatment with metformin. DPP-4 inhibitors are also useful if further weight gain is likely or there is concern about the risk of hypoglycaemia. However, if insulin resistance is a key factor, then treating with a thiazolidinedione may be a better choice. The choice of agent will need to consider the degree of renal impairment, some agents require dose adjustment as renal function deteriorates.

Incretin mimetics

The incretin mimetics, as the name suggests, mimic the effects of incretins. The currently licensed products in the UK, exenatide, liraglutide, dulaglutide and lixisenatide are only available as subcutaneously injectable products. Incretin mimetics have been demonstrated to cause weight loss, which is a particularly beneficial effect in many patients with type 2 diabetes.

Mode of action. The incretin mimetics bind to and activate the glucagon-like peptide-1 (GLP-1) receptor, hence increasing insulin secretion, suppressing glucagon secretion, increasing satiety and slowing gastric emptying. All of these effects help lower blood glucose levels.

Pharmacokinetics. Incretin mimetics have a longer duration of action than endogenous GLP-1. Exenatide is eliminated primarily by renal clearance. However, the specific organ responsible for liraglutide elimination has not been identified.

Adverse effects. All incretin mimetics have been associated with nausea and other gastro-intestinal disturbances. However, once therapy has been established, the incidence of these side effects decreases. Acute pancreatitis has also been rarely reported.

For this reason, both patients and their carers should be advised of the signs and symptoms of this complication and advised to stop taking the drug and seek medical attention immediately if they occur. Because the incretin mimetics cause glucose-dependent insulin release, hypoglycaemia is uncommon and in most cases can be attributed to other agents taken concurrently.

Drug interactions. The potential for drug interactions with the incretin mimetics is low. However, because they can cause a delay in gastric emptying, they may influence the absorption of other medicines administered at the same time. For this reason, it is advised that any narrow-therapeutic-index drugs taken concomitantly are monitored carefully.

Role of incretin mimetics. It is recommended that GLP-1 mimetics be added as third-line therapy for patients who have a BMI of ≥35 kg/m², are of European descent (adjustments to this threshold may be made for other ethnic groups at greater risk of cardiac disease) and have other medical problems associated with increased body weight. Alternatively, they may be used in patients with a BMI less than 35 kg/m² who are not able to take insulin, for example, for occupational reasons, or who have other conditions that would benefit from weight loss. Treatment should only be continued if there has been an HbA$_{1c}$ reduction of at least 1% and a weight loss of at least 3% from starting treatment over a 6-month period (NICE, 2015d).

Insulin therapy in type 2 diabetes

The younger age of onset of type 2 diabetes and tighter glycaemic targets mean that the majority of patients with type 2 diabetes progress to insulin therapy because evidence confirms that long-term glycaemic improvement reduces the risk of both microvascular (Holman et al., 2008) and macrovascular (Turnbull et al., 2009) complications.

It is currently common practice to introduce insulin to an oral medication schedule, although the oral medications may be reduced or stopped. A number of different insulin regimens for use in patients with type 2 diabetes are available, the most common of which include once-daily basal insulin, twice-daily biphasic (premixed) insulin, or prandial insulin, using a rapid/short-acting insulin with meals. Studies suggest that patients who have basal insulin or prandial insulin added to their oral therapy have better HbA$_{1c}$ control than those who receive biphasic insulin. In addition, the basal insulin regimen is associated with fewer hypoglycaemic episodes and less weight gain than the other two regimens (Holman et al., 2009). Basal insulin should be titrated to achieve normal fasting glucose levels, and the patient may be taught this self-titration protocol (Davies et al., 2005).

In a lean patient (BMI <25 kg/m²), significant insulin deficiency is more likely, and therefore insulin treatment with either a basal-bolus or twice-daily regimen may be preferred from the outset.

A-glucosidase inhibitors

Acarbose reduces carbohydrate digestion by interfering with gastro-intestinal glucosidase activity, reducing the post-prandial hyperglycaemic peaks. Acarbose is minimally absorbed in unchanged form from the gastro-intestinal tract.

Adverse effects. The most common adverse effect is abdominal discomfort associated with flatulence and diarrhoea. These symptoms usually improve with continued treatment but can be minimised by starting with a low dose and titrating slowly.

Systemic adverse effects are rare, but high doses have been associated with idiosyncratic elevations of serum hepatic transaminase levels; therefore, patients titrated to the maximum should be closely monitored, preferably at monthly intervals for the first 6 months. If elevated transaminase levels are observed, reduction in dose or withdrawal of therapy should be considered.

Role of acarbose. Acarbose is a therapeutic option in type 2 patients inadequately controlled by diet alone or by diet and other oral hypoglycaemic agents. However, the gastro-intestinal side effects do limit the use of acarbose in clinical practice.

Treating hypertension

The co-existence of hypertension and diabetes dramatically increases the risk of microvascular and macrovascular complications. Most important is the increased risk of cardiovascular disease. Tight control of blood pressure may be a more effective method of preventing complications in patients with type 2 diabetes than tight glycaemic control (UKPDS, 1998b). It is recommended that for patients with type 2 diabetes, the target blood pressure should be less than 140/80 mmHg; for those with pre-existing kidney, eye or cerebrovascular damage, the target should be reduced to less than 130/80 mmHg (NICE, 2015d). First-line blood-pressure-lowering therapy should be a once-daily, generically prescribed ACE inhibitor. Exceptions to this are people of African-Caribbean descent, in whom first-line therapy should be an ACE inhibitor plus either a diuretic or a calcium-channel blocker.

In patients with type 1 diabetes, the blood pressure target is less than 135/85 mmHg. However, if there is abnormal albumin excretion (renal disease), then the blood pressure target should be lowered to 130/80 mmHg with maximal doses of either an ACE inhibitor or ARB as first-line therapy (NICE, 2015c).

Patient care

Annual review

People with diabetes should attend their hospital clinic or primary care practice (if this service is offered locally) for an annual review to screen for diabetic complications. Monitoring and optimising of glycaemic control are also undertaken, although these should be done on a more regular basis, as should review of patients with known complications. In the UK the annual review is increasingly taking place in primary care, with referral to secondary care if required. The typical assessments undertaken at an annual review are described in Box 45.4.

Glycaemic management

The theoretical ideal for all patients with diabetes is to achieve normoglycaemia. Because this is not always possible, the aim is to achieve the best possible control compatible with an acceptable lifestyle for the patient. In some patients, this may mean

---

Box 45.4 Annual review for diabetes

Routine assessment
- Capillary blood glucose level
- Weight, body mass index and waist circumference
- Blood pressure
- Urinalysis for glucose, protein and ketones
- Foot assessment

Laboratory investigations
- Lipid profile
- HbA$_{1c}$
- U&E, creatinine
- Liver function tests
- Urine specimen for albumin/creatinine ratio

Referral, if appropriate
- Retinopathy screening (should be done annually)
- Dietician
- Podiatry
- Exercise programme
- Smoking cessation programme

HbA$_{1c}$, glycated haemoglobin, a definition that identifies the average plasma glucose concentration; U&E, urea and electrolytes (blood test used to assess a patient's fluid status, renal function and electrolyte balance).

---

only symptomatic control; in others this may be tight control. In making this decision, the following factors should be considered: the patient's age, motivation, understanding, likely adherence, co-existing diseases, and ability to recognise hypoglycaemia; the duration of their diabetes; and the presence/absence/severity of diabetic complications.

Targets for pre-meal blood glucose of between 4 and 7 mmol/L and post-meal values of less than 8.5 mmol/L may be set for most patients, provided there is no significant hypoglycaemia risk. An optimal HbA$_{1c}$ target of 48 mmol/mol for most of those with type 2 diabetes has been suggested; however, for patients not adequately controlled on a single agent, polypharmacy puts the individual at risk of hypoglycaemia, so a target of 53 mmol/mol should be encouraged (NICE, 2015d). However, it is recommended that targets should be individualised and that for some, a higher target would be more appropriate, especially if there is a risk of hypoglycaemia at the lower target. For those with type 1 diabetes, the recommended target is less than 48 mmol/mol, but again, this does need to be individualised (NICE, 2015c) (see Table 45.6).

The diabetes treatment goals in older people may be different and more conservative than in younger adults. For example, some elderly patients may have poor vision and limited manual dexterity, which may or may not be linked to a degree of cognitive impairment. Others may have multiple pathology and take a number of other medications. Therefore, the goals of therapy need to be both individual and realistic. In some people, they will involve only the optimisation of body weight, control of symptoms and avoidance of hypoglycaemia, which has an increased risk of brain damage and may occur without the usual warning signs in the elderly. In others, reasonably tight control may be appropriate. There is, therefore, a difficult balance between the use of aggressive treatment with its associated risk of hypoglycaemia and the benefits of reducing complications to maintain an acceptable quality of life.

Monitoring glycaemic control

Clinic monitoring

There are several ways in which glycaemic control can be monitored in primary and secondary care. Estimates of average control are often useful. Glycation of minor haemoglobin components occurs in the blood, with the extent depending on both the amount of glucose present and the duration of exposure of the haemoglobin to glucose. Estimates of glycated haemoglobin (HbA_{1c}) provide an index of average diabetes control over the preceding 2–3 months, that is, the lifespan of a red blood cell. HbA_{1c} can be measured at any time, the patient does not need to be fasted and levels are not normally affected by acute changes in therapy, diet or exercise. However, they may be lower in those with reduced red cell lifespan, for example, in pregnancy, advanced renal failure or sepsis. Serum fructosamine represents the glycation of all serum proteins and gives information about control over the preceding 3 weeks. Because albumin is the major serum protein, hypoalbuminaemia may affect fructosamine levels. However, HbA_{1c} is the preferred marker for average glycaemic control.

Home monitoring

Type 1 diabetes. All patients treated with insulin should be offered home blood glucose monitoring. Capillary blood is applied to a reagent strip which has been impregnated with enzymes, for example, glucose oxidase. Home blood glucose monitoring enables patients and carers to make a direct assessment of the effect of changes in medicines, dietary habits, exercise and patterns of illness. It has the additional benefit that it can detect hypoglycaemia.

Patients with type 1, who are by definition ketosis prone, should also know how and when to test for blood ketones. This test need not be carried out as part of routine monitoring but is essential at times of intercurrent illness, especially when the blood glucose is ≥17 mmol/L.

Type 2 diabetes. NICE (2015d) guidance is that routine blood glucose monitoring is not offered to patients with type 2 unless they are on insulin, there is evidence of hypoglycaemia episodes, they are on an oral agent that may increase risk of hypoglycaemia whilst driving or they are is pregnant or planning to become pregnant. Further information about blood glucose monitoring and a person's fitness to drive is provided by the Driver and Vehicle Licencing Agency (DVLA, 2016).

NICE (2015d) guidance suggests considering short-term monitoring for adults when starting treatment with steroids or to confirm suspected hypoglycaemia. Before continuing self-monitoring, it is important to assess (annually) the person's self-monitoring skills, quality and frequency of testing, interpretation of the results, impact on quality of life and continued benefit. Many people with type 2 diabetes are treated with diet alone or with oral hypoglycaemic agents, and unless they have problems with hypoglycaemia, urine glucose monitoring should be adequate. This is a simple, noninvasive test that can detect hyperglycaemia but not hypoglycaemia. Home blood glucose monitoring is used by some patients with type 2, particularly if control is poor, if they are undergoing medication dose titration, if they are being treated with insulin or if they are prone to hypoglycaemia. It is also recommended that blood glucose monitoring be undertaken before driving and at times of intercurrent illness, when blood glucose levels may be particularly erratic.

Regardless of whether individuals with type 1 or type 2 diabetes are using home blood glucose monitoring or urine testing, it is important they are educated about what to do with the results; otherwise, there is little point in testing.

Case studies

Case 45.1

Mrs SG is a 32-year-old woman who has type 1 diabetes. She is hoping to become pregnant and wishes to talk to you about pre-conception care and diabetes. During the consultation, you discover that she is taking folic acid 400 micrograms daily and has been for the previous 6 months but, until now she has not received any pre-conception diabetes care. Her most recent HbA_{1c} was 57 mmol/mol (7.3%). Her regular medications are ramipril 10 mg daily, simvastatin 40 mg daily, insulin glargine at night and insulin aspart three times daily with meals.

···

Questions

1. Why should women of childbearing age be offered advice about pregnancy?
2. What blood glucose targets should Mrs SG be advised to aim for before and after conceiving?
3. Is Mrs SG taking appropriate dietary supplements before conception?
4. What advice should she be given with respect to her regular medication?

···

Answers

1. Mrs SG should be offered preconception advice before becoming pregnant because glucose control needs to be optimal to reduce the risk of miscarriage, congenital malformation, stillbirth and neonatal death. Preconception advice should also include information for the patient on how diabetes affects pregnancy and how pregnancy affects diabetes, what dietary supplements to take and advice on diabetes-related medicines that are unsafe to take during pregnancy.
2. Mrs SG should aim for an HbA_{1c} target of less than 48 mmol/mol (6.5%) before conceiving and throughout the pregnancy, whilst aiming to avoid significant hypoglycaemia. Her capillary blood glucose targets should be the same as for all people with type 1 diabetes, fasting glucose level 5–7 mmol/L on waking and 4–7 mmol/L before meals at other times of the day. During pregnancy, she should aim for fasting blood glucose levels of 5.3 mmol/L and less than 7.8 mmol/L 1-hour post-prandial levels.
3. Mrs SG is taking the appropriate dietary supplement; however, the recommended dose of folic acid for women with diabetes is 5 mg daily, rather than 400 micrograms daily. The 5 mg strength tablets are available by prescription. This should be taken before pregnancy and until 12 weeks of gestation to reduce the risk of having a baby with neural tube defects.

4. Mrs SG should be advised to stop her ramipril and simvastatin because both have been associated with an increased risk of birth defects. She will need to be assessed for hypertension because if ramipril is being used for its antihypertensive effects in addition to renal protection, then consideration will need to be given to alternative antihypertensive medications.

Case 45.2

Mr RK is a 57-year-old man with type 2 diabetes. He has recently had basal insulin (insulin isophane) added to his other diabetes medicines: metformin 1 g twice a day and gliclazide 160 mg twice a day. Mr RK complains of waking with a headache and feeling 'groggy' and unrested in the morning. His recent blood glucose readings have generally been very good, and his recent HbA$_{1c}$ is much improved since the addition of insulin. Mr RK is worried because he is feeling worse since he started insulin, even though his blood glucose levels are much improved. He has completed a hypoglycaemia awareness questionnaire at his community pharmacy and is concerned that nocturnal hypoglycaemia may be causing his recent symptoms. Mr RK wishes to know more about hypoglycaemia and how he can manage the risk whilst maintaining his recent improved blood glucose control.

Questions

1. What is nocturnal hypoglycaemia?
2. How can the diagnosis of nocturnal hypoglycaemia be confirmed?
3. How should it be managed?

Answers

1. Nocturnal hypoglycaemia is a low blood glucose reading that occurs during the night. Definitions vary, but it is generally accepted that a reading of less than 3.5 mmol/L is 'hypoglycaemia'. Night-time blood glucose levels may be even lower than those detected during the daytime because a more pronounced counter-regulatory hormone is required to wake the person with diabetes. The normal symptoms of hypoglycaemia may be missed if the patient does not wake. However, signs noticed (often by partners) might include restlessness, sweating and nightmares. Symptoms experienced by the patient in the mornings commonly include headache and lethargy.
2. Commonly, nocturnal hypoglycaemia can be confirmed by undertaking a blood glucose reading in the early hours of the morning, that is, between 2 and 3 a.m. This may require the patient to set an alarm to be woken at this time.
3. Nocturnal hypoglycaemia, once confirmed, may be managed by either having a bedtime snack or by reducing the dose of night-time insulin. In the case of Mr RK, stopping his sulfonylurea may also help resolve the problem. The timing of the insulin dose may also be adjusted to ensure that the peak activity is not overnight. If this does not help or is not practical, then a long-acting insulin analogue may be appropriate,

Case 45.3

Mr JS is a 69-year-old man with longstanding type 2 diabetes. He has recently noticed that his left shoe has been rubbing his foot, which he finds confusing because he has been wearing these shoes for 6 months with no problems. His whole left foot now looks red and swollen. When Mr JS inspected it closely, he noticed that there was a weeping sore. However, his foot is not painful, so he does not feel too concerned.

Questions

1. What is the most likely reason that Mr JS did not feel any pain associated with the sore?
2. Why might Mr JS's shoe suddenly have started to rub his foot?
3. Should Mr JS be more concerned?

Answers

1. Mr JS has probably developed sensory neuropathy in his feet. This usually begins with the loss of the sensation of vibration, then inability to feel a monofilament, and then may progressively lead to complete loss of sensation.
2. The shape of the feet of people with diabetes has been observed to change over time. This may be due to the development of neuropathy, which can weaken muscles, causing alterations to the shape of the arch of the foot and toes. In this case, Mr JS has sensory neuropathy because he is unable to feel the pain of the weeping sore. It is likely that Mr JS may also have motor neuropathy. Shoes should be checked by the patient daily because, quite often, patients walk around on foreign bodies (small stones, etc.) without even knowing.
3. Mr JS should be concerned because his lack of sensation does not indicate that the foot injury is not serious. He is at risk of developing an infected ulcer and needs prompt treatment to prevent the problem from becoming severe. If Mr JS does not seek treatment, he may even risk losing his foot through amputation. Diabetes patients with neuropathy and a foot problem should always be seen urgently by a healthcare professional on the same day.

Case 45.4

Miss IL is a 17-year-old teenager with recently diagnosed type 1 diabetes. She has been admitted to hospital with DKA, which was precipitated by a diarrhoea and vomiting bug. Because she was vomiting, she was not eating, and hence she temporarily stopped injecting her insulin. Miss IL is normally well controlled on a basal-bolus insulin regimen comprising insulin glargine (Lantus) at night and insulin glulisine (Apidra) three times daily with meals.

Questions

1. Why was it a mistake for Miss IL not to inject her insulin whilst she was not feeling well enough to eat?
2. What advice should patients on insulin be given regarding glucose management when they are feeling unwell and not able to eat normally?
3. What are the initial management priorities for patients admitted with diabetic ketoacidosis?
4. What is the correct way for subcutaneous insulin to be re-introduced after a patient has been on a continuous intravenous insulin infusion?

Answers

1. This is a common misunderstanding amongst patients and sometimes even healthcare professionals. When a person is unwell, his or her insulin requirements can often increase, despite not eating. This is because of the stress involved and the increase in the production of counter-regulatory hormones, which increase glucose levels.

2. Patients should be counselled on what are commonly referred to as 'sick-day rules' and should be given contact numbers for advice if they are unclear or struggling with management. Generally, patients need to increase the frequency of glucose monitoring to every 2–4 hours and test blood ketones on a regular basis. Carbohydrate intake should be maintained as much as possible using sugary drinks or fruit juice, soups, jelly or snack foods if patients are having difficulty in eating. Fluid intake is important, and patients should be advised to have a glass of water every hour, aiming for 3 L in 24 hours. Depending on the glucose and ketone levels, boluses of quick-acting insulin equivalent to 10–20% of their total daily dose will need to be given every 2–4 hours until ketone levels resolve.

3. Intravenous sodium chloride 0.9% should be started as soon as possible. A fixed-rate intravenous insulin infusion should then be started. Current recommendations are to begin at a rate of 0.1 units/kg. Regular hourly monitoring of blood glucose and ketones should be undertaken along with 2-hourly monitoring of serum potassium for the first 6 hours.

4. When the patient is biochemically stable, the patient may be converted back to subcutaneous insulin. The current national guidelines from the Joint British Societies Inpatient Care Group (2010) recommend that long-acting subcutaneous insulin analogues are continued throughout treatment of diabetic ketoacidosis to prevent rebound hyperglycaemia when the intravenous infusion is stopped. Therefore, Miss IL's glargine should have been continued. Her rapid-acting insulin (Apidra) should be re-introduced at the next meal, and the intravenous insulin infusion should be stopped 30 minutes afterward.

Case 45.5

Mr PG is a 55-year-old man. He smokes 10 cigarettes a day and has smoked for more than 30 years. He is prescribed metformin 1 g twice daily, gliclazide 160 mg twice daily and pioglitazone 30 mg once a day. His primary care doctor started the pioglitazone about 4 months ago because his blood glucose had not been well controlled. His BMI is 36 kg/m^2 and his recent HbA$_{1c}$ was 82 mmol/mol. Mr PG has been admitted to hospital with shortness of breath; he is awaiting a cardiac echo to confirm the suspected diagnosis of heart failure.

Questions

1. What would be your next therapeutic intervention?
2. What medication options remain for managing Mr PG's diabetes?
3. What additional information would you need to help you and Mr PG decide on which medication is appropriate?
4. What lifestyle factors should you discuss with Mr PG?

Answers

1. Due to the potential for worsening heart failure, pioglitazone should not be prescribed in people with heart failure and should therefore be stopped in Mr PG. In the UK, a yellow card (Medicines and Healthcare Products Regulatory Agency [MHRA] report of adverse drug reaction) should be completed because the pioglitazone may have contributed to the heart failure. Metformin should also be suspended if there is renal impairment.

2. The remaining options for managing Mr PG's diabetes are DPP-4 inhibitors, SGLT-2 inhibitors, GLP-1 receptor agonists and insulin.

3. The additional information required includes details about Mr PG's current and baseline renal function because this may impact the choice of antidiabetic agents. Discussion about his job and whether he drives are also important. Mr PG's beliefs about medications and aims of treatment should also be considered, taking into account his comorbidities.

4. The lifestyle factors that should be discussed with Mr PG are smoking cessation and weight management as part of a personal plan. Weight reduction should be part of an individualised plan that involves healthy eating based on the individual's nutritional needs, personal choices, cultural preferences and willingness to change. Because Mr PG is obese, medication options that could be considered are the use of orlistat to reduce the absorption of lipids. In addition, GLP-1 receptor agonists could be used to manage his diabetes; this class of medication has been associated with significant weight loss, leading to further improvements in diabetes control.

Case 45.6

Mrs FR is 77-year-old woman. She is usually very independent and has never taken any regular medication. She was recently prescribed two courses of antibiotics for urinary tract infections. Her daughter visited this morning and called the ambulance because her mother was very confused and looked very unwell. Review in the emergency department identified that Mrs FR is extremely dehydrated; her blood glucose level on the standard machine read 'HI' (>27.8 mmol/L), and the laboratory blood glucose was confirmed at 65 mmol/L. Her sodium is 168 mmol/L (normal range 135–145 mmol/L). Her eGFR is reduced to 13 mL/min from her usual baseline of 26 mL/min.

Questions

1. What is the likely cause of Mrs FR's symptoms and elevated blood glucose?
2. How should Mrs FR be managed?
3. What advice should be given about the long-term management of her blood glucose?

Answers

1. The likely cause of the symptoms is prolonged hyperglycaemia and undiagnosed type 2 diabetes. The glycosuria has caused urinary tract infections, and this acute illness has put further physiological strain on Mrs FR. This in turn has caused further increases in the blood glucose and increased dehydration, culminating in the acute emergency episode of HHS.

2. Initial management is fluid resuscitation with sodium chloride 0.9%. This is required to reverse the extreme dehydration, stabilise the blood pressure, improve circulation and increase urine output. Fixed-rate insulin (0.05 units/kg/h) should be started if blood glucose fails to fall despite adequate fluid replacement. Prophylaxis of thromboembolism is also required.

3. Because Mrs FR has renal impairment, metformin, SGLT-2s and some DPP-4s are not suitable. Pioglitazone is not appropriate due to bone fracture risk in post-menopausal women. The remaining agents should be considered on an individual basis. Sulfonylureas and insulin are clinically effective options and will have an immediate effect. Consideration should also be given to the risk of hypoglycaemia, treatment targets and Mrs FR's confidence in monitoring blood glucose results. A non-renal cleared DPP-4 such as linagliptin may also be appropriate.

Case 45.7

Mr PR is a 42-year-old university lecturer. He was diagnosed with type 2 diabetes when he was 27 years old. He is motivated to self-manage his diabetes. His BMI is 29 kg/m². His regular prescription is Levemir 20 units twice daily and NovoRapid variable dose adjusted to carbohydrate intake. Mr PR was recently prescribed a SGLT-2 inhibitor to improve his blood glucose control and possibly aid weight loss. Today Mr PR has come to hospital because he is feeling very unwell, experiencing abdominal pain and has vomited twice; his breathing is very fast and shallow. When he first started his new medicine, the pharmacist had advised that he should seek urgent medical attention if he had these symptoms, even if his blood glucose were normal. The hospital blood test results are as follows:

Blood glucose 8.2 mmol/L
Blood ketones 4.6 mmol/L
Bicarbonate 13 mmol/L

Questions

1. What is the likely cause of Mr PR's symptoms?
2. What changes should be made to Mr PR's medication?
3. What further action should be taken?

Answers

1. The most likely cause of Mr PR's symptoms is DKA. Ketones are present, and symptoms are typical of DKA. An SGLT-2 inhibitor has recently been started, and MHRA reports a link between DKA and SGLT-2 inhibitors. SGLT-2 inhibitors are licensed for use in type 2 diabetes. Blood glucose levels may be only moderately elevated, which is atypical for DKA. This atypical presentation could delay diagnosis and treatment. Reports indicate that half of the cases occurred during the first 2 months of treatment. Some cases occurred shortly after stopping the SGLT-2 inhibitor.

2. The SGLT medication should be stopped and not restarted because the underlying mechanism for SGLT-2 inhibitor-associated DKA has not been established. Counselling points with Mr PR should include that the medicine has been stopped due to his presenting symptoms being indicative of DKA (e.g. nausea, vomiting, anorexia, abdominal pain, excessive thirst, difficulty breathing, confusion, unusual fatigue or sleepiness), and the blood test for raised ketones confirmed this diagnosis. This is serious side effect, and the medicine should not be restarted.

3. A yellow card report for the potential adverse event to SGLT should be completed and submitted to the MHRA.

Acknowledgments

The authors acknowledge the contribution of E. A. Hackett and S. N. J. Jackson to versions of this chapter which appeared in previous editions.

References

American Diabetes Association, 2013. Genetics of diabetes. Available at: http://www.diabetes.org/diabetes-basics/genetics-of-diabetes.html.

Bogardus, C., 1993. Insulin resistance in the pathogenesis of NIDDM in Pima Indians. Diabetes Care 16 (1), 228–231.

Cheng, V., Kashyap, S.R., 2011. Weight consideration sin pharmacotherapy for type 2 diabetes. J. Obs. 984245. https://doi.org/10.1155/2011/984245.

Chan, J.C.N., Malik, V., Jia, W., et al., 2009. Diabetes in Asia: epidemiology, risk factors, and pathophysiology. JAMA 301, 2129–2140.

Chatenoud, L., Warncke, K., Ziegler, A., 2012. Clinical immunological interventions for the treatment of type 1 diabetes. Cold Spring Harb. Persp. Med. 2 (8), a007716.

DAFNE Study Group, 2002. Training in flexible, intensive insulin management to enable dietary freedom in people with type 1 diabetes: Dose Adjustment for Normal Eating (DAFNE) randomised controlled trial. Br. Med. J. 325, 746–749.

Davies, M., Storms, F., Shutler, S., et al., 2005. Improvement of glycaemic control in subjects with poorly controlled type 2 diabetes. Comparison of two treatment algorithms using insulin glargine. Diabetes Care 28 (6), 1282–1288.

De Zoysa, N., Rogers, H., Stadler, M., et al., 2014. A psychoeducational program to restore hypoglycemia awareness: the DAFNE-HART pilot study. Diabetes Care 37, 863–866.

Diabetes UK, 2014. The cost of diabetes: report. Available at: https://www.diabetes.org.uk/Documenta/Diabetes%20UK%20Cost%20of%20Diabetes%20Report.pfd.

Diabetes UK, 2016. Number of people with diabetes reached over 4 million. Available at: https://www.diabetes.org.uk/About_us/News/Number-of-people-with-diabetes-reaches-over-4-million/.

Diabetes Control and Complications Trial Research Group, 1993. The effect of intensive treatment of diabetes on the development and progression of long-term complications in insulin-dependent diabetes mellitus. N. Engl. J. Med. 329, 977–986.

Dormandy, J.A., Charbonnel, B., Eckland, D.J.A., et al., 2005. Secondary prevention of macrovascular events in patients with type 2 diabetes in the PROactive Study (Prospective Pioglitazone Clinical Trial in Macrovascular Events): a randomised controlled trial. Lancet 366, 1279–1289.

Driver and Vehicle Licencing Agency, 2016. Information for drivers with diabetes treated by non-insulin medication, diet, or both. Available at: https://www.gov.uk/government/uploads/system/uploads/attachment_data/file/561792/inf188x2-information-for-drivers-with-diabetes-treated-by-non-insulin-medication-diet-or-both.pdf.

Elliott, J., Jacques, R.M., Kruger, J., et al., 2014. Educational and psychological issues substantial reductions in the number of diabetic ketoacidosis and severe hypoglycaemia episodes requiring emergency treatment lead to reduced costs after structured education in adults with Type 1 diabetes. Diabetes Med. 31, 847–853.

Ergul, A., Kelly-Cobbs, A., Abdaila, M., et al., 2012. Cerebrovascular complications of diabetes: focus on stroke. Endocr. Metab. Immune. Disord. Drug Targets 2 (2), 148–158.

Gavin, J.R., Alberti, K.G.M.M., Davidson, M.B., et al., 2002. Report of the expert committee on the diagnosis and classification of diabetes mellitus. Diabetes Care 25, S5–S20.

He, F.J., Jiafu, L.J., Graham, A., MacGregor, G.A., 2013. Effect of longer term modest salt reduction on blood pressure: Cochrane systematic review and meta-analysis of randomised trials. Br. Med. J. 346, f1325.

Herold, K.C., Taylor, L., 2003. Treatment of type 1 diabetes with anti-CD3 monoclonal antibodies: induction of immune regulation? Immunol. Res. 28 (2), 141–150.

Holman, R., Paul, S., Bethel, M., et al., 2008. 10-year follow-up of intensive glucose control in type 2 diabetes. N. Engl. J. Med. 359, 1577–1589.

Holman, R., Farmer, A., Davies, M., et al., 2009. Three-year efficacy of complex insulin regimens in type 2 diabetes. N. Engl. J. Med. 361, 1736–1747.

International Diabetes Federation, 2015. Diabetes atlas. Available at: http://www.diabetesatlas.org.

Joint British Societies Inpatient Care Group, 2010. The management of diabetic ketoacidosis in adults. NHS diabetes. Available at: http://www.diabetologists-abcd.org.uk/JBDS/JBDS_IP_DKA_Adults_Revised.pdf.

Joint British Societies Inpatient Care Group, 2012. The management of the hyperosmolar hyperglycaemic state (HHS) in adults with diabetes. Available at: http://www.diabetologists-abcd.org.uk/JBDS/JBDS_IP_HHS_Adults.pdf.

Khan, R., Buse, J., Ferrannini, E., et al., 2005. The metabolic syndrome: time for a critical appraisal: joint statement from the American Diabetes Association and the European Association for the Study of Diabetes. Diabetes Care 28, 2289–2304.

Kohner, E.M., Aldington, S.J., Stratton, I.M., et al., 1998. UK Prospective Diabetes Study 30: diabetic retinopathy at diagnosis of non-insulin-dependent diabetes mellitus and associated risk factors (UKPDS 30). Arch. Ophthalm. 116, 297–303.

Lin, S.F., Lin, J.D., Huang, Y.Y., 2005. Diabetic ketoacidosis: comparison of patient characteristics, clinical presentations and outcomes today and 20 year ago. Chang. Gung. Med. L. 28 (1), 24–30.

Mathers, C.D., Loncar, D., 2006. Projections of global mortality and burden of disease from 2002 to 2030. PLoS Med. 3, e442.

Montesi, L., Caletti, M.T., Marchesini, G., 2016. Diabetes in migrant and ethnic minorities in a changing world. World J. Diabetes 7, 34–44.

National Institute for Health and Care Excellence (NICE), 2008a. NICE technology appraisal guidance [TA151]: continuous subcutaneous insulin infusion for the treatment of diabetes mellitus. Available at: https://www.nice.org.uk/Guidance/TA151.

National Institute for Health and Care Excellence (NICE), 2008b. Continuous subcutaneous insulin infusion for the treatment of diabetes mellitus. Technology Appraisal 57. NICE, London. Available at: https://www.nice.org.uk/guidance/ta151.

National Institute for Health and Care Excellence (NICE), 2013. Neuropathic pain in adults: pharmacological management in non-specialist settings. Clinical Guideline 173. NICE, London. Available at: https://www.nice.org.uk/guidance/cg173.

National Institute for Health and Care Excellence (NICE), 2014. Obesity: identification, assessment and management. Clinical Guideline 189. NICE, London. Available at: https://www.nice.org.uk/guidance/cg189.

National Institute for Health and Care Excellence (NICE), 2015a. Diabetes in pregnancy: management from preconception to the postnatal period. Clinical Guideline NG3. NICE, London. Available at: https://www.nice.org.uk/guidance/ng3.

National Institute for Health and Care Excellence (NICE), 2015b. Cardiovascular disease: risk assessment and reduction, including lipid modification. Clinical Guideline 181. NICE, London. Available at https://www.nice.org.uk/guidance/cg181.

National Institute for Health and Care Excellence (NICE), 2015c. Type 1 diabetes adults – diagnosis and management. Clinical Guideline 17. NICE, London. Available at: https://www.nice.org.uk/guidance/ng17.

National Institute for Health and Care Excellence (NICE), 2015d. Type 2 diabetes in adults: management. Clinical Guideline 28. NICE, London. Available at: https://www.nice.org.uk/guidance/ng28.

National Institute for Health and Care Excellence (NICE), 2015e. Diabetic foot problems: prevention and management. NICE Guideline 19. NICE, London. Available at: https://www.nice.org.uk/guidance/ng19.

Thalange, N., Deeb, L., Iotova, V., et al., 2015. Insulin degludec in combination with bolus insulin aspart is safe and effective in children and adolescents with type 1 diabetes. Pediatr. Diabetes 16, 164–176.

Turnbull, F., Abraira, C., Anderson, R., et al., 2009. Intensive glucose control and macrovascular outcomes in type 2 diabetes. Diabetologia 52, 2288–2298.

UK Prospective Diabetes Study Group, 1998a. Effect of intensive blood-glucose control with metformin on complications in overweight patients with type 2 diabetes (UKPDS 34). Lancet 352, 854–865.

UK Prospective Diabetes Study Group, 1998b. Tight blood pressure control and risk of macrovascular and microvascular complications in type 2 diabetes (UKPDS 38). Br. Med. J. 317, 703–713.

Vetter, M.L., Cardillo, S., Rickles, M.R., et al., 2009. Narrative review: effect of bariatric surgery on type 2 diabetes mellitus. Ann. Int. Med. 150, 94–103.

Wang, J., Williams, D.E., Narayan, K.M., et al., 2006. Declining death rates from hyperglycemic crisis among adults with diabetes, U.S., 1985–2002. Diabetes Care 29 (9), 2018–2022.

World Health Organization, 2006. Definition and diagnosis of diabetes mellitus and intermediate hyperglycemia: report of a WHO/IDF Consultation. Available at: http://www.who.int/diabetes/publications/diagnosis_diabtes2006/en/.

Zinman, B., Wanner, C., Lachin, J., et al., 2015. Empagliflozin, cardiovascular outcomes, and mortality in type 2 diabetes. N. Engl. J. Med. 373, 2117–2128.

Further reading

Choudhary, P., Heller, S., 2008. The Somogyi effect: fact or fiction? Diabetes Prim. Care 10 (6), 335–340. Available at: http://www.diabetesandprimarycare.co.uk/journal-content/view/the-somogyi-effect-fact-or-fiction/.

Diabetes Control and Complications Trial Research Group, 1995. Adverse events and their association with treatment regimens in diabetes control and complications trial. Diabetes Care 18, 1415–1427.

Gerstein, H.C., Miller, M.E., Byington, R.P., et al., 2008. Action to Control Cardiovascular Risk in Diabetes (ACCORD) study group: effects of intensive glucose lowering in type 2 diabetes. N. Engl. J. Med. 358, 2545–2559.

Kahn, R., Buse, J., Ferrannini, E., Stern, M., 2005. The metabolic syndrome: time for a critical appraisal: joint statement from the American Diabetes Association and the European Association for the Study of Diabetes. Diabetes Care 28 (9), 2289–2304.

Patel, A., MacMahon, S., Chalmers, J., et al., 2008. Intensive blood glucose control and vascular outcomes in patients with type 2 diabetes. N. Engl. J. Med. 358, 2560–2572.

Useful websites

The Health Foundation. Patient safety resource centre: http://patientsafety.health.org.uk/area-of-care/diabetes

National Institute for Health and Clinical Excellence. Learning tool – type 1 diabetes: http://elearning.nice.org.uk/enrol/index.php?id=18

WHO diabetes factsheet: http://www.who.int/mediacentre/factsheets/fs312/en/

The Joint British Diabetes Societies clinical guidelines: http://www.diabetologists-abcd.org.uk/JBDS/JBDS.htm

46 Menstrual Cycle Disorders

Kay Marshall and Emma Crosbie

Key points

- Girls can begin experiencing menstrual disorders soon after menarche.
- Up to 95% of women experience changes premenstrually, but severe premenstrual syndrome is more common in the 30- to 40-year age group.
- The aetiology of premenstrual syndrome is multifactorial, the symptomatology complex and treatment options diverse.
- It has been estimated that 50–80% of women of childbearing age will suffer from dysmenorrhoea at some time.
- Treatment options vary according to the type of dysmenorrhoea (primary or secondary) but include non-steroidal anti-inflammatory drugs, combined oral contraceptive pills and progestogen-only preparations.
- Heavy menstrual bleeding (previously known as menorrhagia) affects up to 30% of menstruating women. The management of the condition depends upon the cause and can be either medical or surgical.
- Endometriosis (the presence of extrauterine endometrial tissue) can give rise to an array of symptoms including subfertility. Treatment may be designed to improve fertility and/or manage symptoms. Medical and surgical treatments are available.

Once a girl reaches puberty, various physiological events occur, leading to the onset of menstruation, or the menarche. The average age of the menarche has decreased to around 12.5 years, and a halt in this trend towards earlier menarche is not evident. This decline has been attributed to an improvement in nutrition and overall health. Body weight is linked to menarchal age, and it is possible that as body fat increases so does serum leptin (hormone which influences calorie intake), which in turn may increase the pulsatile release of gonadotrophin-releasing hormone (GnRH). However, the data regarding non-genetic influences remain inconclusive. Early menarche is associated with health problems in later life, and these include predisposition to breast cancer, endometrial cancer, type 2 diabetes and psychological problems.

Menstruation is an event that occurs relatively late in puberty, and 95% of girls experience menarche between the ages of 11 and 15 years. One UK study has shown that one girl in eight begins to menstruate whilst still at primary school. Factors that influence menarcheal age are discussed by Morris et al. (2011). Even before the first ovulatory cycle has taken place, childhood ovarian activity will have gradually increased the production of oestrogen, leading to the development of the secondary sexual characteristics. These events are probably initiated by the central nervous system (CNS), which ultimately triggers the necessary gonadal changes that will eventually lead to the establishment of the menstrual cycle. It may take up to 2 years for the hypothalamic–pituitary–gonadal axis to mature and for regular ovulation to take place. In girls who only start to menstruate when they are older, it may take even longer. This should be considered when taking a patient's medical history.

Menstruation itself occurs as a result of cyclic hormonal variations (Fig. 46.1). During the first half or follicular phase of the menstrual cycle, the endometrium thickens under the influence of increasing levels of oestrogen (most notably estradiol, which at the peak of its preovulatory surge reaches around 2000 pmol/L) secreted from the developing ovarian follicles. Once the serum oestrogen level has surpassed a critical point it triggers, by positive feedback, the anterior pituitary to release, about 24 hours later, a surge of luteinising hormone (up to 50 IU/L) and after 30–36 hours, ovulation follows.

After ovulation, which occurs around day 14 of a 28-day menstrual cycle, and as the luteal phase progresses, the endometrium begins to respond to increasing levels of progesterone. Both progesterone and oestrogen are secreted from the corpus luteum, which is formed from the remains of the ovarian follicle after ovulation. The lifespan of the corpus luteum is remarkably constant and lasts between 12 and 14 days; hence the length of the second half or the luteal phase of the menstrual cycle is between 12 and 14 days. Between days 18 and 22 of a 28-day cycle, both sex steroids peak, with levels of progesterone reaching around 30 nmol/L. Because progesterone has a thermogenic effect upon the hypothalamus, basal body temperature increases by about 1 °C in the second half of an ovulatory cycle (Fig. 46.2). Most ovulatory cycles range from 21 to 34 days.

These synchronised changes mean that about a week after ovulation, the endometrium is prepared for implantation, providing fertilisation has taken place. If conception does not occur, then luteolysis begins and steroid levels fall. This means that the endometrium cannot be maintained, there is a loss of stromal fluid, leucocyte infiltration begins and there is intraglandular extravasation of blood. Finally, endometrial blood flow is reduced, and this leads to necrosis and sloughing, that is, menstruation. Initially, the blood vessels that remain intact after sloughing are sealed by fibrin and platelet plugs; subsequent haemostasis is probably achieved as a result of vasoconstriction of the remaining basal arteries. Nitric oxide may be involved in the initiation and maintenance of

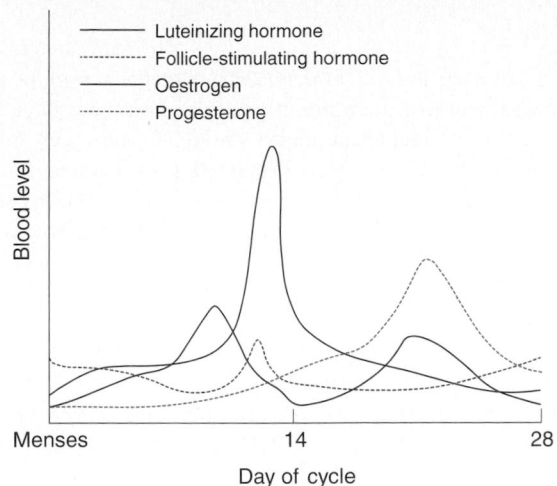

Fig. 46.1 The hormonal events that occur during the menstrual cycle in women.

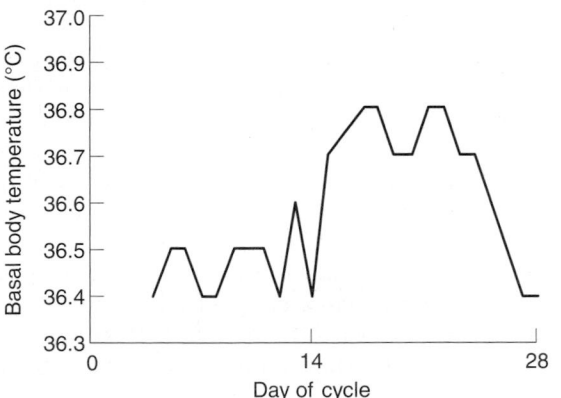

Fig. 46.2 Typical temperature chart from a 28-day ovulatory menstrual cycle.

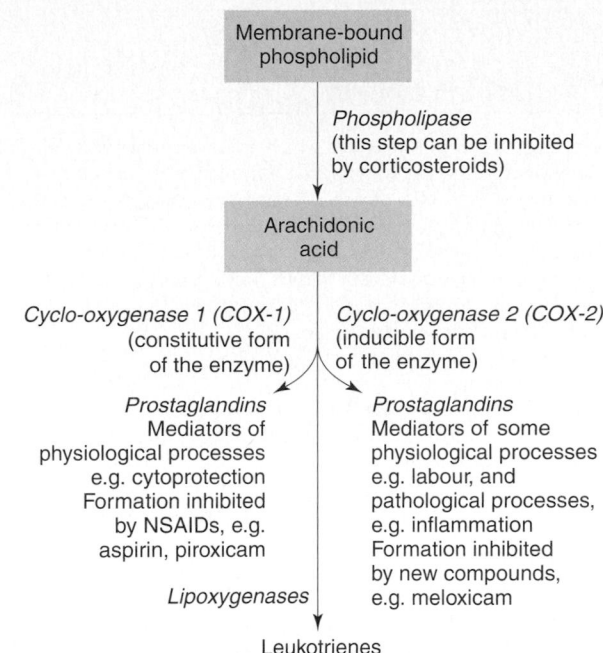

Fig. 46.3 Eicosanoid biosynthesis and inhibition.

menstrual bleeding by promoting vasodilation and inhibiting platelet aggregation. The myometrium is the muscular layer of the uterus that contracts spontaneously throughout the menstrual cycle, the frequency of these contractions being influenced by the hormonal milieu. The myometrium is also more active during menstruation. The average blood loss per period is between 30 and 40 mL.

There is evidence to suggest a physiological and pathological role for the local hormones, known as prostaglandins, in the process of menstruation. Prostaglandins are 20-carbon oxygenated, polyunsaturated bioactive lipids, which are cyclo-oxygenase (COX)-derived products of arachidonic acid. Indeed, both the myometrium and the endometrium are capable of synthesising and responding to prostaglandins. A potential role for another family of autocoids, the leukotrienes, in the regulation of uterine function remains uncertain, although it is known that leukotrienes can also be synthesised from arachidonic acid by lipoxygenase enzymes (Fig. 46.3).

Disorders associated with menstruation are a major medical and social problem for women which also impact upon their families.

Premenstrual syndrome

Premenstrual syndrome (PMS) encompasses both mood changes and physical symptoms. Symptoms may start up to 14 days before menstruation, although more usually they begin just a few days before and disappear at the onset of, or shortly after, menstruation. However, for some women, the beginning of menstruation may not signal the complete resolution of symptoms. Numerous studies have demonstrated that this condition can cause substantial impairment of normal daily activity, including reduced occupational activity and significant levels of work absenteeism. Severity varies from cycle to cycle and may be influenced by other life factors such as stress and tiredness. The most severe form of PMS may be referred to as premenstrual dysphoric disorder (PMDD) as defined by *Diagnostic and Statistical Manual of Mental Disorders, Fifth Edition*, or DSM-V (American Psychiatric Association, 2013). In this edition it is noteworthy that PMDD has been placed in the main text of the manual, thus gaining full diagnostic status. The main criteria are set out in Box 46.1. Other bodies (American College of Obstetricians and Gynecologists, 2000) have published diagnostic criteria for PMS (Box 46.2). There is considerable overlap between PMS and PMDD. The Royal College of Obstetricians & Gynaecologists (2016) 'Green top' guidance for diagnosis and management of PMS was published in 2016. This guidance does include a useful menstrual diary/symptom table.

Epidemiology

Up to 95% of menstruating women experience some changes premenstrually. Clinically relevant PMS occurs in about 15–20% of these women, and PMDD has an estimated incidence rate of 3–8%. It has been estimated that PMS may account for more than 17 million disability-adjusted life years in the European Union. PMS affects young and older women alike and does not appear to be influenced

---

Box 46.1   Summary of DSM-V diagnostic criteria for
premenstrual dysphoric disorder (American
Psychiatric Association, 2013)

One-year duration of symptoms which are present for the
majority of cycles (occur luteal/remit follicular) as evidenced by
prospective daily ratings during at least two consecutive cycles

Five of the following Criteria A symptoms (with at least one of
those marked with an asterisk [*]) must occur during the week
before menses and subside within days of menses.
1. Marked lability (e.g. mood swings)*
2. Marked irritability or anger*
3. Markedly depressed mood*
4. Marked anxiety and tension*
5. Decreased interest in usual activities
6. Difficulty in concentration
7. Lethargy and marked lack of energy
8. Marked change in appetite (e.g. overeating or specific food
cravings)
9. Hypersomnia or insomnia
10. Feeling overwhelmed or out of control
11. Physical symptoms (e.g. breast tenderness or swelling, joint
or muscle pain, a sensation of bloating and weight gain)

Box 46.2   Diagnostic criteria for premenstrual syndrome
(American College of Obstetricians and
Gynecologists, 2000)

Patient reports one or more of the following affective and
somatic symptoms during the 5 days before menses in each of
three prior menstrual cycles.

Affective	Somatic
Depression	Breast tenderness
Angry outbursts	Abdominal bloating
Irritability	Headache
Anxiety	Swelling of extremities
Confusion	
Social withdrawal	

Symptoms relieved within 4 days of menses onset without recurrence until at least cycle day 13

Symptoms present in absence of any pharmacological therapy,
hormone ingestion, or drug or alcohol abuse

Symptoms occur reproducibly during two cycles of prospective
recording

Patient suffers from identifiable dysfunction in social or economic
performance

---

by parity. Severe PMS is more common in the 30- to 40-year age
range, and married women with young children commonly seek
help. Certain events may be linked with the onset of PMS, including
childbirth, cessation of oral contraceptive use (incidence of reported
PMS is lower in pill users), sterilisation, hysterectomy or even
increasing age. PMS may be exacerbated by other stresses, typically
those associated with family life. Women with a body mass index
greater than 30 are more likely to suffer from PMS. There is also
some evidence that crimes, accidents, examination failure, absenteeism and marital disturbances may be more common premenstrually.

Aetiology

PMS is not seen before puberty, during pregnancy or in post-
menopausal women; therefore, the ovarian hormones have been
implicated. The mineralocorticoids, prolactin, androgens, prostaglandins, endorphins, nutritional factors (e.g. pyridoxine, calcium
and essential fatty acids) and hypoglycaemia may be involved.
In addition, changes in CNS function have been implicated
because cerebral blood flow in the temporal lobes is decreased
premenstrually in PMS sufferers, and noradrenergic cyclicity is
disrupted. Because symptoms vary so much from cycle to cycle,
and from individual to individual, it is likely that different aetiological factors apply to different women, all of which may be
affected by extenuating emotional circumstances. There is some
evidence that predisposition to PMDD may be familial.

Hormones

The cyclicity of PMS suggests an ovarian involvement. This is
substantiated by the fact that it is still experienced after hysterectomy if the ovaries are left intact and that it disappears during
pregnancy and after menopause. One theory attributes PMS to
luteal phase progesterone deficiency leading to a progesterone/
estradiol imbalance, but there is no direct clinical evidence to
support this in terms of serum progesterone levels. However,
the problem could lie at the cellular level, that is, a paucity of
functional steroid receptors leading to differential sensitivity to
hormones. One such explanation could include genetic variations
in the oestrogen receptor alpha gene. Alternatively, it could be
a central control defect, because ovarian suppression by GnRH
analogues can alleviate symptoms in some women; however, the
use of these drugs is generally not recommended because of their
unwanted effects associated with production of a hypo-oestrogenic state.

The central actions of the sex steroids or their neuroactive
metabolites are important. Research into the complex relationship between the steroids and the CNS is ongoing, but is progressing with the advent of new tools such as the progesterone
receptor modulators. Estradiol increases neuronal excitability
possibly via increasing the activity of glutamate (an important
excitatory neurotransmitter). Progesterone, and its metabolites,
can bind to the γ-aminobutyric acid A ($GABA_A$) receptor, and
this interaction would induce an effect similar to that evoked by
benzodiazepines. The mineralocorticoid, aldosterone, may be
associated with the increase in fluid retention because serum levels of this hormone are elevated in the luteal phase. However,
no significant difference in blood levels of this mineralocorticoid
has been found between PMS sufferers and non-sufferers. In contrast, one study has found that baseline levels of cortisol were
elevated during the luteal phase in PMS sufferers.

Prolactin is secreted from the decidual cells at the end of the
luteal phase of the menstrual cycle, as well as from the anterior
pituitary. This hormone has a direct effect upon breast tissue, and
hence may be associated with breast tenderness. Prolactin is also
associated with stress and has an indirect relationship with dopamine metabolism and release in the CNS. It promotes sodium,
potassium and water retention. However, there are no consistent
differences in hormone blood levels of prolactin between PMS
sufferers and non-sufferers. Again, the differences could lie at the

receptor level. Local hormones such as the prostaglandins may also be implicated in the aetiology of PMS because synthesis of these autocoids can be affected by the sex hormones, as well as substrate availability. Prostaglandin imbalance is implicated in PMS because increased synthesis of certain prostaglandins, for example, prostaglandin E_2 (PGE_2), has antidiuretic and central sedative effects, as well as promotes capillary permeability and vasodilation. Deficiencies of others, for example, PGE_1, which can attenuate some of the actions of prolactin, may also contribute to the syndrome.

Vitamins and minerals

Pyridoxine phosphate is a cofactor in a number of enzyme reactions, particularly those leading to production of dopamine and serotonin (5-hydroxytryptamine). It has been suggested that disturbances of the oestrogen–progesterone balance could cause a relative deficiency of pyridoxine, and supplementation with this vitamin appears to ease the depression sometimes associated with the oral contraceptive pill. Decreased dopamine levels would tend to increase serum prolactin, and decreased serotonin levels could be a factor in emotional disturbances, particularly depression. There is some evidence that premenstrual mood changes are linked to cycle-related alterations in serotonergic activity within the CNS; therefore, serotonin may be important in the pathogenesis of PMS. There are also data to suggest that a variety of nutrients may play a role in the aetiology of PMS, specifically calcium and vitamin D. Further hydroxylation of 25-hydroxyvitamin D_3 [$25(OH)D_3$)] takes place in target tissues which include the breast and the endometrium. In the Nurses' Health Study II, high total vitamin D intake reduced risk of PMS by almost a third (Bertone-Johnson et al., 2005). Oestrogen influences calcium metabolism by affecting intestinal absorption, as well as parathyroid gene expression and secretion, thus triggering fluctuations throughout the menstrual cycle. Disruption of calcium homeostasis has been associated with affective disorders.

Essential fatty acids

Essential fatty acids, such as γ-linolenic (or gamolenic acid), provide a substrate for prostaglandin synthesis. γ-Linolenic is converted into dihomo-γ-linolenic acid, which forms the starting point for the synthesis of prostaglandins of the 1 series (e.g. PGE_1). It has been suggested that women with PMS are abnormally sensitive to normal levels of prolactin, and that PGE_1 is able to attenuate the biological effects of this hormone. Hence, if there is a γ-linolenic deficiency, then there is less substrate for PGE_1 synthesis. Therefore, the effect of prolactin with respect to breast tenderness, fluid retention and mood disturbances may be exaggerated. Numerous other dietary factors may also be involved, including excess saturated fats and cholesterol, moderate-to-high alcohol consumption, zinc and magnesium deficiencies, diabetes, ageing and viral infections, all of which hinder the conversion of cis-linolenic acid to γ-linolenic. Pyridoxine, ascorbic acid and niacin also increase conversion of γ-linolenic to PGE_1, although there is some evidence to suggest that linolenic acid metabolite levels are reduced in women with PMS.

Psychological factors

PMS may not be wholly explicable in pathophysiological terms, but it should not be regarded as a psychosomatic disorder because there is no simple relationship between its existence, severity and personality. It is not strictly confined to particular types of women, although there is no doubt that PMS interacts with many aspects of life, especially difficult or stressful times. The latter has been termed the 'vulnerability factor' which, although not a function of the menstrual cycle, can affect the way a woman reacts.

Symptoms

Symptoms occur 1–14 days before menstruation begins and disappear at the onset or shortly after menstruation begins. For the rest of the cycle, the woman feels well. Symptoms are cyclical, although they may not be experienced every cycle, and can be either physical and/or psychological (see Boxes 46.1 and 46.2 for symptomatology). The lives of the 5% or so of women who are severely affected may be completely disrupted in the second half of the menstrual cycle. The symptoms of PMS tend to decrease as a woman gets closer to menopause as her ovulatory cycles become less frequent.

Management

The first step in the management of PMS is recognition of the problem and realisation that many other women also suffer. Keeping a menstrual diary is useful and will establish any link between symptoms and menstruation; this also will provide a cornerstone for diagnosis. After a few months, it will allow the patient to make predictions and help her deal with changes when they arrive. The effectiveness of medical intervention depends upon which symptoms are being experienced, underlining the importance of a menstrual diary and experimentation. In terms of treatment, self-help and perseverance will be required in the management of PMS. The wide variety of symptoms may require exploring a number of treatment options before optimal relief can be achieved.

Non-pharmacological strategies

Maintenance of good general health is important, especially with respect to diet and possible deficiencies. Dietary modifications that may be helpful include restricting caffeine and alcohol intake. Smoking can also exacerbate symptoms. Exercise may help, as may learning simple relaxation techniques. If fluid retention is a problem, then reducing fluid and salt intake may be of value. Increasing the intake of natural diuretics such as prunes, figs, celery, cucumber, parsley and foods high in potassium such as bananas, oranges, dried fruits, nuts, soya beans and tomatoes may all be useful. Hypoglycaemia may also be involved in premenstrual tiredness, so eating small, protein-rich meals more frequently may help.

Results from clinical trials involving pyridoxine (vitamin B_6) have shown conflicting results. However, some women do respond to pyridoxine and show improvement, particularly with respect to mood change, breast discomfort and headache. A typical dosage regimen would be 50 mg twice daily after meals or 100 mg after breakfast. The dose should not exceed 100 mg/day. Gastric upset and headaches have been reported at doses greater than 200 mg. High doses over long periods have also been associated with peripheral neuropathies. Pyridoxine should be commenced 3 days before symptom onset and continued for 2 days after menstruation has started.

Calcium supplementation has shown some activity in reducing emotional, behavioural and physical symptoms. In addition, vitamin D and magnesium nutritional status have been found to be compromised in women with PMS. There is limited evidence that supplementation with γ-linolenic acid, found in evening primrose oil, gives relief from physical symptoms, especially breast tenderness.

Pharmacological management

Progestogens. Synthetic progestogens, in preparations such as Cyclogest, have been used in the past. However, because of the lack of convincing trial evidence and the risk of side effects, the use of progestogens is no longer recommended. Possible side effects include weight gain, nausea, breast discomfort, breakthrough bleeding and changes in cycle length. Problems arise because some synthetic progestogens, especially 19-nortestosterone (19-nor) compounds such as norethisterone and levonorgestrel, also display some affinity for glucocorticoid, mineralocorticoid and androgen receptors. The specificity of these synthetic agents is influenced by the substituents present on the steroid nucleus, particularly at C13. For example, the third-generation progestogens that have an ethyl group at C13 (gestodene, desogestrel and norgestimate) have the least androgenic activity of all the 19-nor compounds but are still orally active.

Combined oral contraceptives. Some women are helped by the combined oral contraceptives (COCs) pill because it prevents ovulation from taking place. However, the use of exogenous oestrogen may be contraindicated because it can increase the risk of venous thromboembolism. This occurs because oestrogen decreases blood levels of the potent natural anticoagulant antithrombin III and at the same time increases serum levels of some clotting factors. Women with other risk factors for thromboembolic disease should also avoid this form of therapy. In the March 2016 British National Formulary (Joint Formulary Committee, 2016) the incidence of venous thromboembolism in healthy, non-pregnant women who are not taking an oral contraceptive is cited as 2 cases per 10,000 women per year. For those using COCs that contain second-generation progestogens (e.g. levonorgestrel), this incidence is about 5–7 per 10,000 women per year of use. Some studies have reported a greater risk of venous thromboembolism in women using preparations containing the third-generation progestogens desogestrel and gestodene. The incidence in these women is about 9–12 per 10,000 women per year of use. However, it should be noted that the absolute risk of venous thromboembolism in women using COCs that contain these third-generation progestogens remains very small and well below the venous thromboembolism risk associated with pregnancy.

It is thought that use of third-generation progestogens is associated with increased resistance to the anticoagulant action of activated protein C. Oral contraceptive treatment diminishes the efficacy with which activated protein C downregulates in vitro thrombin formation. This is known as activated protein C resistance and is more pronounced in women using the COC pills that contain desogestrel than in women using those that contain levonorgestrel. However, it has also been recognised that women who do react to third-generation progestogens with venous thromboembolism may be revealing a latent thrombophilia. Several conditions, congenital or acquired, can cause thrombophilic alterations. A genetic factor known as factor V Leiden mutation is the most common inherited cause of thrombophilia, and this mutation results in resistance to the effects of activated protein C. Carriers of this mutation have more than a 30-fold increase in risk of thrombotic complications during oral contraceptive use, although this has been disputed (Farmer et al., 2000) because no increase in risk of venous thromboembolism was found with the third-generation progestogens. In conclusion, if there is a history of thromboembolic disease at a young age in the immediate family, then disturbances of the coagulation system must be ruled out.

The combination of ethinylestradiol with drospirenone is also available as an oral contraceptive and appears to be useful in the management of PMS. Drospirenone is a derivative of spironolactone, with affinity for progesterone receptors, but it also acts as a mineralocorticoid antagonist. This progestogen, therefore, alleviates some of the salt-retaining effects of the ethinylestradiol.

Further comprehensive information on UK Medical Eligibility Criteria for the hormonal contraceptives is available on the Faculty of Sexual and Reproductive Healthcare (2016) website (https://www.fsrh.org).

Antidepressants. The selective serotonin reuptake inhibitors (SSRIs) are becoming more popular in the treatment of PMS-related depression because they are effective and well tolerated (Brown et al., 2009). Several randomised controlled trials using fluoxetine, sertraline, citalopram, fluvoxamine or paroxetine concluded that SSRIs are an effective first-line therapy for severe PMS, and the side effects at low doses are generally acceptable. It is possible that SSRIs increase allopregnanolone levels which enhances GABA-A function. Studies have also found that not only do SSRIs improve behavioural symptoms, but some improvement in physical symptoms has also been noted, and this is being reflected in the increased prescribing of SSRIs (Sammon et al., 2016). Common side effects experienced include headache, nervousness, drowsiness and fatigue, sexual dysfunction and gastro-intestinal disturbances. Other agents such as tricyclic antidepressants and anxiolytics such as buspirone have been used. However, they appear to improve fewer PMS symptoms than the SSRIs. A Cochrane review (Marjoribanks et al., 2013) acknowledged that the overall quality of evidence was low to moderate. However, SSRIs, which could be taken continuously across the cycle or restricted to only the luteal phase, can reduce the symptoms of PMS. Dose-dependent adverse effects are common (e.g. nausea and asthenia). St John's wort has been used to reduce the severity of PMS, but the available evidence is limited.

Other treatments. Bromocriptine stimulates central dopamine receptors, and thus inhibits the release of prolactin. It may be useful for breast tenderness and occasionally has beneficial effects upon fluid retention and mood changes. However, side effects would now be seen as far outweighing the benefits for this particular indication.

Improvements in tension, irritability, depression, headache and general aches and pains can be seen in some women who take prostaglandin synthesis inhibitors. Most of the available information centres upon the use of mefenamic acid at dosages of 250 mg three times a day 12 days before a period is due, increasing to 500 mg three times a day 9 days before the period and continuing until the third day of menstruation. Other inhibitors of prostaglandin synthesis are likely to be just as effective and may be associated with fewer side effects. Some experimental evidence, however, suggests that, in addition to being a COX inhibitor, mefenamic acid also has activity as an antagonist at PGE receptors; therefore, this may be useful if heavy menstrual bleeding is also a problem. For optimum effectiveness, this form of therapy should be started 24 hours before the onset of symptoms. However, this starting point may be difficult to predict for women with irregular cycles.

GnRH analogues, sometimes referred to as gonadorelin analogues, are useful for managing the physical symptoms, but are less effective with respect to emotional symptoms. These agents inhibit the hypothalamic–pituitary–gonadal axis. However, they can be used for only short periods, no more than 6 months, because they induce a hypo-oestrogenic state; therefore, bone loss becomes significant after 6 months of treatment. Should a patient respond well to GnRH analogues for PMS following hysterectomy, because of underlying pelvic pathology, bilateral oophorectomy may also be of benefit.

Dysmenorrhoea

Dysmenorrhoea is usually subdivided into primary and secondary dysmenorrhoea. The former may also be referred to as spasmodic dysmenorrhoea, which is a uterine problem and is predominantly an issue of young women. Secondary dysmenorrhoea is so-called because it occurs secondary to some underlying pelvic pathology such as endometriosis or pelvic inflammatory disease (PID).

Epidemiology

The estimates vary, but epidemiological studies suggest that between 45% and 95% of women will suffer from dysmenorrhoea at some time during their reproductive life, and up to 15% of these women will be seriously debilitated by the condition. However, dysmenorrhoea is still frequently under-diagnosed and under-treated because few women seek medical advice and treatment. This carries social and economic consequences. In the USA, it has been estimated that dysmenorrhoea accounts for the loss of 600 million working hours which equates to more than $2 billion. Such estimates frequently only take into account absenteeism and do not include loss in productivity. Women in Western countries now have fewer pregnancies, and this may be a contributory factor in the increasing prevalence of dysmenorrhoea.

Primary dysmenorrhoea

Aetiology and symptoms

The incidence of primary dysmenorrhoea peaks in women in their late teens and early 20s; the pain coincides with establishment of ovulatory cycles. A typical sufferer will usually describe lower abdominal pain (cramping), which may radiate down into the thighs, and backache. Some women also suffer gastro-intestinal symptoms (nausea, vomiting, diarrhoea), headaches and faintness. Symptoms are intense on the first day of menses but rarely continue beyond day 1 or 2 of the cycle. Factors that appear to increase the severity include young age at menarche, extended duration of menstrual flow (pain can be most severe when the flow is lighter), smoking and parity (the prevalence and severity of dysmenorrhoea is decreased in parous women). Other factors such as weight, length of menstrual cycle or frequency of physical exercise do not influence the condition. However, recurrent menstrual pain as experienced by women with dysmenorrhoea negatively impacts upon quality of life, sleep quality, physical activity and mood, and it may also increase sensitivity to pain (Iacovides et al., 2015).

In terms of aetiology, studies carried out in the 1950s and 1960s first drew attention to the possible role of the prostaglandins. This was followed by many in vivo studies which showed that women suffering from primary dysmenorrhoea do have greater concentrations of prostaglandins, predominantly $PGF_{2\alpha}$, and to some extent PGE_2, in their menstrual fluid compared with matched control subjects. Such a prostaglandin imbalance would favour increased myometrial contractility. The effects of the prostaglandins on human myometrium are now well documented, and increased biosynthesis of prostaglandins may also account for the gastro-intestinal problems encountered by some sufferers. A role for the prostaglandins is substantiated by the fact that women whose diet contains more omega-3 fatty acids tend to suffer less. When eicosapentaenoic acid is the substrate for prostaglandin biosynthesis, prostaglandins of the three series are produced (e.g. PGE_3 and thromboxane A_3). Such local hormones are less potent stimulators of the myometrium and less effective vasoconstrictors. Other potential mediators are the endothelins, vasoactive peptides produced in the endometrium that may play a role in the local regulation of prostaglandin synthesis, and vasopressin, a posterior pituitary hormone that stimulates uterine activity and decreases uterine blood flow. The smaller branches of the uterine arteries are very sensitive to the vasoconstrictor actions of these mediators, and it is these resistance vessels that are important in the control of uterine blood flow. The interrelationship between blood flow and myometrial activity is summarised in Fig. 46.4.

Measurements of intrauterine pressure and myometrial activity have been made for research purposes, but there are no simple objective measurements for dysmenorrhoea.

Secondary dysmenorrhoea

Aetiology and symptoms

Secondary dysmenorrhoea tends to afflict women in their 30s and 40s, and usually occurs as a consequence of some other pelvic pathology such as endometriosis or pelvic inflammation. In

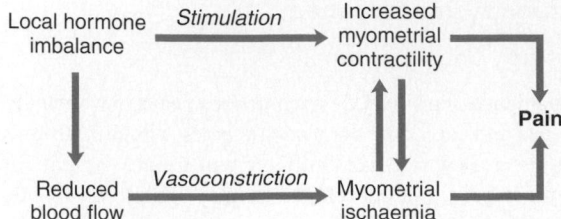

Fig. 46.4 The interactive role of myometrial stimulants and vasoconstrictive agents in the pathway leading to pain in dysmenorrhoea.

terms of symptoms, it differs from primary dysmenorrhoea in that the pain may actually start before menstruation begins, continue for the duration of menses and be associated with abdominal bloating, backache and a general feeling of 'heaviness' in the pelvic area. Women with inflammatory bowel disease also have symptom exacerbation during menses, and it is possible that the prostaglandins are involved in this aspect of pathoaetiology. The intrauterine contraceptive device may also exacerbate menstrual pain, because it causes localised inflammation that triggers the release of prostaglandins. The prostaglandins may also be implicated in the chain of events that lead to pain associated with secondary dysmenorrhoea. For example, if the cause is endometriosis, in which endometrial tissue is found outside the uterine cavity, then this extrauterine tissue can also synthesise prostaglandins, which may in turn disrupt normal uterine function.

Treatment

In terms of analgesia, the most rational choice would be a nonsteroidal anti-inflammatory drug (NSAID) (Zahradnik et al., 2010), because these compounds decrease prostaglandin biosynthesis by inhibiting COX. There is substantive evidence (Marjoribanks et al., 2010) that NSAIDs are effective in the treatment of dysmenorrhoea and are more effective than paracetamol. Differences in anti-inflammatory activity between different NSAIDs are small. There is considerable variation in individual patient tolerance and response, and a lack of response to one particular agent does not mean that a patient would not respond to a different NSAID. However, there is insufficient evidence regarding the comparative efficacy of individual agents in terms of superiority of analgesia or side-effect profile. Further information on when to use a NSAID and more importantly when not to is available in Clinical Knowledge Summaries (National Institute for Health and Care Excellence [NICE], 2015).

Mefenamic acid is frequently used to manage pain caused by dysmenorrhoea. As previously stated, this compound not only inhibits prostaglandin production but also appears to possess some PGE receptor blocking activity which may serve to augment its effect. However, these preparations are not suitable for all women, and some (about 30% of women) will not respond.

The lack of an effect with an NSAID may be explained by pathway diversion, because the arachidonic acid that was to be converted to a prostaglandin via the action of COX can be utilised by an alternative biosynthetic route, leading to increased formation of leukotrienes. Alternatively, the second COX enzyme (COX-2), which is generally induced under pathological conditions, may be involved. Many of the currently available NSAIDs

are relatively poor inhibitors of COX-2, and if some of the prostaglandins in these uterine disorders are produced via the action of this form of COX, then it is not surprising that the NSAIDs are not 100% effective. Celecoxib and etoricoxib have been shown to be effective, although neither is currently licensed for use in dysmenorrhoea.

A small study has investigated the use of the leukotriene receptor antagonist montelukast (Singulair) in the treatment of dysmenorrhoea (Fujiwara et al., 2010). The results suggest blockade of leukotriene receptors alleviate pain and reduce NSAID usage, and this appears to be most effective in women without endometriosis.

It has been estimated that approximately 50% of primary dysmenorrhoea sufferers will gain relief from taking the oral contraceptive pill, although, because this is a condition that afflicts young girls, there may be attitudinal problems to the use of these products either in the patient or her parents. The oral contraceptive pill inhibits ovulation and thereby prevents increased luteal-phase prostaglandin synthesis, thus decreasing uterine contractility. However, not all women are suitable candidates for COC use because of the potential problems associated with exogenous oestrogen. Contraindications include high blood pressure, obesity and a significant personal or family history of venous thromboembolism. Progestogenic preparations (e.g. norethisterone 5 mg three times daily from day 5 to 24 of the cycle) or progestogen-only pills may be useful if they inhibit ovulation. For pain relief, there appears to be no significant difference between the various formulations. Antispasmodics such as hyoscine butylbromide and propantheline bromide have a very limited role in the treatment of dysmenorrhoea, not least because of their poor oral bioavailability. Related compounds such as atropine also have negligible effects upon the human uterus. A summary of the treatment options for dysmenorrhoea is presented in Table 46.1. Future therapy may involve use of vasopressin antagonists. Clinical trials have shown these compounds to be effective and well tolerated, and they do not affect bleeding patterns.

For secondary dysmenorrhoea, the best treatment lies in finding the underlying cause and then taking an appropriate therapeutic route. For example, if some form of PID is diagnosed that can be attributed to a causative organism, then antimicrobial therapy is appropriate. PID is most commonly caused by the presence of a sexually transmitted infection. The most frequent causative organisms are *Chlamydia trachomatis* and *Neisseria gonorrhoeae*. In addition, any procedure that may compromise the mucous barrier of the cervix, for example, insertion of an intrauterine device, may also increase the risk of contracting PID. Treatment of endometriosis will often reduce symptoms of dysmenorrhoea. Surgical treatment for secondary dysmenorrhoea such as hysterectomy is also possible for those women who do not want to become pregnant.

Non-pharmacological management options have been reviewed and include high-frequency transcutaneous nerve stimulation and acupuncture. Both of these therapies showed some potential benefit for acute pain compared with placebo. There is limited evidence to support the use of uterine nerve ablation and presacral neurectomy, to interrupt the sensory nerve fibres near the cervix blocking the pain pathway. Dietary therapies such as vitamin (e.g. vitamin B_1 100 mg daily) and mineral supplementation have also been investigated. One study identified that vitamin B_1

Table 46.1 Summary of treatment options for dysmenorrhoea

Drug	Side effects
NSAIDs	Gastric irritation can be minimised by taking with or after food or selecting an agent with less gastrotoxicity (e.g. ibuprofen). Hypersensitivity reactions, particularly bronchospasm, may occur. Headache, dizziness, vertigo, hearing problems (e.g. tinnitus) and haematuria also may occur. NSAIDs may adversely affect renal function and provoke acute renal failure.
Combined oral contraceptives	Many side effects are dose related and thus the development of the ultra-low-dose preparations (i.e. those containing 20 micrograms ethinylestradiol) is beneficial. An alternative to the oral preparations is the low-dose transdermal combined contraceptive which releases 20 micrograms of ethinylestradiol and 150 micrograms of norelgestromin (active metabolite of the third-generation progestogen, norgestimate). The most serious potential adverse effect is the increased risk of thromboembolism due to a decrease in circulating levels of antithrombin III while increasing serum levels of some clotting factors. This risk increases with age and smoking. Analysis of current data suggests that the risk of breast cancer is not increased for most women who use the combined oral contraceptive for the major portion of their reproductive years. Use of the combined oral contraceptive also conveys several health benefits besides being an effective contraceptive. For progestogenic side effects, see below.
Progestogen-only preparations	Use of these agents may cause menstrual disturbances (e.g. breakthrough bleeding). Other adverse effects relate to the selectivity of the synthetic hormone; e.g. norethisterone is a first-generation progestogen and has some affinity for steroid receptors other than progesterone and so possesses androgenic, oestrogenic and anti-oestrogenic activity. The third-generation progestogens (gestodene, norgestimate and desogestrel) have the least androgenic activity. This should be advantageous because it is the androgenicity of the compounds that correlates with the decrease in high-density lipoproteins.

NSAID, Non-steroidal anti-inflammatory drug.

100 mg daily may be effective in relieving pain. Magnesium supplementation also shows promising results. Unfortunately, evidence is still lacking to support use of other herbal and dietary therapies, for example, omega-3 fatty acids. Some Chinese herbal medicines (e.g. Danggui Shaoyao San) have shown interesting results, but trial quality is poor because of high risk of bias.

Heavy menstrual bleeding

Blood loss is considered to be excessive if it exceeds 80 mL per period, although both women themselves and clinicians find it difficult to objectively quantify blood loss. In practice, it is defined by the woman's subjective assessment of blood loss. Any change in menstruation, whether real or perceived, may be disturbing with respect to social, occupational or sexual activities and can lead to other problems including depression and concern about an undiagnosed problem such as cancer. Physically, excessive blood loss will precipitate iron deficiency anaemia (haemoglobin <12 g/dL) which, if left undiagnosed and untreated, will compound the problems outlined earlier.

If a patient has any intermenstrual or postcoital bleeding, then referral to a gynaecologist for endometrial biopsy is essential in women older than 40 years to exclude intrauterine pathology. Up-to-date cervical cytology is also required. It should also be noted that hormonal contraceptives may cause some irregular spotting or breakthrough bleeding, but this is generally a tolerance effect. Non-oral methods, particularly implants, depots and intrauterine systems, decrease bleeding with continued use. The World Health Organisation recommends a 90-day reference period for reporting vaginal bleeding.

Epidemiology

In the UK about 30% of women report heavy menstrual bleeding, and about 1 in 20 women aged 25–44 years consult their primary care doctor about this problem. In the UK in excess of 800,000 women a year seek help for abnormal menstrual bleeding (Whitaker and Critchley, 2015). Historically, once referred to a gynaecologist, 60% of women could expect to have a hysterectomy within 5 years. Recent changes in the management of women with heavy menstrual bleeding and new treatment options, particularly endometrial ablations and the levonorgestrel intrauterine contraceptive devices (LNG-IUS), have significantly reduced hysterectomy rates to a third of the number in the late 2000s. However, it is estimated that one in three women in the USA, where more than 400,000 hysterectomies are performed each year, will have had a hysterectomy by the age of 60 years. Data suggest that alternatives to hysterectomy are being underused including hormonal and other forms of medical management, operative hysteroscopy, endometrial ablation and use of the LNG-IUS for primary management.

Aetiology and investigation

The aetiology of heavy menstrual bleeding can be divided into three categories: underlying pelvic pathology, systemic disease and dysfunctional uterine bleeding (Box 46.3). The typical symptoms suggestive of underlying pelvic pathology are presented in Box 46.4. Pelvic pathologies associated with heavy menstruation include myomas (fibroids, common benign tumours of the myometrium), endometriosis, adenomyosis (penetration of endometrial tissue into the myometrium), endometrial polyps, polycystic ovary syndrome and endometrial carcinoma. Although endometrial cancer is more typically

Box 46.3 Causes of heavy menstrual bleeding (percentage frequency)

Dysfunctional uterine bleeding (60%); i.e. cause is unknown
Other gynaecological causes (30%):
- Uterine or ovarian tumours
- Endometriosis
- Pelvic inflammatory disease
- Intrauterine contraceptive devices
- Early pregnancy complications

Endocrine and haematological causes (<5%)
- Thyroid disorders, e.g. hypothyroidism
- Platelet problems and clotting abnormalities

Box 46.4 Symptoms suggestive of underlying pelvic pathology

Irregular bleeding
Sudden change in blood loss
Intermenstrual bleeding
Postcoital bleeding
Dyspareunia
Pelvic pain
Premenstrual pain

seen in postmenopausal women, approximately 50% of those patients diagnosed with it premenopausally will have associated heavy menstrual bleeding. Systemic diseases from which heavy menstrual bleeding may stem include hypothyroidism, disorders involving the coagulation system such as elevated endometrial levels of plasminogen activator, and systemic lupus erythematosus. Very few women fall into this group. About 60% of sufferers have no underlying systemic or pelvic pathology and have ovulatory cycles. These patients are said to have dysfunctional uterine bleeding, and local uterine mechanisms appear to be important in the control of menstrual blood loss. Occasionally cycles may be anovulatory, with heavy blood loss because the endometrium has become hyperplastic under the influence of oestrogen. In addition, use of an intrauterine contraceptive device may also increase menstrual blood loss.

Prostaglandins appear to play a role in the aforementioned local mechanisms and have been implicated in heavy menstrual bleeding. Studies have suggested an association between the type and quantity of endometrial prostaglandin synthesis and the degree of menstrual blood loss. In the mid-1970s, it was discovered that women with heavy periods had raised endometrial levels of $PGF_{2\alpha}$ and PGE_2, and that blood loss could be reduced by the use of drugs inhibiting prostaglandin formation. More studies suggested that, in women with heavy menstrual loss, there is a shift towards increased biosynthesis of PGE_2, which is known to dilate uterine vasculature and/or increase the number of membrane receptors for this prostanoid. The availability of arachidonic acid, a substrate for prostaglandin synthesis, is also greater in women with heavy periods. Levels of the vasodilators or their metabolites, PGI_2 and nitric oxide, are also increased in the menstrual blood collected from women with excessive blood loss. It has been suggested that heavy menstrual bleeding is an angiogenesis-related disease associated with changes in the pattern of

vascular fragility involving the upregulation of various vascular endothelial growth factors.

Excessive menstrual blood loss is the most common cause of iron deficiency anaemia in women of reproductive age. In an otherwise healthy, well-nourished woman, it has been estimated that menstrual blood loss would have to exceed 120 mL to precipitate iron deficiency anaemia. Objective measurement of menstrual blood loss is difficult, so measurement of full blood count (including red blood cell indices and serum ferritin levels) and, in particular, haemoglobin concentration gives some indication of blood loss. Thyroid function should also be assessed. If fibroids are suspected, then pelvic ultrasound may be required. Endometrial biopsy is needed in women older than 40 years if there is an associated irregularity of menstruation or if intermenstrual or postcoital bleeding is present. In the case of regular menses, however, investigation of the uterine cavity would usually be required only in women older than 40 years or if medical treatment fails to alleviate symptoms. Young women presenting with dysfunctional uterine bleeding may have underlying coagulopathies such as von Willebrand's disease or Christmas disease, which should be excluded.

The increasing use of inhibitors of activated factor X (factor Xa) has led to reports of heavy menstrual bleeding, particularly with rivaroxaban, compared with the use of vitamin K antagonists or low molecular weight heparins. It remains to be seen whether this is a class effect.

Going forward it is likely that a more structured diagnostic classification framework will be more widely adopted (e.g. FIGO PALM-COEIN) (Munro et al., 2011) which will support the use of treatment modalities optimised for the individual.

Treatment

The management of heavy menstrual bleeding depends upon the cause of the condition and a woman's desire to conceive. Treatment can be either surgical or medical (Table 46.2). The effectiveness of drug therapy is obviously influenced by the accuracy of the diagnosis. Drug treatment is also influenced by a woman's contraceptive needs; for example, COCs can reduce menstrual blood loss by up to 50%, but in women older than 35 years who smoke, this form of therapy would need careful consideration. Low-dose luteal-phase progestogens are no longer recommended for treatment of heavy but regular periods because they increase menstrual blood loss in this situation. However, they may be of value in women with an irregular cycle. Long-term, long-acting progestogens, however, may render a woman amenorrhoeic. Other hormonally based therapies include the GnRH analogues, although their propensity to induce a hypo-oestrogenic state with long-term use may be problematic (a 6-month course would reduce trabecular bone density by 5–6%). Trials of ormeloxifene, a selective oestrogen receptor modulator (similar to raloxifene), 60 mg twice weekly has been used successfully to reduce blood loss and increase haemoglobin levels with relatively few side effects (Dhananjay and Nanda, 2013). The development of selective progesterone receptor modulators such as ulipristal may also increase pharmacological choice because such compounds may decrease uterine blood flow as well as alter endometrial architecture, resulting in reduced blood loss.

Table 46.2 Summary of drug treatment options for heavy menstrual bleeding

Drug	Comments
Combined oral contraceptive	See Table 46.1. These preparations are taken for 21 days with a 7-day pill-free (or placebo) period to allow for a withdrawal bleed
Progestogen-only preparations	See Table 46.1. Compounds such as norethisterone can be used, e.g. 5 mg three times daily or 10 mg twice daily for the latter half of the cycle. Ten days of therapy should be sufficient from day 15 of the cycle in ovulatory cycles. However, if the cycles are anovulatory, then a minimum of 12 days of therapy is more appropriate. Progestogens for 12 days are also required to prevent endometrial hyperplasia in perimenopausal and postmenopausal women who are taking oestrogen. When progestogens such as norethisterone are used, the dosage required is higher than that used in the combined oral contraceptive pill, and the adverse effects associated with the synthetic progestogens, particularly the 19-nortestosterone derivatives, may be more pronounced.
Intrauterine progestogen-only contraceptive	The levonorgestrel-releasing intrauterine device typically releases 20 micrograms of levonorgestrel/24 h. Unlike non-medicated IUCDs, which may increase menstrual blood loss, this device appears to reduce it, as a result of the local endometrial actions of the progestogen. The device also offers contraceptive cover without many of the side effects associated with the non-medicated IUCDs. Progestogen-related side effects should be minimised because of the low dose of levonorgestrel employed. Initially, bleeding patterns may be disrupted, but menstrual blood loss should become lighter within three menstrual cycles
Danazol	Danazol suppress the pituitary–ovarian axis. Side effects include amenorrhoea, hot flushes, sweating, changes in libido, vaginitis and emotional lability. Danazol also causes androgenic side effects such as acne, oily skin and hair, hirsutism, oedema, weight gain, voice deepening and decreasing breast size. Danazol has to be taken daily.
Gonadotrophin-releasing hormone analogues (gonadorelin)	After an initial period of stimulation, these agents suppress the pituitary–ovarian axis. As result of inducing a hypo-oestrogenic state, these compounds should only be used for 6 months because they may decrease trabecular bone density.
Non-steroidal anti-inflammatory drugs	These agents only need to be taken for the first 3–4 days of menses.
Tranexamic acid	This drug appears well tolerated but can produce dose-related gastro-intestinal disturbances. Patients who may be predisposed to thrombosis are at risk if given antifibrinolytic therapy. This compound is usually only taken for the first 3 days of menses.

IUCD, Intrauterine contraceptive device.

Prostaglandins have been implicated in the aetiology of several forms of menorrhagia. Therefore, NSAIDs may be of use in some patients, especially if there is pain associated with menstruation. The NSAIDs can be used with antifibrinolytics.

Women with heavy menstrual bleeding have greater endometrial fibrinolytic activity, hence the use of antifibrinolytic drugs, which are plasminogen activator inhibitors. Tranexamic acid became available for purchase over the counter in UK pharmacies in 2010 as Cyklo-F. This can be sold to women aged 18–45 years old with a history of regular heavy menstrual bleeding over several consecutive menstrual cycles. Tranexamic acid reduces menstrual blood loss by up to 50% (Lethaby et al., 2000), the recommended dose being 1 g three times daily starting on the first day of menses for up to 4 days. Agents such as tranexamic acid carry a risk of unwanted thrombogenesis, but this does not appear to be translated into practice as increased numbers of deep vein thromboses. This class of drugs decreases menstrual blood loss better than NSAIDs and oral luteal phase progestogen (Lethaby et al., 2005). However, tranexamic acid, like NSAIDs, should be stopped if it has produced no benefit after three cycles.

The levonorgestrel intrauterine contraceptive devices (also known as intrauterine systems [LNG-IUSs]) can be left in place for up to 5 years following insertion. They reduce menstrual blood loss by up to 90% after 12 months of use. The LNG-IUS provides relief from dysmenorrhoea, effective contraception and long-term control of heavy menstrual bleeding. In a Cochrane review (Lethaby et al., 2015) of trials, the LNG-IUS was compared with oral medications (norethisterone acetate, medroxyprogesterone acetate, oral contraceptives and mefenamic acid). The authors concluded that the LNG-IUS was more effective in reducing blood loss than the oral treatments but use was associated with more minor side effects. It was less effective than hysterectomy but more cost-effective.

Hysterectomy has been the traditional surgical treatment for heavy periods, with either a laparoscopic or open abdominal or vaginal approach used (Marjoribanks et al., 2016). Newer alternatives to hysterectomy include endometrial ablation, which can be done by electrosurgical, laser, microwave or thermal techniques. Endometrial ablation is less invasive than hysterectomy, but recurrence of heavy bleeding can occur and amenorrhoea cannot be guaranteed. There is evidence that pretreatment with a single dose of a GnRH agonist before the ablation procedure gives a better result. These preparations cause an initial stimulation of gonadotrophin release which then suppresses the hypothalamic–pituitary axis, producing a hypo-oestrogenic state. If circulating levels of oestrogen are low, then endometrial growth will not be stimulated; thus, it will be thinner, making the surgical endometrial destruction more effective.

Endometriosis

Endometriosis is a condition in which endometrial tissue is found outside the uterus. These so-called ectopic endometrial foci have been found outside the reproductive tract in the gastro-intestinal tract, the urinary tract and even the lungs.

Aetiology

Aetiology remains unclear, although retrograde menstruation, when shed endometrial cells migrate up through the fallopian tubes, would appear to be involved. This may occur because abnormalities in uterine innervation cause disruption in the usual patterns of myometrial contractility with consequent loss of the usual fundocervical polarity. Endometriosis is found in women in whom the normal route for the menstrual flow is disrupted, such as when there is some genital tract abnormality. Women who have more frequent and heavier periods also seem to be more likely to suffer from endometriosis. Familial predisposition may also be a factor, and several gene polymorphisms have been identified.

Studies suggest that endometrium from endometriosis sufferers tends to be more invasive. This may reflect either biological or genetic differences in the peritoneal milieu and may be explained by the upregulation of certain types of metalloproteinase responsible for the degradation of basement membrane. Endometrial tissue from women with endometriosis may have aromatase activity which can be stimulated by PGE_2. Therefore, ostensibly the endometriotic lesions have their own oestrogen supply as aromatase converts androgenic precursors into oestrogen and oestrogen stimulates biosynthesis of PGE_2; thus, the cycle is self-perpetuating. In vitro studies have shown that eutopic and ectopic endometrial explants have different lipidomic profiles in terms of their prostaglandin release, and the myometrium from endometriosis sufferers is more contractile during menses. Recent work suggests that the growth factor hypoxia-inducible factor-1α may play a critical role in the development of endometriosis, and thus provide another potential therapeutic target.

Epidemiology

Endometriosis was previously considered to be a disease affecting women in their 30s onwards, but increasing use of laparoscopy has revealed that it can occur at anytime throughout a woman's reproductive life. The condition is dependent upon oestrogen stimulation, and as such, it does not occur before the menarche or after menopause. The exact incidence of the disease is unknown, but it is believed to occur in about 10% in the general female population of reproductive age. One study has found a positive correlation between a menarche before 13 years and increased risk of development of endometriosis.

Symptoms

Although not all women with endometriosis are symptomatic, the pelvis is the most commonly affected site. Consequently, most of the symptoms of endometriosis relate to this region. Symptoms take the form of dysmenorrhoea and pelvic pain. However, the severity of the pain does not necessarily reflect the extent of the disease because women with severe pain may have few lesions, and vice versa. Dyspareunia often with postcoital discomfort is also common. There may also be menstrual irregularities.

The link between endometriosis and infertility is recognised, but the mechanisms involved have not been established. If the ovaries or fallopian tubes themselves are directly affected by the endometriotic lesions, then fertility may be compromised by purely mechanical means. However, the situation is less clear when the endometriosis does not cause any anatomical distortions. In this case, some of the postulated causes of infertility associated with endometriosis include ovulation disorders, such as luteinised unruptured follicle syndrome, anovulation and premature ovulation; hyperprolactinaemia; and changes in the peritoneal environment such as extrauterine endometrial material which, like normal endometrium, is subject to control by the ovarian steroids and, like its uterine counterpart, is also capable of producing prostaglandins. Prostaglandin levels, along with macrophage concentrations, are raised in the peritoneal fluid of women with endometriotic explants, and these may alter tubular and uterine motility within the abdomen.

Outside the reproductive tract, endometrial deposits can be found along the urinary and gastro-intestinal tracts. If the former is involved, then the patient may suffer from cyclical haematuria, dysuria or even ureteric obstruction. If there is gastro-intestinal tract involvement, then symptoms could include dyschezia, cyclical tenesmus and rectal bleeding or even obstruction. Very occasionally, the lesions are found at more distant sites such as the lungs, where they could cause cyclical haemoptysis. A reduction in bone mass in women with endometriosis has also been reported.

Treatment

The aims of treatment in endometriosis are to relieve symptoms and improve fertility if pregnancy is desired. Treatment can be either surgical or medical. Surgery is increasingly performed laparoscopically and can be used to restore normal pelvic anatomy, divide adhesions or ablate endometriotic tissue using either laser treatment or electrodiathermy. Medical treatment utilises the fact that endometriotic tissue is oestrogen dependent, and any drug therapy that will oppose the effects of oestrogen should, among other things, inhibit the growth of the endometriotic tissue. Hence, the choices of drug treatment are as follows.

- GnRH analogues include buserelin, goserelin, leuprorelin and nafarelin. These initially stimulate the hypothalamic–pituitary–ovarian axis but thereafter induce a hypo-oestrogenic state by paradoxically inhibiting follicle-stimulating hormone and luteinising hormone release. GnRH antagonists are currently being evaluated for management of endometriosis. These agents avoid the initial stimulation or 'flare' of the hypothalamic-pituitary-ovarian (HPO) axis. It may be possible to develop a dosing regimen that can be used for long-term pain management that is sufficiently low to avoid bone loss and that does not need an 'add-back' adjuvant.

- Low-dose COC (20–30 micrograms of ethinylestradiol) monophasic preparations have been found to be as effective as GnRH analogues, and they may slow down disease progression in young women and preserve future fertility. Flexible dosing regimens are being trialed where withdrawal bleeds are being eliminated for longer periods. Research shows that half of pill users would prefer not have bleeds at all. However, they remain underused (Nappi et al., 2015), and many women still focus on the side effects rather than the benefits of the hormonal contraceptives.

- Compounds with androgenic activity such as danazol also inhibit pituitary gonadotrophin release by interfering with the negative feedback and cause atrophy of endometrial tissue. Danazol interacts with androgen receptors, but it also has some affinity for the progesterone receptor. It inhibits the pulsatile release of gonadotrophins from the anterior pituitary, and thus abolishes cyclical ovarian activity, leading to amenorrhoea in the majority of women and a subsequent fall in serum oestrogen levels. Side effects relate to the androgenicity of the compound and include nausea, giddiness, muscular pain, weight gain, acne and virilisation. These can be minimised by using locally administered low doses of 200 mg/day.

- Progestogens such as medroxyprogesterone acetate and norethisterone initially cause decidualisation (cellular and vascular changes) of the endometrial tissue followed by glandular atrophy.

- Aromatase inhibitors are still under investigation for use in endometriosis. However, early results suggest that their adverse effect profile, which includes flushes, myalgia, arthralgia, insomnia and decreased libido, is poorer than for the progestogens and oral contraceptives.

None of the aforementioned drug therapies are free from side effects. Use of the GnRH analogues may evoke menopausal symptoms such as hot flushes, decreased libido, vaginal dryness (topical vaginal lubricants may be helpful), mood changes and headache. The problems associated with the hypo-oestrogenic state limit the long-term use of GnRH analogues. Although lipoprotein levels are not affected adversely, bone mass is, and this loss of bone density may not be entirely reversible after cessation of therapy. Various add-back hormone replacement therapies have been successfully used to minimise bone demineralisation, for example, low-dose oestrogen/progestogen combinations used continuously. Such regimens protect against osteoporosis and other hypo-oestrogenic side effects without apparently affecting clinical efficacy. Pain associated with endometriosis was relieved similarly by goserelin and a low-dose oral contraceptive (Prentice et al., 1999). However, side-effect profiles differed, for example, hot flushes and vaginal dryness with the former agent, and headache and weight gain with the latter.

The androgenic compounds, because of their very nature, are associated with hirsutism, weight gain and acne. Side effects associated with synthetic progestogens relate again to androgenicity, although dydrogesterone, like natural progesterone, does not cause virilisation. However, using a levonorgestrel-releasing intrauterine device ensures the low dose of levonorgestrel is delivered locally, and the more direct pelvic distribution may be useful in the management of endometriosis. Recent results

suggest this device causes the downregulation of endometrial cell proliferation and increased apoptotic activity. Longer-term studies, over 5 years, need to be undertaken to determine how long this effect is maintained and also the effectiveness on symptoms such as dyspareunia and dyschezia.

Researchers have also found that certain dietary changes may be beneficial and reduce symptoms. A decreased intake of glycaemic carbohydrates such as sugar, rice and potatoes in addition to reducing/eliminating caffeine and increasing the intake of omega-3 oils such as flax seed oil may also be helpful. In addition, one study found that women with endometriosis tended to have a lower body mass index than those without the condition.

Total pelvic clearance, including the removal of the ovaries, is practical in women who have completed their family. This tends to be a last resort treatment, but it is usually effective. However, surgery may be difficult if multiple lesions are present. There is no evidence that hormonal suppression improves surgical outcome.

Neither surgical nor medical management is effective in all cases. Studies suggest that pain associated with endometriosis responds well to both surgical and medical treatment, but symptoms of recurrence occur in about 50% of patients within 5 years of stopping treatment. Fertility may be increased by the use of surgery to remove endometriotic foci causing anatomical distortion. The same benefit is not associated with medical treatment.

Case studies

Case 46.1

A 13-year-old girl, Miss FL, is brought to her primary care doctor by her mother. She has been struggling with long, heavy periods for 6 months and as a result is missing time at school.

Questions

1. What non-hormonal treatment options would be considered?
2. What other treatments might be an option?

Answers

1. In young girls, it is worthwhile to try non-hormonal treatment options first because they will tend to have a lower side-effect profile than hormonal treatment. Tranexamic acid at a dosage of 1 g three times a day for up to 4 days (maximum 4 g/day) should be taken while bleeding. This is a very simple and effective option with few side effects and a reported 50% reduction in menstrual blood loss. Another option would be to try a non-steroidal preparation such as mefenamic acid (500 mg three times daily from first day of bleeding until period ends), especially if associated dysmenorrhoea is a significant problem. Tranexamic acid and an NSAID can be taken together if required.

2. Cyclical norethisterone (5 mg three times daily for 10 days) can be helpful if the periods are irregular, but it is not recommended for heavy regular periods. Progestogenic side effects such as nausea and bloating can limit use. The COC pill can be very effective at relieving heavy bleeding and dysmenorrhoea, provided that there are no contraindications. Sometimes parents can raise concerns about the use of a contraceptive agent, some parents perhaps believing that it may promote promiscuity.

Case 46.2

A 33-year-old woman, Ms JP, has been diagnosed with endometriosis having presented with severe dysmenorrhoea. She has visited the gynaecology clinic to discuss treatment options but is very concerned about her fertility. Ms JP does not wish to conceive at the present time but would certainly plan to try for a baby in the next couple of years.

Questions

1. What effect does endometriosis and its treatment have on fertility?
2. What treatment options could be considered?

Answers

1. Severe endometriosis with significant distortion of the pelvic anatomy can cause tubal blockage and hence cause tubal factor infertility. Most patients will have much less severe endometriosis which, although not causing any anatomical abnormality, is associated with a reduction in fertility. Such couples tend to take longer to conceive perhaps because the endometrial deposits create an unfavourable milieu for the egg and sperm. Laparoscopic ablation or excision of endometriotic deposits improves conception rates, albeit for a short period. In women who wish to conceive, endometriomas larger than 4 cm in diameter are removed because this improves pregnancy rates. Medical treatments do not improve fertility rates as many treatment options are contraceptive in themselves and should not be used if women wish to try to conceive. In this situation, symptom control with analgesia may be the best option.

2. As this patient is not wishing to conceive, a trial of medical therapy should be considered. Surgery for endometriosis is a highly skilled procedure which has a significant risk of complications. Medical treatment options include the COC pill, a prolonged course of progestogens such as medroxyprogesterone acetate or GnRH analogues. All have different side effects and contraindications but are all equally effective at reducing symptoms of endometriosis. The COC pill can be taken in a conventional way, but anecdotal experience supports tricycling, that is, taking three packets back to back and only having a withdrawal bleed after the third packet. Clearly, the usual contraindications to taking a COC pill apply. Progestogens are often poorly tolerated with

side effects such as bloating and nausea. A 6-month course of a GnRH analogue is generally effective at reducing symptoms and well tolerated. Vasomotor symptoms can be treated with add-back hormone replacement therapy with a continuous combined preparation or tibolone. Treatment is limited to a 6-month course because of the bone loss associated with the GnRH-induced hypo-oestrogenism.

Case 46.3

A 33-year-old, Ms AR, with very heavy and prolonged periods presents to her primary care doctor requesting a hysterectomy. Her mother had a hysterectomy at age 38 and this patient feels that it is her only option.

Questions

1. What treatment options would you offer Ms AR before considering a hysterectomy?
2. What investigations are necessary?

Answers

1. Before considering treatment, Miss AR should have a pelvic examination, primarily to exclude large fibroids which are unlikely to respond to medical therapy. Current advice is to recommend a levonorgestrel-releasing intrauterine device as first line for heavy menstrual bleeding (NICE, 2007). If the patient declines or is not suitable for this, other options would include tranexamic acid and/or an NSAID such as mefenamic acid taken at the onset of the period. The COC pill could be considered if not contraindicated. Cyclical norethisterone may be of benefit if the menstrual cycle is irregular. Endometrial ablative techniques are effective in 80% of women but are recommended only for women who have completed their families. Hysterectomy should be reserved as the last option and if medical therapy fails.

2. If pelvic examination is normal, the only investigation recommended for Miss AR is a full blood count to exclude anaemia. If examination suggests the possibility of a pelvic mass, an ultrasound scan should be organised. Further endometrium investigation, by hysteroscopy or endometrial biopsy, in women younger than 40 years with heavy menstrual bleeding and no intermenstrual bleeding, is not indicated unless medical treatment options fail.

References

American College of Obstetricians and Gynecologists, 2000. Premenstrual syndrome. ACOG Practice Bulletin No 15. ACOG, Washington, DC.

American Psychiatric Association, 2013. Diagnostic and Statistical Manual of Mental Disorders. American Psychiatric Publishing, Arlington, VA.

Bertone-Johnson, E.R., Hankinson, S.E., Bendich, A., et al., 2005. Calcium and vitamin D intake and risk of incident premenstrual syndrome. Arch. Intern. Med. 165, 1246–1252.

Brown, J., O'Brien, P.M.S., Majoribanks, J., et al., 2009. Selective serotonin reuptake inhibitors for premenstrual syndrome. Cochrane Database Syst. Rev. 2009 (2), CD001396. https://doi.org/10.1002/14651858.CD001396.pub2.

Dhananjay, B.S., Nanda, S.K., 2013. The role of Sevista in the management of dysfunctional uterine bleeding. J. Clin. Diagn. Res. 7 (1), 132–134.

Faculty of Sexual and Reproductive Healthcare, 2016. UK Medical Eligibility Criteria for Contraceptive Use UKMEC 2016. Available at: https://www.fsrh.org/standards-and-guidance/documents/ukmec-2016/fsrh-ukmec-full-book-2017.pdf.

Farmer, R.D.T., Williams, T.J., Simpson, E.L., et al., 2000. Effect of 1995 pill scare on rates of venous thromboembolism among women taking combined oral contraceptives: analysis of General Practice Research Database. Br. Med. J. 321, 477–479.

Fujiwara, H., Konno, R., Netsu, S., et al., 2010. Efficacy of montelukast, a leukotriene receptor antagonist, for the treatment of dysmenorrhea: a prospective, double blind, randomized, placebo-controlled study. Eur. J. Obst. Gynecol. Reprod. Biol. 148, 195–198.

Iacovides, S., Avidon, I., Baker, F.C., 2015. What we know about primary dysmenorrhea today: a critical review. Hum. Reprod. Update 21 (6), 762–778.

Joint Formulary Committee, 2016. British National Formulary 71. Br. Med. J. Group and Pharmaceutical Press, London.

Lethaby, A., Farquhar, C., Cooke, I., 2000. Antifibrinolytics for heavy menstrual bleeding. Cochrane Database Syst. Rev. 2000 (4), CD000249. https://doi.org/10.1002/14651858.CD000249.

Lethaby, A., Cooke, I., Rees, M.C., 2005. Progesterone or progestogen-releasing intrauterine systems for heavy menstrual bleeding. Cochrane Database Syst. Rev. 2005 (4), CD002126. https://doi.org/10.1002/14651858.CD002126.pub2.

Lethaby, A., Hussain, M., Rishworth, J.R., Rees, M.C., 2015. Progesterone or progestogen-releasing intrauterine systems for heavy menstrual bleeding. Cochrane Database Syst. Rev. 2015 (4), CD002126. https://doi.org/10.1002/14651858.CD002126.pub3.

Marjoribanks, J., Brown, J., O'Brien, P.M.S., et al., 2013. Selective serotonin reuptake inhibitors for premenstrual syndrome. Cochrane Database Syst. Rev. 2013 (6), CD001396. https://doi.org/10.1002/14651858.CD001396.pub3.

Marjoribanks, J., Lethaby, A., Farquhar, C., 2016. Surgery versus medical therapy for heavy menstrual bleeding. Cochrane Database Syst. Rev. 2016 (1), CD003855. https://doi.org/10.1002/14651858.CD003855.pub3.

Marjoribanks, J., Proctor, M., Farquhar, C., et al., 2010. Nonsteroidal anti-inflammatory drugs for dysmenorrhoea. Cochrane Database Syst. Rev. 2010 (1), CD001751. https://doi.org/10.1002/14651858.CD001751.pub2.

Morris, D.H., Jones, M.E., Schoemaker, M.J., et al., 2011. Determinants of age at menarche in the UK: analyses from the Breakthrough Generations Study. Br. J. Cancer 103 (11), 1760–1764.

Munro, M.G., Critchley, H.O.D., Broder, M.S., et al., 2011. FIGO classification system (PALM-COEIN) for causes of abnormal uterine bleeding in nongravid women of reproductive age. Int. J. Gynecol. Obstet. 113 (1), 3–13.

Nappi, R.E., Kaunitz, A.M., Bitzer, J., 2015. Extended regimen combined oral contraception: a review of evolving concepts and acceptance by women and clinicians. Eur. J. Contracept. Reprod. Health Care 21 (2), 106–115.

National Institute for Health and Care Excellence (NICE), 2007. Heavy menstrual bleeding. Clinical Guideline 44. NICE, London. Available at https://www.nice.org.uk/guidance/CG44.

National Institute for Health and Care Excellence (NICE), 2015. Clinical knowledge summaries NSAIDs: prescribing issues. Available at http://cks.nice.org.uk/nsaids-prescribing-issues.

Prentice, A., Deary, A., Goldbeck-Wood, S., et al., 1999. Gonadotrophin-releasing hormone analogues for pain associated with endometriosis. Cochrane Database Syst. Rev. 1999 (2), CD000346. https://doi.org/10.1002/14651858.CD000346.pub2.

Royal College of Obstetricians and Gynecologists, 2016. Premenstral syndrome, Management (Green-Top Guideline no. 48). Available at https://www.rcog.org.uk/en/guidelines-research-services/guidelines/gtg48/.

Sammon, C.J., Nazareth, I., Petersen, I., 2016. Recording and treatment of premenstrual syndrome in UK general practice: a retrospective cohort study. BMJ Open 6 (3) e010244.

Whitaker, L., Critchley, H.O.D., 2015. Abnormal uterine bleeding. Best Pract. Res. Clin. Obstet. Gynaecol. 34, 54–65.

Zahradnik, H.P., Hanjalic-Beck, A., Groth, K., 2010. Nonsteroidal anti-inflammatory drugs and hormonal contraceptives for pain relief from dysmenorrhea: a review. Contraception 81, 185–196.

Further reading

Bachmann, G., Korner, P., 2009. Bleeding patterns associated with non-hormonal contraceptives: a review of the literature. Contraception 79, 247–258.

Bahamondes, L., Bahamondes, M.V., Shulman, L.P., 2015. Non-contraceptive benefits of hormonal and intrauterine reversible contraceptive methods. Hum. Reprod. Update 21 (5), 640–651.

Barnhart, K.T., Freeman, E.W., Sondheimer, S.J., 1995. A clinician's guide to the premenstrual syndrome. Med. Clin. North. Am. 79, 1457–1472.

Bharadwaj, S., Barber, M.D., Graff, L.A., et al., 2015. Symptomatology of irritable bowel syndrome and inflammatory bowel disease during the menstrual cycle. Gastroenterol. Rep. (Oxf.) 3 (3), 185–193.

Clegg, J.P., Guest, J.F., Hurskainen, R., 2007. Cost-utility of levonorgestrel intrauterine system compared with hysterectomy and second generation endometrial ablative techniques in managing patients with menorrhagia in the UK. Curr. Med. Res. Opin. 23, 1637–1648.

Fall, M., Baranowski, A.P., Elneil, S., et al., 2010. EAU guidelines on chronic pelvic pain. Eur. Urol. 57, 35–48.

Halbreich, U., 2010. Women's reproductive related disorders. J. Affect. Disord. 122, 10–13.

Ismail, K.M.K., O'Brien, S., 2005. Premenstrual syndrome. Curr. Obst. Gynaecol. 15, 25–30.

Kriplani, A., Kulshrestha, V., Agarwal, N., 2009. Efficacy and safety of ormeloxifene in management of menorrhagia: a pilot study. J. Obst. Gynaecol. Res. 35, 746–752.

May, K., Octavia-Iacob, A., Sweeney, C., et al., 2009. Heavy menstrual bleeding annual evidence update. NHS Evidence – Women's Health. Nuffield Department of Obstetrics and Gynaecology, Oxford.

Nothnick, W., Alali, Z., 2016. Recent advances in the understanding of endometriosis: the role of inflammatory mediators in disease pathogenesis and treatment. F1000Res 2016, 5 (F1000 Faculty Rev), 186. https://doi.org/10.12688/f1000research.7504.1.

Oelkers, W., 2004. Drospirenone, a progestogen with antimineralocorticoid properties: a short review. Mol. Cell. Endocrinol. 217, 255–261.

O'Flynn, N., Britten, N., 2000. Menorrhagia in general practice – disease or illness? Soc. Sci. Med. 50, 651–661.

Rapkin, A., 2003. A review of treatment of premenstrual syndrome and premenstrual dysphoric disorder. Psychoneuroendocrinology 28, 39–53.

Yermachenko, A., Dvornyk, V., 2014. Nongenetic determinants of age at menarche: a systematic review. BioMed. Res. Int. 2014, 371583. Available at https://doi.org/10.1155/2014/371583.

Useful websites

Faculty of Sexual and Reproductive Healthcare (FSRH): https://www.fsrh.org

47 Menopause

Kay Marshall and Emma Crosbie

Key points

- Menopause is signalled by the last menstrual period; this cessation of menstruation results from a loss of ovarian follicular activity.

- The problems associated with menopause result from the ensuing loss of the female sex steroid oestrogen.

- On average, 35% of a woman's life is spent in a peri-menopausal or post-menopausal state.

- Declining oestrogen levels can give rise to vasomotor symptoms, localised atrophy of the genitalia, psychological problems, osteoporosis and coronary heart disease.

- In the UK, only about 50% of women seek help for their symptoms.

- The hormonal content of a particular hormone replacement therapy (HRT) regimen is important, as is the route of delivery, in determining the side effects observed.

- Contraindications to HRT include active arterial thrombo-embolic disease and thrombophilic disorders, undiagnosed vaginal bleeding in post-menopausal women or the presence of an oestrogen-dependent tumour.

- For women with an intact uterus, hormone replacement regimens must include a progestogenic component to prevent overstimulation of the endometrium.

- Alternative options to traditional HRT regimens include the use of tibolone, raloxifene and the bisphosphonates.

Menopause

The UK, like many countries in the developed world, has an ageing population; life expectancy is increasing, and women continue to live longer than men, whilst birth rates are declining. Currently, a woman can expect to live about 35% of her life in a post-menopausal state.

Menopause is signalled by a woman's last menstrual period and is defined as the permanent cessation of menstruation resulting from loss of ovarian follicular activity. The occurrence of the last menstruation can only be diagnosed retrospectively and is usually taken as being final if it is followed by a 12-month bleed-free interval; such women are defined as being post-menopausal. The mean age of menopause in the UK is 51 years, and by the age of 54 years, around 80% of women will be post-menopausal. If menopause occurs before 40 years, which happens in approximately 1% of women, it would be classed as a premature menopause. Many women will experience erratic periods before the final cessation due to inadequate ovarian oestrogen secretion; these women are described as being peri-menopausal. This transitional phase usually lasts around 4–5 years. The problems associated with menopause result from oestrogen deprivation, and women should be given information about menopause and concomitant health implications, as well as benefits and risks of treatment.

Menopause is a natural event in the anatomical, physiological and psychological changes that form the female climacteric. Some women will go from the transition of being pre-menopausal to post-menopausal with no symptoms at all. Many will experience the symptoms associated with a lack of oestrogen, whether in the peri-menopausal or post-menopausal phase, which include:

- vasomotor symptoms,
- localised atrophy of urogenital tissues,
- osteoporosis,
- psychological and neurological problems,
- musculoskeletal problems,
- coronary heart disease.

Initially, the symptoms are more likely to include vasomotor symptoms such as hot flushes, night sweats and palpitations, and psychological problems, including mood changes, irritability, sleep disturbance, depression and decreased libido. Many women suffer from vaginal dryness and dyspareunia (painful sexual intercourse), which serve to enhance the loss of libido, and this in turn can adversely affect psychological well-being. The urethral mucosa may become atrophied, leading to an increased incidence of urinary tract infections or urinary incontinence. In some women, the urethra may eventually become fibrosed, leading to dysuria, frequency and urgency (urethral syndrome). The long-term consequences of oestrogen deprivation are often symptomless. There is a significant loss of calcium from the bones, which may give rise to frequent fractures, and there is a change in the blood lipid profile, which is associated with a rise in coronary heart disease.

Physiological changes

Ovarian

The approaching menopause is associated with loss of ovarian follicular activity. Human ovaries contain approximately 700,000 follicles at birth, but these cells have a high mortality rate, and fewer than 500 of them will be ovulated. This number falls progressively with increasing age so that by the time the woman approaches 50 years of age, the number of follicles has fallen to zero or very few. The rate of follicle loss is highest during the decade between 40 and 50 years of age, possibly due to an increase in the rate of degeneration (atresia) of the earliest follicles. Women older than 45 years who are menstruating regularly have been shown to have 10 times as many follicles as those with irregular cycles; those who have not had a period for 12 months have few follicles remaining. Thus, the size of the follicular pool is an important determinant of ovarian function.

Ovarian function includes two major roles: the production of eggs (gametogenesis) and the synthesis and secretion of hormones (hormonogenesis). Both of these functions undergo subtle changes with ageing so that fewer ova are produced and they are less readily fertilised, and the hormone levels become irregular. It is the granulosa cells in the developing follicle that normally secrete estradiol, and a lack of this follicular activity results in diminishing oestrogen secretion. The diminution in the number of active follicles is followed by an increase in follicle-stimulating hormone (FSH) secretion from the anterior pituitary gland as the normal feedback mechanisms between ovarian estradiol secretion and the hypothalamus–pituitary axis become disrupted. It may be that there is an age-related decrease in sensitivity to feedback inhibition that exacerbates this increase in FSH levels. In women who are still bleeding, an FSH level exceeding 10–12 IU/L on day 2 or 3 of the bleed is indicative of a diminished ovarian response. A high FSH level (>30 IU/L) and a low estradiol level (<100 pmol/L) in the plasma characterise menopause. The National Institute of Health and Care Excellence (NICE) Clinical Guideline (NICE, 2015) on menopause includes a chapter on diagnostic testing and concludes that biochemical measurements and ovarian ultrasound are not useful in routine practice and that age and amenorrhoea remain sufficient for routine diagnosis. The low oestrogen level fails to stimulate growth of the uterine endometrium. Because endometrial growth has not occurred, there can be no menstruation (shedding of the endometrium), and this signifies that menopause has arrived. Because ova are not being released, the production of progesterone from the ovary also ceases, and the levels of luteinising hormone (LH) eventually rise. Thus, peri-menopausal and menopausal women are subjected to an increasing ovarian hormone deficiency, as shown in Table 47.1.

When the ovaries are conserved after hysterectomy, they will usually continue to produce some estradiol, but the levels of this hormone will decline up to the age of the natural menopause.

Post-menopausally, in all women, androstenedione (secreted from the adrenal cortex) is converted in adipose tissue and muscle (peripheral conversion) to estrone, which becomes the major circulating oestrogen (but estrone is about 10 times less potent than estradiol). The levels of FSH and LH remain elevated for many years if no HRT is given, but these elevated levels have no effect on the ovary because the follicles are atretic.

The cessation of reproductive function in the woman and the declining oestrogen production from the ovary are not the only physiological events associated with menopause. For many years, oestrogen was considered to be associated only with the genitourinary system, but its effects are more wide ranging, and the major tissues affected include blood vessels, bones and the brain.

Urogenital system

With the failure in ovarian oestrogen production, the number of uterine endometrial oestrogen receptors occupied falls, and endometrial growth is not sustained. Thus, in the post-menopausal woman, the endometrium becomes thin and atrophic. Likewise, in the other target tissues containing oestrogen receptors, the basal layers of the vaginal epithelium are no longer stimulated to maintain the vaginal epithelium and produce natural lubricants from the vaginal glands. The result is vaginal atrophy, and a thin, dry vagina may result in dyspareunia. It is estimated that 50% of post-menopausal women suffer symptoms attributable to vulvo-vaginal atrophy. Because the lower urinary tract and the lower genital tract share a common embryological origin, deprivation of oestrogen can also result in urethral and bladder problems. Often, peri-menopausal and post-menopausal women report an increase in urinary frequency, nocturia and urge incontinence. For some women, these changes may manifest as long as 10 years after menopause.

Bone

Osteoporosis is a systemic skeletal disease characterised by low bone mass and microarchitectural deterioration of bone tissue leading to enhanced bone fragility and a consequent increase in fracture risk. Although the exact magnitude of the problem of osteoporosis is unknown, it has been estimated that it affects 200 million people worldwide. In addition, approximately 30% of women older than 50 years have one or more vertebral fractures compared with 20% of men older than 50 years who will have an osteoporosis-related fracture in their remaining lifetime. The total number of hip fractures in 1950 was 1.66 million, and by 2050, this figure could reach 6.26 million. Twenty percent of people die within 1 year of a hip fracture (Cooper, 1997). Typical morbidities after a vertebral fracture include:

- back pain,
- loss of height,
- deformity (kyphosis, protuberant abdomen),
- reduced pulmonary function,
- diminished quality of life: loss of self-esteem, distorted body image, dependence on narcotic analgesics, sleep disorder, depression or loss of independence.

Table 47.1 Ovarian hormone secretion after the onset of the normal menstrual cycle

	Pre-menopausal (normal cyclic)	Peri-menopausal (irregular cycles)	Post-menopausal (cessation of cycle)
Oestrogens	+++	++	+-⁻-
Progesterone	+++	+	–
Androgens	+	+	+-⁻-

To contextualise risk, the remaining lifetime probability in women at menopause of a fracture at any one of these sites exceeds that of breast cancer (~12%). Also, the likelihood of a fracture at any of these sites is 40% or more in developed countries (Kanis et al., 2000), a figure close to the probability of coronary heart disease. Risk factors for osteoporosis include low body mass index (<19 kg/m²), smoking, early menopause, family history of maternal hip fracture, long-term systemic corticosteroid use and conditions affecting bone metabolism, especially those causing prolonged immobility. Osteoporosis is most common in white women. People with osteoporosis are at risk of fragility fractures, occurring as a result of mechanical forces that would not ordinarily cause fracture. The clinically relevant outcome in evaluating treatments for osteoporosis is the incidence of fragility fracture because otherwise, this condition is asymptomatic and therefore undiagnosed. The most common sites for these fractures are the hip, vertebrae and wrist. In the UK, the cost of hospital care alone for patients with a hip fracture amounts to more than £2 billion per year.

Musculoskeletal system

Musculoskeletal problems are frequently reported by women as they reach menopause. These symptoms could also be attributed to ovarian quiescence and oestrogen deprivation. Muscle mass is inversely correlated with plasma oestrogen levels in women. The mechanism of action by which a decrease in oestrogen level may have a negative effect on muscle mass is not yet understood, but it has been suggested that the decrease in oestrogen concentrations may be associated with an increase in pro-inflammatory cytokines, such as tumor necrosis factor alpha and interleukin-6. It should be noted that skeletal muscle cells do contain oestrogen receptors, ERβ, and hormone replacement improves muscle mass and strength.

Cardiovascular system

Young adult women are protected against the development of hypertension and its deleterious consequences in the cardiovascular system. Levels of low-density lipoprotein cholesterol (LDL-C) and very-low-density lipoprotein cholesterol (VLDL-C) are decreased by oestrogen, and the levels of high-density lipoprotein cholesterol (HDL-C) are increased, thereby giving some protection against atherosclerosis. HDL-C is known to promote cholesterol efflux from macrophages in the arterial wall, thereby reducing atheromatous plaque and conferring a protective effect against heart disease. However, after menopause, this protection is lost, and the incidence of high blood pressure and associated cardiovascular disease increases to levels similar to those found in age-matched men.

Oestrogen has direct beneficial effects in the control of blood pressure, possibly via regulating endothelium-mediated control of arteriolar tone. In women deprived of oestrogen, endothelium-dependent vasodilation is impaired. This dysfunction is largely associated with a reduction in nitric oxide availability. Oestrogen increases nitric oxide availability by stimulating endothelial nitric oxide synthase (eNOS). Oestrogen also stimulates the production of other endothelium-derived relaxing factors, such as prostacyclin (prostaglandin I₂). The role of membrane G-protein-coupled estrogen receptors (GPERs), as opposed to ERα and ERβ, which mediate classical genomic responses, are likely to be involved because they can mediate more rapid responses, which would explain the ability of oestrogen to modulate vascular tone (Prossnitz and Barton, 2014).

Miscellaneous changes

Thinning of the skin, brittle nails, hair loss and generalised aches and pains are also associated with reduced oestrogen levels (Hall and Phillips, 2005). The skin is the largest nonreproductive target on which oestrogen acts. Oestrogen receptors, predominantly of the ERβ type, are widely distributed within the skin. Both types of oestrogen receptor (ERα and ERβ) are expressed within the hair follicle and associated structures. Thus, epidermal thinning, declining terminal collagen content, diminished skin moisture, decreased laxity and impaired wound healing (selective ERα ligands are being investigated for their wound-healing properties) have been reported in postmenopausal women.

In addition, women also show increasing body weight associated with ageing. This weight gain tends to increase or begin near menopause. Body fat redistribution to the abdomen also occurs independent of weight gain. This type of centralised abdominal fat distribution is widely recognised as an independent risk factor for cardiovascular disease in women.

Psychological and neurological changes

Older age at menarche and younger age at menopause are associated with poorer cognitive functioning during ageing. Recent studies have demonstrated that sex steroids have a multifarious and complex relationship with the central nervous system (Hogervorst et al., 2009). For example, there may be a positive correlation between increasing parity and improved executive functioning in response to oestrogen. This temporal relationship between oestrogen deprivation and response to exogenous oestrogen was clearly exemplified in the memory study arm of the Women's Health Initiative (WHI; Coker et al., 2010) and Million Women Study (MWS) studies (Hogervorst and Bandelow., 2010) at the turn of the 21st century.

Depression is twice as common in women as in men and may increase during times of changing hormonal levels such as at menopause. Some aspects of decreased central nervous system function have been related to falling oestrogen levels. Preclinical studies have shown oestrogen to have several positive effects on central nervous system function. Perhaps the most important is the promotion of acetylcholine synthesis and increased synaptogenesis in the hippocampus. ERβ is expressed in this area of the brain, as well as the entorhinal cortex and thalamus, areas crucially involved in explicit memory. Human neuroimaging studies have also indicated that oestrogen influences regional cerebral blood flow in women. In addition, oestrogens may exert neuroprotective actions against excitotoxic neuronal injury by enhancing glutamate transporter levels and their function.

Management

Hormone replacement therapy

Hormone replacement therapy (HRT) is a complicated clinical issue requiring an in-depth risk/benefit assessment. The vast amount of study data is often conflicting, and careful analysis is required. Many factors need to be reviewed before HRT is prescribed. One important factor is age; data have shown that if a woman aged less than 35 has a hysterectomy and a bilateral oophorectomy, her risk of non-fatal myocardial infarction is nearly eight times that of her age-matched counterpart who has retained her ovaries. Age at time of HRT prescription in relation to menopausal age, that is, number of years of oestrogen deprivation before replacement, is also of importance when considering outcomes, and this 'window' for replacing oestrogen is currently subject to close scientific scrutiny. Individual differences in hormone metabolism (both endogenous and exogenous) are also likely to be important because several different cytochrome enzymes metabolise oestrogen and may be affected by inherited polymorphisms. Therefore, some women may produce oestrogenic metabolites possessing considerable oestrogenic activity, whereas others produce metabolites that are relatively non-oestrogenic. Body mass index (BMI) also influences response to HRT, with increased plasma estradiol levels observed in women with higher BMIs.

HRT is effective for symptomatic relief of menopausal symptoms, and its use is justified when symptoms adversely affect quality of life. The publication of major trials, such as the Women's Health Initiative in the USA (Women's Health Initiative, 2002) and the Million Women Study in the UK (Million Women Study Collaborators, 2003) and the interpretation of their findings had a dramatic impact on HRT prescribing. However, the publication of the NICE guidelines in November 2015 may have begun to reverse this. The information in the Box 47.1 is taken from these guidelines.

Contraindications to the use of HRT include undiagnosed vaginal bleeding in post-menopausal women, the presence of an oestrogen-dependent tumour, liver disease (where liver function tests have failed to return to normal), active thrombophlebitis and active or recent arterial thromboembolic disease, for example, angina or myocardial infarction. A history of deep vein thrombosis and pulmonary embolism requires careful evaluation before the use of oestrogen therapy. Use in patients with Dubin–Johnson and Rotor syndromes may also be contraindicated.

Oestrogen therapy

Because the symptoms and long-term effects of menopause are due to oestrogen deprivation, the mainstay of HRT is oestrogen. This may be administered orally or parenterally, but in either case, the oestrogens used are naturally occurring and include the following:

- estradiol,
- estriol,
- estrone,
- estropipate (piperazine estrone sulphate),
- conjugated equine oestrogen (estrone sulphate 40%, equilin sulphate 60%),
- estradiol valerate.

Box 47.1 The importance of patient information
• It is important for healthcare professionals to provide up-to-date, objective and accurate information on the benefits and risks for HRT to help women make an informed choice about which treatment to use for menopausal symptoms. Media reports about HRT have not always been accurate, so providing healthcare professionals and women with a robust source of information is vital.
• Although the Women's Health Initiative found that HRT prevented osteoporotic fractures and colon cancer, it initially reported that HRT increased the risk of having a cardiovascular event as well as the incidence of breast cancer. However, the association between HRT and cardiovascular disease has since been disputed, and the results show that the risk varies in accordance with individual factors.
• HRT dosage, regimen and duration of use should be individualised with yearly appraisals. The NICE (2015) guidelines and consensus statements published by the British Menopause Society (2016) and the International Menopause Society (de Villier et al., 2016) should be used by primary care doctors and other healthcare professionals to enable them to be more confident in prescribing HRT and women more confident in taking it.
• A knowledge gap among some primary care and other healthcare professionals could mean that they are reluctant to prescribe HRT because they overestimate the risks and contraindications and underestimate the impact of menopausal symptoms on a woman's quality of life.

HRT, Hormone replacement therapy.

The use of 'natural' oestrogens reduces the risk of the potentially dangerous oestrogenic effects such as raised blood pressure, alteration in coagulation factors and an undesirable lipid profile, which sometimes occur with the more potent synthetic oestrogens used in the oral contraceptive agents. A 'natural' oestrogen is defined as one that is normally found in the human female and has a physiological effect. Natural oestrogens are less potent (up to 200 times) than synthetic oestrogens. Because they are naturally occurring compounds, the plasma half-life of these oestrogens is similar to that of the ovarian-secreted oestrogens, and the duration of action is shorter than that of the synthetic oestrogens, such as ethinylestradiol, used in many formulations of the contraceptive pill. The plasma ratio of estradiol to estrone is normally about 1:1 to 2:1, and the aim of HRT should be to preserve this ratio.

There are four main routes of administration for oestrogens in HRT:

- oral,
- transdermal (patches/gels/cream),
- subcutaneous (implants),
- vaginal (creams and medicated rings).

The use of oral oestrogen therapy, although convenient for the patient, does mean that the oestrogen will be subjected to conversion to estrone by the liver and the gut, thereby altering the estradiol/estrone ratio in favour of the less active oestrogen, estrone. The oral preparations have different metabolic effects due to first-pass hepatic metabolism. Smoking stimulates metabolism of oestrogens by cytochrome P450 and decreases plasma oestrogen levels by 40–70% in oral oestrogen users. Smoking has no significant effect on plasma oestrogen levels in users of

Table 47.2 Effect of hormone replacement therapy administration route on lipid profile

Oral	Transdermal
↓ Low-density lipoprotein	↓ Low-density lipoprotein
↓ Total cholesterol	↓ Total cholesterol
↑ High-density lipoprotein	↔ High-density lipoprotein
↑ Triglycerides	↓ Triglycerides
↑ Bile cholesterol	↔ Bile cholesterol

transdermal preparations. Oral delivery compared with transdermal delivery (Table 47.2) also has different effects on lipid levels (Vrablik et al., 2008). In addition, orally administered oestrogens undergo first-pass hepatic metabolism, which may result in some reduction in anti-thrombin III, a potent inhibitor of coagulation. Implants and patches show smaller changes in coagulation, platelet function or fibrinolysis.

More constant levels of oestrogen result from the use of transdermal patches containing estradiol, and these have the added advantage of a more physiological estradiol/estrone ratio (Delmas et al., 1999). However, the adhesive used in these transdermal patches and the alcohol base can cause skin irritation. The patch is applied to the non-hairy skin of the lower body, and care should be taken to ensure that it is placed away from breast tissue. The patch is changed either once or twice a week, thus providing a constant reservoir of estradiol to provide a controlled release into the circulation. Estradiol is also available in a gel formulation, applied daily to the skin over the area of a template (to ensure correct dosage), but this formulation may give erratic absorption. The intranasal preparation, administered as a nasal spray, also avoids hepatic first-pass metabolism.

The oestrogen implant gives a constant level of oestrogen from a few days after insertion for up to 6 months. This formulation maintains the best estradiol/estrone ratio and is a convenient method of administration, requiring repeat implants only every 6 months. However, because the levels of oestrogen are constantly raised, there will be some increase in oestrogen receptor numbers, and this can lead to a recurrence of symptoms of oestrogen deficiency due to the presence of unoccupied oestrogen receptors, even in the presence of normal or even high oestrogen levels. This phenomenon, called tachyphylaxis, results in patients becoming symptomatic and requesting repeat implants earlier and earlier. In such cases, it is unwise to treat with additional oestrogen; the patient should receive counselling and perhaps a change of preparation. The disadvantage of the implant is that, once inserted, it cannot be removed readily, and even if it is removed, the oestrogen level will take at least a month to fall. There is also evidence that the uterine endometrium, if present, remains stimulated for some time after removal of the implant.

Both the transdermal and implant preparations avoid the first-pass hepatic effects of oral oestrogens and are less likely to affect liver enzyme systems and clotting factors. Some studies show an increase in the incidence of venous thromboembolism (VTE) in women taking HRT. Therefore, patients who have a history of deep vein thrombosis (DVT) or pulmonary embolism will need careful guidance, with each woman being considered individually, and the relative risks evaluated. Other risk factors include severe varicose veins, obesity or a family history of DVT. If HRT is justified in such patients, transdermal preparations are a better alternative than oral preparations.

Vaginal creams containing oestrogen are available but generally fail to produce the reliable plasma levels required to protect against the long-term effects of oestrogen deprivation. They can be used to provide relief from atrophic vaginitis. An alternative formulation is the vaginal ring, which releases estradiol at a controlled rate in physiological levels for up to 3 months.

The dose of oestrogen used in HRT sufficient to preserve bone density is usually higher than that necessary to alleviate vasomotor symptoms. The doses suggested to protect bone density are estradiol 2 mg/day orally, 50 micrograms/day transdermally and 50 mg every 6 months by implant. If the conjugated equine oestrogens are used, the oral dose should be 0.625 mg/day. The lower doses found in vaginal creams may alleviate the vasomotor symptoms but will not protect against osteoporosis. Current guidelines advise the use of the lowest possible dose of HRT to relieve vasomotor symptoms and recommend alternative treatment to prevent and treat osteoporosis (NICE, 2015).

Oestrogens should be used alone only in women who have undergone a hysterectomy; if the uterus is present, the endometrium will be stimulated, and this increase in endometrial growth may be a precursor to the development of a malignant condition. Current practice is to administer progestogens with oestrogen. In the early 1970s, when oestrogen was used alone, HRT received bad press because in women who had not undergone hysterectomy, there was an increased incidence of endometrial carcinoma. In women who have undergone hysterectomy, oestrogens are usually administered continuously.

Progestogen therapy

The only proven reason for adding a progestogen to oestrogen therapy for HRT in women with an intact uterus is to protect the endometrium from hyperplasia and possible neoplasia. There are many preparations that contain progestogens added to oestrogen for a number of days per month. However, to effectively prevent endometrial hyperplasia, the progestogen must be taken for a minimum of 12 days. The minimum dose of progestogen required to protect against hyperplasia depends on the potency of the compound used.

The progestogens commonly available in HRT preparations are either derivatives of progesterone, such as medroxyprogesterone and dydrogesterone, or 19-nortestosterone substitutes such as norethisterone or levonorgestrel. All these synthetic progestogens are active after oral administration and provide adequate protection of the endometrium against oestrogen stimulation. Some transdermal preparations also incorporate a progestogenic compound in the regimen. As with all semi-synthetic or synthetic hormones, these compounds may act on receptors other than the progesterone receptor, and the long-term consequence of this is not predictable.

Box 47.2 Regimens of combined oestrogen and progestogen therapy for use in hormone replacement therapy

Oestrogen 28 days + progestogen 12 or 14 days, then repeat without interval (bleed every 4 weeks)
Oestrogen 70 days + progestogen 14 days followed by 7 days placebo tablets (bleed every 3 months)
Oestrogen + progesterone continuously (no bleed)
Oestrogen continuously + Mirena IUS (bleed variable, but levonorgestrel likely to reduce bleed and can provoke amenorrhoea)

Progesterone is the only progestogen to act solely on the progesterone receptor, but it has poor oral bioavailability, and so it is difficult to achieve satisfactory plasma concentrations. However, the micronised preparations are better absorbed. Progesterone may also be administered at night in the form of a pessary or suppository, or by injection in the form of a long-lasting subdermal implant. The progestogen in HRT is most commonly administered orally or transdermally, and usually, one of the synthetic progestogens is used.

Oestrogen and progestogen regimens

The monthly withdrawal bleed is perceived by some post-menopausal patients to be an unacceptable side effect of HRT, and this has resulted in the development of a number of regimens in an effort to minimise this effect (Box 47.2). Formulations have been produced with which bleeding only occurs every 3 months instead of every 4 weeks, or it does not occur at all.

The use of the 70-day oestrogen preparation, although being more popular with women because bleeding only occurs every 3 months, needs further evaluation regarding endometrial protection. Bleeding can be avoided altogether if a combination of oestrogen and progestogen is given continuously throughout the treatment (continuous combined HRT). Such a preparation should only be given to women who are at least 12 months post-menopausal and have an atrophied endometrium; otherwise, breakthrough bleeding may occur. Bleeding in the first 6 months (usually just spotting) is not uncommon, but bleeding after this time should be investigated, although the incidence of endometrial hyperplasia is low with this continuous regimen. Others recommend a 28-day interval between courses of treatment to allow the endometrium to become atrophic in patients who are changing from the cyclical therapy to the continuous combined therapy. Patients who commence cyclical HRT before ceasing menstruation should change to a continuous combined preparation only after the age of 54 (when there is an 80% chance that they will be post- rather than peri-menopausal) to reduce the risk of breakthrough bleeding. An alternative option is to use the levonorgestrel-loaded intrauterine system (IUS; e.g. Mirena) in conjunction with oral oestrogen. This option can be particularly useful for women intolerant of the progestogenic side effects associated with systemic dosing.

Not all progestogens have the same pharmacological profile, and these differences have implications for their usage. Two of the most widely used synthetic progestogens are medroxyprogesterone acetate and norethisterone. These are used as the progestogenic component of an HRT regimen in combination with oestrogen but have been shown to increase the risk of breast cancer in long-term HRT users (Women's Health Initiative, 2002; Million Women Study Collaborators, 2003). Structurally, medroxyprogesterone acetate is more similar to natural progesterone than norethisterone. The metabolism of these two compounds is also different; medroxyprogesterone acetate is the major progestogenic compound rather than one of its metabolites. In contrast, the metabolites of norethisterone exhibit significant activity in addition to a wide range of non-progestogenic actions. Norethisterone also binds to sex hormone–binding globulin, whereas medroxyprogesterone acetate does not.

The most notable difference in steroid receptor-binding affinity between the two synthetic progestogens and endogenous progesterone is that although all the compounds have an affinity for the mineralocorticoid receptor, only the natural compound has antagonist activity. As a consequence, the synthetic compounds may be unable to counteract the sodium-retaining and blood pressure–raising effects of the oestrogens used in HRT. Endogenous progesterone affinity for the glucocorticoid receptor is also different, with medroxyprogesterone acetate a more potent antagonist than norethisterone. This may influence their side-effect profiles and impact on inflammation, immune response, adrenal function and bone metabolism.

Tibolone

Tibolone is a synthetic steroid that has oestrogenic, progestogenic and androgenic effects that alleviate menopausal symptoms without a monthly bleed. The oestrogenic effects are weak and should not promote endometrial hyperplasia, but 10–15% of women on this treatment experience breakthrough bleeding. The drug is given continuously but is not suitable for women within 1 year of menopause or immediately after oestrogen therapy because in such cases, breakthrough bleeding is most likely to occur. The evidence suggests that this drug is protective against osteoporosis, but the long-term cardioprotective effects have been debated because there is some evidence of a lowering of HDL-C and thickening of the intima-media in the carotid arteries; however, an epidemiological study (Savolainen-Peltonen et al., 2016) showed reductions in coronary heart disease (CHD) mortality risk if therapy was initiated before 60 years of age. It should also be withdrawn if signs of thromboembolic disease occur. The androgenic action of tibolone tends to increase libido. It has been reported that tibolone does have fewer breast-related adverse effects than oestrogenic or oestrogenic–progestogenic HRT regimens.

Raloxifene

Raloxifene is a non-steroidal benzothiophene that binds to some oestrogen receptors and belongs to a class of drugs referred to as selective oestrogen receptor modulators (SERMs). These compounds act selectively on some oestrogen receptors to increase bone mineral density and antagonise oestrogen-dependent effects on breast and endometrial tissues in post-menopausal women. However, there is a reported increased risk of thromboembolism, particularly in the first 4 months of use. Raloxifene cannot be used to treat vasomotor symptoms in peri-menopausal women. In fact, it is reported to induce hot flushes. It has little or no stimulatory effect on the uterine endometrium and is not associated with uterine bleeding.

In summary, raloxifene is a compound that selectively stimulates one group of oestrogen receptors and may be considered a curative treatment for osteoporosis and a preventive agent in the development of oestrogen-dependent breast tumours.

Clinical monitoring

Before initiating HRT, a detailed patient history and physical examination are essential to eliminate medical disorders and genital malignancy. Bone mineral densitometry can also be helpful to establish a baseline for subsequent measurements. Blood tests should include serum electrolytes and creatinine, liver function tests, haemoglobin, lipids and a full blood count. Urine analysis should also be performed. The history and findings from the physical examination may indicate other tests. The patient should have undergone routine cervical smear examination and, preferably, mammography. In women with an intact uterus, any irregular vaginal bleeding should be investigated to exclude endometrial pathology.

After starting therapy, the woman should be seen within 3 months in the first instance and then at intervals between 6 and 12 months so that symptoms may be assessed and any side effects of therapy can be reported. Blood pressure measurements are undertaken on these routine visits; HRT is usually associated with a fall in blood pressure due to a vasodilator action of oestrogen. Hypertension is not a contraindication to treatment with HRT but does need treatment before starting on oestrogen therapy. Some women may have an elevated blood pressure on oral oestrogen but show no such effect with the non-oral route. Weight gain may occur some months after treatment has been initiated, and the patient should be advised to reduce calorie intake accordingly.

Stopping HRT

Guidelines in the British National Formulary (Joint Formulary Committee, 2016) indicate that there are a number of signs and symptoms suggesting that women should be advised to immediately stop taking HRT, and these include:
- sudden severe chest pain;
- sudden breathlessness or cough with blood-stained sputum;
- unexplained severe pain in calf of one leg;
- severe stomach pain;
- serious neurological effects;
- hepatitis, jaundice, liver enlargement;
- blood pressure above systolic 160 mmHg and diastolic 100 mmHg;
- detection of a risk factor, for example, prolonged immobility after surgery or leg injury.

Once HRT has been stopped, investigation and treatment should be undertaken as appropriate.

Examples of serious neurological effects include unusual severe, prolonged headache. This is especially important if the headache occurs for the first time or it becomes progressively worse. Marked numbness, especially if it suddenly affects one side or part of the body, is important to note. Other neurological effects are sudden partial or complete loss of vision or disturbance of hearing or other perceptual disorders. HRT should also be stopped if the following occur: dysphasia, bad fainting attack or collapse, a first unexplained epileptic seizure/weakness and motor disturbances.

For women who have elected to stop HRT, gradually reducing the dosage may limit recurrence of symptoms in the short-term.

Treatment with hormone replacement therapy
Vasomotor symptoms

Vasomotor symptoms include hot flushes, headaches, insomnia, giddiness and faintness. They occur in about 70–80% of women and result in physical distress in about 50%, lasting for up to 5 years in around one-quarter of the affected women. Flushes and sweats, particularly night sweats, indicate vasomotor instability and probably result from unoccupied oestrogen receptors on blood vessels. Oestrogens cause a rapid rise in blood flow through the blood vessels, and lack of oestrogen will render the oestrogen receptors in these vessels supersensitive to any subsequent rise in oestrogen level. During the peri-menopause and menopause, oestrogen levels tend to fluctuate, and it is suggested that it is these fluctuations that result in vasomotor symptoms. The extreme sensitivity of blood vessel oestrogen receptors tends to mean that a clinical response to vasomotor symptoms is achieved with low doses of oestrogen. There is also likely to be central control via a supra-pituitary mechanism incorporating several chemical pathways involving serotonin, noradrenaline and dopamine. General advice regarding diet, for example, avoiding certain foods and drinks that cause vasodilation, such as hot and spicy foods and alcohol, may be helpful to some women. There is some evidence that regular exercise, which stimulates the production of hypothalamic β-endorphins, may reduce the risk of hot flushes.

Urogenital tract

In the urogenital tract, symptoms include:
- vaginal dryness and dyspareunia;
- vaginal discharge and bleeding;
- urinary incontinence, urgency of micturition and/or recurrent symptoms of cystitis.

Symptoms result from oestrogen deficiency in menopausal women and may be treated either with systemic HRT preparations or with topical applications of oestrogen incorporated into vaginal creams, pessaries and silicone vaginal rings. Such topical routes of administration do result in some systemic absorption of oestrogen through the vaginal mucosa, and because this may be erratic, vasomotor symptoms could ensue. Exogenous oestrogen stimulates blood flow and epithelial thickening and decreases vaginal pH. These changes result in patients reporting less dyspareunia, as well as less irritation and itching. The dose of oestrogen required to stimulate the oestrogen receptors in the vagina and the lower urethra is about 10 micrograms/day, and the efficiency of such low doses has been demonstrated in a number of clinical trials. Local administration is effective in relieving both short- and long-term problems associated with vaginal atrophy, but symptoms will return on cessation of treatment, and women should be told to report any unexpected vaginal bleeding. However, low-dose local administration is safe and has now been assessed as carrying no increased risk of endometrial hyperplasia, so there is no need to add in a progestogenic agent or perform routine endometrial surveillance. The effect of oestrogen on vaginal symptoms is more marked than its effect on urinary symptoms, but the incidence of urinary sensory dysfunction may be improved.

Ospemifene is a selective oestrogen receptor modulator that appears to have oestrogen agonist or antagonist (a partial agonist) effects depending on tissue type. It is used in the treatment of dyspareunia, a symptom of vulvar and vaginal atrophy, due to menopause. The usual oral dose is 60 mg daily with food (approved by the U.S. Food and Drug Administration [FDA], and now licensed in the UK and EU but not yet launched). It is also under investigation in the management of postmenopausal osteoporosis.

Bone

In a woman not treated with HRT, approximately 15% of bone mass is lost within 10 years of menopause, resulting in an increased incidence of fracture, typically of the hip. Such fractures take up at least 10% of orthopaedic beds, and the total cost in terms of morbidity and mortality is high. The effect of oestrogen lack is to increase osteoclastic bone resorption. There is an overall increase in bone turnover, more bone is resorbed than replaced and there is an associated increase in the rate of bone loss, which may continue for 5–10 years. Oestrogens may exert effects on bone through the calcium-regulating hormones such as calcitonin and parathyroid-regulating hormones. Evidence also exists for the effect of oestrogens on the local production of bone growth factors, cytokines, in particular osteoprotegerin, which blocks osteoclastogenesis, and prostaglandin E_2.

The greatest effect of oestrogen on bone is seen with implants, where an approximately 8% increase in vertebral bone density is seen within 1 year of treatment. Estradiol patches are the next most effective route of administration (Fig. 47.1), whereas oral therapy only achieves an increase in bone density of about 2% per annum. However, 5 years of oral oestrogen therapy will still achieve a lifetime reduction in femoral neck fracture of as much as 50%.

Oestrogen improves the quality and quantity of bone in the post-menopausal woman. It may be started at any time after menopause, and the benefit will continue for the duration of treatment. Therefore, HRT does significantly decrease the risk of fragility fracture, and although protection does decrease when treatment is stopped, it may persist for longer if HRT was used for longer. Raloxifene is licensed for the prevention and treatment of osteoporosis as an alternative to HRT. Raloxifene reduces bone loss and increases bone density at the spine and hip

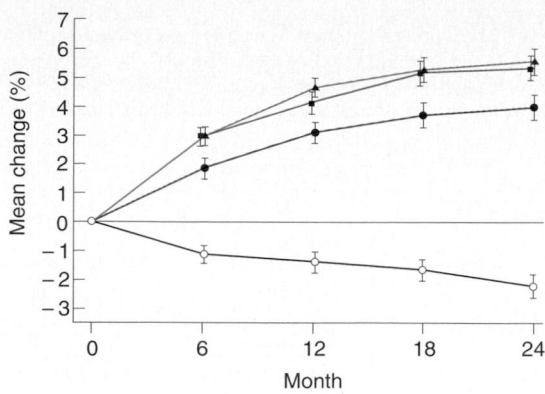

Fig. 47.1 Percentage of change from baseline (mean ± SEM) in lumbar spine bone mineral density in patients receiving placebo (open circles) or transdermal 17β-estradiol 50 micrograms/day (filled circles), 75 micrograms/day (squares) or 100 micrograms/day (filled triangles). (From Delmas et al., 1999.)

in post-menopausal women. With its oestrogen antagonist effect on the breast and endometrium, raloxifene may prove to be an advance over oestrogen treatment in osteoporosis prevention and treatment in post-menopausal women. It does, however, cause hot flushes, which may be unacceptable for some.

Musculoskeletal system

A good body of evidence supports that the decline in muscle mass may be in line with the decrease in oestrogen that characterises the menopausal years. A decrease in muscle strength can play a detrimental role in physical function impairments, such as recovery after imbalance (which in turn could contribute to falls and so fractures). Oestrogen has an anabolic effect on muscle by the stimulation of IGF-1 receptors. The mechanism of this interaction is likely to be complex and could involve gene expression, which is controlled by epigenetic factors, such as DNA methylation, and it is plausible that at least part of the HRT effect is due to changes in the DNA methylation profile. More studies and trials are required to establish a formal relationship, but clinical experience suggests that musculoskeletal symptoms may be improved by HRT.

Cardiovascular system

Coronary heart disease

Women at 45 years are significantly less likely than men to die of coronary heart disease, but by the age of 60 years, the death rate from the disease is similar in both sexes. Oestrogen is probably central to this gender difference because women who experience early loss of endogenous estradiol have an accelerated risk of developing coronary heart disease. Intuitively, it would appear logical that post-menopausal women would gain benefit from receiving exogenous oestrogen. However, there are conflicting views as to whether this is, or is not, the case. Numerous trials have yielded conflicting results and debate around the routes of administration and actual hormone regimens used (particularly

Table 47.3 Estimated impact of hormone replacement therapy formulations and difference in number of breast cancers (per 1000 menopausal women older than 7.5 years, where baseline risk is 22.48 per 1000) using estimations based on randomised control trials or observation

	Current HRT users	Used for more than 5 years	Used for 5 to 10 years	More than 5 years since cessation of HRT
Oestrogen only (RCT)	4 less	No data	No data	5 fewer
Oestrogen only (O)	6 more	4 more	5 more	5 fewer
Combined HRT (RCT)	5 more	No data	No data	8 more
Combined HRT (O)	17 more	12 more	21 more	9 fewer

HRT, Hormone replacement therapy; O, observation; RCT, randomised control trials.
Adapted from NICE (2015).

with respect to the progestogenic component and the androgenicity of this component). The 2015 NICE guidance stressed that all healthcare professionals involved in the care of menopausal women should understand the following:

- HRT does not increase cardiovascular disease risk when started in women aged younger than 60 years.
- HRT does not affect the risk of dying from cardiovascular disease.
- The baseline risk of coronary heart disease and stroke for women around menopausal age varies from one woman to another according to the presence of cardiovascular risk factors.
- HRT with oestrogen alone is associated with no, or reduced, risk of coronary heart disease.
- HRT with oestrogen and progestogen is associated with little or no increase in the risk of coronary heart disease.

Since the NICE (2015) guidance, a large scale (498,105 women with 3.7 million exposure years) epidemiological study focused on the currently popular 'window of opportunity hypothesis' and found that the earlier (<60 years) estradiol-based replacement therapies were started, then the larger the risk reduction of CHD mortality risk; interestingly, the type of progestin (synthetic progestogen) used did not modify the timing effect (Savolainen-Peltonen et al., 2016). It was concluded that timing was important, but the results could not support the window of when or when not to initiate HRT because an increased cardiac mortality risk was not detected when therapy was started in women older than 60 years. Routes of HRT administration are also likely to influence risk factors because transdermal preparations avoid first-pass metabolism. Linked to cardiovascular health, one study found that transdermal but not oral oestrogen replacement therapy significantly reduced the atherogenic index of plasma (Vrablik et al., 2008). This occurred by increasing HDL particle size and therefore improving the antiatherogenic properties.

Venous thromboembolism

It is known that the oestrogen in the combined oral contraceptive pill contributes to thromboembolic disorders, but the dose of oestrogen found in HRT is much lower and more physiological than that in the oral contraceptive pill. All the trials and studies that took into account route of administration of HRT agreed that any increase in risk is attenuated or even obviated with transdermal therapy. Oral oestrogen, in contrast to the transdermal route, undergoes extensive first-pass metabolism. This increases the production of prothrombotic factors in the liver and is associated with a reduction in fibrinogen and factor VII activation, such as von Willebrand's factor and anti-thrombin, and enhanced fibrinolysis. HRT is also associated with increased resistance to activated protein C. Risk disappears after cessation of HRT use. If a woman has had a VTE or has a known thrombophilia such as factor V Leiden mutation, she may still be suitable for HRT but should be referred to a haematologist before commencing therapy.

The SERMs, such as raloxifene, are considered to carry the same risk of thrombosis as oestrogen-containing HRT.

Overall, minimising cardiovascular risk whilst obtaining the benefits of HRT is influenced by the age, body mass index, cardiovascular health and menopausal history of the woman being treated; the timing of initiation of HRT; the formulation of the product used; and polymorphism. Going forward, a better understanding of the non-genomic actions of oestrogen should facilitate the optimisation of therapy by, for example, selectively modulating cardiac non-genomic oestrogen receptor signalling (Knowlton and Korzick, 2014).

Cancer

Details of the estimated influence of HRT on the incidence of cancer are presented in Table 47.3.

Colorectal cancer

Colorectal cancers tend to occur in women older than 50 years, and several studies have indicated that HRT transdermal oestrogen-only therapy may offer more protection than oral, and the benefit appears to be more pronounced with long-term use. The exact mechanism for this protective effect on the colon is unclear, although it has been suggested that oestrogen may decrease the formation of potentially carcinogenic bile acids.

Ovarian cancer

The risk of ovarian cancer is known to be influenced by hormonal events such as the age at menarche and menopause and parity use of exogenous hormones (oral contraceptives and HRT), with a reduced incidence consistently reported in users of oral contraceptives.

A meta-analysis found that risk of ovarian cancer, particularly of the two most common forms, serous and endometrioid tumours, was increased by HRT (Collaborative Group on Epidemiological Studies of Ovarian Cancer, 2015). For example, in women aged 50 who took HRT for 5 years, there was one extra case per 1000 users. This analysis did not take into account formulations or delivery methods. However, a survival benefit relating to epithelial ovarian cancer, particularly in long-term users, has recently been reported in the European Prospective Investigation into Cancer and Nutrition (EPIC) study (Besevic et al., 2015).

Endometrial cancer

Unopposed oestrogen therapy at least doubles the risk of endometrial cancer, but the addition of a progestogen, either in continuous combined or sequential regimens, reduces this risk. Of the two regimens, continuous combined administration is more effective than sequential therapy in reducing the risk of endometrial hyperplasia.

Breast cancer

Breast cancer is the most common cancer in women worldwide, and globally, it is the principal cause of cancer death among women. Over the past 20 years, there has been a growing body of evidence to suggest that progesterone contributes to the development of breast cancer. Evidence to support this came from trials in which the use of combined regimens increased breast cancer risk more than oestrogen alone. This is thought to have occurred because the synthetic progestogens possessed some non-progesterone-like effects that potentiated the proliferating action of oestrogen. In the USA, the most commonly used progestogen in HRT is medroxyprogesterone acetate combined with conjugated equine oestrogen and administered orally. In contrast, in Central and Southern Europe, a wider range of progestogens is used, particularly the 19-nortestosterone derivatives. Studies investigating the use of natural micronised progesterone to improve bioavailability in HRT regimens have demonstrated no increased risk of breast cancer. In vitro studies with medroxyprogesterone have found that it promotes the reproductive transformation of estrone into estradiol by influencing the activity of 17β-hydroxysteroid dehydrogenase. The properties of the synthetic progestogens are outlined in Table 47.4.

The relationship between different HRT regimens and breast cancer is complex (Table 47.4). There are many potential confounders to be considered when interpreting trial data, for example, time of initiation of therapy in relation to menopausal status, body mass index and prior hormone use, among others. Chlebowski et al. (2009) reported on the decline in breast cancer in the USA after a reduction in HRT usage following publication of the 2002 WHI trial. This prompted a response from the president of the International Menopause Society (Sturdee, 2009), summarised as follows: Decline in breast cancer rates started at

Table 47.4 Properties of progestogens and their link to breast cancer

Progestogen	Action
19-Nortestosterone derivatives, medroxyprogesterone acetate	Oestrogenic activity Influence on 17β-hydroxysteroid dehydrogenase
19-Nortestosterone derivatives, medroxyprogesterone acetate	Metabolic effects, opposing those of oestrogen, on insulin sensitivity Hepatic effects, opposing those of oestrogen, i.e. increasing insulin-like growth factor-1; decrease in sex hormone-binding globulin
19-Nortestosterone derivatives	Binding to sex hormone–binding globulin with consequent reduction in capacity to bind oestrogen

Adapted from Campagnoli et al. (2005).

least 3 years before the WHI study was halted (which led to a dramatic drop in HRT use). This implies that decline in breast cancer rates must be independent of the reduction in HRT use.

Breast cancer takes years to develop and at least a decade to reach the detectable stage. If HRT use causes breast cancer, then the drop in breast cancer rates would not be seen for some time. The drop in breast cancer rates could be due to other factors, for example, changes in screening.

Notwithstanding these arguments, the problem on what to advise women contemplating HRT can be problematic, and the NICE (2015) guidance states the following:
- The baseline risk of breast cancer for women around menopausal age varies from one woman to another according to the presence of underlying risk factors.
- HRT with oestrogen alone is associated with little or no change in the risk of breast cancer.
- HRT with oestrogen and progestogen can be associated with an increase in the risk of breast cancer.
- Any increase in the risk of breast cancer is related to treatment duration and reduces after stopping HRT.

Psychological symptoms

Psychological symptoms include:
- depression;
- mood changes and irritability, which may also be associated with other life changes occurring at this time;
- exhaustion;
- poor concentration and memory;
- panic attacks;
- lowered libido, which may be exacerbated by the other symptoms together with dyspareunia linked to lack of oestrogen and falling androgen levels.

The role of HRT in this area has not been clearly defined, although in several studies, surgical menopause has been associated with depression, indicating a correlation with oestrogen lack. Many women experience psychological symptoms around menopause, and although these may be associated with oestrogen deficiency, they may also result from the changes in family life that often occur around this time. The disturbance of sleep pattern and sleep deprivation associated with menopause are likely to contribute to the psychological symptoms. Many women find that treatment with estradiol restores normal sleep, and psychological problems are then reduced. Some of the mood changes will respond to counselling and psychotropic drugs. Treatment with oestrogens at high doses (patches of 100 micrograms or implants of 50 mg) has also been shown to improve depression scores. If a progestogen is added to the regimen, then the results are less predictable because progestogen use is related to mood changes, particularly in women who have previously suffered from the pre-menstrual syndrome. Age negatively influences almost all sexual function domains in a significant manner.

HRT improves some aspects of sexual function during menopause, but it does not appear to improve the domains of desire and arousal. The lowered libido experienced during menopause is associated with reduced levels of circulating androgen resulting from ovarian failure. It has been demonstrated that subcutaneous implants of testosterone, 100 mg every 6 months, will increase the libido in a high proportion of patients, but implants are no longer available in the UK (withdrawn of the grounds of a lack of global profitability). Topical testosterone could be used, but it would be an off-label usage.

Central nervous system

The relationship between oestrogen and neurodegenerative conditions, in particular, Alzheimer's disease (Mulnard et al., 2000), has received attention in the light of an observation that there is an increased incidence of the disease in older women. The development of plaques of amyloid-β, a protein that disrupts nerve cell connections in the brain, occurs more rapidly in the absence of oestrogen. This effect of amyloid-β production results in the symptoms of short-term memory loss and disorientation that occur in Alzheimer's disease (AD). Further studies are essential to clarify the relationship between HRT and Alzheimer's disease. There is some evidence that heavier women, who have higher free estradiol levels, exhibit better cognitive function in several domains. Such women may also have a greater clinical response when using exogenous oestrogen. It should also be noted that conjugated equine oestrogen is composed primarily of oestrone sulphate, and this oestrogen has a much lower affinity for oestrogen receptors than oestradiol. Hence, the findings with respect to exogenous oestrogen and neurological function remain equivocal. The length of oestrogen deprivation before supplementation is also important because early administration of oestrogen for a period of several years may yet be found to be beneficial. Evidence is emerging that the progestogenic component in combined HRT is important, and medroxyprogesterone acetate usage has been associated with negative cognitive outcomes. The potential of SERMs as neuroprotectants has been evaluated in a breast cancer prevention trial which compared tamoxifen with raloxifene (Yaffe et al., 2001). Both agents were found to have similar effects on cognition. Work is also ongoing to develop the so-called neuro-SERMs, designed to provide the neurological benefits of estradiol. It is possible that HRT may

have a neuroprotective effect under certain circumstances in some women, and neuroimaging, for example, using Pittsburgh compound B (PiB; a fluorescent agent) positron emission tomography (PET) scanning, may reveal effects not detectable using cognitive testing. A recent trial using this technique has shown that transdermal 17β-estradiol (used for 4 years) resulted in lower amyloid-β deposition, and this was not seen in women using oral conjugated equine oestrogens. Interpreting trial data has been difficult in this area because it is difficult to control for situational effects such as pre-existing pathologies and genetic polymorphisms (Kantarci et al., 2016).

Alternatives to hormone replacement therapy

HRT (particularly transdermal) remains the most effective treatment for vasomotor symptoms, resulting in 80–90% reduction in hot flushes. Of the non-hormonal agents, serotonin–norepinephrine reuptake inhibitors (SNRIs) such as venlafaxine and its active metabolite desvenlafaxine appear to be useful treatments; clonidine is modestly effective in reducing hot flushes, but these agents are not considered as first-line therapies. In addition, there is limited evidence to support the use of selective serotonin reuptake inhibitors (SSRIs) for anxiety, and they do not appear to improve mood in women who are not clinically depressed. Cognitive behavioral therapy (CBT) may improve mood. CBT, isoflavones and black cohosh may help decrease anxiety. Generally, there is a lack of safety information and high-quality trial data regarding alternative therapies. The same is also true of Chinese medicines. Trials with black cohosh, red clover and soy foods, all of which contain phytoestrogens, have yielded conflicting results and have raised concerns about hepatotoxicity (black cohosh) and interactions with anticoagulants (red clover). An umbrella review by Goldstein et al. (2016) is under way to consider nonpharmacologic management of vasomotor symptoms.

Bisphosphonates such as alendronate, etidronate and risedronate are inhibitors of bone resorption and increase bone mineral density by altering osteoclast activation and function. Bisphosphonates are used with care in women with upper gastro-intestinal problems, and their posology is complex. They are contraindicated in patients with hypocalcaemia. Etidronate is also contraindicated in patients with severe renal impairment. For further information, see NICE technology appraisal guidance TA160, which was updated in 2011 (NICE, 2011). This guidance also includes strontium ranelate, which should only be used for severe osteoporosis because it carries a risk of serious cardiovascular side effects.

Teriparatide, a recombinant human parathyroid hormone, is licensed to treat osteoporosis in post-menopausal women. It stimulates formation of new bone and may increase resistance to fracture. However, it has several contraindications, including hypercalcaemia, severe renal impairment, metabolic bone diseases and unexplained elevations of alkaline phosphatase.

Advances in bone biology may lead to the design of more elegant therapies to deal with osteoporosis. An example would be denosumab, a human monoclonal antibody that binds to the receptor activator of nuclear factor-κβ ligand (RANKL), which is responsible for osteoclast differentiation, activation and survival. Denosumab therefore mimics the function of osteoprotegerin, limiting bone resorption, and is currently used to treat osteoporosis and in the prevention of skeletal-related events in patients suffering from bone metastases due to solid tumours. However, preclinical experiments suggest that the RANKL/RANK pathway plays an important role in primary breast cancer development. Therefore, manipulation of the RANK/RANKL system could serve as a potential target for prevention and treatment of breast cancer.

Some small studies have shown that aerobic exercise can improve cardiovascular parameters and reduce menopausal symptoms in addition to reducing BMI.

Case studies

Case 47.1

A 50-year-old patient, Mrs GY, has been on cyclical combined hormone replacement therapy for 6 months for troublesome hot flushes. Her periods were irregular before starting HRT. The hot flushes have resolved with this treatment, and the withdrawal bleeds are acceptable, but Mrs GY is struggling with the progestogenic side effects. A friend has told her to ask for the 'no-bleed' HRT because she thought this might suit her better.

Questions

1. What is the problem with considering a no-bleed preparation?
2. What other options could you suggest?

Answers

1. No-bleed preparations include continuous combined HRT and tibolone. If these are used in women before they become truly menopausal (rather than just peri-menopausal), they are associated with significant problems of unscheduled bleeding because the dose of hormone in the preparation is insufficient to override any residual ovarian activity. In women who start on HRT while still peri-menopausal, it can be difficult to know when they are truly menopausal. The recommendation therefore is that women should not take continuous combined HRT or tibolone until they are at least 12 months from their last menstrual period or are 54 years of age (when it is estimated that 80% of women will be post-menopausal).
2. Two options could be considered. Tridestra could be used. This is a preparation in which a 14-day course of combined estradiol valerate and medroxyprogesterone acetate is taken after a 70-day course of estradiol valerate. Seven days of inactive tablets follow during which Mrs GY would be expected to have a withdrawal bleed. This means that Mrs GY would only experience a bleed every 3 months rather than monthly. The other option would be to consider using the levonorgestrel IUS as the progestogen component of HRT together with either an oral or transdermal oestrogen preparation. This has the advantage of very few progestogenic side effects and the possibility that Mrs GY will be rendered amenorrhoeic. If the levonorgestrel IUS is used, it should be replaced after 4 years rather than the usual 5 years when used for contraception or as a treatment for menorrhagia.

Case 47.2

A 53-year-old woman, Ms DR, who had a hysterectomy and a bilateral salpingo-oophorectomy for menstrual problems about 6 months ago, has now requested advice about HRT. She had previously refused HRT because she was particularly concerned about the associated cardiovascular risks, but Ms DR has recently found an article that said HRT may actually be safe.

Questions

1. What are the current recommendations relating to HRT and cardiovascular disease?
2. What would be a good HRT regimen for Ms DR?

Answers

1. Reassure Ms DR that the data show that HRT does not increase cardiovascular risk when it is initiated in those younger than 60 years. There is some evidence that there may be an increased risk of stroke (but not haemorrhagic) in menopause, but this is influenced by the preparation, with transdermal regimens carrying less risk than oral dosage forms. It is worth pointing out that recent studies have looked at the administration of HRT in younger women who have started HRT at or around menopause. More recent analyses show that HRT does not affect the risk of dying from cardiovascular disease. The opportunity should be taken to counsel the patient about general risk factors and cardiovascular health. Ms DR should be reassured that her blood pressure will be monitored regularly whilst she is using HRT and be advised of when HRT should be stopped pending further investigations (e.g. unexplained severe pain in the calf of one leg).
2. A suitable regimen for this patient need not contain a progestogen because Ms DR had a hysterectomy and therefore has no endometrium to protect from unopposed oestrogen therapy. Recent data suggest that oestrogen-only treatments are associated with no risk, or reduced risk, of coronary heart disease. She should also be advised that transdermal preparations such as Evorel have less impact on the risk of stroke than oral preparations.

Case 47.3

Ms EC, a 43-year-old woman, was started on cyclical HRT at the age of 37 when she was diagnosed with an early menopause after a 15-month period of amenorrhoea. She has no significant menopausal symptoms and regular light withdrawal bleeds. However, Ms EC has read that HRT should only be continued for 5 years and thinks she might stop HRT now.

Questions

1. Why should Ms EC be advised to continue HRT until the age of 50?
2. What advice would you give Ms EC regarding the dose and type of HRT?

Answers

1. Once a woman enters menopause, the fall in oestrogen levels increases the risk of cardiovascular disease and also increases bone loss, causing a greater risk of osteoporotic fractures. The earlier the menopause, the greater the risk. Concern about breast cancer rates rising with increased HRT was derived from data in women older

than the average age of the natural menopause, that is, in their 50s, 60s and 70s. Therefore, it should not be extrapolated to women who have undergone early menopause. Women with an early menopause should be advised that any increase in the breast cancer risk only becomes important once HRT use continues beyond age 50 years. In addition, the benefits of continuing HRT up to the age of 50 years in terms of cardiovascular and bone health are significant.

2. The current advice is that the lowest dose of HRT to control menopausal symptoms should be used. This can result in the dose of HRT falling below the bone-protective dose, and therefore a risk assessment for osteoporosis should be undertaken. This should

include assessing lifestyle (dietary calcium, weight, weight-bearing exercise, etc.) in addition to a bone densitometry scan. Ms EC may wish to consider treatment with levonorgestrel IUS and oral or transdermal oestrogen because there may be a reduction in breast cancer risk associated with this combination when compared with standard cyclical HRT. This is because of limited systemic progestogen absorption. Ms EC's cardiovascular well-being should be assessed, for example, family history, body mass index, blood pressure, lipids and aerobic exercise, and improved where possible. This would be especially important if, following discussion of the risks and benefits, she still decided to stop HRT.

References

Besevic, J., Gunter, M.J., Fortner, R.T., et al., 2015. Reproductive factors and epithelial ovarian cancer survival in the EPIC cohort study. Br. J. Cancer. 113, 1622–1631.

British Menopause Society, 2016. Summary consensus statement hormone replacement therapy. Available at: https://thebms.org.uk/publications/clinical-statements/consensus-statements/hormone-replacement-therapy/.

Campagnoli, C., Abbà, C., Ambroggio, S., et al., 2005. Pregnancy, progesterone and progestins in relation to breast cancer risk. J. Steroid Biochem. Mol. Biol. 97, 441–450.

Chlebowski, R.T., Kuller, L.H., Prentice, R.L., et al., 2009. Breast cancer after use of estrogen plus progestin in postmenopausal women. N. Engl. J. Med. 360, 573–587.

Coker, L.H., Espeland, M.A., Rapp, S.R., et al., 2010. Postmenopausal hormone therapy and cognitive outcomes: the Women's Health Initiative Memory Study (WHIMS). J. Steroid Biochem. Mol. Biol. 118, 304–310.

Collaborative Group on Epidemiological Studies of Ovarian Cancer, 2015. Menopausal hormone use and ovarian cancer risk: individual participant meta-analysis of 52 epidemiological studies. Lancet 385, 1835–1842.

Cooper, C., 1997. The crippling consequences of fractures and their impact on quality of life. Am. J. Med. 103 (2A), 12S–17S.

de Villier, T.J., Hall, J.E., Pinkerton, J.V., et al., 2016. Revised global consensus statement on menopausal hormone therapy. Climacteric. Available at: https://doi.org/10.1080/13697137.2016.1196047.

Delmas, P.D., Pornel, B., Felsenberg, D., et al., 1999. A dose-ranging trial of a matrix transdermal 17β-estradiol for the prevention of bone loss in early postmenopausal women. Bone 24, 517–523.

Goldstein, K.M., McDuffie, J.R., Shepherd-Banigan, M., et al., 2016. Nonpharmacologic, nonherbal management of menopause-associated vasomotor symptoms: an umbrella systematic review (protocol). Syst. Rev. 5, 56. https://doi.org/10.1186/s13643-016-0232-6.

Hall, G., Phillips, T.J., 2005. Oestrogen and skin: the effects of estrogen, menopause, and hormone replacement therapy on the skin. J. Am. Acad. Dermatol. 53, 555–568.

Hogervorst, E., Bandelow, S., 2010. Sex steroids to maintain cognitive function in women after the menopause: a meta-analyses of treatment trials. Maturitas 66, 56–71.

Hogervorst, E., Henderson, V.W., Gibbs, R.B., et al. (Eds.), 2009. Hormones, Cognition and Dementia: State of the Art and Emergent Therapeutic Strategies. Cambridge University Press, Cambridge.

Joint Formulary Committee, 2016. British National Formulary 71. BMJ Group and Pharmaceutical Press, London.

Kanis, J.A., Johnell, O., Oden, A., et al., 2000. Long-term risk of osteoporotic fracture in Malmo. Osteoporos. Int. 11, 669–674.

Kantarci, K., Lowe, V.J., Lesnick, T.G., et al., 2016. Early postmenopausal transdermal 17β-estradiol therapy and amyloid-β deposition. J. Alzheimer's Dis. 53 (2), 547–556.

Knowlton, A.A., Korzick, D.H., 2014. Estrogen and the female heart. Mol. Cell. Endocrinol. 389, 31–30.

Million Women Study Collaborators, 2003. Breast cancer and hormone-replacement therapy in the Million Women Study. Lancet 362, 419–427.

Mulnard, R.A., Cotman, C.W., Kawas, C., et al., 2000. Oestrogen replacement therapy for treatment of mild to moderate Alzheimer disease. JAMA 283, 1007–1015.

National Institute of Health and Care Excellence (NICE), 2011. Alendronate, etidronate, risedronate, raloxifene and strontium ranelate for the primary prevention of osteoporotic fragility fractures in postmenopausal women. NICE technology appraisal guidance [TA160]. Available at: https://www.nice.org.uk/guidance/ta160.

National Institute of Health and Care Excellence (NICE), 2015. Menopause: diagnosis and management NICE guidelines [NG23]. Available at: https://www.nice.org.uk/guidance/ng23.

Prossnitz, E.R., Barton, M., 2014. Estrogen biology: New insights into GPER function and clinical opportunities. Mol. Cell. Endocrinol. 389, 71–83.

Savolainen Peltonen, H., Tuomikoski, P., Korhonen, P., et al., 2016. Cardiac death risk in relation to the age at initiation or the progestin component of hormone therapies. J. Clin. Endocrinol. Metab. 101 (7), 2794–2801.

Sturdee, D., 2009. President of the International Menopause Society commenting on 'NEJM article on breast cancer and HRT – comment by International Menopause Society'. Available at: http://www.imsociety.org/pages/comments_and_press_statements/ims_press_statement_04_02_09.php.

Vrablik, M., Fait, T., Kovar, J., et al., 2008. Oral but not transdermal estrogen replacement therapy changes the composition of plasma lipoproteins. Metab. Clin. Exp. 57, 1088–1092.

Women's Health Initiative, 2002. Risks and benefits of oestrogen plus progestin in healthy postmenopausal women: principal results from the Women's Health Initiative randomized controlled trial. JAMA 288 (3), 321–333.

Yaffe, K., Krueger, K., Sarkar, S., et al., 2001. Cognitive function in postmenopausal women treated with raloxifene. N. Engl. J. Med. 344, 1207–1213.

Further reading

Bahl, A., Öllänen, E., Ismail, K., et al., 2015. Hormone replacement therapy associated white blood cell DNA methylation and gene expression are associated with within-pair differences of body adiposity and bone mass. Twin. Res. Hum. Genet. 18 (6), 647–661.

Birrer, N., Chinchilla, C., Del Carmen, M., et al., 2016. Is hormone replacement therapy safe in women with a BRCA mutation? A systematic review of the contemporary literature. Am. J. Clin. Oncol. https://doi.org/10.1097/COC.0000000000000269.

Cosman, F., de Beur, S.J., LeBoff, M.S., et al., 2014. Clinician's guide to prevention and treatment of osteoporosis. Osteoporos. Int. 25 (10), 2359–2381.

deGuevara, N.M.L., Galván, C.D.T., Sanchez, A.C., et al., 2016. Benefits of physical exercise in postmenopausal women. Maturitas 93, 83–88.

Gallagher, J.C., 2008. Advances in bone biology and new treatments for bone loss. Maturitas 60, 65–69.

International Menopause Consensus Statement Working Group, 2009. Aging, menopause, cardiovascular disease and HRT. Climacteric 12, 368–377.

Karki, P., Smith, K., Johnson, J., et al., 2014. Astrocyte-derived growth factors and estrogen neuroprotection: role of transforming growth factor-a in estrogen-induced upregulation of glutamate transporters in astrocytes. Mol. Cell. Endocrinol. 389, 58–64.

Kiesel, L., Kohl, A., 2016. Role of the RANK/RANKL pathway in breast cancer. Maturitas 86, 10–16.

Mørch, L.S., Lidegaard, Ø., Keiding, N., et al., 2016. The influence of hormone therapies on colon and rectal cancer. Eur. J. Epidemiol. 31 (5), 481–489.

O'Donnell, S., Cranney, A., Wells, G.A., et al., 2006. Strontium ranelate for preventing and treating postmenopausal osteoporosis. Cochrane Database Syst. Rev. 2006 (4), Art. No. CD005326. https://doi.org/10.1002/14651858.CD005326.pub3.

Pisani, P., Renna, M.D., Conversano, F., et al., 2016. Major osteoporotic fragility fractures: Risk factor updates and societal impact. World J. Orthop. 7 (3), 171–181.

Raz, L., 2014. Estrogen and cerebrovascular regulation in menopause. Mol. Cell. Endocrinol. 389 (1–2), 22–30.

Scott, E.L., Zhang, Q.-G., Vadlamudi, R.K., et al., 2014. Premature menopause and risk of neurological disease: basic mechanisms and clinical implications. Mol. Cell. Endocrinol. 389, 2–6.

Stuenkel, C.A., Davis, S.R., Gompel, A., 2015. Treatment of symptoms of the menopause: an Endocrine Society clinical practice guideline. J. Clin. Endocrinol. Metab. 100 (11), 3975–4011.

Tzur, Y., Yohai, D., Weintraub, A.Y., 2016. The role of local estrogen therapy in the management of pelvic floor disorders. Climacteric 19, 162–171.

Zhu, X., Liew, Y., Liu, Z.L., 2016. Chinese herbal medicine for menopausal symptoms. Cochrane Database Syst. Rev. 2016 (3), Art. No. CD009023. https://doi.org/10.1002/14651858.CD009023.pub2.

48 Drugs in Pregnancy and Lactation

Paula Russell, Laura Yates, Peter Golightly and Sarah Fenner

Key points

Drugs in pregnancy

- Assess risk/benefit ratio for the mother–fetus pair.
- Avoid non-essential drugs.
- Where drug treatment is clinically indicated, select an effective agent with the best safety profile.
- Use the lowest effective dose for the shortest possible time.
- Provide timely and accurate counselling to help avoid unfounded maternal fears about drug safety that may otherwise result in non-adherence with drug therapy or unnecessary pregnancy termination.
- Teratogenic risks of a drug may vary with each trimester of exposure.
- Drug exposure in the second and third trimesters may also result in fetal harm.

Drugs in lactation

- Avoid unnecessary use of drugs.
- Maternal therapy only rarely constitutes a reason to avoid breastfeeding.
- Assess the risk/benefit ratio for both mother and infant.
- Monitor the infant for unusual signs or symptoms.
- Avoid use of new drugs if there is a therapeutic equivalent for which data on use in lactation are available.

Drugs in pregnancy

The use of both prescription and over-the-counter drugs in pregnancy presents a number of challenges to those asked to provide advice to women either pre-conceptually or during pregnancy. This is in part due to the fact that no two cases are the same, and that each enquiry ideally requires an individual risk assessment that takes into account what is known about the drug and its effects on the developing fetus, as well as the woman's personal medical and family history. It is now well recognised that most medicines and/or their metabolites readily cross the placenta, and that some are teratogenic, resulting in harm to the fetus. Robust scientific human data on the effects of many drugs, particularly newer preparations, are, however, frequently lacking.

It is therefore generally accepted that maternal pharmacotherapy should be avoided if not necessary, or minimised where the maternal condition allows. Nevertheless, it has been estimated that more than 80% of expectant mothers take three or four drugs at some stage of pregnancy (Headley et al., 2004), with a significant number of women taking medication at the time their pregnancy is detected. Indications for drug use range from chronic illnesses, such as epilepsy and depression, to those commonly associated with pregnancy, such as nausea and vomiting and urinary tract infections.

Approximately 2–3% of all live births are associated with a congenital anomaly. Although exogenous factors such as drugs may account for only 1–5% of these (affecting <0.2% of all live births), given that drug-associated malformations are largely preventable, they remain an important consideration.

Drugs as teratogens

A teratogen is defined as any agent that results in structural or functional abnormalities in the fetus, or in the child after birth, as a consequence of maternal exposure during pregnancy. Examples of drugs that are known to be human teratogens are listed in Box 48.1. The teratogenic mechanism for most drugs remains unclear but may be due to the direct effects of the drug on the fetus and/or as a consequence of indirect physiological changes in the mother or fetus. Perhaps the best known and most widely studied teratogen is thalidomide, a mild sedative that was widely marketed as a remedy for pregnancy-related nausea and vomiting. In 1961 thalidomide was withdrawn from the UK market after numerous reports of severe anatomical birth defects in infants of mothers who took the drug in early pregnancy. Whereas external congenital anomalies such as limb abnormalities, spina bifida and hydrocephalus may be obvious at birth, some defects may take many years to manifest clinically or be identified. Examples of delayed effects of teratogens are the behavioural and neurodevelopmental disorders associated with in utero sodium valproate exposure and the development of clear-cell vaginal cancer in young women after maternal intake of diethylstilboestrol, used first in the 1930s for the prevention of miscarriage and preterm delivery (Herbst et al., 1971).

Critical periods in human fetal development

The human gestation period is approximately 40 weeks from the first day of the last menstrual period (38 weeks post-conception) and is conventionally divided into the first, second and third trimesters, each lasting 3 calendar months. Another method

Box 48.1   Examples of drugs considered to be human teratogens

Angiotensin-converting enzyme inhibitors
Androgens
Carbamazepine
Carbimazole
Cytotoxics (some)
Danazol
Diethylstilboestrol
Ethanol
Lithium
Methotrexate
Misoprostol
Mycophenolate mofetil
Tetracyclines
Thalidomide
Valproic acid
Vitamin A and derivatives, e.g. isotretinoin
Warfarin

for classifying the stage of pregnancy is according to the stage of embryo-fetal development. This is a more useful approach when assessing the potential risks associated with drug use in pregnancy.

Pre-embryonic stage: weeks 0–2 post-conception

The first 2 weeks post-conception are regarded as the pre-embryonic stage and describe the period up to implantation of the fertilised ovum. Teratogenic exposure during the pre-embryonic stage, sometimes referred to as the 'all-or-nothing' period, is thought to carry a low risk of fetal harm, with most exposures leading either to death of the embryo or complete recovery and normal development of the fetus. Fetal malformations after drug exposure during this period are therefore thought to be unlikely, but robust scientific data to support a low risk of adverse fetal outcome are lacking. Risk to the fetus may also be increased where the half-life of the drug is sufficient to extend exposure into the embryonic stage. A good example of the latter is isotretinoin and related vitamin A derivatives that have half-lives up to a week, and which when used systemically, for example, for the treatment of acne and psoriasis, are recognised teratogens (Nulman et al., 1998).

Embryonic stage: weeks 3–8 post-conception

Organogenesis occurs predominantly during the embryonic stage and, with the exception of the central nervous system (CNS), eyes, teeth, external genitalia and ears, is complete by the end of the 10th week of pregnancy. Exposure to drugs during this critical period therefore represents the greatest risk of major birth defects. For this reason, women are often advised to avoid or minimise all drug use in the first trimester whenever possible. It is important to bear in mind, however, that very few drugs are in fact proven teratogens, and that exposure in the second and third trimesters may still result in fetal harm.

Fetal stage: weeks 9–38 post-conception

During the fetal stage, the fetus continues to develop, grow and mature and, importantly, remains susceptible to some drug effects. This is especially true for the CNS, which can be damaged by exposure to certain drugs, for example, ethanol, at any stage of pregnancy. The external genitalia also continue to form from the seventh week until term; consequently, danazol, which has weak androgenic properties, can cause virilisation of a female fetus if given in any trimester after the eighth week of pregnancy when the androgen receptors begin to form (Rosa, 1984).

Further examples include the angiotensin-converting enzyme inhibitors, which if given in the second and third trimesters can result in fetal renal dysfunction and subsequent oligohydramnios, that is, reduced amniotic fluid volume (Sedman et al., 1995). The non-steroidal anti-inflammatory drugs (NSAIDs) are another important group of drugs that may cause problems, specifically in the third trimester. These drugs inhibit prostaglandin synthesis in a dose-related fashion and, when given late in pregnancy, may result in premature closure of the fetal ductus arteriosus and fetal renal impairment (Koren et al., 2006). NSAIDs should therefore be avoided during the third trimester.

Principles of teratogenesis

In 1959 James Wilson, co-founder of The Teratology Society, proposed several principles of teratogenesis that have since been expanded and modified but remain fundamental in assessing whether a drug or chemical exposure during pregnancy is likely to be associated with reproductive or developmental toxicity. A basic understanding of these factors is essential to both the interpretation of preclinical (animal) reproductive toxicity studies and to enable accurate risk assessment in clinical practice. A subset of Wilson's principles is discussed as follows.

Timing of exposure

The stage of pregnancy at which a drug exposure occurs is key to determining the likelihood, severity or nature of any adverse effect on the fetus. Risk both between and within trimesters may be variable. For example, folic acid antagonists such as trimethoprim have been associated with an increased risk of neural tube defects if exposure occurs before neural tube closure (third to fourth week post-conception), but not after this period (Hernandez-Diaz et al., 2001). It has also been suggested that trimethoprim should be avoided after 32 weeks' gestation in view of the theoretical risk of severe jaundice in the neonate as a result of bilirubin displacement from protein binding, although clinical evidence to support this is lacking (Dunn, 1964). Unfortunately, the precise period of teratogenic risk is known for very few substances. One drug for which this period has been established is thalidomide, where exposure between days 20 and 36 post-conception is associated with a high risk of congenital malformation (Lenz, 1988; Newman, 1986).

Drug dose

A threshold dose above which drug-induced malformations or other adverse effects are more likely to occur has now been demonstrated for certain teratogenic compounds, although for most a 'safe dose' has not been conclusively determined. The likelihood of a dose relationship underlies the recommendation to use the lowest effective dose in pregnancy. For this reason more frequent monitoring of drug levels may be recommended for certain drugs during pregnancy.

Species

Teratogenicity of a drug may be species dependent. Interestingly, preclinical thalidomide studies in mice and rats did not result in congenital malformation in the offspring (Breitkreutz and Anderson, 2008; Miller et al., 2009; Vorhees et al., 2001). Birth defects or other adverse reproductive outcomes observed in animal studies cannot therefore be simply extrapolated to the human situation. Further, the drug dose and route of administration used in early animal studies may not be comparable with clinical use in humans.

Genotype and environmental interaction

Not all fetuses exposed to known teratogenic drugs show evidence of having been affected in utero. It remains undetermined whether this variable susceptibility to teratogenic drugs is a result of genetic differences in the exposed mothers, the fetal genotype, modifying environmental factors or a combination of all three. Malformations are reported to occur in only 20–50% of infants born to mothers exposed to thalidomide during the period of greatest risk of embryopathy, that is, days 20–36 post-fertilisation (Lenz, 1966; Newman, 1985). Similarly, maternal treatment with systemic isotretinoin during the first trimester results in fetal malformation in only 18–35% of the live born infants, with a further 30% of children exhibiting developmental delay in the absence of physical deformity (Benke, 1984; Braun et al., 1984; Hill, 1984).

Pharmacological effect

Pharmacological effects on the fetus are by far the most common drug effects during pregnancy, and the consequences are often minor and reversible compared with the idiosyncratic effects that can lead to major irreversible anomalies. Pharmacological effects are usually dose related and to some extent predictable. Drugs may adversely affect the fetus via effects on the maternal circulation, or they may cross the placenta and exert a direct pharmacological effect on the fetus. Equally, drugs are sometimes administered to pregnant women to treat fetal disorders; for example, flecainide has been used to resolve fetal tachycardia.

The neonate can also be adversely affected by maternal drug therapy (Table 48.1). It is generally only at birth that signs of fetal distress are observed due to in utero drug exposure or the effects of abrupt discontinuation of the maternal drug supply.

Table 48.1 Examples of drugs with pharmacological effects on the fetus or neonate

Drug	Possible adverse pharmacological effect	Notes
Angiotensin-converting enzyme inhibitors	Fetal and neonatal hypoxia, hypotension, renal dysfunction, oligohydramnios and intra-uterine growth retardation	Monitor fetus if long-term therapy in the second or third trimester
β-Blockers, e.g. atenolol	Neonatal bradycardia, hypotension and hyperglycaemia	Neonatal symptoms are usually mild and improve within 48 h; no long-term effects
Benzodiazepines	'Floppy infant syndrome' Withdrawal reactions	Risk if regular use in third trimester Neonatal observation recommended
Corticosteroid (high dose)	Fetal adrenal suppression	Dependent on dose and treatment interval
Non-steroidal anti-inflammatory drugs	Premature closure of the ductus arteriosus (affecting fetal circulation) and fetal renal impairment (decreased urine output)	Avoid repeated use after week 28; if unavoidable, fetal circulation monitored regularly
Opioids	Neonatal withdrawal symptoms Respiratory depression	Risk if used long-term Risk if used near term
Phenothiazines	Neonatal withdrawal and transient extrapyramidal symptoms	Observation for at least 48 h; symptoms may last for several weeks
Tricyclic and selective serotonin reuptake inhibitor antidepressants	Neonatal withdrawal symptoms	Risk if used long-term and/or near term; observation for at least 48 h

Adapted from Schaefer et al. (2014).

The capacity of the neonate to eliminate drugs is reduced, and this can result in significant accumulation of some drugs, leading to toxicity. Neonatal withdrawal effects may require treatment.

Idiosyncratic drug effects in the fetus and neonate are possible but occur rarely compared with pharmacological effects.

Maternal pharmacokinetic changes

Physiological changes in pregnancy induce profound changes to the pharmacokinetic properties of many drugs. These changes,

Table 48.2 Summary of pharmacokinetic changes during pregnancy

	Change during pregnancy
Absorption	
Gastro-intestinal motility	↓
Lung function	↑
Skin blood circulation	↑
Distribution	
Plasma volume	↑
Body water	↑
Plasma protein	↓
Fat deposition	↑
Metabolism	
Liver activity	↑↓
Excretion	
Glomerular filtration	↑
Renal tubule secretion	↑

Adapted from Schaefer et al. (2014).

summarised in Table 48.2, affect absorption, distribution, metabolism, and excretion of drugs, and may also affect their pharmacodynamic properties. Some of the changes that occur in maternal organ systems are secondary to pregnancy-induced hormonal changes, whereas others occur to support the pregnant woman and the developing fetus.

Absorption

Gastric and intestinal emptying time increases by 30–40% in the second and third trimesters (Pavek et al., 2009) and could be important in delaying absorption and time to onset of action for some drugs (Loebstein et al., 1997). There is also a reduction in gastric acid secretion in the first and second trimesters, and an increase in mucous secretion. As a consequence of the increase in gastric pH, the ionisation, and hence absorption, of weak acids and bases can be affected.

Cardiac output and respiratory volume increase during pregnancy, leading to hyperventilation and increased pulmonary blood perfusion. These changes cause higher pulmonary absorption of anaesthetics, bronchodilators, pollutants, cigarette smoke and other volatile drugs.

Distribution

The volume of distribution of drugs may be altered because of an increase of up to 50% in blood (plasma) volume and a 30% increase in cardiac output. Renal blood flow increases by up to 50% at the end of the first trimester, and uterine blood flow increases and

peaks at term (36–42 L/h). There is also a mean increase of 8 L in body water (60% to placenta, fetus and amniotic fluid and 40% to maternal tissues). As a consequence, there may be increased dosage requirements for some drugs to achieve the same therapeutic effect, provided these effects are not offset by other pharmacokinetic changes. Both the total plasma and the free-drug concentrations of phenytoin, carbamazepine and valproic acid decrease during pregnancy, but the free-drug fraction (ratio of free to total plasma concentration) may increase (Pavek et al., 2009).

Protein binding. Albumin is the main plasma protein responsible for binding acidic drugs such as phenytoin and salicylates, whereas α_1-acid glycoprotein predominantly binds basic drugs, including β-blockers and opioid analgesics. As pregnancy progresses the plasma volume increases at a greater rate than the increase in albumin which results in hypoalbuminaemia. In addition, steroid and placental hormones occupy the protein-binding sites. This leads to an increase in the fraction of unbound drug. Clinical effect is related to the concentration of unbound drug, which usually remains unchanged even though the total (bound plus unbound) plasma concentration is decreased. Thus, a decline in the total plasma concentration does not usually require an increase in dose. The α_1-acid glycoprotein concentrations remain the same as those in non-pregnancy.

Phenytoin is bound to albumin and exhibits the effects described earlier, but the situation is further complicated by increased hepatic metabolism that may necessitate a dose increase. Consequently, therapy can only be reliably guided by clinical assessment or measurement of unbound rather than total plasma concentration.

Metabolism

The metabolic activity of cytochrome P450 isoenzymes CYP3A4, CYP2D6, CYP2A6 and CYP2C9 and uridine 5′-diphosphate glucuronosyltransferase (UGT) isoenzymes (UGT1a1, UGT1A4 and UGT2B7) is increased during pregnancy. Drugs metabolised by these isoenzymes may therefore require dose adjustment. This may decrease the amount of the drug available for transfer across the placenta, and thereby influence fetal exposure. In contrast, the metabolic activity of CYP1A2 and CYP2C19 is decreased during pregnancy, and drugs metabolised by these isoenzymes may need dose reduction to minimise toxicity. These changes and their extent depend on the stage of pregnancy, so there may be clinically significant changes in drug concentrations between trimesters (Table 48.3) (Anderson, 2005; Deligiannidis et al., 2014). In general the effects on individual drugs are inconsistent and difficult to predict, but knowledge of the effect of pregnancy on isoenzymes may inform decisions about possible monitoring and/or dose alterations.

Excretion

Within the first few weeks of pregnancy the glomerular filtration rate (GFR) increases by approximately 50%. Consequently, those drugs which are excreted primarily unchanged by the kidneys, for example, lithium, digoxin and penicillin, show enhanced elimination and lower steady-state concentrations. The following

Table 48.3 Summary of pregnancy-induced effects on hepatic metabolism of some drugs

Isoenzyme	Drugs/ probes	Effect on clearance		
		First trimester	Second trimester	Third trimester
CYP1A2	Caffeine	↓ 33%	↓ 50%	↓ 65%
CYP2A6	Nicotine	ND	↑ 54% (combined data)	
CYP2C9	Phenytoin	No effect	No effect	↑ 20%
CYP2C19	Proguanil	ND	↓ 50%	↓ 50%
CYP2D6	Dextro-methorphan[a] Metoprolol	ND	ND	↑ 50%
CYP3A4	Cortisol[a] Nifedipine	ND	ND	↑ Variable[b]
UGT1A4	Lamotrigine monother-apy	↑ 200%	↑ 200%	↑ 300%
	Polytherapy	↑ 65%	↑ 65%	↑ 90%
UGT2B7 (limited data)	Morphine	ND	ND	↑ Variable[b]

[a]Dextromethorphan and cortisol used as probes of CYP2D6 and CYP3A4 activity.
[b]Extent variable depending on the drug studied.
ND, Not detectable.
Adapted from Anderson (2005).

drugs have shown pregnancy-induced increases of 20–65% on their renal elimination (Anderson, 2005):

- ampicillin,
- cefuroxime,
- ceftazidime,
- cefazolin,
- piperacillin,
- atenolol,
- sotalol,
- digoxin,
- lithium,
- dalteparin sodium,
- enoxaparin sodium.

Fetal–placental transfer

Most drugs have a molecular weight less than 600 and diffuse easily across the placenta to enter the fetal circulation to some extent. In general, the fetal/maternal drug concentration ratio is less than 1. Drugs differ in the extent to which they bind to fetal and maternal proteins. For example, fetal and newborn plasma proteins appear to bind ampicillin and benzylpenicillin with less affinity and salicylates with greater affinity than maternal proteins. Maternal albumin gradually decreases during pregnancy and fetal albumin concentrations increase, so different fetal/maternal albumin concentrations occur at different stages of pregnancy. The degree of protein binding of any drug is an important determinant of its movement across the placenta. Drugs that are highly protein bound tend to achieve higher maternal and lower fetal concentrations. Drugs with very large molecular weights such as insulin and heparin have negligible transfer. Lipophilic, un-ionised drugs cross the placenta more easily than polar drugs, and weakly basic drugs may become 'trapped' in the fetal circulation because of the slightly lower pH compared with maternal plasma.

Some other factors such as enzymes or drug efflux transporters in the placenta may facilitate or restrict the transfer of a drug to the fetus. The influence of transporter activity on placental transfer is increasingly recognised. For example, the accumulating evidence about transport mechanisms operating at the placental barrier is expected to be useful in developing techniques to control fetal and placental transfer of antiviral drugs, thus achieving maximum therapeutic benefit while minimising potential fetal toxicity (Tomi et al., 2011).

Maternal pharmacodynamic changes

Pharmacodynamic changes in pregnancy are less well studied than pharmacokinetic changes, but increases in blood pressure and blood glucose associated with corticosteroids may be more common in pregnancy. It is thought that impairment of cell-mediated immunity affects the efficacy of vaccination, particularly late in pregnancy. Sensitivity to the bradycardic effects of β-receptor blocking drugs such as propranolol may also be increased in pregnancy (Rubin et al., 1987). There is currently not a good understanding of pharmacodynamic changes and their clinical implications in pregnancy.

Drug dosing in pregnancy

As a general principle, the dose of a drug given at any stage of pregnancy should be as low as possible to minimise potential toxic effects to the fetus. Drug therapy that is considered essential can be tapered to the lowest effective dose either before conception (ideally) or at the time the pregnancy is diagnosed. Where drug exposure during the third trimester is predicted to have an adverse effect on the neonate postpartum, consideration may be given to slowly reducing the dose towards term to minimise the risks to the baby. Such decisions are, however, not always straightforward. Recommendations to wean an expectant mother off antidepressants and antipsychotics to reduce the likelihood of neonatal withdrawal syndrome (characterised by jitteriness, altered muscle tone, poor feeding and irritability) and, in the case of the selective serotonin reuptake inhibitors (SSRIs), avoid the possible increased risk of persistent pulmonary hypertension of the newborn are now being challenged. Not only are there insufficient data to conclusively demonstrate neonatal benefit or an optimal time of weaning, but also the increased risk of psychiatric problems and relapse in the mother's immediate postpartum period needs to be taken into account.

Many physiological changes occur during pregnancy that may affect the way the body handles drugs. Knowledge of these changes can allow some prediction of the impact on pharmacotherapy while remaining aware that there is variability in the extent of these changes during the pregnancy and high inter-individual variability. The need for changes in dosages is influenced by whether the drug is excreted unchanged by the kidneys or which metabolic isoenzymes are involved in its elimination. Women who are taking drugs with enhanced clearance and for which a good correlation between plasma levels and therapeutic effect exists should have their plasma concentrations closely monitored and dose adjusted to reduce the risk of suboptimal therapy, for example, with phenytoin, carbamazepine, lithium and digoxin. Similarly, highly protein-bound drugs may require free-drug concentration monitoring. However, there is no clear guidance for adjusting doses during pregnancy, and for most drugs, the concentration of free drug, and therefore the effect of that drug, is unchanged.

Pregnancy itself can cause a temporary worsening or improvement of some diseases and in that way influence drug dosages.

Drug selection in pregnancy

Although there are few, if any, drugs for which safe use in pregnancy can be absolutely assured, only a handful of drugs in current clinical use have been conclusively shown to be teratogenic. In general, drugs that have been used extensively in pregnant women without apparent problems are recommended in preference to new drugs for which there is less experience of use. For example, methyldopa is used rarely to treat hypertension in the non-pregnant state but has historically been preferred in pregnancy because of a long history of safe use (National Institute for Health and Care Excellence [NICE], 2011). However, older drugs may be less effective in terms of controlling maternal illness and are often associated with an increased side-effect risk profile.

In most cases the decision whether to commence or continue with a medication in pregnancy will depend on the risk–benefit analysis for that specific mother–infant pair. A frequent error made by health professionals was to apply the recently discontinued US Food and Drug Administration (FDA) pregnancy risk categories (A [*no demonstrable risk*]; B, C, D and X [*teratogenic agents that are considered to be completely contraindicated in pregnancy*]) when considering whether to prescribe a drug in pregnancy. It is now widely accepted that these categories were oversimplified and of little practical help in a clinical setting. More detailed information sheets containing a summary of the fetal risks and the additional maternal factors that need to be taken into consideration are now being used. Consideration also needs to be given to the quality and quantity of both human and animal data, the study design, dose exposure and any reported congenital malformations and/or adverse events (see http://www.fda.gov for up-to-date information).

It is worth noting that standard literature sources often contain unhelpful information such as 'do not use in pregnancy unless the benefits outweigh the risks'. This is understandable from a medico-legal point of view but offers little in terms of risk assessment. The primary literature is frequently inadequate because ethical and legal restraints mean that randomised controlled trials are rarely undertaken in pregnant women. Often the only information that is available is confined to retrospective studies, voluntary reporting schemes and/or animal studies. The rate of anomalies in retrospective studies and voluntary reporting databases may be erroneously elevated due to preferential reporting of abnormal outcomes. Individual case reports are also difficult to interpret because the denominator of drug exposure is unknown, and an abnormal outcome may be coincidental to the drug exposure. More recently, prospective controlled trials have been utilised where the pregnancy outcomes of a defined cohort of women exposed to the drug are compared with outcomes of a matched control group. Complete follow-up of each pregnancy and postnatal monitoring is an essential feature of this type of investigation.

Pre-conception advice

Drug use during the first trimester, in particular, the embryonic stage, carries the greatest risk of malformation because this is when the fetal organs are being formed. Ideally all unnecessary drug therapy should be discontinued prior to conception. However, inadvertent drug exposure frequently occurs, because approximately half of all pregnancies are unplanned. It is thus critical to make careful drug choices when prescribing for women of reproductive potential.

Women with chronic illnesses who require drug treatment should be offered specialist counselling before conception, and the options explored to reduce or change drug therapy to a safer agent if necessary. It is also important to note that many pregnant women become less adherent to their drug therapy out of concern about possible harm to their infant. In many cases, such as asthma, inflammatory bowel disease and epilepsy, inadequate treatment of the underlying disease may be more detrimental to the mother–fetus pair than the drugs used to treat the condition. It is thus essential that women of reproductive potential are given clear and up-to-date information so that unrealistic fears about the risks to their baby do not result in unnecessary pregnancy termination or disease relapse.

All women who are planning a pregnancy should be offered general advice to minimise the risk of congenital anomalies. This includes avoidance of recreational drugs, 'natural' or herbal remedies, alcohol, smoking and vitamin A products; minimisation of caffeine consumption; and beginning daily supplementation with at least 400 micrograms of folic acid to reduce the risk of neural tube defects (NICE, 2014). It is recommended that the daily dose of folic acid be increased to around 5 mg daily in women who have epilepsy (NICE, 2016) or who have had a previous child with a neural tube defect (NICE, 2014). Some infectious diseases may carry important fetal consequences if contracted during pregnancy. For example, rubella infection in the first 20 weeks of pregnancy is associated with an increased risk of miscarriage and a syndrome comprising problems such as deafness, cardiac defects and mental retardation in more than 20% of pregnancies. Women who lack immunity to rubella should be immunised prior to conception.

Post-conception advice

It is important to draw distinction between advice given to women pre-conceptually and that provided to a pregnant woman who has already been exposed to a drug. In the former setting, it may be recommended that an alternative preparation be considered or that a drug treatment be stopped where clinically appropriate. This advice often hinges on the lack of definitive safety data and does not automatically translate to exposure to that drug in pregnancy being an indication for discontinuing the drug, additional fetal monitoring or termination of the pregnancy on the basis of the exposure. Any change to the woman's medication should be based on a careful and individual risk assessment, and include a discussion with the woman to provide her with accurate, up-to-date, evidence-based advice. In many such cases the woman can be reassured that a healthy baby is the most likely outcome, or where appropriate be offered additional prenatal investigation to screen for congenital malformation where the risk to the fetus is considered to be significant.

Teratology information services and pregnancy registries

It is difficult to keep up to date with the published literature. There is an increasing need for summary documents that include and critically appraise all available data, and which enable healthcare providers to have a balanced and informed discussion with patients regarding the risks and benefits of a certain therapy in pregnancy. This is evidenced by the ongoing debate surrounding the teratogenic potential of various antidepressants with conflicting opinion even amongst experts in the field.

Teratology Information Services have been established in several countries across the world and provide evidence-based, up-to-date information and individual case-based risk assessments. In addition to reviewing published literature on drugs, teratology services also have access to specialist online databases and discussion forums. A number routinely collect pregnancy outcome data on the women about whom they receive an enquiry, to enable surveillance for potential teratogens.

For some new drugs, pregnancy registries have been initiated that record all reported drug exposures and follow up the outcome of the pregnancy. These registries are cumulative and work on the basis that specific anomalies would be identified relatively quickly, and that there will eventually be sufficient statistical power to detect the magnitude of any increased risk relative to the general population. These registries may be held by a Teratology Information Service or by independent groups with an interest in a defined area. The 2009 A/H1N1 influenza pandemic provided an example of teratology services across the globe responding to the urgent need for safety data by establishing registries on antiviral and pandemic vaccine exposure during the pandemic.

Drugs in lactation

Breast milk is the best form of nutrition for young infants. It provides all the energy and nutrients required for the first 6 months of life. The World Health Organization (WHO, 2001) and the United Nations Children's Fund recommend exclusive breastfeeding for this period. Benefits of breastfeeding include protection of the infant against infectious diseases (gastro-intestinal, upper and lower respiratory tract, otitis media and urinary tract) and reduction in rates of obesity, types 1 and 2 diabetes, inflammatory bowel disease, childhood leukaemia, asthma, coeliac disease and atopic disease (Eidelman and Schanler, 2012; Kramer and Kakuma, 2012). There is evidence to show that adults who were breastfed as infants have a predisposition to lower blood pressure and cholesterol levels (Horta et al., 2007). Maternal benefits include reduced risk of development of postpartum depression, cardiovascular disease, diabetes (Eidelman and Schanler, 2012), premenopausal breast and ovarian cancer, and delayed resumption of menstrual cycle (Department of Health, 2003; Eidelman and Schanler, 2012). Breastfeeding strengthens the mother–infant bond.

There are few contraindications to breastfeeding; these include galactosaemia in an infant and active untreated tuberculosis and HIV infection in developed countries. However, in the developing world, where mortality is increased in non-breastfeeding infants from a combination of malnutrition and infectious diseases, breastfeeding may outweigh the risk of acquiring HIV infection from human milk.

Reasons for early discontinuation of breastfeeding include problems latching, sore/cracked nipples, engorgement, inconvenience (return to work, feeding in public, lifestyle choices), concerns about inadequate lactation and nutritional adequacy, personal illness and medication, and infant factors (Li et al., 2008).

Breastfeeding mothers frequently require treatment with prescription medicines or may self-medicate with over-the-counter preparations, nutritional supplements or herbal medicines. It is important for health professionals to understand the principles of safe use of medications during lactation to provide appropriate advice.

There are two main goals to consider when formulating advice for nursing mothers. These are to protect the infant from maternal drug-related adverse effects and to allow, whenever possible, necessary maternal medication (Berlin et al., 2009).

Transfer of drugs into breast milk

Most drugs pass into breast milk to some degree, although transfer is usually low. The drug 'dose' ingested by the infant via breast milk only rarely causes adverse effects. Examples of adverse effects observed in breastfed infants exposed to commonly used medicines via breast milk are given in Table 48.4. These examples are of reports that are considered to have a high probability of a direct association between infant exposure in breast milk and maternal ingestion, although not all of these are proven to be directly caused by the drug ingested via breast milk. There are a significant number of reports of possible adverse reactions in breastfed infants due to maternal medication in which the association is less clear, unsubstantiated or anecdotal (Anderson et al., 2003, 2016).

Almost all drugs enter milk by passive diffusion of unionised, unbound drug through the lipid membranes of the alveolar cells of the breast, according to the pH partitioning theory. Several factors influence the rate and extent of passive diffusion.

Table 48.4 Adverse reactions reported in breastfed infants (Anderson et al., 2003, 2016)

Drug	Adverse reaction
Acebutolol	Hypotension, bradycardia, tachypnoea
Aspirin	Metabolic acidosis, thrombocytopenic purpura
Atenolol	Bradycardia, cyanosis, hypotension
Ciprofloxacin	Pseudomembranous colitis
Codeine	Apnoea, bradycardia, death
Cyclophosphamide	Neutropenia, thrombocytopenia
Dapsone	Haemolytic anaemia
Diazepam	Lethargy, sedation, poor suckling
Doxepin	Sedation and respiratory arrest
Erythromycin	Pyloric stenosis
Fluoxetine	Colic, irritability, sedation
Indometacin	Seizures
Lamotrigine	Apnoea, cyanosis
Lithium	Cyanosis, lethargy, T-wave abnormalities, thyroid-stimulating hormone elevation
Mesalazine	Watery diarrhoea
Naproxen	Prolonged bleeding, haemorrhage, anaemia
Oxycodone	Sedation, hypothermia, poor feeding
Paroxetine	Agitation, feeding difficulty
Phenindione	Postoperative haemorrhage
Phenytoin	Methaemoglobinaemia
Sulfasalazine	Bloody diarrhoea
Theophylline	Irritability, poor sleep
Topiramate	Diarrhoea
Yellow fever vaccine	Fever, irritability, convulsions, meningo-encephalitis

These include maternal plasma level, physiological differences between plasma and milk, and the physicochemical properties of the drug. Differences in composition between blood and milk determine which physicochemical characteristics influence diffusion.

Milk differs from blood in that it has a lower pH (7.2 vs. 7.4), less buffering capacity and higher fat content. The following drug parameters affect the extent of transfer into milk:

- pK_a: This is a measure of the fraction of the drug that is ionised at a given pH, for example, physiological pH. Highly ionised drugs tend not to concentrate in milk. For basic drugs (e.g. erythromycin), a greater fraction will be ionised at an acidic pH, so the milk compartment will tend to 'trap' weak bases. In contrast, acidic drugs (e.g. penicillins) are more ionised at higher pH values and will be 'trapped' in the plasma compartment. Drugs with higher pK_a values generally have higher milk/plasma ratios.
- *Protein binding:* Drugs that are highly bound to plasma proteins (e.g. warfarin) are likely to be relatively retained in maternal plasma because there is a lower total protein content in the milk. High protein binding essentially restricts the drug to the plasma compartment because only the free fraction of the drug crosses the biological membrane. Milk concentrations of highly protein-bound drugs are usually low.
- *Lipophilicity:* The alveolar epithelium of the breast is a lipid barrier. Transfer of water-soluble drugs and ions is inhibited by this barrier. CNS active drugs usually have the characteristics required to pass into milk.
- *Molecular weight:* Drugs with low molecular weights (<200) readily pass into milk through small pores in the cell walls of alveolar cells. Drugs with higher molecular weights cross cell membranes by dissolving in the lipid layer which may substantially reduce milk concentrations. Proteins such as heparin or insulin with very large molecular weights greater than 6000 are virtually excluded from milk.

The profile of a drug that passes minimally into milk would therefore be an acidic drug that is highly protein bound and has low-to-moderate lipophilicity (e.g. most NSAIDs). In contrast, a weakly basic drug that has low plasma protein binding and is relatively lipophilic will achieve higher concentrations in the milk compartment (e.g. sotalol).

In the first few days of life, large gaps exist between the alveolar cells. These permit enhanced passage of drugs into milk. By the end of the first week these gaps close under the influence of prolactin (Lawrence and Lawrence, 2016). There is greater passage of drugs into colostrum (early milk) than in mature milk because the former contains more protein and less fat. There is also some variation in fat and protein content of milk between the beginning and end of a feed, but these changes have less influence on drug passage than the physicochemical properties of the drug.

Milk/plasma concentration ratio

Several methods have been proposed to determine the amount of drug transferred to breast milk. The milk/plasma (M/P) ratio is often used as a measure of the extent of drug transfer into breast milk. It is usually obtained from case reports or small clinical studies and may be based on paired concentrations or full area under the concentration–time curve (AUC) analysis. M/P ratios that are based on a pair of milk and plasma samples collected simultaneously may be inaccurate because they

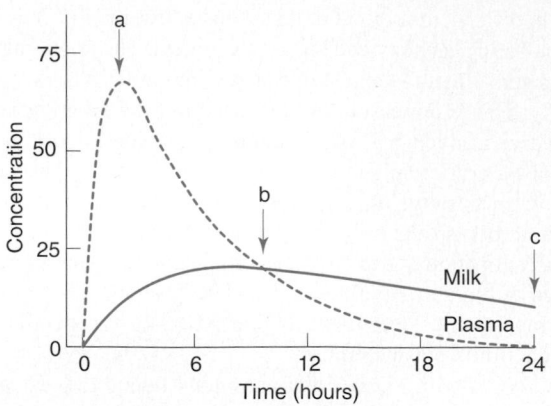

Fig. 48.1 Diagrammatic representation of a drug concentration–time profile in the maternal plasma and milk phases after a single oral dose. The points a, b and c illustrate simultaneous sampling times from both phases. Sampling at (a) would yield an estimated milk/plasma (M/P) ratio of 0.2, at (b) a value of 1.0, and at (c) a value of 9.3. All can be misleading. The true M/P ratio calculated by the area under the concentration–time curve method is 1.2 when extrapolated to infinity.

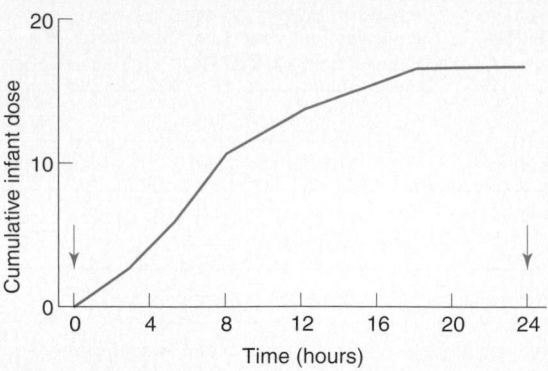

Fig. 48.2 The cumulative dose received by the infant is plotted against time. The arrows represent the maternal dose times. This type of study is undertaken by the mother expressing all the milk, from both breasts, at usual feeding times. An aliquot of milk is taken and assayed for the drug. The volume of milk is measured, and the total amount of drug at each time is calculated as the product of concentration and volume. This type of study must be undertaken at steady state.

assume that the concentrations of drug in milk and plasma are in parallel, which may not be the case. It is better to collect multiple samples of plasma and milk across a dosing interval, or until the drug is cleared from both phases after a single dose, for determination of a M/P ratio based on the respective AUCs (M/P_{AUC}). Fig. 48.1 demonstrates the markedly different estimates of M/P ratio that can be obtained via both sampling methods. The true M/P ratio may vary significantly during the same episode of breastfeeding.

If human-derived M/P ratios are lacking for a particular drug, it may be possible to predict the extent of transfer using known physicochemical properties, for example, pK_a, and a published predictive model (Atkinson and Begg, 1990; Begg et al., 1992; Zhao et al., 2006). M/P ratios obtained from animal studies should not be used for clinical decision making because they may not correlate well with human M/P ratios.

Studies in humans demonstrate that most drugs have an M/P ratio less than 1.0, with the range of reported ratios being from around 0.1–5.0. It is often thought that drugs with high M/P ratios (e.g. 5.0) are unsafe because the concentration in milk exceeds that in plasma, while those with low ratios (<1.0) are believed to be safe. This is not always the case because the M/P ratio often fails to correlate with the 'dose' of drug the infant ingests via milk. The amount of drug transferred into milk is principally determined by the maternal plasma level. Thus, even where the M/P ratio is high, if the maternal plasma level is low, drug transfer is still low. Therefore, the M/P ratio must never be used as the sole measure of drug safety in breastfeeding. However, it can be used to estimate the 'dose' ingested via milk, which is a better predictor of safety.

Calculating the infant 'dose' ingested via milk

Infant plasma drug levels are the most accurate indicator of drug exposure, but these are seldom available.

When using quantitative data from milk analyses, the most accurate estimation of the infant 'dose' is from studies in which the milk is collected over a complete dose interval at steady state and the total dose is calculated (Fig. 48.2). Unfortunately, these studies are seldom performed. Therefore, information must be obtained from less than ideal conditions.

If the M/P ratio is known from published studies, the likely infant dose (D_{inf}) can be calculated as follows, with some assumptions:

$$D_{inf} = Cp_{mat} \times M/P \times V_{milk}$$

where Cp_{mat} is the average maternal plasma concentration, and the M/P_{AUC} should be used in preference to a ratio based on paired concentrations when available. The volume of milk ingested (V_{milk}) is not known but is generally assumed to be around 150 mL of milk per kilogram of body weight per day. The above equation simplifies if the actual milk concentration data are available:

$$D_{inf} = C_{milk} \times V_{milk}$$

The likely infant plasma drug concentration (Cp_{inf}) can be calculated by:

$$Cp_{inf} = F \times D_{inf}/Cl_{inf}$$

where F is oral availability and Cl_{inf} is the infant clearance. Unfortunately, neither F nor Cl_{inf} is known accurately for infants, so estimation of the likely steady-state average plasma drug concentration will be very approximate. Weight-adjusted Cl_{inf} values (i.e. L/h/kg) are often significantly less than adult values in the early stages of life (Table 48.5).

Given the difficulty in estimating infant plasma drug concentrations, the relative infant dose (RID), for example, compared with a therapeutic infant dose, is often used as a surrogate of exposure. To give some basis for comparison, the likely infant dose from milk can be compared with an infant therapeutic dose. This is reasonable for drugs such as paracetamol that are usually administered to infants, but is unsuitable for drugs such as antidepressants that are not. In the absence of a clearly defined range

Table 48.5 Approximate drug clearance by age as percentage of maternal value (Begg, 2000)

Post-conceptual age (weeks)	Approximate drug clearance (%)
24–28	5
28–34	10
34–40	33
40–44	50
44–68	66
>68	100

Box 48.2 Factors that affect infant risk from maternal therapy

- Drug adverse reaction profile
- Relative infant dose
- Oral bioavailability
- Active metabolites
- Half-life
- Gestational age of the infant
- Full maternal drug regimen
- Pharmacogenetic factors

Assessing the risk to the infant

Many factors must be considered when assessing the risk of maternal drug therapy to the breastfeeding infant (Box 48.2).

Pharmacokinetic and pharmacodynamic factors

Inherent toxicity of the drug will be a main factor in determining infant safety. Thus, antineoplastic drugs, radionuclides and iodine-containing compounds would be of concern. Multiple maternal therapy with drugs with similar side-effect profiles, for example, psychotropic drugs or anticonvulsants, is likely to increase the risk to the infant. Oral bioavailability is an indicator of the drug's ability to reach the systemic circulation after oral administration. Drugs with a low oral bioavailability are either poorly absorbed from the gastro-intestinal tract, broken down in the gut or undergo extensive 'first-pass' metabolism in the liver before entering plasma.

The presence of active metabolites (e.g. desmethyldiazepam) may prolong infant drug exposure and lead to drug accumulation, especially where drug clearance is low, such as in the neonatal period. Similarly, drugs with long half-lives (e.g. fluoxetine) may be problematic at this time. Drug clearance by the infant does not reach adult values until 6–7 months (see Table 48.5). A premature infant of 30 weeks' gestational age has a drug clearance value of about 10% of the maternal value. It is important to distinguish between gestational age and time after delivery. A 2-week-old infant born at 28 weeks will have a gestational age of 30 weeks.

The maternal drug regimen can affect infant risk. Single doses or short courses seldom present problems, whereas chronic therapy can be problematic. Topical or inhalation therapy usually results in much lower plasma drug levels and, therefore, lower passage into milk. Multiple maternal medications increase the risk to the infant.

of infant doses, the weight-adjusted maternal dose expressed as a percentage (% dose) is widely used to indicate infant drug exposure.

$$\text{Relative infant dose (RID)} = \frac{D_{\text{inf}} \, (\text{mg/kg/day})}{D_{\text{mat}} \, (\text{mg/kg/day})} \times 100$$

D_{inf} represents dose in infant via milk, and D_{mat} represents dose in mother.

For the great majority of drugs, this calculation yields infant doses in the order of 0.1–5.0% of the weight-adjusted maternal dose expressed as a percentage (% dose). It is generally thought that RID values of less than 10% of the maternal dose are probably safe. However, the inherent toxicity of the drug should be taken into account when using this figure.

To calculate the daily infant drug intake via milk, the standard milk intake of 150 mL/kg/day is multiplied by the concentration of the medication in milk. Some authors use the peak concentration in milk to indicate the maximum infant intake.

$$\begin{aligned} \text{Estimated daily infant intake} &= \text{drug concentration in milk} \\ \text{(micrograms/day)} \quad &\quad (\text{micrograms/L}) \times 0.15 \times \\ &\quad \text{infant weight (kg)} \end{aligned}$$

Variability

To further complicate matters, there will be significant variability between and within individuals in the values used to estimate infant exposure (i.e. D_{inf}, F, Cl_{inf}, where D_{inf} is itself a function of the estimated parameters Cp_{mat}, M/P and volume of milk). Some of this variability will change over time because of developing organ function in the maturing baby, and some will be unexplained variability. In addition to this pharmacokinetic variability, there will be variability in response of the infant to any given concentration of the drug. It is fortunate that most drugs seem to fall readily into a safe range (RID <10%) based on expected exposure. However, care should be taken when using these values to assess drug safety in lactation, when variability in the estimates of the parameters used may impact on the accuracy of prediction of their safety. This is especially true for those circumstances when initial estimates of these parameters are less precise, for example, in neonates.

Pharmacogenetic factors

Recently, attention has been focused on the possible role of pharmacogenetic factors in affecting the safety of breastfed infants exposed to drugs via milk (Madadi et al., 2009). Sedation (and one death) occurred in infants of mothers with rare genotypes of cytochrome P450 CYP2D6. leading to ultrarapid metabolism of codeine to morphine. The incidence of these genotypes varies amongst different populations. The overall percentage of Western Europeans with the CYP2D6 ultrarapid metaboliser phenotype is 5.4% (Ingelman-Sundberg, 2005). Higher percentages have been reported in populations from northeast Africa and the Middle East.

Reducing risk to the breastfed infant

A number of strategies may be adopted to reduce the risk of drug-related side effects in the breastfed infant. One technique that has been recommended for reducing infant exposure is to give the maternal dose immediately after the infant has been fed with the aim of avoiding feeding at peak milk concentrations. However, this is often impractical, especially where young infants are feeding frequently up to 2 hourly. In addition, accurate data on times of peak levels in milk are often unavailable, and it cannot be assumed that times of peak milk levels mirror those in plasma. This technique should be used selectively, where the drug has a short half-life and where peak and trough levels are predictable (e.g. antibiotics, anaesthetics).

Where a single dose of a drug known to be hazardous is given to a breastfeeding mother, for example, a radiopharmaceutical, it will usually be possible to resume breastfeeding after a suitable washout period, calculated as five times the half-life. Where the half-life is very long, the washout period necessary to avoid hazardous exposure to the infant may exceed the period of sustainable lactation.

Breastfeeding mothers should be advised to avoid self-medication. Where drug use is clearly indicated, the lowest effective dose should be used for the shortest possible time. Use of topical therapy, such as eye/nasal drops for hay fever, would reduce drug exposure in comparison with oral antihistamines.

The maternal regimen should be simplified wherever possible. A review of therapy before delivery will help reduce risks to the neonate. New drugs are best avoided if a therapeutic equivalent is available for which data on safe use in lactation exists. All infants exposed to drugs via breast milk should be monitored for any untoward effects. Measures to ensure the safety of the breastfed infant are summarised in Box 48.3.

Some commonly used drugs thought to be safe to use in mothers of full-term, healthy infants are listed in Table 48.6.

Special situations

Neonates and premature infants

Neonates and premature infants are at greater risk of development of adverse effects after exposure to drugs via breast milk. Gastric emptying time is significantly prolonged and, in some cases, may alter absorption kinetics. Protein binding is decreased and values for total body water are higher than for adults. Renal function is limited because the kidney is anatomically and functionally immature (van den Anket, 1996). The neonate's capacity to conjugate drugs in the liver is often deficient.

Glucose-6-phosphate dehydrogenase deficiency

Infants with glucose-6-phosphate dehydrogenase (G6PD) deficiency are susceptible to adverse effects even when only small amounts of certain drugs are present in milk. G6PD is an enzyme present in erythrocytes that is responsible for maintaining the antioxidant compound glutathione in its active form. Deficiency of this enzyme makes the erythrocyte more susceptible to oxidative stress, resulting in haemolysis. Only small amounts of drug are needed to cause such a reaction.

Breastfeeding should be avoided or a safer alternative chosen if the infant has a known or suspected G6PD deficiency and the mother is taking drugs that have been reported to cause oxidative stress (e.g. nitrofurantoin, dapsone).

Allergy

The theoretical possibility exists for an allergic reaction in an infant exposed to a drug in breast milk. Even minimal exposure to the drug could cause an allergic response. However, in practice, such reactions are rare, and only if the infant has already

---

Box 48.3 Measures to ensure the safety of the breastfed infant

- Avoid unnecessary maternal drug use.
- Seek professional advice on the suitability of over-the-counter products.
- Avoid herbal products because of lack of data to support safe use.
- Assess the risk/benefit ratio for both mother and infant.
- Use the minimum clinically effective dose for the shortest possible time.
- Review maternal therapy towards the end of pregnancy.
- Choose a drug regimen and route of administration which presents the minimum of drug to the infant via breast milk.
- Avoid drugs known to cause serious toxicity in adults or children.
- Monitor the infant for unusual signs or symptoms.
- Avoid new drugs if there is a therapeutic equivalent with data to support safe use in lactation.
- Recognise risk factors, e.g. prematurity, infant morbidity and multiple maternal medications.

Table 48.6 Examples of commonly used drugs thought to be safe for use in breastfeeding mothers of full-term, healthy infants

Drug groups	Individual drugs
Antacids	Cetirizine
Bulk laxatives	Chloroquine/proguanil
Cephalosporins	Clotrimazole
Contrast media	Cromoglycate
Inhaled medications (e.g. salbutamol, beclometasone)	Diclofenac
	Fluconazole
Insulins	Heparin (including low molecular weight)
Penicillins	Ibuprofen
Progestogen-only contraceptives	Iron supplements
	Loratadine
Topical formulations (except when applied to breast)	Lactulose
Vaccines (except yellow fever)	Levothyroxine
Vitamins (except high-dose A and D)	Nystatin
	Omeprazole
	Paracetamol
	Paroxetine/sertraline
	Warfarin

This table is to be used as a guide only. Expert advice is required when the maternal dose is high and if the infant is premature, has renal or hepatic disease, or has glucose-6-phosphate dehydrogenase deficiency.

experienced an allergic reaction to a particular drug should maternal use be discouraged or breastfeeding avoided.

Recreational drug use

Accurate background data of maternal use of recreational drugs may be difficult to obtain. Usage may be chronic or sporadic. The role of the healthcare professional in ensuring the safety of the breastfed infant is important, and the advice should be that substances such as cannabis, LSD and cocaine should be avoided whilst breastfeeding.

Significant amounts of alcohol pass into milk, although it is not normally harmful to the infant if the quantity and duration of intake are limited. The occasional consumption of a small alcoholic beverage is acceptable if breastfeeding is avoided for about 2 hours after the drink. Chronic or heavy consumers of alcohol should not breastfeed. High intakes of alcohol decrease milk letdown and disrupt nursing until maternal levels decrease. Heavy maternal use may cause infant sedation, fluid retention and hormone imbalances in breastfed infants.

Nicotine has been suggested to decrease basal prolactin production, although effects may be variable. Ideally mothers should be encouraged not to smoke whilst breastfeeding. Nicotine and its metabolite, cotinine, are both present in milk. Undertaking smoking cessation with a nicotine patch is a safer option than continued smoking. Whilst transdermal nicotine patches produce a sustained lower nicotine plasma level, nicotine gums produce large variations in peak levels. A 2- to 3-hour washout period is recommended before breastfeeding after maternal use of a nicotine gum.

Caffeine appears in breast milk rapidly after maternal intake. Fussiness, jitteriness and poor sleep patterns have been reported in infants of mothers with very high caffeine intakes equivalent to about 10 or more cups of coffee daily. Preterm and newborn infants metabolise caffeine very slowly and are at increased risk of adverse effects.

Drug effects on lactation

Drugs that affect dopamine activity are the main cause of effects on milk production, mainly mediated by effects on prolactin. Early postpartum use of oestrogens may reduce the volume of milk, but the effect is variable and depends on the dose and the individual response. Progestogen only contraceptives are preferred.

Drugs may occasionally be used therapeutically for their effect on lactation. Dopamine agonists such as cabergoline decrease milk production and this effect may be utilised, for example, after an infant death. Dopamine agonists should not be used routinely for relief of the symptoms of postpartum pain or engorgement that can be managed with simple analgesics or breast support. Dopamine antagonists such as domperidone may be used in cases of inadequate lactation that have not responded to first-line methods such as improved technique or milk expression by hand or pump. However, a European and UK regulatory review has recommended restricted use of domperidone because of the risk of cardiac adverse effects (Medicines and Healthcare Products Regulatory Agency, 2014). The use of domperidone to enhance lactation is not specifically covered by the review because it is

an unlicensed ('off-label') indication. However, it is appropriate for the recommendations from the review to apply to its use as a galactagogue. Because there are limited alternative options for the stimulation of lactation, the use of domperidone can be considered provided non-pharmacological options have been unsuccessful. A maternal dosage of 30 mg daily for 1 week should not usually be exceeded, and it should not be used if the mother or infant:

- has conditions where cardiac conduction is, or could be, impaired;
- has underlying cardiac diseases such as congestive heart failure;
- is receiving other medications known to prolong QT interval or are potent CYP3A4 inhibitors;
- has severe hepatic impairment.

If treatment is still required after 1 week, the risks of continuing domperidone must be considered carefully. Alternatively, metoclopramide can be used; however, only for up to 5 days because of the risk of neurological side effects (European Medicines Agency, 2013).

Other drugs may affect lactation as an unwanted side effect, for example, diuretics causing dehydration. When these are used on a long-term basis, infant weight gain should be monitored.

Case studies

Case 48.1

Ms LP is 6 weeks' pregnant and has been diagnosed with depression that warrants pharmacological intervention. She wishes to recommence venlafaxine, which has been helpful in the past. Ms LP is also anxious that the ethanol she consumed around the time of conception may have harmed her baby.

....

Questions

1. What are the safest antidepressants in the first trimester of pregnancy?
2. Is it reasonable for Ms LP to commence venlafaxine?
3. Is there any risk from the ethanol ingestion?

....

Answers

1. The concept of 'safe' needs to take into account the risks of inadequate treatment of the mother, as well as those to the fetus through in utero exposure to a particular antidepressant. Choice of antidepressant in pregnancy will therefore depend on the severity of the maternal depression, the presence of associated symptoms such as anxiety or obsessive-compulsive behaviors, availability and suitability of non-pharmaceutical interventions and, finally, any prior treatment regimens that have been successfully or unsuccessfully used. SSRIs are currently the most commonly prescribed antidepressant group and the most studied in pregnancy. However, human pregnancy data will vary for individual SSRIs. Although not without risk to the fetus, SSRIs are generally prescribed as first-line therapy in preference to tricyclic antidepressants which carry a higher risk of maternal toxicity, especially in overdose, and which are less well studied in human pregnancy.

2. Experience with the use of venlafaxine and many other antidepressants (e.g. moclobemide) in pregnancy is limited. However, in some instances it may be necessary to use an agent such as venlafaxine. For example, if the mother had a history of severe depression that did not respond to multiple trials of other antidepressants, then venlafaxine may be considered the most appropriate choice of antidepressant for that woman. In this case any potential risks associated with venlafaxine are likely to be less than those associated with inadequately treated depression. Discussion of the available data and its limitations with Ms LP is, however, necessary to enable her to make an informed decision.

3. Ethanol is a human teratogen. Fetal alcohol spectrum disorders are characterised by low birth weight, facial dysmorphogenesis and/or delayed development. A 'safe limit' for alcohol consumption in pregnancy has not been defined, and best practice is therefore to avoid all alcohol exposure in pregnancy. In this case Ms LP ingested ethanol at the time of conception. She should be reassured that this is regarded as a relatively low-risk period for fetal harm, but that further ethanol ingestion should be avoided.

Case 48.2

A 30-year-old woman with epilepsy, Ms AD, is currently taking valproic acid 1500 mg daily. She wishes to conceive but is concerned about the possibility of birth defects caused by valproate exposure in pregnancy. Ms AD's seizures have been difficult to control with alternative anticonvulsants.

Questions

1. What are the risks associated with valproate treatment in pregnancy?
2. What advice should Ms AD be given?

Answers

1. Valproate is a human teratogen which has been associated with both structural and lasting neurodevelopmental effects. These may include neural tube defects, craniofacial anomalies such as cleft lip and palate, heart defects, autism, attention deficit hyperactivity disorder and learning difficulties. Recommendations from a European-wide review in 2014 (European Medicines Agency, 2014) advise against valproate use in female children, in female adolescents, in women of childbearing potential and in pregnant women unless other treatments are ineffective or not tolerated. Women of childbearing potential in whom valproate treatment is considered necessary for the treatment of epilepsy are advised to remain on effective contraception during treatment. The MHRA has produced a number of guidance documents for healthcare professionals in the UK, including an openly accessible toolkit for women (https://www.gov.uk/government/-publications/toolkit-on-the-risks-of-valproate-medicines-in-female-patients).

2. It is imperative that Ms AD be advised to request referral to, or review by, a neurologist, ideally with expertise in the treatment of women with epilepsy who become pregnant, and that she continues to use effective contraception until the risks and options available to her have been fully reviewed and discussed. New anticonvulsant therapies that do not appear to carry the same risks as valproate may have become available since Ms AD was last reviewed. Valproate teratogenicity appears to increase with increasing dose. Although no 'safe

dose' has been defined, if this patient needs to remain taking valproate, it may be possible to gradually reduce her daily dose under specialist review. General preconception advice could be given, that is, commence folic acid, optimise weight and general health, etc. It is important that Ms AD understands that folic acid 5 mg daily is advised for all women with epilepsy who are planning a pregnancy (NICE, 2016), but that at present there is no evidence that it prevents or reduces the risk of birth defects or neurodevelopmental impairment caused by valproate.

Case 48.3

A mother, Ms TF, with a history of depression has relapsed and requires treatment with an antidepressant. Ms TF is fully breastfeeding a 2-week old, full-term, fit and healthy baby. In the past she has taken fluoxetine, but stopped this when she found out she was pregnant.

Questions

1. What is the antidepressant of choice during breastfeeding?
2. Ms TF has responded well to fluoxetine previously, so can this be used during breastfeeding?
3. What are the potential risks of using fluoxetine?

Answers

1. Sertraline and paroxetine are the preferred SSRIs for use during breastfeeding because they have shorter half-lives, lower passage into milk and a larger evidence base compared with the other SSRIs. However, it is important that Ms TF has an antidepressant that works for her, so choice of agent should primarily be based on suitability for the patient rather than safety during breastfeeding.

2. If a woman has been successfully treated with an SSRI during pregnancy and requires continued therapy in the postnatal period there is no need to change therapy, provided the infant is full term, fit and healthy, and can be adequately monitored. Although fluoxetine is not a preferred SSRI during lactation, due to its long half-life, because it has proved effective for Ms TF in the past, the balance of benefit to risk will favour use of fluoxetine in this mother.

3. Because fluoxetine has a very long half-life there is a risk of accumulation and, therefore, adverse effects in the breastfed baby. The baby should be monitored for drowsiness, poor feeding, irritability and behavioural effects.

Case 48.4

A mother, Ms CG, is breastfeeding her 20-day-old, full-term, fit and healthy baby. She has postpartum hypertension and has been started on labetalol.

Labetalol does not control Ms CG's hypertension and she is started on nifedipine.

Questions

1. Comment on the suitability of labetalol as a suitable β-blocker for use during breastfeeding.
2. Are there any monitoring requirements?
3. Can Ms CG still continue to breastfeed?

Answers

1. In general, β-blockers that are considered to pose less risk to a breastfeeding infant have, or are predicted to have, lower levels in breast milk, due to a high degree of plasma protein binding, low lipid solubility and a short half-life, and relatively low renal excretion. The risks of available β-blockers vary widely due to these features. Although propranolol is considered to be the β-blocker of choice in breastfeeding, because clinical properties of β-blockers vary widely, propranolol may not always be a suitable clinical choice. Metoprolol and labetalol are also considered to pose low risk. Labetalol would be suitable to use in this situation, with appropriate monitoring.

2. The breastfed infant should be monitored for signs of β-blockade, especially bradycardia. Also consider monitoring for hypotension and hypoglycaemia.

3. Because there will be low levels of nifedipine in breastmilk, amounts ingested by the baby will be small. Nifedipine, including modified-release preparations, is considered compatible with breastfeeding. Therefore, Ms CG can continue to breastfed, but the risk of additive adverse effects in the baby must be remembered.

Case 48.5

A breastfeeding mother, Ms SV, returned to see her midwife 4 weeks after delivery of a full-term, healthy infant. She is complaining of bilateral nipple pain during and after breastfeeding, a problem that was constant for the past 4 days. Ms SV was advised to use miconazole cream 2% to the nipples after each feed. This provided initial relief, but symptoms returned after a few days.

She was given a course of fluconazole 200 mg daily for 10 days for a presumed candidal infection but expressed concern that the medication might affect the infant.

Questions

1. Is this regimen safe to use in lactation?
2. What other therapeutic measures should be taken?

Answers

1. Topical miconazole is effective in treating superficial candidal infections, but oral therapy with fluconazole is needed when the infection spreads to the milk ducts. Fluconazole, after a 200 mg oral dose, produces levels in breast milk similar to those found in maternal plasma. Fluconazole is recommended for use in the treatment of neonates with fungal infections at a dose starting at 3 mg/kg every 72 hours. The calculated dose of fluconazole ingested by an infant feeding at times of peak milk levels of fluconazole would be approximately 0.6 mg/kg/day, which is 60% of the neonatal dose and 20% of the dose for infants aged ≥1 month. Ms SV may be reassured that the amount of drug reaching the infant via milk is a fraction of the dose that would be used to treat an infection in the infant.

2. Candidal infections are easily passed between the mother and the infant, and both should receive treatment. Infants can be treated with nystatin suspension or oral miconazole gel. Miconazole gel is not licensed for use in children younger than 4 months because of the small risk of choking in young babies; this risk can be reduced by using smaller quantities of the gel, applying the gel with a clean finger rather than a spoon and being careful not to touch the back of the infant's throat when applying the gel.

Acknowledgements

The contributions of Stephen B. Duffull, Sharon J. Gardiner, David K. Woods and Elena Grant to previous versions of this chapter which appeared in earlier editions of the textbook are gratefully acknowledged.

References

Anderson, G., 2005. Pregnancy-induced changes in pharmacokinetics: a mechanistic-based approach. Clin. Pharmacokinet. 44, 989–1008.

Anderson, P.O., Pochop, S.L., Manoguerra, A.S., 2003. Adverse drug reactions in breastfed infants: less than imagined. Clin. Pediatr. (Phila.) 42, 325–340.

Anderson, P.O., Manoguerra, A.S., Pochop, S.L., 2016. A review of adverse reactions in infants from medications in breastmilk. Clin. Pediatr. (Phila.) 55, 236–244.

Atkinson, H.C., Begg, J., 1990. Prediction of drug distribution into human milk from physicochemical characteristics. Clin. Pharmacokinet. 18, 151–167.

Begg, E.J., 2000. Clinical Pharmacology Essentials. The Principles Behind the Prescribing Process. Adis International, Auckland.

Begg, E.J., Atkinson, E.J., Duffull, S.B., 1992. Prospective evaluation of a model for the prediction of milk:plasma drug concentrations from physicochemical characteristics. Br. J. Clin. Pharmacol. 33, 501–505.

Benke, P.J., 1984. The isotretinoin teratogen syndrome. JAMA 251, 3267–3269.

Berlin, C.M., Paul, I.M., Vesell, E.S., 2009. Safety issues of maternal drug therapy during breastfeeding. Clin. Pharmacol. Ther. 85, 20–22.

Braun, J.T., Franciosi, R.A., Mastri, A.R., et al., 1984. Isotretinoin dysmorphic syndrome. Lancet 1, 506–507.

Breitkreutz, I., Anderson, K.C., 2008. Thalidomide in multiple myeloma: clinical trials and aspects of drug metabolism and toxicity. Exp. Opin. Drug Metab. Toxicol. 4, 973–985.

Deligiannidis, K.M., Byatt, N., Freeman, M.P., 2014. Pharmacotherapy for mood disorders in pregnancy: a review of pharmacokinetic changes and clinical recommendations for therapeutic drug monitoring. J. Clin. Psychopharmacol. 34 (2), 244–255.

Department of Health, 2003. Infant feeding recommendation. Department of Health, London. Available at: http://webarchive.nationalarchives.gov.uk/20130107105354/http://www.dh.gov.uk/prod_consum_dh/groups/dh_digitalassets/@dh/@en/documents/digitalasset/dh_4096999.pdf.

Dunn, P.M., 1964. The possible relationship between the maternal administration of sulphamethoxypyridazine and hyperbilirubinaemia in the newborn. J. Obstet. Gynaecol. Br. Commonw. 71, 128–131.

Eidelman, A.I., Schanler, R.J., 2012. American Academy of Pediatrics – section on breastfeeding. Breastfeeding and the use of human milk. Pediatrics 129, e827–e841.

European Medicines Agency (EMA), 2013. European Medicines Agency recommends changes to the use of metoclopramide. Changes aim mainly to reduce the risk of neurological side effects. EMA, London. Available at: http://www.ema.europa.eu/docs/en_GB/document_library/Press_release/2013/07/WC500146614.pdf.

European Medicines Agency (EMA), 2014. CMDh agrees to strengthen warnings on the use of valproate medicines in women and girls. Women to be better informed of risks of valproate use in pregnancy and need for contraception. EMA, London. Available at: http://www.ema.europa.eu/docs/en_GB/document_library/Press_release/2014/11/WC500177638.pdf.

Headley, J., Northstone, K., Simmons, H., et al., 2004. Medication use during pregnancy: data from the Avon longitudinal study of parents and children. Eur. J. Clin. Pharmacol. 60, 355–361.

Herbst, A.L., Ulfelder, H., Poskanzer, D.C., 1971. Adenocarcinoma of the vagina. Association of maternal stilbestrol therapy with tumor appearance in young women. N. Engl. J. Med. 15, 878–881.

Hernandez-Diaz, S., Werler, M.M., Walker, A.M., et al., 2001. Neural tube defects in relation to use of folic acid antagonists during pregnancy. Am. J. Epidemiol. 153, 961–968.

Hill, R.M., 1984. Isotretinoin teratogenicity. Lancet 1, 1465.

Horta, B.L., Bahl, R., Martines, J.C., et al., 2007. Evidence On The Long-Term Effects Of Breastfeeding. WHO, Geneva.

Ingelman-Sundberg, M., 2005. Genetic polymorphisms of cytochrome P450 2D6 (CYP2D6): clinical consequences, evolutionary aspects and functional diversity. Pharmacogenomics J. 5, 6–13.

Koren, G., Florescu, A., Costei, A.M., et al., 2006. Non-steroidal anti-inflammatory drugs during third trimester and the risk of premature closure of the ductus arteriosus: a meta-analysis. Ann. Pharmacother. 40, 824–829.

Kramer, M.S., Kakuma, R., 2012. Optimal duration of exclusive breastfeeding. Cochrane Database Syst. Rev. 8, CD003517. https://doi.org/10.1002/14651858.CD003517.pub2.

Lawrence, R.A., Lawrence, R.M., 2016. Breastfeeding. A Guide for the Medical Profession, eighth ed. Elsevier, Philadelphia.

Lenz, W., 1966. Malformations caused by drugs in pregnancy. Am. J. Dis. Child. 112, 99–106.

Lenz, W., 1988. A short history of thalidomide embryopathy. Teratology 38, 203–215.

Li, R., Fein, S.B., Chen, J., et al., 2008. Why mothers stop breastfeeding: mothers' self reported reasons for stopping during the first year. Pediatrics 122 (Suppl. 2), S69–S76.

Loebstein, R., Lalkin, A., Koren, G., 1997. Pharmacokinetic changes during pregnancy and their clinical relevance. Clin. Pharmacokinet. 33, 328–343.

Madadi, P., Ross, C.J., Hayden, M.R., et al., 2009. Pharmacogenetics of neonatal opioid toxicity following maternal use of codeine during breastfeeding: a case control study. Clin. Pharmacol. Ther. 85, 31–35.

Medicines and Healthcare Products Regulatory Agency, 2014. Domperidone: risks of cardiac side effects – indication restricted to nausea and vomiting, new contraindications, and reduced dose and duration of use. Drug Saf. Update 7 (10), A1.

Miller, M.T., Ventura, L., Stromland, K., 2009. Thalidomide and misoprostol: ophthalmologic manifestations and associations both expected and unexpected. Birth Defects Res. A Clin. Mol. Teratol. 85, 667–676.

National Institute for Health and Care Excellence (NICE), 2011. Hypertension in pregnancy: diagnosis and management. Clinical guidance (CG107). NICE, London. Available at: https://www.nice.org.uk/guidance/cg107/.

National Institute for Health and Care Excellence (NICE), 2014. Maternal and child nutrition. Public health guideline (PH11). NICE, London. Available at: https://www.nice.org.uk/guidance/PH11/.

National Institute for Health and Care Excellence (NICE), 2016. Epilepsies: diagnosis and management. Clinical guidance (CG137). NICE, London. Available at: https://www.nice.org.uk/guidance/cg137/.

Newman, C.G., 1985. Teratogen update: clinical aspects of thalidomide embryopathy: a continuing preoccupation. Teratology 32, 133–144.

Newman, C.G., 1986. The thalidomide syndrome: risks of exposure and spectrum of malformations. Clin. Perinatol. 13, 555–573.

Nulman, I., Berkovitch, M., Klein, J., et al., 1998. Steady-state pharmacokinetics of isotretinoin and its 4-oxo metabolite: implications for fetal safety. J. Clin. Pharmacol. 38, 926–930.

Pavek, P., Ceckova, M., Staud, F., 2009. Variation of drug kinetics in pregnancy. Curr. Drug Metab. 10, 520–529.

Rosa, F.W., 1984. Virilization of the female fetus with maternal danazol exposure. Am. J. Obstet. Gynecol. 149, 99–100.

Rubin, P.C., Butters, L., McCabe, R., et al., 1987. The influence of pregnancy on drug action; concentration-effect modelling with propranolol. Clin. Sci. 73, 48–52.

Schaefer, C., Peters, P., Miller, R.K. (Eds.), 2014. Drugs during Pregnancy and Lactation: Treatment Options and Risk Assessment, third ed. Elsevier, Amsterdam.

Sedman, A.B., Kershaw, D.B., Bunchman, T.E., 1995. Recognition and management of angiotensin converting enzyme inhibitor fetopathy. Pediatr. Nephrol. 9, 382–385.

Tomi, M., Nishimura, T., Nakashima, E., 2011. Mother-to-fetus transfer of antiviral drugs and the involvement of transporters at the placental barrier. J. Pharm. Sci. 100, 3708–3718. https://doi.org/10.1002/jps.22642.

van den Anket, J.N., 1996. Pharmacokinetics and renal function in preterm infants. Acta Pediatr. 85, 1393–1399.

Vorhees, C.V., Weisenburger, W.P., Minck, D.R., 2001. Neurobehavioral teratogenic effects of thalidomide in rats. Neurotoxicol. Teratol. 23, 255–264.

World Health Organization (WHO), 2001. 54th World Health Assembly Global Strategy for Infant and Young Child Feeding. The Optimal Duration of Exclusive Breastfeeding. WHO, Geneva. Available at: http://apps.who.int/gb/archive/pdf_files/WHA54/ea54id4.pdf.

Zhao, C., Zhang, H., Zhang, X., et al., 2006. Prediction of milk/plasma drug concentration (M/P) ratio using support vector machine (SVM) method. Pharm. Res. 23, 41–48.

Further reading

Hale, T.W., Rowe, H.E., 2014. Medications and Mothers' Milk, sixteenth ed. Hale Publishing, Amarillo, TX.

Lee, A., 2006. Adverse Drug Reactions, second ed. Pharmaceutical Press, London.

Schaefer, C., Peters, P., Miller, R.K. (Eds.), 2014. Drugs During Pregnancy and Lactation: Treatment Options and Risk Assessment, third ed. Elsevier, Amsterdam.

Thomas, S.H., Yates, L.M., 2012. Prescribing without evidence – pregnancy. Br. J. Clin. Pharmacol. 74, 691–697.

Useful websites

Bumps (Patient Information Leaflets and Online Reporting Facility by UKTIS): Best Use of Medicines in Pregnancy: http://www.medicinesinpregnancy.org

UK Teratology Information Service (UKTIS): http://www.uktis.org

TOXBASE: http://www.toxbase.org

European Network of Teratology Information Services: https://www.entis-org.eu/

American Organisation of Teratology Information Services: OTIS/MotherToBaby: http://mothertobaby.org/

Motherisk (Canadian Teratology information service): http://www.motherisk.org

MHRA Toolkit on the Risks of Valproate Medicines in Female Patients: https://www.gov.uk/government/publications/toolkit-on-the-risks-of-valproate-medicines-in-female-patients

LactMed, National Library of Health: http://toxnet.nlm.nih.gov/cgi-bin/sis/htmlgen?LACT

Medication & Mother's Milk Online, Hale Publishing: http://www.medsmilk.com/ (subscription only).

UK Drugs in Lactation Advisory Service (UKDILAS): https://www.sps.nhs.uk/articles/ukdilas/

49 Prostate Disease

Linda Ross, Ben Challocombe and Sophie Rintoul-Hoad

Key points

Benign prostatic hyperplasia

- Benign prostatic hyperplasia is a common condition that affects only males and increases in prevalence with age.
- A combination of increased adrenergic tone in the prostatic stroma and bladder neck, as well as the anatomical effects of an enlarging prostate, can lead to lower urinary tract symptoms and bladder outflow.
- α-Adrenoceptor blocking drugs are effective in reducing symptoms and increasing flow rates.
- 5α-Reductase inhibitors reduce prostate size, improve symptoms, increase urinary flow rates and reduce the risk of development of complications such as acute urinary retention or the need for prostate surgery.
- Surgical treatments such as transurethral resection of the prostate are effective and commonly used, but other less invasive procedures are also available.

Prostate cancer

- Prostate cancer typically progresses slowly but is influenced by factors such as tumour grade, stage of the disease, comorbidities and life expectancy.
- Aetiology is multifactorial and includes age, race, and family history, with some links to dietary habits.
- Early detection is difficult because no symptoms are specific to prostate cancer, and it starts on the peripheral parts of the prostate away from the urethra.
- A combination of digital rectal examination, serum prostate-specific antigen and magnetic resonance imaging followed by prostate biopsies are used to confirm diagnosis.
- Prostate biopsies can be performed transrectally or transperineally.
- Treatment depends on the grade, volume and stage of tumour, life expectancy and patient choice.
- Curative treatments include radical prostatectomy, brachytherapy and radiotherapy.
- Hormonal treatments arrest prostate and cancer growth, but they are not a cure.

Prostatitis

- Prostatitis is classified as acute bacterial prostatitis, chronic bacterial prostatitis, chronic prostatitis/chronic pelvic pain syndrome and asymptomatic inflammatory prostatitis.
- There is no absolute diagnostic tool for prostatitis. Diagnosis is based on physical examination and clinical history.
- The pathophysiology of prostatitis is poorly understood, and the aetiology is unclear in the majority of patients.
- Prostatitis cases associated with infection or inflammation are treated with antibiotics.

- α-Adrenoceptor antagonists, analgesics and other pain-modulating agents are used for the treatment of chronic prostatitis/chronic pelvic pain syndrome.

Benign prostatic hyperplasia

Epidemiology

Benign prostatic hyperplasia (BPH) is the most common benign tumour in men and is responsible for urinary symptoms in the majority of males older than 50 years. Autopsy studies have revealed the histological presence of BPH in 50–60% of males in their 60s, increasing to 80–90% in those in their 70s and 80s (Roehrborn, 2005). By the age of 80 years, virtually all men exhibit one or more of the symptoms associated with BPH.

BPH is seen in all races, although the overall size of the prostate varies from race to race.

Pathophysiology

The prostate is a part glandular, part fibromuscular structure about the size of a walnut that surrounds the first part of the male urethra at the base of the bladder (Fig. 49.1). In simple terms, the prostate can be divided into a lobular inner zone encapsulated by an external layer. The inner transition zone is where benign hypertrophic changes are generally found, whereas most malignant changes originate in the peripheral zone.

Prostatic hypertrophy is directly related to the ageing process and to hormone activity. Within the prostate, testosterone is converted by 5α-reductase to dihydrotestosterone (DHT). DHT is five times more potent than testosterone and is responsible for stimulating growth factors that influence cell division, leading to prostatic hyperplasia and enlargement.

Histologically, depending on the predominance of the type of prostatic tissue present, prostatic hypertrophy can be stromal, fibromuscular, muscular, fibroadenomatous or fibromyoadenomatous.

As the prostate enlarges, it can compress the urethra (Fig. 49.2) and this, together with increased adrenergic tone, can lead to bladder outflow obstruction and lower urinary tract symptoms.

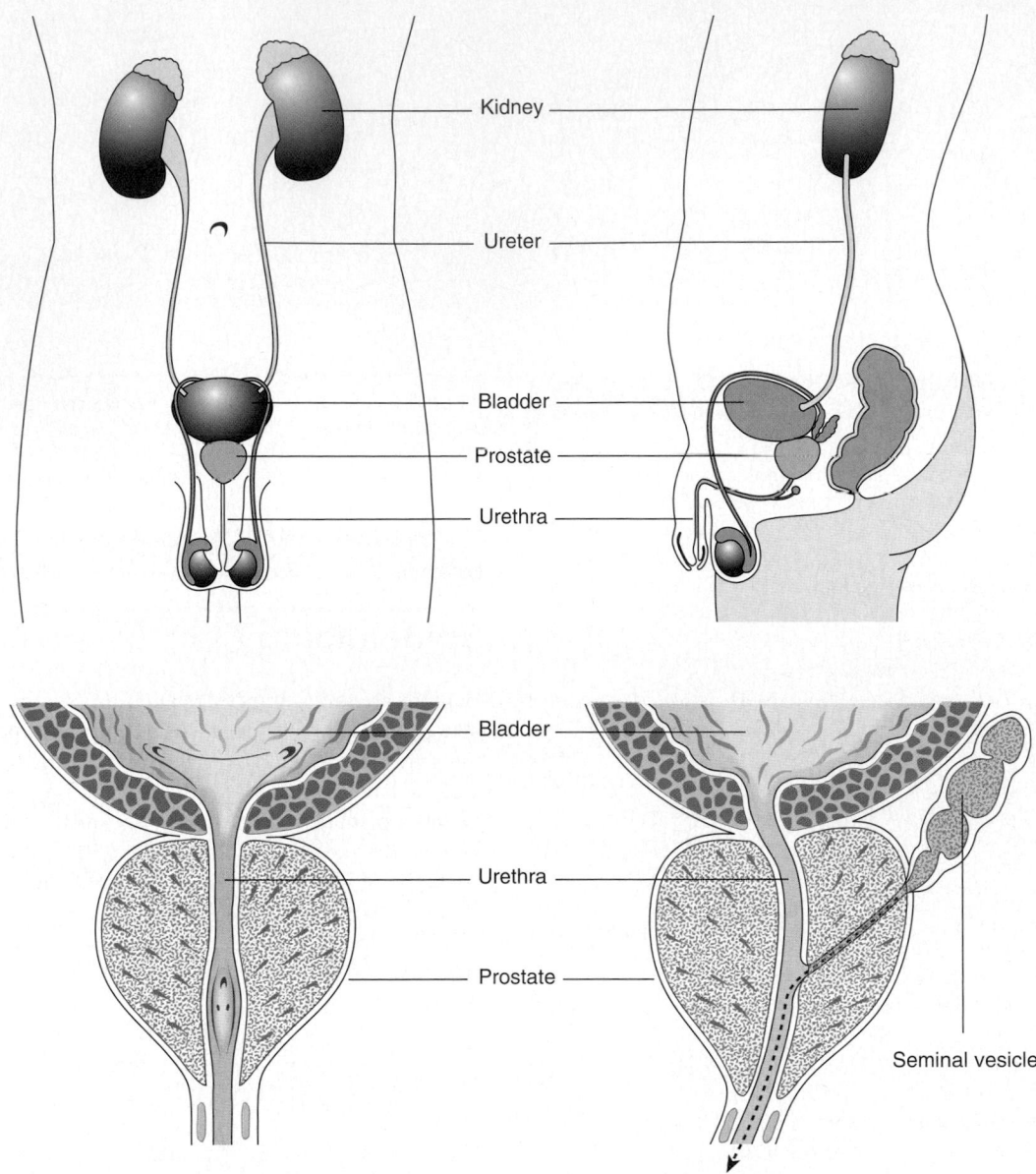

Fig. 49.1 Male urinary system demonstrating the location of the prostate.

However, not all large prostates will cause symptoms. Therefore, the term benign prostatic enlargement is used to describe the clinical features associated with urinary obstruction and lower urinary tract symptoms. BPH should be reserved for describing a histological diagnosis; but for the purpose of this chapter, we will use the term BPH.

Symptoms

Men with BPH can experience bothersome lower urinary tract symptoms that can impact negatively on their quality of life. It is important to emphasise that lower urinary tract symptoms can have different aetiologies, including bladder cancer, bladder stones, overactive bladder (OAB), urinary tract infection (UTI), urethral stricture, among others.

Lower urinary tract symptoms can be divided into symptoms of failure of urine storage (storage) and those caused by failure to empty the bladder (voiding).

Storage symptoms
- Frequency
- Nocturia
- Urgency and urge incontinence

Obstructive symptoms
- Weak urinary flow
- Intermittent stream
- Straining/needing to bear down
- Hesitancy in initiating micturition
- Incomplete emptying
- Terminal dribbling
- Post-micturition dribbling

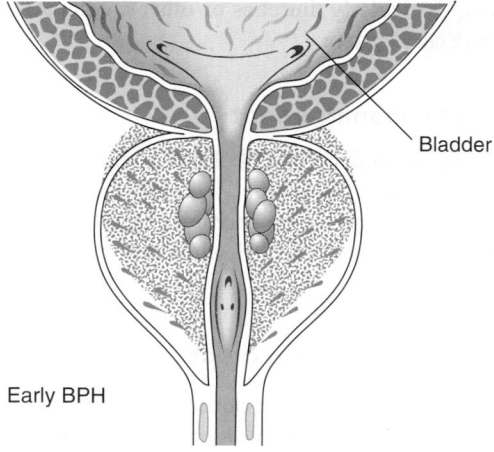

Early BPH

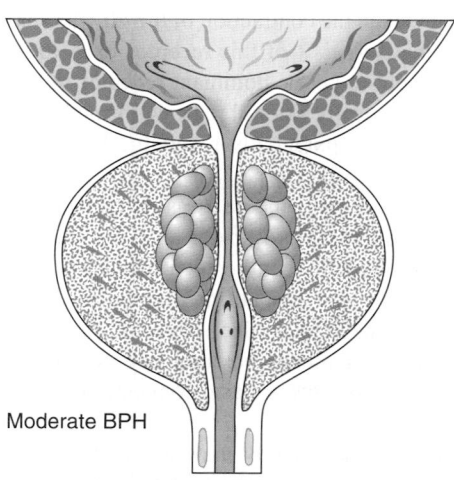

Moderate BPH

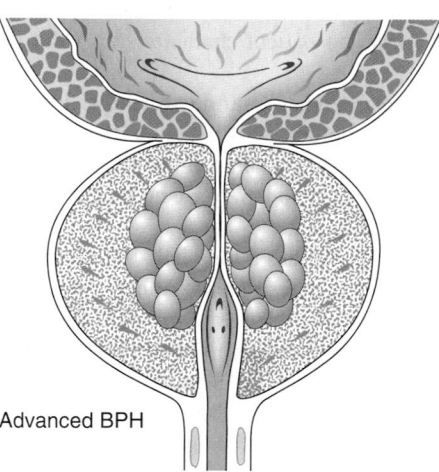

Advanced BPH

Fig. 49.2 Diagrammatic representation of the impact of prostate hyperplasia on the urethra demonstrating overgrowth of cells in the inner zone of the prostate.
BPH, Benign prostatic hyperplasia.

Examination and investigations

A range of investigations and diagnostic tests are available for the evaluation of patients with suspected BPH. Some tests are standard during the assessment of all men with lower urinary tract symptoms. Other investigations are optional and are only performed depending on the patient's presentation and the clinician's judgement.

History

A focused medical history of all men with lower urinary tract symptoms should be taken to elucidate the aetiology of their symptoms. As part of the process, lower urinary tract symptoms should be evaluated using a validated scoring tool such as the International Prostate Symptom Score (IPSS) (Barry et al., 1992) and a bladder voiding diary. This can be used to monitor the severity and progression of the disease, and assess the impact of therapy on lower urinary tract symptoms.

Physical examination

All patients who present with suspected BPH should undergo an abdominal and genital examination and a digital rectal examination (DRE) to evaluate for size, asymmetry and any change in texture, such as areas of generalised or localised firmness (nodules) which could indicate the presence of cancer. A DRE involves the examiner inserting a finger into the anal canal and palpating the prostate through the rectum wall; this assesses a small proportion of the prostate, but the area most likely to harbour cancer, the peripheral zone. It is important that patients give verbal consent for this intimate examination and should be offered the presence of a chaperone; both consent and the offer of a chaperone should be documented.

Investigations

Investigations may be carried out in the clinic to facilitate the diagnostic assessment of patients with lower urinary tract symptoms caused by BPH, and these include urinalysis, urine cultures if infection is suspected, and serum creatinine to assess renal function and establish possible upper urinary tract damage. The measurement of serum prostate-specific antigen (PSA) can be considered after counselling the patient, particularly if DRE reveals a nodular or hard prostate.

Urodynamic studies

Simple non-invasive urodynamic studies provide a surrogate, but objective, measure of bladder outflow obstruction. These include maximum flow rate and post-void residual (PVR). A flow-rate test involves patients passing urine into a specialised machine which measures the speed and volume of urine passed. Slower flow-rate curves than expected may indicate obstruction. After urination the PVR is measured on a simplified, bedside ultrasound scanning machine. Large PVRs of 500 mL, for example, are indicative of bladder dysfunction and predict a poor response to therapy.

Invasive urodynamic studies (used when there is diagnostic uncertainty) involve insertion of a fluid-filled transducer into the bladder and rectum to measure the vesical and abdominal pressures, which can be used to calculate detrusor pressure. These can then be recorded during filling and voiding

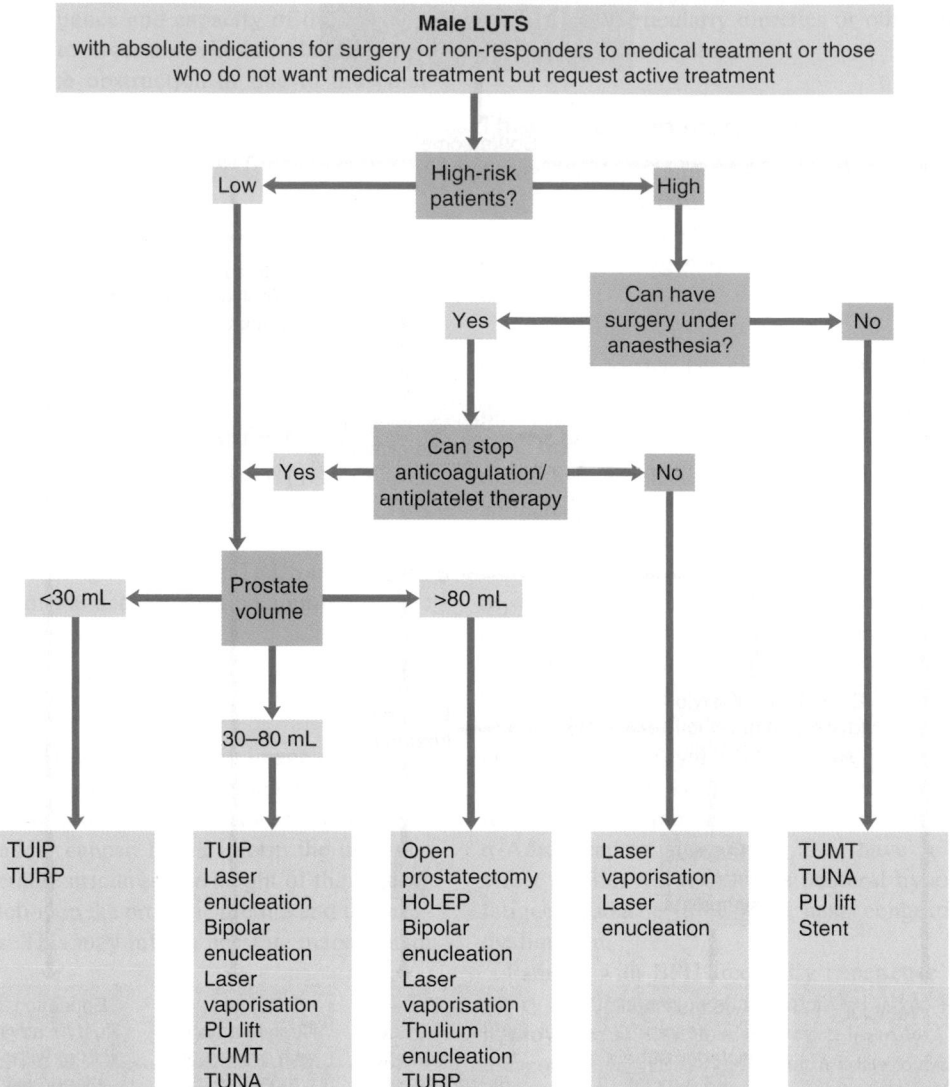

Male LUTS
with absolute indications for surgery or non-responders to medical treatment or those
who do not want medical treatment but request active treatment

High-risk patients?

Low / High

Can have surgery under anaesthesia?

Yes / No

Can stop anticoagulation/ antiplatelet therapy

Yes / No

Prostate volume

<30 mL / 30–80 mL / >80 mL

| TUIP TURP | TUIP Laser enucleation Bipolar enucleation Laser vaporisation PU lift TUMT TUNA | Open prostatectomy HoLEP Bipolar enucleation Laser vaporisation Thulium enucleation TURP | Laser vaporisation Laser enucleation | TUMT TUNA PU lift Stent |

The alternative treatments are presented in alphabetical order.
Notice: Readers are strongly recommended to read the full text that highlights the current
position of each treatment in detail.

Fig. 49.4 Treatment algorithm of bothersome lower urinary tract symptoms (LUTS) refractory to conservative/medical treatment or in cases of absolute operation indications (Gravas et al., 2017). Laser vaporisation includes GreenLight, thulium and diode lasers vaporization. Laser enucleation includes holmium and thulium laser enucleation.
HoLEP, Holmium laser enucleation; TUIP, transurethral incision of the prostate; TUMT, transurethral microwave therapy; TUNA, transurethral needle ablation; TURP, transurethral resection of the prostate.

5α-Reductase inhibitors

The primary androgen responsible for the development and progression of BPH is DHT. There are two isoenzymes of 5α-reductase: type 1 is found in most 5α-reductase-producing tissues such as the liver, skin and hair; type 2 is predominant in genital tissue, including the prostate. 5α-Reductase inhibitors downregulate prostate growth by blocking the conversion of testosterone to the more potent DHT.

The two agents currently available in this group are finasteride and dutasteride. Both have been shown to reduce prostate volume, to improve symptom scores and flow rates, and to reduce the incidence of complications such as acute urinary retention and the need for surgical intervention to treat BPH (Roehrborn et al., 2000, 2002). Improvements in lower urinary tract symptoms are normally seen after the first 6 months of treatment and are sustained during continuous treatment (Lam et al., 2003).

Finasteride. Finasteride is a type 2, 5α-reductase inhibitor that can reduce prostate size, improve symptom scores and increase urinary flow. Those most likely to benefit are men with a prostate larger than 40 mL (Gravas et al., 2017). Side effects

Box 49.1 Advice for the management of lower urinary tract symptoms

- Limit fluid consumption before going out and before going to bed (to reduce urinary frequency and nocturia).
- Reduce alcohol and caffeine intake.
- Schedule toilet visits.
- Manage constipation.
- Review medication (including diuretics and other medicines that can affect the urinary system).
- Attempt bladder training (encourage patient to go longer between voiding and increase the volume voided).
- Use distraction techniques (practice breathing exercises and penile squeezing to control symptoms of irritation).

include decreased libido, impotence, reduced ejaculatory volume and, less commonly, gynaecomastia and breast tenderness. Serum concentrations of PSA may be reduced by 50% in the first year of treatment with finasteride (Gravas et al., 2017), a fact which must be taken into account when attempting to interpret the PSA concentration in men with suspected prostate cancer (PC).

Dutasteride. Dutasteride inhibits both type 1 and type 2 isoenzymes of 5α-reductase. Dutasteride decreases prostate volume and reduces the risk of progression to serious complications of BPH. Lower urinary tract symptoms also improve after 6 months of treatment. Dutasteride is well tolerated, although side effects which include erectile and ejaculatory dysfunction and breast enlargement occur with similar frequency to finasteride.

Antimuscarinic receptor antagonists

The detrusor muscle is stimulated by the parasympathetic nervous system, whose main neurotransmitter is acetylcholine, which stimulates muscarinic cholinoreceptors on the smooth muscle cells. There are five muscarinic receptor subtypes (M1–M5); M2 and M3 are the main ones in the detrusor muscle.

The following agents are currently available for treating storage symptoms: darifenacin, fesoterodine, oxybutynin, propiverine, solifenacin, tolterodine and trospium.

Originally it was believed that prostate-specific drugs should not be used to treat lower urinary tract symptoms in men, and antimuscarinics were therefore mainly tested in females. However, a subanalysis of patients in an open-label trial of tolterodine for OAB showed that age, but not gender, has an impact on urgency, frequency or urgency incontinence (Michel et al., 2002). Tolterodine can significantly reduce urgency incontinence, daytime or 24-hour frequency and urgency-related voiding, and improve patient perception of treatment benefit.

Side effects of these drugs include dry mouth, constipation, micturition difficulties, nasopharyngitis and dizziness.

Phosphodiesterase 5 inhibitors

Whilst phosphodiesterase (PDE) type 5 inhibitors (PDE5Is) increase intracellular cyclic guanosine monophosphate, thus reducing smooth muscle tone of the detrusor, prostate and urethra, they may also reduce chronic inflammation in the prostate and bladder.

Tadalafil, 5 mg once daily, is the only selective oral PDE5I that is currently licensed for the treatment of signs and symptoms of benign hyperplasia and lower urinary tract symptoms in men. Tadalafil is contraindicated in patients prescribed some medicines (e.g. nitrates, nicorandil, doxazosin or terazosin) and in some medical conditions (e.g. unstable angina). Side effects include back pain, dyspepsia, flushing, headache, myalgia, and nausea and vomiting.

β₃-Adrenoceptor agonists

Mirabegron is a β₃-adrenoceptor agonist which activates β₃-adrenoceptors, causing the bladder to relax, which helps it to fill and also to store urine. It is licensed for the treatment of urinary frequency, urgency and urge incontinence associated with OAB syndrome. The usual starting dosage is 50 mg once daily, but this needs to be reduced to 25 mg once daily in patients with mild hepatic impairment and those receiving inhibitors of CYP3A4. The most common side effects are tachycardia and UTIs.

Vasopressin analogue

Desmopressin, an antidiuretic hormone arginine vasopressin, regulates water homeostasis. It can be used for the treatment of nocturia due to nocturnal polyuria. Desmopressin is taken once daily before sleeping. Patients can vary in the dose they require; therefore, it is usually initiated at a low dose and increased gradually. Patients should be informed to avoid drinking fluids at least 1 hour before and for 8 hours after dosing.

Combination therapy

It is well established that α-adrenoceptor antagonists are best for managing acute symptoms but have no impact on reducing the risk of complications such as acute urinary retention or progression to prostate surgery. In contrast, 5α-reductase inhibitors have little impact on short-term acute symptoms but reduce prostate size and improve urinary flow and obstructive symptoms in the long-term. Furthermore, α-adrenoceptor antagonists are effective regardless of prostate volume, whereas the 5α-reductase inhibitors are more suited for the management of lower urinary tract symptoms in men with large prostates. In terms of long-term benefits, continued treatment with 5α-reductase inhibitors decreases the risk of acute urinary retention and BPH-related surgery. Therefore, it appears logical to use a combination of an α-adrenoceptor antagonist and a 5α-reductase inhibitor to manage acute symptoms and reduce progression of BPH.

The benefits of using a combination of doxazosin and finasteride compared with monotherapy have been demonstrated in more than 3000 men (McConnell et al., 2003). Similarly, the CombAT trial (Roehrborn et al., 2010) involved nearly 5000 men with moderate-to-severe symptoms of BPH and prostate enlargement treated with a combination of dutasteride and tamsulosin. This study demonstrated a significant improvement in BPH symptoms over a 4-year period when compared with either agent used alone. The combination was also found to reduce acute urinary retention and progression to BPH-related surgery, and although superior to tamsulosin with respect to these complications, combination therapy was not better than dutasteride. Overall, the adverse events associated with combination therapy were few and treatment was well tolerated.

Combination therapy with an α-adrenoceptor antagonist and a 5α-reductase inhibitor has now been widely adopted into routine practice for the early management of lower urinary tract symptoms and to reduce progression of BPH. A combined preparation of tamsulosin 400 micrograms and dutasteride 500 mg exists in a single tablet.

Combination therapy with an α-adrenoceptor antagonist and muscarinic receptor antagonists has been explored in several randomised controlled trials and prospective studies. It is useful for lower urinary tract symptoms in men with OAB and presumed BPH or as a sequential treatment for storage symptoms persisting whilst on an $α_1$-blocker alone. The risk of urinary retention does not increase whilst using antimuscarinics. The commonest side effect is xerostomia (dry mouth).

Phytotherapy

A number of plant extracts are reputed to be effective in the management of symptoms of BPH. They include saw palmetto berry *(Serenoa repens)*, African plum tree *(Pygeum africanum)*, stinging nettle *(Urtica dioica)* and rye grass pollen. Their mechanism of action remains unclear but may exert an anti-inflammatory effect by inhibition of prostanoid formation and perhaps produce some degree of inhibition of 5α-reductase. Most of the data available to support the use of plant extracts are derived from poorly designed studies. Because evidence to assess efficacy and safety is lacking, phytotherapy remedies are not currently recommended by international guidelines for the management of BPH.

Surgical treatments

Surgical intervention is offered to men with lower urinary tract symptoms caused by BPH that have not successfully responded to medical treatment and are affecting the individual's quality of life. Surgery is also indicated in patients who experience complications such as intractable or recurrent urinary retention, renal impairment, persistent haematuria, recurrent UTIs or bladder stones. BPH can affect men of any age but increasingly affects men of older age who may have serious comorbidities. Therefore, the choice of which surgical intervention to offer must be appropriate for that patient. Clear information should be given to patients who are undergoing surgery regarding the risks, benefits and expected post-operative recovery.

Transurethral resection of the prostate. Transurethral resection of the prostate (TURP) is a common and effective procedure which achieves a high level of improvement in symptoms and flow rate. It is the preferred surgical intervention in men with a prostate volume between 30 and 80 mL. Sections of prostate are removed under vision using electrical wire loops attached to a tubelike telescope (resectoscope) inserted into the urethra. The tissue removed is collected for histological assessment.

There is a small incidence of perioperative mortality associated with TURP, along with complications such as bleeding, UTI and pain on urination. Importantly, there is a risk of electrolyte disturbance as a result of the irrigation solution glycine, resulting in 'TUR syndrome'. Reducing the risks of this includes 1-hour maximum resection time, height of irrigation fluid and education of health professionals to enable early recognition. Long-term complications include stress incontinence, urethral and bladder neck strictures, retrograde ejaculation and erectile dysfunction.

Conventionally, monopolar diathermy is used; however, newer bipolar resection equipment has the advantage of using saline as the irrigating fluid. This has a theoretical advantage of reducing risk of TUR syndrome and ability for longer resection times. Currently, there are no clear differences in outcomes and complications between the two techniques (Hueber et al., 2011).

Open prostatectomy. Open prostatectomy involves the surgical removal of an enlarged prostate. Typically, an incision is made through the lower abdomen, although sometimes the incision is between the rectum and the base of the penis. This procedure is now performed infrequently and is restricted to very enlarged prostate glands (larger than 100 mL) and those with large bladder stones or bladder diverticula (Stoevelaar and McDonnell, 2001). Open prostatectomy requires a longer hospital stay than transurethral resection and is associated with a higher incidence of bleeding and other complications.

Photoselective vaporisation of the prostate. Photoselective vaporisation of the prostate uses an Nd:YAG laser that passes through a specific crystal which doubles the laser's frequency, resulting in green light (Zorn and Liberman, 2011). This high energy vaporises the prostatic tissue and creates a channel. Its advantages include reduced post-operative bleeding leading to early removal of catheter; it can be offered to patients who cannot reduce or stop their anticoagulant medications.

Holmium laser enucleation of the prostate. Holmium laser enucleation of the prostate (HoLEP) technique has evolved to use Holmium:YAG laser to enucleate each lobe of the prostate, then use a morcellator to remove tissue (Aho, 2013). It has been shown to be the preferred method for treating large prostates (>80–100 g), with a very low incidence of recurrence and blood transfusion. It is the current gold standard treatment for men with symptomatic very large BPH.

These newer techniques such as bipolar TURP, photovaporisation of the prostate and HoLEP have shown efficacy outcomes comparable with conventional techniques, yet a reduced complication rate (Cornu et al., 2015). However, they are associated with a surgical learning curve and new equipment; therefore, the standard for many hospitals is monopolar TURP.

Prostate artery embolisation

Prostate artery embolisation (PAE) is a new, minimally invasive technique performed by interventional radiologists; prostatic arteries are selectively embolised (blocked) leading to reduced blood supply and subsequently reduced prostatic volume. PAE does not require a general anaesthetic, there is no

Table 49.1 Common therapeutic problems and proposed management strategies in benign prostatic hyperplasia

Problem	Solution
Patient taking α-blocker still symptomatic after 2 weeks	Patients should be advised that it may take 2–6 weeks before symptomatic treatment relief is seen
Patient taking an α-adrenoceptor blocker complains of cardiovascular adverse effects such as dizziness, syncope, palpitations, tachycardia or angina	These side effects are more likely in elderly patients. They are most common after the first dose and reflect the hypotensive effects of the drugs. They can be reduced by titrating the dose or using more uroselective drugs such as tamsulosin
Sexual dysfunction	Decreased libido or impotence can occur in patients taking finasteride and dutasteride. Abnormal ejaculation can be caused by α-blockers. Tamsulosin in particular can cause a dry climax (retrograde ejaculation). Patients should be forewarned when discussing treatment options
Patient taking finasteride notices breast enlargement	Unilateral or bilateral gynaecomastia is a frequently reported side effect with finasteride and patients need to be counselled accordingly when discussing treatment options
Patient taking finasteride or dutasteride has a sexual partner who is pregnant	Exposure to semen should be avoided as both drugs can cause abnormalities to genitalia in a male fetus. The patient should be advised to use a condom

upper limit of prostatic size that can be effectively treated by PAE and clinical success rates are in the order of 80% when bilateral embolisation is possible (Mirakhur and McWilliams, 2017). However, this is new technology with ongoing multicentre, randomised controlled trials that will hopefully provide the evidence needed to better understand its contraindications and longer-term outcomes.

UroLift

The UroLift system uses adjustable, permanent implants to pull excess prostatic tissue laterally so that it does not narrow or block the urethra (National Institute for Health and Care Excellence (NICE), 2015). In this way, the device is designed to relieve symptoms of urinary outflow obstruction without cutting or removing tissue and aims to avoid sexual dysfunction. It can be used in a day-case setting in men aged 50 years and older and who have a prostate of less than 100 mL without an obstructing middle lobe.

Patient care

Patients generally seek medical help for BPH because of the impact of symptoms on their quality of life. Most men tolerate a high degree of symptoms and impact on daily activities before they seek help. Table 49.1 lists some common therapeutic problems in the management of BPH. Patients should receive information about the management options available, the investigations that they need to undergo and possible treatment outcomes and adverse effects. Patients who are receiving drug therapy should receive specific information about their treatment, including potential benefits, timeline of expected outcomes and possible side effects.

There are two websites which produce particularly useful educational material on prostatic disease: the Men's Health Forum (http://www.menshealthforum.org.uk/) and Prostate Cancer UK section on BPH (http://prostatecanceruk.org/).

Prostate cancer

Epidemiology

PC is the second most common cancer in the world and the most common form of cancer in men. Incidence varies from country to country, with the highest rates in Australia/New Zealand and Northern America and in Western and Northern Europe; they remain low in Eastern and South Central Asia (Globocan, n.d.). In the UK, nearly a quarter of all new male cancer diagnoses are of the prostate. The lifetime risk of PC is 1 in 8 in males in the UK.

The aetiology of PC is multifactorial. Testosterone and DHT have an important role in the disease because PC does not develop in males who undergo castration before puberty. Other factors which can influence the risk of development of PC include age, family history, diet and other factors.

Age

PC is rare before 50 years of age in Caucasians and before 40 years in Africans, but after this age, the incidence and mortality increase exponentially with every passing decade. Most cases are detected around the age of 70 years.

Family history

Presence of PC in a first-degree relative or in multiple family members who need not be first-degree relatives increases the risk. Inheritance of a susceptible gene or polymorphism of gene may be responsible for this.

Diet

Although there is no compelling evidence to prove the direct influence of diet, high intake of fat, red meat and dairy produce, typically the main sources of dietary fatty acids in a Western diet, have individually been linked with PC. The low incidence of PC in China and Japan may be because of their use of soya bean products which contain isoflavones and inhibit protein tyrosine kinases that are responsible for cell proliferation.

Other factors

Other factors include exposure to cadmium (found in cigarette smoke), pesticides, alkaline batteries, radionuclides and heavy metals.

Pathophysiology

The growth and differentiation of cells in the prostate is under androgen control. In the prostate, free testosterone diffuses into the epithelial cells, where it is converted to DHT. Various growth factors are present in stromal cells, and the interaction of these with epithelial cells can play a role in cell proliferation and growth. The development of PC is generally a slow, gradual process where cellular structure changes from normal through dysplastic to cancer. High-grade prostatic intra-epithelial neoplasia represents the precancerous stage of cellular proliferation in prostate cells and can be detected by biopsy. It can predate carcinoma by 10 years or more. There is no link between PC and BPH, but they can co-exist.

Screening

Population-based screening based on PSA levels is prevalent in the USA, and the annual incidence there has doubled due to this. In the UK, screening is not advocated because due to the nature of PC, most patients will not be symptomatic in their lifetime and screening hugely increases the rates of over-treatment with only limited effects on mortality. Targeted testing of at-risk men with a racial or family history is appropriate.

Symptoms

Clinical symptoms of PC are similar to those for BPH, and there are no symptoms which correlate specifically to early PC. As more than 50% of men older than 50 years have prostate-related symptoms, it is difficult to detect early PC. Advanced PC typically presents with symptoms of urethral and bladder outlet obstruction, anaemia, renal failure, weight loss, haematuria or bone pain.

Examination and investigation

Physical examination

A DRE is an important diagnostic tool for PC with an estimated sensitivity of more than 60%. A palpable tumour will have a distinctive texture, but the accuracy of detection may depend on the

Table 49.2 Age-specific levels of prostate-specific antigen

Age (years)	Prostate-specific antigen (ng/mL)
40–49	≤2.5
50–59	≤3.5
60–69	≤4.5
>70	≤6.5

experience of the clinician. False-positive results can occur in the presence of BPH or cysts.

Imaging

A prostate magnetic resonance imaging (MRI) scan is being increasingly used to detect PC. Estimates of the sensitivity of MRI for the detection of cancer vary widely depending on method of analysis used and the definition of significant disease. Estimates using T2-weighted sequences and endorectal coils vary from 60% to 96% (Kirkham et al., 2006). Specificity is not yet good enough to consider the use of MRI in screening but can be used to help target suspicious lesions and in patient follow-up.

Computed tomography (CT) images of the pelvis and isotope bone scan are useful to stage PC, but they are not effective as diagnostic tools.

Prostate-specific antigen

Measurement of PSA is an accurate and clinically useful biochemical marker because it is specific to prostate tissue and produced by the columnar epithelial cells in the prostate gland. Unfortunately, PSA is prostate but not PC specific, and damage to the internal architecture of the prostate can result in its release. As a consequence, it is not a useful tool for diagnosing cancer on its own, but it is useful in monitoring the effect of treatment or tumour progression in untreated patients. Generally, PSA is high in PC, but it can sometimes be low in high-grade malignancy. The standard assay for PSA measures total PSA and includes all molecular forms. The proportion of bound and unbound PSA can be calculated as a percentage; it is thought that a higher proportion of free PSA suggests a lower risk of PC.

Age-specific ranges are available (Table 49.2) and help make it a better predictor, but this is only a rough guide because variations occur due to racial difference. There is no threshold for PSA below which PC cannot be found.

Prostate biopsy

Prostate biopsy is a definitive method to diagnose PC; a sample, or 'core', of the prostate is sent to the laboratory for histological analysis. TRUS-guided biopsy will help obtain samples from the peripheral and transitional zones of the prostate and other suspicious areas. A traditional TRUS-guided biopsy involves random sampling of the prostate with 10–12 biopsies of the peripheral zone. More recently, areas suspicious for PC as seen on TRUS or MRI are the focus of biopsy.

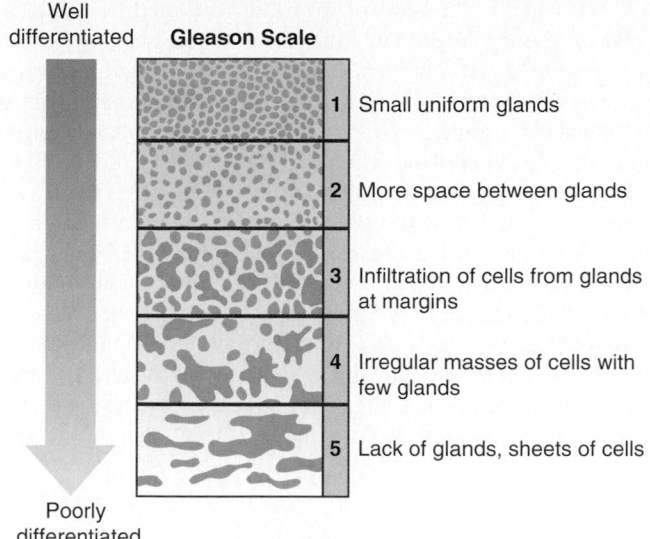

Well differentiated

Gleason Scale

1 Small uniform glands

2 More space between glands

3 Infiltration of cells from glands at margins

4 Irregular masses of cells with few glands

5 Lack of glands, sheets of cells

Poorly differentiated

Fig. 49.5 Gleason scale.

Transperineal biopsies, also known as 'template biopsy', is a new method for performing strategic biopsies of the prostate gland using a 'mapping' grid. This also increases the number of prostate biopsies taken; it is performed under general anaesthetic. It can be advantageous in relation to areas where TRUS biopsy commonly fails to reach. The peripheral zone of the prostate is the location where the majority of the PC occurs. It is difficult to identify PC from transurethral resection of the prostate specimens because not much of it occurs in the transitional zone.

Until 2016 the Gleason scale (Gleason and Mellinger, 1974) was the most widely accepted histological grading system used in the UK, USA and Europe. Histological examination of biopsy tissue is undertaken to identify cancer cells, and these are scored from 1 to 5 depending on the different pattern of glandular tissue (Fig. 49.5). A score of 1 corresponds to well-differentiated cells, whereas a score of 5 corresponds to poorly differentiated cells; the higher the score, the more aggressive the cancer. The number for the two most common types of cell in the sample are added together to get a Gleason score. The score ranges from 2 to 10. The score was used to help predict the future behaviour of the tumour and determine the treatment required.

In 2014 it was recognised that the Gleason scale needed modification. A consensus conference was held and a new scoring system was proposed (Box 49.2) (Epstein et al., 2016) that has also been accepted by the World Health Organization.

Cancer staging

Results from a DRE, biopsy and scan are used to identify the extent of the cancer. The tumour volume, whether there is invasion into or through the capsule, and spread to lymph nodes or bone are all taken into consideration for staging. Staging based on the tumour, node, metastasis system is a classification accepted worldwide (Epstein et al., 2005). Based on the tumour, node, metastasis classification, PC can be classified into: (1) localised disease, (2) locally advanced disease or (3) advanced/metastatic disease.

Box 49.2 Histological definition of new grading system (Epstein et al., 2016)

Grade group 1 (Gleason score ≥6) – only individual discrete, well-formed glands
Grade group 2 (Gleason score 3 + 4 = 7) – predominantly well-formed glands with lesser component of poorly formed/fused/cribriform glands
Grade group 3 (Gleason score 4 + 3 = 7) – predominantly poorly formed/fused/cribriform glands with lesser component of well-formed glands[a]
Grade group 4 (Gleason score 4 + 4 = 8; 3 + 5 = 8; 5 + 3 = 8) – only poorly formed/fused/cribriform glands or predominantly well-formed glands and lesser component lacking glands[b] or predominantly lacking glands and lesser component of well-formed glands[b]
Grade group 5 (Gleason score 9–10) – lacks gland formation (or with necrosis) with or without poorly formed/fused/cribriform glands[a]

[a]For cases with >95% poorly formed/fused/cribriform glands or lack of glands on a core or at radical prostatectomy, the component of <5% well-formed glands is not factored into the grade.
[b]Poorly formed/fused/cribriform glands can be a more minor component.

Treatment

The factors that must be considered to aid the treatment decision relate to the tumour and the patient.

Tumour: staging result, histology, scoring system result and the PSA concentration
Patient: age at diagnosis, life expectancy and the presence of comorbidities such as cardiovascular disease, chronic obstructive pulmonary disease and diabetes

Fig. 49.6 illustrates the site of action of some treatments used in PC.

Localised prostate cancer

Established treatments with curative intent

Active surveillance. It is difficult to distinguish PC which may not cause any problems from that which may grow and spread aggressively. Curative treatment can improve longevity but has side effects which include impotence and incontinence, and can affect the quality of life of the individual. Patients on active surveillance are monitored closely by repeated testing of PSA levels, DRE and biopsy with the intention to make a radical intervention to treat if there is disease progression. A 20-year outcome study following conservative management of localised PC found that the annual mortality rates did not support aggressive treatment (Albertsen et al., 2005). Although active surveillance can spare side effects of treatment without compromising survival, regular biopsies used to monitor the disease can also be uncomfortable and carry a risk of infection. The optimal schedule for measuring PSA and repeating biopsies is unclear.

Radical prostatectomy. Radical prostatectomy is the treatment of choice for localised PC, and the procedure involves

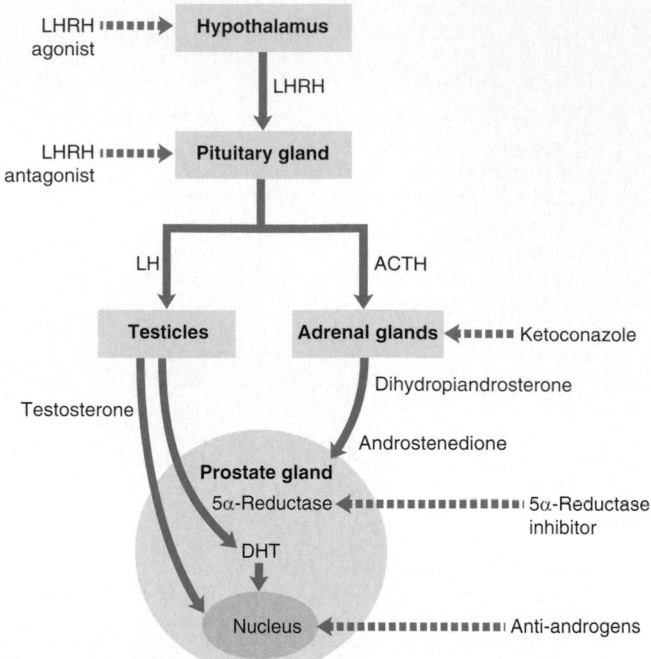

Fig. 49.6 Diagrammatic representation of the site of action of some treatments used in prostate cancer.

the total removal of a prostate, seminal vesicle, distal vasa, ejaculatory ducts and prostatic urethra. In the open procedure it is performed by the retro pubic or perineal approach based on the surgeon's choice. Laparoscopic prostatectomy, and more recently robotic-assisted laparoscopy, have been developed and are now the commonest treatment modalities. The most common complications of prostatectomy are blood loss, post-operative thromboembolism, urinary incontinence, impotence and rectal injury.

Radical external-beam radiotherapy. Radiotherapy is used for locally confined disease and more recently for locally advanced disease state as well. In this treatment high-energy photons produced by a linear accelerator are targeted at the prostate. Sometimes special particles such as protons and heavy ions are used and have advantages over photons in terms of dose distribution. The side effects of radiotherapy include impotence, genitourinary stricture, rectal bleeding, haematuria and incontinence.

Interstitial brachytherapy. With interstitial brachytherapy radioactive isotope seeds are placed in the prostate under ultrasound control. These implants can emit radiation of low energy over several weeks and can be temporary or permanent. This treatment has the potential advantage of less erectile dysfunction than other treatments.

Minimally invasive procedures

Several minimally invasive procedures are in the development stage, and although they may be used in some centres, there are no medium- or long-term follow-up data to prove efficacy. The various procedures are detailed in the following subsections.

Cryosurgical ablation of prostate. Cryosurgical ablation involves freezing the prostate which results in cell death by protein denaturation, direct rupture of cellular membranes and apoptosis. Freezing is achieved by placing 12–15 cryoneedles into the prostate guided by a transrectal ultrasonograph and using the cryoneedles to create freeze–thaw cycles using temperatures of −40 °C.

High-intensity focused ultrasound. In high-intensity focused ultrasound, ultrasound waves from a transducer are focused on the prostate tissue to cause damage to the cells by mechanical and thermal effects. The malignant tissue is subjected to temperatures above 65 °C, and hence is destroyed by coagulative necrosis.

Radiofrequency interstitial tumour ablation. Radiofrequency interstitial tumour ablation involves a needle electrode being placed inside the prostate and radiofrequency waves being delivered through it to heat the tissue up to 100 °C, thereby causing necrosis.

Non-curative intent: 'Watchful waiting'

The 'watching waiting' approach implies that the patient is observed for symptomatic progression and will only receive palliative treatment when clinical symptoms develop. Because the disease often progresses slowly, watchful waiting is an option for patients with early disease because it maintains their quality of life and avoids complications related to surgery or radiation therapy. On the downside, it is not a curative option; the cancer can metastasise, be a source of pain and reduce life expectancy.

Locally advanced prostate cancer

Hormonal therapy/androgen deprivation therapy

In locally advanced disease involving areas outside the capsule, there is an increased risk of relapse and lymph node metastasis after prostatectomy. Testosterone (an androgen) is thought to drive PC; therefore, there are available treatments to reduce available androgens (see Fig. 49.6).

Androgens are produced both in the testes (95%) under the stimulation of luteinising hormone (LH) and luteinising hormone–releasing hormone (LHRH) from the pituitary gland, and in the adrenal glands (5%) under the stimulation of adrenocorticotropic hormone (ACTH). The androgens produced by the adrenal gland are hormone precursors that are enzymatically converted to testosterone and DHT in prostatic and peripheral tissue. Because testosterone is a well-known aetiologic factor associated with PC, it follows that testosterone deprivation can be utilised as part of treatment strategies. In practice this can be achieved by either surgical or medical castration with the period of hormonal control varying from a few months to years.

Medical castration. A number of drugs can be used to reduce the levels of testosterone to those achieved by castration.

Luteinising hormone–releasing hormone agonists. LHRH is released in the hypothalamus and stimulates the secretion of LH by binding to the LHRH receptors in the pituitary. This LHRH receptor complex is normally broken down by enzymes which lead to the release of LH and frees the receptors for further binding with LHRH. LHRH agonists are synthetic analogues that bind to the LHRH receptor, and the complex formed is resistant to enzymatic action. Thus, they maintain a continuous presence on the receptor and render the pituitary gland refractory to hypothalamic regulation compared with the pulsatile release in normal individuals. Continuous administration of LHRH agonists exhibits a biphasic response. There is an initial increase in LH and testosterone release which may cause a 'tumour flare' in metastatic disease followed by a fall over the following 1–2 weeks because of the negative feedback down-regulation and decrease in LHRH release as the receptors are continuously occupied. 'Tumour flare-up' is prevented by first initiating treatment with an anti-androgen before the use of LHRH agonist. The anti-androgen is then continued for a further 2 weeks. Currently available LHRH analogues include buserelin (nasal spray), goserelin, triptorelin and leuprorelin. Goserelin and leuprorelin are administered subcutaneously at monthly or 3 monthly intervals, whereas triptorelin is administered intramuscularly at monthly, 3 monthly or 6 monthly intervals.

Anti-androgens. Anti-androgens competitively inhibit the effect of androgens peripherally by competing with testosterone and DHT for binding sites in the prostate. This results in inhibition of cell growth and apoptosis. Based on their chemical structure, the anti-androgens can be further divided into steroidal agents, which include cyproterone acetate, megestrol acetate and medroxyprogesterone, and non-steroidal agents such as nilutamide, flutamide and bicalutamide.

The steroidal agents also possess progestational activity and inhibit LH secretion by acting centrally on the pituitary, thereby reducing serum testosterone levels. The non-steroidal agents do not possess this additional property. Cyproterone is the most widely used steroidal agent normally administered in two or three daily doses of 100 mg despite having a half-life of 30–40 hours. It can be used to treat the hot flushes associated with LHRH agonists or orchiectomy. Side effects include hepatoxicity, loss of libido and potency, fatigue and depression. Use of medroxyprogesterone and megestrol is limited because of less favourable outcomes in clinical trials compared with cyproterone.

Non-steroidal anti-androgens are used in patients who wish to preserve their quality of life as they do not suppress testosterone and hence preserve libido, physical performance and bone mineral density. The disadvantage of bicalutamide, flutamide and nilutamide is a reduced survival when used as monotherapy because of a gradual rise in testosterone. All three agents have side effects of gynaecomastia, gastro-intestinal upset, idiopathic hepatocellular toxicity and haematuria. Bicalutamide has a better safety and tolerability profile compared with nilutamide and flutamide (Inverson, 2002) and is the commonest one seen in clinical practice. Some trials show that non-steroidal anti-androgens used in combination with surgical castration or LHRH agonists bring about complete or total androgen blockade by also reducing the production of androgens from the adrenal glands, which normally accounts for 5% of the body's production, thereby conferring a small survival advantage.

LHRH agonists and the non-steroidal anti-androgens have been used as neoadjuvant treatment to reduce tumour size before further surgery or other treatment. They can also be used as adjuvant treatment given in addition to primary/initial treatment to reach a treatment goal, or with radiotherapy to improve disease-free and overall survival in patients with locally advanced disease.

Metastatic prostate cancer

Metastatic PC infers the spread of cancer to other areas of the body; it is commonly spread via blood to the bones (90%), lung, liver and adrenals plus via the lymphatic system. Bone metastases commonly appear in the vertebrae and ribs, as well as skull, thorax, pelvis, spine and proximal long bones. X-rays typically show PC metastases as sclerotic lesions, but they appear late. A bone scan or CT/positron emission tomography imaging can be used to detect areas of skeletal metastases, but can have false-positive results. In some patients with vertebral metastases, spinal cord compression can occur and is treated as an oncological emergency.

The following subsections discuss options to arrest PC spread by suppressing the testosterone axis, but these options are not curative and eventually castrate-resistant disease will develop in most patients.

Luteinising hormone–releasing hormone agonists

Patients with metastatic cancer of the prostate usually respond to treatment with LHRH agonists and use is as described earlier for locally advanced disease.

Surgical castration

Surgical castration by bilateral orchiectomy is the treatment of choice for metastatic disease. Advantages include its low cost and morbidity, with testosterone levels falling to castration levels within 5–12 hours of surgery. The disadvantages include psychological trauma, its irreversible nature and the fact that nearly half experience side effects including loss of libido and potency, hot flushes, and bone and muscle loss.

Other palliative treatments

Luteinising hormone–releasing hormone antagonists. LHRH antagonists, which include degarelix and abarelix, work by competitively binding to LHRH receptors in the pituitary, thereby suppressing LH release and creating a rapid and sustained decrease in testosterone levels. They do not cause an initial surge in testosterone levels, and hence there is no risk of 'tumour flare' or need for short-term treatment with anti-androgens, unlike the LHRH agonists. Abarelix requires an induction regimen followed by monthly injections, and use is associated with anaphylactic reactions. Degarelix is given as a monthly depot injection; the most common side effect is a local reaction at the injection site such as swelling and erythema. Degarelix has a place in metastatic PC where the patient is acutely symptomatic with impending spinal cord compression, ureteric obstruction and urinary retention. Degarelix reduces testosterone, LH and PSA levels faster than LHRH agonists and reduces microsurges of testosterone.

Bisphosphonates. Skeletal involvement in PC can be disease related or due to androgen depletion therapy. Bisphosphonates are pyrophosphates that inhibit osteoclast activity in bones, and hence prevent and treat bone lesions. They are administered by intravenous infusion. Pamidronate prevents bone loss, whereas zoledronate not only increases bone mass while on androgen depletion therapy, but also reduces skeletal complications in patients with bone metastasis secondary to PC (Saad and Schulman, 2004).

Bisphosphonates are also recommended for pain relief when analgesics and palliative radiotherapy to bone have failed. Dental examination needs to be carried out before commencing treatment with a bisphosphonate because of the risk of osteonecrosis of the jaw in those with a history of dental trauma, infection or surgery.

Ketoconazole. This anti-fungal can be used at a higher dose than is normal for its anti-fungal effect to inhibit the testicular and adrenal cytochrome P450 enzyme synthesis of sex sterols. It has a rapid onset of action, is usually prescribed at a dosage of 400 mg three times daily and is generally used at the time of acute presentation of metastatic PC. Because it causes adrenal suppression, hydrocortisone supplementation is necessary. Side effects of ketoconazole include drug-induced toxicity, adrenal suppression and hepatotoxicity.

Dexamethasone. Dexamethasone is used if spinal cord compression is suspected and in the palliative setting to improve symptoms and relieve pain.

Castrate-resistant prostate cancer

Androgen deprivation therapy will eventually fail to control disease progression. The reasons for this are unclear but include the clonal selection hypothesis or adaption hypothesis. In the clonal selection hypothesis, the premise is that the basal cells are the stem cells of the prostate and generate secretory epithelial cells. Whilst the secretory epithelial cells undergo apoptosis upon androgen withdrawal, this is not the case with basal or stromal cells. As a consequence, there is selective survival of these androgen-independent cells within the tumour. With the adaption hypothesis, there is the assumption that androgen independence may be an intrinsic, but dormant property of some prostate cells that is activated by androgen deprivation. Whatever the explanation, when there is failure of first-line therapy, quality of life can be improved by using single or combination therapy that includes maximal androgen blockade (by adding an anti-androgen), second-line hormone treatment (oestrogens), corticosteroids, ketoconazole, chemotherapy and bisphosphonates for short-term palliative response.

Oestrogen

Diethylstilboestrol is a synthetic oestrogen which acts by producing negative feedback on the hypothalamus and anterior pituitary, thereby down-regulating the secretion of LHRH, and hence the production of testosterone. Diethylstilboestrol is the least expensive of the synthetic oestrogens and causes fewer hot flushes and psychological trauma compared with the surgical option. Side effects include gynaecomastia, loss of libido and potency, oedema, nausea and vomiting, and significantly increased risk of thromboembolism. It is usually used in a dose of 1 mg once daily to reduce the risk of cardiovascular side effects because it is associated with increased cardiovascular mortality. It is now mainly avoided in practice for this reason.

Corticosteroids

Both prednisolone and hydrocortisone are anti-inflammatory, can alter the body's immune response to various stimuli and are used in combination with other treatments.

Chemotherapy

Chemotherapy inhibits cell growth and proliferation; it has a variable response rate and is used as a last resort.

In the UK, NICE (2006) recommended that docetaxel is used within its licensed indication to treat men with hormone refractory metastatic disease. Repeat courses of treatment are not recommended if the disease reoccurs when the planned course of 10 cycles is complete.

The UK-led STAMPEDE trial is a complex multi-centre randomised controlled trial for patients with locally advanced or metastatic PC who are about to commence androgen deprivation therapy (James et al., 2016). The addition of docetaxel to standard care was associated with increased survival. The trial is still ongoing, but increasing numbers of men are offered upfront chemotherapy as a result.

For the treatment of adult men with metastatic castration-resistant PC whose disease has progressed during, or after, docetaxel therapy, abiraterone (NICE, 2016a), cabazitaxel (NICE, 2016b) and enzalutamide (NICE, 2016c) are approved by NICE.

Abiraterone acetate. Abiraterone acetate is an androgen biosynthesis inhibitor that blocks biosynthesis of extragonadal androgens. Abiraterone leads to a rebound increase in LH and in ACTH, and so it is given with low-dose corticosteroids to normalise mineralocorticoid levels and reduce side effects. Abiraterone is taken orally in combination with prednisolone 5 mg twice daily, on a 28-day cycle. It must not be taken with food. Patients should be advised that taking the dose at night can often minimise the lethargy that is a potential side effect. If toxicity occurs, treatment should be suspended and restarted with the advice of the treating oncologist; there is no evidence to support reducing the dose. The most commonly observed side effects are hypokalaemia, hypertension, lower-limb oedema, diarrhoea and lethargy.

Enzalutamide. Enzalutamide acts on three steps in the androgen receptor signalling pathway: as an androgen receptor antagonist (no agonist activity); by inhibiting translocation of the androgen–receptor complex to the cell nucleus; and by inhibiting receptor binding to DNA in the nucleus and, therefore, preventing cell replication and instigating apoptosis. Enzalutamide is another oral agent and should be swallowed whole with water and can be taken with or without food. If a patient experiences serious toxicity or an intolerable adverse reaction, he will require interruption of enzalutamide therapy and dosing should be withheld for 1 week, or until symptoms improve, then resumed at the same or a reduced dose. The most common side effects are hypertension, hot flushes and headache.

Both abiraterone and enzalutamide can interact with other drugs. Abiraterone may increase exposure of other medicines metabolised by cytochrome P450 (CYP) 2D6, which include metoprolol, propranolol, desipramine, venlafaxine, haloperidol, risperidone, propafenone, flecainide, codeine, oxycodone and tramadol. Enzalutamide is a strong CYP3A4 enzyme inducer. Interactions with medicines that are eliminated via CYP3A4 metabolism are expected, including fentanyl, clarithromycin, cabazitaxel, warfarin, anti-epileptics and calcium channel blockers.

Table 49.3 Common problems associated with prostate cancer

Problem	Solution
Loss of erectile function after prostatectomy	Phosphodiesterase 5 inhibitors such as sildenafil have shown efficacy in prevention and help improve chance of spontaneous erection. If medication fails or is contraindicated a vacuum device, intraurethral inserts or penile prosthesis may be used
Advanced disease with impending spinal cord compression	Treat with oral dexamethasone and either cyproterone or ketoconazole with external-beam radiotherapy. LHRH agonist treatment is not advisable as the tumour flare up in the initial stage can stimulate tumour growth and exacerbate the condition
Bleeding and coagulation disorder	Prostate cancer can cause disseminated intravascular coagulation as a pathological response to the disease. This is a rare condition where small blood clots are formed in the body, disrupt the normal coagulation process and cause bleeding. This can be further complicated if the patient has comorbidities which require treatment with anticoagulants. Prompt treatment of the cancer with hormones and in some cases replacement of blood, platelets and clotting factors may be required
Hot flushes during androgen deprivation therapy	The hypothalamus is the centre for thermoregulation. Orchiectomy and LHRH agonists inhibit some of the peptides involved in thermoregulation. This increases central adrenergic activity and inappropriate stimulation of thermoregulatory centres, causing peripheral body vasodilatation and hot flushes. Low dose cyproterone acetate (100 mg a day) has been used to suppress hot flushes

LHRH, Luteinising hormone–releasing hormone.

Sipuleucel-T

The autologous cellular immunotherapy vaccine sipuleucel-T stimulates the patient's own immune cells to identify and attack PC cells. It is generated from a patient's own peripheral immune cells, obtained via leucopheresis, which are then exposed to a fusion peptide of granulocyte macrophage colony-stimulating factor (serving as immune adjuvant) and pulmonary alveolar proteinosis. It is extremely expensive and available only in a few specialist centres. However, there is renewed interest in immune therapy in oncology; therefore, further trials are expected.

Radium-223

Radium-223 is a radioactive isotope that emits low levels of alpha particle radiation, which causes double-strand breaks in DNA, killing cells. It acts as a 'calcium mimetic' that, like calcium, accumulates preferentially in areas of bone that are undergoing increased turnover, and therefore acts against bone metastases. Patients receiving radium-223 also reported a better quality of life than patients in the placebo group (Parker et al., 2013).

Chemoprevention

Chemoprevention is defined as the administration of micronutrients, dietary products or drugs to prevent or delay the progression of PC.

Diet

There has been interest in a variety of products, and numerous studies have been conducted. Currently in favour are soya-containing foods, green tea, pomegranates and omega-3 fatty acids. Selenium and vitamin E are no longer considered favourable because large, randomised studies showed no benefit and some cardiovascular downsides. Similarly, vitamin D and lycopene found in tomatoes are also out of favour due to the lack of hard positive outcomes.

Drugs

5α-Reductase inhibitors which are currently used in BPH to reduce prostate size due to their inhibitory effect on the production of DHT are thought to have potential for chemoprevention.

Patient care

Treatment options are decided after discussing the various options and side effects with the individual and as part of a multidisciplinary team meeting. Urinary- and sexual function–related problems are common side effects of most treatments in PC and need to be discussed in detail with the patient. Emotional factors like depression may also need to be addressed because they can adversely affect the quality of life of the individual. Clinical nurse specialists are an excellent source of support and information for patients. Some of the common problems associated with PC are listed in Table 49.3. Patients can also be referred to the NHS website (http://www.nhs.uk/prostatecancer) for facts, information and details of choices available in the diagnosis and treatment of PC. Information on how to cope with the disease and live with PC together with details of various support organisations are available online (such as http://www.cancerresearchuk.org/about-cancer/).

Prostatitis

Epidemiology

The term prostatitis comprises a range of disorders that have been defined and classified (Table 49.4) by the International Prostatitis Collaborative Network into four categories (Krieger et al., 1999).

Prostatitis has been estimated to affect up to 16% of adult men. Unlike BPH and PC, which are more prevalent in older men, prostatitis affects men of all ages.

In most instances (between 90% and 95%) the aetiology of prostatitis is unknown with bacteria isolated in only 5–10% of men presenting with prostatitis.

Pathophysiology

Acute bacterial prostatitis is caused by bacterial infection. The most common isolated uropathogen is *Escherichia coli*. Other causative agents include *Proteus* spp., *Klebsiella* spp., *Pseudomonas* spp. and, less commonly, enterococci, *Bacteroides* and *Staphylococcus* spp. Chronic bacterial prostatitis usually involves recurrent bacterial urinary infections caused by the same organism involved in acute bacterial prostatitis. Both syndromes are of infective origin and represent the minority of cases of prostatitis.

In contrast, the aetiology of chronic prostatitis/chronic pelvic pain syndrome is poorly understood. Several possible mechanisms have been proposed including autoimmune disorders, infection, neurogenic inflammation and voiding dysfunction.

Symptoms

In prostatitis, the clinical presentation and symptoms are a strong diagnostic determinant. A validated questionnaire, the Chronic

Table 49.4	International Prostatitis Collaborative Network classification of prostatitis
International Prostatitis Collaborative Network classification	**Comment**
I. Acute bacterial prostatitis	Acute infection of the prostate
II. Chronic bacterial prostatitis	Chronic infection of the prostate
III. Chronic prostatitis/chronic pelvic pain syndrome	No evidence of infection
A. Inflammatory	Leucocytes in prostatic secretions, post-prostate massage urine or semen
B. Non-inflammatory	No evidence of inflammation
IV. Asymptomatic inflammatory prostatitis	Lack of genitourinary symptoms

Prostatitis Symptom Index, quantifies the severity, frequency and location of pain and discomfort. It is also used to assess urinary symptoms and to establish the impact of symptoms on the patient's quality of life.

Patients with acute bacterial prostatitis usually present with symptoms of an UTI which may include dysuria, urinary frequency or urgency, whilst some may present with pain of penile, lower back or perineal origin. Signs and symptoms of systemic infection can be present in some cases and include pyrexia, rigors, malaise and myalgia. Acute bacterial prostatitis can sometimes precipitate acute urinary retention due to prostatic inflammation. A recent history of transrectal biopsies, cystoscopy or catheterisation is common.

In chronic bacterial prostatitis, symptoms of UTI and pain can also be present. Typically, men with chronic bacterial prostatitis remain asymptomatic between infective episodes.

The main feature in chronic prostatitis/chronic pelvic pain syndrome is urological pain (perineum, lower abdomen and back, rectum, penis and testicles). These symptoms are usually present for at least 3 months before a diagnosis can be made. Lower urinary tract symptoms and ejaculatory dysfunction can also affect men with chronic prostatitis/chronic pelvic pain syndrome.

Patients with asymptomatic inflammatory prostatitis have no symptoms. The condition is usually diagnosed when patients undergo investigation to assess other genitourinary complaints. For example, prostatitis may be found in biopsies taken from patients investigated for elevated PSA or when leucocytes are found in semen samples from men being investigated for infertility.

Examination and investigations

If acute bacterial prostatitis is suspected, a urine dipstick and culture are performed to reveal the presence of pathogens and leucocytes. Depending on the clinical picture, a blood culture may be indicated to diagnose concomitant bacteraemia. An ultrasound scan of the bladder can be conducted to evaluate the residual volume of urine and problems with voiding and urinary retention. Rectal examination may reveal an exquisitely tender prostate.

Chronic bacterial prostatitis is diagnosed in men with a history of recurrent or relapsing UTIs. A positive urine dipstick and culture is a common finding during acute episodes. Microscopy and culture of lower tract urinary secretions (urine and prostatic) between symptomatic periods can be performed and will help identify the prostate as the main focus of infection. Imaging of the urinary tract via ultrasound or MRI can be conducted to rule out any structural abnormalities.

Chronic prostatitis/chronic pelvic pain syndrome is a diagnosis of exclusion. Typical disorders which must be excluded include the presence of active urethritis, urogenital cancer, urinary tract disease, functionally significant urethral stricture or neurological disease affecting the bladder (Krieger et al., 1999). The main component of this syndrome is the presence of genitourinary pain. After taking a detailed medical history, the evaluation of symptoms can be done using the Chronic

Prostatitis Symptom Index. Other investigations include a DRE, urinalysis, urine culture and cytology, screening for sexually transmitted diseases, urodynamic studies, prostatic TRUS and serum PSA.

Treatment

Acute bacterial prostatitis can present as a serious infection, and therapy normally includes empirical treatment with parenteral antibiotics. Commonly used agents include broad-spectrum penicillins, fluoroquinolones or third-generation cephalosporins usually in combination with aminoglycosides. Urine culture and sensitivities will inform the choice of future antibiotic treatment, which is recommended to be continued for 2–4 weeks. General supportive measures such as maintenance of appropriate hydration and pain relief are important. Suprapubic catheterisation may be required if acute urinary retention is present.

The treatment of chronic bacterial prostatitis involves long courses (at least 4 weeks) of antibiotics. Fluoroquinolones (e.g. ciprofloxacin, ofloxacin) are used as first-choice agents because of good prostatic penetration, their spectrum of antibacterial activity and favourable safety profile. If infective episodes are frequent, patients can be offered prophylactic antibiotics for several months with periodic follow-up to monitor progress (McNaughton-Collins et al., 2007).

Because the aetiology of most cases of chronic prostatitis/chronic pelvic pain syndrome is unknown, management often involves empirical treatment. Despite not being considered to have an infective nature, up to 50% of patients with chronic prostatitis/chronic pelvic pain syndrome respond to long courses of fluoroquinolones (Nickel et al., 2001), especially men with symptoms of relatively recent onset (a few weeks). Patients with longstanding symptoms refractory to treatment are less likely to benefit from fluoroquinolones. α-Adrenoceptor antagonists are also used alone or in combination with antibiotics in the management of chronic prostatitis/chronic pelvic pain syndrome. The evidence for efficacy is conflicting but remains an option for patients with persistent symptoms. Initially non-steroidal anti-inflammatory drugs (NSAIDs) have a role, as do the neurological pain agents such as gabapentin. There are also limited data describing the use of other therapies in chronic prostatitis/chronic pelvic pain syndrome such as fluoxetine, pollen extract, quercetin, finasteride, mepartricin and pelvic electromagnetic therapy.

No treatment is necessary for patients with asymptomatic inflammatory prostatitis because the condition is characterised by the lack of symptoms.

Patient care

Patients need to be made aware that prostatitis is common, affecting between 1 and 2 out of every 10 men, but very difficult to treat and eradicate. The cause is generally poorly understood,

and it is difficult to diagnose. In chronic cases of prostatitis, symptoms may persist for long periods, although the severity can vary over time. Treatment may involve several therapies. Patients treated with antibiotics must be informed of the importance of completing the prolonged courses necessary to eradicate infection.

The British Prostatitis Support Association's website (http://www.bps-assoc.org.uk) offers information and support to patients.

Case studies

Case 49.1

Mr AT, a 64-year-old man, presents with poor urinary flow and waking at least twice during the night to pass urine. There is no family history of prostate disease, and he is taking no medication.

Question

What investigations are appropriate, and how should Mr AT be managed?

Answer

This patient should be asked to complete a frequency volume chart of voided urine and International Prostate Symptom Score questionnaire, then undergo a full clinical examination, including DRE, abdominal and genital examination. The patient can be offered PSA testing. The PVR volume of urine within the bladder should be measured after micturition.

If the residual volume is low (0–100 mL), the flow rate adequate (>15 mL/s) and the patient's symptoms not bothersome, then he can be reassured and adopt a 'watch and wait' policy. If the PSA is high, then this should be investigated further with imaging as per local hospital policy. Evidence of urinary retention should be managed with catheterisation.

If, however, the patient has slow flow, PVR 100–300 mL and/or has bothersome symptoms, then he can be counselled on medical therapy and offered an α-adrenoceptor antagonist. If he is not hypertensive, a uroselective drug such as tamsulosin can be considered. This should have few systemic side effects and requires no initial titration of dose. If he is hypertensive, a less specific α-blocker may be more appropriate which will serve the dual purpose of an antihypertensive agent, as well as treating his urinary symptoms. Careful dose titration may be necessary initially to counter any potential postural hypotension. The combination of 5α-reductase inhibitor may be considered in patients with larger prostates (>40 g) because this may reduce the risk of progression of BPH.

Case 49.2

Mr CH, a 50-year-old man, requests treatment from his primary care doctor for a 'bladder infection'. On questioning, he describes symptoms of urinary frequency, urgency and urge incontinence, but fever and dysuria are absent.

Question

How should Mr CH be treated?

Answer

The layperson may interpret the symptoms of frequency and urgency as representing an UTI, but in the absence of dysuria this is unlikely. Urinalysis should be performed to assess the presence of leucocytes, blood and nitrites in the urine, which would confirm an infection.

In the absence of infection the patient should be referred for a full clinical assessment which could include urodynamic studies, filling and voiding cystometry, an ultrasound scan of the upper urinary tract, measurement of PSA and assessment of renal function. It is likely the patient has an outflow obstruction which has given rise to secondary instability of the detrusor muscle in the bladder, causing involuntary contractions of the bladder and resulting in incontinence. The other differential is idiopathic detrusor instability or OAB. The obstruction may be caused by either prostate enlargement or a dysfunctional bladder neck. In either case, treatment with an α-adrenoceptor antagonist is appropriate to reduce the outflow resistance. Should the flow be adequate but symptoms of incontinence persist, then concurrent treatment with an antimuscarinic drug such as oxybutynin or tolterodine may be necessary to inhibit the cholinergic-mediated contractions of the detrusor. A combination preparation of tamsulosin and solifenacin (Vesomni) may be preferred.

Case 49.3

Mr IK, a 75-year-old man, presents with acute urinary retention and a history of nocturnal enuresis for the past 2–3 months. His medical history includes a heart valve replacement. He denies any haematuria or dysuria and felt he had a good flow while passing urine. On DRE, the prostate is found to be hard and nodular, and the PSA was 662 ng/mL. He has a palpable bladder to the level of the umbilicus.

The MRI pelvis revealed an enlarged and irregular prostate with intra-vesicle extension of the medial lobe into the bladder neck. Mr IK was confirmed to have adenocarcinoma of the prostate with a Gleason score of 8 and with bone metastasis.

Mr IK's PSA declined from 662 to 130 ng/mL in 5 months and continued to fall to 3.2 ng/mL after 9 months, indicating a good response to hormonal treatment. Although Mr IK wanted to be catheter free, he failed several trials without a catheter and was offered radical radiotherapy and a channel TURP to control local obstructive symptoms.

Questions

1. What investigations are recommended, and how should Mr IK be managed?
2. What treatment choice is available for Mr IK?
3. What are the most likely future complications expected for Mr IK?

Answers

1. Because acute urinary retention can cause renal damage, Mr IK needs to be catheterised to relieve his bladder outflow, and the residual volume and renal function measured. A hard and nodular prostate on DRE together with elevated PSA suggests PC. A high PSA in the context of acute urinary retention does not directly infer PC; if the DRE is normal, then the PSA should be repeated at a later date prior to further investigation. However, with a PSA greater than 100 ng/mL, PC is extremely likely. In view of the suspicious DRE the patient needs to have a range of baseline investigations including a TRUS biopsy and/or MRI of the pelvis and/or isotope bone scan. Although the DRE is suggestive of PC, the TRUS biopsy helps to grade the cancer using the Gleason scale and helps in making the decision about treatment. The bone scan helps identify bone metastasis, which along with the results from MRI is used to stage the cancer based on the tumour, node, metastasis score.

2. Surgical castration can bring down the testosterone levels immediately and is relatively inexpensive but may have a psychological impact on the patient in addition to impotence and hot flushes. Medical castration with LHRH analogues would be effective treatment as well. LHRH agonists can be used to treat systemically, but the concern with this group of drugs is the flare of the disease due to the initial surge in testosterone levels, in addition to the other side effects of decreased libido, hot flush and impotence. Flare can precipitate life-threatening symptoms of the disease if the cancer is close to the spinal cord, where it may cause spinal cord compression and paralysis. If lymph nodes near the ureter are involved, the flare can increase the node size and compress the ureter causing renal impairment. It can also increase bone disease causing severe bone pain. Although initiation of anti-androgens can reduce symptoms of hot flushes associated with flare-up to some extent, the preferred option for patients with increased risk of spinal cord compression would be LHRH antagonist because it can reduce testosterone levels much more quickly with no flare-up. Hormonal treatment was commenced with an LHRH agonist injection together with a 1-month course of bicalutamide to protect against tumour flare.

3. As the disease progresses, Mr IK may develop hormone resistance, and non-hormonal treatment such as chemotherapy with docetaxel and abiraterone/enzalutamide may need to be considered. Osteoporosis is an important potential complication of long-term androgen deprivation therapy and metastatic bone disease, and consequently the patient may experience severe bone pain. Palliative radiotherapy to metastatic bone areas and NSAIDs are recommended to control the symptoms initially, but if pain persists, use of bisphosphonates may be necessary because they are known to inhibit osteoclast activity and relieve bone pain.

Case 49.4

Mr PH, a 35-year-old man, presents with a 3-month history of dysuria, frequency and hesitancy. He also reports pain in the perineum, radiating down the thighs, and discomfort while ejaculating. A DRE reveals the size and shape of his prostate seems to be normal, although it is tender on examination.

Question

What are the various conditions that need to be considered, and what medication will help confirm the diagnosis?

Answer

A urine dipstick and culture is recommended to rule out UTI. PSA can be measured but is raised in BPH, PC and prostatitis, and hence is not a definitive test, so this should be taken into consideration. The symptoms and physical examination are suggestive of chronic prostatitis. A swab should be taken to rule out chlamydia and other sexually transmitted diseases. Prostatitis needs to be confirmed after ruling out other possibilities such as epididymitis, epididymo-orchitis, urethral stricture, renal calculus, PC, bladder cancer and colorectal cancer.

The available evidence suggests a cure or an improvement in symptoms will occur if a quinolone antibiotic is prescribed for 4 weeks. NSAIDs and paracetamol can be used to relieve any associated pain, whilst faecal softeners may be required to reduce discomfort and pain when opening bowels.

Case 49.5

Mr AB, a 43-year-old man, seeks advice from a community pharmacist regarding his difficulty, over the past 3–4 months, when attempting to start urinating and then urinating for a long time. On questioning, he does not have any other significant medical history, and he has no symptoms of a UTI, pain or haematuria.

Questions

1. Is it appropriate to sell over-the-counter tamsulosin to Mr AB?
2. Does the pharmacist need to maintain a record of the sale?

Answers

1. Lower urinary tract symptoms, such as hesitancy and weak stream, indicate BPH which is prevalent in one in four men older than 40 years. Because it is a very sensitive topic for most males, the patient needs to be consulted in a private area to assess the severity of his symptoms by using the International Prostate Symptom Score (IPSS). This is a sum of seven urinary symptoms which include incomplete emptying, frequency, intermittency, urgency, weak stream, straining and nocturia. If these symptoms severely affect the quality of life and there are no contraindications, a supply of tamsulosin 400 micrograms to be taken once daily for 2 weeks initially and then for a further 4 weeks can be made while simultaneously referring the patient to his primary care doctor to confirm diagnosis and to assess his suitability for long-term treatment. If the symptoms do not improve within 14 days or the symptoms worsen, the patient should be asked to discontinue treatment and seek medical advice.

2. Record-keeping is necessary to confirm that the doctor has assessed the patient within 6 weeks of initiating treatment and thereby permits further supply. It is important that the patient's consent is obtained to keep this record.

Acknowledgements

The author would like to acknowledge the contribution of Maria Martinez and Mini Satheesh to previous versions of this chapter which appeared in the previous editions of this book.

References

Aho, T.F., 2013. Holmium laser enucleation of the prostate: a paradigm shift in benign prostatic hyperplasia surgery. Ther. Adv. Urol. 5, 245–253.

Albertsen, P.C., Hanley, J.A., Fine, J., 2005. 20-year outcomes following conservative management of clinically localized prostate cancer. J. Am. Med. Assoc. 293, 2095–2101.

Barry, M.J., Fowler, F.J., O'Leary, M.P., et al., 1992. The American Urological Association symptom index for benign prostatic hyperplasia. The Measurement Committee of the American Urological Association. J. Urol. 48, 1549–1557.

Chaim, M., Hatch, W.V., Fischer, H.D., et al., 2009. Association between tamsulosin and serious ophthalmic adverse events in older men following cataract surgery. J. Am. Med. Assoc. 301, 1991–1996.

Chatziralli, I.P., Sergentanis, T.N., 2011. Risk factors for intraoperative floppy iris syndrome: a meta-analysis. Ophthalmology 118, 730–735.

Cornu, J.N., Ahyai, S., Bachmann, A., et al., 2015. A systematic review and meta-analysis of functional outcomes and complications following transurethral procedures for lower urinary tract symptoms resulting from benign prostatic obstruction: an update. Eur. Urol. 67, 1066–1096.

Epstein, J.I., Allsbrook, W.C., Amin, M.B., et al., ISUP Grading Committee, 2005. The 2005 International Society of Urologic Pathology (ISUP) consensus conference on Gleason grading of prostatic carcinoma. Am. J. Surg. Pathol. 29, 1228–1242.

Epstein, J.I., Egevad, L., Amin, M.B., et al., 2016. The 2014 International Society of Urological Pathology (ISUP) consensus conference on Gleason grading of prostatic carcinoma. Definition of grading patterns and proposal for a new grading system. Am. J. Surg. Pathol. 40, 244–252.

Gleason, D.F., Mellinger, G.T., 1974. Prediction of prognosis for prostatic adenocarcinoma by combined histological grading and clinical staging. J. Urol. 111, 58–64.

Globocan, n.d. Prostate cancer estimated incidence, mortality and prevalence worldwide in 2012. Available at: http://globocan.iarc.fr/old/FactSheets/cancers/prostate-new.asp

Gravas, S., Bach, T., Drake, M., et al., 2017. Treatment of non-neurogenic male LUTS. Available at: http://uroweb.org/guideline/treatment-of-non-neurogenic-male-luts/#1.

Hueber, P.A., Al-Asker, A., Zorn, K.C., 2011. Monopolar vs. bipolar TURP: assessing their clinical advantages. Can. Urol. Assoc. J. 5, 390–391.

Inverson, P., 2002. Antiandrogen monotherapy indications and results. Urology 60 (3 Suppl. 1), 64–71.

James, N.D., Sydes, M.R., Clarke, N.W., et al., 2016. Addition of docetaxel, zoledronic acid, or both to first-line long-term hormone therapy in prostate cancer (STAMPEDE): survival results from an adaptive, multiarm, multistage, platform randomised controlled trial. Lancet 387, 1163–1177.

Kirby, R.S., Andersen, M., Gratzke, P., et al., 2001. A combined analysis of double blind trials of the efficacy and tolerability of doxazosin-gastrointestinal therapeutic system, doxazosin standard and placebo in patients with benign prostatic hyperplasia. Br. J. Urol. Int. 87, 192–200.

Kirkham, P.S., Emberton, M., Allen, C., 2006. How good is MRI at detecting and characterising cancer within the prostate? Eur. Urol. 50, 1163–1174.

Krieger, J.N., Nyberg, L., Nickel, J.C., 1999. NIH consensus definition and classification of prostatitis. J. Am. Med. Assoc. 282, 236–237.

Lam, J.S., Romas, N.A., Lowe, F.C., 2003. Long-term treatment with finasteride in men with symptomatic benign prostatic hyperplasia: 10-year follow-up. Urology 61, 354–358.

MacDonald, R., Wilt, T., 2005. Alfuzosin for treatment of lower urinary tract symptoms compatible with benign prostatic hyperplasia: a systematic review of efficacy and adverse effects. Urology 66, 780–788.

McConnell, J.D., Roehrborn, C.G., Bautista, A.M., et al., 2003. The long-term effect of doxazosin, finasteride, and combination therapy on the clinical progression of benign prostatic hyperplasia. N. Engl. J. Med. 349, 2387–2398.

McNaughton-Collins, M., Joyce, G.F., Wise, M., et al., 2007. Prostatitis. In: Litwin, M.S., Saigal, C.S. (Eds.), Urologic Diseases in America. US Department of Health and Human Services, Public Health Service, National Institutes of Health, National Institute of Diabetes and Digestive and Kidney Diseases. US Government Printing Office, Washington, DC. Available at: http://kidney.niddk.nih.gov/statistics/uda/Prostatitis-Chapter01.pdf.

Michel, M.C., Schneider, T., Krege, S., et al., 2002. Does gender or age affect the efficacy and safety of tolterodine? J. Urol. 168, 1027–1031.

Mirakhur, A., McWilliams, J., 2017. Prostate artery embolization for benign prostatic hyperplasia: current status. Can. Assoc. Radiol. J. 68, 84–89.

National Institute for Health and Care Excellence (NICE), 2006. Docetaxel for the treatment of hormone-refractory metastatic prostate cancer. Technology appraisal guidance (TA101). NICE, London. Available at: https://www.nice.org.uk/guidance/ta101.

National Institute for Health and Care Excellence (NICE), 2015. UroLift for treating lower urinary tract symptoms of benign prostatic hyperplasia. Medical technologies guidance (MTG26). NICE, London. Available at: https://www.nice.org.uk/guidance/mtg26/chapter/2-The-technology.

National Institute for Health and Care Excellence (NICE), 2016a. Abiraterone for treating metastatic hormone-relapsed prostate cancer before chemotherapy is indicated. Technology appraisal guidance [TA387]. NICE, London. Available at: https://www.nice.org.uk/guidance/ta387.

National Institute for Health and Care Excellence (NICE), 2016b. Cabazitaxel for hormone-relapsed metastatic prostate cancer treated with docetaxel. Technology appraisal guidance (TA391). NICE, London. Available at: https://www.nice.org.uk/guidance/ta391.

National Institute for Health and Care Excellence (NICE), 2016c. Enzalutamide for treating metastatic hormone-relapsed prostate cancer before chemotherapy is indicated. Technology appraisal guidance (TA377). NICE, London. Available at: https://www.nice.org.uk/guidance/ta377.

Nickel, J.C., Downey, J., Clark, J., et al., 2001. Predictors of patient response to antibiotic therapy for the chronic prostatitis/chronic pelvic pain syndrome: a prospective multicenter clinical trial. J. Urol. 165, 1539–1544.

O'Leary, M., 2001. Tamsulosin: current clinical experience. Urology 58, 42–48.

Parker, C., Nilsson, S., Heinrich, D., et al., ALSYMPCA Investigators, 2013. Alpha-emitter radium-223 and increased survival in metastatic prostate cancer. N. Engl. J. Med. 369, 213–223.

Roehrborn, C.G., 2005. Benign prostatic hyperplasia: an overview. Rev. Urol. 7 (Suppl. 9), S3–S14.

Roehrborn, C.G., for the ALTESS Study Group, 2006. Alfuzosin 10 mg once daily prevents overall clinical progression of benign prostatic hyperplasia but not acute urinary retention: results of a 2-year placebo-controlled study. Br. J. Urol. Int. 97, 734–741.

Roehrborn, C.G., Bruskewitz, R., Nickel, G.C., et al., 2000. Urinary retention in patients with BPH treated with finasteride or placebo over four years. Eur. Urol. 37, 528–536.

Roehrborn, C.G., Boyle, P.J., Nickel, G.C., on behalf of the ARIA3001, ARIA3002 and ARIA3003 study investigators, 2002. Efficacy and safety of a dual inhibitor or 5-alpha-reductase types 1 and 2 (dutasteride) in men with benign prostatic hyperplasia. Urology 60, 434–441.

Roehrborn, C.G., Siami, P., Barkin, J., et al., 2010. The effects of combination therapy with dutasteride and tamsulosin on clinical outcomes in men with symptomatic benign prostatic hyperplasia: 4-year results from the CombAT study. Eur. Urol. 57, 123–131.

Saad, F., Schulman, C.C., 2004. Role of bisphosphonates in prostate cancer. Eur. Urol. 45, 26–34.

Stoevelaar, H.J., McDonnell, J., 2001. Changing therapeutic regimens in benign prostatic hyperplasia. Pharmacoeconomics 19, 131–153.

Van Dijk, M.M., de la Rosette, J., Michel, M.C., 2006. Effects of α1-adrenoceptor antagonists on male sexual function. Drugs 66, 287–301.

Zorn, K.C., Liberman, D., 2011. GreenLight 180W XPS photovaporization of the prostate: how I do it. Can. J. Urol. 18, 5918–5926.

Further reading

Attard, G., Parker, C., Eeles, R.A., et al., 2016. Prostate cancer. Lancet 387, 70–82.

Useful websites

Men's Health Forum: http://www.menshealthforum.org.uk/
Prostate Cancer UK section on BPH: http://prostatecanceruk.org/
Prostate cancer information for patients: http://www.nhs.uk/prostatecancer and http://www.cancerresearchuk.org/about-cancer/

British Prostatitis Support Association: http://www.bps-assoc.org.uk

50 Anaemia

Niamh McGarry and Anthony Cadogan

Key points

- Anaemia is a common condition. The World Health Organization estimates that the number of people worldwide with anaemia is 2 billion.
- Anaemia is a lack of haemoglobin and is proportional to the oxygen-carrying ability of the red blood cell.
- Anaemia can cause a myriad of symptoms, in part depending on the type of anaemia. The most consistent characteristic is tiredness-related symptoms.
- There are a number of causes, including iron deficiency (iron-deficient anaemia), defective haemoglobin synthesis (macrocytic anaemia and thalassaemia) or overactive destruction of red blood cells (haemolytic anaemia). It is useful to classify them based on the size of red blood cell: microcytic, normocytic or macrocytic anaemia.
- Treatment of anaemia begins with investigations to confirm the cause of the anaemia. There may be more than one cause of anaemia present.

Anaemia can be defined as a reduction from normal of the quantity of haemoglobin in the blood. The World Health Organization (WHO) defines anaemia in adults as haemoglobin levels less than 130 g/L for males and less than 120 g/L for females (WHO, 2011).

Epidemiology

Anaemia has a high prevalence worldwide. It has an impact on almost one-quarter of the population, based on WHO data from 1993–2005. In adults, the lowest prevalence is in men, at 12.7%. The threshold for anaemia in pregnancy is lower, and anaemia is more common in pregnancy. In the most recent WHO data from 2011, which did not include men, the prevalence of anaemia in non-pregnant women was 29% and was highest in pregnant women, at 38.2%. The average prevalence of anaemia in women of reproductive age was 29.4%. The elderly are susceptible to anaemia, with an average world prevalence of 23.9% (WHO, 2015).

There is a much higher occurrence of anaemia in South-East Asian, Eastern Mediterranean and African regions. This is due to a combination of factors, such as higher incidences of sickle cell anaemia and thalassaemias. It also reflects problems associated with sanitation, such as hookworm and schistomiasis (WHO, 2015).

The haemoglobin level varies slightly in different altitudes and is higher in smokers. Haemoglobin is higher in males due to the influence of androgens, which increases haemoglobin production. In the elderly, therefore, the haemoglobin values in men and women are less differentiated. Haemoglobin also has some dependence on the patient's fluid status. In dehydration, due to reduced circulating plasma volume, haemoglobin appears higher. In circumstances of higher plasma volume, such as pregnancy and splenomegaly, it will appear lower. The haemoglobin level does not always correlate with the degree of symptoms experienced by the patient.

Aetiology

The low haemoglobin level that defines anaemia results from two different mechanisms:
- increased haemoglobin loss due to either:
  - haemorrhage (red blood cell loss) or
  - haemolysis (red blood cell destruction).
- reduced haemoglobin synthesis due to either:
  - lack of nutrient or
  - bone marrow failure.

This chapter gives an explanation of the different types of anaemia. It focuses particularly on the types of anaemia that require drug treatment.

Haemopoiesis and erythropoiesis

Haemopoiesis

Haemopoiesis is the formation of blood cells, white blood cells, red blood cells and platelets. Haemopoiesis takes place predominantly in the bone marrow of the central skeleton and in the proximal ends of the long bones. It also takes place in the liver and the spleen, particularly at times of increased need.

All blood cells originate from the pluripotent haemopoietic stem cell. These stem cells have the potential to form any of the blood cells. The red blood cells (erythrocytes) are the most abundant of all the blood cells. Erythrocytes, once matured, do not contain a nucleus. This allows more capacity for the erythrocyte to carry oxygen.

Erythropoiesis

Erythropoiesis is the production line of red blood cells from the stem cells committed to red blood cell production (Fig. 50.1). The stem cell undergoes a complex series of cell divisions and differentiations. The first step is the stem cells proliferating into progenitor cells.

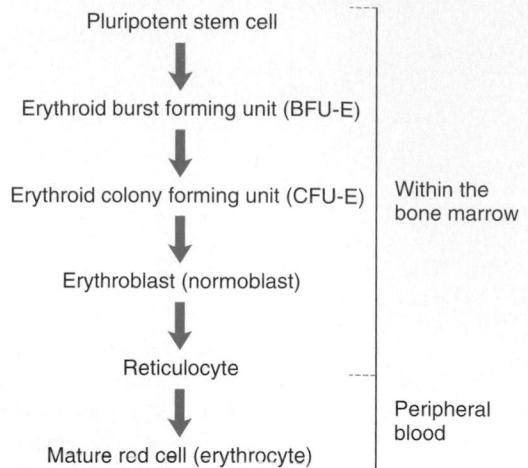

Fig. 50.1 Simplified diagram of some of the stages within erythropoiesis.

Box 50.1 Non-specific signs and symptoms associated with anaemia

- Tiredness
- Pallor
- Fainting
- Exertional dyspnoea
- Tachycardia
- Palpitations
- Worsening angina
- Worsening cardiac failure
- Exacerbation of intermittent claudication

Haemoglobin, deoxyribonucleic acid (DNA) and ribonucleic acid (RNA) become synthesised along the way. Haemoglobin comprises four amino acid chains (globins), described as α_1, α_2, β_1 and β_2, with each chain containing one haem molecule. A haem molecule is formed in mitochondria when a protoporphyrin (pigment) combines with iron in its ferrous state (Fe^{2+}), with pyridoxine acting as a co-factor. Each haem molecule can carry one molecule of oxygen.

The last stage of production in the bone marrow is the formation of the normoblast. A minority of these normoblasts die within the bone marrow without producing red blood cells (e.g. 10–15%). The majority of normoblasts, however, release a large number of reticulocytes into the circulation. Reticulocytes are immature red blood cells constituting a small proportion, 1–3% of all red blood cells. They mature into red blood cells within 48 hours. An increased percentage of reticulocytes is typical after acute blood loss.

Haemopoiesis and erythropoiesis are regulated by growth factors. The most important of these growth factors is erythropoietin. Erythropoietin is a hormone produced by the interstitial cells of the renal cortex. A small percentage, 10%, is produced in the liver and other organs. Erythropoietin production is influenced by the exposure to oxygen in the kidney and is increased in response to reduced oxygen tension. The kidney responds to hypoxia and anaemia by increasing the production of erythropoiesis. Hepcidin is also decreased; this is an inflammatory reactive protein that suppresses iron absorption.

Erythropoietin acts by increasing the number of progenitor cells committed to erythropoiesis. In renal failure, however, the kidney fails to produce sufficient erythropoietin and the patient becomes anaemic. As well as erythropoietin, bone marrow blood cell production requires a number of factors, such as iron, cobalt, vitamin B_1 (thiamine), B_6 (pyridoxine), B_{12}, vitamin C, vitamin E, riboflavin, androgens and thyroxine.

Erythropoietin production is suppressed in many inflammatory and or chronic conditions, such as rheumatoid arthritis, cancer and sickle cell disease. It will also be sensitive to reduced oxygen tension changes due to impaired lung function and cardiovascular function. Each day, approximately 2×10^{11} erythrocytes enter the circulation (Hoffbrand and Moss, 2016).

Normal erythrocytes survive in the peripheral circulation for about 120 days. Abnormal erythrocytes have a shortened lifespan. At the end of their life, the red blood cells are destroyed by the cells of the reticuloendothelial system found in the spleen and bone marrow. Iron is removed from the haem component of haemoglobin and transported back to the bone marrow for reuse. Part of the globin chains is excreted as conjugated bilirubin by the liver.

Clinical manifestations

Anaemia is a manifestation of a condition or more than one condition resulting in a decreased haemoglobin level. It varies widely in its presentation for different anaemia types. A reduction in haemoglobin means the red blood cells have less capacity for delivering oxygen to all the tissues and organs in the body. This results in related symptoms of tiredness, lethargy and exercise intolerance (Box 50.1). Cerebral symptoms such as reduced cognition, confusion, headaches and light-headedness may also be present. In severe or longstanding anaemia, it can progress to further symptoms of oxygen deprivation, such as shortness of breath, angina, tachycardia, palpitations and heart failure.

The speed of onset of anaemia is an important determinant of presentation. A rapid blood loss, for example, haemorrhage, produces shock, with collapse, dyspnoea and tachycardia. Anaemia that develops over a period of time allows the body to partially compensate. As the anaemia becomes worse, more and more signs and symptoms may develop.

Even though in anaemia the amount of haemoglobin is reduced, all the blood that passes through the lungs is fully oxygenated. Increasing the respiratory rate or increasing the FiO_2 (fraction of inspired oxygen) will not improve tissue oxygenation. When the haemoglobin falls to less than 70 or 80 g/L, there is almost always a compensatory increase in cardiac output. Hence, the impact of anaemia on a patient with existing cardiovascular or lung disease will be more profound. The elderly have a lower threshold for cerebral and cardiovascular symptoms than in a younger healthier adult.

Investigations

The diagnosis of anaemia requires a thorough medical history and holistic patient evaluation including noting any medicines the

Box 50.2 Anaemia classified by size and colour of red blood cells

Hypochromic–microcytic
- Iron deficiency
- Sideroblastic
- Anaemia of chronic disease

Normochromic macrocytic
- Folate deficiency
- Vitamin B_{12} deficiency

Polychromatophilic macrocytic
- Haemolysis

Box 50.3 Major causes of iron-deficiency anaemia

- Inadequate iron absorption
  - Dietary deficiency
  - Malabsorption
- Increased physiological demand
- Loss through bleeding

patient is taking and any recent travel which could be linked with hookworm. It is important to be aware of any background of liver disease, chronic renal failure or other haematological history that could help explain laboratory test results and guide the diagnosis.

The investigation into the cause of anaemia begins with a full blood count. Haemoglobin, the mean corpuscular volume (MCV) and the mean cell haemoglobin (MCH) values are of particular interest. The MCV reflects the average size of the red blood cell. It is very useful and indicates microcytic (low MCV), normocytic (MCV in range) or macrocytic anaemia (high MCV). If there are two pathologies, where one causes large cells and other causes small cells, the MCV may appear normal or can be misleading.

The MCH is a similar indicator reflecting the density of the haemoglobin in the red blood cell and typically mirrors the MCV. It has been suggested that it is a more consistently reliable indicator due to the laboratory methods used to measure these indices (Goddard et al., 2011).

If in addition to haemoglobin, white blood cells (leukocytes) and platelet counts are also low this can be an indication of an overall bone marrow suppression (pancytopenia). In such cases, advice should be sought from haematology, and any drug-related causes of bone marrow suppression should be excluded.

Stained blood film allows examination of the morphology of the red blood cells. Box 50.2 is a list of some of the most common anaemias categorised by size. This can give further evidence to the origin of the anaemia. It is particularly useful if there is more than one type of anaemia present.

Other haematinic tests needed for diagnosis are vitamin B_{12}, folate, ferritin, iron and iron-binding capacity/transferrin. Ferritin, iron and iron-binding capacity or variations of this may be referred to as an iron profile. In addition to the liver function tests and renal function tests mentioned, thyroid function tests should be checked because thyroxine is required for healthy bone marrow function. Ultimately, if the cause of the anaemia cannot be elucidated from peripheral blood, a bone marrow aspiration or biopsy will be required.

Iron-deficiency anaemia

Epidemiology

Iron deficiency is described as the most common deficiency state in the world and affects more than 2 billion people worldwide (Camascshella, 2015). A large proportion of this population will have iron-deficiency anaemia (IDA). In developing countries, iron deficiency has a higher association with blood loss due to parasitic worms and insufficient dietary intake. In the developed world, it is attributed to dietary changes (such as veganism) and malabsorption or conditions leading to chronic blood loss. IDA occurs in 2–5% of adult men and postmenopausal women, in the developed world (Goddard et al., 2011). The incidence is always higher in women due to both menstrual blood loss and the high rate of IDA in pregnancy.

Aetiology

In Western societies, the commonest cause of iron deficiency is due to blood loss. In women of childbearing age, this is most commonly due to menstrual loss. Amongst adult males, the most likely cause is gastro-intestinal bleeding. Other causes of blood loss associated with iron-deficiency anaemia include haemorrhoids, nosebleeds or postpartum haemorrhage. The major causes of iron deficiency are listed in Box 50.3.

Pathophysiology

The elimination of iron is not controlled physiologically, so the homeostasis is maintained by controlling iron absorption. Iron is absorbed mainly from the duodenum and jejunum. Absorption itself is inefficient; iron bound to haem (found in red meat) is better absorbed than iron found in green vegetables. The presence of phosphates and phytates in some vegetables leads to the formation of unabsorbable iron complexes, whereas ascorbic acid increases the absorption of iron. In a healthy adult, approximately 10% of the dietary iron intake will be absorbed. Iron is transported around the body bound to a serum protein called transferrin. Normally, this protein is only one-third saturated with iron.

Anaemia may result from a mismatch between the body's iron requirements and iron absorption. The demand for iron varies with age (Table 50.1). Diets deficient in animal protein or ascorbic acid may not provide sufficient available iron to meet the demand.

Iron is an essential micronutrient needed for erythropoietic function. It has further roles in oxidative metabolism and in the cellular immune response. The human body contains around 50 mg/kg of iron. Most of this iron (65%) is stored in haemoglobin. A further 10% is stored in myoglobulin in the muscles and other tissues. The remaining iron is stored in the liver, the reticuloendothelial system of the macrophages and in the bone marrow in the form of iron storage proteins, ferritin and haemosiderin.

Dietary intake is the source of iron. Typically, an adult might consume 15 mg iron daily, in haem (10%) and non-haem (90%) form, in the Western diet. Haem iron is found in meat and fish

Table 50.1 Typical daily requirements of iron

Infant (0–4 months)	0.5 mg
Adolescent male	1.8 mg
Adolescent female	2.4 mg
Adult male	0.9 mg
Menstruating female	2.0 mg
In pregnancy	3.0–5.0 mg
Postmenopausal female	0.9 mg

Table 50.2 Pathological contributors to iron deficiency anaemia in the UK with prevalence as percentage of total (Goddard et al., 2011)

Contributor	Prevalence
Occult GI blood loss	
Common	
Aspirin/NSAID use	10–15%
Colonic carcinoma	5–10%
Gastric carcinoma	5%
Benign gastric ulceration	5%
Angiodysplasia	5%
Uncommon	
Oesophagitis	2–4%
Oesophageal carcinoma	1–2%
Gastric antral vascular ectasia	1–2%
Small bowel tumours	1–2%
Cameron ulcer in large hiatus hernia	<1%
Ampullary carcinoma	<1%
Ancylostoma duodenale	<1%
Malabsorption	
Common	
Coeliac disease	4–6%
Gastrectomy	<5%
Helicobacter pylori colonisation	<5%
Uncommon	
Gut resection	<1%
Bacterial overgrowth	<1%
Non-GI blood loss	
Common	
Menstruation	20–30%
Blood donation	5%
Uncommon	
Haematuria	1%
Epistaxis	<1%

GI, Gastro-intestinal; NSAID, non-steroidal anti-inflammatory drug.

sources and is more easily absorbed than non-haem iron, which is found in non-meat sources such as whole grains, fruits and vegetables. Of our daily iron intake, 1–2 mg may be absorbed, mostly through the duodenum. Iron in its ferrous state, Fe^{2+}, is more readily taken up than iron in its ferric form, Fe^{3+}.

Intake of iron must be sufficient to replace daily iron loss. Each day, 0.5–1 mg iron is lost in faeces, sweat and urine. Over an average of a month, women lose an additional 0.5–1 mg/day in menstruation. In pregnancy, a further 1–2 mg iron is needed daily; therefore, IDA is common in these patient cohorts. The demand for iron also varies with age (see Table 50.1) (Mason, 2008).

The body has no active mechanism of excreting excess iron, so available iron in the body is regulated by the absorption of dietary iron from the duodenum. This must be tightly controlled to avoid IDA. Hepcidin, a regulatory protein, has a key role in inhibiting the uptake of iron from the duodenum.

IDA arises when there is an ongoing imbalance between the body's iron requirements and iron absorption.

The guidelines for the management of anaemia from the British Society of Gastroenterology (Goddard et al., 2011) categorise the causes of IDA into occult gastro-intestinal blood losses, malabsorption problems and non-gastro-intestinal blood losses. Causes of gastro-intestinal occult blood losses include gastric carcinoma, colonic carcinoma and benign gastric ulceration. Malabsorption includes coeliac disease and *Helicobacter pylori* colonisation, which causes iron deficiency (Goddard et al., 2011). Examples of non-gastro-intestinal blood losses most typically include menstruation and blood donation.

Medicines that can cause bleeding can indirectly cause IDA (Table 50.2), with aspirin and non-steroidal anti-inflammatory drugs (NSAIDs) being the main causes. The use of antacid preparations may mask the symptoms of *H. pylori*, which can cause iron deficiency.

Clinical manifestations

In addition to the general symptoms of anaemia, various other features may be present (Box 50.4). The colour of the skin is very subjective and often unreliable. Patients at risk of heart failure may present with breathlessness when anaemic. Koilonychia,

Box 50.4 Features of iron-deficiency anaemia

- Pale skin and mucous membranes
- Painless glossitis
- Angular stomatitis
- Koilonychia (spoon-shaped nails)
- Dysphagia (due to pharyngeal web)
- Pica (unusual cravings)
- Atrophic gastritis

dysphagia and pica are found only after chronic iron deficiency and are relatively rare.

Investigations

As with all anaemias, a full blood count is essential. IDA will show a low MCV and MCH. A stained blood film will also reveal typical IDA red blood cells, which will look microcytic and hypochromic with poikilocytes (often pencil-shaped) and occasional target cells. These are abnormal thin erythrocytes which show a dark centre and peripheral ring when stained.

The most definitive marker of IDA is the level of ferritin. This may be part of an iron profile laboratory tests. A decreased transferrin saturation and a raised total iron-binding capacity reflect a lack of available iron. A low ferritin is expected in IDA, for example, less than 15 micrograms/L. Ferritin is a reactive protein and becomes slightly raised on exposure to inflammatory conditions, infection and cancer. The low ferritin level will therefore be slightly masked and may be as high as 50 micrograms/L and still be consistent with IDA, in the presence of these conditions. A normocytic or microcytic anaemia without a corresponding low level of ferritin is often anaemia of chronic disease in which iron replacement does not provide any benefit clinically or in terms of an increase in haemoglobin. Serum iron is not useful. It exhibits diurnal variation, being higher in the morning and represents a tiny fraction of the total body iron.

Other investigations undertaken are the exclusion of other types of anaemia, the response to iron replacement and a history of IDA.

Treatment

The cause of iron deficiency must be fully elucidated. The treatment for IDA is iron replacement sufficient to restore haemoglobin levels, replenish iron stores, prevent recurrence and matched with an improvement in the patient's overall well-being. Iron replacement is suitable for patients with known ongoing malabsorption problems, for example, inflammatory bowel disease, women with IDA from menstruation, pregnancy and in patients where further investigation of the IDA is not deemed appropriate, such as frail elderly patients.

Iron must be taken long enough to allow the haemoglobin to be normalised and to allow a full-body iron store to be replete. It must be monitored thereafter for early identification of any reoccurrence of IDA. The iron formulation is not critical, but it is generally recommended to use ferrous sulphate,

for example, 200 mg tablets twice or three times daily if tolerated. If this is not tolerated, then ferrous sulphate 200 mg once daily is advised because it has been suggested that the incremental iron absorption is only slightly less with lower doses of iron. Slow-release preparations confer no advantage over regular formulations and may even exacerbate gastro-intestinal effects. Therefore, such preparations should be avoided. Iron can cause gastro-intestinal disturbances such as nausea, abdominal pains and, most typically, constipation, due to the effect iron has on the gut flora.

Patient care

It is important to counsel patients on gastro-intestinal effects and that their stools may appear black. It is important to check that the patient is not taking any medications that interact with iron and, if so, to ensure that they are managed accordingly, for example, having a gap between doses if necessary. If applicable, it may be helpful to remind patients of dietary sources of iron.

Haemoglobin should be checked within 2–4 weeks to assess response to treatment. It should rise by 20 g/L in 4 weeks, and the patient should feel the benefit after 1 week. If haemoglobin has not risen by this amount, the patient's tolerance of and adherence to the medicine should be assessed. The diagnosis should also be re-evaluated because this may be an indication that it is not, in fact, iron-deficiency anaemia. Iron should be continued until the patient's iron stores are replenished, as identified by an adequate ferritin level.

Occasionally, if the patient is severely intolerant of oral iron, treatment with parenteral iron may be necessary. Oral iron should be withheld for at least 7 days after parenteral injection.

Anaemia of chronic disease

Epidemiology

This is the second most common form of anaemia (after iron deficiency). It is associated with a wide variety of inflammatory diseases, including arthritis, malignancies, inflammatory bowel disease, human immunodeficiency virus (HIV) and other infections. It is increasingly being referred to as 'anaemia of inflammation' or 'anaemia of chronic inflammation'.

Aetiology

In anaemia of chronic disease, renal production of erythropoietin is inhibited by inflammatory cytokines. Hepcidin increases in the presence of chronic disease and inflammation. It also has a key role here: it decreases the amount of iron absorption from the gut and reduces the release of iron from body stores. This means that despite the patient having sufficient overall body iron stores, the patient has the symptoms of anaemia because the iron is not being utilised (De Loughrey, 2014).

In malignancies, in addition to the anaemia of chronic disease, the cytotoxic treatments themselves decrease erythrocyte production through their anti-proliferative effects on the bone marrow. Certain cytotoxic agents, such as platinum-based therapies, are more likely to cause anaemia.

In chronic kidney disease and chronic heart failure, the reduced renal blood flow leads to a decreased production of erythropoietin.

Pathophysiology

During infections, inflammation and cancer, the inflammatory cytokines, in particular interleukin-6 released from macrophages, lead to an increased production of hepcidin. Hepcidin, a peptide produced by hepatocytes, plays a key role in iron availability. The hepcidin causes:
- increased uptake of iron by hepatocytes,
- reduced iron absorption,
- reduced release of iron from macrophages.

The reduction of circulating iron is thought to limit this essential nutrient's availability to invading microbes and tumour cells, blocking their proliferation.

In addition, the inflammatory cytokines increase the production of white blood cells, which potentially leads to fewer stem cells being available for red blood cell production.

Clinical manifestations

Patients have the general symptoms of anaemia in addition to their symptoms of the chronic inflammatory condition. Anaemia may lead to a reduced quality of life.

Investigations

The full blood count may reflect a normocytic or microcytic anaemia. It will not be as pronounced as in IDA. See Table 50.3 for a comparison. The ferritin, even allowing for inflammation, will not be low. Other evidence that supports the diagnosis of anaemia of chronic disease is the medical history, for example, heart failure or rheumatoid arthritis. Inflammatory markers may be raised, such as the erythrocyte sedimentation rate (ESR) and C-reactive protein (CRP). It should be considered that anaemia of chronic disease that cannot be attributed to any background conditions may signal an underlying gastro-intestinal malignancy. If anaemia of chronic disease has been mistaken for IDA, the patient will not respond to iron replacement, and the haemoglobin will remain unchanged, thus providing further support for a diagnosis of anaemia of chronic disease.

Table 50.3 Differentiation between iron-deficiency anaemia and anaemia of chronic disease

Test	Iron-deficiency anaemia	Anaemia of chronic disease
Serum iron	Low	Low
Serum ferritin	Low	Normal or high
Serum transferrin	High	Normal or low
Total iron-binding capacity	High	Low

Treatment

Treating the underlying chronic condition is important, where this is possible. If a patient has untreated polymyalgia rheumatica (PMR) with accompanying anaemia of chronic disease, treatment of PMR will reduce the anaemia of chronic disease, although it will never be abolished. Therefore, such patients are likely to always have some degree of anaemia of chronic disease.

Blood transfusions are rarely needed in anaemia of chronic disease. Oral iron therapy is not indicated despite the apparent reduced iron availability because these patients have a functional iron deficiency rather than an actual iron deficiency; also, the raised hepcidin levels reduce the oral absorption of iron.

Patients with chronic renal failure should be referred to a renal specialist. These patients are assessed for erythropoietin deficiency. Intravenous iron in combination with erythropoietin analogues is widely used in chronic kidney disease. The patient's serum ferritin is monitored to check for iron overload.

Patients with inflammatory bowel disease are likely to have IDA and anaemia of chronic disease. They will need iron replacement, and inevitably, intolerance of oral iron will be common in this patient group and necessitate the use of intravenous iron.

There are specialised guidelines for the use of erythropoietins in patients with anaemia induced by cancer treatment (National Institute for Health and Care Excellence [NICE], 2014).

Patient care

It is important to explain to the patient that there are different types of anaemia and that the anaemia they have is not the type that responds to iron therapy. If they are either prescribed iron or buying iron supplements, the patient should be counselled that these will not help.

Sideroblastic anaemias

Epidemiology

In haematopoiesis, there are multiple different steps in the development of the red blood cell in the bone marrow. The erythroblasts are one of the first stages in this process. Sideroblastic anaemia describes a group of anaemias which are characterised by the presence of abnormal erythroblasts, called ring sideroblasts in the bone marrow aspirate. Normal erythroblasts contain some iron granules. Sideroblasts are defective erythroblasts which contain an excess of iron granules in the mitochondrion. (Aclindor and Bridges, 2002). These excess iron granules are arranged in a distinct ring arrangement around the nucleus, hence ring sideroblasts. They are also characterised by impaired haem synthesis, where the body may have sufficient iron stores but is unable to incorporate it into haemoglobin. There are both hereditary and acquired forms of sideroblastic anaemia; the hereditary form of anaemia is comparatively rare.

Aetiology

In the majority of hereditary forms, there is an X chromosome-linked pattern of inheritance. Both autosomal-dominant and autosomal-recessive families have been described. The main defect is a reduced activity of the enzyme 5-aminolevulinate synthase (ALAS), which is involved in haem synthesis. ALAS uses a pyridoxal-6-phosphate co-enzyme to function. There are other rare causes, such as mitochondrial defects.

The more common acquired forms include idiopathic sideroblastic anaemias and those associated with myeloproliferative disorders, for example, a type of sideroblastic anaemia associated with myelodysplasia (bone marrow suppression) called refractory anaemia with ring sideroblasts (MDS-RS, formerly RARS), and forms secondary to the ingestion of drugs (Box 50.5). Its occurrence can be linked to drug toxicity, copper deficiency and, in particular, with alcoholism.

Pathophysiology

A microscopic examination of the bone marrow typically shows cells known as ring sideroblasts. In the hereditary forms, there are low levels of ALAS. This mitochondrial enzyme is involved in the first step in the synthesis of haem and requires pyridoxal phosphate as a cofactor. Pyridoxine is a precursor for pyridoxal. Impaired use of iron by the mitochondria in sideroblastic anaemia has been suggested (Aclindor and Bridges, 2002).

Drugs and toxins

Alcohol can lead to the formation of ring sideroblasts. Alcohol is metabolised to acetaldehyde, which lowers the levels of ALAS and pyridoxal. It is also proposed that folate deficiency may contribute to the sideroblastic anaemia seen in alcoholism.

Isoniazid is a known cause of sideroblastic anaemia. Pyridoxine (vitamin B_6) prophylaxis is therefore usually prescribed for all patients on isoniazid as a prophylactic measure. Chloramphenicol and linezolid are also known putative agents in causing sideroblastic anaemia. This is thought to be due to the inhibition of mitochondrial protein synthesis. Sideroblastic anaemia is associated with copper deficiency, which can be caused by an overdose of medicines used to chelate copper (e.g. penicillamine and trientine

---

Box 50.5 Acquired sideroblastic anaemia

Associated with other disorders
- Myelodysplastic syndromes
- Myeloid leukaemia
- Myeloma
- Collagen diseases

Associated with drugs and toxins
- Alcohol
- Isoniazid
- Chloramphenicol
- Penicillamine
- Pyrazinamide
- Cycloserine
- Progesterone
- Copper deficiency (associated with penicillamine, triethylene tetramine and tetrathiomolybdate)
- Lead
- Zinc

---

used in the treatment of Wilson's disease) or from nutritional deficiency as a result of long-term parenteral nutrition. Hydralazine, theoretically at least, may have the potential for causing sideroblastic anaemia because it is known to reduce pyridoxine levels.

Clinical manifestations

The hereditary forms typically develop in infancy or childhood. The anaemia can be moderate or severe (haemoglobin typically 40–100 g/L). There may be splenomegaly, which can lead to mild thrombocytopenia. The idiopathic acquired forms tend to develop insidiously, usually in middle age or later. Many patients may be asymptomatic for long periods. In the forms associated with other disorders, the clinical picture tends to be dominated by the underlying disease(s). It presents with the typical hallmarks of anaemia, fatigue, reduced exercise tolerance and dizziness. MDS-RS specifically may also present with bleeding tendencies and an increased susceptibility to infection, in common with other myelodysplasias.

Investigations

The common finding in all forms is the presence of sideroblasts in the bone marrow. In the hereditary form, the red blood cells in the peripheral blood are hypochromic and microcytic. Despite this, there are frequently increased iron stores in the bone marrow. The serum iron and ferritin may also be elevated. In the acquired forms, the peripheral blood has hypochromic cells, which may be either normocytic or macrocytic.

Treatment

Treatment is mostly supportive. For acquired forms, it involves eliminating any reversible problems (such as medication) which usually causes the sideroblastic anaemia to resolve. The patient should be investigated for copper and folate deficiency and supplemented if required. In hereditary forms, management will depend on its severity and could include blood transfusions for the most severely affected patients. Some patients with acquired or hereditary sideroblastic anaemia will benefit from pyridoxine therapy (usually 200–600 mg orally daily). Those who respond to pyridoxine therapy have a very positive response and respond quickly (Aclindor and Bridges, 2002). Because pyridoxine is a medicine with comparatively few side effects, it is worth patients being prescribed a course.

Iron deficiency is not associated with sideroblastic anaemia. Ferritin levels are usually raised in sideroblastic anaemia, and it is important that iron overload is avoided because this can contribute to sideroblastic anaemia.

Some patients with severe (hereditary) sideroblastic anaemia may ultimately require frequent blood transfusions. This carries the risk of iron overload.

Patient care

Education about sideroblastic anaemia is important, and healthcare professionals should explain to the patient that it is different from other anaemias, for example, iron-deficiency anaemia, which most people will know about. The patient will need to understand that iron is not helpful in this anaemia and in fact makes the condition worse. Genetic counselling may be appropriate for patients with hereditary sideroblastic anaemia. It is also important to explain to patients commenced on pyridoxine that this medication is not effective in everyone.

Megaloblastic anaemias

The red blood cells in macrocytic anaemia are abnormally large, with a MCV of greater than 95 fl (femtolitres). Macrocytic anaemia encompasses both megaloblastic anaemias and non-megaloblastic anaemias. These are differentiated by the cells having distinctive differences in shape and appearance under microscopic examination, and they also have different causes. This section focuses on the megaloblastic types of macrocytic anaemia and its two main causes, vitamin B_{12} deficiency and folate deficiency.

Epidemiology

WHO has acknowledged that there are no readily available data on the occurrence of vitamin B_{12} deficiency and folate deficiencies, and incidence will vary with the multiple causes of deficiency (WHO, 2008). It could be expected that poor nutrition will be closely correlated, particularly with folate deficiency. Folate levels fall more quickly, with folate body stores becoming depleted in 4 months, whereas it may take vitamin B_{12} 2–3 years to present as a deficiency. Because the main source of vitamin B_{12} in the diet comes from animal sources, vegans will be at higher risk of vitamin B_{12} deficiency. Alcoholism is often accompanied by malnutrition, which can lead to a risk of folate deficiency. The risk of developing deficiency is reputed to increase once the consumption is greater than 80 g alcohol a day (Devalia et al., 2014).

In pregnancy, folate requirements increase in view of increased cell turnover. The risk of B_{12} deficiency and folate deficiency increases with age. One large study estimated that the incidence of vitamin B_{12} and folate deficiency was around 5% in people aged 65–74 years and more than 10% in people 75 or over (Clarke et al., 2004).

Aetiology

Folate is integral in DNA synthesis. There is an increased demand for folate in times of increased cell turnover, which can therefore be associated with folate deficiency (e.g. pregnancy, malignancies and haematological conditions such as haemolytic anaemia). Folate deficiency can also arise if there is increased urinary excretion, for example, in renal dialysis patients. As well as dietary insufficiency, malabsorption can occur, such as in coeliac disease. Some drugs, such as anticonvulsants, are linked with folate deficiency. Trimethoprim and methotrexate are known folate antagonists.

The most common cause of vitamin B_{12} deficiency is pernicious anaemia. Pernicious anaemia is an autoimmune condition causing stomach atrophy, achlorhydria and, ultimately, a lack of intrinsic factor in the stomach. The intrinsic factor is an essential protein, produced by the gastric parietal cells, and it is needed for the uptake of vitamin B_{12} from the gut. The lack of intrinsic factor accounts for the resulting vitamin B_{12} deficiency in pernicious anaemia. It can also occur after gastrectomy surgery where there is a loss of intrinsic factor.

Pathophysiology

Folate is readily absorbed in the gut from folate-containing foods. Main dietary sources are green vegetables, nuts and yeast-containing foods. The daily requirement is 0.1–0.2 mg. Adult folate stores are typically 10–12 mg; this represents enough folate to sustain the body for 3–4 months in the absence of further folate supply. It is present inside the cells in the form of tetrahydrofolate and is critical in the biochemical reactions needed for DNA synthesis. Vitamin B_{12} is needed as a catalyst to convert folate into its active form inside the cell.

Vitamin B_{12} is essential for the neurological system. It is found in animal products such as fish, eggs and dairy products. After ingestion, it binds to intrinsic factor produced in the stomach and is eventually absorbed in the terminal ileum section of the gut. For vitamin B_{12}, the body stores (2–3 mg) are sufficient for 2–4 years (Hoffbrand and Moss, 2016).

Clinical manifestations

Megaloblastic anaemia presents with tiredness-related symptom such as fatigue, lethargy and dyspnea on effort. As with other types of anaemia, these can progress to palpitations and angina, especially if the patient has pre-existing cardiac disease. Further features found specifically with these anaemias are listed in Box 50.6. The patient may not realise he or she has anaemia because the onset is insidious, and it may be picked up when a patient is getting blood tests for another reason.

More serious signs of vitamin B_{12} deficiency are neurological involvement such as unexplained paraesthesia, visual disturbances and cognitive changes such as confusion. Elderly patients may have confusion symptoms with only a slight vitamin B_{12} deficiency. The feature that separates vitamin B_{12} deficiency from other megaloblastic anaemias is progressive neuropathy. It is symmetrical and affects the legs rather than the arms. Occasionally, patients have muscle weakness, have difficulty in walking or experience frequent falls. In folate deficiency, mild peripheral neuropathy and depression may manifest.

Box 50.6 Features of megaloblastic anaemia

- Glossitis (sore, pale, smooth tongue)
- Angular stomatitis
- Altered bowel habit (diarrhoea or constipation)
- Anorexia
- Mild jaundice
- Insidious onset
- Sterility
- Bilateral peripheral neuropathy (mainly vitamin B_{12} deficiency)
- Melanin skin pigmentation (rare)
- Fever (mainly vitamin B_{12} deficiency)

Investigations

A diagnosis of either folate deficiency or vitamin B_{12} deficiency is made from a medical history and clinical examination in combination with a full blood count and a serum folate and vitamin B_{12} level.

A raised mean cell volume is a sign of megaloblastic anaemia. If there are suspicions that the patient may have vitamin B_{12} deficiency, a normal MCV should not exclude further investigation. One source highlighted that 25% of patients presenting with neurological symptoms did not have an elevated MCV (Devalia et al., 2014). If there is a co-existing microcytic anaemia (such as IDA), this may mask megaloblastic anaemia. Leukopenia and thrombocytopenia may also be present, especially in more severe deficiency.

Laboratory reference values vary; however it is generally agreed that a vitamin B_{12} level less than 200 nanograms/L along with a clinical suspicion indicates vitamin B_{12} deficiency (Devalia et al., 2014). This blood test is not costly and easy to perform; however, the specificity of this test is not absolute. A blood film may be required if there are difficulties with ascertaining a diagnosis, in consultation with haematology specialist advice.

A serum folate level less than 3 micrograms/L would be indicative of folate deficiency. Serum folate level is influenced by recent folic acid intake. The gold-standard diagnostic test would be red blood cell folate; however, this is rarely required.

Treatment

It is necessary to establish whether the patient with megaloblastic anaemia has vitamin B_{12} deficiency or folic acid deficiency or both. Replacement therapy with vitamin B_{12} or folate is the mainstay of treatment.

Folic acid is normally administered as 5 mg daily. Four months should be ample duration for the folate to become replete. It should be stopped and then rechecked on an ongoing basis. Some patients may be on folic acid long-term. Folic acid should not be started before a vitamin B_{12} deficiency is excluded. Vitamin B_{12} replacement should ideally be started first if both deficiencies co-exist. Folic acid given alone, without correction of the vitamin B_{12} deficiency, may further the neuropathy symptoms or precipitate a subacute combined degeneration of the spinal cord.

Hydroxocobalamin replacement therapy should follow the schedule in the British National Formulary (BNF) or equivalent local formularies. This is currently five doses of hydroxocobalamin 1 mg given intramuscularly over a period of 2 weeks then 1 mg every 3 months as a maintenance dose (Joint Formulary Committee, 2017).

It is given every 2 months where there is already neurological involvement. Neurological damage may be irreversible. Peripheral neuropathy of recent onset often partially improves, but any spinal cord damage is irreversible even with optimum therapy.

Response to therapy can be seen by an increase in reticulocyte numbers within 3–5 days. More importantly, the patient will start to feel better within 24–48 hours of starting treatment. The haemoglobin will rise slowly at a rate of 20–30 g/L.

Oral cyancobalamin is poorly absorbed. It is used occasionally in mild deficiency related to diet. Hypokalaemia develops in some patients during the initial haematological response because potassium is an intracellular ion used in the production of new cells. Potassium supplements may be needed in the elderly and patients receiving diuretics or digoxin. The serum iron level also falls as it is incorporated into haemoglobin. The more severe the anaemia, the more likely it is to see a fall in the serum potassium or iron level.

Treatment of any reversible or ongoing causes such as previously undiagnosed coeliac disease or tapeworm is also required. Prophylactic folic acid is used in pregnancy, and prophylactic vitamin B_{12} injections are administered in patients after gastrectomy because they will lose intrinsic factor produced by the parietal cells.

Patient care

Folic acid deficiency anaemia

In patients who have a dietary component to their deficiency, appropriate nutritional advice should go alongside their folic acid therapy. If the cause of the deficiency has been eliminated, patients can expect to receive folic acid for approximately 4–6 months. In patients with a continuing requirement, for example, haemolytic anaemia patients can expect lifelong treatment. Those commencing folic acid therapy can anticipate feeling better after a few days but should be informed that their blood count will take much longer to return to normal.

Vitamin B_{12} deficiency anaemia

Patients feel subjectively better very shortly after their first hydroxocobalamin injection. If they have glossitis, it will start to improve within 2 days and return to normal after 2–4 weeks. Patients need to be informed that they need regular injections, usually every 3 months. Surprisingly, some patients say that they feel they are ready for this injection as they approach their appointment time and feel better after their injection.

Patients should be advised to highlight to healthcare staff at appointments and if admitted to hospital that they receive regular vitamin B_{12} injections and when their next injection is due.

Haemolytic anaemias

Normally, there is a natural continuous turnover of erythrocytes. After being produced in the bone marrow, liver or spleen, the new erythrocytes are released into the plasma as immature erythrocytes, reticulocytes. After circulation in the plasma for around 120 days, the erythrocyte gradually degrades and releases haem and globins which are reutilised in the body.

In the haemolytic anaemias, there is a reduced lifespan of the erythrocytes. Anaemia occurs when the rate of destruction of the erythrocytes exceeds their rate of production. Haemolytic anaemias account for 5% of all anaemias. There is a wide range of haemolytic anaemias, with both genetic and acquired disorders (Table 50.4). This section will focus on the main types of autoimmune haemolytic anaemias.

General clinical manifestations

The bone marrow compensates for this overdrive in red blood cell production by an expansion of the bone marrow. In fact, the

Table 50.4 Some examples of haemolytic anaemias	
	Examples
Genetic disorders of	
Haemoglobin	Sickle cell anaemias
	Thalassaemias
Energy pathways	Glucose-6-phosphate deficiency
Membrane	Hereditary spherocytosis
	Hereditary ovalocytosis
Acquired disorders	
Immune	Autoimmune
	Rh or ABO incompatibility
Non-immune	Infections (parasitic, bacterial)
	Drugs and chemicals
	Hypersplenism
ABO, ABO blood groups; Rh, rhesus factor.	

Box 50.7 Drugs associated with autoimmune haemolytic anaemia
• Ciclosporin
• Fludarabine
• Interferon A
• Levodopa
• Mefenamic acid
• Methyldopa
• Penicillin
• Quinine
• Quinidine

enlarged bone marrow can increase the rate of red blood cell production by up to eight times. This compensatory response can mean that symptoms may not present until the erythrocyte production has decreased for 30 days (Hoffbrand and Moss, 2016).

Patients with acute haemolytic anaemia commonly complain of malaise, fever, abdominal pain, dark urine and jaundice. The urine is dark because of excess storage iron (haemosiderin) being excreted in the urine. Jaundice may result from the increased cell turnover causing an increased serum bilirubin. The increased erythrocyte turnover is also reflected in an increased number of reticulocytes. Patients with chronic haemolytic anaemia also usually have splenomegaly. Their anaemia is usually normochromic and normocytic.

General treatment

This increased demand for folate caused by bone marrow hyperplasia may necessitate folate administration. Patients who require frequent transfusions are at risk of iron overload. Any other coexisting types of anaemia should be treated and any offending agents or causes addressed.

Autoimmune haemolytic anaemia

Epidemiology

Autoimmune haemolytic anaemia as the name implies is caused by the body's own immune system. It acts against its own red blood cell antigens. The incidence is described as approximately 1 per 100,000/year (Hill et al., 2017). It can occur at any age; however, it does become more common as people get older. It is divided serologically into two types by the Coombs test, which tests whether the antibody reacts more strongly with red blood cells at a cold temperature or a warm temperature. The result of this test determines how it should be treated. The warm type, called warm autoimmune haemolytic anaemia (WAIHA),

accounts for 65% of this type of anaemia. The cold types, called cold haemagglutinin disease (CHAD) and paroxysmal cold haemoglobinuria, account for 29% and 1%, respectively. The remaining 5% is accounted for by a mixed type (Hill et al., 2017).

Aetiology

In WAIHA, the coating of the red blood cell membrane is rendered defective, making the red blood cell more easily degraded. It is most closely associated with immunoglobulin G (IgG), which attaches to the membrane, mostly in the spleen. It is common for WAIHA to occur in association with other immune-related diseases, such as systemic lupus erythematosus, but it may also occur alone. It typically has a remitting and relapsing course.

In CHAD, it is the IgM antibody that attaches to the red blood cell membrane, in this case, mostly in the peripheral circulation. Primary CHAD can present in middle or older age. It is aggravated by cold temperatures and often associated with intravascular haemolysis. Patients could suffer from cold-induced acrocyanosis (blue discolouration of the peripheries) or Raynaud's disease.

Secondary CHAD can be precipitated by an infection. Certain drugs have also been implicated as leading to immune haemolysis (Box 50.7).

Pathophysiology

The anaemia results from the presence of autoantibodies which agglutinate (clump together) or lyse the patient's own erythrocytes. In WAIHA, the haemolysis is usually extravascular and mediated by IgG. These antibodies react best at body temperature. CHAD is usually mediated by IgM, which attaches to the erythrocytes and causes them to agglutinate at temperatures less than 37 °C. This results in impaired blood flow to the fingers, toes, nose and ears when exposed to cold.

Clinical manifestations

The clinical manifestations of autoimmune haemolytic anaemia have the common signs of anaemia of tiredness-related symptoms but they also vary depending on which subtype is present. The symptoms in WAIHA are related to the severity of the haemolysis and can present as acute or chronic anaemia. The spleen may be enlarged.

In chronic CHAD the patient may present with splenomegaly and mild jaundice. It will generally worsen or become acute during the cold weather. As previously identified, Raynaud's disease or acrocyanosis may occur.

Investigations

A positive direct Coomb's test indicates the presence of antibodies to red blood cells and distinguishes warm and cold subtypes. Drug-induced haemolytic anaemia may be difficult to distinguish from other forms of autoimmune haemolytic anaemia, and a detailed medication history will help. The antibodies produced may react with the red blood cells only in the presence of the drug (or one of its metabolites) or may also react without the drug being present.

Treatment

In WAIHA, the treatment includes removing any underlying cause, such as a drug, if applicable. The British Society of Haematology has produced recommendations on the treatment of autoimmune haemolytic anaemia (Hill et al., 2017). First-line treatment is with steroids, such as prednisolone 1 mg/kg/day. This has a generally good response rate of 80% and can achieve complete remission in two-thirds of patients (Hill et al., 2017). It will usually respond within 3 weeks, and once a haemoglobin of greater than 100 g/L is achieved, the steroid dose can be gradually reduced. Gastroprotection should be prescribed. Rituximab is very effective and can be used alone or as second-line treatment in combination with steroids. Different dosage regimens are used. Ultimately, if necessary, splenectomy is also an effective treatment. Immunosuppressants such as azathioprine and ciclosporin provide further treatment options (Hill et al., 2017).

A different approach is taken in CHAD. Therapeutic intervention should be considered if the patient is symptomatic, especially if the patient has severe symptoms. It is imperative that the patient is proactive in avoiding cold exposure and dresses accordingly. Rituximab may also be used in CHAD, and the addition of fludarabine should be considered if the response to rituximab alone is suboptimal. Steroids do not have a role in CHAD, and splenectomy is usually avoided.

Patient care

Patients will need counselling and support for any of the medicines used. The patient should be informed of the unlicensed use of rituximab and that there is a risk of infusion reactions. Patients will also need advice on the use of corticosteroids, gastroprotection and osteoporosis prophylaxis. If a drug-induced subtype has been identified, they will need to be fully informed about the drug they should avoid and have it listed as an allergy in their medication records. They will need practical advice and support on avoiding cold exposure and maintaining a consistent ambient temperature.

Sickle cell anaemia

Epidemiology

Sickle cell anaemia is so named after the appearance of the red blood cells, which resemble the shape of a sickle, an agricultural tool. Sickle cell disease is a hereditary condition. Several

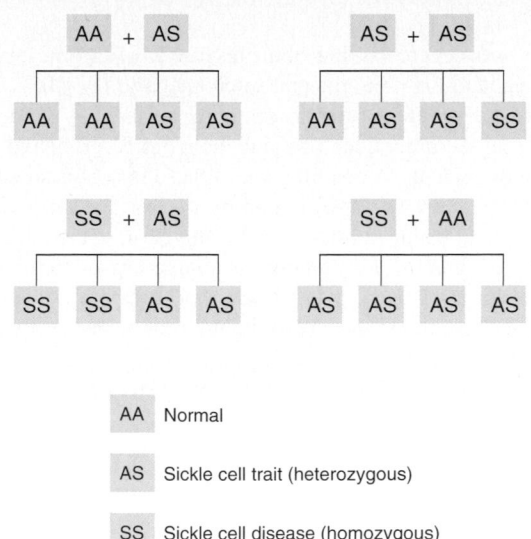

Fig. 50.2 Inheritance patterns in sickle cell trait and sickle cell disease.

different variants of sickle cell disease exist. It is common throughout Africa, the Middle East, parts of India and the Mediterranean. The carrier state is widespread, with a particularly high prevalence in West Africa of up to 30% (Hoffbrand and Moss, 2016).

Aetiology

Patients with sickle cell disease have a different form of haemoglobin. Patients with the most common variant of sickle cell disease have haemoglobin S (HbS). Normal haemoglobin is usually designated haemoglobin A (HbA). HbS has valine substituted for glutamic acid as the sixth amino acid in the β-polypeptide compared with normal haemoglobin. Patients with homozygous haemoglobin S develop many problems, including anaemia.

Sickle cell trait is where a person is a carrier of the gene (heterozygous for the sickle cell gene). These people are usually asymptomatic. Sickle cell trait provides some protection from malaria and is more common in those ethnic groups originating from geographical areas that are endemic for malaria. The offspring from a father with the trait and a mother with the trait has a one in four chance of having sickle cell disease (Fig. 50.2).

Pathophysiology

The membrane of red blood cells containing haemoglobin S is damaged, which leads to intracellular dehydration. In addition, when the patient's blood is deoxygenated, polymerisation of HbS occurs, forming a semisolid gel. These two processes lead to the formation of crescent-shaped cells known as sickle cells. Sickle cells are less flexible than normal cells (flexibility allows normal cells to pass through the microcirculation). The inflexibility leads to impaired blood flow through the microcirculation, resulting in local tissue hypoxia. Anaemia results from an increased destruction (haemolysis) of red blood cells in the spleen.

Clinical manifestations

Patients with severe variants of the disease have chronic anaemia, arthralgia, anorexia, fatigue and splenomegaly. They have crises more frequently than patients with other variants of the disease. A crisis can be precipitated by infection and fever, dehydration, hypoxia or acidosis. A combination of these factors is sometimes present. The clinical manifestation of a crisis can vary with the most common being an infarct crisis. Infarction of the long bones and larger joints or an infarction of a large organ, for example, the liver, lungs or brain, may all occur. Severe pain is a common feature, depending on the site of the infarction. Destructive bone and joint problems are frequently seen.

Infections carry a higher risk of morbidity and mortality due to compromised spleen function.

Investigations

The haemoglobin is typically 60–90 g/L. In healthy adults, there are different variants of haemoglobin; most of our haemoglobin is HbA (96–98%; Hoffbrand and Moss, 2016). The remaining portion consists of small amounts of HbA_2 and haemoglobin-F (HbF). The confirmation tests for sickle cell anaemia are based on the fact that in this condition, patients have a much higher proportion of HbF and have a haemoglobin unique to this condition.

Electrophoresis or high-performance liquid chromatography (HPLC) analysis of the haemoglobin would show HbS 80–99% with no normal. The HbF may also be elevated to about 15%. The background family history is also helpful. The presence of sickle cells in the blood film is also diagnostic. Reticulocytes could be increased as much as up to 10–20%, reflecting the excessive production of red blood cells by the bone marrow.

Treatment

Treatment is based around supportive care, managing pain, preventing infection and modifying HbS production or increasing HbF production and avoiding crises.

To help prevent infections *H. influenzae*, meningococcal and pneumococcal vaccinations are administered. Prophylactic use of penicillin V 250 mg twice a day is usual for adults with erythromycin prescribed for patients allergic to penicillin. Simple measures such as good general nutrition and handwashing are advised. All precipitating factors for a crisis should be avoided as far as possible, such as dehydration. Good daily hydration should be maintained. Folic acid is commonly used because of the high turnover of red blood cells.

Transfusions have been used in severe cases with the aim of suppressing HbS production. Hydroxycarbamide is also an option used in patients who experience frequent crises; it increases HbF, which has a positive effect on reducing symptoms. Erythropoietin may be used occasionally with the same rationale – to increase HbF. However, because erythropoietin levels are not normally low in sickle cell anaemia, its use is limited.

Beyond painful crises, some patients progress to chronic and severe pain. Therefore, such patients also need great attention focused on managing pain and supporting them to maintain a good quality of life.

Sickle cell crises require prompt and effective treatment. Removal of the trigger factor, hydration and effective pain relief are the mainstays of treatment. Appropriate antibiotic therapy should be started at the first signs of infection. Strong opioids are required for pain relief.

Patient care

Patients need to be encouraged to take their prophylactic penicillin and folic acid therapy regularly between crises. During a crisis, some health professionals worry about the patient developing opioid addiction. Although this may happen, it is also important to recognise that crises are extremely painful, and the patient requires effective analgesia.

Thalassaemias

Epidemiology

The thalassaemias are a group of inherited autosomal-recessive diseases. The α thalassaemias are most common in Africa, Afro-Caribbean regions, South and East Asia and in the Eastern Mediterranean. The β thalassaemias occur mainly in populations from around the Mediterranean, North and West Africa, Middle East and the Indian subcontinent.

Aetiology

The thalassaemias are a group of anaemias that result from either a reduced or absent production of one or more of the constituent globin chains in the haemoglobin.

In α thalassaemia the severity is associated with the number of the globin chains which are missing or dysfunctional and the type of deletion or mutation involved. It is generally the result of large deletions within an α globin complex. Haemoglobin Bart's hydrops fetalis is a variant of α thalassaemia and results in stillbirth of a newborn baby, as tissue oxygenation cannot be maintained. More than 100 β thalassaemia mutations have been identified. There are two copies of the β globin gene in each cell. If one is abnormal, this is called β thalassaemia trait. If both genes are affected, it is called β thalassaemia intermedia or major.

Pathophysiology

In β thalassaemias, there is a reduced or absent production of the globin β chain. This leads to a relative excess of α chain which when unpaired becomes unstable and precipitates in the red blood cell precursors. There is ineffective erythropoiesis, and those mature cells that reach the circulation have a shortened lifespan.

In α thalassaemias, the pathology is slightly different. The deficiency of α chains leads to an excess of γ or β chains. This time erythropoiesis is less affected, but the haemoglobin produced (haemoglobin Bart's or haemoglobin H) is unstable. This leads to a shortened lifespan, with the spleen trapping many of the cells.

Clinical manifestations

The anaemia causes erythropoietin production to increase and results in expansion of the bone marrow. In severe disease, this causes bone deformity and growth retardation. The spleen is actively involved in removing the abnormal mature cells from the circulation and becomes enlarged.

Investigations

In α thalassaemia, the MCV and the MCH are decreased and the red blood cell count, as well as reticulocytes, will be increased.

For β thalassaemia, the diagnosis is relatively straightforward: haemolytic anaemia from infancy and ethnicity. Haemoglobin electrophoresis is used to determine the amounts of abnormal haemoglobin. Haemoglobin is reduced but is not usually much less than 100 g/L. The MCV will also be reduced. It is also a microcytic and hypochromic anaemia.

Treatment

For both thalassaemias, there is currently no definitive treatment. Patients with thalassaemia minor (those who carry the thalassaemia gene but still make enough normal haemoglobin) and α thalassaemia usually do not require treatment. Patients with severe forms are dependent on blood transfusions. Iron chelation and avoidance of iron overload, as appropriate, are important. Folate supplementation as well as prompt treatment of infection are also important. Hydroxycarbamide could be used to increase HbF, which is helpful in β thalassaemias.

Patient care

Drug therapy does not currently play a significant role in treatment. If hydroxycarbamide becomes used more frequently, pharmacists will become involved in educating the patient particularly with regard to its cytotoxic effects.

Glucose-6-phosphate dehydrogenase deficiency

Epidemiology

Glucose-6-phosphate dehydrogenase (G6PD) deficiency is a recessive hereditary disease and affects approximately 400 million people worldwide (Nkhoma et al., 2009). There are more than 300 different forms of G6PD deficiency, only some of which cause anaemia. It occurs in West Africa, Southern Europe, the Middle East and South-East Asia. The impact of the deficiency varies between ethnic groups. Typically, the mildest form in black African people and the most severe in Mediterranean people. Severe deficiency occurs occasionally in white people.

Aetiology

Unlike some of the other types, this anaemia can only be genetically derived. The inheritance is sex linked. It is carried by females who show 50% normal G6PD activity and predominantly affects males.

Pathophysiology

A reduced form of glutathione (GSH) confers a protective effect on the cell membranes of haemoglobin and red blood cells from oxidant stress effects. G6PD is needed for the production of nicotinamide adenine dinucleotide phosphate (NADP). This in turn is needed for the production of GSH. In G6DP deficiency, the cells are therefore susceptible to oxidative stress. Exposure to an agent which causes overwhelming oxidative stress precipitates an acute haemolytic anaemia.

Clinical manifestation

Clinically, the two most important types of G6PD deficiency occur in the black population and in people originating from the Mediterranean. The black population has a milder form that results in an acute self-limiting haemolytic anaemia after exposure to an oxidising agent, for example, infection, acute illness, broad beans (fava) beans or drugs (Box 50.8). The haemolytic anaemia is self-limiting because the young cells produced by the bone marrow have higher levels of G6PD activity than old cells. After exposure to the oxidising agent, the old cells are haemolysed but the new cells produced in response are more capable of tolerating the insult until they grow old. In the Mediterranean form of the disorder, the enzyme activity is very low, haemolysis is not usually self-limiting and, indeed, some patients have a chronic haemolytic anaemia despite the absence of an obvious causative factor.

Investigations

The history and the clinical findings steer the diagnosis, which is then confirmed by measuring G6PD activity. Care must be taken during the acute phase because there are increased numbers of young cells with higher levels of activity that may be misleading. The increased numbers of young cells result from the selective destruction of older cells and the increased production of reticulocytes. The full blood count will be normal in between attacks of haemolytic anaemia.

Box 50.8 Common drugs implicated in causing haemolysis in G6PD deficiency

Drugs to be avoided in all variants
- Ciprofloxacin (and probably other quinolones)
- Dapsone
- Methylene blue
- Primaquine (reduced dose may be used in milder variants)
- Nalidixic acid
- Sulfonamides (including co-trimoxazole)

Drugs to be avoided in more severe variants
- Aspirin (low dose used under supervision)
- Chloramphenicol
- Chloroquine (may be acceptable in acute malaria)
- Menadione
- Probenecid
- Quinidine
- Quinine (acceptable in acute malaria)

Treatment

Prevention of haemolysis by avoiding trigger factors (drugs or food) is important. Vaccination against hepatitis A and hepatitis B may reduce attacks. In cases of acute haemolytic anaemia, the causative oxidising agent should be stopped and general supportive measures adopted. In chronic haemolytic anaemia, most patients become reasonably well adjusted to their anaemia. They need to avoid known precipitating factors to prevent acute episodes occurring on top of their chronic haemolytic anaemia.

There is no specific drug treatment. During acute episodes, the patient should be kept well hydrated to ensure good urine output to prevent haemoglobin damaging the kidney. Blood transfusions may be necessary.

Patient care

Patients should be educated and can be given a list of drugs to avoid. It is important that patients remind healthcare professionals of their condition. Pharmacists have a role in keeping healthcare staff informed of the high-risk drugs that can cause G6PD anaemia.

Case studies

Case 50.1

Mr HA, a 60-year-old single unemployed man, was admitted to hospital for investigation of anaemia. He presented with a 6-month history of lethargy, chest pain, dizziness and falls and a past history of having a gastrectomy 26 years ago. The drug history on admission showed that Mr HA was taking diazepam and GTN spray.

Review of systems revealed no vomiting and no melaena. He complained of some indigestion after meals and reported his appetite was fine if someone else cooked. On examination, he was pale, with a blood pressure of 140/80 mmHg, pulse 90 bpm and haemoglobin level of 25 g/L (normal range: 135–180 g/L). Endoscopy and colonoscopy were normal, and a biopsy showed no evidence of coeliac disease. A barium enema was also unremarkable.

Over the first 2 days, he was transfused with 8 units of blood and given furosemide 40 mg with alternate bags. On day 7 he was started on ferrous sulfate 200 mg three times a day, folic acid 5 mg daily and ascorbic acid 200 mg three times a day.

Questions

1. What additional questions should Mr HA have been asked at admission?
2. Comment on the use of vitamin C in Mr HA.
3. How long should Mr HA remain on ferrous sulphate?

Answers

1. Although Mr HA's prescribed drugs were documented, it is possible that he was taking purchased medication. On admission, he complained of indigestion over the last 3 months, and on questioning, he revealed that he was self-medicating with aluminium hydroxide mixture. From a theoretical point of view, antacids may reduce the amount of iron absorbed by increasing the pH of the stomach and by reducing the solubility of ferrous salts. It is unlikely that this contributed significantly to the development of his anaemia, but if he intends to continue using an antacid after discharge, which should be discouraged, it would be better not to take a dose of the antacid within 1–2 hours of his ferrous sulfate. It would also be worth checking to see if he has been self-medicating with a purchased aspirin or ibuprofen-based product; both drugs have been implicated in causing gastro-intestinal blood loss, although in this case his gastro-intestinal investigations were normal.

2. Ascorbic acid increases the absorption of iron in some patients, probably by keeping iron in solution either in the ferrous form or by being a soluble chelate with the ferric form. Its benefit in correcting iron-deficiency anemia is unclear, and it is not routinely recommended. It may be an advantage in Mr HA because he may also benefit from a short course of multivitamins.

3. Mr HA needs to continue iron therapy until he has at least replenished his iron stores. This may take up to 6 months, after which time he should be reassessed. He should be counselled on the importance of an iron-rich diet and referred to a dietician if necessary. In practice, because his iron was dangerously low on admission, it may be quite reasonable to prescribe him iron for the rest of his life.

Case 50.2

Mr WK, a 46-year-old mechanic, is referred to hospital by his primary care doctor. He gave a history of diarrhoea and vomiting a week ago and now was complaining of headaches, abdominal pain and feeling 'lousy'. His doctor had given him metoclopramide and ferrous sulfate because his haemoglobin had dropped. Mr WK was pale but did not appear jaundiced, although he said he had noticed his urine was unusually dark a few weeks ago. On examination, he was obese, with a blood pressure of 120/80 mmHg and a pulse of 80 bpm. Rectal examination revealed black stools. He had a normal gastroscopy with three negative FOBs. His serum biochemistry showed a normal level of alanine transaminase and a slightly raised total bilirubin level. Mr WK's reticulocyte percentage was 13.5% (normal range: 0.5–1.5%). He was diagnosed with having G6PD deficiency, probably triggered by an infection.

Questions

1. How do you explain Mr WK's dark urine and dark stools?
2. Would Mr WK benefit from any medication after admission?
3. Why is it necessary to repeat his red blood cell G6PD levels after 2 months?

Answers

1. Mr WK's dark urine was a consequence of his haemolytic anaemia. Bilirubin is a breakdown product of haemoglobin that is transported to the liver and conjugated before being excreted in the bile. Bacteria in the intestine converts this to urobilinogen, most of which is excreted in the stools. Small amounts of urobilinogen are reabsorbed, and some of this appears in the urine. Urobilinogen is oxidised to urobilin, which is coloured. During episodes of haemolysis, erythrocytes are destroyed faster than normal, and hence there is an increase in the formation of bilirubin and increased excretion of urobilinogen in the urine. Also during haemolysis, free haemoglobin may be released into the blood. If the haemolysis is severe enough, the normal mechanism for removing haemoglobin from the circulation is overcome, and haemoglobin may appear in the urine.

Dark stools may indicate melaena and upper gastro-intestinal bleeding. In Mr WK's case, his gastroscopy was normal, and he had three negative FOBs. His dark stools were therefore likely to be due to the ferrous sulfate prescribed by the primary care doctor before admission.

2. His raised reticulocyte count indicates he is rapidly replacing his lost red blood cells. Erythropoiesis consumes folate and iron, so it may be worth giving him a short course of folate supplements in addition to the oral iron already prescribed, until stores of both are normalised.

3. Young red blood cells tend to have higher levels of enzyme activity than more mature cells. Determining G6PD levels during the acute phase may be misleading because there is a relatively high proportion of young cells. Mr WK's result 2 months later would more accurately represent his normal state.

Case 50.3

Ms PR, a 58-year-old lady, was admitted to the emergency department. She had fallen over and bruised herself but had no broken bones. On examination, it was noted that she appeared pale, with possibly a lemon-yellow tinge to her skin; she was slightly confused and had paresthesiae of the feet and fingers. She has a past history of heart failure. She was admitted for investigation and discovered to have a macrocytic anaemia; pernicious anaemia was suspected. Folate and vitamin B_{12} levels were carried out before commencing treatment.

Questions

1. What are the features that may lead you to consider a diagnosis of pernicious anaemia?
2. Can Miss PR have a blood transfusion after samples have been taken for folate and vitamin B_{12}?
3. The red blood cell folate is reported as 150 mg/L (reference range: 160–640 mg/L). Would Ms PR benefit from folate therapy?

Answers

1. Macrocytic anaemia and paraesthesia are typical features, although not diagnostic, of pernicious anaemia. Patients may be mildly jaundiced, which is often described as lemon-yellow in colour. Interestingly, pernicious anaemia is more common in women than men and is associated with blue eyes and early greying of the hair. Miss PR may have other features of pernicious anaemia, which include glossitis, angular stomatitis and altered bowel habit.
2. Patients with pernicious anaemia develop their anaemia over a long period of time and tend not to tolerate increases in blood volume very well. A transfusion may result in fluid overload and precipitate heart failure. Miss PR already has heart failure, so unless she becomes severely compromised by anaemia, a transfusion should not be given. In patients who have such pronounced anaemia that an urgent transfusion is required, an exchange transfusion of a small volume of packed cells may be appropriate.
3. In vitamin B_{12} deficiency, folate tends to leak from cells, and the red blood cell folate is often low (serum folate is sometimes raised). Many patients initially require both folate and vitamin B_{12} although folate can usually be stopped after a short course. Folate therapy must never be given to patients who have not been fully investigated for vitamin B_{12} deficiency. If vitamin B_{12}–deficient patients are given large doses of folate without hydroxocobalamin, the full blood count may appear to improve, but the peripheral neuropathy from the vitamin B_{12} deficiency progresses.

Case 50.4

Mrs GN, a 76-year-old retired factory worker, was seen by her primary care doctor, complaining of tiredness. She had been seen 2 months earlier and started on ferrous sulfate for microcytic anaemia. Initially, she had felt better, but the tiredness soon returned. A bone marrow aspiration revealed increased erythropoiesis, iron stores and red blood cell precursors.

A diagnosis of sideroblastic anaemia was made, and it was decided to give her monthly transfusions. She was started on pyridoxine 50 mg three times a day in addition to ferrous sulfate.

Questions

1. What are the potential problems with Mrs GN's treatment?
2. After 3 months, there appeared to be little benefit to show from pyridoxine. How might management be improved?

Answers

1. Mrs GN's bone marrow aspiration and serum ferritin level showed that she has high levels of stored iron. Repeated monthly transfusions will also contribute to further iron accumulation; each transfused unit contains around 200–250 mg of iron (Hoffbrand et al., 2012). In sideroblastic anaemia, the bone marrow appears to be inefficient at incorporating the iron into haem. The administration of iron leads to iron overload, which may result in damage to the heart, liver and endocrine organs. The ferrous sulfate must be stopped. If iron accumulation remains a problem, iron chelation therapy using deferoxamine or deferasirox would be necessary.
2. Pyridoxine does not always improve the blood picture in patients with sideroblastic anaemia. In sideroblastic anaemia, the dose of pyridoxine required is usually 400 mg daily. Therefore, in the case of Mrs GN, an increase in dose should be tried. In addition, patients with sideroblastic anaemia may be unaware that pyridoxine is not just a simple vitamin but a specific treatment for anaemia. Counselling the patient would be essential to improve adherence.

Case 50.5

Mrs RO, a 70-year-old retired teacher, presented with a history of increased tiredness over the last 6 weeks. She has a past history of a partial gastrectomy 4 years ago. On questioning, her relevant symptoms included 'pins and needles' in her toes and loose bowels. She said that she had never been a good eater but ate red meat twice a week. On investigation, her serum vitamin B_{12} level was found to be 27 ng/L (range 150–400 ngl/L).

Questions

1. Why was it 4 years after her gastrectomy before Mrs RO developed vitamin B_{12} deficiency?
2. How long will it take for Mrs RO to respond to treatment?
3. What therapy will Mrs RO require?

Answers

1. Vitamin B_{12} requires intrinsic factor produced by the stomach for absorption. Patients with a total gastrectomy and some with a partial gastrectomy malabsorb vitamin B_{12}. Most patients have good body stores, and even if no new vitamin B_{12} enters the body

(e.g. after a total gastrectomy), it will take at least 2 years to deplete the stores.

2. Many patients will feel better within days of starting treatment with hydroxocobalamin and before a change in their haemoglobin concentration can be detected. Mrs RO's blood picture may take a number of weeks to return to normal. However, her 'pins and needles' may be a sign of peripheral neuropathy, which can be irreversible and may not respond to the hydroxocobalamin treatment.

3. Mrs RO will require lifelong replacement therapy. The standard treatment for vitamin B_{12} deficiency is hydroxocobalamin 1 mg intramuscularly three times a week for 2 weeks, then 1 mg every 3 months. If neurological involvement is identified, as in the case of Mrs RO, then a slightly higher dose regimen is recommended of 1 mg on alternate days until no further improvement, followed by 1 mg every 2 months thereafter. Unlike Mrs RO, in patients in whom vitamin B_{12} deficiency is likely to be exclusively diet related, it may be possible to reduce the frequency of injections to twice yearly.

Acknowledgement

The authors acknowledge the contribution of C. Acomb and R. Sanderson to versions of this chapter which appeared in previous editions.

References

Alcindor, T., Bridges, K.R., 2002. Sideroblastic anaemias. Br. J. Haematol. 116, 733–743.

Camaschella, C., 2015. Iron-deficient anaemia. New Engl. J. Med. 372, 1832–1843.

Clarke, R., Grimley-Evans, J., Schneede, J., et al., 2004. Vitamin B_{12} deficiency and folate deficiency in later life. Age Ageing 33 (1), 31–41.

De Loughery, T., 2014. Microcytic anaemia. New Engl. J. Med. 14, 1324–1331.

Devalia, V., Hamilton, M.S., Molloy, A.M., and the British Committee for Standards in Haematology, 2014. Guidelines for the diagnosis and treatment of cobalamin and folate disorders. Br. J. Haematol. 166, 496–513.

Goddard, A.F., James, M.W., McIntyre, A.S., et al., 2011. Guidelines for the management of iron deficiency anaemia. Gut 60, 1309–1316.

Hill, Q., Stamps, R., Massey, E., et al., 2017. The diagnosis and management of primary autoimmune haemolytic anaemia. Guideline. Br. J. Haematol. 176, 395–411.

Hoffbrand, A.V., Taher, A., Cappellini, M.D., 2012. How I treat transfusional iron overload. Blood 120 (18), 3657–3669.

Hoffbrand, V., Moss, P., 2016. Hoffbrand's Essential Haematology, seventh ed. Wiley Blackwell, Oxford.

Joint Formulary Committee, 2017. British National Formulary 73. BMJ Group and Pharmaceutical Press, London.

Mason, P., 2008. Understanding iron requirements. Pharm. J. 281, 47–51.

National Institute for Health and Care Excellence (NICE), 2014. Erythropoiesis-stimulating agents (epoetin and darbepoetin) for treating anaemia in people with cancer having chemotherapy. Available at: https://www.nice.org.uk/Guidance/TA323.

Nkhoma, E.T., Poole, C., Vannappagari, V., et al., 2009. The global prevalence of glucose-6-phosphate dehydrogenase deficiency: a systematic review and meta-analysis. Blood Cells Mol. Dis. 42 (3), 267–278.

World Health Organization (WHO), 2008. Conclusions of a WHO technical consultation on folate and vitamin B_{12} deficiencies. Food Nutr. Bull. 29 (2), 238–244. Available at: http://www.who.int/nutrition/publications/micronutrients/FNBvol29N2supjun08.pdf?ua=1.

World Health Organization (WHO), 2011. Haemoglobin concentrations for the diagnosis of anaemia and assessment of severity. Available at: http://www.who.int/vmnis/indicators/haemoglobin.pdf.

World Health Organization (WHO), 2015. The global prevalence of anaemia in 2011. Available at: http://www.who.int/nutrition/publications/micronutrients/global_prevalence_anaemia_2011/en/.

Further reading

Andro, M., Le Squere, P., Estivin, S., et al., 2013. Anaemia and cognitive performances in the elderly: a systematic review. Eur. J. Neurol. 20, 1234–1240.

Gurasamy, K.S., Nagendran, M., Broadhurst, J.F., et al., 2014. Iron therapy in anaemic adults without chronic kidney disease. Cochrane DB Syst. Rev. 2014 (12), Art. No. CD10649. doi:1002/14651858.CD01064.pou2.

Killick, S., Bown, N., Cavenagh, J., et al., 2016. Guidelines for the diagnosis and management of adult and aplastic anaemia. Br. J. Haematol. 172, 187–207.

Kotze, A., Harris, A., Baker, C., et al., 2015. British Committee for Standards in Haematology Guidelines on the identification and management of pre-operative anaemia. Br. J. Haematol. 171, 322–331.

McGarry, N., 2015. Iron deficiency anaemia. Pharm. J. 294, 280–282.

Polin, V., Coriat, R., Perkin, G., et al., 2013. Iron deficiency: from diagnosis to treatment. Digest. Liver Dis. 45, 803–809.

Useful websites

British Society of Haematology: http://www.b-s-h.org.uk/
Bloodline: http://www.bloodline.net/
BloodMed.com: http://www.bloodmed.com
American Society of Haematology: http://www.hematology.org/

Guideline and Audit Implementation Network, Northern Ireland Transfusion Committee: https://www.rqia.org.uk/RQIA/files/1e/1e2a9adc-7517-4a47-858a-5192b0746456.pdf.

51 Leukaemia

Michelle Lannon and Gail Jones

Key points

- Leukaemias are uncommon malignancies.
- Acute lymphoblastic leukaemia (ALL) is the most common malignancy in childhood.
- With the exception of ALL, leukaemias are more common in the elderly.
- Age is one of the most important prognostic factors in the treatment of leukaemia. With the exception of neonates, older patients are less likely to be cured than younger patients.
- The treatment of leukaemia is continually improving with the introduction of more focused therapy and improvements in supportive care.
- The use of bone marrow transplantation in the treatment of all forms of leukaemia is increasing. Some of the results are exciting, but the short- and long-term problems of this type of intensive treatment need to be considered.

Leukaemias and lymphomas are the commonest forms of haematological malignancy. Although rare, they are of particular interest in that dramatic improvements in the prognosis of patients with these cancers have been achieved through the use of chemotherapy. Cure is now a possibility for many patients.

Many forms of leukaemia exist, but they are all characterised by the production of excessive numbers of abnormal white blood cells. The leukaemias can be broadly divided into four groups:
- acute myeloblastic leukaemia (AML),
- acute lymphoblastic leukaemia (ALL),
- chronic myelocytic leukaemia (CML),
- chronic lymphocytic leukaemia (CLL).

The adjectives *myeloid* and *lymphoid* refer to the predominant cell involved, and the suffixes *-cytic* and *-blastic* to mature and immature cells, respectively. These characteristics can be determined by a combination of cellular appearances, surface antigen expression, cytogenetic features and molecular markers. The international standard for leukaemia classification is the World Health Organization (WHO) system (Swerdlow et al., 2008).

Epidemiology

Haematological malignancies account for only 5% of all cancers; of these, CLL is the most common form of leukaemia. UK incidence data are presented in Table 51.1. CLL mainly affects an older age group: 90% of patients are older than 50 years at diagnosis, and nearly two-thirds are older than 60 years. It rarely occurs in young people and is twice as common in men as in women. CML is primarily a disease of middle age, with the median onset in the 40- to 50-year-old age group, but it can occur in younger people.

Acute leukaemia is rare, with a total annual incidence of approximately 4 per 100,000 population. The most common form of the disease is AML, which accounts for 75% of cases. The incidence of AML rises steadily with age, occurring only rarely in young children. In contrast, ALL is predominantly a childhood disease, with the peak incidence in the 3- to 5-year-old age group, and is the most common childhood cancer.

Aetiology

In common with other cancers, the aetiology of leukaemia is not fully understood. Leukaemia is thought to result from a combination of factors that induce genetic mutations that allow mutated cells to proliferate faster than normal cells and/or to fail to die in response to normal apoptotic signals. Epidemiological studies have, however, identified a number of specific risk factors for the development of leukaemia, which are described as follows.

Radiation

The association between the ionising radiation and the development of leukaemia is evident from nuclear disasters such as Hiroshima and, more recently, Chernobyl. Long-term follow-up of survivors of Nagasaki and Hiroshima has shown an increase in all forms of leukaemia other than CLL. The link is also apparent for patients who received radiotherapy for the treatment of malignant and non-malignant conditions such as Hodgkin's disease or ankylosing spondylitis. The effect of chronic low-level exposure to radiation is less certain.

Exposure to chemicals and cytotoxic drugs

There is a small but definite risk of acute leukaemia occurring in patients successfully treated for other malignancies with cytotoxic and immunosuppressive agents. Combination treatment with chemotherapy, especially alkylating agents such as cyclophosphamide and radiotherapy, presents the highest risk. In addition, topoisomerase II inhibitors, such as etoposide, frequently used in curative treatment for haematological and solid-organ malignancies, pose a risk of therapy-related acute leukaemia. This has practical implications as an increasing number of patients achieve a 'cure' as a result of combination therapy. Occupational exposure of health professionals to these agents is also an area of concern. Occupational exposures to paint, insecticides and solvents, in particular, the aromatic solvent benzene, have all been associated with the development of leukaemia, but it is difficult to be certain whether such exposures genuinely cause the disease.

Viruses

Human T-cell lymphotropic virus, an RNA retrovirus endemic in Japan and the West Indies, has been linked to a rare T-cell leukaemia/lymphoma.

Genetic factors

Down's syndrome, constitutional trisomy of chromosome 21, is associated with an increased risk of leukaemia. Disorders that predispose to chromosomal breaks such as Fanconi's anaemia

and ataxia telangiectasia are also associated with an increased risk of developing acute leukaemia. These alterations may permit the expression of oncogenes, which promote malignant transformation.

Haematological disorders

Many patients with other haematological disorders have a greatly increased risk of developing leukaemia, particularly AML. These disorders include the myelodysplastic syndromes, the non-leukaemic myeloproliferative disorders including myelofibrosis, aplastic anaemia and paroxysmal nocturnal haemoglobinuria.

Pathophysiology

In leukaemia, the normal process of haemopoiesis is altered (Fig. 51.1). Transformation to malignancy appears to occur in a single cell, usually at the pluripotential stem cell level, but it may occur in a committed stem cell with capacity for more limited differentiation. Accumulation of malignant cells leads to progressive impairment of the normal bone marrow function.

Acute leukaemias

In acute leukaemia, the normal bone marrow is replaced by a malignant clone of immature blast cells derived from the myeloid (in AML) or lymphoid (in ALL) series. More than 20% of the cellular elements of the bone marrow are replaced with blasts. This is usually associated with the appearance of blasts in the peripheral circulation accompanied by worsening pancytopenia as a result of the marrow's reduced ability to produce normal blood cells as the proportion of malignant cells increases. In ALL, the blasts may infiltrate lymph nodes and other tissues such as liver, spleen, testis and the meninges, in particular. In AML, blasts tend to infiltrate skin, gums, liver and spleen.

Table 51.1	Incidence 2014 of leukaemia in the UK (Cancer Research UK, 2017)	
	New cases/year	Age-Standardised Incidence per 100,000 of the population
CLL	3515	6.0
CML	748	1.2
ALL	758	1.1
AML	3072	5.2

ALL, Acute lymphoblastic leukaemia; AML, acute myeloblastic leukaemia; CLL, chronic lymphocytic leukaemia; CML, chronic myelocytic leukaemia.

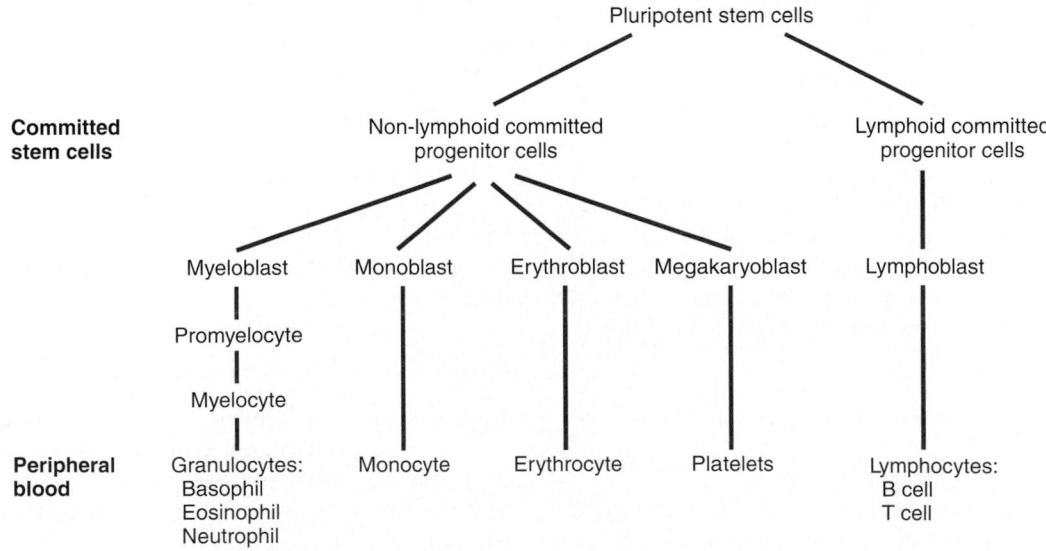

Fig. 51.1 Haemopoiesis.

Table 51.2 World Health Organization classification of acute myeloblastic leukaemia (Swerdlow et al., 2008)

Subgroup	Examples
AML with recurrent genetic abnormalities	Inversion chromosome 16 (inv 16) t(15;17) t(8;21)
AML with multilineage dysplasia	
Therapy-related AML	
AML not otherwise classified	AML without maturation AML with granulocytic maturation AML with granulocytic and monocytic differentiation AML with monocytic differentiation AML with erythroid differentiation AML with megakaryocytic differentiation

AML, Acute myeloblastic leukaemia.

Classification of acute myeloblastic leukaemia

AML has traditionally been classified on the basis of morphological features of the disease. Subtypes displaying granulocytic, monocytic, erythroid and megakaryocytic differentiation can be demonstrated. The WHO has updated this system (Table 51.2). AML is now classified using a combination of morphological, genetic and immunological cell marker features (surface antigen expression) in an attempt to define disease groups of greater prognostic significance (Swerdlow et al., 2008).

Classification of acute lymphoblastic leukaemia

As with AML, the WHO classification system takes account of morphological, genetic and immunological features. The disease is, however, mainly classified immunologically, based on the presence or absence of B- or T-cell markers (Table 51.3). Each subtype displays different clinical presentations, response to treatment and, ultimately, prognosis, with pre-B having the best prognosis and T-ALL the worst. It is worth noting that Burkitt type B-ALL which is associated with translocations of the myc gene located on chromosome 8, seems to be a morphologically and biologically distinct form of leukaemia.

Chronic leukaemias

In chronic leukaemia, the normal bone marrow is replaced by a malignant clone of maturing haemopoietic cells.

Chronic lymphocytic leukaemia

CLL is characterised by a clonal expansion of morphologically mature lymphocytes of B-cell origin. These cells accumulate in

Table 51.3 Classification of acute lymphoblastic leukaemia (Swerdlow et al., 2008)

Pre-B ALL	Possessing the common ALL antigen CD10
B-cell type	B-ALL or Burkitt's type
T-cell type	T-ALL
Null	Non-B, non-T and lacking the common ALL antigen CD10

ALL, Acute lymphoblastic leukaemia.

the peripheral blood and give rise to a lymphocytosis that may be very marked. Lymphocytes accumulate in lymph nodes and can spread to the liver and spleen, which become enlarged. The bone marrow is progressively infiltrated. Although the malignant lymphocytes appear relatively normal morphologically, they are functionally deficient.

Chronic myelocytic leukaemia

The characteristic feature of CML is the predominance of maturing myeloid cells in blood, bone marrow, liver, spleen and other organs. CML was the first cancer to be associated with a specific chromosomal abnormality: the Philadelphia chromosome translocation (Ph) seen in more than 90% of cases. This is a translocation of genetic material between the long arms of chromosome 22 and chromosome 9. This results in the apposition of the BCR gene (chromosome 22) and the ABL gene (chromosome 9). This novel BCR-ABL gene encodes a fusion protein that has tyrosine kinase activity. This genetic event is believed to be crucial in the pathogenesis, or perhaps even to initiate the development, of CML because overactivity of the tyrosine kinase results in the uncontrolled growth characteristic of leukaemic cells (Cilloni and Saglio, 2009).

Clinical manifestations
Acute leukaemia

Most of the clinical manifestations of acute leukaemia are related to bone marrow failure. The disease commonly presents with a short history, and left untreated, it is rapidly fatal. Symptoms of infection, anaemia and bleeding are common and life-threatening presenting problems. Bleeding may be particularly severe in one subtype of AML, acute promyelocytic leukaemia (APL). This condition is most commonly associated with a translocation of genetic material between chromosomes 15 and 17, t(15;17). Disseminated intravascular coagulation (DIC) is commonly the presenting feature of this disease with patients often displaying life-threatening bleeding symptoms at presentation. Some patients with AML develop symptoms and signs due to infiltration of major organs by leukaemic cells.

The involvement of tissues such as spleen, liver, lymph nodes and meninges is more common in ALL than AML. Involvement of the central nervous system (CNS) may give rise to headaches, vomiting and irritable behaviour. CNS disease is rare at presentation but develops in up to 75% of children with ALL unless specific prophylactic treatment is given. Less commonly, patients present with features of hypermetabolism, hyperuricaemia or generalised aches and pains.

Chronic leukaemia

Chronic myelocytic leukaemia

Patients with CML commonly present with non-specific symptoms, such as malaise, weight loss and night sweats. The most common physical sign is an enlarged spleen that may give rise to abdominal discomfort. Hepatomegaly is also detected in approximately 40% of newly diagnosed patients. Neutropenia and thrombocytopenia are uncommon at presentation. Thus, in contrast to the acute leukaemias, patients with CML rarely present with symptoms of infection or haemorrhage. In up to 30% of cases, patients are asymptomatic, and the disease is detected, by chance, as a result of a routine blood test performed for other reasons.

Historically CML was regarded as a triphasic disease. The initial chronic phase typically lasted from months to years, with a median of around 5 years. During this time, treatment was aimed at symptom alleviation with reduction of the white blood cell (WBC) count and spleen size. An accelerated phase typically followed, manifest by the presence of increasing numbers of immature cells in the blood and bone marrow associated with worsening symptoms: unexplained fevers, bone pain and anaemia. Finally, after a period of weeks or months, a blast crisis resembling fulminant acute leukaemia would ensue. In a small number of patients, this occurred abruptly with no prior accelerated phase. Whilst accelerated phase and blast crisis can still occur, the natural history of CML has been profoundly improved by the use of targeted therapies.

Chronic lymphocytic leukaemia

An increasing number of asymptomatic patients are diagnosed as having CLL purely by chance, when a full blood count is performed for an unrelated reason. Symptomatic patients often suffer B symptoms: night sweats, unexplained fever and weight loss. At diagnosis, findings may include generalised lymphadenopathy and some enlargement of the liver and spleen. The course of CLL is variable; in some patients, the disease may remain indolent for many years, whereas others experience a steady deterioration in their health. Survival typically varies from 2 to 20 years depending on the extent of disease. Patients are immunocompromised with a reduction in serum gammaglobulin and are at increased risk of bacterial and viral infections. There is an increased susceptibility to autoimmune disease, particularly immune haemolytic anaemias and thrombocytopenia. With progressive disease, bone marrow failure becomes apparent, resulting in fatigue, infection and bleeding, and the disease becomes less responsive to treatment. Patients with CLL also have an increased risk of developing a more aggressive malignancy, such as high-grade non-Hodgkin's lymphoma (known as Richter's transformation) or prolymphocytic leukaemia (PLL).

Investigations

Traditionally examinations of peripheral blood and bone marrow are the key laboratory investigations carried out in cases of suspected leukaemia. However, some additional investigations can help in the diagnosis and classification of this group of diseases. With the wider general accessibility and understanding of molecular testing, the classification and prognostication of these diseases continue to evolve. Some of the main findings at diagnosis are presented in Table 51.4.

In acute leukaemia, leukaemic blast cells are usually seen on the peripheral blood film. The blasts of ALL and AML are distinguished using morphology, cell surface antigen analysis and cytogenetics. In CML, the principal feature is a leucocytosis with WBC usually ranging from 10×10^9/L to 250×10^9/L and comprising the complete spectrum of myeloid cells from immature to mature. In CLL, it is lymphocytes, in particular, which are increased, with clonal lymphocyte counts exceeding 5×10^9/L. Non-random chromosome abnormalities are increasingly being identified in patients with leukaemia. The information obtained from cytogenetic analysis of bone marrow or peripheral blood cells can be used to confirm the diagnosis and classification of leukaemia and may provide a guide to treatment response and prognosis.

Treatment

Although significant progress has been made in the treatment of leukaemia, work continues to further improve prognosis. As leukaemias are rare malignancies, the most important studies are undertaken on a national or international basis. In addition to the specific anti-leukaemia treatment, general supportive therapy is vital to manage both the disease and the complications of therapy.

Acute leukaemia

At the outset, intensive combination chemotherapy is given in the hope of achieving a complete remission (CR). This initial phase of treatment is termed induction or remission induction chemotherapy. A CR can only be achieved by virtual ablation of the bone marrow, followed by recovery of normal haemopoiesis. If the induction regimen fails to induce CR, an alternative drug regimen can be used. Remission is defined as the absence of all clinical and microscopic signs of leukaemia, less than 5% blast forms in the bone marrow and return of normal cellularity and haemopoietic elements. Despite achieving CR, occult residual disease (also termed minimal residual disease or MRD) will persist, and further intensive therapy is given in an attempt to consolidate the remission. This post-remission consolidation therapy may comprise chemotherapy or a combination of chemotherapy and bone marrow transplantation.

Table 51.4 Findings at diagnosis in leukaemia

	AML	ALL	CML	CLL
WBC	↑ in 60%, may be N or ↓	↑ in 50%, may be N or ↓↓	↑↑ Commonly >100 × 10⁹	Commonly ↑↑
Differential WBC	Mainly myeloblasts	Mainly lymphoblasts	Granulocytes ↑↑, especially neutrophils, myelocytes, basophils and eosinophils <10% blasts present	>5 × 10⁹/L monoclonal lymphocytes
RBC	Severe anaemia	Severe anaemia	Anaemia common	Anaemia in 50% of patients, generally mild
Platelets	↓↓	↓↓	Usually ↑ but may be N or ↓	↓ in 20–30%
Bone marrow aspiration and trephine	Predominantly blasts	Predominantly blasts	Hypercellular Blasts <10%	Lymphocytic infiltration
Cytogenetic analysis	Important abnormalities may be detected but can be N	Important abnormalities may be detected, Ph chromosome detected in 20% of adults	Presence of Ph chromosome	Important abnormalities including p53 deletion or mutation are prognostically significant
Lymphadenopathy	Rare	Common	Rare	Common
Splenomegaly	50%	60%	Usual and severe	Usual and moderate
Other features	DIC, high urate, gum infiltration	High urate, CNS involvement	High urate	Immunoparesis

↓, Reduced; ↑ increased; ALL, acute lymphoblastic leukaemia; AML, acute myeloblastic leukaemia; CLL, chronic lymphocytic leukaemia; CML, chronic myelocytic leukaemia; CNS, central nervous system; N, normal; DIC, disseminated intravascular coagulation; Ph, Philadelphia; RBC, red blood cell; WBC, white blood cell.

Acute lymphoblastic leukaemia

Treatment of ALL in childhood has been one of the success stories of the past three decades. Nearly 90% of children will achieve a remission lasting more than 5 years, and current studies are often focused on trying to identify the 20% of children with poor-risk disease and treating them more aggressively (Pui et al., 2012). Poor risk is defined at presentation based on white cell count, age, underlying genetic conditions (e.g. Down syndrome) and the diagnosis of T-cell ALL. Thereafter, risk is determined by minimal residual disease measurements. This allows for patients with ALL to have risk-adapted therapy in the context of clinical trials.

Unfortunately, the results in adults are less impressive. The combination of vincristine, prednisolone, anthracyclines and asparaginase induces CR in about 90% of children with ALL and 80% of adults, although sadly relapse is far more common in adults. Table 51.5 demonstrates a possible schedule for induction and consolidation therapy for adults with ALL. Given the rarity of the disease, patients should be entered into clinical trials whenever possible where the addition of targeted therapies and comparison of the optimal scheduling of chemotherapy can hopefully be refined.

Patients with ALL are at a high risk of developing CNS infiltration. Cytotoxic drugs penetrate poorly into the CNS, which thus acts as a potential sanctuary site for leukaemic cells. For this reason, all patients with ALL receive CNS prophylaxis. Cranial irradiation, intrathecal methotrexate or high-dose systemic methotrexate can be used in isolation or in combination as part of the treatment schedules for both adults and children.

Maintenance treatment is important to sustain a CR. It is usually less myelotoxic than induction or consolidation chemotherapy but is given for at least 18 months. Treatment usually consists of weekly methotrexate and daily 6-mercaptopurine with intermittent vincristine and prednisolone and in some patients, intrathecal methotrexate.

The treatment of relapsed disease varies with the site of relapse. Isolated CNS or testicular relapse may be successfully treated with radiation and reinduction therapy. Cure can still be achieved for some patients. Bone marrow relapse is much more difficult to cure, especially if it occurs early.

A small proportion of paediatric patients and a larger proportion of adult patients have the Philadelphia chromosome translocation within their ALL blasts. Historically, such patients had a relatively poor prognosis but the use of targeted therapy, such as the tyrosine kinase inhibitor, imatinib, has considerably improved responses. Most adult patients with Philadelphia chromosome positive ALL are assessed for stem cell transplant to further consolidate an initial response.

Acute myeloblastic leukaemia (non-acute promyelocytic leukaemia)

As for ALL, the treatment of AML involves induction and consolidation chemotherapy. In AML therapy, however, the chemotherapy regimens used to achieve remission are typically more myelotoxic, and patients require intensive supportive care to survive periods

Table 51.5 Treatment of acute lymphoblastic leukaemia

	Dose	Route	Regimen
Phase I induction (4-week cycle)			
Daunorubicin	30 mg/m²	i.v.	Weekly for 4 weeks
Vincristine	1.4 mg/m² (max 2 mg)	i.v.	Weekly for 4 weeks
PEGylated Asparaginase	1000 IU/m²	i.v.	Days 4 and 18 of the cycle (only if Ph-negative)
Dexamethasone	10 mg/m²	p.o.	For 4 days each week
Methotrexate	12.5 mg	i.t.	Day 14 of the cycle
Phase II induction (4-week cycle)			
Cyclophosphamide	1000 mg/m²	i.v.	Days 1 and 15 of the cycle
Cytarabine	75 mg/m²	i.v.	Days 2–5, 9–12, 16–19 and 23–26
Mercaptopurine	60 mg/m²	p.o.	Once daily
Methotrexate	12.5 mg	i.t.	Weekly for 4 weeks
Risk assessment – Many will proceed to allogeneic stem cell transplant, but the remainder will continue with consolidation (2 x 4 weekly cycles)			
Cytarabine	75 mg/m²	i.v	Days 1–5 of each cycle
Etoposide	1000 mg/m²	i.v.	Days 1–5 of each cycle
PEGylated Asparaginase	1000 IU/m²	i.v.	Day 5 of cycle 1 only
Methotrexate	12.5 mg	i.t.	Once per cycle
Delayed Intensification I			
Daunorubicin	25 mg/m²	i.v.	Weekly for 4 weeks
Vincristine	1.4 mg/m²	i.v.	Weekly for 4 weeks
PEGylated Asparaginase	1000 IU/m²	i.v.	Day 4 of the cycle
Dexamethasone	10 mg/m²	p.o.	For 4 days each week for 4 weeks
Methotrexate	12.5 mg	i.t.	Days 2 and 17 of the cycle
Cyclophosphamide	1000 mg/m²	i.v.	Day 29 of the cycle
Cytarabine	75 mg/m²	i.v.	Days 30–33 and 37–40 of the cycle
Mercaptopurine	60 mg/m²	p.o.	Days 29–42 of the cycle
Further cycle the same as consolidation (4 weeks)			
Maintenance for 2 years			
Vincristine	1.4 mg/m² (max 2 mg)	i.v.	Once every 3 months
Prednisolone	60 mg/m²	p.o.	For 5 days every 3 monthsw
Mercaptopurine	75 mg/m²	p.o.	Every day
Methotrexate	20 mg/m²	p.o.	Once weekly
Methotrexate	12.5 mg	i.t.	Every 3 months

i.t., Intrathecal; i.v., intravenous; MRC, Medical Research Council; p.o., oral.
Adapted from MRC protocol UKALL 14-2010.

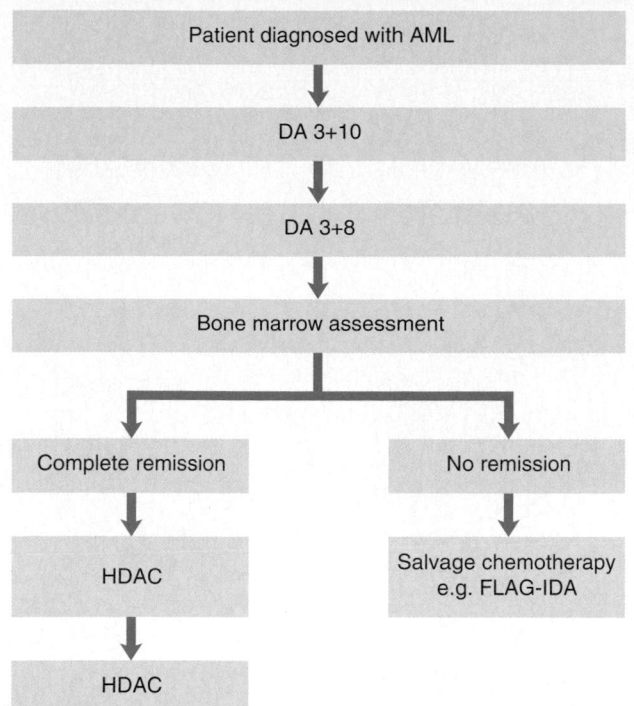

Patient diagnosed with AML

↓

DA 3+10

↓

DA 3+8

↓

Bone marrow assessment

Complete remission | No remission

↓ | ↓

HDAC | Salvage chemotherapy e.g. FLAG-IDA

↓

HDAC

Fig. 51.2 One example of a possible treatment regimen for acute myeloblastic leukaemia (AML). The figure demonstrates that patients are treated with initial induction therapy, then remission is consolidated with at least two courses of chemotherapy. Patients are assessed for the necessity and their suitability for allogeneic stem cell transplant during this treatment. This figure provides a summary only and should not be used as a guide to prescribing or dispensing therapy.
DA 3+10 and DA 3+8 are schedules of daunorubicin and cytarabine; HDAC, high-dose cytarabine; FLAG-Ida, fludarabine, cytarabine and granulocyte colony-stimulating factor combined with idarubicin.

of bone marrow aplasia (Fig. 51.2). The anthracycline, daunorubicin, and the pyrimidine analogue, cytarabine, have formed the backbone of AML therapy for more than 30 years. Sadly, this is an indicator of a lack of progress in the therapy of this disease over the years. Whilst it is possible to achieve 80% remission rates, relapse rates remain high, with 5-year survival of 35–40% in those younger than 60 years at diagnosis and 5–15% in those older than 60 years at diagnosis (Dohner et al., 2015). For this reason, many patients opt for treatment in the context of clinical trials.

For many years, cytogenetic abnormalities in AML blasts have been recognised as having fundamental importance in determining prognosis (Grimwade et al., 2010). They have been used to develop individualised risk-adapted treatment strategies, particularly influencing which patients (i.e. those at highest risk of relapse) potentially have most to gain from allogeneic bone marrow transplant in first remission, for instance. Unfortunately, the largest patient group identified comprised those with a normal karyotype; a standard cytogenetic approach does not allow further risk stratification in this group. Molecular studies, identifying specific gene mutations associated with AML, are now allowing better risk stratification particularly in this normal karyotype group (Grimwade et al., 2016). Molecular technologies are now beginning to aid in the understanding of the biology of AML and the identification potential targets for therapy. It is worth stating,

however, that our ability to detect mutations is improving very quickly; the current challenge is to understand the relative importance of such mutations, given that an individual patient may have several mutations, to be able to best apply this new knowledge for patient benefit. A parallel strand of thinking in AML is to develop robust techniques for MRD monitoring, thus allowing an individualised treatment approach based not on pre-existing molecular or genetic phenotype but on response to treatment. This strategy has been particularly successful in paediatric ALL and is now being better defined in AML (Ivey et al., 2016).

Fig. 51.2 shows a possible treatment schedule for an adult patient with AML. The backbone of daunorubicin and cytarabine remains. For many patients, consolidation chemotherapy, as shown in Fig. 51.2, may be considered the best treatment; an alternative approach to post-remission therapy is stem cell transplantation. In patients younger than 40 years, myeloablative allogeneic bone marrow transplantation has resulted in disease-free survival of 45–65% at 5 years post-transplant. These patients are considered cured of their disease. Only about 10% of patients are suitable for myeloablative allogeneic bone marrow transplants, although reduced-intensity conditioning regimens have a more general applicability. There is little evidence to suggest that autologous stem cell transplantation improves the outcome for patients with AML in first CR. It is always worth remembering that AML is most common in the elderly, and it is not always possible to deliver intensive intravenous chemotherapy regimens to this patient population. Alternative options in the elderly include less intensive, lower-dose daunorubicin and cytarabine, low-dose subcutaneous cytarabine and 5-azacytidine; 5-azacytidine is of recent interest, especially in older patients and those whose disease has evolved from myelodysplastic syndrome (MDS). This agent inhibits DNA methyltransferase, resulting in DNA hypomethylation. This process is thought to increase the activity of some tumour-suppressor genes, resulting in anti-tumour effects. The agent has been shown to slow the rate of progression to AML in patients with high-risk myelodysplastic syndrome and is currently the subject of clinical trials in AML and MDS.

Treatment of AML in relapse is difficult, and the prognosis is generally poor. Whenever possible, patients who enter remission should be offered an allogeneic bone marrow transplant, as chemotherapy alone is unlikely to cure relapsed disease. Encouraging results have been seen using a combination of fludarabine, cytosine arabinoside, idarubicin and granulocyte colony-stimulating factor (G-CSF) as a prelude to allogeneic transplant. Novel approaches in AML therapy are often piloted in this group of poor-risk patients. There are many novel agents currently being investigated in AML; we highlight just a few. Gemtuzumab ozogamicin is a humanised anti-CD33 monoclonal antibody, which targets myeloid blasts, bound to a potent anti-tumour anthracycline antibiotic, calicheamicin (Rowe and Löwenberg, 2013). This antibody, when used in combination with standard chemotherapy, seems to reduce relapse risk in all but the highest-risk patients. Concerns have been raised about possible toxicity in the form of veno-occlusive disease of the liver, and the dosing schedule is not yet optimised. Midostaurin is a multi-targeted FLT3 inhibitor and has been shown to improve survival in the subgroup of patients with FLT3-mutated AML. Increasing numbers of such targeted therapies are likely to be tested in the next few years.

Acute promyelocytic leukaemia

The acute promyelocytic leukaemia subtype of AML deserves special consideration because the approach to treatment and prognosis is quite different from that of other AML variants. APL is associated with the t(15;17) translocation, which involves a genetic translocation of material between chromosomes 15 and 17. The disease is clinically characterised by the presence of DIC at presentation. Because these patients are so prone to life-threatening haemorrhage at diagnosis, the management of a new case of APL is considered a medical emergency. The leukaemic cells are exquisitely sensitive to all-trans retinoic acid (ATRA), which induces blast maturation and can induce remission when used as a single agent (Coombs et al., 2015). Using a combination of ATRA and anthracycline chemotherapy, usually idarubicin, it is now possible to achieve long-term cure in greater than 80% patients. A number of studies have been published demonstrating the efficacy of arsenic trioxide (ATO) in treating relapsed or refractory APL. In the UK, ATO is currently regarded as the standard of care for relapsed APL. It is also effective in first-line therapy, although overall survival of patients treated up front with ATO and ATRA was no different from that of patients treated with anthracycline and ATRA. Given the significant differences in cost between the two regimens, the latter currently remains the standard of care (Burnett et al., 2015).

Chronic leukaemia

Chronic myelocytic leukaemia

Historically, the treatment of CML was essentially palliative in intent, producing modest increases in survival, but with the main aim of keeping patients asymptomatic by normalising the WBC. Traditionally, CML was treated with non-targeted therapies, but these were often poorly tolerated and did not provide a long-term solution. Historically, the only curative option for CML was an allogeneic stem cell transplant, but many patients were not suitable for this intensive treatment due to age and comorbidities.

Hydroxycarbamide was the most widely used drug in the management of CML in chronic phase. Treatment with hydroxycarbamide at a dose of 1.5–2 g/day can be used and usually brings the WBC under control within 1–2 weeks. The dose can then be reduced to a maintenance dose of 0.5–2 g/day. Withdrawing or reducing the dose abruptly can cause a rebound increase in WBC. The side effects of hydroxycarbamide are generally mild but include rashes and gastro-intestinal disturbances.

Interferon can be used to control the symptoms of CML but was also the first agent shown to modify the disease process. It promotes the expression of suppressed normal haemopoiesis at the expense of the malignant clone. Studies have shown that interferon-α therapy prolongs the chronic phase and improves the median survival of CML patients with its effects seemingly enhanced by the addition of low-dose cytarabine (Sawyers, 1999).

Therapeutic options for patients with CML have changed dramatically in the past 10–15 years due to the development of imatinib mesylate. This drug, which belongs to the tyrosine kinase inhibitor (TKI) class of drug, was specifically designed to target

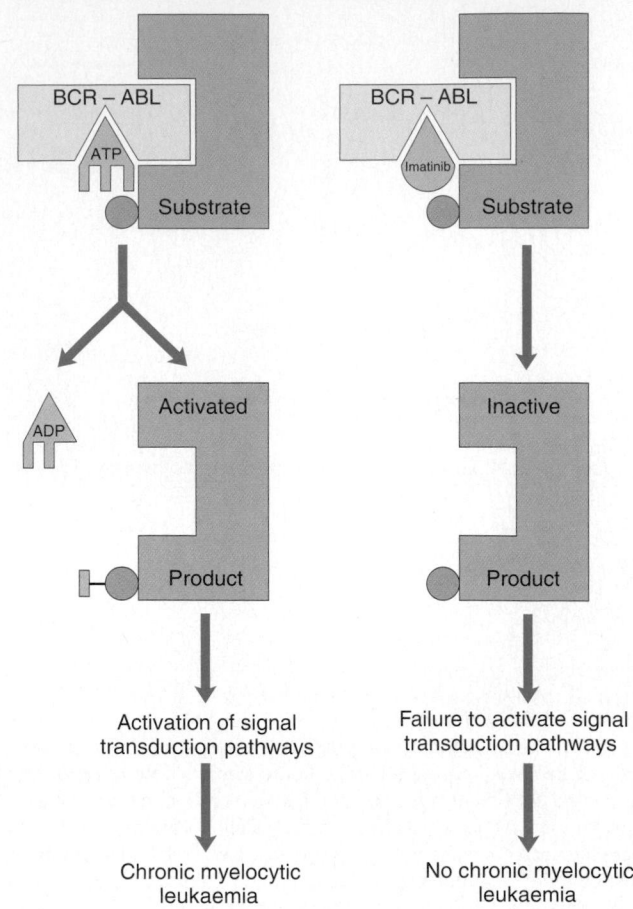

Fig. 51.3 Inhibition of BCR-ABL protein by imatinib. The protein product of the BCR-ABL fusion gene (BCR-ABL protein) acts as a constitutively active tyrosine kinase and uses adenosine triphosphate (ATP), bound within a kinase pocket in the molecule, to phosphorylate tyrosine (o) in a variety of substrates. In doing so, ATP is reduced to adenosine diphosphate (ADP), which falls out of the kinase pocket to be replaced by further ATP. Imatinib prevents the action of the BCR-ABL protein by blocking ATP entry into the kinase pocket.

the abnormal tyrosine kinase product of the BCR-ABL fusion gene (Fig. 51.3). TKIs are now the mainstay of treatment for CML.

In a large randomised controlled trial, patients were randomised to receive imatinib or a combination of interferon-α and cytarabine. Many patients were intolerant of the interferon and cytarabine combination and crossed over to receive imatinib after trial commencement. Despite this problem, progression-free survival at 1 year was 97% in the imatinib arm and 80% in the interferon and cytarabine arm in an intention-to-treat analysis (O'Brien et al., 2003). The Philadelphia chromosome became undetectable in 68% of imatinib recipients compared with 7% of those in the alternative arm (Hughes et al., 2003). However, more sensitive testing methods, such as real-time polymerase chain reaction (PCR), have now shown that many patients who are Philadelphia chromosome negative still possess very low levels of the abnormal BCR-ABL gene produced by the Philadelphia translocation. Complete molecular remission is seen in only a very small proportion of patients. In patients who achieve a cytogenetic or ideally a molecular remission, current studies are underway to determine if TKIs can be stopped and what impact this will have on remission status and survival.

The use of imatinib has inevitably lead to the demonstration of imatinib-resistant clones in some patients; second-generation TKIs are now available, such as nilotinib, dasatinib and bosutinib. In the UK, the National Institute for Health and Care Excellence (NICE) has approved imatinib and nilotinib for first-line therapy for chronic phase CML and dasatinib and nilotinib for the second-line treatment of CML in those who are refractory to or unable to tolerate imatinib (NICE, 2012a).

Due to the effectiveness of imatinib therapy and the development of second-generation agents, allogeneic stem cell transplantation is now rarely used to treat CML, but it is still a potentially curative option for patients with multi-drug-resistant disease.

Transformation of CML into acute leukaemia can be treated in the same manner as de novo acute leukaemia, in an effort to achieve a second chronic phase. Treatment is slightly more successful if transformation is lymphoid rather than myeloid. Imatinib, typically at higher doses than are used in chronic phase disease, can also be used to attempt to return patients to chronic phase disease. In general, remissions are rare, and the median survival is less than 6 months.

Chronic lymphocytic leukaemia

Currently, there is no cure for CLL. All treatment is, therefore, considered palliative. There is no evidence that early treatment of asymptomatic patients improves outcome. Indications for treatment are:

- rapidly increasing WBC,
- increasing or troublesome lymphadenopathy,
- systemic symptoms,
- marrow failure,
- autoimmune complications.

In the last 5 years, there have been very exciting developments in the management of CLL, such as new agents and new combination regimens, that have been adopted successfully into clinical practice.

Formerly, the alkylating agent chlorambucil was the most common agent used in the treatment of CLL. Corticosteroids can reduce the lymphocyte count without contributing to myelosuppression and are used to treat autoimmune phenomena such as haemolytic anaemia and immune thrombocytopenia. The use of purine analogues, particularly fludarabine, marked the beginning of an exciting phase in the treatment of CLL. Although CRs were unusual, good responses were seen even in patients whose leukaemia was resistant to alkylating agents. With regard to initial therapy of CLL, fludarabine-treated patients show a higher response rate than patients treated with chlorambucil. However, no survival advantage for the use of fludarabine has been demonstrated (Rai et al., 2000).

The addition of the anti-CD20 antibody rituximab to fludarabine and cyclophosphamide (FC-R) has been shown in randomised trials to have better overall responses than fludarabine

and cyclophosphamide (FC) alone, with 86% and 73%, respectively (Halleck et al., 2009). This combination of fludarabine, cyclophosphamide and rituximab has been adopted in the UK as the regimen of choice for first-line treatment of CLL as long as patients are considered fit enough and has been used as the comparator to novel drugs and novel combinations for the first-line treatment of CLL.

More recent studies have looked at the use of bendamustine, an intravenous alkylating agent. Studies have shown fludarabine, cyclophosphamide and rituximab (FC-R) and bendamustine and rituximab (BR) to have a similar overall response rate but with better complete responses in those receiving fludarabine, cyclophosphamide and rituximab (Eichhorst et al., 2013). Based on these data, bendamustine can be used as a first-line agent in CLL in those patients not fit for fludarabine, cyclophosphamide and rituximab.

Chlorambucil, alone or in combination with rituximab, remains an excellent choice for patients with significant comorbidities because the treatment is less immunosuppressive. As such, trials are ongoing to look at the effectiveness of chlorambucil in combination with other anti-CD20 agents to try to improve outcomes in the elderly. Obinutuzumab and ofatumumab have both been NICE approved in combination with chlorambucil for first-line treatment for those patients for whom neither fludarabine nor bendamustine is an option for first-line therapy (NICE, 2015a, 2015b).

Alemtuzumab is a humanised monoclonal anti-CD52 antibody. CD52 is present on most lymphocytes including malignant lymphocytes in CLL. Binding of this antibody induces both antibody-mediated and complement-mediated T-cell cytotoxicity against malignant B cells. In relapsed patients, the duration of response to alemtuzumab is relatively short but has shown more promise in those who have difficult to treat disease, namely, those who are found to have a p53 mutation in their CLL clone.

The most recent advance in CLL has been the advent of molecular therapies which target the B-cell signalling pathway. The Bruton kinase inhibitor, ibrutinib, and the PI3K inhibitor, idelalisib, have shown promise. Both of these agents are oral drugs which have targeted action so as to avoid the systemic effects seen with conventional chemotherapy agents.

Splenic complications may necessitate splenectomy or splenic irradiation. Radiotherapy can also be used to control localised painful lymphadenopathy. Combination chemotherapy, such as cyclophosphamide, doxorubicin, vincristine and prednisolone (CHOP; see Chapter 52) used in lymphoma, may be beneficial in advanced disease.

Patients with CLL are very susceptible to infection. Herpes viruses, in particular herpes zoster, can cause significant problems. This susceptibility is increased because many treatments, such as campath-1H, fludarabine and bendamustine, have generalised anti-lymphocyte action and are not absolutely specific for malignant lymphocytes.

Stem cell transplantation

The potential role of stem cell transplantation is increasingly being explored in the management of all types of leukaemia.

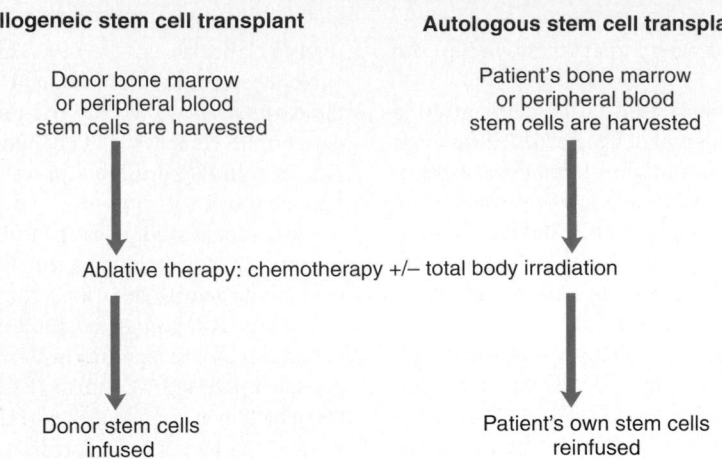

Fig. 51.4 Stem cell transplantation.

The basic principle

This technique provides a means of rescuing the patient from the potentially lethal effects on the bone marrow of ablative therapy given in an attempt to eradicate all traces of disease (Fig. 51.4). The conditioning regimen most commonly used is a combination of high-dose cyclophosphamide and total body irradiation. Other conditioning regimens include high-dose melphalan, fludarabine, busulphan or cytarabine.

After administration of conditioning therapy, 2–3 days elapse to allow its elimination from the body, and then previously harvested stem cells are reinfused peripherally. The stem cells will return to and repopulate the marrow, restoring normal haemopoiesis. Peripheral blood counts recover in 2–4 weeks. Throughout this time, patients require intensive supportive care and the procedure, particularly allogeneic stem cell transplantation, causes significant morbidity and has a mortality rate of 5–30% (Rezvani et al., 2016).

Over the last 30 years it has become clear that cure, after allogeneic bone marrow transplant, is not simply due to the very high doses of chemotherapy that are delivered but is instead an immunological function of a graft-versus-tumour effect that ensues after donor stem cell engraftment.

Allografts and autografts

During allogeneic stem cell transplantation (allograft), stem cells are obtained from a human leucocyte antigen (HLA)-matched donor who may be a sibling or an unrelated donor found through a national/international registry. These stem cells can be removed directly from the bone marrow, under general anaesthetic, or, more commonly, harvested from the peripheral blood. Under certain circumstances, an autologous bone marrow or peripheral blood stem cell transplant (autograft) may be preferred as the best treatment option. During an autologous transplant, the patient donates his or her own bone marrow or peripheral blood stem cells before receiving high-dose conditioning treatment. After conditioning, the patient's own stem cells are re-infused. There is a potential risk that stem cells obtained in this way may contain

undetected, residual disease. Attempts have been made to purge the bone marrow of disease in vitro, but these have generally been unsuccessful. In contrast to allograft recipients, patients receiving an autologous transplant will not benefit from any graft-versus-tumour effect. Autologous transplants are more commonly used to treat myeloma and lymphoma than leukaemia.

Peripheral blood stem cells versus marrow stem cells

Most patients and donors now donate haematopoietic stem cells using a technique of harvesting the cells from the peripheral blood. Donors receive the haematopoietic growth factor G-CSF, either alone or, in the case of patients donating for autologous transplant, after an infusion of high-dose chemotherapy such as high-dose cyclophosphamide. G-CSF is given for a period of about 7 days. This stimulates the release of stem cells into the peripheral circulation. Stem cells are then harvested from the peripheral circulation by a process of cell pheresis. The harvested cells can then be reinfused, fresh, into the patient after conditioning therapy or frozen and stored for later use. Peripheral blood stem cell transplantation offers some advantages over the conventional surgical technique of harvesting haematopoietic stem cells direct from the marrow cavity; collection of peripheral stem cells negates the need for general anaesthesia, and it has been found that the haemopoietic recovery period after transplantation is shortened by several days. This technique can also be used to harvest stem cells from allogeneic donors. In this case, G-CSF is used alone to stimulate stem cell release into the peripheral circulation. It is sometimes impossible to harvest enough stem cells from patients to allow an autologous transplant to be performed. The commonest reason for this is that the patient has been heavily pretreated with chemotherapy or radiotherapy. A new CXCR4 chemokine antagonist, plerixafor, is now available. This agent is thought to reduce the adhesion of stem cells within the bone marrow milieu. It can be given along with G-CSF and allows a proportion of patients who have failed to mobilise stem cells using G-CSF alone to mobilise cells for an autograft.

Complications of allogeneic bone marrow transplantation

Infection is almost inevitable in patients undergoing bone marrow transplantation. Other significant complications of allografting include interstitial pneumonitis and hepatic veno-occlusive disease (VOD), but the major life-threatening complication is graft-versus-host disease (GVHD). The likelihood of graft-versus-host disease occurring increases with recipient age and is one of the factors that explains the higher treatment-related mortality when transplanting older as compared with younger recipients. GVHD is caused by T-lymphocytes in the donated marrow reacting to host tissues. The severity of the reaction ranges from a mild maculopapular rash to multisystem organ failure with a high mortality rate. Acute GVHD is defined as occurring within 100 days of the bone marrow transplantation and typically presents with fever, rash, diarrhoea and liver dysfunction. Prophylactic immunosuppression is routinely given to prevent GVHD and is gradually weaned post-engraftment. The specific regimen depends on the nature of the transplant, but ciclosporin, the anti-CD52 antibody, alemtuzumab, and methotrexate can be used. Should acute GVHD develop, high-dose methylprednisolone, ciclosporin and, more recently, anticytokine monoclonal antibodies, for example, anti–tumour necrosis factor (anti-TNF) or anti-IL-6 antibodies, have been used to treat the condition.

Chronic GVHD is defined as GVHD occurring more than 100 days post-transplant. It is a multisystem disorder associated with chronic hepatitis, severe skin inflammation, gastrointestinal disturbance and profound immunosuppression. Treatment is successful in approximately 50% of patients and consists of immunosuppression with ciclosporin and prednisolone together with prophylactic antibiotics and antifungal agents. Tacrolimus, thalidomide, imatinib and extra-corporeal photopheresis (ECP) have also been used successfully in the treatment of chronic steroid-refractory GVHD. The main cause of death among patients with chronic GVHD is infection.

Reduced intensity allografting

Myeloablative, or full-intensity, allogeneic transplantation is a very intensive procedure associated with significant morbidity and mortality; hence, its application has to be restricted to younger, fitter patients. Attempts have been made to reduce the intensity of transplant conditioning regimens whilst using increased immunosuppression to facilitate marrow engraftment. Although such an approach reduces the intensity of therapy delivered to any residual tumour, the possible downside of this reduction is offset by an immunological graft-versus-tumour effect and by reduced early post-transplant mortality. This form of transplant is often offered to older patients who are considered unfit to receive a standard allograft. The long-term outcomes of this approach are under continual review. Several trials now suggest that the overall survival after myeloablative and reduced intensity transplants may be similar, although the causes of death in the two groups are different. More patients die of disease relapse after reduced intensity transplants, and more die of transplant-related complications in the myeloablative group (Sengsayadeth et al., 2015).

Table 51.6 Indications for allogeneic stem cell transplantation in leukaemia

AML	First remission for those with high-risk genetic or molecular characteristics and is a clinical option for those with standard-risk disease Second remission for relapsed patients
ALL	First remission in most adults Second remission in children
CML	Chronic phase but only if patients are intolerant of or refractory to first- and second-line tyrosine kinase inhibitors
CLL	Generally only considered in the setting of multiple-relapsed disease

ALL, Acute lymphoblastic leukaemia; AML, acute myeloblastic leukaemia; CLL, chronic lymphocytic leukaemia; CML, chronic myelocytic leukaemia.

The place of stem cell transplantation

The place of stem cell transplantation in the management of a particular form of leukaemia depends very much on the prognosis of patients treated with conventional chemotherapy (Table 51.6). For example, the results of intensive chemotherapy in children with ALL are good, and bone marrow transplantation is generally only considered for children who have relapsed and in whom a second remission can be achieved. However, conventional treatment of adults is less successful, and allogeneic bone marrow transplantation may be offered to adults in first remission.

Patient care
Supportive care

The treatment of CLL and CML is largely carried out in a hospital outpatient setting, with patients taking oral medication at home or attending outpatient clinics for injections of chemotherapy. Patients are routinely monitored to follow the progress of disease and to observe treatment-related side effects. Supportive therapy, such as blood transfusions, can also be given on an outpatient basis. In contrast, the intensity of induction and consolidation regimens used in the management of patients with acute leukaemia renders patients severely pancytopenic. Therapy is usually given in an in-patient setting, with patients often remaining in hospital after treatment for 3–4 weeks until their bone marrow recovers sufficiently. Advanced leukaemia, bone marrow transplantation and aggressive chemotherapy for acute leukaemia all result in pancytopenia. Red blood cell transfusions are given to patients to maintain their haemoglobin at a level which prevents significant symptoms. Evidence of bleeding includes petechial haemorrhages in skin and mucous membranes, and patients receiving aggressive treatment must be examined frequently for any of these signs. Platelet concentrates are given to thrombocytopenic patients who have signs of bleeding and are given prophylactically should platelets fall to less than 10×10^9/L, although data are emerging to suggest

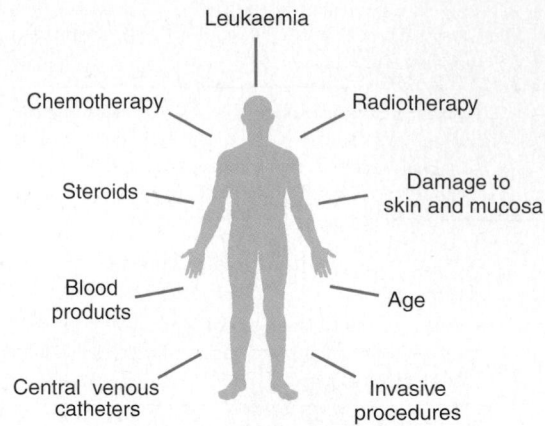

Leukaemia

Chemotherapy

Radiotherapy

Steroids

Damage to skin and mucosa

Blood products

Age

Central venous catheters

Invasive procedures

Fig. 51.5 Infection risk in immunocompromised patients.

that it is safe to transfuse platelets on the basis of symptoms rather than a platelet count per se (Stanworth et al., 2013). The probability of infection developing rises as the WBC count, specifically the neutrophil count, falls. With an absolute neutrophil count of less than 0.5×10^9/L, patients are at high risk of infection, with the risks being even greater if the period of neutropenia is prolonged. Atypical bacterial infections, as well as viral and fungal infections, can be troublesome in patients with prolonged neutropenia.

Chapters 52 and 53 examine many of the non-haematological toxicities which result from the use of cytotoxic drugs, and these are clearly pertinent to haematology patients. The major contributors to morbidity and mortality in patients with leukaemia are relapsed disease and infection.

Infection in the immunocompromised patient

A number of intrinsic and extrinsic factors all contribute to the risk of infection in this vulnerable group of patients (Fig. 51.5).

Although cross-infection can occur via staff, relatives, other patients or contaminated objects, the main sources of infection in this group of patients are endogenous, arising from commensal gut and skin organisms. The normal host defences to infection are broken down; damage to mucous membranes, particularly in the gastro-intestinal tract, occurs with chemotherapy and radiotherapy, allowing infecting organisms to enter the bloodstream. Most infections in neutropenic patients arise from three main sites: the gastro-intestinal and respiratory tracts, and the skin. Table 51.7 lists the main pathogens responsible for infection in this group of patients.

Preventive measures

Oral hygiene. Mouth care is important in all patients receiving chemotherapy but particularly neutropenic patients. Patients are generally asked to use mouthwashes regularly, and prophylactic antifungal therapy may also be given. Although it is important to avoid any sort of trauma to the oral mucosa, teeth should be cleaned regularly using a soft toothbrush. Attention must also be paid to the care of dentures. Patients require careful counselling on mouth care, stressing the importance of oral hygiene.

Table 51.7 Pathogens commonly causing infection in neutropenic patients

Gram-negative bacteria	*Pseudomonas* spp. *Escherichia coli* *Klebsiella* spp. *Enterobacter* spp. *Proteus* spp. *Serratia* spp. *Legionella pneumophilia*
Gram-positive bacteria	*Streptococcus* spp. *Staphylococcus epidermidis* *Staphylococcus aureus*
Anaerobes	*Clostridium difficile* *Clostridium perfringens* *Bacteroides* spp.
Fungi	*Candida* spp. *Aspergillus* spp.
Viruses	Herpes simplex Herpes zoster Cytomegalovirus Epstein–Barr virus Hepatitis
Protozoa	*Pneumocystis carinii*

Table 51.8 Prophylactic anti-infectives

Gram-negative bacteria	Ciprofloxacin
Candidiasis	Nystatin Fluconazole Itraconazole Amphotericin B
Herpes simplex	Aciclovir
Pneumocystis carinii	Co-trimoxazole

Prophylactic anti-infectives. Although it is easy to see the potential advantages in using prophylactic anti-infective agents in severely immunosuppressed patients, the potential complications of drug resistance and, in the case of antibiotics, risks for hospital-acquired infections, such as *Clostridium difficile* and Meticillin-resistant *Staphylococcus aureus* (MRSA), also need to be considered. In the UK, the NICE currently recommends antibiotic prophylaxis for patients who will develop a neutrophil count less than 0.5×10^9/L as a consequence of chemotherapy treatment (NICE, 2012b). Prophylactic antifungal agents are often given, and patients undergoing bone marrow transplantation, patients on therapy for ALL and some patients on therapy for CLL require prophylaxis against herpes virus and *Pneumocystis carinii* (Table 51.8). In patients with ALL, the choice of antifungals should be carefully thought out because the azole class of antifungals is contraindicated in those receiving vincristine due to the potential hepatotoxic effects.

Gut decontamination. Historically, gut decontamination using a combination of non-absorbable oral antibiotics and antifungal agents has been used to reduce the burden of potentially pathogenic organisms in the intestine. One such combination includes neomycin sulphate, colistin sulphate, nystatin and amphotericin. However, opinions are now divided over this practice because gut decontamination can lead to the overgrowth of resistant organisms, so some centres have chosen to avoid gut decontamination.

Growth factors. G-CSF can be used to reduce the time to neutrophil recovery after chemotherapy and has been shown to reduce infection risk and hospitalisation after certain chemotherapy regimens. Current international guidelines suggest that G-CSF should be considered for prophylactic administration if a patient has a risk of greater than 20% of developing febrile neutropenia as a consequence of the chemotherapy (Smith et al., 2015). G-CSF can also be used if patients develop febrile neutropenia and are designated as being at high risk of complications by standard criteria.

Aseptic technique. Careful attention should be paid to the care of intravenous cannulae, particularly central venous catheters. The increased incidence of staphylococcal infection in immunocompromised patients can largely be attributed to their use. Invasive procedures, such as venepuncture, must be carried out using strict aseptic technique. Similarly, urinary catheters are a major source of infection and their use should be avoided if at all possible.

Protective isolation. Reverse barrier isolation during periods of neutropenia, nursing in strict sterile environments and high-efficiency particulate air (HEPA) filtration have been used in an attempt to reduce infection rates. This is extremely demanding for staff and patients alike and is generally only appropriate after bone marrow transplantation.

Treatment of infection

Commonly, neutropenic patients show no signs of focal infection; they are unable to form pus. The only clinical manifestations of septicaemia might be general malaise, fever or hypotension. A patient's condition can deteriorate very rapidly, with collapse occurring within hours of the first signs of infection. Treatment should be instigated as soon as infection is suspected. After a clinically serious febrile episode (temperature: 37.5 °C for more than 1 hour or 38 °C or more on a single reading), samples are taken for culture; these may include blood, urine, sputum and stool cultures along with line and throat swabs. Intravenous antibiotics must be started empirically without delay (Sipsas et al., 2005). Standard empirical therapy varies from unit to unit but commonly comprises an anti-pseudomonal penicillin, such as piperacillin, to provide broad-spectrum bactericidal cover. In penicillin-allergic patients, meropenem may be substituted, but local resistance patterns are of paramount importance. Vancomycin or teicoplanin are often prescribed if an infected central venous catheter is suspected, to provide additional cover against Gram-positive organisms. Microbiological advice should be sought in cases of MRSA infection. Metronidazole may be added to the antibiotic regimen to cover anaerobes if the clinical presentation suggests that the source of the infection may be oral, perineal or gut. Anti-infective therapy should subsequently be modified on the basis of cultures, but in the majority of neutropenic patients, a causative organism is never identified.

If the pyrexia persists for more than 4 days in spite of broad-spectrum antibiotics, or if the patient's condition is deteriorating, systemic fungal infection should be suspected. Empirical antifungal therapy for neutropenic patients with antibiotic-resistant fever reduces mortality and has historically been considered a standard of care. There is no doubt that some patients with persistent fever do have fungal infection, but it's also true that an entirely empiric approach will result in many patients receiving unnecessary treatment. Given the potential side effects of antifungal agents and their cost, many units now have a policy of systematic investigation of patients with ongoing fever including, early high-resolution computed tomography (CT) scanning of the chest and possible use of immunological or molecular tests to detect markers of fungal infection in the blood. This approach aims to target therapy more effectively. A number of broad-spectrum agents are now available for use in this setting, including standard amphotericin, lipid formulation of amphotericin, caspofungin, voriconazole and posaconazole. Intravenous amphotericin is often the first choice to ensure that *Aspergillus* and *Candida* are covered. The main limitation of amphotericin is its toxicity, in particular, nephrotoxicity. Lipid formulations of amphotericin may be appropriate in patients with pre-existing renal impairment or in cases where conventional amphotericin has induced nephrotoxicity. Voriconazole is a useful agent with a similarly broad spectrum of activity. Hepatotoxicity, visual disturbances and prolonged QT interval are the most common side effects of voriconazole. This agent has the advantage of being available as both intravenous and oral preparations, so the conversion from parenteral to oral therapy is straightforward. Posaconazole is only available orally but has a similar broad spectrum of activity.

Although the antifungal activity of the echinocandin caspofungin is more limited than that of amphotericin or voriconazole, it has been shown to be effective for empirical therapy because it has good efficacy against *Candida* and *Aspergillus* spp. It has the advantage of reduced toxicity in comparison with other available agents. The most common side effect is hepatotoxicity. Because this agent has a relatively limited spectrum of activity, it is probably best avoided in the setting of presumed fungal sinus or CNS infection, which are often caused by fungi other than *Aspergillus* or *Candida* spp. Table 51.9 lists some of the common problems encountered in the treatment of the leukaemias.

The following practice points should be used to control infection in immunocompromised patients:
- Measures to prevent infection are important.
- Particular attention should be paid to scrupulous handwashing, mouth care and the use of antifungal, antiviral and antipneumocystis prophylaxis for patients at high risk.
- Treatment of fever in a neutropenic patient is a medical emergency.
- Ongoing fever in neutropenic patients treated with antibiotics should prompt investigation for possible systemic fungal infection.

Table 51.9 Common therapeutic problems in the leukaemias

Problem	Cause	Solutions
Mucositis and oral ulceration	Chemotherapeutic agents directly toxic to mucosal epithelium Radiotherapy is directly toxic to the mucosa and also reduces saliva production by salivary glands Vulnerable mucosa is likely to be attacked by infective agents, e.g. herpes simplex, *Candida*	Regular mouth toilet including the use of antibacterial mouthwash Prophylactic use of antiviral and antifungal agents for patients in whom myelosuppression is likely to be prolonged
Fever in neutropenic patients	Infection predominantly caused by bacteria and/or fungi	Prophylaxis with fluoroquinolone antibiotics for high-risk patients can be considered Broad-spectrum antibiotics must be commenced as soon as blood cultures have been taken A strategy of planned progressive therapy including use of an antifungal agent in non-responsive fever is appropriate alongside diagnostic testing
GVHD	T lymphocytes from the donor react against host tissues	Use a sibling donor if possible Use the donor most closely HLA matched to the patient Consider T-cell depletion of graft (although this may increase the risk of disease relapse) Prophylactic therapy with methotrexate or ciclosporin for example Treat GVHD with corticosteroids, ciclosporin, anti-thymocyte, globulin, anticytokine monoclonal antibodies, imatinib, extra-corporeal photopheresis Irradiate all blood products
Late complications of treatment	Risks of haemopoietic malignancy and non-haemopoietic malignancy are increased post-chemotherapy Late cardiotoxicity secondary to anthracyclines	Aim to tailor therapy to the underlying disease, i.e. do not over-treat and do not under-treat Do not exceed maximum cumulative doses of anthracyclines

GVHD, Graft-versus-host disease; HLA, human leucocyte antigen.

Case studies

Case 51.1

A 30-year-old woman, Ms PL, recently diagnosed with CML, attends the haematology clinic to discuss the options for treatment.

Questions

1. Which treatment options are available?
2. Which treatment is likely to be the best choice for Ms PL?
3. What treatment would be preferable if she was to become pregnant?

Answers

1. There are clearly a number of potential treatment options which need to be explored with the patient. The various treatment options are:
   - active management with targeted drug therapy:
     - imatinib or other tyrosine kinase inhibitors (e.g. nilotinib),
     - treatment as part of a clinical trial, which is likely to involve imatinib or other TKIs in varying doses.
   - allogeneic stem cell transplant:
     - matched sibling donor transplant,
     - matched unrelated donor (MUD) transplantation if a matched sibling is not available.
   - other options:
     - interferon-α +/− cytosine,
     - palliative therapy with hydroxycarbamide to control cell counts.

2. Imatinib or other TKI would be the treatment of choice in a patient presenting at any age, as long as there are no contraindications. Ms PL may be offered treatment in a clinical trial, if available.

   Results with these agents, particularly for patients with newly diagnosed chronic phase disease, are excellent. Complete cytogenetic responses have been seen, although very sensitive quantitative PCR techniques can still detect the abnormal BCR-ABL gene in the vast majority of CML patients in whom the Philadelphia chromosome itself is undetectable. In addition, the drug has been shown to delay progression to accelerated phase disease or blast crisis. It is still not possible, however, to say that imatinib cures patients with CML.

   Although no randomised study has been undertaken, it is clear from historical data that, in the medium term, the mortality associated with allogeneic stem cell transplantation far exceeds that associated with TKIs. In addition to these very encouraging data, which pertain to the effect of the drug on the disease, the side effects of TKIs are generally mild, and patients report this agent far easier to tolerate than interferon-α. The main side effects of imatinib are rash, cytopenias, fluid retention and abnormalities of liver function tests. Second generation TKIs carry some of the same side effect profiles but have other side effects which are unique to them; for example, dasatinib is associated with the development of pleural effusions and reversible pulmonary hypertension. Given the efficacy of imatinib and the fact that the drug is generally very well tolerated, imatinib is regarded as the initial treatment of choice for the vast majority of patients with CML. Ongoing management involves haematological and molecular monitoring of the patient to determine whether he or she has a good response to imatinib. In the event of a good response, the patient continues to take the drug. If at a later stage the molecular response to the agent begins to diminish, then a second-line TKI is considered. If a poor/incomplete response is seen to a second-line agent, then transplantation should be considered.

A purely palliative approach is unlikely to be acceptable to a young patient, thus excluding hydroxycarbamide as a single agent in a patient who is newly diagnosed with CML. Hydroxycarbamide, however, does have a role in the acute setting, where it can be used to control high cell counts before, or during, the commencement of a TKI. There is no doubt that use of interferon-α alone results in cytogenetic remission in a small percentage of patients, and this effect is enhanced by the addition of cytosine. The side effects of interferon-α include flu-like and affective symptoms, and the addition of cytosine increases myelosuppression and risk of mucositis. Although these treatments can induce cytogenetic remission, the duration of such responses is unclear, and only a minority of patients respond completely. The high risk of side effects and the low chance of complete cytogenetic response to interferon-α, with or without cytosine, are likely to make these therapeutic modalities unattractive to Ms PL.

It remains true that allogeneic stem cell transplantation is the only proven curative therapy for patients with CML at present but should be reserved for those who are intolerant of or refractory to multiple TKIs. The fundamental problem with allogeneic transplantation as an approach is that the mortality rate for transplant recipients remains high. The 1-year mortality rate for a 30-year-old patient transplanted using a sibling donor is approximately 10–15%, and this may rise to 20–25% if an unrelated donor has to be used. The major causes of death in this group are GVHD and infection. In addition to the high risk of mortality in the short-term, there is also a risk of long-term morbidity post-allograft. Chronic GVHD can have a significant impact on quality of life for many patients and requires long-term medical follow-up. Ironically, patients with a degree of chronic GVHD are at reduced risk of disease relapse because a GVHD response is associated with a graft-versus-leukaemia effect; some disparity between the immune systems of the transplant donor and recipient is helpful. In addition to these problems, all transplanted patients are at increased risk of a second malignancy as a consequence of the conditioning therapy received as part of the transplant and probably also as a consequence of deficiencies within the transplanted immune system.

Given the problems associated with the various therapeutic strategies discussed earlier, it is not surprising that there was great excitement surrounding the development of the TKI imatinib, and subsequent second-generation TKIs, which remain the agent of choice in first-line therapy.

3. Currently, there are no safety data for the use of TKIs before and during pregnancy. It is therefore more appropriate that disease control is gained with a TKI before pregnancy so that a 'drug holiday' can be undertaken during pregnancy, with the hope of ongoing disease control. If Ms PL required treatment, then safety data are available for the use of interferon-α, and this agent is therefore a reasonable therapeutic option in this rare situation.

Case 51.2

A patient, Mr RB, with AML is currently in first CR and has a fully HLA-matched brother who is medically fit. You have been asked to counsel Mr RB's brother, the potential transplant donor, about stem cell collection.

Questions

1. What methods are available for the collection of stem cells for haemopoietic stem cell transplantation?
2. What are the advantages and disadvantages of each of these stem cell collection methods for the transplant donor?
3. What are the advantages and disadvantages of each of these stem cell collection methods for the transplant recipient, Mr RB?

Answers

1. There are two main methods of collection of haemopoietic stem cells from a sibling donor:
   - Direct harvesting of cells from the bone marrow in the pelvis
   - Collection of circulating peripheral blood stem cells using an apheresis technique after stimulation of the stem cell compartment using G-CSF
2. Direct harvesting of marrow stem cell from the bone marrow is an operative procedure and is performed under general anaesthetic. Clearly, there are risks associated with the use of general anaesthesia, but the risk of death associated with this approach is less than 1 in 10,000 procedures. Marrow harvesting involves a hospital stay, usually for one night postoperatively, but some units also require donors to be admitted the night before surgery. Donors are likely to experience pain around the pelvis, and there is a risk of mechanical back pain in the short to medium term due to pressure applied to the pelvis during repeated needle insertions. This risk is increased in those with a history of back problems before the procedure. Indeed, such potential donors may prefer a peripheral blood stem cell harvesting approach. Donors, such as Mr RB's brother, must be warned about bruising and potential infection at the site of their wounds.

   One of the other potential problems associated with marrow harvesting is that it is impossible to select the type of blood cell harvested, and a large component of the volume of fluid collected comprises red blood cells. This can lead to a degree of anaemia in the donor, who may take several weeks to normalise his or her haemoglobin. It is usually possible to avoid blood transfusion in this situation because it is unusual for donors to be significantly symptomatic. Nonetheless, Mr RB's brother must be warned that the need for allogeneic blood transfusion is a possibility with this procedure.

   Peripheral blood stem cell harvesting has several advantages over direct marrow harvesting from the iliac crests. The procedure can be undertaken during hospital outpatient visits and does not require the use of a general anaesthetic. Because the stem cell harvesting procedure allows selective collection of mononuclear cells, significant anaemia is very unlikely after this procedure. Clearly, red blood cells do circulate within the apheresis circuit, and if the circuit clots off and has to be disconnected from the donor, then red blood cells will be lost. This is unlikely to be of clinical significance unless the donor is a child and hence has a relatively low blood volume.

   Disadvantages of this approach include the need for stimulation of donor haemopoiesis by the G-CSF. Marrow stimulation can result in significant pain especially around the shoulders, back and pelvic girdle. Most donors can manage this pain at home with simple analgesia, but very occasionally hospital admission is required for pain control. Very occasionally patients develop splenic pain, and there have been a couple of reports of splenic rupture in normal donors after G-CSF stimulation, but this is very rare. One difficulty with the use of G-CSF is that it has only been in routine use for the past 20 years. This makes it impossible to categorically reassure potential stem cell donors, such as Mr RB's brother, that use of G-CSF in this way is absolutely safe in the long-term. There is, however, currently no evidence that acting as a peripheral blood stem cell donor increases one's risk of leukaemia development later in life. Some potential donors find this element of uncertainty difficult and prefer to undertake a marrow harvest in which the risks, although present, are better quantified.

The apheresis procedure itself will require Mr RB's brother to lie relatively still with a needle in one or both arms (depending upon the type of apheresis kit used) for approximately 4–5 hours. Some collections can be done in one procedure, but some donors will need to be harvested in two procedures, over 2 days. One prerequisite for peripheral blood stem cell donation is that the potential donor has good enough peripheral veins to allow reliable venous access. If this is not the case and the donor prefers to donate using this method, a temporary central venous line has to be inserted.

Most donors tolerate the apheresis procedure with few problems. One of the most common complications of the procedure is hypocalcaemia which results from calcium binding by the citrate anticoagulant used to prevent clotting within the apheresis circuit. Donors may notice perioral tingling or paraesthesia in other areas and are asked to report this immediately. The problem is easily treated by reducing the concentration of anticoagulant in the circuit and by asking the donor to drink a small amount of milk. If this problem is not picked up early, the consequences can be more severe, with the development of tetany, which would require intravenous calcium replacement.

In summary, Mr RB's brother should be advised that peripheral blood stem cell donation is generally a less invasive and better-tolerated procedure than direct stem cell harvest from the marrow space. However, the associated procedural risks are more easily quantifiable for the latter procedure.

3. There are some potential advantages, to the transplant recipient, in the use of peripheral blood stem cells as opposed to bone marrow stem cells. Engraftment is quicker, so the recipient spends less time in the neutropenic phase, and hence the risk of infection is reduced. Similarly, there is evidence that duration of hospital stay is reduced when peripheral blood stem cells are used. One potential disadvantage of this approach is that the graft includes a larger dose of T-lymphocytes than a graft of stem cells derived directly from the marrow (approximately a 10-fold increase). There is some evidence that rates of chronic GVHD are increased among recipients of peripheral blood stem cells, but this observation has not been borne out in all studies. This potential disadvantage of peripheral blood stem cells is negated if a T-cell-depleted approach is used, as is the case for most matched unrelated procedures.

Case 51.3

A 68-year-old woman, Mrs BG, is admitted with newly diagnosed AML. Once her condition is stabilised, the consultant seeks her consent to start intensive chemotherapy.

....

Questions

1. How should the consultant ensure the consent process is performed as well as possible?
2. What are the treatment options available for Mrs BG?

....

Answers

1. It is vital that consent is taken only after very careful discussions. Consent for such intensive chemotherapy usually requires several

conversations and should be regarded as a process not a single event. The final consent conversation should be done in a quiet private room if possible, and interruptions should be kept to a minimum. Mrs BG should be allowed to have a friend, partner or relative present if she wishes, and ideally, a clinical nurse specialist should be present too. If possible, Mrs BG should be given some written material on chemotherapy before consent even if it is important the treatment is started promptly. Patients should be given a clear explanation of their potential treatment options and should be informed of any clinical trials that may be available to them. It is vitally important to fully inform patients regarding their condition and its prognosis and about treatment options and their potential advantages and disadvantages. Only if patients have all the necessary information can they decide on the treatment option that is most appropriate/acceptable to their individual circumstances.

2. Treatment options for older patients, such as Mrs BG, diagnosed with AML should take into consideration the fitness of the patient, their comorbidities and the characteristics of their leukaemia. These options should be clearly discussed with the patient and their relatives to make the best individualised treatment plan. Broadly speaking, the options are as follows:
   - Intensive therapy:
     - Daunorubicin and cytarabine containing regimens (see Fig. 51.2) may be used in older patients with AML. The decision to treat intensively is largely based on an assessment of the patient's performance status and comorbidities. It must also take into account the disease characteristics and the fitness of the patient for a subsequent transplant procedure. Given that many older patients with AML have disease that displays high risk genetic and molecular characteristics, allogeneic marrow transplantation is often the only potentially curative therapeutic option. Complete remission can be achieved in 50–60% of older patients fit enough to be treated with an intensive approach, but unfortunately, the survival of these patients at 2 years is poor at approximately 15–20% (Lowenberg et al., 2009), due to high relapse rates. Whilst reduced intensity allogeneic transplantation can provide a potentially curative option, only a relatively small number of patients older than 60 years will be fit enough to tolerate this treatment.
     - Ongoing clinical trials are investigating the optimum scheduling, dosing and the addition of targeted therapies to improve the outcome for older patients with AML.
   - Non-intensive therapy:
     - 5-Azacytidine has shown promise in the management of AML with a low disease burden. The 5-azacytidine regimen is delivered on an outpatient basis over 7 days and is less toxic than the intensive in-patient regimens previously described. This treatment may be preferable to those patients wishing for a less intense approach or for those who have comorbidities which may effectively exclude them from a high-dose treatment option. 5-Azacytidine has been shown to deliver complete responses in 18% of patients, with a median overall survival of 10.4 months (Dombret et al., 2015; Fenaux et al., 2010). In addition, this agent has delivered modest responses in reducing the transfusion requirements in those who have a background of myelodysplasia.
     - Low-dose subcutaneous cytarabine is another option which can be delivered in the outpatient setting and is given over 10 days. This option is aimed at reducing toxicity whilst achieving some disease control. Low-dose cytarabine has been shown to deliver complete responses in 18% of patients treated but with a median overall survival of only 5 months (Devillier et al., 2014). This treatment option is best reserved for those who do not have complex/adverse cytogenetics because no benefit has been seen in this group of patients.

- Best supportive care:
  - This approach aims to reduce the disease burden and alleviate symptoms but does not fundamentally alter the overall disease process/natural history. Transfusional support (red blood cells and platelets) is given to reduce the symptoms of anaemia and thrombocytopenia, antimicrobials are used to treat infection and hydroxycarbamide can be administered to reduce the peripheral blood blast percentage and thus minimise symptoms of gum swelling, headache and breathlessness. This treatment option focuses on maximising quality of life, typically over a few months.
  - For palliative management to be effective, regular review of the patient is necessary by team members who are skilled at managing any symptoms which may arise during the palliative phase of the disease.
  - Clinical trials: Mrs BG is in the older AML patient group, which is the focus of current clinical trials because the significant need in this population for effective and better tolerated treatment options is well recognised.

Case 51.4

A 24-year-old patient, Mr TH, with ALL is undergoing chemotherapy and needs intrathecal chemotherapy to prevent relapse in the meninges. Giving drugs by this route is extremely dangerous. Several patients have died as a result of the inadvertent administration of vinca alkaloids into the CSF.

Question

What steps have been taken nationally to try to prevent the inadvertent intrathecal injection of vincristine and other agents not suitable for intrathecal use?

Answer

In the UK, there are now strict guidelines for administration of intrathecal chemotherapy. The procedure can only be performed in hospital units which have been deemed fit for purpose by assessment as part of a rigorous peer-review process. The procedure must be undertaken in a specially designated area which is only used for the purpose of administering intrathecal drugs. To minimise the possibility of the wrong drug being administered, intravenous drugs must not be given in this area. Intrathecal drugs must only be prescribed by a consultant or specialist registrar who has been trained to prescribe or give intrathecal chemotherapy and whose name appears on a locally held register. Drugs for intrathecal administration must only be prescribed on a designated prescription sheet. Once the prescription has arrived in pharmacy, the drugs must be manufactured and checked by pharmacists trained in the manufacture and checking of intrathecal prescriptions. The drugs must be positively labelled 'for intrathecal use only' and must be dispensed by a trained pharmacist. They can only be dispensed once Mr TH has been given any intravenous drugs that are due that day; ideally intrathecal and intravenous chemotherapy should not be given to a patient on the same day. Intrathecal drugs must only be dispensed to a doctor trained and on the register for giving intrathecal drugs who will, in the presence of the dispensing pharmacist, check the details of the drug against the prescription before transporting the intrathecal drugs. The intrathecal drugs must be transported in a specially designated container, and if they need to be stored, then it must be in a separate, specially designated lockable fridge, that is separate from any intravenous chemotherapy. Once the procedure is underway, the intrathecal drugs must be checked by the registered

doctor and by a nurse who has been trained and appears on a register of nurses trained to check intrathecal drugs. The drugs should also be checked by Mr TH or his representative. Intrathecal drugs must not be given in hospitals not approved for the procedure, in non-designated areas, outside office hours or at the weekend unless there are exceptional circumstances. All staff working on oncology or haematology units should be taught about the rules for giving intrathecal therapy.

In addition, to prevent inadvertent vincristine administration into the intrathecal space, hospitals giving intrathecal chemotherapy should follow special rules for labelling vinca alkaloid prescriptions, and vinca alkaloids should be made up in a minimum volume of 20 mL to prevent intrathecal administration. More recent practice has seen hospitals replace their intrathecal syringes with ones which will only lock into intrathecal lumbar puncture needles; this ensures that no other syringes, containing the wrong drugs, can be inadvertently attached or administered.

Case 51.5

A 37-year-old dental technician, Mr SG, presented with acute promyelocytic leukaemia (APL). He had a number of bleeding problems at presentation. Mr SG was commenced on all-trans retinoic acid (ATRA) at presentation but was causing much concern to the treating team because he had a white cell count of 80×10^9/L ($4.0–11.0 \times 10^9$/L) and severe bleeding problems.

Questions

1. Why is ATRA used in this circumstance, and what are its side effects?
2. What options are there for induction management of APL?

Answers

1. APL is a variant of AML which presents with disseminated intravascular coagulation (DIC). This is manifest by coagulation defects, low platelet counts and severe bleeding. Patients, such as Mr SG, are at risk of severe haemorrhage at presentation but have a very good prognosis with chemotherapy if they survive the induction phase. ATRA can rapidly correct the coagulopathy found at presentation by promoting differentiation of the abnormal promyelocytes typical in this condition and thus reducing the trigger for DIC development. ATRA also increases the likelihood of the patient entering remission, when combined with standard high-dose chemotherapy. It is also used as a maintenance agent because it increases the number of patients who remain in long-term remission. In the acute setting, ATRA can cause a severe and life-threatening sterile pneumonitis, otherwise referred to as 'differentiation syndrome'. This causes a rapid onset respiratory distress associated with hypotension and leucocytosis. This normally occurs within 1 week of commencement of ATRA, and it is important to recognise this syndrome quickly because it often responds to withdrawal of the drug and administration of high-dose dexamethasone. If left untreated, differentiation syndrome can lead to respiratory failure and death. The longer-term side effects of ATRA include dry eyes and a dry mouth.
2. Idarubicin and ATRA induction followed by consolidation with idarubicin and mitoxantrone, both combined with ATRA, are the chemotherapy options of choice in the UK at present. A combination of idarubicin and ATRA as induction has been shown to result in a complete response rate of up to 94% (Lo-Coco et al., 2010). This has been used in combination with cytarabine, but a number of

large clinical trials have shown that the addition of cytarabine does not significantly improve the outcomes and is given at the expense of additional toxicity.

Idarubicin, like other anthracyclines, carries the same side-effect profile: anaemia, low platelets resulting in bleeding, neutropenia resulting in severe infections, nausea/vomiting, diarrhoea, hair loss and hepatotoxicity. In addition, there are the long-term toxicities which are of concern, namely, cardio-toxicity and, later, secondary malignancies. Despite very good outcomes in APL, clinical trials have been moving towards using non-chemotoxic agents to minimise toxicity without compromising on response rates and survival.

Arsenic trioxide (ATO) has been the subject of recent clinical trials. When given with ATRA, ATO has been shown to bring about remission in patients who have APL in association with the 15;17 chromosomal translocation and the PML:RARA genetic abnormality. Efficacy has been demonstrated to be non-inferior to idarubicin and ATRA (Burnett et al., 2015), and the need for supportive care was reduced in the ATO group.

Side effects include differentiation syndrome. ATO can cause QT interval prolongation and complete atrioventricular block in some patients. QT prolongation can lead to a torsade de pointes ventricular arrhythmia, which can be fatal. The risk of torsade de pointes is related to the extent of QT prolongation, concomitant administration of QT prolonging drugs, a history of torsade de pointes, pre-existing QT interval prolongation, congestive heart failure, administration of potassium-wasting diuretics or other conditions that result in hypokalemia or hypomagnesemia. Before initiating therapy with ATO, a 12-lead electrocardiogram (ECG) should be performed and serum electrolytes (potassium, calcium and magnesium) and creatinine should be assessed; pre-existing electrolyte abnormalities should be corrected and, if possible, drugs that are known to prolong the QT interval should be discontinued. For QTc greater than 500 ms, corrective measures should be completed and the QTc reassessed with serial ECGs before considering using ATO. ATO is not currently available in the UK for first-line treatment of APL.

Case 51.6

A 57-year-old man, Mr AV, with a 6-year history of CLL presented with a rising white cell count, worsening lymphadenopathy and hepatosplenomegaly. Treatment was commenced with oral fludarabine 40 mg/m² and oral cyclophosphamide 250 mg/m² daily for 3 days with rituximab given on day 1 (FC-R).

....

Questions

1. What additional precautions would you advise the doctor to take and why?
2. Mr AV relapses after 18 months. What treatment options would you discuss with the patient?

....

Answers

1. The combination of fludarabine, cyclophosphamide and rituximab (FC-R) is very powerful for the initial treatment of CLL. It has been used as a second-line therapy, although recent data support its use as a first-line therapy. It has been associated with more frequent and deeper remissions which are typically longer than those attained after single-agent therapy. It is thus currently regarded as the gold standard of treatment in non-p53-mutated CLL patients. It is nonetheless a highly

immunosuppressive combination with activity against both T- and B-cells. Patients treated with this regimen are at high risk of developing *Pneumocystis* pneumonia. It is important that patients are given prophylaxis against this severe infection. Herpes virus infections including herpes simplex and herpes zoster are also common, and most patients are given aciclovir prophylaxis.

As patients are immunosuppressed, they are also at risk of developing transfusion-related GVHD. This is a complication of blood product transfusion, caused by engraftment of lymphocytes from the transfused product. This complication is now very rare in the era of leuco-depleted blood, but where it occurs, it is typically fatal. This complication can be prevented by irradiation of blood products before transfusion. Rituximab is an antibody-based therapy and can be associated with significant reactions which can occasionally be severe and life threatening (see Chapter 52). Paracetamol, chlorphenamine and hydrocortisone are administered to prevent acute reactions to the drug.

Fludarabine-based chemotherapy agents are less effective when used in patients who have deletion or mutations in the p53 gene, and so Mr AV should be tested for this before commencing therapy because it may affect current and future options for therapy.

2. There are many approaches that could be undertaken. The potential treatment options are as follows:

   - Repeat treatment with FC-R. This can be considered given that Mr AV had a reasonable duration of remission with the first course. Again, if any mutations in the p53 gene were detected, then this option would be less favourable.

   - The combination of bendamustine and rituximab (BR) has been shown to be effective in the management of CLL either as first-line or as subsequent therapy. BR has been shown to deliver overall response rates and progression-free survival rates similar to that of FC-R but has achieved higher complete response rates. It is an intravenous treatment delivered as an outpatient and is generally well tolerated. Many of the side effects are shared with FC-R and prophylaxis against *Pneumocystis* pneumonia and herpes viruses should be given.

   - Chlorambucil and rituximab or other novel anti-CD20 agents (e.g. ofatumumab or obinutuzumab) are less intensive regimens which have shown promising results in patients, such as Mr AV, with advancing age or significant comorbidities. Oral chlorambucil in combination with an intravenous anti-CD20 agent is delivered in the outpatient setting. Trial data have shown that progression-free survival for chlorambucil- and obinutuzumab-treated patients exceeds that for chlorambucil- and rituximab-treated patients (median PFS 26 months vs. 16.3 months). The combination of chlorambucil and obinutuzumab has been approved for use in the UK (Goede et al., 2014). Similarly, ofatumumab and chlorambucil have shown enhanced progression-free survival when compared with chlorambucil alone (22 months vs. 13 months) (Hillmen et al., 2013)

   - Alemtuzumab is usually reserved for CLL that is proving difficult to treat, especially in those patients who have p53 mutations/deletions. It is delivered as a subcutaneous injection with dose escalations on the first cycle. Like other agents, alemtuzumab is also associated with increased risk of opportunistic infections; prophylaxis with co-trimoxazole and aciclovir is advised. Patients receiving alemtuzumab should also receive irradiated blood products. Patients are at risk of allergic reactions given that it is a monoclonal antibody, and so prophylaxis to prevent this should be given. In addition, patients are at particular risk of primary cytomegalovirus (CMV) infection or CMV reactivation. It is therefore advised that CMV levels are monitored twice weekly whilst on therapy

- Targeted drug therapies, ibrutinib (Bruton kinase inhibitor) or idelalisib (PI3K inhibitor) should be considered, if available, or in the context of a clinical trial. These agents are oral drugs which effectively target the essential points in the B-cell signalling pathway to block the production of clonal, and other, B cells. Some of the most common, early side effects associated with ibrutinib are diarrhoea, rashes, low platelet counts and an early rise in non-clonal lymphocyte counts which does not seem to be harmful and returns to the normal range after several months of treatment.

- Idelalisib is the only PI3K inhibitor available currently in the UK outside the context of a clinical trial. The main reported side effects are diarrhoea, low blood counts and hepatotoxicity.
- Once started, these drugs should be continued. Their use, although very promising, is expensive. Ongoing studies will be needed to determine the correct sequencing of these highly effective agents.

References

Burnett, A.K., Russell, N.H., Hills, R.K., et al., 2015. Arsenic trioxide and all-trans retinoic acid treatment for acute promyelocytic leukaemia in all risk groups (AML17): results of a randomized, controlled, phase 3 trial. Lancet Oncol. 13, 1295–1305.

Cancer Research UK, 2017. Disease facts. Available at: http://www.cancer researchuk.org/health-professional/cancer-statistics/statistics-by-cancer-type/leukaemia.

Cilloni, D., Saglio, G., 2009. CML: a model for targeted therapy. Balliere's Best Pract. Res. Clin. Haematol. 22, 285–294.

Coombs, C.C., Tavakkoli, M., Tallman, M.S., 2015. Acute promyelocytic leukaemia: where did we start, where are we now, and the future. Blood Cancer J. 5, e304.

Devillier, R., Gelsi-Boyer, V., Murati, A., et al., 2014. Prognostic significance of myelodysplastic-related changes according to the WHO classification among ELN intermediate-risk AML patients. Am. J. Hematol. 13, e22–e24.

Dohner, H., Weisdorf, D.J., Bloomfield, C.D., 2015. Acute myeloid leukaemia. N. Engl. J. Med. 373, 1136–1152.

Dombret, H., Seymour, J.F., Butrym, A., et al., 2015. International phase 3 study of azacitidine vs conventional care regimens in older patients with newly diagnosed AML with >30% blasts. Blood 126, 291–199.

Eichhorst, B., Fink, A., Busch, R., et al., 2013. Chemoimmunotherapy with fludarabine (F), cyclophosphamide (C), and rituximab (R) (FCR) versus bendamustine and rituximab (BR) in previously untreated and physically fit patients (pts) with advanced chronic lymphocytic leukemia (CLL): results of a planned interim analysis of the CLL10 Trial, an international, randomized study of the German CLL Study Group (GCLLSG). Blood 122, 526.

Fenaux, P., Mufti, G.J., Hellstrom-Lindberg, E., et al., 2010. Azacitidine prolongs overall survival compared with conventional care regimens in elderly patients with low bone marrow blast count acute myeloid leukaemia. J. Clin. Oncol. 28, 562–569.

Goede, V., Fischer, K., Busch, R., et al., 2014. Obinutuzumab plus chlorambucil in patients with CLL and coexisting conditions. N. Engl. J. Med. 370, 1101–1110.

Grimwade, D., Hills, R.K., Moorman, A.V., et al., 2010. Refinement of cytogenetic classification in acute myeloid leukemia: determination of prognostic significance of rare recurring chromosomal abnormalities among 5876 younger adult patients treated in the United Kingdom Medical Research Council trials. Blood 116, 354–365.

Grimwade, D., Ivey, A., Huntly, B.J.P., et al., 2016. Molecular landscape of acute myeloid leukemia in younger adults and its clinical relevance. Blood 127, 29–41.

Hallek, M., Fingerle-Rowson, G., Fink, A.M., et al., 2009. First-line treatment with fludarabine (F), cyclophosphamide (C), and rituximab (R) (FCR) improves overall survival (OS) in previously untreated patients (pts) with advanced chronic lymphocytic leukaemia (CLL): results of a randomized phase III trial on behalf of an international group of investigators and the German CLL Study Group. Blood 114, 535.

Hillmen, P., Robak, T., Janssens, A., et al., 2013. Ofatumumab + chlorambucil versus chlorambucil alone in patients with untreated chronic lymphocytic leukemia (CLL): results of the phase III study complement 1 (OMB110911). Blood 122 (21), Abstract 528.

Hughes, T.P., Kaed, J., Branford, S., et al., 2003. Frequency of major molecular responses to imatinib or interferon-alpha plus cytarabine in newly diagnosed chronic myeloid leukaemia. N. Engl. J. Med. 349, 1423–1432.

Ivey, A., Hills, R.K., Phil, D., et al., 2016. Assessment of MRD in standard-risk AML. N. Engl. J. Med. 374, 422–433.

Lo-Coco, F., Avvisati, G., Vignetti, M., et al., 2010. Front-line treatment of acute promyelocytic leukaemia with AIDA induction followed by risk-adapted consolidation for adults younger than 61 years: results of the AIDA-2000 trial of the GIMEMA group. Blood 116, 3171–3179.

Lowenberg, B., Ossenkoppele, G.J., van Putten, W., et al., 2009. High-dose daunorubicin in older patients with acute myeloid leukaemia. N. Engl. J. Med. 361, 1235–1248.

National Institute for Health and Care Excellence (NICE), 2012a. Dasatinib, nilotinib and standard-dose imatinib for the first-line treatment of chronic myeloid leukaemia. Technology Appraisal Guidance TA251. Available at: https://www.nice.org.uk/guidance/ta251.

National Institute for Health and Care Excellence (NICE), 2012b. Neutropenic sepsis: prevention and management in people with cancer. Clinical Guideline 151. Available at: https://www.nice.org.uk/guidance/cg151.

National Institute for Health and Care Excellence (NICE), 2015a. Obinutuzumab in combination with chlorambucil for untreated chronic lymphocytic leukaemia. Technology Appraisal Guidance TA343. Available at: https://www.nice.org.uk/guidance/ta343 .

National Institute for Health and Care Excellence (NICE), 2015b. Ofatumumab in combination with chlorambucil or bendamustine for untreated chronic lymphocytic leukaemia. Technology Appraisal Guidance TA344. https://www.nice.org.uk/guidance/ta344.

O'Brien, S., Guilhot, F., Larson, R.A., et al., 2003. Imatinib compared with interferon and low-dose cytarabine for newly diagnosed chronic-phase chronic myeloid leukaemia. N. Engl. J. Med. 348, 994–1004.

Pui, C., Mullighan, C., Evans, W., 2012. Pediatric acute lymphoblastic leukemia: where are we going and how do we get there? Blood 120, 1165–1174.

Rai, K.R., Peterson, B.L., Appelbaum, F.R., et al., 2000. Fludarabine compared with chlorambucil as primary therapy for chronic lymphocytic leukaemia. N. Engl. J. Med. 343, 1750–1757.

Rezvani, A.R., Lowsky, R., Negrin, R.S., 2016. Hematopoietic cell transplantation. In: Kaushansky, K., Lichtman, M.A., Prchal, J.T., et al. (Eds.), Williams' Hematology, ninth ed. McGraw-Hill Medical Publishing Division, New York.

Rowe, J.M., Lowenberg, B., 2013. Gemtuzumab ozogamicin in acute myeloid leukaemia: a remarkable saga about an active drug. Blood 121, 4838–4841.

Sawyers, C.L., 1999. Medical progress: chronic myeloid leukaemia. N. Engl. J. Med. 340, 1330–1340.

Sengsayadeth, S., Savani, B.N., Blaise, D., et al., 2015. Reduced intensity conditioning allogeneic hematopoietic cell transplantation for adult acute myeloid leukemia in complete remission – a review from the acute leukemia working party of the EBMT. Haematologica 100, 859–869.

Sipsas, N.V., Bodey, G.P., Kontoyiannis, D.P., 2005. Perspectives for the management of neutropenic patients with cancer in the 21st century. Cancer 103, 1103–1113.

Smith, T.J., Bohlke, K., Lyman, G.H., et al., 2015. Recommendations for the use of WBC growth factors: american society of clinical oncology clinical practice guideline update. J. Clin. Oncol. 33, 3199–3212.

Stanworth, S., Phil, D., Estcourt, L.J., et al., 2013. A no-prophylaxis platelet-transfusion strategy for hematologic cancers. N. Engl. J. Med. 368, 1171–1780.

Swerdlow, S.H., Campo, E., Harris, N.L., et al., 2008. WHO Classification of Tumours of Haematopoietic and Lymphoid Tissues, fourth ed. IARC Press, Lyon.

Further reading

Hoffbrand, A.V., Moss, P.A.H., 2015. Essential Haematology, seventh ed. Blackwell Publishing, Oxford.

Howard, M.R., Hamilton, P.J., 2013. Haematology: An Illustrated Colour Text, fourth revised ed. Churchill Livingstone, Edinburgh.

Provan, D., Gribben, J.G., 2010. Molecular Hematology, third ed. Wiley-Blackwell Publishing, Oxford.

Useful websites

BloodMed: http://www.bloodmed.com/home/

TEAMHAEM, Explore Haematology: https://teamhaem.com

52 Lymphomas

Laura Cameron and Catherine Loughran

Key points

- Hodgkin's lymphoma (HL) and non-Hodgkin's lymphoma (NHL) are aggressive diseases that are fatal if untreated.

- In early-stage HL, patients are treated with combined modality treatment usually consisting of two to four cycles of ABVD (doxorubicin [Adriamycin], bleomycin, vinblastine, dacarbazine) and involved field radiotherapy (IFRT) (20–30 Gy); a relapse-free survival rate of 85–90% at 5–10 years is achieved.

- Combination chemotherapy is the current gold-standard regimen for advanced HL, and overall survival at 5 years is 75–80%.

- Low-grade NHL may be treated using R-CVP (rituximab, cyclophosphamide, vincristine, prednisolone) or R-CHOP (rituximab, cyclophosphamide, hydroxydaunorubicin (doxorubicin [Adriamycin]), vincristine [Oncovin], prednisolone) or bendamustine and rituximab (BR) chemotherapy or by adopting a policy of 'watch and wait'.

- R-CHOP chemotherapy is the standard for the treatment of aggressive (intermediate- and high-grade) NHL, curing 60% of patients.

- Relapsed HL and NHL may be treated with further chemotherapy followed by high-dose chemotherapy with bone marrow or peripheral stem cell transplantation.

- Patients receiving chemotherapy for HL and NHL should have full blood count (FBC) and blood biochemistry monitored at frequent intervals.

- Complications such as nausea and vomiting, tumour lysis syndrome (TLS), mucositis and bone marrow suppression may occur as a result of chemotherapy and are significant factors in morbidity.

- Supportive care of the patient undergoing chemotherapy includes appropriate drug therapy to minimise the adverse effects of the treatment.

Lymphoma is cancer of the lymphatic system and accounts for approximately 5% of new cases of cancer reported in the UK each year. The primary cancerous cell of origin is the lymphocyte; as a result, there is often considerable overlap between lymphomas and lymphoid leukaemias. Lymphomas are subdivided into two main categories: Hodgkin's lymphoma (HL) and non-Hodgkin's lymphoma (NHL). Both HL and NHL can be further classified based on histology.

The site of malignancy is usually a lymph node. Extranodal disease, most frequently of the stomach, skin, oral cavity and pharynx, small intestine and central nervous system (CNS), can occur and is more common in NHL than HL.

Hodgkin's lymphoma

Hodgkin's disease, now known as HL, was first described by Thomas Hodgkin in 1832. HL accounts for 13% of all lymphomas, and there are approximately 2000 new cases per year in the UK. HL incidence demonstrates a bimodal age distribution, with the first peak in incidence in young adults aged 20–24 years and a second peak in older men and women. Nearly 50% of patients diagnosed with HL in the UK are aged 45 years and older (Cancer Research UK, 2016a).

Aetiology

The cause of HL is unknown, but a number of risk factors have been identified. Epstein–Barr (glandular fever) virus has been identified in 50% of HL cases and is likely to be associated with an increase in the risk of developing HL. Certain associations have been identified which suggest a genetic link with HL; for example, same-sex siblings of patients with HL have a 10 times higher risk of developing the disease. Patients with reduced immunity, for example, acquired immune deficiency syndrome (AIDS) or those taking immunosuppressants, and those with a history of autoimmune disorders are at increased risk of developing HL.

Pathology

The diagnosis is made by histological examination of an excised lymph node biopsy. HL, as classified by the World Health Organization (WHO), has two distinct entities: classic HL (cHL) and nodular lymphocyte-predominant Hodgkin's lymphoma (NLPHL) (Swerdlow et al., 2008). The characteristic pathological finding in cHL is the identification of Hodgkin and Reed–Sternberg (HRS) cells in an inflammatory background. NLPHL accounts for 5–10% of HL cases and is histologically distinct from cHL with no HRS cells. Reed–Sternberg, but not lymphocyte-predominant (LP) cells express CD-30. Classic Hodgkin's is further subdivided into four histological types:

- nodular sclerosis,
- mixed cellularity,
- lymphocyte depleted,
- lymphocyte rich.

Signs and symptoms

HL usually presents with painless enlargement of lymph nodes, often in the neck. About 25% of patients will present

Table 52.1 Cotswolds modification of the Ann Arbor classification system for Hodgkin's lymphoma (Lister et al., 1989)

Clinical stage	Defining features
I	Involvement of a single lymph node region or lymphoid structure
II	Involvement of two or more lymph node regions on the same side of the diaphragm
III	Involvement of lymph node regions or structures on both sides of the diaphragm: III_1– with or without involvement of splenic, hilar, coeliac or portal nodes III_2– with involvement of para-aortic, iliac or mesenteric nodes
IV	Involvement of extranodal site(s) beyond that designated E

Modifying characteristics:
A: no symptoms
B: fever, drenching sweats, weight loss
X: bulky disease
   >one-third width of the mediastinum
   >10 cm maximal dimension of nodal mass
E: involvement of a single extranodal site, contiguous or proximal to known nodal site
CS: clinical stage
PS: pathological stage

with unexplained fever, drenching night sweats and/or unexplained weight loss (>10% of body weight). These have prognostic significance and are designated B symptoms; others include malaise, itching or pain at the site of enlarged nodes after drinking alcohol. Bone pain may result from skeletal involvement. Primary involvement of the gut, CNS or bone marrow is rare.

If lymph nodes in the chest are involved, patients may present with breathlessness. There is often a disturbance of immune function due to a progressive loss of immunologically competent T-lymphocytes, with patients becoming particularly prone to viral and fungal infections.

Laboratory findings

Laboratory findings include normochromic, normocytic anaemia, a raised erythrocyte sedimentation rate (ESR) and eosinophilia. One-third of patients have a leucocytosis due to an increase in neutrophils. Advanced disease is associated with lymphopenia (lymphocytes $<0.6 \times 10^9$/L). Plasma lactate dehydrogenase (LDH) is raised in 30–40% of patients at diagnosis and has been associated with a poor prognosis.

Investigations and staging

Once the diagnosis has been made on biopsy, further investigations are needed to assess disease activity and the extent of its spread through the lymphoid system or other body sites. This is called staging and is essential for assessing prognosis, with cure rates for localised tumours (stage I or II) being much higher than those for widespread disease (stage IV). The staging of HL is assessed by the Cotswolds modification of the Ann Arbor classification system (Table 52.1). Information about prognostic factors, such as mediastinal mass and bulky disease, is included in the classification system. The tests

required to establish the stage include a complete history, physical examination, full blood count (FBC), urea and electrolytes (U and Es), chest X-ray, positron emission tomography (PET) and computed tomography (CT). Other useful tests include ESR, serum LDH, liver function tests (LFTs) and viral screening for hepatitis B, hepatitis C and human immunodeficiency virus (HIV). After staging, patients are usually classified as having early-stage favourable, early-stage unfavourable or advanced disease (Table 52.2). Advanced-stage disease patients should have their International Prognostic Score (IPS) or Hasenclever score calculated (see Box 52.1). Each risk factor scores 1, with the number of risk factors predicting 5-year freedom from progression (FFP) rates and overall survival (OS). For example, the FFP rate is 84% and OS 89% for patients with a score of 0, whereas FFP is 42% and OS 56% for a score of 5 or more.

Management

HL is potentially curable and, in general, sensitive to both chemotherapy and radiotherapy; therefore, the two main goals of treatment are to maximise the likelihood of cure whilst minimising the risk of late toxicity such as infertility.

Nodular lymphocyte-predominant Hodgkin's lymphoma

Localised NLPHL frequently involves one isolated lymph node, tends to be indolent (slow growing) and can be treated with surgery if resectable. Early-stage patients can be treated with involved-field radiation therapy (IFRT) alone (30 Gy; Eichenauer et al., 2014). Advanced-stage patients should be treated with combination chemotherapy, and because LP cells express CD20, the addition of rituximab can improve the efficacy of treatment (Eichenauer et al., 2014).

Table 52.2 Definition of Hodgkin's lymphoma risk groups according to the European Organisation for Research and Treatment of Cancer /Lymphoma Study Association and the German Hodgkin Study Group (Follows et al., 2014)

	A. Early-stage favourable (patients must have all features)	B. Early-stage unfavourable	C. Advanced disease
European Organisation for Research and Treatment of Cancer disease	Clinical stage 1 or 2 Maximum of three nodal areas involved Age <50 years of age ESR <50 mm/h without B symptoms or <30 mm/h with B symptoms[a] No mediastinal adenopathy	Clinical stage 1 or 2 with one or more of the following: Four or more nodal areas involved Age >50 years of age ESR >50 mm/h without B symptoms or >30 mm/h with B symptoms Large mediastinal adenopathy	Clinical stage 3 or 4
German Hodgkin Study Group	Clinical stage 1 or 2 Maximum of two nodal areas involved No mediastinal adenopathy ESR <50 mm/h without B symptoms or <30 mm/h with B symptoms No extranodal disease	Clinical stage 1 or 2 with one or more of the following: Three or more lymph node sites of involvement Large mediastinal adenopathy ESR >30 mm/h with B symptoms or ESR >50 mm/h without B symptoms Extranodal disease	Clinical stage 3 or 4 or clinical stage 2B with risk factors (large mediastinal mass and extranodal disease)

[a]B symptoms include unexplained fever, drenching night sweats and/or unexplained weight loss (>10% of body weight).
ESR, Erythrocyte sedimentation rate.

Box 52.1 Hasenclever/International Prognostic Score for advanced Hodgkin lymphoma (Hasenclever and Diehl, 1998)

Prognostic risk factors
1. Age >45 years of age
2. Male gender
3. Serum albumin <40 g/L
4. Haemoglobin <10.5 g/dL
5. Stage 4 disease
6. Leucocytosis, i.e. WCC >15 × 10^9/L
7. Lymphopenia, i.e. <0.6 × 10^9/L or <8% of total WCC
    Score 1 for each of the risk factors present at diagnosis.

WCC, White blood cell count.

Classical Hodgkin's Lymphoma

There is no difference in the management of the four subtypes of classical HL. Management is based on risk group and is summarised in Fig. 52.1.

Early-stage (favourable) disease. The cure rate for patients with stages I and IIA disease is greater than 90%. Patients with stages I and IIA disease may be cured with radiotherapy alone (wide or extended field irradiation). However, due to radiation-related late effects, cardiac toxicity and secondary malignancy, most receive combined modality treatment (chemotherapy and radiotherapy). This usually consists of two cycles of ABVD (doxorubicin [Adriamycin]), bleomycin, vinblastine, dacarbazine) chemotherapy followed by IFRT of 20 Gy (Follows et al., 2014). The aim of chemotherapy is to destroy subclinical disease outside the field of radiotherapy. Involved-site radiation therapy (ISRT) is increasingly used as an alternative to IFRT to further minimise the exposure of uninvolved tissue and organs.

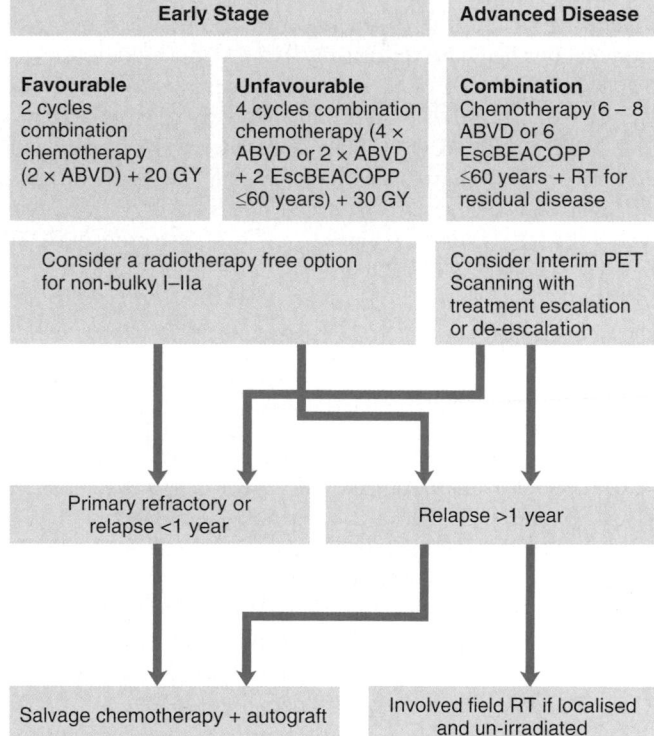

ABVD = Adriamycin (doxorubicin), bleomycin, vinblastine, dacarbazine
EscBEACOPP = escalated bleomycin, etoposide, Adriamycin (doxorubicin), cyclophosphamide,
Oncovin (vincristine), procarbazine, prednisolone
I–IIa = Hodgkin lymphoma stage
GY = gray (unit of ionising radiation dose)
PET = positron emission tomography
RT = radiotherapy

Fig. 52.1 Treatment algorithm for classic Hodgkin lymphoma. (Adapted from Eichenauer et al., 2014.)

894

Box 52.2 Deauville scale (Meignan et al., 2009)

1. No uptake or no residual uptake (when used interim)
2. Slight uptake but below blood pool (mediastinum)
3. Uptake above mediastinal but below or equal to uptake in the liver
4. Uptake slightly to moderately higher than liver
5. Markedly increased uptake or any new lesion (on response evaluation)

Given the high cure rates seen in HL, there has been a drive to minimise radiation toxicity by using chemotherapy alone. The recently published RAPID study investigated whether interim PET scanning after three cycles can identify patients who can avoid radiotherapy and be treated with chemotherapy alone. Those patients with a negative PET scan after three cycles of chemotherapy, as defined by 1 or 2 on the Deauville score (Box 52.2), were randomised to receive IFRT or no further treatment (Radford et al., 2015). At 3-year follow-up, the combined modality group had a lower rate of disease progression, but patients with a negative PET after 3 cycles and no radiotherapy still had an excellent prognosis (3-year progression-free survival 90.8%).

Early-stage (unfavourable) disease. Patients with stage I or II presenting with bulky disease, B symptoms or with more than two sites of disease are considered to be poor risk if treated with radiotherapy alone. These patients are treated with four cycles of combination chemotherapy, usually ABVD, and radiotherapy (30 Gy) to sites of bulky disease (Eichenauer et al., 2014; Follows et al., 2014). The HD14 study compared two cycles of escalated BEACOPP (escBEACOPP; bleomycin, etoposide, doxorubicin [Adriamycin], cyclophosphamide, vincristine [Oncovin], procarbazine, prednisolone) plus two cycles of ABVD with four cycles of ABVD (von Tresckow et al., 2012). The escBEACOPP patients had better disease control and were less likely to relapse but had significant acute toxicities from their chemotherapy. Therefore, escBEACOPP can be considered as a treatment option in younger, fitter patients.

Chemotherapy alone may be considered in selected patients with non-bulky disease to avoid radiation-related late effects, but patients must be counselled on their increased risk of relapse.

Advanced disease. Patients with advanced disease (stages III and IV) are treated with combination chemotherapy. ABVD has been the standard regimen for several decades because 80% of patients will achieve a complete response but experience less toxicity in terms of fertility, haematological toxicity and the development of acute leukaemia and myelodysplasia compared with older regimens, such as MOPP (Mustargen, vincristine [Oncovin], procarbazine, prednisolone) (Table 52.3).

As with unfavourable early-stage disease, escBEACOPP in the advanced setting is associated with fewer progressions and relapses compared with ABVD-based therapy but is more toxic and has not demonstrated an overall survival benefit.

Six to eight cycles of ABVD or six cycles of escBEACOPP is considered the current standard treatment for advanced disease in patients who are 60 years or younger. Patients with a high IPS/Hasenclever score (see Box 52.1) are at a higher risk of relapse and may benefit from more intensive treatment. Recently, the results of the phase 3 HD18 study have been published

Table 52.3 Combination chemotherapy regimens effective in the treatment of Hodgkin's lymphoma

Regimen	Dose and route	Frequency
ABVD (28-day cycle)		
Doxorubicin	25 mg/m² i.v.	Days 1 and 15
Bleomycin	10,000 iu/m² i.v.	Days 1 and 15
Vinblastine	6 mg/m² i.v.	Days 1 and 15
Dacarbazine	375 mg/m² i.v.	Days 1 and 15
BEACOPP escalated (21-day cycle)		
Bleomycin	10,000 iu/m² i.v.	Day 8
Etoposide	200 mg/m² i.v.	Days 1–3
Adriamycin (doxorubicin)	35 mg/m² i.v.	Day 1
Cyclophosphamide	1250 mg/m² i.v.	Day 1
Oncovin (vincristine)	1.4 mg/m² i.v. (max. 2 mg)	Day 8
Procarbazine	100 mg/m² orally	Days 1–7
Prednisolone	40 mg/m² orally	Days 1–14
ChlVPP (28-day cycle)		
Chlorambucil	6 mg/m² orally	Days 1–14
Vinblastine	6 mg/m² i.v.	Days 1 and 8
Procarbazine	100 mg/m² orally	Days 1–14
Prednisolone	40 mg/m² orally (max 60 mg)	Days 1–14
VEPEMB (28-day cycle)		
Vinblastine	6 mg/m² (max: 10 mg) i.v.	Day 1
Endoxan (cyclophosphamide)	500 mg/m² i.v.	Day 1
Prednisolone	30 mg/m² orally	Days 1–5
Procarbazine	100 mg/m² orally	Days 1–5
Etoposide	60 mg/m² orally	Days 15–19
Mitoxantrone	6 mg/m² i.v.	Day 15
Bleomycin	10,000 iu/m² i.v.	Day 15

(Borchmann et al 2018). In this study patients who achieved PET negativity after two cycles of escBEACOPP were assigned to receive either a total of four cycles or a total of 6 or 8 cycles. An impressive 5 year progression free survival of 92% was achieved in the 4 cycle cohort (i.e. after only 12 weeks of treatment) with reduced toxicity compared with a 5-year progression-free survival of 90.8% in the extended treatment arm. This has the potential to become a new standard of care. Patients should be involved in evaluating the risk benefits with respect to efficacy and treatment toxicity. Radiotherapy in advanced disease is given only to those patients with residual disease after chemotherapy (Eichenauer et al., 2014).

For older patients (>60 years), ABVD is the preferred regimen as treatment toxicity is more likely to be tolerated. Options for elderly patients or those unlikely to tolerate ABVD include ChlVPP (chlorambucil, vinblastine, procarbazine, prednisolone) and VEPEMB (vinblastine, cyclophosphamide [Endoxan], prednisolone procarbazine, etoposide, mitoxantrone and bleomycin).

The management of cHL is becoming increasingly individualised to the patient. Studies are ongoing to determine if interim PET scanning after initial therapy may help identify poor responders who are more likely to relapse and require treatment escalation and good responders who can be cured with less intensive therapy (Eichenauer et al., 2014). Recently the Response-Adapted Therapy in Hodgkin Lymphoma (RATHL) study has shown that bleomycin can be omitted, reducing pulmonary toxicity, from ABVD (AVD) in patients achieving a negative PET scan after two cycles of ABVD (Johnson et al., 2016).

Attempts to improve the efficacy of ABVD or reduce the toxicity of escBEACOPP are being made by incorporating new drugs into the backbone of these regimens. For example, brentuximab vedotin, an anti-CD30 monoclonal antibody conjugated to monomethyl auristatin E (MMAE), is being combined with doxorubicin, vinblastine and dacarbazine (A+AVD) and compared with ABVD (Ansell et al., 2014).

Salvage therapy for relapsed disease. Despite advances in HL, 25% of patients progress or relapse. Relapsed disease refers to disease progression after completion of primary treatment which resulted in a complete remission. Depending on previous treatment, options include salvage radiotherapy, salvage chemotherapy or high-dose chemotherapy with autologous stem cell support. In this procedure, stem cells are collected from the patient and returned after high-dose chemotherapy. Patients who relapse after initial radiotherapy alone have a good chance of cure with combination chemotherapy, at least equal to that of patients initially treated with chemotherapy for advanced disease. Occasionally, radiotherapy is used if the disease is localised and previously non-irradiated. Those who relapse after combination chemotherapy have a worse prognosis, although durable remissions can be obtained with further conventional therapy.

Length of remission after first-line chemotherapy influences the success of subsequent salvage therapy, and so the failure of chemotherapy can be used to classify the disease and determine appropriate therapy. If the duration of remission was greater than 12 months (late relapse), then the patient can be re-treated with the initial chemotherapy, salvage regimen or considered for high-dose chemotherapy with autologous transplantation.

Commonly used chemotherapy salvage regimens are listed in Table 52.4. If relapse occurs less than a year after treatment (early relapse), then high-dose chemotherapy with autologous stem cell support should be considered. A patient who has never achieved complete remission (primary refractory disease) should receive high-dose chemotherapy with autologous stem cell support.

Table 52.4 Salvage chemotherapy regimens effective in the treatment of lymphoma

Regimen	Dose and route	Frequency
DHAP		
Cisplatin	100 mg/m² i.v.	Days 1
Cytarabine	2000 mg/m² i.v. 12 hourly	Day 2
Dexamethasone	40 mg orally	Days 1–4
ESHAP		
Etoposide	40 mg/m² i.v.	Days 1–4
Methylprednisolone	500 mg/m² i.v.	Days 1–5
Cytarabine	2000 mg/m² i.v.	Day 1
Cisplatin	25 mg/m² i.v.	Days 1–4
ICE		
Ifosfamide	5000 mg/m² i.v.	Day 2
Carboplatin[a]	AUC 5 i.v.	Day 2
Etoposide	100 mg/m² i.v.	Days 1–3
IVE		
Epirubicin	50 mg/m² i.v.	Days 1
Etoposide	200 mg/m² i.v.	Days 1–3
Ifosfamide	3000 mg/m² i.v.	Days 1–3
IGEV		
Ifosfamide (+ Mesna)	2000 mg/m² i.v.	Days 1–4
Gemcitabine	800 mg/m² i.v.	Days 1 and 4
Vinorelbine	20 mg/m² i.v.	Day 1
Prednisolone	100 mg oral	Days 1–4

[a]Carboplatin dose (mg) = target AUC (mg/mL × min) × (GFR [mL/min] + 25). AUC, Area under the curve; GFR, glomerular filtration rate.

High-dose chemotherapy plus autologous stem cell support is associated with a 40–50% 5-year survival rate. However, the significant toxicity of autologous stem cell transplantation means that it should be reserved for patients in whom there is a clear increase in the chance of cure. Allogeneic transplant is an option in patients relapsing after autologous transplant (Brusamolino et al., 2009).

Brentuximab vedotin is licensed for the treatment of relapsed or refractory CD30+ HL where patients have had an autologous stem cell transplant (ASCT) or at least two prior therapies when ASCT or combination chemotherapy are not treatment options.

New agents

The programmed death 1 (PD-1) pathway serves as an immune checkpoint to dampen T-cell-mediated immune responses. Nivolumab, a monoclonal antibody, which blocks the PD1 protein receptor is an option for treating relapsed or refractory HL (NICE 2017).

Other novel agents under investigation include panobinostat, an oral histone deacetylase (HDAC) inhibitor, and everolimus, a mammalian target of rapamycin (mTOR) inhibitor. Studies are underway to evaluate combinations of novel agents including brentuximab vedotin (Stathis and Younes, 2015).

Non-Hodgkin's lymphoma

The NHLs are a heterogeneous group of lymphoid malignancies ranging from indolent, slow-growing tumours to aggressive, rapidly fatal disease. Paradoxically, the more aggressive NHLs are more susceptible to anticancer therapy. The incidence of NHL in the UK is 23.6 per 100,000 per year for males and 18.6 per 100,000 per year for females. NHL accounts for approximately 4% of all cancers in the UK (Cancer Research UK, 2016b). The disease is rare in subjects younger than 30 years, and the incidence steadily increases with increasing age; the median age at presentation is about 70 years.

Aetiology

The aetiology is unclear, although immunosuppression, for example, after organ transplantation, may predispose to the development of lymphoma. Viruses have been implicated in the pathogenesis of NHL. For example, Burkitt's lymphoma is one of the most common neoplasms to develop in HIV-related immunosuppressed patients; human T-lymphotropic virus type 1 (HTLV-1) is associated with a rare type of T-cell lymphoma, adult T-cell leukaemia/lymphoma (ATLL); and Epstein–Barr virus (EBV) is associated with post-transplant lymphoproliferative disorder (PTLD). Exposure to certain chemicals such as pesticides and solvents can increase the risk of developing NHL. There is an increased incidence of gastro-intestinal lymphomas in patients with inflammatory bowel disease and *Helicobacter pylori* infection.

Signs and symptoms

The most common presentation of NHL is painless lymphadenopathy, frequently in the neck area in the supraclavicular and cervical regions. The spread of disease is haematogenously (via the blood), so extranodal sites may be involved. Signs and symptoms of infection, anaemia or thrombocytopenia may be present in patients with bone marrow involvement. Hepatosplenomegaly may also be present. Patients may also present with any of the following symptoms: unexplained loss of weight, unexplained fever and drenching night sweats. These symptoms are described as B symptoms, and patients without these symptoms are classified as category A. B symptoms are more commonly seen in advanced or aggressive NHL but may be present in all stages and histological subtypes.

Laboratory findings

Laboratory examinations may reveal anaemia, a raised ESR and a raised serum LDH level. There may be a reduction in circulating immunoglobulins, and a monoclonal paraprotein may be seen in a small number of cases. The immune disruption caused by the disease may also result in an increased susceptibility to viral infection or autoimmune haemolytic anaemia or thrombocytopenia. Peripheral blood lymphocytosis (increased lymphocytes) with circulating malignant cells is common in low-grade and mantle cell lymphomas.

Histopathology and classification

There have been many attempts to classify the NHLs into histological categories that have clinical significance. Despite this, many problems and areas of confusion remain. Approximately 85% of NHLs are of B-cell origin, whereas 15% are of T-cell origin or are unclassifiable.

There are two classification systems in common use. The Working formulation, developed in 1982, divides the lymphomas into low, intermediate and high grade. The revised European–American lymphoma (REAL) classification system was developed in 1994 (Table 52.5) and then modified by WHO (Box 52.3)

Table 52.5	Clinical grade and frequency of lymphomas in the REAL classification (Smith et al., 2015)
Diagnosis	% of all cases
Indolent lymphomas	
Follicular lymphoma	22
Marginal zone B-cell, mucosa-associated lymphoid tissue	8
Chronic lymphocytic leukaemia/small lymphocytic lymphoma	7
Marginal zone B-cell nodal	2
Lymphoplasmacytic lymphoma	1
Aggressive lymphomas	
Diffuse large B-cell lymphoma	31
Mature (peripheral) T-cell lymphomas	8
Mantle cell lymphoma	7
Mediastinal large B-cell lymphoma	2
Anaplastic large cell lymphoma	2
Very aggressive lymphomas	
Burkitt's lymphoma	2
Precursor T-lymphoblastic	2
Other lymphomas	7

to further classify lymphomas (Harris et al., 1994; Swerdlow et al., 2008). The REAL/WHO classification incorporates some diagnoses not included in the Working formulation and is a list of lymphomas using morphology, immunophenotype, genotype, molecular and clinical behavior. It recognises the three major categories of lymphoid malignancies: B-cell neoplasms, T-cell/natural killer cell neoplasms and HL. However, in practice, the clinical behaviour of lymphomas informs the treatment strategies employed as these are based on the initial classification into indolent (low-grade) or aggressive (intermediate- and high-grade) NHL. A more biologically relevant classification of lymphoma is done using the WHO modification of the REAL classification together with immunological and molecular characteristics. This increases the diagnostic specificity and improves selection and targeting of therapy (Swerdlow et al., 2008).

Diagnosis

Diagnosis is based on a thorough history, physical examination, laboratory findings and investigation of a lymph node. A definitive diagnosis of NHL can only be made by biopsy of pathological lymph nodes or tumour tissue. An expert histopathologist may need to utilise techniques, such as immunocytochemistry (e.g. CD20) or flow cytometry or a combination of both, to obtain an accurate subclassification. Chromosomal abnormalities are of diagnostic importance. Most translocations involve genes associated with either proliferation (e.g. c-MYC) or apoptosis (e.g. BCL-2).

Investigations are also performed to accurately stage the disease and exclude other disease. Fluorodeoxglucose (FDG)-PET or CT scan of the chest, abdomen and pelvis is the standard for staging. A bone marrow aspirate and trephine are required to exclude leukaemia and will detect bone marrow involvement, which is more common than in HL. Lumbar punctures should be performed for patients at high risk of CNS involvement, for example, Burkitt's lymphoma.

Molecular subtypes

Progress in the knowledge of the molecular pathology of diffuse large B-cell lymphomas (DLBCL) has led to the identification of two molecular subtypes. Studies have shown that the activated B-cell-like (ABC) subtype has a worse prognosis than the germinal center B-cell-like (GCB) subtype. Up to now, patients with DLBCL have been managed in the same way. However, the identification of these subtypes has led to studies investigating whether patients with the ABC subtype benefit from receiving novel agents as part of their treatment (Tilley et al., 2015).

Staging

Determining the extent of disease in patients with NHL provides prognostic information and is useful in treatment planning. Patients with extensive disease usually require different therapy from those with limited disease. The NHLs can be staged according to the Ann Arbor classification (see Table 52.1). In this system, NHL is defined as stage I, II, III or IV, stage I being disease limited to a single lymph node and stage IV being advanced disease, with involvement of extralymphatic sites. The International Prognostic Index (IPI) (Table 52.6) uses the following factors as predictors of poor prognosis: elevated LDH, stage III or IV

Box 52.3	World Health Organization (WHO) modification of the Revised European–American lymphoma classification (REAL/WHO classification) (Swerdlow et al., 2008)

Precursor B-cell neoplasm
- Precursor B-cell acute lymphoblastic leukaemia or lymphoma

Mature (peripheral) B-cell neoplasm
- B-cell chronic lymphocytic leukaemia or small lymphocytic lymphoma
- B-cell prolymphocytic leukaemia
- Lymphoplasmacytic lymphoma
- Splenic marginal zone B-cell lymphoma (with or without villous lymphocytes)
- Hairy cell leukaemia
- Plasma cell myeloma or plasmacytoma
- Extranodal marginal zone B-cell lymphoma (with or without monocytoid B-cells)
- Follicular lymphoma
- Mantle cell lymphoma
- Diffuse large B-cell lymphoma
- Mediastinal large B-cell lymphoma
- Primary effusion lymphoma
- Burkitt's lymphoma or Burkitt cell leukaemia

Precursor T-cell neoplasm
- Precursor T-cell acute lymphoblastic leukaemia or lymphoma

Mature (peripheral) T-cell and natural killer neoplasms
- T-cell prolymphocytic leukaemia
- T-cell granular lymphocytic leukaemia
- Aggressive natural killer cell leukaemia
- Adult T-cell lymphoma or leukaemia
- Extranodal natural killer/T-cell lymphoma
- Enteropathy type T-cell lymphoma
- Hepatoplenic T-cell lymphoma
- Subcutaneous panniculitis-like T-cell lymphoma
- Mycosis fungoides/Sezary syndrome
- Primary cutaneous anaplastic large cell lymphoma
- Peripheral T-cell lymphoma
- Angio-immunoblastic T-cell lymphoma
- Primary systemic anaplastic large cell lymphoma

Table 52.6	International prognostic index for aggressive non-Hodgkin's lymphoma (International Non-Hodgkin's Lymphoma Prognostic Factors Project, 1993)

Factor	Adverse prognosis
Age	≥60 years
Ann Arbor stage	III or IV
Plasma lactate dehydrogenase level	Above normal
Number of extranodal sites of involvement	≥2
Performance status	≥ECOG 2 or equivalent

ECOG, Eastern Co-operative Oncology Group.

disease, greater than 60 years of age, the higher the number of extranodal sites involved and the Eastern Co-operative Oncology Group (ECOG) performance status of 2 or higher. Other prognostic factors include bulky disease, presence of B symptoms and transformation from low- to high-grade disease. Prognostic indicators are important because they inform the treatment plan to avoid over-treating those with good prognosis and under-treating those with poor prognosis.

Treatment

When designing a treatment plan for an individual patient, various factors must be taken into account. These include the patient's age and general health, the extent or stage of the lymphoma and the particular histological subtype. Indolent (low-grade) lymphoma tends to run a slow course, and although it is not curable, patients survive for prolonged periods with minimal symptoms. Aggressive (high-grade) lymphomas result in death within weeks or months if untreated. However, these lymphomas are very responsive to chemotherapy, and up to 50–60% may be cured with combination chemotherapy (Fig. 52.2).

CD20 is essential for cell cycle regulation and cell differentiation. It is expressed on normal B-cells and the majority of malignant B-cell lymphomas. The introduction of rituximab, a monoclonal antibody with specificity for CD20, has changed the way patients with NHL are treated and is now incorporated into most chemotherapy regimens. The mechanism of action of rituximab is not fully understood but is thought to involve complement-mediated lysis of B-cells and antibody-dependent cellular cytotoxicity. Other potential mechanisms include induction of apoptosis and inhibition of cell cycle progression.

Indolent non-Hodgkin's lymphoma

The median age at which patients present with indolent NHLs is 50–60 years, and generally patients have a good performance status. If left untreated, indolent NHL has a comparatively long survival (median: 9 years). Follicular lymphoma is the most common of the indolent lymphomas. Management is summarised in Fig. 52.3. The majority (80%) of patients present with advanced disease (stages II–IV) where the aim of treatment is to reduce disease bulk and offer symptom relief. Bendamustine and rituximab (BR) or the combination of rituximab, cyclophosphamide, vincristine, prednisolone (R-CVP) or R-CHOP (rituximab, cyclophosphamide, doxorubicin, vincristine, prednisolone) is used as the first-line treatment for advanced (stage III or IV) follicular lymphoma. After the response to first-line induction treatment, patients should go on to receive rituximab maintenance (one dose every 2 months) for 2 years.

For patients who are asymptomatic at diagnosis, adopting a policy of 'watch and wait' with active monitoring and initiating treatment when symptomatic is an option.

Relapsed indolent non-Hodgkin's lymphoma. Relapsed patients may be re-treated with rituximab and combination chemotherapy if the time to relapse post-rituximab is greater than 6 months. Assuming response, these patients should receive rituximab maintenance (a dose every 3 months) for 2 years. For some resistant or relapsing patients, particularly if their condition is too poor to merit further radical chemotherapy, palliation will be appropriate. Radiotherapy may be an option in this situation, and this is being evaluated through an ongoing clinical trial. Idelalisib, a small-molecule inhibitor of PI3K, may also have a role in managing patients who are refractory to two lines of treatment.

Aggressive non-Hodgkin's lymphoma

The median age of presentation of aggressive NHL is 60–70 years when 50–60% of patients will present with an advanced stage of the disease. The most common presentation is diffuse large B-cell lymphoma (DLBCL), and therefore the treatment strategies described later refer to this alone. Other aggressive lymphomas, for example, mantle cell, are managed differently. The most important strategy when treating this group of patients is to maintain the dose intensity of chemotherapy and minimise any delay in chemotherapy administration. Treatment is given with curative intent and is summarised in Fig. 52.4.

The treatment for DLBCL is six cycles of the combination of R-CHOP chemotherapy. Doxorubicin can cause cardiotoxicity, and patients with a reduced cardiac ejection fraction may not tolerate R-CHOP. In this situation, doxorubicin may be substituted by gemcitabine (R-GCVP). There is currently an ongoing clinical trial to establish if inotuzumab ozogamicin is an option for this group of patients. For patients with comorbidities or worse performance status, R-mini-CHOP (dose-attenuated R-CHOP) may be used. The addition of bortezomib to R-CHOP in DLBCL is being investigated as a clinical trial, to determine if bortezomib provides any benefit for the ABC or GBC subtypes.

Central nervous system prophylaxis. CNS relapse in patients with DLBCL occurs in approximately 5% of patients. Patients with high IPI, which includes involvement of more than one extranodal site and with an elevated LDH, appear to have a higher risk of CNS relapse. Prophylactic strategies include intrathecal methotrexate or systemic high-dose methotrexate, which are administered in addition to R-CHOP.

National guidance for the safe administration of intrathecal chemotherapy sets out the minimum requirements of a hospital providing an intrathecal chemotherapy service (Department of Health, 2008).

Relapsed aggressive non-Hodgkin's lymphoma. Combination chemotherapy with R-CHOP probably cures 60%. This, therefore, implies that greater than one-third of all patients have refractory disease or relapse after the first treatment.

In younger patients with aggressive NHL, the aim will be to introduce remission with further chemotherapy, using an alternative, salvage regimen, and then to consolidate remission with high-dose therapy (HDT). HDT is usually supported by mobilised peripheral blood stem cells (PBSCs) and an autologous PBSC transplantation (auto-PBSCT). HDT, with autologous stem cell support, is also used as part of primary treatment for younger patients with indolent lymphoma. Patients who receive

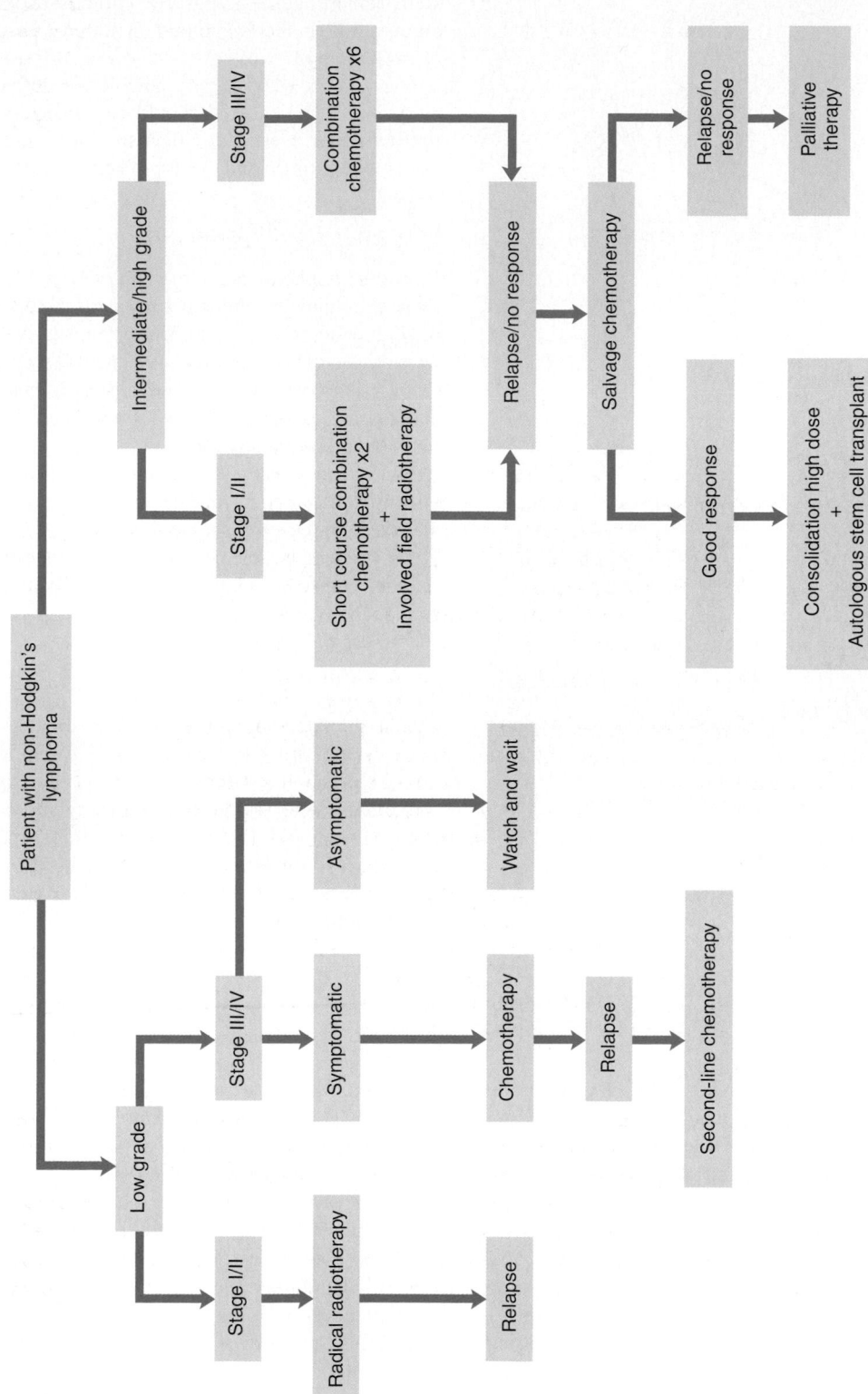

Fig. 52.2 Typical treatment algorithm for non-Hodgkin's lymphoma.

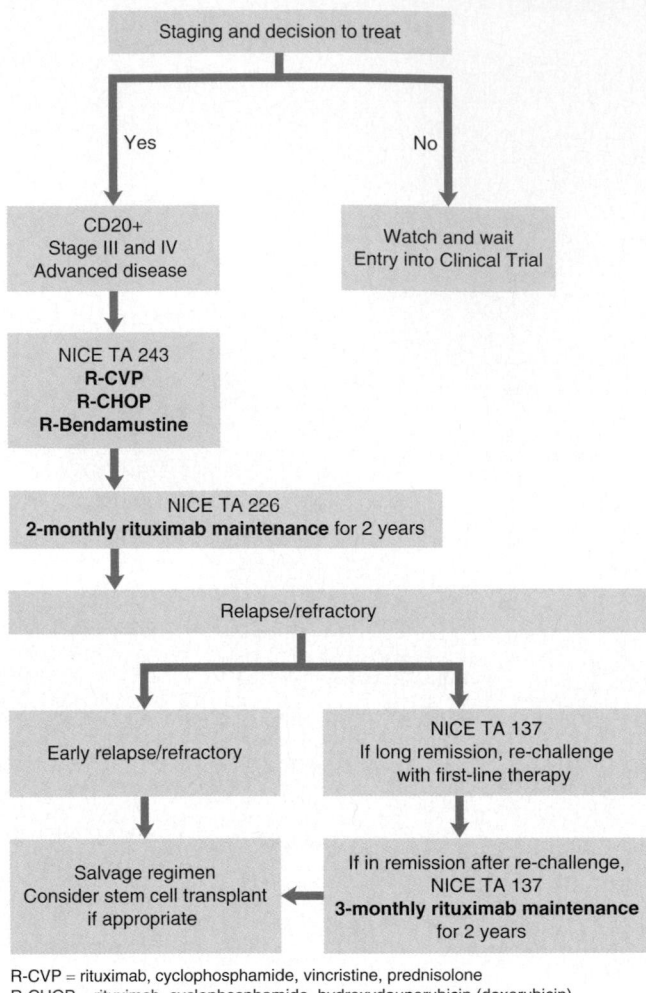

Fig. 52.3 Treatment algorithm for follicular lymphoma.

Within the figure:

Staging and decision to treat

Yes → No

CD20+
Stage III and IV
Advanced disease

Watch and wait
Entry into Clinical Trial

NICE TA 243
R-CVP
R-CHOP
R-Bendamustine

NICE TA 226
2-monthly rituximab maintenance for 2 years

Relapse/refractory

Early relapse/refractory

NICE TA 137
If long remission, re-challenge
with first-line therapy

Salvage regimen
Consider stem cell transplant
if appropriate

If in remission after re-challenge,
NICE TA 137
3-monthly rituximab maintenance
for 2 years

R-CVP = rituximab, cyclophosphamide, vincristine, prednisolone
R-CHOP = rituximab, cyclophosphamide, hydroxydaunorubicin (doxorubicin),
vincristine (Oncovin), prednisolone
R-Bendamustine = rituximab and bendamustine
NICE TA 243 – National Institute for Health and Clinical Excellence 2012
NICE TA 226 – National Institute for Health and Clinical Excellence 2011
NICE TA 137 – National Institute for Health and Clinical Excellence 2008

HDT after their initial treatment can have progression-free survival rates of around 50% at 5 years (Nournier et al., 2012; Philip et al., 1995; Sureda et al., 2015).

To induce a remission in patients with aggressive lymphoma and relapsed disease, it may be reasonable to use the same or a similar regimen as used for front-line chemotherapy. However, in most cases, the regimen chosen introduces new agents that are potentially not cross-resistant with those used in the initial treatment regimen. There are several salvage regimens in use, and they generally have response rates of between 40% and 70%. Examples of salvage regimens are ICE (ifosfamide, carboplatin, etoposide), ESHAP (etoposide, methylprednisolone, cytarabine, cisplatin) and DHAP (cisplatin, cytarabine, dexamethasone) (see Table 52.4). Gemcitabine, a pyrimidine analogue, may be of benefit for patients with relapsed or refractory disease after two lines of treatment. Gemcitabine is used in combination with other agents, such as cisplatin and methylprednisolone. Rituximab can also be added to these salvage regimens. PBSCs are usually harvested after the

second course of the salvage regimen. Patients then receive a high-dose regimen such as BEAM (carmustine, etoposide, cytarabine, melphalan) (Table 52.7) conditioning before stem cell infusion (autograft). Patients should only undergo an autograft if they have demonstrated a response to salvage chemotherapy.

For patients who are not suitable for autologous transplant, entry into a clinical trial should be considered. There are currently studies investigating the use of lenalidomide in combination with rituximab and the use of selinexor.

Very aggressive lymphoma

Burkitt's lymphoma is a rare form of B-cell NHL which occurs most commonly in children and young adults. The median age of adult patients is 30 years. Untreated, survival is measurable in days or weeks, and it is widely accepted that combination chemotherapy should be urgently commenced. Intensive chemotherapy is necessary, together with CNS prophylaxis, and cure is possible in a high proportion of cases.

Multi-agent chemotherapy regimens including high-dose methotrexate, high-dose cytarabine, etoposide and ifosfamide are used. A schedule such as CODOX-M (cyclophosphamide, vincristine, doxorubicin, high-dose methotrexate)/IVAC (ifosfamide, etoposide, high-dose cytarabine) in combination with rituximab is common.

Lymphoblastic lymphomas/leukaemia

Lymphoblastic lymphomas comprise about 2% of adult NHLs. Patients are often treated with the same regimens used in acute lymphoblastic leukaemia (ALL). Despite a very high rate of complete responders, long-term survival remains poor. Patients who fail after first-line chemotherapy have a long-term disease-free survival of less than 10% (Fielding et al., 2007). These cases are subsequently treated as leukaemias (see Chapter 51).

Patient care

The chemotherapy regimens used to treat HL and NHL (see Tables 52.3 and 52.8) are usually administered on a hospital outpatient basis with the patient visiting the clinic regularly for assessment and treatment. The patient is monitored by FBCs carried out before each cycle of chemotherapy and at the 'nadir' between cycles. The nadir is when the blood count is at its lowest point, usually 10–14 days after the first day of chemotherapy. The interval between each cycle of chemotherapy enables normal body cells to recover before the patient receives further treatment. Disease response to treatment is monitored by repeating some of the diagnostic investigations, such as CT, at suitable intervals and the use of PET. If there is little or no response to treatment, a different chemotherapy regimen will be used, or a decision will be made to withdraw from active therapy and provide optimum supportive care.

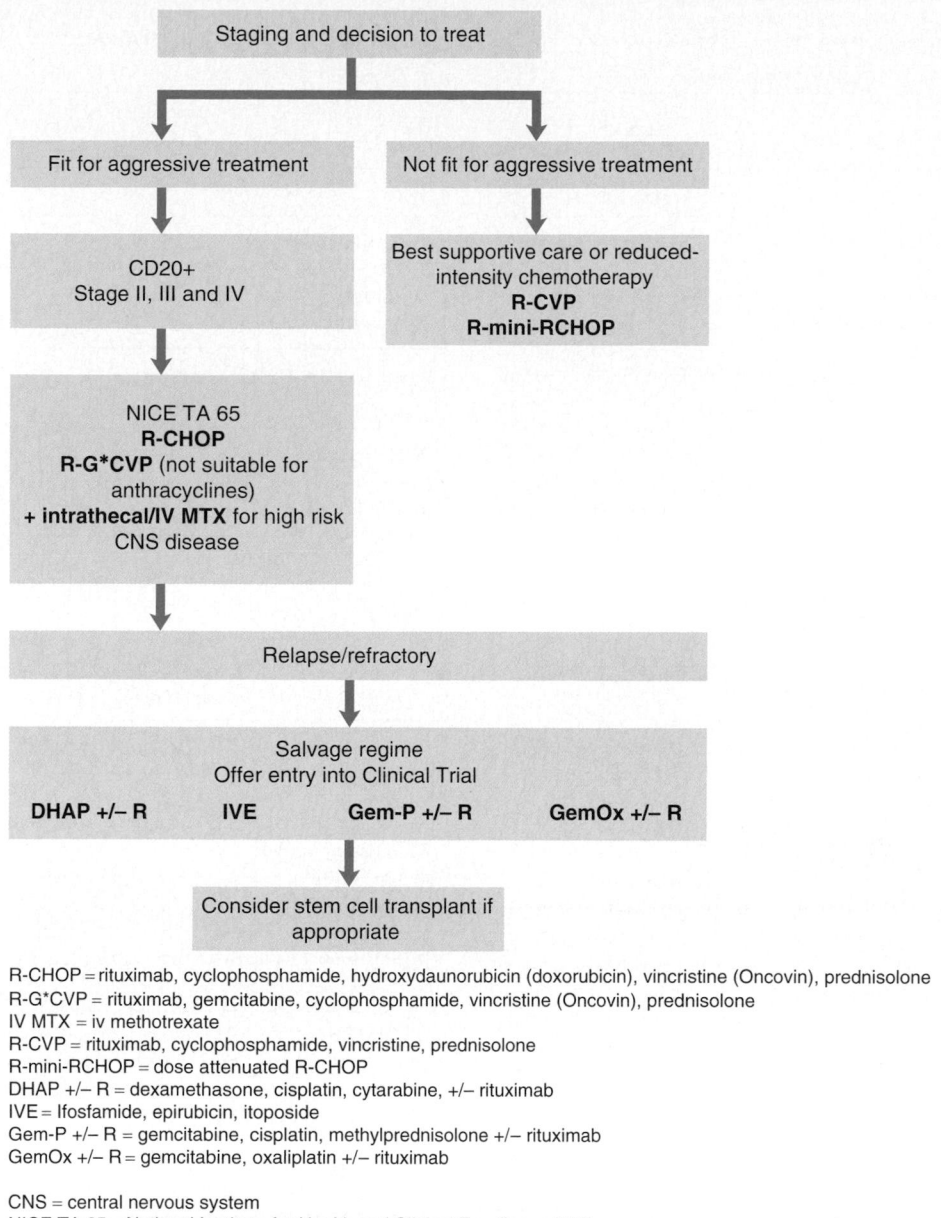

R-CHOP = rituximab, cyclophosphamide, hydroxydaunorubicin (doxorubicin), vincristine (Oncovin), prednisolone
R-G*CVP = rituximab, gemcitabine, cyclophosphamide, vincristine (Oncovin), prednisolone
IV MTX = iv methotrexate
R-CVP = rituximab, cyclophosphamide, vincristine, prednisolone
R-mini-RCHOP = dose attenuated R-CHOP
DHAP +/– R = dexamethasone, cisplatin, cytarabine, +/– rituximab
IVE = Ifosfamide, epirubicin, itoposide
Gem-P +/– R = gemcitabine, cisplatin, methylprednisolone +/– rituximab
GemOx +/– R = gemcitabine, oxaliplatin +/– rituximab

CNS = central nervous system
NICE TA 65 = National Institute for Health and Clinical Excellence 2003

Fig. 52.4 Treatment algorithm diffuse large B-cell lymphoma.

Counselling and support

Counselling is an essential part of the care of the cancer patient and involves not only the explanation of drug therapy and investigations but also the provision of psychological support for the patient and family. Before treatment with chemotherapy, the patient will be counselled by the doctor, chemotherapy nurse and, increasingly, oncology pharmacists and pharmacy technicians. It is necessary to explain how the chemotherapy is to be given and discuss both potential and inevitable side effects. The probability of successful treatment must be weighed against the prospect of serious and life-threatening adverse effects. Patients must be made aware of the long-term complications of chemotherapy and radiotherapy, such as secondary malignancy. If appropriate, patients should discuss options for fertility preservation.

The support available to the cancer patient, to help cope with both the illness and its treatment, has improved dramatically in recent years. Multidisciplinary teams working within specialised units have become skilled in anticipating the problems of lymphomas and their treatment. In addition, many charities provide care, support and advice, such as Macmillan Cancer Support (http://www.macmillan.org.uk) and the Lymphoma Association (http://www.lymphoma.org.uk).

Patient-specific treatment modifications

The selection of appropriate therapy must also take into consideration the individual patient. Factors include the patient's age, renal and hepatic function and underlying medical conditions,

Table 52.7 Conditioning chemotherapy for autologous transplantation

Drug	Dose and route	Day of administration
BEAM		
Carmustine	300 mg/m² i.v.	6 days before reinfusion
Etoposide	200 mg/m² i.v.	5–2 days before reinfusion
Cytarabine	200 mg/m² 12 h i.v.	5–2 days before reinfusion
Melphalan	140 mg/m² i.v.	1 day before reinfusion
Reinfusion of stem cells		Day 0
LACE		
Lomustine	200 mg/m² orally	7 days before reinfusion
Etoposide	1000 mg/m² i.v.	7 days before reinfusion
Cytarabine	2000 mg/m²	6–5 days before reinfusion
Cyclophosphamide	1800 mg/m² i.v.	4–2 days before reinfusion
Reinfusion of stem cells		Day 0

Table 52.8 Chemotherapy regimens effective in the treatment of non-Hodgkin's lymphoma

Drug	Dose and route	Day of administration
R-CHOP (21-day cycle)		
Cyclophosphamide	750 mg/m² i.v.	Day 1
Doxorubicin (hydroxydaunorubicin)	50 mg/m² i.v.	Day 1
Vincristine (Oncovin)	1.4 mg/m² (max 2 mg) i.v.	Day 1
Prednisolone	100 mg orally	Days 1–5
Rituximab	375 mg/m² i.v.	Day 1
R-CVP (21-day cycle)		
Cyclophosphamide	750 mg/m² i.v.	Day 1
Vincristine (Oncovin)	1.4 mg/m² (max 2 mg) i.v.	Day 1
Prednisolone	100 mg orally	Days 1–5
Rituximab	375 mg/m² i.v.	Day 1
FC (28-day cycle)		
Fludarabine	40 mg/m² orally	Days 1–3
Cyclophosphamide	250 mg/m² daily orally	Days 1–3
CHOP (21-day cycle)		
Cyclophosphamide	750 mg/m² i.v.	Day 1
Doxorubicin (hydroxydaunorubicin)	50 mg/m² i.v.	Day 1
Vincristine (Oncovin)	1.4 mg/m² (max 2 mg) i.v.	Day 1
Prednisolone	100 mg orally	Days 1–5
BR (28-day cycle)		
Bendamustine	90 mg/m² i.v.	Days 1–2
Rituximab	375 mg/m² i.v.	Day 1

such as heart disease, diabetes or chronic pulmonary disease. The patient's tolerance of side effects and complications of therapy may then be predicted. The decision is based on an understanding of the pharmacodynamics and pharmacokinetics of the drugs being used, as well as the clinical condition of the patient.

Supportive care

During a course of chemotherapy, the patient requires supportive care to minimise the adverse effects of treatment. The common adverse effects of the chemotherapy regimens discussed in this chapter are outlined in Table 52.9. These will occur to varying degrees depending on the combination of drugs and the doses used, as well as individual patient factors. Practice points to support patient care are described in Box 52.4.

Nausea and vomiting

Nausea and vomiting is the most distressing and most feared adverse effect of chemotherapy. Its effect on the patient should not be underestimated, and its treatment is an important part of supportive care. The severity will depend on the combination of

drugs used. For example, oral chlorambucil is generally well tolerated by almost all patients and requires no antiemetic cover. Regimens such as ABVD, which is highly emetic, will make most patients vomit if no antiemetics are given. Aprepitant, an NK1 receptor antagonist, is licensed for cisplatin chemotherapy regimens and may be useful for managing emesis with DHAP, ESHAP and other regimens. The patient should be counselled on the appropriate use of prescribed antiemetics (see Table 52.9).

Table 52.9 Adverse effects associated with chemotherapy regimens used in the lymphomas with supportive measures and counselling points

Adverse effect	Cytotoxics implicated	Supportive measures	Counselling points
Bone marrow suppression	Chlorambucil Cyclophosphamide Dacarbazine Etoposide Doxorubicin Vinblastine Fludarabine	Blood transfusion Platelet transfusions Mouth care Granulocyte-colony stimulating factor Antibiotic therapy for febrile episodes	Expect tiredness Report bleeding or unusual bruises Adhere to mouth care regimen Avoid people with infections Importance of good personal hygiene Monitor temperature Report febrile episodes or signs of infection immediately
Nausea and vomiting	Doxorubicin Dacarbazine Procarbazine Cyclophosphamide	Antiemetic therapy	Emphasise regular use; a short course is more effective than 'as-required' treatment Report episodes of vomiting (especially if taking oral cytotoxics) For dexamethasone, emphasise short course not to be continued to ensure the patient does not receive repeat prescriptions from primary care doctor Take tablets before meals
Mucositis	Doxorubicin	Mouth care regimen	Importance of good oral hygiene; stress importance of regular mouth care
Tumour lysis syndrome	All cytotoxic drugs and corticosteroids in patients with a high tumour load sensitive to chemotherapy	Hydration, allopurinol, rasburicase	Stress importance of regular allopurinol until appropriate to stop Drink plenty of fluids
Alopecia	Cyclophosphamide Doxorubicin, etoposide	Provision of wig if wanted	Hair usually regrows on completion of therapy
Impaired gonadal function	Alkylating agents Procarbazine, doxorubicin (to a lesser degree)	Sperm storage	Depends on regimen Should be discussed as part of consent to treatment
Neuropathy	Vincristine Vinblastine, Vinorelbine	Reduce dose if continued use of vincristine Because vincristine is more neurotoxic than vinblastine, consider substituting with vinblastine as an alternative to dose reduction	Report tingling sensations or difficulty with buttons, constipation, jaw pain or stiffness
Constipation	Vincristine, bortezomib		Do not self-treat but refer to doctor
Cardiomyopathy	Doxorubicin		Report breathlessness, tiredness
Lung fibrosis	Bleomycin		Report breathlessness

Tumour lysis syndrome

The lymphomas are, in general, highly sensitive to chemotherapy. The resulting lysis of cells which occurs after initiation of chemotherapy may lead to hyperuricaemia, hyperkalaemia and hypocalcaemia in patients with bulky disease and may result in urate nephropathy. There is a high incidence of tumour lysis syndrome (TLS) in tumours with high proliferation rates and tumour burden such as Burkitt's lymphoma and T-lymphoblastic lymphoma. The mainstay of TLS prevention is hydration, with the patient encouraged to maintain a high fluid intake. Hyperuricaemia is controlled with allopurinol and close monitoring of renal function, serum urate levels and electrolytes. Fig. 52.5 describes the purine catabolism pathway and explains the action of allopurinol and rasburicase. Allopurinol must be commenced before chemotherapy and continued until the tumour load has reduced and serum urate levels are normal. In aggressive forms of NHL, rasburicase, a recombinant urate oxidase, may be indicated as prophylaxis.

Rasburicase can also be used to treat TLS but will only correct hyperuricaemia. Treatment of TLS should include hydration at approximately 3 L/m² per day unless the patient has renal insufficiency or oliguria (Cairo et al., 2010). Hypocalcaemia should be corrected if the patient is symptomatic, but this may increase calcium phosphate deposition. Hyperkalaemia and hyperphosphataemia should be corrected; patients may require haemofiltration or dialysis.

Mucositis

Chemotherapy may cause mucositis, which is inflammation of or damage to the surface of the gastro-intestinal tract. In the mouth, this may lead to painful ulceration, local infection and difficulty in swallowing. Dependent on the severity of mucositis, patients may require analgesia ranging from benzydamine mouthwash to systemic opiates. Disruption of the mucosal barrier will give bacteria and fungi easier systemic access. A mouth care regimen should therefore be instituted with myelosuppressive therapy. This involves good oral

---

Box 52.4 Practice points

Neutropenic sepsis
- The usual inflammatory signs of infection (redness, pain, swelling) are often absent due to a lack of neutrophils, and not all patients will present with a fever. Consider neutropenic sepsis in any patient who has received chemotherapy in the past 30 days.
- Neutropenic sepsis is a medical emergency; broad-spectrum antibiotics should be administered within 1 h of presentation. Do not wait for a full blood count to confirm neutropenia.

HL treatment
- Patients with HL should receive irradiated blood products for life.
- HL patients receiving bleomycin should be assessed carefully for signs and symptoms of pulmonary toxicity before each dose.

Tumour lysis syndrome
- Allopurinol should not be prescribed concurrently with rasburicase because it inhibits the production of uric acid, the substrate for rasburicase (see Fig. 52.5).
- Prednisolone and other steroids used to treat lymphoma can also cause tumour lysis syndrome. At-risk patients should receive a hypouricaemic agent before the first dose.
- When treating tumour lysis syndrome, potassium must not be added to the hydration fluid.

HL, Hodgkin's lymphoma.

---

hygiene, for example, gentle brushing with a toothbrush to remove plaque or rinsing with saline to remove debris.

Bone marrow suppression

Myelosuppression is usually the dose-limiting factor with these regimens, and it is necessary to carry out FBCs before treatment to confirm that recovery has occurred. Each chemotherapy protocol should be referred to so as to ensure appropriate management. Generally, if the platelet count is less than $100 \times 10^9/L$ and/or the absolute neutrophil count (ANC) is less than $1 \times 10^9/L$, the subsequent dose may be reduced or treatment delayed by a week.

Anaemia is treated with blood transfusions and thrombocytopenia with platelet transfusions as necessary. Erythropoietin administration reduces blood transfusion requirements and can improve quality of life. However, the evidence suggesting improvement in patient survival is inconclusive.

Neutropenia is the most life-threatening acute toxicity; the neutropenic patient is at constant risk from infections. Seemingly minor infections such as cold sores can spread rapidly, and infections not seen in the normal population (e.g. systemic fungal infections) can occur. Supportive measures involve reducing the risks and the aggressive treatment of any infectious episodes. The patient is counselled to avoid contact with people with infection or those who may be carriers. Most infections, however, are from an endogenous source such as the gut or skin. The patient is educated on the importance of good personal hygiene, mouth care, how to monitor body temperature and to report any febrile episodes immediately. Co-trimoxazole 960 mg once daily may be prescribed as prophylaxis against *Pneumocystis* pneumonia in patients receiving chemotherapy for lymphomas, particularly in those receiving a regimen containing fludarabine or bendamustine. Thorough and frequent handwashing helps prevent the transmission of opportunistic infection to the neutropenic patient.

Neutropenic sepsis

Neutropenic sepsis should be managed as a medical emergency. Susceptibility to infection is likely when the neutrophil count is less than $1 \times 10^9/L$, with increasing risk at levels less than

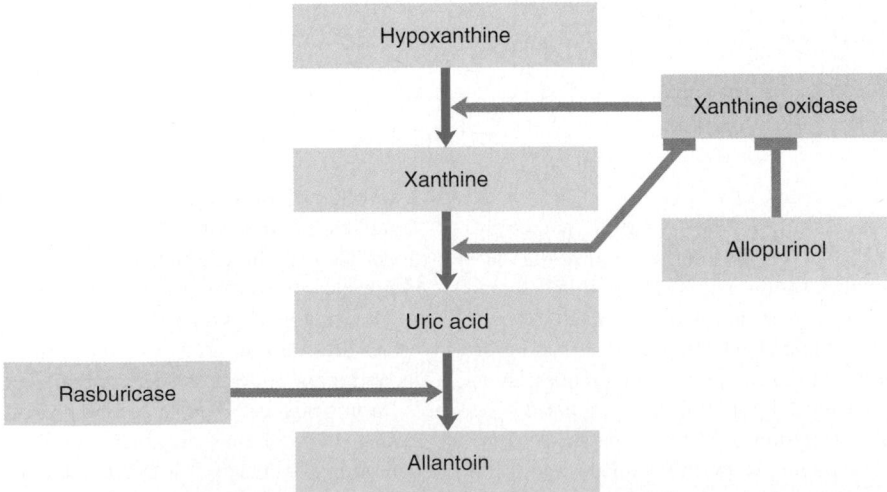

Fig. 52.5 Purine catabolism pathway.

0.5×10^9/L and 0.01×10^9/L. Risk of infection also increases with duration of neutropenia. Fever, usually defined as a temperature greater than 38 °C, may be the only sign of infection. The patient should be assessed to determine the site of infection. Blood cultures from all venous access ports and any other appropriate cultures, for example, midstream urine sample and stool sample, should be taken. Cultures are taken before starting antibiotics to increase the likelihood of obtaining a positive culture. Infection with Gram-negative bacilli, for example, *Escherichia coli*, *Klebsiella pneumoniae* and *Pseudomonas aeruginosa*, and Gram-positive cocci, for example, coagulase-negative staphylococci, β-haemolytic streptococci, enterococci and *Staphylococcus aureus*, is probable in this situation. First-line empiric therapy should cover these common pathogens. Options include carbapenems, a third-generation cephalosporin or antipseudomonal penicillin with or without an aminoglycoside.

Gram-positive infections are becoming more common with the use of indwelling intravenous catheters. If positive microbiological cultures are found, the appropriate antibiotic can be prescribed on the basis of sensitivities; however, if the patient is responding to empiric therapy, the antibiotics should not be changed. Only one-third of suspected infections are ever confirmed, and the pathogen may not be isolated. The febrile episode may not be due to infection; non-infectious causes include blood transfusion, drug administration and underlying disease.

Growth factor support

Patients with persistent neutropenia or those who have repeated admissions for neutropenic sepsis may be supported with granulocyte-colony-stimulating factor (GCSF). There is evidence that patients with lymphomas receiving a reduced dose of chemotherapy as a consequence of myelosuppression have a worse prognosis compared with patients who receive full doses. GCSF is indicated as primary prophylaxis, before any episode of febrile neutropenia, for regimens in which there is a high (>40%) incidence of febrile neutropenia. GCSF has been investigated as a prophylactic measure to increase the dose intensity of chemotherapy in regimens such as CHOP-14 (cyclophosphamide, hydroxydaunorubicin [doxorubicin], vincristine [Oncovin], prednisolone at 14-day intervals).

Case studies

Case 52.1

Mr RB is a 50-year-old man receiving bendamustine and rituximab for follicular lymphoma. He has no other medical problems and has normal renal and hepatic function.

Questions

1. What are the key counselling points for patients receiving bendamustine?
2. What antibacterial agent would you expect to see prescribed with bendamustine?

Answers

1. Immunocompromised patients, for example, those receiving purine analogues, fludarabine, cladribine, pentostatin, and alkylating agents such as bendamustine, are at risk of developing transfusion-associated graft versus host disease (TAGVHD), a rare but usually fatal complication of transfusion. Viable T-lymphocytes in donated blood can recognise the recipient as 'foreign', leading to fever, skin rash, hepatitis and bone marrow involvement. Death occurs in 90% of cases, predominantly due to infection (Kopolovic et al., 2015).

   γ-Irradiation of cellular blood components is the mainstay of TAGVHD prevention. Patients, such as Mr RB, should be given an appropriate patient information leaflet and an alert card. The risk of TAGVHD is minimised by informing transfusion staff and the patient of their need for irradiated blood products.
2. Mr RB should be prescribed co-trimoxazole prophylactically, to prevent *P. carinii* (previously *P. jiroveci*) infection.

Case 52.2

Mrs BC is a 72-year-old widow who has been newly diagnosed with advanced HL. She has been seen in the haematology clinic before starting VEPEMB chemotherapy. She has brought a prescription to the pharmacy for prednisolone, procarbazine, etoposide, and supportive medications. When Mrs BC hands in her prescription, she expresses concern about the side effects of the tablets. The doctor who saw her had spent a lot of time talking to her about her treatment, but she feels confused with all the information given.

Questions

1. What are the side effects of prednisolone, procarbazine and etoposide?
2. How would you counsel Mrs BC?

Answers

1. Prednisolone-related side effects include mood changes, difficulty sleeping, increased appetite, stomach irritation, immunosuppression and hyperglycaemia. Side effects are less common with short courses, but Mrs BC will be taking a moderately high dose (30 mg/m^2 per day).

   The most common side effects of procarbazine are nausea, vomiting and myelosuppression. As procarbazine is a weak monoamine oxidase inhibitor that crosses the blood–brain barrier rapidly, patients can uncommonly suffer with drowsiness, confusion, pins and needles or nightmares.

   Etoposide is associated with dose-limiting myelosuppression which is dose-related. It can cause a sore mouth and hair loss.

   Mrs BC is an elderly patient and is thus more likely to experience toxicity because of deteriorating renal and hepatic function and underlying medical conditions.

   Usually, an H$_2$ antagonist or proton pump inhibitor, 5HT3 antiemetic and anti-infectives (which may include aciclovir, fluconazole, co-trimoxazole and a quinolone) will be prescribed to counteract these side effects.
2. Mrs BC may be distressed by her diagnosis and may not have been able to absorb all the information she was given in the clinic. In addition, VEPEMB is a complicated regimen, and she may also be seeking confirmation of information. Mrs BC should have been allocated a specialist nurse or key worker who will be able to give her ongoing support.

She should be told that she will probably feel tired and be more prone to infection because the tablets lower the blood count and resistance to infection. She should be advised to inform the haematologist or her specialist nurse if she feels unwell.

Other counselling points include the following:

- Complete the course of tablets as prescribed.
- Procarbazine should be swallowed whole with water.
- Avoid drinking alcohol while taking procarbazine (risk of disulfiram-type reaction).
- Etoposide should be swallowed whole on an empty stomach or an hour before food.

Mrs BC should be advised to take her prednisolone with breakfast in the morning to reduce gastric side effects.

Case 52.3

Mr FP is 56-years-old and was diagnosed with stage III high-grade NHL (DLBCL) over 10 weeks ago. Since then, he has received three cycles of R-CHOP and has come to the hospital for his nadir blood count. He complains of painful mouth ulcers and a sore throat. On examination, he has mucositis and oropharyngeal candidiasis. He has a white blood cell count (WCC) of 3.2 (normal range: 3.5–11 × 10^9/L) with an ANC of 0.8 × 10^9/L.

Questions

1. How would you treat Mr FP's candida infection?
2. What advice would you give Mr FP?

Answers

1. Mr FP has an ANC of 0.8 × 10^9/L and is therefore neutropenic (ANC <1.0 × 10^9/L). Localised candida infections can spread rapidly in the immunosuppressed patient, so local therapy with an antifungal mouthwash will be inadequate therapy. A course of fluconazole, 100 mg daily for at least 7 days, should be prescribed. Therapy should continue for a further 7 days if Mr FP is still neutropenic or if the thrush has not completely resolved. Because Mr F is complaining of pain, an analgesic should be added. Benzydamine mouthwash, a locally acting analgesic, could be prescribed initially. If this does not give adequate pain relief, then systemic analgesics should be given.
2. Regular mouth care reduces the risk of infection but does not entirely remove it. It is not necessarily a reflection of how well Mr FP has adhered to his mouth care regimen. The benzydamine mouthwash should be used before meals because Mr FP will probably find eating painful. He should be advised to use a soft toothbrush, to eat soft foods and to avoid hot and spicy dishes. Mr FP may be reassured that once his blood count recovers, his mouth ulcers should resolve and that the fluconazole should relieve his sore throat.

Case 52.4

Mr DG, 38-year-old with advanced HL, is admitted to the haematology ward at the local hospital as an emergency. He had a temperature of 39 °C on the morning of admission and feels generally unwell but has no specific symptoms. It has been 10 days since Mr DG started his second cycle of ABVD.

Blood cultures are taken and piperacillin + tazobactam 4.5 g i.v. three times daily and gentamicin 420 mg i.v. once daily are prescribed, to be commenced immediately. Mr DG weighs 84 kg and is 186 cm tall. His blood biochemistry results are normal; his FBC is as follows:

	Value	Reference range
Haemoglobin	108 g/L	(13.5–18.0 g/dL for men)
White cell count	2.5 × 10^9/L	(3.5–11 × 10^9/L)
Neutrophil count	0.5 × 10^9/L	(1.5–7.5 × 10^9/L)
Platelets	150 × 10^9/L	(150–400 × 10^9/L)

Questions

1. Comment on the rationale for the antibiotic therapy prescribed.
2. How would you monitor this patient?
3. What would be an appropriate second-line regimen if Mr DG remains pyrexial?
4. What modifications would need to be made to subsequent cycles of chemotherapy?

Answers

1. Mr DG's FBC is probably at its nadir after his last course of chemotherapy. He is neutropenic and febrile. Immunosuppression is also a feature of HL and contributes to his susceptibility to infection. Treatment should commence immediately after cultures have been taken because infection can be rapidly fatal in these patients. The antibiotics selected should provide broad-spectrum cover and follow local policy because there are institutional variations in predominant pathogens and antimicrobial sensitivities. Because Gram-negative infections are more rapidly fatal, first-line therapy should be biased towards these infections. Monotherapy with an antipseudomonal agent (e.g. piperacillin+ tazobactam) is sufficient in most cases of uncomplicated neutropenic sepsis. The addition of gentamicin to Mr DG's therapy may be warranted based on local microbial resistance, prior infection history or evidence of severe sepsis (e.g. hypotension). The dose of piperacillin + tazobactam is appropriate. Single-daily-dose gentamicin is at least as effective as multiple dosing and less nephrotoxic; it is more convenient and cost-effective and overcomes deficiencies of the traditional method such as subtherapeutic dosing and inadequate monitoring. The dose is 5–7 mg/kg once daily and has been calculated correctly for Mr DG. He has normal renal function, so no dose modifications are necessary.
2. Monitor Mr DG's temperature, pulse and blood pressure and any symptoms for signs of improvement or deterioration. Blood biochemistry should be checked daily to detect any deterioration in renal function. Microbiology reports should be checked and antibiotics reviewed if any micro-organisms have been cultured. However, no change should be made to antibiotics if Mr DG shows signs of improvement. The administration of gentamicin should be monitored, checking both administration and sampling time for drug levels.
3. If Mr DG remains pyrexial 24–48 hours after the first-line antibiotics have been commenced, but he is clinically stable, empiric antibiotics should not be modified. Consideration should be given to broadening cover, for example, adding vancomycin if the patient has mucositis or evidence of line infection. If blood cultures show growth, found in only 30–40% of neutropenic patients, the choice of antibiotics should be on the basis of sensitivities. Clinical improvement is often seen with the recovery of neutrophil count. Mr DG should recover by day 14, but neutrophil recovery may be delayed by this infection. If Mr DG is still pyrexial at 96 hours, then the likelihood of fungal infection must be considered and an intravenous amphotericin-based product or caspofungin commenced if appropriate.
4. Because Mr DG is being treated with curative intent, it is appropriate to give GCSF and maintain the dose intensity of his chemotherapy.

Case 52.5

Mr RT is 26-year-old man with Burkitt's lymphoma. Mr RT is due to start chemotherapy with rituximab + CODOX-M. His LDH is 960 U/L (normal range 240–480 U/L), and his eGFR is greater than 90 mL/min (normal value ≥90 mL/min per 1.73 m²).

....

Questions

1. Which complications is Mr RT at risk of?
2. How would you treat Mr RT?

....

Answers

1. Mr RT is at high risk of developing tumour lysis syndrome because he has a diagnosis of Burkitt's lymphoma. In addition, his LDH is two times greater than the upper limit of normal.

2. Mr RT should receive prophylactic rasburicase along with appropriate hydration. Hydration should be given at approximately 3 L/m² per day because Mr RT does not have renal insufficiency or oliguria (Cairo et al., 2010). His urine output should be maintained at greater than 100 mL/m² per hour.

   The licensed dose of rasburicase is 0.2 mg/kg for up to 7 days, but a single dose repeated only if clinically necessary has been recommended by a panel of experts (Cairo et al., 2010). Rasburicase metabolises uric acid to allantoin, which is more easily excreted. Allopurinol should not be administered concurrently because this may reduce the efficacy of rasburicase; allopurinol inhibits the production of uric acid, the substrate for rasburicase (see Fig. 52.5).

   Mr RT's urate should be measured daily. The sample must be sent to the laboratory on ice to prevent false assay results because rasburicase will otherwise continue to metabolise the uric acid in the sample tube. His serum creatinine, potassium, calcium, phosphate and uric acid should be checked at baseline and repeated as clinically indicated.

References

Ansell, S.M., Younes, A., Connors, J.M., et al., 2014. Phase 3 study of brentuximab vedotin plus doxorubicin, vinblastine, and dacarbazine (A+AVD) versus doxorubicin, bleomycin, vinblastine, and dacarbazine (ABVD) as front-line treatment for advanced classical Hodgkin lymphoma (HL): Echelon-1 study. J. Clin. Oncol. 32, 5s.

Borchmann, P., Georgen, H., Kobe, C., et al., 2018. PET-guided treatment in patients with advanced-stage Hodgkin's lymphoma (HD18): final results of an open-label, international, randomised phase 3 trial by the German Hodgkin Study Group. The Lancet 390, 2790–2802.

Brusamolino, E., Bacigalupo, A., Barosi, G., et al., 2009. Classical Hodgkin's lymphoma in adults: guidelines of the Italian Society of Hematology, the Italian Society of Experimental Hematology, and the Italian Group for Bone Marrow Transplantation on initial work-up, management, and follow-up. Haematologica 94 (4), 550–565.

Cairo, M.S., Coiffier, B., Reiter, A., et al., 2010. Recommendations for the evaluation of risk and prophylaxis of tumour lysis syndrome (TLS) in adults and children with malignant dis-eases: an expert TLS panel consensus. Br. J. Haematol. 149, 578–586.

Cancer Research UK, 2016a. Hodgkin lymphoma incidence. Available at: http://www.cancerresearchuk.org/health-professional/hodgkin-lymphoma-statistics#heading-Zero.

Cancer Research UK, 2016b. Non-Hodgkin lymphoma incidence statistics. Available at: http://www.cancerresearchuk.org/health-professional/cancer-statisics/statisitics-by-cancer-type/non-hodgkin-lymphoma/incidence#heading-Zero.

Department of Health, 2008. HSC 2008/001: Updated national guidance on the safe administration of intrathecal chemotherapy. Department of Health, London. Available at: http://www.dh.gov.uk/en/Publicationsand statistics/Lettersandcirculars/Healthservicecirculars/DH_086870.

Eichenauer, D.A., Engert, A., André, M., et al., 2014. Hodgkin's lymphoma: ESMO Clinical Practice Guideline. Ann. Oncol. 25 (Suppl. 3), iii70–iii75. Available at: http://www.esmo.org/guidelines/haematological-malignancies/hodgkin-s-lymphoma.

Fielding, A.K., et al., 2007. Outcome of 609 adults after relapse of acute lymphoblastic leukaemia (ALL); an MRC UKALL12/ECOG 2993 study. Blood 109 (3), 944–950.

Follows, G., Ardeshna, K.M., Barrington, S.F., et al., 2014. Guidelines for the first line management of classical Hodgkin lymphoma. Br. J. Haematol. 166, 24–49.

Harris, N.L., Jaffe, E.S., Stein, H., et al., 1994. A revised European-American classification of lymphoid neoplasms: a proposal from the International Lymphoma Study Group. Blood 84, 1361–1392.

Hasenclever, D., Diehl, V., 1998. A prognostic score for advanced Hodgkin's disease. International prognostic factors project on advanced Hodgkin's disease. New Engl. J. Med. 339, 1506–1514.

International Non-Hodgkin's Lymphoma Prognostic Factors Project, 1993. International prognostic index for aggressive non-Hodgkin's lymphoma. New Engl. J. Med. 329, 987–994.

Johnson, P.W., Federico, M., Fossa, A., et al., 2016. Adapted treatment guided by interim PET-CT Scan in advanced Hodgkin's lymphoma. New Engl. J. Med. 370, 2419–2429.

Kopolovic, I., Ostro, J., Tsubota, H., et al., 2015. A systematic review of transfusion associated graft versus host disease (TA-GvHD). Blood 126, 406–414.

Lister, T.A., Crowther, D., Sutcliffe, S.B., et al., 1989. Report of a committee convened to discuss the evaluation and staging of patients with Hodgkin's disease: cotswolds meeting. J. Clin. Oncol. 7, 1630–1636.

Meignan, M., Gallamini, A., Haioun, C., 2009. Report on the First international workshop on interim-PET scan in lymphoma Leuk. Lymphoma 50, 1257–1260.

National Institute for Health and Care Excellence, 2003. Rituximab for aggressive non-Hodgkin's lymphoma. TA 65. NICE, London. Available at: https://www.nice.org.uk/guidance/TA65.

National Institute for Health and Care Excellence, 2008. Rituximab for the treatment of relapsed or refractory stage III or IV follicular non-Hodgkin's lymphoma. TA 137. NICE, London. Available at: https://www.nice.org.uk/guidance/TA137.

National Institute for Health and Care Excellence, 2011. Rituximab for the first-line maintenance treatment of follicular non-Hodgkin's lymphoma. TA 226. NICE, London. Available at: https://www.nice.org.uk/guidance/TA226.

National Institute for Health and Care Excellence, 2012. Rituximab for the first-line treatment of stage III–IV follicular lymphoma. TA 243. NICE, London. Available at: https://www.nice.org.uk/guidance/TA243.

National Institute for Health and Care Excellence, 2017. Nivolumab for treating relapsed or refractory classical Hodgkin lymphoma. TA 462. NICE, London. Available at: https://www.nice.org.uk/guidance/ta462.

Nournier, N., Canals, C., Gisselbrecht, C., et al., 2012. High-dose therapy and autologous stem cell transplantation in first relapse for diffuse large B cell lymphoma in the rituximab era: an analysis based on data from the European Blood and Marrow Registry. Biol. Blood Marrow Transplant. 18, 788–793.

Philip, T., Guglielmi, C., Hagenbeek, A., et al., 1995. Autologous bone marrow transplantation as compared with salvage chemotherapy in relapses of chemotherapy-sensitive non-Hodgkin's lymphoma. New Engl. J. Med. 333, 1540–1545.

Radford, J., Illidge, T., Counsel, T., et al., 2015. Results of a trial of PET-directed therapy for early-stage Hodgkin's lymphoma. New Engl. J. Med. 372, 1598–1607.

Smith, A., Crouch, S., Lax, S., et al., 2015. Lymphoma incidence, survival and prevalence 2004–2014: sub-type analyses from the UK's Haematological Malignancy Research Network. Br. J. Cancer 112, 1575–1584.

Stathis, A., Younes, A., 2015. The new therapeutical scenario of Hodgkin lymphoma. Ann. Oncol. 26, 2026–2033.

Sureda, A., Bader, P., Cesaro, S., et al., 2015. Indications for allo- and auto-SCT for haematological diseases, solid tumours and immune disorders: current practice in Europe, 2015. Bone Marrow Transplant. 50, 1037–1056.

Swerdlow, S.H., Campo, E., Harris, N.L., et al., 2008. WHO Classification of Tumours of Haematopoietic and Lymphoid Tissues, fourth ed. International Agency for Research on Cancer, Lyon.

Tilly, H., Gomes da Silva, M., Vitolo, A., et al., 2015. Diffuse large B-cell lymphomas: ESMO clinical practice guidelines. Ann. Oncol. 26 (Suppl. 5), v116–v125.

von Tresckow, B., Plütschow, A., Fuchs, M., et al., 2012. Dose-intensification in early unfavorable Hodgkin's lymphoma: final analysis of the German Hodgkin Study Group HD14 trial. J. Clin. Oncol. 30, 907–913.

Further reading

American Society of Clinical Oncology, 2006. Guideline for antiemetics in oncology: update 2006. J. Clin. Oncol. 24, 2932–2947.

Gopal, A.K., Kahl, B.S., de Vos, S., et al., 2014. PI3K delta inhibition by idelalisib in patients with relapsed indolent lymphoma. New Engl. J. Med. 370, 1008–1018.

Hesketh, P.J., Bohlke, K., Lyman, G.H., et al., 2016. Antiemetics: American Society of Clinical Oncology. J. Clin. Oncol. 34, 381–386.

Jones, G.L., Will, A., Jackson, G.H., et al., 2015. Guidelines for the management of tumor lysis syndrome in adults and children with haematological malignancies on behalf of the British Committee for Standards in Haematology. Br. J. Haematol. 169, 661–671.

National Institute for Health and Care Excellence, 2016. Non-Hodgkin's lymphoma: diagnosis and management. Guideline 52. Available at: https://www.nice.org.uk/guidance/ng52.

Rummel, M.J., Niederle, N., Mascheye, G., et al., 2013. Bendamustine plus rituximab versus CHOP plus rituximab as first-line treatment for patients with indolent and mantle-cell lymphomas: an open-label, multicenter, randomised, phase 3 non-inferiority trial. Lancet 381 (9873), 1203–1210.

Treleasen, J., Gennery, A., Marsh, J., et al., 2010. Guidelines on the use of irradiated blood components prepared by the British Committee for Standards in Haematology Blood Transfusion Task Force. Br. J. Haematol. 152, 35–51.

Useful websites

Macmillan Cancer Support: http://www.macmillan.org.uk

Lymphoma Association: http://www.lymphoma.org.uk

53 Solid Tumours

Netty (Annette) Cracknell and Alan Lamont

Key points

- Cancer involves a group of relatively normal cells dividing without the controls that usually prevent cells from growing beyond their normal size, site and nutritional base.
- Certain cancers are now considered a long-term illness with many subgroups.
- *Cancer* is a collective term for several diseases, each with its own characteristics and natural history according to where it started. Even for a single site of origin, such as breast cancer, major biological and histological differences can be shown compared with other sites of cancer origin.
- Before treatment, patients must be carefully 'staged' to establish the type and extent of disease.
- Depending on the stage of disease, the aim of treatment may be cure, prolongation of survival or symptom control.
- Cytotoxic chemotherapy remains the main treatment for disseminated disease for most cancers.
- Treatment options depend not only on the 'gold standard' of treatment but also on patient factors and preferences.
- Targeted medical therapies are becoming more common, generally have fewer side effects and are given over a longer-term than conventional chemotherapy

The term *cancer* is used to describe more than 200 different diseases, including those affecting discrete organs (solid tumours) and haematological malignancies (which are not localised in the same way). Whereas some tumours are benign and may be harmless, this chapter focuses on the management of patients with solid malignancies which require some form of treatment. Treatment is generally carried out in specialised cancer centres, cancer units or, for some agents, in the patient's home. Therapy may include surgery, radiotherapy, chemotherapy and biological or targeted therapy as single modalities or in combination. Care of the patient with cancer demands a broad range of services involving a multidisciplinary team working across the hospital, community and hospice network. The cost of systemic anticancer therapeutic agents is now in some cases so high that healthcare systems, such as the UK National Health Service (NHS), are restricting access to funding of individual products or to specific indications.

Epidemiology

Cancer is a common disease, with more than one-third of 1 million people developing cancer each year in the UK (352,197 new UK cancer cases in 2013). This equates to someone in the UK being diagnosed with cancer every 2 minutes. It is predicted that one in two people born after 1960 will be diagnosed with some form of cancer during their lifetime. Of all deaths in the UK, one in four is due to cancer. The most common cancers are lung, breast, bowel and prostate cancers, which make up more than half (53%) of all new cancers in the UK (Cancer Research UK, 2016a).

In 2013 prostate cancer became the most common cancer in men (26%), followed by lung cancer (14%) and bowel cancer (13%). For the same period, in women, breast cancer was the most common (31%), followed by lung cancer (12%) and bowel cancer (11%). However, there are regional variations (Cancer Research UK, 2016a).

Aetiology

The causes of cancer may be categorised as either environmental or genetic, although these may be interrelated, and the causes of some cancers may be multifactorial.

Environmental factors

Increasingly, lifestyle factors play a large part in the development of many cancers. Cigarette smoking has been identified as the single most important cause of preventable disease and premature death in the UK. The beneficial effect of stopping smoking on the cumulative risk of death from lung cancer reduces with increasing age (Doll et al., 2004). Tobacco (both active smoking and environmental tobacco smoke) causes almost one-fifth (19%) of all cancer cases in the UK each year, with the link between tobacco and cancer having been established more than 50 years ago.

The most important lifestyle factor for bowel cancer is diet, whereas cervical cancer is primarily linked to sexual behaviour through the transmissible agent human papilloma virus (HPV) and secondarily to smoking.

Table 53.1 A–K of factors associated with specific cancer sites: An empirical basis for recommending lifestyle changes (Jankowski and Boulton, 2005)

Factor	Associated cancer
Alcohol consumption >3 units a day	Most squamous cancers, especially bladder and oesophagus
Body mass index >25 and certainly >30	All solid cancers
Cigarette smoking at any level (even passive smoking)	Bladder, lung, head and neck, oesophagus and oropharyngeal cancers
Diet, especially one that is high in fat	All solid cancers
Exercising <30 min a day	All solid cancers
Family history of cancer (in at least one first-degree relative and at least three people in two or more generations)	Inherited cancer syndromes, including breast, colorectal, diffuse gastric, ovarian, prostate and uterine cancers
Genital and sexual health (sexually transmitted infections)	Cervical cancer
Health-promoting drugs that may decrease global cancer risks (but need a careful risk/benefit analysis)	Colonic adenomas can be treated with low-dose aspirin but can have serious side effects. Hormone replacement therapy linked with breast cancer
Intense sunburn	Melanoma
Job-related factors	Lung cancer (exposure to asbestos and particulates), skin cancer (contact with arsenic)
Known disease associations	Colorectal cancer has predisposing mucosal pathology – adenomas, coeliac disease, ulcerative colitis

Table 53.1 lists other factors which have been associated with cancer development.

Genetic factors

Some rare tumours are known to be associated with an inherited predisposition, where an individual is born with a marked susceptibility to cancer. This is due to the inheritance of a single genetic mutation which may be sufficient to greatly increase the risk of one or more types of cancer. Examples include the paediatric malignancies, Wilms' tumour of the kidney and bilateral retinoblastoma, a rare cancer of the eye. Some common cancers, such as breast, ovarian and colorectal cancers, may also show a tendency to occur in families, but these represent a small proportion of the overall presentation of common cancers where identifiable risk factors are relevant in only 5–10% of cases, although when the genetic factor is present, the cancers tend to have their onset at a younger age (Garber and Offit, 2005).

Screening and prevention

Screening

Screening programmes aim to detect pre-malignant changes or early-stage cancer in asymptomatic individuals in the general population to provide earlier and thus more effective treatment. Any screening test must be simple, reliable, highly specific (to exclude healthy individuals) and highly sensitive (detection:

90–95%). For a screening programme to be effective in reducing morbidity and mortality, there must also be an available, effective, safe and economically viable treatment that can be applied to the abnormalities detected by the screening test. Screening is well established for cancers of the breast, cervix and bowel. Population screening for prostate cancer using the prostate-specific antigen (PSA) blood test remains more controversial due to the lack of specificity and sensitivity of the test and because of the limited evidence on the viability and effectiveness of the treatment options in early-stage disease. It is currently not recommended for use in screening programmes in the UK but is used in the USA. The evidence base for ovarian cancer screening using the blood test CA 125 and pelvic ultrasound is evolving through clinical trials.

Prevention

The strong association between cancer risk and lifestyle factors means there is great potential for the primary prevention of cancer through:
- avoiding tobacco use, especially exposure to cigarette smoke;
- moderate alcohol consumption;
- healthier eating;
- limiting exposure to sunlight and artificial tanning UV exposure;
- encouraging physical exercise;
- maintaining a healthy body weight;
- maintaining adequate protection from asbestos fibres, radon and other occupational and environmental risk factors.

Chemoprevention

Chemoprevention is the prevention of cancer by using medication. The most common example is tamoxifen (pre-menopausal women) or an aromatase inhibitor (post-menopausal women) prescribed daily for 5 years to reduce the risk of developing breast cancer in high-risk women. However, these treatments are not without their side effects, such as menopausal symptoms and increased risk of thromboembolic events. Therefore, the risk/benefit ratio for each patient needs to be carefully assessed.

Another potential future development is the effect of aspirin as a chemopreventive agent for colorectal cancer. Maximal effect requires long-term use of high-dose aspirin that may increase the risk of gastro-intestinal bleeding. Non-steroidal anti-inflammatory drugs (NSAIDs) and selective cyclooxygenase-2 (COX-2) inhibitors may also be candidates for chemoprevention. However, the regular use of these drugs may also cause gastro-intestinal bleeding and increase the risk of cardiovascular events (Herszényi et al., 2008).

Cancer at the cellular level

Cancer arises from the changes in genes that regulate cell growth. For a normal cell to transform into a cancer cell, genetic changes must occur in the genes that regulate cell growth and differentiation. The nature of the genetic change may be a single-point change to a DNA nucleotide or the complete loss/gain of an entire chromosome. However, the most important factor is that a gene which regulates cell growth and/or differentiation must be altered to allow the cell to grow in an uncontrolled manner. Most cancers require a series of genetic mutations in a cell before an invasive tumour results.

Oncogenes

Oncogenes are where the normal gene, called a proto-oncogene, mutates and is then expressed at inappropriately high levels, therefore increasing the function of that gene. Examples of proto-oncogenes are genes that encode growth factors, signal transducers and transcription factors.

Tumour-suppressor genes

Tumour-suppressor genes are normal genes which have a protective effect against oncogenes and are also known as 'anti-oncogenes'. The tumour-suppressor gene's normal function is usually to control the cell cycle or act as a checkpoint in division. When this function becomes lost due to mutations affecting both copies of the gene in a potentially malignant cell, other genetic mutations have a greater likelihood of progressing to cancer. An example is the *TP53* gene which codes for the suppressor protein product p53.

The p53 protein acts as a regulator of cell growth and proliferation and controls passage from G1 to S phase in cell division (see Fig. 53.1). Agents that damage DNA cause p53 to accumulate. This accumulation of p53 switches off replication in the cell,

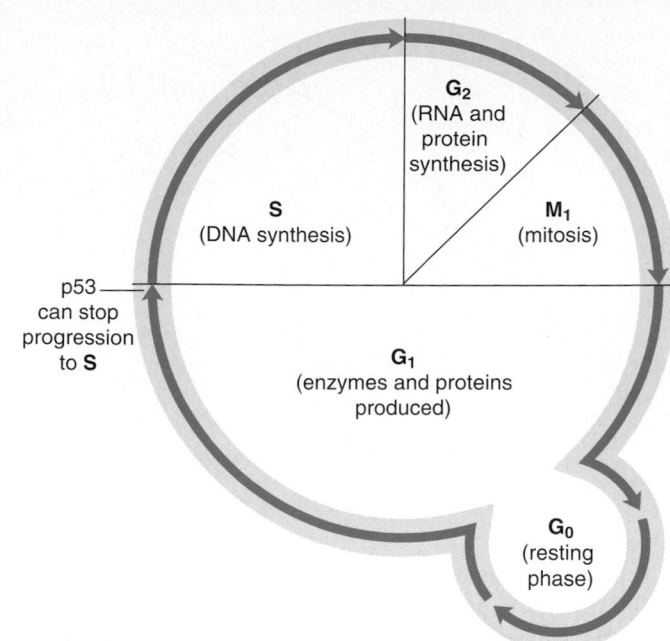

Fig. 53.1 Normal cell cycle.

arresting the cell cycle and allowing time to repair. If repair fails, p53 may trigger cell suicide by apoptosis. Thus, p53 controls and halts the proliferation of abnormal cell growth.

The cancer cell

Cancer cells differ from normal cells in that they function differently. Inherently unstable, they may display different protein or enzyme content and chromosomal abnormalities (such as translocations or deletions), which may be associated with differences in their susceptibility to chemotherapy or radiotherapy. The changes in internal structure and function lead to changes in their appearance which are visible under light microscopy, for example, larger and more varied appearance of the cell nuclei and loss of the appearance of specialised cell functions such as gland formation. This allows them to be easily detected, particularly when these lead to changes in the way clusters of cells form structures as a group and relate to normal cells in a tissue or organ.

Tumour growth

A solid tumour represents a population of dividing and non-dividing cells. The time it takes for a tumour mass to double is known, unsurprisingly, as the doubling time. The latter will vary depending on the type of disease, but for most solid tumours it is about 2–3 months. In most solid tumours, the growth rate is very rapid initially (exponential growth) and then slows as the tumour increases in size and age, a pattern described as Gompertzian growth (Fig. 53.2). The growth fraction is the percentage of actively dividing cells in the tumour, and this decreases with increasing tumour size. Not all of the dividing cells' 'daughters' will continue to grow, divide and add to the cell population of a growing tumour. The balance between the production of new cells and the 'cell loss factor' results in a much lower rate of growth than might be expected from the individual malignant cell's potential for division.

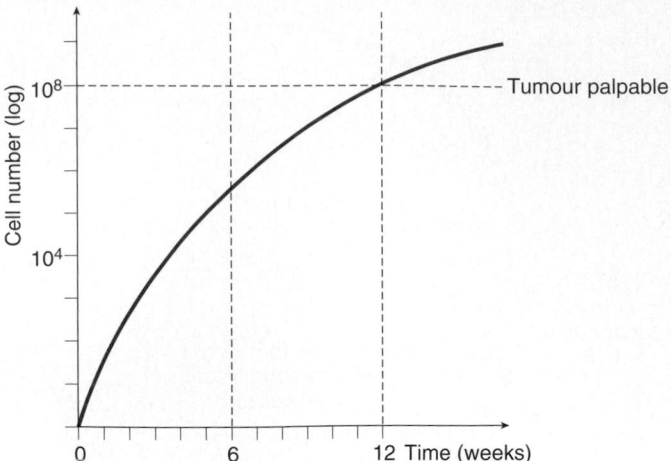

Fig. 53.2 Example of Gompertzian growth of cancer cells.

This pattern of tumour growth kinetics has implications for chemotherapy treatment. Generally, chemotherapy is most successful when the number of tumour cells is low and the growth fraction high, which is the situation in the very early stages of cancer.

Tumour spread

As a primary tumour grows, it both pushes the normal surrounding cells aside and invades between them into normal tissue. It is this property of invasion that characterises a malignant tumour and leads to distant spread of the disease because the abnormal cells often infiltrate through the walls of blood vessels and the lymphatic system. Malignant cells are then released from the infiltrating cluster of tumour cells and are transported by the blood or lymphatic fluid to other organs of the body, where they can subsequently form secondary cancers or metastases. The pattern of spread tends to be predictable for different tumour types, influenced by the anatomy of the primary site and by differences in the local factors affecting the viability of malignant calls when they become deposited elsewhere. For example, breast cancer usually metastasises to the lymph nodes under the arm, lungs and central nervous system, whereas prostate cancer tends to metastasise to bone. Generally, when the primary is first detected, the larger the tumour mass, the more likely that it has metastasised to other sites. It is often possible, using specialised research techniques, to detect circulating tumour cells or DNA in the peripheral blood of patients with even small primary tumours with no evidence of metastatic spread. This is a field of great interest in research for developing methods of early detection of active disease but also indicates that most cells released into the blood by primary tumours do not result in viable secondary tumours.

Patient management

Clinical assessment

Presentation

The clinical features of cancer vary with tumour type. Generally, patients most commonly present with either (1) non-specific complaints, which include weight loss, unexplained anaemia, malaise, lethargy or pain; (2) a specific localising symptom such as bleeding from an identifiable site, a non-healing ulcer, a minor symptom such as a cough or hoarseness not resolving in the usual way or the presence of a painful lump; or more commonly (3) a painless lump. In general, solid tumours are first clinically detectable when there are approximately 10^8–10^9 tumour cells present in a tumour mass in the range of 1–10 g. The patient is usually in the terminal stages of the disease when there are 10^{12} cells present and a tumour burden of around 1 kg. Less commonly, a tumour may be detected by chance during a routine physical examination or by screening or through identification of early symptoms. However, if this does not occur or these symptoms are not present or not recognised, then the disease at presentation is commonly at a stage where there is a high risk that metastatic spread has already occurred at a microscopic level even if that is not clinically detectable.

Before treatment, each patient must undergo a thorough assessment to establish diagnosis, stage of disease and general fitness level. These factors will influence the choice of treatment and give a guide to prognosis.

Diagnosis

An accurate diagnosis is usually made from a tissue sample taken from a suspected primary or secondary tumour, according to the initial clinical investigations. This sampling procedure, known as a biopsy, may be obtained by an open operation, or less invasively by endoscopy or image-guided techniques. Such samples may be obtained, for example, during bronchoscopy when lung cancer is suspected or, as in the case of a patient presenting with a breast lump, aspiration through a fine needle under ultrasound guidance.

Malignant tumours vary in their sensitivity to chemotherapy. For example, there are two major groups of lung cancer: small-cell and non-small-cell lung cancer. Each of these groups is treated with different combinations of surgery, radiotherapy and chemotherapy drugs. Therefore, precise histopathology is important.

Tumour markers

Tumour markers are usually proteins associated with a malignancy and are clinically useful in:

- diagnosing or at least helping indicate a specific tumour;
- monitoring response to treatment;
- estimating prognosis, usually as part of a prognostic index calculation;
- detecting recurrent disease;
- screening a healthy population or a high-risk population for the presence of cancer.

They may be detected in a solid tumour, in circulating tumour cells in peripheral blood, in lymph nodes, in bone marrow or in other body fluids. Some of the tumour markers are presented in Table 53.2.

Staging investigations

Because the cancer is often disseminated at the time of presentation, it is vital that patients undergo thorough staging investigations to establish the extent and nature of disease. This will

Table 53.2 Examples of tumour markers used in detection, diagnosis and monitoring

Tumour marker	Indicative cancer
CA 125	Ovarian cancer, although non-specific
CA 19-9	Upper gastro-intestinal/pancreas though non-specific
CA 15-3	Breast cancer, though limited utility
CEA	Lower gastro-intestinal tumours, although non-specific
α-Fetoprotein β-Human chorionic gonadotrophin	Testicular tumour
5-Hydroxyindole acetic acid, chromogranins A and B	Carcinoid tumours
Thyroglobulin	Thyroid cancer (limited utility unless thyroid-stimulating hormone is suppressed post-thyroidectomy)
α-Fetoprotein	Hepatocellular carcinoma
Prostate-specific antigen	Prostate cancer
Human chorionic gonadotropin	Gestational trophoblastic tumours
β-2-Microglobulin	Myeloma and some related hematological malignancies

Box 53.1 Performance status scales

Karnofsky performance index
100 Normal, no complaints, no evidence of disease
90 Able to carry on normal activity, minor signs or symptoms of disease
80 Normal activity with effort, some signs or symptoms of disease
70 Cares for self, unable to carry on normal activity or do active work
60 Requires occasional assistance but is able to care for most of own needs
50 Requires considerable assistance and frequent medical care
40 Disabled, requires special care and assistance
30 Severely disabled, hospitalisation is indicated, although death is not imminent
20 Very sick, hospitalisation necessary, active supportive treatment is necessary
10 Moribund, fatal processes progressing rapidly

World Health Organization performance scale
0. Able to carry out all normal activity without restriction
1. Restricted in physically strenuous activity but ambulatory and able to carry out light work
2. Ambulatory and capable of all self-care but unable to carry out any work; up and about more than 50% of waking hours
3. Capable of only limited self-care; confined to bed more than 50% of waking hours
4. Completely disabled; cannot carry on any self-care; totally confined to bed or chair

determine the most appropriate treatment offered to the patient. Baseline investigations range from clinical examination, blood tests and liver function tests to diagnostic imaging such as chest and skeletal X-rays, ultrasound, computed tomography (CT), magnetic resonance imaging (MRI) and positron emission tomography (PET), depending on the disease type and likely pattern of spread. Clinical guidelines for staging and management of malignancies of the various body systems have been produced at local and national levels in most developed countries, with relatively minor variations according to local custom and practice. For example, guidelines have been developed by the National Institute for Health and Care Excellence (NICE) in the UK (see http://www.nice.org.uk/ for guidance) and the National Cancer Institute (NCI) in the USA (see http://www.cancer.gov/ for guidance).

Staging classification

Staging is essentially a measure of how far a tumour has progressed in its development at the time of diagnosis, whereas grading is a measure of how aggressive its behaviour is likely to be in future, based on the microscopic appearance of the cells of the tumour. Both measures are relevant to the patient and clinical team in planning the management.

Most tumours are classified according to the TNM (tumour–nodes–metastases) system, where T (0–4) indicates the size of the primary tumour, N (0–3) the extent of lymph node involvement and M (0–1) the presence or absence of distant metastases. Each solid tumour site has a specific grading and staging classification such as Dukes-based staging in colorectal cancer (Cancer Research UK, 2009) and Gleason scoring for grading prostate cancer (Berney, 2007), although these are being superseded by TNM in many healthcare systems, and other prognostic scoring and predictive tools are sometimes used, especially in research trials to stratify into subgroups.

Performance status

The patient's general level of fitness (performance status) at the time of diagnosis is often a surprisingly reliable indicator of prognosis, independent of disease-related factors, and will help determine whether the patient is likely to withstand intensive chemotherapy; this therefore influences the choice of treatment. Various physical rating scales have been devised to assess performance status, including the Karnofsky Performance Index (Karnofsky and Burchenal, 1949) and the World Health Organization (WHO-ECOG) performance scale (Oken et al., 1982) (Box 53.1).

Prognostic factors

Prognostic factors are those that can predict how the disease is likely to behave and determine an outcome in individual patients. For example, Table 53.3 lists prognostic factors in patients with colorectal cancer.

Table 53.3 Prognostic factors in patients with colorectal cancer

Favourable	Unfavourable
Good performance status	Presence of nodal involvement
No penetration of the tumour through the bowel wall	Presence of distant metastases
Absence of nodal involvement	Bowel obstruction and bowel perforation
Absence of distant metastases	

Treatment

Treatment goals

After the diagnosis of cancer has been confirmed and the extent of disease fully investigated, the goals of treatment have to be considered. Depending on the stage of disease, the goal can be the following (and this may change throughout treatment):

- Cure – Patients are said to be 'cured' of cancer when they are completely disease-free and have a normal life expectancy. The smaller the tumour bulk when treatment is given, the greater the potential of achieving cure. A common measure of 'cure' is the 5-year disease-free survival rate.
- Prolong survival while maintaining patient's quality of life.
- Provide palliative relief of symptoms such as pain.

Childhood malignancies, choriocarcinoma and testicular tumours in adults are most responsive to chemotherapy, and these patients are frequently cured, even with advanced disease. However, for most patients treated with chemotherapy, cure is less likely, and treatment will be given to maximise the probability of cure, prolong survival or be purely palliative. The decision is influenced by factors such as the extent of the disease, as well as co-existing symptoms, concurrent medical conditions, performance status and, importantly, the patient's wishes. The possibility of medium- to long-term survival justifies aggressive treatment, but with palliative therapy, it is particularly important that the toxicity of treatment is carefully weighed against the potential benefits.

Treatment guidelines

Consensus on the best approach to managing each particular type of cancer is continually evolving based on the evidence from clinical research, most reliably in the form of randomised controlled trials. National guidelines aim to promote equity for patients and ensure a consistent treatment approach that takes account of the boundaries of affordability for the healthcare system. In the absence of clinical consensus, patients should be encouraged to participate in clinical trials.

Treatment methods

Four main options are available for the treatment of patients with solid tumours: surgery, radiotherapy, conventional chemotherapy and targeted/biological therapies. Each treatment may play a number of roles, either alone or in combination, depending on the disease, stage and grade.

Role of surgery. Surgery can be curative when solid tumours are confined to one primary anatomical site or region as in localised disease. It can also be used to remove isolated metastatic masses with curative intent in rare circumstances or to deal with anatomical consequences of a tumour as a palliative procedure, such as relief of bowel obstruction by defunctioning colostomy. Surgical techniques may be used to support chemotherapy administration when given by continuous infusion or by the intraperitoneal route. Surgery plays a major role in diagnosis through tissue biopsy or in staging to ascertain the extent of tumour involvement such as in ovarian cancer. In the latter, it may also be used to debulk or reduce the size of the tumour to effect pain relief or to improve the effectiveness of subsequent radiation or chemotherapy. However, with more widespread disease, systemic treatment becomes the mainstay of management, with chemotherapy playing a major role

Role of radiotherapy. Radiotherapy can be used to cure cancer, reduce the symptoms of the tumour, reduce the size of the tumour ready for surgery or to prevent re-occurrence of the tumour after surgical removal. It can be used alone or in combination with surgery and/or chemotherapy. A full exposition of the role of radiotherapy is beyond the scope of this chapter, which concentrates on the role of systemic agents. However, the combination of radiotherapy and systemic treatment is becoming increasingly employed as research shows the benefit to disease control and long-term survival, for example, in carcinoma of the uterine cervix (Green et al., 2009).

Systemic therapy. This encompasses cytotoxic chemotherapy, hormonal, biological and targeted therapies, but the term does not usually encompass the modalities of nutritional, complementary, alternative or other 'holistic' interventions, even if employed within a conventional medical environment.

Cytotoxic chemotherapy

Chemotherapy regimen

Although chemotherapy is sometimes administered as a single agent, it is more usual to combine two or more drugs to achieve additive or synergistic effects. Generally, drugs used in combination should have established efficacy as single agents, different mechanisms of action and differing toxicity profiles to allow their use at optimal doses.

Chemotherapy scheduling

Because chemotherapy does not specifically target malignant cells, any actively proliferating normal cell will be at potential risk of damage, in particular the cells of the bone marrow. This causes a fall in the white blood cell count, and with many cytotoxic drugs, the white blood count is at its lowest level (nadir) around 10 days after treatment. Recovery generally occurs by day 20 post-treatment, and therefore chemotherapy treatment is usually repeated every 3–4 weeks. With agents such as mitomycin and lomustine, haematological recovery may be delayed for 42–50 days after treatment, in which case the interval between treatment cycles needs to be increased. In most cases, a course of treatment will comprise a maximum of six cycles of

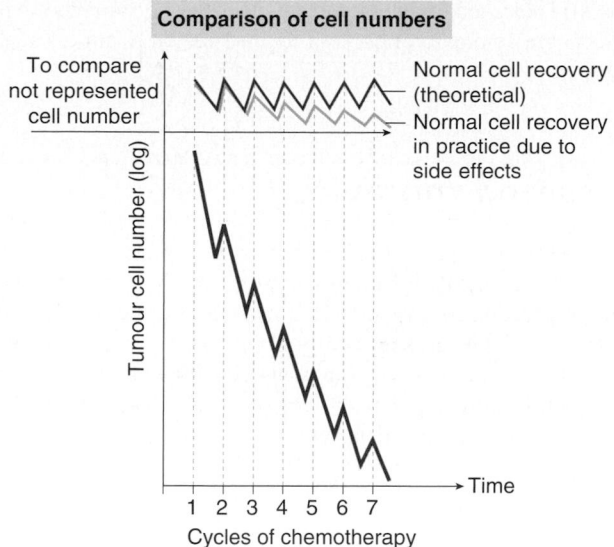

Comparison of cell numbers

To compare not represented cell number

Normal cell recovery (theoretical)

Normal cell recovery in practice due to side effects

Tumour cell number (log)

Time

1 2 3 4 5 6 7

Cycles of chemotherapy

Fig. 53.3 The effect of chemotherapy on tumour mass and healthy cells.

Table 53.4	Example of a chemotherapy regimen FEC–T (fluorouracil, epirubicin, cyclophosphamide, docetaxel [Taxotere]) for breast cancer		
Indication	Adjuvant breast cancer		
Length of cycle	21 days		
No. of cycles	Three cycles of FEC followed by three cycles of Taxotere (Docetaxel)		
FEC			
Fluorouracil	IVB		500 mg/m^2 day 1
Epirubicin	IVB		100 mg/m^2 day 1
Cyclophosphamide	IVB		500 mg/m^2 day 1
T			
Docetaxel	IVI over 1 h		100 mg/m^2 day 1
IVB, i.v. bolus; IVI, i.v. infusion.			

chemotherapy, although in some less common cancers, such as sarcomas, leukaemias and in paediatrics, the regimen may continue with a much longer period of adjuvant or consolidation therapy. Targeted agents may be continued for long periods, in some cases indefinitely until either tolerance is lost or until disease progression.

Fig. 53.3 demonstrates the tumour cell kill for each cycle of chemotherapy together with the healthy normal cell kill. Chemotherapy works in situations where the healthy normal cells recover faster or more completely from the effects of chemotherapy compared with the tumour cells. This allows the tumour cells to be progressively killed off, whilst not having a detrimental effect on the patient.

Chemotherapy dose

The dose of most chemotherapy agents is calculated using the patient's body surface area (BSA) as a surrogate estimate analogous to lean body mass, or weight (kg), and is usually prescribed in the form of milligrams per square metre or per kilogram. Body surface area may be calculated from the height and weight of the patient using a nomogram or standard formula and may need to be recalculated for subsequent cycles of chemotherapy if the patient experiences significant weight changes. Table 53.4 gives an example of a chemotherapy regimen used in breast cancer. The reliability of body surface area as a predictor of the effective safe dose is diminished for patients who are either very thin (cachectic), grossly overweight (morbidly obese) or in the case of limb deformities or loss because it does not then reflect a reasonable estimate of lean body mass.

Adjuvant chemotherapy

Adjuvant chemotherapy means literally 'additional treatment' and is usually given after surgery or radiotherapy when all detectable disease has been removed, but where there remains a statistical risk of relapse due to undetectable disease. Adjuvant therapy is, therefore, used to increase the likelihood of cure. Only patients whose cancers have a high or intermediate risk of recurrence tend to be selected for adjuvant chemotherapy because it is not desirable to expose patients whose disease may already have been cured by surgery or radiotherapy to the toxicity of chemotherapy treatment.

In colorectal cancer, for example, adjuvant chemotherapy provides significant disease-free survival benefit by reducing the recurrence rate and also increases overall survival. This indicates the curative role of chemotherapy in the adjuvant setting (Sargent et al., 2009). Similarly, in breast cancer, adjuvant treatment has been shown to increase recurrence-free survival (Levine and Whelan, 2006), and trials are underway to determine which agents and in what combination further improvements in overall survival will be obtained. One trial has shown that three-weekly AC/T (doxorubicin, cyclophosphamide, docetaxel [Taxotere]) is significantly inferior to CEF (cyclophosphamide, epirubicin, 5-flourouricil) or EC/T (epirubicin, cyclophosphamide, docetaxel [Taxotere]) in terms of recurrence-free survival (Burnell et al., 2010). This is important for development of healthcare system therapeutic management planning because standard treatment choices should move to the superior regimen.

Neo-adjuvant chemotherapy

In neo-adjuvant chemotherapy, chemotherapy is given before local therapy, often preoperatively, to reduce tumour size and facilitate surgical removal. Neo-adjuvant chemotherapy has been of particular value in cases of breast cancer, non-small-cell lung cancer, advanced head and neck cancer, and bone tumours. In Ewing's sarcoma, it allows limb-sparing surgery as an alternative to amputation. It also improves survival with reduced morbidity in osteosarcoma.

Synchronous chemoradiation

In several cancers, chemotherapy alongside radical radiotherapy is now established. Agents such as cisplatin are commonly used as a 'radiosensitiser' in head and neck, oesophageal and cervical cancers. The use of cetuximab in combination with radiotherapy for a certain type of head and neck cancer is also recommended (NICE, 2008). Although in common use, the use of the term *radiosensitiser* in this context is somewhat inaccurate and is distinct from the 'true' radiosensitising drugs such as nimorazole, which interact at a chemical level with very short-lived radiation-induced free radicals, and the effect is more appropriately termed 'combined modality therapy'.

Adverse effects of cytotoxic drugs

Most cytotoxic drugs have been developed because of their effect on dividing cells. Consequently, and as previously mentioned under chemotherapy scheduling, proliferating normal tissue such as bone marrow is at risk. Myelosuppression is frequently the dose-limiting toxicity with these compounds. Neutropenia and thrombocytopenia place patients at risk of life-threatening infection and bleeding, respectively.

The other acute adverse effects occurring most frequently include nausea and vomiting, mucositis, anorexia and alopecia. Individual drugs will also give rise to specific adverse effects, some of which may not be reversible on stopping treatment. Cardiotoxicity, nephrotoxicity and pulmonary toxicity, which are specific to the chemotherapeutic agent or class, may depend on cumulative drug exposure, the schedule of administration and previous therapy. Long-term side effects include infertility due to suppression of ovarian and testicular function and occasionally the induction of a second malignancy.

Chemotherapy-related toxicity is an important issue. Not only can it result in prolonged hospitalisation and a reduction in patients' quality of life, but also successful treatment can be compromised. A reduction in dose intensity, that is, the dose of cytotoxic delivered per unit time, because of dose reductions or treatment delays, can result in reduced response rates and survival. The use of granulocyte-colony-stimulating factors (G-CSFs) to prevent dose-limiting toxicity of myelosuppression can help reduce dose reductions or treatment delays. This is often used in treatments where the dose intensity given is paramount, and the goal of treatment is cure, for example in testicular germ-cell cancer.

Chemotherapy-specific adjunctive treatments

Both ifosfamide and cyclophosphamide are metabolised to the inactive acrolein which is responsible for bladder toxicity. The co-administration of mesna, a sulfhydryl-containing compound which binds to acrolein, has reduced the incidence of haemorrhagic cystitis associated with intravenous regimens of ifosfamide and high-dose cyclophosphamide.

Calcium leucovorin or folinic acid is a reduced form of folic acid and is in effect an 'antidote' to the cytotoxic methotrexate. Folinic acid is effectively used as a form of 'rescue' when high doses of intravenous methotrexate are used, to limit the exposure to the cytotoxic effect to a defined period of time, usually 24 hours.

Targeted therapies

In recent years, there has been a greatly increased understanding of biochemical signalling pathways involved in the growth and progression of tumours. This has allowed the development of therapies targeted specifically at the cell receptors involved. Because they are targeted at tumour cells, they can suppress disease without inflicting the non-selective toxic effects of cytotoxic chemotherapy on the patient.

Epidermal growth factor receptor

The epidermal growth factor receptor (EGFR) is a transmembrane protein with an intracellular tyrosine kinase domain. Extracellular binding of the epidermal growth factor receptor induces tyrosine phosphorylation which activates signal cascade pathways. These ultimately lead to cellular proliferation and metastasis. Epidermal growth factor receptor expression is low in normal tissues, and overexpression is associated with a variety of tumours, including non-small-cell lung cancer, colon cancer and head and neck cancer.

Inhibitors of epidermal growth factor receptor (also known as human epidermal growth factor receptor type 1 [HER1]) include the following:

- Small molecules such as the orally administered erlotinib, gefitinib and adatinib used in the treatment of non-small-cell lung cancer and afatinib used in the treatment of gastrointestinal stromal tumours (GIST) specifically inhibit tyrosine kinase.
- Monoclonal antibodies, such as cetuximab and panitumumab, bind to the epidermal growth factor receptor. Cetuximab has demonstrated synergy when given in combination with irinotecan chemotherapy, offering prolonged survival in selected patients with metastatic colorectal cancer and improved disease control when given in combination with radiotherapy in selected cases of head and neck cancer.

Vascular endothelial growth factor receptor

Angiogenesis is the formation of new blood vessels on which tumour growth depends. Vascular endothelial growth factor (VEGF) is key in angiogenesis, and its overexpression has been associated with increased vasculature, aggressive disease and poor prognosis. The monoclonal antibody bevacizumab inhibits VEGF, thereby reducing new blood vessel growth and interstitial pressure within the tumour, allowing improved chemotherapy access. Studies have demonstrated meaningful survival benefits when bevacizumab is administered in conjunction with chemotherapy in patients with advanced or metastatic colorectal cancer (Hurwitz et al., 2004). Pazopanib is a tyrosine kinase inhibitor and inhibits VEGF. It is used in the treatment of renal cell carcinoma.

Human epidermal growth factor receptor type 2

Overexpression of human epidermal growth factor receptor type 2 (HER2) is associated with a particularly aggressive form of breast cancer (about 20% cases are HER2 positive) and 7–34% of gastric cancers. Trastuzumab, a humanised monoclonal antibody, specifically targets HER2 and is only effective in patients with elevated levels. It is used widely in metastatic and early breast cancer (NICE, 2002, 2006a) and HER2 positive metastatic gastric cancer (NICE, 2010). Pertuzumab, a humanised monoclonal antibody, inhibits dimerisation of HER2 receptors and is used in combination with trastuzumab for breast cancer.

Trastuzumab emtansine is a HER2-targeted antibody–drug conjugate which contains trastuzumab, covalently linked to the microtubule inhibitor DM1. When trastuzumab attaches to the HER2 receptor it releases emtansine into the cancer cell. Emtansine binds to tubulin and inhibits tubulin polymerisation; both DM1 and trastuzumab emtansine cause the cancer cells to arrest in the G2/M phase of the cell cycle, leading to apoptotic cell death.

Capecitabine

Although capecitabine does not target a particular receptor, it is mentioned in this section because it preferentially targets tumour cells.

Capecitabine is a fluoropyrimidine carbamate precursor of 5-fluorouracil (5FU). Given orally, it is converted via enzyme pathways to 5-FU. Because these enzymes are found in higher concentrations in tumour cells, treatment is effectively targeted. Capecitabine has been shown to be at least as effective as intravenous 5-FU (Twelves et al., 2012), and it is widely used in practice. This is of a particular benefit where the total regimen can then be given orally rather than intravenously. Clinical use of capecitabine requires caution because although it is very easy to administer as an apparently simple oral tablet, the toxicity is comparable to intravenous fluoropyrimidine therapy, and a small proportion of the population are exceedingly sensitive due to an inherited defect in the enzyme dihydropyrimidine dehydrogenase (DPD; Cancer Research UK, 2016b).

Management of patients receiving cytotoxic chemotherapy

Prescription verification

Over the years, there has been considerable effort to improve the quality and safety of chemotherapy services for adult patients. In particular, the importance of all chemotherapy prescriptions being checked by appropriately trained and competent pharmacists is now recognised. The British Oncology Pharmacy Association (BOPA) has published standards for pharmacy verification of prescription for cancer medicines (BOPA, 2013). These BOPA standards are summarised in Box 53.2. These were supplemented in 2015 by standards for associated e-prescribing systems (BOPA, 2015).

Box 53.2 Standards for pharmacy verification of prescriptions for cancer medicines (BOPA, 2013)

1. **Check the prescription.**
   - Has the drug or regimen been prescribed in line with legislation and local prescribing policy?
   - Check that the prescriber's details and signature are present, and confirm the prescriber is authorised to prescribe SACT as appropriate
   - Check that the prescription is clear, legible, unambiguous and includes all details required for dispensing, labelling and administration
2. **Check the prescription against the protocol and treatment plan.**
   This will include as appropriate/relevant:
   - Ensuring the regimen has been through local approval processes (e.g. clinical governance and financial approval) and/or is included on a list of locally approved regimens
   - Where there is access to either clinical notes, treatment plan or electronic record on first cycle, check that the regimen is intended treatment and is appropriate for patient's diagnosis, medical history, performance status and chemotherapy history
3. **Check patient details.**
   - Check that patient demographics (age, height and weight) have been correctly recorded on prescription as appropriate
4. **Check administration details.**
   This will include the following as appropriate/relevant:
   - Checking that there are no known drug interactions (including with food) or conflicts with patient allergies and other medication(s)
   - Checking that the timing of administration is appropriate (i.e. interval since last treatment and/or start and stop dates for oral chemotherapy)
   - Checking that appropriate supportive care is prescribed
   - Checking that the method of administration is appropriate
5. **Check calculations: are the BSA and dose calculations correct?**
   - Check that all dose calculations and dose units are correct and have been calculated correctly according to the protocol and any other relevant local guidance (e.g. dose rounding/banding) as appropriate
   - Check that prescribed dose is in line with previous dose reductions
   - Check that BSA is correctly calculated if needed for dose calculation. There should be local agreement for frequency of monitoring and checking patient's weight.
6. **Check laboratory results as appropriate.**
   - Check that laboratory values, FBC, U&Es and LFTs are within accepted limits if appropriate
   - Check that doses are appropriate with respect to renal and hepatic function and any experienced toxicities.
   - Check that other essential tests have been undertaken if appropriate.
7. **Sign and date prescription as a record of verification.**

BSA, Body surface area; FBC, full blood count; LFTs, liver function tests; SACT, systemic anticancer therapy; U&Es, urea and electrolytes.

Cumulative dosing

The use of doxorubicin is limited by a dose-dependent cardiomyopathy. Various other factors have been implicated, including treatment schedule, patient age and pre-existing cardiac disease, but dose is the most important. The maximum recommended cumulative dose is 550 mg/m^2, reducing to 400 mg/m^2

for patients who have received radiotherapy to the mediastinum. Therefore, treatment should be monitored closely to make sure the cumulative dose is not exceeded throughout the patient's lifetime. All other anthracycline antibiotics also have a lifetime cumulative dose limit.

Dose modification or delay

Appropriate investigations must be carried out before each treatment to ensure that patients are fit for chemotherapy. In particular, the patient's haematological, renal and hepatic function should be determined by blood testing and further investigation as indicated. For some cytotoxic drugs, it may be necessary to adjust the dose, or even stop treatment, in the presence of renal or hepatic impairment to ensure that delayed excretion or reduced metabolism does not result in excess toxicity. Therefore, the individual summary of product characteristics (SPC) for the chemotherapy agent should be consulted; SPCs can be found at http://www.medicines.org.uk.

If the bone marrow does not recover sufficiently between cycles of treatment, then a dose reduction or a delay in treatment may be necessary. In general, patients with a neutrophil level less than $1 \times 10^9/L$ or a platelet count less than $100 \times 10^9/L$ should not be given myelosuppressive cytotoxics at full doses (note that different ranges will apply for hematological malignancies and when specified in solid-tumour schedules such as germ-cell malignancy).

Drug interactions

Prescriptions for cancer chemotherapy are often complex, sometimes involving combinations of both parenteral and oral cytotoxic drugs, intravenous fluids and other supportive therapies. The potential for drug interactions to arise is considerable. However, care is required when assessing the clinical significance of potential drug interactions. A documented interaction does not necessarily imply that drugs should not be used in combination but can necessitate close monitoring of the patient.

Patient information and counselling

All patients must be provided with information about their treatment, including any anticipated side effects. Patients should be encouraged by health professionals to ask questions about their treatment.

Patients must understand the different medication, the specific role of each medicine and the duration of treatment. Duration of treatment is particularly important to prevent highly potent medicines from being inadvertently continued beyond their intended course.

Symptom control

Nausea and vomiting

Chemotherapy-induced nausea and vomiting (CINV) is one of the most frequently experienced side effects encountered by chemotherapy patients and is considered to be the most distressing. In extreme cases, poor symptom control can result in patients refusing further treatment.

In selecting an appropriate antiemetic regimen, relevant factors include the emetogenic potential of the chemotherapy drugs prescribed, the putative mechanism(s) of inducing emesis, and the likely onset and duration of symptoms. Individual patient characteristics also have to be taken into consideration. For example, predisposing factors which increase a patient's susceptibility to emesis as a result of chemotherapy treatment are as follows:

- Poor control with prior chemotherapy
- female sex
- younger age <50 years
- a current or prior history of low chronic alcohol intake
- history of sickness: pregnancy/travelling/surgery
- anxiety
- smoking
- radiation to gastro-intestinal tract, liver or brain
- other medications: various medications can cause nausea and vomiting such as anaesthetic agents, antidepressants, antimicrobials, antifungals, iron, levodopa, carbidopa, NSAIDs

Differences in the severity of emesis can also occur between patients receiving the same type of chemotherapy and even between treatment cycles in the same patient; however, modern drug treatment can successfully control CINV for the majority of patients.

The 5-hydroxytryptamine type 3 ($5HT_3$) receptor antagonists, which include dolasetron, granisetron, ondansetron, palonosetron and tropisetron, have become the standard management of acute CINV when treating patients with moderately emetogenic chemotherapy regimens. For highly emetogenic chemotherapy regimens such as those including cisplatinum, the use of the NK_1 inhibitor, aprepitant or netupitant, together with a $5HT_3$ antagonist is becoming the gold standard. These agents are most effective in dealing with acute emesis (duration of <24 hours) when combined with a potent steroid such as dexamethasone.

It is important to achieve optimal control of nausea and vomiting at the outset to avoid subsequent anticipatory symptoms which can prove very difficult to treat.

The route of administration for antiemetics is an important consideration. With intravenous chemotherapy, it may be simpler to administer all treatments by the intravenous route. Alternatives to the oral route may be useful when vomiting occurs and include the rectal and buccal route.

Pain control

Drug therapy remains one of the cornerstones of effective pain management, but it is often underprescribed, thus highlighting the importance of regular patient assessment and appropriate dose or drug treatment changes. For example, patients experiencing intolerable side effects to morphine may be transferred to oxycodone or transdermal fentanyl skin patches. Analgesia should be prescribed both regularly and for breakthrough pain, and stimulant laxatives should be prescribed to prevent opioid-related constipation. Combinations of analgesics which have synergistic activity, for example, opiates plus NSAIDs, can be highly effective whilst minimising the dose-related side effects of each agent.

The route of administration is also important. When patients are unable to manage oral medication, it is important to assess the use of alternative routes such as the rectal, subcutaneous, epidural and transdermal routes.

Table 53.5 National Cancer Institute Common Terminology Criteria for Adverse Events v4.0: anaemia (haemoglobin) (NCI, 2010).

Adverse event, grade	0	1	2	3	4
Haemoglobin (Hgb)	WNL <LLN–100 g/L <LLN–6.2 mmol/L	<LLN–10.0 g/dL 80–<100 g/L 4.9–<6.2 mmol/L	8.0–<10.0 g/dL 65–<80 g/L 4.0–<4.9 mmol/L	6.5–<8.0 g/dL <65 g/L <4.0 mmol/L	<6.5 g/dL <LLN–100 g/L <LLN–6.2 mmol/L

LLN, Lower limit of normal; WNL, within normal limits.

Bone marrow suppression

Myelosuppression after chemotherapy is common, and for some patients profound. The risk of systemic infection can be reduced by good oral hygiene and mouth care using antiseptic mouthwashes and antifungal prophylaxis. Patients must be advised to immediately report symptoms of infection and bruising. Platelet transfusions may be required, but fever or other evidence of infection occurring in a neutropenic patient when the neutrophil count is less than $1.0 \times 10^9/L$ must be aggressively treated with broad-spectrum intravenous antibiotics to prevent overwhelming infection. Most treatment centres will have developed and implemented a local policy for management of suspected 'neutropenic sepsis' with a recommended antibacterial schedule.

The duration and depth of neutropenia can be dramatically reduced by the administration of G-CSFs, which stimulate neutrophil production and, in cases of severe neutropenia, effectively rescue the patient. Once the patient's neutrophil count has recovered sufficiently, their use may be safely discontinued. These agents may also be used prophylactically in patients with a high risk of febrile neutropenia before receiving chemotherapy.

Blood transfusions are commonly required by patients at some stage of their treatment due to anaemia. Alternatively, erythropoietin may be useful in some patients receiving chemotherapy to shorten the period of anaemia and to improve the patient's quality of life where blood transfusions are not possible.

Extravasation

Extreme care must be taken when administering cytotoxic drugs parenterally because of the dangers of extravasation. Extravasation, which is the accidental leakage of an intravenous drug into the surrounding tissue, can cause pain, erythema and severe local necrosis, resulting in permanent tissue damage. The patient must be asked to immediately report any pain or a stinging sensation at the injection site because the degree of damage is determined by the amount of drug extravasated and the speed at which it is detected. If extravasation is suspected, the administration of further chemotherapy must stop, and remedial treatment must commence as soon as possible. The effectiveness of such therapy varies according to the agent extravasated. Most treatment facilities will have developed and implemented a policy for the management of extravasation according to the agent involved.

In-patient or outpatient treatment

The majority of patients receive chemotherapy in the outpatient clinic or day-care setting, where cytotoxics are administered mainly by short intravenous infusion at 3- or 4-week intervals.

Other treatments include monoclonal antibodies, which usually require close monitoring of the patient for several hours in case of anaphylactic reactions. More complex treatments, such as cisplatinum-containing regimens which require prehydration with intravenous fluids, need the patient to attend all day.

Currently, in-patient treatment of chemotherapy only occurs for the small minority of treatments, and this number is declining further as novel ways of administering long infusions are being developed.

Domiciliary treatment

Oral cytotoxic drugs can safely be taken at home so long as the patient is informed and able to monitor side effects. Availability of a 24-hour helpline is essential for these patients should they encounter problems whilst on treatment. In the future, administration of intravenous treatments, such as the monoclonal antibody trastuzumab, may be carried out more frequently in the home setting, particularly when safety permits and where patient preference becomes an influential factor.

Monitoring anticancer therapy

In addition to desirable outcomes, treatment with chemotherapy may result in a variety of undesirable outcomes; both require careful monitoring.

Toxicity

The toxicity resulting from treatment is routinely assessed after each cycle of chemotherapy and may result in therapy being modified on subsequent cycles, for example, a dose reduction, a delay in treatment or, in some cases, an alternative treatment. A number of international rating scales are available for rating predictable acute reactions arising from chemotherapy, including that of the National Cancer Institute Common Toxicity Criteria (NCI, 2010). For an example, see Table 53.5. Standardising the assessment of treatment-related toxicity in this way allows comparison to be made between published reports of clinical trials.

Response to treatment

Throughout treatment, the response to therapy is closely monitored, noting changes in performance status, symptoms and objective measurements of the tumour. This may necessitate repeating some or all of the initial staging investigations. Should the initial treatment prove ineffective, an alternative can then be considered without delay. Assessment of response should be formally documented before proceeding to further therapy.

Definitions of response. Definitions of response have been standardised by WHO:

- *Complete response or remission* (CR). The disappearance of all recognisable tumour masses and/or biochemical changes directly related to the tumour and resolution of symptoms determined by two observations at least a month apart.
- *Partial response* (PR). Decrease by 50% or more in all tumour masses, measured by the product of the longest × the widest perpendicular diameters for at least a month.
- *Stable disease* (SD) *or no change* (NC). Changes smaller than those described for PR or less than for progressive disease for at least a month.
- *Progressive disease* (PD). The occurrence of any new lesion or increase in the longest × widest perpendicular diameters of measurable disease by at least 25%.

Again, this allows comparison of results between different reported studies. An update of the WHO guidelines has been published (Therasse et al., 2000) called Response Evaluation Criteria in Solid Tumours (RECIST). To avoid confusion, it is important to stipulate in trial protocols which system will be used. Although clinical response indicates tumour sensitivity, it may not necessarily predict long-term survival, nor does it measure other benefits such as quality of life.

Case studies

Case 53.1

Mrs BH, a 53-year-old post-menopausal mother of two teenage children, has recently completed six cycles of FEC(100)-T (5-fluorouracil, epirubicin, cyclophosphamide, docetaxel) as adjuvant chemotherapy for her node-positive early breast cancer. She tolerated her chemotherapy well and did not require any dose reductions or delays.

Her receptor status at diagnosis was oestrogen receptor positive and progestogen receptor positive (ER+/PR+); she was also HER2 positive.

Her oncologist has recommended that she commences adjuvant treatment with trastuzumab.

Questions

1. What treatment regimen for trastuzumab should be followed?
2. How long will Mrs BH have to continue treatment with trastuzumab?
3. What other treatments should be considered for this patient?

Answers

1. Trastuzumab targets the epidermal growth factor receptor (EGFR) and is indicated for the treatment of early breast cancer overexpressing HER2 after surgery, chemotherapy (neo-adjuvant or adjuvant) and radiotherapy if applicable as recommended by NICE (2006a). The product license for trastuzumab recommends the dosing schedule used in the HERA study (Piccart-Gebhart et al., 2005), that is loading dose of 8 mg/kg body weight, followed by 6 mg/kg body weight 3 weeks later and then 6 mg/kg repeated at three-weekly intervals administered as infusions over approximately 90 minutes.

2. It is recommended to continue for 12 months, stopping sooner if disease reoccurs, or if unacceptable toxicity appears.
3. In view of her receptor status, this patient should be offered hormonal treatment. Depending on the perceived level of risk of recurrence as estimated using a model such as the Nottingham Prognostic Index (Galea et al., 1992), she should be offered either 5 years' treatment with an aromatase inhibitor or planned sequential treatment with tamoxifen, switching to an aromatase inhibitor after 2–3 years' therapy. The long-term effect on cardiovascular health (tamoxifen) or bone health (aromatase inhibitors) together with the expected level of benefits should be used to guide the choice of treatment. Further information can be found in national guidance for the early management of breast cancer with hormonal treatments (NICE, 2006a).

Case 53.2

Mr BS, a 67-year-old man with a history of localised prostate cancer, is reviewed by his oncologist. Mr BS was previously treated with radical radiotherapy and more recently several lines of hormonal therapy.

His PSA has risen over the last 6 months and is now 80 ng/mL. It was 0.1 ng/mL on completion of radical radiation therapy. He also complains that his longstanding back pain controlled by low-dose NSAIDs has now become much worse and is out of control.

Questions

1. What is the most likely cause of Mr BS's back pain and raised PSA?
2. What treatment options should be discussed with the patient?
3. Why should he be referred for a dental examination before commencing any further treatment?

Answers

1. The fact that the PSA is markedly raised suggests a recurrence of prostate cancer. Moderate rises in the PSA would have warranted a change in hormonal therapy. The elevated PSA together with the increased back pain suggests metastatic bone disease as a result of distant recurrence of his prostate cancer. This could be confirmed with plain film X-rays or by bone scan. The risk of both local and distant recurrence depends on the stage at presentation.
2. Treatment options for recurrent prostate cancer include further hormonal therapy, chemotherapy with or without corticosteroids, and best supportive care. Localised radiotherapy to specific bone lesions could improve his back pain; this would depend on the distribution of treatable lesions identified. The choice of therapy depends on the symptoms, the site of relapse, performance status of the patient and the presence of other comorbidities. Best supportive care can be provided with radiotherapy, bisphosphonates, steroids and analgesics and is the only option for patients who are too ill to tolerate further systemic intervention. Tolerability of chemotherapy is of concern, particularly because most patients with prostate cancer are elderly and many have other medical problems. Mr BS has already received more than one line of hormonal therapy; his tumour is unlikely to respond to further hormonal manipulation. An alternative strategy that is available is the use of radioactive isotopes such as Strontium 89 for systemic treatment of multiple bone metastases. The use of chemotherapy in the treatment of hormone-refractory prostate cancer should be considered in patients with a Karnofsky performance status of 60% or greater. Further information on the use of docetaxel for the treatment of hormone-refractory metastatic prostate cancer is available (NICE, 2006b).

3. Future treatment options for this patient may include the use of bisphosphonates to stabilise his bone lesions and reduce his pain. Long-term use of bisphosphonates has been associated with osteonecrosis of the jaw; the risk is exacerbated by poor dental hygiene, concurrent dental procedures, chemotherapy, corticosteroids and malignant disease. Examination and preventive dental treatment should be considered for patients before commencing therapy with bisphosphonates to avoid any invasive procedures, for instance, dental extraction, during bisphosphonate therapy.

Case 53.3

Mr SG, a 46-year-old patient, was diagnosed with colon cancer several months ago. Since then, he has undergone a left hemicolectomy. He is currently receiving capecitabine monotherapy as adjuvant treatment. He telephones the pharmacy department for advice on how to cope with the side effects he is currently experiencing.

Questions

1. What side effects are commonly associated with capecitabine?
2. How do these differ from those associated with intravenous 5FU?
3. What advice should Mr SG be given?

Answers

1. Side effects most commonly associated with capecitabine treatment are mainly related to the skin and the gastro-intestinal tract:
   - palmar–plantar erythema (hand–foot syndrome), 57%;
   - diarrhoea, 47%;
   - nausea, 35%;
   - stomatitis, 23%;
   - vomiting, 18%;
   - fatigue, 16%;
2. Although capecitabine is converted enzymatically to 5FU, there is a difference in the frequency with which specific side effects are experienced, making it more akin to continuous infusions of 5FU. Patients receiving intermittent bolus therapy with 5FU are more likely to experience the gastro-intestinal side effects, particularly diarrhoea or stomatitis, rather than the cutaneous reactions. Myelosuppression may also infrequently be a problem encountered by these patients.
3. Mr SG should be instructed to contact the emergency telephone number he would have been given with his treatment from the hospital looking after him, especially if there is any reason to suspect infection (e.g. feverishness).
   If detected early, side effects usually improve within 2–3 days. Treatment may be reinstated at the same dose if side effects are moderate, or at a reduced dose if more severe. Symptomatic relief for palmar–plantar erythema may be provided by the use of emollients. There is little evidence to support the use of specific antidotes.

Case 53.4

Mrs PQ, a 59-year-old woman, has non-small-cell lung cancer. She has had a course of gemcitabine combined with carboplatin and now requires second-line chemotherapy. The doctor has suggested erlotinib.

Questions

1. What type of treatment is erlotinib, and how is it given?
2. What common side effects should Mrs PQ be informed about when she is giving consent for treatment?
3. What other treatments should be considered for Mrs PQ?

Answers

1. Erlotinib is an epidermal growth factor receptor/human epidermal growth factor receptor type 1 (EGFR; also known as HER1) tyrosine kinase inhibitor. Erlotinib potently inhibits the intracellular phosphorylation of EGFR. Epidermal growth factor receptor is expressed on the cell surface of normal cells and cancer cells. In non-clinical models, inhibition of EGFR phosphotyrosine results in cell stasis and/or death. It is an oral tablet given once a day until disease progression or unacceptable toxicity.
2. Rash (75%) and diarrhoea (54%) were the most commonly reported adverse drug reactions (ADRs). In general, rash manifests as a mild or moderate erythematous and papulopustular rash, which may occur or worsen in skin areas exposed to the sun. For patients who are exposed to the sun, protective clothing, and/or use of sun screen (with minimum SPF 15, e.g. mineral-containing) may be advisable. The rash generally starts about 8–10 days after starting treatment but usually improves after a few weeks. Diarrhoea is usually mild and can be controlled with anti-diarrhoeal drugs. Fatigue, nausea and vomiting and sore mouth are also quite common. Some people also develop sore, red eyes (conjunctivitis) or dry eyes.
3. Cytotoxic therapy with docetaxel is an alternative second-line treatment currently available for the treatment of non-small-cell lung cancer, although the use of alternative targeted agents may also be available in some health-care systems.

Case 53.5

Mrs GH is a 64-year-old woman with lung cancer. She has had several cycles of chemotherapy and had her third cycle of cisplatin/vinorelbine 7 days ago. She is due her day 8 vinorelbine tomorrow. Mrs GH is feeling 'a bit unwell', and her husband thinks she is not at all her usual self and is, therefore, worried about her.

Questions

1. What side effect may Mrs GH be suffering from?
2. How would you explain to Mrs GH how to take her oral vinorelbine?
3. What are the possible patient safety concerns regarding oral chemotherapy?

Answers

1. Mrs GH may be suffering from neutropenic sepsis. The signs can be difficult to identify with a small elevation in temperature and a general feeling of not being well. If she is suffering from neutropenic sepsis, it is important that Mrs GH is prescribed i.v. antibiotics as soon as possible before she succumbs to an infection. Chemotherapy patients are all at varying degrees of risk of neutropenic sepsis due to the marked decrease in neutrophils in the body due to the chemotherapy. She should also have a blood test to check her neutrophil level, but the administration of antibiotics should not wait for these results. Each hospital will have guidelines or a protocol in place to treat neutropenic sepsis in patients receiving chemotherapy. She will need to call the hospital emergency chemotherapy number.
2. Take the vinorelbine dose on day 8 with a glass of water.

3. Healthcare workers and their staff must be made aware that the prescribing, dispensing and administering of oral anticancer medicines should be carried out and monitored to the same standard as injected therapy. This requires the following:
   - Healthcare organisations are to prepare local policies and procedures that describe the safe use of these oral medicines.
   - Treatment is to be initiated by a cancer specialist.
   - All oral anticancer medicines are to be prescribed only in the context of a written protocol and treatment plan

- Non-specialists who prescribe or administer ongoing oral anticancer medication must have ready access to appropriate written protocols and treatment plans.
- Staff dispensing oral anticancer medicines must be able to confirm that the prescribed dose is appropriate for the patient.
- Patients are to be fully informed and receive verbal and up-to-date written information about their oral anticancer therapy from the initiating hospital.

References

Berney, D.M., 2007. The case for modifying the Gleason grading system. Br. J. Urol. Int. 100, 725–726.

British Oncology Pharmacy Association, 2013. Standards for pharmacy verification of prescriptions for cancer medicines. Available at: http://www.bopawebsite.org/sites/default/files/publications/BOPA%20Standards%20for%20Clinical%20Pharmacy%20Verification%20of%20cancer%20medicine%20prescriptions%20V2.3%20FINAL%209.4.13.pdf.

British Oncology Pharmacy Association, 2015. Standards for reducing risks associated with e-prescribing systems for chemotherapy. Available at: http://www.bopawebsite.org/sites/default/files/publications/Standards_reducing_risks_associated_ePrescribing_systems_chemo2015.pdf.

Burnell, M., Levine, M.N., Chapman, J.A.W., et al., 2010. Cyclophosphamide, epirubicin, and fluorouracil versus dose-dense epirubicin and cyclophosphamide followed by paclitaxel versus doxorubicin and cyclophosphamide followed by paclitaxel in node-positive or high-risk node-negative breast cancer. J. Clin. Oncol. 28, 77–82.

Cancer Research UK, 2009. Dukes stages of bowel cancer. Available at http://www.cancerresearchuk.org/about-cancer/type/bowel-cancer/treatment/dukes-stages-of-bowel-cancer.

Cancer Research UK, 2016a. Cancer stats: cancer statistics for the UK. Available at: www.cancerresearchuk.org/cancer-info/cancerstats.

Cancer Research UK, 2016b. DPD deficiency and fluorouracil. Available at: http://www.cancerresearchuk.org/about-cancer/cancers-in-general/cancer-questions/dpd-deficiency-and-fluorouracil.

Doll, R., Peto, R., Boreham, J., et al., 2004. Mortality in relation to smoking: 50 years' observations on male British doctors. Br. Med. J. 328, 1519. Available at: http://www.bmj.com/content/328/7455/1519.

Galea, M.H., Blamey, R.W., Elston, C.E., et al., 1992. The Nottingham Prognostic Index in primary breast cancer. Breast Can. Res. Treat. 22, 207–219.

Garber, J.E., Offit, K., 2005. Hereditary cancer predisposition syndromes. J. Clin. Oncol. 23, 276–292.

Green, J.A., Kirwan, J.J., Tierney, J., et al., 2009. Concomitant chemotherapy and radiation therapy for cancer of the uterine cervix. Cochrane DB Syst. Rev. 2005 (3), Art. No CD002225. doi:10.1002/14651858.CD002225.pub2.

Herszényi, L., Farinati, F., Miheller, P., et al., 2008. Chemoprevention of colorectal cancer: feasibility in everyday practice? Eur. J. Cancer Prevent. 17, 502–514.

Hurwitz, H., Fehrenbacher, L., Novotny, W., et al., 2004. Bevacizumab plus irinotecan, fluorouracil and leucovorin for metastatic colorectal cancer. N. Engl. J. Med. 350, 2335–2342.

Jankowski, J., Boulton, E., 2005. Cancer prevention. Br. Med. J. 331, 618.

Karnofsky, D.A., Burchenal, J.H., 1949. The clinical evaluation of chemotherapeutic agents in cancer. In: MacLeod, C.M. (Ed.), Evaluation of Chemotherapeutic Agents. Columbia University Press, New York.

Levine, M., Whelan, T., 2006. Adjuvant chemotherapy for breast cancer – 30 years later. N. Engl. J. Med. 355, 1920–1922.

National Cancer Institute, 2010. National Cancer Institute Common Terminology Criteria for Adverse Events (CTCAE) v4.03. Available at: https://evs.nci.nih.gov/ftp1/CTCAE/CTCAE_4.03_2010-06-14_QuickReference_8.5x11.pdf.

National Institute for Health and Care Excellence (NICE), 2002. Guidance on the use of trastuzumab for the treatment of advanced breast cancer. NICE, London. Available at: https://www.nice.org.uk/guidance/ta34.

National Institute for Health and Care Excellence (NICE), 2006a. Trastuzumab for the adjuvant treatment of early-stage HER2-positive breast cancer. NICE, London. Available at: https://www.nice.org.uk/guidance/ta107.

National Institute for Health and Care Excellence (NICE), 2006b. Docetaxel for the treatment of hormone refractory prostate cancer. NICE, London. Available at: https://www.nice.org.uk/guidance/ta101.

National Institute for Health and Care Excellence (NICE), 2008. Cetuximab for the treatment of locally advanced squamous cell cancer of the head and neck. NICE, London. Available at: https://www.nice.org.uk/guidance/ta145.

National Institute for Health and Care Excellence (NICE), 2010. Trastuzumab for the treatment of HER2-positive metastatic gastric cancer. NICE, London. Available at: https://www.nice.org.uk/guidance/ta208/chapter/1-Guidance.

Oken, M., Creech, R., Tormey, D., et al., 1982. Toxicity and response criteria of the Eastern Cooperative Oncology Group. Am. J. Clin. Oncol. 5, 649–655.

Piccart-Gebhart, M.J., Procter, M., Leyland-Jones, B., et al., 2005. Trastuzumab after adjuvant chemotherapy in HER2-positive breast cancer (HERA Study). N. Engl. J. Med. 353, 1659–1672.

Sargent, D., Sobrero, A., Grothey, A., et al., 2009. Evidence for cure by adjuvant therapy in colon cancer: observations based on individual patient data from 20,898 patients on 18 randomized trials. J. Clin. Oncol. 27, 872–877.

Therasse, P., Arbuck, S.G., Eisenhauer, E.A., et al., 2000. New guidelines to evaluate the response to treatment in solid tumours. J. Natl. Cancer Inst. 92, 205–216.

Twelves, C., Scheithauer, W., McKendrick, J., et al., 2012. Capecitabine versus 5-fluorouracil/folinic acid as adjuvant therapy for stage III colon cancer: final results from the X-ACT trial with analysis by age and preliminary evidence of a pharmacodynamic marker of efficacy. Ann. Oncol. 23 (5), 1190–1197. Available at: http://annonc.oxfordjournals.org/content/23/5/1190.

Further reading

Centre for Pharmacy Postgraduate Education, 2015. CPPE cancer. Distance learning released. Available at: https://www.cppe.ac.uk/programmes/l/cancer-p-01/.

Devita, V.T., Lawrence, T.S., Rosenberg, S.A., et al., 2014. DeVita, Hellman, and Rosenberg's Cancer – principles and practice of oncology, tenth ed. Lippincott, Williams and Wilkins, Philadelphia.

Useful websites

British Oncology Pharmacy Association: http://www.bopawebsite.org
Cancer Research UK, cancer statistics: http://www.cancerresearchuk.org/cancer-info/cancerstats
National Extravasation Information Service: http://www.extravasation.org.uk

UK National Screening Committee, What is screening: definition: http://www.screening.nhs.uk/screening

54 Rheumatoid Arthritis and Osteoarthritis

Tina Hawkins

Key points

Rheumatoid arthritis

- Approximately 1% of the population worldwide is affected by rheumatoid arthritis.
- The peak age of onset in the UK is between 40 and 70 years.
- Rheumatoid arthritis is about two to four times more prevalent in women than in men.
- The cause of rheumatoid arthritis remains unclear.
- Disease-modifying anti-rheumatic drugs (DMARDs) should be commenced as soon as a diagnosis is made.
- Disease-modifying drugs include conventional DMARDs (e.g. methotrexate), biologic DMARDs (e.g. tumour necrosis factor inhibitors) and targeted synthetic agents (e.g. baricitinib and tofacitinib).
- Glucocorticoids are initiated while awaiting the onset of action of DMARDs.
- The ideal is clinical remission, or if this is not achievable low disease activity.
- Uncontrolled disease is associated with significant morbidity and early mortality.

Osteoarthritis

- Osteoarthritis is a degenerative disorder of the joints that commonly affects the knee, hip, hands and spine.
- It is the most common musculoskeletal condition in older people.
- The cause of osteoarthritis is unknown.
- Risk factors for the development of osteoarthritis include increasing age, obesity, gender, bone density, joint injury, occupation and genetics.
- No medical treatments are proven to prevent or delay the onset of osteoarthritis.
- Non-pharmacological measures such as weight loss, structured exercise programmes and supportive aids form the cornerstone of management.
- Pharmacological treatments such as paracetamol and topical or oral non-steroidal anti-inflammatory drugs are used as adjuncts to provide moderate symptomatic relief.

Rheumatoid arthritis

Rheumatoid arthritis (RA) is a chronic autoimmune condition characterised by inflammation of the synovium of joints combined with a number of additional systemic effect features resulting from abnormal immune response and secondary inflammation. Common joints affected include the proximal interphalangeal joints (PIPs) and metacarpophalangeal joints (MCPs) of the hands, wrists, knees, ankles and small joints of the feet. It is not purely a disease of the joints; extra-articular manifestations may affect the lungs, skin, blood, eyes and other organs of the body. There is no cure for RA. In early disease, management aims to suppress disease activity and induce remission, prevent loss of function, control joint damage, control pain and enhance self-management. Disease-modifying anti-rheumatic drugs (DMARDs) should be commenced upon diagnosis and adjusted in a timely manner to achieve the aim of clinical remission. In established disease, management should address complications and associated comorbidity, as well as the effect of the condition on the person's quality of life.

Epidemiology

Approximately 1% of the population worldwide is affected by RA. It is estimated that there are around 400,000 people with RA in the UK, and of these, approximately 15% have severe disease (National Institute for Health and Care Excellence [NICE], 2015a). RA is about two to four times more prevalent in women than in men. It can develop at any age, but the peak age of onset in the UK is between 40 and 70 years. Patients with RA have a shortened life expectancy and an increased risk of other diseases including cardiovascular and malignant disease (e.g. lymphoma). A poorer prognosis is associated with a positive rheumatoid factor (RF), raised inflammatory markers, early radiographic joint damage and the presence of tender/swollen joints. Early referral to a rheumatologist is essential.

Aetiology and pathophysiology

The cause of RA remains unclear, with hormonal, genetic and environmental factors playing a key role. Genetic factors contribute 53–65% of the risk of development of this disease. The HLA-DR4 allele is associated with both the development and severity of RA. There is now a large body of work that has identified a link between smoking and the incidence of RA. Smoking has been shown to reduce remission rates in men and women, but it causes a greater reduction in response to treatment in the male RA population (Inoue et al., 2015).

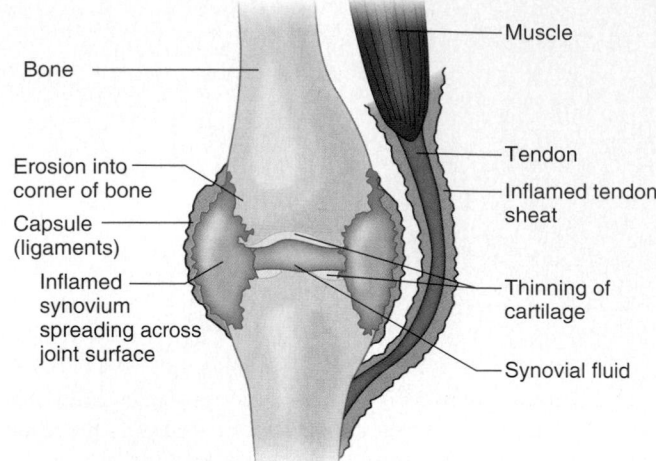

Fig. 54.1 Joint affected by rheumatoid arthritis. The inflamed synovium spread across the joint service forming a 'panus'. There is subsequent thinning of the cartilage and bone erosion. (Reproduced from Arthritis Research UK, with permission.)

More recent research has identified a relationship between periodontal inflammation and RA, although it is unclear whether periodontal disease is a trigger for RA, a propagating factor, a target of circulating autoimmunity or all three of these (Payne et al., 2015). An association has also been found between the microbiome of the gut (and other mucosal areas) and RA activity in Chinese patients; specifically, certain organisms were associated with changes in disease activity (Zhang et al., 2015).

Pathologically, RA is characterised by the infiltration of a variety of inflammatory cells into the joint. The synovial membrane, which is normally acellular, becomes highly vascularised and hypertrophied, creating a so-called pannus formation, as shown in Fig. 54.1. There is proliferation of synovial fibroblasts and an increase in the number of inflammatory cells present within the joint. The inflammatory cells involved in RA include T cells (predominantly CD4 helper cells), B cells, macrophages and plasma cells. Cytokines are released by these cells which cause the synovium to release proteolytic enzymes, resulting in the destruction of bone and cartilage. Key cytokines involved in RA include tumour necrosis factor (TNF)-α, interleukin-1 (IL-1), IL-6 and granulocyte macrophage colony-stimulating factor. These play a crucial role in the pro-inflammatory reaction.

Clinical manifestations

There are different patterns of clinical presentation of RA. The disease may present as a polyarticular arthritis with a gradual onset, intermittent or migratory joint involvement, or a monoarticular onset. In addition, extra-articular manifestations may be present (Box 54.1). Extra-articular features are associated with a poorer prognosis, but they are less commonly encountered now because of earlier diagnosis of the disease and earlier introduction of appropriate DMARD therapy.

Box 54.1 Examples of the extra-articular features of rheumatoid arthritis

- Amyloidosis
- Carpal tunnel syndrome
- Episcleritis
- Felty's syndrome
- Fever
- Lymphadenopathy
- Nodules; may be subcutaneous or within the lungs, eyes or heart
- Osteoporosis
- Pericarditis
- Pleural and pericardial effusions
- Scleritis
- Vasculitis

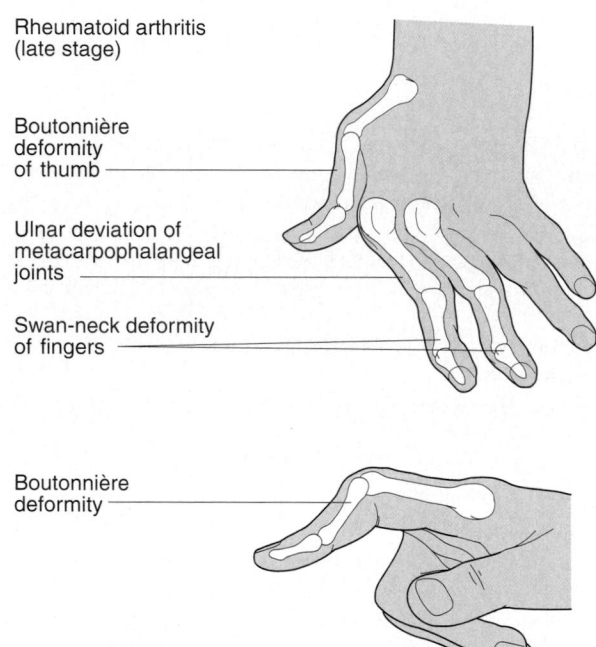

Fig. 54.2 Typical ulnar deviation, swan neck and boutonnière deformities.

Disease onset is usually insidious with the predominant symptoms being pain, stiffness and swelling. Typically, the metacarpophalangeal interphalangeal joints and PIPs of the fingers, interphalangeal joints of the thumbs, the wrists and metatarsophalangeal joints of the toes are affected during the early stages of the disease. RA-associated deformities affecting multiple joints of the hands are shown in Fig. 54.2. Other joints of the upper and lower limbs, such as the elbows, shoulders and knees, are also affected. Morning stiffness may last for 30 minutes to several hours and usually reflects the severity of joint inflammation. Up to one-third of patients also suffer from prominent myalgia, fatigue, low-grade fever, weight loss and depression at disease onset.

RA shows a marked variation of clinical expression in individual patients both in the number and pattern of joints affected, disease progression and the rapidity of joint damage. Disease activity may not abate in 10–20% of cases. Remission has been reported in a small proportion of patients but usually is rare without DMARDs.

Diagnosis

A clinical diagnosis of RA is made based on the patient's history, presenting symptoms and clinical findings. Family history is useful, as well as investigations including blood tests, ultrasound for the presence of synovitis and X-rays. The presence of joint destruction indicates that the disease may have been active for a period of time before a formal diagnosis being made.

Emphasis on early diagnosis and treatment is extremely important to prevent disease activity, duration and ultimately joint destruction. The American College of Rheumatology (ACR) and the European League Against Rheumatism (EULAR) use a score-based algorithm in diagnosing RA. The scoring system consists of four categories, A–D (Table 54.1), and a score of at least 6 out of 10 is required for a classification of RA. Parameters include the number and type of joints affected, the patient's serology (RF and anti-citrullinated antibodies), the presence of raised acute-phase reactants (C-reactive protein [CRP] and erythrocyte sedimentation rate [ESR]) and symptom duration.

Investigations

Inflammatory markers

Inflammatory markers, including CRP and ESR, are usually, but not always, elevated in active disease and are useful for monitoring response to treatment. It should be noted that CRP and ESR are non-specific and may be elevated as a consequence of other pathologies including infection and malignancy.

Serology

RF was the initial defining auto-antibody in RA. It is an antibody against the Fc portion of immunoglobulin G (IgG). RF and IgG combine to form complexes that contribute to the disease process. Although used as a test in the diagnosis of RA, a positive result may be due to another cause and a negative result does not rule out a diagnosis of RA. Approximately 80% of individuals with RA will be positive for RF, and it may precede symptom onset by years. The presence of RF in RA is associated with a poorer prognosis. Other conditions associated with an elevated RF include chronic hepatitis, primary biliary cirrhosis, chronic viral infection, bacterial endocarditis, leukaemia, dermatomyositis, infectious mononucleosis, systemic sclerosis and systemic lupus erythematosus (SLE).

Raised anti-citrullinated peptide antibodies (ACPAs), also referred to as anti-citrullinated protein antibodies (anti-CCPs), are a marker of RA. Post translational modification of arginine residues to citrulline is the antigen recognised, and it has a higher specificity for distinguishing RA from other rheumatic disease. The presence of ACPA/anti-CCP, like RF, often precedes symptom onset by years. The presence of ACPAs/anti-CCPs appears to be highly predictive of the future development of RA in both healthy individuals and patients with undifferentiated arthritis. Individuals who have ACPAs/anti-CCPs tend to have a poorer

Table 54.1 American College of Rheumatology/European League Against Rheumatism scoring algorithm for diagnosing rheumatoid arthritis (Kay and Upchurch, 2012)

Classification criteria for rheumatoid arthritis (score-based algorithm: add score of categories A–D)
A score of 6/10 is needed for classification of a patient as having definite rheumatoid arthritis

A	Joint Involvement	Score
	1 large joint	0
	2–10 large joints	1
	1–3 small joints (with or without involvement of large joints)	2
	4–10 small joints (with or without involvement of large joints)	3
	>10 joints (at least 1 small joint)	5
B	Serology (At Least 1 Test Result Is Needed for Classification)	Score
	Negative RF *and* negative ACPA	0
	Low-positive rheumatoid arthritis *or* low-positive ACPA	2
	High-positive rheumatoid arthritis *or* high-positive ACPA	3
C	Acute-Phase Reactants (At Least 1 Test Result Is Needed for Classification)	Score
	Normal CRP *and* normal ESR	0
	Abnormal CRP *or* abnormal ESR	1
D	Duration of Symptoms	Score
	<6 weeks	0
	≥6 weeks	1

ACPA, Anti-citrullinated protein antibody; CRP, C-reactive protein; ESR, erythrocyte sedimentation rate; RF, rheumatoid factor.

prognosis with an increased level of joint damage and lower remission rates compared with people who are not positive for these antibodies.

Auto-antibodies

Anti-nuclear antibodies (ANAs) are a prominent feature of auto-immune rheumatic diseases. Detection of these antibodies and their differing profiles plays an important part of the diagnostic process. ANAs are a diverse group of antibodies, often directed to large cellular complexes containing protein and nucleic acid components. The most frequently occurring ANAs react with components of deoxyribonucleic acid (DNA)–protein or ribonucleic acid (RNA)–protein complexes. Auto-antibodies are of value in situations where clinical expression of a disease such as SLE is incomplete; the presence of a particular ANA profile can be diagnostic of SLE.

Other blood parameters

Other abnormal laboratory tests include an elevated alkaline phosphatase, an elevated platelet count, raised plasma viscosity, a decreased serum albumin and a normochromic, normocytic anaemia. The white cell count, particularly neutrophils, is elevated in patients with infected joints and is elevated whilst the patient is on corticosteroids.

Disease activity

A patient's level of disease activity can be assessed with the Disease Activity Score of 28 joints (DAS28) (Box 54.2). The value is calculated from the number of tender and swollen joints, the patient's ESR or CRP, and a self-determined patient assessment of general health status according to a 100-mm visual analogue scale. A score >5.1 indicates high disease activity, ≥3.2 and up to 5.1 indicates moderate disease activity, between 3.2 and 2.6 indicates low disease activity, whereas <2.6 indicates remission. The DAS28 score is often used to determine when treatment with a biologic medicine should be commenced and to evaluate the patient's response to that treatment. In the UK the NICE requires the patient's DAS28 to be greater than 5.1

Box 54.2 Summary of DAS28 criteria in the assessment of rheumatoid arthritis

DAS28 is a composite formula. Four parameters are used to calculate a disease severity score:
1. number of swollen joints out of a total of 28 specified joints;
2. number of tender joints out of a total of 28 specified joints;
3. ESR or CRP level;
4. patient's interpretation of well-being, with 0 being at their best and 100 their worst.

Programmed calculators are used to determine the final DAS28. DAS28 does not take into account other features of a patient's disease, such as synovitis and other clinical symptoms.

High disease activity: DAS28 >5.1
Moderate disease activity: DAS28 >3.2–5.1
Low disease activity: DAS28 2.6–3.2
Remission: DAS28 <2.6

---

before treatment is permitted with a biologic therapy (NICE, 2016). However, drawbacks associated with using the DAS28 exist: some patients may not have particularly high inflammatory markers but still have severe disease, different patients may vary in their perception and reporting of their general health status, and secondary non-inflammatory factors such as the presence of degenerative disease can overestimate the DAS28.

The EULAR has developed criteria to assess the degree of change in DAS28 to determine good, moderate or non-response to treatment (Table 54.2). NICE permits continuation of treatment with a biologic therapy only if there is a moderate EULAR response 6 months after starting therapy.

Clinical trials assessing the efficacy of treatments for the management of RA often use the ACR response criteria (Box 54.3). This requires a specified improvement in tender joint count, swollen joint count, global assessments, pain, disability and an acute-phase reactant, for example, ESR or CRP. The ACR20 represents a 20% improvement in the patient's baseline ACR score. This is usually the minimum efficacy criteria for a medicine to achieve in a clinical trial for RA when compared with placebo or a comparative drug therapy. The ACR50 and ACR70 may also be assessed and represent a relative improvement from a baseline of 50% and 70%, respectively.

Treatment

There are four primary goals in the treatment of RA:
- symptom relief including pain control,
- slowing or prevention of joint damage,
- preserving and improving functional ability,
- achieving and maintaining disease remission.

Treatment should be aimed at reaching a target of remission or low disease activity in every patient; ideally this should be achieved within the first 6 months of starting treatment. Clinical remission is indicated by the absence of signs and symptoms of significant inflammatory disease activity. The ACR/EULAR have proposed two definitions for defining remission in RA for utilisation in clinical trials. One is a Boolean-based definition, as shown in Box 54.3; the other is a composite index of RA, the Simple Disease Activity Index (Felson et al., 2015).

A disease activity target should be set in all patients at the start of therapy and adaptations made to achieve this target. It can take up to 6 months to see the full benefit of disease-modifying

---

Table 54.2 EULAR response criteria (Fransen and van Riel, 2005)

DAS28 improvement → Present DAS28 ↓	>1.2	>0.6–1.2	≤0.6
≤3.2	Good response	Moderate response	No response
>3.2–5.1	Moderate response	Moderate response	No response
>5.1	Moderate response	No response	No response

Box 54.3 American College of Rheumatology/European League Against Rheumatism definitions of remission in rheumatoid arthritis clinical trials (Felson et al., 2015)

Boolean-based definition at any time point, patient must satisfy all of the following:
- tender joint count ≤1,
- swollen joint count ≤1,
- CRP ≤1 mg/dL,
- patient global assessment ≤1 (on a 0–10 scale).

A Simple Disease Activity Index score ≤3.3 at any time point: The simple sum of the tender joint count (using 28 joints), swollen joint count (using 28 joints), patient global assessment (0–10 scale), physician global assessment (0–10 scale), and CRP level (mg/dL).

medicines, but assessment of initial response is recommended at the 3-month stage (Smolen et al., 2017). If the individual has had only a minor response or no response at the 3-month stage, then he or she is unlikely to reach the target of remission at 6 months (Aletaha et al., 2016; Smolen et al., 2017).

Patients should have access to a multidisciplinary team (MDT) to address the pharmacological and non-pharmacological aspects of disease management. Education is extremely important because patients cope better if they understand their condition and have realistic expectations of the benefits and disadvantages of their treatment strategies. It is important that any therapeutic decision is jointly agreed with the patient. Shared decision making includes the need to inform the patient of the risks of RA and the benefits of reaching the targeted disease activity states, as well as the advantages and disadvantages of respective therapies. The individual should be empowered to make active decisions about his or her treatment and therapeutic goals in conjunction with the MDT.

Patients may need psychological support and employment counselling to help them adjust to living with their condition. Occupational therapy aims to provide support and aid to allow patients to improve function and limit disability in their activities of daily living. This includes devices to alleviate tasks that may be troublesome for those with restricted manual dexterity, such as twisting lids to open bottles. Physiotherapy involves assessment of function and designing a programme to aid pain relief and rehabilitation. The programme should aim to improve general fitness through regular exercise, and tailor exercises to the individual patient to enhance joint flexibility and muscle strength.

Drug treatment

The term DMARD is used to describe medicines used in the management of RA. For a medicine to be classified as a DMARD it should be able to demonstrate the capacity to inhibit structural damage to cartilage and bone. Historically there was only one category of DMARD, but due to the introduction of biologic medicines that alter the disease process and the newer targeted synthetic agents, there are now three categories of DMARD. The first category is conventional synthetic DMARDs (csDMARDs), such as methotrexate, hydroxychloroquine, sulfasalazine and leflunomide, which have been used for decades to manage RA. The second category of DMARDs is the biologic medicines (bDMARDs), such as the tumour necrosis factor inhibitors (TNFi's), abatacept, rituximab and the IL-6 inhibitors (tocilizumab and sarilumab). More recently a new group of medicines has been introduced (the third category), which inhibit the enzyme JAK-Kinase (baricitinib and tofacitinib). These have been defined as targeted synthetic DMARDs (tsDMARDs).

Low-dose corticosteroids may be used as part of the initial treatment strategy (first 6 months), in combination with csDMARDs, while awaiting the therapeutic onset of the csDMARD(s). The role of non-steroidal anti-inflammatory drugs (NSAIDs) in the management of RA has considerably changed over the last decade. Traditionally the therapeutic pyramid was employed whereby initial treatment was conservative, with the use of NSAIDs for several years and progression on to DMARDs when the disease was not controlled. This approach has been replaced now by early treatment with csDMARDs followed by bDMARDs, because there is evidence that most patients develop joint destruction within the first 2 years of their disease. Despite this, NSAIDs still continue to be prescribed as DMARDs are still not used optimally. Where there is residual inflammatory pain NSAIDs are effective in reducing stiffness and swelling associated with this. It is important that any NSAID use does not mask the need for modification of DMARDs.

Research is ongoing with regard to the dose tapering of DMARDs once the target of disease remission has been achieved. Findings suggest that therapies may be reduced and remission maintained in a subset of patients. If the individual has achieved a prolonged period of remission on combined csDMARDs and bDMARDs, in the absence of glucocorticoids, the dose tapering of the bDMARDs may be considered (Smolen et al., 2017). The rheumatologist in consultation with the patient may agree an individualised tapering plan.

Disease-modifying anti-rheumatic drugs (conventional/synthetic)

Early therapeutic intervention with csDMARDs can improve patient outcomes and reduce disease progression. All patients with a confirmed diagnosis of RA should be commenced on a csDMARD. csDMARDs commonly used in the management of RA include methotrexate, leflunomide, sulfasalazine and hydroxychloroquine (Table 54.3).

csDMARDs do not provide pain relief but do suppress the disease process. They have a delayed onset of action; it can be 4–6 weeks before the patient starts to see a response, and up to 4–6 months before a full response is achieved. The precise mechanism of action of these drugs is unclear. There is good evidence that csDMARDs inhibit the activity of inflammatory cytokines. Methotrexate and leflunomide have been shown to also inhibit T cells.

Practice may differ regarding the use of combination or csDMARD monotherapy following diagnosis. NICE encourages the use of combination csDMARD therapy, including methotrexate, in newly diagnosed RA. Where combination csDMARD therapy is not possible due to comorbidities, csDMARD monotherapy may be initiated with fast escalation to a clinically effective dose (NICE, 2015a). EULAR guidance states that both monotherapy

Table 54.3 Conventional synthetic disease-modifying anti-rheumatic drugs (csDMARDs) used in the treatment of rheumatoid arthritis

Name	Dosage	Adverse reactions	Monitoring Baseline	Long-term	Time period to benefit
Hydroxychloroquine	200–400 mg daily	Ocular toxicity, GI and visual disturbances	FBC eGFR LFT Visual acuity	Annual review with optometrist	2–3 months
Leflunomide	10–20 mg daily Loading dose is not commonly used in practice because of GI side effects	Weight loss, hypertension, GI disturbances, myelosuppression	FBC eGFR LFTs BP Weight	FBC, LFTs and eGFR every 2 weeks until patient has been on a stable dose for 6 weeks. Then monthly for 3 months and thereafter if stable 12 weekly. Monthly blood tests should be continued long-term if co-prescribed with another immunosuppressant or potentially hepatotoxic agent Regular BP and weight checks	8–12 weeks, although longer if the loading dose is not given
Methotrexate	7.5–25 mg once weekly	Hepatotoxicity, myelosuppression, pneumonitis, nausea and vomiting	FBC eGFR LFTs Chest X-ray	FBC, eGFR, LFTs every 2 weeks until methotrexate dose and monitoring stable for 6 weeks, then monthly thereafter until dose and disease stable for 1 year. Following this, reduction in frequency of monitoring may be considered depending on various patient factors, e.g. renal impairment	6 weeks to 3 months
Sodium aurothiomalate (IM gold)	10 mg test dose, then 50 mg weekly until significant response or total dose of 1000 mg has been given	Rash, oral ulceration, proteinuria, myelosuppression	FBC Urinalysis eGFR LFTs	FBC and urinalysis every 4 weeks	Usually when 500 mg cumulative dose has been reached
Sulfasalazine	500 mg to 3 g daily	GI disturbances, myelosuppression, hepatotoxicity	FBC eGFR LFTs	FBC and LFTs monthly for first 3 months, then every 3 months thereafter. Reduce frequency after first year if dose and results are stable	3 months

BP, Blood pressure; eGFR, estimated glomerular filtration rate; FBC, full blood count; GI, gastro-intestinal; IM, intramuscular; LFT, liver function test.

and combination therapy with csDMARDs are effective, and that patient preferences and expectations of adverse events should be considered when discussing treatment options (Smolen et al., 2017). Ideally combination therapy with csDMARDs should include methotrexate, because other combinations have not been sufficiently studied. Whether using combination or monotherapy, it is important that there is frequent monitoring of disease activity, with timely dose titration and the introduction of new therapies to reach the ideal therapeutic target for disease remission.

Methotrexate. Methotrexate is highly effective in the management of RA both as a monotherapy and on the basis of its ability to increase the efficacy of biologic medicines when used in combination. It is therefore considered the 'anchor drug' in RA (Smolen et al., 2014). No other csDMARD has shown superiority in terms of clinical efficacy; meta-analyses have confirmed TNFi monotherapy is not superior to methotrexate in improving signs and symptoms, although they do have a superior effect on radiographic progression (Smolen et al., 2014).

Methotrexate is generally used as a first-line agent, unless comorbidity precludes. It has an onset of action of approximately 1 month and can be given either orally or by subcutaneous or intramuscular injection. It tends to be given by injection when patients are unable to tolerate oral doses because of gastric side effects, or where doses of 25 mg or more weekly are being given.

Box 54.4 Important points to cover when counselling a patient who is receiving methotrexate

- Why the patient is taking methotrexate
- How long it will take for methotrexate to work
- The dose and the frequency
- For oral methotrexate the strength and number of tablets
- The importance of regular blood monitoring
- The side effects including warnings symptoms for urgent referral to the doctor
- Interactions with other medicine, including over-the-counter and herbal remedies
- The need for adequate contraception in males and females
- Inform healthcare professionals that methotrexate is prescribed

The starting dose varies according to clinician preference and patient tolerability. Common starting doses are 10 or 15 mg/week, but where there are concerns about tolerability the lower starting dose of 7.5 mg/week may be prescribed. Ideally the optimal dose of methotrexate (25–30 mg weekly) or maximum tolerated dose should be achieved within a few weeks and maintained for at least 8 weeks, because maximum effect of methotrexate is attained only after 4–6 months. Common side effects include mouth ulcers (stomatitis) and nausea. Methotrexate reversibly inhibits the enzyme dihydrofolate reductase, resulting in a lowering of serum folate; supplementation with folic acid is given to counteract this side effect. Folic acid tends to be given as a 5 mg once-daily dose, although other regimens are used including a once-weekly dose. Most regimens omit the folic acid dose on the day of methotrexate therapy to avoid any potential impact on the latter's efficacy.

The use of methotrexate has been associated with haematological, hepatic and pulmonary toxicity. Because of methotrexate's potential to suppress bone marrow and cause liver toxicity it is essential that certain blood tests be performed regularly on patients who are taking methotrexate. All patients should have the following baseline blood tests: full blood count (FBC), estimate of glomerular filtration rate (eGFR), and albumin and liver function tests (LFTs). These should then be performed regularly throughout the course of treatment (see Table 54.3). Lower doses and slower dose titration are indicated in the presence of moderate renal impairment, and in the presence of severe impairment the use of methotrexate should be avoided.

Although methotrexate is a safe medicine when used appropriately, deaths have occurred as a consequence of patients taking this medicine incorrectly. The patient must understand how and when to take the medicine, plus the need for regular blood monitoring. It must be quite clear that the medicine is taken only once a week. The patient should also be re-counselled every time they are issued with a prescription for methotrexate irrespective of how long they have been receiving treatment (Box 54.4).

The National Patient Safety Agency (NPSA) in England has issued guidance on the prescribing and dispensing of oral methotrexate (NPSA, 2004). The guidance recommends that all patients who are taking methotrexate should be issued with a core patient information leaflet and a handheld methotrexate monitoring booklet. The prescriber should provide the patient with information about the benefits and risks of treatment with methotrexate. The term 'as directed' should not be used on a prescription, and patients should be quite clear on the number of tablets they are taking and on which day of the week. There should also be consistency on the strength of the tablet issued; ideally patients should remain on the 2.5 mg strength to avoid confusion. When issuing the medication to the patient, clearly explain which is the methotrexate container and which is the folic acid container, so the patient is able to differentiate between the two. Patients should be aware of certain signs and symptoms that may suggest toxicity, such as increased breathlessness, a dry, persistent cough, unexplained sore throat, or vomiting and diarrhoea, and who to contact if they experience these side effects. Most rheumatology departments operate a telephone helpline, staffed by specialist nurses, which patients can contact if they are experiencing side effects because of their rheumatology medication.

Leflunomide. In cases of methotrexate contraindications (or early intolerance), leflunomide or sulfasalazine may be considered as alternatives to methotrexate as part of the initial treatment strategy. Both sulfasalazine and leflunomide have shown clinical, functional and structural efficacy, and although methotrexate doses in respective comparative trials may not have been optimal, both have shown efficacies similar to methotrexate (Smolen et al., 2014).

Leflunomide has both immunomodulatory and immunosuppressive characteristics. It inhibits the synthesis of pyrimidine nucleotides in response cells (particularly T cells) and reduces pro-inflammatory cytokines (TNF and IL-6). Studies have shown it to be at least as effective as sulfasalazine and methotrexate, and for quality-of-life measures some evidence suggests superiority. When given as a loading dose of 100 mg daily for 3 days followed by a maintenance dosage of 10–20 mg daily its therapeutic effect starts after 4–6 weeks, and further improvement may be seen for up to 4–6 months. However, many centres do not use this loading dose regimen, because patients are unable to tolerate the gastro-intestinal side effects associated with it. The use of leflunomide has been associated with both haematological and hepatotoxic side effects. FBC, eGFR, albumin and LFTs must be performed before therapy is initiated and then every 2 weeks until on a stable dose for 6 weeks, then once monthly for 3 months and then every 12 weeks (Ledingham et al., 2017). When leflunomide and methotrexate are used in combination extra caution is advised, and patients should be monitored closely because of the increased risk of hepatotoxicity. Leflunomide can also cause hypertension: blood pressure should be checked before commencing leflunomide and periodically thereafter. Both men and women who are taking leflunomide are required to use adequate contraceptive measures during treatment and for at least 2 years after treatment in women and at least 3 months after treatment in men. If the individual plans to conceive before completion of this period, then a washout protocol must be followed. This involves treatment with cholestyramine or activated charcoal and measuring the concentration of the active metabolite. A washout protocol may also be used if a patient develops a toxic side effect caused by treatment with leflunomide or there is a need to switch to a different DMARD.

Sulfasalazine. Sulfasalazine (enteric coated) is indicated in mild-to-moderate disease. It has an onset of action of 6–12 weeks. To reduce the side effect of nausea, the dose is usually titrated upwards from 500 mg daily, increasing at weekly intervals to 1 g twice daily. Haematological abnormalities have occurred rarely with the use of sulfasalazine, and patients should be counselled to report unexplained bleeding, bruising, purpura, sore throat, fever or malaise. Patients should also be warned that sulfasalazine can colour urine red and stain contact lenses. Baseline FBCs and LFTs should be performed on patients taking sulfasalazine and repeated intermittently throughout the course of treatment (see Table 54.3). Sulfasalazine is considered safe in pregnancy when given in combination with folic acid. In males it may cause oligospermia, which can be reversed within 2–3 months of stopping treatment.

Hydroxychloroquine and chloroquine. The antimalarial drugs hydroxychloroquine and chloroquine may be used in milder disease. They show some efficacy as a monotherapy with respect to the signs and symptoms of RA, but they have not been shown to inhibit structural damage sufficiently when compared with other csDMARDs. They are often combined with other csDMARDs in the management of RA (Katz and Russell, 2011). There is a rare risk of retinopathy associated with their use, so patients should have an annual eye check and be informed to report any changes in vision or how they perceive colours.

Other conventional synthetic disease-modifying antirheumatic drugs. Injectable gold (sodium aurothiomalate) has been shown to be efficacious in the management of RA, but its use is limited because of an unfavourable side-effect profile. Due to the risk of anaphylaxis, an initial 10 mg test dose should be given in the first week of treatment followed by a maintenance dose of 50 mg the following week. Administration is by deep intramuscular injection. Patients should be monitored for 30 minutes following each dose. FBC and urine should be checked before giving the next full dose of 50 mg intramuscularly. The maintenance dose of 50 mg every week is given until the first signs of remission occur. At this point the interval between injections is extended to 2 weeks until full remission occurs. The interval between injections can then be increased progressively to 3 weeks, 4 weeks, and then, after 18 months to 2 years, to 6 weeks.

Penicillamine is no longer used in the management of RA because of its poor side-effect profile and lack of efficacy compared with other agents.

Azathioprine and ciclosporin may be used occasionally for progressive disease refractory to other csDMARDs or where a biologic agent is contraindicated. Azathioprine may also be used as a steroid-sparing agent. Azathioprine is an oral purine analogue that inhibits lymphocyte proliferation. It becomes biologically active after metabolism by the liver to 6-mercaptopurine. Bone marrow suppression and liver toxicity are associated with its use, and FBCs and LFTs should be performed during treatment. Renal function should also be monitored because the drug is renally excreted. Ciclosporin works by impairing the function of B and T lymphocytes. Dose-related hypertension and nephrotoxicity are common side effects. FBCs should be performed during treatment, and liver and renal function monitored. Ciclosporin drug levels are not routinely measured when it is used for the management of RA.

Glucocorticoids

Glucocorticoids act by inhibiting cytokine release and give rapid relief of symptoms and decrease inflammation. Depending on the number of affected joints, corticosteroids may be injected directly into the joint (intra-articular), given as an intramuscular depot injection or given as short-term oral therapy. The standard intramuscular dose used is 120 mg methylprednisolone, and oral starting doses can be up to 30 mg once a day of prednisolone. For very severe disease, particularly where there are extra-articular manifestations, pulsed intravenous infusions of methylprednisolone (e.g. 250 mg) may be given in rare instances, but this approach is less common now because of the availability of more modern therapies.

Glucocorticoids are often used as a bridging therapy to reduce symptoms and disease activity when waiting for the therapeutic onset of a csDMARD or when changing from one csDMARD to another. In addition they have been shown to be effective adjunctive treatments with the main csDMARD therapy to more efficiently achieve the desired target (usually clinical remission). Treatment with glucocorticoids should ideally be short-term, and they should be gradually withdrawn as soon as it is clinically feasible according to disease activity. Ideally treatment should be gradually reduced and stopped by 3 months (Smolen et al., 2017). In more refractory cases it may be more difficult to withdraw treatment with glucocorticoids because the individual's disease tends to flare as the dose is reduced. A reducing rate as slow as 1 mg/month may even be necessary in some patients. In rare instances where there is intolerance, contraindications or therapeutic failure with DMARDs, it may be necessary to continue with a small maintenance dose of glucocorticoid.

The long-term side effects of corticosteroids include osteoporosis, peptic ulceration, diabetes mellitus and hypertension. Oral glucocorticoid treatment with greater than 5 mg prednisolone daily can lead to a reduction in bone mineral density and a rapid dose-dependent increase in the risk of fracture (van Staa, 2006). The risks are highest during the initial stages of treatment. In patients exposed to high-dose and/or long-term corticosteroid, consideration should be given to the need for bone protection with a bisphosphonate and calcium plus vitamin D supplementation. Gastric protection, such as a proton pump inhibitor, should be co-prescribed with glucocorticoids in patients with risk factors for peptic ulcer disease, for example, the elderly and concomitant NSAID use. Although hypothalamic–pituitary–adrenal axis suppression may vary greatly from person to person, it should be anticipated in any patient receiving more than 7.5 mg prednisolone or equivalent daily for more than 3 weeks (Cooper and Stewart, 2003). The importance of not stopping glucocorticoid therapy suddenly should be explained to the patient. Health professionals should also consider the need for replacement therapy during acute illness in patients with RA who have received glucocorticoids for a prolonged period.

Non-steroidal anti-inflammatory drugs

NSAIDs are effective in reducing the pain, swelling and stiffness associated with RA; however, it is important that their use does not mask the need for optimisation of DMARD therapy.

The mechanism of action of NSAIDs involves the inhibition of cyclo-oxygenase-1 (COX-1) and/or COX-2. COX-1 catalyses the production of prostaglandins involved in various physiological functions, that is, the maintenance of renal function, mucosal protection in the gastro-intestinal tract and platelet activation. COX-2 is expressed as part of the inflammatory response, resulting in vasodilation, platelet inhibition and inhibition of smooth cell proliferation. The inhibition of COX-2 by NSAIDs plays a role in mediating pain, fever and inflammation. Non-selective NSAIDs inhibit both COX-1 and COX-2 enzymes. Inhibition of COX-1 results in an increased risk of gastro-intestinal bleeding. COX-2 selective NSAIDs were developed to maintain analgesic efficacy while minimising gastro-intestinal side effects associated with COX-1 inhibition. Two licensed COX-2 inhibitors are available in the UK: celecoxib and etoricoxib. Despite the potential gastro-intestinal benefit of COX-2 selective NSAIDs, they have been shown to have a higher risk of cardiovascular events. A large meta-analysis found that compared with placebo, the risk of major vascular events was increased by 33% in patients taking COX-2 selective agents or diclofenac (Bhala et al., 2013). The proposed mechanism of cardiovascular toxicity associated with NSAIDs is inhibition of the cardioprotective prostaglandin I_2 that is generated by COX-2. Naproxen is proposed to have a lower cardiovascular risk compared with the other licensed NSAIDs (Trelle et al., 2011). The use of NSAIDs increases the risk of gastro-intestinal toxicity, such as the development of peptic ulcer disease, upper gastro-intestinal haemorrhage or perforation. The risk of these complications may vary among NSAIDs. Agents such as ibuprofen and celecoxib have a lower relative risk of gastro-intestinal complications, while piroxicam and ketoprofen have been shown to have a higher relative risk (Castellsague et al., 2012). Chronic NSAID use can lead to kidney impairment due to direct and indirect effects on the kidney. The use of NSAIDs can increase blood pressure, cause fluid retention and decrease kidney function in patients with kidney disease. It should also be noted that 10% of total drug-induced hepatotoxicity is NSAID related (Bessone, 2010).

NICE guidance on the management of RA recommends that both non-selective NSAIDs and COX-2 inhibitors are prescribed at their lowest effective dose for the shortest period of time. Whether the NSAID is selective or non-selective, a proton pump inhibitor should always be co-prescribed. As the analgesic effect of NSAIDs is the same, selection should be based upon the patient's individual risk factors. If a person with RA needs to be prescribed low-dose aspirin, prescribers should consider other analgesics before substituting or adding an NSAID or a COX-2 inhibitor (with a proton pump inhibitor) if pain relief is ineffective or insufficient (NICE, 2015a).

Biologic disease-modifying anti-rheumatic drugs

Biologic therapies used in RA target specific immune-mediated pathways involved in the pathophysiology of the condition. They are derived from living cells through highly complex manufacturing processes. Biologic medicines used in RA may exist as a whole antibody (e.g. monoclonal antibody) or a specific fragment of an antibody, usually the binding site portion (e.g. fusion protein). Monoclonal antibodies may also be fully humanised (fully humanised monoclonal antibody) or partially humanised, where they consist of a combination of both animal and human proteins (chimeric monoclonal antibody).

bDMARDs have markedly changed the management and outcome of RA. Current biologic therapies available for the management of RA include the TNFi's, as well as abatacept, tocilizumab and rituximab. These medicines now form part of the standard treatment strategy for RA, and NICE recommends the use of a biologic medicine in patients with a DAS28 greater than 5.1 whose disease has not responded to intensive therapy with a combination of csDMARDs (NICE, 2016).

Biosimilars. As patents for biologic medicines near their expiry, pharmaceutical manufacturers have taken steps to develop medicines with equivalent therapeutic effect to their branded counterparts, but with a considerably lower acquisition cost. These new medicines have been classified as 'biosimilars'. NHS England (2015, p. 5) defines biosimilar medicines as: 'a biological medicine which is highly similar to another biological medicine already licensed for use. It is a biological medicine which has been shown not to have any clinical meaningful differences from the originator biological medicine in terms of quality, safety and efficacy'. Biosimilar medicines have specific European Union (EU) regulatory pathways that differ from the authorisation process applied to generic medicines. The licensing process for biosimilars includes a head-to-head comparison of randomised controlled trial (RCT) data. There should be no clinically significant difference between the biosimilar and the original reference product. Biosimilar medicines are not required to have comparative phase III clinical trial data for all the indications of the original product. The information submitted to the European Medicines Authority (EMA) by the manufacturer of the biosimilar should be of sufficient quality and quantity to allow 'extrapolation' by the EMA to all the indications of the original reference product.

Biosimilar products for the management of RA have already been introduced into the UK market. The TNFi's infliximab and etanercept are now available as biosimilars. Biosimilar medicines are also in clinical development for other biologics including adalimumab and rituximab. Multiple branded products will become available for each biologic medicine. It is important that all prescriptions for a biologic medicine available as both the original reference drug and as a biosimilar specifically state the brand name of the desired product to avoid confusion. Due to the complex nature of these medicines there is a risk that small differences between the products could potentially affect response. Prescribing by brand ensures the patient is maintained on the same product.

Tumour necrosis factor inhibitors. TNF-α and IL-1 are pro-inflammatory cytokines that are present in the synovial fluid and tissue. In RA they are produced in excess. Blocking of TNF-α by TNFi agents results in dampening of the inflammatory cascade and blocking of IL-1 activity. TNFi therapy has been shown to reduce the signs and symptoms of RA, improve physical function and slow the progression of joint damage. Five originator TNFi's are currently available in the UK: adalimumab, certolizumab, etanercept, golimumab and infliximab. At the time of writing this chapter, three biosimilar infliximab products plus two etanercept biosimilar are available (Table 54.4).

Table 54.4 Current licensed tumour necrosis factor inhibitors available in the UK for rheumatoid arthritis

Adalimumab (Humira)	Etanercept (Enbrel, Benepali)	Certolizumab (Cimzia)	Golimumab (Simponi)	Infliximab (Remicade, Inflectra, Remsima, Flixabi)
Humanised monoclonal antibody	P75 fc fusion protein	Fab fragment	Humanised monoclonal antibody	Chimeric human/murine antibody
Dose in RA Subcutaneous injection 40 mg alternate weeks	Dose in RA Subcutaneous injection 50 mg once a week or 25 mg twice a week	Dose in RA Subcutaneous injection 400 mg at weeks 0, 2 and 4 and then 200 mg on alternate weeks	Dose in RA Subcutaneous injection 50 mg once a month increased to 100 mg per month in patients >100 kg	Dose in RA Intravenous infusion 3 mg/kg at weeks 0, 2 and 6, then 8 weekly
RA with or without MTX	RA with or without MTX	RA with or without MTX	RA: must be in combination with MTX	RA: must be in combination with MTX
Licensed for: RA JIA PsA Axial spondyloarthritis AS Crohn's disease UC HS	Licensed for: RA JIA PsA Axial spondyloarthritis AS Plaque psoriasis	Licensed for: RA Axial spondyloarthritis AS PsA	Licensed for: RA + MTX PsA +/ MTX Axial spondyloarthritis AS UC	Licensed for: RA + MTX PsA +/− MTX AS Psoriasis Crohn's disease UC

AS, Ankylosing spondylitis; HS, hidradenitis suppurativa; JIA, juvenile idiopathic arthritis; MTX, methotrexate; PsA, psoriatic arthritis; RA, rheumatoid arthritis; UC, ulcerative colitis.

The market authorisations for adalimumab, etanercept and certolizumab approve use in combination with methotrexate or as monotherapy. However, infliximab and golimumab should be administered in combination with methotrexate for the management of RA. At present TNFi monotherapy has failed to demonstrate superiority over methotrexate alone, whereas combination therapy has. Current European guidance suggests a dosage of 10 mg or more weekly of methotrexate (where not contraindicated) with all TNFi's until additional evidence becomes available (Smolen et al., 2014). NICE permits the use of adalimumab, etanercept, and certolizumab pegol as monotherapy where methotrexate is contraindicated or not tolerated (NICE, 2016).

Adalimumab is a recombinant human monoclonal antibody that binds specifically to TNF-α and neutralises its biological function by blocking its interaction with cell surface TNF-α receptors. Due to it being a fully humanised monoclonal antibody, it is less likely to engender an immune response in the recipient than agents that contain non-human or artificial sequences. It is used in combination with methotrexate in patients with moderate-to-severe active RA who have had an inadequate response to csDMARDs, including methotrexate. Adalimumab is administered as a 40 mg subcutaneous injection every other week. It can be used as monotherapy in patients who are intolerant of methotrexate, or where methotrexate is contraindicated. When given as monotherapy, the dose may be increased to 40 mg once a week where there is a decrease in response.

Certolizumab pegol consists of a portion of a recombinant, humanised monoclonal antibody (fab fragment) bound to polyethylene glycol (PEG). The PEG portion increases the half-life to approximately 14 days, which is that of a whole antibody, and is much longer than the half-life of unconjugated fab fragments. The formulation was developed to address concerns that some of

the toxicity associated with infliximab and adalimumab might be caused by the effects of the Fc portion of the antibody such as complement activation and antibody-dependent cell-mediated cytotoxicity. Certolizumab pegol, in combination with methotrexate, is indicated for the treatment of moderate-to-severe active RA in adult patients when the response to csDMARDs, including methotrexate, has been inadequate. Certolizumab pegol can be given as monotherapy in case of intolerance to methotrexate or when continued treatment with methotrexate is inappropriate. The recommended starting dose of certolizumab pegol for adult patients with RA is 400 mg (as two subcutaneous injections of 200 mg each on one day) at weeks 0, 2 and 4, followed by a maintenance dose of 200 mg every 2 weeks. Full clinical response to certolizumab pegol should be achieved within the first 12 weeks of treatment. If the desired therapeutic response has not been achieved at this point, then treatment with certolizumab pegol should be discontinued.

Etanercept is a recombinant human soluble TNF-α receptor. It competitively inhibits the activity of TNF-α by binding to its cell surface receptors. It can be used as monotherapy or in combination with methotrexate for the treatment of moderate-to-severe active RA. It is given by subcutaneous injection, either 25 mg twice weekly or 50 mg once weekly. The patent for the original reference drug (Enbrel) has now expired, and etanercept is now available as a biosimilar (Benepali and Erelzi). Etanercept should therefore be prescribed according to its brand name.

Golimumab is a human monoclonal antibody that forms high-affinity, stable complexes with both the soluble and transmembrane bioactive forms of human TNF-α, thus preventing the binding of TNF-α to its receptors. It must be administered in combination with methotrexate, and it is licensed for the treatment of moderate-to-severe active RA, following an inadequate response

Box 54.5 Screening tests to be performed before commencing biologic disease-modifying anti-rheumatic drugs

- Full clinical/infection screen to exclude the presence of infection
- Urea and electrolytes plus urinalysis
- FBC
- Chest radiograph to exclude infection, TB or lung fibrosis
- QuantiFERON-TB or T Spot to establish TB status
- Hepatitis B and C screening
- Assess risk factors for HIV and consider screening
- Check vaccination status
- Check family/patient history with regards to demyelinating disease
- Previous history of malignancy
- Antibody profile: ANAs and DNA
- Check blood pressure and review cardiac function

ANA, Anti-nuclear antibodies; DNA, deoxyribonucleic acid; FBC, full blood count; HIV, human immunodeficiency virus; TB, tuberculosis.

Box 54.6 Factors that influence biologic disease-modifying anti-rheumatic drug selection

Perform a risk–benefit assessment taking into account the following factors:
1. Disease characteristics: serological status (RF +ve or −v) and CRP level
2. Concomitant methotrexate or monotherapy
3. Comorbidities: relative versus absolute contraindications to biologics
4. Concomitant immune-mediated inflammatory diseases, e.g. psoriasis and IBD
5. The ability to self-inject

CRP, C-reactive protein; IBD, inflammatory bowel disease; RF, rheumatoid factor.

to csDMARDs or following failure or intolerance to other TNFi's. In RCTs it has demonstrated efficacy in patients with RA who have not responded positively to one to two previous TNFi's. Clinical response is usually seen after 12–14 weeks of treatment. It requires less frequent administration than the other subcutaneous TNFi's and is given once a month. The starting dosage is 50 mg by subcutaneous injection once a month; patients who weigh more than 100 kg should have their dose increased to 100 mg/month if they have not achieved an adequate response after three or four doses. If an adequate response is not achieved following administration of three or four doses of 100 mg, treatment should be discontinued.

Infliximab is a chimeric human–murine monoclonal antibody that binds with high affinity to both soluble and transmembrane forms of TNF-α, leading to inhibition of its functional activity. Infliximab is the only TNFi that is given by intravenous infusion. It must be given concomitantly with methotrexate. The recommended dosage in RA is 3 mg/kg. The initial infusion is given over a 2-hour period; subsequent infusions are given 2 and 6 weeks after the first. The patient is then maintained on 8-weekly maintenance infusions. Due to it being not fully humanised there is a higher risk of the development of human anti-chimeric antibodies (HACAs) against infliximab. The development of HACAs may result in a loss of therapeutic effect and an increased risk of infusion reaction. Methotrexate is co-administered to reduce the risk of development of HACA. Blood tests are now available for determination of infliximab plasma blood levels; a drop in the plasma level may be indicative of the development of antibodies to infliximab. Due to the availability of biosimilar infliximab, all prescriptions for infliximab should include the brand name of the product to avoid inadvertently switching to an alternative product.

Screening and safety issues associated with tumour necrosis factor inhibitors. Before commencing a TNFi, a number of important screening tests should be performed (Box 54.5) and a risk–benefit assessment be made (Box 54.6). The use of TNFi's has been associated with an increased incidence of infection and reactivation of latent tuberculosis (TB). Tests to establish TB immune status (QuantiFERON-TB or T Spot) should be performed in addition to a chest radiograph. A small minority of

patients have experienced lupus-like symptoms while receiving TNFi, and it is important to test for the presence of autoantibodies that may predispose the individual to development of a lupus-type reaction. Live vaccinations are not permitted while receiving TNFi's; therefore, the individual's vaccine status should be evaluated before commencing treatment and appropriate vaccines given. It should be noted that the influenza and pneumococcal vaccines can be administered while receiving treatment with a TNFi because these are non-live vaccines. In rare instances neurological complications have been associated with TNFi use, and it is therefore important to establish any background history of demyelinating disorders before treatment commences.

The presence of infection should be excluded before commencing a patient on a TNFi. In addition, the risks and benefits of commencing TNFi in certain patient groups should be carefully considered. TNFi's may be avoided in circumstances such as patients with chronic leg ulcers, septic arthritis in a native joint within the last 12 months, sepsis in a prosthetic joint in the last 12 months (if the joint remains in situ), persistent or recurrent chest infections, or indwelling urinary catheter and bronchiectasis (associated with frequent chest infection). Although data from RCTs and the British Society for Rheumatology (BSR) Biologic Registry failed to demonstrate an increase in treatment-related serious infections, data from the meta-analysis of RCTs and the German registries suggest that TNFi use is associated with an increased risk of serious infections, particularly early on in the course of therapy (Humphreys et al., 2016). An increased incidence of opportunistic and fungal infections has also been associated with treatment with a TNFi.

There is a well-established increased risk of TB associated with TNFi therapy, with registry data (from the British and French registries) demonstrating a greater risk associated with anti-TNF monoclonal antibodies as opposed to fusion protein (Humphreys et al., 2016). Before commencing treatment with TNFi therapy, all patients should be screened for mycobacterial infection. Active mycobacterial infection needs to be adequately treated before TNFi can be started. Where there is evidence of potential latent TB, the need for prophylactic treatment should be considered. Patients should be continued to be monitored for the development of mycobacterial infections during treatment and for 6 months after stopping.

Conflicting data exist on the role of TNFi and heart failure. Demonstration of worsening of moderate-to-severe heart failure in initial trials that evaluated TNFi for heart failure (Chung et al., 2003; Mann et al., 2004) underlines the need for accurate assessment of cardiac function in all patients with pre-existing heart failure before considering treatment with TNFi. Treatment is contraindicated in moderate-to-severe impairment (New York Heart Association [NYHA] class III/IV) and should be used with caution in patients with mild heart failure (NYHA class I/II). Treatment with anti-TNF should be discontinued in patients who develop new or worsening symptoms of congestive heart failure.

Rare cases of SLE and vasculitis (ANCA associated) have been reported in association with TNFi treatment. SLE symptoms occurred 3–6 months after starting therapy and included fever, malaise, arthritis, discoid lupus rash, erythematous facial rash and hypertension. These resolved 6–14 weeks after stopping therapy. TNFi therapy should be stopped if symptoms of an SLE-like syndrome develop.

There are a number of reports of demyelination and acute neurological complications associated with TNFi therapy (although registry data have not led to a clear signal); nevertheless, because of this, TNFi therapy should not be given to patients with a history of demyelinating disease and should be carefully considered if there is a strong family history of demyelination. Therapy should be stopped if signs or symptoms suggestive of demyelination develop.

Concerns have previously been raised about the increased risk of cancer associated with anti-TNF therapy. It is important to be aware that RA itself and continued disease activity is associated with a greater risk of cancer (particularly lymphoma) than the general population. For TNFi, overall long-term registry data have been reassuring, with no conclusive evidence for an increase in solid tumours or lymphoproliferative disease with the anti-TNF therapies above that which would be expected for the rest of the RA population. However, this continues to be monitored closely (Ding et al., 2010). There does appear to be an increased risk of non-melanoma skin cancers with anti-TNF therapies, and patients should be counselled on appropriate skin protection (Ding et al., 2010).

It should be noted that limited data are available on the newer licensed TNFi, certolizumab pegol and golimumab, but information collected so far suggests that their side-effect profile does not differ significantly from the older agents.

Non-TNFi biologic medicines. Currently, five non-TNFi biologic medicines are available for the management of RA in the UK: abatacept, rituximab, tocilizumab, sarilumab and anakinra (Table 54.5). Tocilizumab and sarilumab are monoclonal antibodies which block the actions of IL-6. Elevated IL-6 levels have been found in the synovial fluid of patients with RA, and the cytokine is thought to play an important role in the inflammation and joint destruction associated with RA. Both IL-6 inhibitors are licensed following treatment failure with csDMARDs. Use is recommended in combination with methotrexate, but monotherapy can be considered where there is intolerance or a contraindication to methotrexate. Abatacept is a fusion protein that modulates T-lymphocyte–dependent antibody responses and inflammation. Use is recommended only in combination with methotrexate. Indications include highly active disease in patients without prior treatment with methotrexate or following treatment failure with one or more csDMARDs (including methotrexate) or a TNFi. Rituximab is a monoclonal antibody that binds specifically to the transmembrane antigen CD20, which ultimately results in B cell lysis. It is available as both the original reference drug and as biosimilar formulations. It is given as an intermittent intravenous infusion in combination with a weekly dose of methotrexate and is used following treatment failure with both csDMARDs and bDMARDs. Anakinra is a human IL-1 receptor antagonist licensed for the management of RA. It is given as a once-daily

Table 54.5 Non–tumour necrosis factor inhibitor biologic medicines licensed in rheumatoid arthritis

Abatacept (Orencia)	Rituximab (MabThera, Rixathon, Truxima)	Tocilizumab (RoActemra)	Sarilumab (Kevzara)
Fusion protein: blocks T cell activation	Monoclonal antibody: CD20 B-cell depletion	Humanised monoclonal antibody against soluble and membrane IL-6 receptor	Human monoclonal antibody selective for soluble and membrane IL-6 receptor
Dose in RA Intravenous infusion: at weeks 0, 2 and 4, then 4 weekly (<60 kg = 500 mg, 60–100 kg = 750 mg, >100 kg = 1000 mg) or Subcutaneous injection: 125 mg once a week	Dose in RA Intravenous infusion: two infusions of 1000 mg given 2 weeks apart, repeat as clinically indicated (no more than 6 monthly) (Only available as an intravenous infusion for RA)	Dose in RA Intravenous infusion: 8 mg/kg 4 weekly (maximum dose 800 mg) or Subcutaneous injection: 162 mg once a week	Dose in RA 200 mg once every 2 weeks by subcutaneous injection
Licensed: Moderate-to-severe RA following csDMARD or TNFi failure (with MTX) Polyarticular JIA	Licensed: RA (with MTX) following csDMARD + TNFi failure GPA with glucocorticoids NHL CLL	Licensed: RA (+/− MTX) following csDMARD failure sJIA (+/− MTX) JIA	Licensed: RA (+/− MTX) following csDMARD failure

CLL, Chronic lymphocytic leukaemia; DMARD, disease-modifying anti-rheumatic drug; GPA, granulomatosis with polyangiitis and microscopic polyangiitis; IL-6, interleukin-6; JIA, juvenile idiopathic arthritis; MTX, methotrexate; NHL, non-Hodgkin's lymphoma; RA, rheumatoid arthritis; sJIA, systemic juvenile idiopathic arthritis; TNFi, tumour necrosis factor inhibitor.

subcutaneous injection in combination with weekly methotrexate. Its use is not supported for the management of RA because it is clinically less effective than the other agents currently available (NICE, 2015a).

Rituximab. Rituximab is a genetically engineered monoclonal antibody which binds to CD20, a protein expressed on B lymphocytes. It is available as the original reference drug MabThera and also as the biosimilar brands Rixathon and Truxima. The three products are licensed in combination with methotrexate for the treatment of severe active RA in patients who have had an inadequate response or intolerance to other DMARDs, including one or more TNFi therapies. Rituximab works by a variety of methods including depleting B cells, affecting B- and T-cell interaction, antigen presentation and cytokine production. In RA, B cells can be found in the synovium. They produce antibodies that contribute to the disease and inflammatory cytokines. B cells also affect the function of other cells involved in inflammation. A course of rituximab consists of 1000 mg by intravenous infusion at week 0 followed by a second 1000 mg intravenous infusion 2 weeks later. Intravenous methylprednisolone is administered with each infusion to prevent infusion reaction along with an antihistamine and oral paracetamol. The need for further courses should be evaluated 24 weeks following the previous course. Available data suggest that clinical response is usually achieved within 16–24 weeks of an initial treatment course. All patients treated with rituximab should be given a patient alert card at each infusion. Contraindications to rituximab include hypersensitivity to rituximab or other murine proteins, active severe infections and severe heart failure (NYHA class IV).

In the UK, NICE recommends treatment with rituximab, in combination with methotrexate, as an option for the treatment of adults with severe active RA who have had an inadequate response to, or are intolerant of, DMARDs, including at least one TNFi (NICE, 2010). Treatment is permitted no more frequently than every 6 months. EULAR guidance on the management of RA states that in the presence of certain contraindications for other biologic medicines, such as a recent history of lymphoma, latent TB with contraindications to the use of chemoprophylaxis, living in a TB-endemic region or a previous history of demyelinating disease, then rituximab may be considered as a first-line biological agent (Smolen et al., 2017). Some rheumatologists also give preference to rituximab in patients with a recent history of any malignancy because there are no indications that rituximab use is associated with the occurrence of cancers (Smolen et al., 2017).

Recently, pooled data from two phase III studies in methotrexate-inadequate responder populations, as well as a substudy from the IMAGE study that evaluated methotrexate-naive patients, have all reinforced the view that seropositive patients (ACPA/anti-CCP, RF or both) demonstrate a more robust response to rituximab (Tak et al., 2011). In the IMAGE study, there was evidence of significantly greater joint protection in the seropositive subpopulation treated with rituximab and methotrexate; whereas in the seronegative group, inhibition of the progression of damage in each treatment group was comparable and generally low even in the placebo/methotrexate group (Tak et al., 2011). As a consequence of this, some rheumatologists may prefer to use an alternative biologic to rituximab in seronegative patients. In seronegative patients with refractory disease who have not responded positively to multiple biologic DMARDs, rituximab may be considered if there are limited treatment options. The SMART study (Sellam et al., 2011) found that those with evidence of erosive disease, those with a high DAS28 (i.e. those with high joint counts and inflammatory markers) had greatest benefit from rituximab. The presence of these factors may override serological status in patients with difficult to treat disease.

There have been a number of reported cases of hepatitis B virus reactivation in oncology patients treated with rituximab, although reports in the RA population are very low. All patients should be screened for hepatitis B (surface antigen and core) and hepatitis C before commencing rituximab. At present, there is no evidence of an increased frequency of TB in patients with lymphoma treated with rituximab, and prescreening for TB is not warranted (Buch et al., 2011). Patients considered for rituximab therapy should receive all indicated vaccines (hepatitis B for at-risk population, pneumococcus, tetanus toxoid every 10 years, influenza annually) before treatment. Ideally, vaccination should be undertaken at least 4 weeks before rituximab therapy.

A reduced baseline level of the IgG has been shown to be a risk factor for severe infections with rituximab (Gottenberg et al., 2010). On all of these grounds, rituximab treatment in patients with RA with hypogammaglobulinaemia (below the lower limit of normal) should be considered with caution. It is recommended that patients have their baseline IgG measured before starting rituximab and before each cycle of rituximab (Buch et al., 2011).

The most frequent adverse event with rituximab is infusion reaction (30–35% with the first infusion with concomitant glucocorticoids). Fewer reactions are observed with the second and subsequent infusions (Buch et al., 2011). In a recent pooled analysis of safety data from rituximab in combination with methotrexate, the rate of adverse events and serious events, including infections and serious infections, remained stable across several courses (van Vollenhoven et al., 2010).

Tocilizumab. IL-6 is a multifunction cytokine that has a wide range of biological activities in various target cells and regulates immune responses, acute-phase reactions, haematopoiesis and bone metabolism (Adachi et al., 2008). Because IL-6 is involved in a number of important physiological roles, deregulated overproduction of IL-6 causes various pathological conditions, including autoimmune, inflammatory and lymphoproliferative disorders. In RA, elevated production of IL-6 is observed in the synovial fluid and blood, with levels correlating with disease activity. Some of the clinical aspects of RA, such as overproduction of acute-phase proteins, raised platelet counts, induction of osteoclasts, production of auto-antibodies and decreased albumin, can be explained by activities of IL-6 (Nishimoto et al., 2008).

Tocilizumab is a monoclonal antibody that binds specifically to both soluble and membrane-bound IL-6 receptors (sIL-6Rs and mIL-6Rs) resulting in the inhibition of sIL-6Rs and mIL-6R–mediated signalling. Tocilizumab is indicated for the treatment of moderate-to-severe RA in patients who have not previously received methotrexate and in patients who have failed or been intolerant to one or more csDMARDs or TNFi's. Its license permits its use in combination with methotrexate or as monotherapy where methotrexate is contraindicated or not been tolerated. It can be administered as a once-weekly 162 mg subcutaneous injection or given as an intravenous infusion of 8 mg/kg (maximum 800 mg) every 4 weeks.

Tocilizumab is the only biologic therapy to repeatedly demonstrate superiority over methotrexate monotherapy or other csDMARDs (Jones et al., 2010; Nishimoto et al., 2007). A study involving 2057 participants with RA assessing changes in Clinical Disease Activity Index and DAS28, as well as the likelihood to be in remission, showed no significant difference whether tocilizumab was used as monotherapy or in combination with csDMARDs (Gabay et al., 2016). However, tocilizumab retention was more prolonged when tocilizumab was prescribed in combination with csDMARDs. EULAR supports the combination of all biologic medicines with methotrexate, but where there is intolerance or a contraindication to use of methotrexate, then preference is given to tocilizumab monotherapy (Smolen et al., 2014).

NICE recommends the use of tocilizumab either in combination with methotrexate or as monotherapy when a patient's DAS 28 is greater than 5.1 and they have not responded to intensive therapy with a combination of csDMARDs (NICE, 2016). It can also be prescribed when csDMARDs and a TNFi have not been effective, the individual cannot have rituximab for medical reasons or because of a bad reaction, or when treatment with rituximab has failed (NICE, 2012).

Due to tocilizumab's mode of action, its use may be associated with a decline in neutrophil and platelet counts, a change in lipid profiles and abnormal LFTs. Its use is also associated with a number of significant drug interactions. Treatment should not be commenced in patients with an absolute neutrophil count (ANC) less than 2×10^9/L. Neutrophils and platelets should be monitored 4–8 weeks after start of therapy and thereafter according to standard clinical practice. The licensed datasheet provides specific recommendations with regards to dosage reduction or delaying treatment according to platelet and neutrophil levels. Elevated lipid levels including total cholesterol, low-density lipoprotein (LDL), high-density lipoprotein (HDL) and triglycerides have been reported in studies following treatment with tocilizumab. Patients receiving tocilizumab should have their lipid parameters checked 4–8 weeks following the initiation of tocilizumab therapy. Patients with raised cholesterol levels should be managed according to local clinical guidelines for the management of hyperlipidaemia. In view of the elevated hepatic transaminases commonly associated with treatment, aspartate transaminase (AST) and alanine transaminase (ALT) levels should be monitored every 4–8 weeks for the first 6 months of treatment followed by every 12 weeks thereafter. Caution should be exercised in commencing treatment in patients whose ALT or AST level is greater than 1.5 × the upper limit of normal (ULN). Consideration should be given to adjusting the dose of methotrexate if AST/ALT level is one to three times the ULN. Persistent elevation following on from this may warrant dose reduction or treatment interruption or termination.

Pro-inflammatory cytokines, such as IL-6, have been associated with suppression of hepatic cytochrome P450 (CYP450) enzymes. Reduction in these cytokines following the administration of a biologic therapy may lead to normalisation of enzyme expression and improved drug metabolism. In vitro studies have shown that IL-6 caused a reduction in CYP1A2, CYP2C9, CYP2C19, and CYP3A4 enzyme expression. These enzymes are responsible for the metabolism of a number of medicines including atorvastatin, calcium channel blockers, theophylline, warfarin, phenytoin, ciclosporin and benzodiazepines. Following the administration of tocilizumab, the function of these enzymes normalised, resulting in the need for a dosage increase of these medicines in some patients. Following discontinuation of tocilizumab, enzyme activity may be affected for a number of weeks because of the long half-life of the drug. Live vaccines should not be administered to people who are receiving treatment with tocilizumab. It is recommended that all patients be brought up to date with all immunisations, in agreement with current immunisation guidelines, before initiating tocilizumab therapy. Annual influenza vaccination and pneumococcal vaccines may be given to patients who are receiving tocilizumab.

Sarilumab. Sarilumab is a subcutaneous IL-6 inhibitor licensed in combination with methotrexate for the treatment of moderately to severely active RA in adult patients who have responded inadequately to, or who are intolerant to, one or more csDMARDs. It can be given as monotherapy in case of intolerance to methotrexate or when treatment with methotrexate is inappropriate. Sarilumab is a fully human monoclonal antibody, whereas tocilizumab is a 'humanised' monoclonal, meaning its protein sequence has been modified to increase its similarity to antibody variants produced naturally by humans. Contraindications, side effects and drug interactions are similar between the two IL-6 inhibitors, and both require regular blood monitoring including neutrophils, platelets and liver transaminases. The recommended dose of sarilumab is 200 mg once every 2 weeks administered as a subcutaneous injection. Dose reduction to 150 mg once every 2 weeks or omission of the drug is recommended according to neutrophil, platelet and liver enzyme levels. NICE recommends the use of sarilumab, with or without methotrexate, in individuals with a DAS28 score of 5.1 or greater despite treatment with combination csDMARDs. It is also approved where other bDMARDs and csDMARDs have failed or are contraindicated and the person cannot have rituximab. Individuals failing to respond to rituximab may also have sarilumab provided they have also been treated with at least one other bDMARD (NICE, 2017c).

Abatacept. Abatacept is a recombinant human fusion protein that binds to proteins naturally expressed on the surface of activated T cells, causing attenuation of T-cell activity by blocking a co-stimulatory signal. T cells are central to the immune response and are found in the synovium of patients with RA. In the synovium, T cells express activation markers, secrete cytokines and stimulate macrophages, thereby contributing to the development of inflammation and joint destruction. Abatacept, in combination with methotrexate, is indicated for the treatment of moderate-to-severe active RA in adult patients who responded inadequately to previous therapy with one or more csDMARDs including methotrexate or TNFi's. Its benefit is not seemingly different between seropositive and seronegative RA, and may therefore be particularly considered in place of rituximab in such patients who have not responded positively to TNFi therapy. It can be administered as an intravenous infusion according to weight (<60 kg = 500 mg; 60–100 kg = 750 mg; >100 kg = 1000 mg). Following the initial infusion it is given 2 and 4 weeks later, then every 4 weeks thereafter. The infusions are generally well tolerated and administered efficiently (30 minutes). Alternatively, it can be administered as a 125 mg subcutaneous injection once a week.

In the UK, abatacept in combination with methotrexate is recommended as a first-line biologic treatment option in patients with a DAS28 greater than 5.1 who have not responded to intensive therapy with a combination of csDMARDs (NICE, 2016). It is also recommended, in combination with methotrexate, as a second-line treatment option for adults with severe active RA who have had an inadequate response to or have an intolerance of other DMARDs, including at least one TNFi, and who cannot receive rituximab therapy because they have a contraindication to it, or when rituximab is withdrawn because of an adverse event (NICE, 2010).

Common adverse reactions (≥10%) among abatacept-treated patients include headache, nausea and upper respiratory tract infections. The frequencies of serious infection and malignancy relative to placebo among abatacept-treated patients older than 65 years were higher than among those younger than 65 years. Because there is a higher incidence of infections and malignancies in the elderly in general, caution should be used when treating elderly patients. Live vaccines should not be given concurrently with abatacept or within 3 months of its discontinuation.

The GDH-PQQ–based glucose monitoring systems may react with the maltose present in abatacept infusion, resulting in falsely elevated blood glucose readings on the day of infusion. When receiving abatacept infusions, patients who require blood glucose monitoring should be advised to consider methods that do not react with maltose, such as those based on glucose dehydrogenase nicotine adenine dinucleotide (GDH-NAD), glucose oxidase or glucose hexokinase test methods.

Targeted synthetic disease-modifying anti-rheumatic drugs

In 2017 a new class of DMARD became available for the management of moderate-to-severe RA, the Janus Kinase Inhibitors (also known as JAK inhibitors or Jakinibs). Due to their differing mode of action to existing oral DMARDs they have been given the classification of tsDMARDs. Janus Kinase Inhibitors inhibit the activity of one or more of the Janus Kinase family of enzymes (JAK1, JAK2, JAK3 and TYK2). These enzymes transduce intracellular signals from cell surface receptors for a number of cytokines and growth factors involved in haematopoiesis, inflammation and immune function. Within the intracellular signalling pathway, JAKs phosphorylate and activate signal transducers and activators of transcription (STATs), which activate gene expression within the cell. Inhibition of the JAK-STAT pathway results in a reduction in cytokine signaling.

Baricitinib (Olumiant) and tofacitinib (Xeljanz) are licensed for the treatment of moderate-to-severe active RA in adult patients who have responded inadequately to or who are intolerant to one or more DMARDs. Use is recommended in combination with methotrexate, but they can also be given as monotherapy where there is a contraindication or intolerance to methotrexate. NICE recommends the use of baricitinib (Olumiant) or tofacitinib (Xeljanz) in patients with a DAS28 greater than 5.1 and where there has been previous treatment failure with a combination of csDMARDs (NICE, 2017a, 2017b). Use is also permitted in patients with a DAS28 greater than 5.1 whose disease has responded inadequately to, or who cannot have, other DMARDs, including at least one biological DMARD and in whom treatment with rituximab is not appropriate. Ideally they should be given in combination with methotrexate, but NICE permits monotherapy

where there is a contraindication or intolerance to methotrexate. All use is under the proviso that the manufacturers provide baricitinib and tofacitinib at a discounted price as per the agreed patient access scheme. EULAR recommends the use of either JAK Kinase inhibitor when there is high disease activity despite treatment with a csDMARD or where treatment with a bDMARD or first JAK kinase inhibitor has failed (Smolen et al., 2017).

Baricitinib (Olumiant) partially inhibits the JAK1 and JAK2 enzymic activity, thus affecting interferon-γ and IL-6 signaling, and consequently T helper cell 1 cell differentiation. A non-inferiority study comparing baricitinib with adalimumab demonstrated baricitinib 4 mg was superior to adalimumab for the ACR20 response (Taylor et al., 2017).

All patients should be screened for TB, hepatitis B and hepatitis C plus the presence of infection before considering treatment with a JAK Kinase inhibitor. It is taken as a 4 mg once-daily dose with or without food. The dose should be reduced to 2 mg once daily in patients older than 75 years or where there is a history of chronic/recurrent infection, or creatinine clearance is between 30 and 60 mL/min. Use is not recommended where the creatinine clearance is less than 30 mL/min or in the presence of severe hepatic impairment. Dose reduction is also recommended in patients who are taking Organic Anion Transporter 3 (OAT3) medicines because these medicines can cause a significant rise in the plasma concentration of baricitinib (Olumiant), for example, probenecid. It should not be used in conjunction with bDMARDs or other JAK Kinase inhibitors because of the risk of increased immunosuppression and risk of infection.

Events of deep venous thrombosis (DVT) and pulmonary embolism (PE) have been reported in patients who are receiving baricitinib (Olumiant). It should be used with caution in patients with risk factors for DVT/PE, such as older age, obesity, a medical history of DVT/PE or patients undergoing surgery and immobilisation. If clinical features of DVT/PE occur, baricitinib (Olumiant) treatment should be temporarily interrupted and patients should be evaluated promptly, followed by appropriate treatment. Regular blood monitoring of haemoglobin, neutrophils, lymphocytes and hepatic transaminases is recommended throughout treatment according to local practice. Use has been associated with abnormal lipid profiles. Lipids should be checked at baseline and 12 weeks after initiation of treatment with any abnormality being managed in accordance with national guidance for the management of hyperlipidaemia.

In human cells, tofacitinib (Xeljanz) preferentially inhibits signalling by heterodimeric cytokine receptors that associate with JAK3 and/or JAK1 with functional selectivity over cytokine receptors that signal via pairs of JAK2. Inhibition of JAK1 and JAK3 by tofacitinib attenuates signalling of ILs (IL-2, -4, -6, -7, -9, -15, -21) and type I and type II interferons, which will result in modulation of the immune and inflammatory response. Clinical trial data showed non-inferiority when tofacitinib with methotrexate was compared with adalimumab in combination with methotrexate (Fleischmann et al., 2017). The standard dosage is 5 mg twice a day orally with or without food. No dose reduction is required in the elderly or in patients with mild-to-moderate renal function (creatinine clearance 30–49 mL/min). In severe renal impairment (creatinine clearance less than 30 mL/min) the dose should be reduced to 5 mg once a day. In moderate hepatic impairment (Child-Pugh B) the dose should be reduced to 5 mg once a day, and use is not permitted in severe impairment (Child-Pugh C). Tofacitinib (Xeljanz) is metabolised through the CYP450 system; the dosage should be reduced to 5 mg once a day in the presence of strong inhibitors of CYP450 3A4 (e.g. ketoconazole). Dosage reduction is also warranted in patients who are receiving one or more concomitant medicinal products that result in both moderate inhibition of CYP3A4, as well as potent inhibition of CYP2C19 (e.g. fluconazole). Co-administration of potent inducers of CYP450 3A4 (e.g. rifampicin) is not recommended because it may result in a loss of clinical efficacy. The manufacturer of tofacitinib (Xeljanz) states that it should not be combined with bDMARDs, other JAK Kinase inhibitors, azathioprine, ciclosporin or tacrolimus because of increased risk of infection when these medicines are combined.

As with baricitinib (Olumiant), the use of tofacitinib (Xeljanz) has been associated with a decline in haemoglobin, neutrophil and lymphocyte levels. An FBC should be performed at baseline, after 4–8 weeks and then regularly at 3-monthly intervals. Abnormal lipid profiles have been observed within 6 weeks of commencing treatment. Assessment of lipid parameters is recommended at baseline and 8 weeks after commencing treatment. Due to adverse events noted in clinical trials, caution should also be exercised in patients with a history of malignancy, chronic lung disease and in patients at increased risk of gastro-intestinal perforation (history of diverticulitis, concomitant use of corticosteroids and/or nonsteroidal anti-inflammatory drugs).

Rheumatoid arthritis treatment pathway

The initial treatment strategy involves the use of csDMARDs in combination with short-term glucocorticoids. In the UK a combined csDMARD approach is recommended (NICE, 2016), whereas EULAR recommends initial csDMARD monotherapy (Smolen et al., 2017). Following treatment failure with combined csDMARDs in patients with a DAS28 greater than 5.1, NICE recommends a combination of methotrexate with either a TNFi or abatacept, tocilizumab or baricitinib (NICE, 2016). Where methotrexate is contraindicated or not tolerated, adalimumab, certolizumab, etanercept, tocilizumab or baricitinib can be used as monotherapy (NICE, 2016). In contrast, EULAR proposes treatment escalation to a bDMARD or tsDMARD, in combination with methotrexate, following treatment failure with the first csDMARD in the presence of poor prognostic factors (e.g. moderate to high disease activity after csDMARD, high acute-phase reactant levels, high swollen joint counts, the presence of RF and/or ACPA, and the presence of early erosions). In the absence of poor prognostic factors, a trial of a second csDMARD is recommended (Smolen et al., 2017) before considering a bDMARD or tsDMARD.

EULAR gives preference to bDMARDs over tsDMARDs because of greater availability of long-term registry data on their safety. None of the bDMARDs are given hierarchical ranking over another by either EULAR or NICE. However, EULAR does propose the use of an IL-6 inhibitor (e.g. tocilizumab) or a tsDMARD (e.g. baricitinib) over a bDMARD when csDMARDs cannot be given in combination (Smolen et al., 2017). The rheumatologist when making a decision in conjunction with the patient will evaluate the individual's risk–benefit profile and propose a particular biologic medicine based on this assessment (see Box 54.6). Factors that will be considered include the patient's serology, comorbidities (e.g. heart disease), history of malignancy, the presence of lung disease, concomitant methotrexate, the presence of other autoimmune diseases (e.g. psoriasis and inflammatory bowel disease [IBD]), auto-antibody status and the ability to self-inject.

The TNFi should be avoided in patients who are positive for auto-antibodies suggestive of an overlying connective tissue disease such as SLE. This is due to the potential risk of worsening pre-existing lupus or triggering a lupus-type reaction. It may therefore be preferable to use tocilizumab or abatacept in individuals who have shown positivity for auto-antibodies linked to lupus. Other immune-mediated diseases, such as psoriasis and IBD, may co-exist with RA. Where the patient suffers from both RA and psoriasis or IBD it may be preferable to use an agent that is licensed for management of both conditions such as a TNFi.

Patients vary in their response to biologic medicines; they may fail to clinically respond to the first biologic they are given defined as a 'primary non-response'. In addition, some patients after initially having a good response to a particular biologic medicine may subsequently lose clinical response; this may be classified as a 'secondary non-response'. There is variation in patient tolerability to different biologic medicines; for example, an individual may experience an adverse reaction to one TNFi leading to discontinuation and then be able to tolerate another TNFi with good clinical effect. To maintain adequate disease control, patients may be switched to an alternative biologic; this is known as biologic sequencing. No comparative studies have been conducted to date offering clear guidance on biologic sequencing in RA (Smolen et al., 2014).

NICE recommends the use of rituximab, in combination with methotrexate, where there has been a primary non-response or a secondary loss of response with the first prescribed biologic medicine (NICE, 2010). Adalimumab, etanercept, infliximab, tocilizumab and baricitinib are recommended as alternatives to rituximab, where there is a contraindication to rituximab or rituximab is withdrawn because of an adverse reaction (NICE, 2010, 2017). The use of rituximab is supported only in combination with methotrexate; where methotrexate cannot be given, then either adalimumab, etanercept, tocilizumab or baricitinib monotherapy can be given. EULAR gives no preference to a particular bDMARD following a primary non-response or secondary loss of response to the first bDMARD. Following treatment failure with the original reference, bDMARD use of its corresponding biosimilar is not recommended.

It should be noted that class adverse drug reactions, such as lupus-type reactions or a neurological side effect with a TNFi, would preclude the use of another TNFi. The same risk–benefit assessment applied to the selection of the first biologic medicine is applied in biologic sequencing. In addition the rheumatologist will consider the therapeutic response to the first biologic medicine. It is important that the patient is involved throughout the decision-making process. NICE also permits the use of tocilizumab following primary treatment failure with rituximab or a loss of response to rituximab (NICE, 2012).

Rheumatoid arthritis and pregnancy

Although disease activity may improve during pregnancy, it is important that pregnant patients with RA are not deprived appropriate disease-ameliorating therapies. Active disease during pregnancy is associated with adverse pregnancy outcomes (Østensen et al., 2015). There is growing drug safety evidence to support shared decision making regarding the safe use of medicines during pregnancy. The BSR deems prednisolone to be compatible with each trimester of pregnancy and during breastfeeding (Flint et al., 2016a). Hydroxychloroquine is the anti-malarial of choice in females planning a pregnancy and should be continued post-conception. Guidance also deems it to be compatible with breastfeeding (Flint et al., 2016a). Sulfasalazine is permitted during pregnancy. Oral sulfasalazine inhibits the absorption and metabolism of folic acid and may cause folic acid deficiency; therefore, folic acid 5 mg once daily should be administered in conjunction with sulfasalazine throughout the pregnancy (Flint et al., 2016a). It is important that the DMARDs methotrexate and leflunomide are not taken by females who are trying to conceive, and both medicines are contraindicated during pregnancy and breastfeeding. Females of childbearing age should be counselled on the importance of not getting pregnant while taking either methotrexate or leflunomide and using appropriate contraceptive measures during treatment with these medicines. Methotrexate should be stopped at least 3 months before conception. Leflunomide has an extended half-life, and female patients should use appropriate contraceptive measures for at least 2 years after stopping leflunomide or undergo an appropriate wash-out regimen and have verification by at least two blood tests that the plasma level of drug has dropped below 0.02 mg/L. It should be noted that males wanting to start a family should also stop leflunomide therapy and undergo an appropriate wash-out regimen, with verification of plasma levels.

The current licensed datasheets for the biologic therapies in RA often do not support continuation during conception and pregnancy. However, more recent evidence from biologic registries support the use of certain biologic medicines during pregnancy in patients whose disease activity warrants continuation. Infliximab may be continued for up to the first 16 weeks of pregnancy, whereas etanercept and adalimumab may be continued until the second trimester. Stopping the TNFi at these time points ensures low or no drug level in cord blood at the time of delivery. If infliximab, etanercept or adalimumab is continued beyond the recommended period, then live vaccinations should not be given to the infant until he or she reaches 7 months of age. Due to reduced placental transfer, certolizumab is deemed appropriate in all three trimesters. Golimumab is unlikely to cause harm in the first trimester. Other biologics such as rituximab, tocilizumab and abatacept should be avoided in pregnancy and breastfeeding at present because there are insufficient safety data to support their use.

BSR recommendations on analgesics support the intermittent use of paracetamol throughout pregnancy. However, regular consumption should be avoided especially during weeks 8–14 of pregnancy because of a small reported risk of cryptorchidism (Flint et al., 2016b). Codeine is compatible pre-conception and throughout pregnancy. Caution is advised with the use of codeine in breastfeeding because of the risk of central nervous system depression in the infant. Discordant findings from retrospective, large studies with population controls on the use of non-selective NSAIDs in the first trimester of pregnancy raise the possibility of a low risk of miscarriage and malformation

(Flint et al., 2016b). Caution is therefore advised with regard to using non-selective NSAIDs in the first trimester. All non-selective NSAIDs should be withdrawn at gestational week 32 to avoid premature closure of the ductus arteriosus. Avoidance of COX-2 inhibitors is recommended throughout pregnancy (Flint et al., 2016b).

Patient care

People with RA should have access to and be offered patient education throughout the course of their disease including as a minimum: at diagnosis, at pharmacological treatment change and when required by the patient's physical or psychological condition (Zangi et al., 2015). The content and delivery of patient education should be individually tailored. Ideally both individual and/or group sessions should be provided through face-to-face or online interactions, and supplemented by telephone calls, written material or multimedia material. Information provided should include knowledge and management of the disease, knowledge of side effects and risk factors, non-pharmacological treatment, pain control and self-help methods, as well as activity regulation, physical exercises and behaviour change. Effective communication and education is essential to enable patients with RA to make correct decisions about their treatment in conjunction with their rheumatologist and other members of the MDT. Medicine information sheets are available from the Arthritis Research UK with further information available on their website (http://www.arthritisresearch uk.org).

Many of the treatments used in the management of RA require regular blood monitoring, and hence the rationale for blood tests and the importance of attending for these tests should be clearly explained to the patient. In addition, patients should be reminded of the warning symptoms that must trigger them to contact a healthcare professional. Shared care agreements between secondary and primary care are often employed for csDMARD therapy. This involves a primary care clinician continuing to prescribe and monitor drug treatment that has been initiated by a hospital specialist. Clear guidelines stating the responsibilities of both parties and the action required in the event of toxicity is defined within the document. The main advantage of shared care is that the patient will not be required to attend regular hospital appointments for blood tests and will be managed in primary care.

Counselling about medication should incorporate the need to inform all healthcare professionals involved in the patient's care about the medicines the individual is taking for his or her RA. This is especially important when seeing healthcare practitioners outside of rheumatology who may wish to initiate a new medicine or when purchasing over the-counter products and herbal/complementary therapies.

Osteoarthritis

Osteoarthritis is a degenerative disorder of the joints that most commonly affects the knee, hip, spine and small joints of the hand. It is the most common musculoskeletal condition in older people (Arthritis Research UK, 2013). The exact aetiology of osteoarthritis is unknown, and at present there are no medical treatments proven to prevent or delay its onset. Risk factors for the development of osteoarthritis include increasing age, obesity, gender, bone density, joint injury, occupation and genetics. Symptomatic presentation does not usually occur until middle age. More than two-thirds of people with osteoarthritis are in constant pain, and it is the 11th highest contributor to global disability (Cross et al., 2014). The diagnosis and management of osteoarthritis is dependent upon the type and number of joints affected. Non-pharmacological measures, such as weight loss, structured exercise programmes and supportive aids, form the cornerstone of management. Pharmacological treatments are used as adjuncts to provide moderate symptomatic relief. Joint replacement surgery may be considered in osteoarthritis of the knee or hip when an individual suffers persistent debilitating symptoms despite appropriate management.

Epidemiology

Osteoarthritis is the most common musculoskeletal condition in older people. It involves inflammation and major structural changes to the whole joint, causing pain and functional disability. In the UK around one-third of people aged 45 years and older have sought treatment for osteoarthritis, an estimated 8.75 million (Arthritis Research UK, 2013). Osteoarthritis is more common in women than men, and the prevalence increases steeply with age.

The knee is the most common site in the body to have osteoarthritis in people aged 45 and older. In the UK nearly one in five adults older than 45 years may have symptoms of osteoarthritis of the knee (Arthritis Research UK, 2013). The global prevalence of radiographically confirmed knee osteoarthritis in 2010 was estimated to be 3.8%. The prevalence of knee osteoarthritis is higher in females than in males, 4.8% versus 2.8%, respectively (Cross et al., 2014). Epidemiological studies suggest the prevalence of knee osteoarthritis peaks at 50 years of age, and there are worldwide geographical variations with the highest prevalence in the Asia Pacific high-income region (Cross et al., 2014).

Hip osteoarthritis is less common than knee osteoarthritis, with the global age-standardised prevalence rate of symptomatic radiographically confirmed osteoarthritis estimated to be 0.85%. In the UK, 8% of people aged 45 and older have sought treatment for osteoarthritis of the hip (Arthritis Research UK, 2013). As with osteoarthritis of the knee, prevalence of hip osteoarthritis has been shown to be higher in females than males. Prevalence increases consistently with age, and hip osteoarthritis has the highest prevalence in North American high-income regions (Cross et al., 2014).

Symptomatic osteoarthritis of the hand affects 8% of people aged 60 years or older, and 26% of women and 13% of men aged 70 years and older (Zhang et al., 2002). More recent research in the UK has shown that 6% of people aged older than 45 years have sought treatment for osteoarthritis of the hand and wrist (Arthritis Research UK, 2013). The most commonly affected joints in the hand are the distal interphalangeal joints and PIPs, followed by the base of the thumb. People with hand osteoarthritis have difficulty in performing daily tasks such as gripping and writing, and functional impairment may be as severe as that associated with RA.

Pathophysiology

In osteoarthritis the whole joint is involved in the pathogenesis. In healthy joints, two bones articulate with one another, and the surface of each bone within the joint is covered by shock-absorbing cartilage. Both the bone and cartilage are important in dissipating the load placed through joints every day. When the bone or cartilage is damaged as a consequence of large loads to the joint or some form of impact, numerous repair mechanisms attempt to restore normal function within the damaged joint to ensure the joint continues to dissipate the load correctly. This includes cell-mediated remodelling within the architecture of the cartilage and subchondral bone tissues (Goldring and Goldring, 2010). When the rate of damage exceeds the rate of repair, degeneration of the bone and cartilage ensues and the joint fails to effectively dissipate the load. This then results in a cycle of biomechanical and biochemical degeneration where the shock-absorbing cartilage is progressively destroyed, thus exposing the bone to a greater load with subsequent bone damage (bone marrow lesions) (Suri and Walsh, 2012). This then leads to further loss of cartilage, bone overgrowth with the formation of bony spurs (osteophytes) and narrowing of the joint space. The joint degeneration results in painful and tender inflammation of the synovial lining of the joint (synovitis) and swelling of the joint (effusion). Synovitis may be present in early cartilage changes to the joint, and there is cellular infiltration with macrophages, activated T and B cells, and accompanying vascular proliferation (Roemer et al., 2015; Yusuf et al., 2011). Inflammatory cytokine levels may also be elevated within the joint, but to a lesser extent than seen with RA.

Aetiology

Osteoarthritis may be classified as either primary or secondary osteoarthritis. In primary osteoarthritis the exact cause is unknown (idiopathic), while in secondary osteoarthritis there is a link to a specific cause such as previous injury to the joint, a pre-existing congenital abnormality (congenital hip dysplasia) or inflammatory arthritis such as gout or RA. Osteoarthritis can affect weight-bearing and non-weight-bearing joints, and may involve single or multiple joints.

The exact aetiology of osteoarthritis is unknown; however, a combination of risk factors may predispose an individual to its development. The main risk factors for osteoarthritis include age, gender, obesity, bone density, joint injury or disease, occupation, joint abnormalities and genetics (Box 54.7). At present there is no validated risk tool for quantitative prediction of the development of osteoarthritis.

Box 54.7 Osteoarthritis risk factors

- Age older than 50 years
- Female sex
- Increased body mass index (>25)
- Bone density
- Joint injury or joint disease (e.g. rheumatoid arthritis and gout)
- Occupation—physically demanding work
- Abnormal joint development (e.g. congenital hip dysplasia)
- Genetic factors

Box 54.8 Management of osteoarthritis

- Appropriate information and education
- Activity and exercise
- Interventions to achieve weight loss
- Pharmacological adjuncts to provide symptomatic relief

Increasing age and female gender have been associated with an increased risk of development of osteoarthritis. The effect of female gender on risk of hand osteoarthritis peaks around menopause, with more than 3.5-fold higher rates in women aged 50–60 years when compared with men of similar age (Prieto-Alhambra et al., 2014). It has been hypothesised that sex hormones may influence the development of hand osteoarthritis in young women (Zhang et al., 2010). However, research involving hormone replacement therapy has failed to support this hypothesis, and studies are required to further evaluate the relationship between female hormones and osteoarthritis. Being overweight increases loading on the joints and the risk of osteoarthritis, especially in the knee (Zhang et al., 2010).

Inheritance studies in twins and other family-based studies have assessed the estimated heritability for osteoarthritis in the range of 40–65% depending on the joint site (Jonsson et al., 2003; Kraus et al., 2007). Genome-wide association studies have identified as least 11 loci associated with osteoarthritis (Evangelou et al., 2014). The effect size of individual identified loci is small, and the genetic architecture of osteoarthritis is likely to consist of multiple variants of similar magnitude (Glyn-Jones et al., 2015).

Diagnosis

The diagnosis of osteoarthritis is based on the combination of typical mechanical pain symptoms and physical joint findings in an individual with risk factors for the development of osteoarthritis. No diagnostic tool for osteoarthritis has been validated for use in routine clinical practice. The individual may present with pain in more than one joint. The pain associated with osteoarthritis is of gradual onset and is worsened by activity; unlike RA there is only a short period of early-morning stiffness. People with osteoarthritis frequently present with muscle wasting around the affected joint(s) due to the avoidance of movement as a consequence of pain (disuse atrophy). In osteoarthritis of the hip people may encounter difficulty when putting on shoes, getting in and out of the car, or going up and down stairs. Pain related to hip osteoarthritis can occur in different locations than the thigh area, including the groin, buttocks and knees. The individual may be not aware that the pain is originating from the hip. The intensity of pain increases when the hip joint is moved. People with osteoarthritis of the knee typically experience activity-related pain, which is often worse towards the end of the day. The pain is relieved by rest, and there is only mild morning or inactivity-related stiffness. Symptoms may be episodic and vary in severity, but as the osteoarthritis of the knee becomes more advanced the pain can become persistent and occur during rest and during the night.

Osteoarthritis of the hand is characterised by Heberden's and Bouchard's nodes. Heberden's nodes are visible hard, bony swellings occurring at the distal interphalangeal joints at the end of the fingers. They are a consequence of bony outgrowths (osteophytes) that form in the articular cartilage as part of the joint repair mechanism. Bouchard's nodes are less common in hand osteoarthritis and are hard, bony outgrowths in the PIP joints.

Occasionally X-rays may be used to aid diagnosis in osteoarthritis. Typical features seen on X-ray include joint space narrowing, bone spurs (osteophytes), subchondral sclerosis and subchondral cysts. There may be poor correlation between the pain experienced by an individual and the extent of change demonstrated on X-ray. Blood tests and X-rays are not required for a diagnosis of osteoarthritis but may be performed to exclude other diseases such as psoriatic arthritis, RA and gout.

Management

The pain and disability associated with osteoarthritis can have significant impact on mood and may impair participation in both work and recreational activities. Patients should be educated about their osteoarthritis and be provided with a tailored self-management plan to maintain physical function and fitness, reduce pain and prevent further deterioration (Box 54.8). Pharmacological treatments are used as adjuncts, and the key to management is lifestyle change. People with osteoarthritis who experience joint symptoms (pain, stiffness and reduced function) that have a substantial impact on their quality of life and are refractory to non-surgical management should be referred for consideration of joint replacement surgery (NICE, 2014).

Non-pharmacological treatment

Weight loss

It is important that overweight patients are encouraged to lose weight because obesity is a known risk factor for the development of osteoarthritis (Bijlsma et al., 2011). Studies in patients with knee osteoarthritis have shown that supervised weight-loss programmes demonstrate small but significant improvements in pain and physical function (Fernandes et al., 2013; McAlindon et al., 2014). Overweight patients with osteoarthritis should be educated on weight loss and provided with support to achieve and maintain their target weight.

Exercise

Exercise can reduce pain and improve overall function in people with hip or knee osteoarthritis. NICE recommends exercise as a core treatment of osteoarthritis irrespective of age, comorbidity, pain severity or disability (NICE, 2015b). Exercise regimens should include local muscle strengthening, for example, quadriceps exercises for knee osteoarthritis, combined with general aerobic exercise. EULAR recommends patients with osteoarthritis perform moderate-intensity aerobic training for at least 30 minutes/day and progressive strength training involving the major muscle groups at least 2 days/week at moderate to vigorous intensity for 10 repetitions (Jordan et al., 2003). The regimen needs to be continued long-term and become part of the patient's usual lifestyle rather than an additional task they are required to perform.

Physical aids

Appropriate footwear can help reduce pain and improve physical function in people with osteoarthritis of the hip and knee. Studies involving patients with knee osteoarthritis have demonstrated that shock-absorbing insoles worn for 1 month reduced pain and improved physical function (Turpin et al., 2012). Athletic shoes with custom-made insoles and conventional athletic shoes have both been found to reduce pain in patients with knee osteoarthritis (Erhart et al., 2010). Specialised footwear is not required; EULAR recommends footwear with no raised heel and thick, shock-absorbing soles with support for the arches and of sufficient size to give comfortable space for the toes (Fernandes et al., 2013).

The Osteoarthritis Research Society International recommends the use of walking sticks in the management of knee osteoarthritis, but states there is a lack of evidence to support their use in multiple joint osteoarthritis (McAlindon et al., 2014). A single RCT concluded that using a walking stick, in comparison with usual disease management, can diminish pain and improve function and some aspects of quality of life in participants with knee osteoarthritis (Jones et al., 2012). In addition to walking sticks EULAR recommends walking frames or wheeled walkers in people with osteoarthritis of the hip or knee. Adaptive measures in the home, such as raising the height of chairs, beds and toilet seats or adding hand rails to stairs, may also be of benefit (Fernandes et al., 2013).

Joint protection is recommended in people with hand osteoarthritis. This consists of using the hands in a different way to avoid adverse pressure on the joints (Hochberg et al., 2012; Zhang et al., 2007). People with osteoarthritis of the hand should avoid gripping things too tightly and also positions that push the joint towards deformity. The Arthritis Research UK website (http://www.arthritisresearchuk.org) provides clear guidance on how to protect the hand joints when performing simple daily activities. Splints may be used for thumb base osteoarthritis.

Joint surgery

Joint surgery can be divided into arthroscopic (keyhole) surgery and joint replacement. Arthroscopic surgery is not recommended as part of osteoarthritis treatment unless a person with knee osteoarthritis has a clear history of true mechanical locking; this is where the knee suddenly cannot be fully straightened from a position of knee bend. This surgery does not otherwise improve clinical outcomes of knee osteoarthritis, even with symptoms of 'giving way' (typically a symptom of muscle weakness) or evidence of loose bodies on X-rays (Zhang et al., 2010). Joint replacement surgery should be considered when a patient with osteoarthritis suffers persistent debilitating symptoms despite treatment (NICE, 2014). Patients with osteoarthritis can be referred for a surgical opinion irrespective of age, gender, comorbidities, obesity and smoking status. Referral should occur before severe pain or established functional limitation develops.

Pharmacological management

The key management strategy for osteoarthritis is lifestyle change. Medication should be seen as an adjunct and not a replacement for appropriate exercise and diet. Paracetamol or topical NSAIDs should be used as first-line pharmacological treatments in patients with hand or knee osteoarthritis. Where either agent alone provides insufficient symptomatic benefit, the two medicines may be used in combination before progressing to the next step of pharmacological management. It is important to confirm that persistent pain is not being caused by non-adherence to a recommended exercise regimen.

Recommended treatments for osteoarthritis

Topical non-steroidal anti-inflammatory drugs. NICE (2014) supports the use of topical NSAIDs in the management of osteoarthritis. None of the current recognised international guidelines on the management of osteoarthritis give preference to a particular topical NSAID. A Cochrane review on the use of topical NSAIDs for chronic musculoskeletal pain in adults concluded that topical NSAIDs provide a good level of pain relief in osteoarthritis (Derry et al., 2016). In the review topical diclofenac solution was found to be equivalent to oral NSAIDs in knee and hand osteoarthritis, but there was no evidence for other painful conditions. For every six participants treated with diclofenac solution in the assessed studies, only one experienced a good level of pain relief over a period of 8–12 weeks. Diclofenac solution was shown to be more effective than diclofenac gel in the review (Derry et al., 2016). Gastro-intestinal side effects for topical NSAIDs did not differ from placebo, but there was an increase in localised skin reaction. Pain relief with topical NSAIDs may not be instant and is likely to increase over a period of several days; treatment should be discontinued if there is a lack of benefit after 4 weeks.

Paracetamol. Paracetamol monotherapy on a as required basis may be tried as an alternative first-line strategy to a topical NSAID in osteoarthritis. If intermittent consumption does not provide sufficient pain relief, then paracetamol may be given on a regular basis. It should be noted that both a systematic review and a meta-analysis have found paracetamol to be less effective in osteoarthritis than originally thought (Towheed et al., 2006; Zhang et al., 2010). In addition, toxicity associated with paracetamol use is greater than previously perceived at upper-end doses, with a dose-related increased incidence of mortality, cardiovascular, gastro-intestinal and renal adverse events (Craig et al., 2012; Roberts et al., 2016). It is important that all patients are advised not to exceed the recommended dose in a 24-hour period.

Oral non-steroidal anti-inflammatory drugs. NICE (2014) recommends the use of oral NSAIDs when initial treatment with a topical NSAID and/or paracetamol has provided no symptomatic relief or the relief provided by using these agents is insufficient. Where there has been no relief with topical NSAID and/or paracetamol these medicines should be stopped and the patient should be commenced on either a non-selective NSAID or a COX-2 inhibitor. Where partial relief has been achieved with the initial therapeutic strategy, it is recommended paracetamol be continued and the topical NSAID be switched to either a non-selective NSAID or a COX-2 inhibitor. No preference is made for either type of NSAID; the choice should be based on any additional comorbidities the patient may have (e.g. cardiovascular disease, renal disease, history of peptic ulcer disease), concomitant medication, patient preference and the side-effect profile of the individual NSAID. A meta-analysis has demonstrated an increased cardiovascular risk in all NSAID users, irrespective of their baseline risk or duration of use (Trelle et al., 2011). A higher risk was demonstrated where there was chronic, high-dose consumption, particularly in the case of COX-2 inhibitors and diclofenac (Bhala et al., 2013). Naproxen was shown to have a lower thrombotic risk compared with other assessed NSAIDs. It is recommended that the lowest effective dose of NSAID should be used and the duration kept to a minimum. Gastric protection in the form of a proton pump inhibitor should be co-prescribed with all NSAIDs including the COX-2 inhibitors in patients with osteoarthritis. Patients vary in their clinical response to NSAIDs; if no clinical response is seen after 3–4 weeks, then it may be beneficial to switch the patient to an alternative NSAID.

Opioid analgesics. In patients with osteoarthritis who are taking low-dose aspirin it may be preferable to use an opioid analgesic in combination with paracetamol in place of an oral NSAID. Opioid analgesics may also be used where there is a contraindication to the use of an oral NSAID and initial management with a topical NSAID and/or paracetamol has been ineffective. NICE (2014) supports the use of opioids in its guidance, but makes no recommendation with regard to the type of opioid analgesic to be used. A Cochrane review evaluating the benefit of oral (excluding tramadol) or transdermal opioids for osteoarthritis of the knee or hip found a small mean benefit, but a significant increase in adverse effects associated with opioid use (da Costa et al., 2014). The ACR guidance on the management of osteoarthritis supports the use of tramadol, but not other opioids (Hochberg et al., 2012).

Care should be taken when prescribing opioids in elderly patients because they are particularly sensitive to the side effects associated with opioid consumption. Laxatives should be provided where appropriate to prevent constipation. The risk of a fall may be increased due to sedation and/or dizziness associated with opioid consumption, especially in the presence of other medicines known to cause sedation. A medication review should be performed and previous tolerance to opioid side effects evaluated before commencing an opioid analgesic in an elderly patient.

Topical capsaicin. Topical capsaicin cream is derived from capsicum extract, which comes from the pepper family of plants. Its mechanism of action is not fully understood, but it has been proposed to exert its analgesic effect by depleting and preventing the re-accumulation of substance P in peripheral sensory neurones. Substance P is thought to be involved in the transfer of pain impulses from the peripheral nervous system to the central nervous system. The 0.025% cream is licensed for the management of osteoarthritis in the UK, and NICE (2014) recommends it as an adjunct therapy for knee and hand osteoarthritis. Its use can be considered at any stage of treatment. It is important that the cream is applied at regular intervals, up to four times a day, to ensure the patient gains tolerance to the burning sensation associated with the initial use of capsaicin. Relief of pain usually starts within the first week of treatment, but this gradually builds if the cream is applied regularly for 2–8 weeks.

Intra-articular corticosteroids. In osteoarthritis of the knee, intra-articular injections of corticosteroids into the joint may relieve inflammation and reduce pain and disability (Bannuru et al., 2009). NICE guidance on the management of osteoarthritis suggests intra-articular corticosteroids should be considered as adjuncts to core treatment for the relief of moderate-to-severe pain (NICE, 2015b).

Other therapies available for osteoarthritis management

Chondroitin and glucosamine. Supplements containing chondroitin and/or glucosamine are proposed to provide relief of pain in musculoskeletal conditions such as osteoarthritis. Chondroitin sulphate belongs to a class of very large molecules called glycosaminoglycans, which are made up of glucuronic acid and galactosamine. It is manufactured from natural sources such as shark and bovine cartilage. The rationale for taking this supplement in osteoarthritis is that chondroitin is found endogenously in the cartilaginous tissues of most mammals and serves as a substrate for the formation of the joint matrix structure. A published meta-analysis showed no statistically significant benefit of chondroitin when compared with placebo (McAlindon et al., 2014). In addition, in a stratified analysis of larger, high-quality trials the effects sizes for pain were small to non-existent for chondroitin (Reichenbach et al., 2007).

Glucosamine is available in three forms: glucosamine hydrochloride, glucosamine sulphate and *N*-acetylglucosamine. Glucosamine is required for the synthesis of mucopolysaccharides; these are carbohydrate-containing compounds found in tendons, ligaments, cartilage, synovial fluid, mucous membranes, structures in the eye, blood vessels and heart valves. Meta-analyses have failed to demonstrate a benefit in terms of pain relief or disease modification (Lee et al., 2010; Wandel et al., 2010).

NICE currently states that glucosamine and chondroitin products should not be offered for the management of osteoarthritis (NICE, 2014). The ACR also does not support the use of glucosamine and/or chondroitin in osteoarthritis of the hip or knee (Hochberg et al., 2012).

Hyaluronic acid intra-articular injections. Hyaluronan is a natural substance found in the body and is present in high amounts in the synovial fluid of joints. It acts as a lubricant and shock absorber within the joint. Synthesised hyaluronic acid is gel-like in nature and is injected intra-articularly into the knee joint to supplement the natural hyaluronan in the joint and reduce the pain associated with osteoarthritis of the knee. The injection may reduce pain over 1–6 months, but there may be an increase in knee inflammation in the short-term. Inconsistent conclusions from meta-analyses and conflicting results regarding safety have led to reluctance to support its use in the management of knee osteoarthritis. A systematic review found a small, but significant effect on knee pain by week 4 and a peak at week 8 (moderate clinical significance), with effect lasting up to 24 weeks (Bannuru et al., 2011). Other reviews have found only moderate benefit (Rutjes et al., 2012). In the UK the routine use of hyaluronic intra-articular injections is not supported (NICE, 2014). Current ACR recommendations support use in people older than 74 years with knee osteoarthritis that is refractory to standard pharmacological treatments (Hochberg et al., 2012).

Future management

Disease-modifying anti-rheumatic drugs. Biopsy studies have demonstrated histological synovitis in the early stages of chondral damage in osteoarthritis with cellular infiltration with macrophages, activated T and B cells, and vascular proliferation. Elevated cytokine levels have been demonstrated, but to a less extent than those seen in RA. Ongoing osteoarthritis methotrexate studies, including the PROMOTE study, are evaluating the benefits of oral methotrexate in knee osteoarthritis (Kingsbury et al., 2015). The analgesic and structural benefit of hydroxychloroquine in osteoarthritis is also being studied (Kingsbury et al., 2013). Current guidance on the management of osteoarthritis does not incorporate the use of DMARDs; further research is required to clearly define their role in osteoarthritis.

In vitro blocking TNF action decreases production of enzymes and pro-inflammatory mediators in osteoarthritis cartilage explants (Kobayashi et al., 2005). The use of TNFi has therefore been proposed in refractory osteoarthritis. A recent French study evaluating the symptomatic efficacy of adalimumab in patients suffering from hand osteoarthritis with a high level of pain and no response to analgesics and NSAIDs failed to show superiority over placebo (Chevalier et al., 2015). Other biologic therapies being evaluated include anti-nerve growth factor (anti-NGF) monoclonal antibodies. They work by selectively targeting, binding to and inhibiting NGF. NGF levels increase in the body as a result of injury, inflammation or in chronic pain states. The NGF monoclonal antibody tanezumab is the first medicine of this kind given US Food and Drug Administration fast-track approval for the treatment of chronic pain in osteoarthritis.

Patient Care

No pharmacological treatments are known to prevent or cure osteoarthritis. Pharmacological treatments are adjuncts that offer at best moderate symptom relief, and the key to

management is promoting lifestyle change. The limited role that medication plays should be explained to the patient, and that it is not a substitution for lifestyle modification. Patients should be encouraged to lose weight and eat a healthy diet. Exercise should become part of their daily routine, and the ideal regimen should include local muscle strengthening (e.g. quadriceps muscle exercise for knee osteoarthritis) combined with general aerobic fitness.

Case studies

Case 54.1

Mrs SM is a 56-year-old woman who has been referred to the hospital rheumatologist by her primary care clinician. Mrs SM has an 8-week history of painful joints in her fingers (mainly the PIP and MCP) and in the joints of her lower limbs. She initially thought her symptoms were due to her working hard in the garden, but they have gradually worsened over the past few weeks despite resting. She also complains of feeling tired all the time. The primary care clinician initially thought it was musculoskeletal pain and prescribed a short course of NSAIDs in combination with paracetamol. However, when her symptoms failed to resolve and there was evidence of swelling in the small joints of her hands he decided to perform some blood tests including inflammatory markers and refer her to a rheumatologist. Blood tests showed a CRP level of 20 mg/L. She has a medical history of hypertension, and current medication consists of amlodipine 5 mg once daily, naproxen 500 mg twice a day and paracetamol 500 mg four times a day. In clinic, the hospital doctor takes a brief medical history from the patient and performs a physical examination. On examination there is active synovitis in the wrists, MCP joints and PIP joints of both hands and synovitis in both ankles. Mrs SM complains of early-morning stiffness persisting for up to 2 hours each morning. Her hands and wrists of both arms have been tender and swollen for the last 2 weeks, and she has found it difficult to walk because of swelling and pain in both knee joints and in her feet. The hospital doctor following blood tests, X-rays and physical examination makes a provisional diagnosis of RA.

Questions

1. What common signs and symptoms of RA does Mrs SM present with?
2. What treatments would be recommended for the initial management of Mrs SM's RA?

Answers

1. Mrs SM presented with swelling and pain in the small joints of the hands (PIPs and MCPs). Examination of the hand joints by the doctor indicated the presence of active inflammation (synovitis). There was also active synovitis in the ankle joints and she had a raised CRP level. Morning stiffness is a common early feature of RA. Mrs SM complained of stiffness lasting up to 2 hours each morning. Patients may experience fatigue and widespread musculoskeletal pain before there is visible swelling of the joints. There is no specific test to confirm the presence of RA. Presenting symptoms, X-ray images and blood tests including non-specific inflammatory markers (CRP, ESR) and auto-antibodies (RF, ACPA) are used in the diagnosis of RA. The presence or absence of these features is used to generate a score using the ACR and the EULAR diagnostic algorithm. A score of at least 6 out of 10 is required for a diagnosis of RA.

2. It is recommended that treatment with either combination or csDMARD monotherapy is commenced as soon as a diagnosis of RA is made. The agent of choice is methotrexate, and it can either be combined with other csDMARDs or given as monotherapy according to clinician and patient preference. Where methotrexate is contraindicated either leflunomide or sulfasalazine may be considered. Hydroxychloroquine tends to be used in mild disease or in combination with other csDMARDs because it has not been shown to inhibit structural damage sufficiently when compared with other csDMARDs. Response to treatment with csDMARD therapy should be closely monitored using a disease activity scoring system such as the DAS28. If there is a lack of clinical response at 3 months, then the therapeutic strategy should be altered. The aim is to achieve the therapeutic target of clinical remission at 6 months or where this is not possible low disease activity.

DMARDs have a delayed onset of action: it may take 4–6 weeks before the patient starts to see a response, and up to 4–6 months before a full response is achieved. The use of low-dose glucocorticosteroids is recommended as part of the initial treatment strategy because they are effective in reducing symptoms and disease activity when waiting for the therapeutic onset of a DMARD. In addition they have been shown to be effective adjunctive treatments with the main DMARD therapy to more efficiently achieve the desired target (usually clinical remission). When oral corticosteroids are used as part of the initial treatment strategy they should be tapered off as rapidly as clinically feasible and ideally within 6 months. Due to the effect of corticosteroids on bone mineral density, the need for calcium and vitamin D supplementation in combination with a bisphosphonate should be considered during treatment with corticosteroids.

Mrs SM is already taking the NSAID naproxen. NSAIDs may be prescribed in addition to csDMARD and glucocorticoids because they can help relieve pain and stiffness. They should be used in short courses at the lowest effective dose to provide symptomatic relief. Persistent pain and stiffness, despite the introduction of csDMARDs, indicates active disease and the need to change or step up treatment with DMARDs. No NSAID has demonstrated superiority over another in RA, but they differ in their side-effect profiles. The basis of selection should be according to patient preference and comorbidities. An increased cardiovascular risk is associated with all NSAIDs, irrespective of their baseline risk, and not only in chronic users. The greatest concern relates to chronic users of high-dose NSAIDS, especially the COX-2 selective agents and diclofenac. Evidence suggests that naproxen is associated with a lower thrombotic risk than the COX-2 selective agents. A gastro-protective agent should be prescribed with an NSAID whether it is non-selective or COX-2 selective.

Paracetamol used in combination with a weak opiate such as dihydrocodeine can be beneficial in providing simple pain relief. Although the combination has no anti-inflammatory properties and will not affect the disease process, simple analgesic combinations such as this do have a place in both early and late stages of the disease.

Case 54.2

Mr PB is a 58-year-old man who was diagnosed as having RA 6 months ago. He has been on combination DMARD therapy with injectable methotrexate 25 mg subcutaneously once a week, and hydroxychloroquine 200 mg twice a day. At his hospital appointment with the rheumatologist he is still symptomatic with active synovitis demonstrated by ultrasound in the small joints of his hand. He reports significant fatigue and feeling unwell. His calculated DAS28 is 5.2. After a discussion with the rheumatologist, a decision is made to start a biologic DMARD.

The rheumatologist discusses the various biologic medicines available with the patient and provides the patient with a number of leaflets about these medicines prepared by Arthritis Research UK. He asks the patient to have a think about which therapy he would prefer while important screening tests are performed.

Questions

1. Does Mr PB meet the UK criteria for commencement of a biologic medicine in RA?
2. What first-line biologic medicines are likely to be offered to Mr PB by his rheumatologist?
3. What blood tests should be performed before Mr PB is commenced on a biologic medicine?

Answers

1. Mr PB's RA has failed to respond to combined treatment with two csDMARDs, methotrexate and hydroxychloroquine. His calculated DAS28 score is also greater than 5.1. Biologic medicines now form part of the standard treatment strategy for RA, and NICE recommends the use of a biologic medicine in RA in patients with a DAS28 greater than 5.1 whose disease has not responded to intensive therapy with a combination of conventional DMARDs (NICE, 2016).

2. In the UK NICE supports the use of adalimumab, etanercept, infliximab, certolizumab pegol, golimumab, tocilizumab and abatacept, all in combination with methotrexate (NICE, 2016). In patients who cannot take methotrexate, adalimumab, etanercept, certolizumab pegol or tocilizumab can be given as monotherapy. At present there is no evidence to support one biologic over another as a first-line option. NICE proposes that the least expensive biologic medicine should be prescribed, but consideration should be given to the patient's preferred mode of administration and treatment schedules which do not interfere with work and home commitments. Other factors which will be considered by the rheumatologist include the presence of comorbidities such as heart disease, lung disease, previous malignancy, co-existing autoimmune diseases (IBD and psoriasis) and the presence of auto-antibodies associated with connective tissue diseases such as SLE.

3. The use of biologic medicines is associated with an increased risk of serious infection including TB and hepatitis B/C. The presence of these diseases must be excluded before a biologic medicine is commenced. Mr PB will be asked to have blood test to evaluate the presence of TB (QuantiFERON-TB) and antibodies associated with past hepatitis B and C infection. An FBC, chest X-ray and urinalysis will be performed to exclude the presence of other types of infections. The TNFi may activate or worsen SLE. Mr PB will be screened for the presence of auto-antibodies which are associated with the development of SLE; this can be done using a simple blood test. Baseline LFT should be performed because the TNFi, abatacept and tocilizumab can cause a rise in transaminases. Particular care should be taken with tocilizumab in patients with elevated ALT or AST greater than 1.5 times ULN because of the increased incidence of significant rises in transaminases associated with the use of tocilizumab. None of the first-line recommended biologics have been studied in moderate-to-severe renal disease, and there are no specific recommendations regarding dose reduction. Renal function should be evaluated at baseline and intermittently throughout treatment. The use of tocilizumab has been associated with abnormal lipid profiles; if Mr PB has a background history of cardiovascular disease the rheumatologist may also assess Mr PB's lipid profile.

Case 54.3

Mrs JT is a 65-year-old woman who is referred by her primary care clinician for progressive left knee pain. She has little morning stiffness and significant swelling towards the end of the day. She is taking paracetamol, but this is not particularly helpful. She has been gaining weight (body mass index is now 36), and more recently her knee is giving way when she is walking.

Questions

What measures would you recommend to manage Mrs JT's symptoms of osteoarthritis?

Answers

The measures to be undertaken as listed below:

- Provide advice and support on achieving weight loss. Weight loss has been shown to have a dose-dependent effect on pain relief, and ideally 10% of body weight should be lost. This may be best achieved by walking in the swimming pool first, so that it is not too painful for Mrs JT.
- Review Mrs JT's analgesia. Mrs JT is already taking paracetamol; a trial of topical capsaicin 0.025% cream four times a day for 1 month or a topical NSAID should be tried. If a trial of topical therapies is not beneficial, then treatment may be stepped up to an oral NSAID provided there are no contraindications.
- Recommend use of a knee brace because this can help reduce pain and further structural damage.
- Encourage exercise and seek the support of the physiotherapy service. They will assess Mrs JT's current muscle strength and provide her with an exercise programme which will include exercises to improve and maintain quadriceps strength. Quadriceps exercises should be maintained lifelong to stabilise the joints and reduce pain.
- If in spite of all of the above recommendations Mrs JT still has persistent activity-related pain that is starting to affect other parts of her body (e.g. shoulders, hips), then referral for knee replacement surgery will be considered.

References

Adachi, Y., Yoshio-Hoshino, N., Nishimoto, N., 2008. The blockade of IL-6 signalling in rational drug design. Curr. Pharm. Des. 14, 1217–1224.

Aletaha, D., Alasti, F., Smolen, J.S., et al., 2016. Extended report: optimisation of a treat-to-target approach in rheumatoid arthritis: strategies for the 3-month time point. Ann. Rheum. Dis 75, 1479–1485.

Arthritis Research UK, 2013. Osteoarthritis in General Practice: Data and Perspectives. Arthritis Research UK, Chesterfield, UK.

Bannuru, R.R., Natov, N.S., Dasi, U.R., et al., 2011. Therapeutic trajectory following intra-articular hyaluronic acid injection in knee osteoarthritise meta-analysis. Osteoarthritis Cartilage 19, 611–619.

Bannuru, R.R., Natov, N.S., Obadan, I.E., et al., 2009. Therapeutic trajectory of hyaluronic acid versus corticosteroids in the treatment of knee osteoarthritis: a systematic review and meta-analysis. Arthritis Rheum. J. 61, 1704–1711.

Bessone, F., 2010. Non-steroidal anti-inflammatory drugs: what is the actual risk of liver damage? World J. Gastroenterol. 16, 5651–5661.

Bhala, N., Emberson, J., Merhi, M., et al., 2013. Coxibs and traditional NSAID Trialists' (CNT) collaboration. Vascular and upper gastro-intestinal effects of non-steroidal anti-inflammatory drugs: meta-analysis of individual participant data from randomised trials. Lancet 382, 769–779.

Bijlsma, J.W., Berenbaum, F., Lafeber, F.P., 2011. Osteoarthritis: an update with relevance for clinical practice. Lancet 377, 2115–2126.

Buch, M.H., Smolen, J.S., Betteridge, N., et al., 2011. Updated consensus statement on the use of rituximab in patients with rheumatoid arthritis. Ann. Rheum. Dis. 70, 909–920.

Castellsague, J., Riera-Guardia, N., Calingaert, B., et al., 2012. Individual NSAIDS and upper gastro-intestinal complications: systematic review and meta-analyses of observational studies (the SOS project). Drug Safety 35, 1127–1146.

Chevalier, X., Ravaud, P., Maheu, E., et al., 2015. Extended report: adalimumab in patients with hand osteoarthritis refractory to analgesics and NSAIDs: a randomised, multicentre, double-blind, placebo-controlled trial. Ann. Rheum. Dis. 74, 1697–1705.

Chung, E.S., Packer, M., Lo, K.H., et al., 2003. Randomized, double-blind, placebo-controlled, pilot trial of infliximab, a chimeric monoclonal antibody to tumor necrosis factor-alpha, in patients with moderate-to-severe heart failure: results of the anti-TNF Therapy Against Congestive Heart Failure (ATTACH) trial. Circulation 107, 3133–3140.

Cooper, M.S., Stewart, P.M., 2003. Corticosteroid insufficiency in acutely ill patients. N. Engl. J. Med. 348, 727–734.

Craig, D.G.N., Bates, C.M., Davidson, J.S., et al., 2012. Staggered overdose pattern and delay to hospital presentation are associated with adverse outcomes following paracetamol-induced hepatotoxicity. Br. J. Clin. Pharmacol. 73, 285–294.

Cross, M., Smith, E., Hoy, D., et al., 2014. The global burden of hip and knee osteoarthritis: estimates from the Global Burden of Disease 2010 study. Ann. Rheum. Dis. 73, 1323–1330.

da Costa, B.R., Nuesch, E., Kasteler, R., et al., 2014. Oral or transdermal opioids for osteoarthritis of the knee or hip. Cochrane Database Syst. Rev. 9, CD003115. https://doi.org/10.1002/14651858.CD003115.pub4.

Derry, S., Moore, R.A., Rabbie, R, 2016. Topical NSAIDs for chronic musculoskeletal pain in adults. Cochrane Database Syst. Rev 4, CD007400. https://doi.org/10.1002/14651858.CD007400.pub3.

Ding, T., Ledingham, J., Luqmani, R., et al., 2010. BSR and BHPR rheumatoid arthritis guidelines on safety of anti-TNF therapies. Rheumatology 49, 2217–2219.

Erhart, J.C., Mundermann, A., Elspas, B., et al., 2010. Changes in knee adduction moment, pain, and functionality with a variable-stiffness walking shoe after 6 months. J. Orthop. Res. 28, 873–879.

Evangelou, E., Kerkhof, H.J., Styrkarsdottir, U., et al., 2014. A meta-analysis of genome-wide association studies identifies novel variants associated with osteoarthritis of the hip. Ann Rheum. Dis. 73, 2130–2136.

Felson, D.T., Smolen, J.S., Wells, G., et al., 2011. American College of Rheumatology/European League Against Rheumatism provisional definition of remission in rheumatoid arthritis for clinical trials. Ann. Rheum. Dis. 70, 404–413.

Fernandes, L., Hagen, K.B., Bijlsma, J.W., et al., 2013. EULAR recommendations for the non-pharmacological core management of hip and knee osteoarthritis. Ann. Rheum. Dis. 72, 1125–1135.

Fleischmann, R., Mysler, E., Hall, S., et al., 2017. Efficacy and safety of tofacitinib monotherapy, tofacitinib with methotrexate, and adalimumab with methotrexate in patients with rheumatoid arthritis (ORAL Strategy): a phase 3b/4, double-blind, head-to-head, randomised controlled trial. Lancet 390, 457–468.

Flint, J., Panchal, S., Hurrell, A., et al., 2016a. BSR and BHPR guideline on prescribing drugs in pregnancy and breastfeeding – part I: standard and biologic disease modifying anti-rheumatic drugs and corticosteroids. Rheumatology 55, 1693–1697.

Flint, J., Panchal, S., Hurrell, A., et al., 2016b. BSR and BHPR guideline on prescribing drugs in pregnancy and breastfeeding – part II: analgesics and other drugs used in rheumatology practice. Rheumatology 55, 1698–1702.

Fransen, J., van Riel, P.L.C.M., 2005. The Disease Activity Score and the EULAR response criteria. Clin. Exp. Rheumatol. 23 (Suppl. 39), S93–S99.

Gabay, C., Riek, M., Lund Hetland, M., et al., 2016. Effectiveness of tocilizumab with and without synthetic disease-modifying antirheumatic drugs in rheumatoid arthritis: results from a European collaborative study. Ann. Rheum. Dis. 75, 1336–1342.

Glyn-Jones, S., Palmer, A.J.R., Agricola, R., et al., 2015. Osteoarthritis. Lancet 386, 376–387.

Goldring, M.B., Goldring, S.R., 2010. Articular cartilage and subchondral bone in the pathogenesis of osteoarthritis. Ann. N. Y. Acad. Sci. 1192, 230–237.

Gottenberg, J.E., Ravaud, P., Bardin, T., et al., 2010. Risk factors for severe infections in patients with rheumatoid arthritis treated with rituximab in the autoimmunity and rituximab registry. Arthritis Rheum. 62, 2625–2632.

Hochberg, M.C., Altman, R.D., April, K.T., et al., 2012. American College of Rheumatology 2012 recommendations for the use of nonpharmacologic and pharmacologic therapies in osteoarthritis of the hand, hip, and knee. Arthritis Care Res. 64, 465–474.

Humphreys, J., Hyrich, K., Symmons, D., 2016. What is the impact of biologic therapies on common co-morbidities in patients with rheumatoid arthritis. Arthritis Res. Ther. 18, 282.

Inoue, Y., Nakajima, A., Tanaka, E., et al., 2015. Effect of smoking on remission proportions differs between male and female patients with rheumatoid arthritis: a study based on the IORRA survey. J. Rheumatol. 42, 1083–1089.

Jones, G., Sebba, A., Gu, J., et al., 2010. Comparison of tocilizumab monotherapy versus methotrexate monotherapy in patients with moderate to severe rheumatoid arthritis: the AMBITION study. Ann. Rheum. Dis. 69, 88–96.

Jones, A., Silva, P.G., Silva, A.C., et al., 2012. Impact of cane use on pain, function, general health and energy expenditure during gait in patients with knee osteoarthritis: a randomised controlled trial. Ann. Rheum. Dis. 71, 172–179.

Jonsson, H., Manolescu, I., Stefansson, S.E., et al., 2003. The inheritance of hand osteoarthritis in Iceland. Arthritis Rheum. 48, 391–395.

Jordan, K.M., Arden, N.K., Doherty, M., et al., 2003. EULAR Recommendations 2003: an evidence based approach to the management of knee osteoarthritis: Report of a Task Force of the Standing Committee for International Clinical Studies Including Therapeutic Trials (ESCISIT). Ann. Rheum. Dis. 62, 1145–1155.

Katz, S.J., Russell, A.S., 2011. Re-evaluation of antimalarials in treating rheumatic diseases: re-appreciation and insights into new mechanisms of action. Curr. Opin. Rheumatol. 23, 278–281.

Kay, J., Upchurch, K.S., 2012. ACR/EULAR 2010 rheumatoid arthritis classification criteria. Rheumatology 51 (Suppl. 6), vi5–vi9.

Kingsbury, S.R., Tharmanathan, P., Adamson, J., et al., 2013. Hydroxychloroquine effectiveness in reducing symptoms of hand osteoarthritis (HERO): study protocol for a randomized controlled trial. Trials 14, 64.

Kingsbury, S.R., Tharmanathan, P., Arden, N.K., et al., 2015. Pain reduction with oral methotrexate in knee osteoarthritis, a pragmatic phase III trial of treatment effectiveness (PROMOTE): study protocol for a randomized controlled trial. Trials 16, 77.

Kobayashi, M., Squires, G.R., Mousa, A., et al., 2005. Role of interleukin 1 and tumour necrosis alpha in matrix degradation of human osteoarthritic cartilage. Arthritis Rheum. 52, 128–135.

Kraus, V.B., Jordan, J.M., Doherty, M., et al., 2007. The Genetics of Generalized Osteoarthritis (GOGO) study: study design and evaluation of osteoarthritis phenotypes. Osteoarthritis Cartilage 15, 120–127.

Ledingham, J., Gullick, N., Irving, K., et al., 2017. BSR and BHPR guideline for the prescription monitoring of non-biologic disease modifying antirheumatic drugs. Rheumatology 56, 865–868.

Lee, Y.H., Woo, J.H., Choi, S.J., et al., 2010. Effect of glucosamine or chondroitin sulfate on the osteoarthritis progression: a meta-analysis. Rheumatol. Int. 30, 357–363.

Mann, D.L., McMurray, J.J., Packer, M., et al., 2004. Targeted anticytokine therapy in patients with chronic heart failure: results of the Randomized Etanercept Worldwide Evaluation (RENEWAL). Circulation 109, 1594–1602.

McAlindon, T.E., Bannuru, R.R., Sullivan, M.C., et al., 2014. OARSI guidelines for the non-surgical management of knee osteoarthritis. Osteoarthritis Cartilage 22, 363–388.

National Institute for Health and Care Excellence (NICE), 2010. Adalimumab, etanercept, infliximab, rituximab and abatacept for the treatment of rheumatoid arthritis after the failure of a TNF inhibitor. Technology appraisal guidance [TA195]. NICE, London. Available at: https://www.nice.org.uk/guidance/ta195.

National Institute for Health and Care Excellence (NICE), 2012. Tocilizumab for the treatment of rheumatoid arthritis. NICE technology appraisal guidance [TA247]. NICE, London. Available at: https://www.nice.org.uk/guidance/ta247.

National Institute for Health and Care Excellence (NICE), 2014. Osteoarthritis: care and management. Clinical guidance [CG177]. Available at: https://www.nice.org.uk/guidance/cg177.

National Institute for Health and Care Excellence (NICE), 2015a. Rheumatoid arthritis in adults: management. NICE guidelines [CG79]. NICE, London. Available at: https://www.nice.org.uk/guidance/cg79.

National Institute for Health and Care Excellence (NICE), 2015b. Osteoarthritis quality standard [QS87]. Available at: https://www.nice.org.uk/guidance/qs87.

National Institute for Health and Care Excellence (NICE), 2016. Adalimumab, etanercept, infliximab, certolizumab pegol, golimumab, tocilizumab and abatacept for rheumatoid arthritis not previously treated with DMARDs or after conventional DMARDs only have failed. Technology appraisal guidance [TA375]. NICE, London. Available at: https://www.nice.org.uk/guidance/ta375.

National Institute for Health and Care Excellence (NICE), 2017a. Baricitinib for moderate to severe rheumatoid arthritis. Technology appraisal guidance [TA466]. NICE, London. Available at: https://www.nice.org.uk/guidance/ta466.

National Institute for Health and Care Excellence (NICE), 2017b. Tofacitinib for moderate to severe rheumatoid arthritis. Technology appraisal guidance [TA480]. NICE, London. Available at: https://www.nice.org.uk/guidance/ta480.

National Institute for Health and Care Excellence (NICE), 2017c. Sarilumab for moderate to severe RA. Technology appraisal guidance [TA485]. NICE, London. Available at: https://www.england.nhs.uk/guidance/ta485.

National Patient Safety Alerts (NPSA), 2004. Towards the safer use of oral methotrexate. NPSA, London.

NHS England, 2015. What is a biosimilar medicine? (Draft 8.3) NHS England. Available at: https://www.england.nhs.uk/wp-content/uploads/2015/09/biosimilar-guide.pdf.

Nishimoto, N., Hashimoto, J., Miyasaka, N., et al., 2007. Study of active controlled monotherapy used for rheumatoid arthritis, an IL-6 inhibitor (SAMURAI): evidence of clinical and radiographic benefit from an x ray reader-blinded randomised controlled trial of tocilizumab. Ann. Rheum. Dis. 66, 1162–1167.

Nishimoto, N., Terao, K., Mima, T., et al., 2008. Mechanisms and the pathologic significances in increase in serum interleukin-6 (IL-6) and soluble IL-6 receptor after administration of an anti-IL-6 receptor antibody, tocilizumab, in patients with rheumatoid arthritis and Castleman's disease. Blood 112, 3959–3964.

Østensen, M., Andreoli, L., Brucato, A., et al., 2015. State of the art: reproduction and pregnancy in rheumatic diseases. Autoimmun. Rev. 14, 376–386.

Payne, J.B., Golub, L.M., Thiele, G.M., et al., 2015. The link between periodontitis and rheumatoid arthritis: a periodontist's perspective. Curr. Oral Health Rep. 2, 20–29.

Prieto-Alhambra, R.D., Judge, A., Kassim Javaid, M., et al., 2014. Incidence and risk factors for clinically diagnosed knee, hip and hand osteoarthritis: influences of age, gender and osteoarthritis affecting other joints. Ann. Rheum. Dis. 73, 1659–1664.

Reichenbach, S., Sterchi, R., Scherer, M., et al., 2007. Meta-analysis: chondroitin for osteoarthritis of the knee or hip. Ann. Intern. Med. 146, 580–590.

Roberts, E., Nunes, V.D., Buckner, S., et al., 2016. Paracetamol: not as safe as we thought? Ann. Rheum. Dis. 75, 552–559.

Roemer, F.W., Kwoh, C.K., Hannon, M.J., et al., 2015. Can structural joint damage measured with MR imaging be used to predict knee replacement the following year? Radiology 274, 810–820.

Rutjes, A.W., Juni, P., da Costa, B.R., et al., 2012. Viscosupplementation for osteoarthritis of the knee: a systematic review and meta-analysis. Ann. Intern. Med. 157, 180–191.

Sellam, J., Hendel-Chavez, H., Rouanet, S., et al., 2011. B cell activation biomarkers as predictive factors for the response to rituximab in rheumatoid arthritis: a six-month, national, multicenter, open-label study. Arthritis Rheum. 63, 933–938.

Smolen, J.S., Landewé, R., Bijlsma, J., et al., 2017. EULAR recommendations for the management of rheumatoid arthritis with synthetic and biological disease-modifying antirheumatic drugs: 2016 update. Ann. Rheum. Dis. 76, 960–977.

Smolen, J.S., Landewé, R., Breedveld, F.C., et al., 2014. EULAR recommendations for the management of rheumatoid arthritis with synthetic and biological disease modifying anti-rheumatic drugs: 2013 update. Ann. Rheum. Dis. 73, 492–509.

Suri, S., Walsh, D.A., 2012. Osteochondral alterations in osteoarthritis. Bone 51, 204–211.

Tak, P.P., Rigby, W.F., Rubbert-Roth, A., et al., 2011. Inhibition of joint damage and improved clinical outcomes with rituximab plus methotrexate in early active rheumatoid arthritis: the IMAGE trial. Ann. Rheum. Dis. 70, 39–46.

Taylor, P.C., Keystone, E.C., van der Heijde, D., et al., 2017. Baricitinib versus placebo or adalimumab in rheumatoid arthritis. N. Engl. J. Med. 376, 652–662.

Towheed, T.E., Maxwell, L., Judd, M.G., et al., 2006. Acetaminophen for osteoarthritis. Cochrane Database Syst. Rev. 1, CD004257. https://doi.org/10.1002/14651858.CD004257.pub2.

Trelle, S., Reichenbach, S., Wandel, S., et al., 2011. Cardiovascular safety of non-steroidal anti-inflammatory drugs: network meta-analysis. Br. Med. J. 342, c7086.

Turpin, K.M., De Vincenzo, A., Apps, A.M., et al., 2012. Biomechanical and clinical outcomes with shock-absorbing insoles in patients with knee osteoarthritis: immediate effects and changes after 1 month of wear. Arch. Phys. Med. Rehabil 93, 503–508.

van Staa, T.P., 2006. The pathogenesis, epidemiology and management of glucocorticoid-induced osteoporosis. Calcif. Tissue Int. 79, 129–137.

van Vollenhoven, R.F., Emery, P., Bingham, C.O., et al., 2010. Longterm safety of patients receiving rituximab in rheumatoid arthritis clinical trials. J. Rheumatol. 37, 558–567.

Wandel, S., Juni, P., Tendal, B., et al., 2010. Effects of glucosamine, chondroitin, or placebo in patients with osteoarthritis of hip or knee: network meta-analysis. Br. Med. J. 341, c4675.

Yusuf, E., Kortekaas, M.C., Watt, L., et al., 2011. Do knee abnormalities visualised on MRI explain knee pain in osteoarthritis? A systematic review. Ann. Rheum. Dis. 70, 60–67.

Zangi, H.A., Ndosi, M., Adams, J., et al., 2015. EULAR recommendations for patient education for people with inflammatory arthritis. Ann. Rheum. Dis. 74, 954–962.

Zhang, W., Doherty, M., Leeb, B.F., et al., 2007. EULAR evidence based recommendations for the management of hand osteoarthritis: report of a Task Force of the EULAR Standing Committee for International Clinical Studies Including Therapeutics (ESCISIT). Ann. Rheum. Dis. 66, 377–388.

Zhang, W., Nuki, G., Moskowitz, R.W., et al., 2010. OARSI recommendations for the management of hip and knee osteoarthritis: part III: changes in evidence following systematic cumulative update of research published through. January 2009. Osteoarthritis Cartilage 18, 476–499.

Zhang, X., Zhang, D., Jia, H., et al., 2015. The oral and gut microbiomes are perturbed in rheumatoid arthritis and partly normalized after treatment. Nat. Med. 21, 895–905.

Zhang, Y., Nui, J., Kelly-Hayes, M., et al., 2002. Prevalence of symptomatic hand osteoarthritis and its impact on functional status among the elderly: the Framingham Study. Am. J. Epidemiol. 156, 1021–1027.

Further reading

Sharma, L., 2016. Osteoarthritis year in review 2015: clinical. Osteoarthritis Cartilage 24, 36–48.

Smolen, J.S., Aletaha, D., McInnes, I.B., 2016. Rheumatoid arthritis. Lancet 388, 2023–2038.

Useful websites

American College of Rheumatology: http://www.rheumatology.org
Arthritis Research UK: http://www.arthritisresearchuk.org

British Society of Rheumatology: http://www.rheumatology.org.uk
European League Against Rheumatism: http://www.eular.org

55 Gout and Hyperuricaemia

Tina Hawkins

Key points

- Gout is the most common inflammatory joint disease in men and is strongly age related.
- The prevalence and burden of gout has increased over recent decades.
- It is caused by the deposition of monosodium urate crystals within articular and periarticular tissue.
- The degree of elevation of uric acid levels above the saturation point for urate crystal formation is a major determinant in precipitating an attack.
- Not all people with hyperuricaemia experience development of gout.
- Gout is normally the result of an interaction between genetic, constitutional and environmental risk factors.
- The aim of long-term therapy is to reduce the serum uric acid level sufficiently so that crystals can no longer form and existing crystals are dissolved.
- Non-pharmacological measures such as lifestyle and dietary modification play an important role in the management of gout.
- Unmanaged recurrent attacks can result in progressive cartilage and bone erosion, deposition of tophi, secondary osteoarthritis and disability.
- Despite the introduction of modern therapies and treatment guidelines, the management of gout remains suboptimal.

The global burden of gout is rising and it is now the most common cause of inflammatory arthritis (Kuo et al., 2015a; Smith et al., 2014). Gout results from the deposition of monosodium urate crystals in peripheral joints and soft tissues due to persistent elevation of uric acid levels above the saturation point for crystal deposition. Chronic hyperuricaemia is associated with disorders of purine metabolism caused by underexcretion or overproduction of uric acid, the final metabolite of endogenous and dietary purine metabolism. Gout usually presents as a monoarthritis in the foot or ankle, especially in the first metatarsophalangeal joint (big toe), and is often referred to as podagra (from the Greek 'seizing the foot'). Subsequent attacks may be in the same or other joints, or involve multiple joints. Other commonly affected joints include the knee, wrist, elbow and finger joints.

Although an acute attack is extremely painful, it is usually self-limiting, resolving spontaneously in 1–2 weeks. Acute attacks are managed with rest, sometimes ice and one or more of the following pharmacological agents: colchicine, non-steroidal anti-inflammatory drugs (NSAIDs), corticosteroids and, in severe refractory disease, the interleukin-1 (IL-1) receptor antagonists. Some patients may only ever experience one attack, but once a second attack occurs (often within 6–12 months), there is an increased risk of subsequent attacks. Patients with recurrent attacks require long-term prophylaxis with drugs that lower the serum urate level. The drug of choice is usually allopurinol; however, a small percentage of patients are unable to tolerate allopurinol and require treatment with an alternative urate-lowering agent, such as febuxostat, or a uricosuric agent such as benzbromarone, lesinurad, sulfinpyrazone or probenecid. Recombinant forms of the enzyme uricase may be used to lower serum urate levels in individuals with severe tophaceous gout. It is essential that pharmacological measures are combined with non-pharmacological measures, such as dietary and lifestyle modification, to prevent recurrent attacks. Inappropriate management of gout can result in chronic tophaceous gout with polyarticular, destructive low-grade joint inflammation, joint deformity and tophi. Gout is not only an inflammatory arthritis of the joints, it is also associated with obesity, hypertension, metabolic syndrome and an increased future risk of major cardiovascular events and premature mortality (Rho et al., 2016).

Epidemiology

Gout is one of the oldest recognised diseases and was identified by the Egyptians in 2460 BC. Hippocrates described it as 'arthritis of the rich' because of the association with certain foods and alcohol. Due to an ageing population and rising obesity, the burden of gout is increasing around the world, especially in high-income countries (Smith et al., 2014). The reported prevalence of gout worldwide ranges from 0.1% to approximately 10%, and the incidence from 0.3 to 6 cases per 1000 person-years (Kuo et al., 2015b). Recent studies have demonstrated both an increase in the prevalence and the incidence of gout in the UK (Kuo et al., 2015a). A study evaluating data up to 2012 has estimated the UK prevalence rate of gout to be 2.49%, with an incidence of 1.77 per 1000 patient-years (Kuo et al., 2015a). Before this, the UK prevalence rate was estimated to be 1.4% and remained fairly static between the period of 1999–2005 (Annemans et al., 2008). Prevalence estimates for Spain and the Netherlands are similar to the UK, whereas Greece has the highest reported prevalence rate of gout in Europe at 4.75% in the adult population. In the USA, gout has overtaken rheumatoid arthritis to become the most common inflammatory arthritis (Smith et al., 2014).

Gout before the age of 20 years is rare, but prevalence progressively increases from the age of 30 regardless of gender and tends to reach a plateau after the age of 70 years. Worldwide the prevalence of gout is significantly higher in men than women, and the male-to-female ratio is estimated to be 3–4:1 (Kuo et al., 2015b). It is important to note that the prevalence of gout is low in females before the age of 45 years, and this is thought to be due to a link between the menopause and gout (Hak et al., 2010).

A genetic predisposition, increasing age and changes in lifestyle have contributed to the increasing prevalence of gout in many developed countries. The Maori population has been shown to have a genetic predisposition to gout, but before 1700 they did not experience this inflammatory joint disease. Maori now have a threefold greater risk of gout than New Zealanders of European descent (Winnard et al., 2012). It is thought that adaptation to a European diet and lifestyle by the Maori has led to the appearance and increasing prevalence of gout in New Zealand.

Pathophysiology

Uric acid is mainly formed as a by-product from the breakdown of cellular nucleoproteins within the body and purine nucleotides synthesised de novo (Fig. 55.1). The remaining third of uric acid production comes from purine ingestion as part of an individual's diet. The enzyme xanthine oxidase catalyses the oxidation of hypoxanthine, the breakdown product resulting from the catabolism of cellular nucleoproteins, dietary purine and purine nucleotides, to xanthine and xanthine to uric acid (see Fig. 55.1). Uric acid, produced as a consequence of this process, is a weak organic acid with a pK_a of 5.75, and at the physiological pH of the extra-cellular compartment 98% of uric acid is in the ionised form of urate. This is mainly present as monosodium urate due to the high concentration of sodium in the extra-cellular compartment. Monosodium urate has a solubility limit of 380 mmol/L; when the concentration exceeds 380 mmol/L, as in hyperuricaemia, there is a risk of precipitation and the formation of monosodium urate crystals.

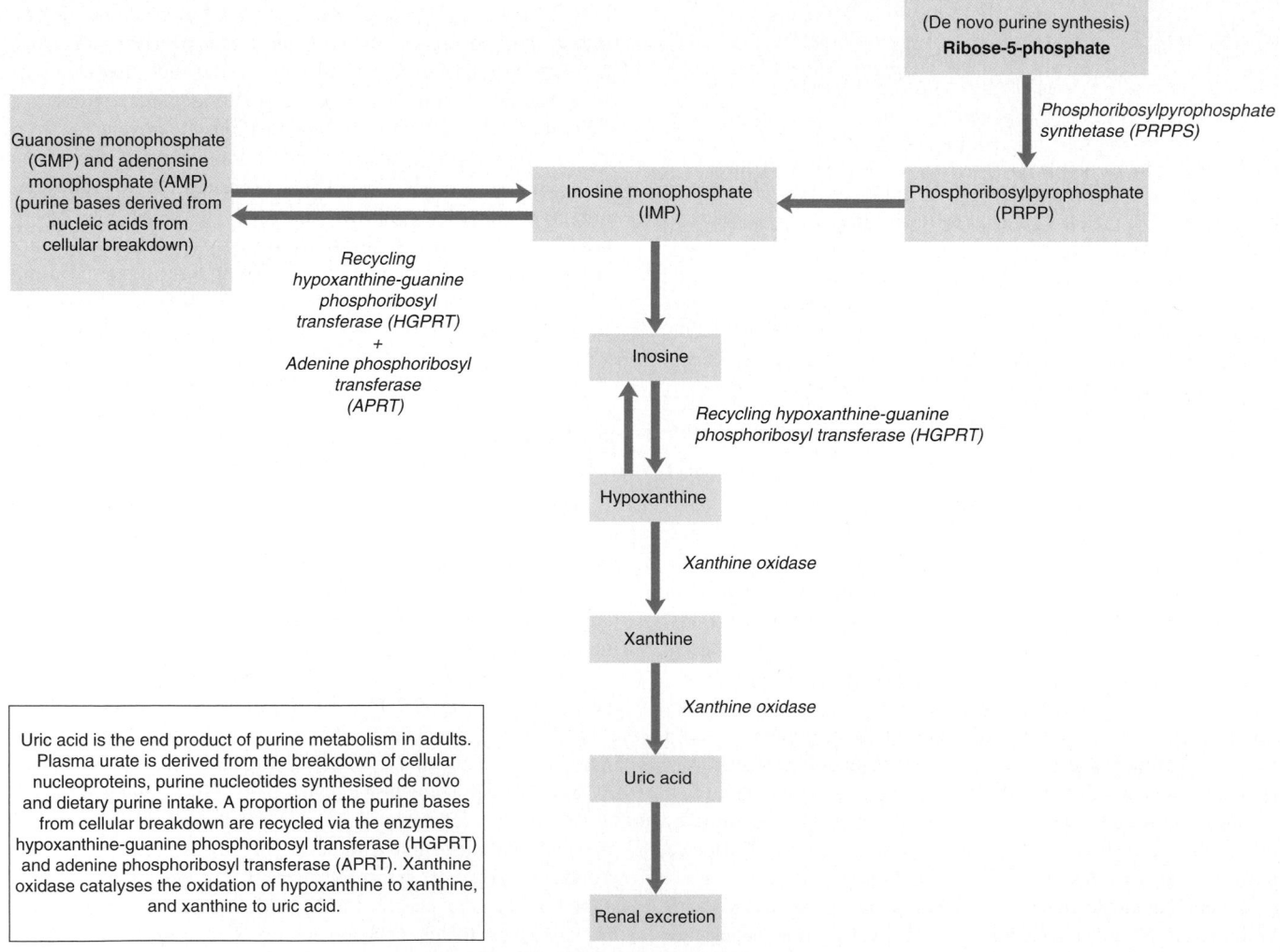

Uric acid is the end product of purine metabolism in adults. Plasma urate is derived from the breakdown of cellular nucleoproteins, purine nucleotides synthesised de novo and dietary purine intake. A proportion of the purine bases from cellular breakdown are recycled via the enzymes hypoxanthine-guanine phosphoribosyl transferase (HGPRT) and adenine phosphoribosyl transferase (APRT). Xanthine oxidase catalyses the oxidation of hypoxanthine to xanthine, and xanthine to uric acid.

Fig. 55.1 Purine pathway.

Urate haemostasis depends upon the balance between production and complex processes of secretion and reabsorption in the kidney tubule and excretion in the intestine. It is estimated that approximately 30% of uric acid excretion is by the intestine, while renal mechanisms account for the other 70% (Roddy and Doherty, 2010). In the human kidney, urate handling involves urate glomerular filtration followed by a complex array of resorptive and secretory mechanisms taking place in the renal proximal tubule. The urate reabsorption pathway involves a number of important anion transport proteins which are located in the renal proximal tubule; these include URAT1, OAT4 and OAT10 (So and Thorens, 2010). The URAT-1 transporter is targeted by a number of drugs including lesinurad, benzbromarone, probenecid, losartan and sulfinpyrazone (Bernal et al., 2016). GLUT9 is a member of the glucose transporter family and is highly expressed in the kidney proximal tubules of humans. Studies have shown that GLUT9 may play an important role in renal urate reabsorption (Matsuo et al., 2016). Renal mechanisms are responsible for the majority of hyperuricaemia in individuals, with overproduction representing less than 10% of patients with gout.

Gout can be classified as primary or secondary, depending on the presence or absence of an identified cause of hyperuricaemia. Primary gout is not a consequence of an acquired disorder, but is associated with rare inborn errors of metabolism and isolated renal tubular defects in the fractional clearance of uric acid. A rare group of enzyme defects result in an increased de novo purine synthesis such as hypoxanthine-guanine phosphoribosyl transferase deficiency (Lesch–Nyhan syndrome), phosphoribosyl pyrophosphate synthetase super activity, glucose-6-phosphatase deficiency and myogenic hyperuricaemia (Table 55.1).

Secondary gout is the consequence of the use of specific drugs or develops as a consequence of other disorders such as chronic kidney disease or cardiovascular disease. Certain diseases are associated with enhanced nucleic acid turnover, for example, myeloproliferative and lymphoproliferative disorders, psoriasis and haemolytic anaemia, and can lead to hyperuricaemia (see Table 55.1).

Risk factors

Hyperuricaemia

Hyperuricaemia is considered the most important risk factor for the development of gout. A community-based, cross-sectional Taiwanese study involving 3185 adults older than 30 years reported an odds ratio for prevalent gout of 3.65 between men with and without hyperuricaemia (Lin et al., 2000a). The 5-year cumulative incidence of gout was 18.8% in the 223 men who had asymptomatic hyperuricaemia at baseline (Lin et al., 2000b). Another study in Germany reported a 32-fold increased risk of gout in patients with hyperuricaemia compared with those with normal serum uric acid (SUA) levels (Duskin-Bitan et al., 2014). The Framingham Heart Study and Normative Aging Study in the USA also reported a relationship between increased SUA and the risk of gout (Campion et al., 1987; Hall et al., 1967). It is important to note that hyperuricaemia alone is not an indicator of gout; a number of contributing factors may result in gout developing in an individual (Box 55.1).

Genetics

The involvement of genetics in the development of gout has been supported by both clinical and epidemiological evidence, combined with recent advances in genetic studies. The varying prevalence of gout worldwide suggests both ethnic and genetic differences. A population study in Taiwan demonstrated an aggregation of gout within families with an inheritability of 35.1% in men and 17% in women (Kuo et al., 2015b). As previously discussed, the urate reabsorption pathway involves a number of important anion transport proteins which are located in the renal proximal tubule. Genome-wide association studies have identified single nucleotide polymorphisms in the genes that encode these transport proteins. The SLC22A12

Table 55.1 Causes of primary and secondary gout

Primary gout	Secondary gout
Idiopathic	**Increased uric acid production**
Rare enzyme deficiencies	Lymphoproliferative/ myeloprofilerative disorders
Hypoxanthine-guanine phosphoribosyl transferase deficiency	Chronic haemolytic anaemias
Phosphoribosyl pyrophosphate synthetase super-activity	Secondary polycythaemia
Ribose-5-phosphate AMP-deaminase deficiency	Severe exfoliative psoriasis
	Gaucher disease
	Cytotoxic drugs
	Glucose-6-phosphate deficiency
	High-purine diet overproduction
	Reduced uric acid secretion
	Renal failure
	Hypertension
	Drugs (diuretics, aspirin, ciclosporin)
	Lead nephropathy
	Alcohol
	Down's syndrome
	Myxoedema
	Beryllium poisoning

Box 55.1 Risk factors for gout

Hyperuricaemia
Genetics
Age, sex and socioeconomics
Renal disease
Comorbidities, e.g. obesity, dyslipidaemia, glucose intolerance, hypertension and osteoarthritis
Diet
Alcohol consumption
Medication

gene codes for the urate transporter 1 (URAT1). URAT1 is important in controlling the reabsorption of uric acid from the proximal renal tubules and is the site of action for a number of drugs including lesinurad, benzbromarone and probenecid. A polymorphism of the SLC22A12 gene has been associated with relative underexcretion of uric acid and hyperuricaemia in German Caucasians (Graessler et al., 2006). The SLC2A9 gene encodes for the glucose and fructose transporter GLUT9, and polymorphisms in these gene have been associated with increased SUA and self-reported gout (Dehghan et al., 2008). Genome-wide studies have also identified a number of other important genes that may be implicated in urate metabolism including ABCG2, which is associated with an urate efflux transporter in the proximal collecting ducts (Matsuo et al., 2016). Ongoing studies are likely to identify other important genes that influence urate levels and the development of gout.

Age, sex and socioeconomics

The prevalence of gout is much higher in men, and the risk of gout steadily increases in men as they age. Females have a low prevalence of gout up to the age of 45 years, but the risk of gout sharply rises after menopause. The rapid rise after menopause is thought to be due to the loss of the uricosuric effects associated with oestrogen. In the Nurse's Health Study, the use of hormone replacement therapy in menopausal women was shown to reduce the risk of the development of gout (Hak et al., 2010). Geographical location may also play a role in the development of gout; European studies have shown that rural residents have a much lower risk of gout compared with their urban counterparts (Kuo et al., 2015b). Historically gout was considered a disease of affluence, but recent research in the UK has demonstrated higher rates of gout in less affluent areas (Kuo et al., 2015a).

Renal disease

Experts have emphasised the importance of screening for renal disease in individuals with gout and/or hyperuricaemia because of the strong association between the two conditions (Sivera et al., 2014). An increased incidence of end-stage renal disease has been found in patients with hyperuricaemia, but gout has not been found to be an independent predictor for this disease (Iseki et al., 2004). However, studies have shown a fourfold increase in mortality due to kidney disease in patients with gout compared with their non-gout counterparts (Hsu et al., 2009). A retrospective study in the USA involving 259,209 patients registered on a renal database found the incidence rate of gout to be 5.4% in the first year of dialysis and 15.4% in the first 5 years (Cohen et al., 2008). UK studies have also demonstrated an increased risk of gout in patients with renal transplant (Mikuls et al., 2005). Men with gout have a twofold greater risk of kidney stones than patients without gout (Jordan et al., 2007). The likelihood of stones increases with serum urate concentration, extent of urinary acid secretion and low urine pH.

Comorbidities

Metabolic syndrome is a multiplex risk factor for atherosclerotic cardiovascular disease that consists of atherogenic dyslipidaemia,

raised blood pressure, increased blood glucose, and both pro-thrombotic and pro-inflammatory states. In the USA, metabolic syndrome is present in 63% of those with gout compared with 25% of those without gout (Choi et al., 2007a). Other studies have shown obesity, weight gain and hypertension all to be independent risk factors for the development of gout (Choi et al., 2005). The skin disease psoriasis, as well as certain types of anaemia (sickle cell anaemia), has also been associated with an increased incidence of gout (Kuo et al., 2015b). Osteoarthritis has been linked to gout rather than being an actual risk factor because of the increased propensity for nucleation and growth of monosodium urate crystals in osteoarthritic cartilage (Roddy and Doherty, 2010).

Diet

Studies have demonstrated that a purine-rich diet increases the risk of gout. In the Health Professional Follow-up Study in the USA the incidence of gout was higher in individuals who consumed greater quantities of meat or seafood (Choi et al., 2004). In contrast, a diet high in purine-rich vegetables does not increase the risk, and the consumption of low-fat dairy products reduces the relative risk of gout with each additional dairy serving. The consumption of soft drinks sweetened with sugar (not diet drinks) has also been linked to an increase in the number of gout cases, particularly in the USA (Choi and Curham, 2008). A study in New Zealand found that the consumption of four sugar-sweetened soft drinks per day was associated with a sevenfold increase in prevalent gout in European descendants and a fivefold increase in Maori (Batt et al., 2014). Fructose contained in commercial sweetened soft drinks increases the degradation of purine nucleotides that act as a substrate for uric acid production. Vitamin C (ascorbic acid) has been shown to have a modest uricosuric effect (Huang et al., 2005), and coffee consumption may reduce the risk of the development of gout (Choi et al., 2007b). The consumption of cherries, but no other fruits, has been shown to decrease uric acid levels (Zhang et al., 2006).

Alcohol

Increased daily consumption of alcohol is associated with a higher risk of gout. Beer carries the greatest risk, probably because of its high purine content, followed by spirits. However, a moderate consumption of wine is not associated with an increased risk of the development of gout (Jordan et al., 2007). The mechanism of action involved is thought to be the metabolism of ethanol to acetyl coenzyme A leading to adenine nucleotide degradation, with resultant increased formation of adenosine monophosphate, a precursor of uric acid. Alcohol also raises lactic acid levels in blood, which inhibits uric acid excretion.

Medication

A number of drugs are associated with increased uric acid levels (Box 55.2). The use of both loop and thiazide diuretics is the most common modifiable risk factor for secondary gout, especially in

Box 55.2 Examples of drugs known to raise serum urate levels

Alcohol
Aspirin
Ciclosporin
Cytotoxic chemotherapy
Diuretics (both loop and thiazide)
Ethambutol
Levodopa
Pyrazinamide
Ribavirin and interferon
Ritonavir
Teriparatide

the elderly. It is thought that loop and thiazide diuretics may precipitate an attack via volume depletion and reduced renal tubular secretion of uric acid. Aspirin has a bimodal effect; low doses inhibit uric acid excretion and increase urate levels, while doses greater than 3 g/day are uricosuric.

The prescribing of ciclosporin in organ transplant patients is an independent risk factor for new-onset gout in this group. The proposed mechanism of action is the interaction of ciclosporin with the hOAT10 transporter that mediates urate/glutathione exchange in the kidney (Bahn et al., 2008). Radiotherapy and chemotherapy in patients with neoplastic disorders can cause hyperuricaemia because of increased cell breakdown; to overcome this, prophylactic treatment may be given with allopurinol, commencing 3 days before therapy. Patients with HIV have been proposed to have a higher risk of gout; this has partly been linked to the use of ritonavir that can cause hyperuricaemia (Creighton et al., 2005).

Presentation and diagnosis

An acute attack of gout has a rapid onset, with pain being maximal at 6–24 hours of onset and spontaneously resolving within several days or weeks. The first attack usually affects a single joint in the lower limbs in 85–90% of cases, most commonly the first metatarsophalangeal joint (big toe). The next most frequent joints to be affected are the mid-tarsi, ankles, knees and arms. The affected joint is hot, red and swollen with shiny overlying skin. Even the touch of a sheet on the affected joint is too painful for the patient to bear. The patient may also have a fever, leukocytosis, raised erythrocyte sedimentation rate or C-reactive protein (CRP), and the attack may also be preceded by prodromal symptoms such as anorexia, nausea or change in mood. After resolution of the attack, there may be pruritus and desquamation of the overlying skin on the affected joint.

Monosodium urate crystals preferentially form in cartilage and fibrous tissues, where they are protected from contact with inflammatory mediators. The deposition of crystals may continue for months or years without causing symptoms; it is only when the crystals are shed into the joint space or bursa that inflammatory reaction occurs precipitating an acute attack of gout. The shedding of crystals can be triggered by a number of factors including direct trauma, dehydration, acidosis or rapid weight loss. The acute-phase response associated with intercurrent illness or surgery may also precipitate an attack; during this phase, there is increased urinary urate excretion with a lowering of SUA that leads to partial dissolution of monosodium urate crystals and subsequent shedding of crystals into the joint space.

The shed crystals are phagocytosed by monocytes and macrophages, activating the NACHT–LRR–PYD-containing protein-3 (NALP3) inflammasome and triggering the release of IL-1β and other cytokines, a subsequent infiltration of neutrophils and the symptoms of an acute attack (Dalbeth and Haskard, 2005). The NALP3 inflammasome (cryopyrin) is a complex of intracellular proteins that is activated on exposure to microbial elements, such as bacterial RNA and toxins. Activation of NALP3 leads to the release of caspase-1, which is required for cleavage of pro-IL-1β to active IL-1β (Richette and Bardin, 2009). IL-1β has been shown to be critically associated with the inflammatory response induced by monosodium urate crystals (Rider and Jordan, 2010).

The presence of hyperuricaemia alone is insufficient to confirm a diagnosis of gout, and approximately one-third of patients will have normal uric acid concentrations during an acute attack of gout because of increased urinary urate excretion. The most appropriate time to measure serum urate for monitoring purposes is when the attack has completely resolved. The gold standard for the diagnosis of gout is the demonstration of urate crystals in synovial fluid or in a tophus by polarised light microscopy (Sivera et al., 2014). Crystals may be found in fluid aspirated from non-inflamed joints, even in those joints that have not previously experienced an attack. The crystals are large (10–20 micrometres) and needle shaped with a strong, intense, characteristic light pattern under polarised light. In contrast, the calcium pyrophosphate dehydrate crystals associated with pseudo-gout are small, rhomboid crystals of low intensity. In some clinical settings it may not be possible to aspirate monosodium urate crystals. Under these circumstances the European League Against Rheumatism (EULAR) recommends a diagnosis based on the classical features of gout such as podagra, tophi and rapid response to colchicine (Sivera et al., 2014). Modern imaging techniques, such as ultrasound and dual-energy computed tomography, can also be used to assist in diagnosis. Gout and septic arthritis may co-exist and to exclude septic arthritis, synovial fluid is sent for Gram staining and culture.

Course of disease

The course of gout follows a number of stages; initially, the patient may be asymptomatic with a raised SUA level (Fig. 55.2). Some patients may only ever experience one attack, but often a second attack occurs within 6–12 months. Subsequent attacks tend to be of longer duration, affect more than one joint and may spread to the upper limbs. Untreated disease can result in chronic tophaceous gout, with persistent low-grade inflammation in a number of joints resulting in joint damage and deformity. The disease is characterised by the

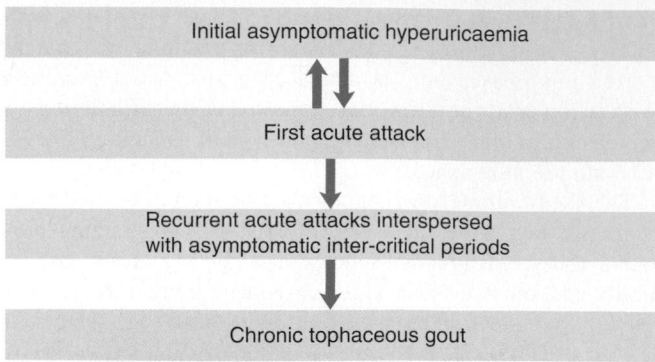

Initial asymptomatic hyperuricaemia

⇅

First acute attack

↓

Recurrent acute attacks interspersed with asymptomatic inter-critical periods

↓

Chronic tophaceous gout

Fig. 55.2   Schematic representation of the stages of gout.

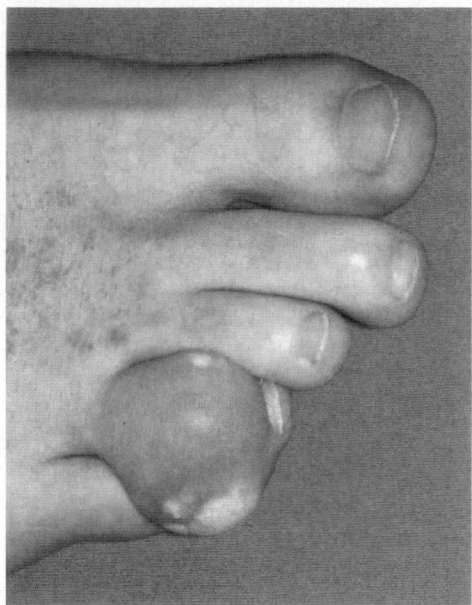

Fig. 55.3   Chronic tophaceous gout.

Box 55.3   Treatment aims in gout

Rapid alleviation of the acute attack
Prevention of future attacks
Lower serum uric acid levels to below saturation point
Reduce risk of comorbidities, e.g. cardiovascular disease
Lifestyle modification

Box 55.4   Lifestyle measures

Things to encourage	• Daily intake of low-fat or non-fat dairy products • Daily intake of fresh vegetables • Regular exercise • Remaining well hydrated (at least 2 L of water per day)
Items to limit	• Limit portion sizes and weekly consumption of beef, lamb and pork • Limit portion sizes and weekly consumption of seafood high in purines (e.g. sardines and shellfish) • Limit servings of naturally sweet fruit juices • Limit table sugar and salt • Limit alcohol consumption, particularly high-purine-type products such as beer
Things to avoid	• Smoking • Overweight • Organ meats high in purine content (e.g. liver, kidney and sweetbreads) • High-fructose corn-syrup-sweetened soft drinks or foods • Alcohol overconsumption (more than 2 units per day for a male and 1 unit per day for a female) • Avoid alcohol completely during an attack or if experiencing frequent attacks • Avoid becoming dehydrated

---

presence of tophi (Fig. 55.3), monosodium urate crystals surrounded by chronic mononuclear and giant-cell reactions. Tophi deposition can occur anywhere in the body, but they are commonly seen on the helix of the ear, within and around the toe or finger joints, on the elbow, around the knees or on the Achilles tendons. The skin overlying the tophi may ulcerate and extrude white, chalky material composed of monosodium urate crystals.

Treatment

The management of gout can be split into the rapid resolution of the initial acute attack and long-term measures to prevent future episodes (Box 55.3).

Gout is often associated with other medical problems including obesity, hypertension, excessive alcohol and the metabolic syndrome of insulin resistance, hyperinsulinaemia, impaired glucose intolerance and hypertriglyceridaemia. This contributes to the increased cardiovascular risk and deterioration of renal function seen in patients with gout. Management is not only directed at alleviating acute attacks and preventing future attacks, but also identifying and treating other comorbid conditions such as hypertension and hyperlipidaemia. Renal function should be measured and the individual's cardiovascular risk evaluated. A recent general population study has suggested that gout may be independently associated with an increased risk of diabetes, and that the magnitude of association is significantly larger in women than men (Rho et al., 2016). It is important that pharmacological measures are combined with non-pharmacological approaches such as weight loss, changes in diet, increased exercise and reduced alcohol consumption (Box 55.4). Patients with gout should remain adequately hydrated at all times, especially those with a history of urolithiasis (kidney stones). At least 2 L of water should be consumed per day, and alkalinisation of urine with potassium citrate (60 mEq/day) should be considered in recurrent stone formers.

Box 55.5 Medicines used in the management of an acute attack of gout

Initially select a single agent based on the patient's characteristics:

- Colchicine
- Oral NSAIDs (non-selective and selective)
- Intra-articular corticosteroids
- Oral corticosteroids
- Intramuscular corticosteroids
- IL-1 inhibitors

If the first agent is ineffective, consider switching to another or combining two agents (colchicine plus NSAID or colchicine and corticosteroids).

These should always be combined with non-pharmacological approaches:

- Rest the joint for 1–2 days.
- Apply ice to help alleviate pain.
- Remove contributing factors – complete a full medication review.
- Recommend lifestyle changes – diet, exercise and alcohol consumption.

NSAID, Non-steroidal anti-inflammatory drug.

Management of an acute attack

Drugs used in the management of an acute attack include colchicine, NSAIDs, corticosteroids (oral and injectable), and IL-1 inhibitors (Box 55.5). Current guidance gives no preference to a particular agent, but recommends selection based on the number plus type of joint(s) affected and individual patient characteristics (Khanna et al., 2012a; Sivera et al., 2014). In severe cases, where treatment with a single agent has been insufficient, it may be necessary to use a combination approach. Suggested combinations include colchicine with an NSAID and colchicine combined with oral or intra-articular corticosteroids (Khanna et al., 2012b). Simple analgesics such as paracetamol and weak opiates (codeine or dihydrocodeine) can also be added to the treatment regimen to provide additional pain relief. Treatment should be commenced as soon as possible and continued until the attack is terminated, usually between 1 and 2 weeks. The affected joints should also be rested for 1–2 days and initially treated with ice, which has a significant analgesic effect during an acute attack.

A complete medication review should be performed, and ideally medication that is likely to have contributed to the attack discontinued. Where loop and thiazide diuretics are being used for the management of hypertension alone, an alternative antihypertensive agent should be considered according to national guidance. Losartan, an angiotensin receptor blocker effective in hypertension, has been shown to have uricosuric properties and is a suitable agent in hypertensive patients with gout (Sica and Schoolwerth, 2002; Takahashi et al., 2003). In patients with heart failure, diuretics are often essential and cannot be discontinued. Although low-dose aspirin (≤325 mg/day) is known to elevate serum urate, its benefits in terms of cardiovascular disease prevention outweigh its modest effect on uric acid levels (Khanna et al., 2012a). Patients who are already taking urate-lowering medicines, such as allopurinol, should continue to take these medicines and should be counselled on the importance of continuing urate-lowering therapies (ULTs) even during an acute attack of gout.

Colchicine

Colchicine is an alkaloid derived from the autumn crocus (colchicum autumnale) and has been reported to have been used in the treatment of gout since the 6th century AD. Colchicine has a slower onset of action than NSAIDs, and it should ideally be commenced within 36 hours of an acute attack. Although the mode of action of colchicine in gout is not fully understood, it is thought to arrest microtubule assembly in neutrophils and inhibit many cellular functions. It suppresses monosodium urate crystal–induced NALP3 inflammasome-driven caspase-1 activation, IL-1β processing and release, and L-selectin expression on neutrophils. Colchicine also blocks the release of a crystal-derived chemotactic factor from neutrophil lysosomes, blocks neutrophil adhesion to endothelium by modulating the distribution of adhesion molecules on the endothelial cells, and inhibits monosodium urate crystal–induced production of superoxide anions from neutrophils (Nuki, 2008).

Although widely used, few studies have demonstrated the efficacy of colchicine. A single, randomised, controlled trial has compared the benefits of colchicine with placebo in acute gouty flare (Ahern et al., 1987). Patients were given 1 mg colchicine followed by 500 micrograms every 2 hours until the attack stopped or they felt too ill to continue taking colchicine. Colchicine was found to be superior to placebo with an absolute reduction of 34% for pain and a 30% reduction in clinical symptoms such as palpation, swelling, redness and pain. The number needed to treat (NNT) with colchicine to reduce pain was 3, and the NNT to reduce clinical symptoms was 2. All participants given colchicine experienced gastro-intestinal side effects such as diarrhoea and/or vomiting. No studies have compared colchicine with either NSAIDs or corticosteroids in an acute flare of gout.

More recent evidence has shown that low-dose colchicine (1.8 mg in 24 hours) is more effective than placebo and as effective as high-dose colchicine with an improved safety profile (Terkrltaub et al., 2008). EULAR guidance recommends a regimen of up to 2 mg daily (500 micrograms four times a day) for the management of an acute flare (Sivera et al., 2014). American College of Rheumatology (ACR) guidance differs in that it incorporates a 1 mg loading dose followed by 500 micrograms 1 hour later and then after 12 hours has elapsed, 500 micrograms three times a day until the acute attack resolves (Khanna et al., 2012a). If the patient has already been taking colchicine as flare prophylaxis (see later) and has received a treatment dose of colchicine in the last 14 days for an acute flare, then an alternative agent should be selected to manage the attack (Khanna et al., 2012a). It should be noted that only the oral formulation of colchicine is now available in the UK; the intravenous formulation is no longer licensed because its use has been associated with a number of fatalities (2% mortality rate).

Common side effects associated with colchicine are abdominal cramps, nausea, vomiting, and rarely bone marrow suppression, neuropathy and myopathy. Side effects are more common in patients with hepatic or renal impairment. The dose of colchicine should be reduced in mild-to-moderate renal impairment, for example, creatinine clearance 10–50 mL/min, and it should not be used in patients with severe renal impairment, for example, creatinine clearance less than 10 mL/min. Care should also be exercised in patients with chronic heart failure because of colchicine's ability to constrict blood vessels and stimulate central vasomotor centres.

Colchicine is metabolised by CYP3A4 and excreted by P-glycoprotein; toxicity can be caused by drugs that interact with its metabolism and clearance, and this includes macrolides, disulfiram, ciclosporin and protease inhibitors. The absorption of vitamin B_{12} may be impaired by chronic administration of high doses of colchicine. It is important to check for potential drug interactions before commencing treatment with colchicine.

Non-steroidal anti-inflammatory drugs

Both non-selective NSAIDs and selective NSAIDs (cyclo-oxygenase-2 inhibitors) are recommended for the management of an acute flare (Khanna et al., 2012b; Sivera et al., 2014). Non-selective NSAIDs act by direct inhibition of COX-1 and COX-2 via blockade of the COX enzyme site. The subsequent inhibition of prostaglandin production not only reduces inflammation, but also results in additional activities on platelet aggregation, renal homeostasis and gastric mucosal integrity. COX-2 inhibitors preferentially inhibit the COX-2 pathway, and their use is associated with a lower incidence of gastro-intestinal side effects. There are no high-quality trials comparing NSAIDs with placebo, and there is no evidence demonstrating superiority of one NSAID over another in the management of an acute flare (Sivera et al., 2014). Selection should be based on the individual and the presence of comorbidities. Recent studies suggest that some increased cardiovascular risk may apply to all NSAID users, irrespective of their baseline risk, and not only to chronic users (Trelle et al., 2011). The highest risk has been associated with the use of the COX-2 inhibitors, while the non-selective NSAID naproxen is proposed to have the lowest risk associated with its use. NSAIDs should be avoided in patients with heart failure, renal insufficiency and a history of gastric ulceration. Care should also be exercised in elderly patients with multiple pathologies.

The maximum recommended dose of an NSAID (selective or non-selective) should be commenced rapidly after the onset of an attack and then tapered 24 hours after the complete resolution of symptoms. The usual treatment period is 1–2 weeks. Gastric protection should be co-prescribed with both selective and non-selective NSAIDs.

Corticosteroids

Corticosteroids are usually considered where the use of an NSAID or colchicine is contraindicated or in refractory cases. They may be given intravenously, intramuscularly or direct into a joint (intra-articular) when only one or two joints are affected. In patients with a monoarthritis, an intra-articular corticosteroid injection is highly effective in treating an attack. The dose of intra-articular corticosteroids is based on the size of the affected

joint; common doses are 80 mg methylprednisolone acetate for a large joint such as a knee, and 40 mg methylprednisolone acetate or 40 mg triamcinolone acetonide for a smaller joint such as a wrist or elbow. In patients who are unable to take oral colchicine or NSAIDs and intra-articular injection is not appropriate, then intramuscular or oral corticosteroids may be considered. Intramuscular triamcinolone acetonide 60 mg has been shown to be as safe and effective as indometacin 50 mg three times daily in treating an acute attack of gout with earlier resolution of symptoms in the steroid group (Alloway et al., 1993). In patients who are nil by mouth and for whom intra-articular corticosteroids are not appropriate, then intramuscular or intravenous corticosteroids may be considered.

Studies have also demonstrated that oral corticosteroids are equally as effective as NSAIDs and have a similar safety profile (Janssens et al., 2008; Man et al., 2007). Oral prednisolone 30 mg daily for 5 days has also been shown to be equally efficacious to indometacin 50 mg three times a day for 2 days or 25 mg three times a day for 3 days plus paracetamol and has fewer adverse events (Man et al., 2007). The ACR recommends prednisolone 0.5 mg/kg/for 5–10 days then stopping, or 0.5 mg/kg per day for 2–5 days and then tapering over 7–10 days (Khanna et al., 2012b). Other oral corticosteroid regimens used in practice include prednisolone 30 mg daily for 1–3 days with subsequent dose tapering over 1–2 weeks. Corticosteroids may have fewer adverse events than other acute treatments when used short-term, particularly in the elderly.

Interleukin-1 inhibitors

IL-1β is critically associated with the inflammatory response induced by monosodium urate crystals (Rider and Jordan, 2010). Canakinumab is a fully humanised monoclonal antibody against IL-1β. Its clinical effectiveness was demonstrated in the β-RELIEVED and β-RELIEVED II studies where it was compared with intramuscular triamcinolone 40 mg in individuals with recent gouty flares (Cavagna and Taylor, 2014). It is licensed in Europe for the symptomatic treatment of adult patients with frequent gouty arthritis attacks (at least three attacks in the previous 12 months) in whom NSAIDs and colchicine are contraindicated, are not tolerated, or do not provide an adequate response, and in whom repeated courses of corticosteroids are not appropriate. The National Institute for Health and Care Excellence (NICE) does not currently support the use of canakinumab in the management of gout (NICE, 2013).

Anakinra, an IL-1 receptor antagonist, has been shown to reduce the pain of gout and bring about complete resolution by day 3 in the majority of patients after a course of three 100-mg subcutaneous injections (McGonagle et al., 2007; So et al., 2007). Anakinra is currently not licensed for the management of gout in Europe.

Rilonacept is an Fc fusion protein that engages both IL-1α and IL-1β, and has demonstrated efficacy in the management of gout flares. Its market authorisation in Europe was withdrawn in 2012 at the request of the market authorisation holder because of commercial reasons.

Due to the considerable cost of the IL-1 inhibitors, compared with other agents used in the management of acute flares, their use tends to be limited to patients with severe, refractory disease who have responded inadequately to standard therapies.

Management of chronic gout

The presence of hyperuricaemia is not an indication to commence prophylactic therapy. Some patients may only experience a single episode, and a change in lifestyle, diet or concurrent medication may be sufficient to prevent further attacks (see Box 55.4). Patients who suffer one or more acute attacks within 12 months of the first attack should normally be prescribed prophylactic ULT (Box 55.6). There are, however, some groups of patients where prophylactic therapy should be instigated after a single attack. These include individuals with uric acid stones, the presence of tophi at first presentation and young patients with a family history of renal or cardiac disease. The criteria for starting prophylactic therapy for the management of gout is detailed in Box 55.6.

The aim of ULT is to maintain the serum urate level below the saturation point for monosodium urate. The British Society Rheumatology proposes a target level of 300 mmol/L or less to prevent further crystal formation and aid the dissolution of existing crystals (Jordan et al., 2007). European guidance recommends a slightly higher level of 360 mmol/L, but in the presence of tophi it suggests a lower cutoff point of 300 mmol/L (Sivera et al., 2014).

It is generally recommended that the initiation of ULT should be delayed until the acute attack has resolved; this is due to the fact that changes in SUA levels caused by ULT can prolong the acute episode or cause a repeat flare. However, the ACR suggests that ULT can be started during an acute attack provided effective anti-inflammatory management is given in conjunction with the ULT (Khanna et al., 2012a). It is important that at whatever point ULT is commenced, appropriate flare prophylaxis is given. On initiation of ULT, SUA levels should be checked regularly during dose titration (every 2–5 weeks). Once the desired SUA level is reached, it is recommended that the level is checked intermittently along with renal function.

ULTs can be classified into three groups according to their pharmacological mode of action (Box 55.7). Xanthine oxidase inhibitors (XOIs; uricostatics) act on the enzyme xanthine oxidase. Xanthine oxidase catalyses the oxidation of hypoxanthine to xanthine and subsequently xanthine to uric acid (see Fig. 55.1). Hypoxanthine comes from the catabolism of cellular nucleoproteins and purine nucleotides. Blocking the action of this enzyme reduces the production of uric acid. Agents in this group include allopurinol and febuxostat.

Allopurinol

Allopurinol is the prophylactic agent of choice in the management of recurrent gout. To become pharmacologically active, allopurinol must be metabolised by the liver to oxypurinol. Oxypurinol has a much longer half-life than allopurinol, 14–16 hours compared with 2 hours. Both allopurinol and oxypurinol are renally excreted, with oxypurinol undergoing reabsorption from the renal tubule. In patients with reduced renal function, the half-life of oxypurinol is increased with the risk of accumulation and toxicity. It is, therefore, essential that a patient's renal function is checked before the prescribing of allopurinol, and the dose carefully titrated according to this.

Historically a treatment algorithm for allopurinol dose reduction in renal impairment was used because of concerns about toxicity and the increased risk of hypersensitivity reactions (allopurinol hypersensitivity syndrome [AHS]) in patients with poor kidney function. However, many patients do not achieve the desired SUA level with these reduced dosage regimens. A specific relationship between higher allopurinol doses in renal impairment and the risk of AHS has not been demonstrated (Stamp et al., 2012). It is proposed that the commencing dose of allopurinol is the critical factor and the rate at which the dose is then increased (Stamp et al., 2012). It has been shown that the dose can be increased above that based on creatinine clearance even in patients with renal impairment (Stamp et al., 2011, 2012).

In patients with normal renal function the staring dose should be no greater than 100 mg/day; in patients with renal impairment (glomerular filtration rate ≤30 mL/min) this should be reduced to 50 mg once a day. The dose should be increased every 2–5 weeks until the desired serum urate level is reached (<300 mmol/L). In patients with normal renal function the recommended dose increment is 100 mg and the maximum recommended daily dose is 900 mg/day. Where there is reduced renal function, the dose should be increased in 50 mg increments, but potentially can be increased to 300 mg/day as long as the patient is appropriately educated and is regularly monitored for signs of drug toxicity, for example, pruritus, rash and

---

Box 55.6 Criteria for starting prophylactic therapy for gout

The presence of one of the following factors indicates the need for a urate-lowering therapies:
- Recurring acute attacks of gout (two attacks per year)
- Identifiable tophi at presentation (palpable or imaged)
- Identifiable joint damage associated with gout
- Renal impairment at presentation (chronic kidney disease stage 2 or worse)
- History of renal stones (urolithiasis)
- First acute attack and unable to discontinue diuretic medication contributing to attack
- Primary gout starting at a young age (particularly in the presence of a family history of renal or cardiac disease)

Box 55.7 Categories of urate-lowering therapies

Selective urate reabsorption inhibitors
Benzbromarone
Probenecid
Sulfinpyrazone
Lesinurad

Xanthine oxidase inhibitors
Allopurinol
Febuxostat

Uricases
Pegloticase
Rasburicase

elevated hepatic enzymes (Khanna et al., 2012a). A decrease in serum urate will occur within a couple of days of introducing allopurinol therapy, with a peak effect at 7–10 days. The dissolution of tophi may take up to 6–12 months with effective therapy.

Approximately 3–5% of patients treated with allopurinol suffer from an adverse reaction; these usually occur within the first 2–3 months of treatment. True AHS is rare, and in the USA the estimated incidence is approximately 1:1000, with a reported mortality rate of 20–25% (Khanna et al., 2012a). The spectrum of AHS includes Stevens–Johnson syndrome and toxic epidermal necrolysis, as well as systemic features such as eosinophilia, vasculitis, rash and major end organ disease. Concurrent use of thiazide diuretics, age and renal impairment has been implicated as a risk factor. Genetic studies have identified an association with HLA-B*5801 positivity and AHS in certain subpopulations. The ACR recommends the testing of HLA-B*5801 in Koreans with stage 3 or worse chronic kidney disease plus Han Chinese and Thai irrespective of renal function (Khanna et al., 2012a). If these individuals are found to be positive it is recommended that allopurinol be avoided. Before the availability of other ULTs, allopurinol desensitisation was attempted in patients with a mild hypersensitivity to allopurinol. This involved starting with a very low dose (50 micrograms daily) and gradually increasing the dose over a period of several weeks to 100 mg daily. Desensitisation is now only considered where the reaction has been mild and there is an absence of alternative treatment options.

There are a number of important drug reactions with allopurinol. Azathioprine and mercaptopurine are metabolised by xanthine oxidase; co-administration of allopurinol reduces the metabolism of these two medicines, leading to accumulation and toxicity. The dose of azathioprine or mercaptopurine should be reduced to approximately one-quarter of the normal dose when co-prescribed with allopurinol. In addition, full blood counts should be performed at regular intervals to identify potential toxicity. High-dose allopurinol (>600 mg/day) increases carbamazepine blood levels by approximately one-third; the same effect is not associated with lower doses of allopurinol (<300 mg/day).

Febuxostat

Febuxostat is a more selective and potent inhibitor of xanthine oxidase than allopurinol, and it has no effect on other enzymes involved in purine or pyrimidine metabolism (Lawrence Edwards, 2009). It is licensed for the treatment of chronic hyperuricaemia in conditions where urate deposition has already occurred, including a history, or presence of, tophus and/or gouty arthritis. It is recommended as a second-line agent in patients who are intolerant of allopurinol or for whom allopurinol is contraindicated.

Febuxostat is more effective than fixed-dose allopurinol 300 mg in lowering uric acid concentrations in trials of up to 40 months in duration (Schumacher et al., 2008, 2009). However, a reduction in the incidence of episodes of acute gout has not been demonstrated.

The recommended starting dosage for febuxostat is 80 mg once daily. If the SUA is greater than 357 mmol/L (6 mg/100 mL)

after 2–4 weeks, the dose should be increased to 120 mg once daily. The increased potency and good oral bioavailability of febuxostat leads to rapid decreases in SUA levels permitting the testing of levels 2 weeks after starting therapy or adjusting the dose. No dosage adjustment is necessary in patients with mild or moderate renal impairment; however, there are no current recommendations for use in patients with severe renal impairment, for example, creatinine clearance less than 30 mL/min. In patients with mild hepatic impairment, the dose should not exceed 80 mg daily; the use of febuxostat has not been studied in patients with severe hepatic impairment. Febuxostat should not be given to patients with ischaemic heart disease or congestive heart failure because of cardiovascular side effects. When initiating therapy with febuxostat, gout flare prophylaxis should be prescribed for at least 6 months.

The most common adverse effects include respiratory infection, diarrhoea, headache and liver function abnormalities. Rare hypersensitivity reactions have been reported, including Stevens–Johnsons syndrome and toxic epidermal necrolysis; these have generally occurred in the first month of treatment. It is recommended that liver function should be tested in all patients before the initiation of therapy and periodically thereafter based on clinical judgement. The use of febuxostat is not recommended in patients concomitantly treated with mercaptopurine or azathioprine and in patients who are taking theophylline.

Selective urate reabsorption inhibitors (uricosuric agents)

Uricosuric agents increase uric acid excretion primarily by inhibiting post-secretory tubular absorption of uric acid from filtered urate in the kidney. They are indicated as second-line agents in those who are urate under-excreters and are dependent on the patient having an adequate level of renal function. These agents should be avoided in patients with urate nephropathy or those who are overproducers of uric acid due to the high risk of development of renal stones. Patients who are receiving an uricosuric agent are required to maintain an adequate fluid intake, and the need for alkalinisation of urine should be considered to prevent urate precipitation.

Benzbromarone

Benzbromarone is a potent uricosuric agent that acts via the renal transporters URAT1 and GLUT9. It has been shown to be effective in lowering serum urate levels and reducing the time to resolution of tophi (Kumar et al., 2005; Reinders et al., 2009). However, its use was associated with hepatoxicity and it was withdrawn from the UK, although it is still possible to obtain benzbromarone on a named patient basis. The risk of hepatotoxicity has been estimated to be 1:17,000 patients. For those who are prescribed benzbromarone, regular liver function tests must be performed during the first 6 months of therapy, and the hepatotoxic risk associated with the medicine should be clearly explained to the patient at the outset.

The dosage ranges from 50 to 200 mg daily. It remains active in mild-to-moderate renal impairment, but is ineffective

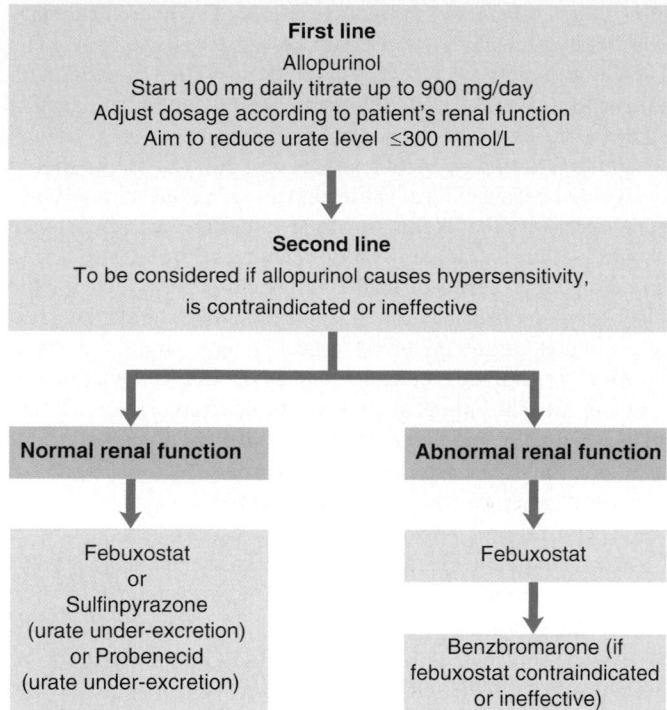

First line
Allopurinol
Start 100 mg daily titrate up to 900 mg/day
Adjust dosage according to patient's renal function
Aim to reduce urate level ≤300 mmol/L

Second line
To be considered if allopurinol causes hypersensitivity,
is contraindicated or ineffective

Normal renal function

Febuxostat
or
Sulfinpyrazone
(urate under-excretion)
or Probenecid
(urate under-excretion)

Abnormal renal function

Febuxostat

Benzbromarone (if
febuxostat contraindicated
or ineffective)

Fig. 55.4 Management of chronic gout in patients who require urate-lowering therapy.

at a creatinine clearance less than 20 mL/min. It should only be used when there is a contraindication to other agents used in the management of gout such as allopurinol and febuxostat (Fig. 55.4). Diarrhoea may be troublesome in approximately 10% of patients.

Sulfinpyrazone

Sulfinpyrazone is effective in reducing the frequency of gout attacks, tophi and plasma urate levels at dosages of 200–800 mg/day. It has the same mode of action on the kidney as benzbromarone and probenecid, all of which inhibit URAT-1 transporter, resulting in reduced urate reabsorption. However, in addition to this, sulfinpyrazone inhibits prostaglandin synthesis resulting in a similar adverse effect profile to NSAIDs, for example, gastrointestinal ulceration, acute renal failure, fluid retention, elevated liver enzymes and blood disorders. The use of sulfinpyrazone is reserved for use in patients with adequate renal function who are underexcretors of uric acid and intolerant or resistant to treatment with allopurinol.

Probenecid

Probenecid monotherapy is less effective than the other agents, and it is generally reserved for those who cannot tolerate or fail to achieve the target serum urate level with XOIs. The combination of allopurinol and probenecid can provide additional urate lowering than either agent alone (Stamp and Chapman, 2014). Dosages of 0.5–2.0 g/day have been used. As with sulfinpyrazone, it is ineffective in renal impairment and is not recommended if the

creatinine clearance is less than 50 mL/min. Dyspepsia and reflux may be troublesome in some patients, and probenecid can interact with renally excreted anionic drugs. Probenecid is no longer marketed in the UK.

Lesinurad

Lesinurad is a new URAT-1 selective uric acid reabsorption inhibitor. It gained a European license in 2016 and is recommended in combination with a XOI in adults with gout who have not achieved the target SUA level with a XOI alone. The recommended dosage is 200 mg once a day, and it should be administered at the same time as the XOI. SUA levels should be measured 4 weeks after commencing treatment. The minimum allopurinol dosage to be given with lesinurad is 300 mg once a day in normal renal function and 200 mg when the glomerular filtration rate 30–59 mL/min. In clinical trials there were a number of adverse renal events, and lesinurad is contraindicated where the creatinine clearance is less than 30 mL/min, in patients undergoing dialysis and in patients with renal transplant. Renal function should be measured at baseline and at least four times a year. It is also not recommended in patients with unstable angina, New York Heart Association class III or IV heart failure, uncontrolled hypertension or with a recent event of myocardial infarction, stroke, or deep venous thrombosis within the last 12 months, due to insufficient data. Because lesinurad is metabolised by the cytochrome P450 enzymes, there are a number of important drug reactions involving substrates for CYP3A (e.g. simvastatin, amlodipine, felodipine and hormonal contraceptives) and CYP2C9 (e.g. inhibitors: fluconazole and amiodarone; inducers: carbamazepine).

Uricolytics (uricases)

In humans and the great apes, uric acid is the end product of purine degradation, but in other mammals, uric acid is further degraded by the enzyme uricase to allantoin, which is highly soluble. Biotechnology processes have been utilised to produce recombinant forms of the enzyme uricase, and current forms include rasburicase and pegloticase. The use of these recombinant products is usually restricted to severe, refractory cases of gout because of the high cost, the need for intravenous administration and the development of neutralising antibodies with subsequent hypersensitivity reactions.

Rasburicase

Rasburicase, a recombinant form of the enzyme urate oxidase (uricase), is derived from a cDNA code from a modified *Aspergillus flavus* strain expressed in a modified strain of *Saccharomyces cerevisiae*. It is licensed to treat tumour lysis syndrome and is given intravenously at a dose of 0.2 mg/kg in short courses for 5–7 days. Rasburicase has a half-life of approximately 19 hours. No dosage adjustment is required in patients with renal or hepatic impairment. Rasburicase is generally well tolerated, but adverse effects include fever, nausea, vomiting, rash, diarrhoea, headache, allergic reactions and the development of auto-antibodies.

Pegloticase

Pegloticase is a polyethylene glycol conjugate of the recombinant enzyme uricase. Its European Market Authorisation is for severe, debilitating, chronic tophaceous gout in adults who may also have erosive joint involvement and who have failed to normalise SUA levels with an XOI at maximum dose or in whom XOIs are contraindicated. It is given as an 8 mg intravenous infusion every 2 weeks, and pre-medication with antihistamines and corticosteroids is required. Although phase III studies have shown it to be highly effective in lowering SUA levels and dissolving tophi, its use is limited by its immunogenicity. The generation of anti-pegloticase antibodies results in infusion reactions and a loss of clinical response. Pegloticase is currently unavailable in the UK and its use is not supported by NICE.

Preventing gout flare when initiating urate-lowering therapy

When prophylactic treatment is commenced, there is a risk of precipitating an acute gout attack, or 'mobilisation flare', for approximately 12 months. Mobilisation flares are thought to be caused by the rapid decrease in serum urate after the initiation of a ULT. When ULT therapy is commenced it is very important that additional medicines are co-prescribed to prevent precipitating an acute flare.

Colchicine

Colchicine is the agent of first choice to prevent the precipitation of a flare when commencing chronic gout treatment. Low doses of colchicine (500 micrograms orally twice a day or once a day) should be prescribed and continued for at least 6 months.

NSAIDs

If there are no contraindications to the use of NSAIDs, they may be considered second line to colchicine in patients who are intolerant to colchicine. NSAIDs should be continued for a maximum of 6 weeks, and gastric protection should be provided.

Corticosteroids

Intramuscular steroid injections (methylprednisolone acetate 80–120 mg) or low-dose oral prednisolone (<10 mg prednisolone/day) may sometimes be used to prevent the precipitation of a flare on initiation of ULT for gout.

Patient care

Patients should be provided with verbal and written information on the causes and consequences of gout, its curable nature, the aims of drug therapy and lifestyle advice. The need for dietary and lifestyle changes should be stressed (see Box 55.4). The UK Gout Society website can assist in providing patients with information about the condition and how it should be managed (http://www.ukgoutsociety.org). In overweight patients, gradual weight loss should be encouraged; very rapid weight loss should be avoided because it can cause ketosis and result in raised uric acid levels with the likelihood of precipitating an attack. Advice should include an 'action plan' for dealing with acute gout, and an emergency supply of medicine should be provided for the management of an acute attack. The patient should be clear on what dose of the medicine to take, when to initiate therapy, how long to take the medication and any possible side effects to look out for. The patient should also be advised to avoid certain over-the-counter medicines that may exacerbate an attack, for example, the use of aspirin as an analgesic.

Patients who are taking long-term prophylactic therapy need to understand the importance of continuing therapy despite being asymptomatic. Patients should be informed that gout flares will abate over time if they remain adherent to their ULT. The importance of not running out of their ULT medication should be stressed, and they should be warned that even a short gap in therapy may precipitate an attack. All patients should be advised to remain well hydrated with a water intake of at least 2 L/day; this is especially important for patients who are receiving uricosuric agents due to the risk of uric acid stone formation in the kidneys.

Case studies

Case 55.1

Mr SC is a 62-year-old man admitted to hospital with a suspected stroke. His medical history includes uncontrolled hypertension and recurrent gout. An ischaemic stroke is later confirmed after imaging. Medication on admission is amlodipine 5 mg once a day, ramipril 10 mg once a day and colchicine 500 micrograms three times a day for acute attacks of gout. The patient has no recorded drug allergies. His estimated glomerular filtration rate is 53 mL/min, he has a raised CRP of 115 mg/dL and his uric acid level is 579 mmol/L. During his recovery in hospital he experiences an acute flare of gout in his left big toe. Fluid aspirated from the joint contains monosodium urate crystals, and on examination the patient has palpable tophi on the toes. The doctor on the ward prescribes a course of colchicine (500 micrograms three times a day). After the third day the patient's symptoms improve, and the doctor stops the patient's colchicine and discusses with the patient the need to start a medicine to lower the patient's SUA level. The patient tells the doctor that he had allopurinol in the past, but it made things worse. He tells the doctor that his son takes febuxostat for his gout and has no problems. The doctor prescribes febuxostat 80 mg once a day. Three days later the patient experiences another acute episode of gout, this time affecting his elbow. The doctor stops the febuxostat during this second acute attack.

Questions

1. Are there any contraindications to use of febuxostat in this patient?
2. What might have been the cause of the second attack of gout after commencement of febuxostat?

3. How could this second flare of gout been prevented?
4. What advice would you give to patients commenced on ULTs?

Answers

1. Febuxostat is recommended for the management of chronic hyperuricaemia in patients with gout who are intolerant of allopurinol or in whom allopurinol is contraindicated. Intolerance to allopurinol is defined as adverse effects that are sufficiently severe to warrant discontinuation or prevent full dose escalation for optimal effectiveness. Mr SC said that allopurinol made things worse in the past, but before excluding the use of allopurinol it is important to verify how Mr SC took his allopurinol and whether he was adherent to treatment. Intermittent use of allopurinol is likely to precipitate recurrent flares and result in non-adherence. Later discussions with Mr SC revealed that when he originally took allopurinol he did not take it regularly as he struggled to attend for blood tests and did not obtain repeat prescriptions from his primary care doctor because he was working away as a lorry driver. Fluctuations in SUA levels due to intermittent use of allopurinol by the patient caused recurrent flares and hence why he felt it made things worse.

   The recommended starting dosage of allopurinol in patients with normal renal function is 100 mg once a day. This should be gradually increased in increments of 100 mg every 2–5 weeks until the desired serum urate level is reached (<300 mmol/L). The maximum recommended dosage in normal renal function is 900 mg/day. In renal impairment (glomerular filtration rate ≤30 mL/min) the recommended starting dosage is 50 mg once a day with increased increments of 50 mg every 2–5 weeks. Failure to appropriately titrate the dose of allopurinol can result in therapeutic failure.

   The patient has a history of uncontrolled hypertension and was admitted to hospital with an ischaemic stroke at the age of 62 years. In the APEX (Schumacher et al., 2008) and FACT (Becker et al., 2005) studies involving febuxostat and allopurinol, a numerically greater incidence of investigator-reported cardiovascular Anti-Platelet Trialists' Collaboration (APTC) events (defined endpoints from the APTC including cardiovascular death, non-fatal myocardial infarction and non-fatal stroke) was observed in the febuxostat total group compared with the allopurinol group (1.3 versus 0.3 events per 100 patient-years). The same profile was not observed in the CONFIRMS studies (Becker et al., 2010). The incidence of investigator-reported cardiovascular APTC events in the combined phase 3 studies (APEX, FACT and CONFIRMS studies) was 0.7 versus 0.6 events per 100 patient-years. In the long-term extension studies the incidences of investigator-reported APTC events were 1.2 and 0.6 events per 100 patient-years for febuxostat and allopurinol, respectively. No statistically significant differences were found, and no causal relationship with febuxostat was established. Identified risk factors among these patients were a medical history of atherosclerotic disease and/or myocardial infarction, or of congestive heart failure. Treatment with febuxostat in patients with ischaemic heart disease or congestive heart failure is not recommended. In view of the patient's recent ischaemic stroke and history of uncontrolled hypertension, it would be preferable to use an alternative ULT.

2. Febuxostat treatment should not be started until an acute attack of gout has completely subsided. Gout flares may occur during the initiation of treatment because of changing SUA levels resulting in the mobilisation of urate from tissue deposits.

3. When initiating treatment with febuxostat, flare prophylaxis should be given for at least 6 months. Medicines recommended for the prevention of gout flares during initiation of ULT include colchicine, NSAIDs and corticosteroids. Colchicine is the agent of choice and should be given at a dose of 500 micrograms once or twice daily for at least 6 months with the febuxostat. It is important that prophylaxis against flare is given on initiation of all ULTs. It is also important that patients stabilised on ULTs do not stop their ULT during an acute flare. The gout flare should be managed concurrently as appropriate for the individual patient.

4. Patients who are taking long-term prophylactic therapy need to understand the importance of continuing therapy despite being asymptomatic. Patients should be informed that gout flares will abate over time if they remain adherent to their ULT. The importance of not running out of their ULT medication should be stressed, and they should be warned that even a short gap in therapy may precipitate an attack. All patients should be advised to remain well hydrated with a water intake of at least 2 L/day; this is especially important for patients who are receiving uricosuric agents because of the risk of uric acid stone formation in the kidneys.

Case 55.2

Mr DW is a 77-year-old man admitted to accident and emergency with a painful swollen right knee. It woke him up in the middle of the night, and there is significant pain and swelling. He is unable to mobilise and cannot tolerate the knee being even lightly touched. He denies any trauma to the knee, and there is no fever or systemic symptoms. On examination there is palpable tophi on his fingers and his knee is swollen, hot and tender to touch. His CRP is 169 mg/dL, estimated glomerular filtration rate is 40 mL/min, urate is 713 mmol/L and he is hypertensive (185/100 mmHg). His medical history includes Charcot's arthropathy of the right foot, type 2 diabetes mellitus, stroke, chronic kidney disease, hypertension and osteoarthritis. Medication on admission is gliclazide 40 mg once a day, ramipril 2.5 mg once a day, clopidogrel 75 mg once a day, atorvastatin 40 mg once at night and lansoprazole 15 mg once a day. He drinks approximately 2 pints of beer per day, but does not smoke. He denies any history of gout. Fluid aspirated from his right knee contains monosodium urate crystals.

Questions

1. What initial therapy would you recommend to treat Mr DW's acute attack of gout?
2. What risk factors could have contributed to the acute attack?
3. Should Mr DW be placed on therapy to prevent further attacks?
4. What lifestyle and dietary advice would you give to Mr DW to assist in preventing further attacks?

Answers

1. Initial therapy should be directed at promptly and safely resolving the pain. Drugs used in the management of an acute attack include colchicine, NSAIDs and corticosteroids. Current guidance (Khanna et al., 2012b) gives no preference to a particular agent, but recommends selection based on the number plus type of joint(s) affected and individual patient characteristics. In view of Mr DW's age and multiple comorbidities including renal impairment and cardiovascular disease, the use of NSAIDs should ideally be avoided. Oral corticosteroids may have fewer adverse events than other acute treatments when used short-term, particularly in the elderly. However, Mr DW has type 2 diabetes mellitus and oral corticosteroids are likely to increase his blood sugars, leading to poor diabetic control. In patients with a monoarthritis, an intra-articular corticosteroid injection is highly effective in treating an attack. The dose of intra-articular corticosteroids is based on

the size of the affected joint; common doses are 80 mg methyl-prednisolone acetate for a large joint such as a knee, and 40 mg methylprednisolone acetate or 40 mg triamcinolone acetonide for a smaller joint such as a wrist or elbow. Intra-articular steroids act locally with less release into the systemic circulation and are therefore not likely to significantly affect Mr DW's diabetic control. However, in addition to the acute flare in the right knee, Mr DW's smaller joints in the left foot are also affected. Intra-articular injection into the right knee (80 mg methylprednisolone acetate) combined with oral colchicine is likely to be suitable in view of the severity of the attack and Mr DW being unable to mobilise his knee. Current guidance (Khanna et al., 2012b) recommends colchicine up to 2 mg/day for the management of an acute flare in patients with normal renal function. The dose of colchicine should be reduced or the interval between doses increased in mild-to-moderate renal impairment (creatinine clearance 10–50 mL/min). The use of colchicine is contraindicated in patients with a creatinine clearance less than 10 mL/min. A preferable dosage in Mr DW would be 500 micrograms twice a day. Before commencing colchicine a review of the patient's medication should be performed to identify any potential drug interactions. Colchicine has a number of important drug interactions; a reduction in colchicine dosage or interruption of colchicine treatment is recommended in patients with normal renal and hepatic function if treatment with a P-glycoprotein (ciclosporin, verapamil or quinidine) or a strong CYP3A4 inhibitor (ritonavir, atazanavir, indinavir, clarithromycin, telithromycin, itraconazole or ketoconazole) is required. Colchicine should not be co-prescribed with these medicines in the presence of hepatic or renal impairment. The patient is taking atorvastatin, and acute myopathy has been reported in patients given colchicine with statins. Mr DW should be advised to report muscle pain or weakness, and he should also stop his colchicine if he experiences diarrhoea or vomiting. Simple analgesics such as paracetamol and weak opiates (codeine or dihydrocodeine) can also be added to the treatment regimen to provide additional pain relief. The affected joints should be rested for 1–2 days and initially treated with ice, which has a significant analgesic effect during an acute attack.

2. Mr DW has a number of risk factors that pre-dispose him to the development of gout. These include being male, increasing age, hyperuricaemia, poor renal function, hypertension, type 2 diabetes mellitus and alcohol consumption.

   The prevalence of gout is much higher in men, and the risk of gout steadily increases in men as they age. Hyperuricaemia is considered the most important risk factor for the development of gout. However, it is important to note that hyperuricaemia alone is not an indicator of gout, and there are a number of contributing factors including genetics and lifestyle which may result in gout developing in an individual. Experts have emphasised the importance of screening for renal disease in individuals with gout and/or hyperuricaemia due to the strong association between the two conditions (Sivera et al., 2014). In addition, men with gout have a twofold higher risk of kidney stones than patients without gout (Jordan et al., 2007). Metabolic syndrome is a multiplex risk factor for atherosclerotic cardiovascular disease that consists of atherogenic dyslipidaemia, raised blood pressure, increased blood glucose, and both prothrombotic and pro-inflammatory states. In the USA, metabolic syndrome is present in 63% of those with gout compared with 25% of those without gout (Choi et al., 2007a). Other studies have shown obesity, weight gain and hypertension all to be independent risk factors for the development of gout (Choi et al., 2005). Increased daily consumption of alcohol is associated with a higher risk of gout. Beer carries the greatest risk, probably because of its high purine content, followed by spirits. However, a moderate consumption of wine is not associated with an increased risk of development of gout (Jordan et al., 2007). The mechanism of action involved is thought to be the metabolism of ethanol to acetyl coenzyme A, leading to adenine nucleotide degradation, with resultant increased formation of adenosine monophosphate, a precursor of uric acid. Alcohol also raises lactic acid levels in blood, which inhibits uric acid excretion. It is recommended that males restrict their alcohol consumption to no more than 14 units/week and females to no more than 7 units/week (Khanna et al., 2012a). Beer, stout, port and fortified wines should be avoided. Alcohol should be avoided during an acute attack of gout.

   Mr DW also has osteoarthritis; this has been linked to gout rather than being an actual risk factor due to the increased propensity for nucleation and growth of monosodium urate crystals in osteoarthritic cartilage.

3. Although Mr DW denies a history of gout, the severity of the attack and the presence of tophi suggest a period of prolonged hyperuricaemia. There may have been other attacks that he has self-managed. His presentation and chronic kidney disease support the initiation of a ULT.

   Guidance (Khanna et al., 2012a) suggests that patients who suffer one or more acute attacks within 12 months of the first attack should normally be prescribed prophylactic ULT. However, for some groups of patients, prophylactic therapy should be instigated after a single attack. These include individuals with uric acid stones, the presence of tophi at first presentation, identifiable joint damage associated with gout, renal impairment (CKD2 or worse), history of renal stones and patients presenting at a young patient age with a family history of renal or cardiac disease.

4. It is also important to stress the importance of lifestyle modification to Mr DW because this can be helpful in preventing further attacks. Moderate physical exercise can be beneficial; however, intense muscular exercise should be avoided because it can lead to a rise in uric acid levels. In overweight patients, gradual weight loss should be encouraged. Rapid weight loss can precipitate ketosis and a subsequent rise in the urate pool. Mr DW should be given appropriate dietary advice. It is the regular consumption of foods containing purines rather than the absolute purine content of a particular food that is important. The UK Gout Society (http://www.ukgoutsociety.org) provides a fact sheet with dietary recommendations and the purine content of various foods for patients. Ideally, total daily purine intake should not exceed 200 mg/day, and foods such as shellfish, offal and sardines should be avoided. Dairy products have been shown to be beneficial in lowering SUA, and even the addition of yoghurt on alternate days has been shown to reduce levels. The consumption of soft drinks sweetened with fructose or sucrose (not diet drinks) should be limited. Cherries, whether sweet, tart, juice or fruit, have a urate-lowering potential. As previously mentioned, Mr DW should moderate his alcohol consumption.

Acknowledgements

The author thanks Professor Philip Conaghan, Leeds Institute of Rheumatic and Musculoskeletal Medicine, University of Leeds, for his invaluable comments regarding the structure and content of this chapter, and Amy Vigar (nee Cunningham) for her valuable contribution in the previous edition.

References

Ahern, M.J., Reid, C., Gordon, T.P., et al., 1987. Does colchicine work? The results of the first controlled study in acute gout. Aust. N. Z. J. Med. 17, 301–304.

Alloway, J.A., Moriarty, M.J., Hoogland, Y.T., et al., 1993. Comparison of triamcinolone acetonide with Indometacin in treatment of acute gouty arthritis. J. Rheumatol. 29, 111–113.

Annemans, L., Spaepen, E., Gaskin, M., et al., 2008. Gout in the UK and Germany: prevalence, comorbidities and management in general practice. Ann. Rheum. Dis. 67, 960–966.

Bahn, A., Hagos, Y., Reuter, S., et al., 2008. Identification of a new urate and high affinity nicotinate transporter, hOAT10 (SLC22A13). J. Biol. Chem. 283, 16332–16341.

Batt, C., Phipps-Green, A.J., Black, M.A., et al., 2014. Sugar-sweetened beverage consumption: a risk factor for prevalent gout with SLC2A9 genotype-specific effects on serum urate and risk of gout. Ann. Rheum. Dis. 73, 2101–2106.

Becker, M.A., Schumacher, H.R., Espinoza, L.R., et al., 2010. The urate-lowering efficacy and safety of febuxistat in the treatment of the hyperuricemia of gout: the CONFRIMS trial. Arthritis Res. Ther. 12 (2), R63. https://doi.org/10.1186/ar2978.

Becker, M.A., Schumacher, H.R., Wortmann, R.L., et al., 2005. Febuxostat, a novel non-purine selective inhibitor of xanthine oxidase: a twenty-eight day, multicenter, phase II, randomized, double-blind, placebo-controlled, dose-response clinical trial examining safety and efficacy in patients with gout. Arthritis Rheumatol. 52, 916–923.

Bernal, J.A., Quilis, N., Andrés, M., et al., 2016. Gout: optimizing treatment to achieve a disease cure. Ther. Adv. Chronic Dis. 7 (2), 135–144.

Campion, E.W., Glynn, R.J., Delabry, L.O., 1987. Asymptomatic hyperuricaemia: risks and consequences in the Normative ageing study. Am. J. Med. 82, 421–426.

Cavagna, L., Taylor, W.J., 2014. The emerging role of biotechnological drugs in the treatment of gout. Biomed. Res. Int. 2014, 264859.

Choi, H.K., Atkinson, K., Karlson, E.W., et al., 2004. Purine rich foods, dairy and protein intake, and the risk of gout in men. N. Engl. J. Med. 350, 1093–1103.

Choi, H.K., Atkinson, K., Karlson, E.W., et al., 2005. Obesity, weight change, hypertension, diuretic use, and risk of gout in men: the health professionals follow-up study. Arch. Intern. Med. 165, 742–748.

Choi, H.K., Curham, G., 2008. Soft drinks, fructose consumption, and the risk of gout in men: prospective cohort study. Br. Med. J. 336, 309–312.

Choi, H.K., Ford, E.S., Li, C., et al., 2007a. Prevalence of metabolic syndrome in patients with gout: the Third National Health and Nutrition Examination Survey. Arthritis Rheum. 57, 109–115.

Choi, H.K., Willet, W., Curhan, G., 2007b. Coffee consumption and the risk of incident gout in men: a prospective study. Arthritis Rheum. 56, 2049–2055.

Cohen, S.D., Kimmel, P.L., Neff, R., et al., 2008. Association of incident gout and mortality in dialysis patients. J. Am. Soc. Nephrol. 19, 2204–2210.

Creighton, S., Miller, R., Edwards, S., et al., 2005. Is ritonavir boosting associated with gout? Int. J. STD AIDS 16 362–362.

Dalbeth, N., Haskard, D.O., 2005. Mechanisms of inflammation in gout. Rheumatology 44, 1090–1096.

Dehghan, A., Kottgen, A., Yang, Q., et al., 2008. Association of three genetic loci with uric acid concentration and risk of gout: a genome-wide association study. Lancet 372, 1953–1961.

Duskin-Bitan, H., Cohen, E., Goldberg, E., et al., 2014. The degree of asymptomatic hyperuricaemia and the risk of gout. A retrospective analysis of a large cohort. Clin. Rheumatol. 33, 549–553.

Graessler, J., Graessler, A., Unger, S., et al., 2006. Association of the human urate transporter 1 with reduced renal uric acid excretion in a German Caucasian population. Arthritis Rheum. 54, 292–300.

Hak, A.E., Curhan, G.C., Grodstein, F., et al., 2010. Menopause, postmenopausal hormone use and risk of incident gout. Ann. Rheum. Dis. 69, 1305–1309.

Hall, A.P., Barry, P.E., Dawber, T.R., et al., 1967. Epidemiology of gout and hyperuricaemia: a long-term population study. Am. J. Med. 42, 27–37.

Hsu, C.Y., Iribarren, C., Mcculloch, C.E., et al., 2009. Risk factors for end stage renal disease: 25 year follow-up. Arch. Intern. Med. 169, 342–350.

Huang, H.Y., Appel, L.J., Choi, M.J., et al., 2005. The effects of vitamin C supplementation on serum concentrations of uric acid: results of a randomized controlled trial. Arthritis Rheum. 52, 1843–1847.

Iseki, K., Ikemiya, Y., Inoue, T., et al., 2004. Significance of hyperuricaemia as a risk of developing ESRD in a screened cohort. Am. J. Kidney Dis. 44, 642–650.

Janssens, H.J., Janssen, M., van dr Lisdonk, E.H., et al., 2008. Use of oral prednisolone or naproxen for the treatment of gout arthritis: double-blind, randomised equivalence trial. Lancet 371, 1854–1860.

Jordan, K.M., Cameron, S., Snaith, M., British Society for Rheumatology and British Health Professionals in Rheumatology Standards, Guidelines and Adult Working Group (SGAWG), 2007. British Society for Rheumatology and British Health Professionals in Rheumatology guideline for the management of gout. Rheumatology (Oxford) 46 (8), 1372–1374.

Khanna, D., Fitzgerald, J.D., Khanna, P.P., et al., 2012a. American College of Rheumatology Guidelines for the management of gout. Part 1: systematic non-pharmacological and pharmacological therapeutic approaches to hyperuricaemia. Arthritis Care Res. 64, 1431–1446.

Khanna, D., Khanna, P.P., Fitzgerald, J.D., et al., 2012b. American College of Rheumatology Guidelines for the management of gout. Part 2: therapy and anti-inflammatory prophylaxis of acute gouty arthritis. Arthritis Care Res. 64, 1447–1461.

Kumar, S., Ng, J., Gow, P., 2005. Benzbromarone therapy in management of refractory gout. N. Z. Med. J. 118, U1528.

Kuo, C.-F., Grainge, M.J., Zhang, W., et al., 2015a. Global epidemiology of gout: prevalence, incidence and risk factors. Nat. Rev. Rheumatol. 11, 649–662.

Kuo, C.-F., Grainge, M.J., Mallen, C., et al., 2015b. Rising burden of gout in the UK but continuing suboptimal management: a nationwide population study. Ann. Rheum. Dis. 74, 661–667.

Lawrence Edwards, N., 2009. Febuxostat: a new treatment for hyperuricaemia in gout. Rheumatology 48 (Suppl. 2), ii15–ii19.

Lin, K.C., Lin, H.Y., Chou, P., 2000a. Community based epidemiological study on hyperuricaemia and gout in Kin Hu, Kinmen. J. Rheumatol. 27, 1045–1050.

Lin, K.C., Lin, H.Y., Chou, P., 2000b. The interaction between uric acid level and other risk factors on the development of gout among asymptomatic hyperuricaemen men in a prospective study. J. Rheumatol. 27, 1501–1505.

Man, C.Y., Cheung, I., Cameron, I., et al., 2007. Comparison of oral prednisolone/paracetamol and oral Indometacin/paracetamol combination therapy in the treatment of acute gout like arthritis: a double blind randomized, controlled trial. Ann. Emerg. Med. 49, 670–677.

Matsuo, H., Yamamato, K., Nakaoka, H., et al., 2016. Genome-wide association study of clinically defined gout identifies multiple risk loci and its association with clinical subtypes. Ann. Rheum. Dis. 75, 652–659.

McGonagle, D., Tan, A.L., Shankaranarayana, S., et al., 2007. Management of treatment resistant inflammation of acute or chronic tophaceous gout with anakinra. Ann. Rheum. Dis. 66, 1683–1684.

Mikuls, T.R., Farrar, J.T., Bilker, W.B., et al., 2005. Gout epidemiology: results from the UK General Practice Research Database 1990–1999. Ann. Rheum. Dis. 64, 267–272.

National Institute for Health and Care Excellence (NICE), 2013. Canakinumab for treating gouty arthritis attacks and reducing frequency of subsequent attacks (terminated appraisal). Technology Appraisal Guidance 281 NICE, London. Available at: https://www.nice.org.uk/Guidance/ta281.

Nuki, G., 2008. Colchicine: its mechanism of action and efficacy in crystal-induced inflammation. Curr. Rheumatol. Rep. 10, 218–227.

Reinders, M.K., Haagsma, C., Jansen, T.L., et al., 2009. A randomised controlled trial on the efficacy and tolerability with dose escalation of allopurinol 300–600 mg/day versus benzbromarone 100–200 mg/day in patients with gout. Ann. Rheum. Dis. 68, 892–897.

Rho, Y.H., Lu, N., Peloquin, C.E., et al., 2016. Independent impact of gout on the risk of diabetes mellitus among women and men: a population based, BMI-matched cohort study. Ann. Rheum. Dis. 75 (1), 91–95.

Richette, P., Bardin, T., 2009. Gout. Lancet 375, 318–328.

Rider, T.G., Jordan, K.M., 2010. The modern management of gout. Rheumatology 49, 5–14.

Roddy, E., Doherty, E., 2010. Epidemiology of gout. Arthritis Res. Ther. 12, 223. Available at: http://arthritis-research.com/content/12/6/223.

Schumacher, H.R., Becker, M.A., Lloyd, E., et al., 2009. Febuxostat in the treatment of gout; 5-yr findings of the FOCUS efficacy and safety study. Rheumatology 48, 188–194.

Schumacher, H.R., Becker, M.A., Wortmann, R.L., et al., 2008. Effects of febuxostat versus allopurinol and placebo in reducing serum urate in subjects with hyperuricaemia and gout: a 28-week, phase III, randomized, double blind, parallel-group trial. Arthritis Rheumatol. 59, 1540–1548.

Sica, A.D., Schoolwerth, A.C., 2002. Part 1. Uric acid and losartan. Curr. Opin. Nephrol. Hypertens. 11, 475–482.

Sivera, F., Andrés, M., Carmona, L., et al., 2014. Multinational evidence based recommendations for the diagnosis and management of gout: integrating systematic literature review and expert opinion of a broad panel of rheumatologists in the 3e initiative. Ann. Rheum. Dis. 73, 328–335.

Smith, E., Hoy, D., Cross, M., et al., 2014. The global burden of gout: estimates from the global burden of disease study. Ann. Rheum. Dis. 73, 1470–1476.

So, A., De Smedt, T., Revas, S., et al., 2007. A pilot study of IL-1 inhibition by anakinra in acute gout. Arthritis Res. Ther. 9, R28.

So, A., Thorens, B., 2010. Uric acid transport and disease. J. Clin. Invest. 120 (6), 1791–1799.

Stamp, L.K., Chapman, P.T., 2014. Urate lowering therapy: current options and future prospects for elderly patients with gout. Drugs Aging 31, 777–786.

Stamp, L.K., O'Donnell, J., Zhang, M., et al., 2011. Using allopurinol above the dose based on creatinine clearance is effective and safe in chronic gout, including those with renal impairment. Arthritis Rheumatol. 63 (2), 412–421.

Stamp, L.K., Taylor, W.J., Jones, P.B., et al., 2012. Starting dose is a risk factor for allopurinol hypersensitivity syndrome: a proposed safe starting dose of allopurinol. Arthritis Rheumatol. 64, 2529–2536.

Takahashi, S., Moriwaki, Y., Yamamoto, T., et al., 2003. Effects of combination treatment using anti-hyperuriaemic agents with fenofibrate and/or losartan on uric acid metabolism. Arthritis Res. Ther. 72, 671–674.

Terkeltaub, R., Furst, D.E., Bennett, K., et al., 2008. Low dose (1.8 mg) vs high dose (4.8 mg) oral colchicine regimens in patients with acute gout flare in a large, multicentre, randomized, double-blind, placebo controlled, parallel group study. Arthritis Rheumatol. 58 (Suppl. 9), 1944.

Trelle, S., Reichenbach, S., Wandel, S., et al., 2011. Cardiovascular safety of non-steroidal anti-inflammatory drugs: network meta-analysis. Br. Med. J. 342, c7086.

Winnard, D., Wright, C., Taylor, W.J., et al., 2012. National prevalence of gout derived from administrative health data in Aotearoa New Zealand. Rheumatology 51, 901–909.

Zhang, W., Doherty, M., Pascual, E., et al., 2006. EULAR evidence based recommendations for gout. Part I: diagnosis. Report of a task force of the EULAR Standing Committee for International Clinical Studies Including Therapeutics (ESCISIT). Ann. Rheum. Dis. 65, 1301–1311.

Further reading

Sivera, F., Andrés, M., Carmona, L., et al., 2014. Multinational evidence based recommendations for the diagnosis and management of gout: integrating systematic literature review and expert opinion of a broad panel of rheumatologists in the 3e initiative. Ann. Rheum. Dis. 73, 328–335.

Khanna, D., Fitzgerald, J.D., Khanna, P.P., et al., 2012. American College of Rheumatology Guidelines for the management of gout. Part 1: systematic non-pharmacological and pharmacological therapeutic approaches to hyperuricaemia. Arthritis Care Res. 64, 1431–1446.

Khanna, D., Khanna, P.P., Fitzgerald, J.D., et al., 2012. American College of Rheumatology Guidelines for the management of gout. Part 2: therapy and anti-inflammatory prophylaxis of acute gouty arthritis. Arthritis Care Res. 64, 1447–1461.

Stamp, L.K., Chapman, P.T., 2014. Urate lowering therapy: current options and future prospects for elderly patients with gout. Drugs Aging 31, 777–786.

Useful websites

Gout Society: http://www.ukgoutsociety.org

56 Glaucoma

Tamara Ahmed Ali and Mark D. Doherty

Key points

- Glaucoma describes a group of conditions characterised by progressive optic nerve damage and is accompanied by characteristic visual field defects.
- Primary open-angle glaucoma (POAG) is a chronic progressive disease of insidious onset.
- The aim of treatment in POAG is to reduce the intraocular pressure (IOP) to a target level, tailored individually to the patient, with the aim of preventing further damage to the nerve fibres and the development and progression of visual field defects.
- A wide range of pharmaceutical agents can be used to treat POAG. Laser treatment or surgery may be undertaken if the target pressure is not attained with medical therapy.
- POAG generally does not cause symptoms until the damage reaches an advanced stage. Adherence with therapy is therefore a critical issue.
- Acute primary angle closure (PAC) is an ophthalmological emergency that must be rapidly treated to prevent irreversible sight loss.
- The role of medical treatment in acute PAC is to reduce the IOP with a view to subsequent laser and/or surgical treatment.
- A range of drugs can provoke an attack of acute PAC in susceptible individuals.

The term 'glaucoma' comprises a number of distinct conditions that have differing clinical features but share a common finding: progressive optic neuropathy (nerve damage) causing characteristic visual field defects. Although glaucoma is frequently associated with raised intraocular pressure (IOP), the diagnosis is often made despite a measured IOP within the 'normal' range. Raised IOP therefore remains the most significant, and is the only modifiable risk factor for glaucoma, but it does not form part of the diagnostic criteria.

Normal IOP is a statistical description of the range of IOP found in the population. Mean IOP is estimated at 15–16 mmHg, and the upper limit of the normal range is calculated as 2 standard deviations above the mean, approximately 21 mmHg.

There is a circadian cycle of IOP, with maximum levels often occurring between 8 and 11 a.m. and minimum levels between midnight and 2 a.m. This may affect IOP readings taken in outpatient clinics at different times of the day. In addition, diurnal variations may be greater in patients with glaucoma. Although elevated IOP is not the only risk factor for glaucoma, it is the only parameter that can currently be modified by pharmacological intervention and, therefore, is central to the evaluation of disease progression and clinical management.

Glaucoma management involves the setting of a target IOP, a value at which disease progression is significantly slowed. In setting the target IOP, a common strategy is to aim for a 25–30% reduction from the initial IOP at which damage occurred. In practice it is a dynamic, clinical judgement, which is frequently adjusted as appropriate to the patient's clinical course and response to treatment. Continuous evaluation of the patient's progress is therefore essential to achieve this objective.

Epidemiology

Glaucoma is the leading cause of irreversible blindness worldwide. In 2013 the number of people aged 40–80 years with glaucoma was estimated to be 64.3 million. This figure is due to increase to 76.0 million in 2020 and 111.8 million in 2040 (Tham et al., 2014). Affected individuals require lifelong monitoring for disease control and detection of progression, to minimise the risk of permanent visual damage.

Primary open-angle glaucoma

Primary open-angle glaucoma (POAG) is a chronic progressive disease of insidious onset, usually affecting both eyes. It is frequently an inherited condition, with a 10-fold increased lifetime risk in patients with a family history (Wolfs et al., 1998). Approximately 10% of UK blindness registrations are ascribed to glaucoma, and around 2% of people older than 40 years have POAG, a figure which rises to almost 10% in white Europeans older than 75 years (National Institute for Health and Care Excellence [NICE], 2009). The prevalence of POAG is higher in people of black African or black Caribbean descent (Sommer et al., 1991). Based on these estimates, around 500,000 people are affected by POAG in England and Wales where more than a million glaucoma-related outpatient visits are made to the hospital eye service annually (King et al., 2013).

Normal tension glaucoma

Normal tension glaucoma (NTG) shares a number of features with POAG, but by definition develops (and often progresses) at an IOP usually regarded as within the 'normal' range. It is unclear

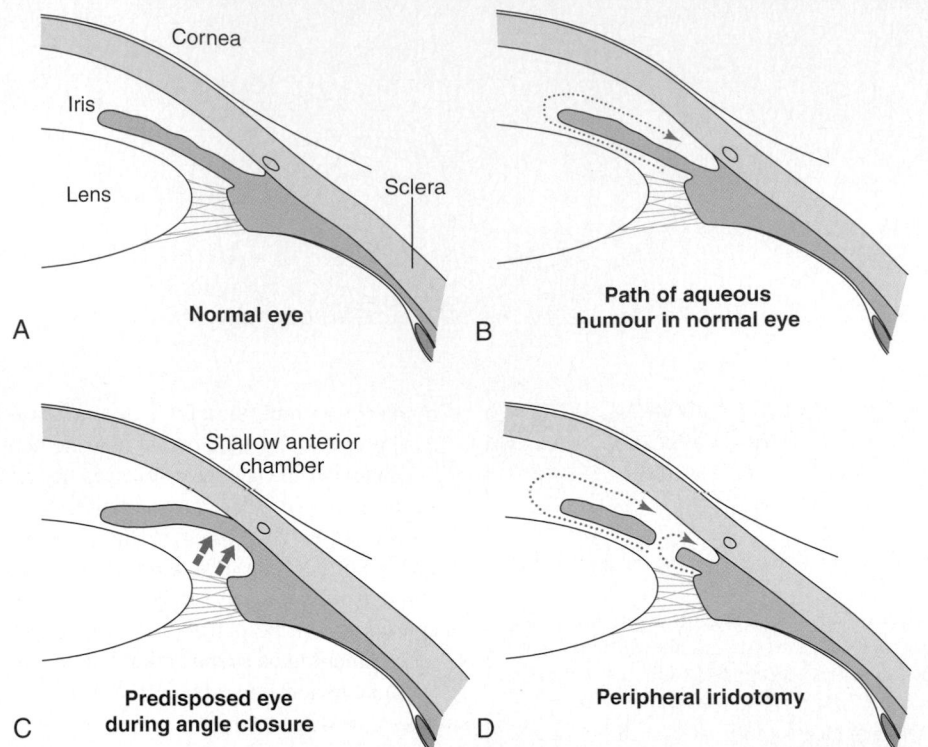

Fig. 56.1 The iridocorneal angle. (A and B) Normal eye. (C) Primary angle closure. (D) After peripheral iridotomy.

whether POAG and NTG are separate conditions or similar entities occurring at opposing ends of the IOP spectrum. It has been reported that up to 24% of patients with glaucoma have NTG.

Ocular hypertension

Ocular hypertension (OHT) is a condition whereby the IOP is elevated in the absence of visual field loss or glaucomatous optic nerve damage. It is estimated that 3–5% of those older than 40 years have OHT, although the prevalence is lower in Indian and Japanese patients, and higher in African or Caribbean patients. OHT represents a risk of future development of POAG, and lowering IOP has been shown to protect against conversion to POAG.

Primary angle-closure glaucoma

Primary angle-closure glaucoma (PACG) is a condition in which closure of the iridocorneal angle results in a reduction in aqueous outflow, usually in predisposed eyes. The disease affects 0.4% of Caucasian adults older than 40 years, with higher rates in patients of Asian or East Asian descent (Day et al., 2012). It occurs in four times as many females as males. Although rarer than POAG, it carries a significantly higher risk of blindness.

Secondary glaucoma

Secondary glaucoma occurs as a result of an instigating condition or clinical circumstance. Examples include corticosteroid therapy, intraocular inflammation, pigment dispersion, pseudoexfoliation, trauma, neovascularisation and developmental abnormalities.

Congenital glaucoma

Congenital glaucoma occurs within the first year of life, typically presenting with watering, light sensitivity and blepharospasm (involuntary tight eyelid closure). The condition is due to an abnormally developed iridocorneal angle. Surgery is the mainstay of treatment. Further details of congenital glaucoma are beyond the scope of this chapter.

Aetiology

The factors that determine the level of IOP are the rate of aqueous humour production and the rate of its outflow. A fine balance between these is necessary to maintain a desirable pressure within the eye. When production exceeds outflow, IOP rises.

Production of aqueous humour occurs in the ciliary epithelium by three mechanisms:

- active secretion (independent of the level of IOP),
- ultrafiltration (influenced by the level of IOP),
- passive diffusion of ions.

Aqueous humour is produced by the ciliary body and passes anteriorly through the pupil into the anterior chamber. Outflow of aqueous humour occurs by two routes. Approximately 80–90% of total outflow is through the trabecular meshwork into the canal of Schlemm and into the venous circulation via the aqueous veins (Fig. 56.1A and B). The uveoscleral pathway, accounting for the remaining 10–20%, describes the outflow of the aqueous humour through the ciliary body, into the suprachoroidal space, finally leaving the eye through the sclera (Fig. 56.2).

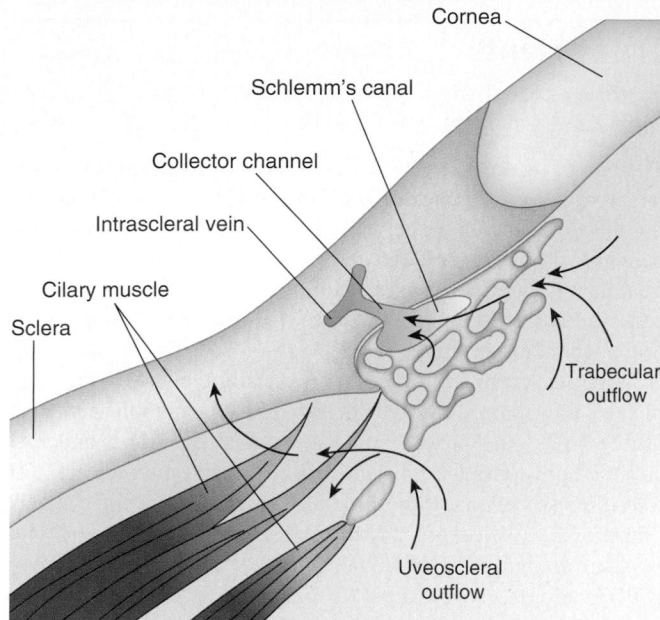

Cornea

Schlemm's canal

Collector channel

Intrascleral vein

Cilary muscle

Sclera

Trabecular outflow

Uveoscleral outflow

Fig. 56.2 Physiological aqueous outflow pathways. (From Alm and Kaufman, Uveoscleral Outflow: Biology and Clinical Aspects. Mosby-Wolfe Medical Publications. Reproduced with permission of Mosby-Wolfe Medical Publications, 1998.)

Pathophysiology

The precise pathophysiology of glaucomatous damage is not entirely understood. Degeneration specifically affects the retinal ganglion cells, whose axons pass across the retina and through the lamina cribrosa to form the optic nerve head. Raised IOP causes deformation of the lamina cribrosa, with damage to retinal ganglion cell axons and subsequent cell death (Weinreb et al., 2014). Other pressure-independent mechanisms, such as impaired vascular supply and low cerebrospinal fluid pressure, may also influence glaucomatous progression. Such factors are perhaps more likely to be more significant in NTG.

In POAG, increased resistance within aqueous drainage channels causes the rise in IOP. It is thought that the main route of resistance to aqueous outflow lies in the dense juxtacanalicular trabecular meshwork and the endothelium lining the inner wall of Schlemm's canal (Stamer et al., 2015). Age-related dysfunction of these structures increases resistance to outflow and subsequent raised IOP.

In PACG, the rise in IOP is caused by a decreased outflow of aqueous humour due to closure of the iridocorneal angle. It occurs in anatomically predisposed eyes with increased lens size, shallower anterior chamber and shorter axial length (see Fig. 56.1C).

The lens continues to grow throughout life, thereby bringing its anterior surface closer to the cornea. Slackening of the zonules compounds this movement. Both factors lead to a gradual and progressive shallowing of the anterior chamber. This effect is more significant in a short hypermetropic eye with a thick and relatively anteriorly located lens. These factors in combination lead to physical obstruction of the trabecular meshwork by the iris. This is a gradual process that can ultimately lead to a sudden escalation in IOP, precipitating

an attack of acute angle closure (see Fig. 56.1C). Alternatively the condition may remain asymptomatic, with the progressive development of scarring adhesions between iris and trabecular meshwork, gradually increased IOP and subsequent glaucomatous damage.

Clinical manifestations

Table 56.1 presents the clinical features of the different glaucoma types.

Primary open-angle glaucoma

POAG is typically characterised by the following:

- IOP greater than 21 mmHg: This is most accurately measured using the Goldmann applanation tonometer attached to the slit lamp. The cornea is anaesthetised and then gently applanated with a disposable tonometer head. The IOP is then read from a scale on the side of the tonometer.
- An open angle: Gonioscopy refers to the examination of the iridocorneal angle at the slit lamp using a specialised contact lens placed onto the cornea. Observations can be made regarding the angle width, the iris features, and the presence or absence of irido-trabecular adhesions (synechiae). An estimation of the angle's likelihood of closure can thereby be made.
- Glaucomatous optic neuropathy: The hallmark sign is cupping, an increase in size of the depressed 'cup' located in the centre of the optic nerve head (optic disc). The cup becomes more prominent as the disease progresses because of ongoing retinal ganglion cell death. This may be accompanied by progressive disc pallor. Disc photography is invaluable in providing a baseline for subsequent comparison in follow-up visits.
- Retinal nerve fibre layer thinning: This can be assessed at the slit lamp and may be facilitated by the use of a green filter. Focal areas of thinning may be apparent on direct observation and may indicate early glaucomatous damage.

Chronic primary angle-closure glaucoma

Chronic PACG is usually associated with raised IOP. The anterior chamber is shallow. Gonioscopy reveals a closed iridocorneal angle, and synechiae may be evident. The disc is cupped, and nerve fibre layer defects may be evident.

Acute primary angle closure

Acute primary angle closure (PAC), an ophthalmic emergency, is caused by sudden closure of the angle and a marked elevation in IOP. The symptoms include rapidly progressive visual impairment and pain frequently with nausea and vomiting. The signs include dilation of the conjunctival blood vessels. The anterior chamber is shallow bilaterally, with the affected pupil fixed in a semi-dilated position. The IOP is elevated, frequently between 60 and 80 mmHg, causing corneal oedema. The optic disc is not usually cupped unless the IOP has been elevated for a protracted period.

Secondary glaucomas

Secondary glaucomas share features common to POAG and PACG, and may be identified by signs indicating the underlying process. Examples include iris transillumination in pigment dispersion, lens deposits in pseudoexfoliation and abnormal iris vessels in neovascularisation.

Investigations
Perimetry (visual field testing)

Visual field loss is usually asymptomatic until it reaches an advanced stage. Perimetry identifies functional deficits at an earlier stage and is a key component in the diagnosis, monitoring and management of glaucoma. The earliest clinically significant field defect is a scotoma, which is an area of depressed vision within the visual field.

Pachymetry

Measurement of central corneal thickness may influence the measured IOP, with a thick cornea causing a falsely high reading. It is considered in assessing an individual's risk of glaucomatous progression, and may also affect the efficacy of certain drug treatments (Johnson et al., 2008).

Nerve fibre analysis

Clinical findings can be augmented with the use of imaging modalities such as optical coherence tomography and laser scanning laser polarimetry. These can assist in the identification of early defects before visual field loss becomes established.

Treatment
Primary open-angle glaucoma
Medical treatment

The aim of treatment in POAG is to reduce the raised IOP to the target value, preventing further damage to the nerve fibres and the development of further visual field defects to maintain the patient's visual function and quality of life. The key to effective treatment is careful and regular follow-up, with continuous reassessment and tailoring of the target IOP in response to evidence of glaucomatous progression.

The initial treatment of POAG is usually medical in the form of topical eyedrops, with a wide range of preparations available (Table 56.2). The prostaglandin analogues (PGAs) latanoprost and travoprost and the prostamide bimatoprost are indicated for first-line use because these produce the greatest decline in IOP (Table 56.3). β-Blockers may then be added in combination with PGAs if the initial effect is inadequate, or used as monotherapy if PGAs are poorly tolerated. Carbonic anhydrase inhibitors are frequently prescribed for patients unresponsive to first-line drugs, in patients in whom the first-line agents are contraindicated or as adjunctive therapy. An α-agonist such as brimonidine may also be used in the same clinical setting. Pilocarpine is rarely used in POAG. Oral therapy with carbonic anhydrase inhibitors is reserved for use as a last resort, usually in patients awaiting surgery.

Guidance on the treatment of people with OHT or suspected POAG has been published (NICE, 2009). The treatment options (Table 56.4) take into account central corneal thickness and age, although age thresholds are appropriate only where vision is normal and the treatment is purely preventative.

Table 56.1 Clinical features of main glaucoma types

	Primary open-angle glaucoma	Normal tension glaucoma	Ocular hypertension	Primary angle closure glaucoma	Secondary glaucoma[a]
When symptoms occur	Late in disease	Late in disease	None	Pain, blurring, nausea in acute setting	Dependent on underlying condition
Mechanism	Inflow of aqueous humour exceeds outflow	Vascular and non-intraocular pressure factors likely to have a more prominent role	Inflow of aqueous humour exceeds outflow	Closed iridocorneal angle preventing adequate outflow of aqueous humour	Dependent on underlying condition
Intraocular pressure	>21 mmHg	≤21 mmHg	>21 mmHg	Any	Any
Angle	Open	Open	Open	Closed	Open or closed, depending on underlying condition
Optic nerve	Cupped	Cupped	Normal	Cupped	Cupped
Other distinguishing features	None	May have disc haemorrhages	None	May have peripheral anterior synechiae	Dependent on underlying condition

[a]Secondary glaucoma is where there is an identifiable cause of increased pressure. For example it may be caused by an eye injury, inflammation, medications or diabetes.

Surgical treatment

The improved control of IOP with PGAs and prostamides has reduced the demand for surgical intervention in glaucoma (Kenigsberg, 2007). A significant number of patients will still require laser or surgical procedures to reach their target pressure.

Laser trabeculoplasty aims to improve the outflow of aqueous fluid through the trabecular meshwork and is a useful modality to reduce IOP without employing incisional surgery. This may be particularly useful for patients with mild glaucoma who require a modest IOP reduction, or in whom topical treatment is ineffective or poorly tolerated. Traditionally this was undertaken with an argon laser. More recently, selective laser trabeculoplasty has been introduced as a procedure that is easier to perform and better tolerated, with a lower complication rate.

There is great interest in the use of minimally invasive glaucoma surgery in the management of early glaucoma. A number of different techniques and devices are available with the aim of surgically reducing IOP without the perceived complication profile of more invasive surgical solutions.

In patients with coexistent POAG and cataract, surgical removal of the latter with insertion of an intraocular lens is a useful technique that is frequently utilised to achieve a modest reduction in IOP.

The most frequently performed surgical procedure for POAG, trabeculectomy, creates a fistula between the anterior conjunctiva and subconjunctival space to act as a new route for aqueous outflow. Where trabeculectomy is undesirable or ineffective, the insertion of a glaucoma drainage device is a useful alternative. The frequency of glaucoma drainage device usage has increased markedly since the 1990s when two new designs were introduced.

Finally, where target IOP has not been achieved, or in eyes with limited visual potential, external cyclophotocoagulation can be a useful means to obtain a lower IOP by the targeted destruction of ciliary processes with a diode laser.

Acute primary angle-closure glaucoma

The medical management of acute PAC aims to relieve symptoms, reduce IOP to a safe level and prepare the eye for laser or surgical treatment. Analgesics and antiemetics are sometimes needed, dependent on symptom severity, to make the patient comfortable. The unaffected eye is usually treated prophylactically with pilocarpine, to protect against a similar attack in the fellow eye.

Paralysis of the iris sphincter usually occurs at an IOP of more than 60 mmHg as a result of ischaemia. Pilocarpine is therefore usually ineffective in the early stages, and the IOP is lowered by aqueous suppressants such as topical timolol 0.5%. An intravenous loading dose of acetazolamide is frequently used, followed by regular oral treatment. Mannitol is now a less frequently used alternative because of a greater perceived risk of

Table 56.2 Drugs used in the treatment of primary open-angle glaucoma

Therapeutic category	Primary mechanism
Topical prostaglandins	Increase aqueous outflow
Topical prostamides	Increase aqueous outflow
Topical β-blocking agents	Decrease aqueous formation
Topical miotics	Increase aqueous outflow
Topical adrenergic agonists	Increase aqueous outflow and decrease aqueous formation
Topical carbonic anhydrase inhibitors	Decrease aqueous formation
Oral carbonic anhydrase inhibitors	Decrease aqueous formation

Table 56.3 Comparison of reduction in intraocular pressure with a range of ocular hypotensive drugs

Drug	Relative IOP change from baseline at trough, % (95% CI)	Relative IOP change from baseline at peak, % (95% CI)
Bimatoprost	−28 (−29 to −27)	−33 (−35 to −31)
Travoprost	−29 (−32 to −25)	−31 (−32 to −29)
Latanoprost	−28 (−30 to −26)	−31 (−33 to −29)
Timolol	−26 (−28 to −25)	−27 (−29 to −25)
Betaxolol	−20 (−23 to −17)	−23 (−25 to −22)
Dorzolamide	−17 (−19 to −15)	−22 (−24 to −20)
Brinzolamide	−17 (−19 to −15)	−17 (−19 to −15)
Brimonidine	−18 (−21 to −14)	−25 (−28 to −22)
Placebo	−5 (−9 to −1)	−5 (−10 to 0)

CI, confidence interval; IOP, intraocular pressure.
Adapted from **van derValk** et al. (2009).

Table 56.4 Treatment of people with ocular hypertension or suspected primary open-angle glaucoma (National Institute for Health and Care Excellence, 2009)

Central corneal thickness	>590 micrometres		555–590 micrometres		<555 micrometres		
Untreated IOP (mmHg)	>21–25	>25–32	>21–25	>25–32	>21–25	>25–32	>32
Age (years)	Any	Any	Any	Treat until 60	Treat until 65	Treat until 80	Any
Treatment	No treatment	No treatment	No treatment	β-Blocker	Prostaglandin analogue	Prostaglandin analogue	Prostaglandin analogue

cardiopulmonary decompensation. The acetazolamide should allow the IOP to drop sufficiently to relieve iris ischaemia and allow the sphincter to respond to pilocarpine therapy.

When the IOP has been reduced medically, both eyes are treated with laser iridotomies, creating an opening in the peripheral iris to allow the flow of aqueous humour through an alternative pathway (see Fig. 56.1D). If unsuccessful, alternatives include laser iridoplasty (a succession of peripheral iris burns causing iris contraction and distraction from the angle), surgical iridectomy (removal of a peripheral section of iris tissue), cataract surgery or diode laser. Filtration surgery may be indicated later if the IOP remains uncontrolled despite these interventions.

Normal tension glaucoma

Treatment is not always required in NTG. A significant proportion of untreated patients (50% at 5 years in the Collaborative Normal-Tension Glaucoma Study Group [CNTGS] study) do not show visual field progression (CNTGS, 1998). Patients with NTG demonstrating progression despite a 'normal' IOP may be commenced on IOP-lowering medications. The treatment regimen employed is usually similar to that of POAG. Some clinicians avoid β-blockers because of their potential for reducing systemic blood pressure, lowering ocular perfusion pressure and increasing susceptibility to glaucomatous progression.

Secondary glaucoma

Treatment of secondary glaucoma initially involves control of the causative factor where possible. Examples include reducing or changing medication in steroid-induced glaucoma, arresting the inflammation in uveitic glaucoma, or retinal laser and anti–vascular endothelial growth factor formulations in neovascular glaucoma. If still required the IOP can then be lowered using a regimen similar to that used in other types of glaucoma.

Drug treatment

The importance of early diagnosis and treatment is essential in slowing disease progression and improving the quality of life for patients with glaucoma (McKean-Cowdin et al., 2008). Topical glaucoma medications are the first choice of therapy; these drugs lower IOP by a variety of mechanisms (see Table 56.2).

There are five main classes of drugs:
- ocular prostanoids (PGAs and prostamides),
- β-blockers (β-adrenoceptor antagonists),
- carbonic anhydrase inhibitors and systemic drugs,
- sympathomimetic agents (α_2-adrenergic agonists),
- miotics (parasympathomimetic).

The PGAs latanoprost, tafluprost and travoprost and the prostamide bimatoprost are indicated for first-line use because these produce the greatest decline in IOP. β-Blockers, which were traditionally the drug of choice, are now often prescribed either in combination with these or as an alternative (NICE, 2009). Carbonic anhydrase inhibitors are frequently prescribed for patients unresponsive to first-line drugs, in patients in whom the first-line agents are contraindicated or as adjunctive therapy. Sympathomimetics are less commonly prescribed in POAG, and miotics are rarely used. Contraindications and drug interactions should be considered before offering any glaucoma treatment.

Ocular prostanoids: prostaglandin analogues and prostamides

PGAs (latanoprost, tafluprost and travoprost) lower IOP by increasing uveoscleral outflow with no significant effect on other parameters of aqueous humour dynamics. The prostamide (bimatoprost) is thought to increase outflow through both trabecular and uveoscleral outflow pathways. However, there is still debate about the precise mechanisms of action of this group (Lim et al., 2008; Toris et al., 2008).

A recent systematic review and network meta-analysis comparing the effectiveness of first-line medications for POAG concluded that drugs in the prostaglandin class (bimatoprost, latanoprost and travoprost) were more efficacious than drugs in other classes in reducing IOP at 3 months. The 'within-class' differences were generally small (Li et al., 2016). In another meta-analysis these drugs have been shown to have a greater effect on both peak and trough readings of IOP than timolol, betaxolol, dorzolamide, brinzolamide and brimonidine, producing declines in IOP of 28–29% at trough and 31–33% at peak as shown in Table 56.3 (van der Valk et al., 2009). They are also known to reduce the IOP fluctuation during the 24-hour period with a maximum effect achieved 3–5 weeks after starting therapy (Bartlett and Jaanus, 2008).

Table 56.5 Ocular prostanoids

	Bimatoprost		Latanoprost	Tafluprost	Travoprost
Trade name	Lumigan		Xalatan	Saflutan	Travatan
Pharmacological class	Prostamide		Prostaglandin analogue	Prostaglandin analogue	Prostaglandin analogue
Strength	0.03%	0.01%	0.005%	0.0015%	0.004%
Preservative		Benzalkonium chloride 0.02%	Benzalkonium chloride 0.02%	None	Polyquaternium-1 0.001%
Storage requirements	≤25 °C	≤25 °C	2–8 °C until opened, then ≤25 °C for a period of use of 4 weeks	2–8 °C until opened, then ≤25 °C for a period of use of 4 weeks	≤25 °C

All the drugs in this class are licensed for the reduction of elevated IOP in POAG and OHT. They are administered once daily in the evening, and systemic side effects are relatively uncommon. The NICE guideline (NICE, 2009) does not differentiate between the PGAs and the prostamide (Table 56.5), but recommends one of this class for the treatment of POAG, certain patients with OHT and certain POAG suspects (see Table 56.4).

The prostanoids have some interesting local side effects (Table 56.6), most commonly increased pigmentation of the iris as a result of increased deposition of melanin in the stromal melanocytes of the iris. This mainly occurs up to 1 year of use in patients with mixed colour (green-brown, yellow-brown or blue/grey-brown) irides. Therefore, before treatment is initiated, patients should be informed of the possibility of a change in eye colour.

An increase in the length and thickness of the eyelashes and pigmentation of the palpebral skin are also known side effects. Use of these drugs may lead to disruption of the blood–aqueous barrier in patients with aphakia (no lens) and pseudophakia (implanted intraocular lens), and increase the risk of development of cystoid macular oedema; they should be used with caution in such patients and patients with known risk factors for macular oedema.

PGAs and prostamides should be used with caution in patients with active intraocular inflammation such as iritis and uveitis. They should not be used in pregnant women because there is a theoretical risk of promoting miscarriage.

Reactivation of herpes simplex infection has been reported with bimatoprost, travoprost and latanoprost; hence these drops are contraindicated in patients with a history of previous infection.

Latanoprost

Latanoprost is an isopropyl ester prodrug, which after hydrolysis is converted to its active free acid on entering the eye. The prodrug is well absorbed through the cornea, and all of the drug that enters the aqueous humour is hydrolysed during the passage through the cornea. In the UK latanoprost is the most prescribed drug in POAG (Connor and Fraser, 2014). It was the first of the prostanoids to be launched in 1996 and remains the current market leader. Like timolol among the β-blockers, latanoprost is the drug in this class against which new drugs or combinations are assessed.

Optimal effect is obtained if latanoprost is administered in the evening. The dosage should not exceed once daily because it has been shown that more frequent administration can decrease the IOP-lowering effect (Schmier et al., 2010).

Latanoprost eye drops as with other prostanoids may gradually change eye colour by increasing the amount of brown pigment in the iris. It also may gradually change eyelashes, causing increased length and thickness; eyelash changes are reversible upon discontinuation of treatment. Among prostaglandins, latanoprost has been reported to have a lower risk of conjunctival hyperaemia (redness) than travoprost and bimatoprost (Li et al., 2016).

Latanoprost is generally very well tolerated; serious adverse drug reactions were reported in only 17 of 3936 (0.43%) patients using latanoprost over a 5-year period (Goldberg et al., 2008). In practice it is well known that patient persistence with latanoprost therapy is better than that with all other frequently used monotherapies (Rahman et al., 2009).

Latanoprost is not heat stable and requires refrigeration; however, it is stable enough to be stored at room temperature for the 4-week in-use period applied in the UK.

The concentration of the preservative benzalkonium chloride in latanoprost eye drops, commonly used as a preservative in ophthalmic products, may limit its use in certain patients. The benzalkonium chloride concentration is 0.02%; this has been reported to cause punctate keratopathy and/or toxic ulcerative keratopathy and eye irritation. Contact lenses may absorb benzalkonium chloride, and these should be removed before applying the drops but may be reinserted after 15 minutes. Latanoprost in a preservative-free formulation as a single unit dose (Monopost) was launched in 2012 for the reduction of elevated IOP in patients with POAG and OHT who have proven sensitivity to benzalkonium chloride.

Travoprost

Like latanoprost, travoprost is an ester prodrug, converted to its active acid form by corneal hydrolytic enzymes as it is absorbed through the eye. It was launched in the UK in 2001, and appears to be generally well tolerated by patients and is relatively free of systemic side effects, although abdominal cramping has been reported.

It contains polyquaternium-1 as a preservative rather than benzalkonium chloride. Travoprost is licensed for the reduction in

Table 56.6 Side effects of prostanoids

Ocular	Systemic
Asthenopia	Abdominal cramp
Allergic conjunctivitis	Asthenia
Blepharitis	Asthma
Blepharospasm	Bradycardia
Browache	Dizziness
Cataract	Dyspnoea
Conjunctival follicles, papillae	Elevated liver function tests
Conjunctival hyperaemia	Headache
Cystoid macular oedema	Hirsutism
Corneal erosion	Hypertension
Conjunctival oedema	Hypotension
Deepening of lid sulcus	Infection (primarily upper respiratory tract infections)
Distichiasis	Peripheral oedema
Eye discharge	Skin rash
Eye pain	
Eyelash changes – increased number, length, thickness, pigmentation, misdirection, poliosis	
Eyelid oedema, eyelid retraction	
Eyelid and periocular skin darkening	
Foreign body sensation	
Increase in vellus hair on eyelids	
Increased iris pigmentation	
Iritis	
Lid margin crusting	
Localised skin reactions on the eyelids	
Ocular burning, dryness, irritation pruritus, fatigue	
Photophobia	
Punctate epithelial erosions	
Retinal haemorrhage	
Tearing	
Uveitis	
Visual disturbance	

IOP for both OHT and POAG in adults and children older than 2 months. Data in the age group 2 months to less than 3 years are limited. As with latanoprost, optimal effect is obtained if the dose is administered in the evening.

Patients treated with travoprost show good diurnal fluctuation control, and an ocular hypotensive effect was shown to exceed 24 hours with a single dose.

Travoprost is a stable compound throughout a range of temperatures, and the commercially available product does not require refrigeration.

Tafluprost

Tafluprost, launched in 2008, was the first of the prostanoids available in a preservative-free form. It was mainly indicated in patients allergic to, or intolerant of, benzalkonium chloride. It needs to be stored in a fridge, but can be kept up to 28 days at room temperature after opening the foil pouch on use.

Bimatoprost

Bimatoprost is a synthetic prostamide which has a potent ocular hypotensive effect. It is a fatty acid amide, which is pharmacologically similar to prostaglandin $F_{2\alpha}$1-ethanolamine (prostamide $F_{2\alpha}$). Several mechanisms of action have been proposed, including activity of bimatoprost or its free acid, 17-phenyl prostaglandin F_{2a}, at the prostaglandin $F_{2\alpha}$-receptor, prostamide mimetic activity, and inhibition of PGF synthase, which leads to an increase in endogenous $PGF_{2\alpha}$. Although the free acid has been found in human eyes, its presence alone does not explain the 24-hour efficacy of bimatoprost or its hypotensive superiority over latanoprost. The pharmacology of bimatoprost itself is not explained wholly by its interaction with known prostaglandin $F_{2\alpha}$-receptors.

Bimatoprost is administered once daily in the evening; more frequent administration may lessen the IOP-lowering effect. It lowers the IOP to a greater extent than any other topical ocular hypotensive (van der Valk et al., 2009). Some studies show it is superior to latanoprost in terms of response rate, decline in IOP and the percentage of patients reaching their target IOP (Simmons et al., 2004). Bimatoprost has also been reported to be as effective as the fixed combination of latanoprost and timolol.

Studies have shown that patients who are not achieving their target IOP while receiving latanoprost achieved lower IOPs when switched to bimatoprost by an additional 10% reduction (Sonty et al., 2008). Therefore, significant long-term IOP-lowering may be achieved by switching to bimatoprost in patients with open-angle glaucoma who are not at target IOP with latanoprost.

Generally, bimatoprost causes similar ocular side effects to latanoprost, tafluprost and travoprost. However, bimatoprost causes hyperaemia more frequently than latanoprost. This may contribute to the higher discontinuation rate seen with bimatoprost therapy (Rahman et al., 2009). To address this issue, in 2010 the manufacturers of bimatoprost introduced a lower-strength (0.01%) version containing a higher concentration of benzalkonium chloride to aid penetration of the drug. In a 12-month study, the bimatoprost 0.01% was equivalent to bimatoprost 0.03% in lowering IOP and demonstrated improved tolerability, including less frequent and severe conjunctival hyperaemia (Katz et al., 2010).

Table 56.7 Ophthalmic β-blockers

Drug	Brand name	Strength (%)	Daily dosage frequency
Betaxolol	Betoptic solution	0.5	2
	Betoptic suspension[a]	0.25	2
Carteolol	Teoptic	1	2
		2	2
Levobunolol	Betagan[a] and generic form	0.5	1–2
Timolol	Timoptol[a] and generic form	0.25	2
		0.5	2
	Timoptol-LA	0.25	1
		0.5	1
	Cosopt[a] and generic form (with dorzolamide 2%)	0.5	2
	Xalacom and generic form (withlatanoprost 0.005%)	0.5	1
	DuoTrav (with travoprost 0.004%)	0.5	1
	Ganfort (with bimatoprost 0.03%)	0.5	1
	Combigan (with brimonidine 0.2%)	0.5	2
	Azarga (with brinzolamide 1%)	0.5	2
	Taptiqom (with tafluprost 0.0015%)	0.5	1

[a]Available in unit dose and multidose forms.

Table 56.8 Pharmacological profile of ophthalmic β-blockers

Drug	Potency[a]	Intrinsic sympatho-mimetic activity	Cardiose-lectivity	Membrane-stabilising activity
Betaxolol	3–10	–	++	+
Carteolol	30	++	–	–
Levobunolol	6	–	–	–
Timolol	5–10	–	–	+

[a]Propranolol = 1.

In 2014 bimatoprost 0.03% preserved drops were discontinued. Bimatoprost 0.03% as single dose unit preservative-free is still available for patients intolerant of 0.02% benzalkonium chloride.

β-Blockers

Ocular hypotensive effects of β-blockers (β-adrenoceptor antagonists) were first evaluated in the 1970s. They reduce the IOP by a blockade of ciliary β-receptors in the ciliary epithelium inhibiting the synthesis of cyclic adenosine monophosphate, causing a reduction in aqueous humour formation as opposed to having an effect on the aqueous humour outflow.

Although there are both β_1- and β_2-receptors in the eye, the latter predominate, and even cardioselective β-blockers are thought to work by blockade of β_2-receptors. Genetic factors have been shown to be important in patients' response to this group of drugs (Sidjanin et al., 2008).

Two types of topical β-blockers are available for use in reducing IOP; non-selective, which block both β_1- and β_2-adrenoceptors, and cardioselective, which block only β_1-adrenoceptors. Of the β-blockers commercially available in the UK for topical administration, timolol, levobunolol and carteolol are non-selective; only betaxolol is cardioselective (Table 56.7).

β-Blockers have a number of important properties in addition to β-adrenoceptor blockade. These include intrinsic sympathomimetic activity (ISA), cardioselectivity and membrane-stabilising activity, which are all of importance when considering the side effects seen with these agents (Table 56.8). The property of membrane stabilisation is relevant to the incidence of ocular side effects.

Ocular β-blockers can cause systemic adverse effects after topical application to the eye; therefore, they are contraindicated in patients with bradycardia, heart block or uncontrolled heart failure (Müller et al., 2006).

All topical β-blockers have been reported to cause bronchospasm; hence 'at-risk' patients with a tendency to airway disease who require therapy for glaucoma should be treated with extreme caution. The precipitation of bronchospasm in susceptible patients can occur with the administration of as little as one drop of timolol. The β-blockers that show cardioselectivity or ISA are less likely to cause bronchoconstriction, and it has been demonstrated that respiratory function improved in patients whose treatment was changed from timolol to betaxolol or an adrenergic agonist.

Ocular β-blockers are generally not contraindicated in diabetes, although a cardioselective agent may be preferable. However, they are best avoided in patients who suffer frequent hypoglycaemic attacks because they may mask the signs and symptoms of acute hypoglycaemia.

The long-term benefits of β-blockers on visual function preservation have been shown to be less than would be expected. This may be because of adverse effects on the ocular microcirculation, whereby the β-blockers interfere with endogenous vasodilation and cause optic nerve head arteriolar vasoconstriction. The various β-blockers demonstrate marked differences in their vasoconstrictive effect, with betaxolol possibly demonstrating the least vasoconstriction.

Non-selective β-blockers are avoided by some clinicians in patients with NTG because of the perceived risk of a nocturnal decline in arterial pressure, causing a reduction in ocular perfusion and subsequent glaucomatous damage (Orgul et al., 2005).

Ophthalmic β-blockers may induce dryness of eyes, hence patients with corneal disease should be treated with caution. Ocular side effects of topically administered β-blockers are shown in Table 56.9.

Table 56.9 Ocular and systemic side effects of topical β-blockers

Ocular	Systemic
Allergic blepharoconjunctivitis	**Central nervous system**
Burning and itching	Anxiety
Blurred vision	Depression
Conjunctival hyperaemia	Fatigue
Corneal anaesthesia	Hallucinations
Dryness	Irritability
Foreign body sensation	Sleep disturbances
Macular oedema	**Endocrine**
Nasolacrimal duct obstruction	Hypoglycaemia (insulin induced)
Pain	**Gastro-intestinal**
Punctate keratitis	Nausea
Uveitis	Diarrhoea
	Vascular
	Arrhythmias
	Bradycardia
	Hypotension
	Peripheral vasoconstriction
	Reduced stroke volume
	Respiratory
	Bronchoconstriction
	Dyspnoea

Timolol

Timolol is a non-cardioselective β-blocker without ISA, which was the first to be introduced, and as such it is the agent against which all newer β-blockers have been compared. It is effective in the long-term treatment of glaucoma, often in conjunction with other antiglaucoma therapies.

Given topically to patients with an increase in IOP, timolol induces a significant and long-lasting ocular hypotensive effect. Studies have shown that IOP is lower early in the course of treatment as opposed to later stages. In addition the IOP in the fellow untreated eye may show a decrease in IOP, which suggests that a consensual effect resulting from systemic absorption can be significant.

Many patients can be placed on once-a-day therapy provided the IOP is maintained at satisfactory levels. The presentation of timolol 0.1% in a prolonged-release formulation Tiopex (a polysaccharide-based, gel-forming solution) leads to a prolonged corneal contact time and increased penetration of timolol into the eye. Therefore, this is the preferred form for once-daily administration.

Timolol eye gel 0.1% has been shown to be as effective as the 0.5% solution administered twice daily. The 0.1% gel has the advantage of a much lower drug load, giving rise to plasma levels of timolol 10 times lower than that achieved after twice-daily dosage of timolol 0.5% eye drops. The concentration of timolol achieved in the aqueous humour after administration of the 0.1% gel formulation, despite being approximately 40% of that after administration of the 0.5% solution, is sufficient to occupy 100% of β_1- and β_2-receptors (Volotinen et al., 2009). Timolol is also available in 0.25% strength, and there is good evidence showing

that it has similar efficacy compared with the 0.5%. Timolol is still considered the first-line choice for the treatment of POAG in third world countries due to cost (Yadav and Patel, 2013).

Levobunolol

Levobunolol is the potent L-isomer of bunolol. It is metabolised to dihydrolevobunolol in the eye, prolonging the drug's half-life and making it one of only two topical β-blockers licensed for once-daily use. It is as effective with once-daily dosing as the usual twice-daily regimen. It is a non-cardioselective drug, showing greater affinity for the β_2-receptor, and does not possess ISA. It is reported to be as effective as timolol 0.5% in lowering IOP and more effective than betaxolol 0.5%. The incidence of allergic contact dermatitis is greater with levobunolol than timolol (Jappe et al., 2006), and a greater percentage of patients receiving levobunolol than timolol or betaxolol discontinued the drug because of adverse effects (Rahman et al., 2009).

Carteolol

It has been suggested that because of the ISA of carteolol, which is attributable to its metabolite 8-hydroxycarteolol found in the plasma, smaller changes are seen in pulmonary and cardiovascular parameters than are seen with the non-cardioselective β-blockers without ISA (timolol and levobunolol). Carteolol appears to be neutral in its effect on serum lipid levels, whereas timolol adversely affects high-density lipoprotein cholesterol and the total cholesterol/high-density lipoprotein cholesterol ratio. Carteolol is generally well tolerated and has been shown to be as effective as timolol at lowering IOP in the majority of patients. It has a greater vasodilator effect on the retinal and choroidal vasculature than timolol and levobunolol, but less than that of betaxolol. It is the least lipophilic of the topical β-blockers and consequently is likely to show a lower incidence of central nervous system side effects.

Betaxolol

In theory, because of its cardioselectivity, betaxolol should have fewer adverse effects on the pulmonary system. It should also have fewer adverse cardiovascular effects because of comparatively lower systemic β-receptor occupancy after ocular administration. Maximum occupancies for β_1- and β_2-receptors after ophthalmic administration were 52% and 88% for carteolol, 62% and 82% for timolol, and 44% and 3% for betaxolol, respectively (Yasuhiko et al., 2001). However, betaxolol is less effective than other β-blockers as an ocular hypotensive agent (van der Valk et al., 2009). On initiation of treatment, the decline in IOP is slower than with other topical β-blockers. The 0.25% suspension is as effective as the 0.5% solution and is better tolerated by the patient (Yalvac et al., 2007). Experimental studies showed the drug reaches the retina after topical administration and displays a voltage-dependent L-type calcium channel-blocking activity, which probably leads to improved retinal perfusion. This effect may explain the significant improvement in visual field performance seen with betaxolol in a comparison study with timolol in

Box 56.1 Side effects of systemic carbonic anhydrase inhibitors

Acidosis
Diarrhoea
Drowsiness
Elevated uric acid
Hypokalaemia
Nausea/vomiting
Malaise complex
Paraesthesia
Sulfonamide crystalluria
Sulfonamide sensitivity
Transient myopia

Table 56.10 Side effects of topical carbonic anhydrase inhibitors

Ocular	Systemic
Blurred vision	Dry mouth
Burning/stinging	Dyspnoea
Conjunctivitis	Headache
Eyelid pain/discomfort	Nausea
Fatigue	Taste perversion
Itching	
Nasolacrimal duct obstruction	
Ocular discharge	
Tearing	

open-angle glaucoma. The significant improvement with betaxolol occurred despite the more effective reductions in IOP with timolol (Araie et al., 2003).

Carbonic anhydrase inhibitors

There are many forms of the carbonic anhydrase isoenzyme in body tissues, three of which (CA-I, CA-II and CA-IV) are present in ocular tissues. Bicarbonate formation is an essential component of aqueous production. In the ciliary epithelium, the inhibition of CA-II slows the formation of bicarbonate ions and their secretion into the posterior chamber of the eye. This reduces the sodium transport into the posterior chamber and decreases aqueous humour production, resulting in lower IOP. Inhibition of other forms of the enzyme results in many side effects. Carbonic anhydrase inhibitors are sulfonamides; although there is little evidence to suggest sensitivity overlap, they are still contraindicated in patients with known hypersensitivity to sulfonamides.

Acetazolamide

Acetazolamide is the only systemic carbonic anhydrase inhibitor available in the UK. Although it is among the most potent ocular hypotensive agents available, it has limited use in the long-term management of glaucoma due to unpleasant and potentially dangerous side effects. It may be added to treatment in POAG and other chronic glaucomas in patients refractory to standard treatment. The systemic side effects are shown in Box 56.1.

Acetazolamide is readily absorbed from the gastro-intestinal tract after oral administration; it attains peak plasma level within 2–4 hours. Peak levels are maintained for 4–6 hours.

Paraesthesia occurs in almost all patients on commencement of therapy, but usually disappears on continued therapy. The malaise complex can include fatigue, depression, weight loss and decreased libido. Chronic use can lead to dangerous electrolyte imbalance such that the monitoring of renal function is mandatory. In the acute setting, acetazolamide is also available in injection form and given intravenously. Plasma levels sufficient to decrease IOP occur only minutes after intravenous administration of acetazolamide. It may be useful in the preoperative treatment of POAG and in the emergency treatment of PAC.

Topical carbonic anhydrase inhibitors

The topical carbonic anhydrase inhibitors dorzolamide and brinzolamide are less effective in lowering IOP than acetazolamide but have a lower potential to produce adverse effects. They are licensed as monotherapy for patients with POAG or OHT resistant to β-blockers or those in whom use of β-blockers is contraindicated. They can also be prescribed in combination with other treatment.

Dorzolamide is also licensed for the treatment of pseudo-exfoliative glaucoma, and limited clinical data in paediatric patients are available. Both drugs are licensed as adjunctive therapy to β-blockers and brinzolamide to PGAs, although there is evidence to suggest that dorzolamide is as efficacious as brinzolamide when added to latanoprost (Nakamura et al., 2009).

Dorzolamide is used either alone three times a day or concurrently with a β-blocker or twice daily with a PGA. Although the license for brinzolamide states that the drug can be used twice a day as monotherapy, some patients may respond better to a three times daily dosage. Mean changes in IOP with brinzolamide administered twice daily and three times daily and dorzolamide administered three times daily are equivalent. However, the decline in IOP achieved with these agents is less than that seen with timolol 0.5% twice daily.

Side effects similar to those of systemic sulfonamides may occur and should be monitored. The most common side effects are shown in Table 56.10. Of the two topical carbonic anhydrase inhibitors, brinzolamide appears to cause less burning and stinging on instillation because of the neutral pH (7.5) of the formulation. This is reflected in a much greater discontinuation rate with dorzolamide (31%) than with brinzolamide (14%) (Rahman et al., 2009). Owing to its form as a more viscous suspension, however, blurring is more common with brinzolamide than with dorzolamide.

Table 56.11 Examples of available ocular products containing sympathomimetic agents

Drug	Trade name	Strength	Daily dosage frequency
Apraclonidine	Iopidine	1%	1h before surgery and on completion
	Iopidine	0.5%	3
Brimonidine	Alphagan	0.2%	2

Table 56.12 Ocular and systemic side effects of topical α_2-agonists

Ocular	Systemic
Ocular pruritus	Dry mouth/nose
Discomfort	Headache
Tearing	Asthenia
Hyperaemia	Bradycardia
Conjunctival and lid oedema	Depression
Lid retraction, conjunctival blanching and mydriasis (reported after perioperative use of apraclonidine)	
Miosis (reported with brimonidine)	
Uveitis	

Sympathomimetic agents

Sympathomimetic agents (α_2-adrenergic agonists) reduce IOP by reducing aqueous inflow via an α-mediated vasoconstriction in the ciliary body and increased outflow due to a dilation of the aqueous and episcleral veins.

The original sympathomimetic drug, adrenaline (epinephrine), and its lipophilic prodrug dipivefrine have been used in the treatment of OHT and POAG since the early 1920s. Both are classed as non-selective α- and β-adrenoreceptor agonist drugs with a relatively high potential for both ocular and systemic side effects, and are no longer used in routine clinical practice. They have been superseded by the more selective sympathomimetics: apraclonidine and brimonidine. Commercially available preparations of sympathomimetic agents are listed in Table 56.11. Ocular and systemic side effects of α_2-agonists are listed in Table 56.12. Sympathomimetics are generally mydriatic; therefore, their use is contraindicated in untreated PAC because of the risk of precipitating acute angle closure.

Apraclonidine

Apraclonidine (a derivative of clonidine) was the first of the selective adrenergic agonists to be introduced. This drug, which acts predominantly on α_2- but also on α_1-receptors, reduces the rate at which aqueous humour is produced due to ciliary vasoconstriction. Eye drops containing apraclonidine 1% are used to control or prevent postsurgical elevation of IOP after anterior segment laser surgery, for example, trabeculoplasty. Eye drops containing a 0.5% solution are licensed for the short-term adjunctive treatment of patients receiving maximally tolerated medical therapy who require additional IOP reduction to delay laser treatment or glaucoma surgery, but the benefit for most patients is less than 1 month.

Apraclonidine 0.5% is as effective in lowering IOP as brimonidine 0.2%, but has less effect on blood pressure and heart rate. Although an off-license use, apraclonidine is sometimes used in children in whom brimonidine is strictly contraindicated (Wright and Freedman, 2009).

Brimonidine

More α_2-selectivity is seen with brimonidine, which results in miosis rather than mydriasis. Vasoconstriction of microvessels is also not seen. It is thought to increase uveoscleral outflow, as well as reducing aqueous production. Brimonidine administered twice daily is almost as effective as timolol twice a day at peak. However, brimonidine is significantly less effective at trough, and some consider it to be more efficacious when administered three times a day, which is the frequency used in the USA.

A database containing details of drug use in 956 patients with glaucoma older than 18 years shows that brimonidine had the highest proportion of discontinuations because of adverse effects (Rahman et al., 2009). It has high allergenicity and may increase the likelihood of allergy to preparations subsequently used.

Brimonidine may be used as monotherapy to lower IOP in patients with POAC or OHT who are intolerant of β-blockers or in whom β-blockers are contraindicated, because there is no effect on pulmonary function and only minimal cardiovascular effect. It may also be used as an adjunctive therapy in those patients whose IOP is not adequately controlled with a single agent because its IOP-lowering activity has been shown to be additive to that of β-blockers and PGAs.

In a 4-month study, the co-administration of latanoprost and brimonidine 0.15% resulted in a greater decline in IOP than the co-administration of latanoprost and brinzolamide or dorzolamide (Bournias and Lai, 2009); this product is not available in the UK. Brimonidine is contraindicated in patients who are receiving monoamine oxidase inhibitors or antidepressants which affect noradrenergic transmission, and there is the possibility of brimonidine potentiating or causing an additive effect with central nervous system depressants.

Topical miotics

Miotics act to increase the outflow of aqueous humour by a stimulation of ciliary muscle and an opening of channels in the trabecular meshwork. Miotics are directly acting parasympathomimetic agents that act at muscarinic receptors. The only such drug

Box 56.2 Ocular side effects of topical pilocarpine

Allergic conjunctivitis
Blurred vision
Ciliary/conjunctival injection
Ciliary spasm
Induced myopia
Lens changes (chronic use)
Lid twitching
Pain
Pigment epithelial cells
Poor night vision
Posterior synechiae
Pupillary block
Retinal tear/detachments
Uveitis
Vitreous haemorrhage

Box 56.3 Systemic side effects of topical pilocarpine

Bradycardia
Bronchial spasm
Browache, headache
Diarrhoea
Hypotension
Lacrimation
Nausea and vomiting
Pulmonary oedema
Salivation
Sweating

does not effectively reduce IOP to within the target range, and treatment with at least two medications from different classes is required (Higginbotham, 2010). Treatment with more than one eye drop has a number of disadvantages: poorer adherence with treatment, increased risk of medication washout and increased exposure to preservatives, for example, benzalkonium chloride.

The combination of two drugs in one topical ophthalmic preparation may improve adherence and result in a reduction in preservative load. For a combination of two medications to be an acceptable alternative to the prescriber, the fixed combination must be more effective than either of the components used alone and at least as effective as the drugs administered separately. In addition, adverse effects of the fixed combination should not exceed those encountered when the components are administered separately.

When compared with prescribing the individual monotherapies, fixed combination therapies offer a simple and convenient dosing regimen, and may result in some cost saving for patients who pay for their prescription. However, fixed combinations also remove the possibility of titrating the individual components both in terms of concentration and timing of administration, and may not provide the same efficacy as the individual components. Furthermore, the use of timolol in the combination at high concentration may lead to additional side effects.

In the past, fixed combination drops all contained timolol; this limited their use in patients with comorbidities that contraindicate β-blockers. In the UK a timolol-free combination product Simbrinza containing brinzolamide 10 mg/mL and brimonidine tartrate 2 mg/mL is now available.

currently available commercially in the UK is pilocarpine. The onset of action of pilocarpine is 20 minutes, but its short duration of action necessitates four times daily dosing. The ocular and systemic side effects of pilocarpine are shown in Boxes 56.2 and 56.3, respectively.

The use of miotics is almost exclusively confined to the treatment of PACG and some secondary glaucomas. They are no longer commonly used for the treatment of POAG and OHT mainly because of poor tolerance of side effects of these drugs and the frequency of instillation. The main side effect is miosis, which is often accompanied by frontal headache (browache), loss of accommodation and blurred vision.

New drugs in development

Inhibitors of Rho kinase have emerged as a new class of IOP-lowering medications designed to increase outflow through the trabecular meshwork and are currently being tested in clinics (Karmel, 2013).

Latanoprostene bunod, a nitric oxide-donating PGA administered once daily, is currently in development. Recent clinical trials have shown it to be more effective than latanoprost (Weinreb et al., 2015).

Combination products

Clinical practice guidelines recommend initiating treatment with one medication; however, in many patients a single medication

Fixed combination of timolol and dorzolamide

A combination of timolol 0.5% and dorzolamide 2% (Cosopt) was the first topical ocular hypotensive combination to be marketed. It is indicated twice daily in the treatment of elevated IOP in patients with open-angle glaucoma or pseudoexfoliative glaucoma when topical β-blocker monotherapy is insufficient. The fixed combination of dorzolamide and timolol is more effective than either timolol or dorzolamide alone, and as effective as its two components administered separately. Fixed combination dorzolamide and timolol is also generally well tolerated. This suggests that fixed combination dorzolamide and timolol may have a beneficial role as a replacement or adjunct therapy in a clinical glaucoma practice setting when the IOP is not adequately controlled with either (Yeh et al., 2008). It has also been reported to be a useful agent when used adjunctively with latanoprost, resulting in a further decline in IOP. Although generally well tolerated, the main problem with Cosopt is burning and stinging on instillation. Although discontinuation of the combination in trials is low, Cosopt has been found to be the third most frequently discontinued eye product in practice (Rahman et al., 2009).

Fixed combination of timolol and latanoprost

A combination of timolol 0.5% and latanoprost 0.005%, marketed as Xalacom, was first launched in the UK in 2001, shortly before the launch of travoprost and bimatoprost.

Xalacom is indicated for the reduction of IOP in patients with open-angle glaucoma and OHT who are insufficiently responsive to topical β-blockers or PGAs alone. It is administered once a day and has been shown to be more effective when administered in the evening than in the morning (Takmaz et al., 2008).

Fixed combination of timolol and travoprost

A fixed combination of travoprost 0.004% and timolol 0.5% (DuoTrav) has been shown to be more effective than either of its components and is as efficacious as the components administered concomitantly, whereas fewer side effects are reported with the combination product (Gross et al., 2007). The fixed combination of travoprost and timolol is indicated to decrease IOP in patients with open-angle glaucoma or OHT who are insufficiently responsive to topical β-blockers or PGAs. Although the Summary of Product Characteristics states that the dose is one drop in the affected eye(s) once daily, in the morning or evening, it has been shown that an evening dose demonstrates better 24-hour pressure control (Konstas et al., 2009).

Fixed combination of timolol and bimatoprost

A fixed combination of bimatoprost 0.03% and timolol 0.5% (Ganfort) is available for the reduction of IOP in patients with open-angle glaucoma or OHT who are insufficiently responsive to topical β-blockers or PGAs. The fixed combination has been shown to be more effective than either of its components used alone and as effective as the components used in their usual dosing regimen (bimatoprost once daily in the evening and timolol twice daily, used concomitantly). Conjunctival hyperaemia has been reported more frequently by patients receiving bimatoprost (39%) than the bimatoprost/timolol fixed combination (23%), with the lowest incidence in those receiving timolol (7%) (Brandt et al., 2008).

Fixed combination of timolol and brimonidine

A combination of timolol 0.5% with brimonidine 0.2% is marketed as Combigan and is indicated for the reduction of IOP in patients with POAG or OHT who are insufficiently responsive to topical β-blockers.

The fixed combination has been shown to be superior in reducing IOP than either brimonidine or timolol alone and is as safe and effective as concomitant treatment with the individual components. Use of the combination product has been shown to result in a 24% decrease in IOP (Papaconstantinou et al., 2009). Use of the brimonidine and timolol combination results in a greater number of side effects than timolol alone, but has fewer side effects than brimonidine alone (Sherwood et al., 2006) and fewer cases of allergy than brimonidine used alone (Motolko, 2008).

Fixed combination of timolol and brinzolamide

A fixed combination of brinzolamide 1% and timolol 0.5% (Azarga) is a topical ocular hypotensive presentation launched in 2009. The combination is indicated to reduce IOP in adult patients with open-angle glaucoma or OHT for whom monotherapy has produced insufficient IOP reduction. It has greater IOP-lowering efficacy than brinzolamide or timolol alone (Kaback et al., 2008).

Brinzolamide/timolol administration leads to a 30–33% decline in IOP at trough and 34–35% at peak and is better tolerated than, and preferred to, the dorzolamide/timolol combination, probably because of the neutral pH (7.2) of the suspension (Manni et al., 2009).

Fixed combination of timolol and tafluprost

A new preservative-free fixed-dose combination product consisting of 0.0015% tafluprost, a PGA, and 0.5% timolol, a β-blocker (Taptiqom), has recently been developed.

Although studies have shown the IOP reduction in POAG and OHT is similar to other prostaglandin-timolol fixed-combination products, this product causes less superficial ocular side effects and less conjunctival hyperaemia. In conclusion, a review of the double-masked, controlled, phase III clinical trials with the fixed-combination products of prostaglandin and timolol revealed that the products yielded a similar reduction in IOP of approximately 32–36% from an untreated baseline IOP of around 24–29 mmHg (Hollo et al., 2014).

Fixed combination of brinzolamide and brimonidine

Formerly fixed combination drops all contained timolol; this limited their use in patients with comorbidities that contraindicate β-blocker therapy. In 2014, a timolol-free combination product was launched, containing brinzolamide 1% and brimonidine 0.2% ophthalmic suspension. Referred to as Simbrinza it is a fixed combination of carbonic anhydrase inhibitor and an α2-adrenergic receptor agonist. It is indicated for the reduction of elevated IOP in patients with POAG and OT in the UK, European Union, and USA.

Hyperosmotic agents

Hyperosmotic agents can be considered for use in the emergency treatment of acute angle closure because of their speed of action and effectiveness. The most commonly used agents are oral glycerol and intravenous mannitol. The mechanism of action is the creation of osmotic shifts of water from the aqueous circulation, thus lowering IOP. The maximal effect of glycerol is seen within 1 hour and lasts for about 3 hours, whereas mannitol acts within 30 minutes with effects lasting for 4–6 hours.

Glycerol

Glycerol is given orally, usually as a 50% solution in water, the dose being 1–1.5 g/kg body weight given as a single dose. It is not a strong diuretic but may cause headaches, nausea and vomiting. Although it is metabolised to glucose in the body, it may be given to individuals with diabetes that is well controlled. All practitioners should be aware of the difference in dose in millilitres required for a 50% solution of glycerol formulated as a 50% w/v solution and one formulated as a 50% v/v solution (Table 56.13).

Mannitol

Mannitol is given as a 20% solution in water for intravenous administration. The dose is 1–2 g/kg body weight up to a maximum of 500 mL given over 30–40 minutes at a rate not exceeding 60 drops/min (see Table 56.13). It is a strong diuretic and as large volumes are required, it may cause problems because of

Table 56.13 Doses of hyperosmotic agents used in the treatment of acute angle-closure glaucoma

| Oral glycerol 50% at 1 g/kg | | | | Intravenous mannitol 20% w/v[a] | | |
| 50% w/v solution | | 50% v/v solution | | | | |
Weight (kg)	Dose (mL)	Weight (kg)	Dose (mL)	Weight (kg)	Dose at 1 g/kg (mL)	Dose at 2 g/kg (mL)
40	80	44.5	70	40	200	400
50	100	50.8	80	50	250	500
60	120	57.2	90	60	300	–
		63.5	100	70	350	–
70	140	69.9	110	80	400	–
		76.2	120	90	450	–
80	160	82.6	130	100	500	–
90	180	88.9	140			
		95.3	150			
100	200	101.7	160			
For each additional 5 kg	Add 10 mL	For each additional 6.4 kg	Add 10 mL			

[a]Maximum dose 500 mL.

cardiovascular overload, pulmonary oedema and stroke. Cerebral dehydration leads to headache, and the patient may experience chills and chest pain. It should therefore be used with great caution.

Patient care

Primary open-angle glaucoma

When the condition is first diagnosed, patients should be told that the disorder cannot be cured but only controlled by the regular use of the prescribed treatment. Because patients are usually unaware of progression of the disease, the result of non-adherence with treatment should be made clear and the importance of regular attendance at clinics stressed.

The existence of a patient self-help group, the International Glaucoma Association (http://www.glaucoma-association.com), should be brought to the patient's attention. They will be able to put the patient in contact with their nearest local support group.

The patient's technique for installing eye drops should be checked and corrected if necessary. Emphasis should be on the dose (one drop), the position of instillation (into the temporal side of the lower conjunctival sac) and the importance of punctal occlusion to minimise systemic side effects.

The preferred times for administration of topical medication should be discussed with the patient. Prostaglandins and prostamides are best administered at bedtime; a 12-hourly regimen should be used for twice-daily drugs, 8-hourly for drugs given three times a day, and as near a 6-hourly regimen as practical for the aqueous formulation of pilocarpine.

β-Blockers given once daily should be administered in the morning. The importance of allowing a reasonable interval between drops should be emphasised. Sometimes the order of instillation of different types of eye drop is important for pharmacological or practical reasons. For example, the instillation of pilocarpine should always precede that of a sympathomimetic to prevent pain in the eye resulting from a strong miosis after a weak mydriasis.

The instillation of aqueous eye drops, which remain in the conjunctival sac for a maximum of 10 minutes, should precede that of viscous eye drops (e.g. hypromellose eye drops) or suspensions (e.g. dexamethasone 0.1% eye drops) where the contact time is prolonged.

Eye drops containing benzalkonium chloride should not be instilled if soft contact lenses are in situ. The patient should be instructed to remove the lens immediately before instillation and replace it approximately 15 minutes later.

Because there is a hereditary component to POAG, patients should be told to advise first-degree relatives to be screened. Such people older than 40 years are entitled to free eye tests by their optometrist.

Primary angle-closure glaucoma

Patients found to have shallow anterior chambers and narrow angles normally undergo laser peripheral iridotomies. In the interim they should be advised of the symptoms of an attack of acute PAC so that medical attention can be sought if necessary.

If peripheral iridotomies are not performed, the patient should be advised that a number of prescription and non-prescription drugs should be avoided (Lachkar and Bouassida, 2007). When visiting the doctor and purchasing medicines from a pharmacy, the patient should always remember to mention their condition, and the prescriber should ensure that the drug is appropriate for a patient prone to angle closure. Examples of drugs contraindicated in this condition are listed in Table 56.14. Note that the absence of a drug from this list does not imply safety.

After an attack of acute angle closure and surgical treatment of the disorder, the patient should be told that the drugs previously contraindicated can be safely taken provided that iridectomy/iridotomy remains patent.

Patient adherence

The patient is more likely to comply with the prescribed treatment if the drug or drugs can be administered according to a simple, infrequent dosage regimen with minimal, local or systemic side effects.

Thus, a patient treated with a once-daily PGA or prostamide or once- or twice-daily β-blocker would be expected to adhere to the regimen better than someone treated with pilocarpine, with its unfortunate side effects and inconvenient four-times-a-day dosage regimen. Common side effects of topical and systemic medication should be fully discussed with the patient so that the hyperaemia encountered with the prostanoids and the paraesthesia with acetazolamide are not unexpected, leading to premature discontinuation of therapy.

Because glaucoma is predominantly a disease of elderly people, physical disability may prevent successful treatment, however conscientious the patient. For example, rheumatoid arthritis may reduce the patient's ability to squeeze the bottle of eye drops, while the tremor of Parkinson's disease can make correct positioning of instillation difficult. Various aids have been introduced to help with correct positioning and squeezing of eye drops, and these should be made available to patients who require such support.

Table 56.14 Drugs contraindicated in primary angle-closure glaucoma

Therapeutic class		Examples
Antimuscarinics	Topical	Atropine, cyclopentolate, homatropine, tropicamide
	Antispasmodic	Atropine, dicycloverine, hyoscine, propantheline
	Motion sickness	Hyoscine, promethazine, cyclizine
	Bronchodilator	Ipratropium, tiotropium
	Urinary retention	Darifenacin, fesoterodine, flavoxate, oxybutynin, propiverine, solifenacin, tolterodine, trospium
Drugs used in anaesthesia		Glycopyrronium, ketamine, suxamethonium
Antidepressants		Amitriptyline, amoxapine, citalopram, clomipramine, dosulepin, doxepin, duloxetine, fluvoxamine, imipramine, lofepramine, maprotiline, mirtazapine, nortriptyline, paroxetine, phenelzine, reboxetine, sertraline, trazodone, trimipramine, venlafaxine
Antipsychotics		Chlorpromazine, clozapine, flupentixol, fluphenazine, olanzapine, pericyazine, perphenazine, promazine, risperidone, sulpiride, thioridazine, trifluoperazine, zuclopenthixol
Antihistamines		Alimemazine, antazoline, cetirizine, chlorphenamine, clemastine, cyproheptadine, diphenhydramine, hydroxyzine, loratadine, pizotifen
Antiarrhythmics		Disopyramide
Antiepileptics		Carbamazepine, topiramate
Sympathomimetics		Adrenaline, cocaine, dipivefrine, ephedrine, isometheptene, naphazoline, phenylephrine, pseudoephedrine, salbutamol, xylometazoline
Drugs used in the treatment of attention deficit hyperactivity disorder		Atomoxetine, dexamphetamine, methylphenidate, ritodrine
Drugs used in the treatment of parkinsonism		Benserazide, carbidopa, entacapone, levodopa, orphenadrine, procyclidine, selegiline, trihexyphenidyl
Non-steroidal anti-inflammatory drugs		Mefenamic acid
Sulfonamide-derived drugs		Acetazolamide, co-trimoxazole, hydrochlorothiazide, sulfasalazine
Miscellaneous		Botulinum toxin, carboprost, paricalcitol, pilocarpine

Table 56.15 Common therapeutic problems in glaucoma

Problem	Comments
Lack of adherence	Treatment perceived to be worse than disease Complex multiple-drug regimens Frequency of dosing Inability to differentiate between different types of medication Inability to instil medication
Contraindication to therapy	Pilocarpine in uveitis β-Blockers in asthma, bradycardia, heart block, uncontrolled heart failure Prostaglandin analogues and prostamides in aphakia Wide range of topical and systemic drugs in shallow anterior chamber α_2-Agonists in depression Carbonic anhydrase inhibitors in renal failure
Intolerance to drug	Miosis and ciliary spasm with pilocarpine Red eye with prostaglandin analogues, bimatoprost Bronchospasm with β-blockers Paraesthesia with acetazolamide
Use outside of licensed indications	Paediatric patients Pregnant women Nursing mothers
Hypersensitivity	To active drug To preservative in multidose formulation

Patients with poor visual acuity can be helped by the colour coding of eye drop labels and supplying bottles labelled with large print. Some manufacturers have endeavoured to enhance adherence by including dose-reminder caps and facilitating instillation by supplying aids to open or position the bottle.

Other manufacturers have made their eye drop containers easier to squeeze or supply aids to squeeze the bottle. A list of such devices, some of which are available on prescription and others free of charge from manufacturers of drugs used in the treatment of glaucoma, is available on the International Glaucoma Association's website (http://www.glaucoma-association.com).

Where self-medication is impossible, a simple infrequent dosage regimen is more likely to be achieved when a relative, a neighbour or the district nursing service can assist with administration of the medication. In these cases, a drug administered once daily, such as a long-acting timolol preparation or a PGA or bimatoprost, has an obvious advantage over one that should be administered at 12-hourly intervals.

Common therapeutic problems in glaucoma are listed in Table 56.15.

Case studies

Case 56.1

A 64-year-old Asian woman, Mrs GV, attended the emergency department suffering from a severe headache, nausea and vomiting. Her right eye was red, and she reported blurred vision. The only new medication she had used recently was some antimotion tablets recommended by her local pharmacist. Her medical history includes type 2 diabetes.

Question

What is the most likely cause of Mrs GV's symptoms, and what investigations and treatment would you expect Mrs GV to have?

Answer

Headache, painful red eye and blurred vison are all signs of an acute PAC attack. PAC is more common in elderly female patients, especially of Asian ethnicity such as Mrs GV. The lens grows with aging and can push the iris forwards, narrowing the angle between the iris and cornea; this will affect the drainage of aqueous humour. Medication with antimuscarinic side effects (antimotion tablets) can precipitate an attack. A previous history of acute PAC is infrequent and this attack is usually the first indication of having this condition. The attack is usually unilateral; however, long-term management will be for both eyes. Acute PAC is an emergency; prompt diagnosis and treatment are essential to prevent damage to the optic nerve and irreversible blindness.

On examination, Mrs GV feels very unwell; her IOP is substantially elevated, greater than 50 mmHg. Slit-lamp findings include shallow anterior chambers in both eyes, closed iridocorneal angle and corneal epithelial oedema. The pupil is fixed and mid-dilated. Mrs GV's initial treatment involves acetazolamide given intravenously with topical glaucoma medications, for example, timolol if not contraindicated. In addition, steroids drops are used to reduce inflammation, as well as pilocarpine, a miotic that causes the pupil to constrict, opening drainage channels and allowing the aqueous humour to leave and the IOP to reduce.

Case 56.2

A 44-year-old man, Mr JT, has been treated for POAG for more than a year. He visited his primary care physician last week having noticed that both of his eyes were markedly red, sore and dry.

Mr JT is currently using:
  latanoprost at night to both eyes,
  timolol 0.5% twice a day to both eyes,
  dorzolamide twice a day to both eyes.

Question

What are the contributing factors for Mr JT's symptoms?

Answer

Red, sore, dry eyes are associated with a number of underlying conditions. For Mr JT the use of three different eye drops increases his exposure to the preservative benzalkonium chloride that can cause eye irritation and, rarely, ulcerative keratopathy. The concentration of benzalkonium chloride in latanoprost eye drops is generally high (0.02%). Changing to a preservative-free formulation for all the above drops can be an option, as can the prescribing of combination products. It might be worthwhile considering travoprost as an alternative to latanoprost because it contains a different preservative and would reduce the cost associated with preservative-free preparations.

References

Alm, A., Kaufman, P.L., 1998. Uveoscleral Outflow: Biology and Clinical Aspects. Mosby-Wolfe Medical Publications.

Araie, M., Azuma, I., Kitazawa, Y., 2003. Influence of topical betaxolol and timolol on visual field in Japanese open-angle glaucoma patients. Jpn. J. Ophthalmol. 47, 199–207.

Bartlett, J.D., Jaanus, S.D., 2008. Clinical Ocular Pharmacology, fifth ed. Elsevier, Chichester, UK.

Bournias, T.E., Lai, J., 2009. Brimonidine tartrate 0.15%, dorzolamide hydrochloride 2%, and brinzolamide 1% compared as adjunctive therapy to prostaglandin analogs. Ophthalmologyo 116, 1719–1724.

Brandt, J.D., Cantor, L.B., Katz, L.J., et al.; Ganfort Investigators Group II, 2008. Bimatoprost/timolol fixed combination: a 3-month double-masked, randomized parallel comparison to its individual components in patients with glaucoma or ocular hypertension. J. Glaucoma 17, 211–216.

Collaborative Normal-Tension Glaucoma Study Group (CNTGS), 1998. The effectiveness of intraocular pressure reduction in the treatment of normal-tension glaucoma. Am. J. Ophthalmol. 126, 498–505.

Connor, A.J., Fraser, S.G., 2014. Glaucoma prescribing trends in England 2000-20012. Eye (Lond) 28, 863–869.

Day, A.C., Baio, G., Gazzard, G., et al., 2012. The prevalence of primary angle closure glaucoma in European derived populations: a systematic review. Br. J. Ophthalmol. 96, 1162–1167.

Goldberg, I., Li, X.Y., Selaru, P., et al., 2008. A 5-year, randomized, open-label safety study of latanoprost and usual care in patients with open-angle glaucoma or ocular hypertension. Eur. J. Ophthalmol. 18, 408–416.

Gross, R.L., Sullivan, E.K., Wells, D.T., et al., 2007. Pooled results of two randomized clinical trials comparing the efficacy and safety of travoprost 0.004%/timolol 0.5% in fixed combination versus concomitant travoprost 0.004% and timolol 0.5%. Clin. Ophthalmol. 1, 317–322.

Higginbotham, E.J., 2010. Considerations in glaucoma therapy: fixed combinations versus their components medications. Clin. Ophthalmol. 4, 1–9.

Hollo, G., Vuorinen, J., Tuominen, J., et al., 2014. Fixed combination of tafluprost and timolol in the treatment of open-angle and ocular hypertension: comparison with other fixed-combination products. Adv. Ther. 31 (9), 932–944.

Jappe, U., Uter, W., Menezes de Pádua, C.A., et al., 2006. Allergic contact dermatitis due to beta-blockers in eye drops: a retrospective analysis of multicentre surveillance data 1993–2004. Acta Derm. Venereol 86, 509–514.

Johnson, T.V., Toris, C.B., Fan, S., Camras, C.B., 2008. Effects of central corneal thickness on the efficacy of topical ocular hypotensive medications. J. Glaucoma. 17, 89–99.

Kaback, M., Scoper, S.V., Arzeno, G., et al.; Brinzolamide 1%/timolol 0.5% Study Group, 2008. Intraocular pressure-lowering efficacy of brinzolamide 1%/timolol 0.5% fixed combination compared with brinzolamide 1% and timolol 0.5%. Ophthalmology 115, 1728–1734.

Karmel, M., 2013. Glaucoma pipeline drugs: targeting the trabecular meshwork. EyeNet Magaine 38–43. Available at: https://www.aao.org/eyenet/article/glaucoma-pipeline-drugs-targeting-trabecular-meshw.

Katz, L.J., Cohen, J.S., Batoosingh, A.L., et al., 2010. Twelve-month, randomized, controlled trial of bimatoprost 0.01%, 0.0125%, and 0.03% in patients with glaucoma or ocular hypertension. Am. J. Ophthalmol. 149, 661–671.

Kenigsberg, P.A., 2007. Changes in medical and surgical treatments of glaucoma between 1997 and 2003 in France. Eur. J. Ophthalmol. 17, 521–527.

King, A., Azuara-Blanco, A., Tuuloner, A., 2013. Glaucoma. Br. Med. J. 346, 29–33.

Konstas, A.G., Tsironi, S., Vakalis, A.N., et al., 2009. Intraocular pressure control over 24 hours using travoprost and timolol fixed combination administered in the morning or evening in primary open-angle and exfoliative glaucoma. Acta Ophthalmol. (Copenh) 87, 71–76.

Lachkar, Y., Bouassida, W., 2007. Drug-induced acute angle closure glaucoma. Curr. Opin. Ophthalmol. 18, 129–133.

Li, T., Lindsley, K., Rouse, B., et al., 2016. Comparative effectiveness of first-line medications for primary open-angle glaucoma: a systematic review and network analysis. Ophthalmology 123, 129–140.

Lim, K.S., Nau, C.B., O'Byrne, M.M., et al., 2008. Mechanism of action of bimatoprost, latanoprost, and travoprost in healthy subjects. A crossover study. Ophthalmology 115, 790–795.

Manni, G., Denis, P., Chew, P., et al., 2009. The safety and efficacy of brinzolamide 1%/timolol 0.5% fixed combination versus dorzolamide 2%/timolol 0.5% in patients with open-angle glaucoma or ocular hypertension. J. Glaucoma. 18, 293–300.

McKean-Cowdin, R., Wang, Y., Wu, J., et al., 2008. Impact of visual field loss on health related quality of life in glaucoma; the Los Angeles Latino Eye Study. Ophthalmology 115, 941e1–948el.

Motolko, M.A., 2008. Comparison of allergy rates in glaucoma patients receiving brimonidine 0.2% monotherapy versus fixed-combination brimonidine 0.2%-timolol 0.5% therapy. Curr. Med. Res. Opin. 24, 2663–2667.

Müller, M.E., van der Velde, N., Krulder, J.W., et al., 2006. Syncope and falls due to timolol eye drops. Br. Med. J. 332, 960–961.

Nakamura, Y., Ishikawa, S., Nakamura, Y., et al., 2009. 24-Hour intraocular pressure in glaucoma patients randomized to receive dorzolamide or brinzolamide in combination with timolol. Clin. Ophthalmol. 3, 395–400.

National Institute for Health and Care Excellence (NICE), 2009. Glaucoma: diagnosis and management of chronic open angle glaucoma and ocular hypertension. Available at: http://guidance.nice.org.uk/CG85.

Orgul, S., Zawinka, C., Gugleta, K., et al., 2005. Therapeutic strategies for normal-tension glaucoma. Ophthalmologica 219, 317–323.

Papaconstantinou, D., Georgalas, I., Kourtis, N., et al., 2009. Preliminary results following the use of a fixed combination of timolol-brimonidine in patients with ocular hypertension and primary open-angle glaucoma. Clin. Ophthalmol 3, 227–230.

Rahman, M.Q., Montgomery, D.M., Lazaridou, M.N., 2009. Surveillance of glaucoma medical therapy in a Glasgow teaching hospital: 26 years' experience. Br. J. Ophthalmol. 93, 1572–1575.

Schmier, J.K., Lau, E.C., Covert, D.W., 2010. Two-year treatment patterns and costs in glaucoma patients initiating treatment with prostaglandin analogs. Clin. Ophthalmol. 4, 1137–1143.

Sherwood, M.B., Craven, E.R., Chou, C., et al., 2006. Twice-daily 0.2% brimonidine-0.5% timolol fixed-combination therapy vs monotherapy with timolol or brimonidine in patients with glaucoma or ocular hypertension: a 12-month randomized trial. Arch. Ophthalmol. 124, 1230–1238.

Sidjanin, D.J., McCarty, C.A., Patchett, R., et al., 2008. Pharmacogenetics of ophthalmic topical beta-blockers. Per. Med. 5, 377–385.

Simmons, S.T., Dirks, M.S., Noecker, R.J., 2004. Bimatoprost versus latanoprost in lowering intraocular pressure in glaucoma and ocular hypertension: results from parallel-group comparison trials. Adv. Ther. 31, 247–262.

Sommer, A., Tielsch, J.M., Katz, J., et al., 1991. Relationship between intraocular pressure and primary open angle glaucoma among white and black Americans. The Baltimore Eye Survey. Arch. Ophthalmol. 109, 1090–1095.

Sonty, S., Donthamsetti, V., Vangipuram, G., et al., 2008. Long-term IOP lowering with bimatoprost in open-angle glaucoma patients poorly responsive to latanoprost. J. Ocul. Pharmacol. Ther. 24, 517–520.

Stamer, W.D., Braakman, S.T., Zhou, E.H., et al., 2015. Biomechanics of Schlemm's canal endothelium and intraocular pressure reduction. Prog. Retin. Eye Res. 44, 86–98.

Takmaz, T., Aşik, S., Kürkçüolu, P., et al., 2008. Comparison of intraocular pressure lowering effect of once daily morning vs evening dosing of latanoprost/timolol maleate combination. Eur. J. Ophthalmol. 18, 60–65.

Tham, Y.C., Li, X., Wong, T.Y., et al., 2014. Global prevalence of glaucoma and projections of glaucoma burden through 2040: a systematic review and meta-analysis. Ophthalmology 121 (11), 2081–2090.

Toris, C.B., Gabelt, B.T., Kaufman, P.L., 2008. Update on the mechanism of action of topical prostaglandins for intraocular pressure reduction. Surv. Ophthalmol. 53 (Suppl. 1), S107–S120.

van der Valk, R., Webers, C.A., Lumley, T., et al., 2009. A network meta-analysis combined direct and indirect comparisons between glaucoma drugs to rank effectiveness in lowering intraocular pressure. J. Clin. Epidemiol. 62, 1279–1283.

Volotinen, M., Mäenpää, J., Kautiainen, H., et al., 2009. Ophthalmic timolol in a hydrogel vehicle leads to minor inter-individual variation in timolol concentration in aqueous humor. Eur. J. Pharm. Sci. 36, 292–296.

Weinreb, R.N., Aung, T., Medeiros, F.A., 2014. The pathophysiology and treatment of glaucoma: a review. JAMA 311 (18), 1901–1911.

Weinreb, R.N., Ong, T., Scassellati Sforzolini, B., et al., 2015. A randomized, controlled comparison of latanoprostene bunod and latanoprost in the treatement of ocular hypertension and open angle glaucoma; the VOYAGER study. Br. J. Ophthalmol. 99, 738–745.

Wolfs, R.C., Klaver, C.C., Ramrattan, R.S., et al., 1998. Genetic risk of primary open-angle glaucoma. Population-based familial aggregation study. Arch. Ophthalmol. 116, 1640–1645.

Wright, T.M., Freedman, S.F., 2009. Exposure to topical apraclonidine in children with glaucoma. J. Glaucoma. 18, 395–398.

Yadav, A.K., Patel, V., 2013. Drug use in primary open angle glaucoma: a prospective study at a tertiary care teaching hospital. Indian J. Pharmacol. 45, 117–120.

Yalvac, J.S., Basci, N.E., Dulger, B., et al., 2007. Penetration of bextaxolol HCL ionic suspension 0.25% and betaxolol HCL ionic suspension 0.50% into the aqueous humour. Eur. J. Ophthalmol. 17, 368–371.

Yasuhiko, Y., Risa, T., Kohtarou, T., et al., 2001. Assessment of systemic adverse reactions induced by ophthalmic β-adrenergic receptor antagonists. J. Ocul. Pharmacol. Ther. 17, 235–248.

Yeh, J., Kravitz, D., Francis, B., 2008. Rational use of the fixed combination of dorzolamide–timolol in the management of raised intraocular pressure and glaucoma. Clin. Ophthalmol. 2, 389–399.

Further Reading

Royal College of Ophthalmologists, 2016. Commissioning Guide: Glaucoma (Recommendations). Available at: https://www.rcophth.ac.uk/wp-content/uploads/2016/06/Glaucoma-Commissioning-Guide-Recommendations-June-2016-Final.pdf.

Useful websites

International Glaucoma Association: http://www.glaucoma-association.com
Putting in your eye drops (patient video): http://www.moorfields.nhs.uk/knowyourdrops

57 Drug-induced Skin Disorders

Sarah Walsh and Daniel Creamer

Key points

- Drug-induced skin reactions are common, accounting for 30% of all reported adverse drug reactions.
- Diagnosis requires a comprehensive drug history and knowledge of likely causative drugs.
- Treatment involves drug withdrawal and general supportive measures.
- All skin eruptions will cause morbidity, but the severe reactions, such as Stevens–Johnson syndrome/toxic epidermal necrolysis, are associated with appreciable mortality.
- Certain individuals are at higher risk of drug eruptions, for example, patients with HIV infection.
- Some types of drug reaction can cause systemic as well as skin involvement, affecting the hepatic, haematological and lymphatic systems.

Adverse drug reactions (ADRs) are an inevitable consequence of modern drug therapy. They are an important cause of iatrogenic illness in terms of morbidity and mortality. ADRs can cause serious harm to the patient, as well as carrying medico-legal and economic consequences. Fortunately, only about 2% of all drug-induced skin reactions are severe, and very few are fatal. However, all drug-induced skin eruptions can cause morbidity and affect the patient's confidence in the prescriber and future adherence with medication. Therefore, it is important that all drug-associated rashes are carefully evaluated and documented. It is essential that the patient is made aware of his or her sensitivity because subsequent exposure to the drug may cause a more severe eruption. At the population level, both reporting of adverse events via the Medicines and Healthcare Products Regulatory Agency (MHRA) 'yellow card scheme' and post-marketing surveillance of new drugs have a role in identifying patterns of drug eruption.

It is important to remember that the potential of an individual drug to cause a skin eruption is variable. Any drug can potentially cause any reaction pattern in the skin. Some drugs, such as ferrous sulphate, seldom produce a rash, whereas others, for example, carbamazepine, penicillin antibiotics and sulfasalazine, are far more likely to precipitate a skin eruption.

Diagnosis

It is often difficult to determine the cause of a drug-induced eruption for the following reasons:

- Almost any drug can affect the skin.
- Unrelated drugs can produce similar reactions.
- The same drug may produce different reaction patterns in different patients.
- Some drug reactions are difficult to distinguish from specific skin diseases such as acne, eczema and psoriasis.

In most cases, diagnosis of a drug-induced skin eruption is based on the history and the temporal association of the onset of the rash to the commencement of the medication. Particular difficulties are presented by the patient taking combined preparations, for example, co-tenidone, which contains both a diuretic and a β-blocker. Excipients contained in medication, such as preservatives, stabilisers or colours, may be the culprit rather than the drug itself. Changes in the brand of medication may, for this reason, provoke a skin reaction in someone who appears to have been established on a drug for some time and suddenly develops a rash. Patients may be taking preparations acquired over the counter (OTC), or from an alternative practitioner, which they may not immediately volunteer when asked about current medication. If a patient presents with a rash and is currently taking, or has recently finished, medication, the following are important steps:

- Take an accurate drug history, including OTC medicines, herbal and homeopathic preparations and any injections. Record both generic and brand names of medicines.
- Ask if the patient has any history of drug sensitivity.
- Ascertain when the eruption started in relation to drug use (the latency of onset of the eruption).

Definitive diagnosis of a drug-induced dermatosis would require drug re-challenge; however, this is not recommended due to the possibility of provoking a more severe reaction on second exposure (Po and Kendall, 2001).

Drug-induced skin disorders

In this chapter, drug reactions are considered under the following headings: drug reactions causing changes in skin function, mild drug-induced skin disorders and severe drug-induced skin disorders.

Box 57.1 Drugs causing light-induced eruptions

Topical preparations
- Topical NSAIDs
- Components of sunscreen, such as para-aminobenzoic acid, benzophenone

Systemic drugs

Phototoxic reactions
- Amiodarone
- Nalidixic acid
- NSAIDs
- Chlorpromazine
- Tetracyclines

Photoallergic reactions
- Griseofulvin
- NSAIDs
- Sulfonamides
- Sulfonylureas
- Thiazide diuretics

NSAIDs, Non-steroidal anti-inflammatory drugs.

Drug reactions causing changes in skin function

Some drugs alter the ability of the skin and associated structures (hair and nails) to perform their functions normally.

Abnormal photosensitivity

Drugs may induce an excessive sensitivity to sunlight. Ultraviolet wavelengths of sunlight (290–400 nm) are able to interact with certain drugs in the skin to provoke abnormal photosensitivity. An eruption occurring on all uncovered skin implicates exposure to a systemic photosensitising agent, for example, a patient who commences bendroflumethiazide and subsequently develops sunburn on a cloudy day. A localised eruption indicates a reaction to a locally applied topical photosensitiser and subsequent exposure to light. This may be seen in individuals who are sensitive to a component of sunscreens such as benzophenone, a chemical sunblock.

Drug-induced photosensitivity can be either phototoxic or photoallergic (Box 57.1). Phototoxic reactions, which are more common, resemble severe sunburn and can progress to blistering. They are dose dependent for both the drug and sunlight; they occur within 5–15 hours of taking the drug and subside quickly on drug withdrawal. Photoallergic rashes are usually eczematous but may be lichenoid, urticarial, bullous or purpuric. They are not dose dependent and occur after exposure to normal amounts of sunlight exposure. The onset can be delayed by weeks or months, and recovery is often slow after drug withdrawal. Rarely, a photoallergic state can persist for years after the drug responsible has been discontinued.

Patients receiving known photosensitising drugs should be advised to avoid strong sunlight. They should also be advised to use a broad-spectrum topical sunscreen, providing both UVA protection (indicated by the 'star rating' on the bottle) and UVB cover (indicated by the sun protection factor, SPF).

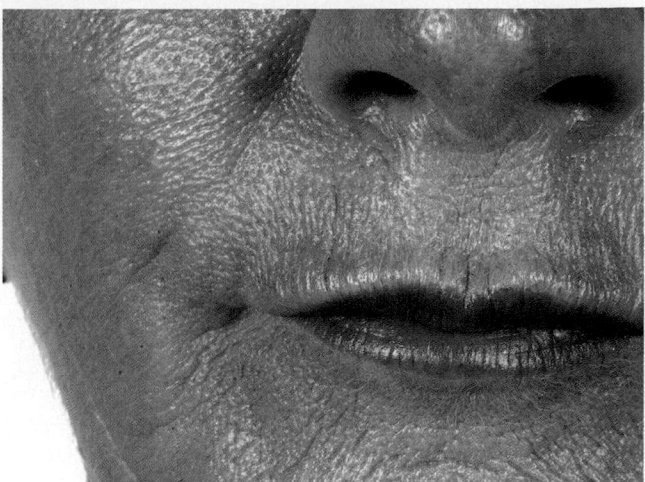

Fig. 57.1 Minocycline pigmentation: this female patient was taking minocycline for 2 years for treatment of rosacea and developed unsightly grey pigmentation around the mouth. This did not respond to stopping the medication.

Pigmentary changes

The skin's colour can be altered by drugs; hyper-pigmentation, hypo-pigmentation and discoloration can all potentially be induced by a variety of medicines (see Fig. 57.1 and Table 57.1). Pigmentary changes can be widespread or localised. The most common examples of localised pigmentation are the facial blue–black pigmentation in individuals on amiodarone or minocycline and melasma facial pigmentation occurring in some women taking the combined oral contraceptive pill. Generalised pigmentary change induced by drugs is rare but can occur with chemotherapeutic agents such as bleomycin. This may have the appearance of generalised hyper-melanosis or may take on a more flagellate appearance with multiple linear areas of hyper-pigmentation.

The mechanism of drug pigmentation is not always known; however, proposed pathogenetic mechanisms are as follows:
- Drug or drug metabolite deposition in the dermis and epidermis. An example of this would be agyria, in which systemic absorption of silver from, for example, topical silver sulfadiazine, causes a slate-grey discolouration of the skin.
- Enhanced melanin production with or without an increase in the number of active melanocytes. This appears to be the pathogenetic mechanism in melasma and also bleomycin-induced pigmentation (Moncada et al., 2009).

Nail changes

The growth and colour of the fingernails and toenails can be modified by drugs. Abnormalities of the texture and architecture of the nail unit can also be drug induced. Blue discoloration of the nails can result from therapy with mepacrine, whereas a blue–black pigmentation may accompany treatment with minocycline and certain cytotoxic drugs such as hydroxyurea. Potassium permanganate solutions will dye nails brown. White nails (leukonychia) can result from treatment with chemotherapy agents, especially cyclophosphamide, doxorubicin and vincristine. Beau's lines, transverse depressions of the nail, represent interruption of the

Table 57.1 Drugs causing skin pigmentation

Drug	Pigmentation
Amiodarone	Blue–grey
Anticonvulsants	Brown
Antimalarials	Blue–grey
β-Blockers	Brown
Imatinib	Hypo-/hyperpigmentation
Imipramine	Blue/grey
Mepacrine	Blue/black
Methyldopa	Brown
Oral contraceptives	Brown spots/patches
Phenothiazines	Brown/blue–grey
Psoralens	Brown
Tetracyclines	Blue–black

Box 57.2 Drugs causing hair disorders

Alopecia
- Acitretin
- Anticoagulants
- Anticonvulsants
- Antithyroid drugs
- β-Blockers
- Cimetidine
- Cytotoxic drugs
- Gold salts
- Interferons
- Isotretinoin
- Leflunomide
- Lithium
- Sodium valproate
- Statins
- Tacrolimus
- Vismodegib

Hirsutism/hypertrichosis
- Acetazolamide
- Anabolic steroids
- Androgens
- Corticosteroids (topical and systemic)
- Ciclosporin
- Danazol
- Minoxidil
- Oral contraceptives
- Penicillamine
- Phenytoin
- Tamoxifen
- Verapamil

normal growth of the nail matrix and are caused by systemic infection, metabolic upset or, occasionally, drugs. In the drug-induced form, the most common cause is again chemotherapy agents, similar to those which cause leukonychia.

Onycholysis is characterised by separation of the nail plate from the underlying nail bed. Any cytotoxic agent may induce onycholysis by direct toxicity to the matrix. Photo-onycholysis describes lifting of the nail plate and is caused by the combination of a photosensitising drug, for example, minocycline or oxytetracycline, and by UVA exposure.

Hair changes

Drugs may exert an effect on the hair follicle itself or on the growth cycle of hair. The cycle of hair growth involves anagen (the growth phase of the hair), catagen (the resting phase) and telogen (the shedding phase). Either loss of hair or excessive growth of hair may result.

Loss of hair. Drug-induced alopecia (Box 57.2) may be partial or complete. The temporal relationship between the introduction of the drug and the subsequent loss of hair depends on the part of the hair cycle with which the drug interferes. Cytotoxic drugs interfere with the 'anagen' or growth phase of the hair cycle, and so loss is rapid and complete; it begins shortly after administration of the drug, and the effect is dose dependent and fortunately reversible, but a delay of several weeks is common before regrowth begins.

Delayed hair loss after the introduction of a drug is a more insidious process and may not be noticed immediately by the patient. In this scenario, the drug is often interfering with the 'telogen' or shedding part of the hair cycle, moving follicles through this phase more quickly. Hair is shed at a rate that exceeds that at which the follicles can produce new hair, resulting in a thinning effect. Given the length of the hair cycle, this type of hair loss can occur 2–4 months after a drug is initiated. Retinoid therapy, including isotretinoin prescribed for acne, or acitretin for psoriasis, may induce a telogen alopecia.

Androgens promote the shrinking of hair follicles and shorten the duration of the growth stage of the hair-follicle cycle (anagen stage). Drugs with androgen activity can induce male-pattern baldness, for example, exogenously administered testosterone, which may be prescribed for hypogonadism in men and occasionally in post-menopausal women as an adjunct to hormone replacement therapy. Oestrogens are known to prolong the anagen stage and counteract androgenetic alopecia. Oestrogenic stimuli may cause the hair follicle to shift into the anagen phase and vice versa. The use of the oestrogen receptor antagonist tamoxifen in women with breast cancer can exacerbate female-pattern hair loss. Tamoxifen competes for the oestrogen receptor and produces an environment with relative hyperandrogenism, which may augment the androgen action on follicles.

Excessive hair. Hirsutism is excessive hairiness, especially in women, in the male pattern of hair growth, whereas hypertrichosis is the growth of hair at sites not normally hairy. Both conditions can be drug induced, and in some cases, the same drug can produce both patterns of hair growth (see Box 57.2). The capacity of minoxidil to produce hypertrichosis was noted during early trials of this drug as an antihypertensive. It is infrequently used for its originally intended purpose because it produces profound

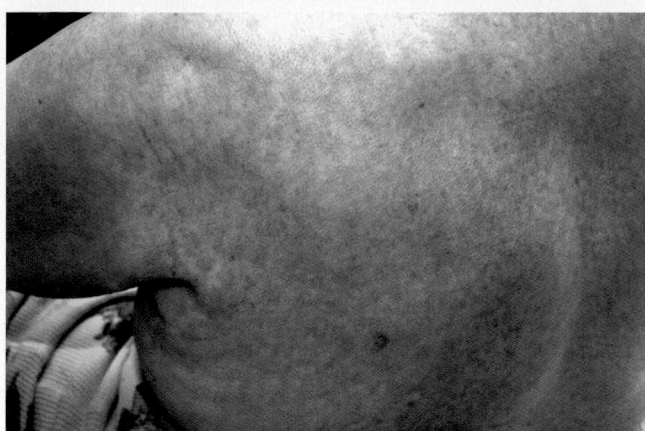

Fig. 57.2 Drug exanthem: maculopapular, itchy eruption appeared 4 days after the introduction of a course of co-amoxiclav for a respiratory tract infection. Note the linear marks indicating excoriation (scratching) on the left posterior shoulder.

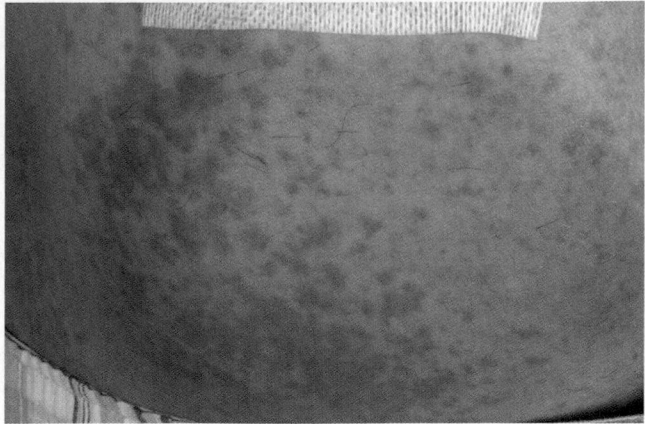

Fig. 57.3 Urticaria: patient developed the classic raised red itchy wheals of urticaria after the commencement of ibuprofen for musculoskeletal pain.

postural hypotension, but its most noticeable side effect has been exploited as a topical preparation for the treatment of male-pattern baldness.

Changes to the skin's immune system and skin malignancy

The skin's innate immune surveillance system detects and repairs UV-induced DNA damage, thus limiting the tendency to cutaneous carcinogenesis. Drug-induced immunosuppression places an individual at an increased risk of skin cancer, notably squamous cell and basal cell carcinomas. As well as a reduction in immune surveillance, immunosuppression increases susceptibility to the human papilloma virus, some strains of which may predispose to the development of squamous malignancy. Patients taking drugs such as azathioprine, ciclosporin, tacrolimus, mycophenolate mofetil and chemotherapeutic agents should be counselled about the importance of sun protection to minimise the risk of the development of malignant and pre-malignant skin cancers. Certain high-risk patients on immunosuppressant drugs, particularly renal transplant recipients, should undergo formal follow-up with skin monitoring by a dermatologist on a yearly basis.

Mild drug-induced skin disorders

Mild drug reaction patterns in the skin are numerous; some of the more commonly seen morphologies are discussed in this section.

Drug-induced exanthems

A drug-induced exanthem (widespread rash) is the most common type of drug reaction in the skin. Exanthems are characterised by erythema (redness) and may be morbilliform (resembling measles) or maculopapular (a mixture of flat and raised areas) (see Fig. 57.2). Less frequently there may be blisters, which may be small (vesicles) or larger (>5 mm, bullae), and the skin may feel hot, burning or itchy.

The proportion of the body surface area (BSA) involved varies from case to case, but when it is severe, involving more than 90% of the BSA, the presentation is referred to as 'erythroderma', which is discussed later. In theory, any drug is capable of producing a drug-induced exanthem in the skin, but in practice, common causes include antibiotics (e.g. sulfonamides, ampicillin, isoniazid), anticonvulsants (e.g. phenytoin, carbamazepine) and antimalarials (chloroquine).

Most drug-induced exanthems begin within 7 days of commencing a drug, the mechanism being a delayed (type IV) hypersensitivity (Griffiths et al., 2016; Hausmann et al., 2012). If the drug can be identified, it should be stopped, and appropriate symptomatic relief should be instituted with antihistamines and topical steroids. A clear record of the reaction should be made in the patient's notes. Both the patient and the primary care doctor should be made aware of the reaction for the purposes of future avoidance.

An exanthematous reaction commonly occurs after administration of ampicillin (or its derivatives, including amoxicillin) to patients suffering from glandular fever (infectious mononucleosis). It does not usually represent a true penicillin allergy but a complex interplay between viral factors (infectious mononucleosis being caused by Epstein–Barr virus) and drug epitopes (Hausmann et al., 2012). This reaction to the drug would not be expected to be seen in the same patient in the absence of the virus.

Urticaria and angioedema

Urticaria, also known as hives, describes the appearance of red, itchy wheals on the skin (Fig. 57.3). Angioedema is a more serious, related condition in which the patient develops deep soft-tissue swellings, most notably on the face. Urticaria and angioedema can be either allergic, a reaction between an antigen and specific mast cell-bound IgE, or non-allergic. Drugs are recognised triggers of urticaria and angioedema (Box 57.3) and can also exacerbate pre-existing urticaria. The most important culprits are the NSAIDs and opiates, both of which lower the threshold for mast cell degranulation. Angiotensin-converting enzyme (ACE) inhibitors and angiotensin receptor blockers (ARBs), for example, candesartan, can provoke angioedema in a susceptible individual.

Box 57.3 Drugs causing urticaria/angioedema

- Antibiotics (particularly penicillins, and especially when given by the parenteral route)
- Barbiturates
- Angiotensin-converting enzyme inhibitors
- Angiotensin receptor blockers
- Levamisole
- Non-steroidal anti-inflammatory drugs
- Opiate analgesics
- Phenolphthalein
- Quinine
- Rifampicin
- Sulfonamides
- Thiopental
- Vancomycin

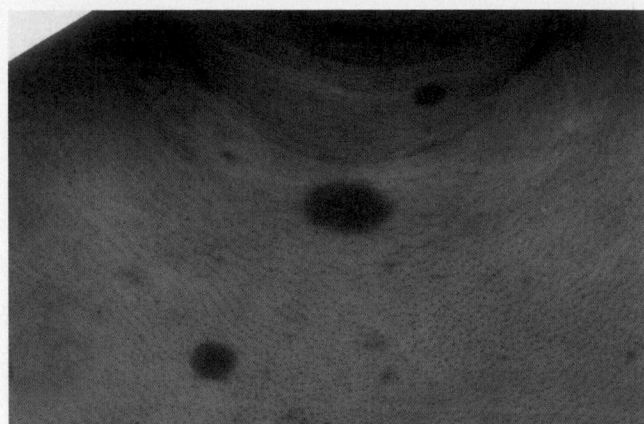

Fig. 57.4 Fixed drug eruption: female patient developed persistent macular inflamed areas on her upper chest wall 2 months after starting a new combined oral contraceptive pill. A fixed drug eruption was suspected, and the lesions resolved after stopping the medicine.

Drug-induced urticaria/angioedema can be a cutaneous manifestation of anaphylaxis, and in this situation, urgent medical attention is needed with the administration of adrenaline, antihistamine and intravenous corticosteroid.

Pruritus

Pruritus (itching) can accompany a drug rash or may be an isolated symptom provoked by a medication. The most common trigger of drug-induced pruritus is the administration of opiate analgesics and their related synthetic derivatives such as tramadol. Opiate-induced pruritus is centrally mediated, rather than by peripheral nerves; therefore, antihistamines do not, in general, ameliorate the itch. This can pose a particular problem in the palliative care setting where opiate analgesics are required regularly.

Fixed drug eruptions

Fixed drug eruption is characterised by one or more inflammatory patches that recur at the same cutaneous or mucosal site(s) each time the patient is exposed to the offending drug (Fig. 57.4). The eruption usually involves the torso, hands, feet, face or genitalia, and is characterised by a deep-red, circular, well-demarcated patch. They take between 2 and 24 hours to develop after drug ingestion. On the first drug exposure, there is usually only one lesion, but subsequent exposure can result in multiple lesions.

The group of drugs with the potential to cause a fixed drug eruption is virtually limitless, but some of the drugs more commonly responsible are listed in Box 57.4.

Once the drug has been stopped, the lesions resolve and may leave an area of post-inflammatory hyperpigmentation. This may be the only physical sign at the time the patient presents. Topical steroids may ameliorate the symptoms.

Acneiform eruptions

Acne may be drug induced or drug exacerbated. One of the most commonly prescribed drugs to produce an acneiform eruption is a corticosteroid, in either topical or oral form. Illicit use of

Box 57.4 Drugs causing fixed drug eruptions

- Ampicillin
- Aspirin
- Barbiturates
- Dapsone
- Metronidazole
- Non-steroidal anti-inflammatory drugs
- Oral contraceptives
- Phenytoin
- Quinine
- Sulfonamides
- Tetracyclines

anabolic steroids by athletes can also produce this effect, occasionally in its most severe form, acne fulminans. Other drugs which may worsen or provoke acne include ciclosporin, lithium and progesterone-only oral contraceptives.

The anticancer drugs classified as endothelial growth factor receptor (EGFR) antagonists, for example, cetuximab, commonly produce an acneiform eruption. The papules and pustules which occur are more monomorphic than those seen in idiopathic acne. Interestingly, studies have shown that there is a positive correlation between the severity of the acneiform eruption and the response of the cancer to the treatment (Susman, 2004). Most drug-induced or drug-exacerbated acne can be managed with the same treatments as used in idiopathic acne, such as topical agents, oral tetracycline antibiotics, erythromycin or, in severe cases, oral retinoids. Examples of drugs which may cause an acneiform eruption are given in Box 57.5.

Psoriasiform eruptions

Drugs can either exacerbate psoriasis in predisposed patients or induce psoriasiform rashes in previously unaffected patients (see Box 57.6). The psoriasiform eruptions mimic psoriasis and are

Box 57.5 Drugs causing acne

- Androgens (in women)
- Corticosteroids (oral and topical) and adrenocorticotropic hormone (including inhaled preparations)
- Ciclosporin
- Epidermal growth factor receptor antagonists (cetuximab)
- Ethambutol
- Haloperidol
- Isoniazid
- Lithium
- Oral contraceptives
- Phenobarbital
- Phenytoin
- Propylthiouracil

Box 57.6   Drugs that exacerbate psoriasis

- Angiotensin-converting enzyme inhibitors
- Antimalarials – chloroquine, mepacrine
- Biological therapy targeting tumour necrosis factor alpha (occasionally – slightly paradoxical given that such drugs are also given to *treat* psoriasis)
- β-Blockers (most frequently atenolol, oxprenolol and propranolol)
- Corticosteroids, e.g. prednisolone
- Granulocyte-colony stimulating factor
- Lithium
- Non-steroidal anti-inflammatory drug

Box 57.7   Drugs causing lichenoid eruptions

- Antimalarials – chloroquine, mepacrine
- Aspirin
- Angiotensin-converting enzyme inhibitors
- β-Blockers
- Calcium channel blockers, e.g. amlodipine, nifedipine
- Carbamazepine
- Ethambutol
- Gold salts
- Imatinib
- Interferon-α
- Lithium
- Methyldopa
- Non-steroidal anti-inflammatory drugs
- Penicillamine
- Phenothiazines
- Quinine
- Sulfonylureas

characterised by itchy, scaly, red patches on the elbows, forearms, knees, legs and scalp. Drugs that have a well-established effect of worsening pre-existing psoriasis include β-blockers, lithium, antimalarials and ACE inhibitors.

Lichenoid eruptions

Drug-induced lichenoid eruptions (see Box 57.7) resemble lichen planus, and occur as flat, mauve lesions. However, they may be atypical, showing scaling and confluence. The lesions can be seen at any site but are found mainly on the forearms, neck and the inner surface of the thighs. The eruption resolves with drug withdrawal, with or without topical steroids, but post-inflammatory hyperpigmentation is often long lasting.

Xerosis, eczematous eruptions and contact dermatitis

Retinoid drugs (such as isotretinoin, acitretin and alitretinoin), EGFR inhibitors (cetuximab, erlotinib, lapatinib) and statins have a drying effect on the skin, termed xerosis. This can exacerbate pre-existing eczema, or precipitate eczema in a susceptible individual. Irritant contact dermatitis may be seen in preparations with an alcohol base, such as topical antibiotics, or with the application of topical preparations, which are inherently irritant such as benzoyl peroxide, tar or dithranol.

Allergic contact dermatitis is a delayed (type IV) hypersensitivity reaction, which can develop to any topical preparation, for example, eye drops in a sensitised individual. Most commonly, this will be a reaction to excipients contained in the preparation, such as preservatives, for example, sodium metabisulfite, fragrances or stabilisers, but may be to the drug itself. In all cases of irritant or allergic contact dermatitis, the patient should be counselled to stop the preparation. Patch testing carried out by a dermatologist is a useful way of investigating patients in whom a diagnosis of allergic contact dermatitis is suspected.

Erythema nodosum

Erythema nodosum is an acute inflammatory reaction with painful subcutaneous nodules, usually but not exclusively found on the shins. Erythema nodosum is usually a complication of infection with, for example, streptococcus or tuberculosis, or is a cutaneous manifestation of an inflammatory condition such as sarcoidosis. In its drug-induced form, it may be caused by oral contraceptives, sulfonamide antibiotics, salicylates, penicillins and gold salts.

Hand–foot reactions

Painful, burning erythema of the hands and feet is a common side effect of some chemotherapeutic agents. This may be termed 'hand–foot syndrome'. It is most frequently caused by 5-fluorouracil, doxorubicin, the EGFR/protein kinase inhibitors (e.g. cetuximab, erlotinib) and BRAF inhibitors (e.g. vemurafenib). The redness may sometimes be accompanied by painful hyperkeratosis (thickening) of the skin of the hands and feet, and in these cases, an emollient containing urea may provide symptomatic relief.

Severe drug-induced skin disorders

Erythema multiforme (EM), Stevens–Johnson syndrome (SJS) and toxic epidermal necrolysis (TEN) are all idiosyncratic, immunologically mediated severe drug eruptions. For our purposes,

Box 57.8 Drugs causing erythema multiforme

- Allopurinol
- Antiretrovirals, e.g. nevirapine
- Barbiturates
- Carbamazepine
- Cimetidine
- Dapsone
- Gold salts
- Isoniazid
- Lamotrigine
- Leflunomide
- Macrolide antibiotics
- Mefloquine
- Non-steroidal anti-inflammatory drugs
- Penicillins
- Phenytoin
- Rifampicin
- Sulfonamides

these diseases may be considered to be on a spectrum, from the mild and self-limiting at one end (EM) to the fulminating severe at the other (TEN).

Erythema multiforme

EM is an eruption of target-like lesions which are characterised by concentric red and pale rings with, in severe cases, central blistering. EM typically occurs on the limbs rather than the trunk, but mucous membrane surfaces, such as the eye, the mouth and the genital tract, may also become involved. A significant proportion of EM cases are caused by infection, particularly herpes simplex virus reactivation; however, in some patients, EM is triggered by a drug (see Box 57.8). Drug-induced EM will usually present within 2 weeks of starting a new medication. Once the responsible drug has been stopped, treatment is symptomatic with paracetamol, topical steroids and appropriate topical therapy for the mouth and other involved mucosal surfaces.

Stevens–Johnson syndrome and toxic epidermal necrolysis

SJS and TEN are terms used to describe a life-threatening, mucocutaneous drug hypersensitivity syndrome characterised by blistering and epidermal sloughing (Fig. 57.5). In SJS, there is epidermal detachment of less than 10% BSA; in TEN, there is detachment of greater than 30% of the BSA, and cases with 10–30% involvement are labelled SJS/TEN overlap. The systemic problems that accompany widespread epidermal loss, such as high losses of heat and fluid, and the heightened risk of infection due to diminished barrier function can cause serious morbidity, similar to extensive burns. TEN carries a mortality rate of approximately 30%, but this can rise to 90% mortality in the presence of co-morbidities. HIV-infected patients and patients with systemic lupus erythematosus (SLE) have an enhanced risk of developing SJS/TEN. Drugs causing SJS/TEN are listed in Box 57.9.

Clinical features. A prodrome of fever, malaise, and upper respiratory tract symptoms may precede the eruption by a few days. Involvement of the mucous membranes of the eyes, mouth, and nose is a prominent early feature. Eye involvement results in blepharitis, haemorrhagic conjunctivitis, mucus secretion, and pseudomembranes. Ophthalmological input is required early if long-term sequelae, such as blindness from corneal opacities and synechiae, are not to occur. Urethral involvement must also be anticipated and the patient catheterised if strictures are not to complicate the disease course. Mouth involvement causes an erosive and haemorrhagic mucositis. On the skin, dusky red macules 1–3 cm in diameter appear at any site and evolve to become confluent. The skin lesions pass through vesicular and bullous phases before epidermal detachment occurs. Shearing pressure to the skin causes detachment of involved epidermis (positive Nikolsky's sign). In TEN, there is widespread epidermal loss and sloughing of the necrotic epidermis, which peels back to leave large areas of exposed dermis. Denuded dermis exudes serum, becomes secondarily infected and readily bleeds. The patient is in severe pain and is usually extremely ill. The visceral manifestations that result from widespread epithelial loss include pneumonia, pancreatitis, thromboembolic disease and renal and hepatic impairment.

The patient with SJS/TEN will require full supportive care, preferably in an intensive care unit. Patients with SJS with less extensive involvement may be managed in a lower-dependency environment but should be monitored closely for signs of progression in the first 48 hours of admission. A multidisciplinary approach, including dermatologists, ophthalmologists and intensive care physicians, is critical to a successful outcome. After drug withdrawal, the management is supportive, including prompt treatment of infection; careful attention to thermoregulation, fluid balance and skin care; and the introduction of appropriate eye and lid care. The literature has failed to identify one treatment which definitively improves outcomes, but agents which have been used include systemic steroids, ciclosporin and intravenous immunoglobulin.

Drug reaction with eosinophilia and systemic symptoms

Drug reaction with eosinophilia and systemic symptoms (DRESS) is sometimes known as drug-induced hypersensitivity syndrome (DIHS) and is a distinct, severe and potentially fatal drug-induced skin disorder. The drugs commonly associated with this syndrome are listed in Box 57.10.

Typically, the dermatosis of DRESS is an extensive, inflammatory, maculopapular exanthem. Other skin signs may also be present, including pustules, purpura, blisters, target-like lesions and facial oedema (Fig. 57.6). To meet the diagnostic criteria, there will also be a haematological abnormality, either a raised eosinophil count ($>1.5 \times 10^9$/L) or the presence of atypical lymphocytes on the blood film. There is prominent systemic involvement in DRESS, most commonly fever, lymph node enlargement and liver function abnormalities. Less typically, there is renal, pulmonary or cardiac involvement.

DRESS is characterised by its long latency of onset, with the syndrome usually presenting between 2 and 8 weeks after commencement of the causative drug. This is an important point to

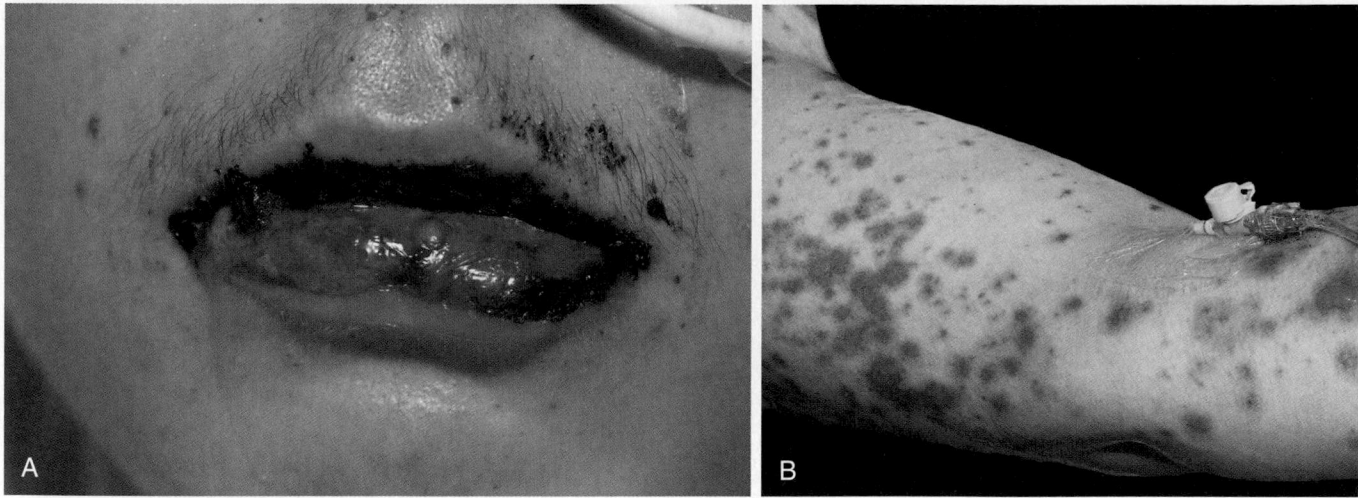

Fig. 57.5 Stevens–Johnson syndrome is a serious, idiosyncratic reaction of the skin (B) and mucous membranes (A) to a drug. It results in blistering and subsequently widespread epidermal loss and can have a high mortality rate.

Box 57.9 Drugs causing Stevens–Johnson syndrome and toxic epidermal necrolysis

- Allopurinol
- Antiretrovirals, e.g. nevirapine
- Carbamazepine
- Co-trimoxazole
- Dapsone
- Gold salts
- Lamotrigine
- Leflunomide
- Non-steroidal anti-inflammatory drugs, e.g. meloxicam, diclofenac
- Penicillins, e.g. amoxicillin, ampicillin
- Phenobarbitone
- Phenolphthalein
- Phenylbutazone
- Phenytoin
- Sulfadiazine
- Sulfasalazine
- Tetracyclines, e.g. doxycycline

Box 57.10 Common causes of Drug Reaction with Eosinophilia and Systemic Symptoms

- Allopurinol
- Antiretrovirals, e.g. efavirenz
- Carbamazepine
- Cotrimoxazole
- Lamotrigine
- Minocycline
- Phenobarbitone
- Phenytoin
- Sulfadiazine
- Sulfasalazine
- Vancomycin

note in the medication history because the drug responsible may often be overlooked if it is considered to have been started 'too long ago'.

DRESS is accompanied by significant morbidity, and the mortality has been estimated at 10%. Systemic steroids are usually administered and may be beneficial, but there are no randomised controlled trials to support their use. Management involves stopping the suspected drug and supportive care dictated by the extent of involvement.

Acute generalised exanthematous pustulosis

Acute generalised exanthematous pustulosis (AGEP) describes a reaction pattern to a drug consisting of widespread sterile, monomorphic pustules studding the skin in a generalised fashion. Such

patients are generally systemically unwell with a fever and the complications of generalised skin inflammation, including excessive heat and fluid loss. The differential diagnosis would include pustular psoriasis. Although the condition is self-limiting, potent topical steroids may accelerate resolution. The drugs which can cause AGEP are summarised in Box 57.11.

Erythroderma and exfoliative dermatitis

Erythroderma is the term used to describe any pattern of drug reaction in the skin where more than 90% of the BSA is involved. This is usually an extension of a severe drug-induced exanthem. The erythrodermic patient often feels shivery and may have lymphadenopathy and fever. The large surface area involved in erythroderma leads to substantial losses of heat and fluid from the body. This puts the patient at risk of electrolyte imbalances, hypothermia and, with the loss of skin barrier function, infection. Admission to hospital is indicated in cases of erythroderma, and management is supportive, with intravenous fluids, warming measures and treatment of infection. Topical corticosteroids are often prescribed but must be used with caution because significant amounts will

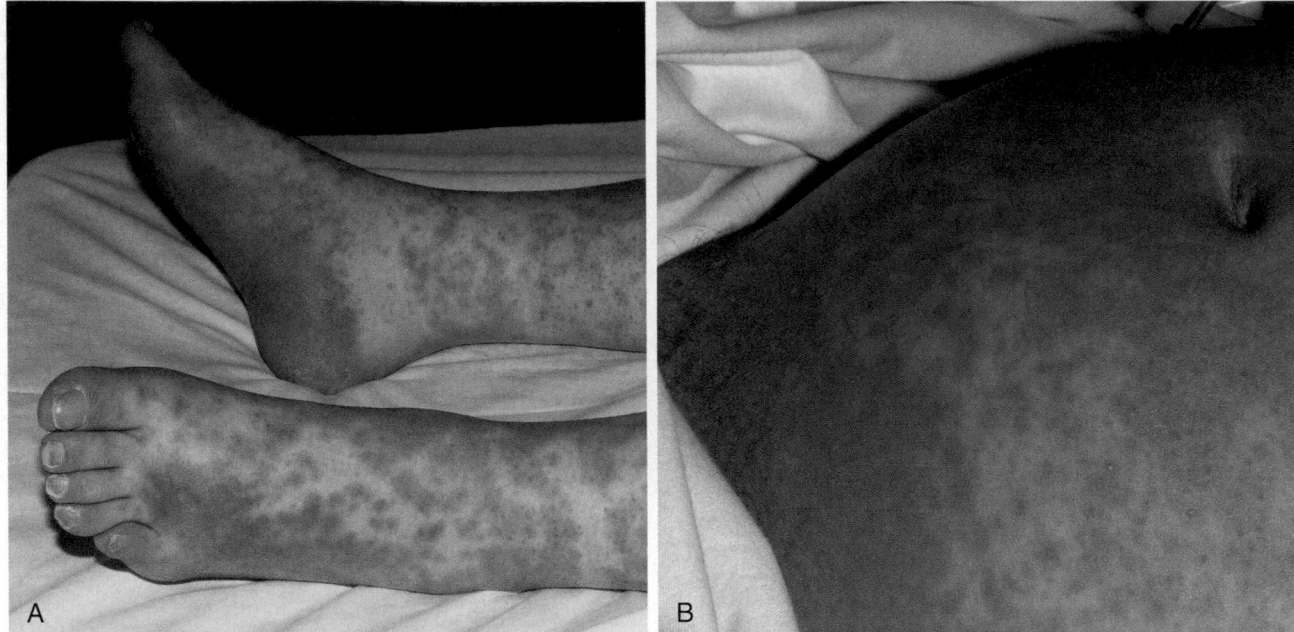

Fig. 57.6 Drug reaction with eosinophilia and systemic symptoms: female patient developed a severe systemic reaction after commencement of phenytoin for seizure prophylaxis after brain surgery. She had an erythematous urticated eruption as seen here accompanied by lymphadenopathy, derangement of liver function and a circulating eosinophilia as seen here (A and B).

Box 57.11	Drugs causing acute generalised exanthematous pustulosis

- Allopurinol
- Amoxicillin
- Carbamazepine
- Cefuroxime
- Co-trimoxazole
- Doxycycline
- Macrolide antibiotics, e.g. erythromycin, pristinamycin
- Metronidazole
- Lamotrigine
- Phenytoin
- Sulfasalazine
- Vancomycin

Box 57.12	Drugs causing exanthemous eruptions

- Amoxicillin
- Ampicillin[a]
- Bleomycin
- Captopril
- Carbamazepine
- Chlorpromazine
- Co-trimoxazole
- Gold salts
- Nalidixic acid
- Non-steroidal anti-inflammatory drug
- Phenytoin
- Penicillamine

[a]Ampicillin rashes do not necessarily indicate penicillin hypersensitivity but may be seen when administered to a patient with glandular fever (see text).

be systemically absorbed across the erythrodermic skin. During recovery, the patient will desquamate, referred to as the exfoliative phase. Drugs commonly provoking this pattern of reaction are similar to those that cause a drug-induced exanthem (Box 57.12).

Lupus erythematosus

Syndromes indistinguishable from lupus erythematosus (LE) may occur after drug administration (see Box 57.13) and can be accompanied by seroconversion to antinuclear antibody (ANA) positivity. Serological clearance of ANA may occur after drug withdrawal, but this may take months or years.

The cutaneous manifestations of drug-induced LE include the characteristic butterfly-shaped rash on the face, photosensitive erythema on dorsal hands and neck and annular lesions on limbs.

Biological therapy targeting tumour necrosis factor alpha (TNF-α), such as infliximab and etanercept, has been found to provoke lupus both in its systemic and limited cutaneous forms.

Vasculitis

Vasculitis is characterised pathologically by inflammation in vessel walls and clinically as palpable purpuric lesions most commonly found on the lower limbs. Cutaneous vasculitis without other organ involvement is the rule, but systemic involvement, such as renal, can occasionally occur. The purpuric areas on the legs may become ulcerated and require specialist dermatology input.

Box 57.13 Drugs causing lupus erythematosus

- Anticonvulsants: phenytoin
- β-Blockers
- Chlorpromazine
- Griseofulvin
- Hydralazine
- Isoniazid
- Lithium
- Methyldopa
- Oral contraceptives
- Penicillamine
- Phenytoin
- Procainamide
- Propylthiouracil
- Sulfasalazine
- Terbinafine
- Biological therapy targeting tumour necrosis factor alpha, e.g. infliximab

Box 57.14 Drugs that may cause cutaneous vasculitic reactions

- Angiotensin-converting enzyme inhibitors
- Allopurinol
- Amiodarone
- Aspirin
- Carbamazepine
- Carbimazole
- Diltiazem
- Erythromycin
- Furosemide
- Gold
- Haematopoietic growth factors (granulocyte-colony stimulating factor and granulocyte-macrophage colony-stimulating factor)
- Hydralazine
- Interferons
- Methotrexate
- Minocycline
- Non-steroidal anti-inflammatory drugs
- Penicillamine
- Propylthiouracil
- Sulfasalazine
- Sulfonamides
- Thiazides
- Thrombolytic agents

Drugs are the cause of approximately 10% of cutaneous vasculitis cases and should be considered in any patient with small vessel vasculitis (Box 57.14). Withdrawal of the causative drug is often sufficient to resolve the clinical manifestations without the need for treatment with systemic corticosteroids or more powerful immunosuppressants.

Skin necrosis

The term *widespread cutaneous necrosis* describes extensive skin infarction, which often heralds a severe systemic coagulopathy. Widespread cutaneous necrosis can be triggered by a reaction to warfarin or, less commonly, to heparin. In warfarin or coumarin skin necrosis, the buttocks and breasts are the most commonly involved sites. Discontinuation of the anticoagulant responsible is essential; however, ongoing management of the coagulopathy is critical, and patients need to be assessed by a haematologist.

Patient care

Withdrawal of the likely offending drug should be the first intervention in cases of suspected drug eruption. This should be done in consultation with the prescribing physician because an alternative drug may be required to control the patient's condition. General methods which will provide symptomatic relief in a mild, limited drug eruption include emollients, soap substitutes and oral antihistamines. A mild topical corticosteroid may also be appropriate. In cases where the eruption is more extensive, or if a mucosal surface is involved, specialist care provided by a dermatologist will be necessary.

Case studies

Case 57.1

A 36-year-old female patient, Ms FG, with a long history of chronic idiopathic urticaria attends her local pharmacy for some advice. Her skin disease is usually well controlled with an occasional dose of cetirizine which she buys OTC. Ms FG has recently begun taking ibuprofen for muscular pain associated with her marathon training, but she has found, to her dismay, that her urticaria has become much worse and is flaring on a daily basis.

....

Questions

1. What is the likely cause of the deterioration in the control of Ms FG's urticaria?
2. What management should be advised?
3. What other group of drugs is likely to produce this effect?

....

Answers

1. NSAIDs are known to increase the frequency of attacks of urticaria in susceptible individuals. It is likely that the self-medicating with ibuprofen has lessened Ms FG's control of her urticaria.
2. In the first instance, the ibuprofen should be stopped. An alternative such as paracetamol could be advised for the musculoskeletal symptoms. An enquiry should be made as to whether or not any symptoms suggestive of angioedema, such as lip/tongue swelling, or difficulty breathing, have accompanied the urticaria, as this would imply a need for medical attention. In the acute phase, regular administration of an antihistamine such as chlorphenamine should help rapidly relieve the symptoms. Ms FG should be warned that the ability of NSAIDs to worsen urticaria is a 'class effect' and that similar symptoms may be produced with drugs such as aspirin, meloxicam and naproxen.
3. Opiate analgesics lower the threshold for mast cell degranulation, which is the most important pathophysiological mechanism in the production of urticaria. Thus, morphine and related products such as codeine should be avoided.

Case 57.2

A 69-year-old male patient, Mr PH, with a history of psoriasis attends the pharmacy looking for advice. In the past, his skin disease has always been well controlled with topical preparations. Mr PH was recently admitted to hospital with a myocardial infarction and has noticed a marked deterioration in his psoriasis control since discharge. During his admission, he was commenced on:
• aspirin 75 mg daily,
• alopidogrel 75 mg daily,
• atorvastatin 80 mg daily,
• bisoprolol 2.5 mg daily,
• ramipril 2.5 mg daily.

Questions

1. What is the likely reason for the exacerbation of Mr PH's psoriasis?
2. How should this be treated?

Answers

1. Mr PH's psoriasis could have worsened due to the stress of his recent illness, but it is probably secondary to the introduction of bisoprolol or ramipril. Both β-blockers and ACE inhibitors have been associated with the worsening of psoriasis.
2. Given the recent myocardial infarct, any interruptions or substitutions to treatment must be made in conjunction with the patient's primary care doctor or cardiologist. The worsening of psoriasis with β-blockers is likely to be a class effect, and therefore substituting a different β-blocker is unlikely to resolve the problem. The treating physician may wish to prescribe a calcium channel blocker. If this does not ameliorate the situation, then the ACE inhibitor may be suspected, and trial stoppage may be considered. An ARB such as candesartan may be acceptable as an alternative.

Case 57.3

A 37-year-old man, Mr AG, presents with swelling of his upper lip. He asks if this could be stress induced because he has had several previous episodes of localised swelling of the face over the last 6–12 months.

Mr AG has been taking bendroflumethiazide and enalapril for hypertension for the last 3 years but has not taken any other medications recently.

Questions

1. What condition does Mr AG's symptoms suggest?
2. Could this be drug induced?
3. How should the condition be treated?

Answers

1. This pattern of localised swelling of the face is characteristic of angioedema.
2. Angioedema is a known adverse effect of ACE inhibitors with an overall incidence of 0.5–1%. Although this commonly occurs in the first week of treatment, delayed-onset angioedema can occur even after many years of treatment.
3. Because angioedema can be life-threatening, any suspect drug should be stopped. There is a very low incidence of this occurring with an ARB, and this may be a suitable alternative for this patient. The acute presentation of angioedema is treated with antihistamine and corticosteroids. If the patient presents with respiratory symptoms, subcutaneous epinephrine (adrenaline) is indicated.

Case 57.4

Miss AF is a 15-year-old renal transplant patient who attends the pharmacy 6 weeks after transplant. She is very distressed about the growth of facial hair and the worsening of acne.

Questions

1. What are the possible causes of Miss AF's skin complaints?
2. What other side effects should be enquired about?
3. How might these conditions be treated?

Answers

1. It is likely that Miss AF is receiving transplant immunosuppression that includes ciclosporin and prednisolone. The ciclosporin is most likely to have caused the growth of facial hair. Both the oral corticosteroid and the ciclosporin may have aggravated pre-existing acne or precipitated new-onset acne.
2. Ciclosporin may cause gingival hyperplasia, tremor, paraesthesia and nausea. Corticosteroids can cause increased appetite/weight gain, alterations of mood (euphoria, depression), sleep disturbance, gastritis and numerous other side effects.
3. Hirsutism is a side effect of ciclosporin that many young transplant patients have to cope with, and depilatory creams are commonly used. Tacrolimus is an alternative long-term immunosuppressant which is less likely to cause acne and hirsutism and which may be used in place of ciclosporin.

Case 57.5

An 85-year-old gentleman with rheumatoid arthritis, Mr DC, attends the local pharmacy with a persistent lesion on his anterior scalp (Fig. 57.7), which has recently been bleeding. For the last 18 years, his rheumatoid arthritis has been treated with methotrexate. You know Mr DC is a retired naval officer, and his skin is severely sun damaged. He tells you he has had a number of skin cancers in the past and is concerned that this may be another.

Questions

1. What is the likely diagnosis?
2. What risk factors does Mr DC have for this diagnosis?
3. How should he be advised?

Answers

1. This is likely to be a squamous cell carcinoma (SCC). Squamous cell carcinomas usually occur on sun-exposed sites and are related to high cumulative levels of sun exposure. They can have a number of different appearances but are generally hyperkeratotic nodules or nodules with a central keratin plug, as in this case.
2. Mr DC has a number of risk factors for developing an SCC:
   • Age: These lesions tend to occur in the older age group, presumably because of their high level of actinic damage accrued over many years. In addition, sunscreen was not as widely used in the mid- to late 20th century as it is today.

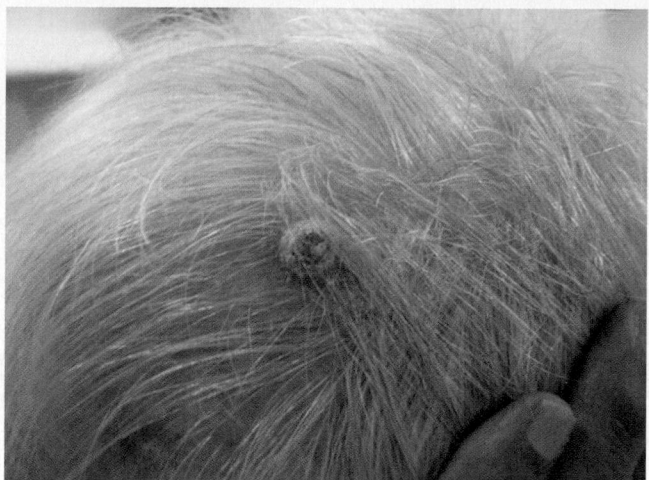

Fig. 57.7 A patient with squamous cell carcinoma.

- Immunosuppressed state: Mr. DC has been on an immuno-suppressant for 18 years, resulting in his tumour surveillance mechanisms being attenuated.
- Occupation: It is likely that Mr DC will have served in some very sunny climates. A history of active service with the Armed Forces should always prompt healthcare professionals to ask about the patient's history of sun exposure.
3. Firstly, Mr DC should be asked to consult his primary care doctor or dermatologist because the lesion will require treatment. If left unattended, squamous cell carcinomas continue to grow and can become locally invasive or can metastasise. Secondly, Mr. DC should be advised of the importance of sun protection, using a high-factor (30 or greater) sunscreen with good UVA protection (as indicated by the star rating system on the back of the bottle). A hat provides excellent cover for the scalp and face. The sun should be avoided completely between the hours of midday and 2 p.m., when the levels of ultraviolet light are at their highest.

Case 57.6

A 56-year-old man, Mr SW, presents to the pharmacy in an alarmed state. In recent months, he has had several episodes of gout and was recently prescribed allopurinol. He has now taken four doses of the drug. Last night, Mr SW developed an unusual rash on his palms and soles, which this morning has developed blisters. The rash has now extended to involve his arms and legs. He also complains of 'mouth ulcers', a gritty feeling in the eyes, and pain on passing urine. Mr SW is not feverish now but had a raised temperature overnight.

Questions

1. What is the likely diagnosis?
2. How should Mr SW be managed?

Answers

1. This patient is developing SJS. He has a blistering eruption which commenced peripherally, which is classical for this disorder. Mr SW now has evidence of mucosal site involvement, including the oral mucosa and conjunctivae, with urethral involvement suggested by his history of dysuria. Allopurinol is a common culprit for this condition.

2. Patients with suspected SJS need urgent dermatological assessment and often require in-patient care. The suspected drug should be withheld. After admission to hospital, a full blood count, urinalysis, blood culture, skin swabs and a chest X-ray should be performed to screen for infection. An ophthalmological opinion should be sought to ensure that no synechiae (scarring) of the eyes forms because this can occasionally arise with the degree of inflammation seen in this patient. Catheterisation is required if urethral mucosal involvement is suspected, to prevent strictures forming due to scarring. Mr SW should not be exposed to allopurinol or related drugs again because recurrence is likely.

Case 57.7

A 24-year-old female, Ms AM, was commenced on the combined oral contraceptive pill last month. Ms AM is concerned because she has noticed the appearance of raised red nodules on both shins, which are tender to touch and have been becoming more numerous over the last 3 days. She has never had any such eruption before. There is no recent travel history, and Ms AM has no rashes elsewhere, nor does she have any arthralgia.

Questions

1. What is your diagnosis?
2. What is the likely cause of Ms AM's eruption, and what are the other possible causes?
3. What is the prognosis?

Answers

1. Ms AM has developed erythema nodosum, an inflammatory condition seen on the anterior legs, usually bilaterally. *Erythema nodosum* is a Latin term meaning 'red lumps', it represents a pathological process in which subcutaneous fat becomes inflamed.
2. The combined oral contraceptive pill is the most likely precipitant in this case. However, a full drug and medical history should be taken because other medicines may cause erythema nodosum, for example, antibiotics or NSAIDs. A very common cause of erythema nodosum in young people is streptococcal throat infection. A travel history is important because the same clinical reaction pattern may be brought about by tuberculosis. Finally, a number of other medical problems, such as ulcerative colitis and Crohn's disease or sarcoidosis, may also produce erythema nodosum.
3. Ms AM should see a dermatologist to have the other causes of erythema nodosum excluded. The management of erythema nodosum is supportive, with regular NSAIDs or paracetamol given for pain. The combined oral contraceptive pill should be stopped, and Ms AM should be switched to a different form of contraception.

Case 57.8

A 17-year-old girl, Miss AW, asks for some advice regarding a widespread itchy rash which has appeared suddenly over the last 24 hours. Miss AW visited her primary care doctor 4 days ago complaining of a sore throat and a productive cough. Having auscultated the chest, the primary care doctor suspected a respiratory tract infection and prescribed amoxicillin. Five days later, Miss AW developed a widespread maculopapular rash. She attends the pharmacy for advice, and you suspect the rash to be drug-induced.

Questions

1. What is the cause of the eruption?
2. How should Miss AW be managed?
3. Should Miss AW be advised to avoid penicillin antibiotics in the future?

Answers

1. This is likely to be an amoxicillin-induced drug eruption.

2. The antibiotic should be stopped, and the clinical indication for an alternative preparation should be assessed by the primary care doctor. An antihistamine and a mild-/moderate-potency topical corticosteroid should provide symptomatic relief. If the patient does not obtain relief with such treatment, if the rash is becoming widespread or if there are any features of a systemic illness such as fever or enlarged lymph nodes, the patient should see the primary care doctor.

3. The reaction may be provoked by any antibiotic in the penicillin group, so the patient needs to be informed of the need to avoid all such antibiotics in the future.

References

Griffiths, C., Barker, J., Bleiker, T., et al., 2016. Drug eruptions. In: Burns, T., Breathnach, S.M., Cox, N., (Eds.), Rook's Textbook of Dermatology, eighth ed. Wiley Blackwell Publishing, Oxford.

Hausmann, O., Schnyder, B., Pichler, W.J., 2012. Etiology and pathogenesis of adverse drug reactions. Chem. Immunology Allergy. 97, 32–46. https://doi.org/10.1159/000335614.

Moncada, B., Sahagún-Sánchez, L.K., Torres-Álvarez, B., et al., 2009. Molecular structure and concentration of melanin in the stratum corneum of patients with melasma. Photodermatol. Photoimmunol. Photomed. 25, 159–160.

Po, A.L.W., Kendall, M.J., 2001. Causality assessment of adverse effects: when is re-challenge ethically acceptable? Drug Saf. 24, 793–799.

Susman, E., 2004. Rash correlates with tumour response after cetuximab. Lancet Oncol. 5 (11), 647.

Further reading

Brockow, K., Przybilla, B., Aberer, W., et al., 2015. Guideline for the diagnosis of drug hypersensitivity reactions: S2K-guideline of the German Society for Allergology and Clinical Immunology (DGAKI) and the German Dermatological Society (DDG) in collaboration with the Association of German Allergologists (AeDA), the German Society for Pediatric Allergology and Environmental Medicine (GPA), the German Contact Dermatitis Research Group (DKG), the Swiss Society for Allergy and Immunology (SGAI), the Austrian Society for Allergology and Immunology (OGAI), the German Academy of Allergology and Environmental Medicine (DAAU), the German Center for Documentation of Severe Skin Reactions and the German Federal Institute for Drugs and Medical Products (BfArM). Allergo J. Int. 24 (3), 94–105.

Litt, J.Z., 2016. Litt's Drug Eruption Reference Manual Including Drug Interactions, twenty-second ed. CRC Press, Boca Raton.

Weller, R.P.J.B., Hunter, H., Mann, M.W., 2015. Clinical Dermatology, fifth ed. Wiley-Blackwell, Oxford.

Useful websites

Drug Eruption Data: http://www.drugeruptiondata.com/

This is a subscription-only online resource linked to the *Litt's Drug Eruption Reference Manual* (cited in Further reading) which updates on a monthly basis all reports of new adverse drug reactions.

58 Eczema and Psoriasis

Richard Woolf and Nemesha Desai

Key points

- Eczema and psoriasis are chronic inflammatory skin diseases that are commonly encountered in clinical practice.

- Eczema and psoriasis manifest as erythematous and pruritic rashes; however, their aetiology, morphology and long-term treatment options differ significantly.

- Emollient therapy is a mainstay of treatment for most types of eczema, with active inflammation commonly treated using topical anti-inflammatory therapies, such as corticosteroids or calcineurin inhibitors.

- Eczematous skin can become secondarily infected, and appropriate recognition of secondary bacterial and viral infections is important.

- Mild-to-moderate psoriasis is often managed with topical therapies alone, such as steroids and vitamin D analogues, in combination with topical emollients.

- Severe psoriasis and severe atopic eczema may require treatment with a systemic agent. This will often be an immunosuppressive medication, such as methotrexate. In psoriasis, additional biologic agents have been developed that target specific inflammatory cytokine pathways. Acute eczema is often treated with systemic corticosteroids, but these should be avoided in patients with psoriasis. Therefore, when choosing a systemic therapy, both careful patient selection and regular monitoring are important.

- These conditions are chronic and have a significant impact on the individual's quality of life. Therefore, patient education and support are extremely important.

Eczema

Eczema refers to a group of conditions that are loosely defined by the development of ill-defined erythematous (red), scaly and pruritic (itchy) patches of skin inflammation. The terms 'eczema' and 'dermatitis' may be used interchangeably and describe the same clinical and histological entity. Although the morphological and histological findings in different eczemas may be similar, their pathologies can be quite different.

Pathology and clinical features

Acute eczema is an inflammatory process that leads to the accumulation of fluid (oedema) in the epidermis. This is seen histologically as epidermal 'spongiosis' and is associated with a predominantly lymphocytic infiltrate in the dermis. Clinically this manifests as a patch of inflamed scaly skin. The epidermal oedema can accumulate and evolve into tiny blisters (histologically intra-epidermal vesicles) that may then coalesce. These may appear as fragile ruptured vesicles at sites of inflammation, or as 'pompholyx' blisters on thicker palmar/plantar skin. Tightly packed keratinocyte cells in the epidermis usually provide a physical barrier that prevents transepidermal fluid loss and the entry of pathogens. This becomes impaired in eczema. A schematic diagram demonstrating the normal skin epidermis and the effects on the barrier function during an acute eczema flare is shown in Fig. 58.1. The main symptom that develops as a result of these pathological processes is itch, which can cause considerable distress to the patient.

In chronic eczema, prolonged scratching and rubbing results in thickening of the epidermis, with an increase in the upper horny cell layer of keratinocytes, which is termed hyperkeratosis. Clinically the skin appears thickened, leathery and 'lichenified', with exaggerated skin markings (Fig. 58.2).

Clinical types

Atopic eczema

The lifetime prevalence rate of atopic eczema is 10–20%, and the majority of cases develop in childhood, making it the commonest skin disorder of children (Deckers et al., 2012). The term 'atopy' describes an increased propensity to form IgE to common allergens. In atopic dermatitis, up to two-thirds of patients will have either elevated serum IgE levels or develop another associated atopic disorder, such as asthma or allergic rhinoconjunctivitis (hay fever). The molecular pathology of atopic eczema is complex and involves a combination of genetic, environmental and immunological factors. Genome-wide association studies (GWASs) have identified more than 30 susceptibility loci, with the strongest known genetic risk factor being a mutation in the gene that encodes the epidermal protein filaggrin, with other loci implicating additional epidermal barrier and immune-mediated mechanisms (Weidinger and Novak, 2016). It is hypothesised that disruption of the epidermal barrier leads to pathological inflammation in the skin, through the activation of keratinocytes, which in turn mediate innate immune responses, Langerhans cell activation, and T-helper type 2 (T_H2) lymphocyte activation. There is increasing evidence that the interaction between the impaired epidermis and this immune environment also facilitates percutaneous allergic sensitisation.

Despite this understanding of the molecular pathology of atopic eczema, it remains a clinical diagnosis. Diagnostic criteria have

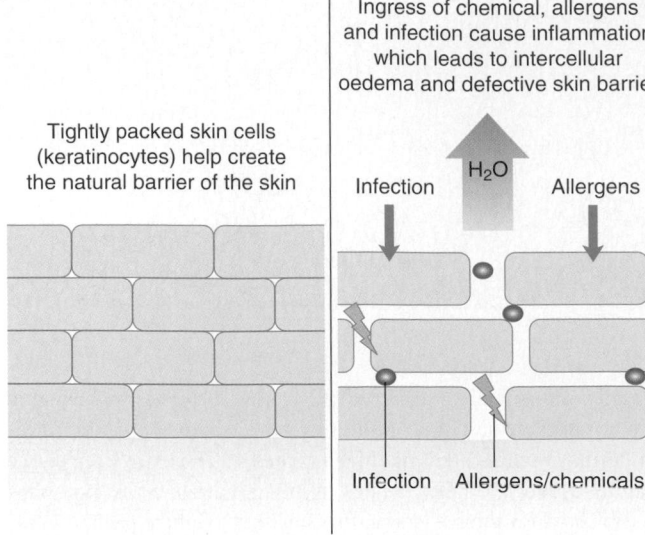

Fig. 58.1 Schematic diagram demonstrating the normal skin epidermis (left) and the effects on the barrier function (right) during an acute eczema flare.

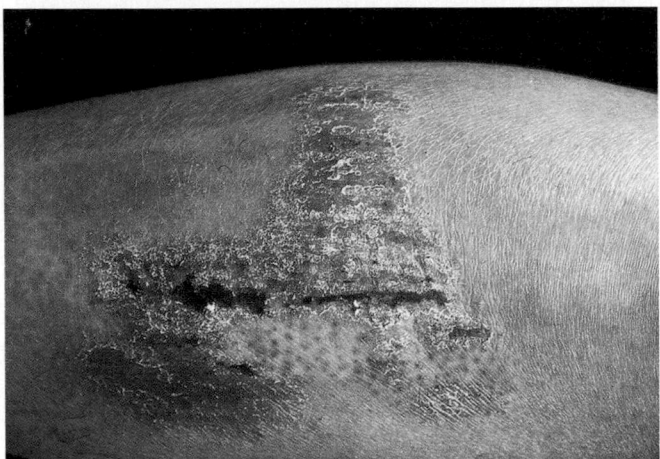

Fig. 58.2 Dry, excoriated, lichenified chronic eczema. (Courtesy of M. Carr.)

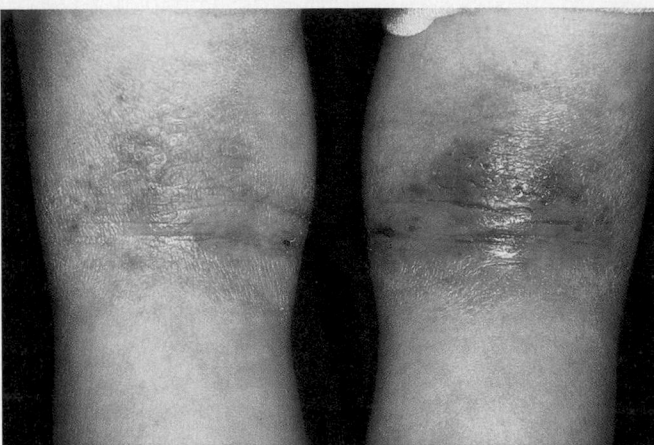

Fig. 58.3 Flexural eczema in childhood. (Courtesy of M. Carr.)

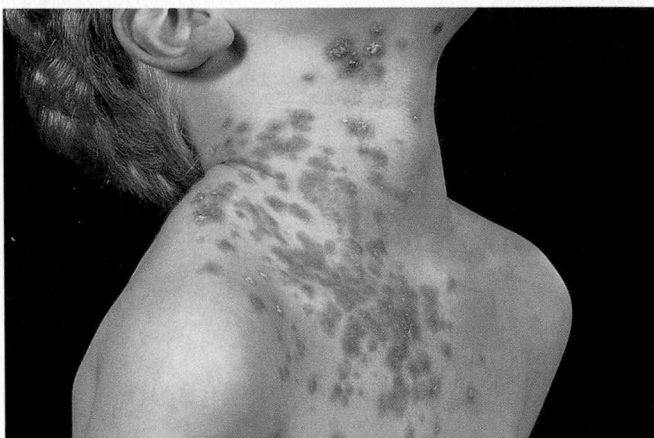

Fig. 58.4 Impetigo complicating atopic eczema. (Courtesy of M. Carr.)

been developed that define key features, such as a chronic relapsing eczema/dermatitis, pruritus, dry skin (xerosis) and a personal or family history of atopy (Brenninkmeijer et al., 2008). The clinical course and typical sites affected change through puberty and adulthood. In infants, common areas involved are the face, neck and limbs. Through childhood, flexural sites, such as folds of the elbows and backs of the knees, are classically affected (Fig. 58.3). In adults, this may go on to involve the hands and neck. Symptoms usually improve with age, and in approximately 60% of individuals atopic eczema resolves by the age of 16 years.

Exacerbating factors

A number of factors can aggravate atopic eczema:

- infection: bacterial or viral;
- irritants: soap, detergents, shower gels, bubble baths and water;
- allergens: contact, food, inhaled and airborne;
- dry environments;
- extremes of temperature;
- stress.

The commonest trigger of exacerbations of atopic eczema in the paediatric population is secondary infection. In atopic eczema there is reduced diversity in the normal skin microbiome, with the skin becoming colonised primarily by the bacterium *Staphylococcus aureus*. This is possibly due to the impaired barrier and aberrant innate and adaptive immune function of the skin of these individuals. *Staphylococcus aureus* can in turn contribute to flares and the chronification of atopic eczema (Fig. 58.4) through their production of proteases, the stimulation of innate immune pathways and the release of enterotoxins that act as T-cell superantigens. In addition, *Staphylococcus aureus* can cause pathological infection of the skin that will require antibiotic therapy. Viral infections, such as herpes simplex, may also complicate atopic eczema. In some cases this may lead to disseminated cutaneous herpes infection, known as eczema herpeticum or Kaposi's varicelliform eruption (Fig. 58.5). This can be a dermatological emergency and requires urgent assessment and treatment with a systemic antiviral agent, such as aciclovir.

In some cases of severe atopic eczema, especially in children, patients are also sensitised to certain foods. This may lead to either

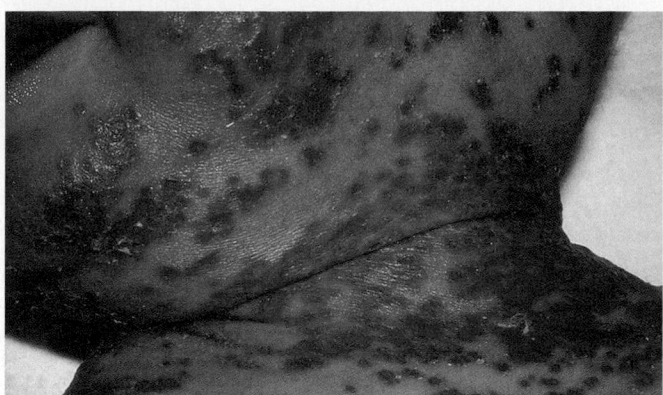

Fig. 58.5 Eczema herpeticum in an infant. (Courtesy of M. Carr.)

Table 58.1	Common locations for allergic contact dermatitis and possible sensitisers
Location	**Possible sensitising agents**
Periorbital	Airborne allergens, cosmetics, contact lens solution
Umbilicus	Nickel hypersensitivity to belt buckle or trouser button
Neck	Antiseptic in soap, cosmetics
Hairline/scalp	p-Phenylediamine in hair dye, hair perming solution
Hands	Latex or rubber accelerators in gloves, nickel, fragrances, protein contact dermatitis in food preparation, irritant contact dermatitis due to water

immediate immunoglobulin E (IgE)-mediated non-eczematous skin reactions, such as urticaria or angioedema, or delayed non-IgE-mediated flares of their eczema. If food allergy is suspected, these cases should be referred to an allergy specialist. Dietary restriction may be required, which should only be done under the supervision of a trained dietician. Although most paediatric food allergies that are associated with atopic eczema tend to resolve with time, allergies to nuts and fish often persist into adulthood.

Contact dermatitis

Contact dermatitis refers to the development of a chemical-induced eczematous rash that is usually limited to the site of cutaneous exposure to that chemical, and can be classified as either an allergic contact dermatitis (ACD) or irritant contact dermatitis (ICD).

Allergic contact dermatitis

ACD describes a delayed-type antigen-specific hypersensitivity reaction that develops upon re-exposure to an allergen to which the host immune system has been previously sensitised. Therefore, symptoms rarely develop on early exposure to the allergen, with the allergic reaction often manifesting months or years after the primary exposure. However, this will depend on when sensitisation or re-exposure occurs.

Many common compounds can lead to ACD:

- metals (e.g. nickel and cobalt),
- medications (e.g. neomycin, a topical antibiotic),
- fragrances (e.g. Balsam of Peru),
- rubber compounds,
- hair dyes (e.g. p-phenylenediamine),
- preservatives (e.g. formaldehyde and formaldehyde-releasing compounds),
- plants (e.g. poison ivy).

The diagnosis of ACD relies heavily on a detailed patient history, as well as recognising the pattern and distribution of the eczematous rash. Although the signs are usually localised to the area exposed to the allergen, a secondary generalised eczema may develop ('autoeczematisation'). When ACD is considered, the standard diagnostic investigation is patch testing, which can differentiate between allergic and irritant causes of contact

dermatitis. This involves the application of a panel of compounds to the patient's back for 48 hours (day 2). A standard panel of potential allergens is tested with and without additional specialised panels for certain allergens (e.g. fragrances), depending on the clinical presentation. This is followed by clinical examination for a cutaneous reaction at days 2 and 4. Identification of the relevant compound allows the patient to avoid the substance in the future, which should reduce symptoms. Common areas of the body affected by ACD, with corresponding potential sensitisers, are listed in Table 58.1.

Irritant contact dermatitis

ICD is the most common form of occupational dermatitis and hand eczema. ICD is not the result of an adaptive immune response to a sensitising agent, but is due to the direct cytotoxic effects of the agent on the skin. This leads to disruption of the epidermal barrier and cutaneous inflammation, which manifests as an acute eczema. Patients with pre-existing epidermal barrier dysfunction, such as atopic eczema, are at higher risk of ICD. Common irritants include detergents, oils, water, inorganic acids, alkalis, alcohols and plastics. Therefore, the occupation of the individual may also be a risk factor, especially those working as builders, hairdressers, gardeners, healthcare workers and chefs. Patch testing may be required to exclude ACD. Management of ICD is primarily with preventative skin care, which includes the use of barriers, such as emollients or cotton gloves, in addition to avoiding suspected irritants.

Discoid eczema

Discoid eczema is a type of disseminated chronic eczema that is also known as nummular dermatitis. It presents with coin-shaped eczematous lesions that are typically intensely pruritic and often on the limbs. Lesions can be very inflamed with vesicles, weep serous fluid and have evidence of secondary bacterial infection. Management is primarily with regular emollients and moderate- to potent-strength topical corticosteroids. Secondary infection should be treated with appropriate topical/systemic antibiotics. If poorly controlled with topical therapy, patients with discoid eczema may require treatment with a systemic agent as in severe atopic eczema.

Dyshidrotic eczema

Dyshidrotic eczema is also known as pompholyx or vesicular palmoplantar dermatitis. It is an eczema that affects the palms and/or soles and is characterised by the development of small and intensely pruritic vesicles, often along the edge of the palms, fingers or soles. These can coalesce to form larger blisters. There is also often thickening of the epidermis, which can become cracked and painful. Management is primarily with regular ointment emollients and moderate- to potent-strength topical corticosteroids.

Stasis eczema

Stasis eczema is also known as stasis dermatitis, gravitational dermatitis or varicose eczema. Clinical features include scaly eczematous plaques confined to the lower legs. Stasis eczema is one component of several clinical changes seen in chronic venous insufficiency, which include varicose veins, peripheral oedema, skin discolouration, subcutaneous fibrotic changes (lipodermatosclerosis) and chronic ulceration. Often multiple topical medications and dressings have been used in this setting, which may also lead to contact dermatitis. Management of the underlying venous stasis should improve the stasis eczema, which can also be symptomatically controlled with regular emollients, soap substitutes and moderate-strength topical corticosteroids.

Asteatotic eczema

Asteatotic eczema usually affects the legs and presents as dry, cracked skin that is likened to 'crazy paving' and is also described as eczema craquelé. Asteatotic eczema can be inflamed and intensely pruritic. It is associated with older age, low humidity and frequent bathing. Management is primarily with regular emollients, soap substitutes and moderate-strength topical corticosteroids.

Seborrhoeic dermatitis

Seborrhoeic dermatitis (syn. Seborrhoeic eczema) is a common disorder that is usually confined to areas with high sebum production. The aetiology is not known but thought to involve an overgrowth of the commensal yeast *Malassezia furfur* (*Pityrosporum ovale*) at these sites. In adults the clinical features are pink-yellow greasy patches of dermatitis with overlying 'greasy' scale, typically in the sebaceous-rich scalp, nasal folds, medial eyebrow, presternal region and flexural sites. In babies, seborrhoeic dermatitis can manifest in the first few months of life as coherent scaling of the scalp with dermatitis and ooze, known as 'cradle cap'. In adults, the symptoms are usually mild with a chronic, relapsing course. More severe seborrhoeic dermatitis is seen in patients with human immunodeficiency virus (HIV) infection or Parkinson's disease. Management usually includes topical antifungals, such as imidazoles (shampoo or cream preparations), and topical anti-inflammatory agents, such as corticosteroids or calcineurin inhibitors.

Treatment

The management of eczema is targeted at improving symptoms and long-term disease control. This involves avoiding exacerbants (which is particularly relevant in contact dermatitis), supporting the barrier function of the skin with regular emollients and soap substitutes, and immunosuppressive medications to limit cutaneous inflammation. Immunosuppressant agents are most commonly used as topical preparations, such as corticosteroids or calcineurin inhibitors; however, severe disease, such as in atopic or discoid eczema, may require a systemic agent. Systemic agents used in atopic eczema include oral prednisolone, methotrexate, ciclosporin, azathioprine or mycophenolate mofetil. Phototherapy may also be of benefit in these patients.

Secondary bacterial infection should be treated with topical/systemic antibiotics; however, these patients have often been exposed to multiple antibiotics, hence bacterial resistance is common. The decision to treat with antibiotics should therefore be carefully considered, and if possible, the choice of agent guided by in vitro bacterial sensitivities as determined by skin swab and culture results. If there is an associated viral infection, this should be confirmed with viral skin swab and polymerase chain reaction assay, and the patient initiated on a systemic antiviral agent, such as aciclovir.

Emollients

Emollients are topical hydrating agents that form a lipid barrier on the surface of the skin, which prevents trans-epidermal water loss and therefore improves hydration of the epidermis. Emollients can be ointment preparations that only contain lipid(s), or lotions and creams that also contain water and emulsifying agents. Emollients are the mainstay of eczema management because a defective skin barrier is central to the pathogenesis and so they are an effective first-line treatment. Regular, liberal use of emollients will reduce physical irritation from dry, scaly skin and can reduce topical corticosteroid requirements. Greasier products that have a higher lipid content have a greater emollient effect; however, they may be less well tolerated by patients and may be impractical for regular use throughout the day. Dry and inflamed skin is often aggravated by soaps and bathing products. Therefore, patients with chronic inflammatory skin conditions, such as eczema, should be advised to use an emollient as a soap substitute for washing.

Emollients are often underused. It is important that patients are educated to use appropriate quantities of emollient and have ongoing access to sufficient amounts. Restoring the barrier function of the skin is important in atopic eczema, and it has been reported that the use of liberal full-body emollients can in fact reduce the risk of development of atopic eczema by up to 50% in high-risk infants (Horimukai et al., 2014; Simpson et al., 2014).

Bandaging

In chronic atopic eczema, occlusion with bandages is useful to prevent scratching and to potentiate the action of ointments and creams on the skin. 'Wet wrapping' involves the application of

Table 58.2 Comparative potencies of topical corticosteroid preparations

UK steroid group	Trade name	Strength	Relative strength compared with hydrocortisone
Hydrocortisone 0.5–2.5%	Hydrocortisone	Mild	1
Fluocinolone acetonide 0.0025%	Synalar 1:10 dilution		
Betamethasone valerate 0.025%	Betnovate RD	Moderately potent	2.5× stronger
Clobetasone butyrate 0.05%	Eumovate		
Fluocinolone acetonide 0.00625%	Synalar 1 in 4 dilution		
Fludroxycortide 0.0125%	Haelan		
Betamethasone valerate 0.1%	Betnovate	Potent	10× stronger
Mometasone furoate 0.1%	Elocon		
Clobetasol propionate 0.05%	Dermovate	Very potent	50× stronger

emollients, with or without topical corticosteroids steroids, under double-layer cotton bandaging to keep the inner layer moist. This approach is more commonly used in children, and parents can be trained to apply these bandages at home. 'Wet wrapping' should not be done if there is concern that the eczema may be secondarily infected because the occlusion may spread the infection.

Topical corticosteroids

Topical corticosteroids are an important agent in the management of acute eczema and form first-line anti-inflammatory treatment. Topical corticosteroids are classified into four main groups according to their strength of action: mild, moderate, potent and very potent (Table 58.2). The choice of topical corticosteroid is dependent on the severity of skin disease and body site where they will be used. Potent and very potent corticosteroids are an effective treatment for the trunk and limbs, but should be avoided on delicate sites such as the face, genitals and flexures, unless under specialist supervision. The periorbital region should be treated with caution because of the thin skin, increasing the likelihood of absorption and risk of cataracts or glaucoma with chronic exposure.

In acute active eczema, patients should be advised to use an appropriate strength topical corticosteroid for that body site once or twice daily. Treatment should be reviewed regularly and tailored accordingly (Hoare et al., 2000). The recommended amount used can be quantified using a fingertip unit (Fig. 58.6), which is the quantity required to cover an area the size of two adult palms. Table 58.3 details the quantities for application to different sites required for twice-daily treatment for 1 week. Under specialist supervision, topical corticosteroids can also be used under occlusion with a dressing or bandage, which will increase absorption and potentiate their actions. There is some evidence in atopic eczema that long-term intermittent application of topical steroid, such as on 2 days of the week, can limit disease relapses (Hoare et al., 2000).

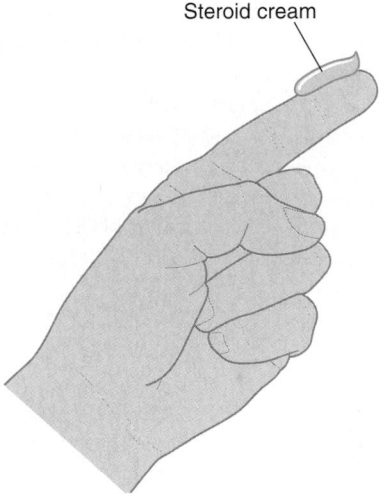

Steroid cream

Fig. 58.6 Recommended amount of a topical corticosteroid corresponding to one fingertip unit. The finger tip unit (FTU) is equivalent to approximately 0.5 grams of cream/ointment and should cover a skin area of about two palms (20 cm²).

Table 58.3 Minimum quantity (grams) of topical application required for twice-daily treatment for 1 week

Age	Whole body	Trunk	Both arms and legs
6 Months	35	15	20
4 Years	60	20	35
8 Years	90	35	50
12 Years	120	45	65
Adult (70 kg)	170	60	90

Courtesy of M. Carr.

Topical corticosteroids are available in a range of preparations that include ointments (oil based), creams (water based) and aqueous/alcohol solutions. In general, ointment preparations are preferable to creams in eczema management because they are absorbed better and have fewer additional preservatives. Alcoholic solutions may lead to irritation and should not be applied to acutely inflamed or broken skin. Foam and shampoo formulations are available for hair-bearing sites, such as the scalp.

Adverse effects of chronic topical corticosteroid use are mainly limited to the sites where the steroid is applied and include hypopigmentation (temporary), epidermal thinning, telangiectasia (visible dilated small blood vessels), bruising, striae (stretch marks) and acneiform rashes. Less common side effects may include poor wound healing, spread or worsening of untreated infections and hypertrichosis. Rarely chronic widespread use of potent or very potent topical corticosteroids can lead to systemic absorption, adrenal suppression and Cushing's syndrome. In addition, patients can become sensitised to topical corticosteroid preparations. Such reactions may be directly to the steroid medication, with some cross-reactivity between different steroids, or a component of the vehicle/base. In patients with chronic eczema that is poorly responsive or possibly exacerbated by topical steroids, patch testing should be considered.

Patients and non-specialists often have high levels of anxiety regarding the potential adverse effects of topical corticosteroids. This commonly leads to undertreatment in adults and children. Local and systemic side effects are rare following the appropriate use and duration of topical corticosteroid treatment. Eczema education programmes are a crucial part of eczema management and should include advice about the safe and effective use of topical corticosteroids.

Antibiotics and corticosteroid combinations

Combination preparations can be useful in treating mild bacterial infection of eczematous skin. Long-term use should be limited because of the risks for sensitisation and antibiotic resistance. In general, invasive bacterial infections are best managed with systemic antibiotics.

Calcineurin inhibitors

Topical calcineurin inhibitors are an anti-inflammatory class of medication that act by blocking the intracellular phosphatase enzyme calcineurin, which is important in lymphocyte activation during inflammatory responses. They offer an alternative to topical corticosteroids and are primarily used as second-line agents, with the aim of avoiding or reducing topical corticosteroid use. Topical pimecrolimus 1% cream is licensed in the UK for mild-to-moderate atopic eczema and is often used to treat the face and neck in children aged 2 years or older. Topical tacrolimus ointment is more effective than pimecrolimus (Paller et al., 2005), is licensed in the UK for moderate-to-severe atopic eczema and is often used in adults (0.03% and 0.1%) and children older than 2 years (0.03%). Topical calcineurin inhibitors also have a role in the long-term prevention of eczema exacerbations with

application to troublesome sites on 2 consecutive days a week reducing flares.

The main side effect of topical calcineurin inhibitors is a burning or stinging sensation after initial application, but this usually improves after a few days, and patients should be advised of this. Rare cases of malignancy (e.g. skin cancer and lymphoma) have been reported in patients treated with these agents. However, a causal relationship has not been established, and although large case-control studies have demonstrated an increased risk of lymphoma associated with increased atopic eczema severity, this was not associated with topical calcineurin inhibitor use (Eichenfield et al., 2014). Therefore, patients should use these agents within licensed indications and be monitored if they use prolonged regimens. Calcineurin inhibitors should be avoided in infected eczema and are generally not as effective as corticosteroids in acutely inflamed eczema. Therefore, their greatest value is in maintenance therapy regimens.

Antihistamines

Pruritus is a prominent and distressing feature of eczema. Oral antihistamines have little direct effect on pruritus in atopic eczema, but may lead to some relief because of their sedating effect, especially overnight. Sedating antihistamines may cause daytime drowsiness, and so caution should be taken if patients are driving or operating machinery or if prescribed to school-aged children.

Coal tar preparations

Tar creams and ointments can be used in the management of hyperkeratotic, lichenified eczema. These are less cosmetically acceptable than other topical preparations, but coal tar is also an effective antipruritic.

Systemic therapies

Corticosteroids

Systemic corticosteroids (e.g. oral prednisolone 0.5 mg/kg) are an effective first-line short-term treatment in the management of severe acute eczema that needs rapid control. Long-term treatment with systemic corticosteroids is now rarely used because of the risk of long-term side effects, including infections, hypertension, diabetes mellitus, osteoporosis and adrenal suppression.

Ciclosporin

Ciclosporin is a calcineurin inhibitor that blocks lymphocyte activation and is used as an oral preparation in the treatment of atopic eczema. It is effective as a short-term bridging therapy in severe chronic adult eczema and is licensed for its treatment. It has a rapid onset of action with an approximate 50% improvement seen by 6–8 weeks of treatment (Schmitt et al., 2007; Roekevisch et al., 2014). Intermittent courses for 3 months at doses of 2.5–5 mg/kg per day are useful in controlling eczema, but dose-related (cumulative) renal nephrotoxicity limits treatment to a maximum duration of 12 months. Other side effects include hypertension and increased risk of malignancy, and a detailed patient history should identify previous skin or cervical malignancy. During treatment with ciclosporin, patients require close monitoring, notably of renal function and blood pressure.

Azathioprine

Azathioprine is a purine analogue that inhibits DNA synthesis. It is used as an unlicensed oral preparation in the treatment of atopic eczema and is effective with a mean 50% improvement seen after 12–24 weeks (Roekevisch et al., 2014). Bone marrow suppression is a major concern. Before azathioprine initiation, patients should have their thiopurine methyltransferase (TPMT) activity determined, because reduced/absent levels are associated with an increased risk of toxicity. Azathioprine should be avoided in individuals with absent TPMT activity, and the dose reduced in those with low TPMT activity. During treatment with azathioprine, patients require close monitoring, notably of full blood count and liver function.

Methotrexate

Methotrexate is an antimetabolite that in its active form inhibits purine and pyrimidine synthesis, required for DNA synthesis, and leads to the accumulation of extracellular adenosine, which has anti-inflammatory effects. It is used as an unlicensed oral or subcutaneous preparation in the treatment of atopic eczema, with some evidence that subcutaneous delivery leads to greater bioavailability. Methotrexate, given once a week, has a similar efficacy to azathioprine at 12–24 weeks of treatment (Roekevisch et al., 2014). The main side effect that patients report with methotrexate therapy is nausea. Concomitant folic acid is often given to reduce toxicity. During treatment with methotrexate, patients require close monitoring, notably of full blood count and liver function. Conception should be avoided during and for at least 3 months after methotrexate treatment in either men or women because of teratogenic risk.

Mycophenolate mofetil

Mycophenolate mofetil prevents T- and B-cell proliferation and is used as an unlicensed oral agent in the treatment of atopic eczema. Although it has a favourable side-effect profile, it is often used as a third-line agent because there is little clinical trial evidence supporting its use in atopic eczema. During treatment with mycophenolate mofetil, patients require close monitoring, notably of full blood count. Conception should be avoided during and for up to 6 weeks (women) or 12 weeks (men) after mycophenolate mofetil treatment because of teratogenic risk.

Phototherapy

Phototherapy can be effective in some patients with atopic eczema, and narrow-band ultraviolet B (UVB) is the therapy of choice (Gambichler et al., 2005; Meduri et al., 2007). Potential adverse events associated with all types of phototherapy include burning, premature ageing and an increased risk of skin cancer that increases with cumulative treatment. A small proportion of patients may have photosensitive eczema, which should be screened for before phototherapy (either a history of photo-aggravated eczema or by formal photo-testing). A treatment course requires a patient to attend two or three times a week for at least 6 weeks.

Patient care

Treatment failure is often due to poor adherence, which can be due to poor information about treatments or inconvenient/impractical regimens. In addition, it is important to recognise that eczema affects many aspects of a patient's life, including social interactions and schooling/work, and can have considerable effects on the family. Additional quality-of-life factors affected in eczema include body image, irritability and loss of sleep due to profound itch (Fig. 58.7). A multidisciplinary approach is often needed in overcoming these issues, and healthcare workers including primary care doctors, dermatologists, specialist nurses and pharmacists may be involved. Treatment regimens should be kept as simple as possible and be tailored to the individual patient, with time taken to clearly explain both the disease process and the treatment goals. Patient and parental education is important because treatments are designed to control and manage the disease. Although atopic eczema is likely to improve throughout childhood, expectations of an immediate cure need to be addressed. Trained nurses or clinical psychologists can provide additional support, and nurse-led clinics improve disease severity and quality-of-life outcomes (Ersser et al., 2014). Patients with eczema should aim to lead as normal a life as possible, and school staff and employers can play an important part in achieving this goal. Advice and support through contact with other patients and their families can be obtained from the National Eczema Society (http://www.eczema.org).

An algorithm for the management of eczema is shown in Fig. 58.8.

Psoriasis

Psoriasis is a chronic inflammatory disorder of the skin that affects approximately 2% of the population in Europe and North America. The usual presentation is with well-demarcated erythematous

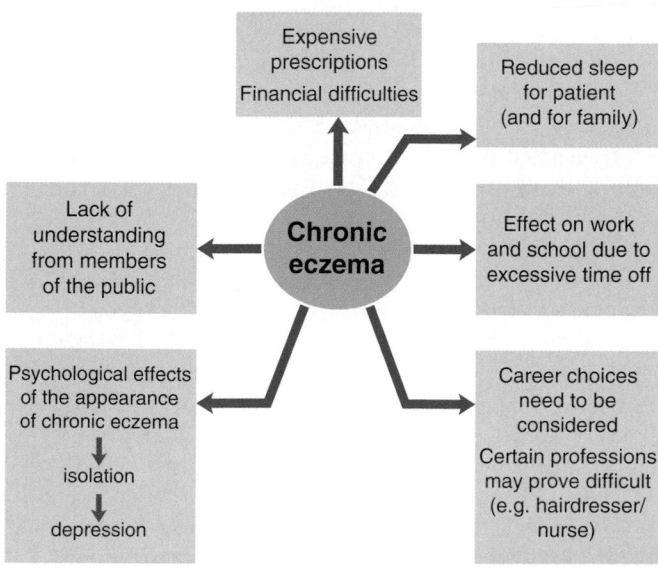

Fig. 58.7 The social and psychological effects of chronic eczema.

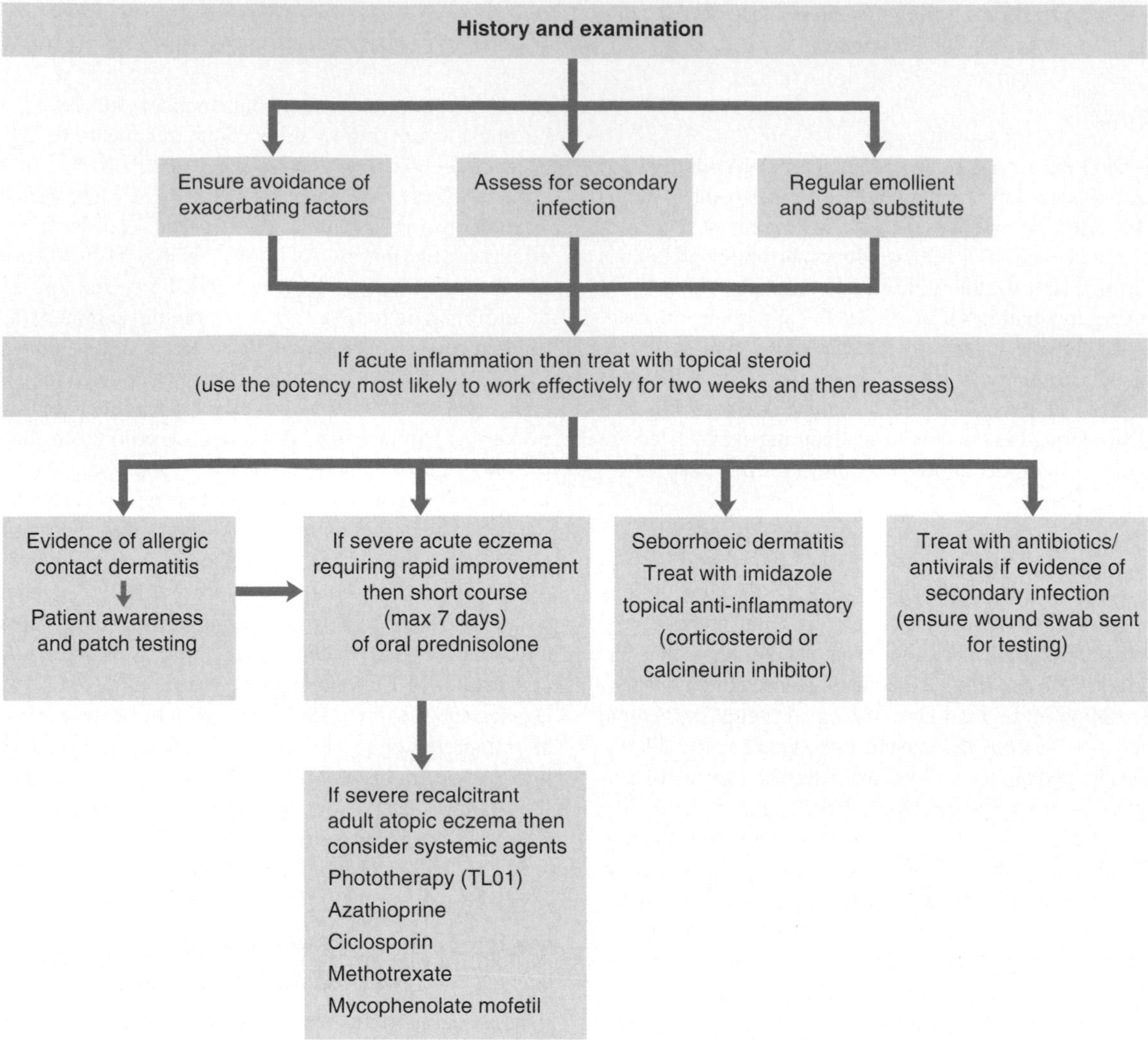

History and examination

- Ensure avoidance of exacerbating factors
- Assess for secondary infection
- Regular emollient and soap substitute

If acute inflammation then treat with topical steroid
(use the potency most likely to work effectively for two weeks and then reassess)

Evidence of allergic contact dermatitis
↓
Patient awareness and patch testing

If severe acute eczema requiring rapid improvement then short course (max 7 days) of oral prednisolone

Seborrhoeic dermatitis
Treat with imidazole topical anti-inflammatory (corticosteroid or calcineurin inhibitor)

Treat with antibiotics/ antivirals if evidence of secondary infection (ensure wound swab sent for testing)

If severe recalcitrant adult atopic eczema then consider systemic agents
Phototherapy (TL01)
Azathioprine
Ciclosporin
Methotrexate
Mycophenolate mofetil

Fig. 58.8 Algorithm for the management of eczema.

plaques with an overlying scale (Fig. 58.9). Common sites affected include the scalp, buttocks, elbows, knees and nails. Although psoriasis is often thought of as limited to the skin, up to 25% of patients also have an associated psoriatic arthropathy (Zachariae, 2003), and moderate-to-severe psoriasis is associated with an increased risk of cardiovascular disease and death (Mehta et al., 2010). In addition, psoriasis causes significant psychosocial morbidity to those affected, resulting in an impaired quality of life.

Pathology and clinical features

The aetiology of psoriasis, as with atopic eczema, is complex and involves a combination of genetic, environmental and immunological factors. Genetic predisposition is important, with a high degree of heritability demonstrated in both linkage and twin studies, and up to 70% of patients report a family history of psoriasis. More recently, GWASs have identified more than 40 susceptibility loci that implicate skin barrier function, innate immunity and adaptive immunity in the disease pathogenesis (Mahil et al., 2015).

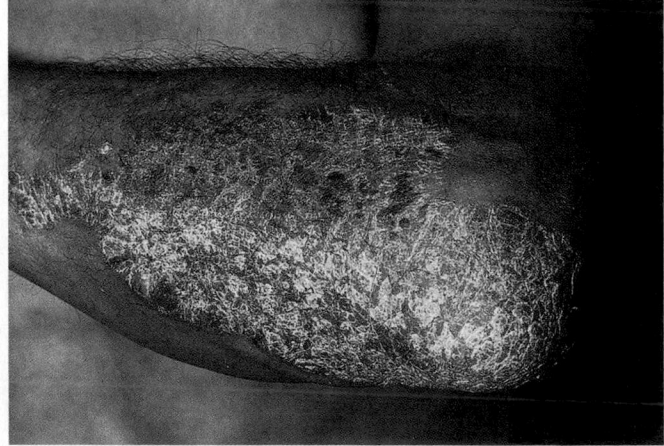

Fig. 58.9 Chronic scaly plaque psoriasis on an elbow. (Courtesy of M. Carr.)

Immune cell activation is central to the pathogenesis of psoriasis, with genetic variation within the major histocompatibility class I region giving the strongest association signal in all GWASs, primarily because of variation in the HLA-Cw6 allele (Mahil et al., 2015). It is hypothesised that, in a predisposed individual, after exposure to uncertain triggers (such as microbial products) there is a complex interaction between cells of both innate and adaptive immunity, including certain dendritic and T-cell subsets (Nestle et al., 2009). These interactions lead to the development of T_H1- and T_H17-mediated immune responses within the skin. As a result, keratinocytes are inappropriately activated, resulting in their hyper-proliferation and the development of a psoriatic plaque. The importance of key inflammatory pathways, such as the cytokines tumour necrosis factor-α (TNF-α), interleukin (IL)-23 and IL-17, has been demonstrated in genetic and immunological studies. This has been confirmed by the response of patients with psoriasis to treatments that either target T cells or specifically block these pro-inflammatory cytokine pathways (Nestle et al., 2009).

Psoriatic plaques are histologically characterised by epidermal hyperplasia (acanthosis), with a thickened upper horny layer (hyperkeratosis), which is reflected by the clinical features of thick, scaly skin. The buildup of scale is due to increased epidermal turnover. The differentiation of cells through the epidermis normally takes approximately 40 days, but in psoriatic skin may be as rapid as 7 days. In the dermis, superficial capillaries proliferate and are dilated, which explains why psoriatic plaques appear erythematous and bleed after minimal trauma/scraping off scale (Auspitz sign). There is a dense dermal lymphocytic infiltrate, with inflammatory cells also migrating up into the epidermis, where granulocytes form microabscesses.

Precipitating factors

Extrinsic factors also have a role in triggering or exacerbating psoriasis in predisposed individuals. These are described as follows.

Infections

It has been hypothesised that bacterial antigens have a role in triggering psoriasis. Streptococcal infections, particularly pharyngitis, frequently precede the onset of guttate psoriasis. In addition, psoriasis in individuals with HIV infection is often more severe.

Drugs

Certain drugs can exacerbate or induce psoriasis in predisposed individuals. The most common agents implicated are lithium, β-blockers, certain antimalarial medications, non-steroidal anti-inflammatory drugs (NSAIDs), tetracyclines and the rapid withdrawal of systemic corticosteroids.

Koebner phenomenon

The Koebner phenomenon refers to the development of psoriatic lesions at sites of skin injury, such as surgical cars, burns and trauma. Certain other inflammatory skin conditions also show koebnerisation.

Alcohol and smoking

Excess alcohol consumption may exacerbate established psoriasis. In addition, psoriasis is associated with high rates of alcoholism, which is thought to be due to the psychological burden of having the condition.

Smoking is strongly associated with palmoplantar psoriasis, with up to 95% of individuals who develop this variant being smokers at its onset. Smoking cessation should be actively discussed with patients because it may improve the psoriasis severity and help reduce the risk of cardiovascular and/or respiratory disease.

Emotional stress

Anecdotal observations and frequent patient reports identify stress as an important trigger factor for psoriasis, with some evidence demonstrating that the onset and severity of psoriasis can correlate with prior stress (Kirby et al., 2008). Furthermore, psoriasis can cause considerable psychological distress and depression.

Clinical types

Psoriasis vulgaris

Psoriasis vulgaris is also known as chronic plaque psoriasis and is the most common subtype of psoriasis, affecting 85–90% of patients. Psoriasis vulgaris most commonly develops in young adults and has a chronic relapsing course. It can, however, develop in individuals of any age, with childhood and late-onset adult variants described. The typical psoriatic lesion is an erythematous well-demarcated plaque with overlying scale. Classically there are multiple lesions that are distributed symmetrically to involve extensor sites, such as the elbows, knees and buttocks. Other sites commonly affected are the sacrum, umbilicus and ears. Involvement of the scalp may be the only manifestation of psoriasis in some patients, which typically affects the anterior hairline or post-auricular scalp but can also be more extensive. Associated hair loss is rare. Psoriatic plaques may itch but not usually to the same extent as eczematous lesions.

Guttate psoriasis

Guttate psoriasis is more commonly seen in children and young adults, and is characterised by a widespread eruption of small (<1 cm) scaly plaques on the trunk and limbs (Fig. 58.10). The presentation is often acute and can appear 10–14 days after a streptococcal upper respiratory tract infection. Topical treatments or UVB phototherapy are usually effective. Guttate psoriasis often resolves; however, it may be the first presentation of psoriasis vulgaris in some individuals.

Generalised pustular psoriasis

Generalised pustular psoriasis is an acute, unstable form of psoriasis that manifests as widespread annular erythematous patches with 'sheets' of tiny sterile pustules, which typically develop towards the edge of the patches. This rare but severe subtype

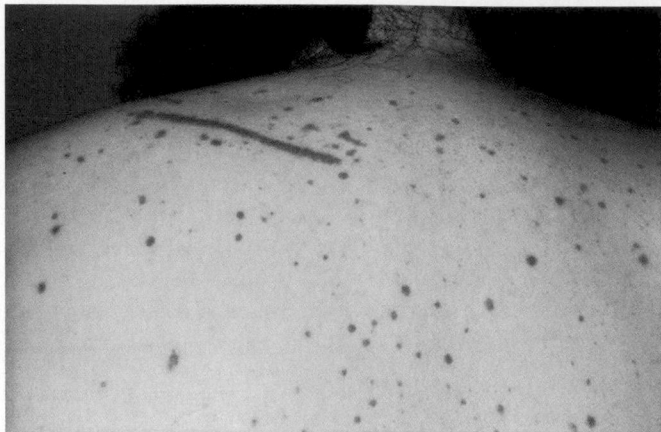

Fig. 58.10 Guttate psoriasis showing Koebner phenomenon in scratch mark. (Courtesy of M. Carr.)

of psoriasis has been shown in genetic studies to have a distinct pathogenesis to psoriasis vulgaris, with the IL-1 pathway and mutations in the *IL36RN* gene implicated (Onoufriadis et al., 2011). Patients with generalised pustular psoriasis can be systemically unwell with fever and general malaise, and their presentation may be a dermatological emergency. Flares of pustular psoriasis can also be precipitated by the withdrawal of systemic or potent topical corticosteroids in patients with known pustular psoriasis or psoriasis vulgaris. Systemic corticosteroids should therefore be avoided in patients with known psoriasis.

Palmoplantar psoriasis

Palmoplantar psoriasis describes psoriasis limited to the palms and soles, where there is sharp demarcation of the involved areas. It can take two forms: either inflamed hyperkeratotic fissured skin, which can be very painful or sterile pustules on an erythematous base which dry to leave small brown macules (palmoplantar pustulosis) (Fig. 58.11). Pustular palmoplantar psoriasis is more common in smokers.

Flexural psoriasis

Psoriasis can occur at flexural sites, such as the axillae, submammary areas, groin, perineum and genitalia. Psoriasis at these sites can differ in appearance from classical psoriasis and although well-demarcated, they tend to be red and shiny, rather than scaly. Secondary infection, particularly with *Candida*, is common. Potent corticosteroids are not advised at these sites because of the risk of skin atrophy. Management is primarily with combined preparations that include mild- to moderate-strength corticosteroids and antifungals, with or without antibiotics.

Erythrodermic psoriasis

Erythroderma, or exfoliative dermatitis, is a severe, potentially life-threatening condition in which greater than 90% of the body surface is erythematous (Fig. 58.12). Erythroderma can occur as a consequence of several different skin conditions, which include psoriasis, as well as eczema, drug eruptions and cutaneous T-cell lymphoma. When large areas of skin are inflamed, its function

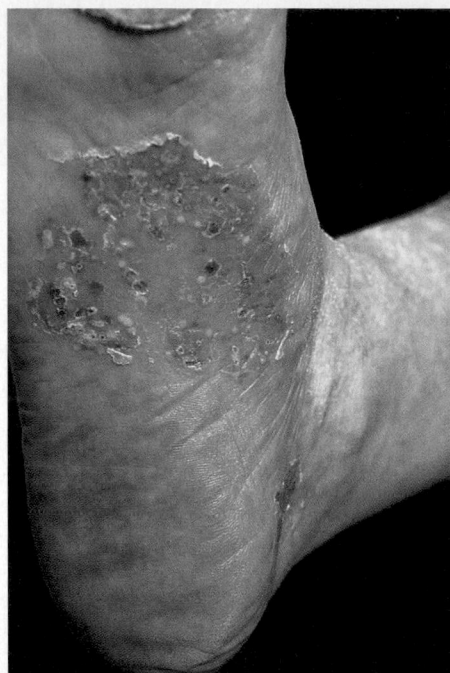

Fig. 58.11 Pustular psoriasis of sole. (Courtesy of M. Carr.)

is significantly impaired and patients suffer dehydration, electrolyte imbalance, temperature dysregulation, and potential serious secondary infection. This is a dermatological emergency, and acutely unwell patients need urgent hospital admission, supportive medical care and topical treatment. Initially, bland emollients (e.g. white soft paraffin) and mild-to-moderate topical corticosteroids should be used. Once a diagnosis is established, often after a skin biopsy, the underlying condition, such as psoriasis, can be treated with appropriate systemic agents.

Psoriatic arthropathy

Up to 25% of patients with psoriasis will also be affected by an associated psoriatic arthropathy (Zachariae, 2003). There are several distinct patterns of psoriatic arthritis that include asymmetrical mono-/oligo-arthritis, symmetrical polyarthritis, distal small joint arthritis, sacroiliitis and arthritis mutilans. Psoriatic arthritis is also associated with enthesitis and tendonitis, and can present as an acutely swollen finger/toe (dactylitis). These patients are rheumatoid factor negative (seronegative), and the arthritis may precede skin findings. Concomitant psoriatic arthritis may indicate the need for systemic treatment and determine the choice of agent, such as methotrexate or biologics that block TNF-α or IL-17. These patients should be jointly managed with a rheumatologist.

Psoriatic nail disease

The nails are frequently affected in psoriasis, and changes seen include nail pitting, nail ridging, onycholysis (separation of the nail from the nail bed), hyperkeratosis under the nail and complete nail destruction. It is thought that some of these changes may represent underlying enthesitis. In a small proportion of patients only the nails are affected with no other skin signs.

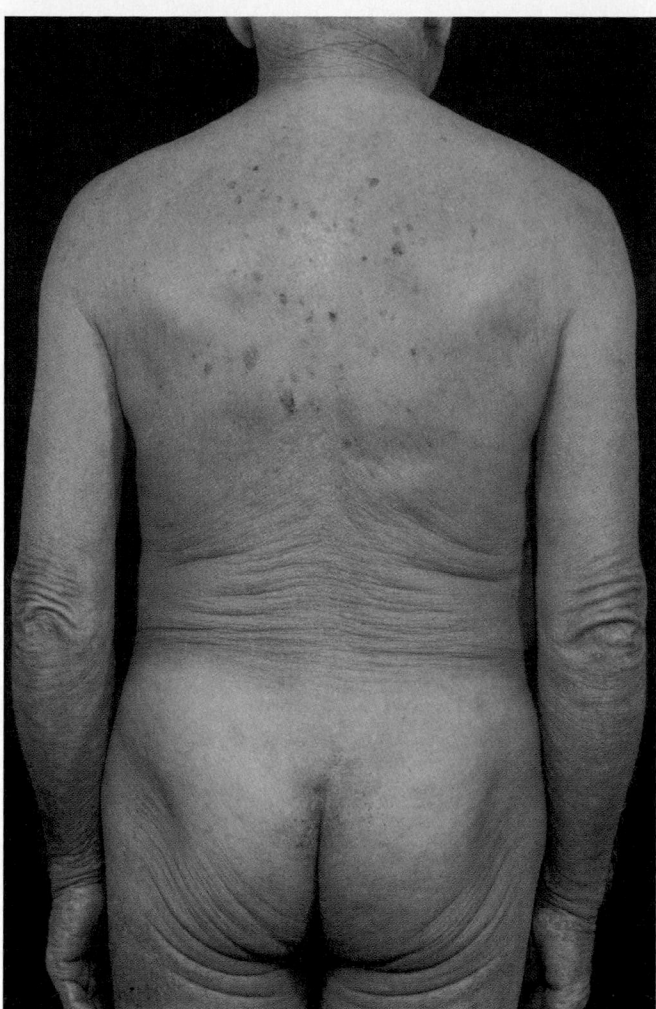

Fig. 58.12 Erythrodermic psoriasis. (Courtesy of St John's Institute of Dermatology, London.)

Psoriatic nail disease can be cosmetically disfiguring, and topical treatments are rarely effective. Systemic treatments such as methotrexate, when prescribed for generalised psoriasis, may improve nail disease.

Treatment

Many patients with psoriasis have only mild localised disease, for example limited to the elbows. This may only require emollient therapy to prevent drying and fissuring of the areas involved. However, a wide range of additional active treatments for psoriasis exists, which range from topical preparations to phototherapy and systemic agents. Psoriasis is a chronic inflammatory condition for which there is no cure, and so treatment decisions should take into account the type and severity of the psoriasis and the impact that it has on the patient's life. Managing the patients' expectation and agreeing on treatment goals will improve patient adherence and treatment outcomes. Other things to consider are patient comorbidities and lifestyle factors, such as their occupation and ability to attend frequent appointments.

Topical therapy

Topical therapies are first-line treatments for mild-to-moderate psoriasis, and can often be used in combination with systemic treatments in more severe psoriasis. In addition to topical active therapies, patients with psoriasis should use regular emollients to hydrate the skin, remove scale and prevent fissuring. When deciding on a topical agent, the prescriber should take into account patient preference, cosmetic acceptability and practical aspects of application such as the extent of psoriasis to be treated. Different formulations should also be discussed with the patient, such as ointment, creams and gels, and the formulation prescribed should be guided by the patient's preference. Some topical treatments are used only in a specialist setting, and some patients benefit from periods of intensive therapy administered by trained staff, such as specialist nurses, in a daycare facility.

Corticosteroids

Topical corticosteroids have an anti-inflammatory effect, and mild-to-moderate strength preparations, when used once or twice daily, are an effective treatment for chronic stable plaque psoriasis. A wide range of corticosteroid preparations are available for psoriasis that are cosmetically acceptable and easy to apply. These include gels, lotions and shampoos for the scalp. Topical corticosteroids are also of great value in acutely inflamed psoriasis. Reducing acute inflammation may also allow subsequent treatment with other agents that would otherwise irritate acutely inflamed plaques, such as vitamin D analogues or coal tar.

Chronic topical corticosteroid use can be limited by irreversible side effects, such as skin atrophy and striae. The use of potent corticosteroids in psoriasis is limited by the risk of systemic absorption and rebound effect (rapid disease relapse) on withdrawal. Potent steroids should only be used on the limbs or trunk under specialist supervision. They are often reserved for localised disease, such as thicker acral sites, and often in combination with salicylic acid if there is hyperkeratosis. Very potent corticosteroids should generally be avoided in psoriasis.

Vitamin D analogues

Vitamin D analogues inhibit keratinocyte differentiation and production, and the most commonly used agent is calcipotriol. Topical calcipotriol applied once or twice daily is an effective treatment for mild localised psoriasis and is commonly used in a primary care setting. Vitamin D analogues can cause some local irritation, and so should not be used, or with caution, on delicate skin sites such as the face and flexures. Hypercalcaemia has been described due to systemic absorption if the maximum weekly dose exceeds 100 g. Efficacy may be enhanced when used in combination with a topical corticosteroid, and some combined corticosteroid and calcipotriol formulations are available.

Coal tar

Coal tar is one of the oldest topical treatments for psoriasis and has anti-inflammatory, antibacterial, antipruritic and antimitotic effects. A variety of preparations are available including bath preparations, shampoos, creams and ointment. Coal tar concentrations of 1–10% can be used; however, higher concentrations should occur in a supervised setting because they can cause local irritation. Coal tar can be used in combination with other products, such as topical corticosteroids or UVB phototherapy (Goeckerman regimen). In addition to being an irritant, coal tar treatment can be limited by its odour and temporary staining of skin and clothing. Although coal tars contain polycyclic aromatic hydrocarbons, epidemiological studies have not demonstrated any association with carcinogenic risk and their topical use.

Dithranol

Dithranol (anthralin in the USA) is a synthetic anthracene derivative that has antiproliferative and anti-inflammatory effects on the skin. It is an effective treatment for psoriasis and, with coal tars, is one of the oldest treatments used. Dithranol can irritate normal skin and stain clothing, with treatment starting at lower concentrations that can be titrated up depending on how well it is tolerated. In current practice it is used in a dermatology daycare setting over several weeks, where it is often used for 'short contact' treatment and washed off after a defined period of time.

Salicylic acid

Salicylic acid is a keratolytic that breaks down the hyperkeratotic component of psoriatic plaques, thereby reducing scale and enabling better penetrance of other topical preparations. Salicylic acid can be used alone or in combination with other topical medications, such as corticosteroids. Higher concentration preparations may be required for particularly hyperkeratotic sites, such as acral sites in palmoplantar psoriasis.

Topical treatment of psoriasis at special sites

Scalp

Scalp psoriasis should first be treated with a potent topical corticosteroid, using an appropriate formulation (shampoo, gel, lotion or foam). Patients should be shown how to effectively use scalp preparations because this can be challenging and lead to poor adherence. If the scalp is scaly, topical corticosteroids should be used in combination with a descaling agent, such as an emollient (e.g. coconut oil or ointment) or a salicylic acid-containing product. Vitamin D analogues, alone or in combination with corticosteroid, are also effective for scalp psoriasis. Coal tar preparations, such as shampoos, are effective in mild disease, but should be used in combination with other treatments for moderate-to-severe scalp psoriasis.

Flexures/Genitals

Flexural and genital regions are prone to irritation and steroid atrophy. These areas should be treated with short courses (1–2 weeks) of mild- to moderate-potency topical corticosteroids. Areas unresponsive to topical corticosteroid can be treated with twice-daily application of a calcineurin inhibitor for up to 4 weeks, which should only be initiated by a specialist.

Nails

Topical treatments are not effective in treating psoriatic nail disease, which may show some response to systemic therapies. When assessing dystrophic nails in a patient with psoriasis, it is also important to exclude fungal infection.

Phototherapy

Many patients with psoriasis will report an improvement in their skin after sunny holidays, with only 10% of patients reporting deterioration in symptoms on sun exposure. Phototherapy with either UVB or photochemotherapy with UVA after psoralen exposure (PUVA) has an immunosuppressive effect on the skin and has been used to treat psoriasis for more than 80 years.

UVB

Narrow-band UVB or TL-01 (311–313 nm) is the most commonly used phototherapy modality for moderate-to-severe psoriasis and is preferable to older broadband UVB (290–320 nm) lamps, due to increased safety and reduced risk of burning. Narrow-band UVB is an effective treatment for getting rapid control of widespread disease, with approximately 75% of patients being clear or nearly clear of psoriasis after a course of treatment (usually two to three treatments a week for approximately 6 weeks) (Dawe et al., 1998).

Photochemotherapy with UVA after psoralen exposure

PUVA also has a role in the treatment of stable moderate-to-severe psoriasis. Psoralens are drugs that are activated by long-wave UV light (320–400 nm), which then act by interfering with DNA synthesis and reducing epidermal turnover. Two psoralens are available in the UK: 8-MOP (methoxypsoralen) and 5-MOP. Usually psoralens are taken orally 2 hours before exposure to UVA to the whole body; however, PUVA can also be given locally for limited disease after topical psoralen application to the affected site, such as the hands or feet. The treatment is usually given twice a week for a 6-week period. The commonest adverse effect is nausea due to systemic psoralens, and the eyes must be photo-protected for at least 12 hours after treatment to reduce the risk of cataracts.

The most serious adverse effect of excessive UV exposure is an increased long-term risk of skin cancer. Therefore, the total number of treatments and cumulative exposure doses need to be carefully monitored. Fair skin types and systemic immunosuppression (past/present) are at greatest risk of skin malignancy after PUVA, and because of these considerations PUVA is generally reserved for patients unresponsive to UVB therapy. Safe exposure limits are considered to be up to 350 treatments for narrow-band UVB therapy and 150–200 treatments for PUVA.

Systemic therapy

Systemic therapy can be used for all types of psoriasis. It is indicated when the psoriasis cannot be controlled with topical therapy alone, is not responsive or rapidly relapses after phototherapy, and the psoriasis is either extensive or localised but associated with significant functional impairment/distress. Objective measures have been developed to measure disease severity; the Psoriasis Area and Severity Index (PASI) is used to measure disease severity based on clinical features of individual lesions and the extent of disease (range 0–72); the Dermatology Quality of Life Index (DLQI) uses a range of questions to grade the impact of the skin condition on daily living (range 0–30). For both indices, scores greater than 10 are considered a marker of severe disease. These measures have been incorporated into national guidelines for certain psoriasis treatments and should be used to assess disease severity before starting a systemic medication, but also at intervals throughout treatment to monitor the patient's response.

When considering initiation of a systemic medication it is important to take into account the psoriasis subtype, treatment history, relevant comorbidities (such as psoriatic arthritis), conceptions plans and the views/goals of the patient. Systemic non-biologic treatments commonly used in psoriasis include methotrexate, ciclosporin, acitretin and hydroxyurea. Drug interactions are important, and a detailed patient drug history is important (Table 58.4). In addition, these treatments require monitoring

Table 58.4 Examples of interactions with drugs used in the treatment of eczema and psoriasis

Interacting drug		Outcome
Methotrexate	Aspirin	Increased plasma concentration and toxicity of methotrexate
	NSAIDs	Increased plasma concentration and toxicity of methotrexate
	Probenecid	Increased plasma concentration and toxicity of methotrexate
	Phenytoin	Increased bone marrow toxicity
	Sulfonamides	Increased toxicity
	Trimethoprim	Increased antifolate effect of methotrexate
	Acitretin	Increased plasma concentration of methotrexate
Azathioprine	Allopurinol	Enhanced effect and toxicity of azathioprine
	Warfarin	Inhibition of anticoagulant effect
	Cimetidine	Enhanced myelosuppression
	Indometacin	Increased risk of leucopenia
Ciclosporin	Non-steroidal anti-inflammatory drugs	Increased risk of nephrotoxicity
	Aminoglycosides	Increased risk of nephrotoxicity
	Co-trimoxazole	Increased risk of nephrotoxicity
	Ciprofloxacin	Increased risk of nephrotoxicity
	Ketoconazole	Increased plasma concentration of ciclosporin
	Itraconazole	Increased plasma concentration of ciclosporin
	Erythromycin	Increased plasma concentration of ciclosporin
	Oral contraceptives	Increased plasma concentration of ciclosporin
	Calcium channel blockers	Increased plasma concentration of ciclosporin
	Phenytoin	Decreased plasma concentration of ciclosporin
	Carbamazepine	Decreased plasma concentration of ciclosporin
	Rifampicin	Decreased plasma concentration of ciclosporin
Acitretin	Methotrexate	Increased plasma concentration of methotrexate

Always check latest British National Formulary or other reference source for specific drug interaction information.

Table 58.5 Common adverse effects and monitoring requirements for systemic treatments of eczema and psoriasis

Therapy	Adverse effects	Monitoring requirements
Methotrexate	Hepatic fibrosis; myelosuppression; nausea; pulmonary fibrosis; teratogenic (contraindicated in both males and females for 4 weeks before and 3 months after treatment)	FBC U&E LFTs Pro-collagen III peptide (P3NP) ± liver biopsy Chest X-ray (screening)
Hydroxyurea/hydroxycarbamide	Myelosuppression; skin reaction; teratogenic; liver toxicity (narrow therapeutic window)	FBC U&Es LFTs
Ciclosporin	Renal nephrotoxicity Hypertension Gingival hypertrophy	FBC U&E LFTs Lipid profile Blood pressure Urinalysis
Acitretin	Teratogenic (including up to 3 years post-treatment) Dryness of mucous membranes and skin Hyperostoses, increased serum triglyceride Occasional hepatotoxic reaction	FBC U&E LFTs Lipid profile
Fumaric acid esters	Gastro-intestinal side effects Flushing Lymphopenia Proteinuria Renal failure	FBC U&E LFTs Urinalysis
Azathioprine	Myelosuppression Deranged liver function Gastro-intestinal effects	TPMT pre-treatment FBC U&E LFTs

FBC, Full blood count; LFT, liver function test; TPMT, thiopurine methyl transferase genetic polymorphism screening; U&E, urea and electrolytes.

for adverse events, with responsibility for treatment being with a specialist centre (Table 58.5). Certain biologic agents, which block specific inflammatory cytokine pathways, are also licensed for the treatment of psoriasis that is unresponsive to standard non-biologic systemic therapy.

Methotrexate

As previously discussed, methotrexate inhibits purine and pyrimidine synthesis, which is required for DNA synthesis, and leads to the accumulation of extracellular anti-inflammatory metabolites. Methotrexate is administered as a weekly oral or subcutaneous dose of usually 15–25 mg, and it is considered the gold standard, first-line systemic agent for moderate-to-severe psoriasis. It is an effective agent with approximately two-thirds of patients treated seeing at least a 50% improvement in psoriasis after 16 weeks of treatment (Heydendael et al., 2003; Saurat et al., 2008). The main side effect that patients report with methotrexate therapy is nausea. Concomitant folic acid is often given to reduce toxicity. Conception should be avoided during and for at least 3 months after methotrexate treatment, in either men or women, because of teratogenic risk.

Patients require close monitoring during treatment with methotrexate, notably of full blood count and liver function, because treatment is associated with myelosuppression and the development of hepatic fibrosis (see Table 58.5). Liver function tests do not reliably predict hepatic fibrosis, and so additional investigations are required. Liver biopsy is the gold standard test to diagnose hepatic fibrosis but is associated with pain, bleeding and a small risk of fatality (0.01–0.1%). Serial blood pro-collagen III peptide measurement has been shown to be an effective screening test to replace/guide routine liver biopsy (Chalmers et al., 2005). Additional non-invasive investigations for hepatic fibrosis, such as liver fibroelastography (FibroScan), are also under investigation for methotrexate-monitoring purposes.

Ciclosporin

Ciclosporin is a calcineurin inhibitor that blocks lymphocyte activation and is used as an oral preparation in the treatment of psoriasis. It is an effective treatment for all clinical subtypes of psoriasis. Ciclosporin is dosed daily, ranging from 2 to 5 mg/kg, and has a similar efficacy to methotrexate at 16 weeks of treatment; however, ciclosporin has a more rapid onset of action that may favour its use in a more acute setting (Heydendael et al., 2003). As with atopic eczema management, ciclosporin treatment is often limited at 12 months because of the increased risk of renal nephrotoxicity with long-term therapy. Adverse events reported include hypertension, hypertrichosis, paraesthesia, tremor and increased risk of infections. There is also a significantly increased risk of skin cancer in patients who have also received multiple courses of phototherapy.

Acitretin

Acitretin is a vitamin A derivative that inhibits epidermal proliferation and is an effective oral agent for disorders of keratinisation, which includes psoriasis, and offers an alternative to immunosuppressive agents. Acitretin is usually initiated at a low dose of 25–30 mg daily for 2–4 weeks, which is subsequently increased as guided by clinical response. In chronic plaque psoriasis it is reported that at higher doses, up to 85% of patients will see at least a 50% improvement in their skin (Ormerod et al., 2010). Common side effects are dry skin/mucous membranes, hair loss and lethargy, and long-term therapy is associated with hyperlipidaemia. Therefore, patients should be monitored whilst on treatment. Conception should be avoided during and for up to 3 years after acitretin treatment because of teratogenic risk (Ormerod et al., 2010).

Hydroxyurea/hydroxycarbamide

Hydroxyurea/hydroxycarbamide is a cytotoxic immunosuppressant drug that inhibits DNA synthesis. It has a similar mode of action to methotrexate, including bone marrow suppression, but it is less hepatotoxic. Hydroxyurea/hydroxycarbamide has been used historically as an unlicensed oral treatment for psoriasis (500–1500 mg/day) and is effective after 6–8 weeks; however, it is now less commonly prescribed. Conception should be avoided during and for up to 12 months after treatment because of teratogenic risk.

Fumaric acid esters

Fumaric acid esters have been used since the early 1960s to treat psoriasis and target both keratinocyte and T-cell activity. Although fumaric acid esters are licensed in Europe for severe chronic plaque psoriasis, they are not licensed in the UK. The main side effects are gastro-intestinal upset and flushing, and rare adverse events include renal impairment and lymphopenia.

Biologic therapy

Biologic therapies or 'biologics' in psoriasis refer to a group of engineered monoclonal antibodies that specifically block pro-inflammatory cytokines, including TNF-α, IL-23 and IL-17, which are central to the disease pathogenesis. Biologics are effective therapies for moderate-to-severe chronic plaque psoriasis, with 50–80% of patients seeing at least a 75% improvement in their disease after 12–16 weeks of treatment and with some patients having very striking responses (Menter et al., 2007; Saurat et al., 2008; Griffiths et al., 2010; Langley et al., 2014). These treatments, however, are expensive, and national registries have also been developed to collect prospective safety data regarding the use of these relatively newer agents. In the UK, biologics are recommended for patients with moderate-to-severe chronic plaque psoriasis (as defined by PASI ≥10 and DLQI >10) who have not responded successfully to at least two standard systemic agents that includes methotrexate (Smith et al., 2009). Before initiating a biologic agent, patients should be screened for infections, including viral hepatitis, HIV and active/latent tuberculosis, with certain additional cautions or contraindications for each agent. Biologics are generally well tolerated, with injection-site reactions sometimes reported. Clinical response should be assessed after 12–16 weeks of treatment, at which point a decision should be made whether to continue the treatment (NICE, 2012).

The following are the licensed dosing regimens for these agents (UK).

TNF-α antagonists

The pro-inflammatory cytokine TNF-α plays a central role in the pathogenesis of psoriasis, and several biologics that block its function have been developed for the treatment of chronic plaque psoriasis. These include adalimumab, infliximab and etanercept, which all have a potent targeted immunosuppressant action. Serious adverse events associated with anti-TNF-α agents include serious infections requiring hospitalisation, in particular reactivation of tuberculosis, exacerbation of severe cardiac failure, demyelinating disease and a potential risk of malignancy, including solid organ tumours and lymphoma. Therefore, careful selection of suitable patients and regular monitoring are important.

Adalimumab. Adalimumab is humanised anti-TNF-α monoclonal antibody. It is administered by subcutaneous injection, initially at a dose of 80 mg, followed by a fortnightly maintenance dose of 40 mg.

Infliximab. Infliximab is a chimeric anti-TNF-α monoclonal antibody. It is administered by intravenous infusion at a dose of 5 mg/kg at weeks 0, 2 and 6 and then a maintenance dose every 8 weeks. Infliximab has been associated with acute infusion-related reactions and delayed hypersensitivity reactions, especially if there has been a break in treatment, and should therefore be administered in a setting with access to appropriate resuscitation equipment and facilities.

Etanercept. Etanercept is an engineered receptor fusion protein that binds to soluble TNF-α with high affinity and blocks its actions. It is administered as a subcutaneous injection at a dose of 25 mg twice weekly.

IL-12/IL-23 antagonists

Ustekinumab. Ustekinumab is a fully human monoclonal antibody licensed in the treatment of moderate-to-severe psoriasis, which acts by binding to and blocking a common subunit of the cytokines IL-12 and IL-23. It is administered as a subcutaneous injection at a dose of 45 mg (or 90 mg if >100 kg) at baseline, week 4, and then every 12 weeks.

IL-17 antagonists

Secukinumab. Secukinumab is a fully human anti-IL-17A monoclonal antibody. It is administered as a subcutaneous

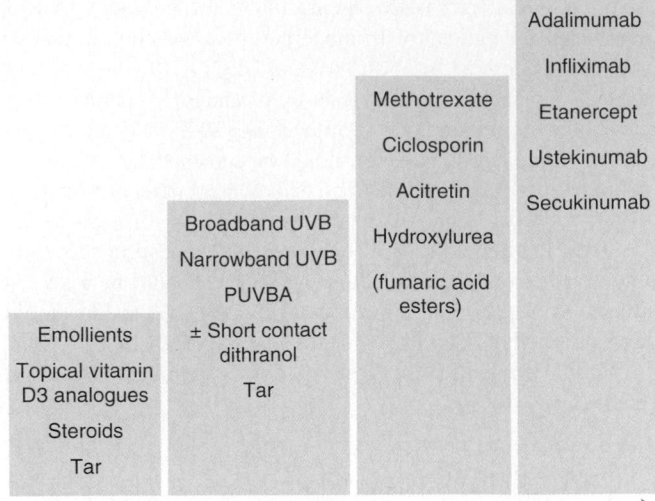

Fig. 58.13 Treatment algorithm for psoriasis. PUVA, psoralen with ultraviolet A; UVB, ultraviolet B.

PASI = Psoriasis area and severity index
DLQI = Dermatology quality of life index

Increasing **PASI** and **DLQI**

injection at a weekly dose of 300 mg for 4 weeks, followed by a 300 mg monthly maintenance dose.

A treatment algorithm for psoriasis is shown in Fig. 58.13.

Patient care

Psoriasis is a chronic disease, and many of the psoriasis treatments are not straightforward. Topical regimens can be time consuming and messy, and systemic treatments require regular blood tests and outpatient consultations. Patients often experience 'treatment fatigue' and frustration with the chronicity of the condition. Psoriasis can also affect many other aspects of patients' lives. Co-existent psoriatic arthritis may cause physical disability that impacts on individuals' ability to perform daily activities, which may also impact on their work or education. Psoriasis is also associated with significant psychosocial morbidity, such as depression, alcohol misuse, negative body image and difficulty with intimate relationships. This is overall associated with a reduced quality of life. Therefore, in the holistic approach to caring for such patients, all of these factors must be considered. It is important that patients are educated about their condition, and that realistic treatment goals are set out with agreement of both the clinical team and patient. Engaging with patients' broader needs and providing support for these can further help to improve their adherence to treatment. Organisations such as The Psoriasis Association (http://www.psoriasis-association.org.uk) provide excellent additional support services for patients, together with practical advice for managing their condition from day to day.

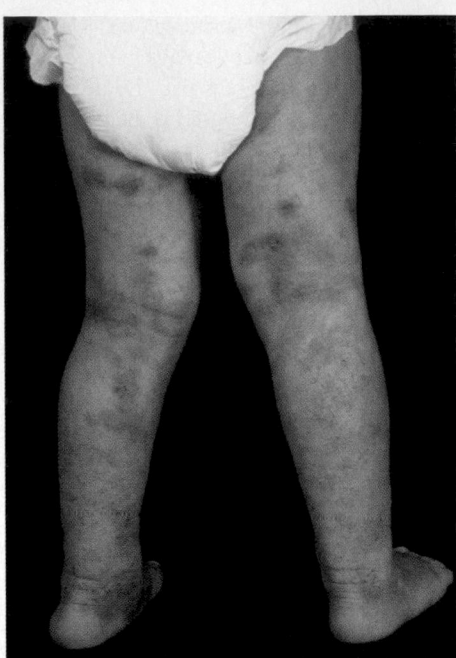

Fig. 58.14 A young child with moderate-to-severe atopic eczema. (Courtesy of St John's Institute of Dermatology, London.)

Case studies

Case 58.1

A 3-year-old child with known atopic eczema is seen in clinic with a widespread, excoriated, dry rash (Fig. 58.14). Her eczema symptoms started at the age of 6 weeks. Her sleep has always been poor because of the marked itch symptoms at night. She has had two recent courses of oral antibiotics for presumed bacterial skin infection. Her normal skin treatment involves hydrocortisone 1% ointment to affected areas twice daily. Her parents are concerned regarding the possible triggers of her eczema flares and are keen to pursue possible allergy testing.

Question

What advice could be given to the child's parents?

Answer

Fig. 58.14 shows a young child with moderate-to-severe atopic eczema. Ill-defined, dry, erythematous patches of eczema are visible. A few of the patches around her ankles appear crusty and eroded. This may represent secondary infection.

Management should include regular topical emollient therapy, and the correct quantities should be emphasised. A regular soap substitute should be prescribed. The skin is excoriated and crusted, and so there may be secondary infection, most likely with *Staphylococcus aureus*. Therefore, when infection is present, wet wrap dressings are not appropriate because they may exacerbate this. Wound swabs should always be taken before prescribing an oral antibiotic for presumed infected eczema.

A moderately potent or potent topical corticosteroid ointment should be administered daily. When a moderately potent or potent topical corticosteroid is prescribed for a child, medical follow-up must be arranged to avoid potential local side effects such as skin atrophy. If the treatment is ineffective, a short admission to hospital or regular dermatology day care should be arranged for further intensive topical treatments or dressings. Time should be spent explaining to the parents the aetiology of atopic eczema. Although atopic eczema is considered a chronic disease with no 'cure', it should also be explained that approximately 60% of children will have minimal or no symptoms after the age of 16 years. Carers of children with atopic eczema commonly request allergy testing. Although allergies are more common in children with eczema, it is not always appropriate. Allergy testing may be indicated if there is a clear history of the hives (urticarial) or swelling (angioedema) after exposure to possible triggers or exacerbations of the eczema. However, triggers to eczema flares are often not allergens and may be environmental irritants, such as soaps, or other factors such as psychological stress. Allergy testing may involve blood tests (RAST tests), skin prick tests and patch testing. Such testing should be done in a specialist paediatric allergy centre because a positive result does not always directly correlate with the effect of allergen avoidance on the course of atopic eczema.

Case 58.2

A 22-year-old male nurse attends outpatients reporting dry, painful eczema affecting his hands. He had previously suffered with childhood eczema and asthma. Since starting his new job, his symptoms have developed, causing severe pain, fissures, itch and dry skin. His finger pulps are particularly affected. He attended occupational health and was then advised to see a dermatologist.

Question

What is the likely cause of his symptoms, and what advice should be given?

Answer

The aetiology of hand dermatitis is often complex and multifactorial. This man has an atopic predisposition, but this also puts him at greater risk of an ICD and/or ACD than the general population. The need for him to regularly wash his hands with soaps and/or antiseptic hand wash is likely to be a major factor.

This man should be advised to use an emollient soap substitute when washing his hands, and some products exist that also contain antiseptic agents, for example, Dermol 500. In addition, to treat the active dermatitis, a potent topical corticosteroid and emollient with a good barrier effect should be prescribed. For fissured areas, overnight application of adhesive tape that is impregnated with corticosteroid (Haelan tape) may also beneficial for local therapy. Patch testing would also be appropriate to ascertain whether there is an allergic contact component to his symptoms.

Atopic eczema predisposes to contact dermatitis. Therefore, young adults with moderate or severe eczema should be made aware of this risk when they are considering certain occupations that are also associated with a higher risk of contact dermatitis, especially ICD. Such careers include hairdressing, domestic cleaning or working in a healthcare environment that requires regular hand washing.

Case 58.3

A 28-year-old male management executive with lifelong atopic eczema has attended clinic with worsening severity of his eczema.

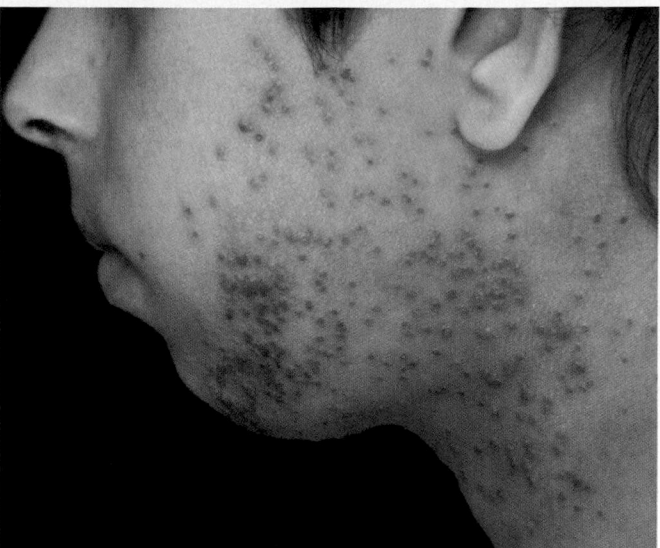

Fig. 58.15 A young patient with eczema herpeticum. (Courtesy of St John's Institute of Dermatology, London.)

He has been using emollients and moderately potent topical corticosteroids for many years and feels that these are no longer effective. Over the past year, he has required two short courses of oral corticosteroids. His sleep is affected and he is concerned at how much time he is taking off work.

Question

What are the treatment options for this patient?

Answer

This patient needs a more effective treatment regimen. Although systemic corticosteroids are an effective short-term treatment for severe flares of eczema, they are not a long-term option. His topical regimen should be explored to ensure that it is optimal. His use of emollients and soap substitutes should be discussed, as well as the quantity and frequency of topical corticosteroids for regular eczema management. In addition, his aims, expectations and other medical issues should be explored with a view to possible systemic treatment.

Ciclosporin would be an appropriate first-line systemic agent, and pre-treatment screening should include blood pressure measurement, urinalysis and blood tests to assess renal function. Although ciclosporin has a more rapid effect than other systemic agents, treatment should be limited to less than 12 months because of the risk of the development of treatment-associated side effects. If longer-term systemic management is anticipated, or second-line agent required after ciclosporin, azathioprine or methotrexate would be potential options, but efficacy would only be evident after approximately 8 weeks of treatment.

Case 58.4

A 12-year-old boy with known atopic eczema presented with a vesicular, blistering eruption over his face and trunk (Fig. 58.15). His mother noticed the blisters 2 days ago and brought him to hospital as he has become systemically unwell and feverish. He has chronic atopic eczema that is usually well controlled with regular emollients and twice-weekly application of calcineurin inhibitors to troublesome sites. His sister has recently been suffering with cold sores.

Question

Fig. 58.15 shows the young patient with eczema herpeticum. What advice would you give this patient and his mother?

Answer

Eczema herpeticum, or Kaposi's varicelliform eruption, is an important and potentially serious complication in patients with atopic eczema and certain other chronic inflammatory skin conditions. This eruption occurs after inoculation of herpes simplex virus to skin damaged by eczema and can spread rapidly to affect the eyes and lungs. Typically, the tiny blisters (vesicles) have an umbilicated appearance and may also develop into 'punched-out' erosions that commonly have a golden crust, which is indicative of secondary staphylococcal infection ('impetigenisation').

Eczema herpeticum can progress rapidly, and therefore should be treated aggressively with systemic antiviral medications, such as aciclovir, and antibiotics, if there is concern of secondary bacterial infection. If the skin is dry or inflamed, aerosolised emollients, such as Emollin spray, can be used which also limit cutaneous spread of infection. Skin swabs should be done to confirm viral infection and test for bacterial antibiotic sensitivities. If systemically unwell, patients may require hospitalisation. If there is a concern that there may be eye involvement, urgent ophthalmological review is required to assess for herpetic corneal ulceration, which can lead to long-term visual complications.

Children with atopic eczema and their parents should be educated to recognise the signs and symptoms of eczema herpeticum.

Case 58.5

A 33-year-old electrician presents to clinic with a 5-month history of a mildly itchy eruption occurring around the nasal area and eyebrows (Fig. 58.16). He describes it as occasionally scaly and is very concerned regarding the cosmetic appearance. On examination, he also has mild scale and erythema affecting the scalp. The dandruff shampoos he usually purchases from his local community pharmacy have been ineffective.

Question

What would you offer as a topical treatment for facial seborrhoeic dermatitis?

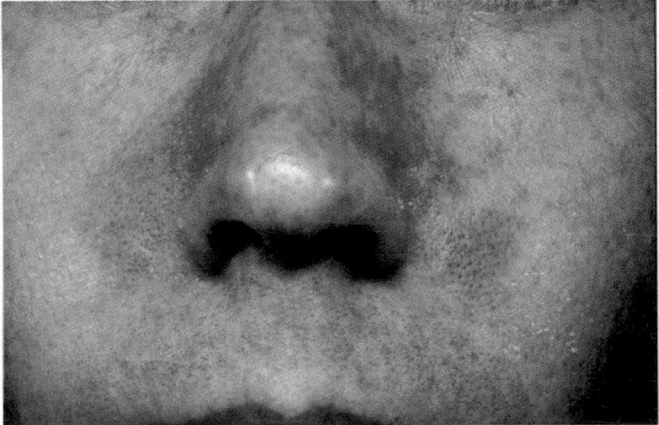

Fig. 58.16 Man with seborrheic dermatitis. (Courtesy of St John's Institute of Dermatology, London.)

Answer

Ketoconazole shampoo and ketoconazole 2% cream will reduce the population of *Pityrosporum ovale* on the skin, which may improve the rash. If there is marked dermatitis and the area is symptomatic (itchy), a mild topical corticosteroid with or without an antifungal or a topical calcineurin inhibitor would be appropriate. In addition, patients should be counselled that seborrheic dermatitis is a common condition that is often chronic, so periodic exacerbations may occur.

Case 58.6

A 55-year-old woman presents with a history of long-standing chronic plaque psoriasis. Since the age of 16 she has used multiple topical treatments with repeated course of UVB phototherapy; however, more recently these have not managed her skin adequately. In addition, for the past 18 months she has developed painful swelling and stiffness over the proximal joints of both hands, which is much worse in the morning. NSAIDs have not alleviated her symptoms, and her function at work is now affected. On examination, she has moderate-to-severe psoriasis and evidence of proximal interphalangeal joint swelling (synovitis) with subtle deformity.

Question

What management options should be offered for this patient?

Answer

This woman has moderate-to-severe psoriasis with evidence of psoriatic arthropathy. Psoriatic arthropathy affects up to 30% of patients with psoriasis, which can manifest as a destructive arthritis leading to significant functional disability. In addition to regular NSAIDs and analgesics to improve symptomatic control, a systemic treatment should be considered, and this woman would optimally be jointly managed by a dermatologist and rheumatologist. Methotrexate is the gold standard systemic medication for both chronic plaque psoriasis and psoriatic arthritis. If methotrexate fails, there should be a low threshold for a biologic medication that would treat both the skin and joint disease, such as an anti-TNF-α agent (e.g. adalimumab) or anti-IL-17 agent (e.g. secukinumab). Systemic corticosteroids should be avoided as an arthritis treatment because there is a significant risk that upon their withdrawal the psoriasis flares and/or develops into a generalised pustular psoriasis.

Case 58.7

A 45-year-old man with psoriasis has been reporting an itchy, scaly scalp for the last 8 months. He has seen his primary care doctor who has prescribed a moderate-strength topical corticosteroid preparation, but this treatment has had little effect. He is troubled by thick scale and severe itch at night.

Question

What treatment options could be considered?

Answer

Treatment of scalp psoriasis often can be challenging and differs from other forms of psoriasis because of the presence of thick hair.

Topical treatments can be difficult and messy to apply, and photo-therapy is not usually effective. Topical preparations should be used in conjunction with a method to reduce the scale, which will increase their efficacy. Oil-based emollients, such as coconut oil or Arachis oil (avoid if peanut allergic), or preparations that contain salicylic acid are effective at softening/lifting scale. These preparations should be left on for approximately 1 hour and then washed off. In addition to de-scaling the scalp, an anti-inflammatory agent is often required, such as coal tar–containing preparations or potent topical corticosteroids. Most topical preparations used to treat psoriasis on the body have equivalent scalp preparations, but these are often in a lotion or gel formulation to improve the ease with which they can be applied to the scalp. As with other body sites, intermittent rather than prolonged use of topical corticosteroids is advised. Education and support from specialist nurses are often invaluable in treating severe scalp psoria-sis because many patients find treatment regimens complicated and time consuming.

Case 58.8

A 45-year-old man has become increasingly limited by his palmo-plantar pustular psoriasis. He has had frequent crops of inflamed pustules on the palms and soles which dry up to form crusts and scaling followed by painful fissuring of the skin. He works as a joiner, and is finding this increasingly difficult, leading to prolonged periods off work. He has tried both regular emollients and intermit-tent topical corticosteroids, but with only temporary relief.

Question

What are the best options for the treatment of this patient?

Answer

This patient should be encouraged to continue using regular emol-lient therapy to the hands and feet, and soap substitutes to wash the affected areas. Topical corticosteroid therapy could be optimised by either using a very potent preparation (e.g. clobetasol propionate 0.05%) in an ointment vehicle, such as propylene glycol, or with sali-cylic acid. In addition, occluding the sites with either cotton garments or cling film can improve corticosteroid penetration into the skin, but this should be done under specialist supervision. Alternatively, a sys-temic therapy may be appropriate, of which either oral acitretin or ciclosporin is an effective therapy for palmopustular psoriasis. Both agents require blood test monitoring during the treatment period. If acitretin or ciclosporin cannot be used, localised hand and foot PUVA is an alternative, but this would require frequent attendance at a specialist centre. Smoking exacerbates palmoplantar psoriasis, and so patients should be advised to either avoid or stop smoking, with some evidence demonstrating that smoking cessation improves disease severity (Michaëlsson et al., 2006).

Case 58.9

A 24-year-old man presents at the clinic with a 10-year history of plaque psoriasis affecting his elbows, knees and sacral area,

with a few small plaques elsewhere. He is otherwise fit and well. He regularly plays football and is embarrassed by the appearance of his skin. He has tried Betnovate RD ointment (0.025%), which smoothed the plaques a little, and calcipotriol ointment, which removed the scale from the plaques but did not clear them.

Question

What treatment could this patient try next?

Answer

Because the patient has only a few localised plaques, topical therapy could be optimised. One option would be to use a more potent topi-cal corticosteroid *in combination* with topical calcipotriol, for which some combined formulations exist (e.g. Dovobet). These are applied once daily to the affected areas until the plaques clear. Alternatively, if the patient is willing to attend his local dermatology department he could either have a course of short contact dithranol or tar therapy or narrow-band UVB phototherapy. Although effective skin-targeted therapy should induce a remission in mild-to-moderate disease, this may not be long lasting, and the patient should be counselled about potential future systemic medications.

Case 58.10

A 35-year-old male patient with chronic plaque psoriasis is being reviewed in the dermatology department. He has used multiple previous treatments, including topicals, UVB phototherapy, and ciclosporin. Most recently he has been established on methotrex-ate – initially orally for the first 4 months and then subcutaneous injections for the last 6 months. Despite this his psoriasis remains poorly controlled and his work and psychological well-being are suffering. He is otherwise well with no significant comorbidities. On examination he has severe plaque psoriasis affecting more than 40% of his body surface area. This is consistent with a PASI of 25 and DLQI of 13.

Question

What treatment options could now be offered?

Answer

This man fulfils the eligibility criteria for biologic therapy in the UK (Smith et al., 2009). He has 'severe disease', which is defined as hav-ing both a PASI and DLQI greater than 10. In addition, he has been unresponsive to standard systemic therapy, which includes methotrex-ate, the gold standard systemic therapy for chronic plaque psoriasis. Before initiating a biologic agent, pre-treatment screening for infec-tion (including active or latent tuberculosis), heart failure, demyelin-ating disease and malignancy is required. Several different classes of biologic therapy are licensed to treat psoriasis in the UK, and agents that target either TNF-α (e.g. adalimumab) or IL-12/23 (e.g. ustekinumab) are used first line.

References

Brenninkmeijer, E.E., Schram, M.E., Leeflang, M.M., et al., 2008. Diagnostic criteria for atopic dermatitis: a systematic review. Br. J. Dermatol. 158, 24–30.

Chalmers, R.J., Kirby, B., Smith, A., et al., 2005. Replacement of routine liver biopsy by procollagen III aminopeptide for monitoring patients with psoriasis receiving long-term methotrexate: a multicentre audit and health economic analysis. Br. J. Dermatol. 152, 444–450.

Dawe, R.S., Wainwright, N.J., Cameron, H., et al., 1998. Narrow-band (TL-01) ultraviolet B phototherapy for chronic plaque psoriasis: three times or five times weekly treatment? Br. J. Dermatol. 138, 833–839.

Deckers, I.A., McClean, S., Linssen, S., et al., 2012. Investigating international time trends in the incidence and prevalence of atopic eczema 1990–2010: a systematic review of epidemiological studies. PLOS One 7, e39803.

Eichenfield, L.F., Tom, W.L., Berger, T.G., 2014. Guidelines of care for the management of atopic dermatitis: section 2. Management and treatment of atopic dermatitis with topical therapies. J. Am. Acad. Dermatol. 71, 116–132.

Ersser, S.J., Cowdell, F., Latter, S., et al., 2014. Psychological and educational interventions for atopic eczema in children. Cochrane Database Syst. Rev. 1, CD004054.

Gambichler, T., Breuckmann, F., Boms, S., et al., 2005. Narrowband UVB phototherapy in skin conditions beyond psoriasis. J. Am. Acad. Dermatol. 52, 660–670.

Griffiths, C.E., Strober, B.E., van de Kerkhof, P., et al., 2010. Comparison of ustekinumab and etanercept for moderate-to-severe psoriasis. N. Engl. J. Med. 362, 118–128.

Heydendael, V.M., Spuls, P.I., Opmeer, B.C., et al., 2003. Methotrexate versus cyclosporine in moderate-to-severe chronic plaque psoriasis. N. Engl. J. Med. 349, 658–665.

Hoare, C., Li Wan Po, A., Williams, H., 2000. Systematic review of treatments for atopic eczema. Health Technol. Assess. 4, 1–191.

Horimukai, K., Morita, K., Narita, M., et al., 2014. Application of moisturizer to neonates prevents development of atopic dermatitis. J. Allergy Clin. Immunol. 134, 824–830.

Kirby, B., Richards, H.L., Mason, D.L., et al., 2008. Alcohol consumption and psychological distress in patients with psoriasis. Br. J. Dermatol. 158, 138–140.

Langley, R.G., Elewski, B.E., Lebwohl, M., et al., 2014. Secukinumab in plaque psoriasis – results of two phase 3 trials. N. Engl. J. Med. 371, 326–338.

Mahil, S.K., Capon, F., Barker, J.N., 2015. Genetics of psoriasis. Dermatol. Clin. 33, 1–11.

Meduri, N.B., Vandergriff, T., Rasmussen, H., et al., 2007. Phototherapy in the management of atopic dermatitis: a systemic review. Photodermatol. Photoimmunol. Photomed. 23, 106–112.

Mehta, N.N., Azfar, R.S., Shin, D.B., et al., 2010. Patients with severe psoriasis are at increased risk of cardiovascular mortality: cohort study using the General Practice Research Database. Eur. Heart J. 3, 1000–1006.

Menter, A., Feldman, S.R., Weinstein, G.D., et al., 2007. A randomized comparison of continuous vs. intermittent infliximab maintenance regimens over 1 year in the treatment of moderate-to-severe plaque psoriasis. J. Am. Acad. Dermatol. 56 (1), 31.e1–31.e15.

Michaëlsson, G., Gustafsson, K., Hagforsen, E., 2006. The psoriasis variant palmoplantar pustulosis can be improved after cessation of smoking. J. Am. Acad. Dermatol. 54, 737–738.

National Institute for Health and Care Excellence, 2012. Psoriasis: assessment and management of psoriasis. Clinical guidelines CG153. Available at: https://www.nice.org.uk/guidance/cg153.

Nestle, F.O., Kaplan, D.H., Barker, J., 2009. Psoriasis. N. Engl. J. Med. 361, 496–509.

Onoufriadis, A., Simpson, M.A., Pink, A.E., et al., 2011. Mutations in IL36RN/IL1F5 are associated with the severe episodic inflammatory skin disease known as generalized pustular psoriasis. Am. J. Hum. Genet. 89, 432–437.

Ormerod, A.D., Campalani, E., Goodfield, M.J., et al., 2010. British Association of Dermatologists guidelines on the efficacy and use of acitretin in dermatology. Br. J. Dermatol. 162, 952–963.

Paller, A.S., Lebwohl, M., Fleischer Jr., A.B., et al., 2005. Tacrolimus ointment is more effective than pimecrolimus cream with a similar safety profile in the treatment of atopic dermatitis: results from 3 randomised, comparative studies. J. Am. Acad. Dermatol. 52, 810–822.

Roekevisch, E., Spuls, P.I., Keuster, B.A., et al., 2014. Efficacy and safety of systemic treatments for moderate-to-severe atopic dermatitis: a systematic review. J. Allergy Clin. Immunol. 133, 429–438.

Saurat, J.H., Stingl, G., Dubertret, L., et al., 2008. Efficacy and safety results from the randomized controlled comparative study of adalimumab vs. methotrexate vs. placebo in patients with psoriasis (CHAMPION). Br. J. Dermatol. 158, 558–566.

Schmitt, J., Schmitt, N., Meurer, M., 2007. Cyclosporin in the treatment of patients with atopic eczema – a systematic review and meta-analysis. J. Eur. Acad. Dermatol. Venereol. 21, 606–619.

Simpson, E.L., Chalmers, J.R., Hanifin, J.M., et al., 2014. Emollient enhancement of the skin barrier from birth offers effective atopic dermatitis prevention. J. Allergy Clin. Immunol. 134, 818–823.

Smith, C.H., Anstey, A.V., Barker, J.N., et al., 2009. British Association of Dermatologists' guidelines for biologic interventions for psoriasis. Br. J. Dermatol. 161, 987–1019.

Weidinger, S., Novak, N., 2016. Atopic dermatitis. Lancet 387 (10023), 1109–1122.

Zachariae, H., 2003. Prevalence of joint disease in patients with psoriasis: implications for therapy. Am. J. Clin. Dermatol. 4, 441–447.

Further reading

Griffiths, C., Barker, J., Bleiker, T., et al., 2016. Rook's Textbook of Dermatology, ninth ed. John Wiley & Sons, Chichester, UK.

Nast, A., Gisondi, P., Ormerod, A.D., et al., 2015. European S3-guidelines on the systemic treatment of psoriasis vulgaris – update 2015 – short version – EDF in cooperation with EADV and IPC. J. Eur. Acad. Dermatol. Venereol. 29, 2277–2294.

Ring, J., Alomar, A., Bieber, T., et al., 2012. Guidelines for treatment of atopic eczema (atopic dermatitis) part I. J. Eur. Acad. Dermatol. Venereol. 26, 1045–1060.

Ring, J., Alomar, A., Bieber, T., et al., 2012. Guidelines for treatment of atopic eczema (atopic dermatitis) part II. J. Eur. Acad. Dermatol. Venereol. 26, 1176–1193.

Sidbury, R., Davis, D.M., Cohen, D.E., et al., 2014. Guidelines of care for the management of atopic dermatitis: section 3. Management and treatment of atopic dermatitis with phototherapy and systemic agents. J. Am. Acad. Dermatol. 71, 327–349.

Useful websites

National Eczema Society: http://www.eczema.org

The Psoriasis Association: http://www.psoriasis-association.org.uk

59 Wounds

Samantha Holloway and Keith Harding

Key points

- Acute wound healing should progress through an orderly sequence of events to re-establish tissue integrity.
- A functional blood vessel network is fundamental for wound healing.
- Changes occur in the repaired tissue for a year or more, with the scar tissue becoming stronger with time.
- A number of intrinsic and extrinsic factors can affect the healing process and include age, diabetes, infection, nutrition, smoking and drugs.
- Wounds are costly to treat, and therefore accurate assessment of a patient and his or her wound is important.
- Assessment should be part of an ongoing process, with opportunity for regular re-assessment.
- Acute wounds such as surgical incisions heal quickly with minimal complications; chronic (non-healing) wounds such as diabetic foot ulcers, leg ulcers and pressure ulcers take longer to heal.
- The management of patients with diabetic foot ulcers needs to include treatment of their diabetes, as well as local wound management and off-loading techniques to reduce foot pressures.
- Venous leg ulcers are the most common cause of ulceration in the population and require the external application of compression therapy (bandages and hosiery) to aid healing. These ulcers can be complicated by gravitational eczema; therefore, treatment of the surrounding skin is of equal importance.
- The majority of pressure ulcers are preventable. Management of patients requires a multidisciplinary approach with the use of pressure redistribution, support surfaces and repositioning as adjunctive measures to ensure appropriate care.

A wound can be thought of as any break in the integrity of the skin (Enoch and Leaper, 2005), although when this is due to minor trauma, it might be termed a cut or an abrasion. Such wounds tend to heal fairly quickly by the process of regeneration of tissue and cells and generally do not pose any long-term problems. However, the time it takes for a wound to heal will depend on a number of factors related to the nature of the wound, the individual and the environment. Many of these factors will be dealt with at different points throughout this chapter.

Structure of the skin

The skin is made up of the epidermis and dermis, below which is the sub-cutis, muscle and bone. Within the epidermis, there are four layers:

- stratum corneum,
- stratum granulosum,
- stratum spinosum,
- stratum basale.

Within the very thin structure of the epidermis, some of the key cells required for healing are present, in particular, keratinocytes, dendritic cells and melanocytes.

The dermis is separated into the papillary and reticular dermis and is thicker than the epidermis. It is joined to the epidermis by structures known as rete ridges or 'pegs'. In uninjured tissue, this arrangement helps the skin maintain its normal function, something which can be affected when a wound occurs or as an individual's skin changes with age. Like the epidermis, the dermis also contains many of the key cells/structures that are required for the normal healing response to occur; these include:

- fibroblasts for the production of collagen;
- endothelial cells to stimulate blood vessel growth;
- leucocytes such as lymphocytes, neutrophils and macrophages;
- smooth muscle cells;
- extracellular matrix.

The functions of the skin and the factors that affect skin condition are listed in Table 59.1. How these roles link to wounds and wound healing will be explored in more detail later.

Wound healing

In adults, a scar is the normal end product of most injuries, with occasionally excessive scarring that is hypertrophic or keloid, complicating matters. However, wound healing can also be scarless, such as in fetal skin or the oral mucosa (Desai, 1997a; Wysocki, 2007). This type of healing presents an interesting concept and may offer some significant developments in the future. There are also many individuals for whom healing is delayed; such wounds are often referred to as 'chronic' or 'non-healing'. Other terminology is used in clinical practice to describe how wounds heal and includes:

- primary intention,
- delayed primary closure,
- secondary intention.

Table 59.1 Functions of the skin and factors affecting skin condition

Functions of the skin	Factors affecting skin condition
Protective covering	Dryness
Moisture retention	Age
Sensation	Environment
Regulation of body temperature	Nutrition
Release of waste	Hydration
Absorption of nutrients, i.e. vitamin D	

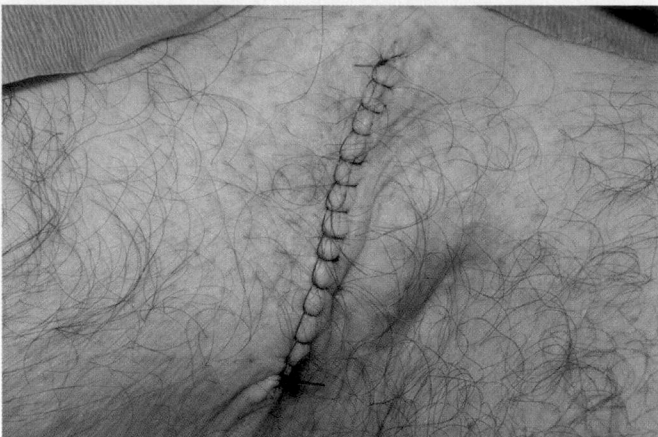

Fig. 59.1 Example of wound healing by primary intention.

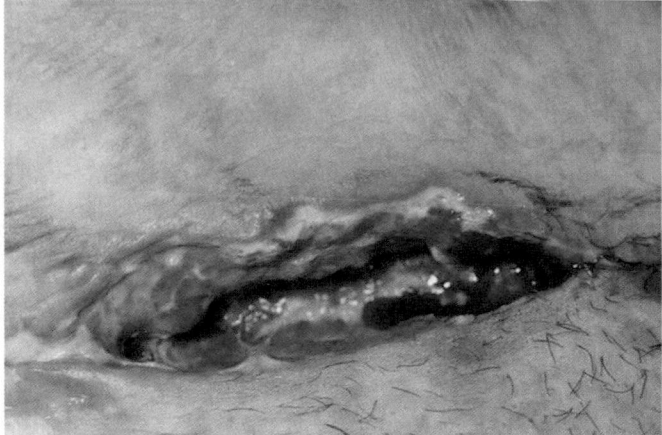

Fig. 59.2 Example of wound healing by secondary intention. Wound bed shows healthy granulation tissue, and epithelial tissue can be seen at the wound edges.

Essentially, healing by primary intention (Fig. 59.1) describes where the wound edges are apposed, that is, brought together by sutures, staples or glue, and wound healing occurs mainly by connective tissue formation. Delayed primary closure is used where there may be a risk of contamination or infection, such as if the patient has undergone emergency abdominal surgery. In this instance, some of the layers of tissue are stitched, and the sutures are placed in readiness for the remainder of the wound to be closed after 48 hours when the risk of infection is less. In contrast, healing by secondary intention (Fig. 59.2) describes a situation in which the wound is left open to heal by the laying down of granulation tissue and wound contraction. This type of healing is relevant to many of the types of wounds that will be discussed later.

Any injury to the skin will result in a sequence of events aimed at repairing the defect. Fig. 59.3 shows the process of wound healing, which is divided into four phases:

- haemostasis,
- inflammation,
- proliferation,
- remodelling or maturation.

An insult to the tissues causes a number of systemic processes to occur simultaneously. Platelets aggregate and adhere to the sub-endothelium; coagulation factors and growth factors are also released. Through changes in the platelet structure and function, thrombin and fibrin are released to aid clot formation and reduce excess blood loss. Once this has occurred, haemostasis is said to have been established. The initial fibrin matrix provides the scaffold for the subsequent structure. This process relies on the individual having a normal clotting response and may be affected by drugs or systemic disease.

After haemostasis, the inflammatory phase extends from day 0 through to about day 10 in normal healing and involves neutrophils (early inflammation) and macrophages (late inflammation). Neutrophils phagocytose bacteria and kill foreign bodies by producing oxygen metabolites such as hydroxyl radicals, hydrogen peroxide and superoxide ion. In normal healing, the numbers of neutrophils decrease in number over time leading to an increase in the number of macrophages present. The key function of macrophages is to digest bacteria, dead tissue and old neutrophils. There is some evidence to suggest that in wounds which are not healing, it may be the inflammatory phase and its related

cells that are at fault. The classic signs of inflammation are well reported and include:

- redness,
- swelling,
- heat,
- pain.

These signs are normal and should not be considered as indicating the presence of infection.

The proliferative phase begins approximately 1 day post-injury and should be resolving by about day 30. There are three main activities that occur during this time:

- granulation tissue formation, which requires new blood vessel formation (known as angiogenesis) and formation of collagen;
- contraction of the wound;
- epithelialisation.

The presence of a functional blood vessel network is fundamental for wound healing to progress. Angiogenesis, the formation of blood vessels, is required to supply oxygen to the wound environment, and it is through the migration of capillaries through the provisional matrix that the vasculature is re-established. Endothelial cells migrate and proliferate to eventually join the existing blood supply to the injured area. Once this has

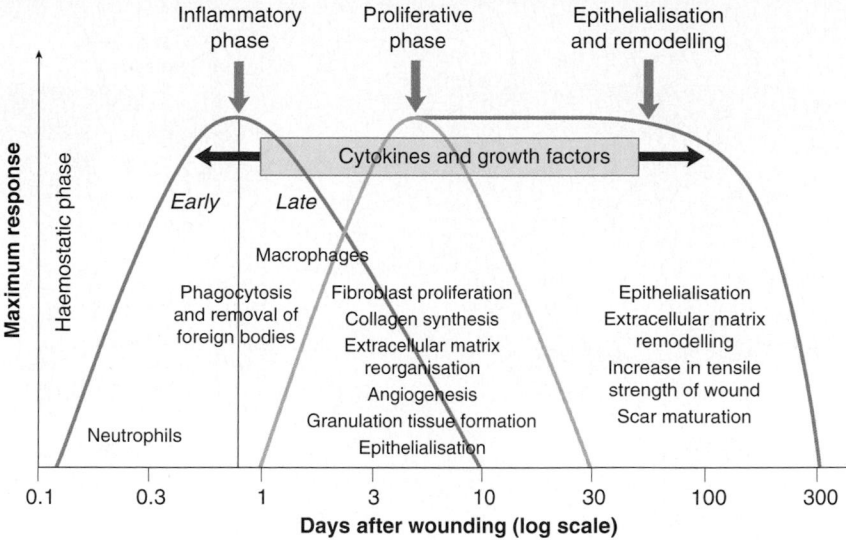

Fig. 59.3 Phases of wound healing. (From Enoch et al., 2008.)

occurred, granulation tissue can form to begin to repair the defect. The provisional tissue laid down (see Fig. 59.2) is made up of fibrin, fibronectin, collagen and glycosaminoglycans. Through the action of fibroblasts, collagen is produced, and the continued presence of macrophages ensures the wound is kept 'clean'. Collagen production is essential for healing to progress, and in particular, types I, III and IV are required.

In conjunction with the laying down of granulation tissue, the wound edges begin to contract at around day 8, and this process assists wound closure. The key cell involved is the myofibroblast, which applies tension to the surrounding matrix to induce contraction. The normal process of contraction should not be confused with contracture, which is an abnormal feature of scarring.

Around the same time, it may also be possible to see signs of epithelialisation occurring (see Fig. 59.2). Keratinocytes, the cell associated with this process, are initiated hours after injury; they migrate from the edge of a wound over the provisional matrix laid down, or they dissect through it. Hair follicles can act as islands of regenerating epithelium in some areas. During the proliferative phase the wound bed can be easily damaged by simple things, such as incorrect dressing choice, causing significant damage. Current clinical practice still reflects the original principles of moist wound healing proposed by Winter (1962) to support the normal physiological process of healing.

The final phase of the healing process is termed remodelling or maturation. During this time, the initial collagen that has been laid down is synthesised by enzymes, ultimately leading to a more ordered network that increases in structure and strength over time. However, this repaired area is never as strong as normal tissue and is always at risk of breakdown. These final changes can take place for up to a year or more after the initial injury.

Factors affecting wound healing

Generally, wound healing should progress as described previously; however, numerous factors that affect healing have been

Table 59.2 Intrinsic and extrinsic factors affecting wound healing

Intrinsic (systemic) factors	Local factors	Extrinsic factors
Age	Blood supply	Nutrition
Uraemia	Changes in oxygen tension	Smoking
Jaundice	Vessel trauma	Radiotherapy
Diabetes	Abnormal scarring	Infection
Anaemia	Haematoma	Drugs
Hormones	Local infection	Iatrogenic influences
Malignant disease		Wound dressings

identified (Grey and Harding, 2008). A summary of these is provided in Table 59.2, some of which include:

- age,
- diabetes,
- infection,
- nutrition,
- smoking,
- drugs.

Age

Younger patients appear to have an increased rate of healing, and there are differences in fetal healing that make the regeneration process superior, with little or no inflammation or scarring (Desai, 1997b). In comparison, wound repair in the elderly is slower (Ashcroft et al., 2002), and management may be more challenging because of concurrent disease processes. This is a particular problem in the proliferative

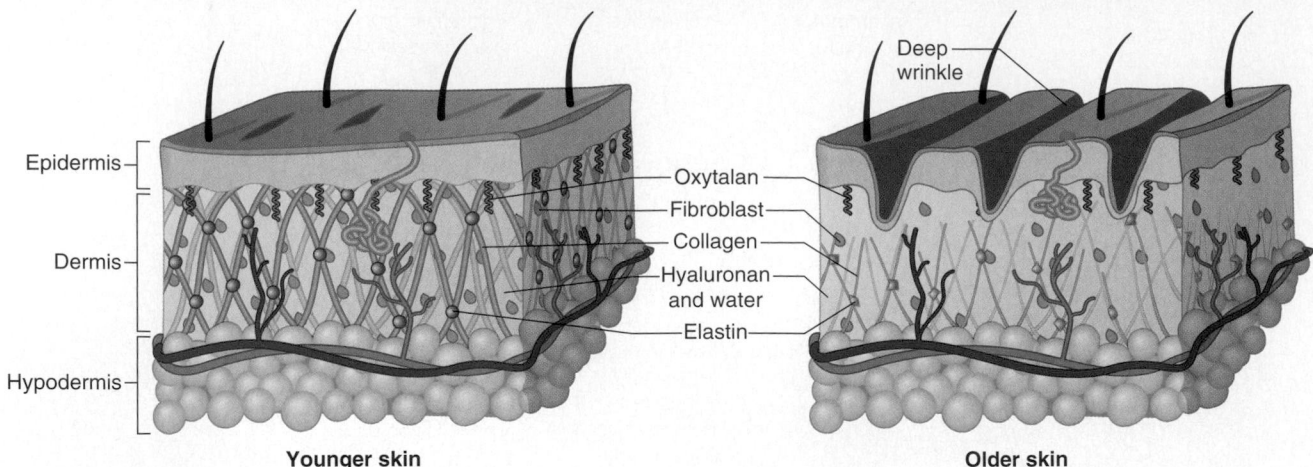

Fig. 59.4 Skin changes that occur with age.

Table 59.3	Complications of diabetes
Peripheral neuropathy	Causes damage to nerves that leads to a lack of the protective pain sensation, but the blood supply remains good. Very common and can lead to foot deformities and abnormal walking patterns. Neuropathy should be considered in terms of sensory, autonomic and motor changes. The foot is usually warm, numb and dry, with palpable foot pulses.
Peripheral arterial disease	Often develops as a result of atherosclerosis but develops at a faster rate in diabetic patients. Can affect the large (macro) and small (micro) vessels, leading to decreased blood flow to the legs and feet, which can ultimately lead to minor or major amputations. The foot is often cool and clammy, with absent or reduced foot pulses.
Neuro-ischaemia	A combination of peripheral neuropathy and peripheral arterial disease.
Infection	More common in diabetic patients, probably because they have an associated defective immunity. The neutrophil and lymphocyte response is slow (partly due to vascular problems); therefore, the inflammatory and subsequent phases are impaired. Hence, these patients have an increased tendency to develop infections.

and remodelling phases, where tissue appears to be more friable and fragile. The overall effects of age on wound healing appear to be:
- decreased inflammatory response,
- delayed angiogenesis,
- decreased collagen synthesis and degradation,
- slower epithelialisation.

There are also changes that affect the skin as we age, for example, the normal epidermal turnover rate is 28 days. This increases by 30–50% by the age of 80. Also, changes in the stratum corneum and reduced lipid content alter the barrier function, as does the slower turnover rate. Decreased amino acids also lead to a decrease in natural moisturising factors, meaning the skin is much more at risk of being dry. The collagen content of the skin decreases by 1% per year and becomes less soluble, and the process of new collagen formation is slowed. Furthermore, delayed angiogenesis leads to changes in the microvasculature and nerve function, leading to atrophic skin (Marcos-Garcés et al., 2014) (Fig. 59.4).

Diabetes

In individuals with diabetes, wound healing can be delayed, and management is often challenging because of concurrent peripheral diabetic neuropathy (PDN), peripheral arterial disease (PAD), neuro-ischaemia and infection (Table 59.3).

Infection

Bacterial invasion of wounds is very common. In fact, any break in the skin integrity places the wound at risk of local contamination or infection and if untreated can lead to systemic infection. The spectrum of infection from colonisation through to infection is demonstrated in Fig. 59.5. The difficulty may be in recognising when such circumstances are present. The normal inflammatory signs were discussed earlier, and these should be borne in mind when examining a patient's wound. However, there are additional local signs that may be present in wounds healing by primary or secondary intention (Fig. 59.6) that suggest an infective process. These include:
- increased pain;
- delayed wound healing;
- wound that bleeds easily;
- friable, fragile tissue;
- pocketing/bridging of tissue;
- wound breakdown (dehiscence).

Infection in a wound can often be diagnosed by clinical signs and symptoms alone, and unless a systemic infection is suspected, that is, the patient complains of flu-like symptoms, it can be treated locally with topical antimicrobial dressings rather than oral antibiotics.

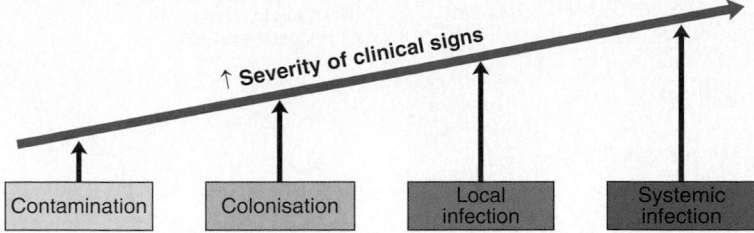

Fig. 59.5 Schematic representation for the outcome of bacterial invasion.

↑ Severity of clinical signs

Contamination Colonisation Local infection Systemic infection

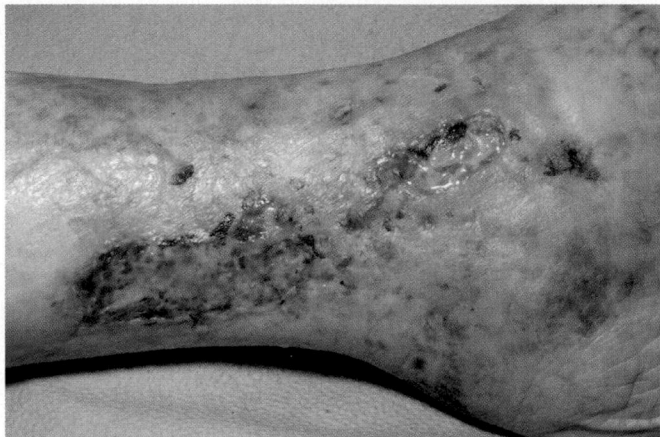

Fig. 59.6 Infection in a granulating wound.

In recent years, there has been increased recognition that bacteria have the ability to build up colonies that present a challenge in terms of the management of bacterial load. Known as biofilms, they have the ability to resist removal and have been implicated in delayed healing of a number of wound types. The removal of dead tissue from the wound bed seems to have some effect in preventing the growth of biofilms (Wolcott and Rhoads, 2008); however, this method is not suitable for all wounds, so other approaches are being sought.

The choice of topical treatment for the management of local wound infection is dealt with in a later section.

Nutrition

The nutritional requirements for wound healing have been the subject of debate, with limited evidence as to the exact dietary components for individual wound types. In general, if the patient has a balanced diet, this should be sufficient for the normal processes to take place. However, a diet that is lacking in vital nutrients can lead to delayed wound healing and wound breakdown. In the extreme, the patient can become malnourished, with surgical patients most at risk of protein-energy malnutrition (PEM). Box 59.1 outlines the nutritional factors that should be considered in the assessment of individuals, many of which have been incorporated in nutritional risk assessment tools. Individuals who are most at risk of nutritional deficiencies are those affected by:

- ill health in old age,
- cancer,
- chronic neurological disease,
- chronic inflammatory bowel disease,
- surgery (pre- and postoperatively),
- stroke,
- acute and chronic pain,
- immunodeficiency disease such as HIV and AIDS.

One of the most commonly used tools to assess nutritional status in clinical practice is the Malnutrition Universal Screening Tool (MUST; British Association for Parenteral and Enteral Nutrition, 2015).

Smoking

Smoking is known to be detrimental to health generally, and in addition, the effect of nicotine and carbon monoxide on skin and muscles is well documented (Ortiz and Grando, 2012). These substances reduce the oxygen levels in the tissues and can lead to

---

Box 59.1 Nutritional assessment and treatment options

General nutritional assessment to include
Current appetite
Food intake
Patient's ability to eat/chew/swallow
Presence of dentures

Specialist nutritional assessment
Anthropometric measurements such as:
Body mass index, % weight loss, haemoglobin, skinfold thickness, grip strength, serum albumin
Gut function
Total energy requirements

Nutrients required for healing
Protein
Zinc
Copper
Iron

Vitamins required for healing
A
B complex
C
E

Treatment options
Modified normal diet: increase high-energy/high-protein foods
Modified normal diet plus nutritional supplementation
Total enteral support
Naso-gastric feeding
Total parenteral nutrition
Percutaneous endoscopic gastrostomy

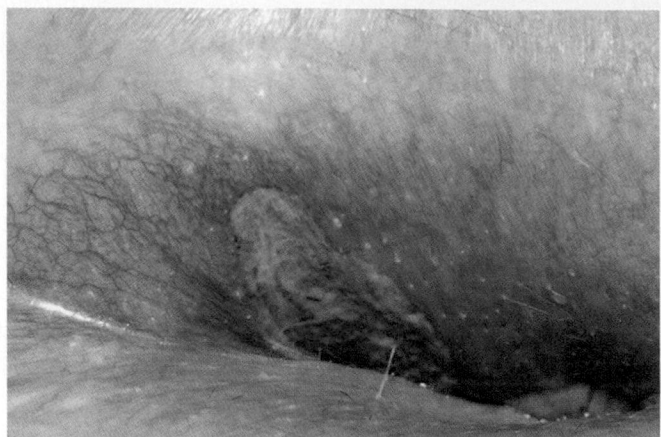

Fig. 59.7 Perianal ulceration associated with administration of nicorandil.

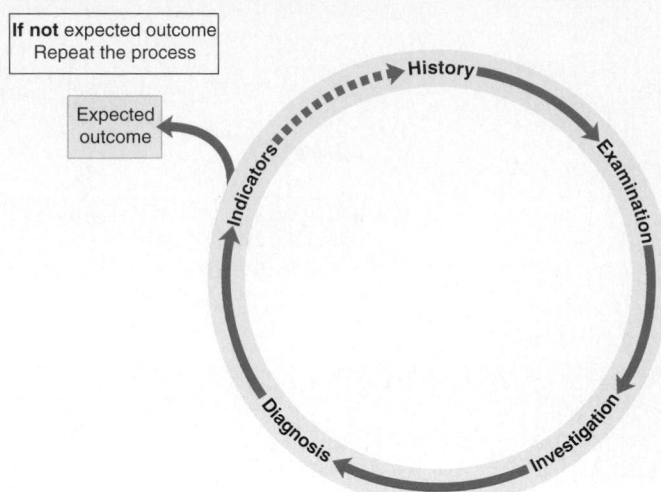

Fig. 59.8 Assessment of a patient with a wound.

the formation of thrombi. A good blood supply and adequate vascularisation are important for normal wound healing. There has been debate about the period of time patients should abstain from smoking to reduce relevant potential complications. This has been suggested to vary from 4 (Sorensen et al., 2003) to 8 weeks (Møller et al., 2002). There is emerging evidence to suggest that offering nicotine replacement to reduce the risk of postoperative complications along with smoking cessation counselling can be helpful (Thomsen et al., 2014).

Drugs

There are certain drugs that are suggested to have an effect on the healing process. These include non-steroidal anti-inflammatory drugs (NSAIDs), corticosteroids and immunosuppressive agents (Grey and Harding, 2008), which affect the inflammatory response, collagen synthesis and mitosis, respectively. Whilst drugs do not generally cause wounds, there have been recent reports that nicorandil (used for the treatment of angina) may cause peri-anal wounds (Fig. 59.7) that resolve on cessation of the medication (Ferner, 2016).

Wound assessment

Wounds are costly to treat (Phillips et al., 2016); therefore, it is important to appreciate the various considerations that need to be taken into account when assessing a patient. Assessment should not be viewed as a one-off occurrence but instead should be undertaken as part of an ongoing process with the emphasis on the patient, not just his or her wound.

A structured approach to the assessment of a patient with a wound is required. The six key elements of the original wound healing matrix are as follows, and the key concepts are depicted in Fig. 59.8:
- Phase of wound healing
- Aetiology:
  - acute, for example, surgical, trauma, burn injuries;
  - chronic, for example, leg ulcers, diabetic foot ulcers, pressure ulcers.
- Clinical manifestation:
  - size;
  - shape;
  - characteristics, that is, exudate, odour, tissue type.
- Environment and care:
  - primary care;
  - secondary care.
- Healthcare system and resources
- Site of the wound

Diabetic foot ulcers
Epidemiology

According to estimated figures, in 2014 the number of individuals diagnosed with diabetes in the UK increased to more than 3.2 million (Diabetes UK, 2014). The cost of treating individuals with diabetes accounts for at least 9% of the acute healthcare costs in the UK. These costs, however, do not take into account the personal cost to the individual, such as a reduction in the ability to work and the time he or she may need to take off work (Waters and Holloway, 2009). Diabetic foot problems are the most common cause for admission, and patients admitted to hospital for in-patient care are often hospitalised for 4–6 weeks, which obviously increases the financial costs considerably.

One of the major risks to patients with diabetic foot disease is that of amputation, which could be minor, that is mid-foot to toe, or major, that is mid-foot and above (Holman et al., 2012). The National Service Frameworks for diabetes introduced by the Department of Health (DH) in 2001 and 2007 sought to address this (DH, 2001, 2007a, 2007b). Of concern is that up to 85% of amputations are preceded by foot ulcers. Therefore, if the incidence of foot ulcers can be reduced, this might lead to a reduction in amputations.

Aetiology

Individuals with diabetes are at risk of a number of systemic complications (see Chapter 45).

Table 59.4 Clinical features of a diabetic foot with neuropathy or arterial disease

Characteristic	Peripheral neuropathy	Peripheral arterial disease
Temperature	Warm	Cool
Foot pulse	Present/'bounding'	Absent/reduced
Pain	Commonly no pain[a]	Pain on walking (intermittent claudication) Depends on degree of neuropathy
Site of ulcers	Toes and metatarsal heads	Lateral (outer) border of foot
Callus (hard skin)	Present	Absent

[a]Painful peripheral neuropathy is a rare but potential feature.

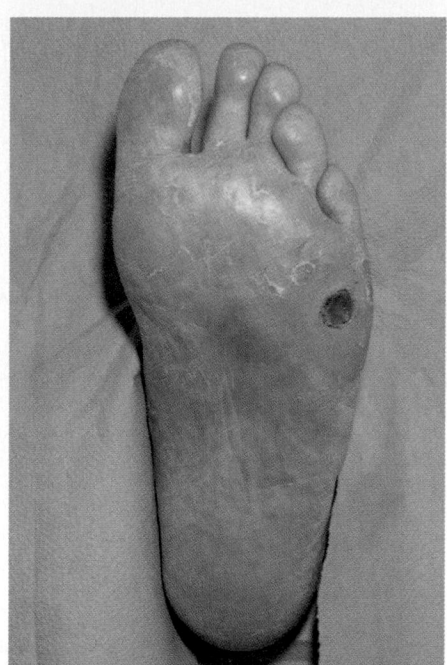

Fig. 59.9 Diabetic foot ulcer caused by peripheral neuropathy.

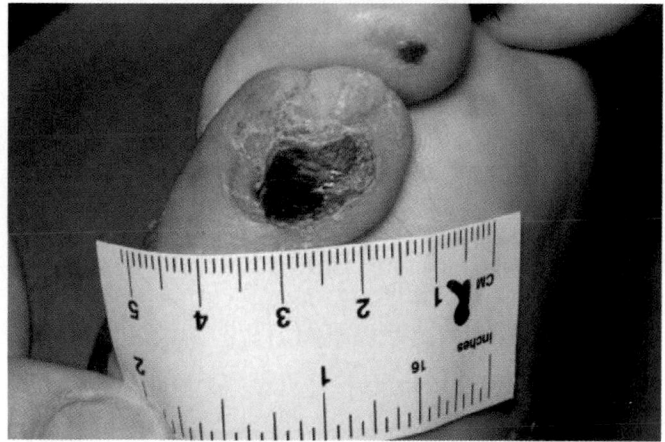

Fig. 59.10 Peripheral arterial disease in a patient with diabetes.

There are two main causes of foot ulceration in patients with diabetes:

- peripheral diabetic neuropathy (PDN),
- peripheral arterial disease (PAD).

PDN causes damage to the nerves that leads to a lack of the protective pain sensation and is present in 75% of patients with diabetes. In this group of individuals, the blood supply to the extremities remains good, but the foot becomes insensate and can subsequently become deformed. This leads to an abnormal walking pattern and potentially tissue breakdown from abnormal pressures placed upon the foot. The characteristics of the diabetic foot are set out in Table 59.4. Unfortunately, the early systemic changes associated with the onset of diabetes may be present for up to 12 years before a diagnosis is made, by which time damage has already begun to occur and is often irreversible.

Neuropathy can be related to lack of sensation (sensory neuropathy) and may also cause atrophy and weakness of muscles in the foot (motor neuropathy). In addition, there are effects on the autonomic nervous system which can cause changes in blood flow and sweat secretion (autonomic neuropathy). Each of these elements needs to be considered as each has significant effects on the lower limb in individuals with diabetes.

PAD usually occurs as a result of atherosclerosis. This often results in a reduction in blood flow to the lower limbs and pain on walking (claudication), pain at rest with possible progression to gangrene and amputation. PAD is common in the elderly and is not just a complication of diabetes, although people who have diabetes are at an increased risk of developing it. Foot ulceration due to PAD is less common, accounting for approximately 5% of cases.

Clinical signs

The clinical features of a diabetic foot with PDN and PAD are summarised in Table 59.4, and their typical presentations are shown in Figs. 59.9 and 59.10, respectively. There are a number of factors that place patients at increased risk of ulceration, including foot deformity; ill-fitting footwear; mechanical injury, for example, treading on a sharp object; thermal injury, for example, heat from a fire, or stepping into a hot bath; and chemical trauma, typically caused by an over-the-counter preparation purchased to remove hard skin. National guidelines outline the processes that should be in place to ensure the monitoring of patients deemed at risk (National Institute of Health and Care Excellence [NICE], 2015a, 2015b). One of the key issues to consider is that the feet of patients with diabetes do not ulcerate spontaneously; instead, any one, or a combination, of the factors discussed could be the cause.

Diagnosis

Initial assessment should include a clinical examination of the foot and may also require objective testing, for example, an

Table 59.5 Examination of the diabetic foot

Clinical examination		Objective test
Shape and deformities	Toe deformities Foot deformities Callus	X-ray
Sensory function	Vibration Protective sensation	Biothesiometry Semmes–Weinstein filament
Motor function	Wasting Weakness Ankle reflexes	Electrophysiological tests
Autonomic function	Reduced sweating Callus Warmth Appearance of veins on the foot	Quantitative sweat test
Vascular status	Foot pulses Temperature Swelling	Non-invasive Doppler studies, ankle brachial pressure index and/or toe pressure indices

X-ray. The key features of this examination are set out in Table 59.5. In addition, further tests such as a full blood count, examination of urine, alternate imaging methods, magnetic resonance imaging, colour duplex scans and angiograms, may be indicated.

Infection in the diabetic foot is a real risk and a common complication. It has been estimated that 20–50% of diabetic ulcers are infected. The severity of the infection will depend on the nature of the bacteria, but commonly cellulitis and osteomyelitis occur in patients with neuropathic ulcers with gangrene being more associated with PAD. Bacterial cultures from ulcers are usually polymicrobial with both Gram-positive and Gram-negative organisms, as well as anaerobic bacteria. There should be concern if any of the following features occur:

- difficulty walking and/or applying shoes;
- swelling in part or all of the foot;
- redness or other discolouration;
- foot becomes hotter than normal;
- discharge or unusual odour;
- open sores or blisters;
- nausea, vomiting or high temperature;
- difficulty maintaining blood glucose control.

Treatment

Infection

The signs of infection are often delayed or insidious in patients with diabetes. Virtually all diabetic foot infections require antimicrobial therapy, but this alone is rarely sufficient. If soft-tissue infection is superficial, then oral, relatively narrow-spectrum antibiotics for 1–2 weeks are indicated for mild infections and 2–3 weeks for moderate to severe infections (Lipsky et al., 2012); however, if there is cellulitis and spreading infection, parenteral antibiotic therapy may be required for up to 4 weeks. In addition to antibiotics, the patient may require hospitalisation if removal of dead tissue (debridement) is required. An X-ray of the foot may also be advisable if the tissue loss is over the bone, and referral to a vascular or orthopaedic specialist may be necessary for surgery.

Other considerations

Treatment of a diabetic foot ulcer should also include:
- podiatry,
- skin and wound care,
- provision of footwear to remove/redistribute weight,
- offloading options to include orthoses/custom-made insoles,
- patient education,
- pain relief,
- control of diabetes,
- multidisciplinary team approach.

The range of treatment options will be determined by whether there is neuropathy and/or PAD present, as well as the presence of ulcers and/or infection. The debridement of callus and dead tissue is essential because it enables the true dimensions of the ulcer to be established (Edmonds and Foster, 2000). Dressings are important but should not be viewed in isolation from the other essential aspects of treatment listed previously. Key aspects in the choice of dressing for diabetic foot ulcers are how it will perform in a shoe, whether it will withstand pressure and shear forces, how well it will absorb any fluid from the wound, how often the dressing needs to be changed and the cost effectiveness of the dressing.

Prevention of recurrence

Many of the considerations discussed previously are also important in terms of preventing a recurrence of ulceration and should be borne in mind when planning the management of individuals with diabetes. Ideally, ulceration should be prevented via intensive screening programmes, although unfortunately, this is not always achievable. In addition, the maintenance of tight control over blood glucose and blood pressure is required. Guidelines (NICE, 2015a, 2015b) recommend the following:
- blood pressure ≤140/80 mmHg or ≤130/80 mmHg if there is kidney, eye or cerebrovascular damage;
- blood glucose 48 mmol/mol (6.5%) or 53 mmol/mol (7%) for adults on a drug associated with hypoglycaemia.

Leg ulcers
Epidemiology

The prevalence of leg ulcers in the Western world is 0.11–0.18% (Briggs and Closs, 2003). There is a preponderance of 2.8:1 female to male ratio, with venous disease being the main cause of ulceration. The risk of leg ulceration increases with age.

The estimated cost in the UK of all leg ulcers is between £200 million and £600 million, with the costs of individual ulcer treatment between £557 and £1366 over a year (Tennvall and Hjelmgren, 2005). Between 60% and 90% of patients are managed in the community.

Aetiology

Leg ulcers can be classified as follows:
- venous;
- arterial;
- mixed, that is ulcers that have a venous and arterial component;
- diabetic, typically on the foot, rather than the leg;
- autoimmune, for example, rheumatoid arthritis.

Venous ulcers

Ulcers of venous origin account for the majority of all leg ulcers. There are a number of reasons why they occur, including failure of the calf muscle pump to work effectively, which leads to pooling of fluid in the lower limb and oedema. This can lead to high pressures in the lower limb on walking, known as venous hypertension. This swelling can lead to poor oxygenation of the tissues and trapping of harmful substances such as growth factors and enzymes. Ultimately, this can lead to tissue breakdown precipitated by simple trauma such as knocking the leg.

The calf muscle pump relies on an adequate level of mobility; therefore, anything that might affect this, such as increasing age, obesity and trauma, predisposes the individual to a sequence of events if the individual also has poor venous return.

Risk factors associated with the development of venous ulcers include deep vein thrombosis (DVT), varicose veins, and surgery/trauma to the leg.

Clinical signs

Venous disease. As a result of venous hypertension and leakage of fluid, red blood cells are deposited in the tissues, causing discolouration known as haemosiderin. This can often be seen on the lower limb and may be red or brown in colour. Varicose veins may also be visible as will oedema (swelling) and a characteristic change known as lipodermatosclerosis (LDS). Over time, the limb may develop a typical inverted 'champagne bottle' appearance. Venous ulcers are typically shallow and develop in the gaiter area (Fig. 59.11). Patients may also have associated gravitational eczema.

Diagnosis

The key element is the accuracy of the assessment, which should include:
- clinical history,
- clinical investigation,
- assessment of the limb,
- assessment of the ulcer.

Table 59.6 summarises the key aspects of the assessment of an individual with a leg ulcer.

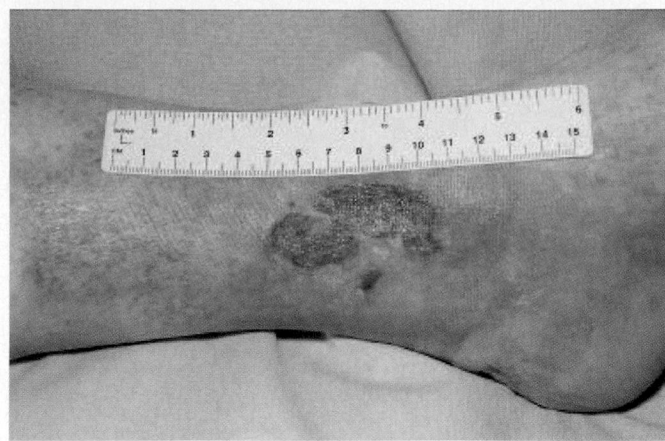

Fig. 59.11 Venous leg ulceration.

Assessment of ankle brachial pressure index (ABPI). The use of a hand-held Doppler device is used to assess the arterial blood flow. Ideally, this test should be undertaken on any patient presenting with a leg ulcer. Furthermore, it should be carried out on first presentation and at subsequent intervals depending on whether the ulcer is improving or not. Essentially, the ABPI compares the patient's brachial (arm) and ankle systolic pressures:

$$ABPI = \frac{\text{highest ankle systolic pressure}}{\text{highest brachial systolic pressure}}$$

The patient should rest for 20 minutes before the assessment, and the pressures should be measured supine (lying down). Two measurements should be taken from the foot and the highest value used in the calculation.

The ABPI is not a definitive measure of arterial status but merely serves as an indicator of blood flow. Other clinical signs and symptoms such as the colour and temperature of the limb, the presence/absence of pulses and pain also need to be taken into account.

As a general principle, the ABPI or ratio should be ≥1.0 in individuals with no arterial disease (Al-Qaisi et al., 2009) (Table 59.7). However, this should not be relied upon in the presence of diabetes because calcification of arteries can occur and lead to falsely high ABPI readings. In this instance, a Duplex scan would be a more reliable indicator of vascular status. Furthermore, both hypo- and hypertension can affect the readings.

Treatment

The mainstay of treatment for confirmed venous ulceration is compression therapy (bandages and hosiery). Known as graduated compression, specific bandage systems are used to apply external pressure to aid venous return. The ABPI must be ≥0.9 for this treatment to be used. Although there is much debate about which bandage system is preferable, the choice should be based on an individual patient assessment and may include (Wounds International, 2013):
- bandage components or layers wrapped around the leg (either full leg or below knee),
- compression hosiery (e.g. compression stockings).

Table 59.6 Factors to be taken into account in the assessment of an individual with a leg ulcer

Clinical history	Clinical investigations	Assessment of both limbs	Assessment of the ulcer
Family history	Blood pressure	Oedema	Year first ulcer occurred
Varicose veins	Ankle brachial pressure index	Site of ulcer	Site of ulcer/previous ulcers
Deep vein thrombosis/pulmonary embolus	Full blood count	Depth of wound	Size of ulcer(s)
Phlebitis		Appearance of wound bed	Number of previous episodes
Surgery or fracture of the leg		Surrounding skin	Time free of ulcers
Heart disease/stroke		Perfusion of feet	Past treatment (successful or not)
Diabetes		Presence of pulses	Previous/current uses of compression bandaging
Peripheral arterial disease		Ankle brachial pressure index	
Chest pain/angina			
Smoker			
Rheumatoid arthritis			
Medication			
Allergies			

Table 59.7 Ankle brachial pressure index or ratio (Andriessen et al., 2017)

ABPI[a]	Arterial status	Compression therapy
>1.3	Is usually indicative of non-compressible blood vessels	
>1.00–1.3	Considered to be normal	Indicated
= 0.8–1.0	Mild peripheral disease	Use with caution
≤0.8–0.6	Significant arterial disease	Modified compression may be used with caution – specialist referral required
<0.5	Critical ischaemia may be associated with rest pain, ischaemic ulceration or gangrene	Compression contraindicated. Urgent referral to a vascular specialist required

[a]ABPI, Ankle brachial pressure index – should be used in conjunction with a comprehensive clinical assessment.

The aim of most systems is to create pressures of 40 mmHg at the ankle decreasing up to the knee to assist in venous return. In addition to bandaging, the patient should be encouraged to keep mobile, which could be as simple as undertaking ankle exercises to improve blood flow. Leg elevation and rest should also form part of overall management.

Even where arterial disease has been excluded as a complication, the patient should be monitored carefully for signs of compromised blood flow because serious injury, such as skin necrosis, can occur. This is a potentially serious complication that in the extreme can lead to significant circulatory compromise and amputation.

Other treatment options may include antibiotics if systemic infection is suspected or topical antimicrobial dressings for local infection, which include iodine- or silver-based products.

Intermittent pneumatic compression, surgery, skin grafting, bioengineered skin and pharmacological treatments such as oxpentifylline have all been suggested as adjuvant therapies to compression therapy (Scottish Intercollegiate Guideline Network, 2010).

General wound care should include cleansing of the ulcerated area with saline or tap water to maintain cleanliness and hygiene, as well as debridement of any dead tissue. Dressings should be simple and as low adherent as possible because they have to perform well under the compression system chosen. There is a need to be aware of the potential of contact sensitivity to the dressings, bandages or skin treatments used.

Gravitational eczema is commonplace in patients with venous disease and is related to the changes caused by venous hypertension (Fig. 59.12). The patient may complain of intense itching, and scratch marks may be visible on examination. It is important to distinguish eczema from contact sensitivity and cellulitis because each of these requires a different treatment. Treatment of eczema will include a combination of a topical corticosteroid

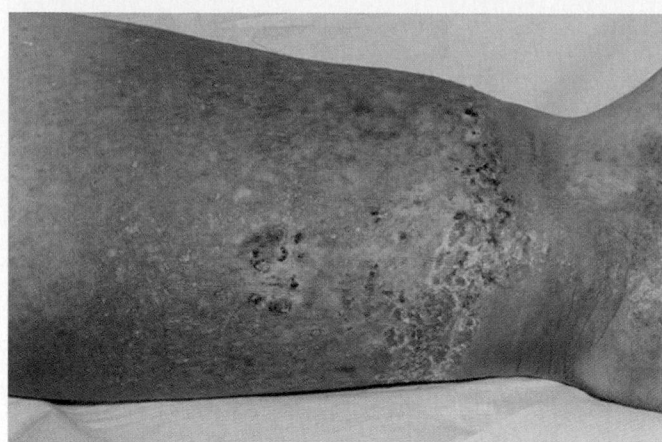

Fig. 59.12 Venous leg ulceration and gravitational eczema.

Table 59.8 British National Formulary compression values for hosiery

Compression class	Level of support	Compression hosiery (British Standard)
Class 1	Light	14–17 mmHg[a]
Class 2	Medium	18–24 mmHg[a]
Class 3	Strong	25–35 mmHg[a]

[a]Compression provided at the ankle.

such as clobetasone butyrate (Eumovate) or mometasone furoate (Elocon) ointments and emollients such as Epaderm or similar mixtures of soft white paraffin and liquid paraffin to manage this inflammatory condition.

Prevention of recurrence

Once a venous ulcer is healed, compression hosiery (in the form of stockings) is required. This hosiery is classed as 1, 2 or 3 depending on the level of pressure applied. Class 3 stockings and tights provide strong support (25–35 mmHg at the ankle) and are the preferred choice to prevent recurrence of venous ulcers. Table 59.8 provides the compression values for hosiery. Ideally, they will need to be worn for life or at least a minimum of 5 years. Unfortunately, recurrence is common, often because of the inconvenience associated with the wearing of stockings. Patient education and follow-up are essential. Community leg ulcer clinics have been established in many areas of the UK and have shown to be effective in supporting patients (Lindsay, 2013).

Arterial ulcers

Arterial ulceration is commonly associated with atherosclerosis and peripheral arterial occlusive disease (PAOD), much of which has been discussed previously in relation to diabetic foot disease. Both macro-disease (large vessel) and micro-disease (small vessel) may be present.

Clinical signs

The classic clinical features of arterial insufficiency are:
- intermittent claudication/rest pain;
- colour changes, for example, pallor;
- muscle atrophy/weakness;
- poor perfusion, for example, cool limb;
- loss of skin hair;
- thickening/hardening of the nails;
- ulceration;
- gangrene.

Arterial ulcers often appear 'punched out' (Fig. 59.13) and have a pale wound bed. The significant feature is pain, with many patients reporting pain on walking known as intermittent

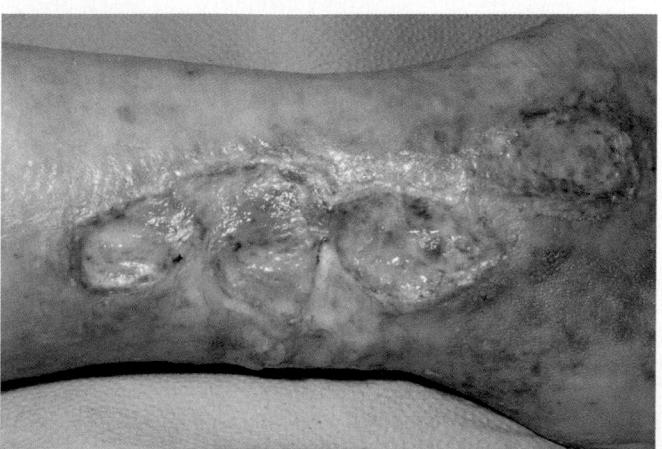

Fig. 59.13 Arterial leg ulceration.

claudication. As the disease progresses, patients may also report that their pain is worse at rest, particularly when their legs are elevated. This feature affects their ability to sleep, eat and keep mobile, which can ultimately mean they are unable to leave the house.

Diagnosis

A simple test known as Buerger's test (see Glossary) is normally used to look for positive signs of disease. If it is possible, a Doppler test should also be undertaken to calculate the patient's ABPI. Typically, an ABPI of 0.5–0.8 indicates a moderate degree of arterial disease, whereas a value of ≤0.5 is considered to be indicative of severe disease (Al-Qaisi et al., 2009). In addition, a colour Duplex scan is usually required to ascertain the extent of the disease. If treatment is required, angiography will usually be undertaken to examine the affected vessels.

Treatment

An angioplasty may be carried out to improve the blood supply. Where this is not possible, vascular reconstruction may be advised to try and prevent further progression. Treatment should also include pain relief, prevention of infection and nutritional support. In addition, smoking cessation advice may be needed as might pharmaceutical intervention for cholesterol or lipid-lowering purposes.

Table 59.9 Incidence of pressure ulcers in UK (Clark et al., 2004)

	Grade[a] distribution	Annual incidence
Grade I	34.9%	140,000
Grade II	41.2%	170,000
Grade III	12.9%	50,000
Grade IV	11.0%	50,000

[a]Grade is the same as category/stage in the new NPUAP et al. (2014) guidelines.

Prevention of recurrence

The main risk of individuals with arterial disease is amputation (minor or major). The patient plays a key role in prevention because many of the predisposing factors are lifestyle issues such as giving up smoking, eating a healthy diet and exercise.

Mixed ulcers

Although the term 'mixed ulceration' is used in clinical practice to describe ulcers with an element of venous and arterial disease, technically, it is not a diagnosis. Patients present with symptoms of venous and arterial disease, for example, skin discoloration and skin changes, as well as intermittent claudication. The ABPI is likely to be between 0.6 and 0.8. Treatment is directed at the symptoms causing the most concern, with compression therapy only used under very close supervision. The management options are as discussed previously for venous and arterial ulcers, with the degree of arterial compromise being the most significant factor determining management.

Pressure ulcers

Epidemiology

Previously referred to as 'bed sores' or 'pressure sores', this wound type is now generally referred to as a pressure ulcer (National Pressure Ulcer Advisory Panel [NPUAP] et al., 2014) and defined as follows:

A pressure ulcer is localized injury to the skin and/or underlying tissue usually over a bony prominence, as a result of pressure, or pressure in combination with shear. A number of contributing or confounding factors are also associated with pressure ulcers; the significance of these factors is yet to be elucidated.

(NPUAP et al., 2014, p. 12)

The prevalence of pressure ulcers across five European countries was previously estimated at 18.1% (Clark et al., 2004). There is no national method for collecting data on the occurrence of pressure ulcers; however, Table 59.9 provides a summary of the most recent data on incidence (Clark et al., 2004).

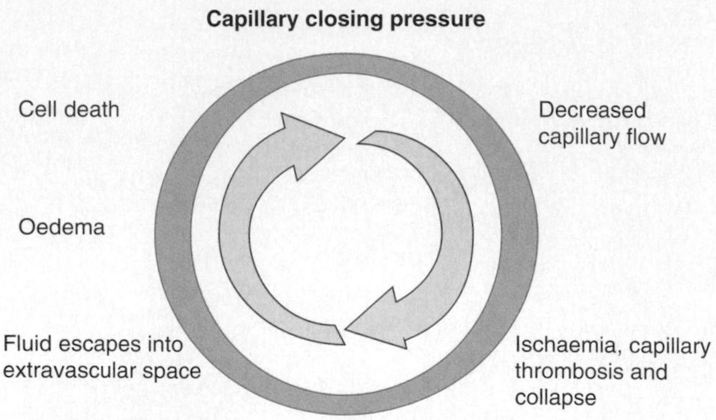

Fig. 59.14 Effect of external pressure on the capillaries.

Common sites of pressure ulcers

Pressure ulcer damage can occur anywhere on the body but is most common over bony prominences, including:

*   sacrum,
*   heels,
*   buttock,
*   trochanter.

Sacral damage often occurs from the patient slipping down the bed or whilst sitting in a chair, with shear forces causing the most damage. Injury to other areas is more likely to be due to direct pressure over a bony prominence. In acutely ill patients, medical devices and equipment such as nasal cannula can even cause pressure damage to the nose.

Aetiology

As the name implies, this sort of wound is caused by external pressure on the tissues, which, if sustained, leads to decreased capillary flow, ischaemia and capillary thrombosis. In turn, fluid escapes from the vasculature into the surrounding tissues causing oedema, accumulation of metabolic waste and cell death (Fig. 59.14).

There are different types of pressure that may be implicated in the onset of damage, and it is both the type and duration of pressure that is of importance. The types of pressure are listed as follows:

*   capillary closing pressure,
*   vertical pressure,
*   tissue interface pressure,
*   shear and friction forces.

In addition to pressure, other factors that may influence the development of the damage include:

*   reactive hyperaemia,
*   reperfusion injury,
*   patient age: extremes of age most at risk,
*   nutritional status: extremes of weight most at risk,
*   mobility status,
*   condition of peripheral circulation,
*   continence status.

Clinical signs

Early signs of damage may present as a red area on the skin that remains even after the pressure has been relieved (referred to as non-blanching erythema), or damage may present as broken skin or an abrasion. Pressure ulcers are now classified using six categories or stages based on the NPUAP et al. (2014) guidelines, as described in the following sections.

Category/stage I: non-blanchable erythema

These pressure ulcers have intact skin with non-blanchable redness of a localised area usually over a bony prominence. Darkly pigmented skin may not have visible blanching; its color may differ from the surrounding area.

The area may be painful, firm, soft and warmer or cooler compared with adjacent tissue. Category/stage I may be difficult to detect in individuals with dark skin tones. This may indicate 'at-risk' individuals (a heralding sign of risk).

Category/stage II: partial skin loss

These pressure ulcers have partial-thickness loss of dermis presenting as a shallow open ulcer with a red–pink wound bed, without slough. This may also present as an intact or open/ruptured serum-filled blister. Presents as a shiny or dry shallow ulcer without slough or bruising. Bruising indicates suspected deep tissue injury. This category/stage should not be used to describe skin tears, tape burns, perineal dermatitis, maceration or excoriation.

Category/stage III: full-thickness skin loss

These pressure ulcers have full-thickness tissue loss. Subcutaneous fat may be visible, but bone, tendon or muscle is not exposed. Slough may be present but does not obscure the depth of tissue loss. This may include undermining and tunnelling. The depth of a category/stage III pressure ulcer varies by anatomical location. The bridge of the nose, ear, occiput and malleolus do not have subcutaneous tissue, and category/stage III ulcers can be shallow. In contrast, areas of significant adiposity can develop extremely deep category/stage III pressure ulcers. Bone/tendon is not visible or directly palpable.

Category/stage IV: full-thickness tissue loss

These pressure ulcers have full-thickness tissue loss with exposed bone, tendon or muscle. Slough or eschar may be present on some parts of the wound bed. The wound often includes undermining and tunnelling. The depth of a category/stage IV pressure ulcer varies by anatomical location. The bridge of the nose, ear, occiput and malleolus do not have subcutaneous tissue, and these ulcers can be shallow. Category/stage IV ulcers can extend into muscle and/or supporting structures (e.g. fascia, tendon or joint capsule), making osteomyelitis possible. Exposed bone/tendon is visible or directly palpable.

Unstageable: depth unknown

These pressure ulcers have full-thickness tissue loss in which the base of the ulcer is covered by slough (yellow, tan, grey, green or brown) and/or eschar (tan, brown or black) in the wound bed. Until enough slough and/or eschar is removed to expose the base of the wound, the true depth, and therefore category/stage, cannot be determined. Stable (dry, adherent, intact without erythema

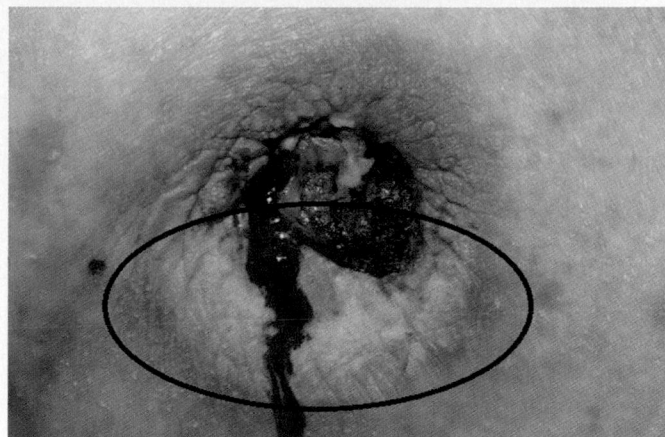

Fig. 59.15 Category III pressure ulcer showing presence of undermining.

or fluctuance) eschar on the heels serves as 'the body's natural (biological) cover' and should not be removed.

Suspected deep tissue injury: depth unknown

These pressure ulcers have a purple or maroon localised area of discoloured intact skin or blood-filled blister due to damage of the underlying soft tissue from pressure and/or shear. The area may be preceded by tissue that is painful, firm, mushy, boggy and warmer or cooler compared with adjacent tissue. Deep tissue injury may be difficult to detect in individuals with dark skin tones. Evolution may include a thin blister over a dark wound bed. The wound may further evolve and become covered by thin eschar. Evolution may be rapid exposing additional layers of tissue even with optimal treatment.

Diagnosis

Pressure ulcers are usually diagnosed on clinical appearance and presenting history. Using the classification system outlined previously, it is also possible to determine the severity of the ulcer.

X-rays of the ulcer may be required, especially if it is over a bony area, to exclude any underlying infection in the bone (osteomyelitis). In addition, blood tests to examine inflammatory markers, such as C-reactive protein (CRP) and erythrocyte sedimentation rate (ESR), may also be useful in determining the presence of infection.

If undermining or tunnelling is present (Fig. 59.15), further ultrasound scans may be required to examine the full extent of the wound and to identify any collection of fluid.

Treatment

The care of patients with pressure ulcers will depend on the severity of the damage, but there are interventions common to all patients, and these include (NPUAP et al., 2014):
- nutrition,
- repositioning and early mobilisation,
- support surfaces,
- classification of pressure ulcers,
- assessment of pressure ulcers and monitoring of healing,
- pain assessment and treatment,
- wound care: cleansing,

- wound care: debridement,
- assessment and treatment of infection and biofilms,
- wound dressings,
- growth factors,
- biophysical agents,
- surgery.

Prevention of pressure ulcers

The majority of pressure ulcers are preventable. Important considerations in terms of prevention include:
- patient repositioning,
- use of equipment,
- skin care,
- nutritional support.

An individual's potential risk of developing damage should be assessed with a view to identifying those that are vulnerable. Once an individual is deemed to be at risk of skin breakdown, the aim should be to improve tissue tolerance, which can be achieved using the elements described previously.

Principles of wound management

There are a number of principles to wound management, including:
- knowledge of wound healing physiology,
- assessment of the patient,
- assessment of the wound/ulcer,
- assessment of the tissue type,
- recognition of factors affecting healing,
- knowledge of dressings available,
- availability of resources.

The healthcare professional needs to be clear about the aim of management, and the expected outcome before the most appropriate treatment can be selected. Table 59.10 outlines the main considerations to be taken into account. Whilst wound healing is often viewed as the eventual outcome, in some instances this may not be feasible; therefore, alternative aims should be identified to demonstrate success.

Assessment of the tissue type should include examination of the following:
- dead tissue, that is, slough (yellow or grey), necrosis (black);
- infected tissue (bright red, bleeds easily, green discolouration);
- granulating, that is, presence of pink tissue in the wound bed;
- epithelial tissue, that is, pink, silvery tissue at the edges of a wound.

Once this information has been established, the selection of a dressing will depend on:
- treatment objective,
- stage of healing,
- tissue type,
- site and size of the wound,
- frequency of the dressing change,
- comfort/cosmetic appearance,
- where/by whom the dressing is to be changed,
- if the dressing is available.

Box 59.2 lists the main types of dressings available. Dressings alone will not heal a wound, and other aspects of care may need to be taken into account, including:

Table 59.10 Criteria to consider in choosing appropriate wound management

Aim	Criteria
Protect from	Drying out Infection Further damage
Debride using	Autolytic methods Mechanically Sharp/surgical
Control	Larvae Bleeding Exudate Pain Odour

Box 59.2 Wound management products

Basic wound contact dressings, that is, knitted viscose/polymer dressings
Low-adherence dressings – indicated for clean granulating wounds with a light amount of exudate. Note: Dressing may stick, so be cautious of trauma on removal
Absorbent dressings – are also low adherence and suitable for mild and moderate (but not viscous) exudate

Advanced wound dressings
Hydrogel – generally donates liquid to aid autolytic debridement of sloughy, necrotic wounds. Available in amorphous or sheet form depending on the size and shape of the wound. Choice will depend on the amount of exudate present.
Vapour permeable films and membranes – also allow the passage of water vapour and oxygen but remain impermeable to water and bacteria. They allow viewing of the wound and are flexible and conform to awkward wound shapes. Mainly suitable for partial-thickness wounds and formulated with and without an absorbent pad for exudate management. Use would be avoided in infected and highly exuding wounds.
Soft polymer – often with added silicone. Designed to be non-adherent and are useful if the skin/wound is fragile and where further damage is to be avoided. They can be used on wounds that have light to moderate exudate but may require a secondary absorbent dressing if large amounts of exudate are present.
Hydrocolloids – semi-permeable to water vapour and oxygen and to gel in the presence of exudate. Promote autolytic debridement and are also useful on granulating wounds because they can be left in place for a number of days. Generally, these dressings are indicated for moderate to heavy exudate; careful monitoring for maceration of the wound edges and surrounding skin would be important.
Foam – suitable for most types of wounds but requires a moist wound interface. Can absorb various levels of exudate, with some having better fluid-handling capacity than others. Presented in adhesive and non-adhesive forms, the choice of which is often based on the integrity of the patient's surrounding skin.

Box 59.2 Wound management products—cont'd

Alginate – usually fibrous dressings, made from seaweed; some have haemostatic properties. Require moisture so are not suitable for dry wounds. They are suitable for exuding wounds and can aid autolytic debridement. Available as packing material (ropes) or flat sheets, the choice of which depends on the size and shape of the wound. May require a secondary dressing to hold in place.

Capillary action – contraindicated in bleeding wounds but useful for exuding wounds, particularly when slough is present. Absorbent core absorbs and contains the exudate, which minimises the risk of maceration. A secondary dressing is also required.

Odour absorbent – utilise activated charcoal to absorb odour from wounds. Some require a suitable primary contact layer, whereas others are layered and provide a non-adherent wound contact interface. The cause of the odour should always be established because underlying infection may require additional treatment.

Antimicrobial – used to treat local rather than spreading or systemic infection. Can be used to reduce the levels of bacteria in the wound. The amount of exudate should be a consideration when choosing an antimicrobial dressing.

Honey – medical honey is anti-inflammatory as well as antimicrobial and can aid with debridement of the wound and combating odour. Caution should be exercised in diabetic patients and its use should be avoided if a patient is allergic to bees/bee stings.

Iodine – available as povidone-iodine or cadexomer-iodine, preparations are useful in clinically infected wounds. Iodine is effective against a wide range of bacteria, but its effect can be diluted if large amounts of exudate are present. Cadexomer-iodine is effective at debriding wounds. Iodine can cause sensitivity, and systemic absorption can occur, especially from large wounds or prolonged use.

Silver – used when infection is suspected. Available in different presentations and can be used on all wound types that have clinical signs of infection and where exudate is present. Skin discoloration and systemic absorption can occur; therefore, use is contraindicated in pregnancy and neonates.

Other antimicrobials – including preparations such as chlorohexidine, Flaminal and Prontosan.

Specialised dressings

Protease-modulating matrix – acts on the proteolytic enzymes in chronic wounds and re-establishes normal enzymatic activity. Can be used on non-healing wounds that do not seem to be progressing.

Silicone keloid dressings – used to reduce hypertrophic and keloid scarring and therefore are not appropriate for open wounds. A staged approach to application is advised, with increasing wear time being indicated. Dressings can be washed and re-used.

Adjunct dressings and appliances

Surgical absorbents – useful as secondary layer over a primary wound contact layer. Absorb exudate but allow leakage of exudate ('strike-through'). Can adhere to the wound bed, and fibres may be shed; therefore, should be used cautiously.

Wound drainage pouches – use when other exudate-absorbing dressings are not sufficient to manage the fluid levels; wound drainage bags may be useful as a means of containing the leakage.

Physical debridement pads – used for the debridement of superficial wounds containing loose slough or debris. Can also be used to remove hyperkeratosis.

Complex adjunct therapies

Topical negative pressure therapy – useful for acute and chronic cavity wounds and shallower wounds healing by secondary intention; topical negative pressure or vacuum-assisted closure aims to stimulate angiogenesis, remove excess exudate, reduce the bacterial burden and stimulate the production of granulation tissue.

Bandages

Compression (multi-layer) – provide compression for treatment of venous ulcers. Correct application of bandage is essential because the incorrect application technique can be hazardous. A Doppler assessment to establish the patient's ankle brachial pressure index (ABPI) is essential before application. Systems include high compression, short stretch and multi-layer (four layers and two layers). Choice is often dependent on patient preference.

Compression hosiery – prevents recurrence of venous ulcers but also now used in the treatment of active ulceration. ABPI should be established prior to application. Class III is preferred.

Compression garments – for management of lymphoedema. Used in conjunction with intermittent pneumatic compression systems.

Skin care

Skin barriers that protect the peri-wound area are important because wound exudate contains enzymes that can cause damage to tissues. Simple silicone-based creams or petroleum-based ointments can be useful in providing a protective layer for fragile skin.

Refer to the British National Formulary for more detailed information (http://www.evidence.nhs.uk/formulary/bnf/current/a5-wound-management-products-and-elasticated-garments).

- compression therapy for patients with venous ulcers,
- pressure-relieving equipment for individuals with or at risk of pressure ulcers,
- footwear and off-loading devices for patients with diabetic foot disease,
- devices such as negative pressure wound therapy (NPWT) for wounds healing by secondary intention,
- nutritional supplementation,
- drugs to influence healing,
- surgical interventions.

Case studies

Case 59.1

A 75-year-old man, Mr DL, was admitted to hospital after a stroke. Over the proceeding few days, Mr DL developed a sore area between his buttocks (Fig. 59.16). The area is very moist and there is loss of the epidermis, but the ulcer is shallow.

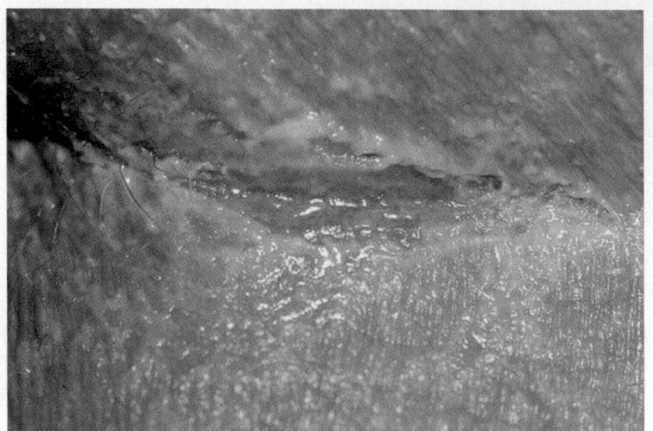

Fig. 59.16   A shallow wound between the buttocks of a patient.

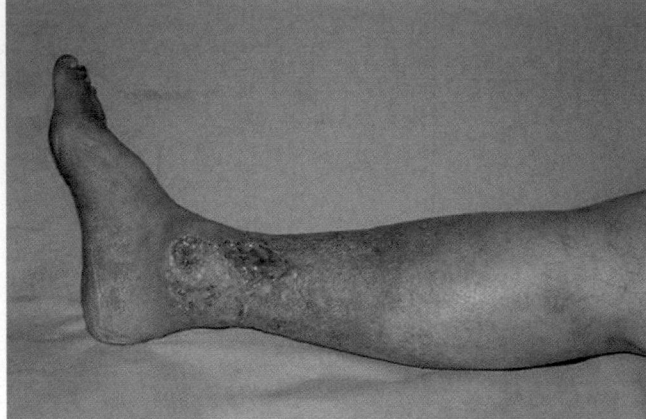

Fig. 59.17   A wound on the medial malleolar area.

Questions

1. What is the most likely cause of the ulceration?
2. How should the wound be managed?
3. How can this damage be prevented?

Answers

1. Whilst from the position and appearance of the wound it looks like a category II pressure ulcer, it is in fact a 'moisture lesion'. A moisture lesion is defined as being caused by urine and/ or faeces and perspiration which is in continuous contact with intact skin of the perineum, buttocks, groins, inner thighs, natal cleft or skin folds and where skin is in contact with skin. Moisture lesions cause superficial loss of epidermis and/or dermis, which may be preceded by areas of erythema on intact skin (All Wales Tissue Viability Nurse Forum and All Wales Continence Forum, 2014).
2. If Mr DL is incontinent the skin should be cleansed carefully. However, care must be taken to avoid damaging the skin further with harsh cleansers; therefore, a pH-balanced skin cleanser should be used. Skin barrier products can also be used to protect the skin from excessive moisture. These are topical preparations that are available as a cream, spray, foam applicator or wipes. Creams can be applied to dry, intact skin, whereas sprays, wipes or applicators can be applied to broken and/or intact skin.
3. Assessment and management of continence issues is the main way to prevent moisture lesions from occurring. In addition, there are other areas that need attention, such as the following: skin monitoring and good skin care; ensuring the patient has a good nutritional status; maintaining an optimal microclimate; repositioning immobile patients; providing adequate pressure relief.

Case 59.2

A 78-year-old man, Mr AT, presents with ulceration to his lower limb (Fig. 59.17). He has signs of venous disease, for example, haemosiderin staining and lipodermatosclerosis, and has been treated with compression therapy previously. Mr AT now reports having increased pain in his lower leg, particularly when walking. The primary care nurse has undertaken a Doppler, and his ABPI is 0.8.

Questions

1. What is the likely cause of Mr AT's ulcers?
2. How should Mr AT be managed?
3. What treatment should be avoided, and why?

Answers

1. Mr AT has signs and symptoms of venous disease but also reports pain on walking. This is known as intermittent claudication because the pain is relieved by rest. Mr AT's ABPI result suggests the presence of arterial disease; that is, 0.8 suggests only 80% blood flow in the lower limb. Given the presenting symptoms, Mr AT would be deemed to have 'mixed ulcers'.
2. Mr AT should be referred to a vascular surgeon, where he is likely to have a Duplex scan and may then require angiography and/or surgery to improve the blood supply to the lower limb.
3. Mr AT should not have compression therapy. The blood flow to his lower limb is reduced, and application of compression could reduce that further. The risk to the patient is the loss of a limb if the circulation is compromised further.

Case 59.3

A 58-year-old woman, Mrs SG, presents with a raised scar to her sternum (Fig. 59.18). She underwent cardiac surgery 12 months previously. Mrs SG is worried about the appearance as the scar is raised and itchy.

Questions

1. Is this the normal appearance of a scar at 1 year post-surgery?
2. What name is given to this sort of scarring?
3. What treatment is required?

Answers

1. The remodelling phase of wound healing takes place up to 1 year after injury. The initial collagen that is laid down is changed, so the scar should be thinner, flatter and also paler.

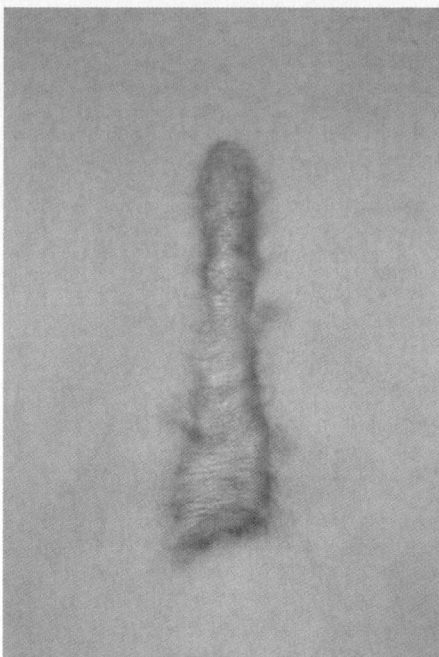

Fig. 59.18 Scar tissue 12 months post cardiac surgery.

2. This type of scarring is known as hypertrophic scarring. A hypertrophic scar is a red, raised scar that forms along a wound and can have the following characteristics for around 2–5 years:
   - It can restrict movement because scar tissue is not as flexible as the original skin.
   - It heals within the size of the original wound.
   - The healing tissue is thicker than usual.
   - It is red and raised initially, becoming flatter and paler with time.
3. Treatment might include the use of silicone gel sheets such as CICA-CARE (Smith & Nephew), which is thought to occlude the skin to hydrate the scar area. This results in increased moisture around the scar, reducing the blood supply and deposit of collagen. The patient may require referral to a dermatologist or plastic surgeon if the scarring does not resolve. Further treatment might include the use of pressure garments, intra-lesional corticosteroid injections or surgery.

References

All Wales Tissue Viability Nurse Forum and All Wales Continence Forum, 2014. Prevention and management of moisture lesions. Wounds UK, London. Available at: http://www.wounds-uk.com/supplements/awtvnf-prevention-and-management-of-moisture-lesions.

Al-Qaisi, M., Nott, D.M., King, D.H., et al., 2009. Ankle Brachial Pressure Index (ABPI): an update for practitioners. Vasc. Health Risk Manage. 5, 833–841.

Andriessen, A. Apelqvist, J., Mosti, G., et al., 2017. Compression therapy for venous leg ulcers: risk factors for adverse events and complications, contraindications – a review of present guidelines. J. Europ. Acad. Dermatol. Venereol. 31 (9), 1562–1568.

Ashcroft, G.S., Mills, S.J., Ashworth, J.J., 2002. Ageing and wound healing. Biogerontology 3, 337–345.

Briggs, M., Closs, S.J., 2003. The prevalence of leg ulceration: a review of the literature. Eur. Wound Manage. Assoc. J. 3, 14–20.

British Association for Parenteral and Enteral Nutrition, 2015. Malnutrition Universal Screening Tool. Available at: http://www.bapen.org.uk.

Clark, M., Defloor, T., Bours, G., 2004. A pilot study of the prevalence of pressure ulcers in European hospitals. In: Clark, M. (Ed.), Pressure Ulcers: Recent Advances in Tissue Viability. Quay Books, Salisbury, pp. 8–22.

Department of Health, 2001. National Service Framework for Diabetes: Standards. DH, London.

Department of Health, 2007a. Working Together for Better Diabetes Care. DH, London.

Department of Health, 2007b. The Way Ahead: The Local Challenge Improving Diabetes Services. DH, London.

Desai, H., 1997a. Ageing and wounds part 1: fetal and post-natal healing. J. Wound Care 6, 192–196.

Desai, H., 1997b. Ageing and wounds part 2: healing in old age. J. Wound Care 6, 237–239.

Diabetes UK, 2014. Number of people diagnosed with diabetes reaches 3.2 million. Available at: https://www.diabetes.org.uk/About_us/News/Number-of-people-diagnoses-with-diabetes-reaches-32-million/.

Edmonds, M., Foster, A., 2000. The Ulcerated Foot. Managing the Diabetic Foot. Blackwell Science, London.

Enoch, S., Grey, J.E., Harding, K.G., 2008. Recent advances and emerging treatments. In: Grey, J.E., Harding, K.G. (Eds.), ABC of Wound Healing. BMJ Books. Blackwell Publishing, Oxford.

Enoch, S., Leaper, D.J., 2005. Basic science of wound healing. Surgery 23, 37–42.

Ferner, R.E., 2016. Ulceration from nicorandil. Adverse Drug Reaction Bull. 296, 1143–1146.

Grey, J.E., Harding, K.G., 2008. ABC of Wound Healing. BMJ Books. Blackwell Publishing, Oxford.

Holman, N., Young, R.J., Jeffcoate, W.J., 2012. Variation in the recorded incidence of amputation of the lower limb in England. Diabetologia 55, 1919–1925.

Lindsay, E., 2013. Lindsay Leg Clubs: clinically effective, cost effective. J. Commun. Nursing 27, 5–8.

Lipsky, B.A., Berendt, A.R., Cornia, P.B., et al., 2012. Infectious Diseases Society of America clinical practice guideline for the diagnosis and treatment of diabetic foot infections. Clin. Infect. Dis. 54 (12), e132–e173. https://doi.org/10.1093/cid/cia346.

Marcos-Garcés, V., Molina Aguilar, P., Bea Serrano, C., et al., 2014. Age-related dermal collagen changes during development, maturation and ageing – a morphometric and comparative study. J. Anatomy 225 (1), 98–108. https://doi.org/10.1111/joa.12186.

Møller, A., Villebro, N., Pedersen, T., et al., 2002. Effect of preoperative smoking interventions on postoperative complications: a randomised clinical trial. Lancet 359 (9301), 114–117.

National Institute for Health and Care Excellence, 2015a. Diabetic foot problems: prevention and management. Available at: https://www.nice.org.uk/guidance/ng19.

National Institute for Health and Care Excellence, 2015b. Type 2 diabetes in adults. Available at: http://www.nice.org.uk/guidance/ng28.

National Pressure Ulcer Advisory Panel, European Pressure Ulcer Advisory Panel and Pan Pacific Pressure Injury Alliance, 2014. Prevention and treatment of pressure ulcers: quick reference guide. In: Haesler, E. (Ed.). Cambridge Media, Perth.

Ortiz, A., Grando, S.A., 2012. Smoking and the skin. Int. J. Dermatol. 51, 250–262.

Phillips, C.J., Humphreys, I., Fletcher, J., et al., 2016. Estimating the costs associated with the management of patients with chronic wounds used linked routine data. Int. Wound J. 13 (6), 1193–1197.

Scottish Intercollegiate Guideline Network, 2010. Management of chronic venous leg ulcers. Available at: http://www.sign.ac.uk/guidelines/fulltext/120/recommendations.html.

Sorensen, L.T., Karlsmark, T., Gottrup, F., 2003. Abstinence from smoking reduces incisional wound infection: a randomized controlled trial. Ann. Surg. 238, 1–5.

Tennvall, G.R., Hjelmgren, J., 2005. Annual cost of treatment for venous leg ulcers in Sweden and the United Kingdom. Wound Repair Regen. 13, 13–18.

Thomsen, T., Villebro, N., Møller, A.M., 2014. Interventions for preoperative smoking cessation. Cochrane DB Syst. Rev. 27 (3), CD002294. https://doi.org/10.1002/14651858.CD002294.pub4.

Waters, N., Holloway, S.L., 2009. Personal perceptions of the impact of diabetic foot disease on employment. Diabetic Foot J. 12, 119–131.

Winter, G.D., 1962. Formation of the scab and the rate of epithelialization of superficial wounds in the skin of the young domestic pig. Nature 193, 293–294.

Wolcott, R.D., Rhoads, D.D., 2008. A study of biofilm-based wound management in subjects with critical limb ischaemia. J. Wound Care 17, 145–155.

Wounds International, 2013. Principles of compression in venous disease: a practitioner's guide to treatment and prevention of venous leg ulcers. Available at: http://www.woundsinternational.com/media/issues/672/files/content_10802.pdf.

Wysocki, A.B., 2007. Anatomy and physiology of the skin and soft tissue. In: Bryant, R.A., Nix, D.P. (Eds.), Acute and Chronic Wounds: Current Management. Mosby, St Louis, pp. 39–55.

SECTION 4

APPENDICES

Medical Abbreviations

25 OHD	25-hydroxy vitamin D	**AFB**	acid-fast bacillus
5-ASA	5-aminosalicylic acid	**AFP**	α-fetoprotein
5-HIAA	5-hydroxyindolacetic acid	**AGEP**	acute generalised exanthematous pustulosis
5-HT	5-hydroxytryptamine (serotonin)	**AGL**	acute granulocytic leukaemia
A & E	accident and emergency	**AGN**	acute glomerulonephritis
A & O	alert and oriented	**AHA**	autoimmune haemolytic anaemia
A & P	anterior and posterior auscultation and percussion	**AHD**	autoimmune haemolytic disease
A & W	alive and well	**AIDS**	acquired immune deficiency syndrome
AAA	abdominal aortic aneurysm	**AIP**	asymptomatic inflammatory prostatitis
	acute anxiety attack	**AIT**	amiodarone-induced thyrotoxicosis
AAAAA	aphasia, agnosia, apraxia, agraphia and alexia	**AK**	above knee
Ab	antibody	**ALA**	amino laevulinic acid
ABCD	amphotericin B colloidal dispersion	**ALAS**	5-aminolevulinate synthase
ABD	amphotericin B deoxycholate	**ALD**	alcoholic liver disease
abd.	abdomen (abdominal)	**ALF**	acute liver failure
	abduction	**ALG**	antilymphocyte globulin
ABE	acute bacterial endocarditis	**ALL**	acute lymphocytic leukaemia
ABG	arterial blood gases	**ALP**	alkaline phosphatase
ABMT	autologous bone marrow transplant	**ALT**	alanine transaminase
ABP	acute bacterial prostatitis		argon laser trabeculoplasty
ABVD	Adriamycin (doxorubicin), bleomycin, vinblastine, dacarbazine	**AMA**	against medical advice
		AMI	acute myocardial infarction
ACAT	acylcholesterol acyltransferase	**AML**	acute myeloid leukaemia
ACBS	aortocoronary bypass surgery	**AMP**	adenosine monophosphate
ACD	allergic contact dermatitis	**ANA**	anti-nuclear antibody
	anaemia of chronic disease	**ANC**	absolute neutrophil count
ACE	angiotensin-converting enzyme	**ANF**	antinuclear factor
acid phos.	acid phosphatase	**ANP**	atrial natriuretic peptide
ACPA	anti-citrullinated peptide antibodies	**Anti-HbAb**	anti-hepatitis B antibody
ACR	albumin/creatinine ratio	**Anti-CCP**	anti-citrullinated protein antibodies
ACS	acute coronary syndrome	**AOB**	alcohol on breath
ACT	activated clotting time	**AP**	alkaline phosphatase
ACTH	adrenocorticotrophin hormone		angina pectoris
AD	Alzheimer's disease		antepartum
ADC	AIDS dementia complex		anterior pituitary
	anaemia of chronic disease		anteroposterior
ADE	adverse drug event		aortic pressure
ADH	antidiuretic hormone		apical pulse
ADL	activities of daily living		appendectomy
ADP	adenosine diphosphate		artificial pneumothorax
ADR	adverse drug reaction	**APB**	atrial premature beat
ADT	androgen deprivation therapy	**APC**	activated protein C
ADU	acute duodenal ulcer		atrial premature contraction
AED	antiepileptic drug	**APD**	action potential duration
AF	atrial fibrillation	**APKD**	adult polycystic kidney disease

APP	amyloid precursor protein		BM	bowel movement
APSAC	anisoylated plasminogen streptokinase-activated complex		BMI	body mass index
			BMT	bone marrow transplant
APTT	activated partial thromboplastin time		BNO	bowels not open
AR	aortic regurgitation		BOR	bowels open regularly
	apical/radial (pulse)		BP	bypass
ARB	angiotensin receptor blocker			blood pressure
ARBD	alcohol-related brain damage		BPA	British Paediatric Association
ARDS	adult respiratory distress syndrome		BPD	bronchopulmonary dysplasia
ARF	acute renal failure		BPE	benign prostatic enlargement
ARV	antiretroviral		BPH	benign prostatic hyperplasia
AS	aortic stenosis		BPS	bipolar spectrum disorder
	arteriosclerosis		BS	blood sugar
A–S attack	Adams–Stokes attack			bowel sounds
ASB	asymptomatic bacteriuria			breath sounds
ASC	acute severe colitis		BSA	body surface area
ASCA	anti-*Saccharomyces cerevisiae* antibodies		BUN	blood urea nitrogen
ASD	atrial septal defect		BW	body water
ASLO titre	antistreptolysin-O titre			body weight
AST	aspartate transaminase		Bx.	biopsy
ATG	antithymocyte globulin		C	complement
ATN	acute tubular necrosis		C & P	cystoscopy and pyelogram
ATO	arsenic trioxide		C & S	culture and sensitivity
ATP	adenosine triphosphate		c/o	complains of
ATRA	all-trans retinoic acid		$C_1, C_2, \ldots$	cervical vertebrae 1, 2, …
AUC	area under the curve		CA	cancer
AUR	acute urinary retention			carcinoma
AV	aortic valve			cardiac arrest
	atrioventricular			coronary artery
A-V	arteriovenous		Ca	carcinoma
AVNRT	atrioventricular nodal re-entry tachycardia		CABG	coronary artery bypass graft
AVR	aortic valve replacement		CAD	coronary artery disease
	augmented V lead, right arm (ECG)		CAH	chronic active hepatitis
AVRT	atrioventricular re-entry tachycardia		CAP	community-acquired pneumonia
AVS	arteriovenous shunt		CAPD	continuous ambulatory peritoneal dialysis
AXR	abdominal X-ray		cART	combination antiretroviral therapy
B Bx.	breast biopsy		CAT	computed axial tomography
BACUP	British Association of Cancer United Patients		CAVH	continuous arteriovenous haemofiltration
BA-MDI	breath-actuated metered-dose inhalers		CBA	cost–benefit analysis
BAPEN	British Association of Parenteral and Enteral Nutrition		CBP	chronic bacterial prostatitis
			CBT	cognitive behaviour therapy
BBB	bundle branch block		CC	chief complaint
BBBB	bilateral bundle branch block (ECG)			current complaint
BCAA	branched-chain amino acid		CCB	calcium channel blockers
BCC	basal cell carcinoma		CCF	congestive cardiac failure
BCG	bacille Calmette–Guérin		CCU	coronary care unit
BDA	British Diabetic Association		CDAI	Crohn's Disease Activity Index
bDMARDs	biologic disease modifying anti-rheumatic drugs		CEA	cost-effectiveness analysis
BE	base excess		CF	cardiac failure
BEACOPP	bleomycin, etoposide, Adriamycin (doxorubicin), cyclophosphamide, Oncovin (vincristine), procarbazine, prednisolone			complement fixation
				cystic fibrosis
			CFT	complement fixation test
BEAM	carmustine, etoposide, cytarabine, melphalan		CGL	chronic granulocytic leukaemia
BG	blood glucose		CGN	chronic glomerulonephritis
BHS	beta-haemolytic streptococci		CHAD	cold haemagglutinin disease
BIA	bioelectrical impedance analysis		CHB	complete heart block
BJ protein	Bence-Jones protein		CHD	coronary heart disease
BKA	below knee amputation		CHF	congestive heart failure

CHM	Commission on Human Medicines
CHO	carbohydrate
CHOP	cyclophosphamide, hydroxydaunorubicin (doxorubicin), Oncovin (vincristine), prednisolone
CHOP-R	cyclophosphamide, hydroxydaunorubicin (doxorubicin), Oncovin (vincristine), prednisolone, rituximab
CI	cardiac index
	cerebral infarction
	confidence interval
CINV	chemotherapy-induced nausea and vomiting
CIVA	centralised intravenous additive
CK	creatine kinase (same as CPK)
CKD	chronic kidney disease
CL	clubbing
Cl$_{Cr}$	creatinine clearance
CLD	chronic liver disease
	chronic lung disease
CLL	chronic lymphocytic leukaemia
CMA	cost minimisation analysis
CML	chronic myelocytic leukaemia
CMV	cytomegalovirus
CNS	central nervous system
	coagulase-negative staphylococci
CO	cardiac output
CoA	coenzyme A
COC	combined oral contraceptive
COD	cause of death
COG	closed-angle glaucoma
COMT	catechol-*o*-methyl transferase
COP	capillary osmotic pressure
COPD	chronic obstructive pulmonary disease
COX	cyclo-oxygenase
CP	chronic prostatitis
	cor pulmonale
	creatine phosphate
CPA	cardiopulmonary arrest
	cerebellar pontine angle
CPAP	continuous positive airway pressure
CPD	continuous peritoneal dialysis
CPK	creatine phosphokinase
CPM	central pontine myelinolysis
CPN	chronic pyelonephritis
CPPS	chronic pelvic pain syndrome
CPPV	continuous positive pressure ventilation
CPR	cardiopulmonary resuscitation
CPSI	chronic prostatitis symptom index
CPZ	chlorpromazine
CR	cardiorespiratory
	clot retraction
	colon resection
	complete remission
	conditional reflex
	crown-rump
CRD	chronic renal disease
CRF	chronic renal failure
	corticotrophin-releasing factor
CRP	C-reactive protein

CSAP	cryosurgical ablation of prostate
csDMARD	conventional synthetic disease modifying anti-rheumatic drug
CSF	cerebrospinal fluid
	colony stimulating factor
CSH	chronic subdural haematoma
CSM	carotid sinus massage
	cerebrospinal meningitis
CSP	carotid sinus pressure
CSR	Cheyne–Stokes respiration
	correct sedimentation rate
CSS	carotid sinus stimulation
	central sterile supply
CSU	catheter specimen of urine
CT	circulation time
	clotting time
	computed tomography
	Coombs' test
	coronary thrombosis
cTnI	cardiac troponin I
cTnT	cardiac troponin T
CTPA	computed tomography pulmonary angiogram
CTZ	chemoreceptor trigger zone
CUA	cost–utility analysis
CUG	cystourethrogram
CV	cardiovascular
	central venous
	cerebrovascular
	contingent valuation
CVA	cerebrovascular accident (stroke)
	costovertebral angle
CVD	cardiovascular disease
CVP	central venous pressure
CVVH	continuous venovenous haemofiltration
Cx	cervical
	cervix
CXR	chest X-ray
Cys-C	cystatin C
d	dead
	deceased
D & C	dilation and curettage
D & V	diarrhoea and vomiting
D/C	discontinue
D/S	dextrose and saline
D$_5$W	dextrose 5%
DAD	delayed after depolarisation
DAFNE	(insulin) dose adjustment for normal eating
DALY	disability-adjusted life-year
DAS	disease activity score
DBP	diastolic blood pressure
DD	dyssynergic defecation
DDx.	differential diagnosis
DES	diethylstilboestrol
DEXA	dual energy X-ray absorptiometry
DH	drug history
DIC	disseminated intravascular coagulation
DILD	drug-induced liver disease
DILI	drug-induced liver injury

DIP	drug-induced parkinsonism	**ELISA**	enzyme-linked immunosorbent assay
DIT	di-iodotyrosine	**EM**	ejection murmur
DKA	diabetic ketoacidosis		erythema multiforme
DLBCL	diffuse large B-cell lymphoma	**EMEA**	European Medicines Evaluation Agency
DLE	discoid lupus erythematosus	**EMG**	electromyogram
	disseminated lupus erythematosus	**EN**	erythema nodosum
DLQI	Dermatology Quality of Life Index	**ENDR**	endoscopy negative reflux disease
DM	diabetes mellitus	**ENT**	ears, nose and throat
	diastolic murmur	**EP**	ectopic pregnancy
DMARD	disease-modifying antirheumatic drug	**EPSE**	extra pyramidal side effects
DNA	did not attend (outpatients)	**ER**	oestrogen receptor
DOA	dead on arrival	**ERCP**	endoscopic retrograde cholangiopancreatography
DOAC	direct oral anticoagulant	**ERP**	effective refractory period
DOB	date of birth	**ESA**	erythropoietin-stimulating agent
DOD	date of death	**ESBL**	extended spectrum beta-lactamase
DOE	dyspnoea on exertion	**ESHAP**	etoposide, methylprednisolone, cytarabine, cisplatin
DOTS	Directly Observed Treatment	**ESM**	ejection systolic murmur
DPI	dry powder inhalers	**ESN**	educationally subnormal
DPP-4	inhibitors dipeptidyl peptidase inhibitors	**ESP**	end-systolic pressure
DRE	digital rectal examination	**ESR**	erythrocyte sedimentation rate
DRESS	drug rash with eosinophilia and systemic symptoms	**ESRF**	end-stage renal failure
DROP	dyslipidaemia, insulin resistance, obesity and high blood pressure	**ET**	endotracheal tube
			essential tremor
DSM	*Diagnostic and Statistical Manual of Mental Disorders*	**ETT**	exercise tolerance test
DTI	direct thrombus imaging	**FAS**	fetal alcohol syndrome
DTP	diphtheria, tetanus, pertussis (vaccine)	**FB**	finger breadths
DTs	delirium tremens	**FBC**	full blood count
DU	diagnosis undetermined	**FBS**	fasting blood sugar
	duodenal ulcer	**FCE**	finished consultant episode
DUB	dysfunctional uterine bleeding	**FDA**	US Food and Drug Administration
DUE	drug use evaluation	**FeNa**	fractional excretion of sodium
DUP	drug use process	**FEV**	forced expiratory volume
DVT	deep vein thrombosis	**FEV$_1$**	forced expiratory volume in 1 second
Dx.	diagnosis	**FFA**	free fatty acid
DXT	deep X-ray therapy	**FFP**	fresh frozen plasma
E/I	expiration–inspiration ratio	**FH**	familial hypercholesterolaemia
EAD	early after depolarisation		family history
EBV	Epstein–Barr virus	**FHH**	familial hypocalciuric hypercalcaemia
ECBV	effective circulating blood volume	**FMD**	fludarabine, mitoxantrone, dexamethasone
ECF	extracellular fluid	**FOB**	faecal occult blood
ECFV	extracellular fluid volume	**FP**	frozen plasma
ECG	electrocardiogram	**FRC**	functional reserve capacity
ECHO	echocardiogram		functional residual capacity
	echoencephalogram	**FSH**	follicle-stimulating hormone
ECMO	extracorporeal membrane oxygenation	**FSNGN**	focal segmental necrotising glomerulonephritis
ECP	extra-corporeal photopheresis	**FT$_4$**	free thyroxine
ECT	electroconvulsive therapy	**FTI**	free thyroxine index
EDD	expected date of delivery	**FUO**	fever of unknown origin
EDTA	ethylenediaminetetra-acetic acid	**FVC**	forced vital capacity
EDV	end-diastolic volume	**Fx.**	fracture
EEG	electroencephalogram	**G6PD**	glucose-6-phosphate dehydrogenase
EENT	eyes, ears, nose and throat	**GA**	general anaesthesia
EF	ejection fraction		general appearance
eGFR	estimated glomerular filtration rate	**GABA**	γ-aminobutyric acid
EGFR	epidermal growth factor receptor	**GABA$_A$**	γ-aminobutyric acid A
ELBW	extremely low birth weight	**GAD**	glutamic acid decarboxylase
			generalised anxiety disorder

gamma-GT	γ-glutamyl transferase		**HER2**	human epidermal growth factor receptor type 2
GB	gallbladder		**HF**	heart failure
	Guillain–Barré (syndrome)		**HHV**	human herpes virus
GBM	glomerular basement membrane		**Hib**	*Haemophilus influenzae* type b
GBS	Glasgow–Blatchford score		**HIE**	hypoxic-ischaemic encephalopathy
G-CSF	granulocyte-colony-stimulating factor		**HIFU**	high-intensity focused ultrasound
GDM	gastro-intestinal diabetes mellitus		**HIT**	heparin-induced thrombocytopaenia
GF	glomerular filtration		**HIV**	human immunodeficiency virus
	gluten-free		**HLA**	human lymphocyte antibody
GFR	glomerular filtration rate		**HMD**	hyaline membrane disease
GGT	γ-glutamyl transpeptidase (transferase)		**HMMA**	4-hydroxy-3-methoxymandelic acid
GI	gastro-intestinal		**hMPV**	human metapneumovirus
GIK	glucose, insulin and potassium		**HONK**	hyperosmolar non-ketotic hyperglycaemia
GLA	γ-linolenic acid		**HPEN**	home parenteral and enteral nutrition
GM seizure	grand mal seizure		**HPI**	history of present illness
GM-CSF	granulocyte macrophage-colony-stimulating factor		**HPN**	home parenteral nutrition
GN	glomerulonephritis		**HPRT**	hypoxanthine-guanine phosphoribosyl transferase deficiency
GNDC	Gram-negative diplococci		**HPV**	human papillomavirus
GnRH	gonadotrophin-releasing hormone		**HR**	heart rate
GORD	gastro-oesophageal reflux disease		**HRS**	hepatorenal syndrome
grav.	gravid (pregnant)			Hodgkin and Reed-Sternberg
GRE	glycopeptide-resistant enterococci		**HRT**	hormone replacement therapy
GS	general surgery		**HS**	half strength
	genital system			Hartmann's solution
GTN	glyceryl trinitrate			heart sounds
GTT	glucose tolerance test		**HSA**	human serum albumin
GU	gastric ulcer		**HSCT**	haematopoietic stem cell transplantation
	genitourinary		**HSV**	herpes simplex virus
	gonococcal urethritis		**HT, HTN**	hypertension
GUS	genitourinary system		**HUS**	haemolytic uraemic syndrome
GVHD	graft-versus-host disease		**HVA**	homovanillic acid
GWAS	genome wide association studies		**HVD**	hypertensive vascular disease
H & L	heart and lungs		**Hx.**	history
h/o	history of		**IADHS**	inappropriate antidiuretic hormone syndrome
HAA	hepatitis-associated antigen		**IBC**	iron binding capacity
HACAs	human anti-chimeric antibodies		**IBD**	inflammatory bowel disease
HAP	hospital-acquired pneumonia		**IBS**	irritable bowel syndrome
HAS	human albumin solution		**IC**	intercostal intracerebral intracranial
HAV	hepatitis A virus		**ICA**	islet cell antibody
HB	heart block		**ICD**	*International Classification of Diseases*
Hb (Hgb)	haemoglobin			implantable cardioverter-defibrillator
HbA$_{1c}$	glycated haemoglobin			impulse control disorder
HbA$_2$	haemoglobin found in β-thalassaemia carriers			irritant contact dermatitis
HBAg	hepatitis B antigen		**ICE**	ifosfamide, carboplatin, etoposide
HBD, HBDH	hydroxybutyrate dehydrogenase		**ICF**	intracellular fluid
HBGM	home blood glucose monitoring		**ICH**	intracerebral haemorrhage
HBI	Harvey–Bradshaw Index		**ICM**	intracostal margin
HbS	sickle haemoglobin in sickle cell disease		**ICS**	intercostal space
HBsAG	hepatitis B surface antigen			inhaled corticosteroids
HBV	hepatitis B virus		**ICU**	intensive care unit
HCAI	healthcare-associated infections		**ID**	intradermal
Hct. (hct.)	haematocrit		**IDA**	iron deficiency anaemia
HCV	hepatitis C virus		**IDL**	intermediate-density lipoprotein
HDL	high-density lipoprotein		**IDL-C**	intermediate-density lipoprotein cholesterol
HDL-C	high-density lipoprotein cholesterol		**IDP**	intradialytic parenteral nutrition
HDT	high-dose therapy		**IEP**	immunoelectrophoresis
HEPEF	heart failure with preserved ejection fraction		**IFRT**	involved field radiotherapy
HER1	human epidermal growth factor receptor type 1			

Ig	immunoglobulin		**LBW**	low birth weight
iGAS	invasive group A streptococcal infection		**LCAT**	lecithin-cholesterol acyltransferase
IGT	impaired glucose tolerance		**LCT**	long-chain triglyceride
IHC	immunohistochemistry		**LD, LDH**	lactate dehydrogenase
IHD	ischaemic heart disease		**LDL**	low-density lipoprotein
IHR	intrinsic heart rate		**LDL-C**	low-density lipoprotein cholesterol
IID	infectious intestinal disease		**LDS**	lipodermatosclerosis
IMP	impression		**LE**	lupus erythematosus
INI	integrase inhibitors		**LFT**	liver function test
INR	international normalised ratio		**LH**	luteinising hormone
IOP	intraocular pressure		**LHRH**	luteinising hormone-releasing hormone
IPCN	International Prostatitis Collaborative Network		**LIF**	left iliac fossa
IPF	idiopathic pulmonary fibrosis		**LK**	left kidney
IPI	International Prognostic Index		**LKKS, LKS**	liver, kidneys, spleen
IPP	intermittent positive-pressure inflation with oxygen		**LL**	left leg
IPPB	intermittent positive-pressure breathing			left lower
IPPV	intermittent positive-pressure ventilation			lower lobe
IPS	International Prognostic Score		**LLL**	left lower lobe
IRDS	idiopathic respiratory distress syndrome			left lower lid
ISA	intrinsic sympathomimetic activity		**LLQ**	left lower quadrant
ISDN	isosorbide dinitrate		**LMN**	lower motor neurone
ISI	International Sensitivity Index		**LMP**	last menstrual period
ISMN	isosorbide mononitrate		**LMWH**	low molecular weight heparin
IT	intrathecal(ly)		**LN**	lymph node
ITT	insulin tolerance test		**LNG-IUS**	levonorgestrel intrauterine system
IUCD	intrauterine contraceptive device		**LNMP**	last normal menstrual period
IUD	intrauterine death		**LOM**	limitation of movement
	intrauterine device		**LP**	lumbar puncture
i.v.	intravenous		**Lp(a)**	lipoprotein a
IVD	intervertebral disc		**LPA**	left pulmonary artery
IVH	intraventricular haemorrhage		**LS**	left side
IVP	intravenous push			liver and spleen
	intravenous pyelography			lumbosacral
IVSD	interventricular septal defect			lymphosarcoma
IVU	intravenous urography		**LSD**	lysergic acid diethylamide
J	jaundice		**LSK**	liver, spleen, kidneys
JVD	jugular venous distension		**LSM**	late systolic murmur
JVP	jugular venous pressure		**LT**	leukotriene
KA	ketoacidosis		**LTBI**	latent tuberculosis infection
KCCT	kaolin-cephalin clotting time		**LTC**	long-term care
KLS	kidney, liver, spleen		**LTOT**	long-term oxygen therapy
KS	Kaposi's sarcoma		**LUL**	left upper lobe
KUB	kidneys, ureters, bladder		**LUQ**	left upper quadrant
L	left		**LV**	left ventricle
	lower		**LVDP**	left ventricular diastolic pressure
	lumber		**LVE**	left ventricular enlargement
L & A	light and accommodation		**LVEDP**	left ventricular end-diastolic pressure
L & U	lower and upper		**LVEDV**	left ventricular end-diastolic volume
L & W	living and well		**LVET**	left ventricular ejection time
L$_1$, L$_2$, …	lumbar vertebrae 1, 2, …		**LVF**	left ventricular failure
LA	left arm		**LVH**	left ventricular hypertrophy
	left atrium		**LVP**	left ventricular pressure
	local anaesthesia		**M**	male
LABA	long-acting β$_2$-adrenoceptor agonist			married
LAD	left anterior descending			metre
LADA	latent autoimmune diabetes in adults			mother
LAMA	long-acting antimuscarinic			molar
LBBB	left bundle branch block			murmur
LBM	lean body mass			

M:P	milk-to-plasma ratio	MRA	magnetic resonance angiography
MA	marketing authorisation	MRCP	magnetic resonance cholangiopancreatography
MABP	mean arterial blood pressure	MRD	minimal residual disease
MAC	*Mycobacterium avium* complex	MRDM	malnutrition-related diabetes mellitus
MAI	*Mycobacterium avium-intracellulare*	MRI	magnetic resonance imaging
MALT	mucosal-associated lymphoid tissue	MRP	medication-related problem
MAMC	mid-arm muscle circumference	MRSA	meticillin-resistant *Staphylococcus aureus*
MAO-A	monoamine oxidase A	MS	mitral stenosis
MAO-B	monoamine oxidase B		multiple sclerosis
MAOI	monoamine oxidase inhibitor		musculoskeletal
MAP	mean arterial pressure	MSL	midsternal line
MARS	molecular adsorbent recycling system	MSM	men who have sex with men
MBC	minimum bactericidal concentration	MSSA	meticillin-sensitive *Staphylococcus aureus*
MBP	mean blood pressure	MSU	midstream urine specimen
MCH	mean corpuscular cell haemoglobin	MTB	*Mycobacterium tuberculosis*
MCHC	mean corpuscular cell haemoglobin concentration	MTI	minimum time interval
		MTP	metatarsophalangeal
MCI	mild cognitive impairment	MUD	matched unrelated donor
MCP	metacarpophalangeal (joint)	MV	minute volume
MCT	medium-chain triglycerides		mitral valve
MCV	mean corpuscular cell volume	MVP	mitral valve prolapse
MD	mitral disease	MVPP	mustine, vinblastine, procarbazine, prednisolone
	muscular dystrophy	MVR	mitral valve replacement
MDI	metered-dose inhaler	MWH	moist wound healing
MDM	mid-diastolic murmur	N	normal
MDMA	methylenedioxymethamphetamine, ecstasy	N & T	nose and throat
MDRD	modification of diet in renal disease formula for GFR estimation	N & V	nausea and vomiting
		NAAT	nucleic acid amplification techniques
MDRST	multidrug-resistant *Salmonella enterica* serovar typhi	NAD	no appreciable disease
			normal axis deviation
MDR-TB	multidrug-resistant tuberculosis		nothing abnormal detected
MDS	myelodysplastic syndrome	NADPH	nicotinamide adenine dinucleotide phosphate hydrogen
MEN	multiple endocrine neoplasia		
MERS	Middle East respiratory syndrome	NAFLD	non-alcoholic fatty liver disease
MERS-CoV	Middle East respiratory syndrome coronavirus	NAG	narrow-angle glaucoma
met.	metastatic (metastasis)	NAI	neuraminidase inhibitor
MGN	membranous glomerulonephritis	NAPQI	*N*-acetyl-*p*-benzoquinoneimine
MH	medical history	NARI	noradrenergic reuptake inhibitor
	menstrual history	NARTI	nucleoside analogue reverse transcriptase inhibitor
MHPG	methoxyhydroxyphenylglycerol		
MHRA	Medicines and Healthcare products Regulatory Agency	NASH	non-alcoholic steatohepatitis
		NaSSA	noradrenergic and specific serotonergic antidepressant
MI	myocardial infarction		
	mitral incompetence	NBM	nil by mouth
MIC	minimum inhibitory concentration	NEC	necrotising enterocolitis
MID	multi-infarct dementia	NG	nasogastric
MIRU	mycobacterial interspersed repetitive unit typing	NHL	non-Hodgkin's lymphoma
MIT	monoiodotyrosine	NIV	non-invasive ventilation
ML	middle lobe midline	NKHA	non-ketotic hyperosmolar acidosis
MMR	measles, mumps, rubella	NLPHL	nodular lymphocyte-predominant Hodgkin's lymphoma
MMSE	mini-mental state examination		
MODY	maturity-onset diabetes of the young	NMR	nuclear magnetic resonance
MOPP	mustine, Oncovin (vincristine), procarbazine, prednisolone	NMS	neuroleptic malignant syndrome
		NNRTI	non-nucleoside reverse transcriptase inhibitor
MOTT	mycobacteria other than tuberculosis	NOAC	non-warfarin oral anticoagulants
MPJ	metacarpophalangeal joint		novel oral anticoagulants
MR	mitral regurgitation		non-vitamin K antagonists oral anticoagulant
MRCF	medication-related consultation framework	NOF	neck of femur

NS	nephrotic syndrome	**PC**	presenting complaint
	nervous system		prostate cancer
	normal saline	**PCA**	patient-controlled analgesia
	no specimen	**PCAS**	patient-controlled analgesia system
NSAID	non-steroidal anti-inflammatory drug	**PCC**	prothrombin complex concentrate
NSFTD	normal spontaneous full-term delivery	**PCI**	percutaneous coronary intervention
NSR	normal sinus rhythm	**PCO$_2$**	partial pressure of carbon dioxide
NSTEMI	non-ST-elevated myocardial infarction	**PCR**	polymerase chain reaction
NSU	non-specific urethritis		protein creatinine ratio
NT	nasotracheal (tube)	**PCS**	portocaval shunt
NTS	nucleus tractus solitarius	**PCV**	packed cell volume
NVD	nausea, vomiting, diarrhoea	**PD**	Parkinson's disease
NYHA	New York Heart Association		peritoneal dialysis
O	oedema	**PDA**	patent ductus arteriosus
O & A	observation and assessment	**PE**	physical examination
O & E	observation and examination		pleural effusion
O/A	on admission		pulmonary embolism
O/E	on examination	**PEARLA**	pupils equal and react to light and
OA	osteoarthritis		accommodation
OAB	overactive bladder	**PEF**	peak expiratory flow
OAG	open-angle glaucoma	**PEFR**	peak expiratory flow rate
OB	occult blood	**PEG**	percutaneous endoscopic gastrostomy
OCD	obsessive compulsive disorder	**PEJ**	percutaneous endoscopic jejunostomy
OD	overdose	**PEM**	prescription event monitoring
OGTT	oral glucose tolerance test		protein energy malnutrition
OH	occupational history	**PEP**	post-exposure prophylaxis
OHT	ocular hypertension	**PERLA**	pupils equal, react to light and accommodation
OI	opportunistic infection	**PERRLA**	pupils equal, round, react to light and accommo-
OKGA	ornithine salt of α-ketoglutaric acid		dation
OLT	orthoptic liver transplantation	**PET**	position emission tomography
OPA	outpatient appointment	**PF**	peak flow
OPD	outpatient department	**PF4**	platelet factor 4
ORS	oral rehydration solution	**PFR**	peak flow rate
OSAHS	obstructive sleep apnoea hypopnoea syndrome	**PFT**	pulmonary function test
OT	occupational therapy	**PG**	prostaglandin
P & A	percussion and auscultation	**P-gp**	P-glycoprotein
P & V	pyloroplasty and vagotomy	**PH**	past history
PA	pernicious anaemia		patient history
	pulmonary artery		personal history
PAAP	personal asthma action plan		prostatic hypertrophy
PACG	primary angle-closure glaucoma		pulmonary hypertension
PaCO$_2$	arterial carbon dioxide tension	**PHI**	primary HIV infection
PAD	peripheral arterial disease	**PI**	present illness
PAF	platelet-activating factor		protease inhibitor
PAH	pulmonary artery hypertension	**PICC**	peripherally inserted central catheter
pANCA	perinuclear anti-neutrophil cytoplasmic antibody	**PID**	pelvic inflammatory disease
PaO$_2$	arterial oxygen tension	**PIL**	patient information leaflet
PAPS	primary antiphospholipid syndrome	**PIN**	prostatic intra-epithelial neoplasia
PAS	*p*-aminosalicylic acid	**PIP**	proximal interphalangeal joint
	pulmonary artery stenosis	**PIVD**	protruded intervertebral disc
PASI	Psoriasis Area and Severity Index	**PJB**	premature junctional beat
PAT	paroxysmal atrial tachycardia	**PJC**	premature junctional contraction
PAWP	pulmonary artery wedge pressure	**PJP**	*Pneumocystis jiroveci* pneumonia
PB	premature beat	**PKU**	phenylketonuria
PBC	primary biliary cirrhosis	**PL**	product licence
PBI	protein-bound iodine	**PLL**	prolymphocytic leukaemia
PBSCT	peripheral blood stem cell transplantation	**PMDD**	premenstrual dysphoric disorder

pMDI	pressurised metered-dose inhaler	**PV**	vaginal examination (per vagina)
PMH	past medical history	**PVB**	premature ventricular beat
PMI	past medical illness	**PVC**	premature ventricular contraction
PMN	polymorphonucleocyte	**PVD**	peripheral vascular disease
PMR	polymyalgia rheumatica	**PVP**	pulmonary venous pressure
PMS	premenstrual syndrome	**PVR**	post-void residual
	postmenopausal syndrome	**PVT**	paroxysmal ventricular tachycardia
PMT	premenstrual tension	**Px.**	past prognosis
PMV	prolapsed mitral valve	**QALY**	quality-adjusted life-year
PN	parenteral nutrition	**R**	respiration
	percussion note	**RA**	renal artery
	peripheral nerve		rheumatoid arthritis
	peripheral neuropathy		right arm
PND	paroxysmal nocturnal dyspnoea		right atrial (atrium)
	postnasal drip	**RANKL**	receptor activator of nuclear factor-κβ ligand
PO₂	partial pressure of oxygen	**RARS**	refractory anaemia with ring sideroblasts
POAG	primary open-angle glaucoma	**RAST**	radio-allergosorbent test
POMR	problem-oriented medical record	**RAT**	rapid antigen test
PONV	postoperative nausea and vomiting	**RBBB**	right bundle branch block
PPAR-γ	proliferative-activated receptor-γ	**RBC**	red blood cell
PPD	purified protein derivative		red blood (cell) count
PPH	postpartum haemorrhage	**RBS**	random blood sugar
PPHN	persistent pulmonary hypertension of the neonate	**R-CVP**	rituximab, cyclophosphamide, vincristine, prednisolone
PPI	proton pump inhibitor	**RDS**	respiratory distress syndrome
PPNG	penicillinase-producing *Neisseria gonorrhoeae*	**REMS**	rapid eye movement sleep
PPV	positive-pressure ventilation	**Re-PUVA**	PUVA treatment with retinoids
PR	per rectum	**RF**	renal failure
	progestogen receptor		rheumatic fever
PRCA	pure red cell aplasia		rheumatoid factor
PREP	pre-exposure prophylaxis	**RFT**	respiratory function tests
PROM	premature rupture of membranes	**Rh factor**	rhesus factor
PS	pulmonary stenosis	**RHF**	right heart failure
	pyloric stenosis	**RHL**	right hepatic lobe
PSA	prostate-specific antigen	**rhuEPO**	recombinant human erythropoietin
PSC	primary sclerosing cholangitis	**rhuGM-CSF**	recombinant human granulocyte-macrophage colony-stimulating factor
PSG	presystolic gallop		
PSGN	poststreptococcal glomerulonephritis	**RIF**	right iliac fossa
PSVT	paroxysmal supraventricular tachycardia	**RIMA**	reversible inhibitor of monoamine oxidase type A
PT	parathyroid		
	paroxysmal tachycardia	**RITA**	radiofrequency interstitial tumour ablation
	physical therapy	**RK**	right kidney
	physical training	**RL**	right leg
	posterior tibial		right lung
	prothrombin time	**RLC**	residual lung capacity
PTC	percutaneous cholangiogram	**RLD**	related living donor
PTH	parathyroid hormone	**RLL**	right lower lobe (lung)
PTLD	post-transplant lymphoproliferative disorder	**RLQ**	right lower quadrant (abdomen)
PTSD	post-traumatic stress disorder	**RP**	radial pulse
PTT	partial thromboplastin time	**RPGN**	rapidly progressive glomerulonephritis
PTTK	partial thromboplastin time kaolin	**RPI**	resting pressure index
PTU	propylthiouracil	**RQ**	respiratory quotient
PU	pass urine	**RR**	respiratory rate
	per urethra	**RR & E**	round, regular and equal (pupils)
	peptic ulcer	**RRT**	renal replacement therapy
PUCAI	Paediatric Ulcerative Colitis Activity Index	**RS**	respiratory system
PUD	peptic ulcer disease	**RSF**	rheumatoid serum factor
PUO	pyrexia (fever) of unknown origin	**RSV**	respiratory syncytial virus
PUVA	psoralen and ultraviolet A radiation		

RTA	road traffic accident	**SV**	stroke volume
rt-PA	recombinant tissue plasminogen activator	**SVI**	stroke volume index
RUL	right upper lobe	**SVT**	supraventricular tachycardia
RUQ	right upper quadrant	**SWS**	slow-wave sleep
RV	residual volume	**Sx.**	symptoms
	right ventricle	**T**	temperature
RVH	right ventricular hypertrophy	**T & C, T & X**	type and cross-match
RVOT	right ventricular outflow tract	**T₃**	tri-iodothyronine
SA	sinoatrial (node)	**T₄**	thyroxine
	Stokes–Adams (attacks)	**TAGvHD**	transfusion-assisted graft-versus-host disease
	surface area	**TB**	tuberculosis
SAH	subarachnoid haemorrhage	**TBA**	to be administered
SARS	severe acute respiratory syndrome		to be arranged
SARS CoV	severe acute respiratory	**TBG**	thyroid-binding globulin
	syndrome-associated coronavirus	**TBI**	total body irradiation
SB	seen by	**TBM**	tuberculous meningitis
	shortness of breath	**TBW**	total body weight
SBE	subacute bacterial endocarditis	**TC**	total capacity
	shortness of breath on exertion		total cholesterol
SBO	small-bowel obstruction		tricarboxylic acid cycle
SBP	spontaneous bacterial peritonitis	**TCA**	tricyclic antidepressant
SCCAI	simple clinical colitis activity index	**TD**	tardive dyskinesia
SCID	severe combined immunodeficiency syndrome	**TDM**	therapeutic drug monitoring
sCr	serum creatinine	**TEN**	toxic epidermal necrolysis (Lyell's syndrome)
sCT	spiral computed tomography	**TENS**	transcutaneous electrical nerve stimulation
SCU, SCUF	slow continuous ultrafiltration	**TF**	tissue factor
SDD	selective decontamination of the digestive tract	**TFT**	thyroid function test
SEM	systolic ejection murmur	**TGF**	tubuloglomerular feedback
SERM	selective oestrogen receptor modulator	**TG**	triglyceride
SGLT2s	sodium-glucose co-tansporter-2 inhibitors	**TH**	thyroid hormone (thyroxine)
SGOT	serum glutamate-oxaloacetate transaminase	**THA**	tetrahydroaminoacridine
SGPT	serum glutamate-pyruvate transaminase	**THC**	tetrahydrocannabinol
SH	social history	**TIA**	transient ischaemic attack
SIADH	syndrome of inappropriate antidiuretic hormone	**TIBC**	total iron-binding capacity
SIDS	sudden infant death syndrome	**TIMP**	tissue inhibitor of metalloproteinases
SJS	Stevens–Johnson syndrome	**TIPSS**	transjugular intrahepatic portosystemic shunting
SLE	systemic lupus erythematosus	**TKI**	tyrosine kinase inhibitor
SMI	soft mist inhalers	**TLC**	total lung capacity
SNRI	serotonin-noradrenaline reuptake inhibitor		tender loving care
SOA	swelling of ankle(s)	**TLCO**	transfer factor of the lung for carbon monoxide
SOAP	subjective, objective, assessment, plan	**TLS**	tumour lysis syndrome
SOB	short of breath	**TNF**	tumour necrosis factor
SOBOE	short of breath on exertion	**TNF-α**	tumour necrosis factor alpha
SOL	space-occupying lesion	**TNM**	tumour node metastasis
SP	systolic pressure	**TP & P**	time, place and person
SPA	suprapubic aspiration	**t-PA**	tissue plasminogen factor
SPC, SmPC	Summary of Product Characteristics	**TPMT**	thiopurine methyltransferasethiopurine
SR	sinus rhythm		methyltransferase testing
	sustained release	**TPN**	total parenteral nutrition
SS	serotonin syndrome	**TPR**	temperature, pulse, respiration
SSI	surgical site infection	**tPSA**	total prostate-specific antigen
SSRI	selective serotonin reuptake inhibitor	**TRAB**	thyroid receptor antibody
ST	sinus tachycardia	**TRH**	thyrotrophin-releasing hormone
stat.	immediately (Latin: *statim*)	**TRUS**	transrectal ultrasonography
STEMI	ST elevated myocardial infarction	**tsDMARDs**	targeted synthetic disease modifying anti-rheumatic drugs
STD	sexually transmitted disease		
STS	sodium tetradecyl sulphate	**TSF**	triceps skinfold thickness
	serological tests for syphilis	**TSH**	thyroid-stimulating hormone

TTA	transtracheal aspiration
TTO	to take out (to take home)
TUIP	transurethral incision of the prostate
TUMT	transurethral microwave heat treatment
TUR	transurethral resection
TURB	transurethral resection of the bladder
TURP	transurethral resection of the prostate
TV	tidal volume
TVN	tissue viability nurse
TWOC	trial without catheter
Tx.	transfusion treatment
UA	unstable angina
U & E	urea and electrolytes
UBIC	unsaturated iron-binding capacity
UC	ulcerative colitis
UCEIS	ulcerative colitis endoscopic index of severity
UFH	unfractionated heparin
UPCR	urine protein creatinine ratio
URTI	upper respiratory tract infection
US	ultrasound
UTI	urinary tract infection
UVA	ultraviolet A
UVB	ultraviolet B
VaD	vascular dementia
VAP	ventilator associated pneumonia
VAS	visual analogue score
VC	vital capacity
	vulvovaginal candidiasis
VD	venereal disease
VDRL	Venereal Disease Research Laboratory (test for syphilis)
VEGF	vascular endothelial growth factor

VF	ventricular fibrillation
VHD	valvular heart disease
VKA	vitamin K antagonist
VLBW	very low birth weight
VLDL	very low-density lipoprotein
VMA	vanillylmandelic acid
VNTR	variable number of tandem repeats typing
VP	venous pressure
VPC	ventricular premature contraction
V/Q	ventilation/perfusion ratio
VS	vital signs
VT	ventricular tachycardia
VTE	venous thromboembolism
VTEC	verotoxin-producing *Escherichia coli*
VUR	vesicoureteric reflux
VVC	vulvovaginal candidiasis
VZV	varicella zoster virus
WAIHA	warm autoinmune haemolytic anaemia
WBC	white blood cell
	white blood count
WCC	white cell count
WHO	World Health Organization
WPW	Wolff–Parkinson–White (syndrome)
WR	Wassermann reaction
WTA	willingness to accept
WTP	willingness to pay
XDR-TB	extensively drug-resistant tuberculosis
ZE	Zollinger–Ellison (syndrome)
ZIG	zoster immune globulin
ZPP	zinc protoporphyrin

Glossary

Acanthosis nigricans: Diffuse, velvety acanthosis with grey, brown or black pigmentation, chiefly in axilla and other body folds, occurring in an adult form, often associated with an internal carcinoma and in a benign, nevoid form, more or less generalised.

Achlorhydria: Absence of hydrochloric acid from maximally stimulated gastric secretion.

Acral: Pertaining to or affecting a limb or other extremity.

Acropachy: Clubbing of the fingers and toes with distal periosteal bone changes and swelling of the overlying soft tissues.

Addisonian crisis: The symptoms that accompany an acute onset or worsening of Addison's disease, including fatigue, nausea and vomiting, loss of weight, hypotension, fever and collapse.

Adenomyosis: Penetration of endometrial tissue into the myometrium.

Agenesis: Absence of an organ.

Agyria: Congenital malformation or absence of the convolutions of the cerebral cortex.

Alloimmunity: Immunity to an alloantigen.

Alport's syndrome: Hereditary disease of the kidneys that primarily affects men. Heterogeneous group of conditions may manifest, including glomerulonephritis, haematuria, proteinuria, hypertension, nephrotic syndrome, end-stage renal disease, and variably accompanied by sensorineural deafness, coloured urine, swelling, cough and poor vision. Eventually, kidney dialysis or transplant may be necessary.

Amphipathic: Molecules containing groups with characteristically different properties, for example, both hydrophilic and hydrophobic properties.

Amphoteric: Having opposite characters, that is, capable of acting as an acid and a base.

Anoxaemia: Reduction of blood oxygen content below physiological levels.

Anthropometry: The science which deals with the measurement of the size, weight and proportions of the human body.

Anuria: Non passage of urine.

Aphakia: No lens.

Aphasia: Language disorder where people have problems speaking.

Aplasia cutis: Localised failure of development of skin.

Apnoea: Cessation of breathing.

Apoptosis: Programmed destruction of cells; mechanism that keeps cell numbers in check by eliminating senescent cells or those without useful cell function.

Arachnoiditis: Inflammation of the arachnoidea, a delicate membrane interposed between the dura mater and the pia mater.

Ataxia telangiectasia: Hereditary disorder with severe progressive cerebellar ataxia, associated with oculocutaneous telangiectasia, sinopulmonary disease with frequent respiratory infections and abnormal eye movements.

Atelectasis: Incomplete expansion of a lung.

Atretic: Without an opening; characterised by atresia.

Auspitz's sign: Removal of a yellow-white, sharply demarcated plaque of psoriasis, results in pinpoint haemorrhage.

Azoospermia: Absence of spermatozoa in the semen, or failure of formation of spermatozoa.

Bacteriuria: The presence of bacteria in the urine.

Barrett's oesophagus: A precancerous condition in which normal cells lining the oesophagus are replaced with abnormal cells that may develop into an adenocarcinoma.

Basal nucleus of Meynert: Formed in the brain by a group of cells in the substantia innominate.

Beau's lines: Transverse depression of the nail that represents interruption to the normal growth of the nail matrix.

BK virus: A human polyomavirus that causes widespread infection in childhood and remains latent in the host; believed to cause haemorrhagic cystitis and nephritis in immunocompromised patients.

Bronchiectasis: Characterised by dilation of the small bronchi and bronchioles, associated with the presence of chronic pulmonary sepsis. It presents as a chronic cough, often with the production of large amounts of purulent, foul-smelling sputum, and may eventually lead to repeated episodes of pneumonia and respiratory failure.

Bronchoalveolar lavage: A procedure performed during bronchoscopy in which the bronchial tree is literally washed (lavaged) with a small volume of sterile saline. The saline is then collected and sent for microbiological or cytological examination.

Bronchoscopy: The procedure in which a flexible fibreoptic endoscope is inserted into the bronchial tree to allow direct visualisation of the bronchi and, if required, the collection of specimens for microbiology or histology.

Brugada syndrome: A genetic disease characterised by an abnormal electrocardiogram and an increased risk of sudden cardiac death. More prevalent in those from South East Asia.

Bruxism: Tooth grinding.

Budd–Chiari syndrome: Symptomatic obstruction or occlusion of the hepatic veins, usually of unknown origin but probably caused by neoplasms, strictures, liver disease, trauma, systemic infections or haematological disorders.

Buerger's test: Two-part test to assess adequacy of the arterial supply to the leg.

Bullae: A bulla (plural bullae) is a fluid filled blister of more than 5 mm in diameter with thin walls.

Cachectic: A profound and marked state of general ill health and malnutrition.

Cardiogenic emboli: Emboli originating from the heart; caused by abnormal function of the heart.

Carpal tunnel syndrome: A complex of symptoms resulting from compression of the median nerve in the carpal tunnel, with pain and burning or tingling paraesthesias in the fingers and hand, sometimes extending to the elbow.

Catamenia: Term used to designate age at onset of menses.

Cataract: An opacity of the crystalline lens of the eye.

Cavitation: Formation of cavities – for example, in the lungs when the liquefied centre of a tuberculous lesion drains (usually into a bronchus).

Charcot's arthropathy: A destructive arthropathy (disease of any joint) with impaired pain perception or position sense.

Cholelithiasis: The presence or formation of gallstones.

Chondrocyte: A mature cartilage cell embedded in a lacuna (a small pit or hollow cavity) within the cartilage matrix.

Christmas disease: Haemophilia B.

Churg–Strauss syndrome: Allergic granulomatosis.

Chvostek's sign: Spasm of the facial muscles elicited by tapping the facial nerve in the region of the parotid gland, seen in tetany.

Coarctation of the aorta: A localised malformation characterised by deformity of the aortic media, causing narrowing (usually severe) of the lumen of the vessel.

Cognitive: Pertaining to cognition; that operation of the mind by which we become aware of objects of thought or perception; it includes all aspects of perceiving, thinking and remembering.

Corneal arcus: Crescentic deposition of lipids in the cornea.

Cor pulmonale: Persistent lung damage, eventually leads to increased blood pressure in the pulmonary arteries (pulmonary hypertension), which in turn leads to stress on the right ventricle, right ventricular hypertrophy and heart failure. This process is known as cor pulmonale.

Cryptogenic: Obscure, doubtful or unascertainable origin.

Cytotoxin: A toxin or antibody that has a specific toxic action upon cells of special organs.

Denudation: Removal of the epithelial covering from any surface.

Diarthrodial joint: A joint characterised by mobility in a rotary direction.

D-Dimer: D-dimer is a product formed in the body when blood is broken down.

Dimorphic: Occurring in two distinct forms.

Disseminated intravascular coagulation (DIC): In this condition vigorous activation of the clotting cascade causes widespread intravascular deposition of fibrin and consumption of clotting factors and platelets. There are numerous potential triggers for this process, including severe sepsis, burns, massive transfusion and placental abruption.

Diverticulosis: The presence of circumscribed pouches or sacs of variable size called diverticula that occur normally or are created by herniation of the lining mucous membrane through a defect in the muscular coat of a tubular organ such as the gastrointestinal tract.

Ductopenia: Absence/shortage of ducts; typically absence of interlobular bile ducts.

Dubin–Johnson syndrome: Familial chronic form of non-haemolytic jaundice due to a defect in the excretion of conjugated bilirubin and other organic anions.

Dupuytren's contracture: Shortening, thickening and fibrosis of the palmar fascia, producing a flexion deformity of a finger. The term also applies to a flexion deformity of a toe.

Dyschezia: Difficult or painful evacuation of faeces from the rectum.

Dyskinesia: Impairment of the power of voluntary movement, resulting in fragmentary or incomplete movements.

Dyspareunia: Difficult or painful intercourse.

Dyspnoea: Difficult or laboured breathing.

Dystonia: Disordered tonicity of muscle.

Dysuria: Painful or difficult urination.

Eclampsia: Convulsions and coma occurring in a pregnant or puerperal woman, associated with hypertension, oedema and/or proteinuria.

Electrodiathermy: Heating of the body tissues due to their resistance to the passage of an electric current.

Elliptocytosis: A hereditary disorder in which the majority of erythrocytes are elliptical in shape and characterised by varying degrees of increased red cell destruction and anaemia.

Emphysema: A state in which the alveoli of the lung become dilated, possibly with destruction of the alveolar walls, leading to large, empty air spaces which are useless for gas exchange. It is often seen accompanying chronic bronchitis but may be caused by inherited disorders such as α_1-antitrypsin deficiency.

Encephalopathy: Any degenerative disease of the brain.

Endophthalmitis: Inflammation involving the ocular cavities and their adjacent structures.

Enterostomy: The formation of a permanent opening into the intestine through the abdominal wall.

Enterotoxin: A toxin arising in the intestine.

Enthesitis: Inflammation of the entheses, the sites where tendons or ligaments insert into the bone.

Episcleritis: Inflammation of the loose connective tissue forming the external surface of the sclera.

Epstein–Barr virus: A herpes virus originally isolated from Burkitt lymphomas and believed to be the aetiological agent in infectious mononucleosis or closely related to it.

Euthymic: Normal state of thymus.

Exanthema: Widespread rash usually occurring in children caused by toxins, drugs, micro-organisms or autoimmune disease.

Faecal: Occult blood in the stools. Called 'occult' because it is partly digested and therefore no longer red in colour. Usually detected by means of a chemical test.

Faecal microbionta transplantation: Administration of a solution of faecal matter from a donor into the intestinal tract of a recipient in order to directly change the recipient's gut microbial composition and confer a health benefit.

Fanconi's anaemia: A rare hereditary disorder, transmitted in a recessive manner and having a poor prognosis, characterised by pancytopenia, hypoplasia of the bone marrow, and patchy brown discoloration of the skin due to the deposition of melanin, and associated with multiple congenital anomalies of the musculoskeletal and genitourinary systems.

Fastidious organism: An organism that will only grow with specialist culture media or under certain physiological conditions.

Feculent: Having dregs or a sediment.

Felty's syndrome: Combination of chronic rheumatoid arthritis, splenomegaly, leucopenia and pigmented spots on the skin of the lower extremities.

Fibroadenoma: Benign tumour that is made of glandular and fibrous tissue and typically occurs in breast tissue.

Fibromuscular: Composed of fibrous and muscular tissue.

Fistula: An abnormal passage or communication, usually between two internal organs or from an internal organ to the surface of the body.

Foreign body giant cells: Giant cells resembling Langhans giant cells, having clusters of nuclei scattered in an irregular pattern throughout the cytoplasm, characteristic of granulomatous inflammation due to invasion of the tissue by a foreign body.

FRAX score: Diagnostic tool used to assess the 10-year risk of a hip or osteoporotic fracture.

Gastroschisis: Congenital fissure of the abdominal wall not involving the site of insertion of the umbilical cord, and usually accompanied by protrusion of the small and part of the large intestine.

Gaucher's disease: A group of hereditary disorders of glucocerebroside metabolism characterised by accumulation of glucocerebroside in the spleen, liver, lungs, bone marrow and sometimes the brain leading to splenomegaly, hepatomegaly, erosion of the cortices of the long bones and pelvis, and central nervous system impairment.

Glasgow–Blatchford score: Screening tool to assess likelihood that a patient with an acute upper gastro-intestinal bleed will require medical intervention.

Glomerulonephritis: Nephritis characterised by inflammation of the capillary loops in the glomeruli of the kidney.

Glossitis: Inflammation of the tongue.

Goeckerman regimen: Combination of coal tar and ultraviolet B light to bombard the skin with anti-psoriasis treatment.

Gonioscopy: Estimate of the width of the eye chamber angle, measured using a slit lamp.

Goodpasture's disease: Autoimmune disease characterised by glomerulonephritis and haemorrhaging from the lung.

Granuloma: A tumour-like mass or nodule of granulation tissue, with actively growing fibroblasts and capillary buds; it is due to a chronic inflammatory process associated with infectious disease or with invasion by a foreign body.

Guillain–Barré syndrome: Acute febrile polyneuritis.

Haematuria: Blood in the urine.

Haem(at)opoiesis: The formation and development of blood cells.

Harris Benedict equation: Equation first developed in 1919 to predict basal energy expenditure.

Hasenclever score: Prognostic score for Hodgkin's disease.

Haustral: Pertaining to the haustra of the colon, denoting sacculations in the wall of the colon produced by adaptation of its length.

Heberden's nodes: Gelatinous cysts or bony outgrowths on the dorsal aspects of the distal interphalangeal joints.

Heinz bodies: Inclusion bodies in red blood cells resulting from oxidative injury to and precipitation of haemoglobin, seen in the presence of certain abnormal haemoglobins and erythrocytes with enzyme deficiencies.

Henoch–Schönlein purpura: An acute or chronic vasculitis primarily affecting skin, joints and the gastro-intestinal and renal systems.

Hepatorenal syndrome: Development of renal failure secondary to liver disease.

Hirschsprung's disease: Congenital megacolon.

Horner's syndrome: Sinking in of the eyeball, ptosis of the upper eyelid, slight elevation of the lower lid, constriction of the pupil, narrowing of the palpebral fissure, anhidrosis and flushing of the affected side of the face; caused by paralysis of the cervical sympathetic nerves.

Horton's syndrome: Migrainous neuralgia; also called paroxysmal nocturnal cephalalgia.

Huntington's chorea: A rare hereditary disease characterised by chronic progressive chorea and mental deterioration terminating in dementia. The age of onset is variable but usually occurs in the fourth decade of life.

Hyaline membrane: A layer of eosinophilic hyaline material lining the alveoli, alveolar ducts and bronchioles, found at autopsy in infants who have died of respiratory distress syndrome of the newborn.

Hypermelanosis: Excessive deposition of melanin.

Hypersplenism: A condition characterised by exaggeration of the inhibitory or destructive functions of the spleen, resulting in deficiency of the peripheral blood elements, singly or in combination, hypercellularity of the bone marrow and usually splenomegaly.

Hypertrichosis: Growth of hair at sites not normally hairy.

Hypophonic: Reduced volume of speech.

Hypovolaemia: Abnormally reduced volume of circulating fluid in the body/plasma.

Ileus: Obstruction or lack of smooth muscle tone in the intestines.

Immunoblastic: Pertaining to or involving the stem cells (immunoblasts) of lymphoid tissue.

Index case: The first detected case in a particular series that prompts investigation into other patients.

Interstitial nephritis: Inflammation of the renal interstitial tissue resulting from arterial, arteriolar, glomerular or tubular disease which destroys individual nephrons.

Intussusception: The prolapse of one part of the intestine into the lumen of an immediately adjoining part.

Involved-site radiation therapy: Radiation therapy aimed only at the lymph nodes which originally contained lymphoma.

Jod–Basedow syndrome: Thyrotoxicosis produced in a patient with goitre, when given a bolus of iodine.

Kayser–Fleischer ring: A grey-green to red-gold pigmented ring at the outer margin of the cornea, seen in progressive lenticular degeneration and pseudosclerosis.

Koebner phenomenon: Induction of new psoriasis skin lesions following local trauma or injury to the skin.

Koilonychia: Dystrophy of the fingernails, in which they are thin and concave, with edges raised.

Kussmaul's respiration: Air hunger.

Kwashiorkor: Insufficient protein provision.

Kyphosis: Abnormally increased convex curvature of the spinal column.

Labyrinthitis: Inflammation of the labyrinth; otitis interna.

Lacunar syndrome: Small infarct or small cavity in brain tissue that develops after the necrotic tissue of a deep infarct is resorbed.

Laminectomy: Excision of the posterior arch of a vertebra.

Laparoscopy: Examination of the interior of the abdomen by means of a laparoscope.

Lesch–Nyhan syndrome: Rare disorder of purine metabolism due to deficiency of the enzyme hypoxanthine-guanine phosphoribosyl-transferase and characterised by physical and mental retardation, self-mutilation of fingers and lips by biting, choreo-athetosis, spastic cerebral palsy and impaired renal function.

Leucocytosis: Total white cell count in excess of 11×10^9/L.

Leuconychia: White nails.

Lewy bodies: Abnormal protein aggregates which develop inside neurons.

Lichenoid: Resembling the skin lesions designated as 'lichen' – the name applied to many different kinds of papular skin.

Liddle's syndrome: Autosomal dominant disorder in which the kidneys excrete potassium but retain too much sodium and water, leading to high blood pressure diseases in which the lesions are typically small, firm papules that are usually set very close together.

Lipaemia retinalis: Retinal deposition of lipid.

Lipohypertrophy: Thickening of subcutaneous tissues at injection sites because of recurrent injections in the same area.

Livedo reticularis: A peripheral vascular condition characterised by a reddish blue net-like mottling of the skin and extremities.

Lyme disease: A multisystem tick-borne disorder caused by the spirochaete *Borrelia burgdorferi*. Clinical manifestation includes an erythematous macule followed by systemic disorders, such as arthralgias, myalgias and headache, followed by neurological manifestations, cardiac involvement and a migratory polyarthritis.

Lymphadenopathy: Disease of the lymph nodes.

Lymphoblastic: Pertaining to a lymphoblast.

Maculopapular: An eruption consisting of both macules (areas distinguishable by colour from their surroundings, e.g. spots) and papules (small circumscribed, superficial, solid elevations of the skin).

Malleolus medialis: The rounded protuberance on the medial surface of the ankle joint.

Mallory-Weiss tear: Occurs in the mucus membrane at the junction of the lower part of the oesophagus and the upper part of the stomach.

Malrotation: Abnormal or pathological rotation.

Marasmus: Insufficient energy provision.

Melaena: The passage of dark stools stained with blood pigments or with altered blood.

Menorrhagia: Excessive and prolonged uterine bleeding occurring at the regular intervals of menstruation.

Microalbuminuria: Small amounts of albumin present in the urine.

Miliary: Literally, resembling small, round millet seeds. Miliary tuberculosis is so called because the chest radiograph usually shows miliary speckling.

Morbilliform: Resembling the eruption of measles.

Mucositis: Inflammation of a mucous membrane.

Mycosis fungoides: A rare, chronic, malignant, lymphoreticular neoplasm of the skin and, in the late stages, the lymph nodes and viscera, marked by the development of firm, reddish, painful tumours that ulcerate.

Myelofibrosis: Replacement of the bone marrow by fibrous tissue occurring in association with a myeloproliferative disorder or secondary to another disorder.

Myoclonus: Shock-like contractions of a group of muscles.

Myoglobulinuria: Presence of myoglobin in the urine.

Myomas: Fibroids, common benign tumours of the myometrium.

Myometrium: The muscular layers of the uterus that contract spontaneously throughout the menstrual cycle.

Myopathy: Unexplained muscle soreness or weakness.

Myositis: Inflammation of a voluntary muscle.

Necrobiosis lipoidica: A dermatosis usually occurring in individuals with diabetes characterised by necrobiosis (swelling and distortion of collagen bundles in the dermis) of the elastic and connective tissue of the skin, with degenerated collagen occurring in irregular patches, especially in the upper dermis.

Nephrolithiasis: Formation of uric acid calculi in the kidneys.

Nikolsky's sign: Easy separation of the outer portion of the epidermis from the basal layer on exertion of firm sliding pressure by the finger or thumb.

Nocturia: Waking at night to pass urine.

Nosocomial: Originally taking place in a hospital, or acquired in a hospital, used particularly in reference to an infection.

Nystagmus: Involuntary rapid movement of the eyeball, which may be horizontal, vertical, rotatory or mixed.

Obligate intracellular pathogen: An organism that cannot be cultured using artificial media because it requires living cells for growth.

Oligohydramnios: Presence of less than 300 mL of amniotic fluid at term.

Oliguria: Diminished urine output.

Onycholysis: Separation of the nail from its bed.

Oophorectomy: Removal of an ovary or ovaries.

Ophthalmopathy: Any disease of the eye.

Opsonisation: The rendering of bacteria and other cells subject to phagocytosis.

Orchiectomy: Excision of one or both testes.

Orosomucoid: α_1-Acid glycoprotein, a glycoprotein occurring in blood plasma.

Orthopnoea: Difficult breathing except in an upright position.

Orthoptic: Correcting obliquity of one or more visual axes.

Osler's nodes: Small, raised, swollen tender areas, about the size of a pea and often bluish, but sometimes pink or red, occurring most commonly in the pads of the fingers or toes, in the palm or the soles of the feet.

Osteomalacia: Reduced mineralisation.

Osteophyte: A bony or osseous outgrowth.

Pallidotomy: A stereotaxic surgical technique for producing lesions in the globus pallidus or extirpation of it by other means.

Palmar striae: Yellow raised streaks across the palms of the hands.

Pancytopenia: Deficiency of all cell elements of the blood.

Panmyelopathy: A pathological condition of all the elements of the bone marrow.

Paroxysmal nocturnal dyspnoea: Difficult or laboured breathing at night that recurs in paroxysms.

Pericarditis: Inflammation of the fibrous sac (pericardium) that surrounds the heart and the roots of the great vessels.

Petechial: Characterised by pinpoint, non-raised, round, purplish red spots caused by intradermal or submucous haemorrhage.

Phaeochromocytoma: A tumour of chromaffin tissue of the adrenal medulla or sympathetic paraganglia. The cardinal symptom that represents the increased secretion of adrenaline and noradrenaline is hypertension, which may be persistent or intermittent.

Phagocytosis: The engulfing of micro-organisms, cells and foreign particles by phagocytes.

Phlebitis: Inflammation of a vein.

Pica: A craving for unnatural articles of food.

Pneumaturia: Passage of urine charged with air.

Polyangiitis: Previously known as Churg-Strauss syndrome is a type of systemic necrotising vasculitis.

Polycythaemia rubra vera: A myeloproliferative disorder in which the abnormal bone marrow overproduces red blood cells (white cells and platelets may also be raised).

Polymorphic: Occurring in several or many forms.

Polyp: A protruding growth from a mucous membrane.

Pompholyx: A skin eruption on the sides of the fingers, toes, palms or soles, consisting of discrete round intraepidermal vesicles 1 or 2 mm in diameter, accompanied by intense itching and occurring in repeated self-limited attacks lasting 1 or 2 weeks.

Porphyria: Any of a group of disturbances of porphyrin metabolism, characterised by a marked increase in formation and excretion of porphyrins or their precursors.

Pouchitis: Inflammation of the ileal pouch which will have been surgically formed from ileal tissue.

Pretibial myxoedema: Localised myxoedema associated with preceding hyperthyroidism and exophthalmus, occurring typically on the anterior (pretibial) surface of the legs where mucin deposits as plaques and papules.

Priapism: Persistent, abnormal erection of the penis, usually without sexual desire, and accompanied by pain and discomfort.

Prinzmetal's angina: A variant of angina pectoris in which the attacks occur during rest.

Proptosis: A forward displacement or bulging, especially of the eye.

Pseudophakia: False lens.

Pyruvate kinase deficiency: A deficiency in the glycolytic (metabolic) pathway of red blood cells that results in haemolysis.

Pyuria: Presence of pus in the urine.

Raeder's syndrome: A syndrome consisting of Horner syndrome but without loss of sweating on the affected side of the face.

Reed–Sternberg cells: Giant histiocytic cells, typically multinucleate, most often binucleate; the nuclei are enclosed in abundant amphophilic cytoplasm and contain prominent nucleoli.

Retinopathy: Any non-inflammatory disease of the retina.

Retroperitoneal fibrosis: Deposition of fibrous tissue in the retroperitoneal space, producing vague abdominal discomfort, and often causing blockage of the ureters with resultant hydronephrosis and impaired renal function.

Retrosternal: Situated or occurring behind the sternum.

Reiter's syndrome: Triad of non-gonococcal urethritis, conjunctivitis, and arthritis frequently with mucocutaneous lesions.

Reye's syndrome: An acute and often fatal childhood syndrome of encephalopathy and fatty degeneration of the liver, marked by rapid development of brain swelling and hepatomegaly, and by disturbed consciousness and seizures.

Rhabdomyolysis: Dissolution of muscle associated with excretion of myoglobin in the urine.

Rockall score: Scoring system to identify patients at risk of adverse outcome following acute upper gastro-intestinal bleed.

Roth's spots: Round or oval white spots sometimes seen in the retina early in the course of subacute bacterial endocarditis.

Rotor's syndrome: Chronic familial non-haemolytic jaundice differing from Dubin–Johnson syndrome in the lack of liver pigmentation.

Sarcoidosis: A chronic, progressive, generalised granulomatous reticulosis of unknown aetiology, involving almost any organ or tissue.

Schofield equation: An equation to predict basal metabolic rate; may be used to estimate the total calorie intake required to maintain current body weight.

Scleral icterus: A yellowing of the white of the eye.

Sclerotherapy: The injection of sclerosing solutions in the treatment of haemorrhoids or varicose veins.

Scotoma: An area of depressed vision within the visual field, surrounded by an area of less depressed or of normal vision.

Sézary syndrome: Generalised exfoliative erythroderma produced by cutaneous infiltration of reticular lymphocytes and associated with intense pruritus, alopecia, oedema, hyperkeratosis, pigment and nail changes.

Shy–Drager syndrome: Orthostatic hypotension, urinary and rectal incontinence, anhidrosis, atrophy of the iris, external ophthalmoplegia, rigidity, tremor, loss of associated movements, impotence, atonic bladder, generalised weakness, fasciculations and neuropathic muscle wasting.

Sickle cell anaemia: A hereditary haemolytic anaemia occurring almost exclusively in black people, characterised by arthralgia, acute attacks of abdominal pain, ulcerations of the lower extremities and sickle-shaped erythrocytes in the blood.

Sjögren's syndrome: A symptom complex of unknown aetiology, usually occurring in middle-aged or older women, in which keratoconjunctivitis is associated with pharyngitis sicca, enlargement of the parotid glands, chronic polyarthritis and xerostomia.

Sloughing material: Soft, gel-like material often found in ulcer bases. Composed of tissue exudate and cellular debris.

Spherocytosis: The presence of spherocytes (thick, almost spherical red blood cells) characterised by abnormal fragility of erythrocytes, jaundice and splenomegaly.

Splinter haemorrhages: Linear haemorrhages beneath the nail.

Steatosis: Fatty degeneration.

Stenosis: Narrowing or stricture of a duct or canal.

Stevens–Johnson syndrome: A severe form of erythema multiforme in which the lesions may involve the oral and anogenital mucous membranes in association with constitutional symptoms, including malaise, prostration, headache, fever, arthralgia and conjunctivitis.

Stromal keratitis: Immune-mediated non-suppurative stromal inflammation with an intact epithelium usually linked to a causative disorder such as Epstein–Barr virus, herpes zoster and simplex, mumps, measles, Lyme disease and tuberculosis.

Subchondral: Beneath a cartilage.

Subluxation: An incomplete or partial dislocation.

Substantia nigra: Basal ganglia structure located in the midbrain.

Supranuclear palsy: Pseudobulbar paralysis.

Sweet's syndrome: Acute febrile neutrophilic dermatosis.

Sympathetic ileus: Failure of gastro-intestinal motility secondary to acute non-gastro-intestinal illness, for example, hyaline membrane disease or septicaemia.

Tamponade: Surgical use of the tampon; also pathological compression of a part, as compression of the heart by pericardial fluid.

Tau neurofibrillary tangles: These insoluble proteins are a primary marker of Alzheimer's.

Telangiectasia: Prominent surface blood vessels.

Tendon xanthomas: Yellow papules or nodules or lipids deposited in tendons.

Tenesmus: Straining, especially ineffectual and painful straining at stool or in urination.

Tenosynovitis: Inflammation of a tendon sheath.

Thalassaemia: A heterogeneous group of hereditary haemolytic anaemias that have in common a decreased rate of synthesis of one or more haemoglobin polypeptide chains, which are classified according to the chain involved (a, b, g). The homozygous form (thalassaemia major) is incompatible with life. The heterozygous form (thalassaemia minor) may be asymptomatic or marked by mild anaemia.

Thrombocytopenia: Decrease in the number of blood platelets.

Thrombocytosis: Increased number of platelets in blood.

Thrombophilia: A tendency to the occurrence of thrombosis.

Thromboplastin: Phospholipid-protein extract of tissue that promotes the activation of factor X by factor VIII.

Tonometry: Measurement of intraocular pressure.

Tophi: Deposits of monosodium urate crystals, typically in subcutaneous and periarticular areas.

Trephine: Biopsy examination of an intact core of tissue (e.g. liver, bone marrow) obtained through a wide-bore needle.

Tropical sprue: A malabsorption syndrome occurring in the tropics and subtropics. Protein malnutrition is usually precipitated by the malabsorption, and anaemia due to folic acid deficiency is particularly common.

Trousseau's sign: Spasmodic contractions of muscles provoked by pressure upon the nerves which go to them; seen in tetany.

Tuberoeruptive xanthomas: Groups of flat or yellowish raised nodules on the skin over joints, especially the elbows and knees.

Tuberous sclerosis: Congenital familial disease characterised by tumours on the surfaces of the lateral ventricles and sclerotic patches on the surface of the brain and marked clinically by progressive mental deterioration and epileptic convulsions.

Tubular cast: A cast formed from gelled protein precipitated in the renal tubules and moulded to the tubular lumen; pieces of these casts break off and are washed out with the urine.

Uraemic frost: Crystalline area deposited on the skin.

Urethral: Pertaining to the urethra, the membranous canal conveying urine from the bladder to the exterior of the body.

Variant angina: *See* Prinzmetal's angina.

Volvulus: Intestinal obstruction due to a knotting and twisting of the bowel.

Von Willebrand's disease: A lack of or a defective plasma protein (von Willebrand factor) necessary for the adhesion of platelets to vascular elements when a blood vessel is damaged.

Wernicke–Korsakoff syndrome: The co-existence of Wernicke's disease (acute onset of mental confusion, nystagmus, ophthalmoplegia and gait ataxia, due to thiamine deficiency) with Korsakoff's syndrome (a gross disturbance in recent memory, sometimes compensated for by confabulation).

West's syndrome: A form of myoclonus epilepsy with onset in infancy or early childhood and characterised by seizures involving the muscles of the neck, trunk and limbs, with nodding of the head and flexion and abduction of the arms. Mental retardation is common.

Wilson's disease: Characterised by progressive accumulation of copper within body tissues, particularly erythrocytes, kidney, liver and brain, and associated with liver and lenticular degeneration.

Xanthelasma: Yellow plaques or nodules of lipids deposited on eyelids.

Xenotransplantation: Transplantation of tissue from another species.

Xerosis: Dry skin.